Find surgical videos for *Atlas of Neurosurgical Techniques: Spine and Peripheral Nerves, Second Edition* online at MediaCenter.thieme.com!

> Simply visit MediaCenter.thieme.com and, when prompted during the registration process, enter the code below to get started today.
>
> ME58-92R7-JA3L-9FU2

	WINDOWS	MAC	TABLET
Recommended Browser(s)**	Recent browser versions on all major platforms and any mobile operating system that supports HTML5 video playback ** *all browsers should have JavaScript enabled*		
Flash Player Plug-in	Flash Player 9 or Higher* * *Mac users: ATI Rage 128 GPU does not support full-screen mode with hardware scaling*		Tablet PCs with Android OS support Flash 10.1
Recommended for optimal usage experience	Monitor resolutions: • Normal (4:3) 1024×768 or Higher • Widescreen (16:9) 1280×720 or Higher • Widescreen (16:10) 1440×900 or Higher DSL/Cable internet connection at a minimum speed of 384.0 Kbps or faster WiFi 802.11 b/g preferred.		7-inch and 10-inch tablets on maximum resolution. WiFi connection is required.

Find us on Facebook — *Connect with us on Facebook® for exclusive offers.*

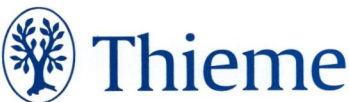

Atlas of Neurosurgical Techniques

Spine and Peripheral Nerves

Second Edition

Richard G. Fessler, MD, PhD
Professor
Department of Neurosurgery
Rush University Medical Center
Chicago, Illinois

Laligam N. Sekhar, MD, FACS, FAANS
Professor and Vice-Chairman
Department of Neurological Surgery
Professor of Radiology
Director, Cerebrovascular Surgery
Director, Skull Base Surgery
University of Washington School of Medicine
Harborview Medical Center
Seattle, Washington

Associate Editors:

Nader S. Dahdaleh, MD
Assistant Professor
Department of Neurological Surgery
Northwestern University Feinberg School of Medicine
Chicago, Illinois

Zachary A. Smith, MD
Assistant Professor
Department of Neurological Surgery
Northwestern University Feinberg School of Medicine
Chicago, Illinois

Lacey E. Bresnahan, PhD
Distributor Principal
BioTek Medical Products
Chicago, Illinois

1155 figures

Thieme
New York • Stuttgart • Delhi • Rio de Janeiro

Executive Editor: Timothy Hiscock
Managing Editor: Sarah Landis
Editorial Assistant: Nikole Connors
Director, Editorial Services: Mary Jo Casey
International Production Director: Andreas Schabert
Vice President, Editorial and E-Product Development: Vera Spillner
International Marketing Director: Fiona Henderson
International Sales Director: Louisa Turrell
Director of Sales, North America: Mike Roseman
Senior Vice President and Chief Operating Officer: Sarah Vanderbilt
President: Brian D. Scanlan
Illustrations: Markus Voll, Karl Wesker, and Andy Evansen
Production Editor: Barbara Chernow
Compositor: Carol Pierson, Chernow Editorial Services, Inc.

Library of Congress Cataloging-in-Publication Data

Names: Fessler, Richard G., editor. | Sekhar, Laligam N., editor.
Title: Atlas of neurosurgical techniques. Spine and peripheral
  nerves / [edited by] Richard G. Fessler, Laligam N. Sekhar.
Other titles: Spine and peripheral nerves
Description: Second edition. | New York : Thieme, [2016] | Includes
  bibliographical references and index.
Identifiers: LCCN 2016003242| ISBN 9781626230545 (alk. paper) |
  ISBN 9781626230552 (eISBN)
Subjects: | MESH: Spinal Nerves—surgery | Neurosurgical
  Procedures | Peripheral Nerves—surgery | Atlases
Classification: LCC RD593 | NLM WL 17 | DDC 617.4/800222—dc23
LC record available at http://lccn.loc.gov/2016003242

Important note: Medicine is an ever-changing science undergoing continual development. Research and clinical experience are continually expanding our knowledge, in particular our knowledge of proper treatment and drug therapy. Insofar as this book mentions any dosage or application, readers may rest assured that the authors, editors, and publishers have made every effort to ensure that such references are in accordance with **the state of knowledge at the time of production of the book.**

Nevertheless, this does not involve, imply, or express any guarantee or responsibility on the part of the publishers in respect to any dosage instructions and forms of applications stated in the book. **Every user is requested to examine carefully** the manufacturers' leaflets accompanying each drug and to check, if necessary in consultation with a physician or specialist, whether the dosage schedules mentioned therein or the contraindications stated by the manufacturers differ from the statements made in the present book. Such examination is particularly important with drugs that are either rarely used or have been newly released on the market. Every dosage schedule or every form of application used is entirely at the user's own risk and responsibility. The authors and publishers request every user to report to the publishers any discrepancies or inaccuracies noticed. If errors in this work are found after publication, errata will be posted at www.thieme.com on the product description page.

Some of the product names, patents, and registered designs referred to in this book are in fact registered trademarks or proprietary names even though specific reference to this fact is not always made in the text. Therefore, the appearance of a name without designation as proprietary is not to be construed as a representation by the publisher that it is in the public domain.

Copyright © 2016 by Thieme Medical Publishers, Inc.
Thieme Publishers New York
333 Seventh Avenue, New York, NY 10001 USA
+1 800 782 3488, customerservice@thieme.com

Thieme Publishers Stuttgart
Rüdigerstrasse 14, 70469 Stuttgart, Germany
+49 [0]711 8931 421, customerservice@thieme.de

Thieme Publishers Delhi
A-12, Second Floor, Sector-2, Noida-201301
Uttar Pradesh, India
+91 120 45 566 00, customerservice@thieme.in

Thieme Publishers Rio de Janeiro, Thieme Publicações Ltda.
Edifício Rodolpho de Paoli, 25º andar
Av. Nilo Peçanha, 50 – Sala 2508
Rio de Janeiro 20020-906 Brasil
+55 21 3172 2297

Printed in China by Everbest Printing Investment   5 4 3 2 1

ISBN 978-1-62623-054-5

Also available as an e-book:
eISBN 978-1-62623-055-2

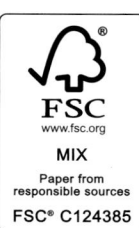

This book, including all parts thereof, is legally protected by copyright. Any use, exploitation, or commercialization outside the narrow limits set by copyright legislation without the publisher's consent is illegal and liable to prosecution. This applies in particular to photostat reproduction, copying, mimeographing or duplication of any kind, translating, preparation of microfilms, and electronic data processing and storage.

This book is dedicated to the memory of my mentors, Dr. Sean Mullan and Dr. Albert Rhoton, Jr. Their patience and commitment to teaching created generations of thoughtful and skilled surgeons. Perhaps more importantly, observing their kindness to patients, colleagues, and families, instilled in us the gift of being compassionate physicians.

R.G.F.

Contents

Video Contents xiii
Foreword xv
Preface xvii
Contributors xix

Section I Occipital-Cervical Junction
Section Editor: Zachary A. Smith

A. Pathology
1. Abnormalities of the Craniovertebral Junction 3
   Brian J. Dlouhy, Raheel Ahmed, and Arnold H. Menezes
2. Rheumatologic and Degenerative Disease of the Craniovertebral Junction 13
   Brian J. Dlouhy, Raheel Ahmed, and Arnold H. Menezes
3. Tumors of the Occipital-Cervical Junction 21
   Mohamad Bydon, Rafael De la Garza-Ramos, Ziya L. Gokaslan, and Jean-Paul Wolinsky
4. Trauma of the Occipital-Cervical Junction 28
   George M. Ghobrial, Ahmed J. Awad, Christopher M. Maulucci, and James S. Harrop

B. Anterior Approach
5. Transoral Approaches to the Craniovertebral Junction 37
   Brian J. Dlouhy, Raheel Ahmed, and Arnold H. Menezes
6. Transoral Odontoidectomy 42
   Brian J. Dlouhy, Raheel Ahmed, and Arnold H. Menezes
7. Extended Transoral Approaches 48
   Brian J. Dlouhy, Raheel Ahmed, and Arnold H. Menezes
8. Transoral Closure 52
   Brian J. Dlouhy, Raheel Ahmed, and Arnold H. Menezes
9. Minimally Invasive Endoscopic Approaches to the Upper Cervical Spine 56
   Mohamad Bydon, Mohamed Macki, Ali Ozturk, and Jean-Paul Wolinsky
10. Extended Maxillotomy Approach for High Clinical Pathology 63
    Raj P. TerKonda and Lawrence J. Marentette

C. Anterolateral Approach
11. Retropharyngeal Approach to the Occipital-Cervical Junction, Part 1 70
    John R. Vender, Steven J. Harrison, and Dennis E. McDonnell
12. Retropharyngeal Approach to the Occipital-Cervical Junction, Part 2 79
    John R. Vender, Steven J. Harrison, and Dennis E. McDonnell

D. Posterior Approach
13. Posterior Suboccipital and Upper Cervical Exposure of the Occipital Cervical Junction 84
    Gregory Hawryluk and Dean Chou
14. Suboccipital Craniectomy and Cervical Laminectomy for Chiari Malformation 91
    Lee A. Tan, Robert G. Kellogg, Carter S. Gerard, and Lorenzo F. Muñoz
15. Occipital-Cervical Encephalocele: Surgical Treatment 96
    Sandi K. Lam and Andrew Jea
16. Occipital Plating and Occipital-Cervical Fusion 100
    Manish K. Kasliwal, Ricardo B.V. Fontes, and Vincent C. Traynelis
17. Exposure of C1 and C2 106
    Manish K. Kasliwal, Ricardo B.V. Fontes, and Vincent C. Traynelis
18. Atlantoaxial Wiring and Arthrodesis 109
    Manish K. Kasliwal, Ricardo B.V. Fontes, and Vincent C. Traynelis
19. C1-C2 Transarticular Fixation Technique 118
    Ricardo B.V. Fontes, Manish K. Kasliwal, and Vincent C. Traynelis
20. C1 Lateral Mass–C2 Pars, Pedicle, and Translaminar Fixation Techniques 123
    Ricardo B.V. Fontes, Manish K. Kasliwal, and Vincent C. Traynelis
21. Odontoid Screw Placement 129
    Christopher M. Maulucci, George M. Ghobrial, Ahmed J. Awad, and James S. Harrop

Section II Midcervical Spine
Section Editor: Zachary A. Smith

A. Pathology

22 Congenital Osseous Anomalies of the Mid- to Lower Cervical Spine.. 137
Jeffrey C. Wang and Dmitri Sofianos

23 Cervical Spine Degenerative Disease and Cervical Stenosis 146
Michael G. Fehlings and Newton Cho

24 Intramedullary Tumors of the Spinal Cord 153
Paul C. McCormick

25 Extramedullary Tumors of the Spinal Cord.. 161
Paul C. McCormick

26 Vertebral Bone Tumors.. 167
Rakesh Ramakrishnan and William F. Lavelle

27 Trauma of the Mid- and Lower Cervical Spine.. 173
Daniel K. Resnick, Christopher D. Baggott, Bennie W. Chiles III, and Paul R. Cooper

B. Anterior Approach

28 Cervical Spine: Anterior Approach, Diskectomy, and Corpectomy... 186
Rueben Nair, Marco C. Mendoza, and Wellington K. Hsu

29 Cervical Arthroplasty 193
Manish K. Kasliwal and Zachary A. Smith

30 Transcorporeal Tunnel Approach for Unilateral Cervical Radiculopathy 201
Gun Choi and Alfonso García Chávez

C. Posterior Approach

31 Cervical Spine: Posterior Exposure 206
Sean Christie and Janet Martin

32 Cervical Laminectomy 213
Sean Christie and Janet Martin

33 Posterior Cervical Foraminotomy and Diskectomy 217
Sean Christie and Janet Martin

34 Minimally Invasive Posterior Cervical, Diskectomy, Laminectomy, and Foraminotomy for Stenosis................... 221
Trent L. Tredway

35 Cervical Laminoplasty 228
Takashi Kaito and Kazuo Yonenobu

36 Gardner-Wells Tong or Crown-Halo Reduction for Cervical Facet Dislocations 234
Joshua Bakhsheshian, Nader S. Dahdaleh, and Zachary A. Smith

37 Posterior Approach for the Treatment of Locked Cervical Facets 239
Ricardo B.V. Fontes, Manish K. Kasliwal, and Vincent C. Traynelis

38 Subaxial Cervical Lateral Mass Screw Fixation 243
Joshua Bakhsheshian, Nader S. Dahdaleh, Richard G. Fessler, and Zachary A. Smith

39 Subaxial Cervical Pedicle Screw Fixation.. 247
Alexander A. Theologis, Sang-Hun Lee, Justin K. Scheer, Shane Burch, and Christopher Pearson Ames

40 C7 Pedicle Subtraction Osteotomy 253
Justin K. Scheer, Vedat Deviren, and Christopher Pearson Ames

D. Combined Anterior-Posterior Approach

41 Combined Anterior-Posterior Approach for Complete Vertebral Resection in the Midcervical Spine.................. 257
Mohamad Bydon, Rafael De la Garza-Ramos, Jean-Paul Wolinsky, and Ziya L. Gokaslan

Section III Cervicothoracic Junction
Section Editor: Zachary A. Smith

A. Anterior Approach

42 Supraclavicular Approach to the Cervicothoracic Junction 263
Zachary A. Smith, Joshua Bakhsheshian, and Nader S. Dahdaleh

43 Transmanubrial-Transclavicular and Transsternal Approach to the Cervicothoracic Junction 268
Joshua Bakhsheshian, Nader S. Dahdaleh, and Zachary A. Smith

44 Cervicothoracic Corpectomy... 274
Robert F. Heary and John C. Quinn

45 Anterior Reconstruction Following Cervicothoracic Corpectomy 280
Robert F. Heary and John C. Quinn

B. Posterior Approach

- 46 Posterior Cervicothoracic Instrumentation and Fusion 283
  Robert F. Heary and John C. Quinn

Section IV Thoracic and Thoracolumbar Spine
Section Editor: Zachary A. Smith

A. Pathology

- 47 Congenital Abnormalities of the Thoracic and Thoracolumbar Spine 291
  Sandi K. Lam, Jared Fridley, Christina N. Sayama, Bradley Daniels, and Andrew Jea
- 48 Disk Disease of the Thoracic and Thoracolumbar Spine 310
  Tobias A. Mattei, Alisson R. Teles, Kristin Huntoon, and Ehud Mendel
- 49 Tumors of the Thoracolumbar Spine 315
  Jonathan N. Sellin, Laurence D. Rhines, and Claudio E. Tatsui
- 50 Trauma of the Thoracic and Thoracolumbar Spine 325
  Nader S. Dahdaleh and Zachary A. Smith
- 51 Thoracic Epidural Abscess and Osteomyelitis 333
  E. Emily Bennett and Edward C. Benzel
- 52 Vascular Malformations of the Spine 340
  Bruno C. Flores, Daniel R. Klinger, Jonathan A. White, and H. Hunt Batjer

B. Antero/Anterolateral Approach

- 53 Open Lateral Transthoracic Approach 356
  Tobias A. Mattei, Victoria Shunemann, and Ehud Mendel
- 54 Open Lateral Transthoracic Diskectomy and Vertebrectomy 361
  Tobias A. Mattei and Ehud Mendel
- 55 Endoscopic Lateral Transthoracic Approach 369
  Justin C. Clark and Curtis A. Dickman
- 56 Endoscopic Thoracic Sympathectomy 378
  Justin C. Clark and Curtis A. Dickman
- 57 Endoscopic Lateral Transthoracic Diskectomy and Vertebrectomy 385
  Roque Fernandez, Inge Preissl, and Daniel Rosenthal
- 58 Lateral Transthoracic and Retropleural MIS Approaches 391
  Jason M. Paluzzi, Michael S. Park, and Juan S. Uribe
- 59 Lateral Transthoracic MIS Diskectomy and Vertebrectomy 395
  Michael S. Park and Juan S. Uribe
- 60 Lateral Graft and Plate Reconstruction 400
  Michael S. Park and Juan S. Uribe
- 61 Open Thoracoabdominal Approach 404
  Hasan R. Syed and Faheem A. Sandhu
- 62 MIS Thoracoabdominal Approach 408
  Shane V. Abdunnur and Daniel H. Kim
- 63 Open Retroperitoneal Approach 412
  Hasan R. Syed and Faheem A. Sandhu
- 64 Minimally Invasive Retroperitoneal Lateral Lumbar Interbody Fusion 416
  Alexander Tuchman, Martin H. Pham, and John C. Liu
- 65 Minimally Invasive Retroperitoneal Vertebrectomy 423
  Alexander Tuchman, Christina Yen, and John C. Liu
- 66 Thoracoabdominal/Retroperitoneal Graft and Lateral Plating 431
  Shane V. Abdunnur and Daniel H. Kim

C. Posterolateral Approach

- 67 Open Costotransversectomy 435
  Robert Andrew Rice, Rocky Felbaum, and Jean-Marc Voyadzis
- 68 MIS Costotransversectomy 440
  Justin K. Scheer, Nader S. Dahdaleh, and Zachary A. Smith

D. Posterior Approach

- 69 Thoracic Laminectomy 443
  Andrew James Grossbach, Stephanus Viljoen, and Patrick W. Hitchon
- 70 Thoracic Laminoplasty 450
  Andrew James Grossbach, Sami Al-Nafi, and Patrick W. Hitchon
- 71 Transpedicular Thoracic Diskectomy 455
  David M. Benglis, Jr., Richard G. Fessler, and Regis Haid, Jr.

72 Intradural Extramedullary Tumor Resection 461
    Paul C. McCormick

73 Intramedullary Tumor Resection 467
    Paul C. McCormick

74 Open Anterolateral Cordotomy 476
    Joshua M. Rosenow

75 Commissural Myelotomy 478
    Joshua M. Rosenow

76 Thoracic DREZ Operation 480
    Joshua M. Rosenow

77 Caudalis DREZ 482
    Joshua M. Rosenow

78 Shunt Placement for Syringomyelia 485
    Ulrich Batzdorf and Langston T. Holly

79 Posterior Approach and In-Situ Fusion of the Thoracic Spine 492
    Hai Le, Rishi Wadhwa, and Praveen V. Mummaneni

80 Pedicle Screw Instrumentation of the Thoracic Spine 496
    Hai Le, Rishi Wadhwa, and Praveen V. Mummaneni

81 Open Scoliosis Correction 500
    Patrick A. Sugrue and Lawrence G. Lenke

82 Minimally Invasive Correction of Spinal Deformity 518
    Nader S. Dahdaleh, Praveen V. Mummaneni, and Zachary A. Smith

83 Minimally Invasive Thoracic Decompression for Multilevel Thoracic Pathology 523
    Cort D. Lawton, Nader S. Dahdaleh, Michael J. Harvey, Richard G. Fessler, and Zachary A. Smith

Section V   Lumbar and Lumbosacral Spine
Section Editor: Nader S. Dahdaleh

A.   Pathology

84 Spondylolysis and Spondylolisthesis in Children 529
    Andrew J. Pugely and Stuart L. Weinstein

85 Lumbar Degenerative Disk Disease 538
    Ricardo B.V. Fontes, Josemberg S. Baptista, and John E. O'Toole

86 Tumors of the Lumbosacral Spine 545
    Mohamad Bydon, Rafael De la Garza-Ramos, Jean-Paul Wolinsky, and Ziya L. Gokaslan

87 Trauma of the Lumbar Spine and Sacrum 552
    Robert G. Kellogg

B.   Anterior Approach

88 Anterior Approach to the Lumbosacral Junction 558
    Randall B. Graham, Nader S. Dahdaleh, and Tyler R. Koski

C.   Anterolateral Approach

89 Anterolateral Retroperitoneal Approach to the Lumbosacral Spine 563
    Jared J. Marks, H. Louis Harkey III, Timothy M. Wiebe, and Michael P. Schenk

D.   Posterior Approach

90 Open Posterior Lumbar Approach 569
    Joseph S. Cheng and Scott L. Zuckerman

91 Open Posterior Lumbar Foraminotomy 576
    Joseph S. Cheng and Nikita Lakomkin

92 Open Posterior Lumbar Hemilaminectomy 579
    Joseph S. Cheng and Peter Morone

93 Open Posterior Lumbar Microdiskectomy 583
    Joseph S. Cheng and Scott L. Zuckerman

94 Open Posterior Lumbar Laminectomy 587
    Joseph S. Cheng and Michael D. Dewan

95 MIS Posterior Lumbar Approach 593
    Russell G. Strom and Anthony K. Frempong-Boadu

96 MIS Posterior Lumbar Foraminotomy 600
    Russell G. Strom and Anthony K. Frempong-Boadu

97 MIS Posterior Lumbar Hemilaminectomy 604
    Russell G. Strom and Anthony K. Frempong-Boadu

98 MIS Posterior Lumbar Diskectomy 608
    Russell G. Strom and Anthony K. Frempong-Boadu

| 99 | MIS Posterior Lumbar Decompression of Stenosis | 612 |

Russell G. Strom and Anthony K. Frempong-Boadu

| 100 | Microdiskectomy for Foraminal or Far Lateral Disc Herniations | 615 |

Olatilewa O. Awe, Andrew James Grossbach, and Patrick W. Hitchon

| 101 | Far Lateral MIS Diskectomy | 621 |

Hani R. Malone and Alfred T. Ogden

| 102 | Transverse Process Fusion | 628 |

Byron C. Branch and Charles L. Branch, Jr.

| 103 | Open Placement of Pedicle Screws: Lumbar, Sacral, and Iliac Screws | 634 |

Eli M. Baron, Neel Anand, and Doniel Drazin

| 104 | Minimally Invasive Transforaminal Lumbar Interbody Fusion | 642 |

Kurt M. Eichholz

| 105 | MIS Placement of Pedicle Screws: Lumbar, Sacral, and Iliac Wing Screws | 650 |

Michael Y. Wang

| 106 | Lumbar Osteotomies | 654 |

Manish K. Kasliwal, Lee A. Tan, and Richard G. Fessler

| 107 | Cortical Trajectory Screws | 664 |

Byron C. Branch and Charles L. Branch, Jr.

| 108 | MIS Facet Screw | 669 |

Carter S. Gerard and Richard G. Fessler

| 109 | Transacral Approach | 673 |

William D. Tobler

| 110 | Repair of Cerebrospinal Fluid Leaks | 684 |

Reid Hoshide, Erica Feldman, and William R. Taylor

| 111 | Lumboperitoneal Shunt | 687 |

Sergei Terterov, Dustin M. Harris, and Marvin Bergsneider

| 112 | Dorsal Rhizotomy of the Lumbosacral Nerve Roots for the Treatment of Spastic Diplegia in Cerebral Palsy Patients | 690 |

Marc Sindou, George Georgoulis, and Andrei Brinzeu

| 113 | Resection of Cauda Equina Ependymomas | 707 |

R. Shane Tubbs and W. Jerry Oakes

| 114 | Release of the Tethered Spinal Cord | 711 |

R. Shane Tubbs and W. Jerry Oakes

| 115 | MIS Release of the Tethered Spinal Cord | 716 |

Mena Kerolus, Bledi Brahimaj, and Richard G. Fessler

| 116 | Implantation of Spinal Cord Stimulators | 720 |

Erika A. Petersen and Konstantin V. Slavin

| 117 | Placement of an Intrathecal Drug Delivery System | 730 |

Erika A. Petersen and Konstantin V. Slavin

| 118 | Vertebroplasty and Kyphoplasty | 738 |

Ricardo B.V. Fontes and Richard G. Fessler

| 119 | Resection of Lumbosacral Lipomas | 746 |

Carter S. Gerard, Lee A. Tan, Robert G. Kellogg, and Lorenzo F. Muñoz

| 120 | Repair of Myelomeningoceles | 753 |

Lorenzo F. Muñoz

| 121 | Excision of Spinal Congenital Dermal Tract/Dermoid | 757 |

Robert G. Kellogg, Carter S. Gerard, Lee A. Tan, and Lorenzo F. Muñoz

| 122 | Resection of Sacrococcygeal Teratoma | 763 |

David Jimenez and Byron C. Branch

| 123 | Surgical Management of Spinal Dysraphism | 769 |

Mena Kerolus, Ravi Nunna, and Lorenzo F. Muñoz

| 124 | Repair of Diastematomyelia | 790 |

Sandi K. Lam and Andrew Jea

| 125 | Sacral Agenesis | 796 |

David Jimenez and Asif Maknojia

| 126 | Iliac Crest Bone Grafting | 799 |

Lee A. Tan and Richard G. Fessler

Section VI Peripheral Nerves
Section Editor: Lacey E. Bresnahan

A. Pathology of the Brachial Plexus

| 127 | Neoplasms of Peripheral Nerves | 807 |

Carlos E. Restrepo Rubio and Robert J. Spinner

128. Traumatic Peripheral Nerve Injuries...813
Zarina S. Ali, Gregory G. Heuer, and Eric L. Zager

129. Compressive Lesions of the Peripheral Nerve..818
Shane V. Abdunnur and Daniel H. Kim

B. Surgery of the Brachial Plexus

130. Supraclavicular Approach to Brachial Plexus Surgery..826
Shane V. Abdunnur and Daniel H. Kim

131. Infraclavicular Approach to Brachial Plexus Surgery..831
Shane V. Abdunnur and Daniel H. Kim

132. Surgical Approach to the Spinal Accessory Nerve...836
Tene A. Cage, Arnau Benet, Erron W. Titus, and Michel Kliot

133. Surgical Approach to the Axillary Nerve...843
Arnau Benet, Tene A. Cage, and Michel Kliot

134. Surgical Treatment of the Musculocutaneous Nerve...849
Angela M. Bohnen, Joseph Weiner, and Aruna Ganju

135. Open and Endoscopic Decompression of the Median Nerve...854
Ahmed Alaqeel, Albert M. Isaacs, and Rajiv Midha

136. Decompression of the Ulnar and Radial Nerve..861
Ahmed Alaqeel, Albert M. Isaacs, and Rajiv Midha

C. Pathology of the Lumbosacral Plexus

137. Trauma to the Lumbosacral Plexus...870
Debora Garozzo

138. Tumors of the Lumbosacral Plexus...881
Carlos E. Restrepo Rubio, Scott P. Zietlow, and Robert J. Spinner

D. Surgery of the Lumbosacral Plexus

139. Approach to the Nerves of the Lower Extremity..886
Jonathan D. Choi and Allan H. Friedman

140. Exposure and Biopsy of the Sural Nerve..899
Ahmed Alaqeel and Rajiv Midha

141. Approach to the Lumbosacral Plexus..903
Debora Garozzo and Stefano Ferraresi

E. Other Nerves

142. The Intercostal Nerves..912
Allan D. Nanney III, Karina Nieto, and Aruna Ganju

143. Surgical Treatment of Ilioinguinal Neuralgia..917
Angela M. Bohnen, Joseph Weiner, and Aruna Ganju

144. Surgical Treatment of Genitofemoral Neuralgia...922
Randall B. Graham, Gurvinder Kaur, and Aruna Ganju

145. Lateral Femoral Cutaneous Nerve..925
James A. Stadler III, Casey Richardson, and Aruna Ganju

146. Peripheral Nerve Grafting and Harvesting Techniques...928
Amit Ayer, Omar Arnaout, Chandan G. Reddy, and Aruna Ganju

147. Superficial Peroneal Nerve Biopsy..932
Brian D. Dalm and Chandan G. Reddy

Index...939

Video Contents

Video 6.1   Transoral approach: A 5-year-old with Down syndrome with a dystopic os odontoideum and dorsal displacement of the hypoplastic dens with instability between the craniocervical region and C2. At an outside institution, she underwent two previous posterior approaches including posterior decompression with instrumentation and fusion. However, proper reduction was not achieved. She was unable to stand and walk and use her arms after her second operative procedure due to severe cervicomedullary compression. Given her pathology and occipitocervical fusion, the reduction was unable to be performed. Therefore, a ventral transoral-transpalatopharyngeal approach and decompression with removal of the anterior arch of C1, os odontoideum, and odontoid process was performed. The patient did well postoperatively and regained significant strength.

Video 8.1   Transoral closure: A proper closure after a transoral-transpalatopharyngeal approach is essential to minimizing complications. Proper closure reestablishes a barrier between the posterior pharyngeal space created by the approach and bony resection and the oropharyngeal space, eliminating dead space, therefore preventing abscess and hematoma formation. Proper closure also enables proper swallowing and prevention of velopharyngeal incompetence.

Video 11.1   High anterior cervical retropharyngeal surgical approach.

Video 28.1   Anterior cervical approach, diskectomy, and instrumented fusion: The video demonstrates the anterior approach to the cervical spine, with diskectomy, grafting, and instrumentation at the C6-C7 level. Video authorship: Anay R. Patel.

Video 30.1   Motion-preserving transcorporeal cervical forminotomy: The video demonstrates a short version of two surgical case examples: in the first case, a right-sided C6 transcorporeal foraminotomy, and in the second, a two-level left C5 and C6. Note that in both cases the disk is spared and a complete decompression is successfully achieved.

This technique is done through a regular anterior Smith-Robinson approach. One major difference between the surgical access for an anterior cervical diskectomy and fusion (ACDF) and the tunnel technique is that in the latter, exposure of only the target disk and proximal vertebral body is required, without the exposure of the inferior vertebral body. The level is confirmed at this stage, and an operating microscope is brought into the field. Before drilling is begun, indigo-carmine dye is injected in the affected disk to facilitate the orientation of disk space while drilling. The position of the drill hole is 4 to 6 mm above the lower border of the proximal vertebra, at the level of the medial border of the longus coli muscle. Drilling is done using a 4-mm diamond bur initially and a 3-mm bur later. At approximately one-third depth of the drilling, we can see the bluish discoloration of the stained disk and we can safely continue to drill further, keeping the blue-stained material in the center of the hole so as to maintain the direction of the trajectory.

After the desired depth is achieved, a blunt probe is used to palpate the base of the tunnel so that the thin ivory-white shell of the posterior vertebral wall can be carefully lifted with a fine bone punch or curette. The posterior longitudinal ligament still acts as a protective barrier between the instruments and the neural structures. Bone wax can be used to stop the bleeding from the spongy bone, and epidural bleeds can be managed with thrombin-soaked Gelfoam or FloSeal. The use of bipolar coagulation is strongly discouraged at this step.

The adequacy of the decompression can be confirmed by observing the bulging nerve root with cerebrospinal fluid (CSF) flow and palpating the superior and inferior pedicles along the course of the nerve root using a root probe.

Wound closure is the same as ACDF with a Hemovac drain for aspiration of postoperative hematoma.

Video 34.1   Tredway cervical microendoscopic foraminotomy.

Video 35.1   Cervical laminoplasty for cervical spondylotic myelopathy (C3–C6: left open door; C7: partial laminectomy of the cranial third): A dorsal skin incision is made from the caudal C2 to C6 spinous process. An avascular plane between the right and left paraspinal muscles is divided at the midline. While preserving the muscles attaching to C2 and C7, the spinous processes from C3 to C6 and to the inner half of where the lateral mass is exposed. Then, the spinous processes of C3 through C6 are cut at the base with a Liston bone-cutting forceps, and the C6 spinous process is set aside for later use as a bone graft. A trough is made across each lamina using a high-speed drill with a 4-mm steel bur. Continuous irrigation is maintained to prevent thermal damage to the surrounding tissue and aid visualization of the bottom of the trough. The drilling continues until the epidural venous plexus at the cranial half of the lamina and yellow ligament at the caudal half of the lamina can be visualized through the thinned inner cortex. A 10-mm raspatory is inserted into the trough and twisted (the lamina makes a snapping sound and moves). The trough for the hinge side is subsequently made in the same manner. When drilling down to the surface of the inner cortex of the lamina at the hinge side, the springiness of the laminae should be checked frequently to prevent laminar fracture of the hinge side. The laminae are elevated starting from C6 (with the cranial third of C7) to C3. Hemostasis from the epidural venous plexus is achieved by bipolar cauterization. The autologous spinous processes from C6 is reshaped and implanted as a supporting strut with a nonabsorbable 2-0 suture. A hydroxyapatite spacer specially made for open-door laminoplasty is used at C4 with the same nonabsorbable 2-0 suture. After sufficient irrigation of the wound with saline, retractors are removed, hemostasis is achieved, and a drainage tube is placed at the hinge side. The fascia is closed with 2-0 Vicryl suture.

Video 55.1   Endoscopic lateral transthoracic approach: This approach is a powerful surgical tool that provides access to the anterior thoracic spine for treatment of a wide range of spinal pathologies. The video demonstrates the key steps involved in safely and effectively utilizing this approach. (Courtesy of Barrow Neurological Institute, Phoenix, Arizona.)

Video 56.1   Endoscopic technique for thoracic sympathectomy: This is an effective surgical strategy for treating hyperhidrosis syndromes. The video outlines the surgical steps involved in treating palmar and plantar hyperhidrosis syndromes via the endoscopic thoracic sympathectomy technique. (Courtesy of Barrow Neurological Institute, Phoenix, Arizona.)

Video 64.1   Minimally invasive retroperitoneal lateral lumbar interbody fusion: The video demonstrates the steps necessary to perform this fusion utilizing the "shallow docking" technique.

Video 72.1 Removal of an intradural schwannoma: This video illustrates the techniques of removal of an intradural schwannoma arising from the proximal caudal equina.

Video 78.1 Syrinx to subarachnoid space shunt placement.

Video 81.1 Open posterior pedicle screw construct correction of an idiopathic scoliosis deformity.

Video 95.1 Right L4-L5 microdiskectomy performed through a tubular retractor.

Video 107.1 Cortical bone screw fixation technique: The video demonstrates the use of this technique with a bilateral posterior lumbar interbody fusion (PLIF) in the treatment of degenerative spondylolisthesis at L3-L4. The video also demonstrates the hybrid mini-open techniques using the Minimal Access Spinal Technologies (MAST) retractor and illumination system (Medtronic, Memphis, TN).

Video 111.1 Lumboperitoneal shunt placement.

Video 112.1 Dorsal rhizotomies for cerebral palsy: This is an efficient and safe technique because of the accuracy of its radicular identification and root sectioning quantification. To optimize accuracy and selectivity while minimizing invasiveness, we developed a tailored interlaminar procedure targeting directly and individually the radicular levels involved in the harmful components of spasticity. In each patient, two to three interlaminar spaces, preselected based on preoperative planning, were enlarged in a "keyhole" fashion, respecting the spinous processes and interspinous ligaments.

The procedure is based on neurophysiological recordings. Ventral root stimulation identifies the radicular level (anatomic mapping). Dorsal root stimulation evaluates its implication in the hyperactive segmental circuits (physiological testing), helping quantify the percentage of rootlets to be cut.

Keyhole interlaminar dorsal rhizotomy (KIDr) offers direct intradural access to each of the ventral/dorsal roots, thus maximizing the reliability of anatomic mapping and enabling individual physiological testing of all targeted roots. The interlaminar (enlarged) approach minimizes invasiveness by respecting the posterior spine structures.

Video 114.1 Identification of the midline filum terminale: Following a midline S1 laminectomy, the dura mater is opened and the midline filum terminale identified. Without tension, the filum is coagulated at two points and then transected with microscissors.

Video 115.1 Intraoperative video of a minimally invasive tethered cord release using a Medtronic X-tube.

Video 128.1 Oberlin's procedure: ulnar to musculocutaneous nerve transfer: The video demonstrates Oberlin's procedure, which involves nerve transfer, or neurotization, for restoration of elbow flexion after brachial plexus injury. This surgical approach is ideally suited to cases of nerve root avulsion or severe intraplexal injury. We transfer the donor ulnar nerve fascicle, providing redundant hand function to the recipient biceps branch of the musculocutaneous nerve in an end-to-end fashion. Neurophysiological testing is used to identify a suitable donor fascicle. The major advantage of this procedure is the decreased distance to the target muscle for regenerating motor axons. (Courtesy of Dr. Ron Ron Cheng.)

Video 135.1 Open decompression of the median nerve at the carpal tunnel: The video demonstrates a step-by-step intraoperative approach to performing this technique.

Video 136.1 Decompression of the ulnar nerve at the elbow: The video demonstrates a step-by-step intraoperative approach to performing this technique.

Foreword

It is indeed a pleasure to write a foreword for this magnificent second edition of the *Atlas of Neurosurgical Techniques: Spine and Peripheral Nerves,* edited by Dr. Richard G. Fessler and Dr. Laligam N. Sekhar. The book is a true compendium of information designed for both the seasoned spine and peripheral nerve surgeon and the novice. Virtually all conceivable spine operations are covered, resulting in an encyclopedic volume that serves as a refresher guide, a reference for hard-to-find information, and an aide to mastering the art of spine surgery.

During their distinguished careers in neurosurgery, Dr. Fessler and Dr. Sekhar developed many new techniques and procedures and trained thousands of residents and clinicians around the globe in these and other techniques. The effort they have put into editing the *Atlas of Neurosurgical Techniques: Spine and Peripheral Nerves* is commendable. Their commitment to driving our specialty forward is an example to those of us who practice spine and peripheral nerve surgery.

I offer the following recommendation to all spine and peripheral nerve surgeons: Keep this book at your bedside and read from it every night. When finished, start over and read it again.

Edward C. Benzel, MD
Chairman, Department of Neurosurgery
Neurological Institute
Cleveland Clinic
Cleveland, Ohio

Preface

In the preface to the first edition of the *Atlas of Neurosurgical Techniques: Spine and Peripheral Nerves,* I commented on the value of updating the seminal text *Operative Neurosurgery* by Dr. Ludwig Kempi. His step-by-step illustrations of neurosurgical operations offered a brilliant introduction to teaching the necessary sequence of individual surgical procedures, and we wanted to emulate his approach. But I also noted that such a task was relatively overwhelming due to the broad expansion in the variety of neurosurgical procedures since his text was published.

Our approach to the text of the first edition of the *Atlas* included the creation of a uniform and consistent format. In addition to the step-by-step illustrations, each section was organized into two types of chapters: The first several summarized common pathologies found in a specific region of the spine; subsequent chapters each detailed a specific operative technique for that region. The operative chapters emphasized accurate and detailed illustrations and photographs of the specific surgical technique and were accompanied by concise descriptions of the procedures, as well as highlighted tables of the indications/contraindications and advantages/disadvantages of that specific technique. This format was intended to enable the student, resident, or surgeon to rapidly review the surgical technique without "wading through" lengthy discussions of the disease processes, etiologies, differential diagnoses, and so on, while still providing that information in the introductory chapters to each section for study when desired. Where numerous procedures utilized the same initial and concluding surgical techniques, redundancy was minimized by detailing them only once and referencing the reader back to the appropriate correlated chapter.

Our efforts on the text were rewarded. In addition to the many positive comments we received from colleagues, the first edition of the *Atlas* was awarded the Association of American Publishers Best Book in Clinical Medicine award in 2006. We were humbled by this acknowledgment, but proud that this text did, indeed, accomplish the goal of being a foundational educational tool for our discipline.

We have maintained the same organizational scheme for this second edition of the *Atlas of Neurosurgical Techniques: Spine and Peripheral Nerves*. During the ten years since the first edition was published, neurosurgical techniques and technology have continued to evolve at a staggering pace. For example, the number of spine procedures performed via minimally invasive technique has dramatically increased. Furthermore, the spine pathology treated by neurosurgeons has progressed, particularly in the arena of deformity. Consequently, the chapters included in this edition have also evolved. Several chapters on techniques that are now performed infrequently have been omitted. Chapters on surgery for spinal deformity have been added. (These chapters cover only the fundamentals, since these techniques are the material for books in and of themselves.) Finally, the "open" and "minimally invasive" surgical techniques can be found side-by-side for each specific operation in which either technique is currently utilized.

It is our hope that, once again, this organization will provide the reader with an up-to-date, easy-to-use reference with minimal redundancy that details current surgical technique through clearly focused text and ample drawings as well as immediately accessible indications, contraindications, advantages, and disadvantages, while still providing specific content on pathology etiology and differential diagnosis.

Richard G. Fessler, MD, PhD

Contributors

Shane V. Abdunnur, MD
Resident, Department of Neurosurgery
University of Texas Health and Science Center at Houston
Houston, Texas

Ahmed Alaqeel, MD, PhD
Department of Clinical Neurosciences
Division of Neurosurgery
University of Calgary
Alberta, Canada
Department of Surgery
Division of Neurosurgery
College of Medicine, King Saud University
Riyadh, Saudi Arabia

Raheel Ahmed, MD
Fellow, Department of Pediatric Neurosurgery
The Hospital for Sick Children
University of Toronto
Toronto, Canada

Zarina S. Ali, MD
Chief Resident, Department of Neurosurgery
University of Pennsylvania
Philadelphia, Pennsylvania

Sami Al-Nafi, MD
Sub-Specialty Consultant, Departments of Neurosurgery and Spine
National Neuroscience Institute
King Fahad Medical City
Riyadh, Saudi Arabia

Christopher Pearson Ames, MD
Professor of Clinical Neurological Surgery and Orthopedic Surgery
Director of Spine Tumor & Spinal Deformity Surgery
Co-director, Spinal Surgery and UCSF Spine Center
Director, Spinal Biomechanics Laboratory
University of California, San Francisco
San Francisco, California

Neel Anand, MD
Director, Department of Orthopedic Spine Surgery
Cedars-Sinai Institute for Spinal Disorders
Los Angeles, California

Omar Arnaout, MD
Chief Resident, Department of Neurological Surgery
Northwestern Memorial Hospital
Chicago, Illinois

Ahmed J. Awad, MD
Associate Researcher, Department of Neurosurgery
Icahn School of Medicine at Mount Sinai
New York, New York
Faculty of Medicine and Health Sciences
An-Najah National University
Nablus, Palestine

Olatilewa O. Awe, MD
Resident, Department of Neurosurgery
University of Iowa Hospitals and Clinics
Iowa City, Iowa

Amit Ayer, MD
Resident, Department of Neurological Surgery
Northwestern Memorial Hospital
Chicago, Illinois

Christopher D. Baggott, MD
Resident, Department of Neurosurgery
University of Wisconsin
Madison, Wisconsin

Joshua Bakhsheshian, MD, MS
Resident, Department of Neurological Surgery
University of Southern California
Keck School of Medicine
Los Angeles, California

Josemberg S. Baptista, PhD
Associate Professor, Departments of Human Anatomy and Morphology
Universidade Federal do Espirito Santo
Vitória, ES, Brazil

Eli M. Baron, MD
Associate Professor of Neurosurgery
Spine Surgeon
Cedars-Sinai Medical Center
Los Angeles, California

H. Hunt Batjer, MD, FACS
Lois C.A. and Darwin E. Smith Professor and Chair
Department of Neurological Surgery
University of Texas Southwestern Medical Center
Dallas, Texas

Ulrich Batzdorf, MD
Professor, Department of Neurosurgery
David Geffen School of Medicine at University of California, Los Angeles
Los Angeles, California

Arnau Benet, MD
Director, Skull Base & Cerebrovascular Laboratory
Assistant Professor, Departments of Neurosurgery and Otolaryngology HNS
University of California, San Francisco
San Francisco, California

David M. Benglis, Jr, MD
Neurosurgeon, Atlanta Brain and Spine Care
Atlanta, Georgia

E. Emily Bennett, MD
Resident, Department of Neurosurgery
Neurological Institute, Cleveland Clinic
Cleveland, Ohio

Contributors

Edward C. Benzel, MD
Chairman, Department of Neurosurgery
Neurological Institute, Cleveland Clinic
Cleveland, Ohio

Marvin Bergsneider, MD
Professor in Residence, Department of Neurosurgery
University of California, Los Angeles
Los Angeles, California

Angela M. Bohnen, MD
Resident, Department of Neurosurgery
Northwestern University Feinberg School of Medicine
Chicago, Illinois

Bledi Brahimj, MD
Resident, Department of Neurosurgery
Rush University Medical Center
Chicago, Illinois

Byron C. Branch, MD
Resident, Department of Neurosurgery
University of Texas Health Science Center at San Antonio
San Antonio, Texas

Charles L. Branch, Jr., MD
Professor and Chair, Department of Neurological Surgery
Eben Alexander Jr, MD, Endowed Chair
Wake Forest Baptist Health System
Winston-Salem, North Carolina

Andrei Brinzeu, MD, MSc
Department of Neurosurgery
Lyon 1 University
Pierre Wertheimer Neurological Hospital
Lyon, France

Shane Burch, MD
Associate Professor in Residence, Department of Orthopaedic Surgery
University of California, San Francisco
San Francisco, California

Mohamad Bydon, MD
Assistant Professor
Departments of Neurologic Surgery, Orthopedic Surgery, and Health Sciences Research
Mayo Clinic
Rochester, Minnesota

Tene A. Cage, MD
Resident, Department of Neurological Surgery
University of California, San Francisco
San Francisco, California

Joseph S. Cheng, MD, MS, FAANS
Associate Professor, Department of Neurosurgery
Director, Neurosurgery Spine Program
Department of Neurosurgery
Vanderbilt University
Nashville, Tennessee

Ron Ron Cheng, MD
Research Fellow, Department of Neurosurgery
University of Pennsylvania
Philadelphia, Pennsylvania

Bennie W. Chilies III, MD, FACS
Physician, Westchester Spine and Brain Surgery, PLLC
Hartsdale, New York

Newton Cho, MD
Resident, Division of Neurosurgery
University of Toronto
Toronto, Canada

Gun Choi, MD, PhD
Chairman of Pohang Wooridul Hospital
Honorary Chairman of Seoul Gimpo Airport Wooridul Hospital
President of World Congress of Minimally Invasive Spine Surgery and Techniques (WCMISST)
Executive director of Asia Congress of Minimally Invasive Spine Surgery and Techniques (ACMISST)
President of Spinal Therapeutic Technology Related Link(STTeL)
Vice president of Korea Medical Service Society
Member of World Federation of Neurosurgical Societies (WFNS) Spine Committee
Soul Gimpo Airport Wooridul Spine Hospital
Seoul, Korea

Jonathan D. Choi, MD
Physician, Monterey Spine and Joint
Monterey, California

Dean Chou, MD
Professor of Neurosurgery
The University of California, San Francisco Spine Center
University of California, San Francisco
San Francisco, California

Sean Christie, MD, FRCSC, FAANS
Associate Professor, Department of Surgery (Neurosurgery) and Medical Neurosciences
Vice-Chair, Division of Neurosurgery
Director of Research, Division of Neurosurgery
Director, Neurosurgery Spine Program
Dalhousie University
Halifax, Nova Scotia, Canada

Justin C. Clark, MD
Division of Neurological Surgery
Barrow Neurological Institute
Phoenix, Arizona

Paul R. Cooper, MD
Clinical Professor
Departments of Neurosurgery and Orthopaedic Surgery
New York University Medical Center
New York, New York

Nader S. Dahdaleh, MD
Assistant Professor, Department of Neurological Surgery
Northwestern University Feinberg School of Medicine
Chicago, Illinois

Brian D. Dalm, MD
Fellow Associate, Department of Neurosurgery
University of Iowa
Iowa City, Iowa

Bradley Daniels, BS
Medical Student, Department of Neurosurgery
Baylor College of Medicine
Houston, Texas

Rafael De la Garza-Ramos, MD
Research Fellow, Department of Neurosurgery
John Hopkins University School of Medicine
Baltimore, Maryland

Vedat Deviren, MD
Professor, Department of Orthopaedic Surgery
University of California, San Francisco
San Francisco, California

Michael C. Dewan, MD
Resident, Department of Neurological Surgery
Vanderbilt University Medical Center
Nashville, Tennessee

Curtis A. Dickman, MD
Division of Neurological Surgery
Barrow Neurological Institute
Phoenix, Arizona

Brian J. Dlouhy, MD
Assistant Professor, Department of Neurosurgery
University of Iowa Children's Hospital
University of Iowa Hospitals and Clinics
Iowa City, Iowa

Doniel Drazin, MD, MA
Chief Resident, Department of Neurosurgery
Spine Center
Cedars-Sinai Medical Center
Los Angeles, California

Kurt M. Eichholz, MD, FACS
Surgeon
St. Louis Minimally Invasive Spine Center
St. Louis, Missouri

Michael G. Fehlings, MD, PhD, FRCSC, FACS
Professor, Division of Neurosurgery
Halbert Chair in Neural Repair and Regeneration
Vice Chair, Research Department of Surgery
University of Toronto
Toronto, Canada

Rocky Felbaum, MD
Resident, Department of Neurosurgery
MedStar Georgetown University Hospital
Washington, DC

Erica Feldman, BS
MD/MPH Candidate, University of Miami Miller School of Medicine
Miami, Florida

Roque Fernandez, MD
Neurosurgical Associates and Spine Section
Hochtaunuskliniken
Bad Homburg, Germany

Stefano Ferraresi, MD
Chief, Department of Neurosurgery
Ospedale S. Maria della Misericordia
Rovigo, Italy

Richard G. Fessler, MD, PhD
Professor, Department of Neurosurgery
Rush University Medical Center
Chicago, Illinois

Bruno C. Flores, MD
Chief Resident, Department of Neurological Surgery
University of Texas Southwestern Medical Center
Dallas, Texas

Ricardo B.V. Fontes, MD, PhD
Assistant Professor, Department of Neurosurgery
Rush University Medical Center
Chicago, Illinois

Anthony K. Frempong-Boadu, MD, FACS, FAANS
Associate Professor, Department of Neurosurgery
Director, Division of Spinal Surgery
New York University–Langone Medical Center
New York, New York

Jared Fridley, MD
Resident, Department of Neurosurgery
Baylor College of Medicine
Houston, Texas

Allan H. Friedman, MD
The Guy L. Odom Professor of Neurological Surgery
Department of Neurosurgery
Duke University Health System
Durham, North Carolina

Aruna Ganju, MD
Associate Professor, Department of Neurological Surgery
Northwestern University Feinberg School of Medicine
Chicago, Illinois

Alfonso García Chávez, MD
Orthopedic Surgeon, Minimally Invasive Spine Surgeon
Wooridul Spine Hospital
Pohang, South Korea

Debora Garozzo, MD
Neurosurgeon, Department of Neurosurgery
Santa Maria della Misericordia Hospital
Rovigo, Italy
Neurospinal Hospital Dubai
United Arab Emirates

George Georgoulis, MD
Neurosurgeon, Department of Neurosurgery
Lyon 1 University
Pierre Wertheimer Neurological Hospital
Lyon, France

Carter S. Gerard, MD
Resident, Department of Neurosurgery
Rush University Medical Center
Chicago, Illinois

George M. Ghobrial, MD
Resident, Department of Neurological Surgery
Thomas Jefferson University
Philadelphia, Pennsylvania

Contributors

Ziya L. Gokaslan, MD, FAANS, FACS
Gus Stoll, MD Professor and Chair, Department of Neurosurgery
The Warren Alpert Medical School of Brown University
Neurosurgeon-in-Chief, Rhode Island Hospital and The Miriam Hospital
Clinical Director, Norman Prince Neurosciences Institute
President, Brown Neurosurgery Foundation
Rhode Island Hospital
Department of Neurosurgery
Norman Prince Neurosciences Institute
Providence, Rhode Island

Randall B. Graham, MD
Resident, Department of Neurological Surgery
Northwestern University Feinberg School of Medicine
Chicago, Illinois

Andrew James Grossbach, MD
Chief Resident, Department of Neurosurgery
University of Iowa Hospitals and Clinics
Iowa City, Iowa

Regis Haid, Jr., MD
Surgeon, Atlanta Brain and Spine Care
Atlanta, Georgia

H. Louis Harkey III, MD
Professor, Department of Neurosurgery
University of Mississippi Medical Center
Jackson, Mississippi

Dustin M. Harris, BS
Medical Student
David Geffen School of Medicine at University of California Los Angeles
Los Angeles, California

Steven J. Harrison, MSMI, PhD, CMI, FAMI
Professor Emeritus, Department of Medical Illustration
Georgia Health Sciences University
Atlanta, Georgia

James S. Harrop, MD, FACS
Professor, Departments of Neurological and Orthopedic Surgery
Director, Division of Spine and Peripheral Nerve Surgery
Neurosurgery Director of Delaware Valley SCI Center
Thomas Jefferson University
Philadelphia, Pennsylvania

Michael J. Harvey, MD
Resident, Department of Orthopaedic Surgery
University of Missouri–Kansas City
Kansas City, Missouri

Gregory Hawryluk, MD, PhD, FRCSC
Assistant Professor of Neurosurgery
Adjunct Assistant Professor of Neurology
Director of Neurosurgical Critical Care
Department of Neurosurgery
University of Utah
Salt Lake City, Utah

Robert F. Heary, MD
Professor, Department of Neurological Surgery
Rutgers New Jersey Medical School
Newark, New Jersey

Gregory G. Heuer, MD, PhD
Assistant Professor, Division of Neurosurgery
University of Pennsylvania
Children's Hospital of Pennsylvania
Philadelphia, Pennsylvania

Patrick W. Hitchon, MD
Professor, Departments of Neurosurgery and Biomedical Engineering
University of Iowa Carver College of Medicine
Department of Neurosurgery
University of Iowa Hospitals and Clinics
Iowa City, Iowa

Langston T. Holly, MD
Professor, Departments of Neurosurgery and Orthopaedics
Vice Chair of Clinical Affairs
David Geffen School of Medicine at University of California Los Angeles
Los Angeles, California

Reid Hoshide, MD, MPH
Resident
Department of Neurosurgery
University of California, San Diego
San Diego, California

Wellington K. Hsu, MD
Clifford C. Raisbeck Distinguished Professor of Orthopaedic Surgery
Director of Research, Department of Orthopaedic Surgery
Northwestern University Feinberg School of Medicine
Chicago, Illinois

Kristin Huntoon, MD
Resident, Department of Neurological Surgery
Ohio State University
Columbus, Ohio

Albert M. Isaacs, BSc, MD
Division of Neurosurgery
Department of Clinical Neurosciences
University of Calgary
Calgary, Alberta, Canada

Andrew Jea, MD, FAANS, FACS, FAAP
Associate Professor, Department of Neurosurgery
Baylor College of Medicine
Staff Neurosurgeon
Director, Neuro-Spine Program
Director, Educational Programs
Texas Children's Hospital
Houston, Texas

David Jimenez, MD, FACS
Professor and Chairman, Department of Neurosurgery
University of Texas Health Science Center at San Antonio
San Antonio, Texas

Takashi Kaito, MD
Assistant Professor, Department of Orthopedic Surgery
Osaka University Graduate School of Medicine
Yamadadaoka, Japan

Manish K. Kasliwal, MD, MCh
Chief Resident, Department of Neurosurgery
Rush University Medical Center
Chicago, Illinois

Gurvinder Kaur, MD
Resident, Department of Neurosurgery
Northwestern University Feinberg School of Medicine
Chicago, Illinois

Robert G. Kellogg, MD
Resident, Department of Neurosurgery
Rush University Medical Center
Chicago, Illinois

Mena Kerolus, MD
Resident, Department of Neurosurgery
Rush University Medical Center
Chicago, Illinois

Daniel H. Kim, MD, FAANS, FACS
Professor, Director of Spinal Neurosurgery
Reconstructive Peripheral Nerve Surgery
Director of Microsurgical Robotic Lab
Department of Neurosurgery
University of Texas
Houston, Texas

Daniel R. Klinger, MD
Resident, Department of Neurological Surgery
University of Texas Southwestern Medical Center
Dallas, Texas

Michel Kliot, MD
Professor, Department of Neurological Surgery
Northwestern University Feinberg School of Medicine
Northwestern Memorial Hospital
Chicago, Illinois

Tyler R. Koski, MD
Associate Professor, Department of Neurological Surgery
Northwestern University Feinberg School of Medicine
Chicago, Illinois

Nikita Lakomkin, MD
Resident, Vanderbilt University
Nashville, Tennessee

Sandi K. Lam, MD, MBA
Assistant Professor, Department of Neurosurgery
Baylor College of Medicine
Division of Pediatric Neurosurgery
Texas Children's Hospital
Houston, Texas

William F. Lavelle, MD
Associate Professor, Orthopedic Spine Surgeon
Department of Orthopedic Surgery
State University of New York Upstate Medical University
Syracuse, New York

Cort D. Lawton, MD
Resident, Department of Orthopedic Surgery
Northwestern University Feinberg School of Medicine
Chicago, Illinois

Hai Le, MD
Resident, Department of Orthopedic Surgery
Massachusetts General Hospital
Boston, Massachusetts

Sang-Hun Lee, MD, PhD
Professor, Department of Orthopaedic Surgery
Spine Center, Kyung Lee
University Hospital at Gangdong
Seoul, Korea

Lawrence G. Lenke, MD
Professor of Orthopedic Surgery
Chief, Division of Spinal Surgery
Director, Spinal Deformity Surgery
Co-Director, Adult and Pediatric Comprehensive Spine Surgery Fellowship
Columbia University Department of Orthopedic Surgery
Surgeon-in-Chief, The Spine Hospital
New York-Presbyterian/Allen
New York, New York

John C. Liu, MD
Professor, Department of Neurosurgery
Co-Director, University of California Spine Center
University of Southern California
Los Angeles, California

Mohamed Macki, MD
Resident, Department of Neurosurgery
Henry Ford Hospital
Detroit, Michigan

Asif Maknojia, MD
Resident, Department of Neurosurgery
University of Texas Health Science Center at San Antonio
San Antonio, Texas

Hani R. Malone, MD
Fellow, Department of Neurological Surgery
Columbia University
New York, New York

Lawrence J. Marentette, MD, FACS
Professor, Department of Otolaryngology–Head and Neck Surgery
University of Michigan Health System
Ann Arbor, Michigan

Jared J. Marks, MD
Assistant Professor, Department of Neurosurgery
University of Mississippi Medical Center
Jackson, Mississippi

Janet Martin, BSc
Medical Student, Dalhousie Medical School
Halifax, Nova Scotia, Canada

Tobias A. Mattei, MD
Surgeon, Department of Neurosurgery
Brain & Spine Center
Invision Health/Kenmore Mercy Hospital
Buffalo, New York

Christopher M. Maulucci, MD
Assistant Professor, Department of Neurological Surgery
Tulane University
New Orleans, Louisiana

Paul C. McCormick, MD, MPH, FAANS
Gallen Professor of Neurological Surgery
Columbia University College of Physicians and Surgeons
New York, New York

Dennis E. McDonnell, MD, FACS, FANNS
Emeritus, Department of Neurosurgery
Gundersen Medical Center
La Crosse, Wisconsin

Marco C. Mendoza, MD
Resident, Department of Orthopaedic Surgery
Northwestern University Feinberg School of Medicine
Chicago, Illinois

Ehud Mendel, MD, FACS
Justine Skestos Endowed Chair
Professor of Neurosurgery, Oncology, Orthopedics and Systems Engineering
Vice Chair Clinical/Academic Affairs
Clinical Director- OSU Spine Research Institute and Biodynamics/Ergonomics Lab
Director-Spine program, Complex/Oncological Fellowship Program
The Ohio State University-Wexner Medical Center
The James Cancer Hospital
Columbus, Ohio

Arnold H. Menezes, MD
Professor and Vice Chairman, Department of Neurosurgery
University of Iowa Hospitals and Clinics
Iowa City, Iowa

Rajiv Midha, MSc, MD, FRCSC, FAANS
Professor and Head
Department of Clinical Neurosciences Calgary Zone
Alberta Health Services Scientist
Hotchkiss Brain Institute Cumming School of Medicine
University of Calgary
Calgary, Alberta, Canada

Peter Morone, MD
Resident, Department of Neurosurgery
Vanderbilt University
Nashville, Tennessee

Praveen V. Mummaneni, MD
Professor and Vice Chairman, Department of Neurosurgery
University of California, San Francisco
San Francisco, California

Lorenzo F. Muñoz, MD, FAANS
Associate Professor, Department of Neurosurgery
Rush University Medical Center
Chicago, Illinois

Rueben Nair, MD
Resident, Department of Orthopaedic Surgery
Northwestern University Feinberg School of Medicine
Chicago, Illinois

Allan D. Nanney III, MD
Chief Resident, Northwestern University Feinberg School of Medicine
Chicago, Illinois

Karina Nieto, MD
Resident, Departments of Obstetrics and Gynecology
Loyola University Medical Center
Chicago, Illinois

Ravi Nunna, MD
Resident, Department of Neurosurgery
Rush University Medical Center
Chicago, Illinois

W. Jerry Oakes, MD
Professor, Departments of Neurosurgery and Pediatrics
University of Alabama Birmingham
Birmingham, Alabama

Alfred T. Ogden, MD
Assistant Professor of Neurological Spine
Director of Minimally Invasive Spine Surgery
Columbia University Medical Center
The Neurological Institute, Columbia University
New York, New York

John E. O'Toole, MD, MS
Associate Professor, Department of Neurosurgery
Rush University Medical Center
Chicago, Illinois

Ali Ozturk, MD
Assistant Professor, Department of Neurosurgery
Pennsylvania Hospital
Philadelphia, Pennsylvania

Jason M. Paluzzi, MD
Resident, Department of Neurosurgery and Brain Repair
Morsani College of Medicine
University of South Florida
Tampa, Florida

Anay R. Patel, MD
Resident, Department of Orthopaedic Surgery
Northwestern University Feinberg School of Medicine
Chicago, Illinois

Michael S. Park, MD
Resident, Department of Neurosurgery and Brain Repair
Morsani College of Medicine
University of South Florida
Tampa, Florida

Erika A. Petersen, MD, FAANS
Assistant Professor, Associate Residency Program Director
Department of Neurosurgery
University of Arkansas for Medical Sciences
Little Rock, Arkansas

Martin H. Pham, MD
Resident, Department of Neurosurgery
University of Southern California
Los Angeles, California

Inge Preissl, MD
Neurosurgical Associates and Spine Section
Hochtaunuskliniken
Bad Homburg, Germany

Andrew J. Pugely, MD
Visiting Adjuvant Professor
Department of Orthopedic Surgery
University of Iowa
Iowa City, Iowa

John C. Quinn, MD
Resident, Department of Neurological Surgery
Rutgers New Jersey Medical School
Newark, New Jersey

Rakesh Ramakrishnan, MD
Departments of Orthopaedic and Spine Surgery
Michigan Orthopaedic Specialists
Clinical Instructor
Wayne State University
Detroit, Michigan

Chandan G. Reddy, MD
Assistant Professor, Department of Neurosurgery
University of Iowa Hospitals and Clinics
Iowa City, Iowa

Daniel K. Resnick, MD, MS
Professor and Vice Chairman
Program Director
Department of Neurosurgery
University of Wisconsin School of Medicine and Public Health
Madison, Wisconsin

Carlos E. Restrepo Rubio, MD
Fellow, Department of Neurologic Surgery
Mayo Clinic
Rochester, Minnesota

Laurence D. Rhines, MD
Professor and Director, Spine Program
Department of Neurosurgery
The University of Texas MD Anderson Cancer Center
Houston, Texas

Robert Andrew Rice, MD
Resident, Department of Neurosurgery
Georgetown University Hospital
Washington, DC

Casey Richardson, MD, BSFS
Resident
St. John's Hospital
Detroit, Michigan

Joshua M. Rosenow, MD, FAANS, FACS
Director of Functional Neurosurgery
Associate Professor of Neurosurgery, Neurology and Physical Medicine and Rehabilitation, Northwestern University Feinberg School of Medicine
Chicago, Illinois

Daniel Rosenthal, MD
Neurosurgical Associates and Spine Section
Hochtaunuskliniken
Bad Homburg, Germany

Faheem A. Sandhu, MD, PhD
Director, Spine Surgery
Department of Neurosurgery
Medstar Georgetown University Hospital
Washington, DC

Christina N. Sayama, MD, MPH
Assistant Professor, Department of Neurosurgery
Division of Pediatric Neurosurgery
Oregon Health & Science University
Portland, Oregon

Justin K. Scheer, BS
Medical Student
University of California, San Diego, School of Medicine
San Diego, California

Michael P. Schenk, MS, CMI (F)
Director, Biomedical Illustration Services
University of Mississippi Medical Center
Jackson, Mississippi

Laligam N. Sekhar, MD, FACS, FAANS
Professor and Vice-Chairman
Department of Neurological Surgery
Professor of Radiology
Director, Cerebrovascular Surgery
Director, Skull Base Surgery
University of Washington School of Medicine
Harborview Medical Center
Seattle, Washington

Jonathan N. Sellin, MD
Resident, Department of Neurosurgery
Baylor College of Medicine
Houston, Texas

Victoria Shunemann, MD
Resident, Department of Neurological Surgery
Ohio State University
Columbus, Ohio

Marc Sindou, MD, PhD
Surgeon, Department of Neurosurgery
Lyon 1 University
Pierre Wertheimer Neurological Hospital
Lyon, France

Konstantin V. Slavin, MD, FAANS
Professor, Department of Neurosurgery
University of Illinois at Chicago
Chicago, Illinois

Zachary A. Smith, MD
Assistant Professor, Department of Neurological Surgery
Northwestern University Feinberg School of Medicine
Chicago, Illinois

Dmitri Sofianos, MD
Physician, Department of Orthopaedics
Chatham Orthopaedic Associates
Savannah, Georgia

Robert J. Spinner, MD
Chair, Department of Neurologic Surgery
Burton M. Onofrio, MD Professor of Neurosurgery
Professor of Orthopedics and Anatomy
Mayo Clinic
Rochester, Minnesota

James A. Stadler III, MD
Resident, Department of Neurosurgery
Northwestern University Feinberg School of Medicine
Chicago, Illinois

Russell G. Strom, MD
Clinical Fellow, Department of Orthopaedic Surgery
University of California, San Francisco
San Francisco, California

Patrick A. Sugrue, MD
Assistant Professor, Department of Neurological Surgery
Northwestern University Feinberg School of Medicine
Chicago, Illinois

Hasan R. Syed, MD
Resident, Department of Neurosurgery
Georgetown University Hospital
Washington, DC

Lee A. Tan, MD
Resident, Department of Neurosurgery
Rush University Medical Center
Chicago, Illinois

Claudio E. Tatsui, MD
Assistant Professor, Department of Neurosurgery
The University of Texas MD Anderson Cancer Center
Houston, Texas

William R. Taylor, MD
Professor, Department of Neurosurgery
University of California, San Diego Medical Center
San Diego, California

Alisson R. Teles, MD
Clinical Fellow, Spine Program
Montreal Neurological Institute
McGill University
Montreal, Canada
Associate Researcher, Department of Neurosurgery
Laboratory of Clinical Studies and Basic Models of Spinal Disorders
University of Caxias do Sul
Caxias do Sul, Brazil

Raj P. TerKonda, MD
Facial Plastic Surgeon
Department of Otolaryngology
Obgai Skin Health Institute
Beverly Hills, California

Sergi Terterov, MD
Resident, Department of Neurosurgery
University of California, Los Angeles
Los Angeles, California

Alexander A. Theologis, MD
Resident, Department of Orthopedic Surgery
University of California, San Francisco
San Francisco, California

Erron W. Titus, BA
Medical Student, University of California, San Francisco
San Francisco, California

William D. Tobler, MD
Professor, Department of Neurosurgery
University of Cincinnati
Mayfield Brain and Spine
Cincinnati, Ohio

Vincent C. Traynelis, MD
Professor, Department of Neurosurgery
Rush University Medical Center
Chicago, Illinois

Trent L. Tredway, MD
Surgeon, Departments of Neurological Surgery and Orthopedic Surgery
Tredway Spine Institute
Seattle, Washington

R. Shane Tubbs, PhD
Chief Scientific Officer
Seattle Science Foundation
Seattle, Washington

Alexander Tuchman, MD
Resident, Department of Neurosurgery
University of Southern California
Los Angeles, California

Juan S. Uribe, MD
Professor and Director, Spine Section
Department of Neurosurgery
University of South Florida
Tampa, Florida

John R. Vender, MD, FACS, FAANS
Professor and Vice Chair, Department of Neurosurgery
Medical Director, Georgia Regents Gama Knife Center
Co-Director, Center for Cranial Base Surgery at Georgia Regents University
Medical College of Georgia, Georgia Regents University
Augusta, Georgia

Stephanus Viljoen, MD
Fellow, Department of Neurosurgery
University of Iowa Hospitals and Clinics
Iowa City, Iowa

Jean-Marc Voyadzis, MD
Professor, Department of Neurosurgery
Co-Director of the Center for Minimally Invasive Spine Surgery
MedStar Georgetown University Hospital
Washington, DC

Rishi Wadhwa, MD
Assistant Clinical Professor
Complex and Minimally Invasive Spine Surgery
General Neurosurgery
Department of Neurosurgery, Marin
UCSF Spine Center, San Francisco
San Francisco, California

Jeffrey C. Wang, MD
Chief, Orthopedic Spine Service
Professor of Orthopedic Surgery and Neurosurgery
University of Southern California Keck School of Medicine
Los Angeles, California

Michael Y. Wang, MD, FACS
Professor, Departments of Neurological Surgery and Rehab Medicine
University of Miami Miller School of Medicine
Miami, Florida

Joseph Weiner, BS
Medical Student, Northwestern University Feinberg School of Medicine
Chicago, Illinois

Stuart L. Weinstein, MD
Ignacio V. Ponseti Chair and Professor of Orthopaedic Surgery
Professor of Pediatrics
Department of Orthopedic Surgery
University Hospital
Iowa City, Iowa

Jonathan A. White, MD
Professor, Department of Neurosurgery
University of Texas Southwestern Medical Center
Dallas, Texas

Timothy M. Wiebe, MD
Physician
Bakersfield Memorial Hospital
Bakersfield, California

Jean-Paul Wolinsky, MD
Professor of Neurosurgery and Oncology
Department of Neurosurgery
John Hopkins University
Baltimore, Maryland

Christina Yen, MD
Resident, Department of Neurosurgery
University of Southern California
Los Angeles, California

Kazuo Yonenobu, MD, DMSc
Professor, Department of Orthopedic Surgery
Graduate School of Health Sciences, Jikei Institute
Osaka, Japan

Eric L. Zager, MD
Professor, Department of Neurosurgery
University of Pennsylvania
Philadelphia, Pennsylvania

Scott P. Zietlow, MD
Associate Professor of Surgery
Mayo Clinic College of Medicine
Department of Education Administration
Consultant, Division of Trauma, Critical Care, and General Surgery
Department of Surgery
Mayo Clinic
Rochester, Minnesota

Scott L. Zuckerman, MD
Resident, Department of Neurosurgery
Vanderbilt University Medical Center
Nashville, Tennessee

Section I Occipital-Cervical Junction

A. Pathology

1 Abnormalities of the Craniovertebral Junction

Brian J. Dlouhy, Raheel Ahmed, and Arnold H. Menezes

The craniovertebral junction (CVJ), also known as the craniocervical junction (CCJ), is composed of the occipital bone that surrounds the foramen magnum, the atlas vertebrae, the axis vertebrae, and their associated ligaments and musculature. The CVJ houses the transition of the central nervous system from the intracranial compartment and the neurovascular structures of the brain to the spinal cord, providing motor and sensory function to the body. The musculoskeletal organization of the CVJ is unique and complex, resulting in a wide range of congenital, developmental and acquired pathology.[1] Early anatomic descriptions of CVJ abnormalities date back to the second quarter of the 19th century. However, the clinical significance of radiographic osseous abnormalities was not described until 1939 by Chamberlain[2] and subsequently by Carl List in 1941. It was List who pointed out that cranial skeletal traction could reduce longstanding cervical dislocation.

Up until the mid-1970s, treatment of CVJ abnormalities consisted of posterior decompression and enlargement of the foramen magnum with removal of the posterior arch of the atlas vertebrae with or without occipitocervical or atlantoaxial fusion. However, for patients with irreducible lesions with ventral cervicomedullary compression, there was considerable morbidity and mortality associated with such treatment. It was not until the late 1970s that the senior author (A.H.M.) refined the transoral approach to the ventral CVJ, minimizing complications that previously plagued the approach.[3,4] In Menezes's 1980 report,[4] nine of 17 patients underwent a transoral approach for congenital, developmental, and acquired CVJ pathology.[3] No postoperative infections occurred, and complications were minimal.

The refinement of the transoral approach enabled the development of the first treatment algorithm by the senior author utilizing a surgical approach for abnormalities of the CVJ.[3,4] The surgical approach is based on an understanding of CVJ dynamics and a determination of the site of encroachment, the type of lesion, and the stability of the CVJ.[5] The pathology of these abnormalities is complex and extensive. There is a wide variety of congenital, developmental, and acquired abnormalities at the CVJ; one or more abnormality can occur in a patient. Since 1977, over 6,000 patients with abnormalities of the CVJ have been evaluated at the University of Iowa Hospitals and Clinics, many undergoing surgical treatment **(Table 1.1)**.[6–16]

Table 1.1 Craniovertebral Junction Pathology that Has Required Surgical Treatment at the University of Iowa Hospitals and Clinics from 1977 to 2014

Location	Congenital	Developmental and Acquired	Primary Neoplastic	Secondary Neoplastic
Clivus/foramen magnum	1. Occipital sclerotome segmentation failures 2. Neurenteric cysts 3. Osteopetrosis 4. Foramen magnum stenosis (achondroplasia)	1. Basilar invagination 2. Basilar impression (Paget's, rickets, osteogenesis imperfecta) 3. Cranial settling (rheumatoid arthritis) 4. Paramesial basilar invagination (achondroplasia) 5. Atlanto-occipital dislocation	1. Eosinophilic granuloma 2. Fibrous dysplasia 3. Chordoma 4. Chondroma 5. Chondrosarcoma 6. Plasmacytoma	1. Metastasis 2. Nasopharyngeal malignancy 3. Ectopic pituitary
Atlas vertebra	1. Atlas assimilation with associated segmentation failures 2. Atlas stenosis (achondroplasia)	1. Chronic C1–2 dislocations from Down syndrome, Morquio syndrome, rheumatoid arthritis, and arthropathies 2. Spontaneous and traumatic C1–2 dislocations/ligamentous instability 3. C1–2 rheumatoid pannus 4. C1–2 calcium pyrophosphate deposition disease (CPDD) pannus	1. Chordoma 2. Chondroma 3. Giant cell tumor 4. Osteoid osteoma 5. Osteoblastoma	1. Metastasis 2. Plasmacytoma 3. Local malignancy extensions
Axis vertebra	1. C2–3 segmentation failure 2. Os odontoideum 3. Neurenteric cysts	1. Basilar invagination 2. Basilar impression (Paget's, osteogenesis imperfecta, skeletal dysplasias, hyperparathyroidism, and arthropathies) 3. Cranial settling (rheumatoid arthritis) 4. C2 fractures 5. C1–2 rheumatoid pannus 6. C1–2 CPDD pannus 7. Osteomyelitis	1. Aneurysmal bone cyst 2. Plasmacytoma 3. Chordoma 4. Giant cell tumor 5. Osteoblastoma 6. Chondroma	1. Metastasis 2. Local tumor extension

Classification

The classification of CVJ abnormalities has been divided into the categories of congenital, developmental, and acquired disorders, and further classification can be made based on pathophysiological mechanisms (**Box 1.1**).

Diagnosis

The most interesting feature of CVJ abnormalities is the diversity of patient presentation. A constellation of symptoms and signs may occur as a result of compromise of the lower brainstem, upper cervical spinal cord, lower cranial nerves, upper cervical nerve roots, and the vascular supply to these structures, as well as resulting from hindbrain herniation and blockage of normal cerebrospinal fluid (CSF) pathways.[7,9] Each of these pathophysiological processes presents with its own characteristic features. A list of the pathological states affecting the CVJ is extensive, and these abnormalities may vary in the magnitude of neurologic dysfunction.

The symptoms of CVJ dysfunction may be insidious and at times may present with false localizing signs. A rapid neurologic progression occurs in rare instances and may be followed by

Box 1.1 Classification of Craniovertebral Junction Abnormalities

I. Congenital abnormalities and malformations of the craniovertebral junction
   A. Malformations of the occipital bone
      1. Manifestations of occipital vertebra
         a. Clivus segmentations
         b. Foramen magnum remnants
         c. Atlas variants
         d. Dens segmentation anomalies
      2. Basiocciput hypoplasia
      3. Condylar hypoplasia
      4. Atlas assimilation (occipitalization of the atlas)
      5. Osteopetrosis
      6. Foramen magnum stenosis (achondroplasia)
   B. Malformations of the atlanto-occipital junction
      1. Atlas assimilation (occipitalization of the atlas)
   C. Malformations of the atlas
      1. Atlas assimilation (occipitalization of the atlas)
      2. Atlantoaxial fusion
      3. Aplasia of atlas arches
   D. Malformations of the atlantoaxial junction
      1. Basilar invagination
   E. Malformations of the axis
      1. Irregular atlantoaxial segmentation
      2. Dens dysplasias
         a. Persistent ossiculum terminale
         b. Os odontoideum
         c. Hypoplasia-aplasia
      3. Segmentation failure of C2/C3

II. Developmental and acquired abnormalities of the craniovertebral junction
   A. Foramen magnum/occipital bone associated abnormalities
      1. Secondary basilar invagination
         a. Basilar impression (e.g., Paget's disease, rickets, osteogenesis imperfecta)
         b. Cranial settling (rheumatoid arthritis)
   B. Atlanto-occipital junction abnormalities
      1. Atlanto-occipital dislocation (AOD)
   C. Atlantoaxial instability
      1. Basilar invagination (primary)
      2. Errors of metabolism (e.g., Morquio's syndrome)
      3. Down syndrome
      4. Infections (e.g., Grisel's syndrome)
      5. Inflammatory (e.g., rheumatoid arthritis)
      6. Traumatic atlantoaxial dislocation; os odontoideum
      7. Tumors (e.g., neurofibromatosis, syringomyelia)
      8. Miscellaneous (e.g., fetal warfarin syndrome, Conradi's syndrome)
   D. C1/C2 pannus formation
      1. Rheumatoid arthritis
      2. Calcium pyrophosphate deposition disease (CPDD)

---

sudden death. Often, an antecedent history of minor trauma triggers a pattern of symptoms and signs that may progress at a rapid pace (**Box 1.2**).

Neuroradiological Investigation

The factors that are considered in determining the appropriate treatment of CVJ osseous, ligamentous, and soft tissue lesions are (1) the reducibility of the lesion; (2) the direction and the mechanics of encroachment and compression of neural structures; (3) the etiology of the abnormality; (4) the presence of abnormal ossification centers and anomalous growth and development of the CVJ; and (5) the presence of associated lesions such as vascular abnormalities, Chiari malformation, and syringohydromyelia.[3–5,7,9]

The word *reducible* refers to the ability to achieve normal osseous alignment, thereby relieving compression on neural structures. To achieve this, maneuvers such as flexion, extension, traction, disimpaction, and reduction distraction are utilized (**Fig. 1.1**). In regard to the direction of encroachment on neural structures, the lesion is either ventral to the cervicomedullary junction or dorsal and may be superior as well as lateral in location to the foramen magnum (**Fig. 1.2**). Associated neural

Box 1.2 Signs and Symptoms of Craniovertebral Abnormalities (Insidious or Rapid in Onset)

- Head tilt
- Short neck, low hairline, limitation of neck motion
- Web neck
- Scoliosis
- Features of skeletal dysplasias
- Neck pain and posterior occipital headache
- Basilar migraine
- Hand or foot isolated weakness
- Quadriparesis/paraparesis/monoparesis
- Sensory abnormalities
- Nystagmus—usually downbeat and lateral gaze
- Sleep apnea
- Repeat aspiration pneumonia, dysphagia
- Tinnitus and hearing loss
- Vertigo

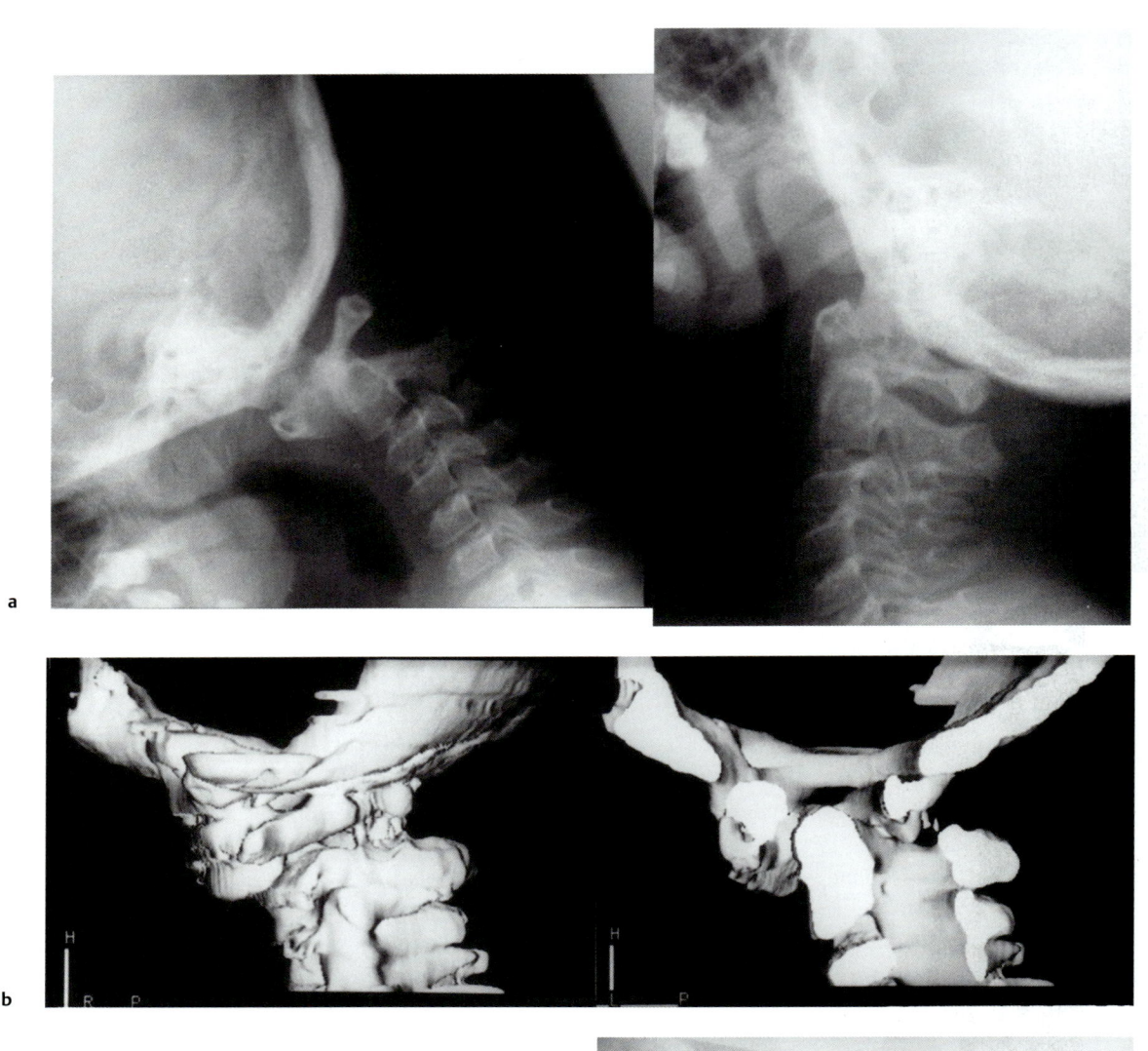

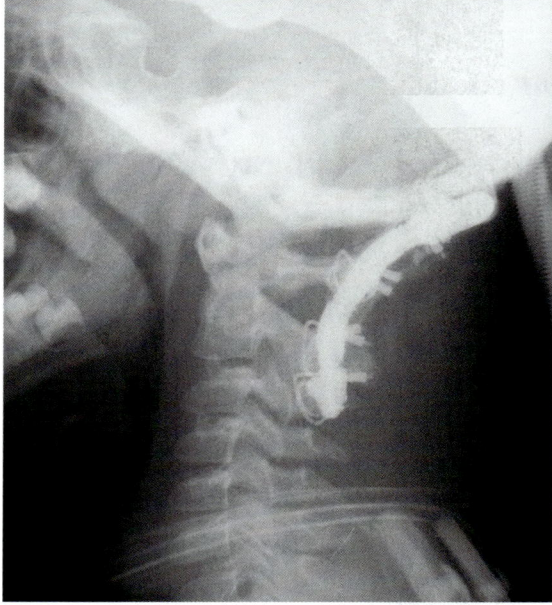

Fig. 1.1 **(a)** Composite of lateral cervical spine radiograph in the flexed *(left)* and the extended *(right)* position in a 7-year-old child with Down syndrome. Note the atlantoaxial dislocation, possible os odontoideum and the anterior atlantal arch sliding forward in extension. **(b)** Composite of lateral three-dimensional (3D) view of the craniovertebral junction (CVJ) *(left)* and a midsagittal section of the 3D reconstruction *(right)*. There is an atlantoaxial dislocation with bifid anterior and posterior arches to the atlas, as well as an os odontoideum. **(c)** Lateral radiograph taken 3 months following a dorsal occipitocervical fixation utilizing custom contoured threaded titanium loop instrumentation with autologous rib graft. The CVJ alignment is maintained.

1 Abnormalities of the Craniovertebral Junction

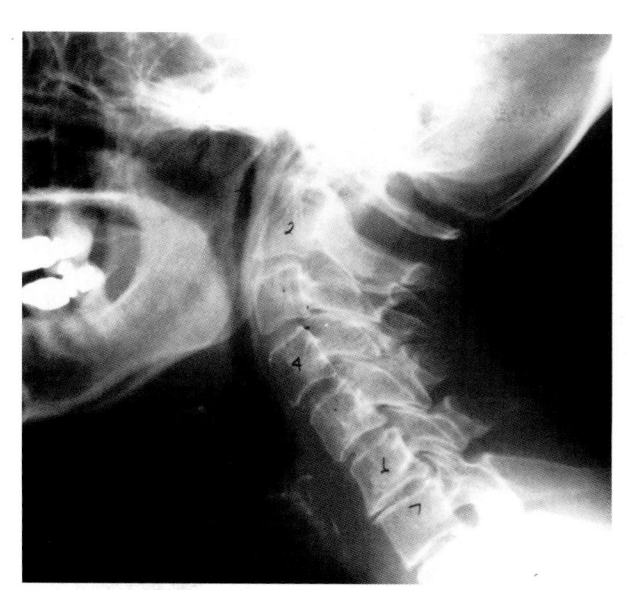

Fig. 1.2 (a) Plain lateral radiograph of posterior fossa and cervical spine in a 68-year-old woman with a diagnosis of basilar migraine who presented with difficulty swallowing, slurred speech, nasal regurgitation, and poor hand and leg coordination. The anterior arch of C1 is not visible, and the odontoid process is well above a line joining the hard palate and the posterior rim of the foramen magnum. There is a marked thinning of the squamous-occipital bone. (b) Midsagittal T2-weighted gadolinium-enhanced magnetic resonance imaging (MRI) of the posterior fossa and cervical spine. There is atlas assimilation with marked foreshortening of the true clivus. The clivus-odontoid angle is less than 90 degrees. There is indentation of the medulla and the basilar artery. (c) Axial T1-weighted gadolinium-enhanced MRI through the plane of the lower medulla. Note the flattening of the medulla in the anteroposterior dimension. (d) Composite of midsagittal T1- and T2-weighted MRI after ventral decompression of the lower clivus, anterior atlas, and the odontoid and axis body. Posterior decompression and dorsal occipitocervical fixation has been performed. There is significant decompression of the pons and medulla as well as the hindbrain herniation.

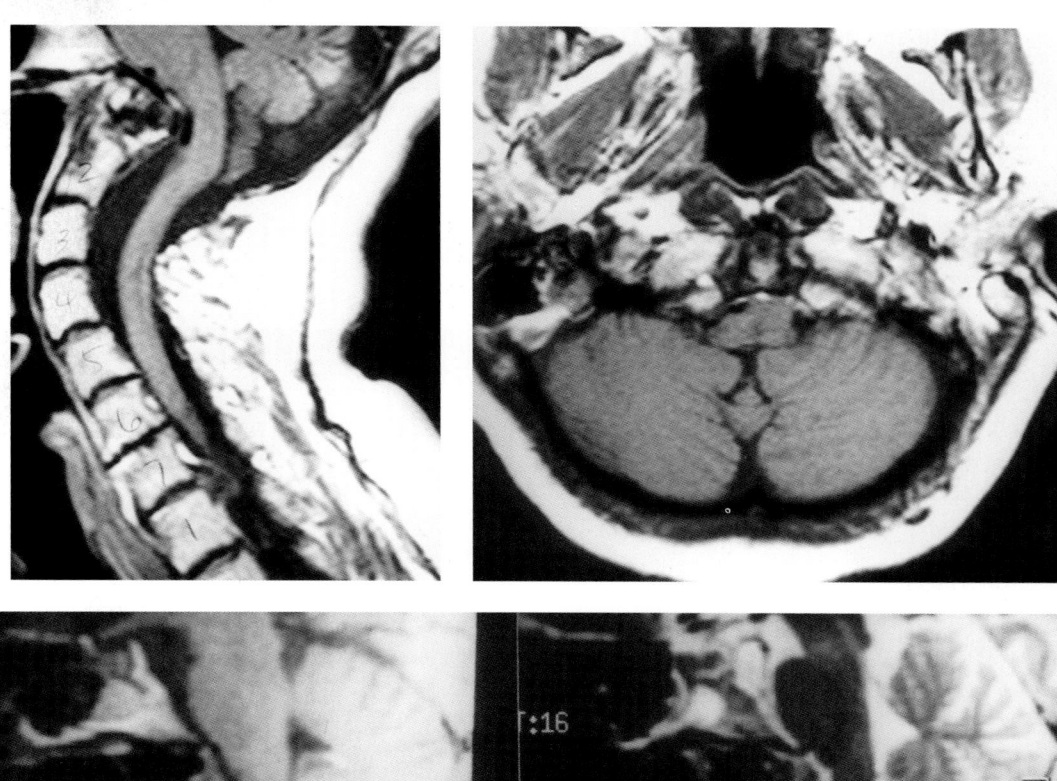

8   I   Occipital-Cervical Junction

abnormalities, such as a Chiari malformation, must be taken into consideration in guiding the primary treatment (**Fig. 1.3**).

Radiographs of the CVJ are usually done as the initial study in the workup of a patient to determine the presence of instability; radiographs are especially preferred in young children, to avoid the higher radiation dose of computed tomography (CT) screening. Radiographs should include a lateral view of the skull showing the spine, and the anterior open-mouth view and oblique views of the cervical spine. Supplementary views such as a Towne's view and the anteroposterior projection into the foramen magnum are done as necessary. High-resolution CT with reformatted two-dimensional (2D) or preferably three-dimensional (3D) imaging is done to clearly define the relationship and the dimensions of the CVJ. These studies can be done with the patient in the flexed and extended position to demonstrate the biomechanics. Magnetic resonance imaging (MRI) with the CVJ in flexed and extended positions defines the relationship of the bony abnormalities with the neural structures and helps with identifying any associated neural abnormalities. However, the bony anatomy must be precisely outlined with CT and 3D CT scanning (**Fig. 1.4**). With all imaging techniques, dynamic studies are necessary to assess the stability and the osseous-angular relationships to the neural structures. This provides information regarding the reducibility as well as the position of

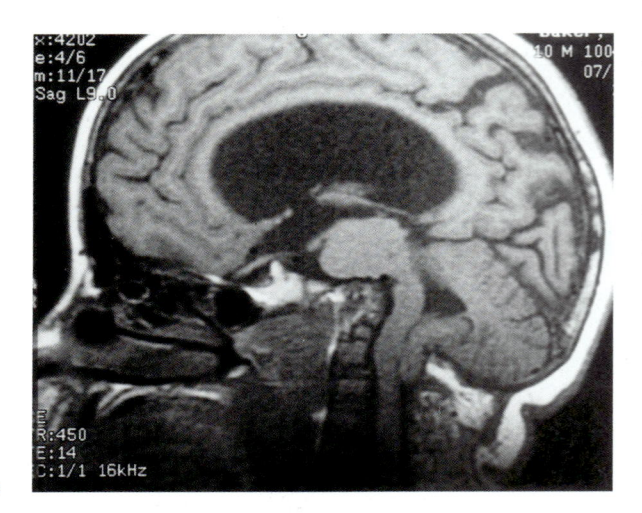

Fig. 1.3 (a) Mid-sagittal T1-weighted MRI in a 12-year-old child with osteogenesis imperfecta. There is a secondary basilar invagination (basilar impression) with a pontomedullary flexure of less than 90 degrees. The clivus and upper cervical articulation is acute in angulation, indenting the pontomedullary junction. A secondary aqueductal stenosis has led to significant hydrocephalus. The vertical height of the posterior fossa is reduced by an upward invagination of the squamous-occipital bone. Note the acquired hindbrain herniation with cerebellar tonsils at the C3 vertebral level. (b) Composite of axial T2-weighted MRI through the plane of the upper clivus *(left)* and above the dorsum sellae *(right)*. There is an invagination of the upper cervical spine and skull base into the cranium. The basilar artery is horizontal and is visualized in its entirety. The hydrocephalus is clearly seen.

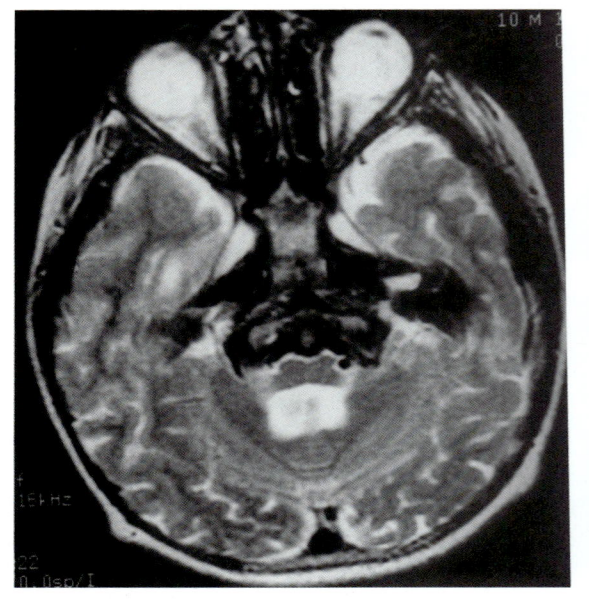

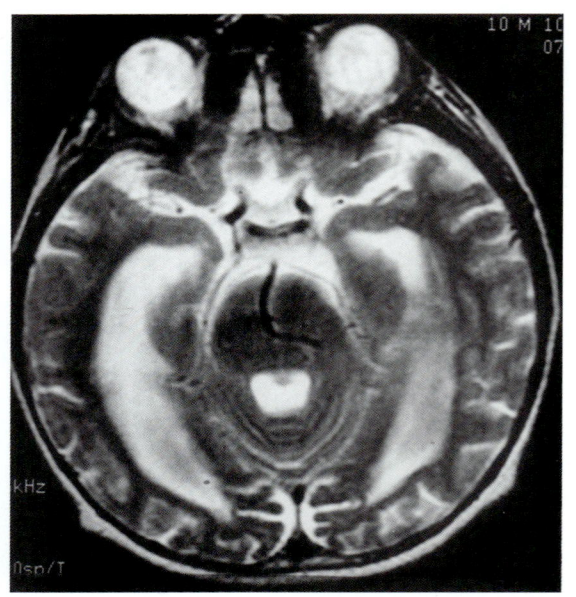

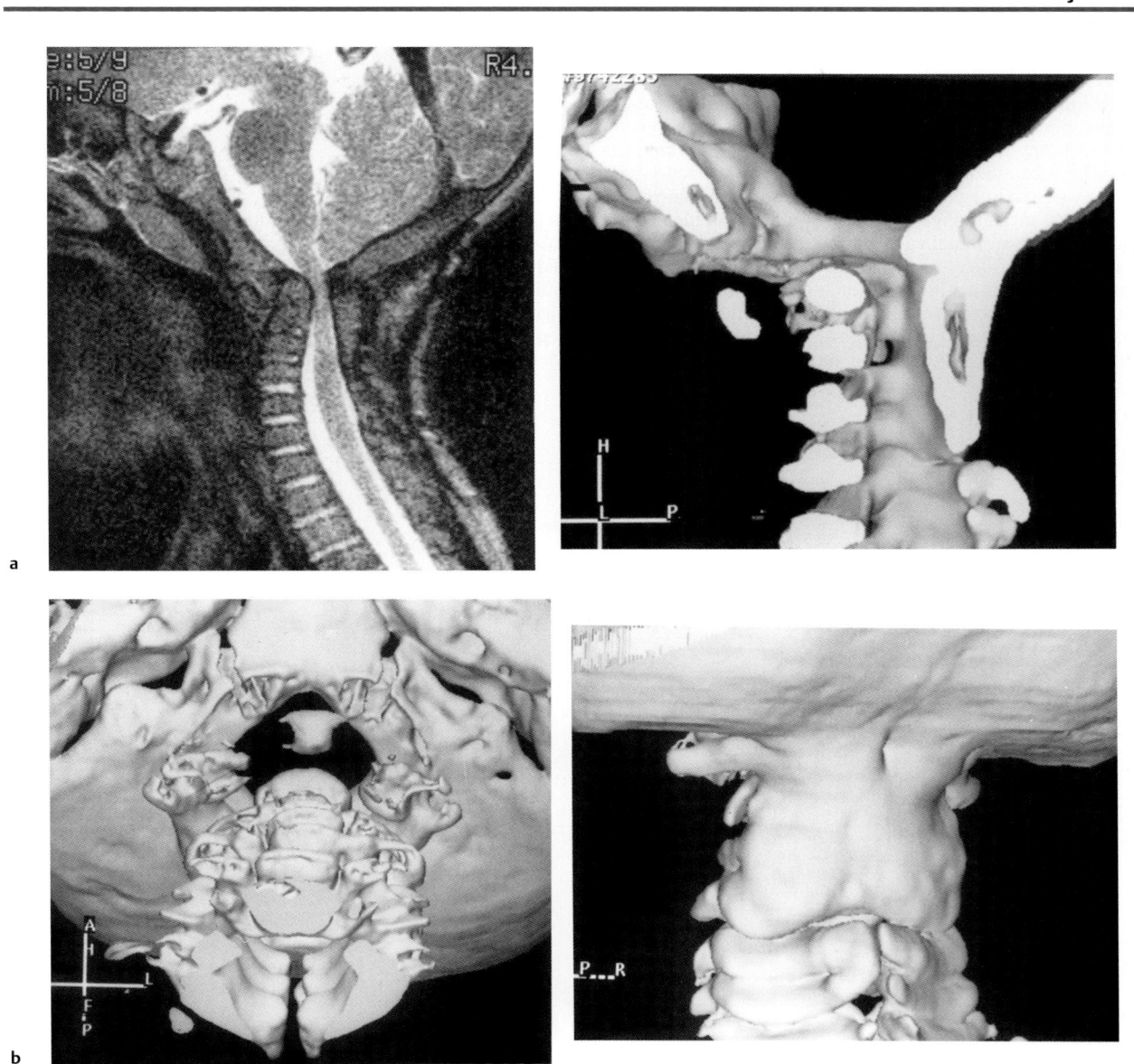

1 Abnormalities of the Craniovertebral Junction

Fig. 1.4 **(a)** Composite of a midsagittal T2-weighted MRI of the posterior fossa and upper cervical spine *(left)* and a 3D midsagittal reconstruction of the posterior fossa and upper cervical spine *(right)* in a child who had undergone a C1 laminectomy with a dorsal occiput-C4 fusion with progressive quadriparesis. It appears that the dorsal occipitocervical fusion is complete. However, there is a fixed atlantoaxial dislocation with an upward migration of the body of C2 indenting into the ventral cervicomedullary junction. **(b)** Composite of 3D computed tomography (CT) of the skull base and upper cervical spine viewed from the frontal and basal position *(left)* and dorsally *(right)*. Note the atlantoaxial dislocation with the absence of the anterior atlantal arch components. The dorsal occipitocervical fusion is complete.

fixation and fusion, should this be essential (**Fig. 1.5**). The effects of cervical traction must be documented not only with plain radiographs but also with intraoperative CT or MRI to confirm the relief of neural compromise and restoration of relationships of the CVJ. Any unexplained neurologic symptom or sign that cannot be accounted for by the previously mentioned studies requires vascular imaging with magnetic resonance angiography (MRA) or CT angiography (CTA), both of which can identify obstruction to the vertebral vessels with rotated head position or as a result of deformity and malignancy. In individuals with atlas assimilation and basilar invagination, a rotary subluxation of the atlas on the axis vertebrae can result in vertebral artery distortion, and occlusions are common. Imaging to determine the position of these critical vessels and the possible distortion that may occur with position change should be done prior to surgical treatment.

Treatment Strategy

Neurodiagnostic imaging[17] should be done to demonstrate the direction and mechanics of compression and associated abnormalities as well as to define the reducibility of the lesion. Reducible osseous pathology needs primary stabilization. Ligamentous reducible pathology such as with inflammatory states or recent trauma should be given a trial of immobilization. A treatment algorithm for problems in this region was first published by the senior author in 1980 and was recently updated by Dlouhy and Menezes. The updated version is shown in **Fig. 1.6**.

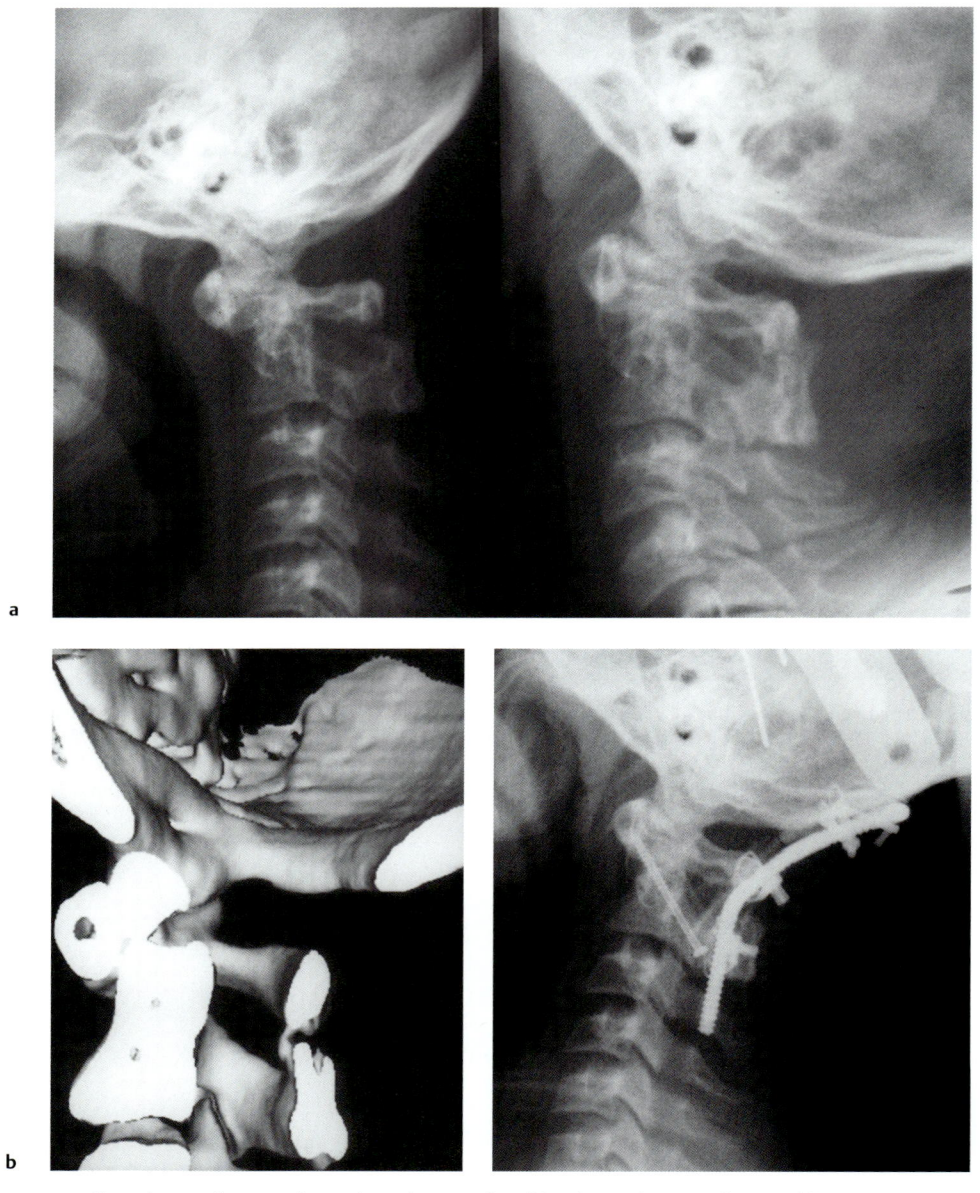

Fig. 1.5 (a) Composite of lateral cervical spine radiographs in the neutral and extended position. This 13-year-old boy with Down syndrome underwent a dorsal atlantoaxial arthrodesis a year previously that failed. There is evidence of os odontoideum with an unstable atlantoaxial articulation. (b) Midsagittal section of 3D CT of the CVJ. Note the os odontoideum. (c) Lateral cervical radiograph taken 6 weeks following transarticular C1-C2 screw fixation (one side) with dorsal occipitocervical fixation and utilizing titanium loop and rib grafts. This patient had gross occipito-atlantoaxial instability.

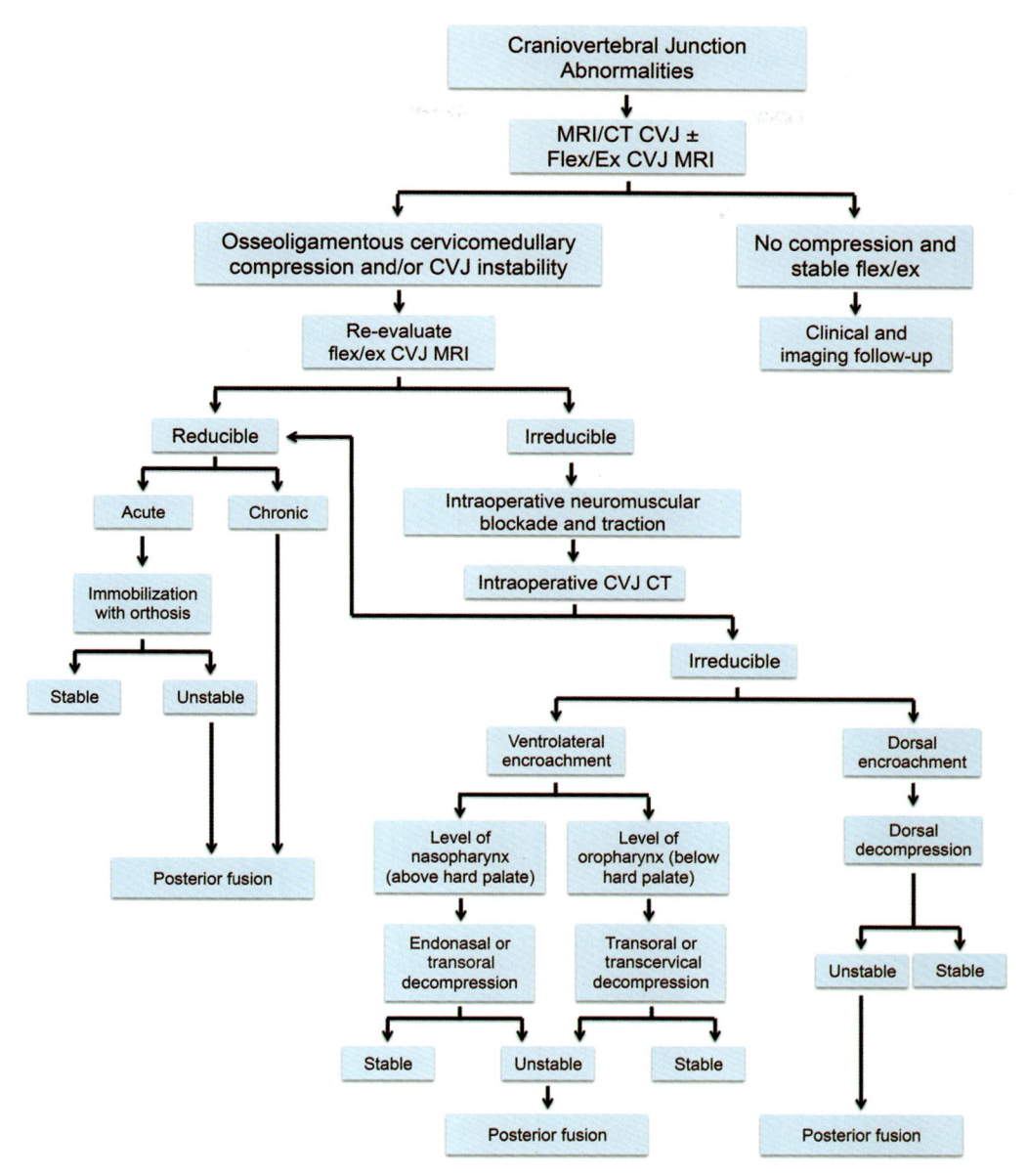

1 Abnormalities of the Craniovertebral Junction

Fig. 1.6 An updated treatment algorithm for osseoligamentous CVJ pathology that results in craniovertebral instability (atlanto-occipital instability, atlantoaxial instability, or a combination of both) or cervicomedullary compression. Advancements in understanding CVJ pathology, ventral approaches, and reduction strategies have been incorporated in the algorithm. CVJ abnormalities can often be associated with a Chiari malformation. Additional treatment of the Chiari may be needed in such cases. Flex/ex, flexion/extension.

Irreducible ventral pathology can be decompressed via a transoral approach, endoscopic endonasal approach, or anterolateral/lateral extrapharyngeal route. This most often is accompanied by a dorsal CVJ stabilization. We have utilized screw-and-rod constructs as well as custom contoured threaded titanium loops for occipitocervical fixation with autologous rib graft for the osseous construct. Postoperative immobilization is essential for osseous integration and fusion. **Box 1.3** lists the surgical approaches to the foramen magnum. A variety of skull base approaches have expanded from the basic anterior, lateral, and posterior routes to the foramen magnum. Irreducible dorsal or lateral encroachment is approached dorsally or laterally, respectively. In either circumstance, if instability is present, posterior instrumentation with fixation and fusion is often necessary.

Box 1.3 Surgical Approaches to the Craniovertebral Junction

Ventral
- Midline
  - Standard transoral
    - Transoral-transpharyngeal
    - Transoral-transpalatopharyngeal
  - Extended transoral
    - Median labiomandibular with or without glossotomy
    - Le Fort I osteotomy with down-fracture of the maxilla
    - Le Fort I osteotomy with palatal split
    - Le Fort II osteotomy
    - Transpalatal
  - Endoscopic endonasal
- Lateral
  - Lateral transcervical extrapharyngeal

Lateral
- Lateral or extreme lateral transcervical transcondylar

Dorsal
- Midline
  - Suboccipital with posterior fossa and cervical midline decompression
- Lateral
  - Far lateral or lateral suboccipital transcondylar

References

1. Menezes AH, Traynelis VC. Anatomy and biomechanics of normal craniovertebral junction (a) and biomechanics of stabilization (b). Childs Nerv Syst 2008;24:1091–1100
2. Chamberlain WE. Basilar impression (platybasia): a bizarre developmental anomaly of the occipital bone and upper cervical spine with striking and misleading neurologic manifestations. Yale J Biol Med 1939;11:487–496
3. Menezes AH, Graf CJ, Hibri N. Abnormalities of the cranio-vertebral junction with cervico-medullary compression. A rational approach to surgical treatment in children. Childs Brain 1980;7:15–30
4. Menezes AH, VanGilder JC, Graf CJ, McDonnell DE. Craniocervical abnormalities. A comprehensive surgical approach. J Neurosurg 1980;53:444–455
5. Menezes AH, VanGilder JC. Transoral-transpharyngeal approach to the anterior craniocervical junction. Ten-year experience with 72 patients. J Neurosurg 1988;69:895–903
6. Menezes AH. Craniovertebral junction anomalies: diagnosis and management. Semin Pediatr Neurol 1997;4:209–223
7. Menezes AH. Craniovertebral junction database analysis: incidence, classification, presentation, and treatment algorithms. Childs Nerv Syst 2008;24:1101–1108
8. Menezes AH. Pathogenesis, dynamics, and management of os odontoideum. Neurosurg Focus 1999;6:e2
9. Menezes AH. Primary craniovertebral anomalies and the hindbrain herniation syndrome (Chiari I): data base analysis. Pediatr Neurosurg 1995;23:260–269
10. Menezes AH. Specific entities affecting the craniocervical region: Down's syndrome. Childs Nerv Syst 2008;24:1165–1168
11. Menezes AH, Fenoy KA. Remnants of occipital vertebrae: proatlas segmentation abnormalities. Neurosurgery 2009;64:945–953, discussion 954
12. Menezes AH, Ryken TC. Craniovertebral abnormalities in Down's syndrome. Pediatr Neurosurg 1992;18:24–33
13. Menezes AH, VanGilder JC, Clark CR, el-Khoury G. Odontoid upward migration in rheumatoid arthritis. An analysis of 45 patients with "cranial settling". J Neurosurg 1985;63:500–509
14. Menezes AH, Vogel TW. Specific entities affecting the craniocervical region: syndromes affecting the craniocervical junction. Childs Nerv Syst 2008;24:1155–1163
15. Ryken TC, Menezes AH. Cervicomedullary compression by separate atlantal lateral mass. Pediatr Neurosurg 1993;19:165–168
16. Sawin PD, Menezes AH. Basilar invagination in osteogenesis imperfecta and related osteochondrodysplasias: medical and surgical management. J Neurosurg 1997;86:950–960
17. Smoker WR, Khanna G. Imaging the craniocervical junction. Childs Nerv Syst 2008;24:1123–1145

2 Rheumatologic and Degenerative Disease of the Craniovertebral Junction

Brian J. Dlouhy, Raheel Ahmed, and Arnold H. Menezes

A host of inflammatory conditions can affect the craniovertebral junction (CVJ), also known as the craniocervical junction (CCJ), with devastating consequences. The best described of these diseases is rheumatoid arthritis (RA). This chapter discusses the effects of RA and other inflammatory conditions on the CVJ.

Rheumatoid Arthritis

Epidemiology and Natural History

Rheumatoid arthritis is a chronic, systemic, inflammatory disorder that affects multiple joints, including those of the CVJ and subaxial cervical spine. The advancements in disease-modifying antirheumatic drugs (DMARDs) beginning in the 1990s have altered the natural history of RA by preserving the integrity and function of the joints.[1,2] Thus, the incidence and severity of rheumatologic spinal disorders has decreased over the past 25 years.

The prevalence of RA in adolescents over the age of 15 and in adults is ~ 1%, with the peak incidence occurring in the fourth through sixth decades of life.[3] Studies demonstrate a female predominance, with females being affected twice as often as males. Involvement of the cervical spine, and more specifically the CVJ, is second in incidence only to that of the hands and feet. Various studies estimate that 59 to 88% of patients with RA develop cervical disease. The abnormalities most frequently described are cranial settling and acquired basilar invagination (BI), retro-odontoid pannus formation, and atlantoaxial instability (AAI) and atlantoaxial subluxation (AAS). There are few large, population-based studies that have examined the incidence of RA affecting the CVJ. In a meta-analysis of 1,749 patients in the published literature, Casey and Crockard[4] found that 32% (range, 5.5–73%) had AAS, whereas 4.2% (range, 1.2–32%) had BI. Over half of those affected in this analysis (17%) had neurologic symptoms or signs. Although significant subaxial cervical disease does occur, it is less common than, and usually found in association with, disease affecting the CVJ. Intervertebral disks are often spared from the inflammatory process. Therefore, subaxial subluxation is usually a late manifestation of the disease.

In a prospective study of 100 patients with RA, Winfield et al[5] found AAS to be an early complication. At 5-year follow-up, 12 patients had documented AAS > 7 mm, whereas three patients had evidence of BI. More than 80% of the patients with AAS had developed it within 2 years of diagnosis of RA. Pellicci et al[6] reported on 106 patients over 5 years and found that, of patients with AAS, 80% worsened over the follow-up period. This same study reported a mortality rate of 17% for patients with RA compared with 9% for an age-matched cohort. In a postmortem study of 104 patients with RA, Mikulowski et al[7] found AAS with cervicomedullary compression in 11 patients; seven of the 11 had succumbed to a sudden death. In a report of 31 patients with RA and myelopathy, 19 patients died, with 15 of those deaths occurring within 6 months of presentation. All 19 patients were either untreated or managed conservatively in a cervical collar. Only fusion provided a reasonable chance for survival. These studies and others strongly suggest that, once cervical myelopathy is established in patients with rheumatoid cervical spine disease, the natural history without surgical intervention is grave, and mortality is more common than previously believed. Additionally, the incidence of cervical myelopathy and therefore mortality from myelopathy is likely underestimated in rheumatoid patients. Progressive pain, immobility, and weakness are often attributed to exacerbation of the systemic disease process rather than to neural compression.

A history of corticosteroid use, seropositivity for rheumatoid factor, the finding of rheumatoid subcutaneous nodules, and the presence of mutilating peripheral articular disease are all predictive of greater progression of cervical instability and neurologic injury. Similarly in a prospective study, Corbett et al[8] have clearly documented that the development of AAS is a predictor of eventual poor functional outcome.

Systemic Clinical Presentation

The clinical manifestations of RA include constitutional symptoms, arthritis, and, in some individuals, extra-articular complications. The systemic manifestations include subcutaneous rheumatoid nodules, ocular inflammatory conditions, pericarditis, pleural effusions, pulmonary nodules, and Felty's syndrome (neutropenia and splenomegaly). Fatigue is common and may be severe. Arthritis is characteristically accompanied by morning stiffness. Joint involvement is generally symmetrical and polyarticular. Joints that ultimately develop severe destruction usually become symptomatic within the first year of disease onset. Additional neurologic involvement not referable to the cervical spine includes compression neuropathies such as carpal tunnel syndrome, diffuse sensorimotor neuropathies, and mononeuritis multiplex. A mild inflammatory myopathy may occur as well. Presentation of patients as related to specific CVJ pathology is discussed in the following sections.

Pathogenesis

Although the etiology of RA is unknown, it is postulated to develop following an environmental exposure, such as an infection, in genetically predisposed people. In fact, there is an association between RA and the class II human leukocyte antigen (HLA) DR4. Despite an extensive search for an infectious agent, none has been found.

The abnormalities seen in the CVJ and cervical spine are the direct result of rheumatoid destruction of bone, cartilage, and supporting ligaments of the involved joints. These changes are due to the same host of inflammatory cells and mediators that causes destruction of the joints in the appendicular skeleton. Although the inciting cause of inflammation is unclear, the inflammatory process itself is well described. Initially, lymphocytes proliferate in the synovium, and polymorphonuclear leukocytes (PMNs) predominate in the synovial fluid. The PMNs release hydrolytic enzymes, oxygen radicals, and arachidonic acid metabolites that induce inflammation and cause tissue damage. Lymphokines, secreted by mononuclear cells, stimulate antibody production and the release of additional degradative products. The influx of combined fluid and inflammatory mediators produces the pain, swelling, and erythema that characterize rheumatoid synovitis.

Granulation tissue known as rheumatoid pannus then forms in the affected joint as a result of proliferating fibroblasts and inflammatory cells. The pannus produces collagenase and other proteolytic enzymes, resulting in damage to adjacent cartilage, tendons, and bone. The ensuing destruction leads to cartilage loss, bony erosions, cranial settling, tendon ruptures, and ligamentous laxity. Subsequent neurologic injury secondary to compression of the spinal cord, nerve roots, or vertebral arteries can result from direct impingement by the proliferating synovitic pannus or from repetitive bony compression due to vertebral subluxation and instability.

The CVJ and cervical spine are at high risk for involvement with the rheumatoid process because of the large number of synovial joints present. As opposed to osteoarthritis, in the rheumatoid process, lesions from the joints of Luschka extend into the disk spaces and vertebral bodies without osteophytosis. Thus, mobility is retained and subluxations are common. Because there is a strong correlation between the severity of cervical disease and that of peripheral erosive disease, cervical subluxation is more likely in those patients with progressive peripheral periarticular erosions.

Craniovertebral Junction Clinical Entities

Cranial settling, retro-odontoid (occiput-C1-C2) pannus formation, and atlantoaxial instability and subluxation can occur singly or in combination in patients with RA.

Cranial Settling

Cranial settling is another form of basilar impression (acquired basilar invagination or secondary basilar invagination), which results from erosion of bone and compression of the lateral mass of the atlas vertebrae with subsequent rostral migration of the axis vertebrae that can result in compression of the ventral cervicomedullary junction by the odontoid process (**Fig. 2.1**).[9] The lateral atlantal mass may fracture, with lateral displacement of the bone fragments. Additional destructive changes are often severe. The occipital condyles may completely erode through the lateral masses of the atlas, separating them into anterior and posterior pieces. The anterior component may migrate caudally over the axis body, whereas the posterior component usually shifts upward.

Cranial settling, most frequently presents with occipital or suboccipital pain, often with radiation toward the vertex. In the large series compiled by the senior author (A.H.M.), such pain was present in 90% of cases, whereas progressive difficulty with ambulation associated with cervical myelopathy was present in 76%. Limb paresthesias, vertigo, diplopia, and transient blackout spells were complaints in 55% of patients with cranial settling. Abnormal neurologic signs such as hyperreflexia and Babinski responses were presents in 80% of patients. A central cord–like syndrome was found in 30% and a similar number had a neurogenic bladder. Evidence of brainstem dysfunction such as internuclear ophthalmoplegia, facial diplegia, downbeat nystagmus, and sleep apnea was found in 20%. The cranial nerves most affected were the hypoglossal, glossopharyngeal, and trigeminal nerves. If lower cranial nerve impairment is seen, swallowing and vocal cord function should be formally evaluated.

In adults, the upper tip of the odontoid process normally lies 1 cm below the anterior margin of the foramen magnum. Several methods exist to evaluate vertical translocation of the dens on lateral cervical radiographs (**Fig. 2.2**). McRae's line connects the anterior and posterior margins of the foramen magnum (basion to opisthion). The dens should not project above this line. Chamberlain's line is drawn from the posterior margin of the hard palate to the opisthion. The tip of the odontoid process commonly lies below or just tangent to Chamberlain's line. The dens should not project more than 3 mm above this line, and 6 mm is pathological. The margins of the foramen magnum may be difficult to identify precisely on plain radiographs, however, making these measurements often inaccurate. McGregor's line, which connects the posterior margin of the hard palate to the most caudal point

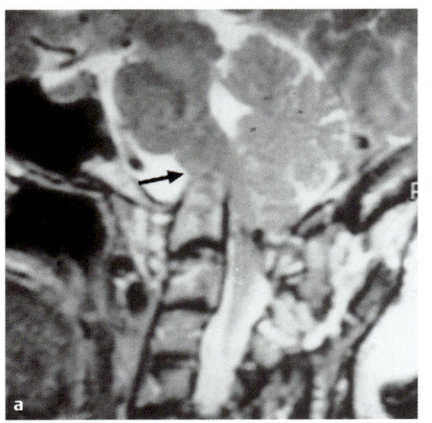

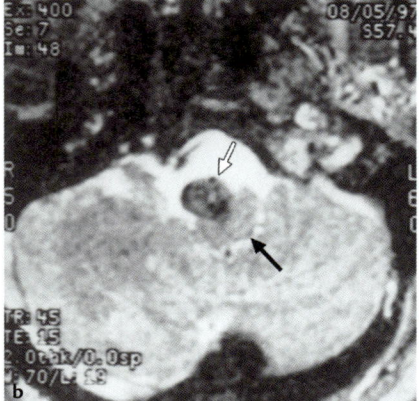

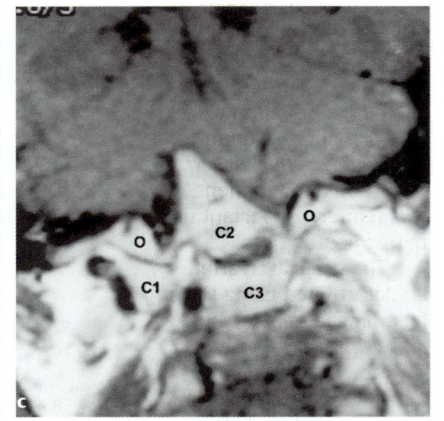

Fig. 2.1 Sagittal **(a)**, axial T2-weighted **(b)**, and coronal T1-weighted **(c)** magnetic resonance imaging (MRI) sequences displaying basilar invagination with ventral cervicomedullary compression. The medulla (*black arrow*) and dens (*white arrow*) are shown. Note also the displaced lateral mass of C1 next to the C3 vertebral body.

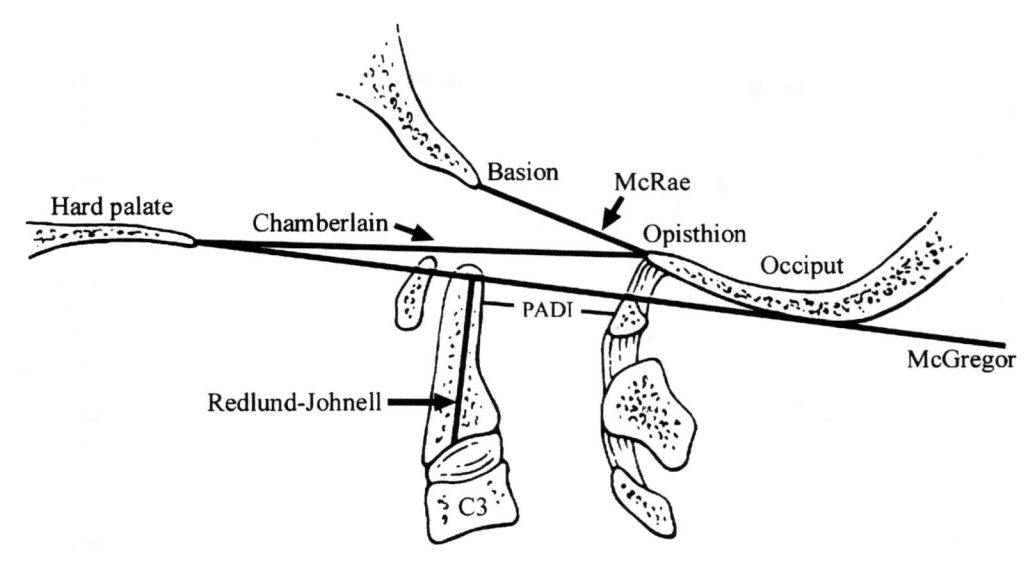

Fig. 2.2 Lateral view of the occipital-cervical junction demonstrating the common methods used to determine the presence of basilar invagination. The posterior atlantodental interval (PADI) is also shown.

of the occiput, may be easier to draw and thus may be more reliable. The tip of the dens should not project more than 4.5 mm above McGregor's line. Fishgold also described a measurement, on an open-mouth anteroposterior (AP) radiograph of the dens, in which the tip of the dens should be 1 cm or more below the digastric line.

Because the tip of the odontoid process may be difficult to identify in rheumatoid patients, another method, in which the tip is not used as a landmark, was described by Redlund-Johnell. This method calculates the perpendicular distance from the central part of the end plate of the C2 vertebral body to McGregor's line. Vertical migration of the dens is present if this measurement is less than 34 mm in men and less than 29 mm in women.

If cranial settling is suspected on plain radiographs, magnetic resonance imaging (MRI), including flexion/extension views, should be done to further assess the vertical migration of the odontoid process, possible craniovertebral instability, as well as neural compression. Breedveld et al[10] have shown that distortion of the spinal cord on MRI evaluation correlates with the signs of myelopathy, and Bundschuh et al[11] have shown that a brainstem cervicomedullary angle of less than 135 degrees (normal 135–175 degrees) on MRI also correlates with cervical myelopathy.

Cranial settling implies occipitoatlantoaxial instability. Conservative treatment of this entity in patients with signs and symptoms of neural compression carries the risk of progressive neurologic impairment and sudden death and is usually contraindicated. Age, severity of disease, and the overall medical condition of the patient, including nutritional status, are all factors that are important for deciding whether surgery should be performed.

The surgical treatment of rheumatoid cranial settling should be determined using the algorithm first developed by Menezes for management of CVJ pathology.[12] Dlouhy (primary author) and Menezes recently updated this algorithm (see **Fig. 1.6** in Chapter 1), incorporating advances in the treatment of CVJ abnormalities over the past 40 years.

Preoperative halo traction is used to reduce the vertical odontoid subluxation and decompress the ventral cervicomedullary junction. In 2007, at the University of Iowa Hospitals and Clinics, we developed and established an intraoperative but preoperative approach to reduce CVJ pathology that obviates the need for prolonged bedside skeletal traction, eliminates the concern for needing a 540-degree procedure, and enables confirmation of reduction prior to committing to an anterior or posterior approach. This method is discussed in detail in Chapter 6. In general, intraoperative traction is performed with the patient under general anesthesia and neuromuscular blockade. A crown halo should be used to apply the traction and initially a 7-lb weight is used, which can be increased as needed to a maximum of 12 lb. Imaging to verify reduction is performed with intraoperative three-dimensional (3D) computed tomography (CT) imaging of the CVJ.

The definitive treatment of rheumatoid cranial settling is dorsal occipitocervical fusion. A variety of techniques have been used to achieve fusion in these patients, including plate, screw-and-rod constructs, bent Luque rectangle, custom-made titanium loops, and wire or cable fixation. Careful analysis of the anatomy with CT is necessary before surgery. The inflammatory process may have destroyed large portions of the CVJ. Preoperative CT is also important for determining the course of the vertebral artery in reference to proposed screw trajectories.

Autogenous bone provides a better fusion substrate than allograft. It is recommended, therefore, that autograft be used in these individuals. This may be obtained from rib with very little morbidity, which is what we prefer. Others have used posterior iliac crest. Rheumatoid patients who have been treated with a dorsal occipitocervical fusion should be managed postoperatively in an orthosis. The type of orthotic employed is chosen on an individual basis depending on the patient's overall condition.

Patients with irreducible rheumatoid cranial settling require decompression (**Fig. 2.3**). The decompression should be directed toward the region of compromise, which is usually ventral. The types of approaches available and the indications for each are described in later chapters in this section of the book. Following ventral decompression, it is important to perform a fusion in these patients. The fusion may be performed immediately following the ventral decompression or, alternatively, these procedures may be staged. The details of the dorsal fusion have already been discussed.

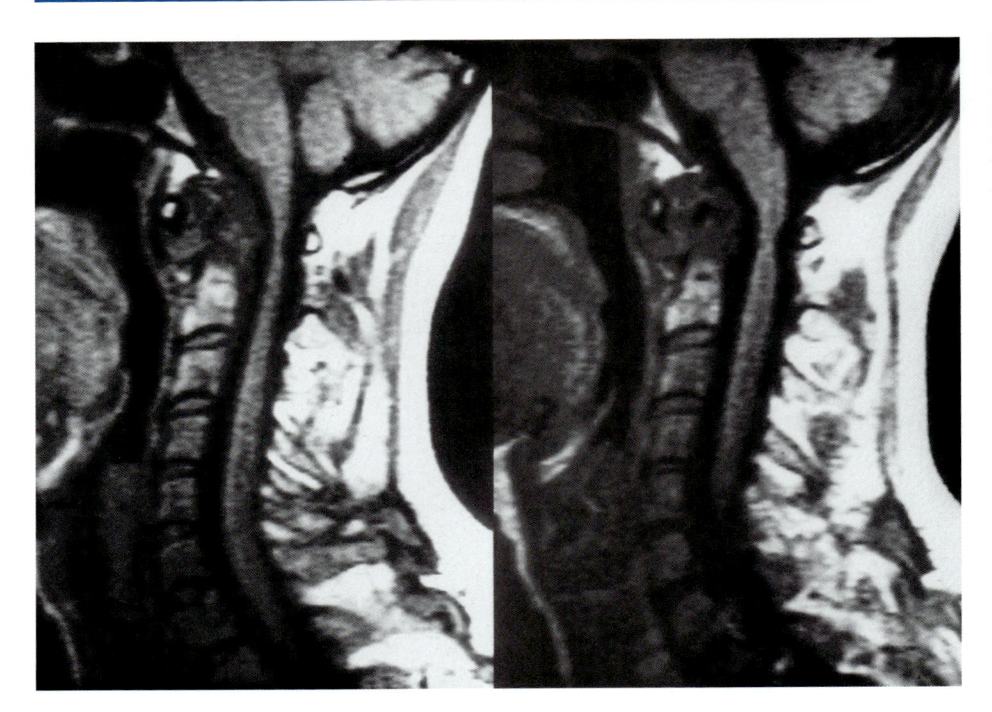

Fig. 2.3 Sagittal T1-weighted MRI before *(left)* and after *(right)* traction revealing irreducible cervicomedullary compression secondary to a large rheumatoid pannus. Patient required transoral decompression and posterior occipitocervical fusion.

Retro-Odontoid (Occiput-C1-C2) Pannus Formation

Rheumatoid cranial settling is often also accompanied by excessive proliferation of granulation tissue and occipitoatlantoaxial pannus formation. This pannus itself or together with the superiorly displaced odontoid process can produce ventral cervicomedullary compression. The pannus cannot be reduced. Therefore, in cases of cervicomedullary compression and progressive neurologic deficit, a ventral approach and decompression is often necessary.

Atlantoaxial Subluxation

In 1951, Davis and Markley[13] published the first case report of AAS in association with RA. AAS is now recognized as the most common type of cervical subluxation, accounting for 65% of all subluxations in patients with RA. Anterior subluxation makes up the majority of these cases, whereas lateral subluxation may occur in ~ 20% and posterior subluxation in fewer than 10%. Rotatory subluxation, although previously reported only infrequently in association with RA, was found in 10% of patients with AAS in a large series reported by the senior author (A.H.M.).

Atlantoaxial subluxation is the result of erosive synovitis in the atlantoaxial and atlanto-occipital joints and in the synovial lined bursa between the atlas, the odontoid process, and the transverse ligament. Ligamentous laxity is also implicated. The atlantoaxial complex depends on the transverse and alar ligaments and to a lesser degree on the apical ligaments for stability. Bony changes to the dens also contribute to instability and include loss of volume, osteoporosis, angulation of the softened bone, and occasional fracture.

Anterior AAS may result in compression of the cervical spinal cord between the dens and the posterior arch of the atlas. Even with minimal abnormal motion, exuberant pannus formation around the odontoid may be sufficient to impinge on the spinal cord. The cervical cord is particularly vulnerable to compression when the neck is flexed because C1 slides forward on C2.

The clinical manifestations of C1-C2 instability may arise from compression of the medulla, the upper cervical spinal cord, and occasionally the vertebral arteries. Compression of the spinal cord at the C1-C2 level may also produce ischemia in more caudal portions of the cervical cord, particularly in the anterior horn. The corticospinal tracts, lateral sensory tracts, second cervical nerve roots, and spinal tract of the trigeminal nerve are among the significant structures at risk with AAS.

The most frequent complaint of patients with C1-C2 subluxation is pain, which is present in 60% of cases. The pain is often greatest in the upper neck and frequently radiates to the occiput or vertex. The pain associated with C1-C2 subluxation is usually increased with neck flexion and rotation and is occasionally accompanied by a "clunking" sensation or a feeling of the head falling forward with flexion and rotation motions. Paresthesias in the C2 dermatome should also alert the clinician to AAS. Neurologic symptoms are multiple and may be vague, ranging from paresthesias in the hands to Lhermitte's phenomenon, especially with neck flexion. With advancing spinal cord or medullary compression, these patients may complain of weakness or incoordination of the arms or legs, vertigo, gait abnormalities, and, rarely, bowel or bladder problems. Additional symptoms of vertebrobasilar insufficiency, including drop attacks, may also be experienced, especially when AAS is combined with basilar impression.

Although objective clinical findings often corroborate a patient's complaints, the examination of the rheumatoid patient may be difficult, and typical signs of myelopathy are often masked by severe peripheral rheumatoid involvement.

Atlantoaxial instability is easily demonstrated on plain radiography (**Fig. 2.4**). Lateral cervical radiographs obtained with the patient in both flexion and extension are used for initial evaluation as well as screening purposes. The anterior atlantodental interval (ADI) measured from the midposterior margin of the anterior ring of the atlas to the anterior surface of the dens has been the most commonly cited measurement for quantitating the amount of subluxation. The upper limit of normal is 3 mm in adults and 4 mm in children. An ADI of more than 10 to 12 mm implies complete disruption of the entire atlantoaxial ligamentous complex. This interval is generally accentuated with neck flexion and diminished with extension. The difference in ADI between flexion and extension is thought to carry more clinical relevance than any single measurement alone. It has become increasingly evident, however, that the ADI is unreliable at identifying which patients have neurologic deficits and which are at risk to incur them. The posterior atlantodental interval (PADI) measured from the posterior aspect of the dens to the anterior margin of the C1 lamina has been found to be more reliable (**Fig. 2.2**). The ADI and PADI were compared in a cohort of rheumatoid patients followed over 20 years.[14] In evaluating the presence of paralysis, use of the PADI with a cutoff of ≤ 14 mm yielded a sensitivity of 97%, a specificity of 52%, and a negative predictive value of 94%. In other words, the ability of this measurement to detect paralysis was 97%, and if the PADI was > 14 mm, there was a 94% chance that the patient was not paralyzed. These values compared very favorably with those for the ADI, which, with an ADI ≥ 8 mm, were a sensitivity of 59%, a specificity of 58%, and a negative predictive value of 56%. It is important to note, however, the PADI does not represent the space available for the cord in a rheumatoid patient who may have a pannus extending behind the dens that is invisible on plain radiography.

Magnetic resonance imaging (MRI) can demonstrate cord compression directly as well as identify other soft tissues such as ligaments and pannus. CT provides less information about soft tissues but displays better bony detail. These studies are invaluable in patients with a neurologic deficit and for preoperative evaluation. MRI obtained with the patient in flexion and extension enables visualization of dynamic cord compression. A spinal cord diameter of less than 6 mm leaves the patient susceptible to myelopathy.

Although the diagnosis of AAS is straightforward, the decision to intervene surgically is complex. The treatment of AAS must be based on a clear understanding of the patient's overall health, the severity of symptoms, and the presence of neurologic findings. Two indications for surgical management are severe or unremitting pain and the presence of neurologic deficits. In patients with deficits, surgery should be performed as soon as neural dysfunction is recognized.

No clear guidelines exist for surgical intervention in patients with asymptomatic atlantoaxial instability. The mere presence of C1-C2 subluxation is not an indication for surgery. Although many surgeons in the past based the decision to operate on measurements of the anterior ADI (ADI ranging from 6 to 10 mm), this, as already mentioned, has not proven reliable. Instead, it is recommended that these patients undergo thorough baseline clinical evaluation including neurophysiological testing. If no abnormalities are found and the PADI is greater than 14 mm on plain radiography, expectant management may be appropriate. Regularly scheduled annual checkups with repeat thorough in-

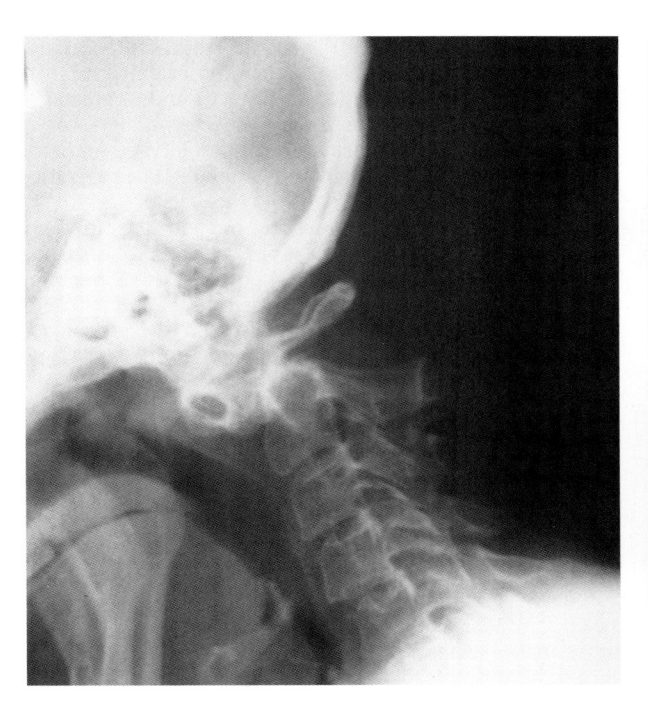

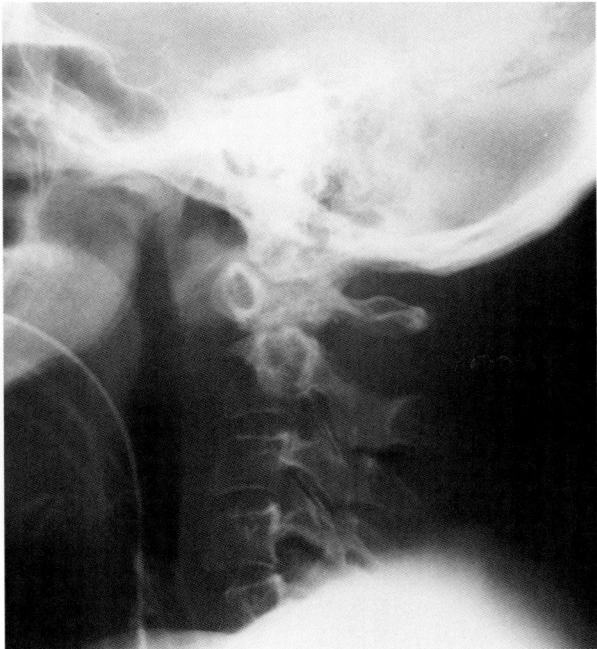

Fig. 2.4 Lateral cervical radiograph before **(a)** and after **(b)** traction demonstrating reducible C1-C2 dislocation. Sagittal T1-weighted MRI after traction also demonstrated partially reducible cranial settling and cervico-medullary compression. Patient presented with high cervical myelopathy and dysfunction of cranial nerves IX, X, and XII. Symptoms were ameliorated with posterior occipitocervical fusion.

vestigations are imperative for timely intervention. Progressive radiographic subluxation with a PADI less than 14 mm, a cervicomedullary angle less than 135 degrees, or a cord diameter less than 6 mm are all indications for arthrodesis because these patients are at risk for myelopathic deterioration. Of note, patients with asymptomatic AAS and any significant degree of cranial settling may warrant a more aggressive approach.

The most common surgical procedure employed for stabilization of AAS is posterior arthrodesis, which can be accomplished by several techniques (**Fig. 2.5**). Ideally, proper spinal alignment is obtained prior to surgery. When that is not possible and there is a fixed subluxation, a C1 laminectomy may be required if the canal is stenotic. Traditionally, C1-C2 arthrodesis has been achieved using screw-and-rod constructs. This essentially eliminates rotatory motion across this joint thereby increasing the likelihood of fusion. Careful preoperative planning is necessary before performing this procedure, especially in rheumatoid patients, to make sure that the lateral mass of the atlas will accept a screw.

In general, atlantoaxial arthrodesis should be employed cautiously in patients with RA because this is a progressive systemic disorder. As such, patients are at risk for developing cranial settling, and fusion at C1-C2 may theoretically hasten this event. If there is any evidence of early settling, or the occipitoatlantal joint is radiographically abnormal, strong consideration should be given to performing a dorsal occipitocervical fusion. The increased use of internal fixation has improved the fusion rate with these operations, and extending the atlantoaxial fusion to the occiput only results in a modest additional loss of flexion/extension motion. Likewise, patients with atlantoaxial instability must be assessed for subaxial instability and, if present, it should be addressed appropriately. A detailed description of the aforementioned procedures can be found in subsequent chapters.

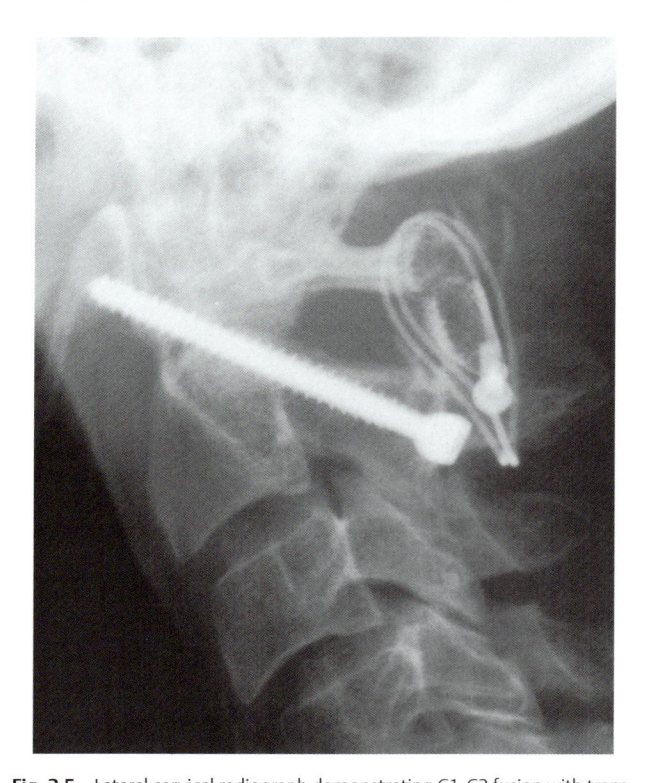

Fig. 2.5 Lateral cervical radiograph demonstrating C1-C2 fusion with transarticular screws and posterior cable and bone construct in a patient with neck pain and progressive radiographic atlantoaxial subluxation.

Posterior Atlantoaxial Subluxation

Posterior C1-C2 subluxation occurs infrequently. It is generally a result of erosion or fracture of the odontoid process and may result in myelopathy secondary to spinal cord compression. Because of their high degree of instability, all posterior AASs should be surgically stabilized.

Atlantoaxial Rotatory Subluxation

Atlantoaxial rotatory subluxation occurs from the same destructive rheumatoid synovitis at the occipitocervical and atlantoaxial joints, allowing rotation at the occiput-C1 and C1-C2 joints. This type of subluxation is progressive and may result in a fixed torticollis occurring over a period of 1 to 6 months. If not recognized and corrected, this deformity will become permanent and will be a continued source of pain.

Cervical and occipital pain in addition to various neurologic signs and symptoms are the usual clinical findings. Many clinicians may underestimate the incidence of C1-C2 rotatory subluxation because of the difficulties in making the diagnosis. Weissman et al[15] found that C1-C2 rotatory subluxation accounted for 21% of all AASs in their series, whereas Menezes reported an incidence of 10% in his series.

The diagnosis is suspected clinically in patients who present with posterior cervical or suboccipital pain and a head tilt. There may be hypesthesia or hypalgesia in the C2 dermatome.

The diagnosis is confirmed radiographically. Atlantoaxial rotatory subluxation has been defined as more than 2 mm of subluxation of the C1 lateral masses on C2. This is associated with a rotational deformity and can be best visualized on CT, both with and without 3D reconstruction of the occipitoatlantoaxial complex. Using CT, Dvorak et al[16] suggested that axial rotation between C1 and C2 greater than 56 degrees is abnormal. Also, a right-left difference in rotation between C1 and C2 greater than 8 degrees represents excessive motion. Such findings may constitute clinically significant rotatory instability. Asymmetry of the lateral masses on AP plain radiography is also suggestive of rotation.

Treatment consists of reduction using intraoperative crown halo traction with neuromuscular blockade and confirmation of reduction by intraoperative 3D CT. A posterior C1-C2 or occipitocervical fusion can then be performed. All of the precautions taken in patients with cranial settling should be exercised. These patients are maintained in a halo vest for 10 to 12 weeks postoperatively and then placed in a soft collar for an additional 6 to 8 weeks.

Outcomes

The goal of surgical management in patients with RA involving the CVJ is to relieve pain, reduce deformity, and prevent neurologic deterioration. This goal may be achieved by posterior arthrodesis combined with a decompressive procedure when needed. Although lack of uniform outcome measures in the literature makes generalizations about prognosis difficult, several factors have been shown to correlate with decreased potential for neurologic recovery after surgical stabilization. These include preoperative PADI of less than 10 mm, subluxation accompanied by BI, poorer Ranawat class, and postoperative pseudarthrosis.[14] In a meta-analysis of 492 patients, only 25% of Ranawat class IIIB patients improved to class II. This group had a 15% perioperative mortality, which rose to 60% at 15 months. In contrast, when all rheumatoid patients were taken together, the average mortality was 6%. Although improved operative techniques and perioperative care are decreasing morbidity and mortality rates, RA of the CVJ remains a challenging problem for the surgeon. Maximal benefit can be realized when patients are treated early in the disease process.

Miscellaneous Inflammatory Conditions Affecting the Craniovertebral Junction

The seronegative spondyloarthropathies are a group of related disorders that cause inflammation and ossification of the entheses or sites of ligamentous/tendinous insertion into the bone. They commonly affect the spine and sacroiliac joints, as well as the peripheral joints. Rheumatoid factor is generally not detected in the serum of patients with these diseases but there is an association with the specific genetic marker HLA-B27. Ankylosing spondylitis (AS), psoriatic arthropathy, reactive arthritis (Reiter's syndrome), and the enteropathic arthropathies (Crohn's disease and ulcerative colitis) all fit under this designation. Whereas these enthesopathies typically result in stiffening or fusion of the involved joints (spondylitis), the associated arthritis can cause severe erosive changes in the ligaments and associated joints.[17,18] When this occurs in the craniovertebral region, significant instability can result.[17,19]

Although the primary pathological process in AS usually involves the subaxial spine, the atlantoaxial region can be involved secondarily. Fusion of the subaxial spine can lead to excessive dynamic loading of the CVJ, resulting in subluxation and promoting secondary BA. In a review of 39 patients with AS, atlantoaxial instability was demonstrated in nearly one third of those who also had associated psoriasis, Reiter's syndrome, or inflammatory bowel disease. Type II odontoid process fractures and hangman's fractures have also been seen in patients with AS in whom spontaneous occipitoatlantal fusion had previously occurred.

Psoriatic arthropathy affects 7% of patients with psoriasis. The spine is eventually involved in 20% of these individuals, with CVJ involvement occurring in much the same way as in AS.

Reiter's syndrome (arthritis, urethritis, and uveitis) may be associated with an acute inflammatory synovitis and has been reported in association with AAS.

Rheumatologic complications have been described in up to 30% of patients with inflammatory bowel disease. Although infrequent, these complications include severe erosive arthritis that involves the CVJ. In 1969, Newman and Sweetnam,[20] in describing their technique for occipitocervical fusion, reported a case of AAS in a 25-year-old woman with ulcerative colitis. In 1986, Jordan et al[17] reported a similar case in a patient with Crohn's disease and indicated that in addition to spondylitis, which is relatively common in patients with seronegative arthritides, inflammatory bowel disease could cause an erosive arthritis similar to that in RA. They concluded that inflammatory bowel disease should be added to the differential diagnosis of patients who present with isolated atlantoaxial instability.

Calcium pyrophosphate deposition in the synovial joints of the CVJ has also been described. This phenomenon has been termed "pseudogout" and may present with compression of the cervicomedullary junction (**Fig. 2.6**).

Although the etiologies may be different, the same principles applied to craniovertebral pathology in cases of RA appear to be appropriate to guide management decisions in these unusual cases.

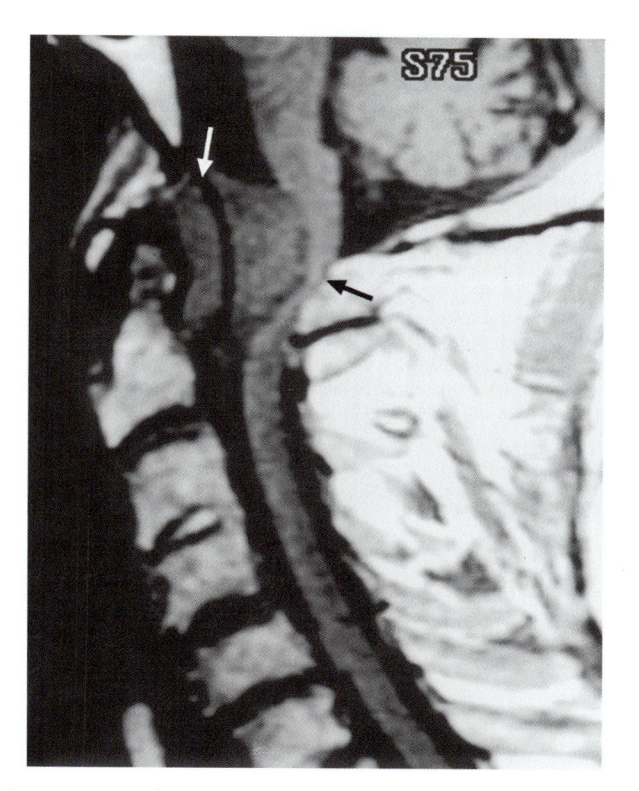

Fig. 2.6 T1-weighted sagittal MRI demonstrating cervicomedullary junction compression (black arrow) secondary to a large mass posterior to the dens. Note the hypointense mass both anterior and posterior to the tectorial membrane (white arrow).

References

1. Kauppi MJ, Neva MH, Laiho K, et al; FIN-RACo Trial Group. Rheumatoid atlantoaxial subluxation can be prevented by intensive use of traditional disease modifying antirheumatic drugs. J Rheumatol 2009;36:273–278
2. Neva MH, Kauppi MJ, Kautiainen H, et al; FIN-RACo Trail Group. Combination drug therapy retards the development of rheumatoid atlantoaxial subluxations. Arthritis Rheum 2000;43:2397–2401
3. Zikou AK, Alamanos Y, Argyropoulou MI, et al. Radiological cervical spine involvement in patients with rheumatoid arthritis: a cross sectional study. J Rheumatol 2005;32:801–806
4. Casey ATH, Crockard HA. Rheumatoid arthritis. In: Dickman CA, Spetzler RF, Sonntag VKH, eds. Surgery of the Craniovertebral Junction. New York: Thieme; 1998:151–174
5. Winfield J, Cooke D, Brook AS, Corbett M. A prospective study of the radiological changes in the cervical spine in early rheumatoid disease. Ann Rheum Dis 1981;40:109–114
6. Pellicci PM, Ranawat CS, Tsairis P, Bryan WJ. A prospective study of the progression of rheumatoid arthritis of the cervical spine. J Bone Joint Surg Am 1981;63:342–350
7. Mikulowski P, Wollheim FA, Rotmil P, Olsen I. Sudden death in rheumatoid arthritis with atlanto-axial dislocation. Acta Med Scand 1975;198:445–451
8. Corbett M, Dalton S, Young A, Silman A, Shipley M. Factors predicting death, survival and functional outcome in a prospective study of early rheumatoid disease over fifteen years. Br J Rheumatol 1993;32:717–723
9. Menezes AH, VanGilder JC, Clark CR, el-Khoury G. Odontoid upward migration in rheumatoid arthritis. An analysis of 45 patients with "cranial settling." J Neurosurg 1985;63:500–509

10. Breedveld FC, Algra PR, Vielvoye CJ, Cats A. Magnetic resonance imaging in the evaluation of patients with rheumatoid arthritis and subluxations of the cervical spine. Arthritis Rheum 1987;30:624–629

11. Bundschuh C, Modic MT, Kearney F, Morris R, Deal C. Rheumatoid arthritis of the cervical spine: surface-coil MR imaging. AJR Am J Roentgenol 1988;151:181–187

12. Menezes AH, VanGilder JC, Graf CJ, McDonnell DE. Craniocervical abnormalities. A comprehensive surgical approach. J Neurosurg 1980;53:444–455

13. Davis FW Jr, Markley HE. Rheumatoid arthritis with death from medullary compression. Ann Intern Med 1951;35:451–454

14. Boden SD, Dodge LD, Bohlman HH, Rechtine GR. Rheumatoid arthritis of the cervical spine. A long-term analysis with predictors of paralysis and recovery. J Bone Joint Surg Am 1993;75:1282–1297

15. Weissman BN, Aliabadi P, Weinfeld MS, Thomas WH, Sosman JL. Prognostic features of atlantoaxial subluxation in rheumatoid arthritis patients. Radiology 1982;144:745–751

16. Dvorak J, Hayek J, Zehnder R. CT-functional diagnostics of the rotatory instability of the upper cervical spine. Part 2. An evaluation on healthy adults and patients with suspected instability. Spine 1987;12:726–731

17. Jordan JM, Obeid LM, Allen NB. Isolated atlantoaxial subluxation as the presenting manifestation of inflammatory bowel disease. Am J Med 1986;80:517–520

18. Ryken T, Menezes A. Inflammatory bowel disease and the craniocervical junction. Neurosurg Focus 1999;6:e10

19. Suarez-Almazor ME, Russell AS. Anterior atlantoaxial subluxation in patients with spondyloarthropathies: association with peripheral disease. J Rheumatol 1988;15:973–975

20. Newman P, Sweetnam R. Occipito-cervical fusion. An operative technique and its indications. J Bone Joint Surg Br 1969;51:423–431

3 Tumors of the Occipital-Cervical Junction

Mohamad Bydon, Rafael De la Garza-Ramos, Ziya L. Gokaslan, and Jean-Paul Wolinsky

The occipital-cervical junction (OCJ) is composed of the clivus, foramen magnum, and upper two cervical vertebrae (atlas and axis). Tumors in this region may arise from osseus, soft tissue, or neural elements.[1-3] Due to the relatively large size of the subarachnoid space at the OCJ, symptoms caused by a tumor in this region usually appear late, after the tumor has grown to a considerable size.[4]

Symptoms of tumors in the OCJ are usually caused by neural compression or traction.[4] Other effects such as syringomyelia, hydrocephalus, or vascular compromise may be seen,[5,6] and Meyer et al[7] reported a mean time of 2.5 years between onset of symptoms and diagnosis.

This chapter reviews tumors in the OCJ, with emphasis on the pathological features, diagnosis, and treatment of these lesions.

Classification of Occipital-Cervical Junction Tumors

Tumors of the OCJ may arise from any of the osseus structures in this region, but also from soft tissues or neural elements (**Fig. 3.1**). Moreover, they can be classified as either primary benign (eosinophilic granuloma, fibrous dysplasia, chondroma, giant cell tumor, osteoid osteoma, meningioma, and neurofibroma) or primary malignant (chordoma, chondrosarcoma, and plasmacytoma) tumors.

Primary Benign Tumors

Eosinophilic Granuloma

Eosinophilic granulomas are a form of histiocytosis (proliferation of activated dendritic cells and macrophages). They most commonly present in children and adolescents,[4] but cases have also been reported in adults.[8] Eosinophilic granuloma is part of Langerhans cell histiocytosis, which in turn can be subdivided into three clinical entities: eosinophilic granuloma (solitary osseus lesion), Hand-Schuller-Christian disease (eosinophilic granuloma plus lytic bone lesions, diabetes insipidus [from pituitary stalk infiltration] and exophthalmos), and Letter-Siwe disease (malignant disseminated granulomas).[8,9] When these lesions involve the spine, they most commonly occur in the thoracolumbar region, but the upper cervical spine and clivus may also be involved.[4]

The most common presenting symptoms are neck pain and muscle spasm.[10] Neurologic symptoms are caused by vertebral collapse, producing torticollis at the OCJ.[4] On conventional X-rays, eosinophilic granulomas appear as osteolytic lesions with sclerotic rims, and may be accompanied by vertebral collapse and flattening (i.e., vertebra plana).[4] Following X-rays, complementary imaging studies such as computed tomography (CT) scans, magnetic resonance imaging (MRI), or bone scans (to detect more widespread variants of the disease) can be performed.

Diagnosis can be made via a CT-guided biopsy or open biopsy.[4,11] Patients with mild symptoms can be observed and treated with cervical immobilization and systemic treatment of the underlying disease process, but neurologic deficits or intractable pain warrant surgical management.[8] Given that eosinophilic granulomas involve the vertebral body or OCJ, tumoral resection requires adequate preoperative planning and possibly anterior/posterior reconstruction techniques.

Low-dose radiation has also proven effective in the treatment of these lesions,[12] but care must be taken in children, because radiation could potentially destroy endochondral plates and injure the spinal cord.[10]

Aneurysmal Bone Cyst

Aneurysmal bone cysts (ABCs) are highly vascularized lesions with an expansile nature; they occur more frequently in females during the first and second decade of life.[13,14] They can occur as primary lesions or in conjunction with a giant cell tumor, fibrous dysplasia, osteosarcoma, or osteoblastoma.[4,15] Of all spinal ABCs, the atlas (C1 vertebra) is involved in only 1% of cases.[4] Histologically, these tumors are composed of large cavernous blood-filled spaces separated by trabeculae or osteoid tissue. Due to their expansile nature, they may cause swelling, pain, bone destruction, and fractures.[16]

Although histologically benign, these tumors are fast-growing and tend to recur spontaneously even after resection. On CT scans, ABCs appear as multiloculated expansile lesions with fluid-fluid levels.[16] On MRI, ABCs, appear with varying degrees of intensity on both T1- and T2-weighted images; after administration of contrast, these lesions appear with heterogeneous enhancement.

The best treatment in terms of prognosis is complete resection with preoperative embolization. Some patients have been reported to be cured with embolization alone,[17] and other treatments such as radiation have been explored.[18] However, the treatment of choice is biopsy followed by serial direct tumoral embolization with calcitonin and steroids. If this fails, then resection and reconstruction are warranted.[19]

Fibrous Dysplasia

Fibrous dysplasia is characterized by the replacement of the medullary cavity of bones with fibrous tissue. This entity may involve only one bone (monostotic) or many bones (polyostotic), best exemplified by McCune-Albright syndrome. Monostotic fibrous dysplasia of the spine is rare, with equal incidence in men and women.[20]

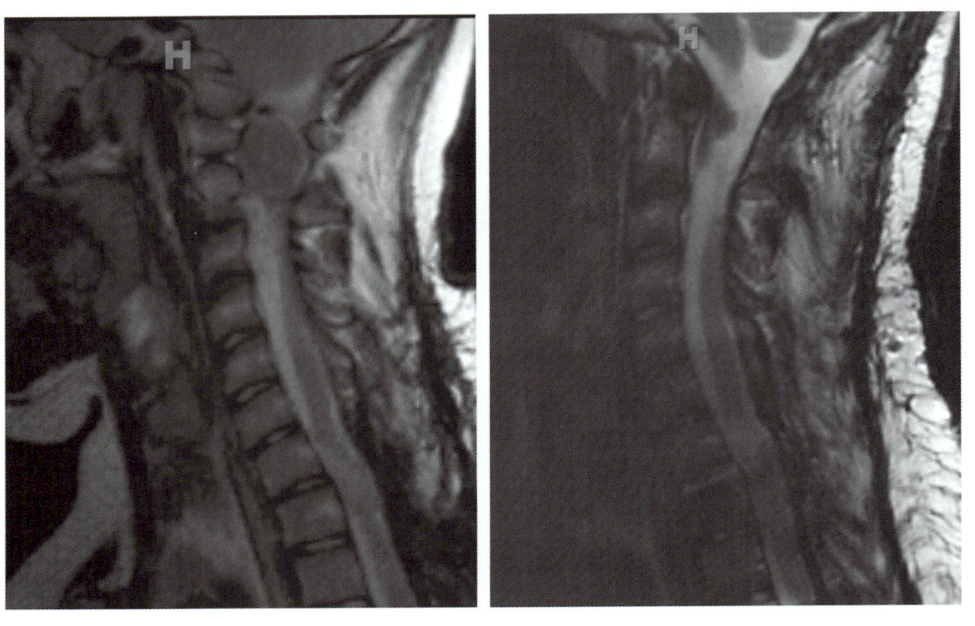

Fig. 3.1 This patient presented with an intradural lesion at the occipital cervical junction, consistent with a meningioma. **(a)** Preoperative sagittal T2-weighted magnetic resonance imaging (MRI). **(b)** Postoperative sagittal T2-weighted MRI.

The most common presenting symptom is neck pain, and conventional X-rays may demonstrate a lytic lesion.[20] On CT-scans, fibrous dysplasia lesions appear as expansile lesions with a "blown-out" cortical shell or as a lytic lesion with sclerotic rims.[21]

Surgery is indicated for patients with neurologic deficits, and for diagnosis confirmation, deformity correction, or intractable pain.[20] The surgical approach and technique are tailored to the patient, but it is important to remember that the bone may be very fragile.[22] For this reason, some surgeons have advocated open vertebroplasty as a treatment modality.[20]

Osteoid Osteoma and Osteoblastoma

Osteoid osteoma and osteoblastoma are blastic lesions that commonly affect the posterior elements of the cervical vertebrae.[23] Osteoid osteomas are usually < 2 cm in diameter, which distinguishes them from the larger osteoblastomas.[24] These tumors are more likely to occur in males and in 50% of cases in the second decade of life.[25–27]

Histologically, these bone-forming tumors are "characterized by a nidus that may originate in the cortical, cancellous, or subperiosteal regions".[24] The cortical (classical) type is the most common in the C1 and C2 vertebrae.[24]

The most common presenting symptom of these tumors is neck pain, which may be accompanied by muscular spasm or torticollis.[24] The pain produced by these tumors is caused by the presence of nerve endings within the tumor and the increased production of prostaglandins inside the nidus, which explains the relief of symptoms with administration of nonsteroidal anti-inflammatory drugs.[28] The best imaging modality for these lesions is CT, which may adequately detect the lesion's nidus; these tumors appear as expansile lesions with reactive sclerosis in the adjacent bone.[24] The best treatment modality is complete surgical resection, which can be achieved via piecemeal excision, curettage, and drilling.[24]

Meningioma

Meningiomas of the OCJ are rare, accounting for 1.8 to 3.2% of all meningiomas.[29] Although these tumors are histologically benign, when they occur in the OCJ they tend to be relatively large and compress adjacent neurovascular structures.[30,31] Initial symptoms include suboccipital headache and upper neck pain.[30] Nonetheless, the average time from symptom onset to diagnosis is over 30 months,[32] and by this time patients often present with irreversible neurologic deficits.[30]

The best imaging modality for these tumors is MRI. T1-weighted images usually show a lesion with varying degrees of intensity compared with the brain parenchyma. T2-weighted images show the lesion as a hypointense mass (**Fig. 3.1**), and sometimes an arachnoid plane can be detected between the tumor, brainstem, and spinal cord.[30] Additionally, the use of gadolinium contrast may help define the dural attachment site of the tumor.[30]

Although surgical resection is the treatment of choice, these lesions are challenging, and a thorough discussion with the patient on the risks and benefits is encouraged. Some patients may be monitored and others may be candidates only for subtotal resection.[30]

Solitary Fibrous Tumor

Solitary fibrous tumors (SFTs) are rare spindle cell neoplasms that occur most commonly in adults. Occurrence in the spine is rare, and few case reports have described SFTs in the OCJ.[33] SFTs appear isodense on CT scans, but show enhancement after contrast administration. They appear as isointense lesions on T1-weighted MRI (**Fig. 3.2**) and hyperintense on T2-weighted MRI. Angiography may demonstrate any major feeding vessels that can be embolized prior to surgery.[33]

Although most SFTs are considered benign tumors, there is malignant potential in 13 to 23% of cases.[33] An attempt should be

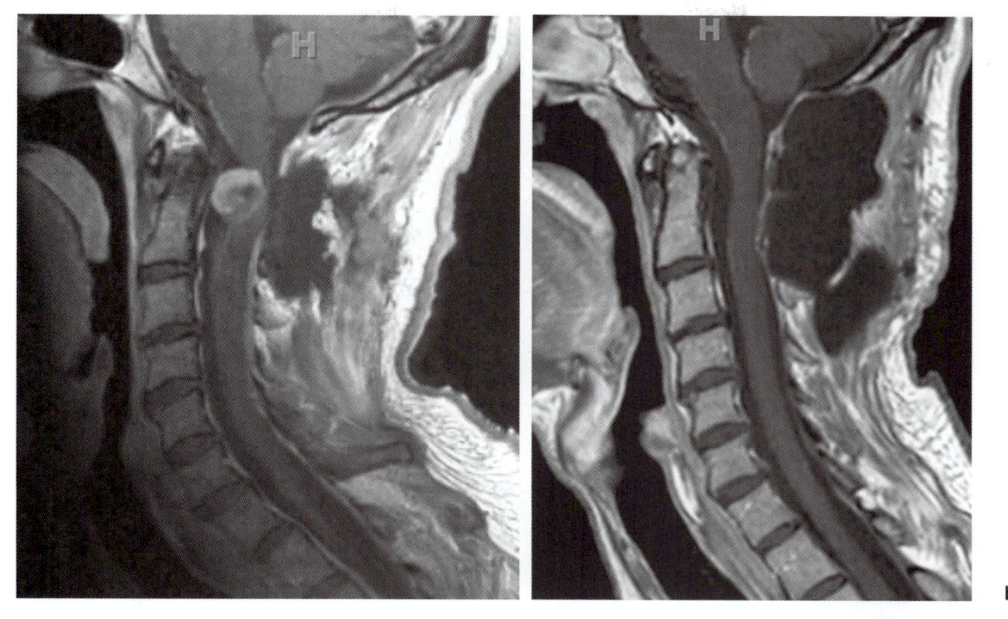

Fig. 3.2 This patient presented with a solitary fibrous tumor of the occipital cervical junction. **(a)** Preoperative sagittal T1-weighted MRI. **(b)** Postoperative sagittal T1-weighted MRI.

made to obtain complete tumor excision, which often may require sacrifice of an involved artery or nerve root.[33]

Hemangiopericytoma

Hemangiopericytomas are a rare neoplasm arising from capillary pericytes. These tumors are most commonly found outside the central nervous system, and when they occur in the spine (uncommonly) they tend to be extradural tumors.[34] These lesions appear hyperintense on CT scans and isodense on T1- and T2-weighted MRI.[35] They enhance heterogeneously and may contain flow voids.[36]

Gross total resection provides the best long-term prognosis and greatest survival.[37] Metastases are a concern with these tumors, and have been reported in 29% of cases.[35] When en-bloc resection is not feasible, hemangiopericytomas may be treated with embolization and debulking.[35]

Neurofibroma

Neurofibromas are intradural extramedullary tumors that arise from nerve sheaths, and in the OCJ they most often occur in the C2 nerve root.[38] Most cases are associated with neurofibromatosis type 1, and patients are often of young age and have multiple tumors.[39] The median time from symptom onset to diagnosis is 24 months, and patients usually present with weakness and poor coordination.[4]

Although MRI is the imaging modality of choice, plain X-ray or CT scan may reveal enlargement of the intervertebral foramen.[4] On MRI, neurofibromas appear hypointense on T1-weighted images and hyperintense on T2-weighted images (**Figs. 3.3 and 3.4**).[4]

Schwannoma

Schwannomas that involve the OCJ may arise from lower cranial nerves or rarely from the C1 nerve root.[40] Patients may present with "hemisensory deficits secondary to brainstem compression at the level of the foramen magnum."[40] Schwannomas may often be mistaken for meningiomas, but there are several key features that differentiate them. On CT scans, schwannomas may show thinning of the C1 lamina, which meningiomas do not show. Schwannomas enhance heterogeneously on MRI, whereas meningiomas are more homogeneous. A dural tail is most commonly found in meningiomas rather than in schwannomas.

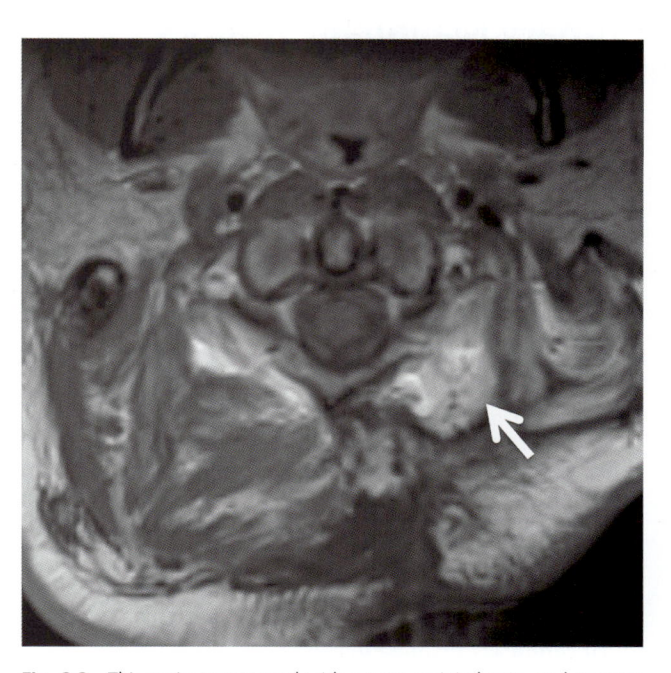

Fig. 3.3 This patient presented with severe occipital pain, and imaging demonstrated a large left paraspinal/suboccipital mass *(arrow)*, which later proved to be a neurofibroma.

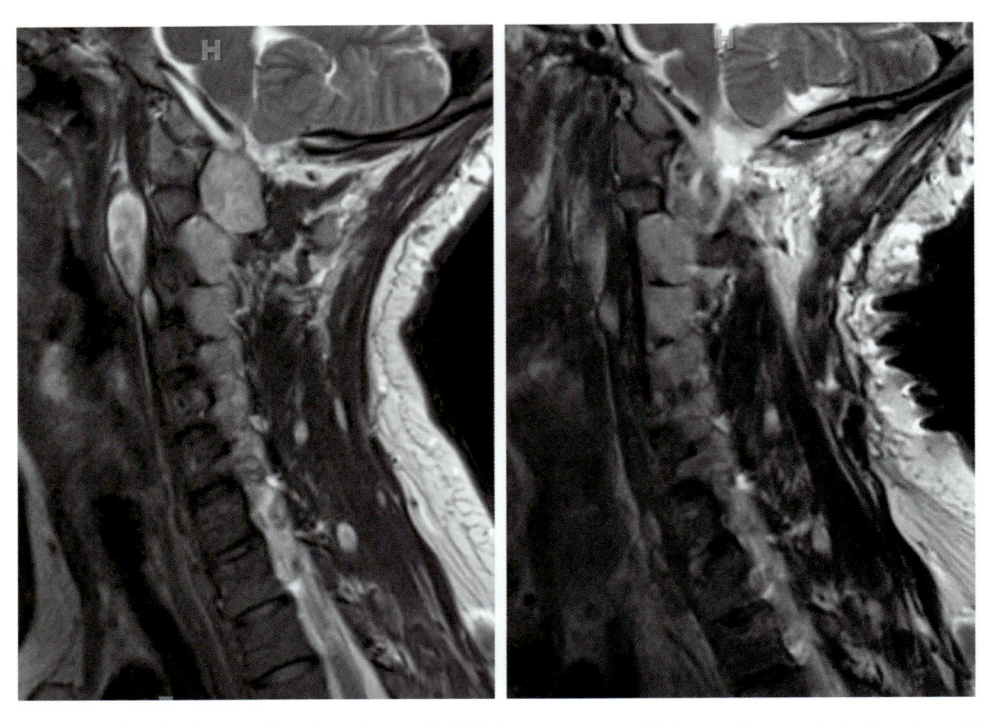

Fig. 3.4 This patient presented with suboccipital, neck, and arm pain. MRI demonstrated multiple neurofibromas, including a large C2 tumor. **(a)** Preoperative sagittal T2-weighted MRI. **(b)** Postoperative sagittal T2-weighted MRI.

Lastly, cranial nerve invasion is possible with meningiomas but is very rare with schwannomas.[40] The most direct route for resection is the far lateral approach, which avoids the need for neural retraction.[40]

Primary Malignant Tumors

Chordoma

Chordomas are slow-growing but aggressive tumors that arise from notochord remnants most commonly in the cranium, cervical spine, and sacrum.[41] They occur more frequently in men,[42] with incidence increasing with age.[41] Although the overall incidence of these tumors is estimated to be 0.2 to 0.5 per 100,000 persons per year, chordomas are the most common extradural tumors of the clivus and craniovertebral junction.[4] Approximately 5 to 40% of all chordomas metastasize,[43–45] and median estimated survival is 6 to 8 years.[46–48]

Histologically, chordomas consist of large and round cells with a vacuolated cytoplasm.[47] Chordoma cells stain positive for epithelial membrane antigen, S-100, and brachyury (nuclear transcription factor).[49,50] On CT scans, chordomas appear as expansile midline lesions with a lytic component; they have irregular borders and most commonly infiltrate the surrounding soft tissues.[51] On postcontrast MRI, enhancement is usually heterogeneous.[52]

When present in the OCJ, patients usually have a chronic history of headache and neck pain.[4] Nonetheless, once the tumor grows to a considerable size, compression of the brainstem and spinal cord leads to alterations in cerebrospinal fluid flow or neurologic deficits.[4] Overall, the most common presentation is pain in the C2 distribution, and this condition may resemble torticollis.[4] Other symptoms include paresthesias of the face and extremities.[4] Elsberg and Strauss[53] considered an abnormal cold sensation of the lower extremities as a pathognomonic sign of a high cervical lesion. Extension of the tumor laterally may cause unilateral deficits such as hypoglossal nerve palsy; anterior and cranial growth may cause symptoms in the pharynx, nasal cavity, or paranasal sinuses.[4]

En-bloc resection with negative margins yields the best long-term disease-free survival and possible cure.[54] Because most chordomas are anterior midline tumors in the OCJ, "most can be approached by midline transoral and extended transoral techniques (transmaxillary and transmandibular), as well as high anterolateral retropharyngeal and lateral approaches to the upper cervical spine, and subtemporal or lateral petrous approaches for clival tumors."[54] For lesions in the C2 vertebra and lower, en-bloc resection is usually an option. For lesions arising in the clivus and C1 body, intralesional resection is performed.

An analysis of 132 operations in 97 patients with OCJ chordomas found the following complications: tumor recurrence in 25% of cases, cerebrospinal fluid leak in 6.2%, chest infection in 4.1%, meningitis in 3.1%, velopharyngeal incompetence in 3.1%, and new cranial palsies in 2.1%, among others.[54] The 5- and 10-year survival for all patients was 55% and 36%, respectively.

Due to the high morbidity of surgery, other potential therapies such as chemotherapy and proton beam therapy have been explored. Chemotherapeutic agents have a small role in the management of chordomas, mainly due to the difficulty of establishing adequate tumor cell lines and consequently the lack of preclinical data.[55] Nonetheless, agents such as rapamycin (sirolimus; inhibitor of interleukin-2) have shown promising results in vitro.[55] Imatinib is a tyrosine-kinase inhibitor that has a potential role in the treatment of advanced platelet-derived growth factor β-positive chordoma. In the largest phase II trial to date, 50 patients were treated with this agent, with one partial response and 35 patients with stable disease.[56] The authors of the report on this trial concluded that it "confirms anecdotal ev-

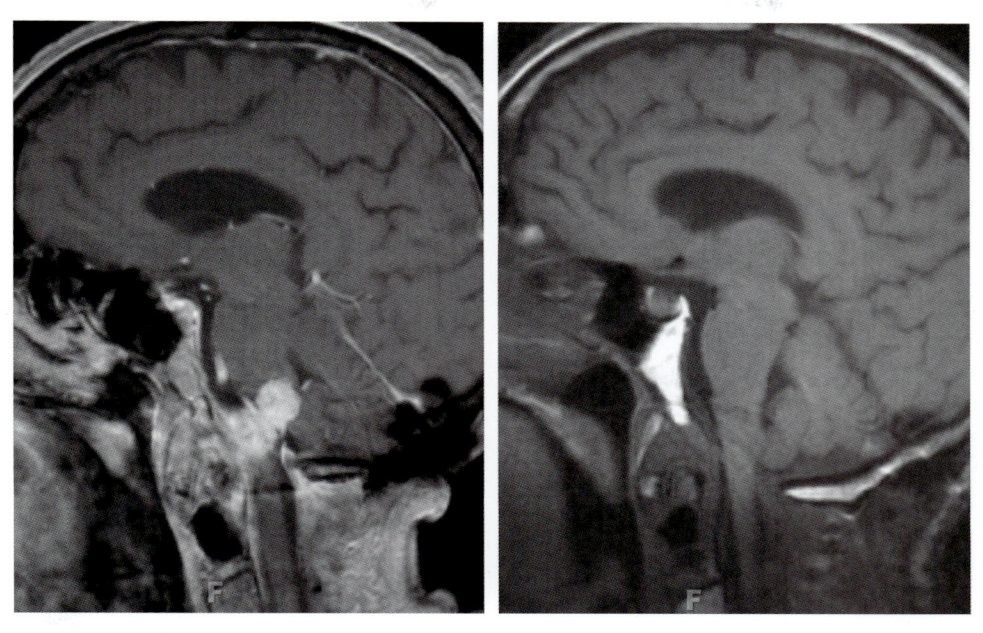

Fig. 3.5 This patient presented with a recurrent chordoma of the occipital cervical junction. **(a)** Preoperative sagittal T1-weighted postcontrast MRI. **(b)** Postoperative sagittal T1-weighted MRI.

idence that imatinib has antitumor activity in this orphan disease, and therefore, it is worth further investigation."[56]

Proton beam therapy utilizes high-energy protons to cause DNA damage to cells, and has the advantage over photons of being able to spare most of the surrounding healthy tissue from radiation damage.[57] A recent study by Deraniyagala et al[58] reported outcomes on 33 patients treated with proton beam therapy for skull base chordomas, with a 92% survival rate at 2 years. The authors reported an 18% rate of unilateral hearing loss and an 86% local control rate. However, this follow-up time is exceptionally short, and with longer follow-up times most patients may tend to suffer a recurrence (**Fig. 3.5**).

Chondrosarcoma

Chondrosarcomas may arise de novo or as secondary transformation from osteochondromas.[51] These tumors are more common in men in young adulthood.[59] Chondrosarcoma cells are binucleated, with increased cellularity and nuclear pleomorphism indicating more aggressiveness.[51]

On CT scans, chondrosarcomas appear as large expansile masses with cortical bone thickening.[51] These tumors appear hyperintense on T2-weighted MRI, and "an enhancement pattern of rings and arcs on gadolinium-enhanced MRI reflects the lobulated growth pattern of these cartilaginous tumors."[51]

A study by Colli and Al-Mefty[60] analyzed prognostic factors of survival in 63 patients with OCJ tumors—53 with chordomas and 10 with chondrosarcomas. Patients most commonly presented with neuro-ophthalmologic symptoms and headaches. All 10 patients with chondrosarcoma underwent surgical excision via transcondylar, transoral, and anterior cervical approaches, among others.[60] The authors reported a 5-year recurrence-free survival rate of 100%.

Chondrosarcomas of the skull base and OCJ can be treated with intralesional resection and postoperative proton beam irradiation, with control rates of 95% at 15 years.[61] However, tumors in the mobile spine tend to recur at higher rates, and tumoral control is achieved via en-bloc resection with negative margins.[62]

Plasmacytoma

Plasmacytomas belong to the spectrum of B-cell lymphoproliferative diseases along with multiple myeloma.[4] A solitary plasmacytomas has a 60% 5-year survival, but multiple or disseminated plasmacytomas behave much like multiple myeloma and 5-year survival decreases to 18%.[4,63] In the OCJ, plasmacytomas arise from the vertebral body, and their expansile nature may destroy the bone cortex. Moreover, these tumors may engulf vertebral vessels and expand into the pedicles in 20% of cases.[4]

Menezes[4] recommends preoperative embolization with tumor excision and stabilization. This can be achieved via a transoral-transpalatopharyngeal approach or from a lateral extrapharyngeal-transcervical approach. However, occipital-cervical instrumented fusion with radiation therapy may be an alternative option.[4]

Conclusion

Tumors of the OCJ are rare, and diagnosis is usually delayed due to the large size of the subarachnoid space in this region. Approaches to the OCJ are challenging to surgeons, and although complete tumoral resection provides the best long-term prognosis, this feat is not always achieved. Future studies into adjuvant treatment modalities such as biologic agents and radiotherapy are needed.

References

1. Jung SH, Jung S, Moon KS, Park HW, Kang SS. Tailored surgical approaches for benign craniovertebral junction tumors. J Korean Neurosurg Soc 2010;48:139–144
2. Maurya P, Singh K, Sharma V. C1 and C2 nerve sheath tumors: analysis of 32 cases. Neurol India 2009;57:31–35
3. Refai D, Shin JH, Iannotti C, Benzel EC. Dorsal approaches to intradural extramedullary tumors of the craniovertebral junction. J Craniovertebr Junction Spine 2010;1:49–54

4. Menezes AH. Tumors of the craniovertebral junction. In: Winn R, ed. Youmans Neurological Surgery. Philadelphia: Saunders; 2011:3114–3130
5. al-Mefty O, Borba LA. Skull base chordomas: a management challenge. J Neurosurg 1997;86:182–189
6. Beatty RA. Cold dysesthesia: a symptom of extramedullary tumors of the spinal cord. J Neurosurg 1970;33:75–78
7. Meyer FB, Ebersold MJ, Reese DF. Benign tumors of the foramen magnum. J Neurosurg 1984;61:136–142
8. Bang WS, Kim KT, Cho DC, Sung JK. Primary eosinophilic granuloma of adult cervical spine presenting as a radiculomyelopathy. J Korean Neurosurg Soc 2013;54:54–57
9. Kilborn TN, Teh J, Goodman TR. Paediatric manifestations of Langerhans cell histiocytosis: a review of the clinical and radiological findings. Clin Radiol 2003;58:269–278
10. Bertram C, Madert J, Eggers C. Eosinophilic granuloma of the cervical spine. Spine 2002;27:1408–1413
11. Jiang L, Liu ZJ, Liu XG, et al. Langerhans cell histiocytosis of the cervical spine: a single Chinese institution experience with thirty cases. Spine 2010;35:E8–E15
12. Richter MP, D'Angio GJ. The role of radiation therapy in the management of children with histiocytosis X. Am J Pediatr Hematol Oncol 1981;3: 161–163
13. Leithner A, Windhager R, Lang S, Haas OA, Kainberger F, Kotz R. Aneurysmal bone cyst. A population based epidemiologic study and literature review. Clin Orthop Relat Res 1999;363:176–179
14. Vergel De Dios AM, Bond JR, Shives TC, McLeod RA, Unni KK. Aneurysmal bone cyst. A clinicopathologic study of 238 cases. Cancer 1992;69:2921–2931
15. Hu H, Wu J, Ren L, Sun X, Li F, Ye X. Destructive osteoblastoma with secondary aneurysmal bone cyst of cervical vertebra in an 11-year-old boy: case report. Int J Clin Exp Med 2014;7:290–295
16. Rajput D, Tungaria A, Jaiswal A, Jain V. Aneurysmal bone cyst of clivus and C1 C2: case report and review of literature. Turk Neurosurg 2012;22: 105–108
17. Mohit AA, Eskridge J, Ellenbogen R, Shaffrey CI. Aneurysmal bone cyst of the atlas: successful treatment through selective arterial embolization: case report. Neurosurgery 2004;55:982
18. Campanacci M, Capanna R, Picci P. Unicameral and aneurysmal bone cysts. Clin Orthop Relat Res 1986;204:25–36
19. Amendola L, Simonetti L, Simoes CE, Bandiera S, De Iure F, Boriani S. Aneurysmal bone cyst of the mobile spine: the therapeutic role of embolization. Eur Spine J 2013;22:533–541
20. Kotil K, Ozyuvaci E. Fibrous dysplasia in axis treated with vertebroplasty. J Craniovertebr Junction Spine 2010;1:118–121
21. Ropper AE, Cahill KS, Hanna JW, McCarthy EF, Gokaslan ZL, Chi JH. Primary vertebral tumors: a review of epidemiologic, histological, and imaging findings, Part I: benign tumors. Neurosurgery 2011;69:1171–1180
22. Hu SS, Healey JH, Huvos AG. Fibrous dysplasia of the second cervical vertebra. A case report. J Bone Joint Surg Am 1990;72:781–783
23. Marcove RC, Heelan RT, Huvos AG, Healey J, Lindeque BG. Osteoid osteoma. Diagnosis, localization, and treatment. Clin Orthop Relat Res 1991; 267:197–201
24. Amirjamshidi A, Roozbeh H, Sharifi G, Abdoli A, Abbassioun K. Osteoid osteoma of the first 2 cervical vertebrae. Report of 4 cases. J Neurosurg Spine 2010;13:707–714
25. Hastings DE, Macnab I, Lawson V. Neoplasms of the atlas and axis. Can J Surg 1968;11:290–296
26. Molloy S, Saifuddin A, Allibone J, Taylor BA. Excision of an osteoid osteoma from the body of the axis through an anterior approach. Eur Spine J 2002;11:599–601
27. Raskas DS, Graziano GP, Herzenberg JE, Heidelberger KP, Hensinger RN. Osteoid osteoma and osteoblastoma of the spine. J Spinal Disord 1992; 5:204–211
28. Ghanem I. The management of osteoid osteoma: updates and controversies. Curr Opin Pediatr 2006;18:36–41
29. Arnautović KI, Al-Mefty O, Husain M. Ventral foramen magnum meningiomas. J Neurosurg 2000;92(1, Suppl):71–80
30. Boulton MR, Cusimano MD. Foramen magnum meningiomas: concepts, classifications, and nuances. Neurosurg Focus 2003;14:e10
31. Bydon M, Ma TM, Xu R, et al. Surgical outcomes of craniocervical junction meningiomas: a series of 22 consecutive patients. Clin Neurol Neurosurg 2014;117:71–79
32. George B, Lot G, Boissonnet H. Meningioma of the foramen magnum: a series of 40 cases. Surg Neurol 1997;47:371–379
33. Hirakawa A, Miyamoto K, Hosoe H, Nishimoto Y, Shimokawa K, Shimizu K. Solitary fibrous tumor in the occipitocervical region: a case report. Spine 2004;29:E547–E550
34. Shirzadi A, Drazin D, Gates M, et al. Surgical management of primary spinal hemangiopericytomas: an institutional case series and review of the literature. Eur Spine J 2013;22(Suppl 3):S450–S459
35. Drazin D, Shweikeh F, Bannykh S, Johnson JP. Hemangiopericytoma invading the craniovertebral junction: First reported case and review of the literature. J Craniovertebr Junction Spine 2013;4:32–34
36. Sheehan J, Kondziolka D, Flickinger J, Lunsford LD. Radiosurgery for treatment of recurrent intracranial hemangiopericytomas. Neurosurgery 2002;51:905–910, discussion 910–911
37. Ecker RD, Marsh WR, Pollock BE, et al. Hemangiopericytoma in the central nervous system: treatment, pathological features, and long-term follow up in 38 patients. J Neurosurg 2003;98:1182–1187
38. Ozawa H, Kusakabe T, Aizawa T, Nakamura T, Ishii Y, Itoi E. Tumors at the lateral portion of the C1-2 interlaminar space compressing the spinal cord by rotation of the atlantoaxial joint: new aspects of spinal cord compression. J Neurosurg Spine 2012;17:552–555
39. Goel A, Muzumdar D, Nadkarni T, Desai K, Dange N, Chagla A. Retrospective analysis of peripheral nerve sheath tumors of the second cervical nerve root in 60 surgically treated patients. J Neurosurg Spine 2008;8: 129–134
40. Helms J, Michael LM II. Large dumbbell-shaped C1 schwannoma presenting as a foramen magnum mass. J Neurol Surg Rep 2012;73:32–36
41. McMaster ML, Goldstein AM, Bromley CM, Ishibe N, Parry DM. Chordoma: incidence and survival patterns in the United States, 1973–1995. Cancer Causes Control 2001;12:1–11
42. Smolders D, Wang X, Drevelengas A, Vanhoenacker F, De Schepper AM. Value of MRI in the diagnosis of non-clival, non-sacral chordoma. Skeletal Radiol 2003;32:343–350
43. Bjornsson J, Wold LE, Ebersold MJ, Laws ER. Chordoma of the mobile spine. A clinicopathologic analysis of 40 patients. Cancer 1993;71:735–740
44. Chambers PW, Schwinn CP. Chordoma. A clinicopathologic study of metastasis. Am J Clin Pathol 1979;72:765–776
45. McPherson CM, Suki D, McCutcheon IE, Gokaslan ZL, Rhines LD, Mendel E. Metastatic disease from spinal chordoma: a 10-year experience. J Neurosurg Spine 2006;5:277–280
46. Baratti D, Gronchi A, Pennacchioli E, et al. Chordoma: natural history and results in 28 patients treated at a single institution. Ann Surg Oncol 2003;10:291–296
47. Bergh P, Kindblom LG, Gunterberg B, Remotti F, Ryd W, Meis-Kindblom JM. Prognostic factors in chordoma of the sacrum and mobile spine: a study of 39 patients. Cancer 2000;88:2122–2134
48. York JE, Kaczaraj A, Abi-Said D, et al. Sacral chordoma: 40-year experience at a major cancer center. Neurosurgery 1999;44:74–79, discussion 79–80
49. Crapanzano JP, Ali SZ, Ginsberg MS, Zakowski MF. Chordoma: a cytologic study with histologic and radiologic correlation. Cancer 2001;93: 40–51
50. Jambhekar NA, Rekhi B, Thorat K, Dikshit R, Agrawal M, Puri A. Revisiting chordoma with brachyury, a "new age" marker: analysis of a validation study on 51 cases. Arch Pathol Lab Med 2010;134:1181–1187
51. Ropper AE, Cahill KS, Hanna JW, McCarthy EF, Gokaslan ZL, Chi JH. Primary vertebral tumors: a review of epidemiologic, histological and imaging findings, part II: locally aggressive and malignant tumors. Neurosurgery 2012;70:211–219, discussion 219
52. Sung MS, Lee GK, Kang HS, et al. Sacrococcygeal chordoma: MR imaging in 30 patients. Skeletal Radiol 2005;34:87–94
53. Elsberg CA, Strauss I. Tumors of the spinal cord which project into the posterior cranial fossa. Arch Neurol Psychiatry 1929;21:261–263
54. Choi D, Melcher R, Harms J, Crockard A. Outcome of 132 operations in 97 patients with chordomas of the craniocervical junction and upper cervical spine. Neurosurgery 2010;66:59–65, discussion 65
55. Ricci-Vitiani L, Runci D, D'Alessandris QG, et al. Chemotherapy of skull base chordoma tailored on responsiveness of patient-derived tumor cells to rapamycin. Neoplasia 2013;15:773–782
56. Stacchiotti S, Longhi A, Ferraresi V, et al. Phase II study of imatinib in advanced chordoma. J Clin Oncol 2012;30:914–920

57. Orecchia R, Vitolo V, Fiore MR, et al. Proton beam radiotherapy: report of the first ten patients treated at the Centro Nazionale di Adroterapia Oncologica (CNAO) for skull base and spine tumours. Radiol Med (Torino) 2014;119:277–282
58. Deraniyagala RL, Yeung D, Mendenhall WM, et al. Proton therapy for skull base chordomas: an outcome study from the university of Florida proton therapy institute. J Neurol Surg B Skull Base 2014;75:53–57
59. Chi JH, Bydon A, Hsieh P, Witham T, Wolinsky JP, Gokaslan ZL. Epidemiology and demographics for primary vertebral tumors. Neurosurg Clin N Am 2008;19:1–4
60. Colli B, Al-Mefty O. Chordomas of the craniocervical junction: follow-up review and prognostic factors. J Neurosurg 2001;95:933–943
61. Baehring JM, Piepmeier J, Duncan C, Ogle E, Kim J, Liebsch N. Chondrosarcoma of the skull base. J Neurooncol 2006;76:49
62. Boriani S, De Iure F, Bandiera S, et al. Chondrosarcoma of the mobile spine: report on 22 cases. Spine 2000;25:804–812
63. McLain RF, Weinstein JN. Solitary plasmacytomas of the spine: a review of 84 cases. J Spinal Disord 1989;2:69–74

4 Trauma of the Occipital-Cervical Junction

George M. Ghobrial, Ahmed J. Awad, Christopher M. Maulucci, and James S. Harrop

The occipital-cervical junction (OCJ) is an anatomic region that includes the occipital bone, sphenoid bone surrounding the foramen magnum, the C1 and C2 vertebrae, as well as associated ligaments and neurovascular structures. Over the past few decades, there have been significant developments in the methods of stabilizing an unstable OCJ, as well as agreed upon classifications of injury morphology. The high force that is associated with unstable OCJ injuries, such as with an atlanto-occipital dislocation (AOD), has historically carried a high mortality, with the majority of patients dying prior to hospital arrival. However, improvements in resuscitation, emergency medical services, and triage have enabled more patients with these injuries of the OCJ to survive and seek a surgical consultation. This chapter discusses the clinical presentation, diagnosis, management, and outcome of each disease process in the spectrum of OCJ injuries.

Relevant Anatomy and Biomechanics

Understanding the unique anatomy of the OCJ is key in having an understanding of OCJ biomechanics and neck stability. Important ligaments providing stability to the craniovertebral junction (CVJ) are divided into two groups: those that attach the skull to the axis, and those that attach to the atlas, which provides the majority of the stability to the CVJ.

One important ligament attaching the skull to the atlas is the anterior atlanto-occipital ligament or membrane, which is an anatomic extension of the anterior longitudinal ligament. This ligament is fixed to the ventral surface of the anterior arch of the atlas and terminates on the skull base, ventral to the basion. The corresponding dorsal ligamentous attachment to the opisthion, on the dorsal aspect of the foramen magnum, is the posterior atlanto-occipital ligament (or membrane). This ligament is much thinner and less structural, articulating with the rostral aspect of the posterior arch of the atlas. A bilateral defect in this membrane transmits the vertebral arteries and suboccipital nerves. The cruciate ligament receives its name from its cross-like shape, consisting of the transverse ligament of the atlas and fibers that transmit laterally in a rostral and caudal fashion.

Ligaments that attach the skull to the axis are more numerous and provide the majority of spinal stability to the CVJ.[1] The tectorial membrane is an extension of the posterior longitudinal ligament, joining the dorsal odontoid to the ventral basion and serving as a ventrally located membrane that resists forces of hyperextension.[2] The alar ligament is composed of atlantal and occipital segments that connect the tip of the odontoid process to the occipital condyles and lateral masses, respectively. The alar ligament serves multiple functions, mainly by restricting neck movements. Historically, the alar ligament was commonly referred to as the "check ligament" as it limits maximum axial rotation at the atlantoaxial joint, and to a much lesser extent limits anteroposterior translation and lateral neck flexion.

Further stability of the CVJ is attributed to the facet capsule at the occiput-C1 and C1-C2 junctions as well as the adherent ligaments. Posteriorly, the posterior ligamentous complex (PLC) comprises the atlanto-occipital membrane, interspinous ligament, obliquus capitis superior and inferior muscles, rectus capitis posterior major and minor muscles, and the ligamentum nuchae.[3]

In the absence of a competent anterior tectorial membrane, the maximum range of neck extension can be exaggerated. Ultimately, occiput movement is limited in extension by the posterior arch of the atlas. Similarly, in the absence of a competent posterior atlanto-occipital membrane, the odontoid tip limits hyperflexion by intersection with the opisthion.

Ligamentous Injuries and Resulting Pathologies

Atlanto-Occipital Dislocation

Atlanto-occipital dislocation (AOD) is the consequence of disruption of the ligamentous structures between the occiput and atlas. These injuries often result in severe dysfunction of the brainstem, cranial nerves, spinal cord, or spinal nerve roots.[1,4] They are usually caused by high-velocity motor vehicle accidents where extreme forces are produced by hyperextension, hyperflexion, lateral flexion, or a combination of these forces.[5,6] It is associated with 6 to 8% of traumatic motor vehicle accident fatalities and is the most common cervical spine injury found during autopsies after these accidents.[5,7] The incidence of such injuries is particularly increased in children due to the susceptible anatomy of the pediatric craniovertebral junction.[8] In addition to the biomechanical instability of articulation in this age group, the ligaments are less stiff in children compared with adults, and the CVJ is subjected to greater stress because of a larger ratio of head size to body size.

Atlanto-occipital dislocations have been classified by Traynelis et al[9] into three types: type I, anterior; type II, longitudinal; and type III, posterior. It is less important to know the type and more important to have a heightened suspicion for this injury in the appropriate clinical setting.

Transverse Ligament Injuries

Transverse ligament disruption is an unstable injury, and should be identified promptly, especially in hyperflexion injuries where a higher index of suspicion should be maintained. Radiographically, insufficiency in the transverse ligament is suggested on lateral plain films by evidence of translation > 3 mm of C1 on C2 in adults and > 5 mm in children. On axial magnetic resonance imaging (MRI) the transverse ligament sometimes can be identified and a disruption diagnosed. However, MRI has a low sensitivity and arguably is not a cost-effective measure if the sole purpose is to identify a transverse ligament rupture.[10] Rarely, with computed tomography (CT) imaging, a fracture or avulsion of the C1 tubercle of the transverse ligament is indicative of C1-C2 instability.

Rotatory C1-C2 Dislocation

Rotatory C1-C2 dislocation, otherwise known as atlantoaxial rotatory subluxation (AARS), is rare in adults, almost always resulting from high-velocity trauma. In children, the more common etiologies of AARS are underlying congenital or inflammatory conditions that cause incompetence in the transverse ligament and alar ligaments, both key ligaments in limiting rotation. Up to 60% of the 90-degree range of rotational motion to either side occurs at the atlantoaxial joint (AAJ).[11] With > 60% range of rotational motion (60 degrees), there are several anatomic considerations. First, the atlantoaxial facets are at risk for dislocation, and there is a higher risk of canal compromise. Also, in an unstable neck allowing higher rotational motion, the ipsilateral vertebral artery is stenosed at the transverse foramen and stretched contralaterally.[12,13] CT imaging is the primary means of identifying a rotated atlas over the axis, and is further aided by three-dimensional imaging. This modality is also useful in ruling out an occipital-atlantal rotatory dislocation, which is sometimes seen in trauma with disruption of the ligaments and soft tissue structures of the neck.[14]

In children, Grisel's syndrome refers to AARS caused by hematogenous spread of an infectious head and neck process to the craniocervical junction, resulting in inflammation and subsequent laxity of the ligamentous structures of the neck. Children often present without neurologic deficits, but with mainly a painful torticollis and recent history of respiratory tract infection. This syndrome is often reducible, not requiring surgery.

Isolated Fractures

Occipital Condyle Fractures

The occipital condyle articulates with the lateral masses of the atlas and is susceptible to fracture due to the relatively high range of mobility at this articulation. However, due to the strength from supporting ligaments and musculature, these injuries are seen only with a high-energy mechanism.[15] Maserati and colleagues[16] reviewed nearly 25,000 trauma patients, finding only 100 patients (0.4%) with occipital condyle fractures. The most widely known classification system for occipital condyle fractures is that of Anderson and Montesano, which entails a gradation of increasing severity.[17] Type I fractures are typically comminuted fractures with minimal if any axial loading. Type II fractures represent further comminution with minimal displacement and the simultaneous extension of the fracture or fractures into the skull base. The hypoglossal canal may be disrupted in comminuted fractures of the occipital condyle due to its proximity, often necessitating a cranial nerve examination checking for tongue deviation, which is a rare finding.[18] Unilateral type I and II fractures can be typically treated with orthosis and do not require surgery. A CT angiogram of the head may be considered to search for arterial dissection, a rare finding when basilar skull fractures in a type II injury traverse the carotid canal. Type III fractures represent the addition of a lateral flexion or rotatory component to the axial vector seen with type I and II fractures. This results in avulsion of the occipital condyle by the alar ligament and represents the most severe of the three types in this grading scheme. Overall, in Maserati's series, the vast majority of patients with craniocervical junction stability and the absence of neural element compression had a good outcome with nonoperative management.[16]

Atlas Fractures

The atlas, or first cervical vertebra, has the most flexibility of any level of the cervical spine, enabling it to serve as the transitional vertebra from the occiput to the cervical spine. Most often, transitional segments between spinal regions have a relatively greater range of flexibility that confers a vulnerability to trauma.[3] As a result, atlas fractures account for 25% of all CVJ trauma[19]; they occur as a result of motor vehicle accidents 85% of the time.[20] Although isolated fractures of the atlas are commonly encountered during the appropriate workup, up to 40% are associated with a concomitant axis fractures.[21–23]

Atlas fractures are most often a result of an axial load plus an additional vector of compressive force.[24] This is unsurprising because the atlas is the primary load-bearing vertebra to the rostrally articulating occiput. The wedge-shaped orientation of the superior and inferior articular facets results in a net outward moment in the setting of axial compression on the C1 ring. When this outward force exceeds the integrity of the C1 neural arch, the classic Jefferson fracture occurs. This is a burst fracture of the anterior and posterior arches and is relatively uncommon. Associated distraction forces raise the risk of a lateral mass fracture.

In the process of deciding whether the neck is stable or not in an isolated C1 fracture, thin-cut CT axial imaging is needed to assess the presence of a fracture through the medial tubercles of the transverse ligament. In the absence of evidence of transverse tubercle fractures, flexion-extension films can be performed to search for subluxation of C1 on C2, with the knowledge that an atlantodental interval should not exceed 5 mm in children or 3 mm in adults. The gradient-echo sequence of an axial MRI is particularly useful for assessing the competency of the transverse ligament, which can be unstable even in the setting of nondisplaced fractures.[25] Furthermore, in the event of a combined spread of the lateral masses and separation ≥ 7 mm on an open-mouth radiograph view, the transverse ligament is considered to be disrupted, helping to diagnose an unstable cervical injury.

Odontoid Fractures

Odontoid fractures are the most common fractures of the axis.[26] Due to the ample anteroposterior diameter of the cervical canal, with roughly one third of available space being occupied by cerebrospinal fluid (CSF), most fractures present without neurologic deficits, regardless of the patient's age.[27,28] Early case series have described odontoid fracture fixation as entailing a high morbidity and mortality.[29–33] More modern fixation techniques have led to a dramatic improvement in surgical outcomes.[34] The commonly accepted system of classification was developed in 1974 by Anderson and D'Alonzo[35] for odontoid fractures. There are three types of fractures diagnosed by location of the fracture line, which is most easily visualized on coronal CT reconstructions. Type I fractures are through the odontoid peg, most commonly a result of an avulsion fracture of the alar ligament.

Type II fractures are the most commonly seen fracture morphology, occurring at the junction of the odontoid process with the body. Type III fractures involve the anterior body of the axis. Type IIA odontoid fractures were later added to the Anderson and D'Alonzo classification to account for further instability and a greater relative risk of nonunion from additional fragmentation of the base of the dens.[36]

In general, the Anderson and D'Alonzo classification can be useful in managing these odontoid fractures. Type III fractures and the less common type I fractures have a high fusion rate with external immobilization. Management of type II odontoid fractures is widely debated,[37] mainly because of the relatively greater frequency with which they are encountered in tandem with the growing number of treatment options,[38] and the lower quality of evidence in the literature.[39]

The increasing age of the type II odontoid fracture population has a direct impact on the need to treat. In one retrospective study evaluating arthrodesis rates from cervical immobilization by a hard collar or halo orthosis, the fusion rate was only 38% in patients 60 years of age or older, whereas in patients younger than 40, a much rarer population, the fusion rate was 82%. The authors also found no significant difference in fusion rate regardless of orthosis.[40] One argument against the use of halo vest orthosis is that it entails a higher morbidity in the elderly population, as do cervical collars, which carry a risk of pressure ulcer from prolonged use. A study by Tashjian et al[41] found a 42% and 20% mortality rate in the halo-treated and non–halo-treated groups, respectively. A recent multicenter prospective study compared surgical treatment with orthosis for type II dens fractures in patients older than 65 years of age and found no difference in the overall rate of complications. However, the surgical group had a significantly lower rate of nonunion (5% versus 21%) and a lower mortality than the group that was nonsurgically managed.[42]

Hangman's Fractures

A condition of bilateral fractures of the pars interarticularis resulting in spondylolisthesis of the dorsal arch of the axis is known as the hangman's fracture.[43] This condition is relatively common for cervical fractures, second in frequency to odontoid fractures for C2 injuries. "Judicial hanging" refers to a different mechanism of hangman's fracture, whereby a submentally placed knot in a hangman's noose causes hyperextension and distraction. In motor vehicle accidents, force is delivered in a pattern that causes hyperextension and compression, typically resulting in sparing of the C2–3 disk space and ligamentous structures, decreasing the lethality. Over time there have been many classification schemes, and in 1981 a three-pattern system became widely accepted, reported first by Effendi and colleagues.[44] In the Effendi system, type I fractures were originally described as isolated hairline fractures of the ring of the axis without C2 body displacement. Type II fractures involved displacement anteriorly of the anterior C2 fragment with minimal retrolisthesis of C2 on C3. Type III fractures involved further angulation or flexion of the C2 body, with C2-C3 dislocation and locking of the facets.

Combination Atlas-Axis Fractures

Combined C1-C2 fractures are usually a result of trauma and are best demonstrated by axial CT imaging with coronal and sagittal reconstructions. As expected, C1-C2 fractures entail a relatively greater risk of instability than an isolated fracture of either the atlas or axis, and a higher index of suspicion for instability should be maintained clinically. Many of the prior methods of C1-C2 posterior fixation such as the Brooks-Gallie methods, Halifax clamping, or other variants of interspinous and posterior column fusions require intact posterior elements. More modern techniques using segmental instrumentation, such as pars, pedicle, lateral mass, laminar, or transarticular screws, have supplanted these older techniques and have enabled the surgeon to match the anatomy to the technique and to provide the patient with a higher rate of fusion.

Clinical Presentation

Although these injuries used to entail a high rate of mortality, improvements in care and triage have enabled a higher survival rate. AOD still entails a high mortality, and those that survive have high morbidity and a high incidence of neurologic deficit, particularly due to brainstem and upper cervical cord injury at the time of dislocation.[45]

Patients with occipitocervical junction injuries in general present with a wide range of minor to severe neurologic deficits. Many patients commonly have hemiparesis due to a unilateral pyramidal injury. Cranial nerves VI, IX, X, XI, and XII are commonly affected. Patients may present with bilateral weakness of hands and arms without significant involvement of the lower extremities, known as Bell's cruciate paralysis.[2,46] Hand weakness gradually improves from proximal to distal.

Radiographic Presentation

Although lateral radiographs can be initially useful in recognizing severe dislocations, they usually fail to diagnose less severe injuries. Radiographs are very useful in studying overall alignment, but are far less sensitive and specific than CT imaging for fracture evaluation.

Atlantal-Occipital Dislocation

Radiographic criteria have been implemented to describe disorders of the CVJ, and in particular atlanto-occipital stability. The Wackenheim line is drawn to extend along the dorsal surface of the clivus in the midsagittal plane (**Fig. 4.1a**). This line should be tangential to the tip of the dens and is not altered by flexion or extension. The line intersects the dens only if the occiput is displaced anteriorly. Power's ratio is the ratio between two lines, one that connects the basion to the posterior atlantal arch (BC), and one that connects the opisthion to the anterior atlantal arch (OA) (**Fig. 4.1b**). Normally, BC/OA is less than 0.77; however, a ratio of 1.0 is fairly indicative of atlantal dislocation.[47] The basion-dental interval (BDI) (**Fig. 4.1c**) is a measure from the tip of the dens to the basion, and is also known as the Wholey dens-basion method of measurement in a neutral neck.[48] The cutoffs of 15 and 12 mm are the limits of normal in adults and children, respectively. Dublin's method (**Fig. 4.1d**) is a measurement of the posterior aspect of the ramus of the mandible to the anterior edge of C1 and C2. Although normal distances of the mandible to C1 range from 2 to 5 mm and 9 to 12 mm for C1 and C2, respectively, this is the least reliable of the above methods, as the measurements must be obtained with imaging 72 cm away from

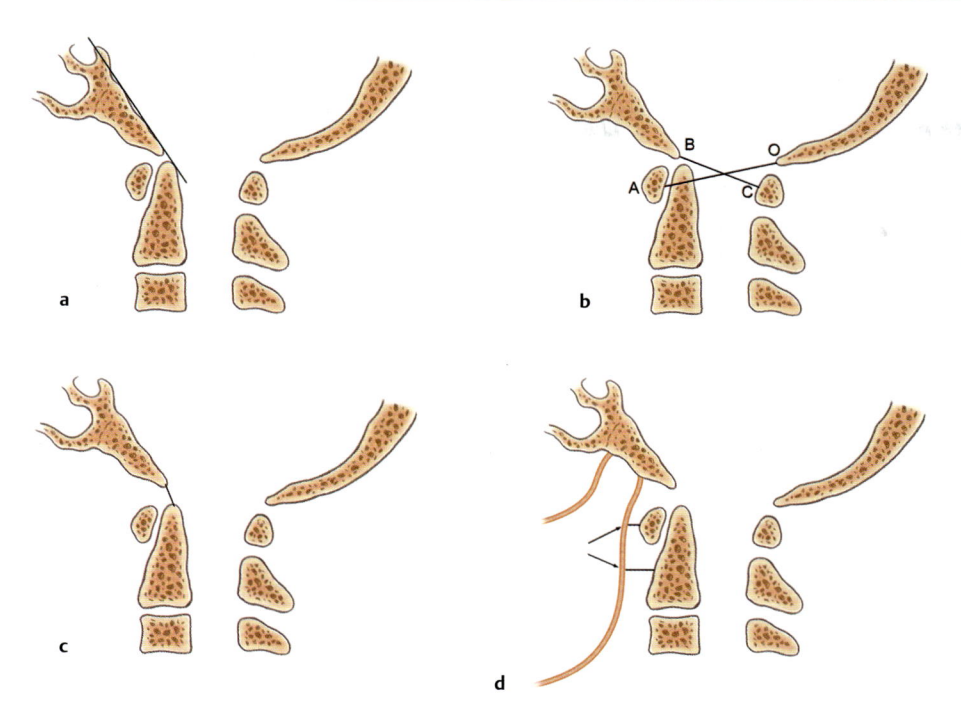

Fig. 4.1 Lateral radiographic criteria for the diagnosis of atlanto-occipital dislocations. **(a)** Wackenheim's line. **(b)** Power's ratio. **(c)** Basion–dental interval. **(d)** Dublin's method. (From Dickman CA, Douglas RA, Sonntag VKR. Occipitocervical fusion: posterior stabilization of the craniovertebral junction and upper cervical spine. BNI Q 1990;6:2–14. Reproduced with permission.)

a closed mouth laterally, and much error can be introduced. Wackenheim's line and the BDI are the most sensitive methods to use with plain radiographs.

Transverse Ligament Disruption

C1-C2 subluxation can occur with or without the disruption of the transverse atlantal ligament. However, C1-C2 subluxation occurs most commonly from odontoid fractures, which less commonly involve disruption of the transverse ligament. Os odontoideum is also a cause of C1-C2 subluxation but is relatively less common, being an uncommon congenital finding. The atlantodental interval (ADI) can be measured on lateral radiographs; flexion ≥ 3 mm is concerning for ligamentous disruption in an adult, and 5 mm is the acceptable cutoff in children. An MRI gradient-echo sequence can be used to best assess the transverse ligament, but thin-cut axials are needed at the C1 region to capture the transverse ligament.[49] Transverse ligament injuries have several classifications. In one system, type I is a disruption of the transverse ligament itself **(Fig. 4.2a)**, and type II involves an avulsion or fracture of the bony tubercle of the transverse ligament **(Fig. 4.2a)**. Type I and type II variants occur less commonly.

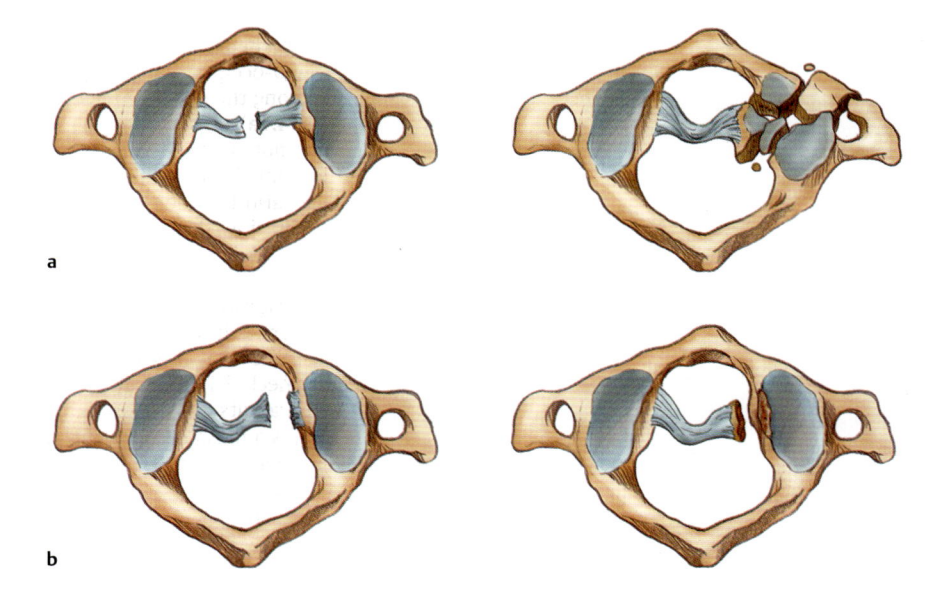

Fig. 4.2 Classification of injuries to the transverse atlantal ligament. **(a)** Type I injuries disrupt the ligament substance in its midportion (type IA) or at its periosteal insertion (type IB). **(b)** Type II injuries disconnect the tubercle for insertion of the transverse ligament from the C1 lateral mass involving a comminuted C1 mass (type IIA) or avulsing the tubercle from an intact lateral mass (type IIB). (Courtesy of the Barrow Neurological Institute.)

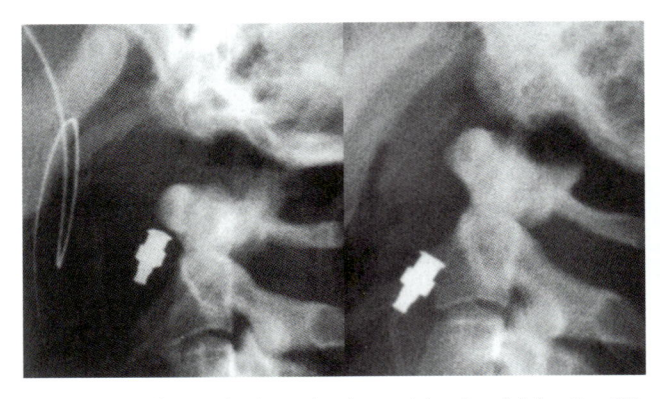

Fig. 4.3 Lateral cervical radiographs of an occipitoatlantal dislocation. This patient arrived in the emergency department with a Philadelphia collar that was applied at the scene of the accident *(right)*. The collar reproduced the distractive mechanism of injury and can cause decompensation of this highly unstable injury. The relative position of the occipital condyles and C1 was immediately improved by removing the cervical collar and immobilizing the head in a neutral position on a spine board *(left)*.

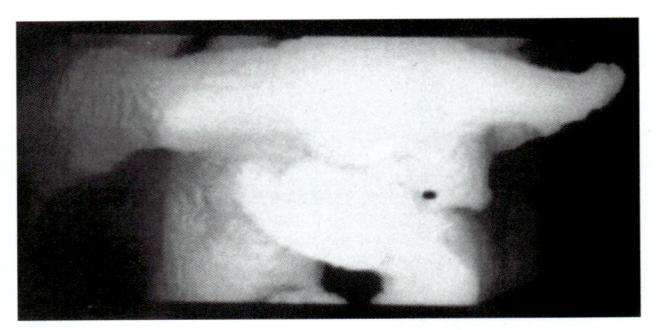

Fig. 4.4 Three-dimensional computed tomography (CT) reconstruction of a C1–C2 rotatory dislocation injury.

Atlantoaxial Rotatory Subluxation

Atlantoaxial rotatory subluxation is more commonly seen in children and adolescents (**Fig. 4.3**). As mentioned previously, CT is a superior modality to plain radiographs in fracture evaluation (**Fig. 4.4**). Moreover, rotational injury, as with AARS, is subtle on radiography, but can be clearly seen with CT imaging, as well as being confirmatory in the case of facet dislocation.

Treatment Options

The initial management of these injuries is focused on the general principles of basic trauma management, including establishing and maintaining a clear airway, breathing, and circulation, and carefully immobilizing and transferring the patient to a treatment facility.[50] To properly manage such injuries, it is very important to know the extent of injuries to bones and ligaments. This is important because disrupted ligaments cannot be repaired. Hence, they usually require surgery to restore stability and preserve the functional integrity of the spine.[51,52] As a result, neutral radiographs are obtained to evaluate alignment, as well as CT imaging for fracture and joint evaluation, and MRI to evaluate the spinal canal, as well as any ligamentous, disk, or soft tissue injury.

Isolated Fractures

Isolated fractures of C1 or C2 can commonly occur. Most of these fractures are nondisplaced and can therefore heal with an orthosis. Displacement is an indirect indicator of ligamentous disruption, and as a result most ascending grading scales relate instability to displacement. Isolated atlas fractures heal in most cases with an orthosis, except in the case of disruption of the tubercle (**Figs. 4.2, 4.5, 4.6, 4.7**) or extensive comminution of the lateral mass. Management of isolated fractures of the axis is less straightforward, due to the various fracture subtypes: odontoid, hangman's, or miscellaneous C2 fractures.

Combined C1 and C2 Fractures

Combined atlantoaxial fractures are also common, but entail a higher rate of neurologic dysfunction and instability due to the relatively higher kinetic energy delivered than with an isolated fracture. Fracture displacement is a major determinant in the decision to perform internal fixation. Displacement of the dens > 5 mm, an associated type III dens fracture, hangman's fracture, or C1 ring fracture as well as with combined displacement of the lateral masses > 7 mm on an open-mouth radiograph are all common features associated with transverse ligament disruption and hence instability. Internal fixation should then be considered in these cases. Many combined nondisplaced fractures will heal in a brace and can be followed in the office with serial radiographs, including flexion-extension views.

Atlantal-Occipital Dislocation

A confirmed atlantal-occipital dislocation is an unstable injury, as the force involved in a dislocation is associated with significant ligamentous injury. Traction and closed reduction should be undertaken under fluoroscopic guidance, preferably in the operating room with neurophysiological monitoring. Disrupted ligaments causing AOD require as little as only 5 lb of traction to achieve reduction, and should only be done by an experienced surgeon.

Transverse Ligament Disruption

Type I or Ia disruptions of the transverse ligament will not heal and therefore require surgery because of the inability of the transverse ligament to repair itself. Type II fractures are avulsions of the tubercle, and may heal in a halo brace, at a rate of 74%.[25]

Rotatory C1-C2 Subluxation

The AARS injuries predominantly occur in children and adolescents. Evaluation by CT in the axial plane demonstrates rotation of C1 on C2 > 45 degrees in almost all cases of dislocation. As previously mentioned, this is successfully treated nonsurgically in most cases, and can be reduced with traction followed by immobilization with a cervical collar for 12 weeks, and occasionally requiring the use of halo placement. In the event of additional transverse ligament disruption, internal fixation may also be required, depending on whether the disruption involves the ligament alone (type I) and is not an avulsion of the tubercle (type II) (**Fig. 4.8**).

Conclusion

Occipitocervical junction trauma can often be lethal, and at best, carries a high morbidity. There are many unique fracture patterns that can be encountered in this region that all require

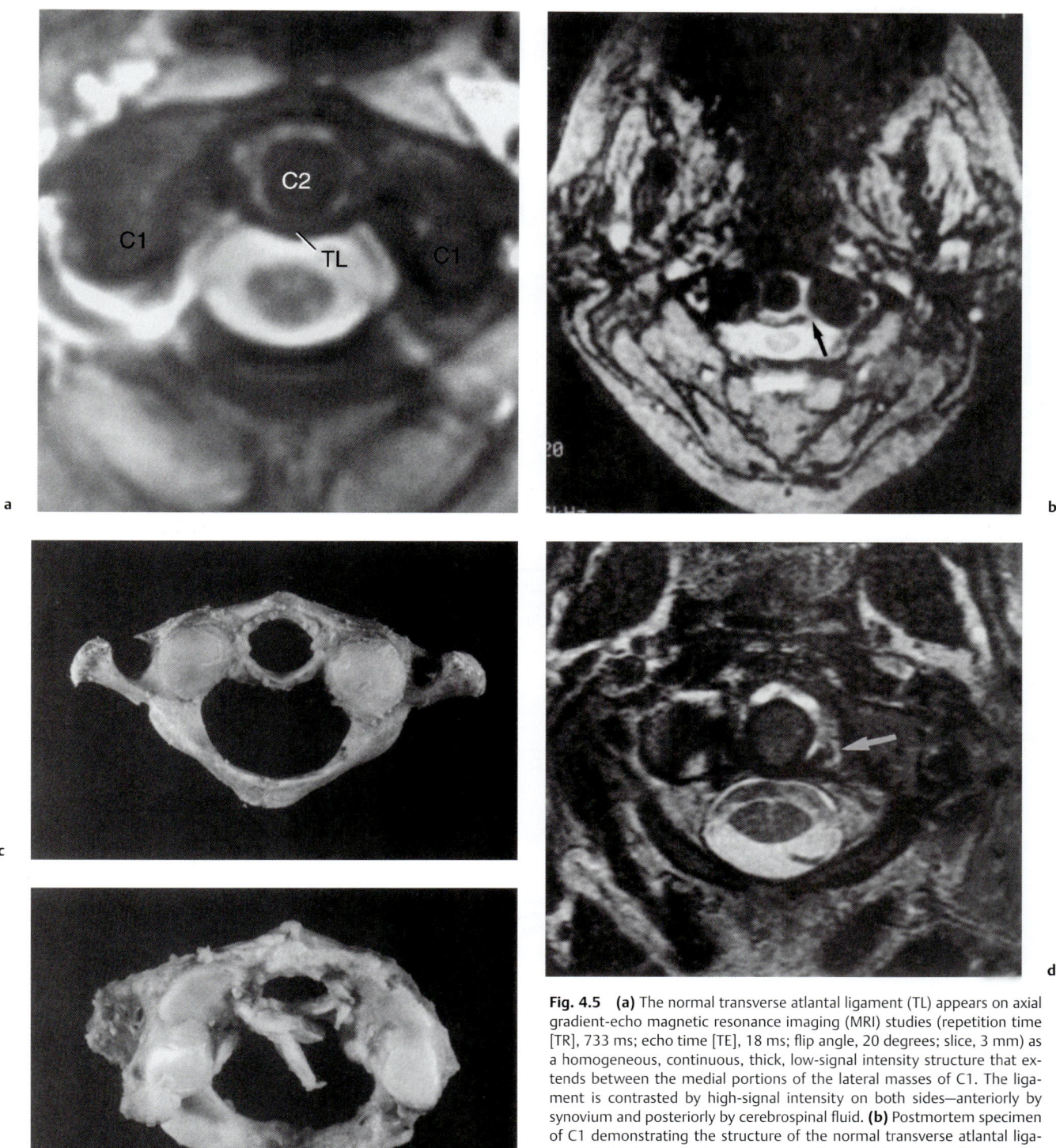

Fig. 4.5 **(a)** The normal transverse atlantal ligament (TL) appears on axial gradient-echo magnetic resonance imaging (MRI) studies (repetition time [TR], 733 ms; echo time [TE], 18 ms; flip angle, 20 degrees; slice, 3 mm) as a homogeneous, continuous, thick, low-signal intensity structure that extends between the medial portions of the lateral masses of C1. The ligament is contrasted by high-signal intensity on both sides—anteriorly by synovium and posteriorly by cerebrospinal fluid. **(b)** Postmortem specimen of C1 demonstrating the structure of the normal transverse atlantal ligament. **(c)** Autopsy specimen demonstrating a midsubstance disruption of the transverse atlantal ligament (type IA injury). **(d,e)** MRI studies of type IB injuries in which the transverse ligament is torn from its periosteal insertion on the C1 tubercle. The disrupted ligaments demonstrate high-signal intensity within the ligament, loss of anatomic continuity, and blood at the insertion of the ligament *(arrows)*.

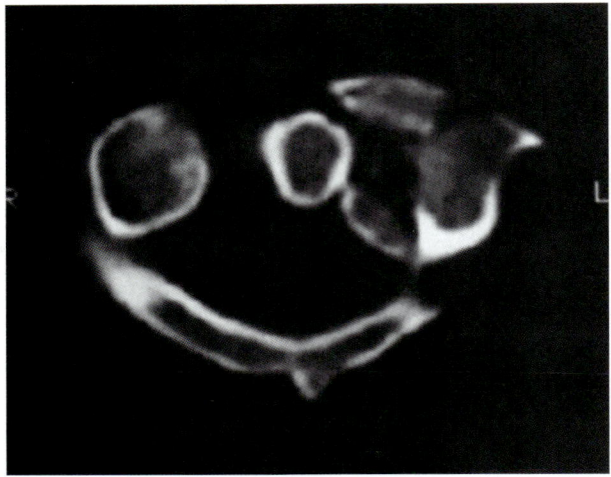

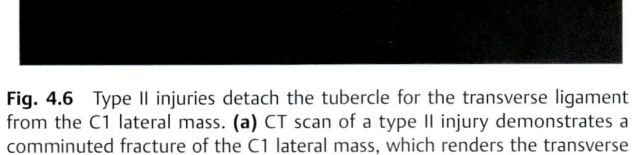

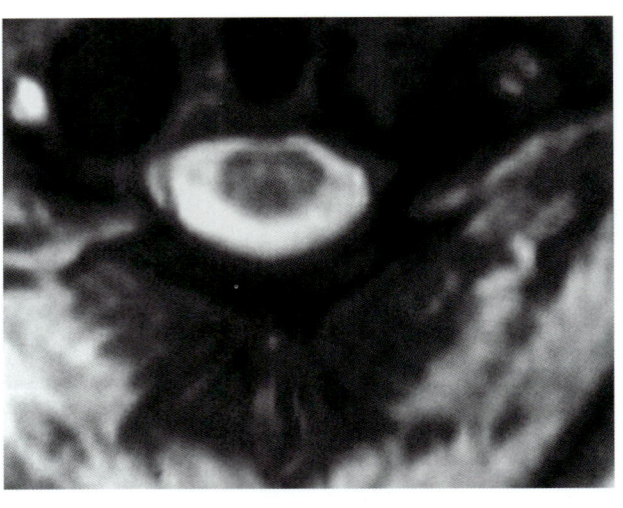

Fig. 4.6 Type II injuries detach the tubercle for the transverse ligament from the C1 lateral mass. **(a)** CT scan of a type II injury demonstrates a comminuted fracture of the C1 lateral mass, which renders the transverse ligament physiologically incompetent. **(b)** MRI corresponding to the CT demonstrates that the soft tissue structure of the transverse ligament is preserved.

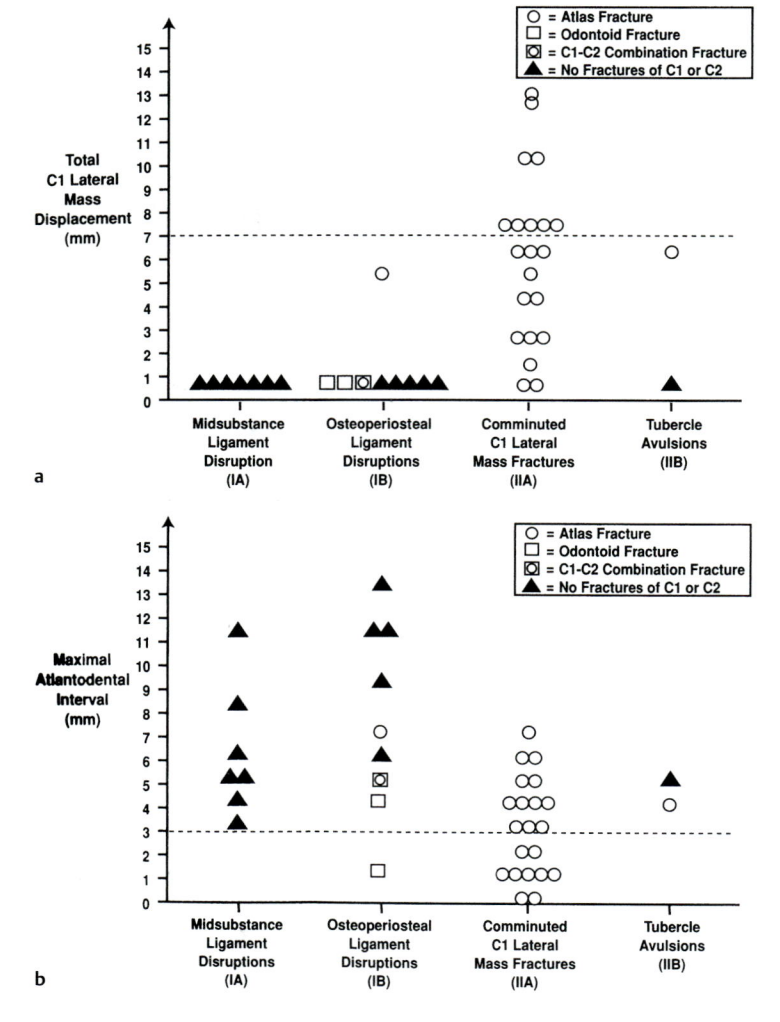

Fig. 4.7 Correlation of plain radiographic findings, with the pathoanatomy of the injury patterns to the bones and ligaments, as visualized using CT and MRI. **(a)** The type of ligamentous injury in relation to the total amount of displacement of the C1 lateral masses on open-mouth views of C1–C2. If a 7.0-mm criterion is used to assume transverse ligament disruption, more than half of the unstable atlas fractures would have been missed. Spence's 7.0-mm rule does not accurately predict the status of the transverse atlantal ligament after an atlas fracture. **(b)** The type of ligament and bone injury in relation to the maximal atlantodental interval on preoperative lateral cervical radiographs. If a 3.0-mm cutoff is used to assume a disrupted transverse atlantal ligament, 10 of the 39 injuries (26%) would not have been detected. Fewer than 10% of the type I injuries, but almost 40% of the type II injuries, would have been missed. (Courtesy of the Barrow Neurological Institute.)

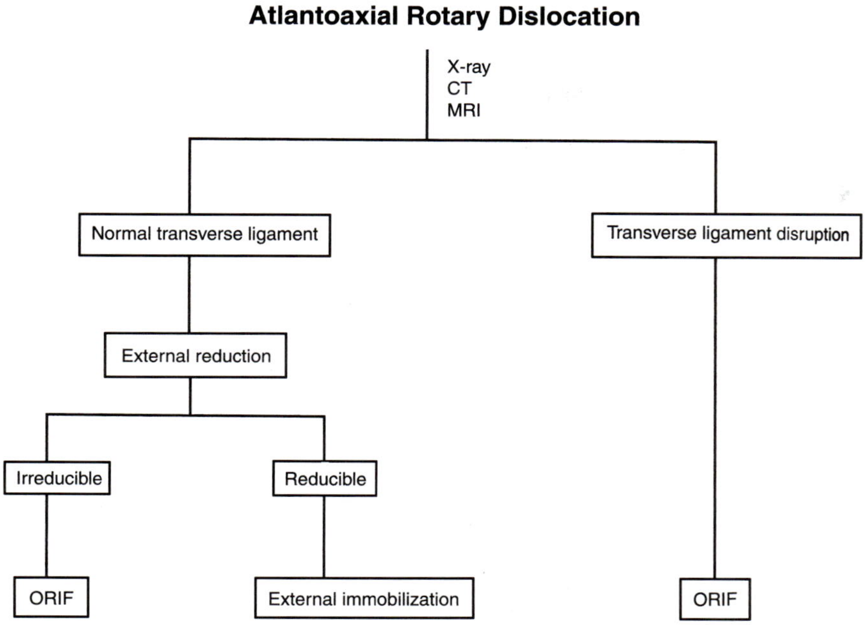

Atlantoaxial Rotary Dislocation

```
              X-ray
              CT
              MRI
        ┌──────┴──────┐
Normal transverse    Transverse ligament
    ligament              disruption
        │                      │
External reduction           ORIF
    ┌───┴───┐
Irreducible  Reducible
    │           │
  ORIF    External immobilization
```

Fig. 4.8 Treatment algorithm for C1–C2 rotatory dislocations. The majority of patients are treated successfully with reduction and immobilization without surgery. ORIF, open reduction and internal fixation. (From Sonntag VKH, Dickman CA. Treatment of upper cervical spine injuries. AANS 1992. Reproduced with permission of the American Association of Neurological Surgeons.)

knowledge of the unique anatomy to consistently identify. Furthermore, the care of each fracture type varies. Therefore, an awareness of the clinical presentation, underlying anatomy, radiographic features, and the implications of each type of injury are vital in achieving a successful outcome for the patient.

References

1. Bucholz RW, Burkhead WZ. The pathological anatomy of fatal atlanto-occipital dislocations. J Bone Joint Surg Am 1979;61:248–250
2. Schneider RC, Cherry G, Pantek H. The syndrome of acute central cervical spinal cord injury; with special reference to the mechanisms involved in hyperextension injuries of cervical spine. J Neurosurg 1954;11:546–577
3. Kakarla UK, Chang SW, Theodore N, Sonntag VK. Atlas fractures. Neurosurgery 2010;66(3, Suppl):60–67
4. Levine AM, Edwards CC. Traumatic lesions of the occipitoatlantoaxial complex. Clin Orthop Relat Res 1989;239:53–68
5. Alker GJ Jr, Oh YS, Leslie EV. High cervical spine and craniocervical junction injuries in fatal traffic accidents: a radiological study. Orthop Clin North Am 1978;9:1003–1010
6. Davis D, Bohlman H, Walker AE, Fisher R, Robinson R. The pathological findings in fatal craniospinal injuries. J Neurosurg 1971;34:603–613
7. Bucholz RW, Burkhead WZ, Graham W, Petty C. Occult cervical spine injuries in fatal traffic accidents. J Trauma 1979;19:768–771
8. Dickman CA, Papadopoulos SM, Sonntag VK, Spetzler RF, Rekate HL, Drabier J. Traumatic occipitoatlantal dislocations. J Spinal Disord 1993;6:300–313
9. Traynelis VC, Marano GD, Dunker RO, Kaufman HH. Traumatic atlanto-occipital dislocation. Case report. J Neurosurg 1986;65:863–870
10. Findlay JM. Injuries involving the transverse atlantal ligament: classification and treatment guidelines based upon experience with 39 injuries. Neurosurgery 1996;39:210
11. Moore KR, Frank EH. Traumatic atlantoaxial rotatory subluxation and dislocation. Spine 1995;20:1928–1930
12. Lefebvre Y, Babin SR, Clavert P, et al. [Traumatic bilateral rotatory C1-C2 dislocation in an adult: case report and review of the literature]. Rev Chir Orthop Repar Appar Mot 2002;88:613–619
13. Robertson PA, Swan HA. Traumatic bilateral rotatory facet dislocation of the atlas on the axis. Spine 1992;17:1252–1254
14. Born CT, Mure AJ, Iannacone WM, DeLong WG Jr. Three-dimensional computerized tomographic demonstration of bilateral atlantoaxial rotatory dislocation in an adult: report of a case and review of the literature. J Orthop Trauma 1994;8:67–72
15. Karam YR, Traynelis VC. Occipital condyle fractures. Neurosurgery 2010;66(3, Suppl):56–59
16. Maserati MB, Stephens B, Zohny Z, et al. Occipital condyle fractures: clinical decision rule and surgical management. J Neurosurg Spine 2009;11:388–395
17. Anderson PA, Montesano PX. Morphology and treatment of occipital condyle fractures. Spine 1988;13:731–736
18. Yoon JW, Lim OK, Park KD, Lee JK. Occipital condyle fracture with isolated unilateral hypoglossal nerve palsy. Ann Rehabil Med 2014;38:689–693
19. Hadley MN, Dickman CA, Browner CM, Sonntag VK. Acute traumatic atlas fractures: management and long term outcome. Neurosurgery 1988;23:31–35
20. Levine AM, Edwards CC. Fractures of the atlas. J Bone Joint Surg Am 1991;73:680–691
21. Ryken TC, Aarabi B, Dhall SS, et al. Management of isolated fractures of the atlas in adults. Neurosurgery 2013;72(Suppl 2):127–131
22. Ryken TC, Hadley MN, Aarabi B, et al. Management of acute combination fractures of the atlas and axis in adults. Neurosurgery 2013;72(Suppl 2):151–158
23. Dickman CA, Hadley MN, Browner C, Sonntag VK. Neurosurgical management of acute atlas-axis combination fractures. A review of 25 cases. J Neurosurg 1989;70:45–49
24. Sköld G. Fractures of the neural arch and odontoid process of the axis: a study of their causation. Z Rechtsmed 1978;82:89–103
25. Dickman CA, Sonntag VK. Injuries involving the transverse atlantal ligament: classification and treatment guidelines based upon experience with 39 injuries. Neurosurgery 1997;40:886–887
26. Greene KA, Dickman CA, Marciano FF, Drabier JB, Hadley MN, Sonntag VK. Acute axis fractures. Analysis of management and outcome in 340 consecutive cases. Spine 1997;22:1843–1852
27. Frangen TM, Zilkens C, Muhr G, Schinkel C. Odontoid fractures in the elderly: dorsal C1/C2 fusion is superior to halo-vest immobilization. J Trauma 2007;63:83–89
28. Harrop JS, Sharan AD, Przybylski GJ. Epidemiology of spinal cord injury after acute odontoid fractures. Neurosurg Focus 2000;8:e4
29. Corner EM. Fractures of the odontoid process of the axis. Med Chir Trans 1907;90:637–665

30. Fineschi G. [Fractures of the odontoid process of the axis by posterior dislocation of the atlas]. Arch Ortop 1950;63:231–240
31. Blockey NJ, Purser DW. Fractures of the odontoid process of the axis. J Bone Joint Surg Br 1956;38-B:794–817
32. Massardier J. [Fractures of the odontoid process]. Lyon Chir 1963;59:766–767
33. Martini M, Essafi Z. [Our experience with fractures of the odontoid process of the axis]. Tunis Med 1964;42:515–523
34. Hadley MN, Browner C, Sonntag VK. Axis fractures: a comprehensive review of management and treatment in 107 cases. Neurosurgery 1985;17:281–290
35. Anderson LD, D'Alonzo RT. Fractures of the odontoid process of the axis. J Bone Joint Surg Am 1974;56:1663–1674
36. Hadley MN, Browner CM, Liu SS, Sonntag VK. New subtype of acute odontoid fractures (type IIA). Neurosurgery 1988;22(1 Pt 1):67–71
37. Harrop JS. Type II odontoid fractures: what to do? World Neurosurg 2013;80:313–314
38. Fassett DR, Harrop JS, Maltenfort M, et al. Mortality rates in geriatric patients with spinal cord injuries. J Neurosurg Spine 2007;7:277–281
39. Harrop JS, Hart R, Anderson PA. Optimal treatment for odontoid fractures in the elderly. Spine 2010;35(21, Suppl):S219–S227
40. Polin RS, Szabo T, Bogaev CA, Replogle RE, Jane JA. Nonoperative management of Types II and III odontoid fractures: the Philadelphia collar versus the halo vest. Neurosurgery 1996;38:450–456, discussion 456–457
41. Tashjian RZ, Majercik S, Biffl WL, Palumbo MA, Cioffi WG. Halo-vest immobilization increases early morbidity and mortality in elderly odontoid fractures. J Trauma 2006;60:199–203
42. Vaccaro AR, Kepler CK, Kopjar B, et al. Functional and quality-of-life outcomes in geriatric patients with type-II dens fracture. J Bone Joint Surg Am 2013;95:729–735
43. Garber JN. Abnormalities of the atlas and axis vertebrae–congenital and traumatic. J Bone Joint Surg Am 1964;46:1782–1791
44. Effendi B, Roy D, Cornish B, Dussault RG, Laurin CA. Fractures of the ring of the axis. A classification based on the analysis of 131 cases. J Bone Joint Surg Br 1981;63-B:319–327
45. Eismont FJ, Bohlman HH. Posterior atlanto-occipital dislocation with fractures of the atlas and odontoid process. J Bone Joint Surg Am 1978;60:397–399
46. Bell HS. Paralysis of both arms from injury of the upper portion of the pyramidal decussation: "cruciate paralysis". J Neurosurg 1970;33:376–380
47. Lee C, Woodring JH, Goldstein SJ, Daniel TL, Young AB, Tibbs PA. Evaluation of traumatic atlantooccipital dislocations. AJNR Am J Neuroradiol 1987;8:19–26
48. Papadopoulos SM, Dickman CA, Sonntag VK, Rekate HL, Spetzler RF. Traumatic atlantooccipital dislocation with survival. Neurosurgery 1991;28:574–579
49. Dickman CA, Mamourian A, Sonntag VK, Drayer BP. Magnetic resonance imaging of the transverse atlantal ligament for the evaluation of atlantoaxial instability. J Neurosurg 1991;75:221–227
50. Walters BC, Hadley MN, Hurlbert RJ, et al; American Association of Neurological Surgeons; Congress of Neurological Surgeons. Guidelines for the management of acute cervical spine and spinal cord injuries: 2013 update. Neurosurgery 2013;60(Suppl 1):82–91
51. Myklebust JB, Pintar F, Yoganandan N, et al. Tensile strength of spinal ligaments. Spine 1988;13:526–531
52. Frank C, Amiel D, Woo SL, Akeson W. Normal ligament properties and ligament healing. Clin Orthop Relat Res 1985;196:15–25

B. Anterior Approach

5 Transoral Approaches to the Craniovertebral Junction

Brian J. Dlouhy, Raheel Ahmed, and Arnold H. Menezes

The craniovertebral junction (CVJ) contains the cervicomedullary junction and its associated blood supply—the ascending vertebral arteries that pass through the foramen magnum and form the basilar artery. The cervicomedullary junction is the crossroads of the central nervous system as the brainstem transitions to the upper cervical spinal cord. The medulla contains the nuclei required for breathing and cardiovascular function, and the cervicomedullary junction contains the descending motor fibers to the spinal cord and ascending sensory fibers. Therefore, the CVJ houses the essential functions of life.

The complex musculoskeletal organization of the CVJ is unique in comparison to the rest of the cervical spine with regard to bony anatomy and joint configuration, shape, and orientation.[1] This sophisticated arrangement of structures is critical to allow complex movements of the head and neck and provide protection of the critical areas of the brainstem and upper cervical spinal cord. However, this complexity also creates the potential for a wide range of congenital, developmental, and acquired pathology.[2] Given the critical neural structures contained within the CVJ, pathology creating bony and ligamentous instability or mass effect causing compression of these neural structures can result in significant impairment. Direct surgical access to the CVJ is paramount for decompression and establishing stability.[3]

Evolution of Craniovertebral Junction Treatment and Transoral Approaches

The treatment of CVJ pathology has undergone remarkable evolution and advancements over the past 100 years. Depending on the location of pathology, the surgical approaches to the CVJ are categorized as ventral, lateral, and dorsal (see **Box 1.3** in Chapter 1).[4] As borne out by the evolution of CVJ treatment, multiple CVJ case series, and anatomic cadaver studies, the most direct approach to the ventral CVJ (lower clivus, atlas, and axis) is via the mouth and posterior pharynx. Therefore, transoral approaches are ideal ventral approaches for decompression of irreducible ventral bony abnormalities as well as extradural bony and soft tissue masses of the CVJ causing compression of the cervicomedullary junction.[3,5] In very rare cases, intracranial intradural tumors may be resected. However, significant complications of cerebrospinal fluid (CSF) leak and infection have led some surgeons to abandon this approach.[6,7]

The transoral approaches for decompression of irreducible ventral pathology at the CVJ have become a mainstay of treatment. In the last 10 years, the emergence of endoscopic endonasal approaches[8] has provided more options for decompression of irreducible ventral CVJ pathology. Additionally, various reduction strategies have evolved. The ability to properly reduce ventral CVJ lesions and avoid a ventral approach has increased over the past 40 years due to improvements in occipitocervical instrumentation,[2,9] preoperative and intraoperative imaging,[10,11] and a better understanding of CVJ pathology. Over the past 40 years at the University of Iowa Hospitals and Clinics, over 6,000 children and adults have been treated for wide-ranging CVJ pathology, and over 800 transoral procedures have been performed for irreducible ventral CVJ pathology. This chapter discusses the transoral approaches.

Transoral Approaches to the Craniovertebral Junction: Historical Beginnings

Recognizing that a lateral approach would not provide adequate access to remove a bullet lodged between the atlas and the clivus and that the most direct approach to the ventral CVJ (lower clivus, atlas, and axis) was via the mouth and posterior pharynx, Kanavel[12] in 1917 was the first to describe the transoral-transpharyngeal approach to the CVJ. In 1957, Southwick and Robinson[13] resected an osteoma of the body of the axis through a transoral-transpharyngeal approach. However, it was not until 1962 that Fang and Ong[14] described the approach in detail, utilizing it in five cases of chronic irreducible atlantoaxial dislocations and one case of tuberculosis of the atlas and axis. In this small series, the complication rate was high, with four cases resulting in infection and one infection leading to death. However, in their discussion of the approach, Fang and Ong suggested that infection could be reduced with meticulous closure of the posterior pharyngeal wall, proper preoperative oral preparation, and preoperative and postoperative antibiotics. Despite this suggestion, the approach was reported only sporadically in case series in the 1960s[15,16] and early 1970s.[17,18] In these reports, refinement of the procedure and the development and widespread availability of the operating microscope helped limit complications, and the approach proved effective for lesions at the ventral CVJ.

It was not until the late 1970s that the senior author (A.H.M.) further refined the transoral approach using extensive preoperative oropharynx preparation; preoperative and postoperative antibiotics; thorough perioperative management; precise microscopic dissection through the soft palate, posterior pharyngeal wall, and longus colli and longus capitis muscles; and a meticulous multilayered posterior pharyngeal wall and soft palate closure.[3,5] In Menezes et al's[3] 1980 report, nine of 17 patients underwent a transoral approach for congenital, developmental, and acquired CVJ pathology.[5] No postoperative infections occurred and complications were minimal. This was the first large series that demonstrated that the transoral approach was not fraught with complications, as suggested by the series from Fang and Ong.[14] This was found to be true in both children[5] and adults.[3] This report also ignited a new era in CVJ treatment. In this same report, Menezes et al proposed an algorithm for CVJ pathology based on the stability and motion dynamics of the craniovertebral junction as well as the reducibility and site of encroachment, incorporating the transoral approach for treatment of irreducible ventral CVJ pathology. This algorithm continues to be used today and is often referred to when discussing treatment of CVJ pathology.

In 1988, Menezes reported on 72 transoral cases over a period of 10 years—the largest series at that time. Given the minimal complications (only one pharyngeal infection treated with antibiotics) and substantial neurologic improvement in these 72 children and adults, the transoral approach became a mainstay in treating irreducible ventral CVJ pathology.[19] It also established the operative nuances for C1 anterior arch resection and odontoidectomy, key principles used today in both transoral and endoscopic endonasal odontoidectomies. Subsequently, the report of 14 transoral cases by Crockard et al[20,21] in 1985 and 53 transoral cases by Hadley et al[22] in 1989 helped solidify the support for this approach.

The transoral approaches are categorized as standard and extended, and each variation provides a different degree of exposure (**Table 5.1**). The standard transoral approach, as popularized by the pioneers cited above, includes the transoral-transpharyngeal approach and the transoral-transpalatopharyngeal approach (see **Box 1.3** in Chapter 1).

Transoral-Transpalatopharyngeal Approach (Standard Transoral)

Degree of Craniovertebral Junction Exposure

The transoral-transpharyngeal approach provides exposure from the clivus to the C2–3 interspace and laterally for 2 cm to either side of the midline (**Table 5.1**). Laterally situated lesions may involve the occipital condyles, as well as the lateral portions of the posterior fossa, the transverse processes of the atlas, and the axis vertebrae. A midline ventral approach enables exposure of the anterior 45 degrees of the circumference of the foramen magnum, to either side of the midline, thus providing a 90-degree exposure.

We prefer to divide the soft palate (transoral-transpalatopharyngeal) when necessary, as it increases exposure superiorly to the inferior one third of the clivus (**Table 5.1**). Many other surgeons have suggested that elevation and retraction of the soft palate provides similar access to dividing the soft palate. However, with normal clival anatomy we have found that elevation and retraction of the soft palate usually only provides rostral access to the inferior tip of the clivus. Additionally, in congenital pathological states, such as with a foreshortened clivus or basioccipital hypoplasia, the clivus tends to be more horizontal in position than vertical. Thus, it becomes essential to divide the soft palate (transoral-transpalatopharyngeal approach) and at times resect the posterior-inferior portion of the posterior hard palate to gain clival exposure.[23] In this manner, the upper portion of the clivus can be visualized. Anatomic studies have confirmed our clinical findings. In an anatomic cadaver study by Balasingam et al,[24] division of the soft palate provided nearly 1 cm of clival exposure. In contrast, retraction of the soft palate into the nasopharynx did not provide adequate exposure of the clivus superior to the foramen magnum, but did provide adequate exposure of the atlantoaxial complex. In general, it is imperative to review the imaging studies preoperatively to determine the adequacy of a clival exposure with or without a soft palate split and to determine whether this exposure is even needed for ventral decompression.

The inferior extent of the exposure, which is limited by the degree of depression of the tongue, is the C2–3 interspace. The lateral extent of the exposure is limited by the condylar canals of the hypoglossal nerve, the eustachian tubes, and the vertebral arteries before they enter the intradural space. However, when a tumor, such as a chordoma, is present, the tumor displaces normal anatomy, creating working space and greater exposure than normal.

Indications

The initial algorithm for the treatment of CVJ pathology continues to be used even 35 years after publication.[3,5] It helps determine when to utilize a transoral or other appropriate anterior approach for ventral CVJ decompression. Reduction pertains to the reestablishment of anatomic alignment to relieve compression of neural structures.[3] If the ventral lesion is irreducible, an

Table 5.1 Exposure Provide by Standard/Extended Transoral Approaches and Endoscopic Transnasal

Approach	Rostral Exposure	Caudal Exposure
Standard transoral		
Transoral-transpharyngeal	Inferior tip of clivus	C2–3 interspace
Transoral-transpalatopharyngeal	Inferior one third of clivus	C2–3 interspace
Extended transoral		
Median labiomandibular	Inferior one third of clivus	C3–4 interspace
Median labiomandibular with glossotomy	Inferior one third of clivus	C4–5 interspace
Le Fort I osteotomy with down-fracture of maxilla	Superior aspect of clivus	C1
Le Fort I osteotomy with palatal-split	Superior aspect of clivus	C2–3 interspace
Endoscopic endonasal	Anterior fossa floor/sella/superior clivus	Determined by nasopalatine line

anterior approach is required for decompression, which then often necessitates posterior instrumentation and fusion.[3] If the lesion is reducible, a ventral transoral approach can be avoided, and dorsal instrumentation and fixation can be performed in the reduced position with or without a posterior decompression.[3] In the last 40 years, transoral procedures have been performed for a variety of irreducible ventral CVJ pathology,[23] such as congenital and developmental basilar invagination,[25] basilar impression, cranial settling,[26] proatlas segmentation abnormalities,[27] os odontoideum, tumors, and other rare congenital bony abnormalities.[23,28]

Limitations

In some young children, the ability to sufficiently open the mouth is extremely limited. A working distance of 2.5 to 3 cm between the upper and lower incisor teeth is necessary. This is further assessed once the child is asleep and paralysis induced by the anesthesiologist. An extended transoral approach via the transmandibular route can be used in such extreme cases, but this is rare (see next section).[28]

Extending the Transoral Approach

The emergence of the transoral approach provided exposure to a previously inaccessible region. Although this approach enabled proper decompression and treatment of a variety of CVJ pathology, it was still limited in its exposure below the C2–3 interspace and above the inferior one third of the clivus. Combining the standard transoral approach with previously described techniques of craniofacial osteotomies that split the mandible and divided the tongue[29,30] or opened the maxilla and divided the hard palate[31] enhances access inferiorly to the C4–5 interspace and superiorly to the upper aspect of the clivus, respectively (**Table 5.1**). We consider these to be "extended" transoral approaches.[32] The transmandibular approaches specifically include variations of the median labiomandibular approach, which consists of a mandibulotomy (division of the mandible) with or without a glossotomy (division of tongue).[29,30] The transmaxillary approaches include the Le Fort I osteotomy with down-fracture of the maxilla and the Le Fort I osteotomy with palatal split. Other approaches, which are rarely used in practice but have been described in the literature,[33] include the transnasomaxillary approach, which uses a Le Fort II osteotomy, and a transpalatal approach in which a circumferential palatal osteotomy is performed. The purpose of these extended technical variations is to extend the standard transoral approach and the empty anatomic spaces of the mouth and pharynx for greater rostral and caudal exposure of the CVJ.

Transmandibular–Median Labiomandibular Approach and Variations

Degree of Craniovertebral Junction Exposure

A combined transoral-transpalatopharyngeal approach with a median mandibulotomy (median labiomandibular approach) provides increased caudal exposure to the C3–4 interspace and maintains the superior exposure to the inferior third of the clivus. Dividing the tongue in the midline further increases the caudal exposure to the C4–5 interspace (median labiomandibular glossotomy [MLG] approach)[28,34–37] (**Table 5.1**).

Indications

The MLG approach to augment exposure of the craniocervical junction and the upper cervical vertebrae is used when the interincisor opening distance is less than 2.5 cm and when access to C3–C5 is required. In children as well as adults, adequate access to the craniocervical junction and upper cervical vertebrae can usually be achieved with a transoral–transpalatopharyngeal route. In some children, however, young age or small size preclude adequate exposure with a soft palatal split alone. Therefore, additional exposure can be gained with the median labiomandibular glossotomy approach. However, this is rarely used. Tracheotomy provides an unobstructed view of the oral cavity and posterior pharyngeal wall and prevents upper airway obstruction secondary to tongue and pharyngeal edema in the perioperative phase. The general advantages of the MLG include a wider surgical field in both transverse and sagittal dimensions. By splitting the mandible, the surgeon also has a shorter working distance to the spine.

Limitations

Disadvantages or risks in addition to the standard transoral risks include unfavorable facial scarring, oral incompetence, injury to developing permanent dentition, malocclusion, dysphagia, limited tongue mobility and sensation, mandibular duct injury, and complications of tracheostomy. However, these outcomes are uncommon, and their risk is justified by the severity of the patient's neurosurgical condition. In general, with proper closure and good surgical technique, the facial scarring is minimal.

Transmaxillary–Le Fort I Osteotomy with Down-Fracture of the Maxilla

Degree of Craniovertebral Junction Exposure

The Le Fort I osteotomy (maxillotomy) with down-fracture of the maxilla is an approach onto itself rather than an extension of the standard transoral approaches.[38–40] A sublabial incision enables a horizontal osteotomy and down-fracture or inferior mobilization of the maxilla and hard palate to be performed. Others have referred to this approach as the "drop-down" maxillotomy approach.[41] This approach provides access to the sphenoid sinus and superior and middle clivus, which is much greater superior exposure than what can often be achieved with a transoral-transpalatopharyngeal approach. However, the inferior displacement of the hard palate obstructs caudal access to C1–2.

Indications and Limitations

The Le Fort I maxillotomy approach is indicated for extensive lesions that are too wide and too inferior for an endoscopic endonasal approach and too rostral for a standard transoral approach. The major limitation of this approach is the inability to proceed lower than the plane of the hard palate. An endoscopic endonasal approach can provide similar access above the hard palate without the morbidity of this approach. However, the Le Fort I osteotomy with down-fracture has advantages over the endoscopic endonasal approach in that it provides wider exposure as well as more inferior viewing past the plane of the hard palate. With advancements of the endoscopic endonasal approach, the use of a Le Fort osteotomy is becoming increasingly rare.

Transmaxillary–Le Fort I Osteotomy with Palatal Split

Degree of Craniovertebral Junction Exposure

The major limitation of the Le Fort I osteotomy with down-fracture is that the inferior displacement of the hard palate obstructs caudal access to C1–2. As mentioned above, this approach is not really an extended transoral approach, as the extension from the mouth is not used to gain exposure. However, the Le Fort I osteotomy with palatal split is truly an extended approach.[42] A horizontal osteotomy is performed along with a midline split of the hard and soft palate.[42,43] This divides the maxilla in the midline, enabling it to be mobilized laterally and extending the standard transoral-transpalatopharyngeal approach. Others have described this as the transmaxillary palatal split approach or the extended "open-door" maxillotomy.[44] It is essentially a Le Fort I osteotomy, and instead of down-fracturing the maxilla, it is divided in the midline and lateralized. This approach provides rostral exposure of the sphenoid sinus and superior and middle clivus while maintaining the inferior exposure provided by the standard transoral approaches to the C2–3 interspace.

Indications and Limitations

The Le Fort I osteotomy with palatal split is indicated for extensive lesions from the superior aspect of the clivus to the body of C2. However, again, with advancements in the endoscopic endonasal approach, the use of a Le Fort osteotomy is becoming increasingly rare. Even in rare cases of such an extensive lesion, an extended endoscopic endonasal approach is effective. The endoscopic endonasal approach is limited by the hard palate, but for extensive lesions from the top of the clivus to the body of C2 and below the nasopalatine line, a combined endoscopic endonasal approach with a standard transoral approach would provide adequate exposure and limit the morbidity of a Le Fort I osteotomy with palatal split.

Transoral Approaches for Intradural Pathology

With popularization of the transoral approach for extradural bony decompression in the late 1980s, some surgeons expanded the indications of the approach to include resection of purely intradural tumors located ventrally at the level of the clivus or foramen magnum.[6,7] In the only series to date, in 1991 Crockard and Sen[7] reported seven patients who underwent a transoral approach for intradural pathology. There were substantial complications, including CSF leak and infection. A watertight closure of the clival dura is difficult or nearly impossible. Therefore, all cases had CSF leak, which required CSF diversion, packing, and reconstruction. Even with these steps, five cases ultimately required lumboperitoneal shunting. The posterolateral–far lateral transcondylar approach to the ventral foramen magnum and upper cervical spine is a classic approach that limits CSF leak and provides adequate visualization for resection of intradural pathology located ventrally and ventral-laterally at the level of the foramen magnum and upper cervical spine.[45] With these results, the use of the transoral approach for intradural pathology was mostly abandoned.

Complications Associated with Transoral Approaches

In the hands of experienced surgeons, transoral complications are minimal.[23] In the senior author's (A.H.M.) series of 280 children younger than 16 years of age who underwent the transoral approach to the posterior pharyngeal wall, there was no occurrence of CSF leak or meningitis.[23] A pharyngeal wound dehiscence occurred in two children (0.7%) In the first case, the incision was reopened by inadvertent handling of a Yankour suction 10 days after surgery. In the second case, infection occurred requiring intravenous antibiotics and drainage into the pharynx. Both of these cases occurred before 1990. Velopalatine incompetence (VPI) was encountered in five children (1.8%) and was a particular problem seen in young children and usually occurred 3 to 6 months after a transoral operation in which the palate had been split. It was thought to be secondary to fibrosis that took place in the soft palate or in the pharyngeal wall. Endoscopy identified the cause. Pharyngeal retraining in three children and an obturator in the other two circumvented the problem. In one child, fat emulsion was injected into the posterior pharyngeal wall to bring it forward and close off the incompetence. This had to be repeated on two occasions. There were no deaths.

Similar complication rates have been seen in other series. In Choi and Crockard's[46] series of 411 standard transoral approaches, pharyngeal wound infection occurred in 0.6 to 1.1% of cases and dysphagia in 2.2 to 3.3% of cases. CSF leak occurred in 0.3 to 1.1% of cases. Velopharyngeal incompetence was higher in this series, occurring in 1.3 to 14.3% of cases, with the higher percentage occurring in cases in which the soft palate was split.

References

1. Menezes AH, Traynelis VC. Anatomy and biomechanics of normal craniovertebral junction (a) and biomechanics of stabilization (b). Childs Nerv Syst 2008;24:1091–1100
2. Menezes AH, Vogel TW. Specific entities affecting the craniocervical region: syndromes affecting the craniocervical junction. Childs Nerv Syst 2008;24:1155–1163
3. Menezes AH, VanGilder JC, Graf CJ, McDonnell DE. Craniocervical abnormalities. A comprehensive surgical approach. J Neurosurg 1980;53:444–455
4. Menezes AH, Traynelis VC, Gantz BJ. Surgical approaches to the craniovertebral junction. Clin Neurosurg 1994;41:187–203
5. Menezes AH, Graf CJ, Hibri N. Abnormalities of the cranio-vertebral junction with cervico-medullary compression. A rational approach to surgical treatment in children. Childs Brain 1980;7:15–30
6. Crockard HA. Transoral surgery: some lessons learned. Br J Neurosurg 1995;9:283–293
7. Crockard HA, Sen CN. The transoral approach for the management of intradural lesions at the craniovertebral junction: review of 7 cases. Neurosurgery 1991;28:88–97, discussion 97–98
8. Kassam AB, Snyderman C, Gardner P, Carrau R, Spiro R. The expanded endonasal approach: a fully endoscopic transnasal approach and resection of the odontoid process: technical case report. Neurosurgery 2005; 57(1, Suppl):E213, discussion E213
9. Menezes AH. Craniocervical fusions in children. J Neurosurg Pediatr 2012;9:573–585
10. Dahdaleh NS, Dlouhy BJ, Menezes AH. Application of neuromuscular blockade and intraoperative 3D imaging in the reduction of basilar invagination. J Neurosurg Pediatr 2012;9:119–124
11. Dahdaleh NS, Dlouhy BJ, Menezes AH. One-step fixation of atlantoaxial rotatory subluxation: technical note and report of three cases. World Neurosurg 2013;80:e391–e395

12. Kanavel AB. Bullet located between the atlas and the base of the skull—technic of removal through the mouth. Surg Clin Chicago 1917;1:361–366
13. Southwick WO, Robinson RA. Surgical approaches to the vertebral bodies in the cervical and lumbar regions. J Bone Joint Surg Am 1957;39-A:631–644
14. Fang HSY, Ong GB. Direct anterior approach to the upper cervical spine. The J Bone Joint Surg 1962;44:1588–1604
15. Bonney GL, Laurence M. Malignant destruction of the axis. Two-year survival. Proc R Soc Med 1969;62:585–586
16. Greenberg AD, Scoville WB, Davey LM. Transoral decompression of atlanto-axial dislocation due to odontoid hypoplasia. Report of two cases. J Neurosurg 1968;28:266–269
17. Bonney G. Stabilization of the upper cervical spine by the transpharyngeal route. Proc R Soc Med 1970;63:896–897
18. Thompson H. Transpharyngeal fusion of the upper cervical spine. Proc R Soc Med 1970;63:893–896
19. Menezes AH, VanGilder JC. Transoral-transpharyngeal approach to the anterior craniocervical junction. Ten-year experience with 72 patients. J Neurosurg 1988;69:895–903
20. Crockard HA. The transoral approach to the base of the brain and upper cervical cord. Ann R Coll Surg Engl 1985;67:321–325
21. Crockard HA, Essigman WK, Stevens JM, Pozo JL, Ransford AO, Kendall BE. Surgical treatment of cervical cord compression in rheumatoid arthritis. Ann Rheum Dis 1985;44:809–816
22. Hadley MN, Spetzler RF, Sonntag VK. The transoral approach to the superior cervical spine. A review of 53 cases of extradural cervicomedullary compression. J Neurosurg 1989;71:16–23
23. Menezes AH. Surgical approaches: postoperative care and complications "transoral-transpalatopharyngeal approach to the craniocervical junction". Childs Nerv Syst 2008;24:1187–1193
24. Balasingam V, Anderson GJ, Gross ND, et al. Anatomical analysis of transoral surgical approaches to the clivus. J Neurosurg 2006;105:301–308
25. Goel A, Bhatjiwale M, Desai K. Basilar invagination: a study based on 190 surgically treated patients. J Neurosurg 1998;88:962–968
26. Menezes AH, VanGilder JC, Clark CR, el-Khoury G. Odontoid upward migration in rheumatoid arthritis. An analysis of 45 patients with "cranial settling". J Neurosurg 1985;63:500–509
27. Menezes AH, Fenoy KA. Remnants of occipital vertebrae: proatlas segmentation abnormalities. Neurosurgery 2009;64:945–953, discussion 954
28. Brookes JT, Smith RJ, Menezes AH, Smith MC. Median labiomandibular glossotomy approach to the craniocervical region. Childs Nerv Syst 2008;24:1195–1201
29. Martin H, Tollefsen HR, Gerold FP. Median labiomandibular glossotomy. Trotter's median (anterior) translingual pharyngotomy. Am J Surg 1961;102:753–759
30. Scaramella LF. Median labiomandibular glossotomy. Laryngoscope 1964;74:1561–1569
31. Drommer RB. The history of the "Le Fort I osteotomy". J Maxillofac Surg 1986;14:119–122
32. Youssef AS, Sloan AE. Extended transoral approaches: surgical technique and analysis. Neurosurgery 2010;66(3, Suppl):126–134
33. Lawton MT, Beals SP, Joganic EF, Han PP, Spetzler RF. The transfacial approaches to midline skull base lesions: a classification scheme. Operative Techniques in Neurosurgery 1999;2:201–217
34. Arbit E, Patterson RH Jr. Combined transoral and median labiomandibular glossotomy approach to the upper cervical spine. Neurosurgery 1981;8:672–674
35. Delgado TE, Garrido E, Harwick RD. Labiomandibular, transoral approach to chordomas in the clivus and upper cervical spine. Neurosurgery 1981;8:675–679
36. Moore LJ, Schwartz HC. Median labiomandibular glossotomy for access to the cervical spine. J Oral Maxillofac Surg 1985;43:909–912
37. Wessberg GA, Hill SC, McBride KL. Median labiomandibular glossotomy. Int J Oral Surg 1981;10:333–337
38. Sasaki CT, Lowlicht RA, Astrachan DI, Friedman CD, Goodwin WJ, Morales M. Le Fort I osteotomy approach to the skull base. Laryngoscope 1990;100(10 Pt 1):1073–1076
39. Uttley D, Moore A, Archer DJ. Surgical management of midline skull-base tumors: a new approach. J Neurosurg 1989;71(5 Pt 1):705–710
40. Wood GD, Stell PM. Osteotomy at the Le Fort I level. A versatile procedure. Br J Oral Maxillofac Surg 1989;27:33–38
41. Liu JK, Couldwell WT, Apfelbaum RI. Transoral approach and extended modifications for lesions of the ventral foramen magnum and craniovertebral junction. Skull Base 2008;18:151–166
42. Sandor GK, Charles DA, Lawson VG, Tator CH. Trans oral approach to the nasopharynx and clivus using the Le Fort I osteotomy with midpalatal split. Int J Oral Maxillofac Surg 1990;19:352–355
43. Williams WG, Lo LJ, Chen YR. The Le Fort I-palatal split approach for skull base tumors: efficacy, complications, and outcome. Plast Reconstr Surg 1998;102:2310–2319
44. James D, Crockard HA. Surgical access to the base of skull and upper cervical spine by extended maxillotomy. Neurosurgery 1991;29:411–416
45. Menezes AH. Surgical approaches: postoperative care and complications "posterolateral-far lateral transcondylar approach to the ventral foramen magnum and upper cervical spinal canal". Childs Nerv Syst 2008;24:1203–1207
46. Choi D, Crockard HA. Evolution of transoral surgery: three decades of change in patients, pathologies, and indications. Neurosurgery 2013;73:296–303, discussion 303–304

6 Transoral Odontoidectomy

Brian J. Dlouhy, Raheel Ahmed, and Arnold H. Menezes

Congenital, developmental, and acquired pathology of the craniovertebral junction (CVJ) can result in ventral compression of the cervicomedullary junction. This compression is often caused by the odontoid process or disease associated with the odontoid, such as with basilar invagination, basilar impression, cranial settling, calcium pyrophosphate dihydrate deposition (CPDD), atlantoaxial subluxation/dislocation, or odontoid tumors. Other pathological conditions such as proatlas segmentation abnormalities, atlantoaxial tumors, clival tumors, and rare congenital osseous abnormalities can also result in ventral cervicomedullary compression. Irreducible ventral cervicomedullary compression requires ventral decompression, and the most direct route to the ventral CVJ is via the mouth and posterior pharynx through the oropharynx. The transoral approach has been a mainstay for the treatment of irreducible ventral CVJ pathology since the late 1970s.

Indications

In cases of irreducible ventral CVJ compression, a transoral approach is indicated. For example, in irreducible basilar invagination, the ventral transoral–transpalatopharyngeal route to the craniocervical junction[1-3] enables removal of the superiorly displaced odontoid process and therefore ventral decompression of the cervicomedullary junction.[4,5] With this ventral decompression, a posterior occipitocervical fusion is often required.[6]

The initial algorithm for the treatment of CVJ pathology, which we published in 1980,[4,5] continues to be used today. If the pathology at the ventral CVJ is reducible, a dorsal approach may be taken without the need for a ventral approach.[4,5] We have established an intraoperative but preoperative approach to evaluate the reducibility (see below) that obviates the need for prolonged bedside skeletal traction and enables confirmation of reduction prior to committing to an anterior or posterior approach.[7,8] Intraoperative posterior distraction techniques[9-11] can be used for additional reduction of basilar invagination. Committing to a posterior-only approach necessitates proper reduction prior to occipital cervical fusion. Instrumentation with fusion without proper reduction and ventral decompression can be catastrophic (**Fig. 6.1**). Proper intraoperative imaging must provide evidence of reduction and decompression. If reduction cannot be achieved, a 540-degree procedure may be necessary in some cases (depending on the pathology), whereby the posterior approach and incision is temporarily closed and the patient is moved to a supine position for a ventral decompression followed by reopening of the posterior incision and posterior fixation.

Endoscopic endonasal approaches to the CVJ can be effective for resection of an invaginated odontoid.[12] However, one must study the anatomy and trajectory utilized in an endoscopic endonasal approach.

Contraindications

In some children and adults, the ability to sufficiently open the mouth is extremely limited. A working distance of 2.5–3 cm between the upper and lower incisor teeth is necessary. However, this is further assessed once the patient is under general anesthesia and paralysis induced by the anesthesiologist. A transmandibular route can be used in such extreme cases, but this is rare.[13,14]

Preoperative Planning

Imaging

Imaging is critical to determining whether a ventral CVJ decompression is warranted.[1,15] Computed tomography (CT) with three-dimensional (3D) reconstructions of the CVJ is an integral part of assessing the bony pathology. CT confirms the location of the occipital condyles, the lateral atlantal and axis masses, and the odontoid process, thus providing a "road map" for the treating surgeon. T1- and T2-weighted magnetic resonance imaging (MRI) of the CVJ in neutral, flexed, and extended positions is also utilized and provides information about the neural structures and their relationship to the osseous abnormalities and vascular structures. The flexed and extended positions provide a dynamic view of the bony anatomy in relationship to the neural structures, specifically the medulla and upper cervical spine. In the neutral position, ventral compression may not be present, but when the neck is flexed, compression from the odontoid process may be much more evident. MR angiography (MRA) of the CVJ in neutral, flexed, extended, and rotated positions is performed when there is neurologic dysfunction that cannot be explained. This can determine if vascular occlusions occur when the patient changes neck position.

Nutritional Status, Preoperative Evaluation, and Oropharynx Preparation

Nutritional status is particularly important in children who have had difficulty in swallowing as well as failure to thrive.[1] Brainstem involvement and lower cranial nerve dysfunction can affect the nutritional status. Therefore, in these patients, preoperative nutritional support is provided. It is thought that failure to do so

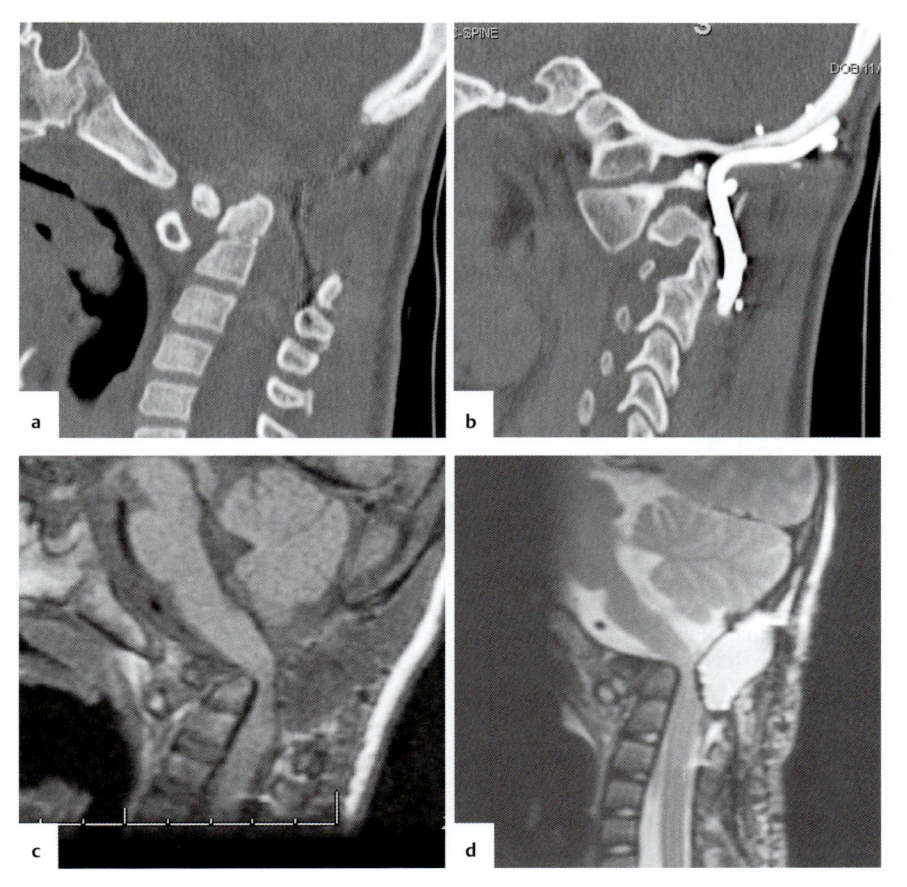

Fig. 6.1 Illustrative case, part 1 (see text). Preoperative imaging after previous posterior fusion by an outside institution demonstrating irreducible and severe cervicomedullary compression. **(a)** Midsagittal cervical computed tomography (CT) demonstrated a dystopic os odontoideum with dorsal displacement of the hypoplastic dens. **(b)** Parasagittal cervical CT demonstrated previous occipital cervical fusion by another institution. Midsagittal cervical **(c)** T1-weighted magnetic resonance imaging (MRI) and **(d)** T2-weighted MRI showed severe compression by the dens at the cervicomedullary junction.

could result in wound dehiscence and also nonfusion. Dental hygiene is addressed to remove causes of bacterial contamination such as dental caries and gingivitis in the operative field. Dental guards are made to protect the upper and lower dentition during surgery. Abnormalities of the brainstem and the lower cranial nerves (IX, X, and XII) are evaluated, and their effects on the pulmonary function documented. Sleep apnea is likewise documented. In one study, loss of vagal, hypoglossal, and glossopharyngeal nerve function mandated a tracheostomy at the start of the operation in 12 patients.[1]

Oropharyngeal cultures are obtained from the nasal passages as well as the oropharynx 4 days prior to the surgical intervention. No antibiotics are administered if normal nasal flora are present. As a precaution, nystatin rinses and Peridex gargles are performed three times a day 2 days before the operative procedure. Mupirocin nasal ointment is used in the nasal passages for 2 days prior to the operative procedure.

Preoperative Reduction via Craniocervical Traction

"Reduction" through skeletal traction is attempted in children, because 80% of children younger than 12 to 14 years of age with atlantoaxial dislocation or basilar invagination can be reduced, thereby relieving compression on neural structures and thus avoiding a ventral procedure.[1] If the lesion is reducible, a transoral approach can be prevented. A dorsal occipitocervical fixation can then be performed in the reduced position with or without decompression. If it is irreducible, then both the ventral and dorsal procedures are performed.

An MRI-compatible crown-halo device (Bremer, Depuy Spine Inc., Raynham, MA) is used for skeletal traction and to assess the reducibility of the lesion. Prior to 2007 at the University of Iowa Hospitals and Clinics (UIHC), we placed the patient in crown-halo traction 4 days prior to the planned surgical procedures.[1] This was performed under mild intravenous sedation and topical and local anesthesia. In this approach, the child is placed in the supine position with a pad underneath the shoulders and head. A crown halo is positioned at the equator of the cranium (pins placed above this plane have a tendency to pull out). Local anesthetic is administered at the pin sites. The frontal pins are placed 2.5 cm above the supraorbital bar, and the retromastoid pins are placed one on either side. In children of ages 8 to 16 years, a total of four pins are utilized, two pins on each side, and they are tightened to 6 to 8 lb of pressure. In children of ages 4 to 6 years, six to eight pin fixation is used under general anesthesia. The maximum tightening pressure for a 6-year-old is 5 to 6 lb and for a 4-year-old is 4 lb. Preoperative traction is maintained with mild elevation of the head—15 to 20 degrees above the horizontal. Cervical traction is started at 5 to 6 lb in an 8-year-old and increased to 9 lb by the end of the first day. Lateral radiographs are obtained to assess reduction. At 48 hours, an MRI is performed with the patient in cervical traction to assess the neural osseous relationships and reduction. In the child in whom an operative procedure is being done for a tumor or a noncongenital abnormality, the crown-halo traction is applied intraoperatively.

Neuromuscular Blockade, Intraoperative Traction, and Three-Dimensional Computed Tomography for Craniovertebral Junction Reduction

Since 2007 at UIHC, we have implemented an additional method of preoperative reduction for basilar invagination by using general anesthesia, intraoperative crown-halo traction, neuromuscular blockade, and intraoperative CT (O-arm, Medtronic Inc., Minneapolis, MN).[7] In this approach, the patient is brought to the operating room, and fiberoptic intubation is performed and general anesthesia is induced. Neuromuscular blockade is achieved using rocuronium and somatosensory evoked potential (SSEP) monitoring is utilized. The crown halo is applied with the patient in the supine position and the head placed on a horseshoe headrest with 8 lb of traction. Using the O-arm, an intraoperative 3D CT of the craniocervical junction is obtained in traction, and the amount of reduction and decompression at the cervicomedullary junction along with the new clivus canal angle and new alignment are evaluated. If there is adequate reduction and decompression in proper alignment, a transoral resection of the odontoid process is not needed. The patient is then placed prone, and another intraoperative 3D CT is obtained to verify adequate reduction, distraction of the odontoid process from the basiocciput, and an appropriate clivus canal angle. If this is satisfactory, a dorsal occipitocervical fusion is performed. We have described dorsal occipitocervical fusion and its variations in a previously published report.[16]

Surgical Technique

Positioning and Preparation

The patient, either child or adult, is brought to the operating room with a cervical collar in place as a precaution during intubation, maneuvers, and positioning. All adults and children 10 to 18 years of age undergo awake fiberoptic oral endotracheal intubation. However, in children younger than 10 years of age or in an older child who cannot tolerate the procedure, general anesthesia is utilized and fiberoptic intubation is performed through the mask.

The patient is positioned supine on the operating table with the head and crown halo resting on a horseshoe headrest with traction being maintained at 5 to 7 lb in children and 7 lb in adults. The endotracheal tube is secured to the skin overlying the mandible with suture, and the nasal passages anesthetized with topical cocaine. A throat pack is used to occlude the laryngopharynx, and oral preparation is performed with 10% povidone-iodine and hydrogen peroxide. The Dingman mouth retractor is then set in place. This retractor has been used for decades for intraoral surgery. It consists of a frame with coiled springs for fastening stay sutures for retraction of tissue, tongue depressors of varying sizes, two cheek retractors movable in any direction, and two movable upper dental hooks. This retractor provides self-retaining exposure of the oral cavity and oropharynx. Although other retractors have been used for the transoral approach, all are a modification or variation of the Dingman retractor. If needed, the mandible can be dislocated under general anesthesia to provide a greater oral opening.

Approach

After proper positioning of the Dingman retractor, the entirety of the procedure is performed under the operating microscope and at high power (see Video 6.1). The soft palate is split in procedures that involve the foramen magnum and the inferior clivus. To prepare the soft palate, it is anesthetized with 0.5% Xylocaine solution with 1:200,000 epinephrine. To divide the soft palate, an incision is made starting at the right of the uvula and extends along the median raphe up to the hard palate. Stay sutures that are attached to the edge of the palate divide and fastened between the coiled springs of the Dingman retractor hold apart the exposure. At times, it is necessary to remove a portion of the hard palate to gain exposure of the high nasopharynx. Large adenoid tissue in the nasopharynx in some cases also requires removal.

After retraction or split of the soft palate (**Fig. 6.2a,b**), the posterior pharyngeal wall (**Fig. 6.2c**) is topically anesthetized with 2% cocaine and the median raphe infiltrated with 0.5% Xylocaine solution with 1:200,000 epinephrine. An ultra-sharp angled monopolar cautery (Stryker Colorado Needle, Stryker Inc, Kalamazoo, MI) is used to incise the posterior pharyngeal wall longitudinally in the midline over the inferior clivus, C1 arch, and C2 vertebral body in the case of an odontoidectomy. The mucosa is incised (**Fig. 6.2d**), and dissection with monopolar cautery proceeds through the midline raphe between the pharyngeal muscles (**Fig. 6.2e**) and the anterior longitudinal ligament to bone. The longus colli and longus capitis muscles are detached from their medial origin on the ventral surface of the cervical vertebrae and mobilized laterally in a subperiosteal fashion using bipolar electrocuting cautery and blunt dissection (**Fig. 6.2f**). These muscles can be held in place with tooth-bladed lateral pharyngeal retractors if needed or held in place with stay sutures (**Fig. 6.2g**). The midline is marked by the tubercle of the anterior arch of C1 and should be identified for orientation (**Fig. 6.2g–i**).

Odontoidectomy

After dissection of soft tissue from the anterior arch of C1 centered over the tubercle of C1 (**Fig. 6.2i**), a high-speed drill with cutting and diamond burs (**Fig. 6.3a**) along with curettes (**Fig. 6.3b**) are used to resect 15 mm of the midline of the anterior arch of the atlas (**Fig. 6.3c**). This provides access to the odontoid. The odontoid process is cored out, leaving an eggshell-thin layer of outer cortical bone (**Fig. 6.3d–f**). The remaining eggshell-thin odontoid process is removed with the drill, curettes, or rongeurs (**Fig. 6.3g**). In cases with congenital and abnormal bony anatomy such as with proatlas segmentation abnormalities or os odontoideum, these abnormal bony protuberances are resected (**Fig. 6.3d,e**). The inferior portion of the clivus is removed when indicated using a diamond bur and fine Kerrison rongeurs. The lateral extent of the exposure is dictated by the amount of de-

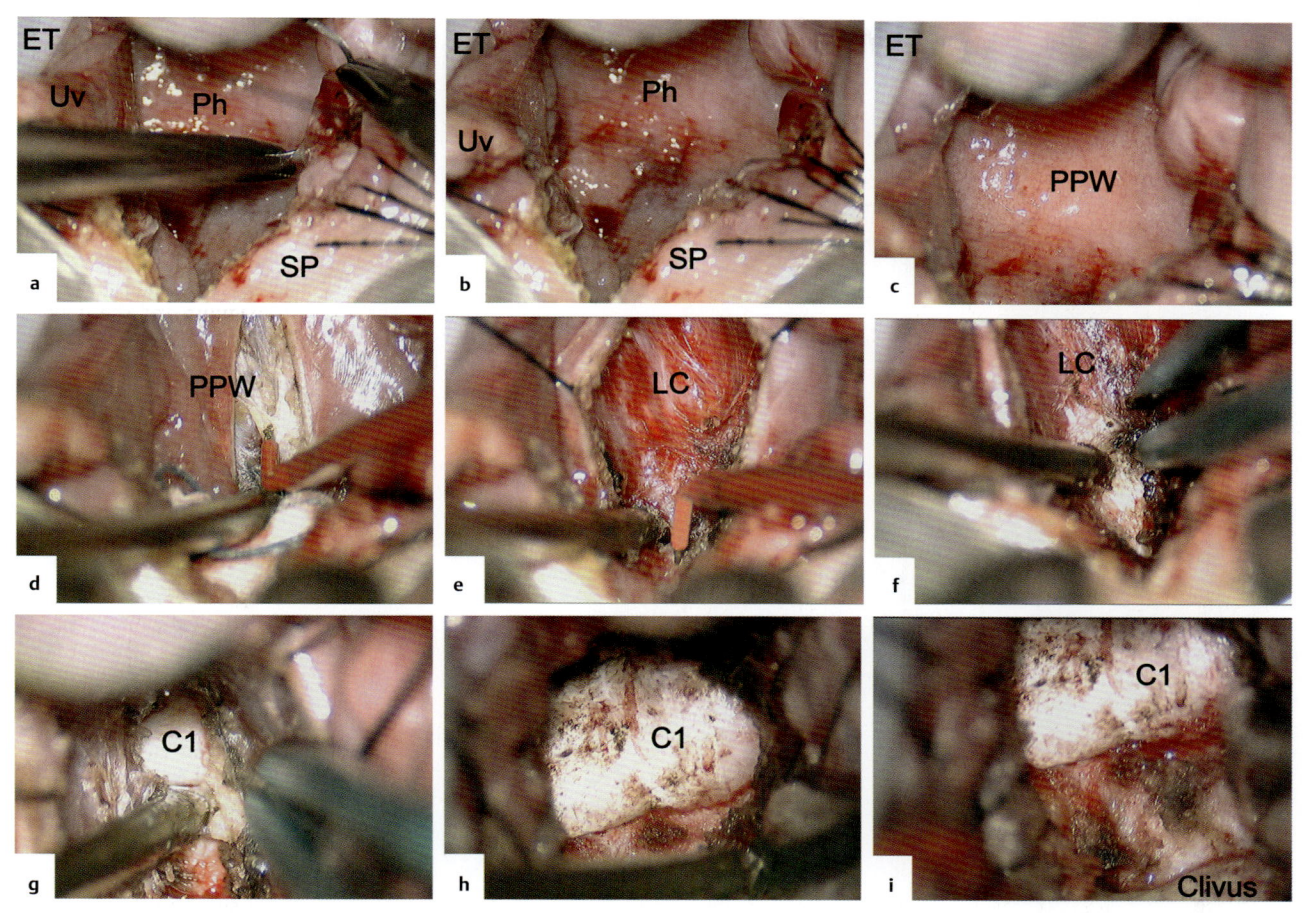

Fig. 6.2 Illustrative case, part 2. Transoral-transpalatopharyngeal approach to C1: microscope views from the surgeon's perspective at the top of the head. **(a)** The Dingman retractor was properly positioned and the endotracheal tube (ET) positioned out of the way of the operative corridor in the corner of the left aspect of the oral cavity and pharynx (Ph). The soft palate (SP) was divided to the right of the uvula (Uv), and stay sutures were placed. **(b)** After placement of multiple stay sutures at the division of the soft palate, the pharynx was opened. **(c)** The posterior pharyngeal wall (PPW) was widely exposed. **(d)** The PPW was sharply divided using monopolar cautery and the mucosa is divided. The divided edges of the PPW were held in place with stay sutures. **(e)** The longus capitis and longus colli (LC) muscles were divided in the midline and **(f)** dissected laterally in a subperiosteal manner. This provided exposure of the **(g)** anterior arch of C1. With further dissection, **(h)** the tubercle of C1 was exposed. Typically, the tubercle of C1 indicated the midline. However, in this case, given the previous fusion, the C1 arch was slightly rotated. **(i)** The clivus was exposed superiorly.

compression required by the preoperative neurodiagnostic images. The cruciate ligament is usually visualized after bony removal. During the operation, cervical traction is maintained for inherent, potential, or iatrogenic instability. The tectorial membrane is not removed. The completion of decompression and resection is evident by the visualization of the transverse ligament, tectorial membrane, and the dura as well as the cruciate ligament inferiorly (**Fig. 6.3h,i**).

Illustrative Case

A 5-year-old girl with Down syndrome presented with a dystopic os odontoideum and dorsal displacement of the hypoplastic dens with instability between the craniocervical region and C2 (**Figs. 6.1, 6.2, 6.3, 6.4, 6.5**) (Video 6.1). At an outside institution, she underwent two previous posterior approaches including posterior decompression with instrumentation and fusion. However, proper reduction was not achieved. She was unable to stand or walk or use her arms after her second operative procedure due to severe cervicomedullary compression. Given her pathology and occipitocervical fusion, she was unable to be reduced. Therefore, a ventral transoral-transpalatopharyngeal approach and decompression with removal of the anterior arch of C1, os odontoideum, and odontoid process was indicated. The patient did well postoperatively and regained significant strength.

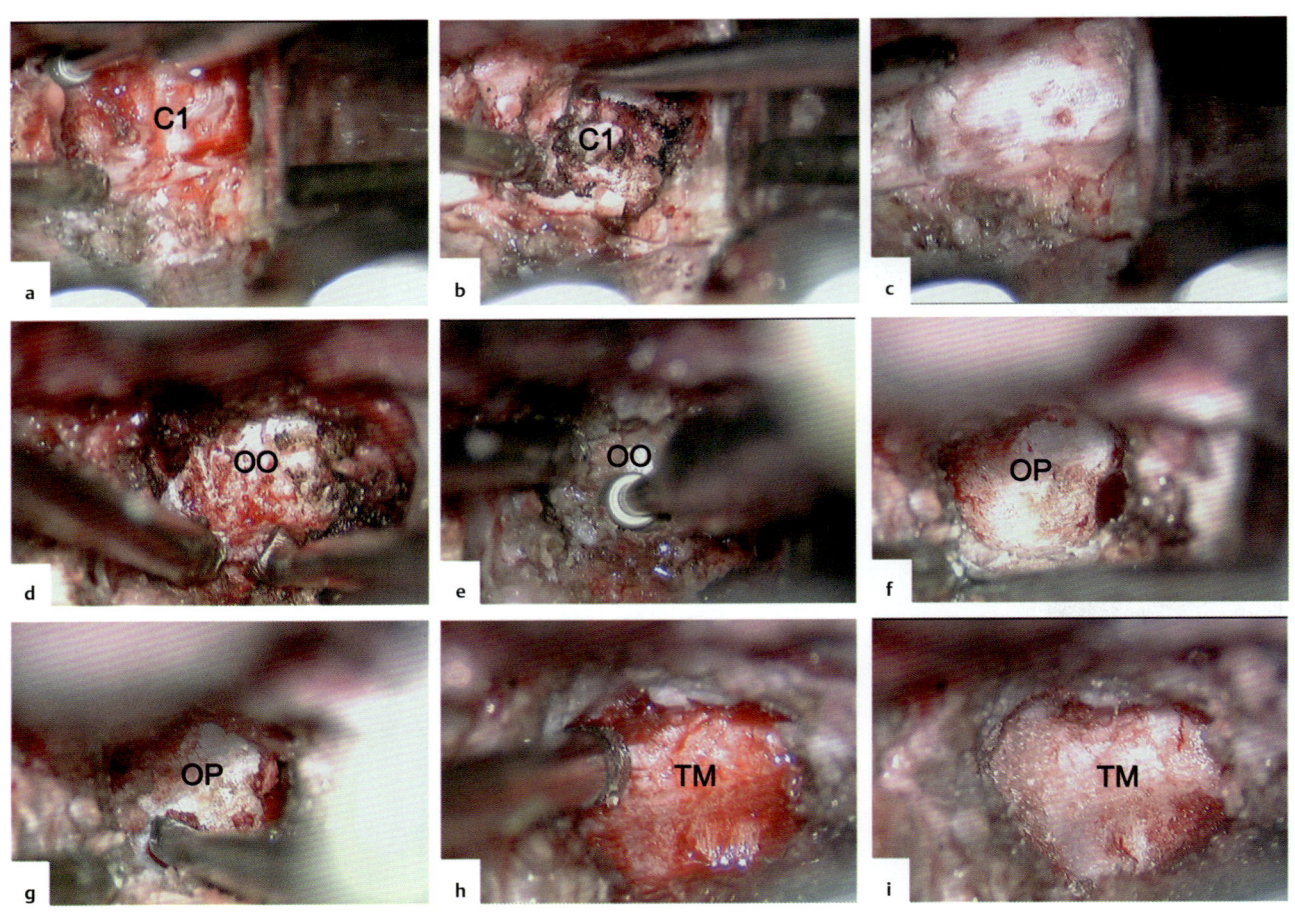

Fig. 6.3 Illustrative case, part 3. Transoral-transpalatopharyngeal odontoidectomy: microscope views from the surgeon's perspective at the top of the head. **(a)** The anterior arch of C1 was cored out with a high-speed drill. **(b)** The posterior aspect of C1 was removed with a curette to **(c)** complete the removal of the medial aspect of the anterior arch of C1—18 mm in this case. **(d)** This allowed exposure of the dystopic os odontoideum (OO). **(e)** The OO was removed using a high-speed drill and curettes to provide exposure of **(f)** the odontoid process (OP). **(g)** The odontoid process (OP) is removed using curettes and a high-speed drill. **(h,i)** After complete removal of the odontoid process, the tectorial membrane (TM) was visualized. Pulsations of the tectorial membrane and ligaments should be visualized demonstrating cervicomedullary decompression.

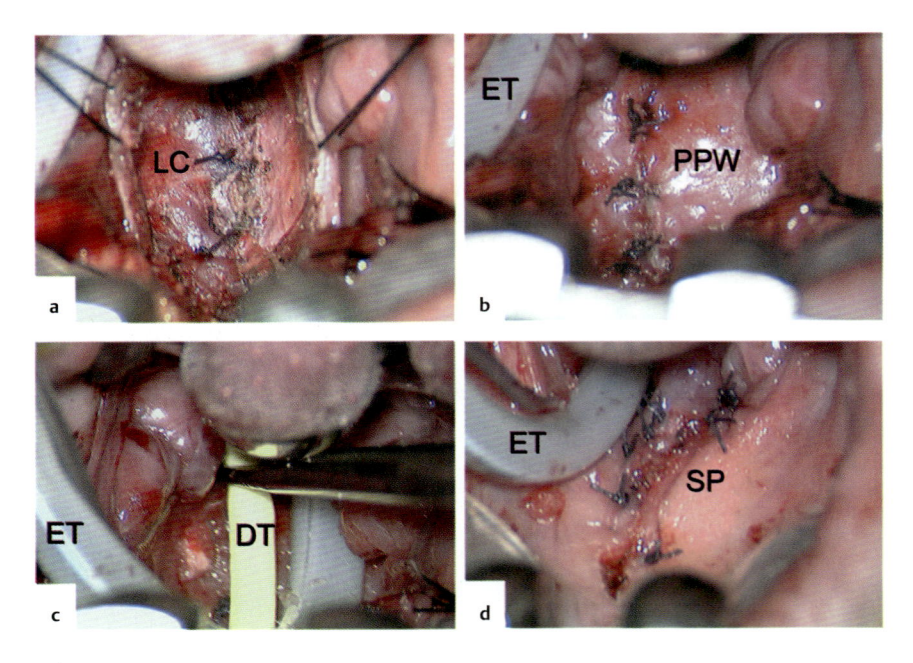

Fig. 6.4 Illustrative case, part 4. Transoral-transpalatopharyngeal closure: microscope views from the surgeon's perspective at the top of the head. **(a)** After satisfactory decompression, the longus capitis and longus colli (LC) muscles were reapproximated in the midline using Vicryl sutures. **(b)** The posterior pharyngeal wall (PPW) was reapproximated using Vicryl sutures. **(c)** A Dobhoff tube (DT) was placed under direct visualization prior to soft palate closure. **(d)** The soft palate (SP) was reapproximated using Vicryl sutures.

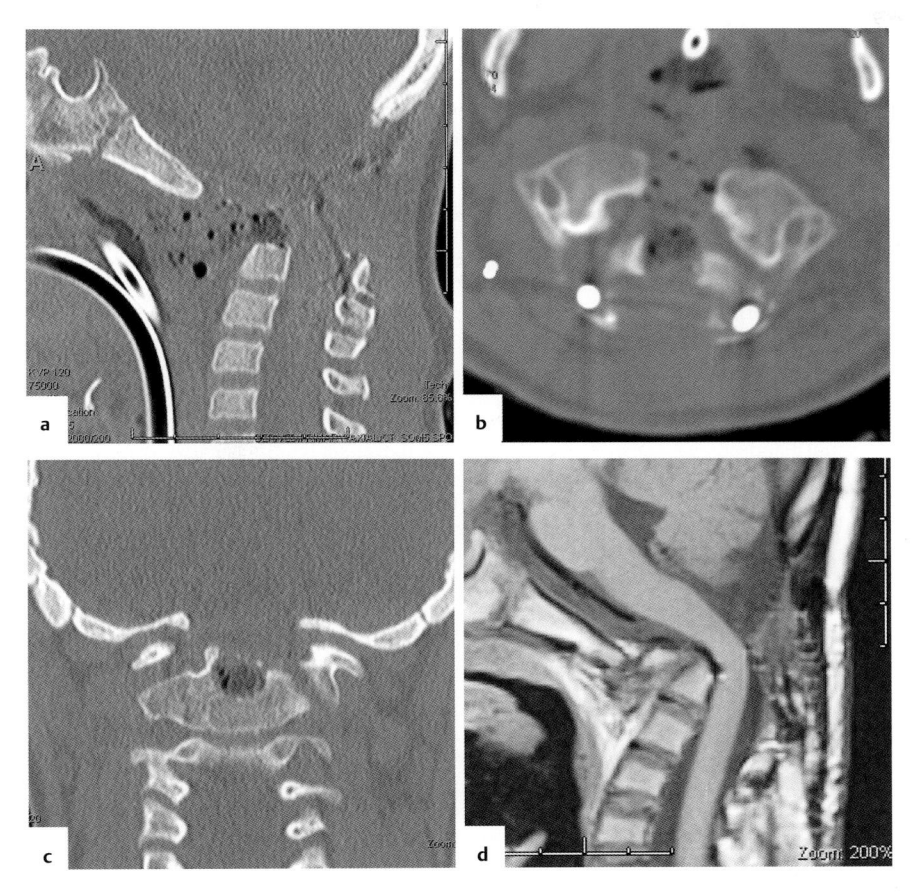

Fig. 6.5 Illustrative case, part 5. Postoperative imaging after transoral-transpalatopharyngeal resection of the anterior arch of C1, dystopic os odontoideum, and odontoid process closure. **(a)** Midsagittal cervical CT, **(b)** axial cervical CT, and **(c)** coronal cervical CT demonstrated satisfactory resection of the anterior arch of C1, the dystopic os odontoideum, and the odontoid process. **(d)** Midsagittal cervical T1-weighted MRI demonstrating decompression of the cervicomedullary junction.

References

1. Menezes AH. Surgical approaches: postoperative care and complications "transoral-transpalatopharyngeal approach to the craniocervical junction." Childs Nerv Syst 2008;24:1187–1193
2. Menezes AH, Traynelis VC, Gantz BJ. Surgical approaches to the craniovertebral junction. Clin Neurosurg 1994;41:187–203
3. Menezes AH, VanGilder JC. Transoral-transpharyngeal approach to the anterior craniocervical junction. Ten-year experience with 72 patients. J Neurosurg 1988;69:895–903
4. Menezes AH, Graf CJ, Hibri N. Abnormalities of the cranio-vertebral junction with cervico-medullary compression. A rational approach to surgical treatment in children. Childs Brain 1980;7:15–30
5. Menezes AH, VanGilder JC, Graf CJ, McDonnell DE. Craniocervical abnormalities. A comprehensive surgical approach. J Neurosurg 1980;53:444–455
6. Ahmed R, Traynelis VC, Menezes AH. Fusions at the craniovertebral junction. Childs Nerv Syst 2008;24:1209–1224
7. Dahdaleh NS, Dlouhy BJ, Menezes AH. Application of neuromuscular blockade and intraoperative 3D imaging in the reduction of basilar invagination. J Neurosurg Pediatr 2012;9:119–124
8. Dahdaleh NS, Dlouhy BJ, Menezes AH. One-step fixation of atlantoaxial rotatory subluxation: technical note and report of three cases. World Neurosurg 2013;80:e391–e395
9. Jian FZ, Chen Z, Wrede KH, Samii M, Ling F. Direct posterior reduction and fixation for the treatment of basilar invagination with atlantoaxial dislocation. Neurosurgery 2010;66:678–687, discussion 687
10. Hsu W, Zaidi HA, Suk I, Gokaslan ZL, Wolinsky JP. A new technique for intraoperative reduction of occipitocervical instability. Neurosurgery 2010;66(6, Suppl Operative):319–323, discussion 323–324
11. Menezes AH. Craniocervical fusions in children. J Neurosurg Pediatr 2012;9:573–585
12. Wolinsky JP, Sciubba DM, Suk I, Gokaslan ZL. Endoscopic image-guided odontoidectomy for decompression of basilar invagination via a standard anterior cervical approach. Technical note. J Neurosurg Spine 2007;6:184–191
13. Arbit E, Patterson RH Jr. Combined transoral and median labiomandibular glossotomy approach to the upper cervical spine. Neurosurgery 1981;8:672–674
14. Brookes JT, Smith RJ, Menezes AH, Smith MC. Median labiomandibular glossotomy approach to the craniocervical region. Childs Nerv Syst 2008;24:1195–1201
15. Smoker WR, Khanna G. Imaging the craniocervical junction. Childs Nerv Syst 2008;24:1123–1145
16. Ahmed R, Traynelis VC, Menezes AH. Fusions at the craniovertebral junction. Child's Nerv Syst 2008;24:1209–1224

7 Extended Transoral Approaches

Brian J. Dlouhy, Raheel Ahmed, and Arnold H. Menezes

The most direct approach to the ventral craniovertebral junction (CVJ) (lower clivus, atlas, and axis) is via the mouth and posterior pharynx.[1–3] Therefore, transoral approaches are ideal ventral approaches for decompression of irreducible ventral bony abnormalities as well as extradural bony and soft tissue masses of the CVJ causing compression of the cervicomedullary junction. The transoral approaches are categorized as standard and extended, and each variation provides a different degree of exposure.[2,4] The standard transoral approaches include the transoral-transpharyngeal approach and the transoral-transpalatopharyngeal approach.[2] The corridor of exposure provided by the standard approaches is generally limited by the extent to which patients can open their mouth. The location of the hard palate relative to the craniovertebral junction limits superior exposure, whereas the mandible and base of the tongue limit the inferior exposure. In most cases, exposure can be obtained from the inferior third of the clivus to the C2–3 interspace.[5]

Combining the standard transoral approach with previously described techniques of craniofacial osteotomies that open the maxilla and divide the hard palate or split the mandible and divide the tongue enhance access superiorly to the upper aspect of the clivus and inferiorly to the C4–5 interspace.[6,7] The transmandibular approaches specifically include variations of the median labiomandibular approach, which consists of a mandibulotomy (division of the mandible) with or without a glossotomy (division of tongue).[6] The transmaxillary approaches include the Le Fort I osteotomy with down-fracture of the maxilla and the Le Fort I osteotomy with palatal split.[8] The purpose of these extended technical variations is to extend the standard transoral approach and the empty anatomic spaces of the mouth and pharynx for greater rostral and caudal exposure of the CVJ.[8]

Median Labiomandibular Approach with or without Glossotomy

Indications

A combined transoral-transpalatopharyngeal approach with a median mandibulotomy (median labiomandibular approach) provides increased caudal exposure to the C3–4 interspace and maintains the superior exposure to the inferior third of the clivus.[6] Dividing the tongue in the midline further increases the caudal exposure to the C4–5 interspace (median labiomandibular glossotomy approach). Indications to use the median labiomandibular approach to augment exposure of the craniocervical junction and the upper cervical vertebrae include an inter-incisor opening distance of less than 2.5 cm and when access to C3–C5 is required. In children as well as adults, adequate access to the craniocervical junction and upper cervical vertebra can usually be achieved with a transoral–transpalatopharyngeal route. In some children, however, young age or small size precludes adequate exposure with a soft palatal split alone. Therefore, additional exposure can be gained with the median labiomandibular glossotomy approach.

Surgical Technique

The patient, either child or adult, is brought to the operating room with a cervical collar in place as a precaution during intubation, maneuvers, and positioning. All adults and children 10 to 18 years of age undergo awake fiberoptic oral endotracheal intubation. In children younger than 10 years of age or in an older child who cannot tolerate the procedure, general anesthesia is utilized and fiberoptic intubation is performed through the mask.

The patient is positioned supine on the operating table. Depending on the pathology, a crown halo may be applied for traction and the patient placed in traction at the beginning of the procedure. Then a tracheotomy is performed, using a modified oral Ring–Adair–Elwyn endotracheal tube trimmed just beyond the curvature of the tube to provide adequate intubation of the trachea when the tube is sutured flush to the chest wall. At the conclusion of the procedure, the tube is replaced with an age-appropriate tracheostomy tube. The patient's face, neck, and anterior chest are prepared and draped in a sterile fashion. If a costal cartilage graft is to be harvested, this portion of the procedure is performed using a separate operative field and separate instruments.

The skin incision is made full thickness in the midline at the lip and sublabial crease, utilizing a notch to aid relocation at the vermillion border, and the incision is carried around the mental protuberance, in a line of relaxed skin tension, and over the lower border of the mandible and back to the midline; it extends inferiorly to the level of the hyoid. To expose the mandible, the labial sulcal incision must deviate from the midline toward the osteotomy site; the incision continues in the midline on the lingual surface at the alveolar ridge. After the stair-step osteotomy is marked, rigid fixation plates are molded to the midline mandible inferiorly and superiorly and secured in place. They are then removed and preserved for reconstruction during closure. This step preserves occlusal relationships postoperatively. Following the mandibular osteotomy, the soft tissue dissection within the floor of the mouth is continued in the midline between the submandibular ducts and carried into the intrinsic tongue musculature. Special care is taken to preserve the submandibular ducts bilaterally. Dissection of the midline tongue is then carried posteriorly along the median raphe to expose the lingual surface of the epiglottis to the level of the hyoid. Additional oropharyngeal exposure can be achieved with a tonsillectomy. If further rostral exposure of the clivus is required, a midline split of the soft palate to one side of uvula can be performed. Additionally, removal of a portion of the posterior hard palate can be removed as well for even greater rostral exposure of the clivus. At this point the mandible can be widely separated. Fluoroscopy is used to confirm the cervical level inferiorly.

An ultra-sharp angled monopolar cautery (Stryker Colorado Needle, Stryker Inc, Kalamazoo, MI) is used to incise the posterior pharyngeal wall longitudinally in the midline over the inferior clivus, C1 arch, and C2 vertebral body, and inferiorly to the inferior aspect of the pathology. The mucosa is incised, and dissection with monopolar cautery proceeds through the midline raphe between the pharyngeal muscles and the anterior longitudinal ligament to bone. The longus colli and longus capitis muscles are detached from their medial origin on the ventral surface of the cervical vertebrae and mobilized laterally in a subperiosteal fashion using bipolar electrocautery and blunt dissection. These muscles can be held in place with stay sutures. The midline is marked by the tubercle of the anterior arch of C1 and should be identified for orientation. A costal cartilage graft can be placed after bony decompression if needed for anterior vertebral body reconstruction. Meticulous closure is performed using the longus colli muscles, pharyngeal musculature, and mucosa. Layered closures of the tongue and soft palate are followed by mandibular reconstruction using the prefashioned rigid fixation plate and tension band. When closing the floor of mouth, care must be taken to cover the osteotomy site intraorally. Layered closure of the anterior neck soft tissue and skin is performed with careful reapproximation of the vermilion–cutaneous junction. A nasogastric feeding tube is placed beyond the posterior pharyngeal incision under direct visualization and secured at the nose. After removal of traction, cervical spine precautions are maintained with placement of a cervical collar through which the tracheostomy tube is positioned.

Le Fort I Osteotomy with Down-Fracture of the Maxilla

Indications

The Le Fort I maxillotomy approach is indicated for extensive lesions that are too wide and too inferior for an endoscopic endonasal approach and too rostral for a standard transoral approach.[9] The clivus becomes accessible from the middle ethmoid sinuses to the foramen magnum and the anterior arch of the atlas of the CVJ. The major limitation of this approach is the inability to proceed lower than the plane of the hard palate. An endoscopic endonasal approach can provide similar access above the hard palate without the morbidity of this approach. However, the Le Fort I osteotomy with down-fracture has advantages over the endoscopic endonasal approach in that it provides wider exposure as well as more inferior viewing past the plane of the hard palate. With advancements in the endoscopic endonasal approach, the use of a Le Fort osteotomy is becoming increasingly rare.

Surgical Technique

The patient, either child or adult, is brought to the operating room with a cervical collar in place as a precaution during intubation, maneuvers, and positioning. All adults and children 10 to 18 years of age undergo awake fiberoptic oral endotracheal intubation.

A sublabial incision is made above the mucogingival reflection along the upper alveolar margin extending from one maxillary tuberosity to the other. The gingival mucosa is elevated subperiosteally over the maxilla to expose the anterior maxilla up to the level of the infraorbital nerves. Once the piriform aperture is identified, the nasal mucosa is elevated from the nasal floor and nasal septum up to the level of the inferior nasal turbinates. Titanium plates and screws are secured over both sides of the intended Le Fort I osteotomy line prior to division to ensure an exact fit when the maxilla is returned to its anatomic position at the time of closure and reduce the risk of malocclusion. They are then removed and preserved for reconstruction during closure. The maxilla is then divided horizontally with a reciprocating or oscillating saw, staying above the roots of the teeth to avoid dental injury (bilateral Le Fort I osteotomies). The nasal septum and the lateral nasal walls are divided with osteotomes, and the pterygoid plates are separated from the maxilla by means of a curved osteotome. The hard palate is down-fractured and mobilized inferiorly into the oral cavity. A Dingman retractor is inserted to keep the maxilla displaced downward. The remainder of the operation is similar to a standard transoral approach as described previously. At the time of closure, maxillary reconstruction is performed using the prefashioned rigid titanium fixation plates. The sublabial gingival mucosa is reapproximated with interrupted absorbable sutures.

Le Fort I Osteotomy with Palatal Split

Indications

The major limitation of the Le Fort I osteotomy with down-fracture is that the inferior displacement of the hard palate obstructs caudal access to C1–2. As mentioned above, the Le Fort I osteotomy with down-fracture is not really an extended transoral approach, as the extension from the mouth is not used to gain exposure. However, the Le Fort I osteotomy with palatal split is truly an extended approach.[10] A horizontal osteotomy is performed along with a midline split of the hard and soft palate.[10,11] This divides the maxilla in the midline, allowing it to be mobilized laterally, extending the standard transoral-transpalatopharyngeal approach. Other surgeons have described this as the transmaxillary palatal split approach or the extended "open-door" maxillotomy.[12] It is essentially a Le Fort I osteotomy, and instead of down-fracturing the maxilla, it is divided in the midline and lateralized. This approach provides rostral exposure of the sphenoid sinus and superior and middle clivus while maintaining the inferior exposure provided by the standard transoral approaches to the C2–3 interspace. The lateral limits of this exposure are the cavernous carotid arteries, the occipital condyles, and the lateral masses of the C1–C2 complex. The major disadvantages of this approach are extended operating time and the complexity of reconstruction and wound closure.

Surgical Technique

A Le Fort I osteotomy is initially performed as described above. The mucosa is incised over the hard palate slightly off the midline, continuing posteriorly through the soft palate, staying on one side of the uvula. Using the same oscillating or reciprocating saw used to the divide the maxilla in the Le Fort I osteotomy, the hard palate is divided in the midline starting between the front incisors. The osteotomy traverses around the anterior nasal spine and continues posteriorly in the sagittal plane. Each hemimaxilla is rotated outward and retracted laterally. The remainder of the operation is similar to a standard transoral approach as described previously. At the time of closure, each hemimaxilla is restored to its anatomic location and fastened with prefashioned rigid titanium fixation plates and screws. The posterior pharyngeal wall and soft palate and mucosa over the hard palate is meticulously reapproximated as described in Chapter 8.

Illustrative Case

A transoral approach with median labiomandibular glossotomy (MLG) for rare congenital CVJ bone abnormality was used in a 4-year-old boy with severe spondyloepiphyseal dysplasia who had severe ventral cervicomedullary compression secondary to retroflexion of the odontoid process and upper cervical bone abnormalities at C2 with cervical kyphosis and craniocervical instability (**Figs. 7.1, 7.2, 7.3, 7.4, 7.5**). The standard transoral-transpalatopharyngeal approach would not provide sufficient exposure due to inadequate caudal exposure and to the patient's young age and small size. Therefore, a transoral approach with median labiomandibular glossotomy and rib graft for C2–3 anterior cervical fusion was performed. Occipital cervical fusion was performed at a later date.

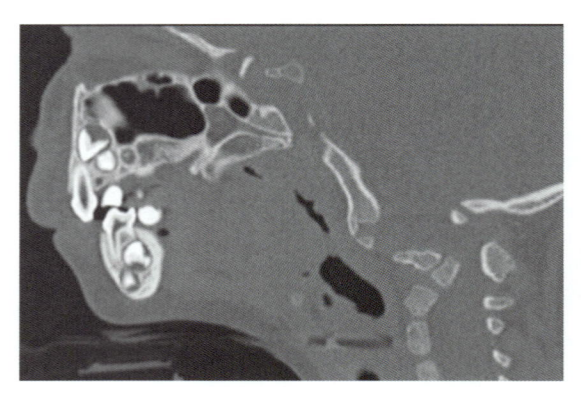

Fig. 7.1 Illustrative case, part 1. Preoperative radiographs demonstrating extensive craniovertebral junction (CVJ) pathology from the clivus to C4 necessitating an extended transoral approach. Lateral CVJ spine radiograph demonstrating craniocervical instability with occiput-C1 subluxation on C2 and abnormal bone formation of C2 with retroflexed odontoid and severe compression of the cervical spine cord.

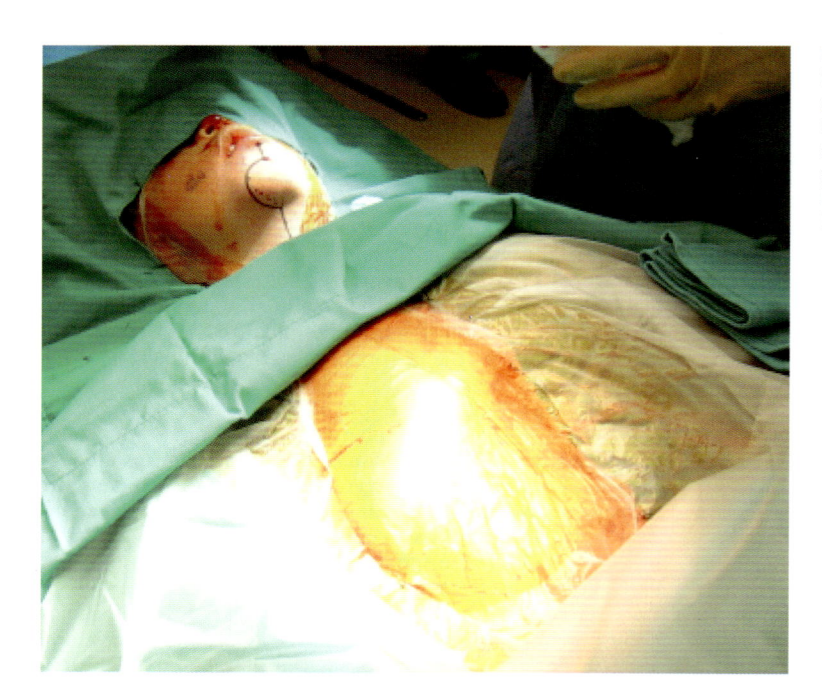

Fig. 7.2 Illustrative case, part 2. Site and skin preparation for the transoral approach with median labiomandibular glossotomy (MLG) and rib graft. The skin incision is made full thickness in the midline at the lip and sublabial crease and is carried around the mental protuberance, in a line of relaxed skin tension, and over the lower border of the mandible, back to the midline; it extends inferiorly to the level of the hyoid.

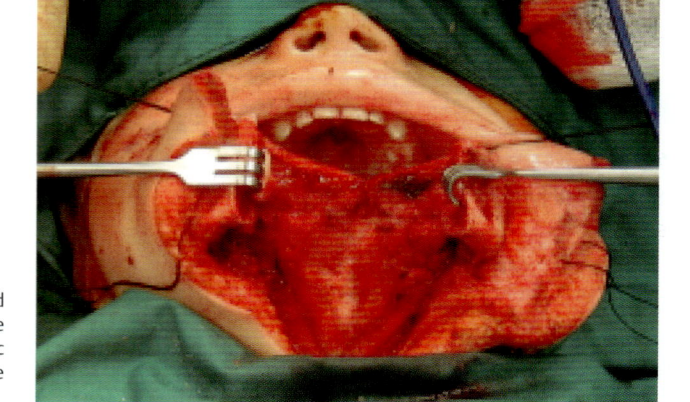

Fig. 7.3 Illustrative case, part 3. A mandibular osteotomy is performed and soft tissue dissection within the floor of the mouth is continued in the midline between the submandibular ducts and carried into the intrinsic tongue musculature to expose the lingual surface of the epiglottis to the level of the hyoid.

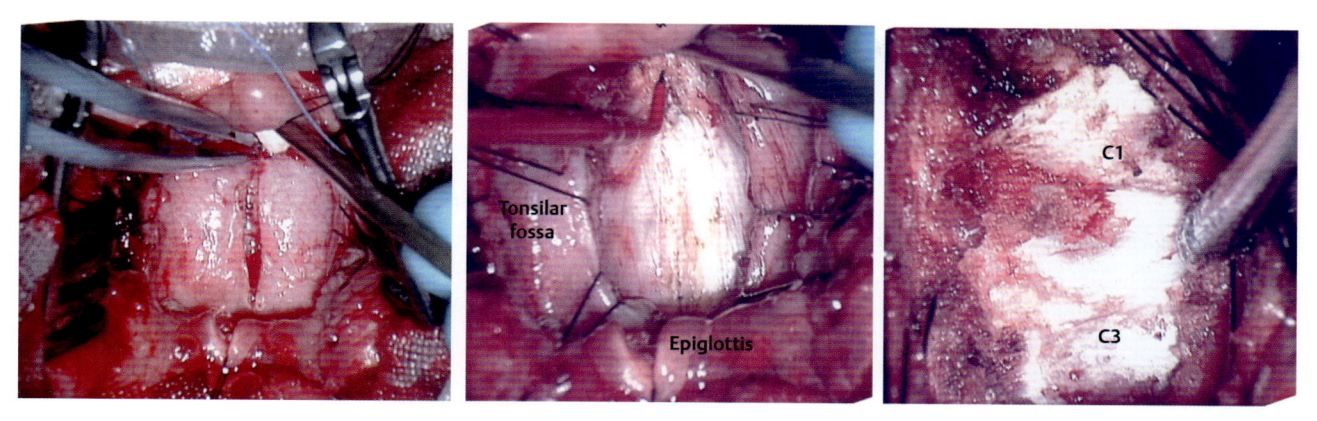

Fig. 7.4 Illustrative case, part 4. Posterior pharyngeal wall dissection. The posterior pharyngeal wall is divided in the midline and the C1–C3 anterior vertebral bodies are exposed.

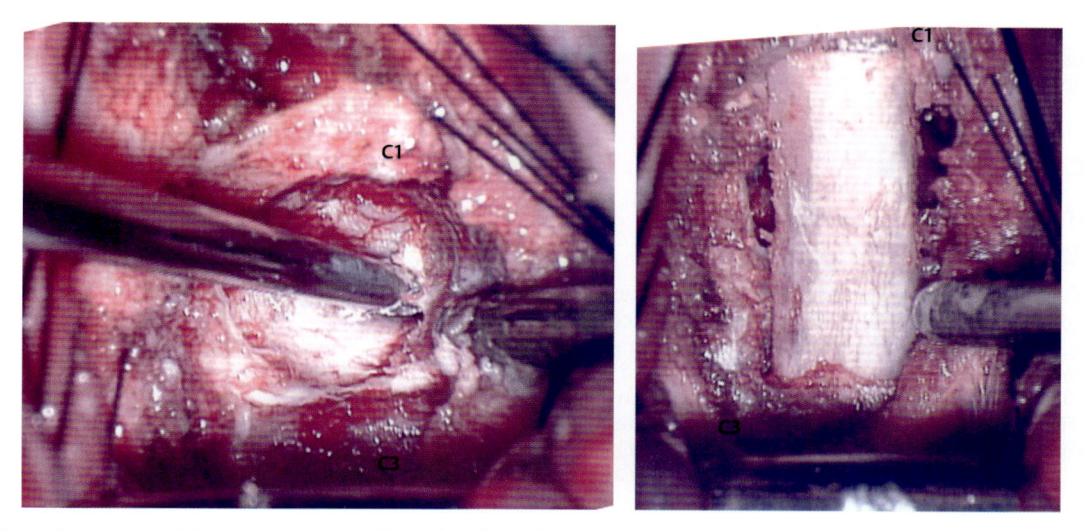

Fig. 7.5 Illustrative case, part 5. Bony reconstruction of CVJ. The odontoid process and body of the odontoid is removed, and harvested rib is used for interbody fusion.

References

1. Menezes AH, Graf CJ, Hibri N. Abnormalities of the cranio-vertebral junction with cervico-medullary compression. A rational approach to surgical treatment in children. Childs Brain 1980;7:15–30
2. Menezes AH, VanGilder JC. Transoral-transpharyngeal approach to the anterior craniocervical junction. Ten-year experience with 72 patients. J Neurosurg 1988;69:895–903
3. Menezes AH, VanGilder JC, Graf CJ, McDonnell DE. Craniocervical abnormalities. A comprehensive surgical approach. J Neurosurg 1980;53:444–455
4. Youssef AS, Sloan AE. Extended transoral approaches: surgical technique and analysis. Neurosurgery 2010;66(3, Suppl):126–134
5. Menezes AH. Surgical approaches: postoperative care and complications "transoral-transpalatopharyngeal approach to the craniocervical junction." Childs Nerv Syst 2008;24:1187–1193
6. Brookes JT, Smith RJ, Menezes AH, Smith MC. Median labiomandibular glossotomy approach to the craniocervical region. Childs Nerv Syst 2008; 24:1195–1201
7. Liu JK, Couldwell WT, Apfelbaum RI. Transoral approach and extended modifications for lesions of the ventral foramen magnum and craniovertebral junction. Skull Base 2008;18:151–166
8. Lawton MT, Beals SP, Joganic EF, Han PP, Spetzler RF. The transfacial approaches to midline skull base lesions: a classification scheme. Operative Techniques in Neurosurgery 1999;2:201–217
9. Drommer RB. The history of the "Le Fort I osteotomy." J Maxillofac Surg 1986;14:119–122
10. Sandor GK, Charles DA, Lawson VG, Tator CH. Trans oral approach to the nasopharynx and clivus using the Le Fort I osteotomy with midpalatal split. Int J Oral Maxillofac Surg 1990;19:352–355
11. Williams WG, Lo LJ, Chen YR. The Le Fort I-palatal split approach for skull base tumors: efficacy, complications, and outcome. Plast Reconstr Surg 1998;102:2310–2319
12. James D, Crockard HA. Surgical access to the base of skull and upper cervical spine by extended maxillotomy. Neurosurgery 1991;29:411–416

8 Transoral Closure

Brian J. Dlouhy, Raheel Ahmed, and Arnold H. Menezes

A proper closure after a transoral-transpalatopharyngeal approach is essential to minimizing complications (see Video 8.1).[1,2] Proper closure reestablishes a barrier between the posterior pharyngeal space created by the approach and bony resection and the oropharyngeal space, eliminating dead space, and therefore preventing abscess and hematoma formation.[1] Proper closure also enables proper function of the soft palate and prevention of velopalatine incompetence.[1]

Surgical Procedure

Transoral Transpalatopharyngeal Closure

After satisfactory decompression at the craniocervical junction, aerobic and anaerobic cultures are obtained, and bacitracin powder is placed in the wound. FloSeal, Surgicel (Johnson & Johnson, New Brunswick, NJ), and Avitene may be placed in the resection cavity to help eliminate dead space and help with hemostasis (**Fig. 8.1**). The longus colli and longus capitis muscles are approximated using interrupted 3-0 Vicryl sutures (**Fig. 8.2**) (Video 8.1). Next, the constrictor muscles of the pharynx are approximated, along with the mucosa of the posterior pharyngeal wall in a separate layer (**Fig. 8.3**). The throat pack is removed. A nasogastric tube is placed under direct visualization for postoperative nutritional care (**Fig. 8.4**). The anesthesiologist auscultates over the abdomen while air is insufflated to ensure proper position of the tube. The tubing is secured to the midline columella using 2-0 Nurolon (**Fig. 8.4**).

The soft palate is closed in two layers. The nasal part of the palate is approximated with interrupted inverted sutures of 3-0 Vicryl. The oral mucosa together with the muscular layer is approximated with interrupted horizontal mattress sutures of 3-0 Vicryl (**Fig. 8.5**). The mouth retractor is removed, the oral mucosa is smeared with hydrophilic ointment with hydrocortisone (1%), and the tongue is massaged. Dorsal occipitocervical fusion combined with posterior fossa decompression is usually mandated and performed under the same anesthetic. The patient remains orotracheally intubated postoperatively.

Postoperative Care

Nasogastric tube feedings are maintained for the first 5 days. A clear liquid diet is then started. Over several days, it is advanced to a full liquid diet and, subsequently, to a soft diet. Postoperatively, the endotracheal intubation is maintained until swelling of the oral tissues, including the tongue, has receded. The endotracheal tube is left in place 3 to 4 days in most patients. Nystatin and Peridex are maintained in the oral cavity for 2 weeks postoperatively. In the event that the dura is opened, broad-spectrum intravenous antibiotics and spinal drainage are maintained

8 Transoral Closure 53

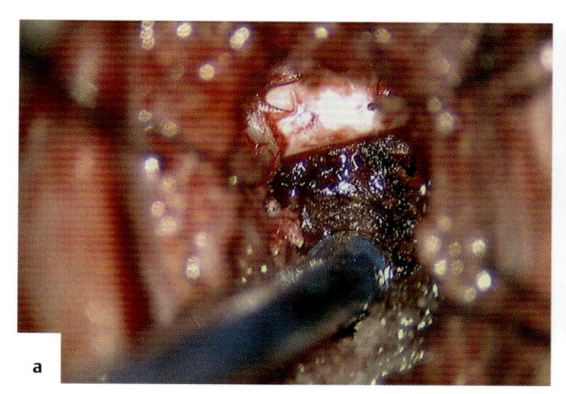

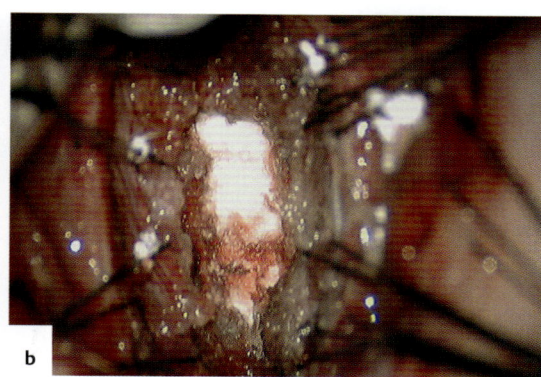

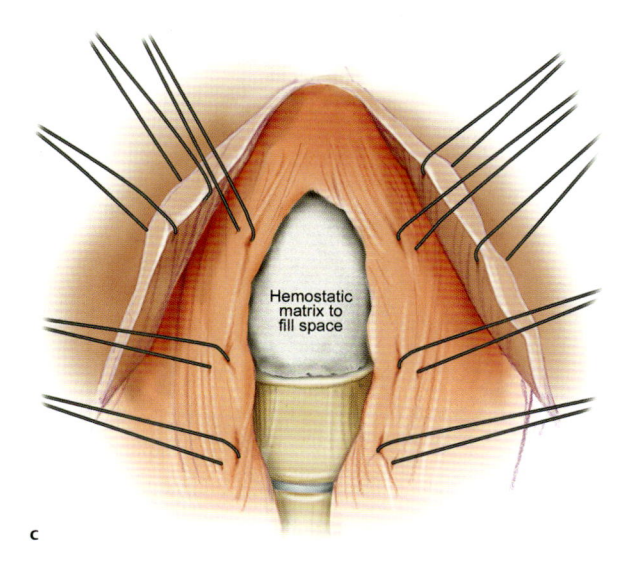

Fig. 8.1 Postresection cavity: obtaining hemostasis and obliterating dead space. **(a)** Postresection cavity after bony removal. **(b,c)** Use of FloSeal, Surgicel, and Avitene along with bacitracin powder to obtain hemostasis and eliminate dead space.

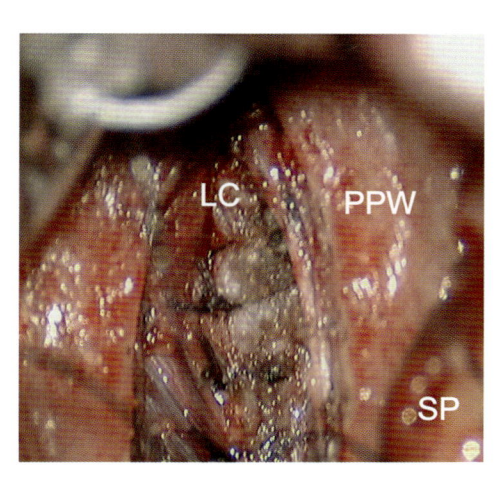

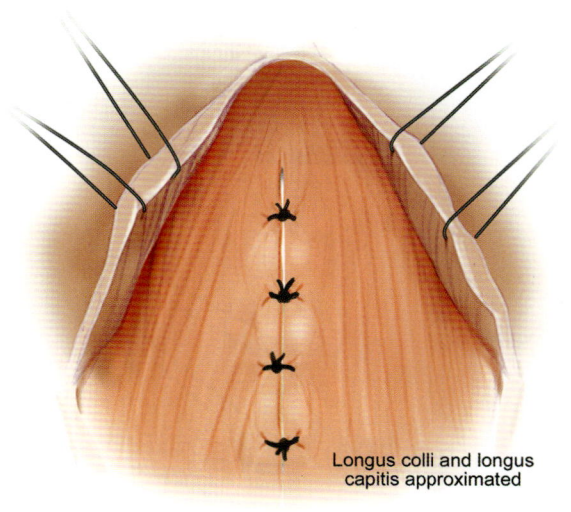

Fig. 8.2 Closure of longus colli and longus capitis muscles. Vicryl sutures are used to reapproximate the longus colli and longus capitis (LC) muscles along the anterior aspect of the upper cervical spine. PPW, posterior pharyngeal wall; SP, soft palate.

54 I Occipital-Cervical Junction

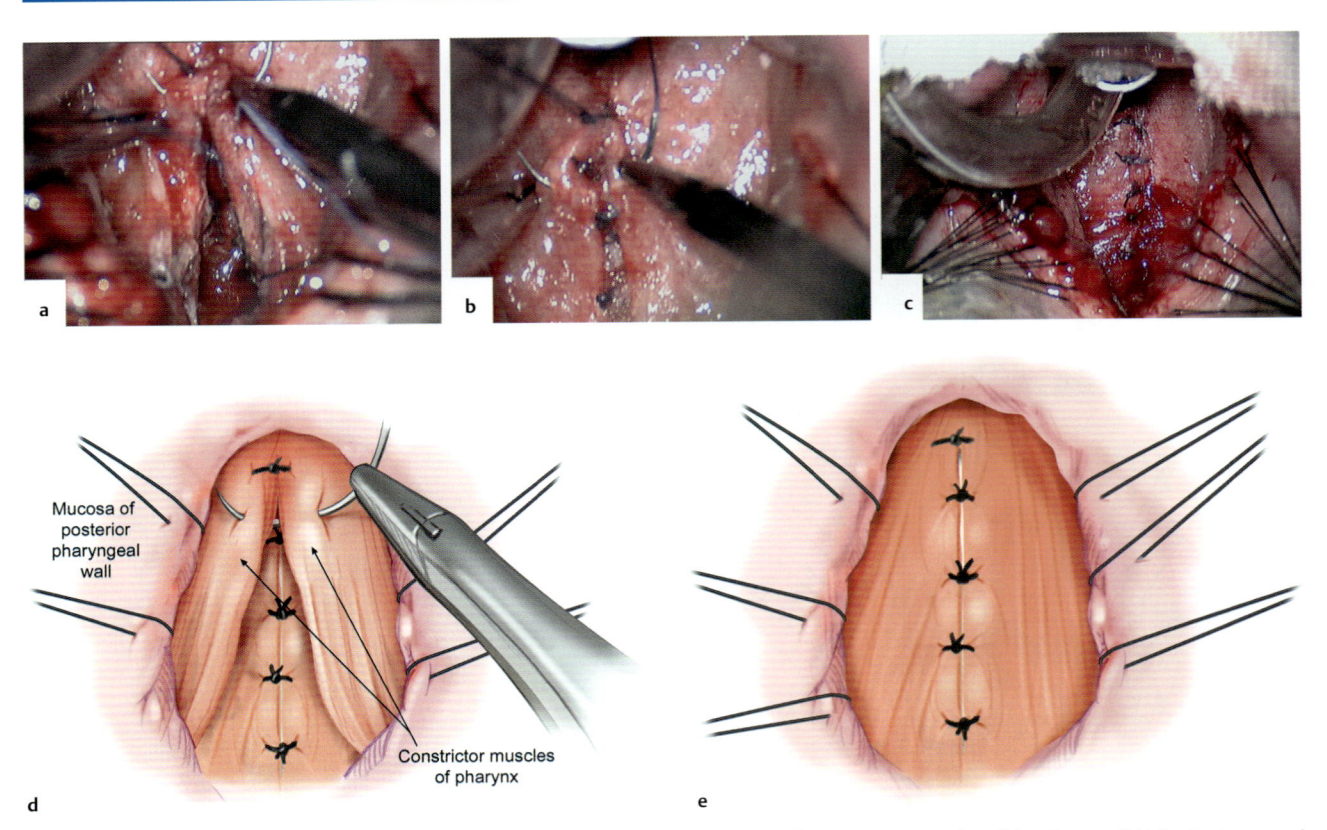

Fig. 8.3 Closure of the posterior pharyngeal wall. **(a)** Vicryl sutures used to reapproximate the constrictor muscles of the pharynx. **(b)** Vicryl sutures used to reapproximate the mucosa of the posterior pharyngeal wall. **(c)** Final closure of the posterior pharyngeal wall. **(d,e)** Illustrative views.

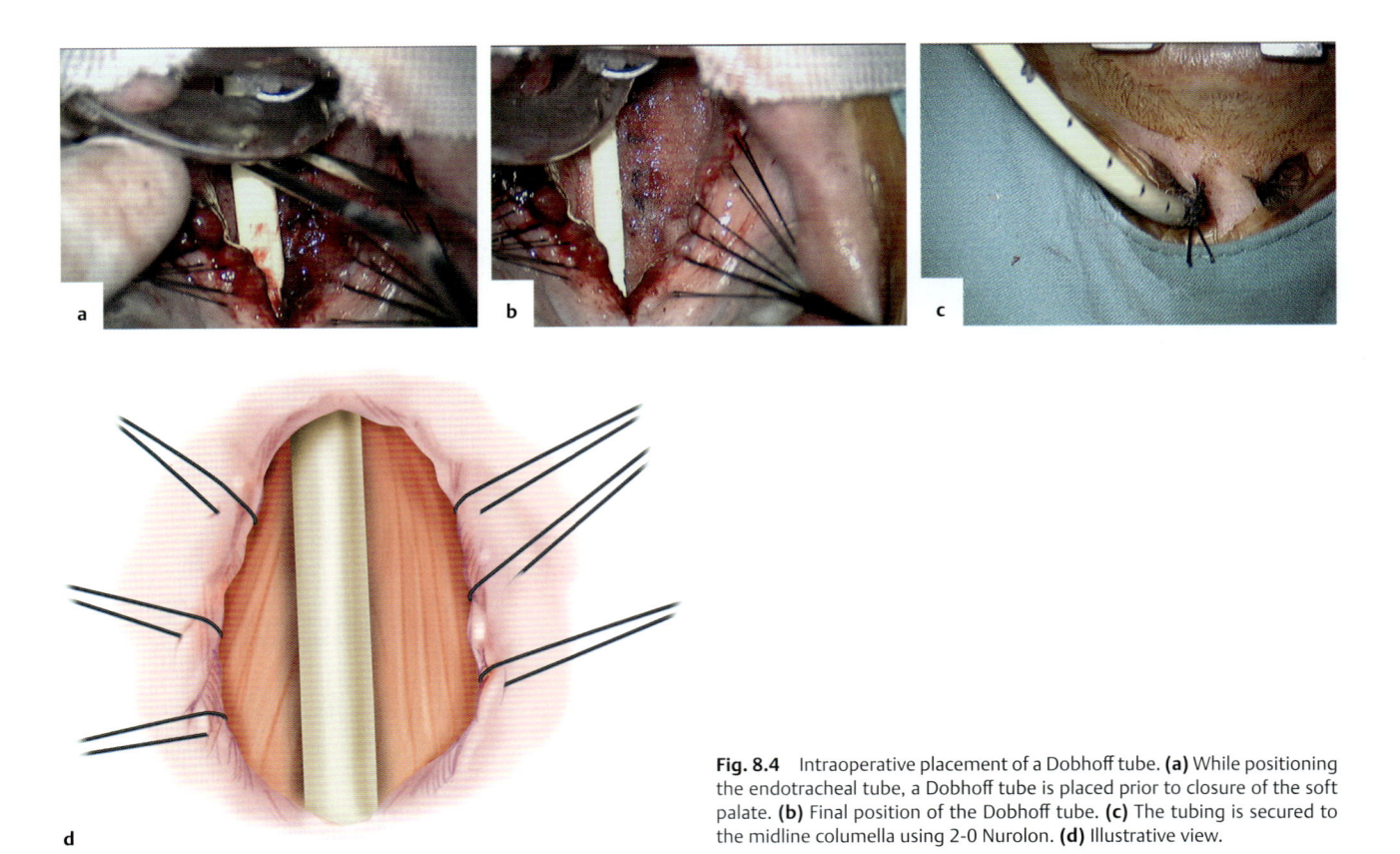

Fig. 8.4 Intraoperative placement of a Dobhoff tube. **(a)** While positioning the endotracheal tube, a Dobhoff tube is placed prior to closure of the soft palate. **(b)** Final position of the Dobhoff tube. **(c)** The tubing is secured to the midline columella using 2-0 Nurolon. **(d)** Illustrative view.

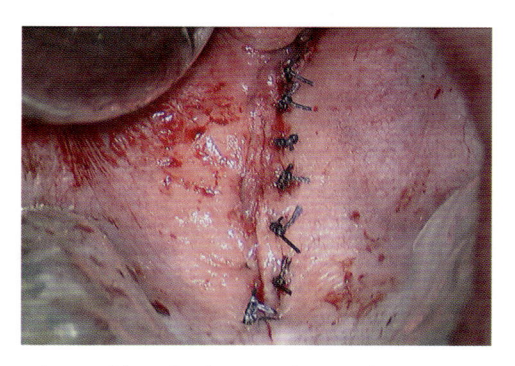

Fig. 8.5 Closure of the soft palate using horizontal mattress sutures.

for 10 days after the operation. Previously, adults and children who had undergone a dorsal fixation after the anterior procedure were ambulated in a halo vest. Currently, this is done with a custom-fitted occipitocervical Minerva-type brace or an Aspen-Minerva brace.

References

1. Menezes AH. Surgical approaches: postoperative care and complications "transoral-transpalatopharyngeal approach to the craniocervical junction." Childs Nerv Syst 2008;24:1187–1193
2. Menezes AH, VanGilder JC. Transoral-transpharyngeal approach to the anterior craniocervical junction. Ten-year experience with 72 patients. J Neurosurg 1988;69:895–903

9 Minimally Invasive Endoscopic Approaches to the Upper Cervical Spine

Mohamad Bydon, Mohamed Macki, Ali Ozturk, and Jean-Paul Wolinsky

Endoscopic surgery has become a leading technique in minimally invasive surgery. In the field of neurosurgery, in particular, accessing deep-seated brain lesions was the primary impetus for the development of the endoscopic technique.[1] The approach was hailed for its accuracy and favorable results. The decreased surgical trauma has led to lower complication rates, shorter hospital stays, and fewer emotional consequences for the patient.[2] Over the past decade, the endoscope has also revolutionized the surgical management of anterior upper cervical pathologies. Indeed, since Frempong-Boadu[3] et al first described the endoscopic transoral technique in 2002, minimally anterior approaches to the upper cervical spine via the endoscope have changed patient outcomes and the prospects for spine surgery.[4] Today, minimally invasive endoscopic procedures have afforded spine surgeons unique entry points and creative techniques to access even the most hard-to-reach areas of the upper cervical spine.

This chapter discusses three minimally invasive endoscopic techniques for the surgical management of upper cervical spine pathologies:

1. Endoscopic transoral approach[3]
2. Endoscopic endonasal approach[5]
3. Endoscopic transcervical approach[6]

Patient Selection

Patient selection depends on the type of disease, the location of the pathology, and the extensions of the lesion. Clival, midline, or paramedian lesions may be accessed with the endoscopic endonasal approach. Patients with significant basilar impression or a high-rising odontoid may also be managed with the endonasal operation. However, caudal extension may make the endonasal exposure unnecessary, as a downward trajectory may be limited by the nasal bone and the cartilaginous soft tissue superiorly. Inferiorly, this approach may reach 1 cm above the base of the C2 vertebral body.[7]

Most pathologies at the craniocervical junction can be accessed with the endoscopic transoral and transcervical approaches, which enable a surgical trajectory. In particular, the transoral approach is well suited for lesions at the base of the clivus, in the odontoid process, or within 2 cm of the midline of the anterior C1 ring or the upper cervical vertebrae. Of note, patients with significant basilar impression may require resection of the anterior arch of C1 with the transoral technique, whereas a more rostral reach with the transoral technique may preclude C1 manipulation for an odontoidectomy. Protecting the C1 arch not only maintains structural stability but also protects medially coursing carotid arteries at the atlas level.

The endoscopic transcervical approach provides wide axial exposure from the distal clivus through the entire cervical spine.[7] With the exception of cranial applications and true basilar invagination (osteogenesis imperfecta), the transcervical operation precludes a resection of the C1 ventral arch for upper cervical lesions. The approach also avoids a surgical incision through the nasopharyngeal and oral mucosa, lowering the risks associated with surgical-site infection.

Preoperative Imaging

Computed tomography (CT) with or without angiography should be done preoperatively, so that it can be used for frameless stereotactic image guidance during the operation.[5] The image guidance is registered with a fiducial array adjusted to less than 2 mm error. Maximal accuracy should be focused on the cervicomedullary junction. Reports have also described the role of the intraoperative Iso-C system with preoperative fluoroscopy used for frameless stereotactic image guidance.[6,8] The imaging modality can be used to evaluate the anterior decompression following bony resection.

Endoscopic Transoral Approach

With the advent of specialized intraoperative instruments, the transoral approach with direct access to the upper cervical spine was popularized by Fang and Ong[9] in 1962. In the ensuing decades, with advances in intraoperative fluoroscopy, endotracheal tubes, and high-speed drills, the transoral technique was modified to decrease the risk of cerebrospinal fluid (CSF) fistula, contamination with oropharyngeal flora, and meningitis.[10,11] In 1985, Crockard[12] refined the transoral operation so that it became minimally invasive surgery with the application of the microscope (details provided in Chapter 6). Briefly, the patient undergoes fiberoptic orotracheal intubation and is placed in the supine position, with the head fixed in mild extension. The technique utilizes a specialized transoral system with a self-retaining mouth retractor, tongue depressor, and retractors for the soft palate and endotracheal tube. The oral cavity is sterilized and draped in a standard fashion. Surgical instruments with extended arms facilitate access to the posterior oral cavity. A microscope is brought into the surgical field for magnification and illumination. A 2- to 3-cm vertical incision is made on the posterior aspect of the pharyngeal mucosa. The underlying muscles, including the longus colli and capitis, are swung laterally with a pharyngeal retractor. The underlying pathology is then addressed. The minimally invasive microscopic transoral approach was later modified with endoscopic applications. In 2002, Frempong-Boadu et al[3] described the endoscopic transoral technique, which provides superior visualization and illumination in the operative field.

Advantages and Disadvantages

The minimally invasive endoscopic transoral technique provides the same access as the standard transoral approach for anterior spinal lesions confined by the pterygoid plates superiorly and the eustachian tubes, hypoglossal canals, and the vertebral and carotid arteries laterally.[7] Of the anterior operations indicated for upper cervical pathologies, the endoscopic transoral exposure provides an anatomic orientation that is well known to most surgeons. In addition, the endoscope confers several benefits over other transoral approaches. In perhaps the greatest advantage, the endoscope includes an angled lens that provides superior visualization through the restricted transoral corridors without extended incisions into the soft palate.[2] Moreover, the endoscope brings the light source and the objective of the visual apparatus deep into the surgical field. This approximation may improve visualization into the operative corridors in comparison to the microscope.[13] However, with expansile or diffusely infiltrating pathologies, access to the lesion may require a transmandibular approach, resection of the hard palate, and/or Le Fort osteotomies.[2,6] These extensile techniques would increase operative time and the rates of surgical-site infection, perioperative morbidity, and postoperative disability.

Indications

As with the standard (microscopic) transoral approach, the endoscopic transoral technique is similarly indicated for pathologies within the anterior bony landmarks at the craniocervical junction, including the clivus, the anterior arch of the atlas, the odontoid process, and the upper cervical vertebrae. Thus, the approach enables exploration of extradural lesions causing compression or instability anywhere from the level of the interpeduncular fossa to the level of the spinomedullary junction.[13] The technique has been described in patients with retrodental panni, dens subluxation, degenerative stenosis of the foramen magnum, and atlantoaxial tumors.

Contraindications

Although the minimally invasive transoral technique provides excellent exposure from the lower third of the clivus to the inferior aspect of C2, endoscopy is technically restricted to anterior pathologies. Lesions that extend beyond 2 cm from the midline or rostral to the lower clivus are difficult to access. The operation should be avoided in patients with temporomandibular joint pathology, oropharyngeal infections, or fixed flexion deformities of the cervical spine.[7] Furthermore, medially located carotid arteries ("kissing" carotids) are a relative contraindication. Although the risk of velopharyngeal incompetence is lower than with the standard microscopic technique, postoperative dysphagia and dysphonia should be distinguished from cranial nerve injury. Intradural pathologies are a relative contraindication for both the traditional transoral approach using the microscope and the transoral approach using the endoscope.

Surgical Procedure

The endoscopic transoral operation follows the technique described by Frempong-Boadu et al.[3] The patient is placed in the supine position on the operating table. A malleable endotracheal tube is inserted via awake, fiberoptic oral intubation. The head is placed in skull traction with a Mayfield three-point apparatus, and the neck is mildly extended with a shoulder roll. General anesthesia is initiated, and gauze is placed in the throat to prevent the digestion of surgical debris. Somatosensory evoked responses are established and monitored throughout the procedure. The oropharyngeal compartment is cleansed and draped. The mouth is opened a moderate amount with a Dingman self-retaining retractor with a tongue blade and soft palate retractor. The tongue blade is temporarily released every half hour to prevent congestion of the venous and lymphatic flow. Lidocaine and epinephrine are injected into the posterior pharyngeal wall. A right-angled endoscope is then placed into the oral cavity for illumination and visualization. Guided with lateral fluoroscopy, a midline incision is made along the posterior pharyngeal wall from the approximation of the base of the clivus to the superior aspect of C3. The retropharyngeal and prevertebral tissues and muscles, including the longus colli and longus capitis, are dissected off the underlying bone. The exposure should not extend beyond 15 mm laterally to protect the eustachian tubes, hypoglossal nerves, and carotid arteries. Placement of self-retaining retractors ~ 15 mm from the midline provides adequate exposure of the lower clivus and atlantoaxial levels. The endoscope is then advanced through the incision. Under endoscopic assistance, the drill is used to remove the anterior arch (and possibly the inferior aspect of the clivus) to exposure the dens. The intended operation may now be performed. After the procedure is completed and hemostasis is achieved, the Valsalva maneuver is artificially induced to exclude any CSF leak. The pharyngeal wall is closed in two layers via a paraendoscopic technique.[13] The Dingman self-retaining retractors are removed, and a feeding tube is applied. The application of a synthetic corticosteroid cream on the tongue and surrounding oral cavity reduces pressure-induced swelling.

Endoscopic Endonasal Approach

The endoscopic transnasal approach provides access to the upper cervical spine via the nasal cavity. In 2002, Alfieri et al[14] discussed the anatomic feasibility in a cadaveric study. They adopted the endoscopic endonasal approach to the craniocervical junction from the endoscopic endonasal skull-base surgeries.[15] With the advent of endoscopic technology, endonasal approaches to the pituitary and parasellar structures have rapidly expanded. In 2005, Kassam et al[5] described the first endoscopic endonasal approach to the craniocervical junction for a retrodental rheumatoid pannus.

Advantages and Disadvantages

Owing to the direct anatomic trajectory, the endoscopic endonasal approach provides direct exposure of the craniocervical junction. The endonasal endoscopic operation also obviates aggressive manipulation of the oropharyngeal cavity. Without tongue retraction and subsequent postsurgical glossal edema, the more rostral endonasal approach may enable rapid extubation and earlier mobilization. Postoperatively, the surgical incision site is less likely to become infected with food or saliva, in comparison to the endoscopic transoral approach. This allows for earlier oral feeding.

Consultation with an otolaryngologist may be necessary not only during the operation but also in the postoperative management, as nasal crusting and rhinorrhea may ensue.[7] Also, as the endoscope follows an upward trajectory through the nose, the inferiormost visualization of the endoscopic endonasal approach is limited by the superior migration of the nasal bone. Thus, caudal dissections may only reach up to ~ 1 cm above the base of the C2 vertebral body.[7]

Indications

The endoscopic endonasal approach is indicated for lesions medial to the paraclival carotid artery, pterygoid plate, and eustachian tube. Unlike the endoscopic transoral and transcervical techniques, this approach provides visualization of the entire rostrocaudal aspect of the clivus.[7] The endonasal operation particularly provides direct access to the foramen magnum and upper cervical spine. Similar to the endoscopic transoral technique, patients with retrodental panni, dens subluxation, degenerative stenosis of the foramen magnum, or atlantoaxial tumors have been treated with the endoscopic endonasal operation.[4] For suspicious lesions, some authors recommend preoperative imaging to identify intradural extensions, as intradural pathologies may be challenging to address via endoscopic techniques.[7]

Contraindications

The endoscopic endonasal approach alone is not recommended in patients with laterally situated lesions. Other lateral skull base approaches should be used in conjunction with the endonasal operation, such as the transpterygoid approach for extensions to the pterygopalatine fossa, Meckel's cave, or petrous apex,[16,17] as well as the transmaxillary approaches for extensions to the hypoglossal canal and medical occipital condyle.[18] The approach should be avoided in patients with medially located carotid arteries ("kissing" carotids). Finally, as with other minimally invasive endoscopic techniques, intradural pathologies are relatively contraindicated.

Surgical Procedure

The endoscopic endonasal operation follows the technique described by Kassam et al.[5] Fourth-generation cephalosporins are administered for preoperative prophylaxis. In the operating room, the patient is placed in the supine position. After endotracheal intubation, the patient's head is placed in the neutral position and fixed with Mayfield pins. Somatosensory evoked responses are established and monitored throughout the procedure. The nares are prepped in a standard sterile fashion. A 0-degree endoscope with an irrigation sheath in placed in the right nares and the surgical instruments in the left nares. Because of the limited surgical corridors within the nasal cavity, the endoscopic endonasal technique entails the following special considerations. First, a bilateral endonasal approach provides somewhat more space than the limited surgical window in which surgical resections are performed. Second, an interdisciplinary surgical team that includes an otolaryngologist specializing in sinus surgery and a neurosurgeon is appropriate. To that end, instead of an endoscopic holder, dynamic movement of the endoscopic between the two disciplines will help establish a three-dimensional orientation of the narrow operative window. This will also prevent loss of visualization due to the close contact of the endoscope with the mucosa. Third, a specialized long angled drill is necessary to traverse the long nasal passage, particularly in operations at the cervicomedullary junction. Similarly, a long angled attachment is placed on the ultrasonic aspirator. Fourth, bayoneted handheld instruments provide greater ease for the surgeon during the operation.

The procedure begins in the right nares with removal of the middle turbinate. Wide bilateral sphenoidotomies are performed through the right nares. Generous osteotomies are required for two reasons: (1) to identify the rostral anatomic landmarks, including the carotid canals, medial pterygoid plates, and the pterygoid canal and vidian nerve (nerve of the pterygoid canal); and (2) to take advantage of the deeper position of the endoscope, which enables identification of the boundaries within the fossa of Rosenmüller (pharyngeal recess): the nasopharyngeal mucosa posteriorly, the floor of the sphenoid rostrally, the soft palate caudally, and the eustachian tubes laterally. Next, the left middle turbinate is displaced laterally, but not resected. Less than 1 cm of the posterior aspect of the nasal septum is removed to facilitate bilateral access of the surgical instruments by moving the endoscope. An inverted U-shaped flap in the nasopharyngeal mucosa is created from the level of the sphenoidotomy rostrally to the soft palate caudally. The flap is reflected down to the soft palate to expose the sphenoid floor. A diamond bur is used to create an opening in the sphenoid floor. Using an electrocautery device, the paraspinous muscles are removed from their C1 attachment to expose the arch of C1. Image guidance is an important adjunct at this stage because the surgical plane must remain medial to the eustachian tubes, behind which the retropharyngeal carotid artery travels. The intended operation may now be performed. The trajectory of the endoscopic endonasal approach frequently requires resection of the distal clivus and anterior arch of C1 to gain access to the odontoid. In significant basilar impression, a large portion of the clivus may need to be resected to gain access to the intracranial odontoid. After the surgical indication has been addressed, the posterior nasopharyngeal incision is not reapproximated. Rather, the defect is covered with fibrin glue. The surgical site and surrounding nasal cavity is irrigated, and septal splints are inserted to prevent postoperative synechiae.

Endoscopic Transcervical Approach

Unlike the transoral and endonasal approaches through the contaminated naso-oropharyngeal mucosa, the endoscopic transcervical approach provides a unique surgical corridor through the neck (**Figs. 9.1 and 9.2**). Described by Wolinsky et al[6] in 2007, the technique provides a third option in treating ventral lesions of the upper cervical spine. The minimally invasive transcervical approach utilizes a tubular retractor with a beveled tip, designed to protect the surrounding neurovascular structures, the esophagus, and the trachea. When combined with an endoscope, the technique provides favorable visualization from the distal clivus through the entire cervical spine.[4] Thus, the endoscopic transcervical approach provides superior exposure relative to the other two minimally invasive alternatives, which are limited to the atlantoaxial vertebrae caudally. Moreover, with the exception of cranial applications and true basilar invagination (osteogenesis imperfecta), the transcervical operation precludes a resection of the C1 ventral arch for upper cervical lesions. Therefore, the anteriorly situated carotid arteries and accompanying sympathetic nerves have a decreased risk of injury. Lastly, because the retractor has a trajectory from an inferior insertion point, high-lying odontoid lesions do not require surgical manipulation of the clivus.

Advantages and Disadvantages

Perhaps the primary advantage of the transcervical approach over the transoral and endonasal alternatives is the avoidance of the contaminated nasopharyngeal and oral mucosa. Thus, the technique is thought to decrease the risk of surgical-site infections.[6,7] As the transcervical approach provides access through sterile corridors, the risk of CSF fistulas resulting in meningitis is decreased.[6,7] Skin incisions heal much better and faster than incisions in the moist and contaminated environment of the mu-

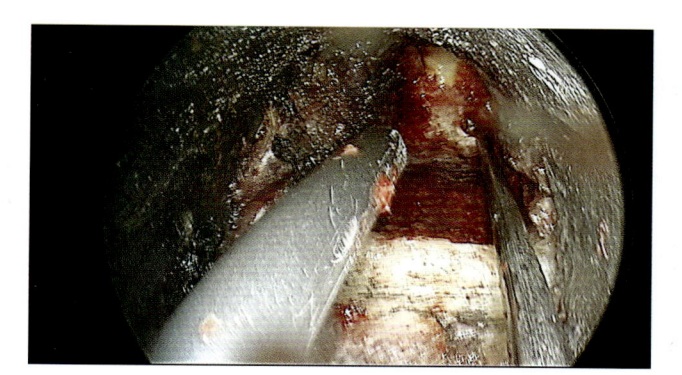

Fig. 9.1 (a) Endoscopic photo of the C1-C2 junction. (b) The endoscope allows ample illumination in the beveled-tip tubular retractor. (c) The setup of the endoscopic transcervical operation.

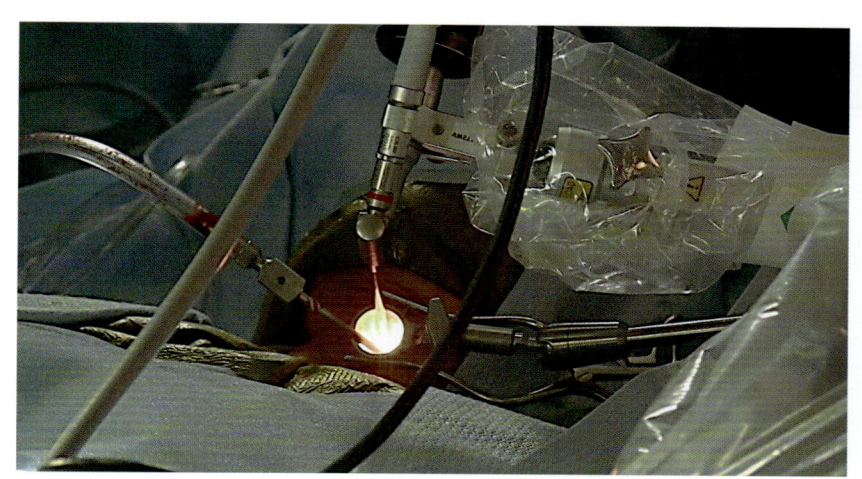

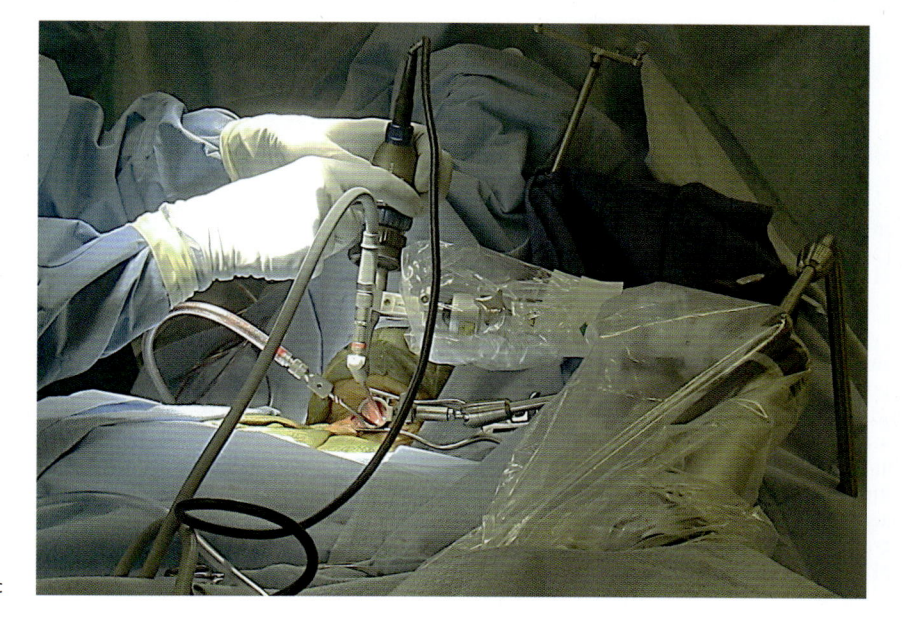

cosal cavity.[7] By bypassing the pharynx, the endoscopic transcervical operation also precludes the need for tracheostomy and postoperative enteral feeding. Patients subsequently experience decreased pain and require shorter hospital stays.[6]

A disadvantage of the minimally invasive endoscopic transcervical approach is the steep learning curve. Because the surgeon operates from an indirect surgical entry point in the transcervical technique, familiarity with the three-dimensional anatomic relationships and landmarks of the upper cervical spine is essential.[7]

Indications

The endoscopic transcervical approach is indicated for lesions located from the lower clivus through the foramen magnum to the C7 level. The approach is appropriate for localized abnormalities,

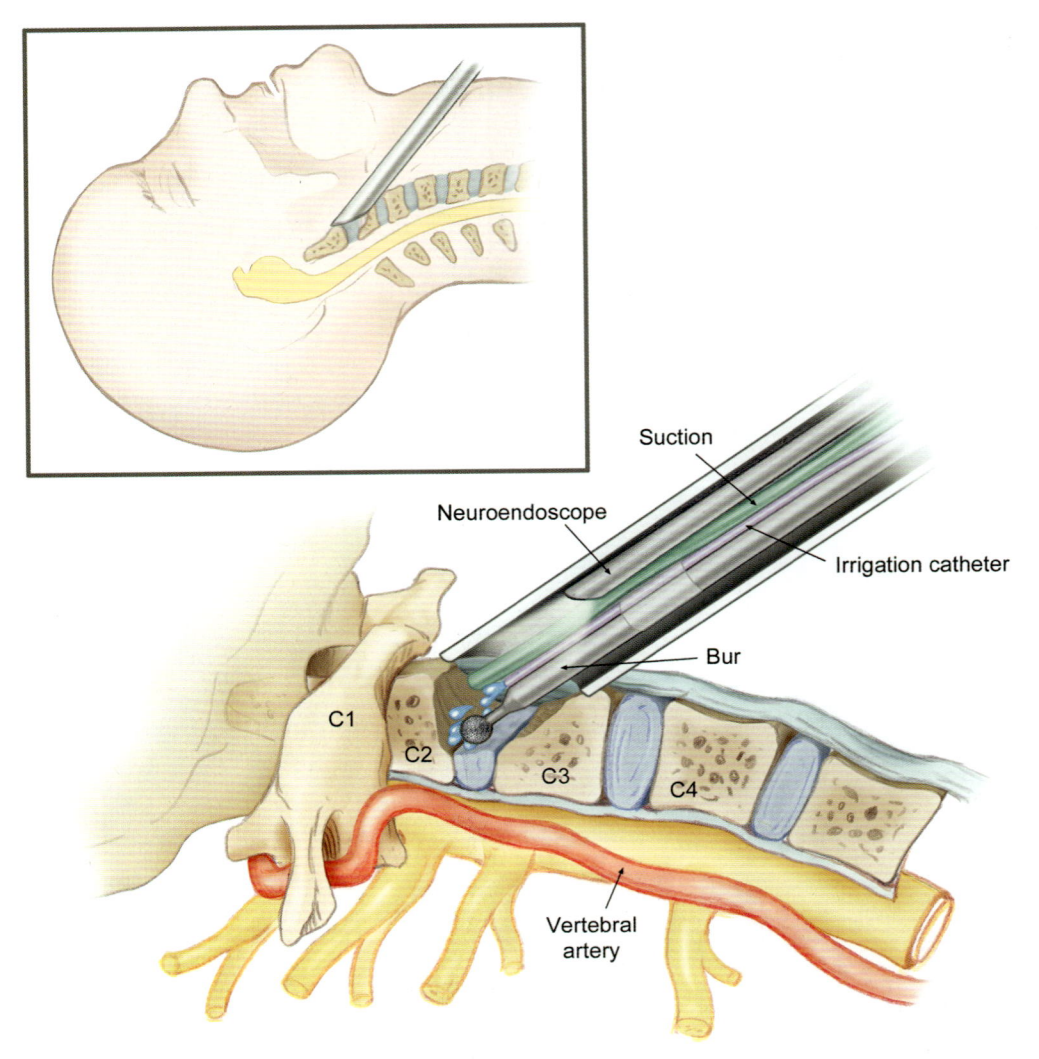

Fig. 9.2 Artist rendition of the endoscopic transcervical operation. The tubular retractor, placed against the anterior cervical spine, acts as a channel for the endoscope and instruments. (Adapted from Wolinsky JP, Sciubba DM, Suk I, Gokaslan ZL. Endoscopic image-guided odontoidectomy for decompression of basilar invagination via a standard anterior cervical approach. Technical note. J Neurosurg Spine 2007;6:184–191.)

multiple noncontiguous lesions, and diffusely infiltrative pathologies. Even the deepest basilar invaginations may be decompressed with the endoscopic transcervical. Significant basilar impression with the odontoid well into the skull base (> 35 mm above McGregor's line) can also be reached through this approach. Through a single incision in the neck, the transcervical technique also enables caudal vertebral body resection and long fusion constructions, especially instrumentation extended into the subaxial vertebral bodies. In fact, cervical tumors, odontoid trauma, atlantoaxial rheumatoid diseases, and degenerative basilar invagination have all been described with the minimally invasive transcervical technique.[6,7]

Contraindications

Although the endoscopic transcervical approach has had excellent success rates, the technique has a steep learning curve and requires a three-dimensional understanding of the upper cervical spine anatomy. The endoscopic transcervical approach is limited in patients suffering from morbid obesity or severe kyphosis, or in patients with barrel chests. The long tubular tools necessary for the minimally invasive technique limit its application with highly vascular lesions. Lastly, the risk of recurrent laryngeal nerve palsy is equivalent to that in other cervical approaches,[6] and intradural pathologies are a relative contraindication to surgery.

Surgical Procedure

The endoscopic transcervical operation follows the technique described by Wolinsky et al.[6] In the operating room, the patient is placed in the supine position on the operating table. The skull is placed in traction with a halo ring connected to a Mayfield halo adapter, and the neck is mildly extended with a shoulder roll. The patient undergoes nasotracheal intubation with a cuffed endotracheal tube. Somatosensory evoked responses are established and monitored throughout the procedure. A fixed retractor and endoscope are mounted on the side of the table that is contralateral to the surgeon and caudal to the surgical field.

The lateral neck is sterilized and prepped in a standard fashion (right side for right-handed surgeons). The operation begins with a standard Smith-Robinson approach with a transverse in-

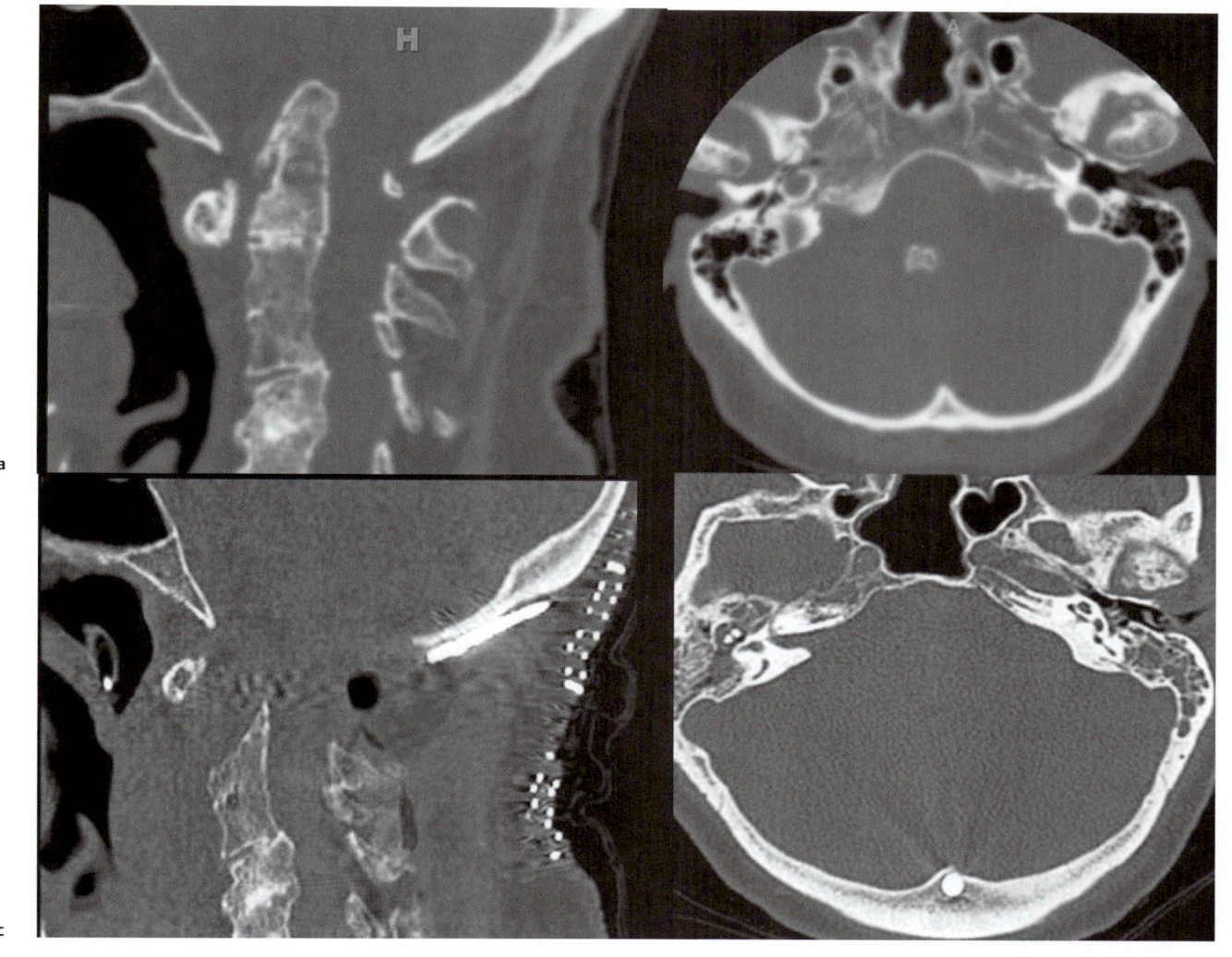

Fig. 9.3 (a) Sagittal and (b) axial computed tomography (CT) demonstrates significant basilar impression extending well beyond the craniocervical junction. (c) Postoperative sagittal and (d) axial CT demonstrates odontoid resection performed by the transcervical endoscopic approach.

cision starting at approximately C4, just off the midline and extending laterally for 3.5 to 4.0 cm.[19] Blunt dissection is used to isolate and then swing the sternocleidomastoid and carotid sheath laterally and the esophagus and trachea medially. The cuffed endotracheal tube enables tracheal movement with minimal resistance, and esophageal retraction is maintained with a handheld retractor. Dissection of the loose connective tissue ventral to the spine provides exposure of the cervical spine at the anterior tubercle of C1. The rostral end of the beveled retractor is then advanced to the C1 tubercle, and the location is confirmed with intraoperative navigation. With the beveled-tip retractor, the longus colli muscles are retracted away from the spine. However, care should be taken between the C2 transverse process and the C2-3 interspace, where the anatomy can be variable. The vertebral arteries may course medially at the level of C2-C3 before traversing laterally. After careful dissection at the upper cervical spine, the tubular retractor is then placed up against the diseased vertebrae. A 30-degree, 4-mm endoscope attached to the endoscope arm is positioned inside the retractor for visualization throughout the procedure. For bone resection, the drill is calibrated and used with the neuronavigation system. The apical ligaments, posterior longitudinal ligaments, and transverse ligaments provide a natural barrier between the osseous resection and the underlying dura; therefore, these ligaments and/or panni should not be resected until after osseous drilling is complete. Instability from osseous resection may require stabilization. After the indicated procedure is completed, the endoscope and tubular retractors are carefully removed. The surgical incision is closed in a standard multilayer fashion, and the wound thoroughly cleansed (**Fig. 9.3**).

Postoperative Course

Because of the limited incision and surgical dissection, patients undergoing minimally invasive endoscopic operations have favorable outcomes. Depending on the amount of bony resection and decompression, atlantoaxial spinal instability may ensue, for which the patient is placed in a halo external orthosis and repositioned for a posterior instrumented fusion.[20] Following the operation, patients are extubated on the day of surgery.[7] Patients undergoing the endoscopic transoral technique are placed on oral intake restrictions to protect the surgical site from infection. In the endonasal and transcervical counterparts, patients may resume oral intake on postoperative day 1. However, all patients should have swallowing functions evaluated prior to advancing to an oral diet.

Postoperative Complications and Precautions

In the event of a CSF leak, the surgical defect is covered with a fascial graft and sealed with fibrin glue. A tunneled lumbar drain is also necessary to prevent submucosal fluid collections and to monitor daily fluid outputs. Patients are placed on prophylactic antibiotics and oral intake restrictions until healed.

The risks of other complications may vary with the endoscopic approach. Patients undergoing the transoral and the transcervical operation run the risk of lower cranial nerve dysfunction, velopharyngeal incompetence, and pharyngeal wall injury.[7] Rarely, in the event of tracheopharyngeal dysfunction, these patients may require enteral nutrition or a tracheal tube for airway secretions. These complications may be prevented in the endoscopic transoral technique by restricting the incision to the posterior oral cavity, without extension to the soft palate. The endoscopic endonasal and transoral approaches may entail an increased propensity for surgical-site infections, owing to the moist mucosal lining and natural flora. Similar to CSF leaks, these patients may be managed with lumbar drains, antibiotics, and oral intake restrictions until healed.

Conclusion

The endoscopic techniques in spine surgery offer unique entry points for hard-to-reach lesions without the morbidity associated with wide surgical exposures. This chapter focused on three minimally invasive endoscopic approaches to the upper cervical spine: the endoscopic transoral approach, the endoscopic endonasal approach, and the endoscopic transcervical approach. The transoral and endonasal routes provide direct trajectories to the upper cervical pathologies. However, this approach should be balanced with the risks of traversing the contaminated naso-oropharyngeal mucosa. On the other hand, the endoscopic transcervical approach provides sterile surgical corridors through the neck to the entire cervical spine via a beveled-tip tubular retractor.

References

1. Crockard HA, Johnston F. Development of transoral approaches to lesions of the skull base and craniocervical junction. Neurosurg Q 1993;3:61–82
2. Husain M, Rastogi M, Ojha BK, Chandra A, Jha DK. Endoscopic transoral surgery for craniovertebral junction anomalies. Technical note. J Neurosurg Spine 2006;5:367–373
3. Frempong-Boadu AK, Faunce WA, Fessler RG. Endoscopically assisted transoral-transpharyngeal approach to the craniovertebral junction. Neurosurgery 2002;51(5, Suppl):S60–S66
4. Fraser JF, Nyquist GG, Moore N, Anand VK, Schwartz TH. Endoscopic endonasal transclival resection of chordomas: operative technique, clinical outcome, and review of the literature. J Neurosurg 2010;112:1061–1069
5. Kassam AB, Snyderman C, Gardner P, Carrau R, Spiro R. The expanded endonasal approach: a fully endoscopic transnasal approach and resection of the odontoid process: technical case report. Neurosurgery 2005; 57(1, Suppl):E213, discussion E213
6. Wolinsky JP, Sciubba DM, Suk I, Gokaslan ZL. Endoscopic image-guided odontoidectomy for decompression of basilar invagination via a standard anterior cervical approach. Technical note. J Neurosurg Spine 2007;6:184–191
7. Haertl R, Korge A. Minimally Invasive Spine Surgery: Techniques, Evidence, and Controversies: AOSpine. New York: Thieme Medical; 2012
8. Laufer I, Greenfield JP, Anand VK, Härtl R, Schwartz TH. Endonasal endoscopic resection of the odontoid process in a nonachondroplastic dwarf with juvenile rheumatoid arthritis: feasibility of the approach and utility of the intraoperative Iso-C three-dimensional navigation. Case report. J Neurosurg Spine 2008;8:376–380
9. Fang HS, Ong G. Direct anterior approach to the upper cervical spine. J Bone Joint Surg Am 1962;44A:1588–1604
10. Menezes AH. Surgical approaches: postoperative care and complications "transoral-transpalatopharyngeal approach to the craniocervical junction." Childs Nerv Syst 2008;24:1187–1193
11. Tuite GF, Veres R, Crockard HA, Sell D. Pediatric transoral surgery: indications, complications, and long-term outcome. J Neurosurg 1996;84:573–583
12. Crockard HA. The transoral approach to the base of the brain and upper cervical cord. Ann R Coll Surg Engl 1985;67:321–325
13. de Divitiis O, Conti A, Angileri FF, Cardali S, La Torre D, Tschabitscher M. Endoscopic transoral-transclival approach to the brainstem and surrounding cisternal space: anatomic study. Neurosurgery 2004;54:125–130, discussion 130
14. Alfieri A, Jho HD, Tschabitscher M. Endoscopic endonasal approach to the ventral cranio-cervical junction: anatomical study. Acta Neurochir (Wien) 2002;144:219–225, discussion 225
15. Jho HD, Carrau RL. Endoscopic endonasal transsphenoidal surgery: experience with 50 patients. J Neurosurg 1997;87:44–51
16. Hofstetter CP, Singh A, Anand VK, Kacker A, Schwartz TH. The endoscopic, endonasal, transmaxillary transpterygoid approach to the pterygopalatine fossa, infratemporal fossa, petrous apex, and the Meckel cave. J Neurosurg 2010;113:967–974
17. Kassam AB, Vescan AD, Carrau RL, et al. Expanded endonasal approach: vidian canal as a landmark to the petrous internal carotid artery. J Neurosurg 2008;108:177–183
18. Schwartz TH, Fraser JF, Brown S, Tabaee A, Kacker A, Anand VK. Endoscopic cranial base surgery: classification of operative approaches. Neurosurgery 2008;62:991–1002, discussion 1002–1005
19. Robinson RA, Southwick WO. Surgical approaches to the cervical spine. Instr Course Lect 1960;17:299–330
20. Dickman CA, Locantro J, Fessler RG. The influence of transoral odontoid resection on stability of the craniovertebral junction. J Neurosurg 1992; 77:525–530

10 Extended Maxillotomy Approach for High Clinical Pathology

Raj P. TerKonda and Lawrence J. Marentette

The extended maxillotomy approach to the skull base provides unparalleled exposure of the midline craniovertebral junction via an anterior approach. This approach provides the neurosurgeon access from the superior clivus to the body of the third cervical vertebra (C3). Removal of the bony nasal septum extends the access superiorly to the sphenoid sinus. Routine transoral approaches with palatal retraction provide access only to the inferior clivus to the superior body of C3 (**Fig. 10.1**). When compared with the transoral approach, the extended maxillotomy approach is technically more difficult, extends the operative time by about 6 hours, and has greater potential morbidity. It is critical that the surgeons identify the exact extent of the lesion preoperatively to determine the appropriate approach.

The procedure consists of a horizontal osteotomy of the maxilla (Le Fort I), splitting the hard and soft palate, and vertical pharyngotomy. The term *extended maxillotomy* is confusing because there are at least three different approaches to the skull base with the same name.[1-3] The technique detailed in this and the next chapter was first described by James and Crockard.[2] This procedure is based on maxillofacial techniques and is more appropriately termed "two-piece Le Fort I osteotomy with palatal split."[4] The single-piece Le Fort I osteotomy without palatal split (Crawford's "unextended" transmaxillary approach) provides access only to the clivus and not the cervical spine.[5]

Indications

- Congenital craniovertebral junction abnormalities with basilar invagination (e.g., osteogenesis imperfecta)
- Rheumatoid arthritis with odontoid displacement
- Fracture dislocation of the odontoid process
- Midline extradural tumors of the clivus and upper cervical spine
- Basilar aneurysms

Contraindications

- Intradural tumors
- Extradural tumors with lateral extension
- Acute sinusitis
- Severe trismus
- Poor dentition

Advantages

- No facial incisions
- Excellent exposure of clivus, C1, and C2, and excellent ventral exposure from the rostral clivus to the body of C3
- Dentition preserved
- Removal of the nasal septum extends exposure to the sphenoid sinus.

Disadvantages

- Technically difficult and prolonged
- Only appropriate for midline lesions
- Significant blood loss
- Increased risk of morbidity

Objective

- To gain access to the midline clivus and upper cervical spine via an anterior approach

Preoperative Planning

This approach should be performed by a facial surgeon familiar with maxillary osteotomies, such as a facial plastic and reconstructive surgeon with otolaryngology training, an oral maxillofacial surgeon, or a general plastic surgeon. Both magnetic resonance imaging (MRI) and computed tomography (CT) scans are required to determine the extent of the lesion. A thorough dental examination is obtained to rule out periapical abscesses and other dental problems that may interfere with the osteotomies. A Panorex of the mandible and maxilla, and anteroposterior (AP) and lateral cephalograms are reviewed. Dental impressions are mandatory on all patients in the unfortunate event of maxillary necrosis. An interdental splint is made from the dental impressions by a prosthodontist to prevent malocclusion postoperatively. The patient should be typed and crossed for two units of packed red blood cells. Preoperative culture of the oral and nasal flora is not routinely performed[5] (**Box 10.1**).

Box 10.1 Preoperative Planning
Computed tomography and magnetic resonance imaging scans of skull base and cervical spine
Panorex of the mandible and maxilla
Anteroposterior/lateral cephalograms
Possible angiogram
Dental consultation
Dental impressions
Interdental splint
Typed and crossed for two units of packed red blood cells

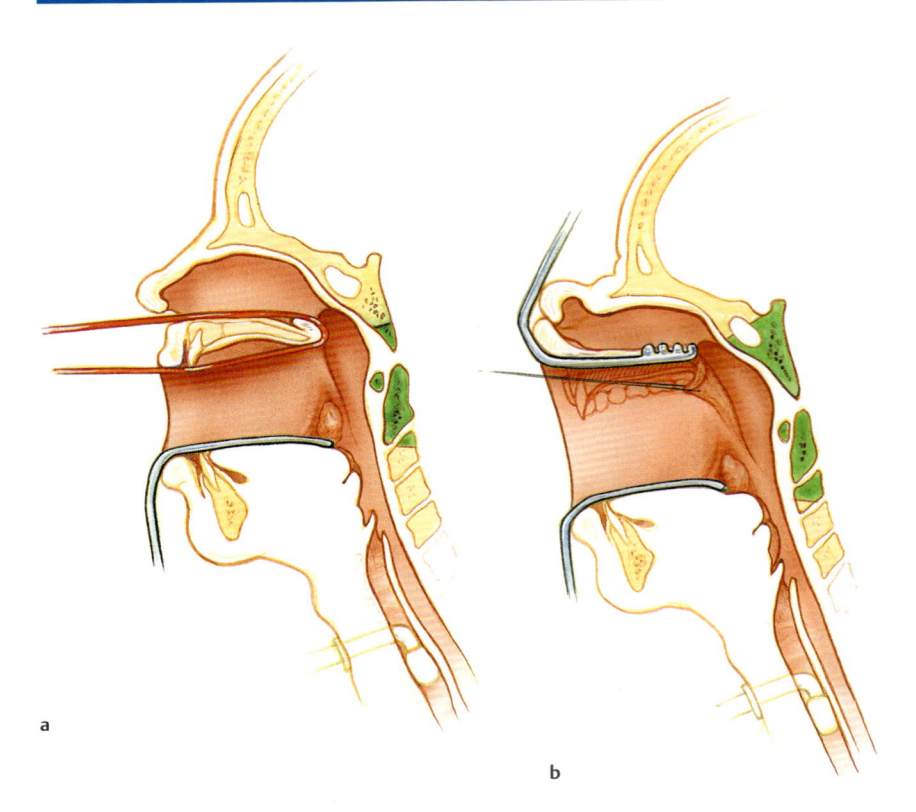

Fig. 10.1 Extent of exposure for the **(a)** routine transoral approach and **(b)** extended maxillotomy approach.

Surgical Techniques

Tracheostomy

An elective tracheostomy is performed at the beginning of the procedure. If the patient is at risk for brainstem/spinal cord compression with neck extension, an awake tracheostomy is performed under local anesthesia. Otherwise, the patient is routinely intubated prior to tracheostomy.

Elective tracheotomy has several advantages. The tracheostomy precludes the interference by a nasal endotracheal tube. Interdental fixation is required at the end of the procedure; therefore, an oral endotracheal tube is not an option. A patient with a tracheostomy is unable to perform a Valsalva maneuver, thereby decreasing the risk of dehiscence of the pharyngotomy suture line and cerebrospinal fluid (CSF) leakage. If the patient requires posterior cervical stabilization at a later date, the tracheostomy allows the patient to be anesthetized easily for this second procedure. If not, the tracheostomy is removed as soon as mechanical ventilation is not required.

Patient Positioning

After tracheostomy, the bed is rotated 180 degrees. During stabilization with a Mayfield head holder, the patient may be awakened to assess worsening of brainstem/spinal cord compression symptoms during positioning. If the patient has a stable cervical spine, a shoulder roll is placed to aid neck extension. A C-arm fluoroscope is positioned over the chest; this will be moved superiorly after the maxillary osteotomies and pharyngotomy are completed. Cottonoids soaked with oxymetazoline are placed in each nasal cavity for decongestion. The face is prepped with Betadine solution only, and a Betadine-soaked sponge is place intraorally.

Exposure of Maxilla and Nasal Cavity

Erich arch bars are anchored to the maxilla and mandible with 24-gauge wires. The arch bars are used to place the teeth in interdental fixation at the end of the procedure. The maxillary gingivobuccal sulcus, nasal floor and septum, and palate are injected with 1/2% lidocaine with epinephrine 1:200,000. Leaving a 1-cm cuff, an incision is made with a guarded needlepoint cautery in the gingivobuccal sulcus between the left and right second premolars (**Fig. 10.2**). The parotid duct papillae are carefully avoided.

The soft tissues of the maxilla are elevated superiorly in the subperiosteal plane to the level of the infraorbital nerves, which should be clearly identified (**Fig. 10.3**). Posterolaterally, the dissection is performed to the maxillary tuberosity. Using Cottle and curved Freer elevators, the nasal mucosa is elevated from the inferior meatus, nasal floor, maxillary crest, and nasal septum bilaterally. This prevents lacerating the nasal mucosa during osteotomies and decreases the risk of nasal airway problems postoperatively. The nasal septum is separated from the maxillary crest using a flat or U-shaped osteotome (**Fig. 10.4**). Alternatively, the cartilaginous septum can be reflected laterally ("swinging door" technique), and the bony septum can be removed for access to the sphenoid sinus.

Preparation for Le Fort I Osteotomy

The markings for the Le Fort I osteotomy are made above the level of the dental roots. The canine root is easily palpated and the Panorex of the maxilla will aid in placement. The marking extends bilaterally from the piriform aperture just below the attachment of the inferior turbinate to the lateral (zygomaticomaxillary) buttress of the midfacial skeleton.

Titanium miniplates with 2.0-mm screws are used for rigid fixation of the osteotomies during closure. Typically, four-hole

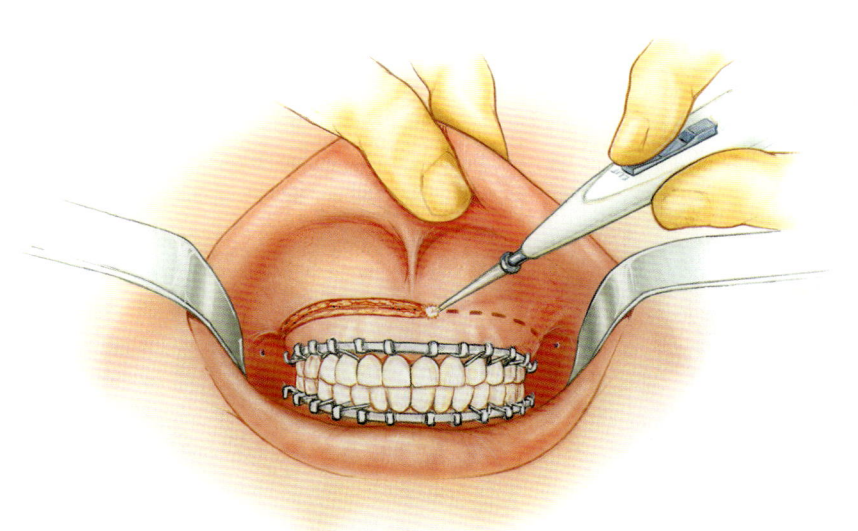

Fig. 10.2 Gingivobuccal incision for maxillary exposure. Note arch bars and location of parotid duct papilla.

Fig. 10.3 Exposure of maxilla with preservation of infraorbital nerves. The nasal mucosa is carefully elevated. The *dashed line* represents the location of the Le Fort I osteotomy.

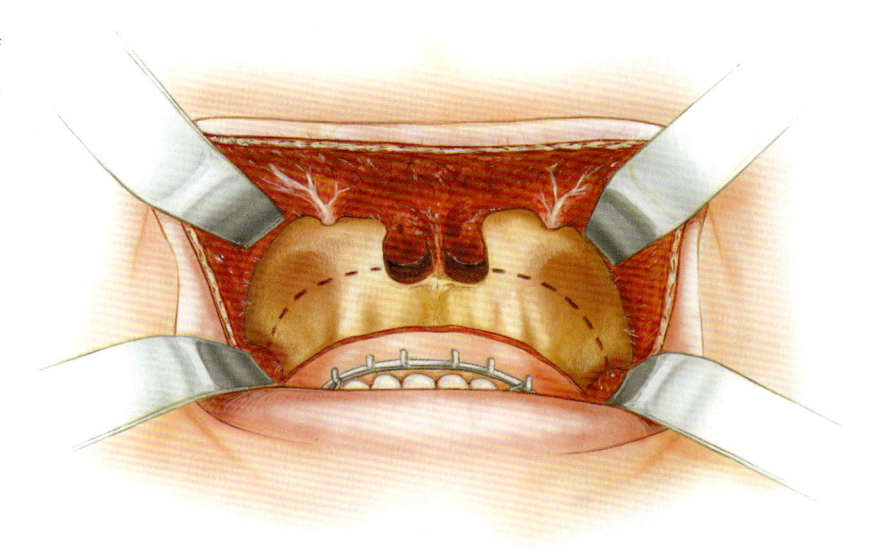

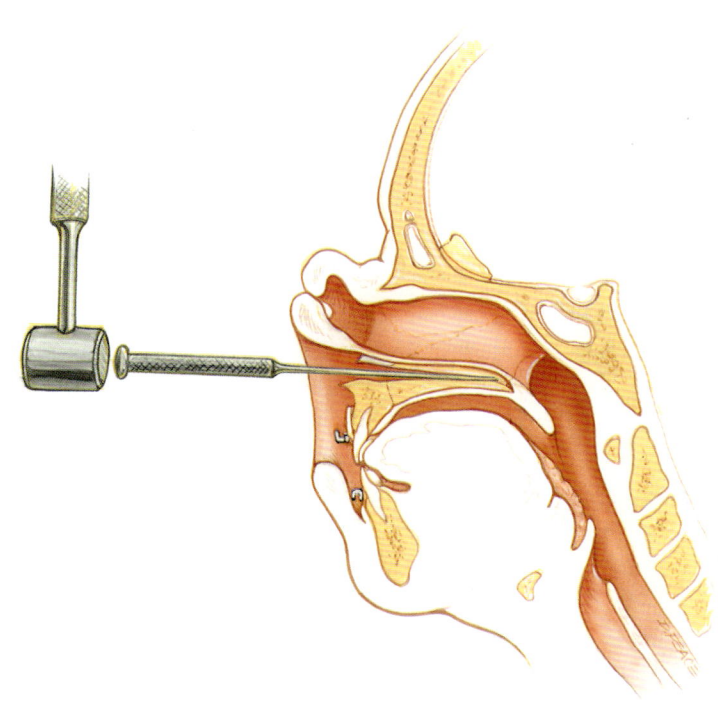

Fig. 10.4 The cartilaginous and bony nasal septum is separated from the maxillary crest with an osteotome.

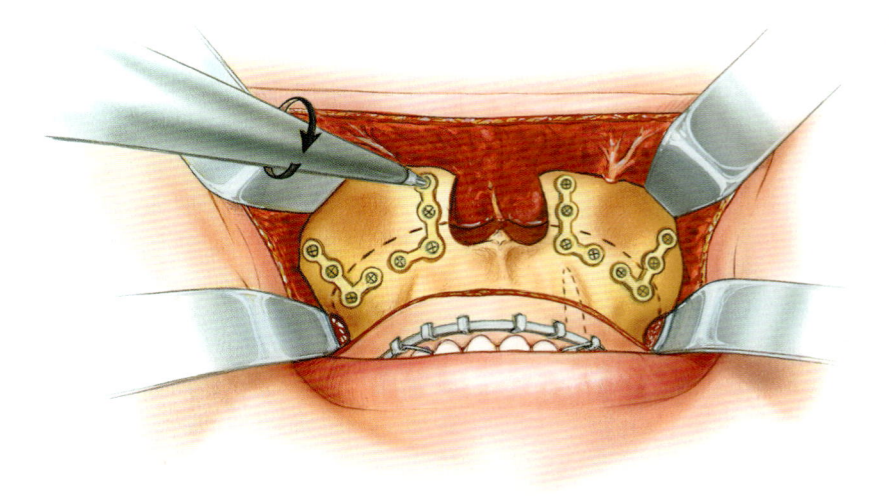

Fig. 10.5 Preplating of medial and lateral buttresses prior to osteotomy. Depending on the anatomy of the tooth roots, the orientation of the medial buttress plates may vary.

L-shaped plates are placed over the medial and lateral buttresses, the structural "beams" of the face (**Fig. 10.5**). To maintain exact dental occlusion postoperatively, the plates and screws are placed into position prior to osteotomy and then removed. It is important to keep the screws and plates in exact orientation on the back table. The reciprocating saw used for osteotomy will remove 1 to 2 mm of bone. If the edges are touching at the end of repair, malocclusion may occur. Preplating the horizontal osteotomy ensures that the small gap will be maintained for perfect occlusion postoperatively.

Palatal Split

The hard and soft palate is split prior to Le Fort osteotomy while the maxilla is stable. A Dingman retractor is placed to open the oral cavity (**Fig. 10.6**). An incision is marked in the midline hard and soft palate. It deviates laterally to either side of the uvula to maintain the shape of this delicate structure. A full-thickness incision with a No. 11 blade is made in the soft palate to the posterior aspect of the hard palate (**Fig. 10.7**). The incision is continued anteriorly in the oral mucosa of the hard palate to the medial incisors. The oral mucosa is elevated a few millimeters from the hard palate bilaterally to prevent maceration during midline osteotomy. As the nasal mucosa is retracted, a midline osteotomy is made in the hard palate using a reciprocating saw from posterior to anterior up to the medial incisors (**Fig. 10.8**). To avoid damage to the tooth roots, a fine osteotome is used to complete the osteotomy between the medial incisors to the piriform aperture (**Fig. 10.9**).

Le Fort I Osteotomy

The Le Fort I osteotomy is also performed with the reciprocating saw. Again, the nasal mucosa is protected. The saw is place along

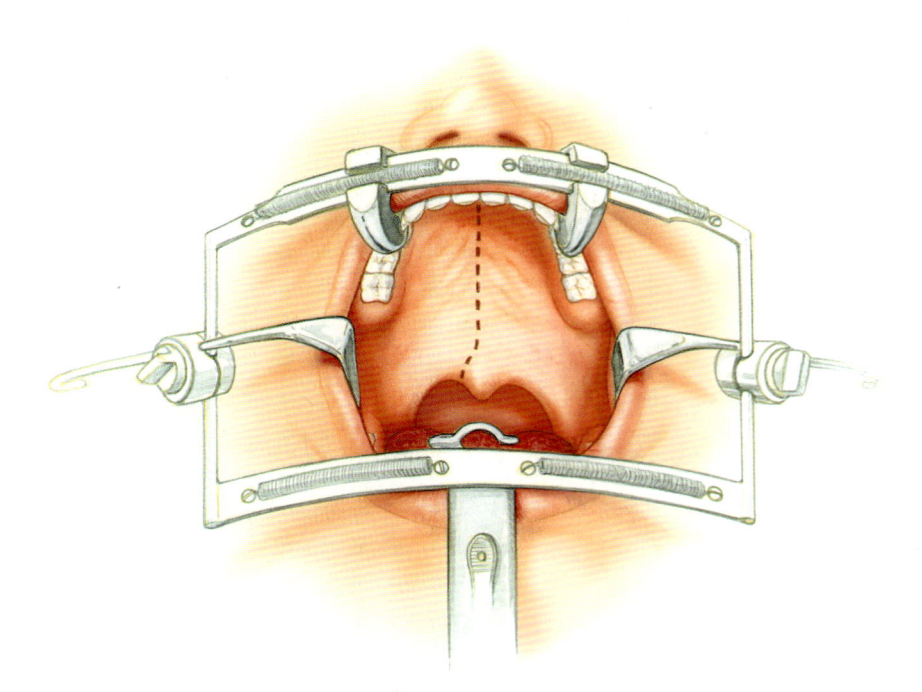

Fig. 10.6 Intraoral exposure with Dingman retractor. The *dashed line* indicates the palatal incision.

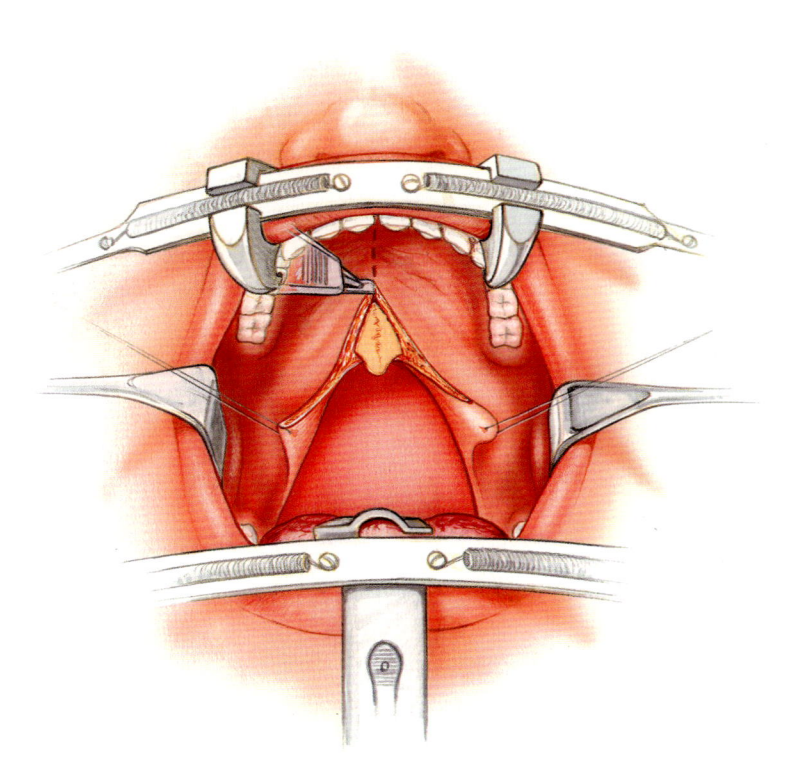

Fig. 10.7 Palatal incision with all three layers of the soft palate incised.

the posterolateral wall of the maxilla, and the osteotomy is performed in a medial direction to the piriform aperture (**Fig. 10.9**). It is very important to make the cut exactly on the markings and between the drill holes for the titanium screws.

Each maxillary half remains attached to the skull base via the pterygoid plates. A wide curved osteotome is placed posteriorly between the maxillary tuberosity and pterygoid plates, and detachment from the skull base is performed. An index finger of the opposite hand is placed intraorally in the retromolar area to palpate completion of the osteotomy (**Fig. 10.10**). Each maxillary half is then down-fractured with Rowe maxillary disimpaction forceps to complete the skull base separation and fracture the posterior maxillary sinus wall (**Fig. 10.11**). The maxillary halves are gently retracted laterally; their only blood supply is the greater palatine arteries. An angled Crockard pharyngeal retractor is used to separate the maxillary halves. This provides exposure of the nasopharynx and posterior pharyngeal wall (**Fig. 10.12**).

Vertical Pharyngotomy

The tubercle of C1 is palpated, and positioning is confirmed by fluoroscopy. A midline linear pharyngotomy is made in the posterior nasopharyngeal and oropharyngeal mucosa to the body of C3. The incision is carried to the level of the white, shiny prevertebral fascia. At this point, C1, C2, and the clivus are covered with several ligaments (**Fig. 10.13**). Exposure is verified with fluoroscopy, and the case is turned over to the neurosurgery team.

Conclusion

The extended maxillotomy approach to the skull base provides excellent exposure of the midline craniovertebral junction from the superior clivus to the body of the third cervical vertebra (C3). Access can be extended superiorly to the sphenoid sinus by

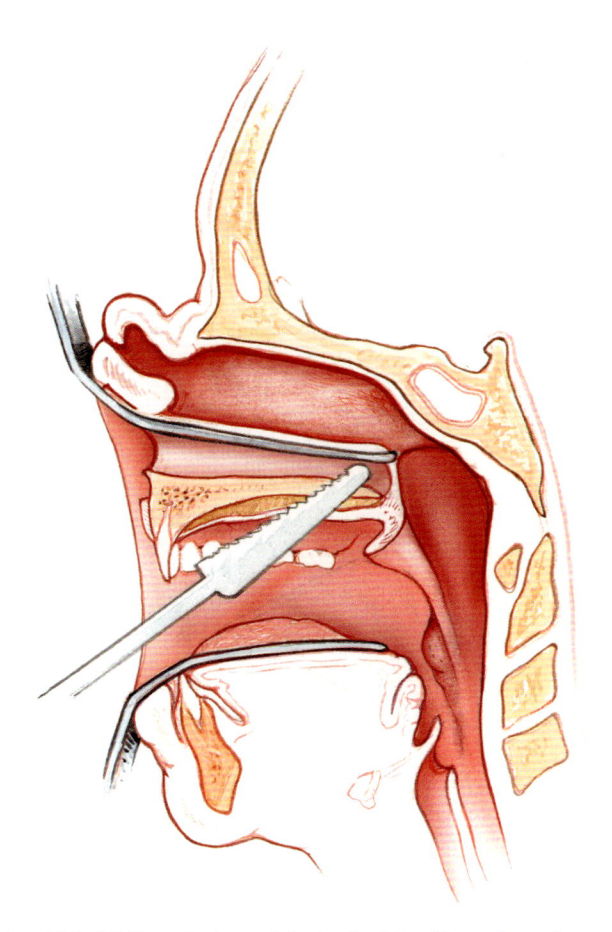

Fig. 10.8 Midline osteotomy of the hard palate with a reciprocating saw. Note protection of the nasal mucosa with a retractor.

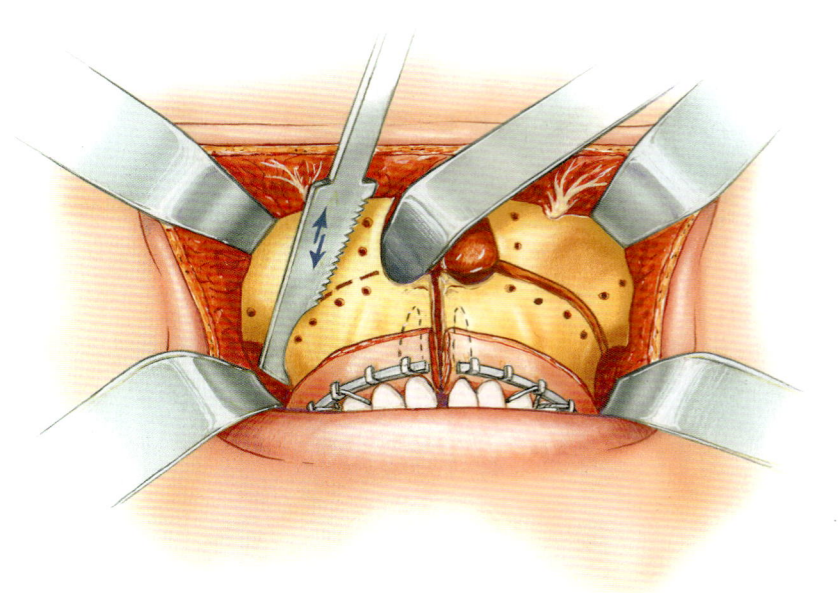

Fig. 10.9 Le Fort I osteotomy performed after midline palatal split.

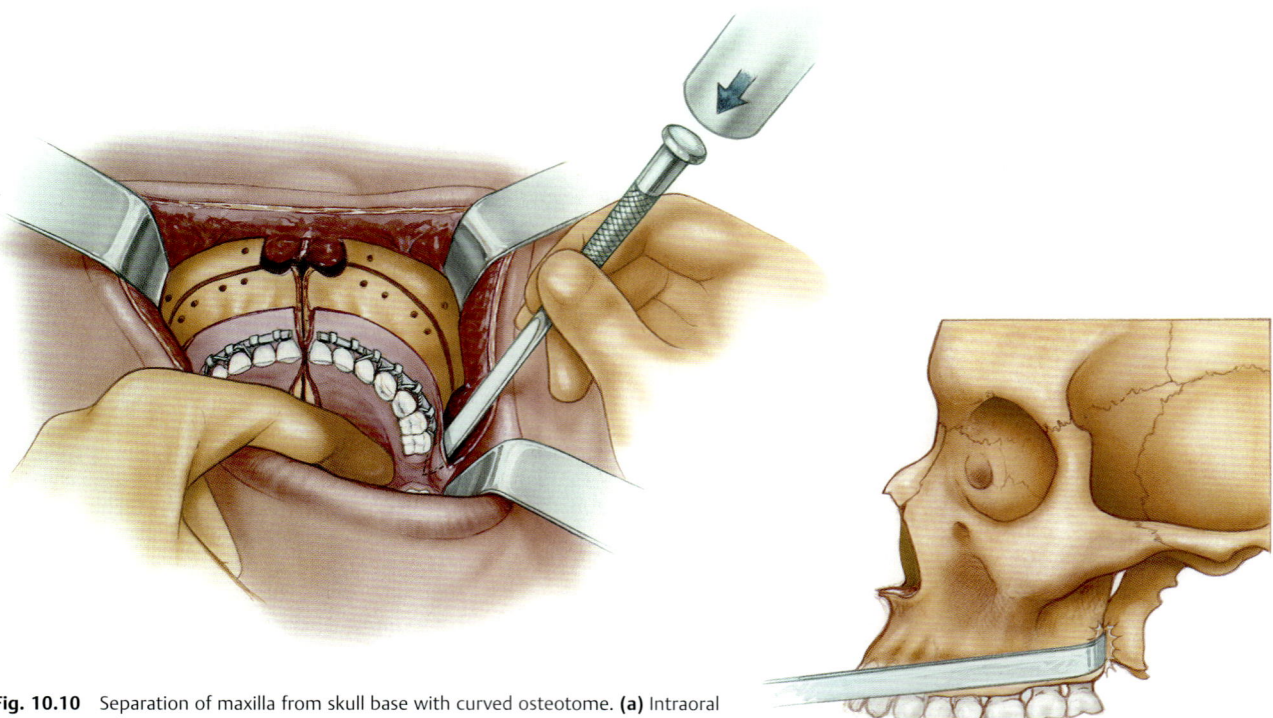

Fig. 10.10 Separation of maxilla from skull base with curved osteotome. **(a)** Intraoral view. **(b)** Lateral view.

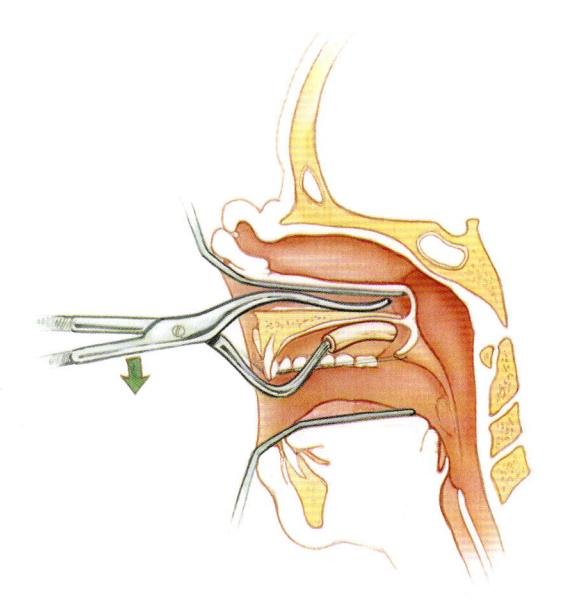

Fig. 10.11 Placement of Rowe maxillary disimpaction forceps for down-fracture of each maxillary half.

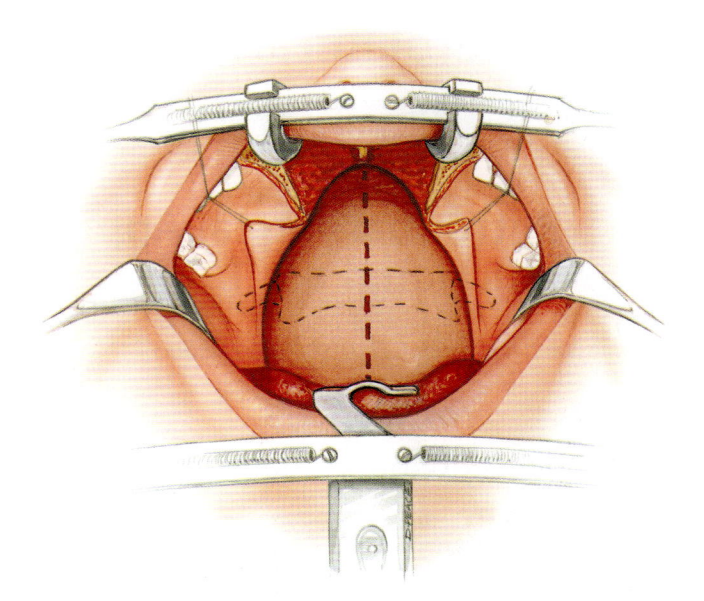

Fig. 10.12 Separation of maxillary halves with exposure of posterior pharynx and nasopharynx.

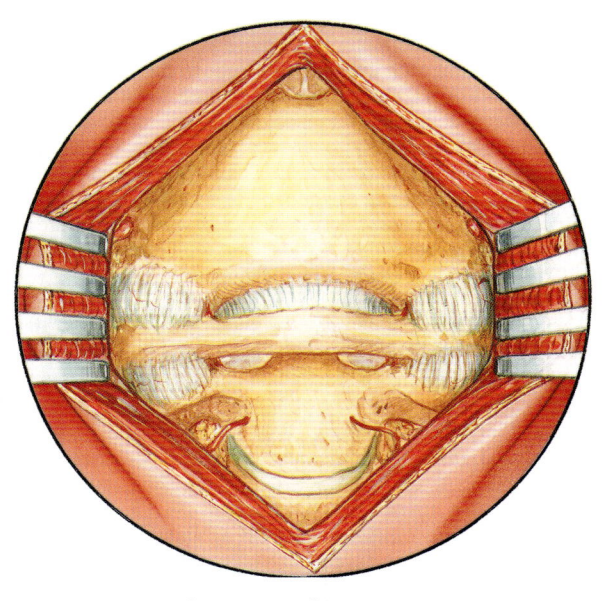

Fig. 10.13 Exposure after posterior pharyngotomy.

removing the bony nasal septum. When compared with the transoral approach, the extended maxillotomy approach is technically more difficult, extends the operative time by about 6 hours, and has greater potential morbidity. It is critical that the surgeons identify the exact extent of the lesion preoperatively to determine the appropriate approach.

References

1. Cocke EW Jr, Robertson JH, Robertson JT, Crook JP Jr. The extended maxillotomy and subtotal maxillectomy for excision of skull base tumors. Arch Otolaryngol Head Neck Surg 1990;116:92–104
2. James D, Crockard HA. Surgical access to the base of skull and upper cervical spine by extended maxillotomy. Neurosurgery 1991;29:411–416
3. Catalano PJ, Biller HF. Extended osteoplastic maxillotomy. A versatile new procedure for wide access to the central skull base and infratemporal fossa. Arch Otolaryngol Head Neck Surg 1993;119:394–400
4. Williams WG, Lo LJ, Chen YR. The Le Fort I–palatal split approach for skull base tumors: efficacy, complications, and outcome. Plast Reconstr Surg 1998;102:2310–2319
5. Crockard HA. The transmaxillary approach to the clivus. In: Sekhar LN, Janecka IP, eds. Surgery of Cranial Base Tumors. New York: Raven; 1993: 235–244

C. Anterolateral Approach

11 Retropharyngeal Approach to the Occipital-Cervical Junction, Part 1

John R. Vender, Steven J. Harrison, and Dennis E. McDonnell

The high anterior cervical retropharyngeal approach provides an alternative to the transoral approach to the ventral occipital-cervical junction (OCJ). It is designed to expose the basiocciput of the clivus, the anterior rim of the foramen magnum, and the rostral cervical segments of C1–C4. This option avoids the bacterially contaminated environment of the oral cavity and pharynx. This exposure provides direct access for the relief of compression from basilar impression, the resection of neoplastic lesions, and the repair of chronic fractures and pannus with broader and safer latitudes than those available via the transoral route. Indications and contraindications for this procedure, pathological processes, anatomic perspectives, technical aspects, and complications of this approach along with the authors' clinical experience are discussed in this and the following chapter.

Patient Selection

Patients with anteriorly or anterolaterally situated craniocervical junction lesions involving the clivus rostrally to the upper cervical spine caudally amenable to an anterior approach are candidates for a high anterior retropharyngeal procedure. If anterior decompression is necessary, either the transoral or parapharyngeal approach can be used.[1,2] The parapharyngeal approach is preferable if the lesion requires exposure of the C1-C2 lateral masses, is caudal to the mid-clivus, requires corpectomy caudal to C2, or requires opening of the dura.

Indications

The high anterior retropharyngeal approach is an effective surgical option for treating basilar impression, occipitocervical osseous anomalies (e.g., odontoid agenesis, os odontoideum), rheumatoid arthritis, pyogenic retropharyngeal abscesses, ventral foramen magnum, clival, or upper cervical spinal cord/spinal tumors (e.g., chordomas, meningiomas, neurofibromas), and chronic fractures.

The natural history of basilar impression is progressive myelopathy that leads to quadriparesis and respiratory paralysis and ultimately death. This sad course can be averted by surgical decompression and stabilization of the OCJ. The pathological compressive lesion may be posterior or anterior to the cervicomedullary junction of the neural axis. Chronic "glacial" instability is also an integral part of the pathological process. The etiology may be developmental, genetic, or acquired. Acquired lesions are inflammatory, neoplastic, or traumatic in origin.[3] These are dynamic anatomic abnormalities that are diagnosed clinically and by radiographs, computed tomography (CT), and magnetic resonance imaging (MRI) of the OCJ.[4–6]

Occipitocervical osseous anomalies of developmental origin arise from defective segmentation in embryonic precursors of the first four sclerotomes. Hypoplasia of the dens, atlantoaxial instability, and chronic dislocation may occur as developmental abnormalities in congenital conditions such as Down syndrome (trisomy 21). Neurodysgenetic lesions such as Chiari I and syringomyelia may be seen upon diagnostic imaging of developmental osseous abnormalities in this region.

Rheumatoid arthritis is the most common inflammatory condition affecting this region. The inflammatory dissolution of craniovertebral support ligaments, including the transverse ligament, which secures the dens to the anterior arch of the atlas, leads to instability. Concomitant bone erosion of atlantoaxial lateral masses and occipital condyles leads to cranial settling and rostral migration of C2 into the foramen magnum and more ventral impingement on the neural axis.[7,8] Osteoporosis also accelerates subluxation of these bone structures and impedes surgical attempts of arthrodesis to treat this condition. Pyogenic retropharyngeal abscesses can cause bone and ligament destruction, resulting in ventral neural compression. Usually the compressive process is due to bone destruction, instability, and cranial settling, but chronic granulomatous lesions and pannus also produce direct mass effect upon the neural axis.[9]

Neoplasms can cause neural compression either by direct tumor extension or through bone destruction and pathological fracture in this region. These may be primary or metastatic tumors of the bone or neural tumors, which can be extra-axial or intra-axial. Chordomas tend to occur in this location as well as destructive metastatic tumors to the vertebral body of C2 or adjacent segments. Meningiomas arising from the clivus, anterior rim of foramen magnum, or ventral spinal canal are treacherous in this region. Neurofibromas of Recklinghausen's disease causing ventral neural compression in this location also challenge the patient with progressive paralysis.

Fractures tend to occur because the occipitoatlantoaxial complex is a transition zone and accounts for half of head movement in flexion, extension, and rotation. Fractures involve ligamentous support structures as well as bony elements, leading to craniovertebral instability. Nonunion fractures of the dens and subluxation of the atlas on the axis may result in ventral compression of the neural axis causing chronic pain and progressive myelopathy.

The os odontoideum is an independent bone rostral to the body of C2 but separated from it and located in the position of the dens. It is a chronic unstable condition due either to nonunion of an odontoid fracture, which occurred in childhood, or a congenital failure of the ossification centers of the dens to assimilate with the body of the axis. The orthotopic type is in the normal position of the dens; the dystopic type is more rostrally located and related to the clivus.[3]

Symptoms and signs of neural compression at the OCJ are multiple and varied. They are due to direct compression of the medulla, spinal cord, cranial nerves, cervical roots, or vascular structures (arterial, capillary, or venous) that supply these structures. Congenital lesions may be associated with external physical characteristics such as short neck, cervical web, low hairline, torticollis, and limited neck movement.

Myelopathy is usually present but of variable severity. It can be manifested by early fatigue in ambulation to monoparesis, hemiparesis, or quadriparesis. Central cord myelopathy is a common presentation with upper extremity weakness and relative sparing of lower extremity strength. Gait disturbance with clumsiness and stumbling is frequent. Hyperreflexia, clonus, extensor planter responses, and a Hoffmann response are also frequent findings. Posterior column disturbance with impaired joint and position sense is much less common than numbness and hypalgesia unless the process is advanced. Dysesthesias and cold sensations in the hands are noticed early in the process.[10] Urinary hesitancy and frequency imply myelopathic bladder disturbance. Respiratory disturbance and intermittent sleep apnea occur and are particularly ominous. Periods of acute apnea may herald rapid neurologic deterioration and are life threatening. Cranial nerve dysfunction can result in dysphagia, palatal paralysis, shoulder weakness, and loss of hearing. Nystagmus can occur from brainstem compression. The most common symptom is suboccipital pain that radiates to the vertex. Characteristically, head movement aggravates the pain. Pain is particularly severe for patients with rheumatoid cranial settling and patients with traumatic or neoplastic lesions compromising the ligamentous structures and causing instability or bone destruction.[11]

Patients presenting with findings that suggest a lesion in the OCJ should have plain X-rays of the skull and cervical spine, including an open-mouth view. Bone assimilation defects, platybasia, basilar invagination, dens defects, cranial settling, and spinal segmentation defects can all be suggested with these simple studies. MRI is the diagnostic procedure of choice because this technology allows direct imaging of the neural axis. MRI can demonstrate compressive distortion, demyelination, syringomyelia, and presence of neural tissue abnormalities, such as Chiari malformation.[4,6] Surgical treatment is tailored to the pathology of each patient as determined by these diagnostic studies.[12,13]

Contraindications

This approach is contraindicated in patients with lesions that extend rostral to pharyngeal tubercle, lesions that extend too caudally, severe spinal instability, poor wound healing capacity, and systemic instability.

The rostral limit of this exposure is the pharyngeal tubercle, which is the origin attachment of the superior pharyngeal constrictor muscle. This is on the ventral surface of the clivus at the symphysis between the basisphenoid and basiocciput. If the pathological lesion extends rostral to the pharyngeal tubercle, another route of approach should be chosen. The caudal extent of the lesion is of less concern because the approach can be modified to address lesions in the middle to lower cervical spine. However, this results in a longer segment of decompression with increased biomechanical demands on the fusion. An alternative approach or a combined retropharyngeal/posterior arthrodesis and instrumentation option should be considered. The options for arthrodesis in this region may not be mechanically adequate for severe spinal instability as a stand-alone construct. Consideration of an alternative approach or use of an adjuvant posterior fusion is appropriate. The neurologic decline is often insidious in onset, and problems in this area are typically characterized by a delay in diagnosis, resulting in patients with advanced medical and neurologic conditions. Patients with poor wound healing or severe systemic diseases may not be candidates for this approach. Would healing issues are particularly important if an intradural lesion is present or if a stand-alone anterior fusion construct is anticipated.

Advantages

- The approach provides exposure of the basiocciput of the clivus, anterior rim of foramen magnum, and rostral cervical segments of C1–C4.
- Compared with the transoral approach, this approach provides broader, more extensive exposure.
- The approach fosters better wound healing than the transoral incision because there are more tissue layers.
- Any lesion involving the ventral craniocervical junction that is approachable by the transoral route can be approached by the transcervical retropharyngeal approach.
- This is a noncontaminated route offering an advantage in avoiding infection.
- This is a safer approach for managing ventral intradural lesions at the basion and rostral cervical region, avoiding lower cranial nerves and controlling the cerebrospinal fluid (CSF). Preemptive placement of a lumbar subarachnoid drain will help to avoid CSF fistula and retropharyngeal pseudomeningocele.
- This approach enables a C1 anterior arch arthrodesis to C3 using structural support graft and instrumental screw/plate fixation for a one-stage stabilization following odontoidectomy.
- This approach offers wider exposure of the lateral mass articulations of C1 and C2 laterally and the basiocciput rostrally, which is preferable for neoplastic spinal lesions here.
- This approach is a straightforward procedure that can be mastered by any spinal surgeon familiar with the anatomy and following wide fascial exposure of sequential anatomic landmarks.
- This approach does not require specialized instruments. Most hospitals and surgeons performing anterior cervical procedures already have access to the usual retraction devices for anterior cervical spinal surgery, an operating microscope, a pneumatic high-speed drill, surgical laser, and fluoroscope.

Disadvantages

- This approach is technically more difficult than the transoral approach.
- This is a less direct approach for select pathologies (e.g., lesion of C2 dens).
- More anatomic structures are at risk during the approach.
- Most surgeons are not familiar with this approach and have reservations about using it for uncommon lesions.
- Midline orientation may be confusing because the patient's head is rotated contralateral to the perpendicular midsagittal orientation familiar to the surgeon. Attention to anatomic landmarks helps to avoid such disorientation.
- The hypoglossal nerve is usually impaired, causing speech and swallowing dysfunction for a variable period of time.

- Retraction of the superior pharyngeal constrictor muscle can lead to protracted dysphagia that may require tube feeding for up to several weeks.
- The superior laryngeal nerve is vulnerable to traction injury that can lead to voice hoarseness and risk of aspiration. This is almost always temporary but may also require transabdominal gastrojejunal tube feeding.

Choice of Operative Approach

The transoral approach has steadily gained popularity and is a viable option in many cases. This approach exploits the natural approach corridor of the oral cavity and provides an excellent surgical angle for lesions of C2. This option is not optimal, however, in cases with more laterally placed lesions or with lesions extending below C2. Also, if intradural surgery or arthrodesis and instrumentation are planned, the high anterior retropharyngeal approach is preferable. The high anterior retropharyngeal approach has been described by many authors.[14-20] Although the approach appears complex and intimidating, the skills required are similar to those needed for any anterior cervical surgery. The key to the procedure is wide, cadaveric dissection of each cervical fascial plane. This provides access to the subsequent layer with minimal retraction. These planes, when divided into layers identified by familiar structures that serve as guides, become avenues of access to the ventral OCJ and make the dissection and approach straightforward.[21,22]

Preoperative Testing

Standard preoperative testing, imaging, and appropriate medical clearances are required when planning surgery. Because many patients are significantly compromised medically and neurologically, careful attention to nutritional and respiratory issues prior to surgery will help ameliorate problems after surgery. Supportive devices, such as a surgical feeding tube or tracheostomy, can be placed electively prior to the day of the procedure. Because caloric supplementation can improve both immune function and wound healing, patients feeding access and supplemental nutritional support can be started in severely malnourished patients days or weeks prior to surgery. Patients with chronic misalignment causing compression are given a trial of cranial traction to determine if the misalignment is reducible or not. Because patients will need a halo vest postoperatively, the halo head ring can be used instead of cranial tongs. Either device can be applied after the induction of anesthesia to serve as the anchor point for traction. It is applied under local anesthesia with the patient supine, the cervical spine in extension, and the trajectory of traction dictated by specific abnormality. Achieving normal alignment usually decompresses the neuraxis. In these cases an occipitocervical fusion in the position of normal alignment is all that is needed. If traction is not successful in reducing misalignment, or reduction does not yield adequate decompression, then the anterior retropharyngeal approach is used.

Surgical Procedure

Anesthesia

Awake intubation under local topical anesthesia and fiberoptic airway visualization is recommended to avoid excessive movement of the head and neck during tracheal intubation and induction of anesthesia. If ventilator support is required for several days, an elective tracheotomy offers an early advantage in management of such patients due to pharyngeal swelling and upper airway obstruction that often accompany this procedure. Intravenous antibiotics are infused 1 hour prior to the incision and then redosed every 3 hours during the surgery.

Positioning

The patient is placed in the supine position with the head on a sponge support or horseshoe headrest and in skull traction if necessary. The head is rotated 30 degrees away from the surgeon and in extension. This head position raises the mandible up and away from the surgeon's line of sight to the field. The fluoroscope is positioned for lateral projection, and the operating microscope with laser shutter attachment is draped and available (see Video 11.1).

Incision

Various incisions have been proposed, but most cases can be adequately exposed through a transverse incision 2 cm below and parallel to the mandible, extending from the angle of the mandible to beyond the midline, taking care to avoid injuring the marginal mandibular branch of the facial nerve, which supplies the mental muscles of the lower lip (**Fig. 11.1**).[21,22]

Approach

There are three major layers of fascia in the anterior cervical area: superficial, middle, and deep. The middle and deep layers split into superficial, middle, and deep subdivisions.[23,24] The retropharyngeal approach requires dissection of these fascial planes in the submandibular triangle rostral to the hyoid bone and adjacent to the superior pharyngeal constrictor muscle, ultimately accessing the space between the vertebral bodies and the prevertebral fascia, which is limited laterally by the transverse processes and extends from the skull base to the coccyx. The key to adequate exposure is wide, "cadaveric," sharp dissection of each fascial plane, beginning with development of a wide subcutaneous flap on each side of the incision superficial to the platysma muscle (**Fig. 11.2**).[25,26] Anatomic landmarks identify each plane and guide the way. Each landmark is dissected free of its fascial sheath and preserved both anatomically and functionally. The fascia is kept taut with countertraction, using pickup forceps, as the dissection continues; this helps to define the fascial layer that is being dissected. When lifted and opened, the areolar fibrous texture of the fascia becomes evident. Its transparency provides a view of the structures it contains. Wide opening of each fascial layer in a sequential, methodical manner ensures adequate exposure of the deeper structures while preserving the intervening ones. The skin flaps can now be retracted to expose the superficial surface of the platysma muscle.

Platysma Muscle

The medial edge of the platysma is elevated in the midline, and a hole is cut in the medial fascial raphe (linea alba) to pass though the superficial to the middle fascial layer. Vertical dissection determines this layer in a cephalocaudal direction. The fascial sheet thus formed is cut longitudinally in the midline for 6 cm from the mandibular symphysis to the median notch of the superior thyroid cartilage (**Fig. 11.3**). This defines the medial edge of the platysma muscle and initiates vertical access to allow easier retraction of deeper structures. The medial edge of the platysma muscle is now elevated to dissect and free the undersurface of the platysma. This maneuver opens the middle (visceral) layer and superficial layer of the deep fascia. The platysma is then transected, in line with the primary incision. The platysma flaps thus formed are retracted.

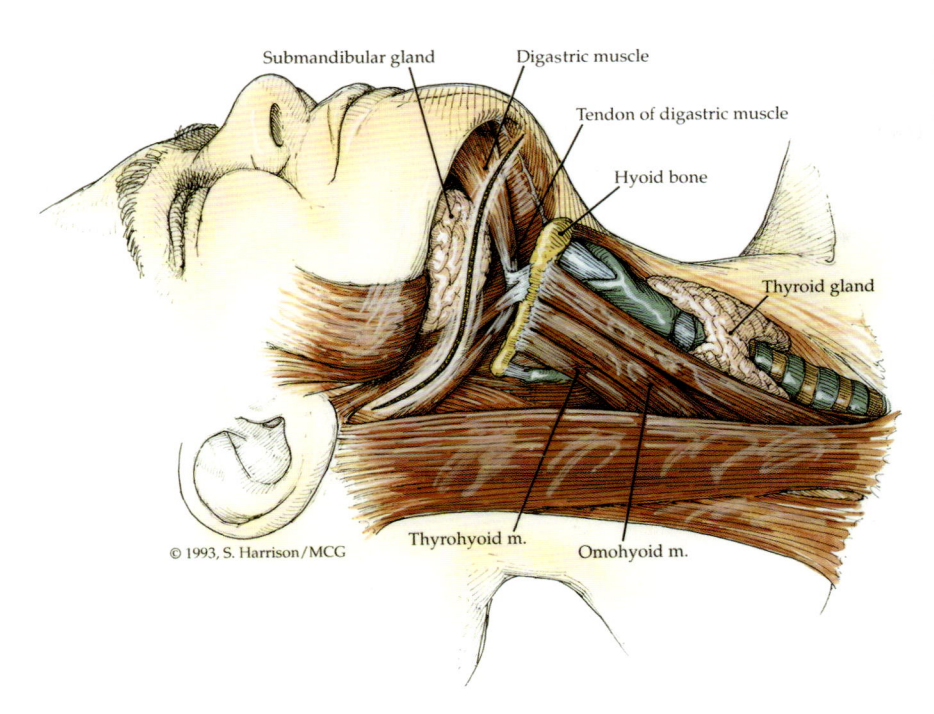

11 Retropharyngeal Approach to the Occipital-Cervical Junction, Part 1

Fig. 11.1 The patient's position is oriented with the head extended and rotated contralateral to the side of approach. The curvilinear incision is 2 cm below and parallel to the lower edge of the mandible.

Submandibular Gland

The next fascial layer is identified by the submandibular gland, which bulges under the superficial layer of the deep cervical fascia (**Fig. 11.4**). The inferior edge of the gland is elevated. The fascial capsule is opened, undermined, and dissected in line with the incision. The facial artery and vein are dissected along their course. This maneuver further opens this fascial plane. The facial vein is transected. The facial artery is preserved. Dissection of the facial artery proximally leads to the reflection of the alar fascia as it forms the carotid sheath and the lateral limit of this exposure. The facial artery is dissected and retracted with the submandibular gland superiorly to expose the next landmark—the tendon of the digastric muscle.

Digastric Muscle and Tendon

The tendon of the digastric muscle is identified as a glistening white cord running parallel to the course of the incision beneath the inferior edge of the submandibular gland. This leads to the

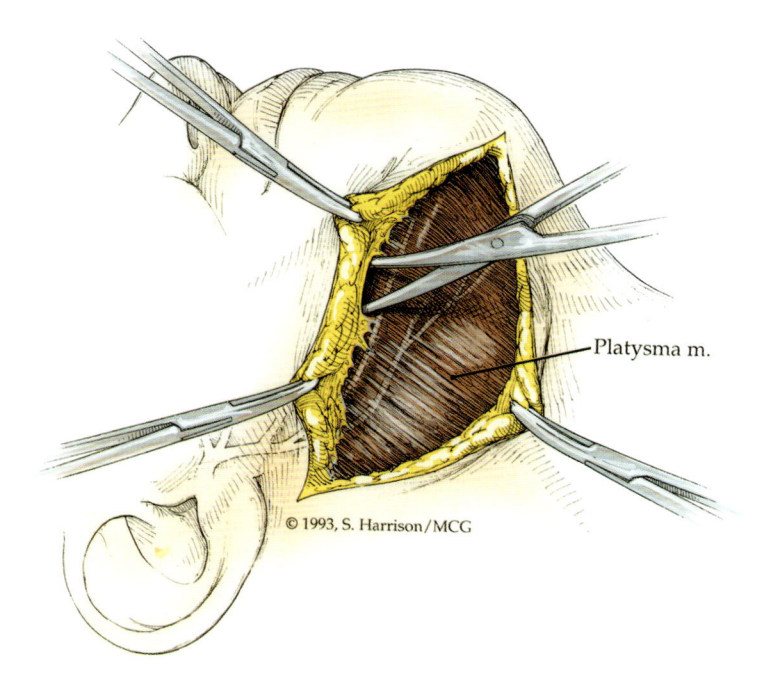

Fig. 11.2 Wide dissection of the subcutaneous layer opens the most superficial layer of the cervical fascia, exposing the outer surface of the platysma muscle. Care is taken to avoid injury to the mental branch of the facial nerve, which can cause a droop of the ipsilateral lower lip.

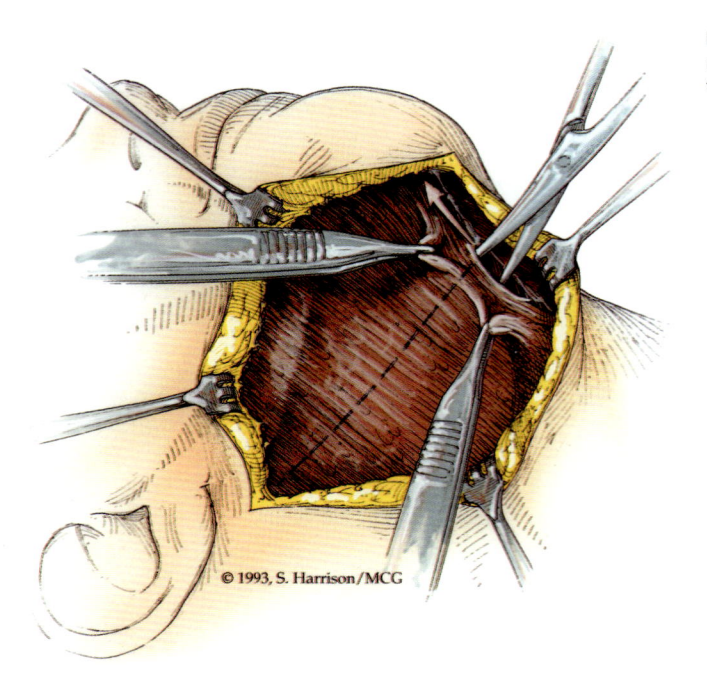

Fig. 11.3 The medial border of the platysma muscle is found at the midline and split vertically from the mental symphysis to the notch of the thyroid cartilage; this initiates access to the next fascial layer.

next fascial layer. A fascial sling tethers this tendon to the greater wing of the hyoid bone. By transecting this fascial sling along the course of the tendon, the tendon is freed and retracted rostrally toward the mandible. This retraction is facilitated by freeing the undersurface of the anterior and posterior digastric muscle bellies. This then exposes the next fascial plane. The hypoglossal nerve comes into view coursing just deep, slightly inferior, and parallel to the digastric tendon.

Hypoglossal Nerve

The hypoglossal nerve is gently dissected along its course and is carefully preserved (**Fig. 11.5**). Posterolaterally the dissection is carried along the nerve trunk toward the descending hypoglossal ramus, which is another guide to the region of the carotid artery. Again, it is not necessary to dissect along the medial border of the carotid sheath unless segments caudal to C4 are to be

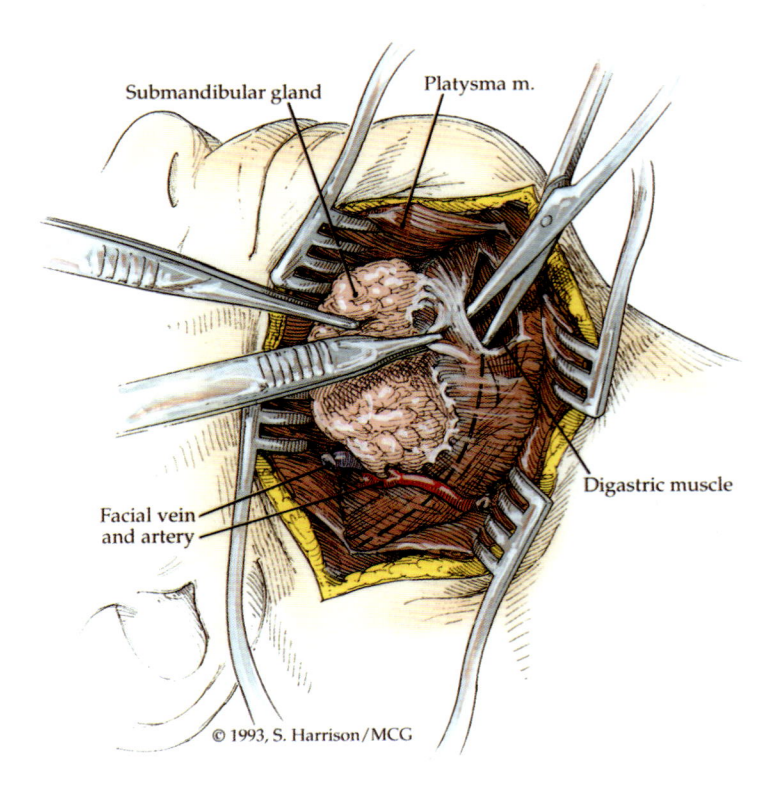

Fig. 11.4 The platysma muscle is transected; lifting the tissues with grasping forceps and applying countertraction assists with the dissection. This exposes the next fascial layer. Retraction of the platysma flaps exposes the submandibular gland as well as the facial artery and vein. Dissection of these structures opens the next layer of cervical fascia. The anterior belly of the digastric muscle is exposed when the facial vein is transected and the submandibular gland is elevated and retracted superiorly.

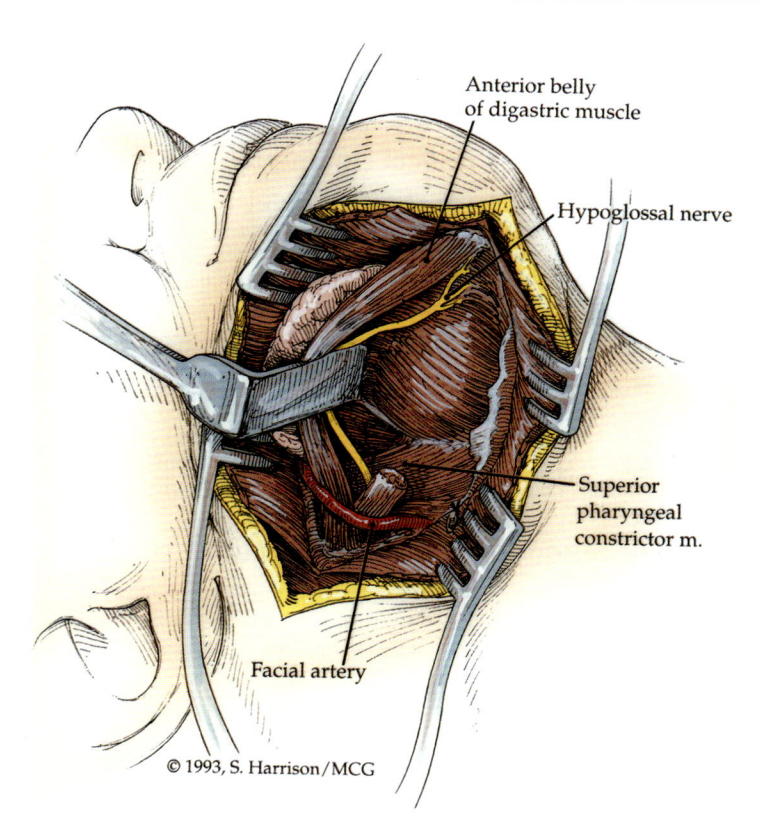

Fig. 11.5 Transecting the fascial investment of the digastric muscle exposes and frees the next landmark and opens the next layer of cervical fascia. The digastric tendon is separated from its fascial sling at the hyoid bone and retracted superiorly. This exposes the hypoglossal nerve, the next landmark, and the next layer of cervical fascia. Dissection of the hypoglossal nerve opens this layer of cervical fascia and enables retraction of the nerve to expose the next landmark, the greater cornu of the hyoid bone. Opening the fascia along the hyoid bone exposes the lateral wall of the superior pharyngeal constrictor muscle.

exposed. Thus freed, the hypoglossal nerve is retracted superiorly, exposing the hyoglossus muscle. The greater cornu of the hyoid bone now comes into view.

Hyoid Bone

The greater cornu of the hyoid bone can now be seen and palpated. The fascia overlying it is opened along the course of the hyoid bone to the carotid sheath. The carotid artery is easily palpated and is the lateralmost limit of this dissection. It is retracted laterally. This maneuver opens the retropharyngeal space. It is not necessary to cut any muscles, nerves, or vessels. The superior laryngeal nerve (SLN) is vulnerable to injury at this juncture. The SLN courses deep to the internal carotid artery along the middle pharyngeal constrictor muscle toward the superior cornu of the hyoid bone and adjacent to the superior pharyngeal constrictor muscle. The SLN is not seen in the dissection of this approach. However, the SLN can be injured by stretch from retraction. Wide dissection of the fascial planes as described here should tend to protect the SLN from retraction injury because less force is required to separate the tissues that are freed by wide fascial dissection. The SLN is not involved in the soft tissues retracted superiorly for this exposure. It would be more vulnerable to injury if the deep cervical fascia were opened inferiorly in the lateral exposure. If access below C2 is needed, the SLN is identified and preserved; a separate approach to the lower cervical segments is then made.

Superior Pharyngeal Constrictor Muscle

The pharyngeal constrictor muscles are retracted medially by a deep, right-angled retractor. The retropharyngeal areolar tissue, comprising the alar and prevertebral fasciae, is opened with scissors. The anterior surfaces of C2 and C3 are easily palpated. The prominence of the anterior tubercle of C1 is palpated and is the focus of rostral orientation. The midline of the cervical spine orients the midsagittal plane identified between the longus colli and longus capitis muscles (**Fig. 11.6**).

Longus Colli–Capitis Muscles

The converging medial boarders of the longus colli muscles are cauterized and elevated from the anterolateral surfaces of C2 and C3 by sharp dissection. The retractor blade engaged along the dissected muscle border is used to separate the longus colli muscles. This preliminary soft tissue retraction initiates access to deep structures. The microscope is adjusted to the field. A quick glimpse with the fluoroscope in the lateral projection will assist the surgical orientation. The potassium titanium oxide phosphate (KTP 586) or CO_2 laser is advantageous, but not mandatory, in separating the longus colli and longus capitis muscles from their medial attachments. Laser dissection facilitates the exposure of the anterior arch of C1 and the atlas and axis lateral mass articulations. It enables muscle separation up to the pharyngeal tubercle of the basiocciput (**Fig. 11.7**). View of these most rostral structures requires rostral retraction using a deep, narrow, right-angled retractor blade. This retraction is critical for exposure and access. The medial half of the C1 and C2 lateral masses and anterior rim of the foramen magnum and the basiocciput rostral to the anterior arch of C1 should be in view before proceeding.

Median Tubercle C1 Anterior Arch

The C1 anterior tubercle is a guide, which helps to maintain orientation with the midsagittal plane. The surgeon's perspective to the field is upward and angled 45 degrees. The C1 arch, base of dens, pre-dens space, and lateral mass articulations are seen

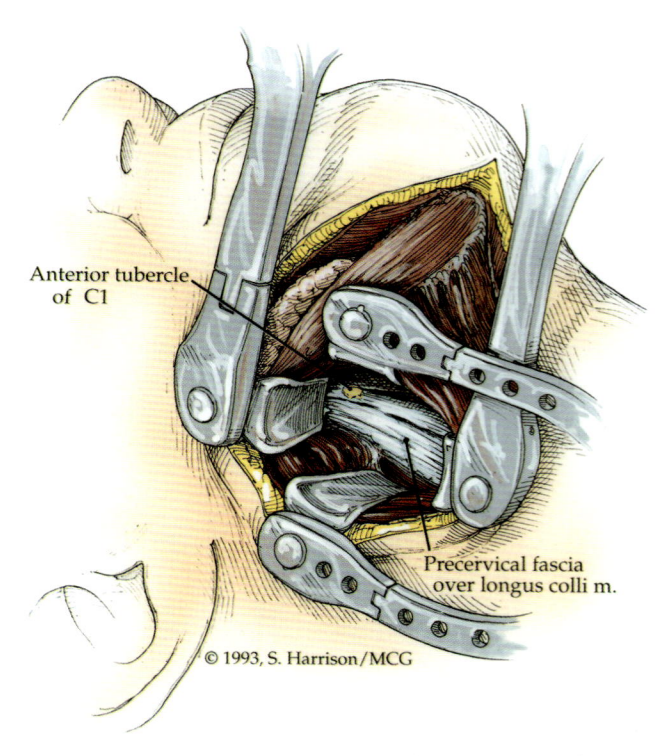

Fig. 11.6 Retraction of the superior pharyngeal constrictor opens the retropharyngeal space and exposes the alar fascia, precervical fascia, and longus colli muscles. The anterior tubercle of C1 identifies the midline.

(**Fig. 11.8**). Laser removal of overlying soft tissue clears the view. The dens, body of C2, and atlantotransverse ligament can be removed without removing the anterior arch of C1 if so desired.

Transverse Cervical Ligament

The transverse ligament is a tough, rather thick, delineated, pale yellow, ligamentous belt behind the dens. The ligament comes into view after the dens has been resected (**Fig. 11.9**). It is a guide after the C1 arch and odontoid have been removed because they may be obscured by the destructive changes of disease. The dura may be densely adherent to the posterior surface of the transverse ligament and adjacent tectorial membrane. Sharp microdissection of the tectorial membrane is necessary to separate it from the underlying dura. Active bleeding from epidural veins can be troublesome but is ultimately controlled by bipolar coagulation and packing with topical hemostatic material. The dura is vulnerable to laceration at this juncture.

Anterior Rim Foramen Magnum

The anterior rim of the foramen magnum and caudal basiocciput can be palpated and seen between the attachments of the longus capitis muscles. These attachments can be separated to expose the bony elements for removal if required.

Clival/Pharyngeal Tubercle

The pharyngeal tubercle is the rostral limit of this exposure. A hole drilled into the clivus rostral to the anterior rim can serve as an anchor site for rostral soft tissue retraction, as illustrated in

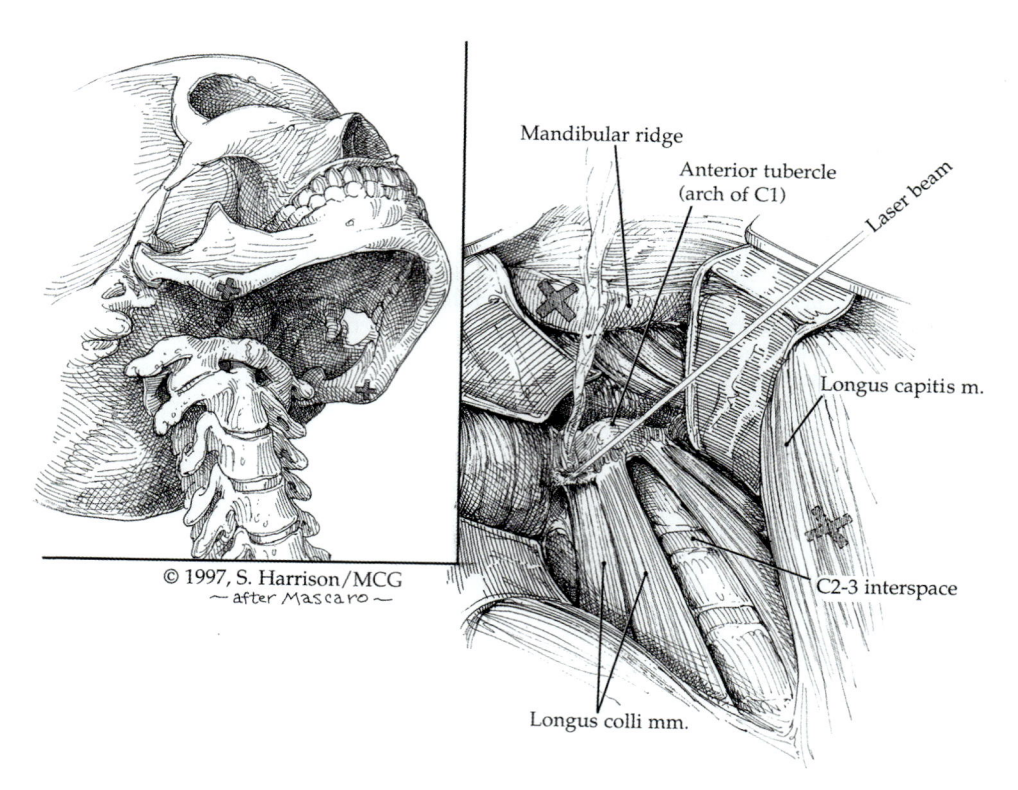

Fig. 11.7 The longus colli muscles are dissected from the arch of C1 and the anterior surface of C2 and C3. The laser, controlled through the microscope attachment, facilitates this dissection. The surgeon's perspective is rotated 30 degrees and in a rostrally oblique direction, and constant attention to this is required to maintain correct orientation.

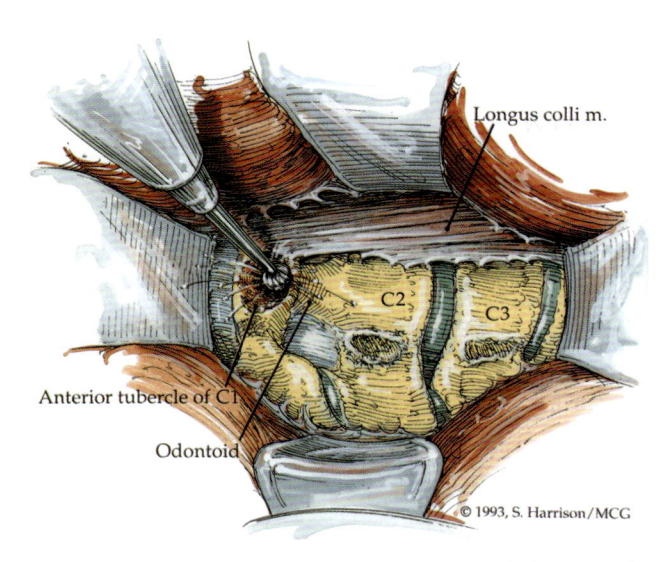

Fig. 11.8 The anterior arch of C1 is being removed, which exposes the dens. The dens is best drilled away from its apex toward its base.

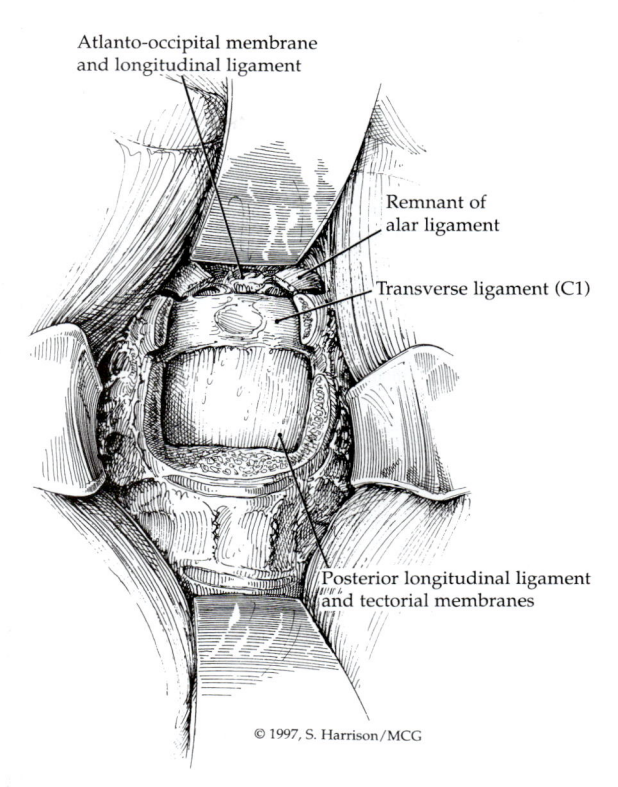

Fig. 11.9 The transverse ligament is the next landmark. It is identified as a thick fibrous transverse band. It may be obscured by chronic inflammation and scarring. The transverse ligament along with the posterior longitudinal ligament must be removed to adequately decompress the neural axis.

the next chapter. This bone ridge can also be drilled away if necessary for lesion exposure or neural decompression.

Bone Resection: C2 Corpectomy with or Without Resection of the Anterior Arch of C1

With this approach, the rotated and extended head position can confuse the surgeon's orientation. The ipsilateral C1-C2 lateral mass articulation is more forward and can be mistaken for the anterior arch of C1, leading to disorientation. The surgeon must keep these perspectives in mind while using this approach. The anatomy of this region has been well described and must be familiar to the surgeon.[27] A high-speed, pneumatic drill with cutting bur is used to begin the bone removal for the C2 corpectomy (**Fig. 11.8**). The dens is removed beginning at the apex, working caudally, keeping the base intact for control and orientation. Otherwise the tip of the dens can become disconnected and the freely mobile bone could cause injury to underlying structures while being removed.

After the bone has been thinned like an eggshell, a diamond bur can then be used to complete the removal and reduce the risk of injury of adjacent tissues. The medial wall of the lateral masses can be removed to widen the ventral exposure; this is helpful if the lesion is intradural. If the anterior arch of C1 is involved in the pathological process, it can be removed prior to the corpectomy to enhance visualization. However, the caudal-to-rostral trajectory of the surgeon's perspective offered by this approach enables the resection of the deep landmark structures described to be accomplished and still preserve the anterior arch of C1. This orients the midline and can buttress a strut graft between the C1 arch and the superior epiphysis of C3. In select cases, removing just the inferior edge of the anterior arch of C1 can enhance the view of the dens and adjacent articulations. Partial removal of the arch of C1 can be done with caution. Overzealous partial resection of the arch of C1 can undermine its mechanical integrity and prevent its use as the superior anchor point for a C1–C3 arthrodesis. The C2-C3 disk must also be removed. Care must be taken to ensure that the cartilaginous end plate is completely resected. A dental mirror can help with visualization because the superior end plate of C3 angles away from the surgeon's line of site. If additional levels require removal, then they would be resected at this time. The transverse ligament is identified for orientation (**Fig. 11.9**).

Transverse Ligament and Tectorial Membranes

The transverse ligament combines the tectorial membrane along with the apical bursa, cruciform, and tectorial ligaments to form a composite of the posterior longitudinal ligament. This must be separated from the dura and removed. The laser allows "no-touch" removal of these structures. These ligaments and pannus can be thick, tough, and adherent in cases of long-standing instability at C1-C2. The anterior rim of the foramen magnum can now be removed if needed.

The surgical procedure, postoperative care, and potential complications and precautions are discussed in the next chapter.

References

1. Hadley MN, Spetzler RF, Sonntag VKH. The transoral approach to the superior cervical spine. A review of 53 cases of extradural cervicomedullary compression. J Neurosurg 1989;71:16–23
2. Miller E, Crockard HA. Transoral transclival removal of anteriorly placed meningiomas at the foramen magnum. Neurosurgery 1987;20:966–968

3. VanGilder J, Menezes A, Dolan K, eds. The Craniovertebral Junction and Its Abnormalities. Mount Kisco, NY: Futura; 1987
4. Han JS, Benson JE, Yoon YS. Magnetic resonance imaging in the spinal column and craniovertebral junction. Radiol Clin North Am 1984;22:805–827
5. Hinck VC, Hopkins CE, Savara BS. Diagnostic criteria of basilar impression. Radiology 1961;76:572–585
6. Smoker WRK, Keyes WD, Dunn VD, Menezes AH. MRI versus conventional radiologic examinations in the evaluation of the craniovertebral and cervicomedullary junction. Radiographics 1986;6:953–994
7. Stevens JM, Kendall BE, Crockard HA. The spinal cord in rheumatoid arthritis with clinical myelopathy: a computed myelographic study. J Neurol Neurosurg Psychiatry 1986;49:140–151
8. Santavirta S, Slätis P, Kankaanpää U, Sandelin J, Laasonen E. Treatment of the cervical spine in rheumatoid arthritis. J Bone Joint Surg Am 1988;70:658–667
9. Menezes AH, VanGilder JC, Clark CR, el-Khoury G. Odontoid upward migration in rheumatoid arthritis. An analysis of 45 patients with "cranial settling". J Neurosurg 1985;63:500–509
10. Meyer FB, Ebersold MJ, Reese DF. Benign tumors of the foramen magnum. J Neurosurg 1984;61:136–142
11. Phillips E, Levine AM. Metastatic lesions of the upper cervical spine. Spine 1989;14:1071–1077
12. Menezes AH, VanGilder JC, Graf CJ, McDonnell DE. Craniocervical abnormalities. A comprehensive surgical approach. J Neurosurg 1980;53:444–455
13. Hsu W, Wolinsky JP, Gokaslan ZL, Sciubba DM. Transoral approaches to the cervical spine. Neurosurgery 2010;66(3, Suppl):119–125
14. de Andrade JR, Macnab I. Anterior occipito-cervical fusion using an extrapharyngeal exposure. J Bone Joint Surg Am 1969;51:1621–1626
15. Grieshaber DC, Ball EA, Summers LE, Dafford KC, Melgar MA. Retropharyngeal/anterolateral approach for C2 corpectomy. J La State Med Soc 2009;161:160–164
16. Lesoin F, Autricque A, Franz K, Villette L, Jomin M. Transcervical approach and screw fixation for upper cervical spine pathology. Surg Neurol 1987;27:459–465
17. McAfee PC, Bohlman HH, Riley LH Jr, Robinson RA, Southwick WO, Nachlas NE. The anterior retropharyngeal approach to the upper part of the cervical spine. J Bone Joint Surg Am 1987;69:1371–1383
18. Park SH, Sung JK, Lee SH, Park J, Hwang JH, Hwang SK. High anterior cervical approach to the upper cervical spine. Surg Neurol 2007;68:519–524, discussion 524
19. Singh H, Harrop J, Schiffmacher P, Rosen M, Evans J. Ventral surgical approaches to craniovertebral junction chordomas. Neurosurgery 2010;66(3, Suppl):96–103
20. Whitesides TE Jr, McDonald AP. Lateral retropharyngeal approach to the upper cervical spine. Orthop Clin North Am 1978;9:1115–1127
21. Vardiman AB, Dickman CA, Sonntag VKH. The modified anterolateral retropharyngeal approach to the craniovertebral junction: anatomic and practical considerations. BNI Q 1994;10:26–34
22. McDonnell DE, Harrison SJ. Lateral approach to the craniocervical complex. Tech Neurosurg 1998;4:306–318
23. Grodinsky M, Holyoke E. The fasciae and fascial spaces of the head, neck, and adjacent regions. Am J Anat 1938;63:367–408
24. Pernkopf E. Topography of the neck. In: Ferner H, ed. Atlas of Topographical and Applied Human Anatomy, vol 1. Philadelphia: WB Saunders; 1963:232–273
25. Haller JM, Iwanik M, Shen FH. Clinically relevant anatomy of high anterior cervical approach. Spine 2011;36:2116–2121
26. Russo VM, Graziano F, Russo A, Albanese E, Ulm AJ. High anterior cervical approach to the clivus and foramen magnum: a microsurgical anatomy study. Neurosurgery 2011;69(1, Suppl Operative):ons103–ons114, discussion ons115–ons116
27. de Oliveira E, Rhoton AL Jr, Peace D. Microsurgical anatomy of the region of the foramen magnum. Surg Neurol 1985;24:293–352

12 Retropharyngeal Approach to the Occipital-Cervical Junction, Part 2

John R. Vender, Steven J. Harrison, and Dennis E. McDonnell

The high anterior cervical approach provides the option to place a fusion mass and anterior plate-and-screw instrumentation. Arthrodesis can be performed between the anterior arch of C1 or the clivus and the superior epiphysis of C3. Arthrodesis can also extend below C3 if more caudal levels of decompression are required. This is advantageous in many cases because the instability resulting from the pathological process or the decompression can be addressed in the same setting via the same surgical approach. If the spine has already been stabilized posteriorly, then only a decompression is required. In either case, the closure of the high anterior cervical retropharyngeal wound is very straightforward because only fascial planes are opened. Soft tissue structures resume normal anatomic alignment when the retraction is removed. However, there are several preemptive steps in the closure that can reduce the risk of the complications that can accompany this approach.

Indications

General indications for the high anterior cervical approach were discussed in Chapter 11. The option of also performing an arthrodesis and instrumentation during the same surgical session must be considered based on specific patient-related issues and the pathological process. An anterior arthrodesis is appropriate in patients with chronic or glacial instability rather than gross instability, in patients without medical conditions or therapies that undermine bone fusion, and in patients with adequate C1 arch structure to support fusion. Conditions such as occipitocervical osseous anomalies of developmental origin, primary or metastatic neoplasm, fractures, cranial settling, and some inflammatory conditions can be consistent with successful anterior arthrodesis.

Contraindications

Contraindications to anterior arthrodesis include extensive lesions that compromise or destroy the arch of C1, and cases where there is limited bone access for fusion if extensive lesions or gross instability are present. Advanced osteoporosis and inflammatory conditions such as rheumatoid arthritis limit the option of a C1–C3 fusion in some cases. Decisions can be made intraoperatively as to whether or not adequate structure exists to safely perform an arthrodesis. An infected field (i.e., retropharyngeal abscess) is a relative contraindication. Although instrumentation can be placed into infected fields, the limited amount of bone structure, the large volume of graft (sequestrum), and the adjacent cervicomedullary junction increase the risk of problems with this approach.

Advantages

- This approach provides exposure of the basiocciput of the clivus, anterior rim of foramen magnum, and rostral cervical segments of C1–C4.
- Compared with the transoral approach, this approach provides broader, more extensile exposure.
- This approach fosters better wound healing than the transoral incision because more layers are involved.
- The noncontaminated field helps to avoid infection—a distinct advantage if the dura has been entered or if there is a cerebrospinal fluid (CSF) leak.
- The dura can be closed more directly with this approach; a fibrin glue closure will not be diluted by exposure to saliva or other oral secretions.
- Direct C1 to C3 arthrodesis using a structural strut graft between the anterior arch of C1 (preserved by using this approach) and the superior epiphysis of C3 can be placed and internally fixed using a screw/plate construct through the anterior arch of C1 and the body of C3.
- This approach offers the possibility of a single-stage closure and internal fixation of an unstable craniovertebral junction in the context of destabilizing pathology or following a surgically destabilizing procedure.

Disadvantages

- This approach is technically more difficult than the transoral approach.
- It is a less direct approach for some pathologies (e.g., lesion of C2 dens).
- More anatomic structures are at risk during this approach.
- Upper airway edema can cause mechanical obstruction, interfering with adequate ventilation so that intubation with mechanical ventilator support may be required for several days.
- Superior constrictor dyspraxia can result in debilitating dysphagia that requires tube feeding of liquid formula to maintain adequate nutrition.
- Hypoglossal nerve, superior laryngeal nerve (SLN), and glossal pharyngeal nerve dysfunction can occur from retraction and may persist for several weeks. Such functional sequelae are almost always temporary but can be a serious debilitating addition to the patient's overall condition.

Surgical Procedure
Complete Neural Decompression

For neurologic function to recover from mechanical compression, the compression has to be effectively removed. Adequate neuraxis decompression is ensured when the ventral surface of the dura bulges into the opened corpectomy defect (**Fig. 12.1**). The dura may be transparent enough to reveal pial surface vessels and cord pulsation. As a further confirmatory measure, contrast can be injected into the corpectomy defect, and a lateral fluoroscopic image can confirm that there are no filling defects, thus providing confirmation that all compression has been addressed. Bleeding from dural venous sinuses and epidural veins in this region can be particularly challenging. The usual techniques of bipolar electrocoagulation, topical collagen fiber, thrombin and gelatin foam, gentle tamponade with cotton pledgets, and patience are used for hemostasis.

Retraction

Adequate retraction is required to efficiently accomplish the goals, and fully exploit the advantages, of this approach. Criticisms of this approach refer to the deep, narrow, off-midline access, which can be overcome by retraction and the surgical microscope. A narrow 90-degree angled retractor helps to lift the soft tissues rostrally initially. The deep blades of the Cloward (Codman, Randolph, MA) or Caspar (Aesculap, San Francisco, CA) self-retaining retraction systems are adequate for retraction of the longus capitis muscles. The table-mounted Thompson-Farley (Thompson, Traverse City, MI) retraction system is a useful alternative instrument for retraction of rostral and medial soft tissues.[1] We prefer a modified Taylor-type retractor that is secured in an anchor hole drilled into the clivus just rostral to the anterior rim of the foramen magnum (**Fig. 12.1**). The handle of this retractor is secured to the surgical drapes using elastic bands with a Kocher forceps gripping the sheets through an ether screen support mounted at the table head. The retractor can also be seated against the superior surface of the anterior arch of C1. This may need to be done early in the dissection before the clivus is adequately visualized. However, the downward force of the retractor against C1 will reorient the arch inferiorly enough to impair visualization when the corpectomy and other decompressive procedures are being performed. To avoid needless resection of the inferior part of the arch of C1, the retractor can be relocated to the clivus.[2,3]

Dural Closure

The dura usually cannot be closed primarily here.[4] An autograft fascia lata or allograft fascia is tacked to the dural edge at multiple sites using a rigid, semicircular cutting needle. The P-2 Ethicon needle (Johnson & Johnson, Somerville, NJ) or the PR-1 needle (Davis and Geck, Wayne, NJ) is useful for suturing in tight spaces. The suture size is 5-0 polydioxanone, which is used for traction suture and dural patch closure. This can also be supplemented with fibrin glue or any commercially available dural sealant. Cryoprecipitate can be applied topically over the graft, which is then sprayed with thrombin. This produces a thick coagulum that augments the dural repair seal.[4,5] Composite baffles of fascia lata and a small bone plate have also been described in successfully closing the defect transorally by wedging the bone plate behind the cranial spinal bone defect.[6]

Intraoperative Craniovertebral Stabilization

Spinal stabilization is important to consider in preoperative planning because all patients have stability issues due to either the pathological process or the decompressive procedures performed. Intraoperative cranial traction is best achieved with the use of the halo head ring because conversion to a halo orthosis is anticipated after surgery. However, if the surgeon prefers, standard cranial tongs can be also be used prior to the procedure. Light traction with 5 to 10 lb is maintained throughout the procedure. Care must be taken when determining how much weight is required because craniovertebral junction stability is often compromised. A rope attached to the traction device is hung over an ether screen support frame and the angle adjusted, as the surgeon requires. In cases where stability remains a concern postoperatively, traction can be maintained as a temporizing measure after the procedure until the final posterior stabilization is achieved. The option of placing an osseous fusion in situ is one of the advantages of this approach. Several anterior fusion and instrumentation options have been developed. The C1-C2 lateral masses can be exposed and are available for interarticular arthrodesis by bone graft insert or transarticular screw. An intact C1 anterior arch can be used as an anchoring site for a notched strut graft to purchase (**Fig. 12.2**). These alternatives imply that the atlanto-occipital articulation is intact, and this must be determined prior to fashioning the fusion construct. Otherwise the occiput must be included in the arthrodesis, which can be tenuous from this anterior approach for lack of a solid anchoring site rostrally into the clivus.[7–9] Occipitocervical arthrodesis is performed as a subsequent procedure if there is occipitocervical instability.

Primary C1 Arch to C3 Strut Arthrodesis

The lateral retropharyngeal approach enables complete resection of the C2/odontoid complex, including the adjacent ligaments, while maintaining the anterior arch of C1. This still leads to in-

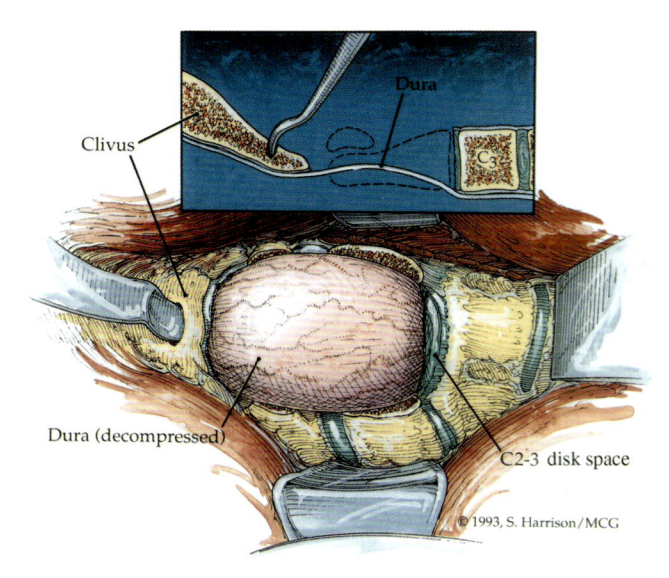

Fig. 12.1 Bulging of the dura into the resection site ensures adequate decompression. Note the position of the retractor point that has been inserted into a drill hole within the clivus. The area surrounded by the dashed lines represent the anterior arch of C1 and the odontoid and vertebral body of C2 that are resected during this approach.

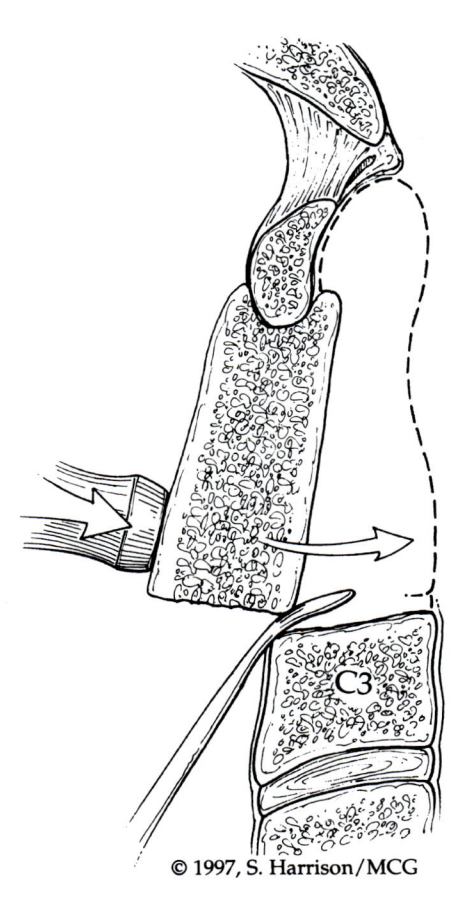

Fig. 12.2 A tricorticate bone graft from the iliac crest is measured and notched transversely across the rostral end so that it will accept the anterior arch of C1. The caudal end of the graft is wedged into position over the superior epiphysis of C3 using a 5-mm curved osteotome as a prying lever and a bone mallet to position the graft.

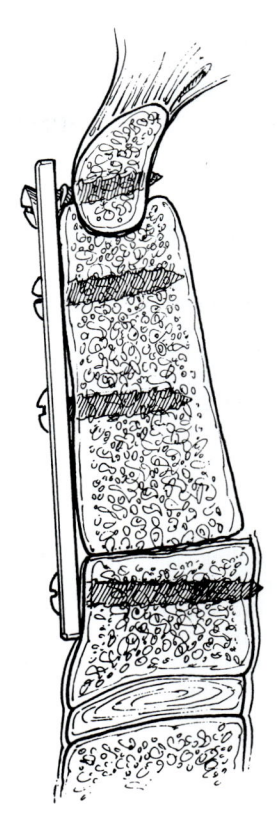

Fig. 12.3 A Caspar titanium plate is positioned and secured using bicorticate screw purchase into the anterior arch of C1 and body of C3. An autograft or allograft of iliac bone crest can be used as the strut graft between C1 and C2.

herent instability that must be addressed.[10] The interval between the inferior edge of the anterior arch of C1 and the superior end plate of C3 is measured with a caliper. Because the arch of C1 is typically mobile, it is important to size the graft with the arch in a neutral position to avoid under- or oversizing the graft. A tricorticate iliac crest strut or allograft humerus strut is notched at the cephalic end so that the notch engages the anterior C1 arch. The flat caudal end of the graft is then levered into position over the superior epiphyseal surface of the C3 body. A narrow curved osteotome can serve as the lever and be worked like a shoehorn to position the lower end of the graft to effect a "press fit" of the construct (**Fig. 12.2**). Manual traction on the mandible or skull tongs can assist in placement of the graft. This is then secured with a screw-plate fixation device. Nonrigid bicortical screw fixation through the graft and C1 arch and C3 body is preferred because the screws can be angled as needed. The Caspar plate (Aesculap, San Francisco, CA) has been used with success (**Fig. 12.3**). Either autograft or allograft bone can be used depending on individual patient requirements. Allograft tibia or humerus has been found to be about the correct dimensional width and affords circumferential cortical bone to bolster the strength of the support strut. The medullary cavity is first cleared of trabecular bone and packed with autogenous bone from the resected C2 body, if appropriate, or iliac crest to facilitate bone fusion.[11]

Postoperative Care

Airway Management

Awake tracheal intubation under local anesthesia is frequently required to avoid manipulation of the patient's neck and the risk of further neurologic injury. Preemptive tracheotomy is the preferred tactic when the patient is immobilized by myelopathic quadriparesis. Upper airway obstruction caused by soft tissue swelling in the postoperative period is a major consideration with this procedure, particularly with myelopathic and debilitated patients. To ensure a competent upper airway, endotracheal intubation may be required for several days with the patient in a head-up position until the edema resolves. A positive end-expiratory pressure of 5 cm H_2O on the ventilator tends to prevent atelectasis. Nursing the patient in a rotokinetic bed can assist with pulmonary drainage in selected patients.

Nutritional Support

Optimal nutrition is important to the recovery of any stressed patient. Often patients who have chronic myelopathy are already nutritionally depleted. The pharyngeal and upper airway edema that occurs following this procedure impedes swallowing for several days or even weeks. Maintenance of the metabolic balance is facilitated by preoperative placement of a feeding gastrostomy/jejunostomy to ensure enteric alimentation. Effectively supplying nutritional support helps to avoid mucosal bacterial translocation and sepsis; it also helps to promote earlier rehabilitation of these patients. With patients who are already debilitated by their disease prior to surgical treatment, preemptive placement of some form of enteric access is advisable. This would enable enteric nutritional support from the very beginning of the patient's convalescence.

Cerebrospinal Fluid Diversion

In cases where intradural surgery is planned a lumbar drain can be placed prior to positioning to control CSF intraoperatively to facilitate the surgery as well as to provide CSF diversion postoperatively. If a durotomy occurs during the surgery, it is recommended to place a drain postoperatively to reduce the risk of pseudomeningocele or CSF fistula. The catheter can be placed percutaneously via a Tuohy needle. By tunneling the catheter several centimeters using the Tuohy needle, the life span of the drain can be dramatically extended. CSF diversion into an external collection system is an effective prophylaxis for pseudomeningocele and external CSF cutaneous fistula as well as to enhance wound healing. The drainage can be controlled by volume or pressure regulation at the discretion of the treating surgeon. Excessive drainage of CSF can lead to intracranial hypotension and headache. Inadequate drainage can increase CSF pressure against the dural repair and create a CSF fistula. CSF drainage should be monitored closely to avoid complications of this maneuver. One alternative that has enhanced the success of drainage in our patients is the use of closed, continuous drainage. This is performed using a computerized intravenous (IV) pump to remove a predetermined amount of CSF per hour while avoiding the "peaks and valleys" of CSF pressure and volume inherent in traditional drainage methods. Drainage via this technique is started at 8 mL per hour and then gradually titrated over the first day to 12 to 14 mL per hour. In most patients this is well tolerated. Low-pressure headache may require reduction in hourly drainage volume to meet the patient's tolerance level. This technique of CSF diversion has all but eliminated lumbar CSF drainage complications.[12]

Spinal Stabilization

In patients in whom an anterior decompression was not immediately followed by either an anterior or posterior arthrodesis, traction can be used as a temporizing measure in the neurologic intensive care unit (ICU), pending a second posterior procedure. External orthoses, such as a halo brace, are usually not adequate as the sole source of stability after this procedure. In cases where arthrodesis is performed and instrumentation is placed, the halo head ring is connected to the halo vest. Halo orthosis supplemental stabilization is continued for 3 months. Anteroposterior and lateral radiographs are taken monthly to confirm the stability of the construct. At 3 months the head ring is released from the vest, and flexion/extension radiographs are taken. If there is no movement, then the halo is removed and the patient is managed in a rigid cervical collar for 6 weeks. If movement is present, then the vest is reattached to the head ring and the patient undergoes 6 additional weeks of stabilization. If instability persists at that point, then the patient undergoes an elective posterior cervical or occipitocervical fusion.

Potential Complications and Precautions

Complications associated with the high anterior retropharyngeal approach include dysphagia, CSF leak/pseudomeningocele, non-union of the arthrodesis, fracture of the arch of C1, deep wound infection, hypoglossal nerve palsy, and hoarseness of the voice. All patients complain of dysphagia to some degree immediately postoperatively; it clears spontaneously within 1 to 2 weeks of surgery in most patients. Persistent dysphagia requires long-term gastrojejunal enteric tube feeding. Persistent dysphagia is ascribed to dysfunctional contractility of the upper pharynx and probably a stretch injury to the SLN. This risk can be minimized with wide release of the fascial planes, thus minimizing the degree and force of retraction needed for visualization. Prolonged dysphagia will ultimately resolve as well, and the feeding access can be removed after a caloric intake assessment confirms adequate oral intake. CSF fistula and pseudomeningoceles are usually successfully controlled with the use of the lumbar subarachnoid drain. In refractory cases a lumboperitoneal shunt can provide long-term control. Nonunion is a particular concern in patients with abnormal bone physiology due to advanced inflammatory conditions as well as ongoing immunolytic and steroid medical therapies.

Some patients complain of persistent pain or regression toward their preoperative neurologic baseline. Close clinical and radiographic observation will identify the problem. In these cases a posterior fusion and instrumentation procedure is the solution. Fracture of the arch of C1 occurs in rare cases when the arch, although preserved, is not structurally adequate, resulting in rostral migration of the strut. This emphasizes the importance of avoiding or minimizing resection of the inferior portion of the arch during exposure. Removal of the strut is required and a posterior fusion and instrumentation can be performed, typically at the same session. The use of implanted or exogenously applied bone stimulation devices can be used at the discretion of the surgeon.

Deep wound infections are uncommon. They can be managed with irrigation and debridement followed by a course of closed irrigation, with the placement of a closed wound irrigation system in conjunction with intravenous antibiotics. The closed wound irrigation technique is very effective in clearing infection while preserving the fusion mass and instrumentation.[13]

Most patients will develop an ipsilateral hypoglossal nerve palsy with hemiglossal atrophy. This will improve but will remain evident on clinical examination even after several years. However, it is unusual for patients to complain of glossal dysfunction. Voice hoarseness caused by SLN dysfunction can occur but typically resolves in most patients. Careful dissection leading to reduced retraction force is the best way to minimize this injury.[14] Patients are referred to an otolaryngologist for assessment of aspiration risk and to determine if any procedures are warranted.

Conclusion

The retropharyngeal approach to the occipitocervical junction is predicated on careful and complete dissection of sequential layers of cervical fascia investing the submandibular triangle. Intraoperative use of the operative microscope and lateral projection fluoroscopy improves the surgeon's vision and orientation throughout this procedure. This procedure offers a wider exposure with more versatility and safety than the transoral route to this region. Laser facilitates dissection of the thick ligaments and muscle/tendon insertions that otherwise add to the difficulty of surgically exposing the deep structures available with this approach. The complication of dural CSF leakage is easily managed by a shunting procedure, with minimal risk of infection or meningitis. Potential complications can be reduced by preemptive measures such as preoperative tracheostomy, placement of transcutaneous enteric access, anterior stabilization utilizing the preserved C1 anterior arch, and preoperative percutaneous lumbar CSF drainage. Chronic rheumatoid arthritis and long-term immunosuppressive drug therapy are conditions that put patients at higher risk for complications with this procedure. These patients should probably undergo posterior occipital cervical arthrodesis rather than an anterior fusion procedure due to osteoporosis, poor bone quality, and the need to continue medical therapies that impair fusion.

References

1. Borges LF. Thompson-Farley spinal retraction system. [review] Neurosurgery 1993;33:160–163
2. McDonnell DE, Harrison SJ. Transcervical approach to the craniovertebral junction. In: Menezes AH, Sonntag VKH, eds. Principles of Spinal Surgery. New York: McGraw-Hill; 1996
3. McDonnell DE, Harrison SJ. Lateral approach to the craniocervical complex. Tech Neurosurg 1998;4:306–318
4. Hadley MN, Martin NA, Spetzler RF, Sonntag VK, Johnson PC. Comparative transoral dural closure techniques: a canine model. Neurosurgery 1988; 22:392–397
5. Shaffrey CI, Spotnitz WD, Shaffrey ME, Jane JA. Neurosurgical applications of fibrin glue: augmentation of dural closure in 134 patients. Neurosurgery 1990;26:207–210
6. Bonkowski JA, Gibson RD, Snape L. Foramen magnum meningioma: transoral resection with a bone baffle to prevent CSF leakage. Case report. J Neurosurg 1990;72:493–496
7. de Andrade JR, Macnab I. Anterior occipito-cervical fusion using an extrapharyngeal exposure. J Bone Joint Surg Am 1969;51:1621–1626
8. Kansal R, Sharma A, Kukreja S. An anterior high cervical retropharyngeal approach for C1-C2 intrafacetal fusion and transarticular screw insertion. J Clin Neurosci 2011;18:1705–1708
9. Koller H, Kammermeier V, Ulbricht D, et al. Anterior retropharyngeal fixation C1-2 for stabilization of atlantoaxial instabilities: study of feasibility, technical description and preliminary results. Eur Spine J 2006;15: 1326–1338
10. Dickman CA, Locantro J, Fessler RG. The influence of transoral odontoid resection on stability of the craniovertebral junction. J Neurosurg 1992; 77:525–530
11. Vender JR, Harrison SJ, McDonnell DE. Fusion and instrumentation at C1-3 via the high anterior cervical approach. J Neurosurg 2000;92(1, Suppl): 24–29 (spine I)
12. Houle PJ, Vender JR, Fountas K, McDonnell DE, Fick JR, Robinson JS. Pump-regulated lumbar subarachnoid drainage. Neurosurgery 2000;46: 929–932
13. Vender JR, Hester S, Houle PJ, Choudhri HF, Rekito A, McDonnell DE. The use of closed-suction irrigation systems to manage spinal infections. J Neurosurg Spine 2005;3:276–282
14. Mehra S, Heineman TE, Cammisa FP Jr, Girardi FP, Sama AA, Kutler DI. Factors predictive of voice and swallowing outcomes after anterior approaches to the cervical spine. Otolaryngol Head Neck Surg 2014;150: 259–265

D. Posterior Approach

13 Posterior Suboccipital and Upper Cervical Exposure of the Occipital-Cervical Junction

Gregory Hawryluk and Dean Chou

Indications

The posterior craniocervical junction is commonly exposed by neurosurgeons for various pathologies. Careful exposure of this region is critical because of the exquisitely vital regional structures and the important structural support provided by the posterior bony anatomy and ligaments. This approach can be employed for posterior fossa lesions, or it can be used to perform a decompression or fusion involving the occiput and cervical spine. Pathologies requiring this approach include the following:

- Chiari malformation
- Cranial settling
- Atlanto-occipital dislocation
- Basilar invagination
- Craniocervical instability secondary to rheumatoid arthritis
- Severely unstable traumatic C1-C2 injuries
- Unstable occipital condyle fractures (rare)
- Posterior fossa tumors (commonly metastases)
- Tumors causing C1-C2 destruction

Patient Selection, Preoperative Counseling, and Contraindications

Patients should not undergo surgeries in the region of the posterior craniocervical junction if there is an unfavorable risk/benefit ratio or if the sequelae of the specific procedure are not acceptable to the patient. In preoperative discussions with the patient, the risks inherent to operating specifically in this area should be emphasized. In addition to the risk of injury to the spinal cord, brainstem, and nerve roots, risk of injury to the vertebral artery needs to be discussed. Other key issues include marked restriction in neck range of motion with fusion procedures and sequelae of C2 nerve root sacrifice, should it be required for C1 lateral mass screw placement.

The vertebral artery can be injured in numerous ways during surgery in this region. A unilateral vertebral artery injury is unlikely to lead to an infarct in the posterior cerebral circulation unless the contralateral artery is hypoplastic, but the risk of stroke must be discussed with the patient. Potential need for long-term antiplatelet or blood thinning agents if vertebral dissection is encountered should also be discussed. The risk of a delayed infarct from a thromboembolism must also be considered, and the patient should also be warned about possible procedures with interventional radiology should there be a vertebral artery injury. Moreover, injury to the vertebral artery may preclude completion of the planned operation.

Restriction of neck range of motion must also be discussed. A fusion at C1-C2 markedly reduces neck mobility because the C1-C2 articulation provides approximately half of the neck's rotation.[1] The restriction is even greater for those undergoing occipitocervical fusion, and these patients must be counselled extensively regarding the implications. The problems of driving a car, because of the difficulty of checking the blind spot, and the need to buy new car mirrors should be discussed with the patient. The problems that the patient will encounter in performing activities of daily living with a fused occipitocervical region should be discussed and documented. The patient needs to understand that this is a profound, life-altering operation that is irreversible. If the patient's occupation is critically dependent on neck mobility, then the patient must understand that a high cervical or occipitocervical fusion may be career altering or even career ending. Such a risk may not be worth it to some patients.

Another issue specific to surgery in this region is that the C2 nerve roots sometimes must be sacrificed to facilitate placement of C1 lateral mass screws (**Fig. 13.1d**), and this is associated with numbness or other sensory changes at the back of the head. If the C2 nerve roots are not sacrificed, their manipulation, coagulation of the nearby venous plexus, or irritation from the C1 screws may result in severe neuropathic pain, and patients should be warned of this possibility.

The typical risks of spine surgery must also be discussed, such as the risk of postprocedural kyphosis or instability necessitating a fusion if a decompression alone is performed. If a fusion is performed, the risk of pseudarthrosis, the need for screw repositioning, and adjacent segment degeneration should be discussed. In addition, a durotomy may necessitate a lumbar drain or reoperation. The patient should also be warned of the risk of peripheral nerve issues or pressure sores that may result from positioning. Meralgia paresthetica can be seen postoperatively if a Jackson table is used with padding over the anterior superior iliac spine. Likewise, caudal retraction of the shoulders risks brachial plexus stretch if too much force is applied. Long operations with the patient in the prone position can result in pressure sores and abrasions.

Advantages and Disadvantages of Operative Approach and Patient Positioning

The approach to the posterior craniocervical junction can be performed with the patient in the prone, decubitus, or sitting positions. The sitting position should theoretically portend less blood loss from decreased venous pressure, but it entails the risk of air embolism. The decubitus position is awkward for the sur-

13 Posterior Suboccipital and Upper Cervical Exposure of the Occipital-Cervical Junction

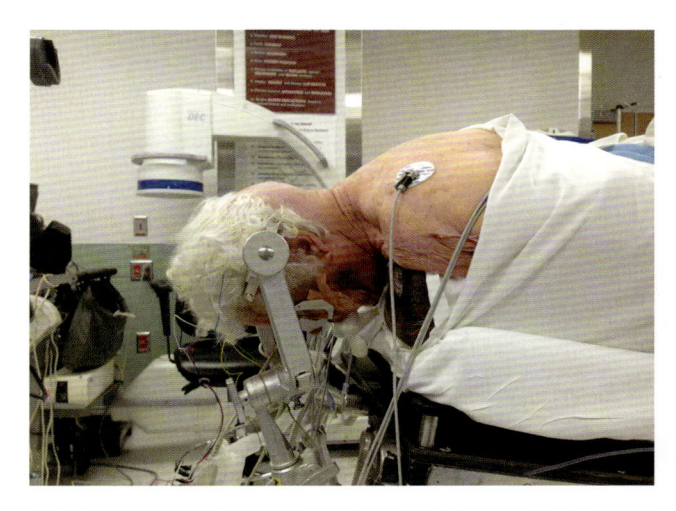

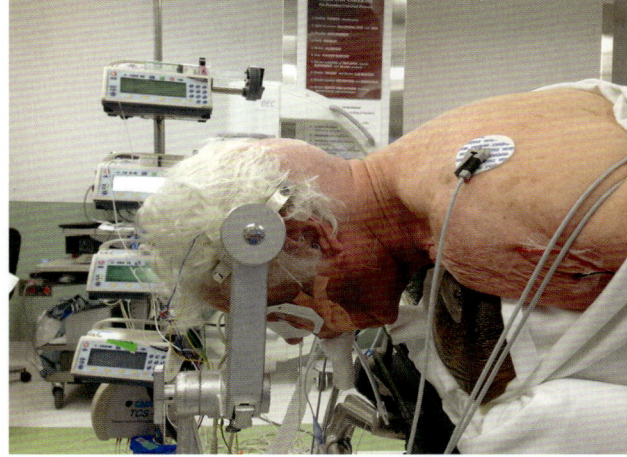

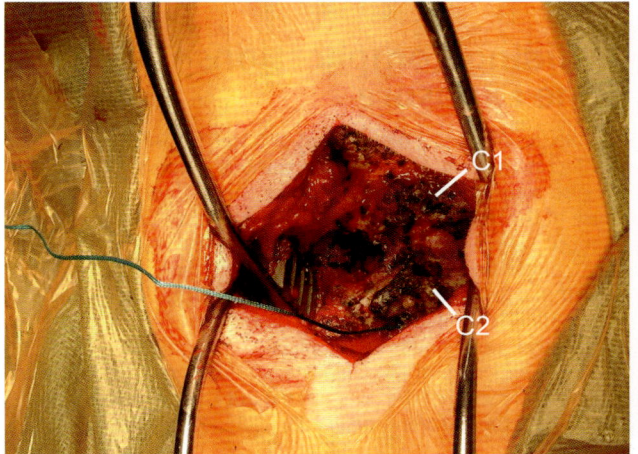

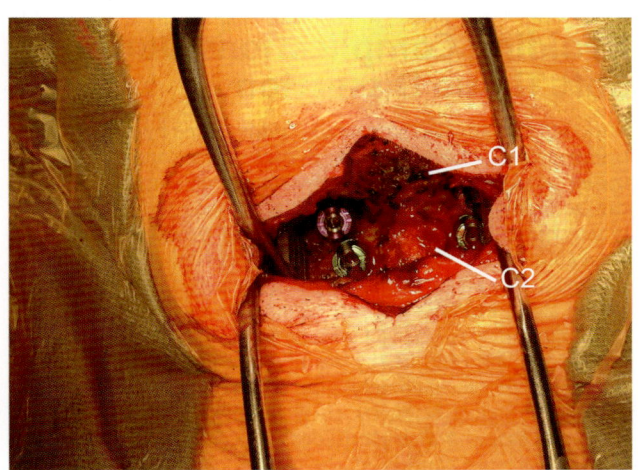

Fig. 13.1 (a, b) Patient about to undergo a C1–2 fusion. The head is secured with a Mayfield head frame and care is taken to ensure that the head is not rotated. **(a)** Slight head flexion which facilitates more facile exposure and screw placement. Intra-operatively the patient's head can then be extended to a more neutral position as shown in **(b)** prior to placement of the rod. **(c)** The typical appearance of C1 and C2 after exposure has been completed. Here the C1 posterior arch and C2 spinous process are clearly seen. **(d)** The same view after C1 lateral mass (purple) and C2 pars screws have been placed. The rods have not yet been placed.

geon and limits an assistant's access to the surgical field, but this may be useful for far lateral approaches or other intracranial pathologies. The prone position is most commonly employed but can be associated with abdominal compression that increases venous pressure and ooze. This is especially problematic for obese patients. A Jackson table or efforts to minimize pressure on the abdomen can reduce this risk. If the patient is positioned on either a Wilson frame or chest bolsters, be sure that the padding is over the iliac crests to raise the abdomen off the table.

With the prone position, the patient's head is generally fixed to the table rigidly with a head frame to prevent movement during surgery. Flexion can improve exposure of the occipital-cervical junction (**Fig. 13.1a**). If a fusion is to be performed, however, it is best to ensure that the patient's head is in a neutral position, especially for long fusions, when placing the rods (**Fig. 13.1b**). It is critical that the patient's chin be free from compression against the edge of the bed to prevent a pressure sore. A wide margin is safest because the patients can slide over the course of a procedure even when the head is bolted. The Mayfield head holder should also have plenty of clearance from the nose. The Mayfield can also shift during surgery and can press against the nose, causing a serious abrasion without attention to this issue. We routinely have the anesthesiologist examine the nose, the chin, and the eyes to ensure that no pressure occurs over these spots during the course of the surgery.

For patients undergoing a C1-C2 fusion, it is important that the patient is in the neutral position in the axial plane to prevent fixation with a rotatory component. This can be double checked by noting that the ears are level, and the nose is perpendicular to the floor. If the patient is undergoing an occipitocervical fusion, it is critical that the patient is neutral in both the axial and sagittal planes so that the patient can look forward and walk. Moreover, it is important that the patient's head not be translated dorsally (as in the classic "military tuck" position); such a dorsal translation will prevent the patient from being able to properly swallow. It is generally favorable to allow the patient to be fixed in a relaxed neutral position, and in many cases, this includes slight forward translation of the head because of the upper thoracic kyphosis.

In many cases it may be difficult to perform the operation or place instrumentation without flexion of the head. In such cases, the patient's head can be flexed, the implants placed, and then when the rods are ready to be placed, the patient's head is released from its flexion into its desired neutral position (**Fig. 13.1a,b**). During this maneuver, one surgeon stays scrubbed while the other is unscrubbed. Both surgeons coordinate so that the scrubbed surgeon holds the Mayfield while the unscrubbed surgeon releases the Mayfield. The patient is then gently extended into a neutral and slightly forward translated position to account for the thoracic kyphosis. The unscrubbed surgeon should then view the patient from a lateral position by looking under the sterile drapes to ensure that the patient appears neutral relative to the torso. The scrubbed surgeon maintains control of the head during manipulation and also views the wound during extension. If too much extension is induced, the surgical field may be so small that it makes placing the rods too difficult. During rod placement for C1-C2 or occipitocervical fusion, it is important not to place a rod that extends significantly cephalad to the C1 screws as this prevents the occiput from fully extending. Here contact between skull and the protruding rod can further reduce the patient's ability to look up.

Avoiding Complications During Soft Tissue Dissection

Although C2 and C7 can generally be identified by palpation, intraoperative imaging is critical in confirming appropriate localization and reducing the risk of wrong-level surgery. Surgeons can be fooled into thinking subaxial spinous processes are C2, when the patient simply has large spinous processes in the subaxial spine. Moreover, large spinous processes of C6 can mimic C7, and it may be hard to distinguish between C7 and T1 by palpation alone. Perhaps the only time when intraoperative imaging is not critical is when C1 and the occiput are clearly identified intraoperatively (**Fig. 13.1c**). We advocate preoperative localization and a skin incision only large enough to identify a spinous process with electrocautery. Then a clamp is placed on the spinous process, and a single fluoroscopic image is taken. After proper levels are confirmed, the incision is then opened to the appropriate size. This makes the skin incision only as large as necessary, and it also prevents inadvertent dissection of the large muscles off of C2 or inadvertent dissection of the C7-T1 ligament, helping to prevent kyphosis.[2–4] Caudal retraction of the shoulders by taping or manual traction can assist in visualizing lower cervical levels, especially in patients with large shoulders, but care must be taken not to pull too hard, or else the patient may develop a brachial plexus stretch injury.

Many times the dissection of the posterior occipitocervical region is done without regard to the actual muscles, ligaments, and their function. Numerous large and small muscles are found at the craniocervical junction posteriorly. Most superficial is the trapezius, which attaches to the superior nuchal line of the skull, the spine of the scapula, and the spinous processes of the cervical and thoracic vertebrae. Beneath that is the obliquely oriented splenius capitis muscle. Deeper yet is the semispinalis capitis muscle, which is oriented in a more sagittal plane. The deepest muscular layer contains numerous small muscles that attach to the inferior nuchal line. Although these muscles undoubtedly serve to fine-tune neck movements, it is believed that proprioception may be their most important function.[5] The rectus capitis posterior minor attaches to the posterior tubercle of C1. The more lateral rectus capitis posterior major muscle attaches to the spinous process of C2. The obliquus capitis superior muscle attaches to the transverse process of C1. The obliquus capitis inferior muscle spans from the transverse process of C1 to the spinous process of C2.

The ligamentum nuchae is found in the midline of the neck posteriorly and it offers an essentially bloodless plane for the surgeon seeking to expose this area. Palpation of the external occipital protuberance and the cervical spinous processes will help ensure that the incision and subsequent soft tissue dissection is performed in the midline. C2 has the most prominent spinous process in the upper cervical spine. Gentle palpation of the local osteology becomes easier as the exposure deepens; even the posterior arch of C1 can be readily felt. Knowledge of the underlying osteology is key to using monopolar cautery safely and avoiding inadvertent durotomy or injury to local nerves or vessels. This is especially true when approaching the foramen magnum (**Fig. 13.2**). The atlanto-occipital membrane can be inadvertently pierced with monopolar cautery, despite it being very tough and fibrous to dissect and remove away from the dura. This is because the dura will slope dorsally when it passes cephalad to C1 toward the foramen magnum, just as the dura slopes dorsally at the lower lumbar spine at L5-S1. Congenital fusions and bony defects are best recognized preoperatively with computed tomography (CT). Midline bony defects are not uncommon and portend a risk of dural or neural injury (especially with monopolar cautery) if their presence is not anticipated.

Avoiding Complications During Bone Exposure

It is best to minimize the amount of bone exposed. The numerous ligaments that attach to the spinous process of C2 should only be stripped off if necessary for the intended surgery because of the risk of kyphosis. Likewise the facet joints should be exposed only when needed, and when they must be exposed care, should be taken to avoid injury to facet capsules not included in a fusion to reduce the risk of destabilizing the spine.[6,7] Generally one should not expose more than half of the facets bilaterally if no fusion is taking place.[6]

Bony exposure of the C1 posterior arch must be done with great care because of the unprotected dura above and below, and because of the vertebral artery laterally (**Figs. 13.2** and **13.3**).

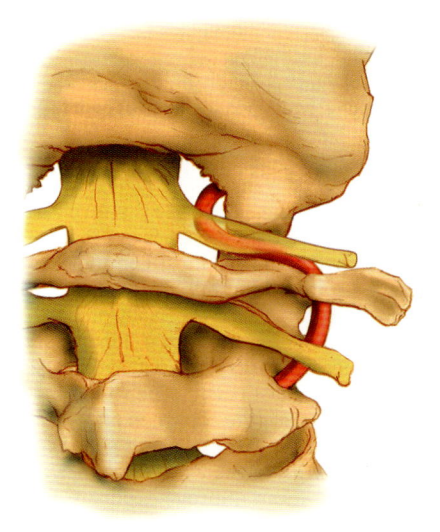

Fig. 13.2 The anatomy of the posterior craniocervical junction is shown. It is noteworthy that the C2 nerve roots emerge from the dura dorsal to the facet joints in distinction with those elsewhere in the spine. As is clearly seen, the dura between the occipital bone and the posterior arch of C1) lacks the bony cover typical at other levels. It is thus vulnerable to an unintentional durotomy during exposure. The dura between the posterior arch of C1 and the C2 lamina is similarly vulnerable. The illustration illustrates why the C2 nerve root must sometimes be sacrificed to facilitate placement of C1 lateral mass screws.

Here blunt dissection with a Penfield No. 4 is preferable to the use of monopolar cautery, which is more likely to injure the vertebral artery. If it is critical to use monopolar cautery at C1, we turn the current on at an extremely low setting for more gentle and accurate dissection. It is commonly thought that exposure of the posterior arch of C1 1.5 cm from the midline on either side bears less risk of vertebral artery injury.[8]

The vertebral artery is usually surrounded by a venous plexus that may bleed upon initial dissection. This can be stopped with a Gelfoam/thrombin slurry. However, if the actual vertebral artery injury has occurred, Gelfoam/thrombin slurry is contraindicated because it can be directly squirted into the posterior circulation of the brain, causing infarct. If a vertebral artery injury is suspected, multiple patties should be placed on top of the bleeding site; direct, constant pressure is required to achieve hemostasis if it is indeed injured.

To dissect cephalad under the ring of C1, one should use an up-going curette after initial dorsal exposure with electrocautery. If preoperative magnetic resonance imaging (MRI) demonstrates compression under the ring of C1, the ring can be amputated on either side of the cord with a high-speed bur. Then using an instrument to hold the posterior arch away from the cord, the dura can be dissected away safely. This will gently strip away the atlanto-occipital membrane and identify the dura below the arch of C1.

During placement of C1 lateral mass screws, the C1-C2 facet joint must be exposed. Significant venous ooze can be encountered during this approach. Subperiosteal dissection can minimize hemorrhage. One trick to reduce bleeding from the venous plexus is to first identify the plexus and begin cauterizing it with bipolar cautery medially over the spinal cord itself. Once coagulated, the plexus can be divided using microscissors until the C2

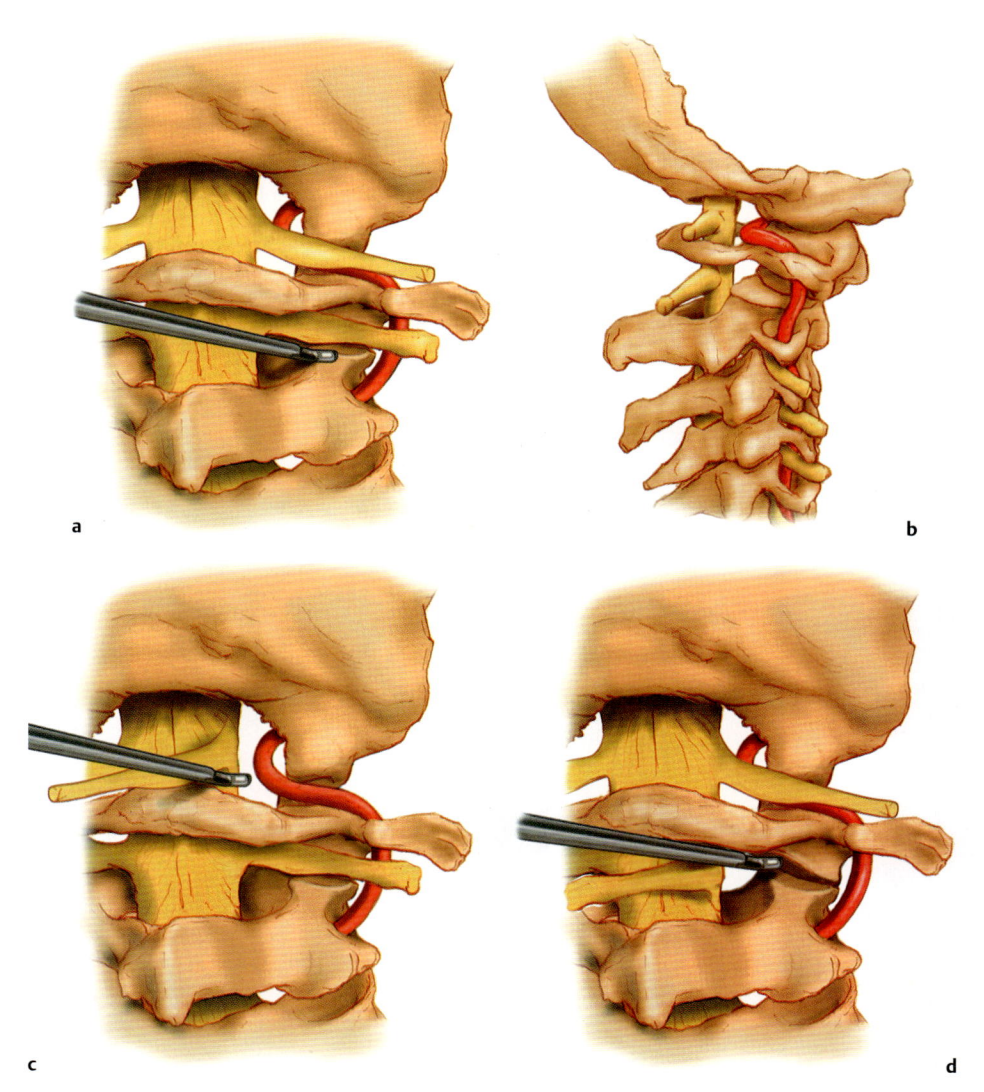

Fig. 13.3 The posterior craniocervical junction is shown. **(a, b)** demonstrate posterior and lateral views, respectively. Note that the C2 nerve roots emerge posterior to the facet joints. The vertebral artery is vulnerable to injury above the C1 arch where it can be injured by dissecting too laterally or by a paramedian approach to this region. Dissection 1.5 cm on either side of the midline is generally safe but the possibility of an abnormally tortuous vertebral artery should be considered. **(c)** and **(d)** more clearly demonstrate the course of the right vertebral artery ventral to the C2 nerve root.

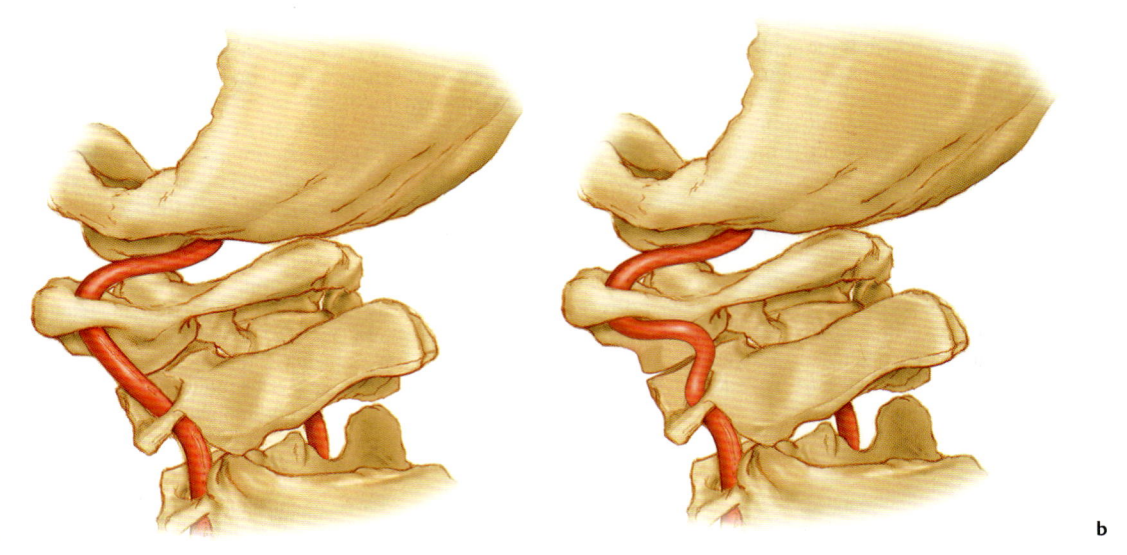

Fig. 13.4 The course of the vertebral artery is demonstrated on a second model devoid of neural elements. **(a)** demonstrates the normal course of the vertebral artery; **(b)** demonstrates a tortuous vertebral artery which is at higher risk of injury during exposure of the C2 pars. The vertebral artery can actually be dorsal to the C2 pars in these cases. This highlights the importance of careful sub-periosteal dissection during this approach.

nerve, the C1 lateral mass, and the C1-C2 facet are identified. Once the plexus begins to uncontrollably bleed (which it invariably will), packing with hemostatic agents and dissecting the contralateral side can be an effective approach. This back-and-forth packing and dissecting usually enables the dissection ultimately to be performed. Elevating the head relative to the heart can also substantially reduce venous ooze, but the surgeon must be judicious with the use of this technique because excessive elevation risks air embolism.

Care should be taken to minimize lateral dissection on C2 where the vertebral artery can be injured (**Fig. 13.4**). In some elderly patients, the vertebral artery can be so tortuous that it rides dorsal to the pars, precluding safe use of monopolar cautery in this region (**Fig. 13.5b**). Dissection with a blunt dissector

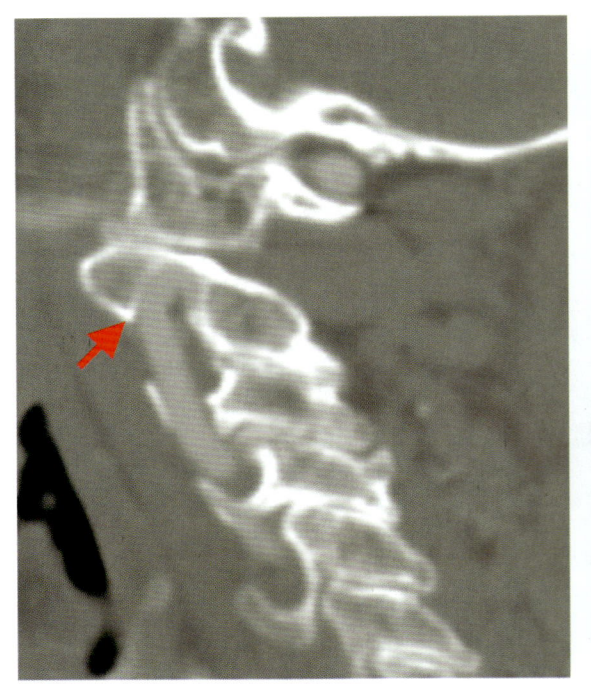

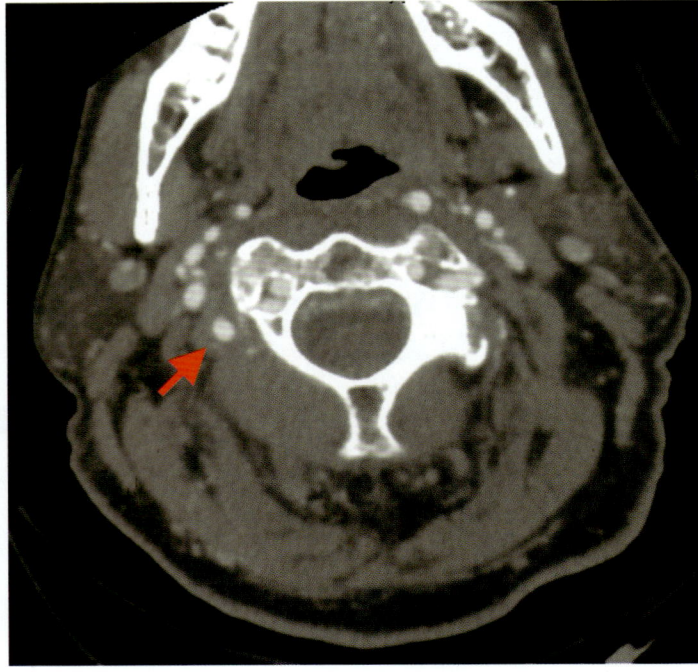

Fig. 13.5 **(a)** demonstrates a tortuous, high riding vertebral artery (denoted by red arrow) which precludes placement of a transarticular screw for C1–2 fusion. **(b)** demonstrates a tortuous subaxial vertebral artery dorsal to the pars and facet of C2 (denoted by red arrow). This is vulnerable to injury during exposure of the lateral aspect of C2. Recognition on pre-operative imaging is important and should prompt careful dissection during exposure.

such as a Penfield No. 4 may thus be safer in elderly patients.[9,10] A preoperative CT angiogram may help the surgeon to prevent such an injury.

When the C2 nerve root must be sacrificed to facilitate lateral mass screw placement, it is generally preferable to perform the transection proximal to the dorsal root ganglion to reduce the risk of neuropathic pain. We try to avoid taking the C2 nerve root, but sometimes the surgery is simply not feasible without its removal. Moreover, removal of the C2 nerve root facilitates easier access into the C1-2 joint space, facilitating good decortication and packing of graft material into the joint itself. In elderly patients, there is good evidence showing that C2 nerve root sacrifice does not result in significant morbidity.[11] Although there are many techniques to sacrifice the C2 nerve root, we find that tying off the root is the least reliable given the small working space. We generally bipolar the C2 nerve root proximal to the dorsal root ganglion and cut with microscissors if the root must be sacrificed. We then remove the C2 ganglion distally to facilitate access the joint space.

Vertebral Artery Anatomy

The vertebral artery enters the foramen transversarium at the C6 level in at least 85% of cases.[12] The left-sided vertebral artery is considered dominant in 50 to 70% of patients.[12,13] The vertebral artery courses straight rostrally in the transverse foramen of the subaxial spine until it reaches the transverse foramen of C2 where it heads ventral to the C2 pars and laterally to facilitate entry into the transverse foramen of C1 (**Fig. 13.3**). After passing through the transverse foramen of C1, the vertebral artery then courses medially immediately apposed to the rostral surface of the posterior arch of C1 in a groove referred to as the sulcus arteriosus. It then curls medially around the occipital condyle as it heads ventrally to pierce the dura and ascend anterolaterally into the brainstem. At the base of the pons, the vertebral arteries unite to ascend as the basilar artery.

The vertebral artery can be injured at multiple points during dissection of the craniocervical junction. The vertebral artery is very vulnerable to injury during dissection laterally above the C1 posterior arch and during lateral dissection at the C1-C2 facet joint. Venous ooze from the perivertebral venous plexus generally warns the surgeon that dissection is being conducted near the vertebral artery. Preoperative imaging demonstrating enlarged foramina transversaria should alert the surgeon to the possibility of a tortuous vertebral artery and the need for extra caution. The vertebral artery is also at risk of injury during placement of most types of screws in the cervical spine. A lateral trajectory is important for avoiding vertebral artery injury during subaxial lateral mass screw placement. Placement of C2 pars screws with a trajectory that is too caudal or too lateral also jeopardizes the vertebral artery (**Fig. 13.6**). A high-riding vertebral artery should be excluded prior to placement of transarticular screws, and a high-riding vertebral artery may also necessitate a short pars screw into C2 (**Fig. 13.5a**). The relationship of the vertebral artery to these screw trajectories can be assessed by preoperatoive CT imaging, and if there is any significant abnormality seen on CT, a CT angiogram may be obtained.

Ponticulus posticus is an anatomic variant that should be familiar to spine surgeons. In approximately half of cases the anomaly is complete, meaning that a vertebral artery is encased in a bony foramen circumferentially as it passes above C1; in incomplete cases, bony outgrowth downward from the superior articulating surface of C1 or upward from the posterior arch is seen that that does not enclose the artery circumferentially.[14] A recent meta-analysis of 21,879 patients demonstrated that the overall prevalence of this anomaly is 16 to 19% depending on the means of detection.[14,15] Ponticulus posticus is more commonly unilateral than bilateral.[14] Failure to recognize this anomaly can lead to vertebral artery injury during C1 lateral mass screw placement. Thus, a preoperative CT scan to evaluate the bony anatomy is critical before instrumentation in this region; a CT angiogram is also helpful if there is any suspicion of abnormal anatomy based on other preoperative imaging or clinical findings.

If the vertebral artery is injured during surgery, expedient diagnosis and subsequent surgical and nonsurgical management can minimize the sequelae of this complication. The sequence of management priorities should aim first to achieve local hemostasis, then to prevent immediate vertebrobasilar ischemia, and lastly to prevent future thromboembolic cerebrovascular complications.[16] When the vertebral artery injury occurs at the depths of a hole intended for screw placement, placing the screw generally provides acceptable hemostasis. Placement of a screw that is shorter than intended should prevent complete occlusion

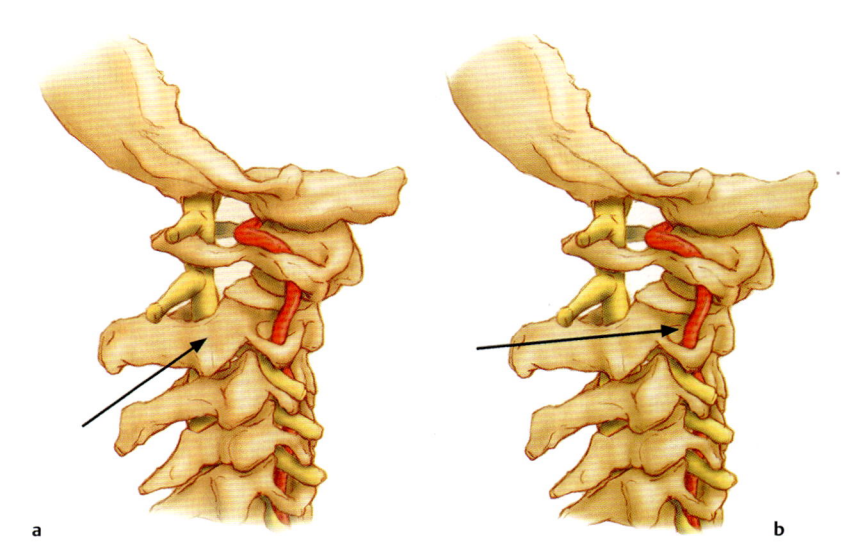

Fig. 13.6 (a) demonstrates the proper rostral angle for placement of a pars screw in C2. The vertebral artery can be injured with an inappropriately caudal or lateral trajectory, as shown in (b).

of the artery and reduce the risk of cerebral infarct. If the vertebral artery is injured during dissection, attempts should be made to tamponade the hemorrhage and the event should be communicated promptly to the anesthesia team, which must prepare for rapid resuscitation. The surgeon can attempt to expose and repair the vessel or to sacrifice it based on intraoperative findings. Seeking the assistance of a vascular surgeon is a very reasonable approach. Emergent endovascular approaches have several advantages in this context, if available, because they involve a lower risk to local nerve roots and they provide information on collateral flow. Stenting and vessel sacrifice may be options depending on the size and flow of the vessel. Patients with intimal injury are at risk for subsequent embolic strokes in the posterior cerebral circulation. Antiplatelet or anticoagulant therapies are typically employed to reduce this risk of these significant adverse events. When a unilateral vertebral artery injury occurs, placement of contralateral screws is contraindicated because it risks bilateral vertebral artery injury and a high probability of brainstem infarction. This may mean that a unilateral fusion must be tolerated and perhaps combined with a Brooks or Gallie fusion, and/or a halo.

Postoperative Care

Postoperative care is tailored to the specific pathology addressed at surgery. A postoperative MRI will demonstrate the results of a surgery addressing soft tissues, whereas CT will demonstrate the results of bone work and its instrumentation. Flexion-extension films are helpful for assessing postoperative instability, which can develop in delayed fashion after spinal surgery.

Conclusion

Exposure of the posterior craniocervical junction is routine for many surgeons but requires thorough planning, exquisite knowledge of the anatomy and anatomic variations specific to each patient, and meticulous surgical technique. Careful patient selection and preoperative discussion play an important role in postsurgical patient satisfaction. Preoperative detection of anatomic variants can prevent surgical misadventure and debilitating complications. Surgeons operating in this area must be familiar with the recommended strategies for handling such complications and have a familiarity with the resources at their institution that may assist them.

References

1. Panjabi M, Dvorak J, Duranceau J, et al. Three-dimensional movements of the upper cervical spine. Spine 1988;13:726–730
2. Takeshita K, Seichi A, Akune T, Kawamura N, Kawaguchi H, Nakamura K. Can laminoplasty maintain the cervical alignment even when the C2 lamina is contained? Spine 2005;30:1294–1298
3. Seller K, Jäger M, Krämer R, Krauspe R, Wild A. [Occurrence of a segmental kyphosis after laminectomy of C2 for an aneurysmatic bone cysts—course and treatment strategy]. Z Orthop Ihre Grenzgeb 2004;142:83–87
4. McLaughlin MR, Wahlig JB, Pollack IF. Incidence of postlaminectomy kyphosis after Chiari decompression. Spine 1997;22:613–617
5. McPartland JM, Brodeur RR, Hallgren RC. Chronic neck pain, standing balance, and suboccipital muscle atrophy—a pilot study. J Manipulative Physiol Ther 1997;20:24–29
6. Zdeblick TA, Abitbol JJ, Kunz DN, McCabe RP, Garfin S. Cervical stability after sequential capsule resection. Spine 1993;18:2005–2008
7. Zdeblick TA, Zou D, Warden KE, McCabe R, Kunz D, Vanderby R. Cervical stability after foraminotomy. A biomechanical in vitro analysis. J Bone Joint Surg Am 1992;74:22–27
8. Gupta T. Quantitative anatomy of vertebral artery groove on the posterior arch of atlas in relation to spinal surgical procedures. Surg Radiol Anat 2008;30:239–242
9. Molinari R, Bessette M, Raich AL, Dettori JR, Molinari C. Vertebral artery anomaly and injury in spinal surgery. Evid Based Spine Care J 2014;5:16–27
10. Peng CW, Chou BT, Bendo JA, Spivak JM. Vertebral artery injury in cervical spine surgery: anatomical considerations, management, and preventive measures. Spine J 2009;9:70–76
11. Hamilton DK, Smith JS, Sansur CA, Dumont AS, Shaffrey CI. C-2 neurectomy during atlantoaxial instrumented fusion in the elderly: patient satisfaction and surgical outcome. J Neurosurg Spine 2011;15:3–8
12. Wakao N, Takeuchi M, Kamiya M, et al. Variance of cervical vertebral artery measured by CT angiography and its influence on C7 pedicle anatomy. Spine 2014;39:228–232
13. Hong JM, Chung CS, Bang OY, Yong SW, Joo IS, Huh K. Vertebral artery dominance contributes to basilar artery curvature and peri-vertebrobasilar junctional infarcts. J Neurol Neurosurg Psychiatry 2009;80:1087–1092
14. Elliott RE, Tanweer O. The prevalence of the ponticulus posticus (arcuate foramen) and its importance in the Goel-Harms procedure: meta-analysis and review of the literature. World Neurosurg 2014;82:e335–e343
15. Young JP, Young PH, Ackermann MJ, Anderson PA, Riew KD. The ponticulus posticus: implications for screw insertion into the first cervical lateral mass. J Bone Joint Surg Am 2005;87:2495–2498
16. Park HK, Jho HD. The management of vertebral artery injury in anterior cervical spine operation: a systematic review of published cases. Eur Spine J 2012;21:2475–2485

14 Suboccipital Craniectomy and Cervical Laminectomy for Chiari Malformation

Lee A. Tan, Robert G. Kellogg, Carter S. Gerard, and Lorenzo F. Muñoz

Chiari malformations were first described in 1891 by the Austrian pathologist Hans Chiari in his paper titled "Concerning Alterations in the Cerebellum Resulting from Cerebral Hydrocephalus."[1] Chiari I malformation is characterized by caudally displaced cerebellar tonsils herniating through the foramen magnum into the spinal canal. This was thought to be due to a mismatch of the posterior cranial fossa volume and its contents, which can be derived from congenital or acquired causes. Chiari I malformations are estimated to be present in more than 0.5% of the general population and are often asymptomatic. Symptomatic patients with Chiari I malformations often present with suboccipital headaches that worsen with Valsalva-like maneuvers, neck pain, blurred vision, dysphagia, cranial nerve deficits, as well as sensorimotor disturbances in the extremities when an associated syringomyelia is present. Syringomyelia is estimated to be present in more than half of the patients with Chiari I malformation,[2] and the percentage can be much higher if signs of spinal cord dysfunction are present.

Several theories exist for the pathophysiology of syringomyelia formation in Chiari I malformation. In 1958, Gardner and Angel[3] proposed the hydrodynamic theory, in which cerebrospinal fluid (CSF) outflow obstruction in the fourth ventricle forced CSF into the central canal of the spinal cord, thus creating syringomyelia by a "water hammer" effect. This theory subsequently led to the practice of obex plugging for syringomyelia treatment. In 1969, Williams[4] proposed the craniospinal pressure dissociation theory, which postulated that venous pulsations from respiration resulted in a craniospinal pressure gradient responsible for syrinx formation. In 1972, Ball and Dayan[5] proposed that the herniated cerebellar tonsils through the foramen magnum act as a one-way valve preventing outward movement of CSF from the foramina of Luschka and Magendie; instead, the CSF is transmitted into the syrinx during systole by the pressure gradient generated by the heart through the Virchow-Robin space in the spinal cord. This theory is supported by studies utilizing modern dynamic magnetic resonance imaging (MRI).[6-8]

Regardless of the exact pathophysiology, surgical decompression of the posterior fossa is an effective treatment for symptomatic patients with Chiari I malformation. A high percentage of these patients show improvement in their clinical symptoms along with regression of the associated syringomyelia. The main surgical approach for treatment of Chiari I malformation consists of a suboccipital craniectomy. Cervical laminectomies, typically limited to C1, may be needed depending on the extent of tonsillar herniation. Duraplasty, arachnoid dissection, and tonsillar resection are often used in conjunction with suboccipital craniectomy. Intraoperative ultrasound is often used by some surgeons to assess the extent of posterior fossa decompression and to determine if duraplasty is necessary.[9] Some surgeons may even elect to leave the dura open without duraplasty, although this approach may potentially increase the incidence of postoperative CSF leak. The preferred surgical treatment may vary greatly by institution and by surgeon, and it remains a topic of controversy.

Patient Selection

Not all patients with radiographic diagnosis are symptomatic. The symptom onset in Chiari I patients is usually slow and progressive. However, there have been reports of asymptomatic patients presenting with abrupt neurologic deterioration including weakness, respiratory failure, and acute hydrocephalus.[10] Radiology and pathology studies have shown that Chiari I malformation can be present in > 0.5% of the general population but not all patients with Chiari I malformation require surgery.[1] In general, most neurosurgeons agree that surgical candidates are symptomatic patients with evidence of foramen magnum crowding on MRI and evidence of disruption of normal CSF dynamics (e.g., presence of hydrocephalus, syringomyelia, or abnormal dynamic MRI; **Fig. 14.1**). The goal of surgery is posterior fossa decompression with emphasis on the posterior foramen magnum and expansion of the cisterna magna to restore normal CSF dynamics. We often use the analogy of "a cork in a bottle neck" when explaining the anatomy to patients.

Indications

- Chiari I malformation

Contraindications

- Craniocervical junction instability
- Basilar invagination
- Secondary acquired Chiari I malformation (treat primary etiology first, e.g., idiopathic or induced intracranial hypertension)
- Pseudotumor cerebri (increased risk for postoperative CSF leak)

Advantages

- Familiar approach for most neurosurgeons
- Easy access to pericranium and ligamentum nuchae for duraplasty

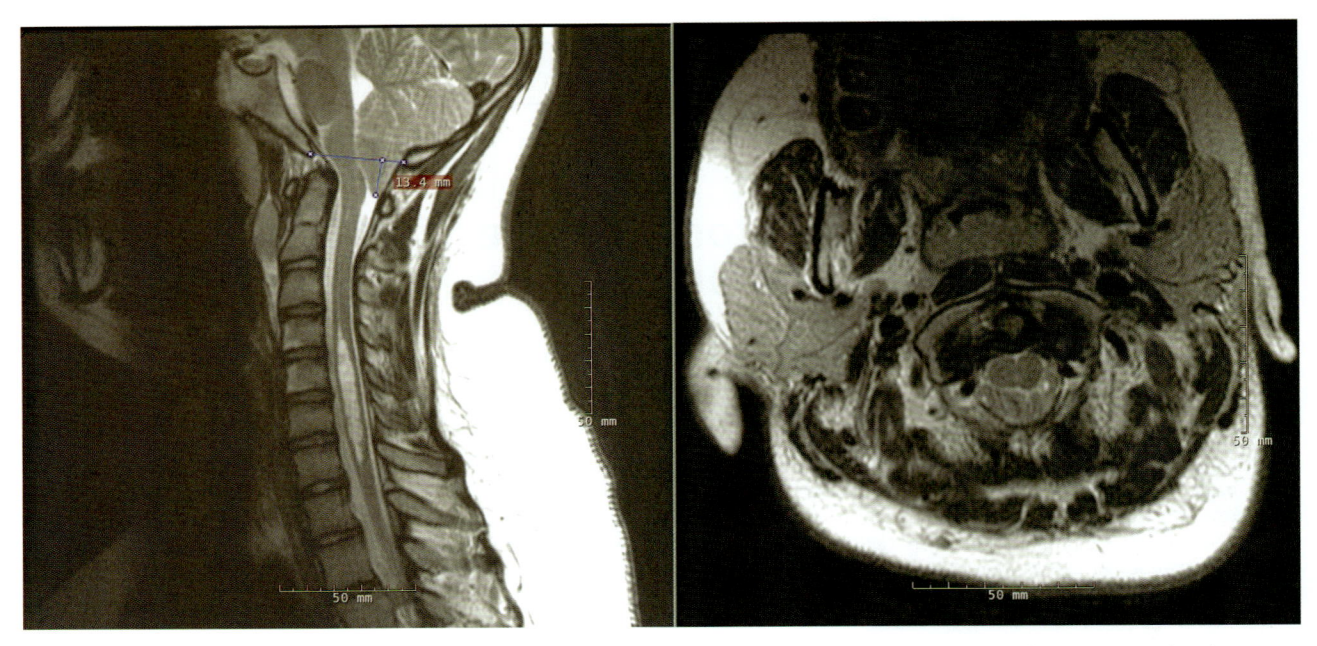

Fig. 14.1 Magnetic resonance imaging (MRI) demonstrating a Chari I malformation characterized by **(a)** cerebellar tonsillar herniation with an large syringomyelia in the cervical spinal cord and **(b)** crowding in at the level of the foramen magnum.

Disadvantages

- Potential injuries to vertebral and posterior inferior cerebellar arteries
- Potential for spinal cord injury during C1 laminectomy
- CSF leak if dural closure is not watertight

Preoperative Tests

A history and physical examination in symptomatic patients often reveal suboccipital headaches that worsen with Valsalva, neck pain, blurred vision, dysphagia, cranial nerve deficits, as well as sensorimotor disturbances in the extremities when associated syringomyelia is present. An MRI of the brain and cervical/thoracic spine should be obtained preoperatively to assess the degree of tonsillar herniation and whether associated syringomyelia is present. The commonly accepted radiographic criteria are tonsil herniation > 6 mm below the foramen magnum in children, 5 mm in adults, and 4 mm in the elderly. These differences in cutoff values account for the upward displacement of the cerebellar tonsils with aging and brain atrophy.

Surgical Procedure

After general endotracheal tube anesthesia, the patient is placed in the prone position in a Mayfield head holder with the head slightly flexed **(Fig. 14.2)**. Perioperative antibiotics are given prior to starting the procedure. Hair in the suboccipital region may be shaved, and a midline skin incision is marked from the inion to the C2 spinous process **(Fig. 14.3)**. Local anesthetic is used to infiltrate the skin along the planned incision. If pericranial graft harvesting is planned for duraplasty, the incision can be extended ~ 3 cm above the inion. Alternatively, ligamentum nuchae can also be harvested as an autograft for duraplasty. Various allografts from different manufacturers are also available for duraplasty. The senior author (L.F.M.) prefers using pericranium for duraplasty, given its malleability and the lack of potential aseptic meningitis.

After the patient is prepped and draped in a standard sterile fashion, a No. 10 blade is used to make the midline skin incision. Further tissue dissections are performed in layered fashion with a monopolar cautery. The cervical fascia can be opened with a linear or a Y-shaped incision; the Y-shaped incision is preferred by some surgeons because it can be used to reattach the suboccipital muscles during closure. Deeper dissections are carried down the midline vascular plane. Monopolar cautery is used to detach the suboccipital muscles from the inion to the foramen magnum in a subperiosteal fashion to expose the occipital bone **(Fig. 14.4)**. The soft tissue dissection should be performed lateral enough to facilitate adequate suboccipital decompression. The venous plexus are often encountered during soft tissue dissection around this area, and gentle pressure with Gelfoam often is adequate for hemostasis. The C1 posterior tubercle is palpated, and then the soft tissue overlying the C1 posterior arch is also detached. A bifid C1 posterior arch may be present infrequently, and it is imperative to keep this in mind during dissection to avoid inadvertent injury to the spinal cord.

Once the suboccipital and paraspinal muscles have been mobilized from the occiput and C1, respectively, and although some surgeons place bur holes as far lateral as the transverse-sigmoid junction, we find that a 4 × 4 cm bony decompression will suffice. To that end, the bur holes need not overlie the transverse sinus **(Fig. 14.5a)**. The suboccipital craniectomy is then completed using a combination of the drill, craniotome, and Kerrison punches **(Fig. 14.5b)**. The senior author prefers using an M8 drill instead of the craniotome to complete the craniectomy because it gives the surgeon more control, as the craniotome sometimes does not fit in the surgical field. The final reflection of the bone flap from the foramen magnum is often associated with vigorous bleeding from the adjacent venous plexus and circular sinus at the craniocervical junction; hemostasis can usually be achieved by gentle pressure with the aid of Gelfoam. The C1 laminectomy is completed with either a drill or Kerrison punches in a standard fashion.

14 Suboccipital Craniectomy and Cervical Laminectomy for Chiari Malformation

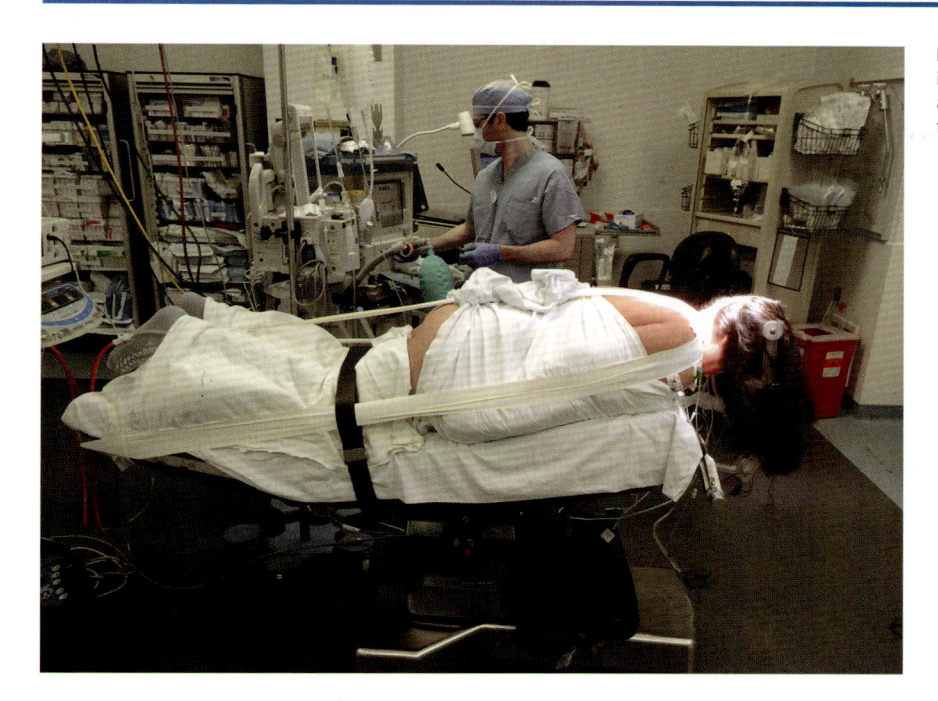

Fig. 14.2 Intraoperative photograph showing the patient placed in the prone position in a Mayfield head holder with the head slightly flexed.

Ultrasound can be used after the craniectomy and before the dural opening to assess the degree of tonsilar herniation and to tailor the extent of tonsilar resection.[9] The dura is then opened in a Y-shaped fashion with a No. 15 blade and scissors. It is important to leave enough dura cuffs during dura opening to account for possible dura edge retraction during hemostasis with bipolar cautery. Care is taken to avoid opening the underlying arachnoid layer in the interest of preventing the undue trickling of blood into the subarachnoid space. The lower limb of the incision should extend down at the midline to C1 (**Fig. 14.5c**). The important thing here is to see the distal tip of the tonsils. If they extend beyond the C1-2 interspace, then a C2 or even a C3 laminectomy may be required; if the tonsillar herniation extends beyond C3, then a tonsillar corticectomy can be performed by hollowing out the tonsils and pulling them up to achieve decompression. Further resection will be tailored to avoid residual mass effect in the area. The expansion of the posterior craniocervical junction should be apparent after the dura is opened. The

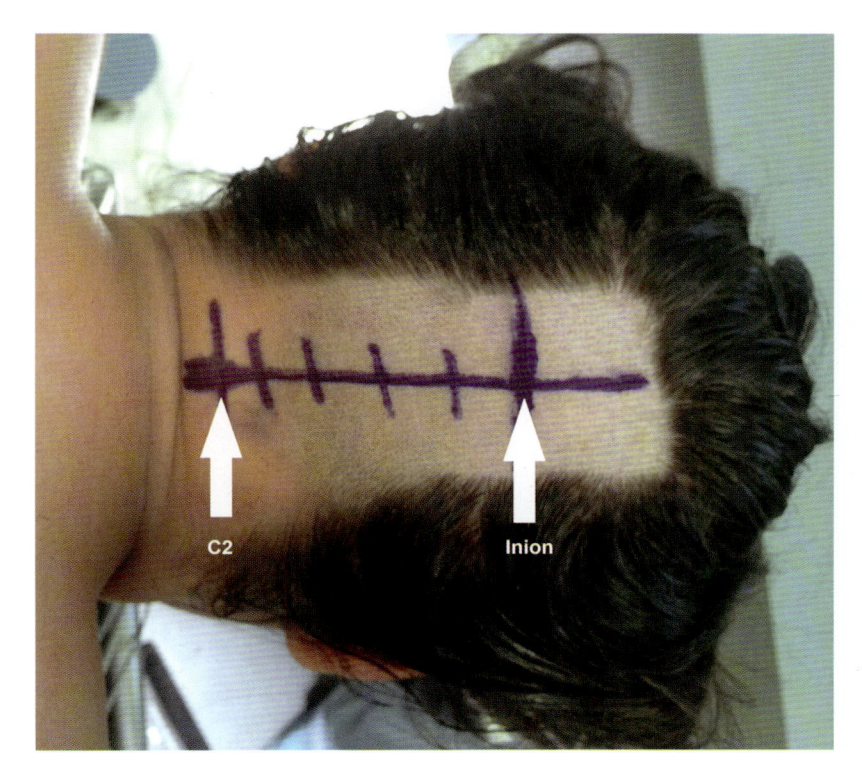

Fig. 14.3 A typical midline incision used for Chiari decompression extending from the inion to C2 spinous process; the incision can be extended 3 cm above the inion if pericranium graft harvesting is planned.

94 I Occipital-Cervical Junction

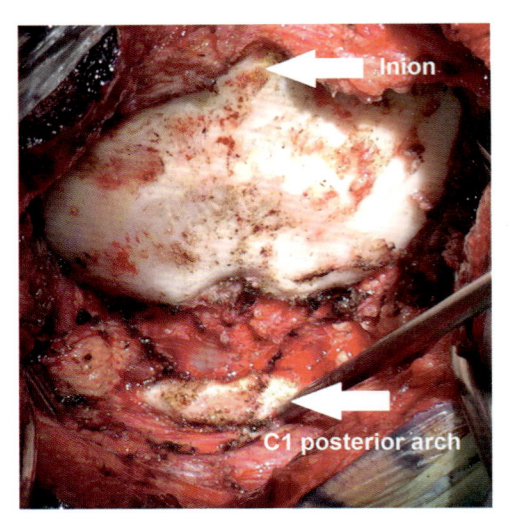

Fig. 14.4 Intraoperative photograph demonstration the extent of soft tissue and paraspinal muscle dissection in the suboccipital and upper cervical region.

pericranial autograft or dura substitute allograft can be used for duraplasty and expansion of the posterior fossa. The pericranium graft should be harvested before opening the dura to prevent blood getting into the arachnoid space. The patch can be sutured in place with either 4-0 Nurolon or 6-0 Gore-Tex (**Fig. 14.5d**). Some surgeons advocate the use of interrupted stitches because running stitches in theory may loosen over time.[11] To verify that the duraplasty is completed in a watertight fashion, a Valsalva-procedure ranging from 40 to 60 mm Hg can be done by the anesthesia team. Dural closure can also be augmented with fibrin glue if needed, although we have not found this to be critical. The incision is then closed in a layered fashion. If a Y-shaped fascia incision was used originally, the suboccipital paraspinal muscles can be reattached to the occiput by suturing to the tissue cuff.

The key operative steps are summarized in **Box 14.1**.

Postoperative Care

The patient is typically monitored in the neurosurgical intensive care unit overnight. A postoperative CT is often obtained to establish the baseline for the ventricle size in case of delayed hydrocephalus. Muscle relaxants should be prescribed to help to

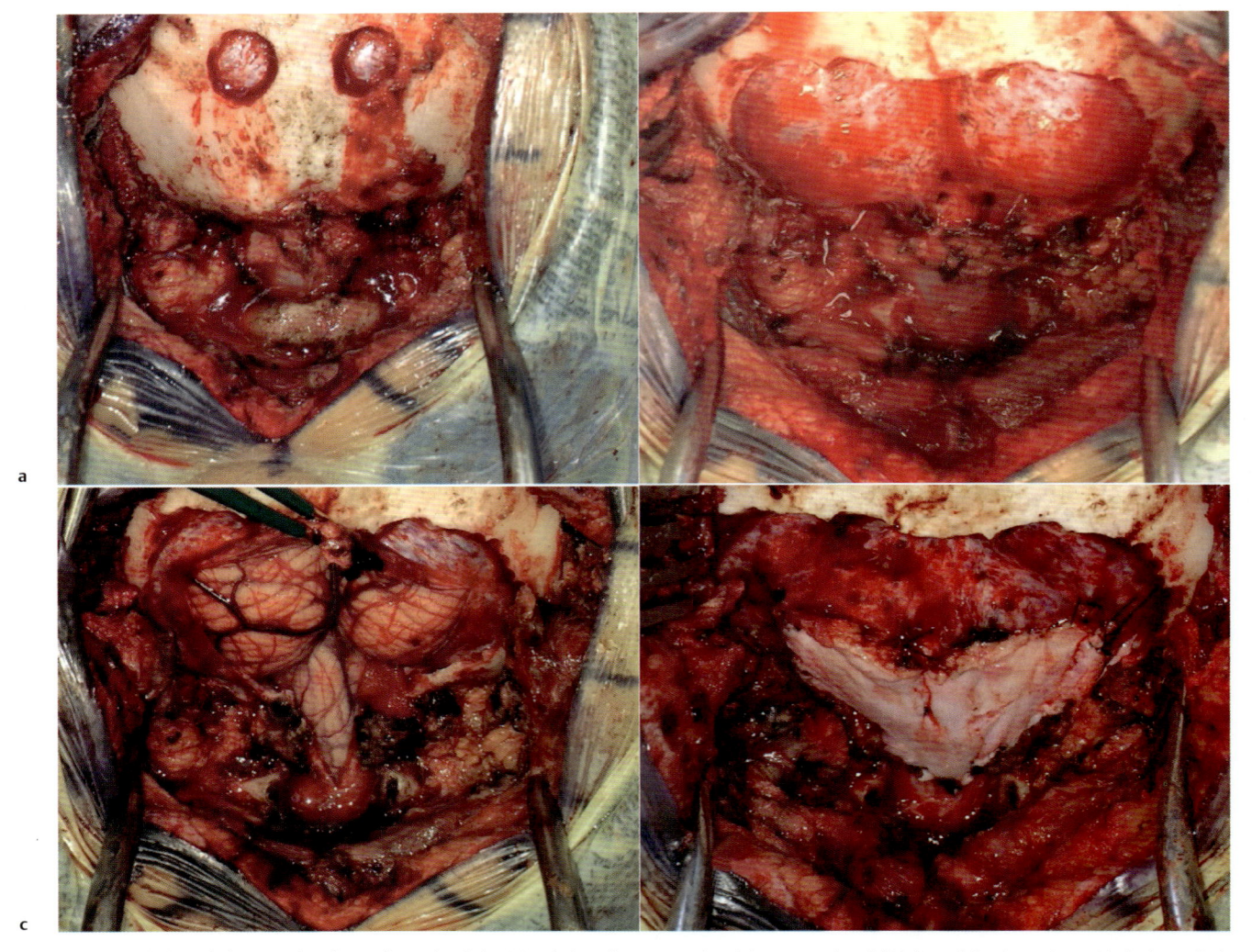

Fig. 14.5 (a) Bur holes are placed at either side of the inion below the transverse sinus for suboccipital craniectomy. (b) Completed suboccipital craniectomy and C1 laminectomy demonstrating the extend of bony removal and decompression. (c) Y-shaped dural opening, with the lower limb of the incision extending down to the upper cervical level. (d) Duraplasty with pericranial autograft and expansion of the cistern magnum.

> **Box 14.1 Key Operative Steps**
>
> - Secure the patient's head in a Mayfield head holder.
> - Perform sufficient soft tissue dissection and bony removal to ensure adequate foramen magnum decompression.
> - Avoid potential injury to the transverse and sigmoid sinuses.
> - Use a large piece of pericranial autograft or dural substitute for expansion of the posterior fossa and cisterna magnum.
> - Perform meticulous dural closure and soft tissue closure to avoid postoperative CSF leak.
> - Prescribe muscle relaxant postoperatively to reduce pain related to muscle spasm and to reduce narcotics use.

relieve muscle spasms, which are common in these patients postoperatively. The patient can be transferred to a general medical ward on postoperative day 1. After adequate ambulation is demonstrated and pain control is established, the patient can be discharged with a follow-up appointment in 2 weeks to check the wound healing.

Potential Complications and Precautions

Common postoperative complications may include CSF leak, postoperative hemorrhage, aseptic meningitis, wound infection, failure to restore normal CSF flow, and cerebellar subsidence from excessive bony decompression. Many of these complications can be avoided by meticulous surgical technique and careful hemostasis. Acquired Chiari I malformations can occur in patients with pseudotumor cerebri (often after lumboperitoneal shunt) or other supratentorial lesions. In these cases the need of posterior fossa decompression can be eliminated by addressing the primary pathologies.[12] There may be a high risk of postoperative CSF leak in pseudotumor patients if the increased intracranial pressure is not adequately addressed before the posterior fossa decompression. If a CSF leak occurs postoperatively, possible causes may include (1) poor closure technique, (2) underlying hydrocephalus/pseudotumor cerebri, and (3) infection precluding tissue healing. It is often helpful to conduct a funduscopic exam and to look closely at the sella on an MRI preoperatively to rule out papilledema or the presence of the "empty sella sign" that may indicate increased intracranial pressure. Excessively large craniectomies have been reported to cause cerebellar sagging postoperatively. A typically craniectomy with a 3- to 4-cm width is adequate for cerebellar decompression; however, some surgeons have also reported the routine use of wide bony decompression expanding from one transverse-sigmoid junction to the other with good results.[13]

Conclusion

Despite being a disease process that was first described over 120 years ago, the diagnosis and management of Chiari I malformation remain controversial today. The technological advancement of a cine flow MRI is a useful tool for pre- and postoperative evaluation of the adequacy of posterior fossa decompression and restoration of normal CSF dynamics.[14] The surgical procedure undertaken should be tailored to the individual patient's symptomatology, with the goal of restoring normal CSF flow.

References

1. Bejjani GK. Definition of the adult Chiari malformation: a brief historical overview. Neurosurg Focus 2001;11:E1
2. Alzate JC, Kothbauer KF, Jallo GI, Epstein FJ. Treatment of Chiari I malformation in patients with and without syringomyelia: a consecutive series of 66 cases. Neurosurg Focus 2001;11:E3
3. Gardner WJ, Angel J. The mechanism of syringomyelia and its surgical correction. Clin Neurosurg 1958;6:131–140
4. Williams B. The distending force in the production of "communicating syringomyelia". Lancet 1969;2:189–193
5. Ball MJ, Dayan AD. Pathogenesis of syringomyelia. Lancet 1972;2:799–801
6. Schroth G, Klose U. Cerebrospinal fluid flow. I. Physiology of cardiac-related pulsation. Neuroradiology 1992;35:1–9
7. Schroth G, Klose U. Cerebrospinal fluid flow. II. Physiology of respiration-related pulsations. Neuroradiology 1992;35:10–15
8. Schroth G, Klose U. Cerebrospinal fluid flow. III. Pathological cerebrospinal fluid pulsations. Neuroradiology 1992;35:16–24
9. Milhorat TH, Bolognese PA. Tailored operative technique for Chiari type I malformation using intraoperative color Doppler ultrasonography. Neurosurgery 2003;53:899–905, discussion 905–906
10. Massimi L, Della Pepa GM, Tamburrini G, Di Rocco C. Sudden onset of Chiari malformation type I in previously asymptomatic patients. J Neurosurg Pediatr 2011;8:438–442
11. Baisden J. Controversies in Chiari I malformations. Surg Neurol Int 2012; 3(Suppl 3):S232–S237
12. Payner TD, Prenger E, Berger TS, Crone KR. Acquired Chiari malformations: incidence, diagnosis, and management. Neurosurgery 1994;34:429–434, discussion 434
13. Chotai S, Kshettry VR, Lamki T, Ammirati M. Surgical outcomes using wide suboccipital decompression for adult Chiari I malformation with and without syringomyelia. Clin Neurol Neurosurg 2014;120:129–135
14. Alperin N, Kulkarni K, Loth F, et al. Analysis of magnetic resonance imaging-based blood and cerebrospinal fluid flow measurements in patients with Chiari I malformation: a system approach. Neurosurg Focus 2001; 11:E6

15 Occipital-Cervical Encephalocele: Surgical Treatment

Sandi K. Lam and Andrew Jea

Encephalocele is the protrusion of the cranial contents beyond the normal confines of the skull through a defect in the calvarium. Congenital cranial anomalies are relatively rare, occurring in 1 to 3 per 10,000 live births.[1] Encephalocele is a congenital anomaly characterized by herniation of the brain and meninges through a defect along the midline of the cranial vault or at the base of the skull. The most common sites of encephalocele are occipital (75%) and frontoethmoidal (13 to 15%). Occipital encephalocele (**Fig. 15.1**) is more common in the Western Hemisphere, whereas anterior encephaloceles are more often encountered in Southeast Asia.[2,3]

The embryological abnormalities in encephaloceles are thought to occur with neurulation, resulting in mesodermal defects because of separation failure between the surface ectoderm and the neuroectoderm.[4] The extracranial herniations range from small to extensive, with major abnormalities involving the brain and upper spinal cord. The contents of the protruded sac may include tissue of the occipital lobe, cerebellum, brainstem, or cervical spinal cord. Encephalocele lesions can be diagnosed prenatally with ultrasound. About 80% of encephaloceles occur in the occipital region, with a female preponderance in this area. Large and extensive craniocervical herniations are rare and can be associated with other neural tube defects.[2,5]

Hydrocephalus can occur in a majority of cases, either at presentation or after encephalocele repair. The contents of the occipitocervical sac can vary, ranging from meninges only with cerebrospinal fluid (CSF) to herniation of major brain structures including the cerebral cortex and hindbrain. The prognosis is thus directly proportional to the amount of brain within the defect as well as the association of other congenital cranial or multisystem abnormalities.[6]

Patient Selection

The risk of mortality for infants with this condition is highest in the perinatal period. The prognosis is based on the clinical characteristics, including the site of the defect, the contents of the encephalocele sac, low birth weight, and associated congenital anomalies. In addition to neurologic deficits, airway anomalies and respiratory distress may pose additional challenges. The absence of brain tissue within the sac is the single most favorable prognostic factor for survival.[7,8]

Risk factors for poor cognitive outcome include the presence of hydrocephalus and of other brain abnormalities, such as dysgenesis of the corpus callosum, heterotopias, and cerebral dysgenesis.[5]

Indications and Contraindications

The goal of treatment is the closure of the defect. Most lesions are skin-covered without CSF leakage. The timing of the repair is elective unless the lesion is open. Surgery is usually accomplished soon after birth when the infant is medically stable to reposition the bulging brain back into the skull, remove any dysplastic brain tissue/sac-like protrusion, and correct the skull deformity. The goals are to repair the occipital encephalocele while maintaining the integrity and function of the vascular and neural structures contained inside, if they are functional. If the contents of the encephalocele consist of gliotic, fibrous, or dysplastic nonfunctional tissue, the mass may be removed. The amount of available tissue coverage for closure should be evaluated, and, if needed, plans for coverage should be made prior to proceeding to operation. Hydrocephalus is managed with CSF diversion and ventriculoperitoneal shunting. Hydrocephalus, if present, should be addressed, as CSF leakage after encephalocele repair may be a complication in the face of untreated hydrocephalus. Medical instability, such as with sepsis, or a grim neurologic prognosis, such as with anencephaly, would preclude operative intervention.[2]

Choice of Operative Approach

The surgical approach is dictated by the location, size, and anatomy of the specific lesion. The appropriate treatment depends on the encephalocele anatomy, including the amount and type of functional/dysplastic neural structures involved, the arterial and venous patterns, the bony anatomy, the soft tissue coverage, and the presence of hydrocephalus.

Preoperative Testing

Magnetic resonance imaging (MRI) is recommended to evaluate the contents of the encephalocele. Prenatal ultrasound can provide the diagnosis, but MRI of the brain is superior in terms of providing detail for surgical planning. It is vital to understand the relationship of the encephalocele anatomy, the protruding brain tissue, the arterial supply, and the venous drainage. MRI of the brain and neuraxis also demonstrates the presence of other cerebral and congenital anomalies, which are necessary to identify prior to the decision is made for intervention. Computed tomography (CT) may be helpful in evaluating the bony structures for surgical planning, especially when bony reconstruction needs to be considered.[9]

Neonatology/pediatrics and anesthesiology assessment and input are important in evaluating systemic fitness and medical optimization prior to the planned surgery.

Surgical Procedure
Positioning

The encephalocele is repaired with the infant positioned prone, overlying two well-padded gel chest rolls (the lateral position

15 Occipital-Cervical Encephalocele: Surgical Treatment

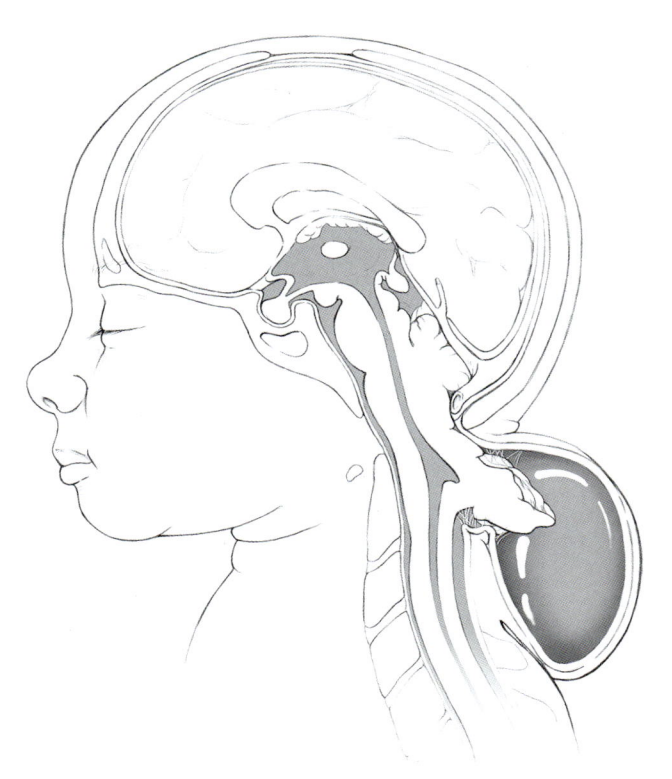

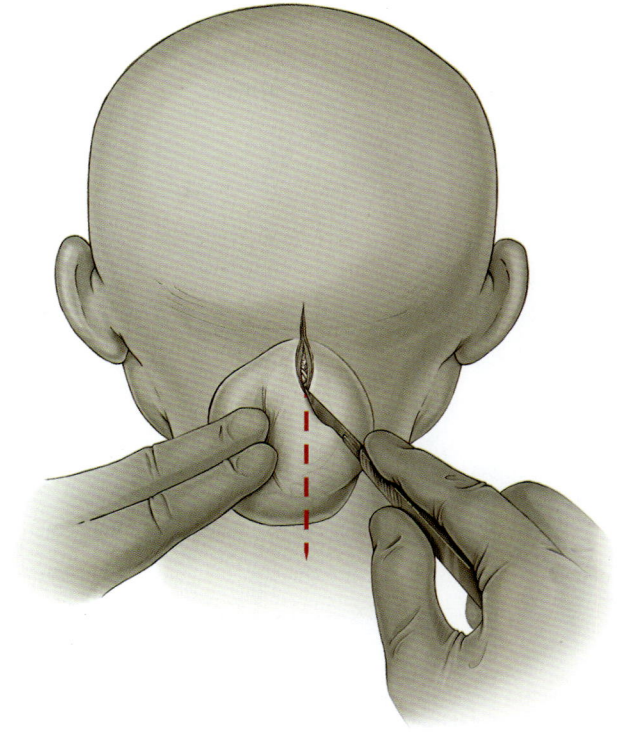

Fig. 15.1 Drawing of an occipital-cervical encephalocele. This lesion consists of herniated neural tissue and meninges through the bony defect.

Fig. 15.2 An incision through the skin is made, staying outside of the dura at this stage.

has also been described). The head is placed face down in the prone position onto a well-padded horseshoe gel headrest. Care must be taken to prevent pressure on the eyes. The neck is flexed as needed to obtain adequate exposure of the encephalocele, and the occipitocervical region is prepped and draped in sterile fashion. The encephalocele sac may need to be elevated or repositioned during prepping to ensure complete skin cleansing. Care must be taken when manipulating the sac to prevent injury to the structures within. Care also must be taken to prevent prep fluid from getting into the patient's eyes in the prone position.

Incision

The incision is planned to enable primary skin closure at the end of the surgery, such as longitudinally, or a vertical ellipse if needed (**Fig. 15.2**). In cases of dysplastic skin covering, the skin incision is made at the junction of the normal and dysplastic skin. Care should be taken to prevent premature entrance into the intradural encephalocele contents at skin incision.

Exposure

Exposure can be done with careful electrocautery, which minimizes blood loss. This is especially important in small patients. A plane is developed between the dura and the subcutaneous tissues. The dura is exposed. The bony defect is circumferentially exposed at all edges, defining the stalk/neck of the lesion.

For cervical and low-lying occipital encephaloceles, the sac is opened vertically to provide access to both the upper cervical spine and the posterior fossa.

When the encephalocele arises entirely from a defect in the upper cervical spine, it is repaired by a midline posterior approach, with the dissection beginning at normal cervical spine levels both rostral and caudal to the defect. Limited laminectomies or osteoplastic laminectomies both above and below the level of the defect can be undertaken.

The bony defect surrounding the encephalocele stalk may have to be widened to provide better exposure of the encephalocele stalk. If possible, the sac should not be entered at this stage of the operation. Dissection is performed to separate the skin from the underlying dura until the neck of the sac and the margins of the skull defect can be delineated circumferentially.

Dural Opening

The dura is entered sharply near its dome to expose the interior of the sac (**Fig. 15.3**).

Encephalocele Contents

The contents of the sac are carefully examined to determine the proper surgical approach.[10] The extent to which an encephalocele can be corrected depends on the size of the malformation and the amount and type of herniated brain tissue. Herniated brain tissue, if functional, is typically not reduced back into the intracranial compartment.[11]

If there is no neural tissue present (as in the case of a simple meningocele), the redundant skin and dura are excised, leaving enough dura at the base that is primarily closed in watertight fashion. If neural tissue is present in the sac, the surgeon must decide whether to resect or preserve this tissue. In cases where there is a large amount of functional extracranial tissue, the tissue cannot be reduced. In many cases, the extracranial neural tissue is severely dysplastic and ischemic, with few viable neurons.

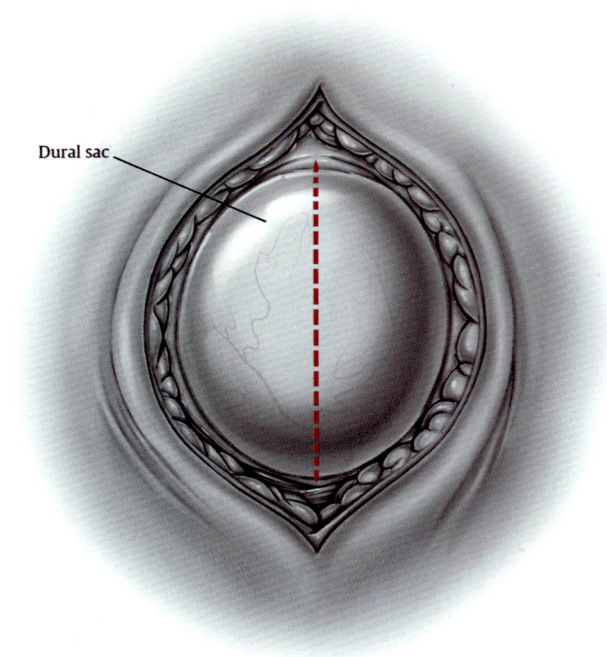

Fig. 15.3 The edges of the bony defect are exposed, defining the neck of the encephalocele. The bone edges should be defined all around the defect before entering the dura for intradural exploration.

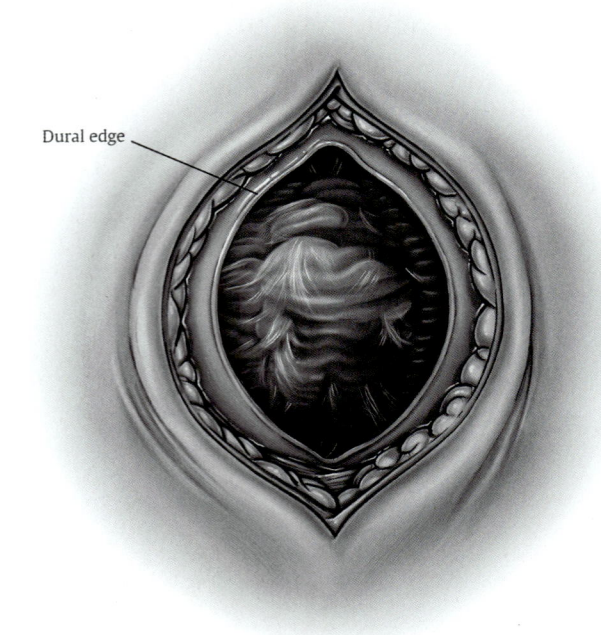

Fig. 15.4 The dura mater is incised. The herniated tissue is inspected. If it consists of fibroglottic scar, then the nonfunctional tissue is transected at its base. If it consists of functional tissue, a dural graft and protective reconstruction are undertaken.

If the extracranial neural tissue is deemed nonfunctional, it can be excised flush with the skull defect (**Fig. 15.4**). Blunt dissection and bipolar cautery are used to circumferentially isolate the neural tissue from the dura at the base of the sac, and the herniated tissue is then transected at its base. Large arterial and venous vascular channels are often found coursing through the tissue and must be thoroughly clipped and/or cauterized prior to excising the tissue. Meticulous hemostasis is achieved, and the dura is closed in watertight fashion. A dural patch graft may be necessary (**Fig. 15.5**).

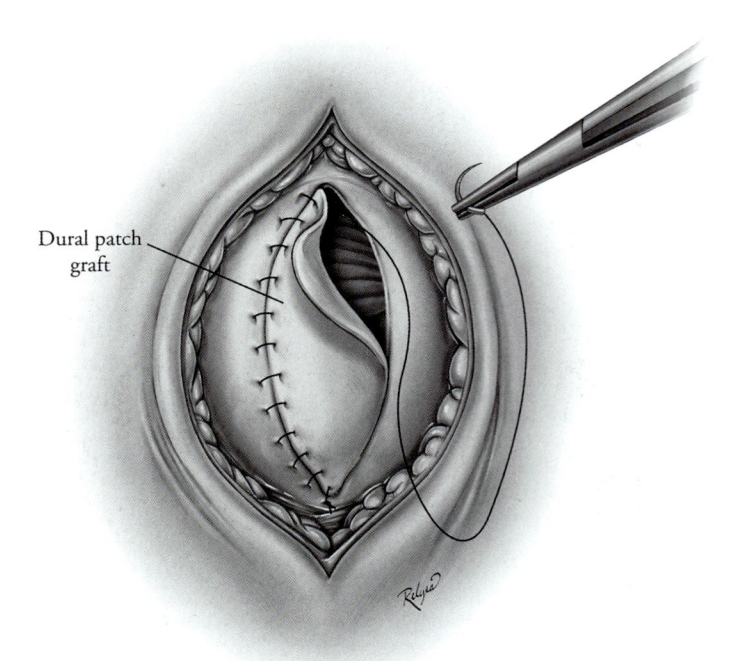

Fig. 15.5 The dura mater can be closed primarily or reinforced with a dural patch graft.

In patients with functional extracranial neural tissue, the herniated tissue should not be excised. A dural patch graft and expansion cranioplasty may be undertaken to close the defect around the herniated contents. In select cases, CSF diversion may encourage regression of the tissue into the cranium/cervical spinal canal and facilitate delayed closure.[12]

Closure: Bony Coverage

In patients with occipitocervical encephaloceles with a large skull defect associated with a large amount of herniated tissue, different techniques can be used to close the skull defect. In young infants capable of new bone regeneration, a full-thickness calvarial graft can be harvested from adjacent normal skull to cover the skull defect, accompanied by surrounding barrel stave expansile osteotomies.[13] Encephaloceles can also be repaired in a staged fashion, with duraplasty followed by delayed cranioplasty, with a split-thickness autologous bone graft performed at a later date when the bone has grown thicker. A three-dimensional computed tomography (CT) custom-fitting polymer implant is another option, although many prefer repair with autologous bone in young children. In patients with hydrocephalus at presentation, initial treatment may involve placement of an external ventricular drain or ventriculoperitoneal shunt to encourage regression of the encephalocele sac contents back into the cranial vault/cervical spinal canal and subsequent delayed closure of the occipitocervical encephalocele.[12]

Closure: Skin Coverage

To close the skin, excess full- or partial-thickness skin (if present) is trimmed away. In other cases, blunt dissection within the subgaleal space may be needed to mobilize sufficient skin for a tension-free closure.[10] The skin is then closed in layers: the galea is closed with buried interrupted 3-0 or 4-0 resorbable sutures followed by closure of the skin with a running 4-0 or 5-0 monofilament suture.

Postoperative Care

The wound should be kept free of pressure. Hydrocephalus should be treated; this would also minimize the risk of wound breakdown with a CSF leak. If not shunted at the outset, the patient should be followed postoperatively for development of hydrocephalus after encephalocele repair.

Multidisciplinary care is needed for continued welfare of the child, as many children have associated congenital anomalies with occipitocervical encephalocele. A majority have physical or mental impairment, although a minority with minimal brain tissue involvement in isolated small defects may attain a normal level of development and function.

Potential Complications and Precautions

The complications associated with the repair of occipitocervical encephaloceles include injury to underlying neural structures, extensive blood loss, CSF leakage, and infection. All of these potential outcomes can be minimized with adequate preoperative visualization and planning, as well as careful surgical technique. Because over half of these patients may have hydrocephalus, early CSF diversion is critical in preventing CSF leakage, symptomatic hydrocephalus, and infection.

Conclusion

The outcome and the surgical care of these complex congenital lesions are directly proportional to their size, extent of brain herniation, and associated anomalies. The surgical closure of these lesions may be technical challenging. In smaller lesions, favorable outcomes can be achieved.

Key Points

- Anatomy and contents of the encephalocele are major predictors of functional outcome.
- Specific lesion anatomy dictates the surgical treatment plan. Herniated brain structures, arterial supply, and venous drainage may all be anomalous; patient-specific anatomic details are important to address with careful preoperative planning.
- Hydrocephalus is often present before or after encephalocele repair. Patients should be monitored closely for hydrocephalus after surgery. CSF diversion prior to encephalocele repair may facilitate delayed closure if viable tissue is herniated into the protruded sac.

References

1. Wiswell TE, Tuttle DJ, Northam RS, Simonds GR. Major congenital neurologic malformations. A 17-year survey. Am J Dis Child 1990;144:61–67
2. McLone DG. Encephaloceles. Pediatr Neurosurg 2000;33:56
3. Shokunbi T, Adeloye A, Olumide A. Occipital encephalocoeles in 57 Nigerian children: a retrospective analysis. Childs Nerv Syst 1990;6:99–102
4. Smith JL, Schoenwolf GC. Neurulation: coming to closure. Trends Neurosci 1997;20:510–517
5. Albright A, Pollack I, Adelson P, eds. Principles and Practice of Pediatric Neurosurgery, 3rd ed. New York: Thieme; 2014
6. Chapman PH, Caviness VS. Subtorcular occipital encephaloceles. Concepts Pediatr Neurosurg 1988;8:86–96
7. Brown MS, Sheridan-Pereira M. Outlook for the child with a cephalocele. Pediatrics 1992;90:914–919
8. Lo BW, Kulkarni AV, Rutka JT, et al. Clinical predictors of developmental outcome in patients with cephaloceles. J Neurosurg Pediatr 2008;2:254–257
9. Alexiou GA, Sfakianos G, Prodromou N. Diagnosis and management of cephaloceles. J Craniofac Surg 2010;21:1581–1582
10. Cheek WR, ed. Atlas of Pediatric Neurosurgery. Philadelphia: WB Saunders; 1996
11. Anson J, Benzel E, Awad I, eds. Syringomyelia and the Chiari Malformations: Neurosurgical Topics. Park Ridge, IL: American Association of Neurological Surgeons; 1997
12. Snyder WE Jr, Luerssen TG, Boaz JC, Kalsbeck JE. Chiari III malformation treated with CSF diversion and delayed surgical closure. Pediatr Neurosurg 1998;29:117–120
13. Pang D, Dias MS. Cervical myelomeningoceles. Neurosurgery 1993;33:363–372, discussion 372–373

16 Occipital Plating and Occipital-Cervical Fusion

Manish K. Kasliwal, Ricardo B.V. Fontes, and Vincent C. Traynelis

Instability at the occipital-cervical junction (OCJ) may result from a myriad of disorders that, if left untreated, can lead to severe neurologic morbidity or even mortality. Significant loss of structural integrity of the craniovertebral junction (CVJ) may be due to trauma, rheumatoid arthritis, infection, tumor, congenital deformity, and degenerative processes.[1] This junctional area is challenging in terms of fixation. The anatomic and biomechanical characteristics of this region make internal fixation difficult, and early attempts at surgical stabilization were met with high rates of failure.[2,3] Additionally, these pioneering procedures often required cumbersome and prolonged postoperative external immobilization with either a halo vest or Minerva jacket to obtain acceptable fusion rates.[2,3] The development of rigid fixation has led to increasingly successful outcomes and a concomitant decrease in the need for postoperative immobilization. Wire or cable fixed rods or loops represented an advance over prior techniques, but such constructs only provided semirigid fixation. Modern segmental screw-based constructs enable rigid short-segment fixation and provide adequate stability to achieve successful fusion in over 90% of patients.[3-8] This chapter describes the technique of rigid occipitocervical fixation.

Patient Selection

The OCJ can be affected in a wide variety of conditions such as trauma, inflammation, infection, congenital or neoplastic.[1] The availability of modern rigid occipitocervical instrumentation has obviated the need of postoperative halo immobilization with a very high fusion rate.[3-8] Patients with a neurologic deficit or meeting the radiographic criteria for instability in this region, regardless of the cause, often require and are amenable to occipitocervical plating and arthrodesis. Nevertheless, patients selection remains the key for successful outcome, and occipitocervical plating should be avoided in patients with irreducible symptomatic anterior compression and significant medical comorbidities precluding general anesthesia administration. Similarly, although atlantoaxial instability can be treated with occipitocervical fusion, it should primarily be treated with atlantoaxial fusion.

Advantages

- Provides immediate rigidity to the spine, thus eliminating postoperative halo vest immobilization
- Avoids passage of sublaminar wire with its attendant complications

Disadvantages

- Fixed hole-to-hole distance may not match every patient's anatomy, preventing optimal screw placement.
- Plate bulk can limit the space available for placement of graft material.
- Occipital plate fixation may limit the ability to place occipital screws along the midline, the thickest and strongest bone area in the occiput.

Choice of Operative Approach

A successful occipitocervical fusion can provide a favorable outcome in both acute and chronic types of craniocervical instability. There are a variety of techniques to obtain a fusion varying from onlay grafts, wiring, plates, and most recently plate–rod constructs.[2,9] The screw–rod and screw–plate constructs have been shown to provide improved neurologic status postoperatively, decreased instrumentation failure rates, and few postoperative complications.[2,5,9] Rigid occipital fixation has been combined with a variety of screw anchor options in the cervical spine to provide great flexibility in terms of managing simple and complex pathology. These constructs are biomechanically superior to previous nonrigid fixation techniques and are very efficacious from a clinical perspective.

Indications

Occipitocervical instability can be acute, which is usually precipitated by trauma (**Fig. 16.1**) or chronic secondary to causes such as degenerative, inflammatory/autoimmune, infectious, neoplastic (metastatic or primary), and congenital processes.[5,10,11] The indications for occipitocervical fusion include occipitocervical instability and atlantoaxial instability where the patient is not a candidate for atlantoaxial fusion or has failed previous attempts at C1-C2 fusion. Indications for occipitocervical fusion include the following:

- Trauma: occipitoatlantal dislocation
- Occipitocervical kyphotic deformity
- Cranial settling with brainstem compression
- OCJ instability (iatrogenic/osteomyelitis/rheumatoid arthritis /tumor)
- Congenital CVJ lesion causing brainstem compression
- Atlantoaxial instability (not a candidate for atlantoaxial fusion or has failed previous attempts at C1-C2 fusion)

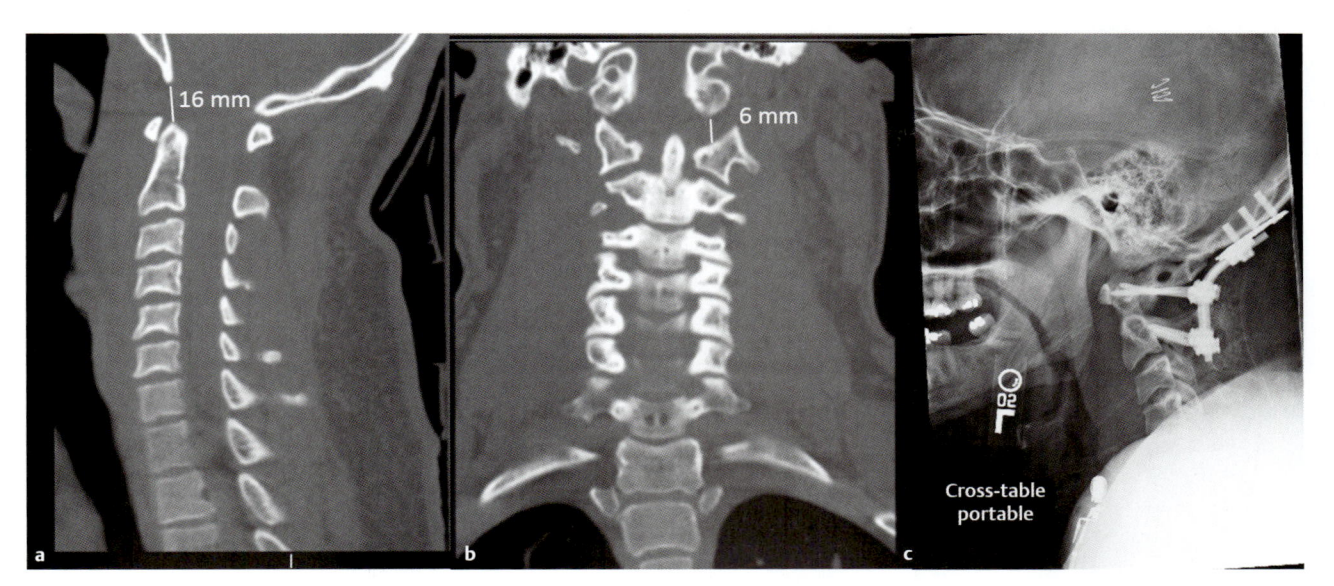

Fig. 16.1 Lateral **(a)** and anteroposterior **(b)** reconstructed computed tomography (CT) scans demonstrating a case of traumatic occipitoatlantal dislocation as exemplified by an increased basion dental interval (16 mm) and condyle-C1 interval (6 mm). **(c)** A occipitocervical plating and fusion was performed. Also noted on the X-ray is an incidental ponticulus posticus.

Contraindications

- Irreducible symptomatic anterior compression
- Significant medical comorbidities precluding general anesthesia administration
- Occipital bone defects (involving the target fixation site): relative as occipital-cervical fusion may still be performed by placement of occipital condyle screws.[12]

Preoperative Imaging

- Radiographs: anteroposterior (AP) and lateral cervical spine with or without dynamic films depending on pathology
- Computed tomography (CT) scan with sagittal and coronal reconstructions
- Magnetic resonance imaging (MRI) of the cervical spine to determine degree and severity of spinal cord compression
- CT myelogram if MRI is not available or is contraindicated

Relevant Surgical Anatomy

Stabilization of the OCJ requires a comprehensive understanding of the regional anatomy. The thickness of the bone in the suboccipital region varies depending on location, with anatomic studies demonstrating that the external occipital protuberance is the thickest in the midline and decreases laterally to inferiorly.[13] In the midline, the internal occipital crest contributes to a mean thickness of 8.3 mm at the level of the inferior nuchal line, increasing to a mean of 13.8 mm at the external occipital protuberance. Lateral bone is thinner, ranging from a mean of 3.7 mm at the level of the inferior nuchal line and increasing to a mean of 8.3 mm at the level of the superior nuchal line. Screw fixation is preferred below the level of the superior nuchal line to avoid a transverse sinus injury and along the dense midline ridge below the external occipital protuberance (**Fig. 16.2**). Additionally, the soft tissue coverage above the nuchal line is very poor, and extending the instrumentation above this level places the patient at risk for exposure of the hardware due to scalp breakdown (**Fig. 16.3**). The quality of and depth of the midline bone is optimal and this region is the ideal point for occiput screw fixation.

For atlantoaxial instrumentation and fixation, multiple fixation methods may be used, including transarticular screws, C1 lateral mass screws, or C2 pedicle, pars, or translaminar screws. Transarticular screws require a drill trajectory that starts at the C7-T1 region. Thus, excessive kyphosis precludes the ability to obtain the approach angle. Generally, the presence of an irreducible C1-C2 subluxation, deficient C2 bony pars, or aberrant medialized vertebral artery excludes this option.[14] These anatomic variations must be evaluated as part of the preoperative plan. The details of regional anatomy and specific instrumentation techniques involving the atlas, axis, and the subaxial cervical spine is discussed in Chapters 17 to 20, 31, and 38. These fixation points are precisely defined, whereas the occiput represents a relatively large target for screw implantation. For this reason the cervical screws should be placed prior to moving to the occiput.

Surgical Technique

Positioning and Preparation

Patients are intubated in a carefully controlled manner, maintaining the alignment of the cervical spine at all times. The patient is positioned prone with the head fixed either with Mayfield pins, which is the senior author's (V.C.T.) preference, or tong traction. Tong traction should not be used in patients with vertical displacement injuries to avoid further distraction. It is critical to

102　I　Occipital-Cervical Junction

Fig. 16.2 Schematic diagram demonstrating the area *(shaded triangle)* for optimal screw placement in the occipital bone.

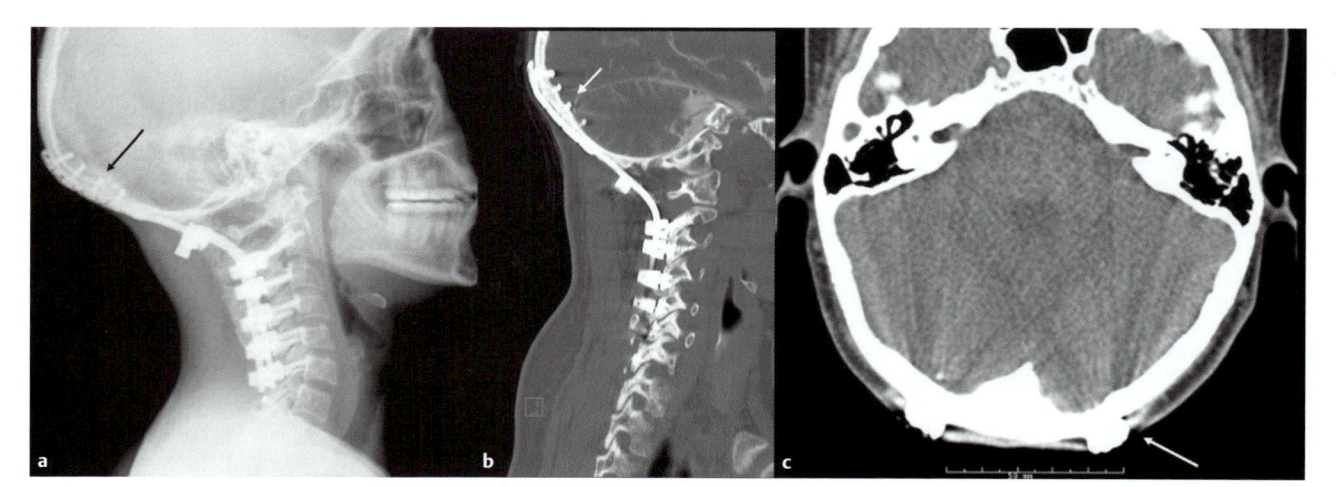

Fig. 16.3 Lateral X-ray **(a)** and reconstructed sagittal CT **(b)** of a female patient who underwent occipital-cervical fusion at an outside institution, demonstrating a very high riding occipital plate extending above the inion/superior nuchal line *(arrow)* with the left-sided plate eroding through the skin as demonstrated on the axial CT **(c)**. She underwent reexploration surgery and removal of occipital instrumentation. The screws were inserted too deep as can be seen on the CT, with one of them penetrating the transverse sinus *(arrow)*. Caution should be exercised to keep the instrumentation below the level of the superior nuchal line to avoid a transverse sinus injury and along the dense midline ridge below the external occipital protuberance to obtain good fixation. This also provides good soft tissue coverage and avoids skin-related complication.

optimize the patient's head alignment because fixation in an extended or flexed position can lead to significant postoperative morbidity. Radiographic studies should be performed to confirm satisfactory anatomic alignment prior to starting the procedure. Evoked potential monitoring may be useful in highly select situations. If such monitoring is employed, baseline studies with the patient in the supine position are necessary to compare with the potentials in the prone position. Long-acting paralytic agents and nitrous oxide may blunt motor evoked potentials (MEPs) and somatosensory evoked potentials (SSEPs), respectively.[6] It is important to maintain an adequate mean arterial pressure, particularly when there has been a spinal cord injury or when there is significant spinal cord compression.

Exposure

The incision is midline and extends from the inion to the lowest level to be incorporated into the fusion construct. At a minimum, lateral masses to C3 are usually exposed. Subperiosteal dissection with exposure of the suboccipital bone and dorsal elements of the cervical spine is performed using the Bovie electrocautery to minimize blood loss. Care is taken to note any aberrant vertebral artery loops on preoperative scans to avoid injury to these structures during the exposure. If a suboccipital decompression is performed the bone should be saved to use as autograft. The details relative to the exposure and fixation of the axis, atlas, and subaxial cervical spine are described in Chapters 17 to 20, 31, 38, and 39.

Instrumentation

Once adequate exposure is accomplished, decompression is performed if necessary, and ideally screw fixation of the caudal regions is accomplished. Currently, the most commonly used suboccipital fixation method is bicortical screw fixation into the midline suboccipital keel and paramedian cranium. The screws may be placed through a plate that is then connected to the longitudinal supporting members of the construct (most often rods), or the longitudinal rods can be secured to the skull with small connectors that each accommodate a single screw (**Fig. 16.4**). The senior author prefers the latter because the technique offers the most flexibility in screw placement, usually enables fixation with six screws, and leaves more posterior occipital bone exposed for grafting. Drilling, tapping, and screw insertion is the same for both techniques.

Plate fixation starts with choosing an appropriately sized plate. The plate should be contoured to fit snugly against the skull. Bicortical holes are drilled though the apertures of the plate using a hand-held power drill (**Fig. 16.5**). A 6-mm drill guide is used to start. The hole is drilled and probed. The drilling depth is increased by 2-mm increments until the hole is bicortical. The skull is so hard that it is mandatory that the hole be fully tapped (**Fig. 16.5**). The angle to correctly place screws can be extreme, in which case angled instruments may be needed to obtain the appropriate trajectory. On occasion, a small amount of cerebrospinal fluid or slow venous bleeding may emanate from the pilot holes. This stops when a bicortical screw is placed. A rod is used to connect the occiput to the cervical bone screws (**Fig. 16.6**). It is possible to bend a straight rod into the proper configuration, but it is more efficient to use either a pre-bent rod or articulated rod. It is our preference to place 3.5-mm cobalt chrome rods because of their strength. The rod is contoured to lie flat on the occiput and does not pass the superior nuchal line. In-situ benders can be very useful in terms of fine tuning the rod geometry. Attention to head position for fusion should avoid extension, flexion, or rotation, and maintain a neutral occipitocervical angle as mentioned earlier. The rod is then connected to cervical fixation points directly or with offset connectors if required (**Fig. 16.7**).

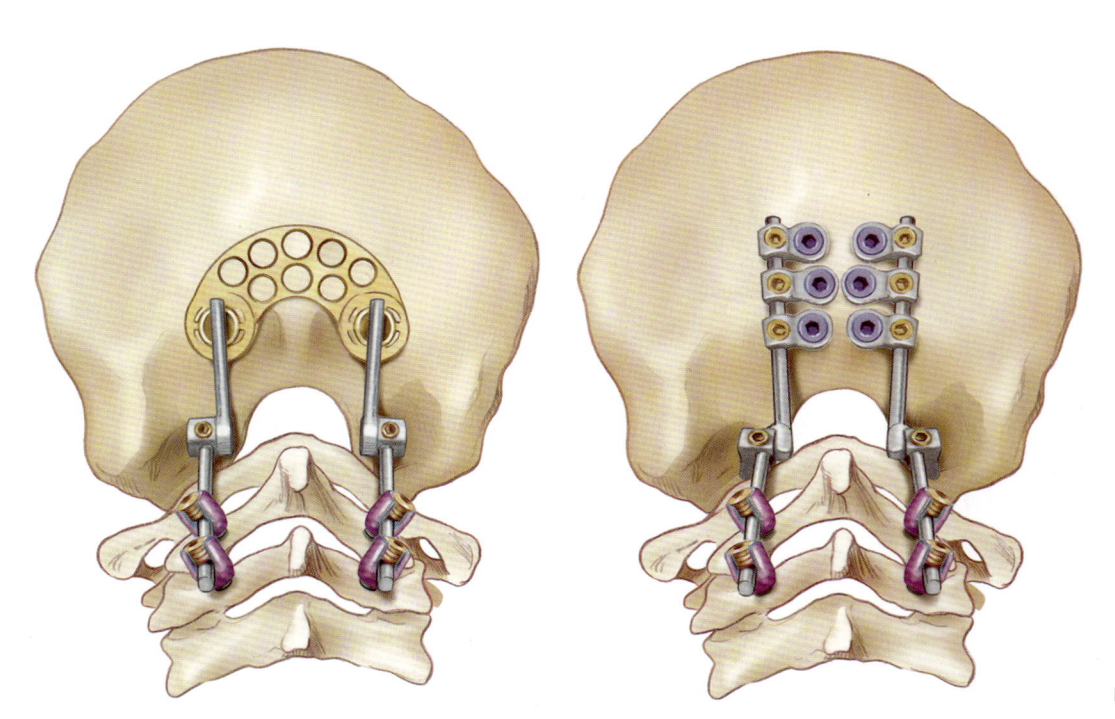

Fig. 16.4 Schematic diagrams showing the two types of rigid occipital-cervical fusion constructs in which the screws may be placed either through a plate that is then connected to the rod (**a**) or the longitudinal rods can be secured to the skull with small connectors that each accommodate a single screw (**b**).

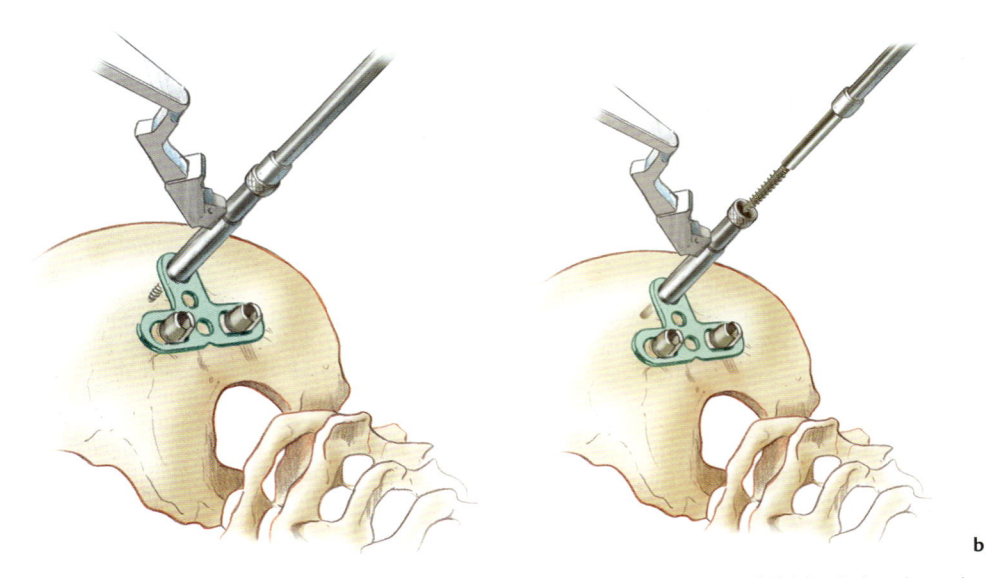

Fig. 16.5 Illustrations showing drilling of a hole through the aperture of the plate using a hand-held power drill **(a)**, which is then subsequent tapped. **(b)** The drilling depth is increased by 2-mm increments until the hole is bicortical.

Arthrodesis

Subsequent to the placement of instrumentation, an optimal environment for fusion is prepared by decortication using a high-speed bur, and bone graft is placed underneath and lateral to the rod construct. If decompression is performed, it is important to avoid graft placement into the defect and on the dura. Many options exist for bone graft; however, autograft remains the gold standard in most cervical fusions despite associated morbidity of harvest sites including the iliac crest. We use autogenous rib bone graft for occipital-cervical fusion and place strips of bone graft bridging the space between the suboccipital cranium onto bony portions of the cervical spine. Nevertheless, with rigid internal fixation, occipitocervical pseudarthrosis is extremely rare even with local bone graft and graft extenders and any of those may be used depending on the surgeon's preference.[5,8,9] A subfascial drain is placed and the wound is closed in anatomic layers.

Postoperative Care and Outcome

The patient is allowed to ambulate the same day or the day after surgery, and is usually placed in a hard collar for 6 to 12 weeks with radiographic follow-up. After 6 to 12 weeks, flexion/extension

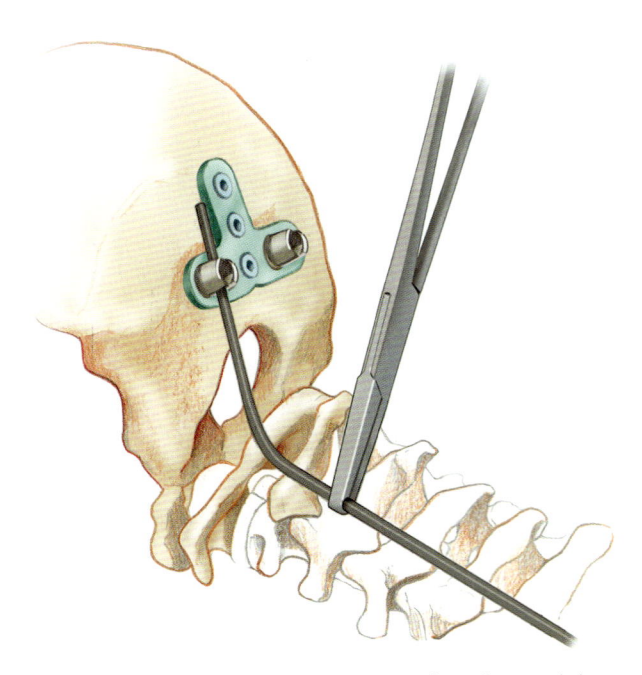

Fig. 16.6 A template can be used to determine the rod size and shape needed to connect the occipital plate and cervical screws.

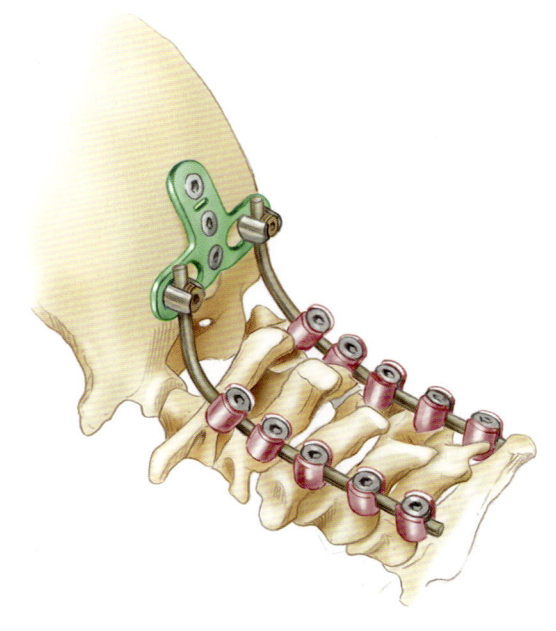

Fig. 16.7 Schematic diagram demonstrating the final occipitocervical construct after placement of bilateral rods.

views should be obtained to determine if fusion is noted radiographically. Serial radiographs should be obtained, and the occurrence of the fusion should be confirmed, which generally occurs by the end of 1 year. A CT may be necessary to assess fusion in some cases. Screw fixation technologies have demonstrated better relief of cervical pain and correction of malalignment and high fusion rates, with recent large series showing a fusion rate of 94 to 97% with the use of screw–rod or screw–plate constructs.[1,2,4,5]

Potential Complications and Precautions

Minor complications include wound infection, hematoma formation, dural tear, and cerebrospinal fluid leak.[2,4–6,8,15] Although postoperative rigidity and lack of neck movement is an expected outcome and goal of the procedure, the limitations secondary to it should be clearly emphasized and discussed with the patient before the surgery.[16,17] To avoid further morbidity related to the postoperative mobility, it is important to avoid excessive flexion at the OCJ, as it can lead to upper-airway obstruction and dysphagia.[16] Fixation of the patient's neck in exaggerated extension and flexion may limit activities of daily living and should be avoided by carefully aligning the patient on the operating table. The occiput-C2 angle has been shown to be a practical intraoperative radiological parameter and should be kept the same as or slightly greater than the preoperative occiput-C2 angle to avoid inadvertent postoperative dyspnea or dysphagia.[17] There are emerging data on the use of local vancomycin powder to reduce the risk of postoperative wound infections. Major potential complications include spinal cord injury, nerve root injury, cerebellar injury resulting from occipital screw penetration, posterior fossa hematoma, meningitis, vertebral artery injury from errant screw placement, and pseudarthrosis requiring reoperation.[2,4–6,8,15] Most of these can be avoided by careful assessment of preoperative imaging studies and adhering to proper anatomy during the exposure and when performing instrumentation. For patients with poor bone quality, postoperative halo fusion can be considered to reduce the risk of pseudarthrosis and instrumentation failure.

Conclusion

The craniocervical junction presents anatomic and biomechanical challenges that subject any instrumentation construct to significant stress. The evolution of occipitocervical fixation with the availability of rigid fixation technology has allowed firm anchorage at each level of the OCJ, with the elimination of rigid external orthoses, and still enabling bony fusion to occur in close to 100% of patients. Regardless, there is no substitute for a thorough understanding of the relevant cervical bony and soft tissue anatomy to avoid complications and achieve a successful clinical outcome.

References

1. Steinmetz MP, Mroz TE, Benzel EC. Craniovertebral junction: biomechanical considerations. Neurosurgery 2010;66(3, Suppl):7–12
2. Garrido BJ, Myo GK, Sasso RC. Rigid versus nonrigid occipitocervical fusion: a clinical comparison of short-term outcomes. J Spinal Disord Tech 2011;24:20–23
3. Vender JR, Rekito AJ, Harrison SJ, McDonnell DE. The evolution of posterior cervical and occipitocervical fusion and instrumentation. Neurosurg Focus 2004;16:E9
4. Abumi K, Takada T, Shono Y, Kaneda K, Fujiya M. Posterior occipitocervical reconstruction using cervical pedicle screws and plate-rod systems. Spine 1999;24:1425–1434
5. Garrido BJ, Sasso RC. Occipitocervical fusion. Orthop Clin North Am 2012; 43:1–9, vii
6. Lu DC, Roeser AC, Mummaneni VP, Mummaneni PV. Nuances of occipitocervical fixation. Neurosurgery 2010;66(3, Suppl):141–146
7. Martin MD, Bruner HJ, Maiman DJ. Anatomic and biomechanical considerations of the craniovertebral junction. Neurosurgery 2010;66(3, Suppl): 2–6
8. Winegar CD, Lawrence JP, Friel BC, et al. A systematic review of occipital cervical fusion: techniques and outcomes. J Neurosurg Spine 2010;13: 5–16
9. Oda I, Abumi K, Sell LC, Haggerty CJ, Cunningham BW, McAfee PC. Biomechanical evaluation of five different occipito-atlanto-axial fixation techniques. Spine 1999;24:2377–2382
10. Ahmed R, Traynelis VC, Menezes AH. Fusions at the craniovertebral junction. Childs Nerv Syst 2008;24:1209–1224
11. Sonntag VK, Dickman CA. Craniocervical stabilization. Clin Neurosurg 1993;40:243–272
12. Le TV, Vivas AC, Baaj AA, Vale FL, Uribe JS. Optimal trajectory for the occipital condyle screw. J Spinal Disord Tech 2014;27:93–97
13. Zipnick RI, Merola AA, Gorup J, et al. Occipital morphology. An anatomic guide to internal fixation. Spine 1996;21:1719–1724, discussion 1729–1730
14. Jacobson ME, Khan SN, An HS. C1-C2 posterior fixation: indications, technique, and results. Orthop Clin North Am 2012;43:11–18, vii
15. Fehlings MG, Cadotte DW. Occipital cervical fusion: an evolution of techniques. J Neurosurg Spine 2010;13:3–4, author reply 4
16. Ota M, Neo M, Aoyama T, et al. Impact of the O-C2 angle on the oropharyngeal space in normal patients. Spine 2011;36:E720–E726
17. Miyata M, Neo M, Fujibayashi S, Ito H, Takemoto M, Nakamura T. O-C2 angle as a predictor of dyspnea and/or dysphagia after occipitocervical fusion. Spine 2009;34:184–188

17 Exposure of C1 and C2

Manish K. Kasliwal, Ricardo B.V. Fontes, and Vincent C. Traynelis

The posterior approach to the C1-C2 region is a very common procedure performed for various indications.[1-3] This approach provides exposure of the posterior elements of C1 and C2, which enables performing several procedures that involve treating atlantoaxial instability.

Patient Selection

Posterior exposure of the atlantoaxial region is often indicated for patients with atlantoaxial instability resulting from congenital, traumatic, inflammatory, or neoplastic processes. The indications for posterior exposure of the atlantoaxial region are very robust, and considering the availability of newer instrumentation and various fixation options available, posterior exposure and subsequent instrumentation and arthrodesis enables the treatment of most of the pathologies involving this region of the spine.

Indications

- Fractures of the odontoid (type II and III)
- Adjacent fractures of C1 and C2
- Rotatory subluxation
- Rheumatoid arthritis
- Os odontoideum
- Postodontoidectomy without basilar invagination
- Tumors involving the posterior elements of atlas and axis

Advantages

- Familiarity
- Enables performing decompression and stabilization in a single approach
- Associated with decreased morbidity as compared with anterior transoral approaches

Disadvantages

- Lateral dissection places vertebral artery at risk.

Choice of Operative Approach

Posterior exposure of the atlantoaxial region is very useful for addressing atlantoaxial instability resulting from congenital, traumatic, inflammatory, or neoplastic processes. Following exposure of the C1-C2 region, the options available for fixation and arthrodesis have evolved over decades from wiring to more sophisticated screw-based constructs. The choice of exact operative approach following exposure depends on the need to do a decompression, the bone quality, and the presence/absence of vertebral artery anomalies.

Preoperative Imaging

- Dynamic X-rays of the cervical spine to determine the presence of instability, unless the injury pattern noted on computed tomography (CT) or magnetic resonance imaging (MRI) clearly identifies an unstable situation
- MRI of the cervical spine (especially with myelopathy to determine degree and severity of spinal cord compression)
- CT myelogram, if MRI is not available or contraindicated

Surgical Technique

Positioning

Patients with documented or suspected atlantoaxial instability should undergo a careful intubation so as to not produce or worsen a preexisting neurologic deficit. It is imperative that excessive neck flexion and extension be avoided. The use of intraoperative electrophysiological monitoring depends on the surgeons' preference but is not mandatory. When monitoring is performed, nondepolarizing paralytic agents and nitrous oxide should be avoided, as they blunt the motor evoked potentials (MEPs) and somatosensory evoked potentials (SSEPs), respectively. Avoiding hypotension is critical when treating patients with severe canal stenosis or myelopathy.

The major purpose of monitoring in such cases is to provide another means of detecting ischemia, so monitoring should not be necessary in the setting of anesthetic diligence. Our group prefers to request a mean arterial pressure (MAP) of 90. Although this is higher than what is usually used, it provides a "cushion" that theoretically would increase safety.

The posterior exposure of C1 and C2 is performed with the patient in the prone position, and it is our preference to rigidly fix the head in a Mayfield device (**Fig. 17.1**). Other surgeons use continuous traction, and this is also reasonable. The torso is supported on firm rolls that are positioned longitudinally from the shoulder to the waist. The thoracic cage and abdomen are left as free as possible to enable maximal ventilation and minimal venous back-pressure, so as to avoid excessive intraoperative bleeding. The pressure points should be well padded. In females, the breasts should be between the rolls placed to stabilize the torso. In males, the penis and scrotum should be free of compression. In obese patients, the shoulders can be retracted caudally using tape or other methods to improve radiographic imaging and decrease the neck skin folds. If the procedure is expected to last more than 2 hours or involve significant blood loss,

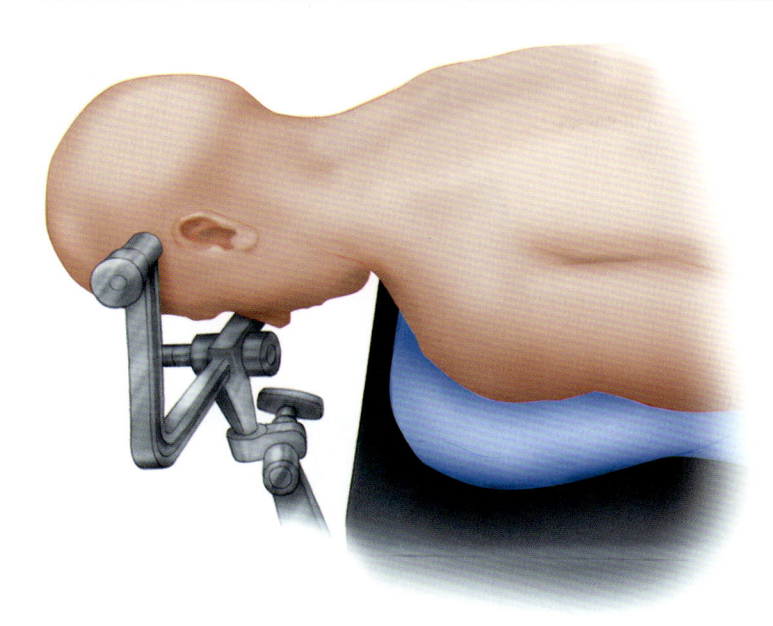

Fig. 17.1 The patient is placed in the prone position on chest rolls, with the shoulders and arm retracted caudally and the neck in neutral position.

Foley catheter placement should be considered to monitor urine output during the procedure. The patient's hair is clipped as deemed appropriate. Usually the C2 spinous process can be palpated beneath the skin, which can be an aid in planning the incision. Local anesthetic in combination with epinephrine may be infiltrated along the incision site; the infiltration should be limited to the dermal and subdermal levels and ideally is performed more than 5 minutes prior to making the skin incision to optimize the vasoconstrictive properties of epinephrine. Prior to infiltration of the local agent, the anesthesiologist should be informed so that he or she can be vigilant in monitoring the patient's cardiovascular status.

Exposure

Following incision of the skin with a knife, self-retaining retractors are placed and unipolar electrocautery is used until the fascia is identified (**Fig. 17.2**). It is imperative to stay in the midline to maintain an avascular plane. After division of the medial fascia of the trapezius muscle, the spinous processes are encountered. The bifid spinous process of C2 and posterior tubercle of C1 are useful landmarks during dissection, but the muscular and ligamentous attachments to the large C2 spinous process should not be released unless the laminae of the atlas needs to be exposed. Although this chapter deals with the exposure of C1 and C2, in which case it is usually necessary to expose all of the axis, it is important to note that maintaining the soft tissue attachments to C2 is critical in terms of minimizing the development of postoperative C2-C3 kyphosis and should always be preserved unless C2 is the surgical target. The posterior tubercle of the atlas is identified, and subperiosteal dissection of the arch ensues (**Fig. 17.3**). Initially the dissection should be performed over the posterior and inferior regions of the atlas, which are relatively remote from the vertebral artery. Superior lateral dissection increases the risks of vertebral artery injury and should be performed very carefully, especially when extending the exposure more than 15 mm lateral to the midline. Next, the muscular attachments to C2 and C3 are released from medial to lateral until the facets are defined. The self-retaining retractors are inserted deeper to maintain the exposure for the subsequent primary focus of the procedure, which is dictated by the pathology (**Fig. 17.4**).

One important anomaly, ponticulus posticus, is important to recognize on preoperative imaging and while performing the posterior C1 and C2 exposure.[4-6] A ponticulus posticus has been reported to be present in 5.1 to 37.8% of the population in the

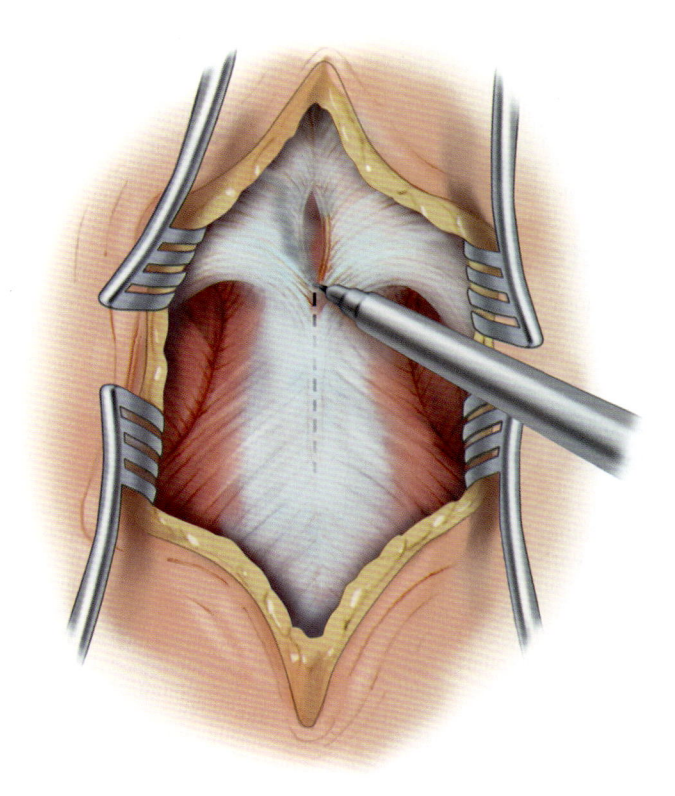

Fig. 17.2 Schematic diagram showing posterior exposure of the fascia. A knife or electrocautery can be used to perform the subperiosteal dissection.

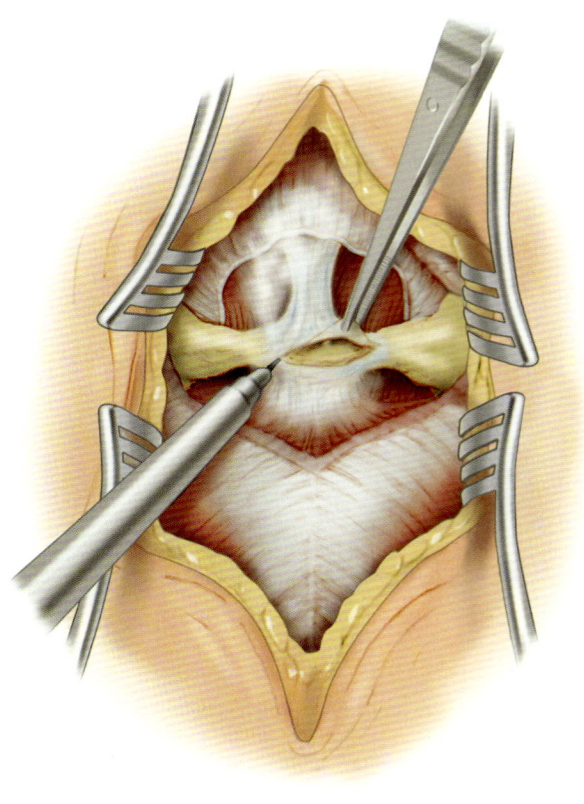

Fig. 17.3 Schematic diagram demonstrating subperiosteal dissection of C1.

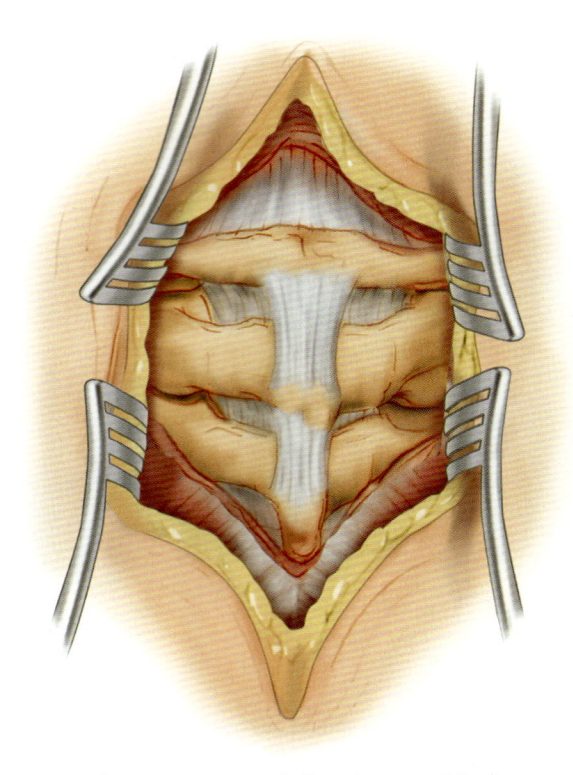

Fig. 17.4 Following exposure to the lateral margin of the facet complex at C2-C3, self-retaining retractors are inserted deeper to maintain the exposure.

Western Hemisphere and is defined as an abnormal small bony bridge that is formed between the posterior portion of the superior articular process and the posterolateral portion of the superior margin of the posterior arch of the atlas.[4-6] It has also been termed sagittale foramen, atlantal posterior foramen, arcuate foramen, a variant of Kimmerle's anomaly, upper retroarticular foramen, canalis vertebralis, retroarticular vertebral artery ring, retroarticular canal, and retrocondylar vertebral artery ring.

Postoperative Care

The postoperative care depends on the exact operative technique performed and is discussed in Chapters 16 and 18 to 20 in this textbook.

Potential Complications and Precautions

Excessive neck flexion and extension should be avoided while positioning the patient. It is critical to avoid hypotension in patients with severe canal stenosis and/or myelopathy, with maintenance of MAP ≥ 90 to reduce the risk of spinal cord ischemia. Care should be taken to avoid injury to the C2-C3 facet capsule during exposure. The muscular and ligamentous attachments to the large C2 spinous process should not be released unless the laminae of the atlas need to be exposed. The vertebral artery is at risk of injury during exposure, and the dissection should be limited to ≤ 1.5 cm laterally from the midline for wiring-based techniques, and a superior lateral approach should be performed very carefully, especially when extending the exposure > 15 mm lateral to the midline.

Conclusion

Posterior exposure of C1-C2 needs to be performed for a myriad of pathologies affecting the atlantoaxial region. Identical to the exposure of all other portions of the spine, it is best to meticulously maintain the dissection in the subperiosteal plane, which decreases both muscle injury and bleeding. This is most critical when addressing the atlantoaxial segment, which is encased with a dense venous network. Although one cannot always remain within the subperiosteal plane, if this dissection plan can be accomplished, the surgeon will be rewarded with a bloodless field, which is well worth the investment in time and effort.

References

1. Dickman CA, Crawford NR, Paramore CG. Biomechanical characteristics of C1-2 cable fixations. J Neurosurg 1996;85:316–322
2. Hott JS, Lynch JJ, Chamberlain RH, Sonntag VK, Crawford NR. Biomechanical comparison of C1-2 posterior fixation techniques. J Neurosurg Spine 2005;2:175–181
3. Jacobson ME, Khan SN, An HS. C1-C2 posterior fixation: indications, technique, and results. Orthop Clin North Am 2012;43:11–18, vii
4. Chitroda PK, Katti G, Baba IA, et al. Ponticulus posticus on the posterior arch of atlas, prevalence analysis in symptomatic and asymptomatic patients of Gulbarga population. J Clin Diagn Res 2013;7:3044–3047
5. Elliott RE, Tanweer O. the prevalence of the ponticulus posticus (arcuate foramen) and its importance in the Goel-Harms procedure: meta-analysis and review of the literature. World Neurosurg 2014;82:e335–e343
6. Young JP, Young PH, Ackermann MJ, Anderson PA, Riew KD. The ponticulus posticus: implications for screw insertion into the first cervical lateral mass. J Bone Joint Surg Am 2005;87:2495–2498

18 Atlantoaxial Wiring and Arthrodesis

Manish K. Kasliwal, Ricardo B.V. Fontes, and Vincent C. Traynelis

Atlantoaxial instability may be induced by traumatic, congenital, neoplastic, infectious, rheumatologic, degenerative, and iatrogenic etiologies. The common result of each of these entities is a narrowed spinal canal that can produce intermittent or chronic impingement of the neural elements or structural changes causing neurologic deterioration, deformity, or pain. Instability in the upper cervical spine is defined in terms of the atlantodental interval (ADI), with an ADI greater than 5 mm generally accepted as a sign of an unstable C1-C2 articulation in adults.[1] Application of a halo alone, although able to reduce motion in the subaxial cervical spine, does not provide effective immobilization in the upper cervical spine, and internal fixation is usually recommended to treat atlantoaxial instability because it enables early patient mobilization and has been associated with improved fusion rates.[2-5] Thorough knowledge of the atlantoaxial anatomy as well as of the articulations and associated neural and vascular anatomy is essential for a safe, effective exposure and subsequent instrumentation. The first step in performing any atlantoaxial fusion surgery involves adequate exposure of C1 and C2 to enable performing the technique to be used, followed by placement of the instrumentation and fusion substrate. Most surgeons use one of three common posterior stabilization options: sublaminar wiring, laminar clamps, and screw fixation.[2,6,7] This chapter describes the various surgical techniques of atlantoaxial wiring and fusion.

One of the earliest reports of posterior cervical wiring of the lamina of C1 and C2 was by Mixter and Osgood,[8] who in 1910 treated an odontoid fracture in a 15-year-old boy using a braided silk loop passed below the C1 arch and around the C2 spinous process. Gallie[9] subsequently described in 1939 his technique of posterior atlantoaxial wiring, which was supplemented with an H-shaped bone graft to aid in arthrodesis. This technique remained popular for several decades. It was not until almost 40 years later that Brooks and Jenkins[10] offered an alternative method of posterior C1-C2 laminar wiring. Dickman and Sonntag et al[11] reported their further modification of the posterior wiring technique in 1991.

Posterior atlantoaxial wiring biomechanically acts primarily as a tension band, and as such provides outstanding resistance to flexion. Placement of a graft between the dorsal elements of C1 and C2 serves to limit extension while axial rotation is resisted mostly by friction between the cable and posterior elements. C1-C2 wiring has been used to treat several pathological conditions.[9-11]

Patient Selection

Most patients with atlantoaxial instability resulting from congenital, traumatic, inflammatory, or neoplastic processes are potential candidates for posterior C1-C2 wiring techniques, provided that the posterior elements are intact and the bone quality adequate.[7,9-11]

Indications

Atlantoaxial wiring can be performed to eliminate instability for the following indications:

- Fractures of the odontoid (type II and III)
- Select fractures of C1 and C2
- Rotatory subluxation
- Rheumatoid arthritis
- Os odontoideum
- Postodontoidectomy without basilar invagination

Contraindications[2,7,10-13]

- Absent posterior element of either C1 or C2
- Atlas assimilation
- Severe osteoporosis

Advantages

- Simple and inexpensive procedure
- Relatively easy exposure
- Very low or no risk of vertebral artery injury in patients with ectatic vertebral artery
- May be useful in patients with hypoplastic pars interarticularis

Disadvantages[7,10,14,15]

- Requires an intact posterior arch of C1 and C2 and cannot be performed if there are fractures of the C1 or C2 posterior elements (including hangman's or Jefferson's fracture)
- Cannot be performed when posterior decompression of the C1-C2 complex is required or in the presence of significant osteoporosis
- Potential for injury to the dura or spinal cord during sublaminar passage of a cable, especially in patients with significant stenosis
- Fixation is only semirigid and it is least effective for axial rotation.
- Postoperative bracing is necessary (rigid orthosis or optimally a halo vest) to optimize the fusion rate.

Choice of Operative Approach

Posterior atlantoaxial wiring enjoyed great popularity for atlantoaxial arthrodesis after Gallie popularized a technique of midline wiring using a modified H-graft dorsal to the arch of the atlas.[9] Various wiring techniques were subsequently described and remained the mainstay of atlantoaxial fusion before the availability of modern screw-based constructs.[3-5,10,11,14] Even though the posterior wire-based techniques provided good fusion rates, they often were supplemented with halo-vest immobilization to increase the chances of successful fusion.[10,11] Also, the posterior wiring techniques require an intact posterior arch of C1 and C2 and cannot be utilized if there are fractures of the C1 or C2 posterior elements (including hangman's or Jefferson's fracture), or if posterior decompression of the C1-C2 complex is required, or in the presence of significant osteoporosis.[9-11] Even though these wiring techniques can be performed in a stand-alone fashion for C1-C2 arthrodesis, the frequent need of halo immobilization following surgery along with the availability of newer screw-based techniques have dampened enthusiasm for wire- or cable-based techniques. Although relatively inexpensive and easy to perform, posterior wiring currently is most often employed as an adjunct to screw-based fixation techniques of the atlantoaxial segment to increase the stiffness of the construct.[16] These wiring techniques are still important adjuncts to screw fixation, as they can improve sagittal plane stability and facilitate solid graft support.

Preoperative Imaging

- Dynamic X-rays of the cervical spine to assess for instability unless the injury pattern noted on computed tomography (CT) or magnetic resonance imaging (MRI) clearly defines an unstable situation.
- MRI of the cervical spine (especially with myelopathy to determine degree and severity of spinal cord compression)
- CT myelogram, if MRI is not available or contraindicated

Relevant Surgical Anatomy

The first cervical vertebra (C1) consists of an anterior arch, a posterior arch, and two lateral masses, which sum to produce a ring like structure[17] (**Fig. 18.1**). The anterior tubercle serves as an attachment site for the longus colli muscle, and posteriorly the fovea dentis serves as the articulation point for the odontoid process of the second cervical vertebra (C2). The posterior arch provides a smooth edge for the attachment of the posterior atlanto-occipital membrane. The sulcus arteriae vertebralis is present behind each superior articular process and represents the superior vertebral notch. The vertebral artery and the first spinal nerve reside within this sulcus. The undersurface of the posterior arch provides an attachment surface for the posterior atlantoaxial ligament. The lateral masses of C1 have an inferior

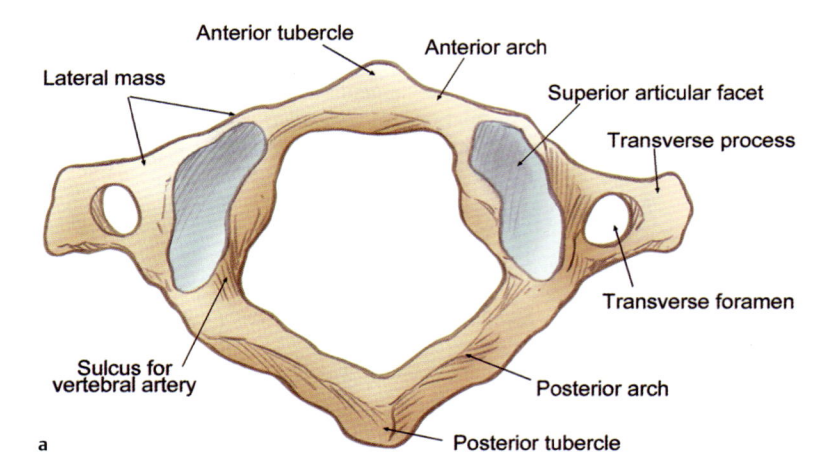

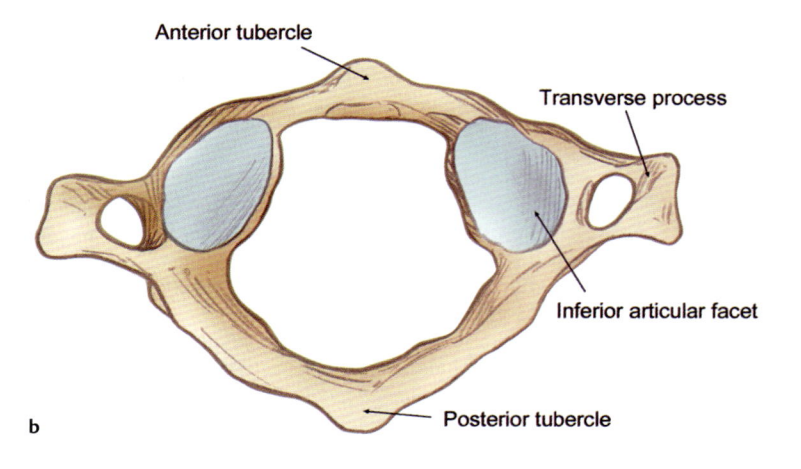

Fig. 18.1 Superior (**a**) and inferior (**b**) views showing the anatomy of the atlas vertebrae.

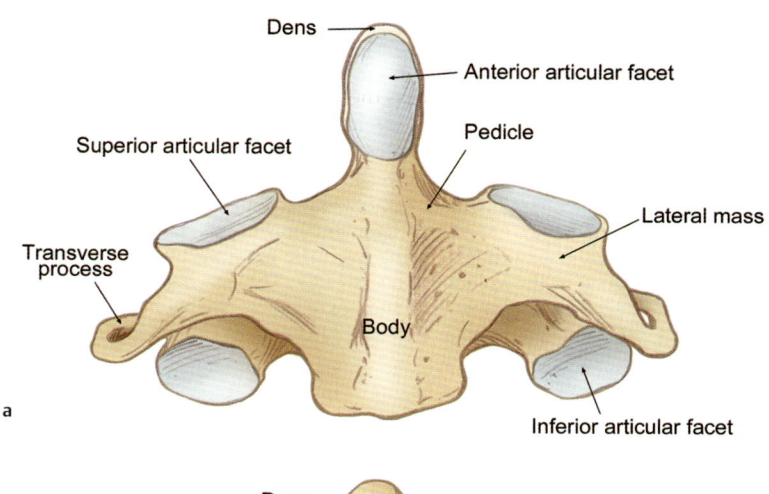

Fig. 18.2 Anterior (**a**) and posterior (**b**) views demonstrating the anatomy of the axis vertebrae.

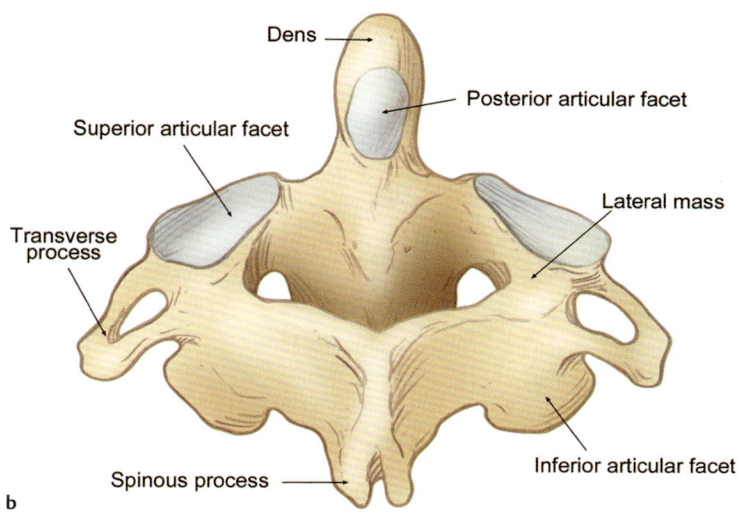

and a superior articular facet; the superior facet surface forms a cuplike articulating surface for the corresponding condyle of the occiput.

The second cervical vertebra (C2) or axis forms a pivot around which the first vertebra rotates (**Fig. 18.2**). The C2 spinous process is large and bifid. The superior articular process of C2 does not extend superiorly, but rather sits on the body of C2. It artic-ulates with the inferior facet surface of C1 to permit rotation of the head. Anteriorly, at the level of the superior facet, the important transverse atlantal ligament (a component of the cruciate ligament) traverses the C1 ring, dividing the vertebral foramen into an anterior part, which encases the dens, and a posterior part, which contains the spinal cord (**Fig. 18.3**). The odontoid process projects upward and articulates with the posterior part

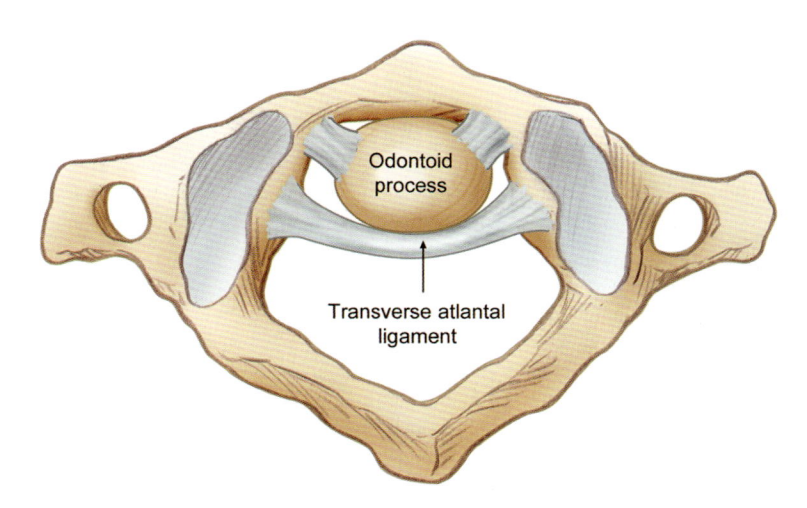

Fig. 18.3 Superior view demonstrating the anatomy at the level of the transverse atlantal ligament.

of the anterior arch of the atlas, where a synovial joint is present. Therefore, there are three atlantoaxial joints: two lateral mass articulations and the atlantodental joint.[17] There are no intervertebral disks between the occiput, atlas, and axis, and all joints are synovial. In some cases, the sulcus for the vertebral artery on the dorsal aspect of the atlas may be completely covered by an anomalous ossification, termed the ponticulus posticus.[18] The relevance of this finding is that some surgeons have advocated the starting point of a C1 lateral mass screw to be at the dorsal aspect of the posterior arch instead of the base of the lateral mass. The presence of an unidentified ponticulus posticus may lead to iatrogenic injury to the vertebral artery. The dens has an apex and neck at which it joins the body. An oval facet on its anterior surface enables articulation with the atlas. Posteriorly, the neck of the dens is the insertion site of the transverse atlantal ligament. The apical odontoid ligament attaches along the apex, and caudally, along either side of the neck, the alar ligaments attach, which connect the odontoid process to the occiput. The pedicles essentially are covered by the superior articular surfaces that articulate with C1.

Various ligaments stabilize the bony anatomy in this region (**Fig. 18.4**).[17] The large ligamentum nuchae spans multiple motion segments extending from the external occipital protuberance to the spinous process of C7. The ligamentum nuchae is a posterior tension band that resists excessive cervical flexion. The ventrally located anterior longitudinal ligament is referred to as

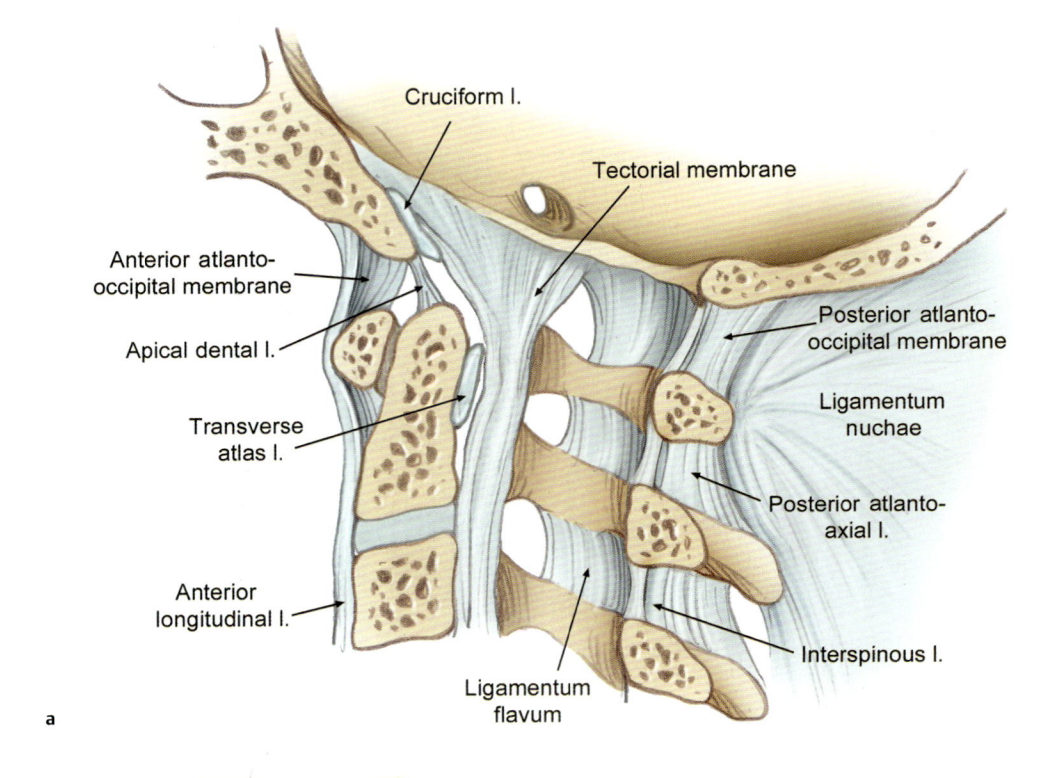

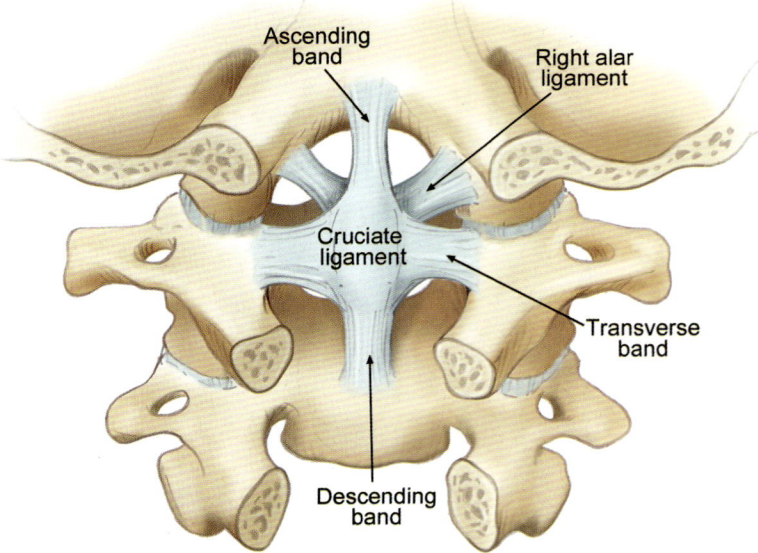

Fig. 18.4 Lateral (**a**) and dorsal (**b**) views demonstrating various ligaments in the occipitocervical region.

the anterior atlanto-occipital membrane once it traverses superior to C2 to attach between C1 and the occiput. The apical ligament attaches the tip of the dens to the basion of the occiput. The cruciate ligament has both vertical and transverse segments that are important in stabilizing the atlantoaxial articulation. However, it is the transverse portion of this ligament, also known as the transverse atlantal ligament, that attaches to the medial borders of the lateral masses of the atlas and provides the strongest resistance to posterior displacement of the odontoid process relative to the anterior arch of the atlas. Two other important stabilizing ligaments are the alar ligaments that attach the lateral apex of the dens to the occipital condyles. Finally, the apical ligament arises from the tip of the dens and attaches to the foramen magnum and is considered a notochordal remnant. The alar ligaments limit lateral rotation, and, similar to the transverse atlantal ligament, they also resist posterior translation of the dens. Anterior translation is blocked by the arch of C1.

The transverse processes of the cervical vertebra each contain a central aperture, the foramen transversarium, through which the vertebral artery ascends, usually beginning at C6. After exiting the foramen transversarium of the axis, these arteries track laterally prior to coursing through the foramen transversarium of the atlas.[19] The vertebral arteries are directed posteromedially along the superior aspect of the atlas in the vertebral notch before entering the dura.[19] One of the vertebral arteries is clearly dominant in two thirds of patients. The importance of understanding the anatomy of the vertebral artery and various anomalies cannot be overemphasized, especially with the increasing use of atlantoaxial screw fixation. It is critical to carefully review a cervical spinal CT scan before placing instrumentation at these levels, particularly at the axis, as an anomalous vertebral artery course may preclude safe screw placement into certain structures (transarticular, C2 pedicle, etc.).

Surgical Technique

Great care is required when intubating patients with documented or suspected atlantoaxial instability, and frequently these individuals are managed with an awake, fiberoptic intubation. The use of intraoperative electrophysiological monitoring depends on surgeon preference and is not always necessary. Standard vascular access should be obtained using sterile techniques, and the degree of monitoring required depends on the patient's comorbidities. It is important to maintain the mean arterial pressure (MAP) at 80 in patients with severe stenosis and if possible we prefer this value to be 90, which provides an extra margin of safety.

Positioning

Once the patient is intubated, vascular access is established, and the monitoring devices are in place, the patient is placed in the prone position. A Mayfield clamp is preferred by our group, although many surgeons use traction. The endotracheal tube is secured in place and three-point head fixation is applied. The head is held in a neutral position as the patient is rolled from supine to prone; in highly unstable situations a rigid cervical orthosis may also remain in place during the turn. A fluoroscopic image is obtained immediately to evaluate the sagittal alignment of the craniovertebral junction. The head can be manipulated using the Mayfield so that the atlantoaxial alignment is neutral or as close to neutral as possible. A small amount of capital flexion opens the space between C1 and the occiput, which facilitates access for sublaminar fixation. If neuromonitoring is performed, the evoked potentials are promptly compared with the preintubation and prepositioning baselines.

The torso is supported on firm jelly-rolls placed longitudinally from shoulder to waist. The thoracic cage and abdomen are left as free as possible to enable maximal ventilation and minimal venous back-pressure, so as to avoid excessive intraoperative bleeding. The pressure points should be well padded. In females, the breasts should be between the rolls placed to stabilize the torso. In males, the penis and scrotum should be free of compression. In most of these procedures a Foley catheter is placed to evaluate urine output during the procedure. The patient's hair is shaved as deemed appropriate. Usually, the incision is marked from one or two fingerbreadths below the external occipital protuberance to the C3 level and should be confirmed with intraoperative X-ray. Local anesthetic in the form of a 1% lidocaine/epinephrine mixture in a ratio of 1:200 is infiltrated along the incision site. Prior to infiltration of the local agent, the anesthesiologist is informed of its imminent administration so that he or she can observe any cardiovascular changes.

Exposure

The incision is usually marked from about one to two fingerbreadth below the external occipital protuberance to at least the spinous process of the third cervical vertebra. The incision is made in the midline and carried down through the soft tissue with Bovie electrocautery. Staying in the midline enables the exposure to be obtained through the avascular plane that separates the posterior cervical muscles, thereby limiting blood loss and soft tissue trauma. Electrocautery is used to detach the muscles from the bone in a subperiosteal manner. Knowledge of muscle layer anatomy is useful while performing exposure in the posterior cervical spine.

The superficial layer of the posterior cervical musculature contains the splenius capitis and cervicalis muscles (**Fig. 18.5**). The ligamentum nuchae lies in the midline and is in the plane of the trapezius muscle. Traversing this structure exposes the fascia separating the two splenius capitis muscles. These muscles are relevant in the exposure of the lower cervical spine and extend from the lower portion of the ligamentum nuchae and the spinous processes of C7–T4 proceeding laterally to attach to the mastoid process and the lateral part of the superior nuchal line and are generally not encountered during exposure of the C1 and C2. The splenius cervicalis has an origin similar to that of the splenius capitis but inserts on the posterior tubercles of the transverse processes of C1 through C4. The rectus capitis posterior major muscle attaches to the C2 posterior elements superomedially, whereas the inferior oblique muscle attaches superolaterally.

The intermediate layer consists of the erector spinae muscle groups, all of which originate along the iliac crest, sacrum, and lower lumbar vertebrae and form three columns: the spinalis group medially, the longissimus group in the middle, and the iliocostalis laterally (**Fig. 18.6**). The spinalis group inserts onto the spinous processes of the cervical spine, whereas the longissimus muscle and iliocostalis group insert onto the mastoid process of the temporal bone and posterior tubercles of the transverse processes of C4 through C6 vertebra, respectively.

The deepest muscle layer does not exist above the axis and consists of the semispinalis, multifidis, and rotators (**Fig. 18.6**). The semispinalis capitis groups originate from the transverse processes of T1 through T6 and insert on the suboccipital bone. The semispinalis cervicalis has an origination similar to that of the semispinalis capitis but inserts on the cervical spinous processes, especially C2. The C2 has a large and bifid spinous process with the attachment of the semispinalis cervicis muscles at its inferior edges. The multifidis group lies beneath the semispinalis and consists of short muscles spanning one to three segments from the lamina inferiorly to the spinous process superiorly. The

114 I Occipital-Cervical Junction

Fig. 18.5 Anatomy of the superficial muscular layer in the posterior cervical region.

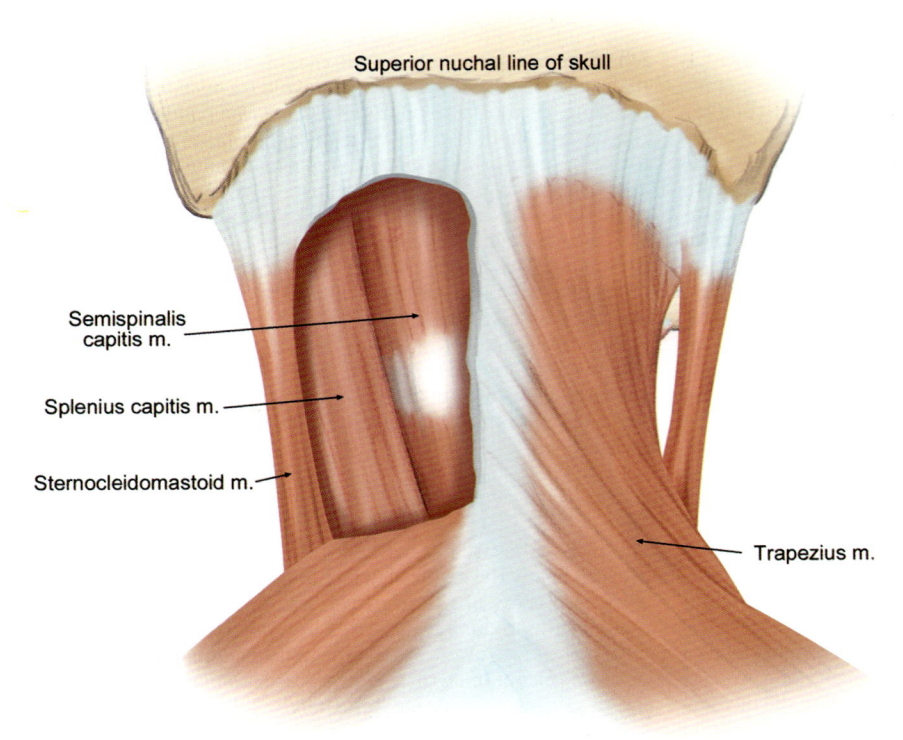

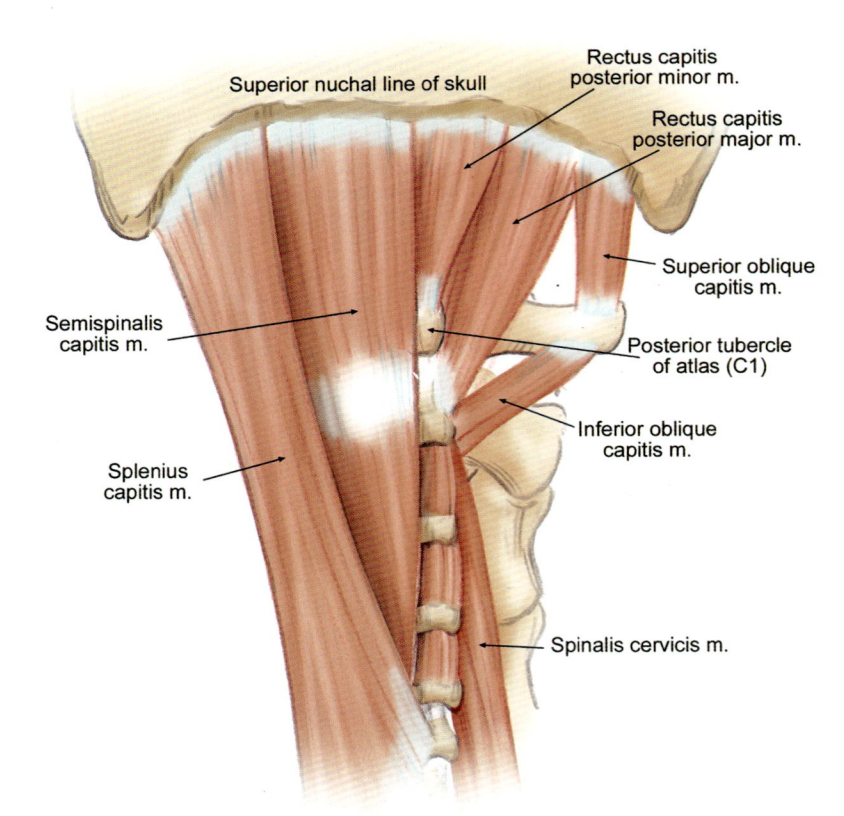

Fig. 18.6 Middle and deep muscular anatomy of the posterior cervical region.

rotator muscle group arises from the transverse processes and inserts at the base of the spinous process one level rostrally.

The suboccipital area has a set of muscles that do not exist below C2 and that lie deep to the semispinalis layer[20] (**Fig. 18.6**). The rectus minor muscle originates from the posterior tubercle of C1 and from the C2 spinous process and attaches laterally to the suboccipital bone. The inferior oblique muscles arise from the posterior tubercle of the axis and attach to the transverse process of the atlas. The superior oblique muscles span the transverse processes of the atlas and attach to the suboccipital bone. The suboccipital triangle consists of the inferior oblique muscle inferiorly, the superior oblique laterally, and the rectus major muscle superiorly. The suboccipital nerve and vertebral artery pass through the suboccipital triangle as they perforate the posterior atlanto-occipital membrane and are important references during surgical exposures.[20] The key to minimizing blood loss is to strictly maintain the dissection in the subperiosteal plane.

Atlantoaxial Wiring and Arthrodesis

If the C1 posterior arch is intact, then the use of cable fixation from C1 to C2 is a viable option. Three basic cable/wire fixation techniques—the Gallie, the Brooks, and the interspinous technique—are commonly used for C1-C2 fixation.

Gallie's Method

Gallie[9] first described in 1939 posterior C1-C2 sublaminar wire fixation with the use of steel wire. Following exposure of the C1-C2 region, a meticulous sublaminar dissection at C1 and C2 is performed after removal of the occipitoatlantal membrane and ligamentum flavum. Ensuring free access of the wire between the lamina and dura minimizes the risk of dural tears. The graft usually consists of a corticocancellous iliac crest bone measuring ~ 1.5 cm by 3 cm and notched inferiorly in the midline to dock onto the C2 spinous process. The graft is placed over the C2 spinous process and leaned against the posterior arch of C1. In this technique a single 20-gauge steel wire is passed underneath the C1 lamina from inferior to superior, which holds the graft in place and then wraps around the spinous process of C2. Passage of the sublaminar wire under the lamina of C2 is avoided to decrease the risk of neural or dural injury. These wires are tightened, compressing the bone graft over the arch of C1 and to the lamina of C2 (**Fig. 18.7**). The Gallie fusion provides good stabilization in flexion but very poor stabilization during extension and rotational maneuvers. Consequently, the rate of nonunion with the Gallie fusion has been reported to be as high as 25%.[7] The Gallie technique is difficult to apply to an irreducible, posteriorly displaced C1 ring. This technique has been almost completely replaced with other methods, but it is still found in the literature and so it is appropriate to understand the procedure.

Brooks Method

In 1978, Brooks and Jenkins[10] refined the Gallie technique by utilizing sublaminar wires at C1 and C2 with an interlaminar wedge bone graft. Biomechanically, this fixation technique is superior to that of the Gallie, but there is additional risk because it involves the passage of wire beneath two laminae. The superior portion of the C2 lamina is fashioned to receive the grafts on each side of the midline to minimize translation during compression of the wires. In the Brooks-Jenkins fusion technique, unlike the Gallie fusion technique, two separate iliac crest autografts are placed between C1 and C2. Each autologous iliac crest graft is beveled superiorly and inferiorly and wedged in between the C1

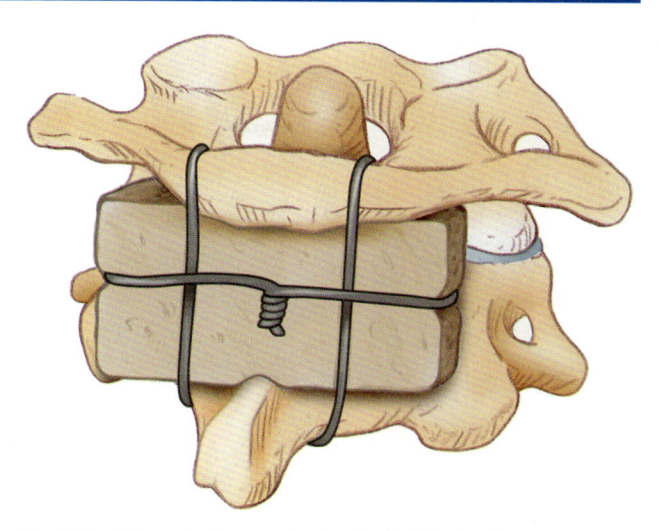

Fig. 18.7 Schematic diagram showing the Gallie's C1-C2 posterior wiring construct.

and C2 lamina on each side of the midline. The original description detailed the passage of two wires on each side (**Fig. 18.8a**) but currently most surgeons who use this technique pass a single sublaminar cable on each side of the midline under both the C1 and C2 arches (**Fig. 18.8b**). The cables are then tightened around the grafts and secured and crimped in place. The Brooks-Jenkins fusion technique provides more rotational stability than does the Gallie technique, and it has stability in flexion and extension that is similar to that of the Gallie fusion technique. The rate of fusion after this technique has been reported to be as high as 93%, and achievement of the optimal rates requires postoperative halo immobilization. One disadvantage of the Brooks-Jenkins fusion technique is the need for passage of bilateral sublaminar cables beneath both C1 and C2.

Interspinous C1-C2 Technique

The Gallie technique was modified by Volker Sonntag in the early 1990s in such a manner that the rotational stability was improved without the need for bilateral sublaminar C1-C2 cables as in the Brooks-Jenkins technique.[11] Sonntag called this the interspinous technique, although it is more frequently referred to as the Sonntag technique. Fixation is accomplished by passing a sublaminar cable under the posterior C1 arch from inferior to superior. This requires a two-handed process, simultaneously feeding and pulling the wire to avoid anterior displacement of the wire and compression of the dorsal aspect of the spinal cord. The senior author (V.C.T.) prefers to first place a 0 Vicryl suture beneath the arch of C1. This can be relatively easily passed by sliding the blunt end of the needle beneath the lamina. The suture is tied to the cable and is used to pull the cable under the C1 lamina from a superior to inferior direction. A notch is created at the spinolaminar junction bilaterally at C2 with a Kerrison rongeur, providing a slot for seating the wire at the C2 level.

Next, a carefully cut autograft (iliac crest or rib) is placed between the dorsal elements of C1 and C2 after first decorticating the spinal regions that contact the graft. The cable is next looped over the autograft and placed into a notch created on the inferior aspect of the C2 spinous process, trapping the graft between C1 and C2. Various multistranded titanium braided cables are available (ATLAS® Cable System, Medtronic, Minneapolis, MN; Sof'wire Cable System, Codman, Johnson and Johnson Professional, Raynham, MA; and Songer cable system, Synthes Spine,

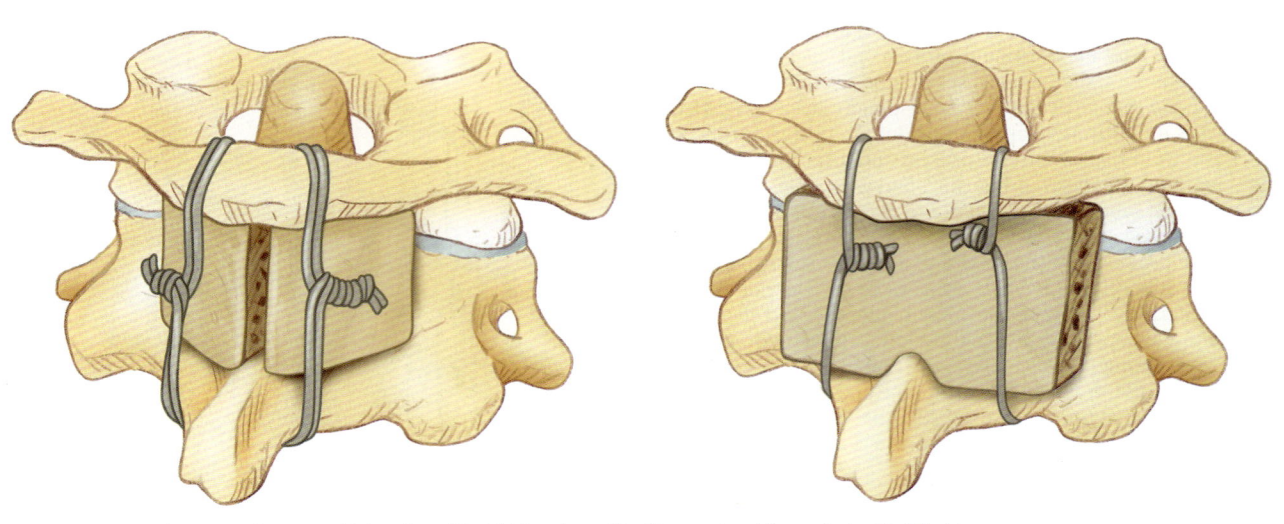

Fig. 18.8 Figure illustrating the original **(a)** and modified **(b)** Brooks and Jenkins construct for posterior C1-C2 wiring.

West Chester, PA), and have replaced the stainless steel monofilament wire that was commonly used in the past. These systems have a variable angle eyelet crimp at one end that allows passing the other end through it. Each system has a slightly different method of applying tension to the cable and fixing it in place. The maximum recommended tension for stainless steel cables is 60 pounds and for titanium alloy cables is generally 35 pounds. Once set to the appropriate tension, the cable is tightened and crimped, and this not only secures the spine but also places the graft under compression (**Fig. 18.9**). It should be kept in mind that, in the spine, the cables can fail not by breaking but by cutting through bone. Additional cancellous graft can be placed over the entire construct. The wound is then closed in a multilayer fashion.

Postoperative Care

Following each of the above operations, it is optimal to immobilize the patient in a halo-vest orthosis for 6 to 12 weeks after surgery. Then, flexion and extension radiographs should be obtained to assess the fusion. If there is no motion, the halo can be removed. The patient should be followed clinically and radiographically until fusion has occurred. Although a rigid orthosis may be used instead of a halo, the fusion rate will suffer. In patients treated with only the interspinous technique and no other instrumentation, Sonntag recommended the use of a halo to immobilize patients for 3 months after surgery and the use of a rigid cervical collar for an additional 1 to 2 months after that, demonstrating a 97% fusion rate with the technique.[11,14]

Potential Complications and Precautions

Complications of dorsal wiring techniques are rare. Nonunion is a well-known complication of any arthrodesis procedure and may occur in up to 30% of cases.[2,15,21,22] Furthermore, the construct is biomechanically inferior to other available techniques now, and the advantages and disadvantages of this wiring technique as against newer options should be considered in selecting the best surgical option. Other complications following atlantoaxial wiring are iatrogenic fracture of the posterior arch during wire tensioning, necessitating extension of the fusion construct; risk of dural tear; and neurologic injury while passing sublaminar wires.[9,10,14]

Conclusion

C1-C2 posterior wiring techniques are relatively less challenging as compared with other newer screw-and-rod–based techniques. Even though the wiring techniques are not as rigid as screw-based techniques, they do offer higher rates of fusion when combined with halo immobilization. However, they require an intact posterior arch of C1 and C2, which is not always available.

References

1. Martin MD, Bruner HJ, Maiman DJ. Anatomic and biomechanical considerations of the craniovertebral junction. Neurosurgery 2010;66(3, Suppl): 2–6
2. Jacobson ME, Khan SN, An HS. C1-C2 posterior fixation: indications, technique, and results. Orthop Clin North Am 2012;43:11–18, vii

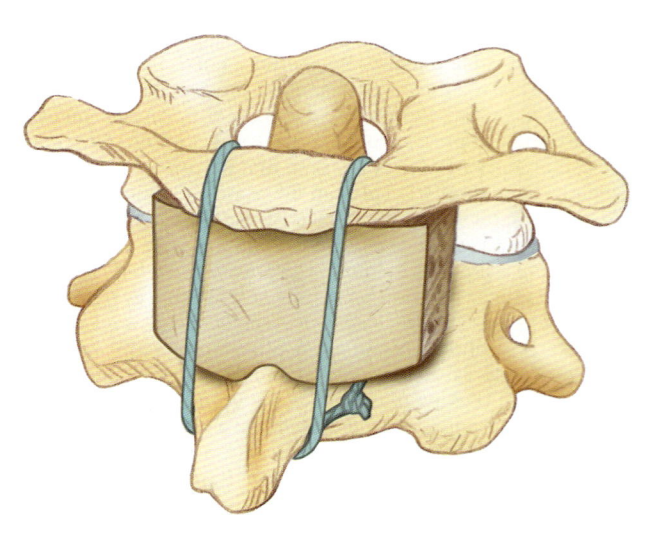

Fig. 18.9 Schematic diagram demonstrating the interspinous C1-C2 posterior wiring technique. See text for details.

3. Aryan HE, Newman CB, Nottmeier EW, Acosta FL Jr, Wang VY, Ames CP. Stabilization of the atlantoaxial complex via C-1 lateral mass and C-2 pedicle screw fixation in a multicenter clinical experience in 102 patients: modification of the Harms and Goel techniques. J Neurosurg Spine 2008;8:222–229
4. Harms J, Melcher RP. Posterior C1-C2 fusion with polyaxial screw and rod fixation. Spine 2001;26:2467–2471
5. Grob D, Magerl F. [Surgical stabilization of C1 and C2 fractures]. Orthopade 1987;16:46–54
6. Hott JS, Lynch JJ, Chamberlain RH, Sonntag VK, Crawford NR. Biomechanical comparison of C1-2 posterior fixation techniques. J Neurosurg Spine 2005;2:175–181
7. Mummaneni PV, Haid RW. Atlantoaxial fixation: overview of all techniques. Neurol India 2005;53:408–415
8. Mixter SJ, Osgood RB. IV. Traumatic lesions of the atlas and axis. Ann Surg 1910;51:193–207
9. Gallie WE. Fractures and dislocations of the cervical spine. Am J Surg 1939;46:495
10. Brooks AL, Jenkins EB. Atlanto-axial arthrodesis by the wedge compression method. J Bone Joint Surg Am 1978;60:279–284
11. Dickman CA, Sonntag VK, Papadopoulos SM, Hadley MN. The interspinous method of posterior atlantoaxial arthrodesis. J Neurosurg 1991;74:190–198
12. Gallie WE. Skeletal traction in the treatment of fractures and dislocations of the cervical spine. Ann Surg 1937;106:770–776
13. Waddell JP, Reardon GP. Atlantoaxial arthrodesis to treat odontoid fractures. Can J Surg 1983;26:255–257, 260
14. Dickman CA, Crawford NR, Paramore CG. Biomechanical characteristics of C1-2 cable fixations. J Neurosurg 1996;85:316–322
15. Dickman CA, Sonntag VK. Posterior C1-C2 transarticular screw fixation for atlantoaxial arthrodesis. Neurosurgery 1998;43:275–280, discussion 280–281
16. Härtl R, Chamberlain RH, Fifield MS, Chou D, Sonntag VK, Crawford NR. Biomechanical comparison of two new atlantoaxial fixation techniques with C1-2 transarticular screw-graft fixation. J Neurosurg Spine 2006;5:336–342
17. Steinmetz MP, Mroz TE, Benzel EC. Craniovertebral junction: biomechanical considerations. Neurosurgery 2010;66(3, Suppl):7–12
18. Young JP, Young PH, Ackermann MJ, Anderson PA, Riew KD. The ponticulus posticus: implications for screw insertion into the first cervical lateral mass. J Bone Joint Surg Am 2005;87:2495–2498
19. Peng CW, Chou BT, Bendo JA, Spivak JM. Vertebral artery injury in cervical spine surgery: anatomical considerations, management, and preventive measures. Spine J 2009;9:70–76
20. Youssef AS, Uribe JS, Ramos E, Janjua R, Thomas LB, van Loveren H. Interfascial technique for vertebral artery exposure in the suboccipital triangle: the road map. Neurosurgery 2010;67(2, Suppl Operative):355–361
21. Haid RW Jr, Subach BR, McLaughlin MR, Rodts GE Jr, Wahlig JB Jr. C1-C2 transarticular screw fixation for atlantoaxial instability: a 6-year experience. Neurosurgery 2001;49:65–68, discussion 69–70
22. Naderi S, Crawford NR, Song GS, Sonntag VK, Dickman CA. Biomechanical comparison of C1-C2 posterior fixations. Cable, graft, and screw combinations. Spine 1998;23:1946–1955, discussion 1955–1956

19 C1-C2 Transarticular Fixation Technique

Ricardo B.V. Fontes, Manish K. Kasliwal, and Vincent C. Traynelis

The treatment of C1-C2 instability underwent a major revolution with the introduction of screw-based posterior segmental instrumentation. The first of these techniques was the C1-C2 transarticular screw fixation, which was reported in 1979 by Magerl.[1] Transarticular screw fixation was originally described in conjunction with the placement of interspinous or interlaminar grafts and posterior wiring, but it may be performed as a stand-alone technique in situations in which the posterior arch of C1 or the C2 lamina are not competent. Biomechanically, C1-C2 transarticular fixation offers significantly greater resistance to lateral bending and axial rotation than any posterior wiring or clamping technique, even when performed as a stand-alone construct.[2-4] C1-C2 transarticular fixation greatly stiffens the C1-C2 segment when compared with normal; its main weakness as a stand-alone construct is its resistance to flexion and extension, which has been reported as equal to or slightly worse than that of posterior wiring techniques.[3-5] It is uncertain, however, if this minimal disadvantage in flexion/extension results in a clinical difference in outcome or even fusion rates; the biomechanical disadvantage in flexion/extension disappears if posterior wiring techniques are combined with C1-C2 transarticular fixation.[3] Overall, reported fusion rates of C1-C2 transarticular fixation are far superior to those of the posterior wiring techniques, even when the latter techniques were combined with the use of postoperative halo-type orthoses.[6]

Patient Selection

Most patients with atlantoaxial instability (AAI) caused by degenerative, traumatic, neoplastic, or infectious processes are potential candidates for C1-C2 transarticular fixation, provided that the anatomy of the C2 pars interarticularis accommodates the screw, the C1 lateral masses are preserved, the vertebral artery anatomy is not aberrant, the C1-C2 alignment can be achieved for optimal screw trajectory, and access is not precluded from the upper thoracic region. C1-C2 transarticular screw placement has been reported in patients from 1 to 98 years of age.[7] Approximately 20 to 25% of patients have at least one anatomic contraindication to the placement of a transarticular screw in one of the C2 pars.[8,9]

Indications

C1-C2 transarticular screw fixation is indicated for AAI caused by the following:

- Complex, combined C1 and C2 fractures[6,10]
- Type II odontoid fractures with contraindications for direct anterior repair (**Fig. 19.1**)[11,12]
- Type III odontoid fractures that are either not appropriate for or have failed nonoperative management[11]
- Neoplastic or infectious compromise of anterior axis structures such as the odontoid process or transverse ligaments (e.g., Grisel syndrome)
- Postodontoidectomy without basilar invagination
- Os odontoideum
- Rheumatoid arthritis[13]
- Down syndrome
- Other congenital anomalies

Contraindications

- Aberrant vertebral artery or C2 pars anatomy[8,9]
- Destruction of C1 lateral masses due to tumor or rheumatoid arthritis
- Inability to obtain C1 lateral mass–C2 pars alignment for screw trajectory
- Severe osteoporosis[14]
- Inability to obtain needed trajectory due to upper thoracic anatomic variations

Advantages and Disadvantages

The fundamental advantage of C1-C2 transarticular fixation is the immediate stability of the C1-C2 articulation, with excellent potential for fusion without the use of halo-type orthoses. As described above, it is a very solid construct from the biomechanical standpoint when combined with posterior wiring and graft and still considerably stiffer than the intact segment when used as a stand-alone device. C1-C2 transarticular fixation is also more stable than C1 lateral mass–C2 translaminar screw construct, with significantly better fusion rates.[3,15]

Although C1 lateral mass–C2 pars (or pedicle) constructs may offer a similar or slightly better biomechanical profile, C1-C2 transarticular constructs obviate the need for dissection of the C1-C2 joint if posterior grafting is utilized. Transarticular screw placement, however, is technically demanding, and the complications associated with it can be serious; a thorough preoperative understanding of the vertebral artery course is imperative.

Choice of Operative Approach

Once the decision to treat AAI is made, the initial choice of operative approach is between an anterior or a posterior technique. Our group still considers anterior C1-C2 stabilization a procedure to be performed only in exceptional circumstances, given the multiple posterior options that are available and familiar to most surgeons and the ability to decompress the canal if necessary.[16,17] Once the posterior approach is selected, C1-C2 transarticular fixation in our hands has been the fastest and easiest way to accomplish C1-C2 stabilization and is therefore the technique of

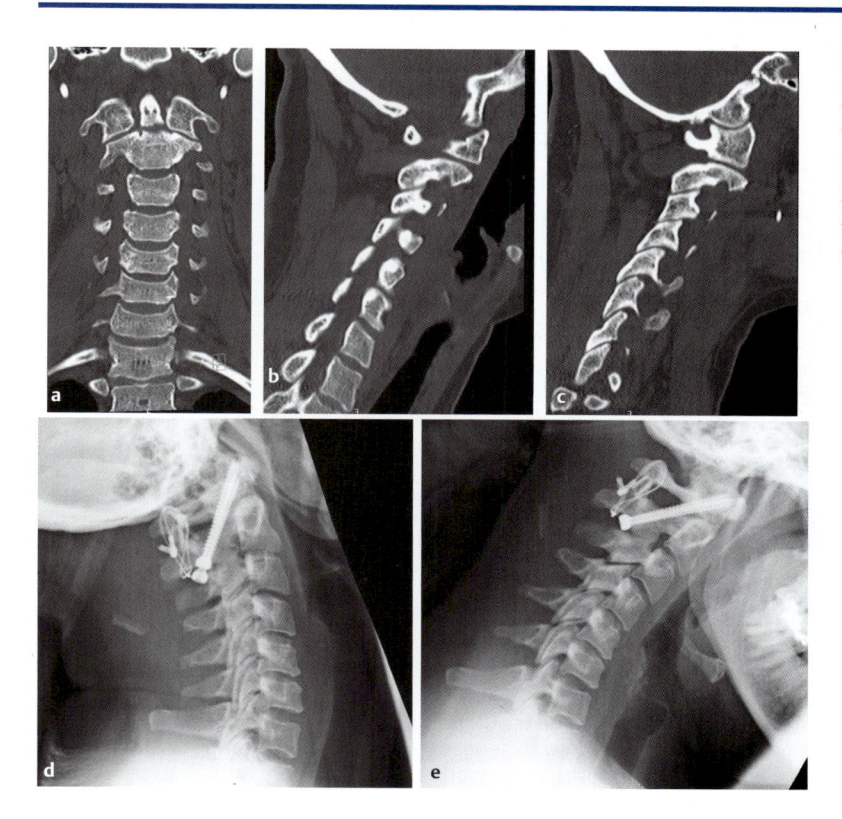

Fig. 19.1 Case example. A 37-year-old woman sustained a type II odontoid fracture that was treated nonoperatively with a halo vest 6 months before arriving at our service with persistent neck pain. **(a)** Computed tomography (CT) demonstrates a nonhealed type II odontoid fracture. **(b,c)** Pars anatomy is amenable to transarticular fixation; this was complemented with posterior wiring and rib interspinous autograft. **(d,e)** Six-month postoperative radiographs demonstrate solid fusion and absence of motion.

choice, unless one of the contraindications listed above is present. The necessary equipment for C1 lateral mass–C2 pars fixation should always be made available in case it is determined that a C1-C2 alignment is not ideal for transarticular fixation once the patient is positioned on the operating table.

Preoperative Imaging

Every patient should have a computed tomography (CT) scan to delineate the bony anatomy involved in C1-C2 transarticular fixation. The size of each C2 pars and relation to the foramen transversarium is noted. It has been our practice not to attempt the placement of C1-C2 transarticular screws if the space for bony purchase between the cortex of the foramen transversarium and the pars interarticularis is smaller than 4 mm. The size of the C1 lateral mass can also be approximated. This is important in cases of advanced rheumatoid arthritis in which the C1 lateral mass may be so destroyed that solid screw purchase is not possible, in which case a craniocervical fusion is required. Patients in whom there is no concern about an extreme instability that may produce neurologic deficits may also be evaluated with flexion and extension cervical radiographs. Most patients will also undergo magnetic resonance imaging (MRI) of the cervical spine to assess the need for neural element decompression. If aberrant vertebral anatomy is suspected, vascular imaging such as CT angiography, MR angiography, or conventional digital subtraction angiography may be considered. However, it is usually best just to alter the operative plan to either a unilateral screw or fixation using other purchase points (C1 lateral mass–C2 pars, pedicle, or laminae).

Surgical Procedure

Patient preparation and positioning is performed as described in Chapter 17. Unless severe cord compression is present preoperatively in the context of AAI, we do not routinely perform intraoperative neurophysiological monitoring with somatosensory evoked potentials (SSEPs) or motor evoked potentials (MEPs). Briefly, the patient is positioned prone with gel bolster chest support and appropriate padding of pressure points, and the head is immobilized with the Mayfield three-point skeletal fixation device (**Fig. 19.2**). The patient is positioned in a slight "chin tuck" position, with posterior translation and slight flexion of the head. As soon as the patient is turned, proper alignment is verified with lateral fluoroscopy.

Following preparation and exposure as described in Chapter 17, the C2 posterior elements and pars are completely exposed. The posterior arch of C1 is exposed for wire/cable fixation or decompression, depending on the situation. The entry point of the C1-C2 transarticular screw is slightly lateral (3 mm) to the caudal part of the C2 lamina–inferior articular process junction, and 3 mm cranial to the inferior articular surface of C2 (**Fig. 19.3**). We perform all steps of screw placement on one side before proceeding to the other, so that the procedure for the second side can be aborted if there is a vertebral artery injury (see below). The entry point is marked and decorticated with a high-speed bur. A 2.5-mm drill bit is placed in neutral orientation in the lateromedial plane and 25 to 30 degrees cranially, aiming at the anterior tubercle of the atlas on lateral fluoroscopy (**Fig. 19.1**). Although some surgeons have described a medial angulation with the drill (5–10 degrees) we prefer a straight parasagittal orientation as described above. Prior exposure of the cranial and medial surfaces of the C2 pars also provides additional cues to the craniocaudal and mediolateral trajectories. The medial cortical wall of the C2 pars is always palpated and a Penfield dissector to verify the position of the spinal canal prior to drilling. The correct sagittal orientation of the drill results in an angle that often necessitates caudal exposure of the cervical-thoracic junction. Alternatively, separate stab incisions around T1 can be made.

A trocar is then tunneled into the surgical exposure, and the drilling, tapping, and screw placement is accomplished through

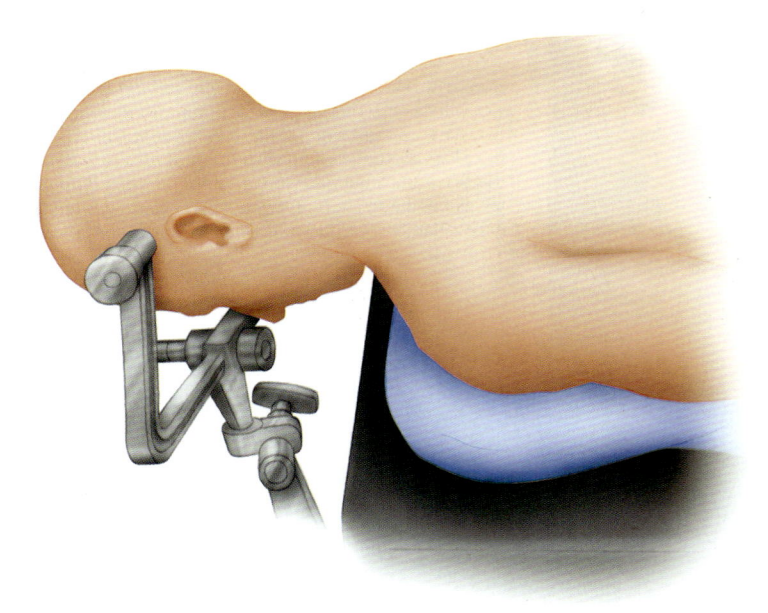

Fig. 19.2 The patient is placed in the "chin tuck" position. The projected trajectory of the C1-C2 transarticular screw is shown. The entry point in the skin is normally around C7.

this working channel. Sometimes holding the C2 spinous process with a bone clamp and gently moving it posteriorly may facilitate drill orientation. The drill bit is advanced manually under fluoroscopic guidance until the joint is encountered. The joint is difficult to traverse by hand because cortical bone is very hard, and at this point power is used to complete the drilling. Using the hand technique initially provides tactile feedback, so the surgeon is more likely to stay within the cancellous bone of the pars. Once the joint is encountered, the vertebral artery is not at risk and power drilling is much more efficient. Ultimately, the surgeon should feel the passage of the drill through three cortical surfaces—the C2 superior facet, the C1 inferior facet, and the anterior surface of the atlas—carefully following along on lateral fluoroscopy so as not to over-drill and injure any of the skull base structures, particularly the jugular vein, carotid artery, and the hypoglossal nerve.[18] Alternatively, all steps of this procedure may be performed under navigation.[19,20]

Some systems employ a cannulated drill in which case the original tract is made with a long Kirschner wire (K-wire), although cannulated drill bits can bind to the K-wire, forcing it to advance further than intended. Frequent fluoroscopic checks are necessary to prevent this from happening. After the guide hole has been drilled, the entire trajectory is tapped. It is our practice to determine the screw length using the calibrations on the tap. Generally, fully threaded 4.0- or 4.5-mm screws are placed; although some surgeons use a lag screw, there is no evidence to suggest this is more effective, and the key is to have proper alignment prior to beginning to drill.[21]

Posterior C1-C2 wiring with placement of interspinous graft is then accomplished as described in Chapter 18. Our choice of autograft is rib, which can be readily harvested while the cervical exposure is being performed, with minimal postoperative morbidity. In the case of removal of the C1 posterior arch or C2 lamina for cord decompression, the C1-C2 joint can be prepared and packed as described above before drilling.[21] Several authors have combined the transarticular fixation technique with polyaxial screws with some sort of C1 fixation, either a hook or a lateral screw.[5,22] We feel this added fixation is unnecessary in most cases, given the excellent biomechanical profile.

Postoperative Care

Unless the C1-C2 fixation is being performed as a more complex procedure, the patient is extubated in the operating room and transferred to a regular hospital room. We utilize a rigid cervical collar, such as the Aspen or Miami J, for the initial 6 weeks, which will have the main effect of restricting flexion and extension. Ambulation is started immediately after surgery, and the patient can be discharged on the first postoperative day, after anteroposterior, open-mouth odontoid, and lateral cervical radiographs are obtained. The patient is seen in the clinic at 2, 6, 12, and 24 weeks post op. At the patient's 48-week visit, a CT scan is obtained.

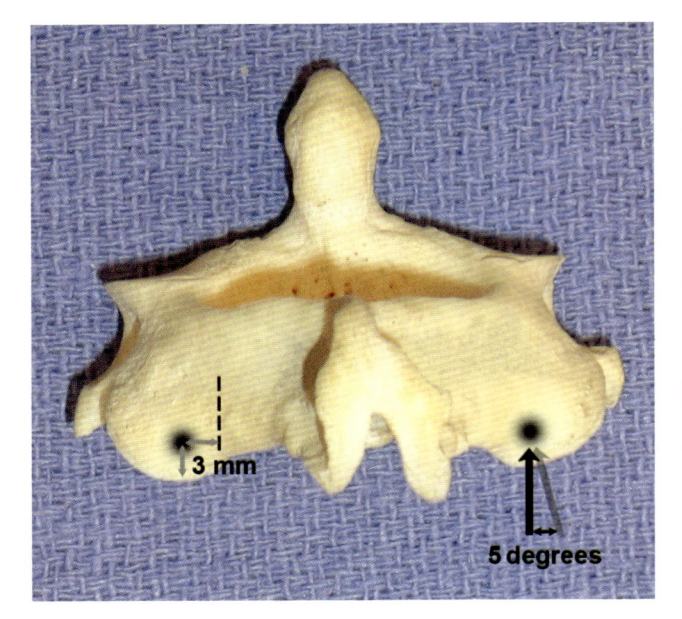

Fig. 19.3 C2 entry point and orientation for C1-C2 transarticular screw placement. The *dashed line* marks the lamina–articular process junction. The favored neutral lateromedial trajectory is shown as well as the 5-degree medial alternative.

Potential Complications and Precautions

Careful planning can prevent the most dangerous complication of C1-C2 transarticular fixation—injury of the vertebral artery. If this injury happens during the exposure, the injury is invariably distal to the C1 foramen transversarium, and every attempt should be made to repair the injury because the vessel is accessible. On the other hand, if the injury happens during drilling or tapping, the surgeon will note high pressure pulsatile blood exiting the drill hole, in which case the screw should be placed as described and the procedure aborted on the contralateral side. Posterior wiring and placement of a graft should complement the procedure, if possible. Though suboptimal from the biomechanical standpoint, unilateral transarticular fixation has been reported with fusion rates of upward of 90%.[23] After surgery is concluded, the patient should be maintained under anesthesia and immediately transferred to the interventional suite for a conventional four-vessel cerebral angiography. Both arteriovenous fistulas and pseudoaneurysms have been reported, though the best method (occlusion versus stenting) and timing (immediate versus delayed) for endovascular treatment of stable (nonbleeding) injuries is still debated.[24-26]

Other vascular and nervous injury can happen if the screw is advanced beyond the anterior cortex of the C1 lateral mass; ideally, it should be just tricortical.[18,27] If such injury is detected postoperatively, screw removal and replacement is necessary. Pseudarthrosis has not been a frequent concern, given reported fusion rates of better than 95%.[6,28] Revision strategies usually involve extension of fusion to the occiput.[6]

Box 19.1 Key Operative Points and Avoiding Complications

- Use general anesthesia. The patient is placed in the prone position with the head in a Mayfield clamp and the chin tucked.
- Use lateral fluoroscopy confirmation and guidance throughout the surgery; navigation is also an option.
- Map the midline posterior incision on the skin.
- Expose the C1 posterior arch and the C2 lamina and pars.
- Perform cord decompression and packing of the C1-C2 joint, if necessary.
- Mark the C2 entry point with a bur, 3 mm lateral to the lamina-articular process junction, and 2 mm cranial to the inferior articular facet.
- Insert the drill through the lower cervical stab incisions, in a neutral lateromedial orientation, 25 to 30 degrees cranially; aim at the C1 anterior tubercle.
- Drill under radiological guidance, using the "three cortices" technique.
- Tap the entire trajectory and measure the length.
- If a vertebral artery injury occurs, insert a screw and abort the contralateral side.
- Insert a screw.
- Perform posterior wiring and an interspinous graft, if possible.

Conclusion

Box 19.1 summarizes the main points of the chapter. C1-C2 transarticular screw fixation is a very useful technique that can be successfully employed by most spine surgeons. It offers immediate stability and excellent clinical results. Most complications can be avoided with careful preoperative planning, and patients will certainly appreciate not having to wearing a halo vest postoperatively.

References

1. Grob D, Magerl F. [Surgical stabilization of C1 and C2 fractures]. Orthopade 1987;16:46-54
2. Chittiboina P, Wylen E, Ogden A, Mukherjee DP, Vannemreddy P, Nanda A. Traumatic spondylolisthesis of the axis: a biomechanical comparison of clinically relevant anterior and posterior fusion techniques. J Neurosurg Spine 2009;11:379-387
3. Härtl R, Chamberlain RH, Fifield MS, Chou D, Sonntag VKH, Crawford NR. Biomechanical comparison of two new atlantoaxial fixation techniques with C1-2 transarticular screw-graft fixation. J Neurosurg Spine 2006;5:336-342
4. Hott JS, Lynch JJ, Chamberlain RH, Sonntag VKH, Crawford NR. Biomechanical comparison of C1-2 posterior fixation techniques. J Neurosurg Spine 2005;2:175-181
5. Guo X, Ni B, Zhao W, et al. Biomechanical assessment of bilateral C1 laminar hook and C1-2 transarticular screws and bone graft for atlantoaxial instability. J Spinal Disord Tech 2009;22:578-585
6. Gluf WM, Schmidt MH, Apfelbaum RI. Atlantoaxial transarticular screw fixation: a review of surgical indications, fusion rate, complications, and lessons learned in 191 adult patients. J Neurosurg Spine 2005;2:155-163
7. Gluf WM, Brockmeyer DL. Atlantoaxial transarticular screw fixation: a review of surgical indications, fusion rate, complications, and lessons learned in 67 pediatric patients. J Neurosurg Spine 2005;2:164-169
8. Madawi AA, Casey AT, Solanki GA, Tuite G, Veres R, Crockard HA. Radiological and anatomical evaluation of the atlantoaxial transarticular screw fixation technique. J Neurosurg 1997;86:961-968
9. Paramore CG, Dickman CA, Sonntag VK. The anatomical suitability of the C1-2 complex for transarticular screw fixation. J Neurosurg 1996;85:221-224
10. Guiot B, Fessler RG. Complex atlantoaxial fractures. J Neurosurg 1999;91(2, Suppl):139-143
11. Anderson LD, D'Alonzo RT. Fractures of the odontoid process of the axis. J Bone Joint Surg Am 1974;56:1663-1674
12. Kuntz C IV, Mirza SK, Jarell AD, Chapman JR, Shaffrey CI, Newell DW. Type II odontoid fractures in the elderly: early failure of nonsurgical treatment. Neurosurg Focus 2000;8:e7
13. Casey AT, Madawi AA, Veres R, Crockard HA. Is the technique of posterior transarticular screw fixation suitable for rheumatoid atlanto-axial subluxation? Br J Neurosurg 1997;11:508-519
14. Bambakidis NC. Surgery of the Craniovertebral Junction. New York: Thieme; 2012. Available at: http://search.ebscohost.com/login.aspx?direct=true&scope=site&db=nlebk&db=nlabk&AN=534258. Accessed April 11, 2014
15. Sciubba DM, Noggle JC, Vellimana AK, et al. Laminar screw fixation of the axis. J Neurosurg Spine 2008;8:327-334
16. Cavalcanti DD, Agrawal A, Garcia-Gonzalez U, et al. Anterolateral C1-C2 transarticular fixation for atlantoaxial arthrodesis: landmarks, working area, and angles of approach. Neurosurgery 2010;67(3, Suppl Operative):ons38-ons42
17. Li W-L, Chi Y-L, Xu H-Z, et al. Percutaneous anterior transarticular screw fixation for atlantoaxial instability: a case series. J Bone Joint Surg Br 2010;92:545-549
18. Ebraheim NA, Misson JR, Xu R, Yeasting RA. The optimal transarticular C1-2 screw length and the location of the hypoglossal nerve. Surg Neurol 2000;53:208-210
19. Moses ZB, Mayer RR, Strickland BA, et al. Neuronavigation in minimally invasive spine surgery. Neurosurg Focus 2013;35:E12
20. Uehara M, Takahashi J, Hirabayashi H, et al. Computer-assisted C1-C2 transarticular screw fixation "Magerl technique" for atlantoaxial instability. Asian Spine J 2012;6:168-177

21. Jeanneret B, Magerl F. Primary posterior fusion C1/2 in odontoid fractures: indications, technique, and results of transarticular screw fixation. J Spinal Disord 1992;5:464–475
22. Vergara P, Bal JS, Hickman Casey AT, Crockard HA, Choi D. C1-C2 posterior fixation: are 4 screws better than 2? Neurosurgery 2012;71(1, Suppl Operative):86–95
23. Song GS, Theodore N, Dickman CA, Sonntag VK. Unilateral posterior atlantoaxial transarticular screw fixation. J Neurosurg 1997;87:851–855
24. Choi J-W, Lee J-K, Moon K-S, et al. Endovascular embolization of iatrogenic vertebral artery injury during anterior cervical spine surgery: report of two cases and review of the literature. Spine 2006;31:E891–E894
25. Daentzer D, Deinsberger W, Böker D-K. Vertebral artery complications in anterior approaches to the cervical spine: report of two cases and review of literature. Surg Neurol 2003;59:300–309, discussion 309
26. Prabhu VC, France JC, Voelker JL, Zoarski GH. Vertebral artery pseudoaneurysm complicating posterior C1-2 transarticular screw fixation: case report. Surg Neurol 2001;55:29–33, discussion 33–34
27. Estillore RP, Buchowski JM, Minh V, et al. Risk of internal carotid artery injury during C1 screw placement: analysis of 160 computed tomography angiograms. Spine J 2011;11:316–323
28. Haid RW Jr. C1-C2 transarticular screw fixation: technical aspects. Neurosurgery 2001;49:71–74

20 C1 Lateral Mass–C2 Pars, Pedicle, and Translaminar Fixation Techniques

Ricardo B.V. Fontes, Manish K. Kasliwal, and Vincent C. Traynelis

The introduction in 1979 of rigid posterior fixation for the treatment of atlantoaxial instability (AAI) with C1-C2 transarticular screws provided immediate internal stabilization of the atlantoaxial segment that was so robust that it negated the need for postoperative halo immobilization.[1] Despite offering the best biomechanical profile of all C1-C2 fixation techniques and a relatively easy exposure, a significant number of patients are not eligible for this technique. Up to 25% of patients may have a vertebral artery course that precludes insertion of a transarticular screw on at least one side.[2] Additionally, anatomic alignment of C1 relative to C2 is required, and therefore transarticular fixation is not feasible in those patients with irreducible anterior, posterior, or rotatory subluxations.[3] Until the advent of C1 lateral mass–C2 pars (C1L-C2P) fixation, these patients frequently had to be treated with posterior wiring techniques, almost all of which required immobilization in an halo vest for at least 12 weeks to optimize the fusion.[4]

Insertion of screws into the pedicles of C2 was first described by Leconte[5] in 1964 for the treatment of traumatic spondylolisthesis of the axis. Borne et al[6] in 1984 reported perfect results in a series of 18 patients without morbidity; these authors reported that the screw trajectory is best described as "pars-pedicle." Utilization of this technique for AAI, however, still required the development of a favorable means of C1 fixation. Goel and Laheri[3] in 1994 first reported the C1-C2 fixation technique utilizing a screw-plate construct. Harms and Melcher[7] modified this technique to incorporate a polyaxial screw–rod construct in 2001, which greatly added to its ease of implantation and versatility, allowing for the addition of transversal connectors in cases of C1 burst fractures.[8] Its utilization with the addition of joint "spacers," again first described by Goel, has become a very useful adjuvant in the treatment of basilar invagination and confers added stiffness to the reconstructed segment, frequently obviating the need for an anterior transoral decompression.[9] C2 translaminar fixation was introduced in 2004 by Wright.[10] Despite the obvious disadvantage of not being feasible when cord decompression is necessary, translaminar screw placement does not place the vertebral artery at risk and is performed under direct vision.

An initial comment is necessary on the transitional anatomy of C2. The vertebral pedicle, by definition, connects structures derived from anterior ossification centers to those derived from posterior ossification centers. The pars interarticularis, as the term implies, is the osseous structure located between the two vertebral articular processes, but this term is not found in either the Latin or English versions of the *Terminologia Anatomica*.[11] A posteriorly placed "pedicle" screw, therefore, necessarily traverses the pars into the vertebral body.[11–13] Placement of a true "pedicle" screw, however, is also complicated by the presence of a high-riding vertebral artery in a manner similar to transarticular fixation, though the risk for injury is slightly lower; Yeom et al[14] calculated that a C2 pedicle screw would risk a vertebral artery injury in 18% of cadavers they studied. Elliott et al[15] performed a literature meta-analysis and calculated the incidence of vertebral artery injury at 1.68% for transarticular versus 1.09% for C2 pedicle fixation, a statistically significant difference. On the other hand, if a shorter C2 pars screw is placed and remains completely posterior to the vertebral artery course, the risk of injury is virtually zero.[15] This is the technique that we prefer; the biomechanical difference between transarticular, C1 lateral mass–C2 pedicle, and C1 lateral mass–C2 pars techniques is very small and unlikely to produce any significant difference in fusion rates or clinical outcome, particularly if a posterior tension band and atlas/axis wiring is performed.[15–18]

Patient Selection

Most patients with AAI caused by degenerative, traumatic, neoplastic, congenital/developmental, or infectious processes are potential candidates for C1-C2 fixation, provided that the anatomy allows for safe insertion of screws and solid fixation. The position of the vertebral artery is indirectly assessed through analysis of the foramen transversarium in C1 and C2 and the ponticulus posticus in C1. We have utilized this technique in patients up to 94 years of age with good results.

Indications

This technique is indicated for AAI caused by the following:

- Complex, combined C1 and C2 fractures[19,20]
- Type II odontoid fractures with contraindications for direct anterior repair (**Fig. 20.1**)[21,22]
- Type III odontoid fractures that have failed to respond to nonoperative treatment (**Fig. 20.2**)[21]
- Traumatic rupture of the transverse ligament
- Neoplastic or infectious compromise of anterior axis structures such as the odontoid process or transverse ligaments (e.g., Grisel syndrome)
- Postodontoidectomy
- Indirect reduction of basilar invagination or impression
- Os odontoideum
- Rheumatoid arthritis[23]
- Down syndrome
- Other congenital anomalies

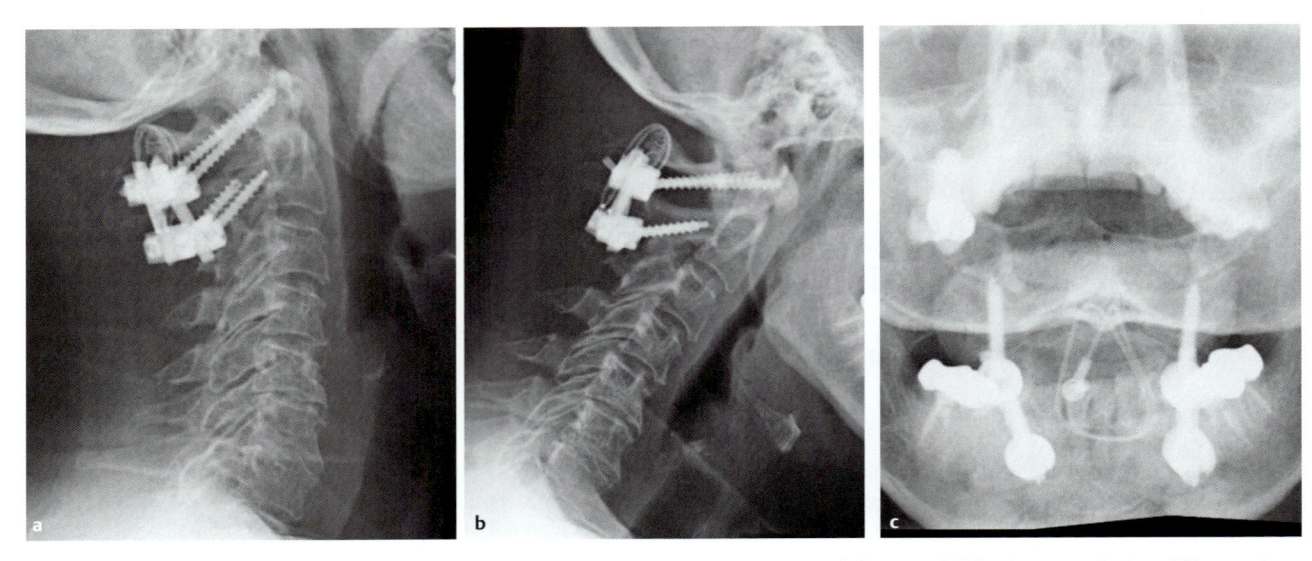

Fig. 20.1 Case example of C1 lateral mass–C2 pars fixation supplemented by posterior wiring and rib autograft following a type II odontoid fracture in an elderly patient. **(a)** extension, **(b)** flexion, and **(c)** transoral view.

Contraindications

- Destruction of C1 lateral masses or both the C2 pars interarticularis and pedicle due to tumor or rheumatoid arthritis
- Destruction or absence of the C2 lamina (translaminar technique only)
- Severe osteoporosis[24]

Advantages and Disadvantages

The greatest advantage of screw-based fixation is its versatility, which is afforded by the multiple fixation options. Rigid fixation provides immediate stability of the C1-C2 articulation, and this is associated with excellent fusion rates that may be accomplished without the use of halo-type orthoses. From the biomechanical standpoint, it is as rigid or just slightly less rigid than transarticular fixation but no difference is found in fusion rates.[25,26] If a C1 and/or C2 laminectomy is necessary, axially loaded grafts can still be placed within the joint, a technique that is also useful to indirectly reduce basilar invagination or impression.

The greatest disadvantage of C1-C2 fixation is related to the exposure of the posterior surface of the C1 lateral mass. Despite reports of insertion of C1 screws through the posterior arch to obviate such dissection, this technique provides a much more restricted screw pathway, may result in a fracture or at least compromise of the integrity of the posterior arch of C1 (which would preclude placement of a tension band), and increases the risk of injuring the vertebral artery. Vertebral artery injury is much more likely to occur when a ponticulus posticus is present; it may occur in up to 5.1 to 37.8% of normal individuals.[27,28] Screw placement in the C1 lateral mass has also been associated with postoperative C2 neuralgia.[3,7] Partially threaded screws have been utilized to minimize the risk of C2 root irritation, although there is no high-quality evidence that this is helpful.[7] Some authors advocate routine sectioning of the C2 root to minimize this complication, improve visualization, and facilitate hemostasis, placement of the instrumentation, and decortication of the joint space for arthrodesis.

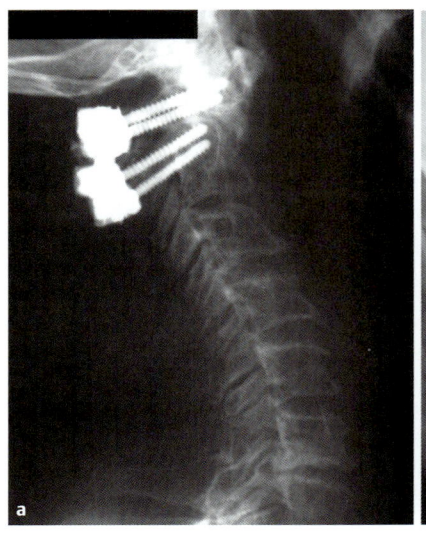

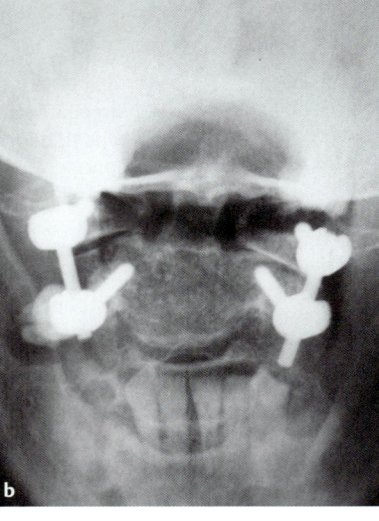

Fig. 20.2 Case example of C1 lateral mass–C2 pedicle fixation following an unstable type III odontoid fracture. Note the longer screws and more medial trajectory of the C2 pedicle screws as compared with pars fixation. **(a)** lateral view and **(b)** transoral view.

Dewan et al[29] and Hamilton et al[30] each reported small series of C2 transection with no cases of postoperative neuralgia; even though numbness was present in approximately half the patients, it did not impact outcome negatively. Yeom et al[28,31] experienced the opposite with worse outcomes following C2 root transection, including persistent neuralgia at long follow-up periods (up to 80 months). The same group also advocated placing the C1 screw through the posterior arch to minimize irritation of the C2 root, but a few patients still developed this complication despite Yeom et al's utilizing this technique, and it was associated with a relatively high incidence of C1 arch fracture. In our practice, we have encountered neither complication. Our C2 transection rate has been slightly less than 50%, and we have encountered neither persistent neuralgia nor painful numbness of the "anesthesia dolorosa" type negatively impacting outcome. Our technique has thus been to attempt to preserve the C2 root and minimize coagulation around the root ganglion; if bleeding from the venous plexus poses a problem or visualization is impaired, the C2 root is transected.

C2 translaminar fixation has the advantage of not placing the vertebral artery at risk (although this could happen if one drills lateral to the C2 pars), but also has the relative disadvantage of being the most recently developed technique. Over 95% of the normal population has a laminar thickness of 3.5 mm or more, which can accommodate a translaminar screw.[32] C2 translaminar fixation does not have the historical efficacy profile of other techniques. Biomechanically, C2 translaminar fixation is less rigid than the other two forms of fixation described in this chapter and definitively less rigid than transarticular fixation.[18,33,34] It appears to be equivalent in sagittal plane flexion/extension to C2 pars or pedicle fixation but may be less restrictive for axial rotation and lateral bending (**Fig. 20.3**). Whether these biomechanical findings will translate into a clinically significant difference is not clear at this time. The original author of the technique reported a fusion rate of 97.6%, which is similar to that of other techniques for all translaminar fusions (axial and subaxial), but this was accomplished in conjunction with significant (40%) off-label utilization of recombinant human bone morphogenetic protein 2 (rhBMP-2).[32] In a separate study, Parker et al[35] reported an increased rate of revision for subaxial fusions when compared with C2 pedicle constructs. Results for AAI from both studies were very good, and no revisions were needed. Dural violation was rare (2–8%) but present in both series. Our personal experience with C2 translaminar fixation in C1-C2 fusions in the setting of an odontoid fracture is suboptimal, with a quarter to a third of patients developing a nonunion. A nonunion rate of < 5% was found in this population with pars/pedicle/transarticular screws. When there is failure in this group of patients, the C2 screws have large halos around them. We have not seen this problem with subaxial screw fixation extending to C2, but many of these patients had anterior C2-C3 diskectomies and fusions, and this group of patients did not have marked instability.

Choice of Operative Approach

As described in the Chapter 19, the initial choice is between a posterior and an anterior approach; the latter has been utilized only in exceptional cases (such as a hangman's fracture, which is usually treated successfully with a C2-C3 diskectomy and instrumented anterior fusion). Our preferred technique for posterior C1-C2 stabilization has been transarticular fixation with posterior wiring and placement of an interspinous rib autograft because it is faster and does not require dissection of the C1-C2 joint space. However, if C1 or C2 laminectomy is necessary or any of the previously discussed anatomic or alignment concerns are present, C1-C2 segmental fixation is chosen. Usually when a C1-C2 transarticular screw cannot be placed for anatomic reasons, our group opts for screw fixation in the C1 lateral mass and the C2 pars. The placement of a pars screw is very similar to that of a transarticular screw, which has driven our decision-making process. If the pars is unacceptable, the C2 pedicle is examined with computed tomography (CT), and, if appropriate, a screw is placed into this structure.

Preoperative Imaging

Ideally, every patient should be evaluated with flexion and extension cervical radiographs and CT to accurately delineate the bony anatomy. The size of the C2 pars and pedicles must be determined as well as their relation to the foramen transversarium. It has been our practice not to attempt the placement of C2 pars or pedicle screws if the space for bony purchase is less than 4 mm (**Fig. 20.4**). The specific anatomy and size of the C2 laminae is noted when C2 translaminar fixation is required. Almost all patients are assessed with magnetic resonance imaging (MRI) of the cervical spine to evaluate the need for neural element

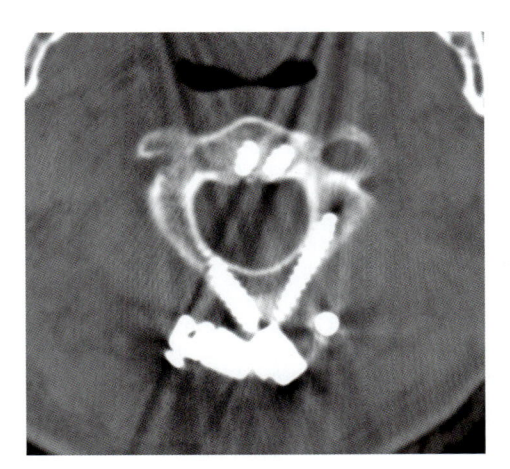

Fig. 20.3 Axial computed tomography (CT) image demonstrating C2 translaminar screw fixation as part of an anterior-posterior cervical construct.

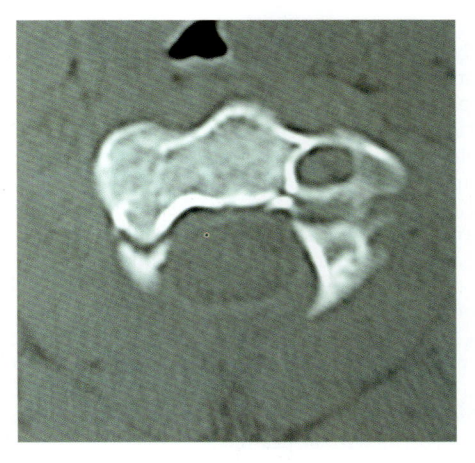

Fig. 20.4 Example of a large foramen transversarium precluding pedicle insertion on the left side of C2 in another patient with an unstable type III fracture.

decompression. If an aberrant vertebral anatomy is suspected by a standard MRI, vascular imaging may be obtained. Unlike the transarticular technique, vertebral artery anatomy distal to the C1 foramen transversarium is also important, considering the additional cranial exposure. The location of the carotid artery anterior to the lateral mass of the atlas should be reviewed.

Surgical Procedure

Patient preparation and placement in a "chin tuck" position is performed as described in Chapters 17 and 19. It is our preference to use fluoroscopy when placing the screws, but some surgeons prefer to rely on navigation guidance, and a smaller subset use neither technique.[36] The surgeon needs to be aware of the presence of clefts in the posterior arch of the atlas, which may be present in 1 to 3% of the population. Failure to recognize these clefts will increase the risk of creating a dural violation early in the procedure.[37] Care should be taken to avoid injury to the vertebral artery, and it is usually safest to expose the inferior portion of the C1 lamina first and dissect laterally over the superior edge of this structure with caution. Localization of the lateral mass of C1 is facilitated by first identifying the medial border of the pars interarticularis of C2. Exposure of the posterior surface of the C1 lateral mass is accomplished via a subperiosteal dissection, which results in minimal blood loss. The C2 nerve root can often be reflected caudally along with the venous plexus. If the venous plexus is entered, brisk bleeding may occur, which is best controlled by tamponade. If this is unsuccessful strong consideration should be given to C2 root transection. C2 exposure is performed as described previously for transarticular fixation.

Arthrodesis is often achieved by placing bone graft substrate dorsal to the posterior elements of C1 and C2, but it also may be accomplished with intraarticular grafts. The C1-C2 joint is cleaned of cartilage with curettes or rasps of increasing height. The space is filled with morselized bone, machined allografts (4–6 × 8 × 10 mm), or a small cage. The entry point for the C1 lateral mass screw is roughly the center of the lateral mass or, if possible, slightly more cranial where the arch joins the lateral mass.[24] It is marked with a high-speed bur or awl, and the position is confirmed under fluoroscopy (**Fig. 20.5**). The drill is aimed slightly medial (10 degrees) and cranial (10 degrees), so that on lateral fluoroscopy it seems to be aiming at the anterior tubercle of C1. The drill is then advanced carefully under fluoroscopy until the anterior cortex is penetrated. The senior author (V.C.T.) creates the aperture initially with a Kirschner wire (K-wire) and then enlarges it with the drill. The trajectory is tapped, and a 3.5- or 4.0-mm-diameter screw is inserted. Total screw length is usually in the 34- to 40-mm range. Fully or partially threaded screws may be placed.

C2 pars screw placement is basically identical to that of a transarticular screw; the entry point is slightly lateral (3 mm) to the lamino-inferior articular process junction, and 2 to 3 mm cranial to the inferior articular facet of C2 (**Fig. 20.5**). Sagittal orientation is sharply cranial in the 25- to 30-degree range and can be confirmed by visual inspection of the cranial surface of the C2 pars or by lateral fluoroscopy. Mediolateral orientation is neutral to up to 10 degrees medial; this is again facilitated by palpation of the medial wall of the C2 pars with a small dissector. If a C2 pedicle fixation is desired, then a more lateral starting point is employed—about 6 mm lateral from the lamino-articular junction (**Fig. 20.5**)—and the trajectory is angled medially 25 to 30 degrees and cranially ~ 25 degrees. Once the starting point is marked, it is drilled to the desired length—16 to 20 mm for a pars trajectory, and 24 to 28 mm for a pedicle screw—so that it is just past the posterior wall of the vertebral body on lateral fluoros-

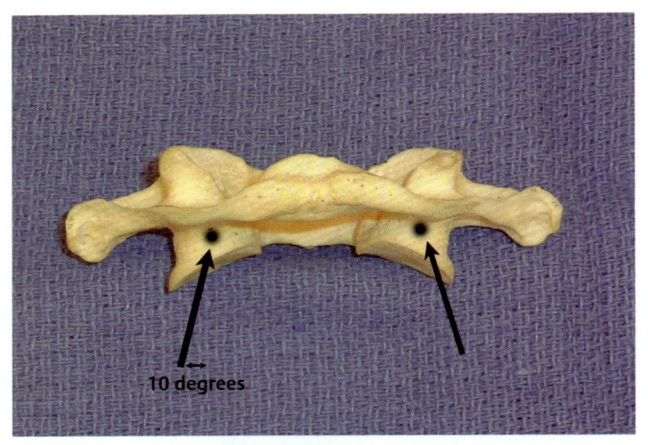

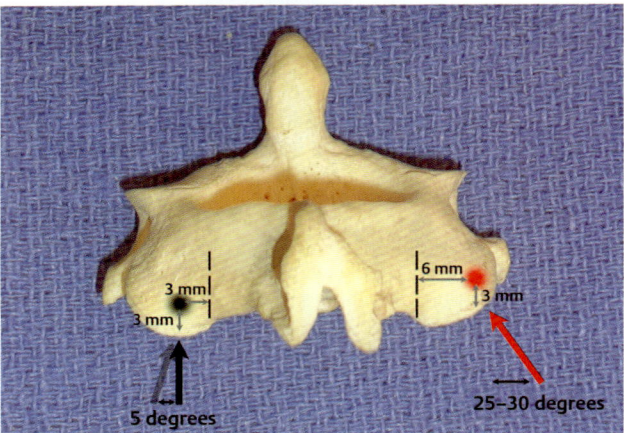

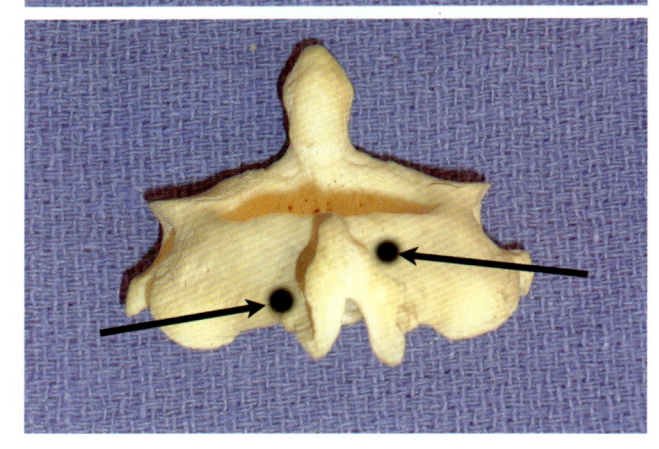

Fig. 20.5 Starting points for C1 lateral mass (**a**), C2 pars (*black mark, left side*) and pedicle (*red mark, right side*) (**b**), and C2 translaminar screws (**c**). C2 pars trajectory demonstrates our suggested neutral angulation (*solid line*) as well as the 5-degree medial alternative. The *dashed line* marks the lamina-articular process junction.

copy (**Figs. 20.1 and 20.2**). Once again, all steps are performed on one side before proceeding to the other, so that if the vertebral artery is injured, fixation of the contralateral side can be aborted.

If C2 translaminar screws are planned, the base of the C2 spinous process is cleared of all soft tissue, and the superior and inferior borders of the laminae are well defined. The C2-C3 supra- and interspinous ligaments are left intact. The starting points for the translaminar screws are staggered within the spinous process in the sagittal plane. The cranial and caudal edges of the lamina are exposed, and the entry points are marked with a bur on each side just above the base of the spinous process. A hand drill is aimed contralaterally at a 25- to 30-degree angle so that it matches the visualized anatomy of the lamina (**Fig. 20.5**). We prefer to drill the trajectory by hand with a 2.4-mm drill bit to a length of 20 to 26 mm, and the screw is placed in the usual manner; only the first 2 mm of the trajectory is tapped to allow for a strong cortical grip around the screw. Probing the tract is particularly important to avoid violations of the vertebral canal.

C1 and C2 screws are connected with a rod of the appropriate length and capped; a cross-link connector may be added over the C1 screws if a C1 burst fracture (Jefferson) is being repaired. Posterior C1-C2 wiring with placement of interspinous graft may be also added.

Postoperative Care

Unless C1-C2 fixation is being performed as part of a more complex procedure, the patient is extubated in the operating room and transferred to a regular hospital room. We utilize a rigid cervical collar, such as the Aspen or Miami J, for the initial 6 weeks, which has the main effect of restricting flexion and extension. Ambulation is started immediately after surgery and the patient can be discharged on the first postoperative day, after anteroposterior and lateral radiographs are obtained. The patient is seen in the clinic at 2, 6, 12, and 24 weeks post op. At the patient's 48-week visit, a CT scan is obtained.

Potential Complications and Precautions

C1-C2 fixation appears to have a better safety profile than transarticular fixation, but care still needs to be exercised to avoid vertebral artery injury while exposing C1 and placing the screws. If this injury happens during the exposure phase, cranial to C2, every attempt should be made to repair the injury because the artery should be visible in the field. On the other hand, if the injury happens during the drilling phase, repair is much more difficult. This may occur if the drill skips laterally over the C1 articular mass or when drilling the pars or pedicle of C2. In the former situation, the vessel needs to be identified and repaired or ligated. Injury from drilling or tapping into C2 is controlled by screw placement. If either occurs, the procedure is aborted on the contralateral side. Posterior wiring and placement of a graft should complement the procedure, if possible. Unilateral C1-C2 fixation has not been reported in the literature, but there is no reason to believe fusion rate should be significantly different from that of unilateral C1-C2 transarticular fixation.[38] After surgery is concluded, the patient with suspected arterial injuries should be immediately transferred to the interventional suite for an angiography. Both arteriovenous fistulas and pseudoaneurysms have been reported, though the best method (occlusion versus stenting) and timing (immediate versus delayed) for endovascular treatment of stable (nonbleeding) injuries is a subject of debate.[39–41]

C1 lateral mass fixation also has the potential for injuring anterior structures such as the carotid artery, jugular vein, and the hypoglossal nerve. Should a patient present with hypoglossal nerve palsy postoperatively, screw position should be assessed with a CT and revised if necessary.[42,43] Pseudarthrosis has not been a frequent concern, given reported fusion rates of better than 95%.[9] Revision strategies usually involve extension of fusion to the occiput.

Conclusion

Box 20.1 summarizes the main points of the chapter. C1 lateral mass–C2 pars screw fixation is a safe and versatile technique with rare anatomic contraindications precluding its application. Exposure is more elaborate than transarticular fixation, and meticulous dissection should be performed to avoid vertebral artery injuries. If performed successfully, the procedure typically has an excellent fusion rate without the need for halo orthoses.

Box 20.1 Key Operative Points and Avoiding Complications

- Use general anesthesia. The patient is placed in the prone position with the head in a Mayfield clamp and the chin tucked.
- Use lateral fluoroscopy confirmation and guidance throughout the surgery; navigation is also an option.
- Map the midline posterior incision on the skin.
- Expose the C1 posterior arch and the C2 lamina and pars.
- Expose the C1 lateral masses from medial to lateral. Transect the C2 nerve root if necessary.
- Perform cord decompression and packing of the C1-C2 joint, if necessary.
- C1 screw insertion: mark the entry site at the center of the lateral mass. Aim 10 degrees cranial, 10 degrees medial; aim for the anterior tubercle on lateral fluoroscopy.
- Drill C1 until it is bicortical. Tap and insert a partially-threaded screw.
- Mark the C2 pars screw entry point with a bur, 3 mm lateral to the lamina-articular process junction, and 3 mm cranial to the inferior articular facet.
- Drill the C2 pars trajectory: neutral to 10 degrees medial orientation, 25 to 30 degrees cranially. Follow the visual cues (top of the C2 pars; the medial wall of the pars is palpated with a Penfield dissector).
- Drill under radiological guidance to 16 to 20 mm; tap and insert a screw.
- C2 pedicle entry point: 5 to 6 mm lateral to the lamino-articular junction, 3 mm cranial to the inferior articular facet. Aim 25 to 30 degrees medial, 25 to 30 degrees cranial. Tap and insert the screw.
- If a vertebral artery injury occurs, insert a screw and abort the contralateral side or opt for translaminar fixation.
- C2 translaminar fixation: staggered the insertion points; aim contralaterally parallel to the laminar surface. Drill to 18 to 20 mm and tap only the initial 2 mm. Insert the screw to 20 to 26 mm.

References

1. Grob D, Magerl F. [Surgical stabilization of C1 and C2 fractures]. Orthopade 1987;16:46–54
2. Paramore CG, Dickman CA, Sonntag VK. The anatomical suitability of the C1-2 complex for transarticular screw fixation. J Neurosurg 1996;85:221–224
3. Goel A, Laheri V. Plate and screw fixation for atlanto-axial subluxation. Acta Neurochir (Wien) 1994;129:47–53

4. Dickman CA, Sonntag VK, Papadopoulos SM, Hadley MN. The interspinous method of posterior atlantoaxial arthrodesis. J Neurosurg 1991;74: 190–198

5. Leconte P. Fracture et luxation des deux premieres vertebres cervicales. In: Judet R, ed. Luxation Congenitale de la Hanche. Fractures du Cou-depied Rachis Cervical. Actualites de Chirurgie Orthopedique de l'Hopital Raymond-Poincare, vol 3. Paris: Masson et Cie; 1964:147–166

6. Borne GM, Bedou GL, Pinaudeau M. Treatment of pedicular fractures of the axis. A clinical study and screw fixation technique. J Neurosurg 1984; 60:88–93

7. Harms J, Melcher RP. Posterior C1-C2 fusion with polyaxial screw and rod fixation. Spine 2001;26:2467–2471

8. Aryan HE, Newman CB, Nottmeier EW, Acosta FL Jr, Wang VY, Ames CP. Stabilization of the atlantoaxial complex via C-1 lateral mass and C-2 pedicle screw fixation in a multicenter clinical experience in 102 patients: modification of the Harms and Goel techniques. J Neurosurg Spine 2008;8:222–229

9. Goel A, Shah A, Gupta SR. Craniovertebral instability due to degenerative osteoarthritis of the atlantoaxial joints: analysis of the management of 108 cases. J Neurosurg Spine 2010;12:592–601

10. Wright NM. Posterior C2 fixation using bilateral, crossing C2 laminar screws: case series and technical note. J Spinal Disord Tech 2004;17:158–162

11. Carazzo CA, Guirado VM de P, Meluzzi A, et al. Características morfológicas da pars de C2 de humanos. Coluna/Columna 2009;8:279–285. doi: 10.1590/S1808-18512009000300008

12. Ebraheim NA, Fow J, Xu R, Yeasting RA. The location of the pedicle and pars interarticularis in the axis. Spine 2001;26:E34–E37

13. Federative Committee on Anatomical Terminology. Terminologia anatomica: international anatomical terminology. Stuttgart; New York: Thieme; 1998

14. Yeom JS, Buchowski JM, Kim H-J, Chang B-S, Lee C-K, Riew KD. Risk of vertebral artery injury: comparison between C1-C2 transarticular and C2 pedicle screws. Spine J 2013;13:775–785

15. Elliott RE, Tanweer O, Boah A, et al. Comparison of screw malposition and vertebral artery injury of C2 pedicle and transarticular screws: meta-analysis and review of the literature. J Spinal Disord Tech 2014;27:305–315

16. Hott JS, Lynch JJ, Chamberlain RH, Sonntag VKH, Crawford NR. Biomechanical comparison of C1-2 posterior fixation techniques. J Neurosurg Spine 2005;2:175–181

17. Melcher RP, Puttlitz CM, Kleinstueck FS, Lotz JC, Harms J, Bradford DS. Biomechanical testing of posterior atlantoaxial fixation techniques. Spine 2002;27:2435–2440

18. Sim HB, Lee JW, Park JT, Mindea SA, Lim J, Park J. Biomechanical evaluations of various c1-c2 posterior fixation techniques. Spine 2011;36:E401–E407

19. Gluf WM, Schmidt MH, Apfelbaum RI. Atlantoaxial transarticular screw fixation: a review of surgical indications, fusion rate, complications, and lessons learned in 191 adult patients. J Neurosurg Spine 2005;2:155–163

20. Guiot B, Fessler RG. Complex atlantoaxial fractures. J Neurosurg 1999; 91(2, Suppl):139–143

21. Anderson LD, D'Alonzo RT. Fractures of the odontoid process of the axis. J Bone Joint Surg Am 1974;56:1663–1674

22. Kuntz C IV, Mirza SK, Jarell AD, Chapman JR, Shaffrey CI, Newell DW. Type II odontoid fractures in the elderly: early failure of nonsurgical treatment. Neurosurg Focus 2000;8:e7

23. Casey AT, Madawi AA, Veres R, Crockard HA. Is the technique of posterior transarticular screw fixation suitable for rheumatoid atlanto-axial subluxation? Br J Neurosurg 1997;11:508–519

24. Bambakidis NC. Surgery of the craniovertebral junction. New York: Thieme; 2012. Available at: http://search.ebscohost.com/login.aspx?direct=true&scope=site&db=nlebk&db=nlabk&AN=534258. Accessed April 11, 2014

25. Härtl R, Chamberlain RH, Fifield MS, Chou D, Sonntag VKH, Crawford NR. Biomechanical comparison of two new atlantoaxial fixation techniques with C1-2 transarticular screw-graft fixation. J Neurosurg Spine 2006;5: 336–342

26. Sciubba DM, Noggle JC, Vellimana AK, et al. Laminar screw fixation of the axis. J Neurosurg Spine 2008;8:327–334

27. Elliott RE, Tanweer O. The prevalence of the ponticulus posticus (arcuate foramen) and its importance in the Goel-Harms procedure: meta-analysis and review of the literature. World Neurosurg 2014;82:e335–e343

28. Yeom JS, Kafle D, Nguyen NQ, et al. Routine insertion of the lateral mass screw via the posterior arch for C1 fixation: feasibility and related complications. Spine J 2012;12:476–483

29. Dewan MC, Godil SS, Mendenhall SK, Devin CJ, McGirt MJ. C2 nerve root transection during C1 lateral mass screw fixation: does it affect functionality and quality of life? Neurosurgery 2014;74:475–480, discussion 480–481

30. Hamilton DK, Smith JS, Sansur CA, Dumont AS, Shaffrey CI. C-2 neurectomy during atlantoaxial instrumented fusion in the elderly: patient satisfaction and surgical outcome. J Neurosurg Spine 2011;15:3–8

31. Yeom JS, Buchowski JM, Kim H-J, Chang B-S, Lee C-K, Riew KD. Postoperative occipital neuralgia with and without C2 nerve root transection during atlantoaxial screw fixation: a post-hoc comparative outcome study of prospectively collected data. Spine J 2013;13:786–795

32. Gorek J, Acaroglu E, Berven S, Yousef A, Puttlitz CM. Constructs incorporating intralaminar C2 screws provide rigid stability for atlantoaxial fixation. Spine 2005;30:1513–1518

33. Hong JT, Takigawa T, Udayakunmar R, et al. Biomechanical effect of the C2 laminar decortication on the stability of C2 intralaminar screw construct and biomechanical comparison of C2 intralaminar screw and C2 pars screw. Neurosurgery 2011;69(1, Suppl Operative):ons1–ons6, discussion ons6–ons7

34. Dorward IG, Wright NM. Seven years of experience with C2 translaminar screw fixation: clinical series and review of the literature. Neurosurgery 2011;68:1491–1499, discussion 1499

35. Parker SL, McGirt MJ, Garcés-Ambrossi GL, et al. Translaminar versus pedicle screw fixation of C2: comparison of surgical morbidity and accuracy of 313 consecutive screws. Neurosurgery 2009;64(5, Suppl 2):343–348, discussion 348–349

36. Moses ZB, Mayer RR, Strickland BA, et al. Neuronavigation in minimally invasive spine surgery. Neurosurg Focus 2013;35:E12

37. Kwon JK, Kim MS, Lee GJ. The incidence and clinical implications of congenital defects of atlantal arch. J Korean Neurosurg Soc 2009;46:522–527

38. Song GS, Theodore N, Dickman CA, Sonntag VK. Unilateral posterior atlantoaxial transarticular screw fixation. J Neurosurg 1997;87:851–855

39. Choi J-W, Lee J-K, Moon K-S, et al. Endovascular embolization of iatrogenic vertebral artery injury during anterior cervical spine surgery: report of two cases and review of the literature. Spine 2006;31:E891–E894

40. Daentzer D, Deinsberger W, Böker D-K. Vertebral artery complications in anterior approaches to the cervical spine: report of two cases and review of literature. Surg Neurol 2003;59:300–309, discussion 309

41. Prabhu VC, France JC, Voelker JL, Zoarski GH. Vertebral artery pseudoaneurysm complicating posterior C1-2 transarticular screw fixation: case report. Surg Neurol 2001;55:29–33, discussion 33–34

42. Ebraheim NA, Misson JR, Xu R, Yeasting RA. The optimal transarticular c1-2 screw length and the location of the hypoglossal nerve. Surg Neurol 2000;53:208–210

43. Estillore RP, Buchowski JM, Minh V, et al. Risk of internal carotid artery injury during C1 screw placement: analysis of 160 computed tomography angiograms. Spine J 2011;11:316–323

21 Odontoid Screw Placement

Christopher M. Maulucci, George M. Ghobrial, Ahmed J. Awad, and James S. Harrop

Fractures of the odontoid account for up to 18% of all cervical spine fractures.[1] This type of fracture may result in a devastating neurologic injury. It has been estimated that up to 40% of people who sustain an odontoid fracture die at the scene of the accident.[2] However, for those who survive, few have any immediate neurologic impairment. If left untreated, though, signs and symptoms of myelopathy or bulbar dysfunction may develop.[2] The most often used classification system for these injuries was proposed by Anderson and D'Alonzo[1] in 1974. It consists of three fracture categories: type I, through the upper part of the odontoid process; type II, extending to the base of the odontoid; and type III, through the body of the atlas and into the lateral masses. A type II fracture, at the base of the odontoid peg, is considered unstable. The resultant atlantoaxial instability requires treatment via either external bracing or internal fixation. This region of the neck is responsible for ~ 50% of the rotatory motion of the cervical spine.[3] Immobilization of the atlantoaxial joint via posterior fusion results in a most noticeable loss of range of motion for the patient.

The most common cervical spine fracture in patients 65 years of age or older is a type II odontoid fracture.[4] In patients over the age of 80, this fracture pattern is more common than all cervical fractures combined.[5] In this often comorbidity-laden patient population, an external orthosis, such as a halo vest, is an attractive option given its minimal risk to the patient. However, a mortality rate of up to 40% has been reported in elderly patients placed in a halo vest, perhaps as a result of respiratory compromise,[6] and nonunion rates of up to 41% have also been reported.[7] Therefore, surgical fixation of type II odontoid fractures in elderly patients who are well enough to tolerate general anesthesia should be considered.[4] Studies have shown that elderly patients treated with surgery have significantly better outcomes with regard to pain and the successful union of the fracture.[4]

Patient Selection: Indications and Contraindications

Treatment of a type II odontoid fracture with anterior screw fixation provides immediate stability and preserves motion at the atlantoaxial joint. Patients should be quickly mobilized postoperatively to reduce the risk of complications attributed to prolonged bed rest. However, careful patient selection is necessary before proceeding.

The morphology of the fracture is the primary determinant of whether anterior screw fixation should be attempted. A comminuted fracture is an absolute contraindication to anterior screw placement. The most advantageous fracture pattern courses from the anterosuperior to the posteroinferior part of the dens (**Fig. 21.1a**).[8] This pattern enables insertion of a screw perpendicular to the fracture. A screw may then be used to engage the fractured odontoid and bring the gragment down to the body of C2 in an anatomic position. A fracture that courses from anteroinferior to posterosuperior is a contraindication to anterior fixation, as the screw would parallel the fracture, potentially pulling the odontoid anteriorly, with resultant misalignment and nonunion (**Fig. 21.1b**). Horizontal fractures, as long as they do not involve the vertebral body, may also be treated with an anterior screw (**Fig. 21.1c**). This fracture pattern enables the odontoid screw to engage the fragment at an acute angle that is still favorable for achieving anatomic alignment. Type III odontoid fractures are typically not considered for anterior screw fixation, as the vertebral body involvement may result in poor proximal screw fixation.[8]

The integrity of the transverse ligament must also be evaluated before electing to proceed with odontoid screw fixation. Disruption of the ligament is an absolute contraindication. The ligament is well delineated on magnetic resonance imaging (MRI) as its imaging characteristics contrast with those of the surrounding structures.[9] The transverse ligament may also be indirectly assessed through measurement of the atlantodental interval (> 3 mm denotes instability).

The quality of the bone should also be taken into account. Osteopenic or osteoporotic bone is often present in the elderly. Although this is not an absolute contraindication, the screw purchase should be examined, and if it is deemed questionable, an external brace may be necessary.

Anatomic features not related to the fracture should be assessed preoperatively as well, as they may affect the surgeon's ability to direct a screw in the proper trajectory. Patients with a barrel chest, a cervical kyphotic deformity, or an inability to extend the neck may not be ideal candidates for anterior odontoid screw fixation. Obese patients or those with a barrel chest pose a challenge as the instrument handles, such as those of the drill and screw inserter, may encounter the chest wall before they have been angled cranially enough to aim for the tip of the odontoid.

A relative contraindication is advanced patient age. Elderly patients develop dysphagia due to reduction in muscle mass and loss of connective tissue elasticity. An anterior cervical procedure necessitating manipulation of the esophagus may result in severe dysphagia.[10]

Fractures older than 6 months or those with sclerotic margins have a lower fusion rate of 25%.[11] In these patients, posterior instrumented fusion may be considered. Patients with os odontoideum or other developmental anomalies may not be candidates either.

Advantages and Disadvantages

The advantages of odontoid fixation with an anterior screw include immediate stability, usually without the need for an external orthosis; preservation of atlantoaxial rotation; and a high fusion rate in properly selected patients. Anterior odontoid screw fixation achieves excellent stability and a low mechanical failure rate during short-term and long-term follow-up.[12] The fusion

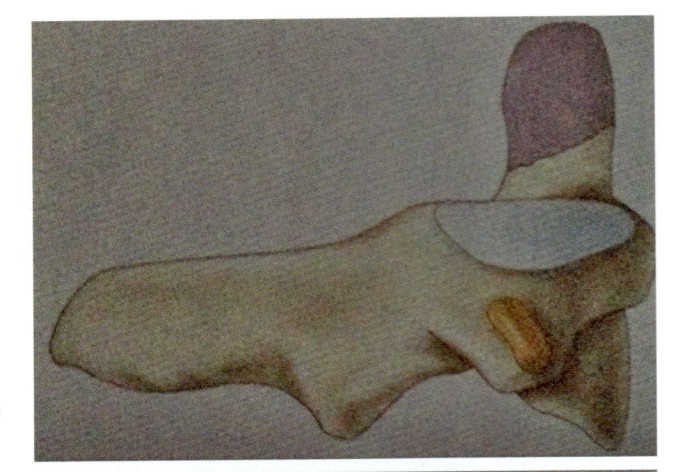

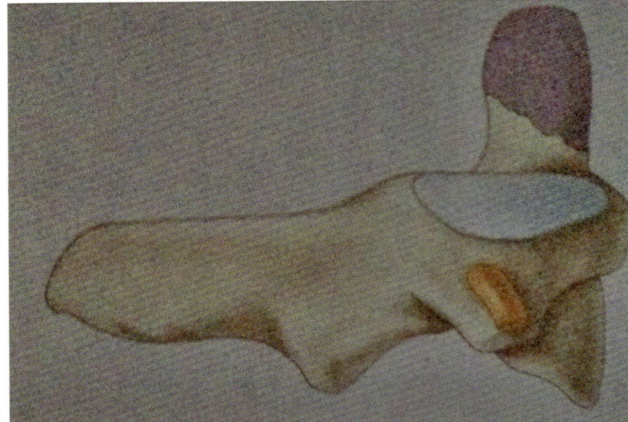

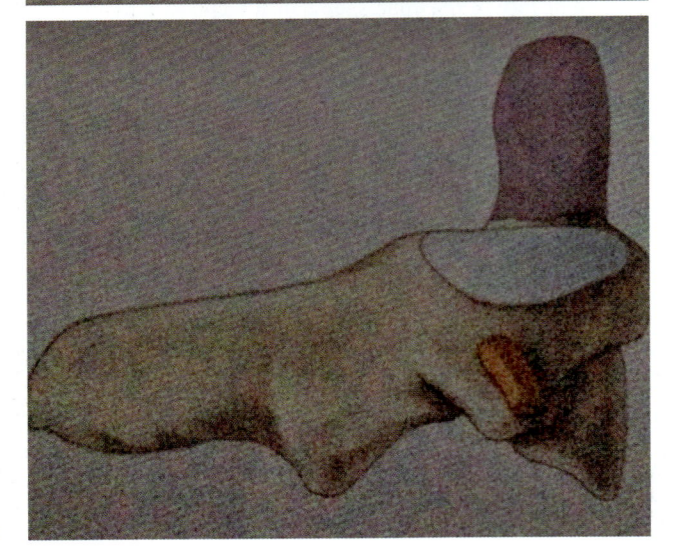

Fig. 21.1 (a) Posterior oblique (anterior superior to posterior inferior) fracture that is appropriate for screw fixation. The screw path is roughly perpendicular to the fracture line. (b) Anterior oblique fracture (posterior superior to anterior inferior), which can make screw fixation difficult due to the fracture's course parallel to the screw's course. (c) Horizontal type II odontoid fracture. (Reproduced with permission from Vaccaro AR, Baron EM. Operative techniques-spine surgery. Philadelphia: Elsevier; 2008:43.)

rate for anterior odontoid fixation for all patient populations is ~90%.[13] No disadvantages have been noted in the literature.

Preoperative Imaging

Conventional radiographs of the cervical spine may be obtained as part of the evaluation of a patient with a suspected cervical spine fracture. Lateral, anteroposterior, and open-mouth anteroposterior views provide information on spinal alignment and may possibly demonstrate fractures. Computed tomography (CT) sagittal and coronal reconstructed views give detailed information on bone quality, potential ligamentous injury, and the fracture pattern of the odontoid. MRI demonstrates injury to ligaments and neural elements.

Surgical Procedure

Anesthesia

If extension of the neck produces abnormal motion of the fracture fragment, an awake nasotracheal or fiberoptic intubation can be used. Lateral projection fluoroscopy can be used before, during, and after intubation to ensure that there has not been compromise of the central canal. Neuromonitoring with motor evoked potentials (MEPs) may also be used before and after intubation to evaluate for changes in spinal cord activity.

Positioning

The patient is positioned supine on a radiolucent table. The head may be gently extended with a support beneath the shoulders if the fracture reduces with extension. Otherwise, the head is kept neutral. The head is immobilized with 10 lb of halter traction. A radiolucent bite block should be inserted, opening the jaw as much as possible. If available, two C-arm fluoroscopic units should be positioned for lateral and anteroposterior projections (**Fig. 21.2**). If only one C-arm is available, the draping should be arranged to allow for frequent repositioning of the fluoroscopic unit.

Approach

A standard anterior cervical approach to the C5-C6 level should be performed, either from the left or right side (**Fig. 21.3**). Right-handed surgeons may find a right-sided approach preferable. Once the prevertebral fascia has been divided, blunt dissection is used cranially up to the C1 region. The longus colli muscles are elevated, and self-retaining retractor blades are firmly seated beneath the muscle. A superiorly directed retractor blade is then inserted to retract the pharyngeal tissues away from the upper cervical spine. Biplanar fluoroscopy is then used to confirm the proper level as well as the midline at the anterior inferior aspect of the C2 body. If the surgical plan is to place one screw, then a Kirschner wire (K-wire) should be placed at the C2 midline and impacted 3 to 5 mm into the entry site (**Fig. 21.4**). If two screws are to be used, then a paramedian site 2 to 3 mm from midline should be selected.[7] Once the K-wire is in place, a hollow-core drill is placed over the K-wire and advanced under biplanar fluoroscopy until the apex of the odontoid is penetrated. This step is crucial; if the cortical apex of the odontoid is not penetrated, the screw may not effectively align the fragment with the C2 body. Attention must be paid to the K-wire while drilling to ensure that it does not advance cranially into the foramen magnum. The drill is removed and a hollow-core tap is inserted over the K-wire along the entirety of the previously drilled path. After removal of the tap, a hollow-core lag screw is inserted with fluoroscopy along the same path. As the threads of the screw engage the apical cortex of the odontoid, the fracture fragment should be pulled toward the C2 body. The head of the screw should be countersunk into the C2-C3 annulus or the C2 body (**Fig. 21.5**). A second screw may then be placed repeating the above steps. However, there is no evidence that two screws provide fixation that is superior to that of one screw.[7] Halter traction is then removed. Stability of the fracture may be confirmed by flexing and extending the patient's neck under fluoroscopy.[14]

A fully-threaded screw may be used in cases where fracture reduction is not necessary.[15] This reduces the need to engage the apical cortex of the odontoid as there is excellent bone-screw interfacing all along this type of screw. For patients with low bone density, augmentation of the C2 body may be achieved with the use of polymethylmethacrylate (PMMA) cement (**Fig. 21.6**).[16] Newer technologies that enable surgical navigation, such as isocentric three-dimensional fluoroscopy[17] and other imaging systems, can also be used instead of biplanar fluoroscopy.

Postoperative Care

Patients should be monitored overnight for acute complications such as respiratory compromise. Most patients can quickly resume normal low-impact activities of daily living. Barring swallowing dysfunction and other trauma-related issues, the typical postoperative stay in the hospital is 1 to 2 days. A soft cervical collar may be provided for comfort. A rigid orthosis can be used in cases of questionable bone density. Postoperative fracture union is assessed by serial radiographs and CT if there is question as to the presence of a nonunion.

Potential Complications and Precautions

To ensure proper screw trajectory, a straight instrument can be placed alongside the neck under fluoroscopy to plan the incision.[14] Proper elevation of the longus colli is needed to fix the retractors firmly. After retractor placement, the endotracheal tube can be deflated and then reinflated to center it within the larynx.[18] After drilling and tapping under biplanar fluoroscopy, an image with the tap in place should be saved and used as a guide for screw placement, again under biplanar fluoroscopy. If the fragment alignment is suboptimal, the head may be manipulated with fluoroscopic guidance to align the odontoid. The distal cortex of the odontoid should be engaged by the screw to pull the fracture fragment toward the body.

Conclusion

Anterior odontoid screw fixation is an effective and safe method for treating odontoid fractures. It confers immediate stability, potentially preserves C1-C2 rotatory motion, and provides optimum conditions for bony fusion. Fracture anatomy and patient body habitus should be taken into account before proceeding with surgery. The timing of surgery for odontoid fractures is important, as there is an increased risk of nonunion more than 6 months after injury.

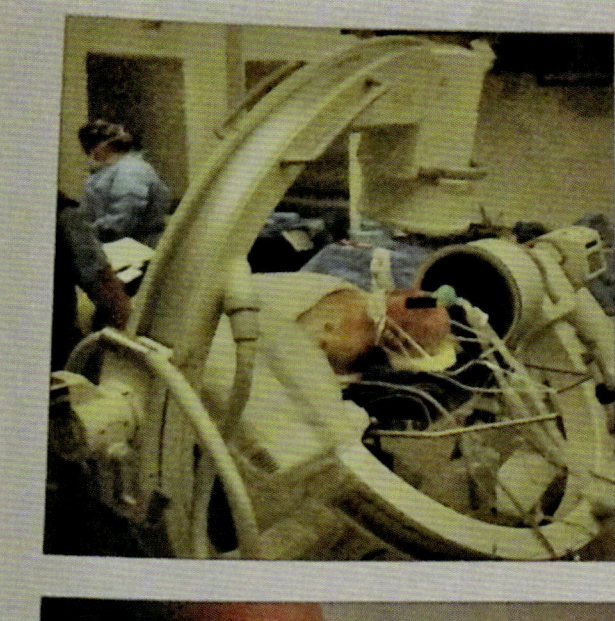

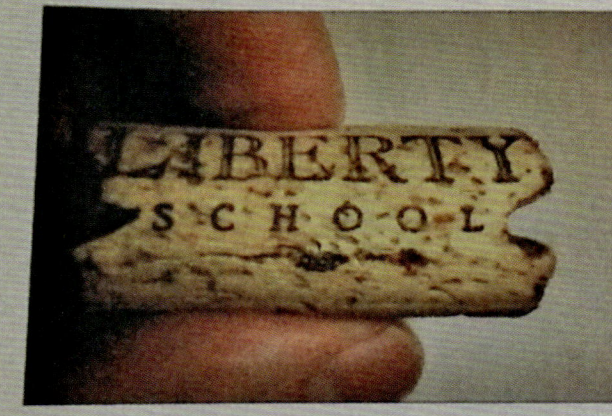

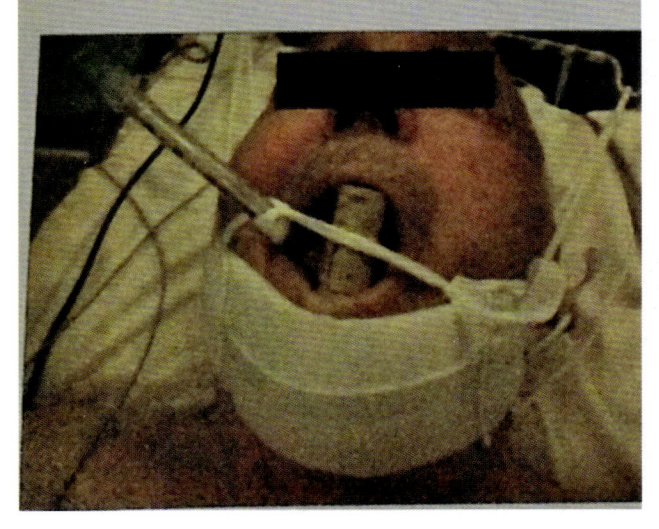

Fig. 21.2 Operating room setup for odontoid screw placement. **(a)** Biplanar fluoroscopy in place before draping. **(b)** a radiolucent bite block, such as a cork, can be used to effectively hold the mouth open. Other radiolucent materials may also be used. **(c)** In a neutral head position, 10 lb of halter traction is applied. (Reproduced with permission from Vaccaro AR, Baron EM. Operative techniques-spine surgery. Philadelphia: Elsevier; 2008:43.)

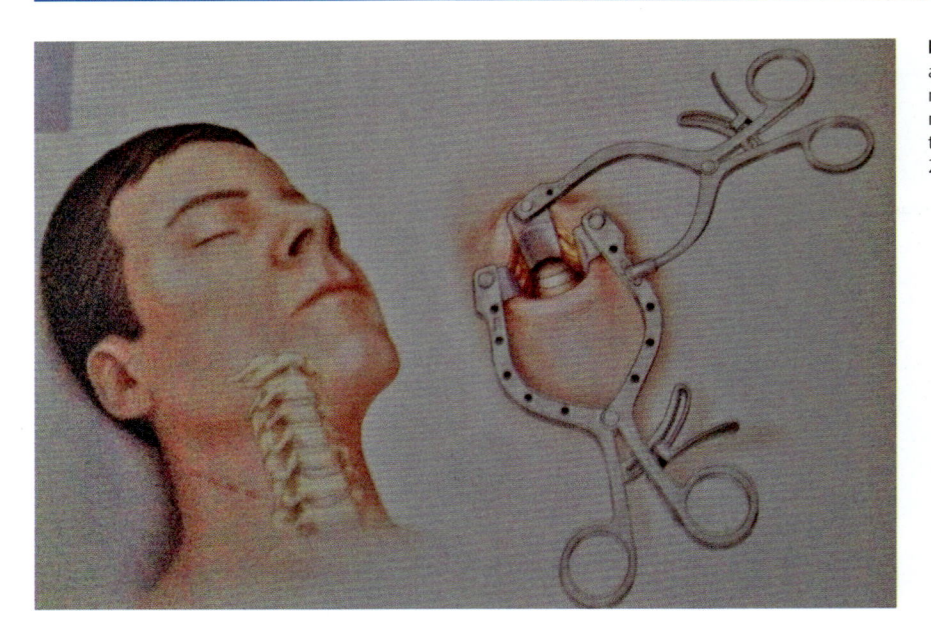

Fig. 21.3 A transverse skin incision overlying approximately C5 is planned, and self-retaining retractors are placed. (Reproduced with permission from Vaccaro AR, Baron EM. Operative techniques-spine surgery. Philadelphia: Elsevier; 2008:43.)

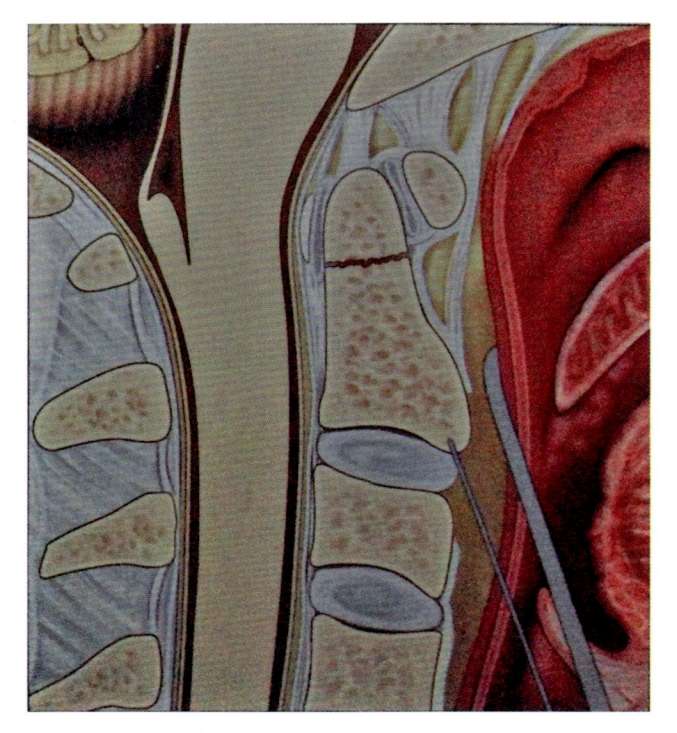

Fig. 21.4 The Kirschner wire (K-wire) is positioned at the anterior inferior edge of the C2 body. (Reproduced with permission from Vaccaro AR, Baron EM. Operative techniques-spine surgery. Philadelphia: Elsevier; 2008:43.)

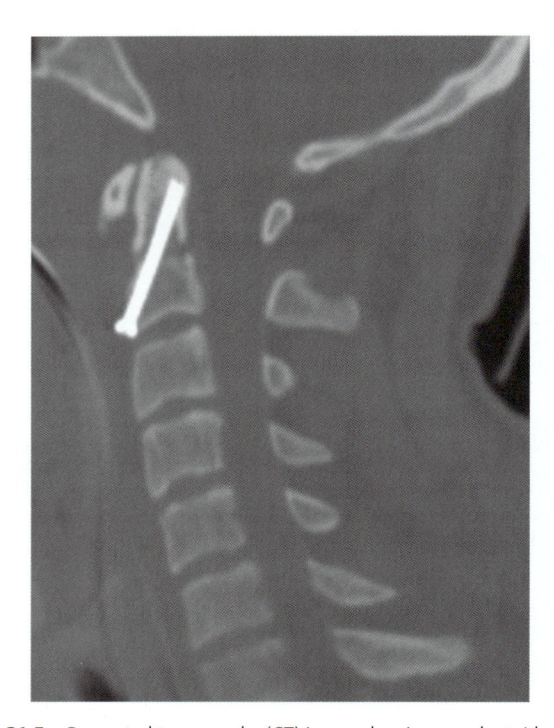

Fig. 21.5 Computed tomography (CT) image showing an odontoid screw in which the head of the screw is countersunk into the end plate of C2 and the screw engages the cortex of the odontoid. Anatomic cervical alignment is maintained.

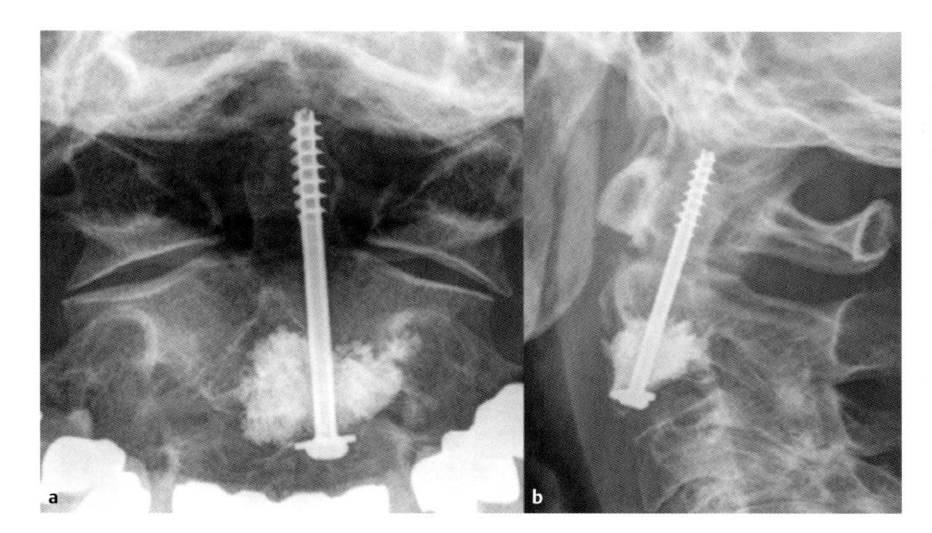

Fig. 21.6 Anteroposterior **(a)** and lateral **(b)** radiographs of odontoid screw fixation with cement augmentation in the body of C2. (Reproduced with permission from Kohlhof H, Seidel U, Hoppe S, Keel MJ, Benneker LM. Cement-augmented anterior screw fixation of Type II odontoid fractures in elderly patients with osteoporosis. The Spine Journal 2013; 13(12):1858–1863.)

References

1. Anderson LD, D'Alonzo RT. Fractures of the odontoid process of the axis. J Bone Joint Surg Am 1974;56:1663–1674
2. Crockard HA, Heilman AE, Stevens JM. Progressive myelopathy secondary to odontoid fractures: clinical, radiological, and surgical features. J Neurosurg 1993;78:579–586
3. White AA, Panjabi MM. Clinical Biomechanics of the Spine. Philadelphia: Lippincott; 1990
4. Vaccaro AR, Kepler CK, Kopjar B, et al. Functional and quality-of-life outcomes in geriatric patients with type-II dens fracture. J Bone Joint Surg Am 2013;95:729–735
5. Ardeshiri A, Asgari S, Lemonas E, et al. Elderly patients are at increased risk for mortality undergoing surgical repair of dens fractures. Clin Neurol Neurosurg 2013;115:2056–2061
6. Majercik S, Tashjian RZ, Biffl WL, Harrington DT, Cioffi WG. Halo vest immobilization in the elderly: a death sentence? J Trauma 2005;59:350–356, discussion 356–358
7. Jenkins JD, Coric D, Branch CL Jr. A clinical comparison of one- and two-screw odontoid fixation. J Neurosurg 1998;89:366–370
8. Mazur MD, Mumert ML, Bisson EF, Schmidt MH. Avoiding pitfalls in anterior screw fixation for type II odontoid fractures. Neurosurg Focus 2011; 31:E7
9. Dickman CA, Mamourian A, Sonntag VK, Drayer BP. Magnetic resonance imaging of the transverse atlantal ligament for the evaluation of atlantoaxial instability. J Neurosurg 1991;75:221–227
10. Sura L, Madhavan A, Carnaby G, Crary MA. Dysphagia in the elderly: management and nutritional considerations. Clin Interv Aging 2012;7:287–298
11. Apfelbaum RI, Lonser RR, Veres R, Casey A. Direct anterior screw fixation for recent and remote odontoid fractures. J Neurosurg 2000;93(2, Suppl): 227–236
12. Fountas KN, Kapsalaki EZ, Karampelas I, et al. Results of long-term follow-up in patients undergoing anterior screw fixation for type II and rostral type III odontoid fractures. Spine 2005;30:661–669
13. Patel AA, Lindsey R, Bessey JT, Chapman J, Rampersaud R; Spine Trauma Study Group. Surgical treatment of unstable type II odontoid fractures in skeletally mature individuals. Spine 2010;35(21, Suppl):S209–S218
14. Vaccaro AR, Baron EM. Operative Techniques—Spine Surgery. Philadelphia: Elsevier; 2008
15. Magee W, Hettwer W, Badra M, Bay B, Hart R. Biomechanical comparison of a fully threaded, variable pitch screw and a partially threaded lag screw for internal fixation of type II dens fractures. Spine 2007;32:E475–E479
16. Kohlhof H, Seidel U, Hoppe S, Keel MJ, Benneker LM. Cement-augmented anterior screw fixation of type II odontoid fractures in elderly patients with osteoporosis. Spine J 2013;13:1858–1863
17. Martirosyan NL, Kalb S, Cavalcanti DD, et al. Comparative analysis of isocentric 3-dimensional C-arm fluoroscopy and biplanar fluoroscopy for anterior screw fixation in odontoid fractures. J Spinal Disord Tech 2013; 26:189–193
18. Apfelbaum RI, Kriskovich MD, Haller JR. On the incidence, cause, and prevention of recurrent laryngeal nerve palsies during anterior cervical spine surgery. Spine 2000;25:2906–2912

Section II Midcervical Spine

A. Pathology

22 Congenital Osseous Anomalies of the Mid- to Lower Cervical Spine

Jeffrey C. Wang and Dmitri Sofianos

In general, congenital anomalies of the cervical spine, especially the subaxial cervical spine, are uncommon. Most affected individuals are asymptomatic or notice only a mild restriction of neck motion. If symptoms do occur in the mid- to lower cervical spine, it is usually in adult life secondary to degenerative arthritis in the segments adjacent to the congenitally fused segments.[1] In fact, the presence of a congenital osseous cervical spine anomaly is most significant in that it often is an indication of other underlying congenital systemic malformations. This factor is of paramount importance to the treating physician, whose main attention may be directed solely toward the patient's neck. The topic of congenital osseous anomalies of the cervical spine is dominated by the subject of Klippel-Feil syndrome. Thus, most of this chapter focuses on the diagnostic workup, including physical and radiographic examination of the syndrome itself and of the various congenital systemic malformations that are known to occur in conjunction with Klippel-Feil syndrome. Various other genetic conditions that can present with congenital osseous anomalies are also discussed, along with specific treatment options.

In 1912, Klippel and Feil[2] published the first description of the clinical and pathological aspects of cervical spine deformities in a patient with complete fusion of the cervical spine. They noted the unusual findings of marked shortening of the neck, a low posterior hairline, and severe restriction of neck motion. In its present usage, the term *Klippel-Feil syndrome* refers to congenital fusion of the cervical vertebrae. The problems unique to fusions of the craniovertebral and atlantoaxial junction are beyond the scope of this chapter.

The prevalence of Klippel-Feil syndrome is unknown because the majority of individuals who have this condition are asymptomatic and may not have any other associated anomalies. In a study of the skeletal specimens of 1,400 cervical spines, Brown et al[3] found that only 10 of the 75 fused segments discovered below the second cervical vertebrae were congenital in nature. In the majority of series, the most common site of fusion is between the second and third cervical vertebrae, with fusion of the fifth and sixth cervical vertebrae seen next most commonly. These two sites of fusion may be inherited in an autosomal dominant or autosomal recessive fashion, respectively.[4]

Classification

Various classification schemes have been offered in the literature, many of which are variations of other schemes. Some are only descriptive, whereas others attempt to correlate anatomic and radiographic findings with clinical pictures. Some classifications were designed to predict future neurologic status based on radiographic findings. Klippel and Feil[2] classified the syndrome into three groups based on the site and extent of the fusion.

Type I is fusion of the cervical and upper thoracic vertebrae. Type II is fusion isolated to the cervical spine. Type III is fusion of the cervical vertebrae associated with lower thoracic or lumbar fusions. No clinically relevant correlations have been made with this classification, although many authors continue to use it.

Hensinger[1,5] has popularized a classification based on a variation of the findings made by McRae[6] that described three patterns of potentially unstable fusions. Pattern 1 is fusion of C2 and C3 with occipitalization of the atlas. Pattern 2 is a long fusion with an abnormal occipitocervical junction. Pattern 3 is a single open interspace between two fused segments.

Nagib et al[7] categorized the patients in their series who had neurologic deficits into three groups based on the most significant anomaly and the probable mechanism of injury. Type I is an unstable fusion pattern, such as two long segments of block vertebrae with an intervening open disk space. Type II is craniovertebral anomalies. Type III is congenital fusion associated with spinal stenosis. Patients with type I and II patterns were advised to avoid contact sports; if any neurologic symptoms or deformity developed, operative stabilization was recommended. Patients with type III patterns were advised to avoid strenuous physical activity, and were further advised to undergo a decompression and stabilization if neurologic symptoms developed.

Three patterns of fusion were observed in the series of Guille et al.[8] Type I is isolated block vertebrae anywhere in the cervical spine. Type II is two segments of block vertebrae separated by one isolated unfused vertebra with open disk spaces on either end. Type III is two segments of block vertebrae separated by an open disk interspace. No correlation was seen between the type of fusion pattern and the later presence of signs or symptoms that could be attributed to the syndrome.

Pizzutillo et al[9] described a functional classification. Class I is normal range of motion in the upper and lower cervical spine with no translational instability. Class II is intersegmental hypermobility of the upper cervical spine, basilar impression, or iniencephaly. Class III is intersegmental hypermobility of the lower cervical spine, or spondylosis. Class IV is a combination of class II and class III. Treatment recommendations were based on this classification. Asymptomatic patients in class I should be followed with serial observation. Class II patients should be followed annually, or more frequently if necessary. These patients should avoid contact sports. Class III patients should be treated symptomatically for spondylosis. Class IV patients should be treated similarly to the patients in classes II and III. This study concluded that patients with hypermobility of the upper cervical spine are at increased risk for neurologic problems, whereas those with involvement of the lower cervical spine are likely to develop early degenerative disease.

Phenotypic Features

The original description of the Klippel-Feil syndrome included the triad of decreased range of neck motion, a short neck, and a low hairline. This triad has been reported in approximately half of the patients with the syndrome, partly due to the subjective nature of what is considered a short neck or low hairline (**Fig. 22.1**).[10,11] The most consistent finding in these patients is limited range of motion of the neck, especially lateral side bending. If fewer than three vertebrae are fused or if only the lower cervical segments are fused, the patient generally has no detectable limitation that is usually due to compensation. Flexion and extension, which occur primarily at the occipitocervical junction, and rotation, which occurs primarily at the atlantoaxial junction, are usually preserved unless these levels are fused or anomalous. Some authors have observed that if less than three vertebral levels are fused, loss of motion may be unnoticeable, and much of neck motion may be compensated for at adjacent unfused levels.

Torticollis

Torticollis is often a clinical manifestation of congenital osseous cervical spine anomaly, usually cervicothoracic scoliosis or a hemivertebra. Tumors of the posterior fossa or infection may also create the picture of torticollis. The deformity is characterized by a lateral tilt of the head with rotation of the face.

Often the deformity is mild and is compensated for unconsciously by the patient. Facial asymmetry, which may be permanent, can occur in long-standing, untreated situations. When there is no fixed bony deformity, the condition responds well to stretching; tenotomy of the sternocleidomastoid may be required in recalcitrant states and yields good results if it is performed when the patient is young. If the etiology is of a bony nature, a unilateral hemiepiphysiodesis or fusion could be performed on the convex side of the curve in a young child in the hope that continued growth on the concave side would provide correction. Of course, there has to be the assumption that growth potential exists on the concave side, as demonstrated by open disk spaces and pedicle shadows. Cervical spine radiographs should be taken in children who present with torticollis to rule out osseous etiologies. Surgical correction of the bony deformity by direct means, such as wedge osteotomy, is not recommended.[1]

Pterygium Colli

Patients with Klippel-Feil syndrome may have pterygium colli, which is various degrees of webbing of the skin from the side of the neck to the shoulders (**Fig. 22.2**).[12] When pterygium exists bilaterally, it gives the appearance of a short neck; when unilat-

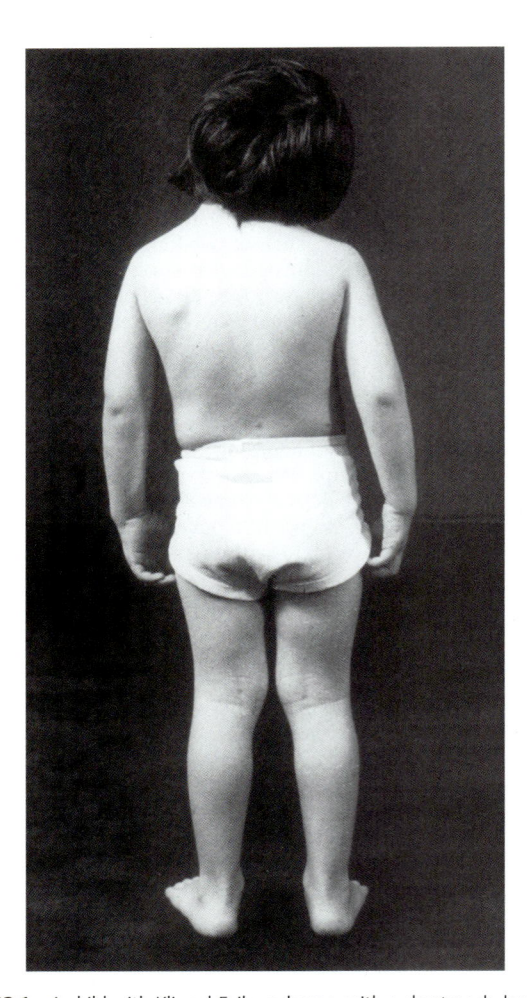

Fig. 22.1 A child with Klippel-Feil syndrome, with a short neck, low hairline, torticollis, and a Sprengel's deformity on the left side.

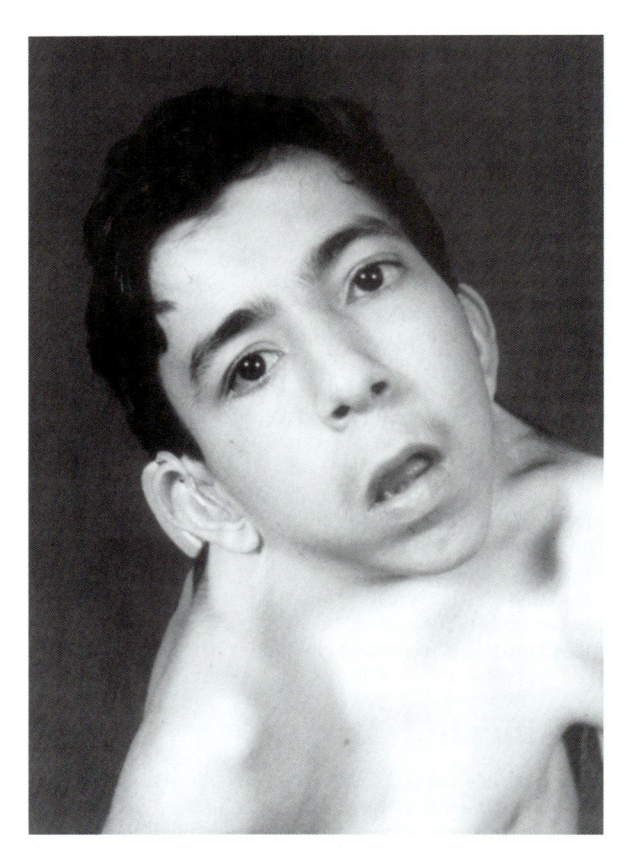

Fig. 22.2 A child with Klippel-Feil syndrome showing bilateral pterygium colli and torticollis. Note the hearing aid.

eral, it can give the appearance of torticollis. Pterygium colli is commonly seen in girls with Turner's syndrome. Various techniques describing Z-plasties and rotational flaps have been described to address the deformity in carefully selected patients. Rarely, however, do these procedures improve range of motion of the neck. These cosmetic deformities are usually referred to a plastic surgeon for further consideration. Hensinger[1] has cautioned that cosmetic treatment of the torticollis posture has been met with limited success. Occasionally, it can be improved with bracing; however, this requires long-term application and excellent patient cooperation.

Facial and Ocular Deformities and Hearing Deficits

Patients with congenital cervical spine problems should be inspected for abnormal facies and ear anomalies.[13] Facial asymmetry may be secondary to long-standing torticollis. Congenital cervical spine anomalies have been associated with Apert's syndrome and Crouzon's disease. Oculoauriculovertebral dysplasia, also known as Goldenhar's syndrome, is a rare congenital defect characterized by incomplete development of the ear, nose, lip, mandible, and occasionally the spine, and is a variant of hemifacial microsomia. In the spine it can manifest as underdeveloped, absent, or fused vertebrae mostly in the cervical and thoracic areas. Cervico-oculo-acoustic dysplasia, or Wildervanck syndrome, typically affects females and manifests as Klippel-Feil syndrome along with abducens nerve paralysis, retraction of the eyeball, and deafness. A history of hearing impairment should be sought and a basic hearing test performed in all of these patients.[14–16] Hearing loss has been reported to occur in 30% of patients with Klippel-Feil syndrome. The ossicles may be congenitally malformed, with resultant conductive hearing impairment. An awareness of these problems is especially important for the otolaryngologist because there have been several cases with operative complications, including stapes gushers, which are a sudden profuse flow of cerebrospinal fluid after opening the vestibule of the inner ear.[17]

Sprengel's Deformity

Congenital elevation of the scapula, also known as Sprengel's deformity, is seen in 25 to 35% of patients with Klippel-Feil syndrome (**Fig. 22.3**). Clinically, the appearance is that of uneven shoulder heights, and bilateral Sprengel's deformity can give the appearance of a short neck. The diagnosis is often made early because of unaesthetic disfigurement (shoulder asymmetry) or functional difficulties (limited abduction). Normally the scapula descends to its normal thoracic position by the age of 8 weeks. In Sprengel's deformity, not only does the scapula fail to descend to its usual location, but the body of the scapula is often hypoplastic and malrotated. This may or may not be seen in association with an omovertebral bone, which is a bony or fibrous band of tissue spanning from the cervical or upper thoracic vertebrae to the medial border of the scapula that acts as a tether to scapular descent and shoulder motion. An omovertebral bone should not be confused with a cervical rib, which can occur in up to 15% of patients, especially women (**Fig. 22.4**).[18,19] Cervical ribs are usually asymptomatic, although a cervical rib at the seventh cervical vertebra can cause thoracic outlet syndrome.[20] If the elevation of the scapula is cosmetically unacceptable and if the range of motion of the shoulder is decreased, the scapula can be operatively released from its muscular attachments and reattached in a more anatomic position by either the Woodward or Green procedure.

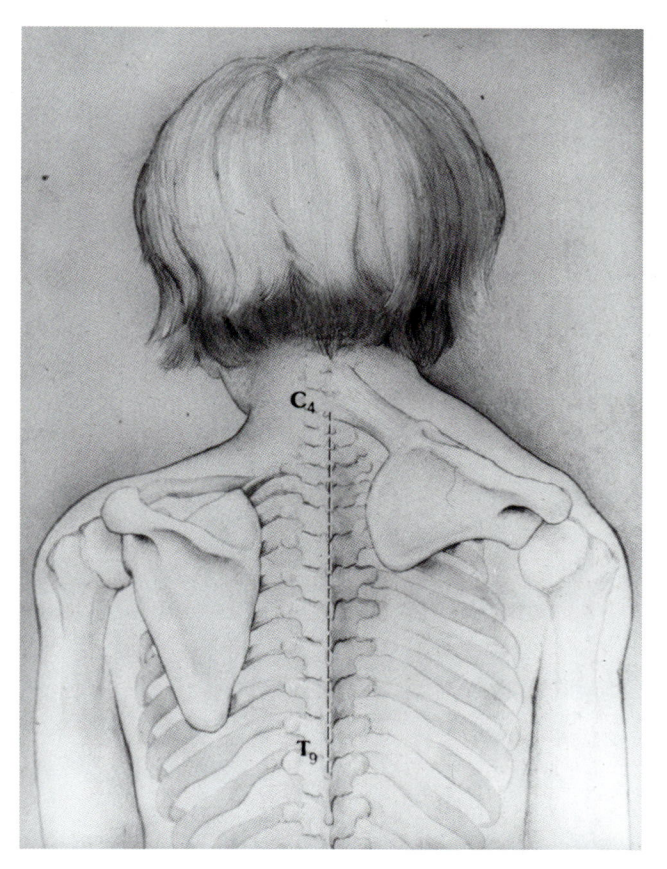

Fig. 22.3 Congenital elevation of the scapula (Sprengel's deformity) on the right side with an omovertebral bone at the level of the fourth cervical vertebra.

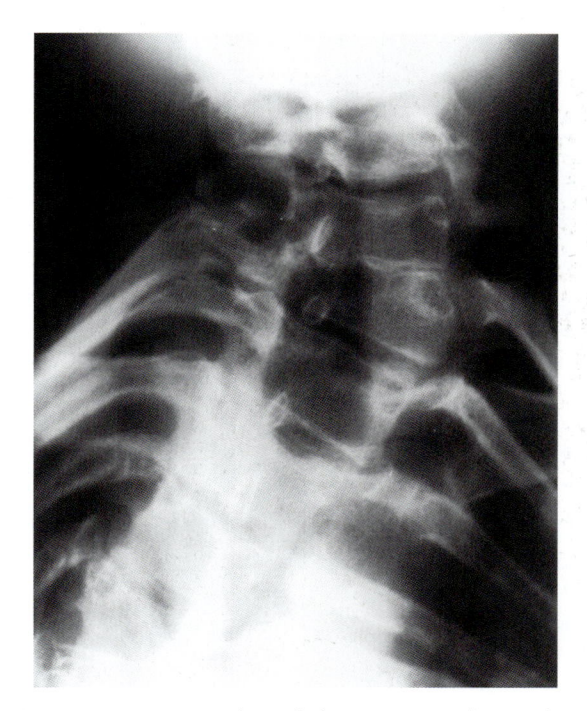

Fig. 22.4 Anteroposterior radiograph showing congenital cervicothoracic scoliosis and cervical ribs.

Table 22.1 Associated Anomalies Reported with Klippel-Feil Syndrome

Musculoskeletal System	Peripheral/Central Nervous System	Genitourinary System	Cardiovascular/Pulmonary System	Gastrointestinal System
Facial/palate/eye/ear deformities	Synkinesia	Agenesis/dysgenesis of kidney (unilateral > bilateral)	Ventricular/atrial septal defects	Megacolon
Torticollis	Cranial nerve palsy	Duplication of collecting system	Patent ductus arteriosus	Neurenteric cysts
Pterygium colli	Horner's syndrome	Bladder deformities	Truncus arteriosus	Situs inversus
Sprengel's deformity	Ptosis	Horseshoe kidney	Coarctation of the aorta	Tracheoesophageal fistula
Scoliosis	Nystagmus	Tubular ectasia	Dextrocardia	Hepatic deformities
Vertebral anomalies	Duane lateral rectus contracture	Renal ectopia	Aortic stenosis	
Cervical ribs/rib anomalies	Lateral rectus palsy	Hydronephrosis	Valvular malformations	
Syndactyly/polydactyly	Deafness	Vaginal agenesis	Conduction defects	
Thumb anomalies	Microtia	Ovarian agenesis	Agenesis or hypoplasia of lung	
Supernumerary digits	Absent auditory canal	Uterine anomalies	Pulmonary stenosis	
Carpal and metacarpal fusion	Speech retardation	Hypospadias		
Short phalanges		Cryptorchidism		
Clinodactyly				
Congenital dislocation of radial head				
Radial/ulnar aplasia or hypoplasia				
Radioulnar synostosis				
Pectus excavatum/carinatum				
Pectoralis muscle asymmetry				
Pterygium				
Hip dysplasia				
Lower limb asymmetry				
Cavus foot/club foot				

If the decision is made to treat surgically, then the omovertebral bone or supernumerary structure must be resected. If no omovertebral bone is detected on X-rays, then an ultrasound exam may be useful for detecting a fibrous or cartilaginous structure.[21]

Congenital Scoliosis, Kyphosis, and Lordosis of the Thoracolumbar Spine

Congenital scoliosis, kyphosis, and lordosis, individually or in combination, can occur with congenital cervical spine fusions in more than half of patients.[5,9,22–24] The exact prevalence is unknown because many studies combine all types of deformities, and much of the research has come from tertiary referral centers that specialize in these problems. What is known is that these deformities can be severe and of such a magnitude as to require operative treatment. Theiss et al,[22] in their series of 120 patients with Klippel-Feil syndrome of whom 65 had scoliosis, found that no particular fusion pattern put the patient at risk for neurologic symptoms, and that neither the number of vertebrae fused nor the levels fused were predictive of symptomatology.

Clinically, the most relevant of these deformities for the present discussion is cervicothoracic scoliosis.[25] A cervicothoracic curve, by definition, has its apex at the cervicothoracic junction, with a hemivertebra often found at this level. The curve may have a congenital component or it may be a compensatory curve above another curve. Outwardly, this deformity may be manifested by uneven shoulder heights, rotation of the upper thorax, and torticollis. Ideally, these deformities should be addressed early because cosmetic improvement is often a challenge. Bracing has been shown to be ineffective in controlling congenital spinal deformities, especially in the cervicothoracic region, and spinal arthrodesis is often the only option.

Sagittal Plane Deformities of the Cervical Spine

Congenital osseous anomalies of the cervical spine can also create lordosis and kyphosis in the sagittal plane. Severe lordosis is usually seen in patients with iniencephaly. Iniencephaly is characterized by a short immobile neck with a hyperextension deformity of the head.[26] Congenital cervicothoracic kyphosis is rare, with a high incidence of neurologic problems, especially if the deformity is the result of a failure of formation. For curves less than 50 degrees, posterior spinal arthrodesis in situ is usually sufficient, and the potential exists for continued correction with growth if anterior growth centers exist. Larger deformities are best treated with combined anterior and posterior arthrodesis.

Other Congenital Musculoskeletal Anomalies

Other congenital musculoskeletal anomalies have been described, but with less frequency. They are listed in **Table 22.1**.

Cardiopulmonary Defects

Congenital anomalies of the cardiovascular system are said to occur in 4.2 to 14% of patients with Klippel-Feil syndrome, especially girls.[11,27,28] A ventricular septal defect has been the most common anomaly reported in most series. Atrial septal defects, dextrocardia, aortic stenosis, and patent ductus arteriosus also have been reported. The cardiopulmonary tree is a common site for anomalous development, with reports of pulmonary aplasia and hypoplasia and pulmonary stenosis. Signs of heart failure can include cyanosis, dyspnea, short stature, and fingernail clubbing. A baseline electrocardiogram is warranted for all patients with a known fusion in the cervical spine, and an echocardiogram if surgical intervention is planned.

Genitourinary Defects

The prevalence of genitourinary defects in patients with Klippel-Feil syndrome has ranged from 2 to 64%.[10,11,29] The most common anomaly is unilateral renal agenesis, which is said to occur 400 times more frequently in patients with Klippel-Feil syndrome than in the general population. The second most commonly seen anomaly is malrotation of a normally functioning kidney. Renal pelvic and ureteral duplication occurs 25 times more frequently in these patients than in the general population. Pelvic renal ectopia is usually unilateral and involves a normally functioning kidney (**Fig. 22.5**). Renal dysgenesis occurs 40 times more often in patients with Klippel-Feil syndrome than in the general population and may predispose these patients to uremia. All patients with Klippel-Feil syndrome should have an ultrasound evaluation of the renal system. An intravenous pyelogram need only be done if abnormalities are found on the sonogram or if the study is inconclusive.[30] If the sonographic study reveals abnormalities in the renal system, the internal female reproductive organs should be scanned as well.

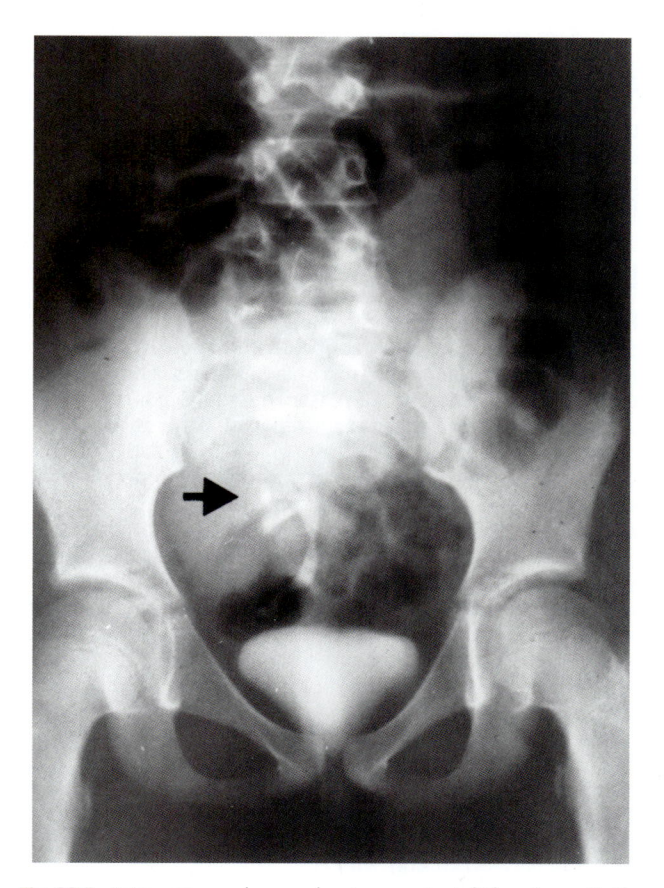

Fig. 22.5 Intravenous pyelogram showing an ectopic kidney (arrow) in the confines of the pelvis.

Radiological Evaluation

Radiographs

The standard cervical spine series is the first set of radiographic studies to obtain, including an anteroposterior view, an open-mouth odontoid view, and lateral neutral, flexion, and extension views.[31]

Hemivertebrae are best seen on the anteroposterior view. The three lateral views provide the most information. The levels of fusion are easily identified on the neutral view. If there is a question about whether two levels are fused, the flexion and extension views will demonstrate a change in the distance between the spinous processes. Translational instability is best seen comparing the flexion and extension views. Measurement of spinal stenosis is done on the lateral films as well.

Standing posteroanterior and lateral radiographs of the thoracolumbosacral spine should be done to determine the presence of any other congenital spinal deformity. Aside from being fused, the vertebrae are often widened and flattened. The vertebrae may assume a wasp-waist appearance, with the anterior and posterior cortices concave toward the center of the vertebral body. The neural foramina should be inspected for osteophytes, which may be present in older individuals with degenerative changes. Disk spaces may be absent or narrowed. It has been shown by magnetic resonance imaging (MRI) that protrusion of disk material may occur in levels thought to be fused on radiographs.[8] In general, fusion of the posterior elements parallels fusion of the vertebral bodies. However, in young children, careful attention should be paid to the laminae and posterior elements because these areas may ossify before the intervertebral spaces.[32]

Computed Tomography

Computed tomography (CT) may be done to better define osseous anatomy and determine the presence of intraspinal anomalies. CT is only undertaken when necessary, given the concern for excess radiation in the child or young adult.

Magnetic Resonance Imaging

It is important to remember that any congenital spine deformity can be associated with a high incidence of spinal dysraphism, ranging from a tethered cord to a Chiari malformation with associated syringomyelia. For this reason, the spinal axis (spinal cord and brainstem) needs to be evaluated in all patients with a congenital spine deformity. The advent of MRI has greatly enhanced our ability to evaluate the soft tissue anatomy in patients with congenital fusions of the cervical spine. Intraspinal lesions such as syringomyelia, meningioma, and lipoma are clearly identified (**Fig. 22.6**). Evaluation of the intervertebral disks by MRI can show disk desiccation, herniation, and protrusion (**Fig. 22.7**). In the series of Guille et al,[8] degenerative changes of the disks were seen in all of the patients, as demonstrated by a low-intensity signal on the T2-weighted images. Nineteen of their 22 patients (86%) had abnormal findings on the MRI scans, including disk protrusion, osteophytes, and narrowing at the craniovertebral junction. Four patients had a cervical syringomyelia. No spinal stenosis or instability was documented in their patients at an average age of 35 years (range, 26–57 years). This is in contrast to Ritterbusch et al,[33] who documented stenosis of 9 mm or less in five of 20 patients (25%) and subluxation > 5 mm in five of 20 patients (25%) on MRI. Four cord abnormalities were seen in three patients: one hydromyelia, one Arnold-Chiari I malformation, and two diplomyelia. Ulmer et al[34] reported the findings of 24 patients evaluated by MRI and CT studies. Ten of the 24 patients (42%) had cervical spondylosis, most commonly seen in the lower cervical spine, or disk herniation. Five patients had cervical cord dysraphism or diastematomyelia and two patients had an Arnold-Chiari type I malformation.

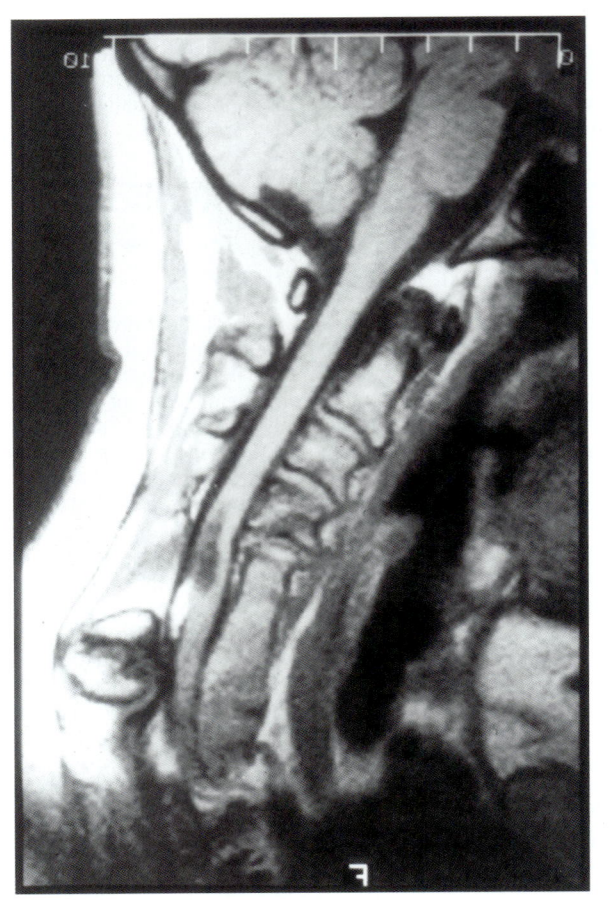

Fig. 22.6 Magnetic resonance image of the cervical spine showing an intraspinal lesion.

Evaluation of Stenosis and Instability

Different authors have used different criteria to evaluate spinal canal stenosis and vertebral instability.

These measurements are notoriously difficult to make secondary to the congenitally dysplastic vertebrae and, unfortunately, assumptions or extrapolations are often made. The sagittal diameter of the canal is measured on the neutral lateral view, from the midpoint of the posterior aspect of the vertebral body to the nearest point on the line representing the junction of the laminae and spinous process. Normal values vary according to the age of the patient, vertebral level, and target distance.[35,36] Generally, in the subaxial cervical spine an osseous canal less than 12 mm is considered stenotic. The Torg-Pavlov ratio, which is the ratio of the spinal canal to the vertebral body, is another method to evaluate spinal stenosis.[37] The ratio is determined by measuring the distance from the midpoint of the posterior aspect of the vertebral body to the nearest point on the corresponding spinolaminar line divided by the anteroposterior width of the vertebral body. A ratio less than 0.8 is considered abnormal.

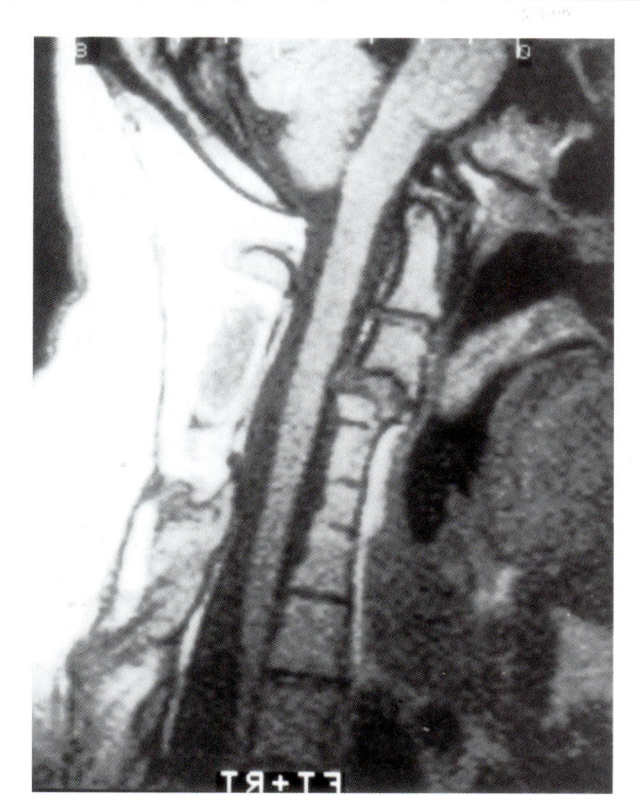

Fig. 22.7 Magnetic resonance image of the cervical spine showing marked degenerative changes. Note that the disk is approaching the cord, but there is no bony stenosis of the cervical canal.

Anterior or posterior translation of one vertebral body relative to another of greater than 5 mm may signify instability, especially if associated with neurologic findings. Flexion and extension of the cervical spine may exacerbate this relationship between the vertebrae. The combination of radiographic findings and neurologic signs makes the diagnosis easier to make. It is difficult to determine what to do with an individual with radiographic findings alone. Prediction of future neurologic risk based on positive radiographic findings in an asymptomatic patient is important, yet difficult to perform.

Neurologic Problems

No specific symptoms can be attributed directly to congenital fusions in the cervical spine. Patients may have nonspecific complaints such as headaches, syncope, weakness, and numbness. Radiculopathies are usually the result of nerve root irritation or impingement from osteophytes at the hypermobile segments adjacent to the fused vertebrae.

Long-tract signs may develop from long-standing spinal cord compression. A widely held belief is that the magnitude of symptoms is related to the location and extent of the congenital fusion; however, many investigators have found little basis for this belief. Neurologic problems have been reported in patients with isolated fusions of only two vertebrae.[38] Synkinesia is a phenomenon in which mirror movements are observed, most often in the upper extremities.[39] The etiology is unknown, but a central nervous system anomaly is suspected. The condition is more common in younger children and tends to improve with age.[5] Individuals who exhibit synkinesis should be referred to an occupational therapist as early as possible for rehabilitation.

Trauma to an individual with a congenital cervical spine anomaly can be catastrophic, as has been demonstrated in many reports.[7,40–43] Most of these reports, however, describe patients who had congenital anomalies of the upper cervical spine. Torg et al[37] noted an association between neuropraxia of the cervical spinal cord in football players with congenital fusion and a decreased anteroposterior diameter of the bony canal. They recommend that players with stenosis and a congenital anomaly should be treated and counseled on an individual basis because no guidelines have been established for this subset of patients.

Spinal Stenosis and Instability

Spinal stenosis and instability of the cervical spine in individuals with Klippel-Feil syndrome is a debated issue. First, it must be determined if the stenosis is congenital and part of the syndrome or secondary to degenerative changes. Therefore, the levels in question must be defined. Some authors believe that primary spinal stenosis in this patient population is uncommon, and some authors have even found the canal to be enlarged.[8,40] Ritterbusch et al[33] found that stenosis occurred in both the regions of the congenital fusion as well as at the level of hypermobile segments, as seen on MRI. They also found evidence of vertebral subluxation > 5 mm on the radiographs in five of their 20 patients. What is known is that coexisting spinal stenosis and vertebral subluxation are an unfortunate combination.

Basic Surgical Principles

As discussed previously, an MRI of the spinal axis is indicated in all patient with a congenital osseous anomaly of the cervical spine. Additional imaging studies may be required on a case-by-case basis. Often the use of CT scan with three-dimensional (3D) reconstructions may give better osseous definition and enable the surgeon to study patient anatomy and plan accordingly. If the decision is made to proceed with surgery, there should be good communication with the anesthesia team. The anesthesiologist should be comfortable performing a Stagnara wake-up test in the event a suspected change in spinal cord function has occurred. Neurologic monitoring is required for any congenital deformity patient undergoing surgical intervention.[44]

In general, anterior arthrodesis alone should be avoided in very young children but may be an option for older children. For severe cases of cervical kyphosis or in rigid deformities, consideration of circumferential decompression and fusion should be considered. For arthrodesis, titanium implants are usually preferred over stainless steel because they allow for clear imaging with MRI of the spinal cord in the future. Given the osteogenic potential for the pediatric population and the success of allograft in these patients, it is rare to need to harvest autogenous iliac crest bone graft. Local harvested graft can be used along with supplemental freeze dried corticocancellous allograft.[45]

Treatment in General

There are few reports in the literature of operative treatment of congenital mid- to lower cervical spine conditions.[7,46–49] It is difficult to evaluate the results of most of these series because patients with upper cervical spine fusions have been included. Some series report the entire surgical management of these patients, including release of pterygium colli, correction of Sprengel's deformity, and spinal arthrodesis for scoliosis. Regardless of the underlying condition, the anatomic deformity in the cervical spine must be identified and addressed with standard principles applied.[40] Before proceeding with surgery, a thorough preoperative workup should be undertaken and include screening for other organ system anomalies including screening ultrasound of the genitourinary system and a screening electrocardiogram and echocardiogram.

Genetic Syndromes with Cervical Spine Anomalies and Treatment

Klippel-Feil Syndrome

As discussed earlier, there are no specific treatment guidelines for patients with Klippel-Feil syndrome. The indications and timing of stabilization are not clearly defined. However, neurologic compromise and sudden death have been reported. This risk must be weighed against the disadvantage of losing additional motion segments with a stabilization procedure.

Larsen Syndrome

Larsen syndrome typically presents with multiple joint dislocations, distinct facial anomalies, clubfoot, heart defects and cleft palate. Cervical kyphosis and instability in this syndrome will progress with time. For this reason surgical intervention is usually required. Anterior fusions alone are generally not recommended in young children because of the risk of spinal cord injury from arrest of anterior growth and continued kyphosis from posterior growth. Posterior fusion is indicated in patients with mild and flexible kyphosis. However, in severe or rigid kyphosis or myelopathic symptoms, anterior decompression and circumferential fusion is indicated with consideration of a postoperative halo vest.[50]

Diastrophic Dysplasia

Diastrophic dysplasia (DD) manifestations include cauliflower ear, hitchhiker's thumb, clubfoot, cleft palate, short-limbed stature and spinal anomalies such as cervical kyphosis, cervical spina bifida, and scoliosis. Midcervical kyphosis is unique to DD from vertebral body wedging, ligamentous laxity, and spina bifida. Curves ≤ 60 degrees typically resolve spontaneously before age 6, but careful observation and close follow-up is required. In cases with kyphosis > 60 degrees or in cases in which the apex vertebra are rounded, triangular, or displaced, then progression is likely. In these cases, decompression and circumferential fusion is indicated.[50]

Fibrodysplasia Ossificans

Fibrodysplasia ossificans (FOP) is characterized by progressive heterotopic ossification with resulting cervical stenosis. Neck stiffness is an early finding. Characteristic anomalies of the cervical spine include large posterior elements, tall narrow vertebrae, enlarged pedicles, and fusion of the facets from C2 to C7. There is no fusion between the vertebral bodies or between the occiput and C2. This helps differentiate FOP from Klippel-Feil syndrome.

Early diagnosis of FOP is important to avoid unnecessary or counterproductive surgical intervention. Currently, there is no effective surgical or medical treatment to stop the progression, so the treatment is generally preventive and supportive. Preventive measures include fall prevention, avoidance of intramuscular injection, and influenza prophylaxis.[50]

Conclusion

It is imperative to perform a complete review of systems and a thorough physical examination in all patients with a congenital osseous anomaly of the cervical spine. Because the majority of the associated findings are reproducible and consistent, a systematic approach should be undertaken. Aside from physical examination, associated tests need to be ordered when indicated. MRI is the modality of choice when certain subtleties cannot be appreciated on plain radiographs. To date, no classification scheme can accurately identify those individuals at risk for neurologic injury or those who may benefit from early elective surgical intervention. Each patient's treatment options must be considered individually and only after a comprehensive informed discussion with the patient and family.

Preoperative workup should include screening for other organ system anomalies, and an MRI of the entire spinal cord and brainstem. A 3D CT scan should be considered to provide a thorough understanding of the patient's anatomy. As with all complex patients, attention to detail and proper education provide the best chance at successful nonoperative or operative intervention.

References

1. Hensinger RN. Congenital anomalies of the cervical spine. Clin Orthop Relat Res 1991;264:16–38
2. Klippel M, Feil A. Un Cas d'absence des vertebres cervicales avec cage thoracique remontant jasqua la base due crance. Nouv Iconogr Salpetriere. 1912;25:2–3
3. Brown MW, Templeton AW, Hodges FJ III. The incidence of acquired and congenital fusions in the cervical spine. Am J Roentgenol Radium Ther Nucl Med 1964;92:1255–1259
4. Gunderson CH, Greenspan RH, Glaser GH, Lubs HA. The Klippel-Feil syndrome: genetic and clinical reevaluation of cervical fusion. Medicine (Baltimore) 1967;46:491–512
5. Hensinger RN, MacEwen GD. Congenital Anomalies of the Spine. Philadelphia: WB Saunders; 1982
6. McRae DL. Bony abnormalities in the region of the foramen magnum: correlation of the anatomic and neurologic findings. Acta Radiol 1953; 40:335–354
7. Nagib MG, Maxwell RE, Chou SN. Identification and management of high-risk patients with Klippel-Feil syndrome. J Neurosurg 1984;61:523–530
8. Guille JT, Miller A, Bowen JR, Forlin E, Caro PA. The natural history of Klippel-Feil syndrome: clinical, roentgenographic, and magnetic resonance imaging findings at adulthood. J Pediatr Orthop 1995;15:617–626
9. Pizzutillo PD, Woods M, Nicholson L, MacEwen GD. Risk factors in Klippel-Feil syndrome. Spine 1994;19:2110–2116
10. Gray SW, Romaine CB, Skandalakis JE. Congenital fusion of the cervical vertebrae. Surg Gynecol Obstet 1964;118:373–385
11. Hensinger RN, Lang JE, MacEwen GD. Klippel-Feil syndrome: a constellation of associated anomalies. J Bone Joint Surg Am 1974;56:1246–1253
12. McElfresh E, Winter R. Klippel-Feil syndrome. Minn Med 1973;56:353–357
13. Sherk HH, Uppal GS. Congenital Bony Anomalies of the Cervical Spine. New York: Raven; 1991
14. Miyamoto RT, Yune HY, Rosevear WH. Klippel-Feil syndrome and associated ear deformities. Am J Otol 1983;5:113–119
15. McLay K, Maran AG. Deafness and the Klippel-Feil syndrome. J Laryngol Otol 1969;83:175–184
16. Stark EW, Borton TE. Hearing loss and the Klippel-Feil syndrome. Am J Dis Child 1972;123:233–235
17. Daniilidis J, Maganaris T, Dimitriadis A, Iliades T, Manolidis L. Stapes gusher and Klippel-Feil syndrome. Laryngoscope 1978;88(7 Pt 1):1178–1183
18. Roos DB. Congenital anomalies associated with thoracic outlet syndrome. Anatomy, symptoms, diagnosis, and treatment. Am J Surg 1976;132:771–778
19. Resnick D. Additional Congenital or Heritable Anomalies and Syndrome. Philadelphia: WB Saunders; 1988

20. Sherk HH. Klippel-Feil syndrome and other congenital anomalies of the lower cervical spine. In: Company CM, ed. AAOS Instructional Course Lectures, vol 27. 1978:191–194
21. Guillaume R, Nectoux E, Bigot J, et al. Congenital high scapula(Sprengel's deformity): four cases. Diagn Interv Imaging 2012;93:878–883
22. Theiss SM, Smith MD, Winter RB. The long-term follow-up of patients with Klippel-Feil syndrome and congenital scoliosis. Spine 1997;22:1219–1222
23. Winter RB, Moe JH, Lonstein JE. The incidence of Klippel-Feil syndrome in patients with congenital scoliosis and kyphosis. Spine 1984;9:363–366
24. Thomsen MN, Schneider U, Weber M, Johannisson R, Niethard FU. Scoliosis and congenital anomalies associated with Klippel-Feil syndrome types I–III. Spine 1997;22:396–401
25. Smith MD. Congenital scoliosis of the cervical or cervicothoracic spine. Orthop Clin North Am 1994;25:301–310
26. Sherk HH, Shut L, Chung S. Iniencephalic deformity of the cervical spine with Klippel-Feil anomalies and congenital elevation of the scapula; report of three cases. J Bone Joint Surg Am 1974;56:1254–1259
27. Nora JJ. Klippel-Feil syndrome with congenital heart disease. Am J Dis Child 1961;102:110–117
28. Morrison SG, Perry LW, Scott LP III. Congenital brevicollis (Klippel-Feil syndrome) and cardiovascular anomalies. Am J Dis Child 1968;115:614–620
29. Moore WB, Matthews TJ, Rabinowitz R. Genitourinary anomalies associated with Klippel-Feil syndrome. J Bone Joint Surg Am 1975;57:355–357
30. Drvaric DM, Ruderman RJ, Conrad RW, Grossman H, Webster GD, Schmitt EW. Congenital scoliosis and urinary tract abnormalities: are intravenous pyelograms necessary? J Pediatr Orthop 1987;7:441–443
31. Brinker MR, Weeden SH, Whitecloud TSI. Congenital Anomalies of the Cervical Spine. Philadelphia: Lippincott-Raven; 1997
32. Fietti VG Jr, Fielding W. The Klippel-Feil syndrome: early roentgenographic appearance and progression of the deformity. A reprot of two cases. J Bone Joint Surg Am 1976;58:891–892
33. Ritterbusch JF, McGinty LD, Spar J, Orrison WW. Magnetic resonance imaging for stenosis and subluxation in Klippel-Feil syndrome. Spine 1991;16(10, Suppl):S539–S541
34. Ulmer JL, Elster AD, Ginsberg LE, Williams DW III. Klippel-Feil syndrome: CT and MR of acquired and congenital abnormalities of cervical spine and cord. J Comput Assist Tomogr 1993;17:215–224
35. Keats TE. Atlas of Roentgenographic Measurement. St. Louis: Mosby Yearbook; 1990
36. Hinck VC, Hopkins CE, Savara BS. Sagittal diameter of the cervical spinal canal in children. Radiology 1962;79:97–108
37. Torg JS, Pavlov H, Genuario SE, et al. Neurapraxia of the cervical spinal cord with transient quadriplegia. J Bone Joint Surg Am 1986;68:1354–1370
38. Lee CK, Weiss AB. Isolated congenital cervical block vertebrae below the axis with neurological symptoms. Spine 1981;6:118–124
39. Gunderson CH, Solitare GB. Mirror movements in patients with the Klippel-Feil syndrome. Neuropathologic observations. Arch Neurol 1968;18:675–679
40. Prusick VR, Samberg LC, Wesolowski DP. Klippel-Feil syndrome associated with spinal stenosis. A case report. J Bone Joint Surg Am 1985;67:161–164
41. Karasick D, Schweitzer ME, Vaccaro AR. The traumatized cervical spine in Klippel-Feil syndrome: imaging features. AJR Am J Roentgenol 1998;170:85–88
42. Hall JE, Simmons ED, Danylchuk K, Barnes PD. Instability of the cervical spine and neurological involvement in Klippel-Feil syndrome. A case report. J Bone Joint Surg Am 1990;72:460–462
43. Sherk HH, Dawoud S. Congenital os odontoideum with Klippel-Feil anomaly and fatal atlanto-axial instability. Report of a case. Spine 1981;6:42–45
44. Mooney JF III, Bernstein R, Hennrikus WL Jr, MacEwen GD. Neurologic risk management in scoliosis surgery. J Pediatr Orthop 2002;22:683–689
45. Hedequist DJ. Instrumentation and fusion for congenital spine deformities. Spine 2009;34:1783–1790
46. Ducker TB. Clinical opinion. J Spinal Disord 1988;1:94, discussion 95–99
47. Van Kerckhoven MF, Fabry G. The Klippel-Feil syndrome: a constellation of deformities. Acta Orthop Belg 1989;55:107–118
48. Baba H, Maezawa Y, Furusawa N, Chen Q, Imura S, Tomita K. The cervical spine in the Klippel-Feil syndrome. A report of 57 cases. Int Orthop 1995;19:204–208
49. Bonola A. Surgical treatment of the Klippel-Feil syndrome. J Bone Joint Surg Br 1956;38-B:440–449
50. McKay SD, Al-Omari A, Tomlinson LA, Dormans JP. Review of cervical spine anomalies in genetic syndromes. Spine 2012;37:E269–E277

23 Cervical Spine Degenerative Disease and Cervical Stenosis

Michael G. Fehlings and Newton Cho

The cervical spine provides stability and mobility to the neck, and over time it can succumb to various degenerative changes collectively referred to as cervical spondylosis. Cervical spondylosis includes all the degenerative changes associated with aging that affect the vertebral bodies, intervertebral disks, facet joints, and spinal ligaments.[1] It can be associated with significant morbidity, ranging from pain to paraplegia/quadriplegia. This chapter reviews the anatomy and biomechanics of the cervical spine, as well as the clinical presentation, evaluation, and treatment options for cervical spondylosis and stenosis.

Anatomy

The cervical spine is composed of seven vertebrae, but there are eight cervical nerve roots. In general, the cervical vertebrae other than C1 and C2 share similar features. In terms of bony anatomy, ventrally, the cervical vertebra is composed of a vertebral body connected to a posterior neural arch that together enclose the vertebral foramen, which includes the spinal cord.[2] The vertebral body is the main axial load-bearing structure consisting of cancellous bone surrounded by cortical bone.[3] The neural arch is composed of a spinous process, usually bifid (except for C7), in the midline connected laterally by laminae to transverse processes on each side.[2] The transverse processes are then connected anteriorly to the vertebral body by pedicles. The space between the pedicles of adjacent vertebrae form the intervertebral foramen through which cervical nerve roots pass. The lamina and pedicle on each side of the vertebrae join to an inferior and superior articular process (lateral mass), each of which articulates with the vertebrae below and above the vertebra, respectively. Each cervical vertebra has a foramen transversarium, which is located in the transverse process and harbors the vertebral artery, its associated sympathetic nerve fibers, and a vertebral venous plexus, except for C7, which does not include the vertebral artery. The posterior bar of bone that projects from the pedicle behind the foramen ends in the posterior tubercle. Similarly, the anterior bar of bone that projects from the body in front of the foramen ends in the anterior tubercle. These tubercles are connected by an intertubercular lamella.[2] In terms of the relationship of the vertebral artery and nerves to the bony anatomy, one cadaveric study found that the cervical nerve roots from C3 to C8 are midway between the posterior midpoints of the lateral masses above and below (at least 3 mm from the posterior midpoint).[4] The vertebral artery at C3 to C5 is located medial to the posterior midpoint of the lateral mass and anterior to the midpoint at C6. Clinically, this suggests that starting at the posterior midpoint of the lateral mass can be considered safe in posterior cervical instrumentation to avoid injury to the cervical nerve roots and vertebral artery.

C1 (atlas) and C2 (axis) have several distinct features that distinguish them from the rest of the cervical spine. C1 does not have a body; instead, it has an anterior arch that forms an anterior tubercle at its apex.[2] The anterior arch is then joined laterally to a lateral mass on each side that then joins to a posterior arch that forms a posterior tubercle at its apex. A transverse process extends from each lateral mass, and each transverse process has a foramen that contains the vertebral artery. C2 is characterized by the odontoid process (dens), which projects upward from the body between two lateral masses. A transverse process extends from each lateral mass with a foramen directed upward and outward to direct the vertebral artery laterally to the foramen transversarium of C1, which is located lateral to that of C2 and the rest of the cervical spine. C2 has thick laminae that join to form a large spinous process that forms an inverted U at its tip.[2]

Several joints connect successive vertebrae both anteriorly and posteriorly. Adjacent vertebral bodies are held together by an intervertebral disk and anterior and posterior longitudinal ligaments.[2] Hyaline cartilage covers the superior and inferior end plates of each vertebral body, and these end plates of adjacent vertebrae are connected by a ring of collagenous tissue, fibrocartilage, and islands of hyaline cartilage called the annulus fibrosus, which contains a semiliquid gelatinous substance called the nucleus pulposus.[2,5] Clinically, the nucleus pulposus is present at birth, but by 40 years of age it disappears, making it impossible to herniate the nucleus pulposus, strictly speaking, at this age, although the nucleus pulposus is replaced by ligamentous fibrocartilage tissue that could herniate.[5] Cadaveric studies are divided in terms of the anatomic relation of the intervertebral disk to the nerve roots in the cervical region. One study reports that distal to C3-C4, the nerve roots exit at sites 4 to 8 mm below the intervertebral disk, making it less likely that disk herniation could compress the nerve roots.[5] However, another more recent study found that at the entrance zone to the intervertebral foramina, the C4-C5 disk is anterior to the C5 nerve root, whereas the C5-C6 and C6-C7 disks are axillary to the C6 and C7 nerve roots, respectively, with disk degeneration and nerve root impingement being most common at the C5-C6 and C6-C7 levels.[5,6] The anterior longitudinal ligament (ALL) extends from the occiput of the skull to the sacrum, firmly attaching the ventral periosteum of the vertebral bodies and broadening as it descends caudally.[2,5] In contrast, the posterior longitudinal ligament (PLL) extends from the dorsal aspect of the body of C2 down to the sacrum, firmly attaching to the intervertebral disks and narrowing as it descends caudally.[2,5] It is also serrated to enable basivertebral veins to exit from the posterior surface of the vertebral body.[2] With increasing age, especially over the age of 45, osteophytes form at the level of the intervertebral disks that may compress the cord, but because of the nature of attachment of the ALL and PLL, osteophytes tend to be larger and more common anteriorly than posteriorly because the disk is firmly attached to the PLL.[5]

The articular processes of adjacent vertebrae attach via synovial joints called zygapophyseal joints (facet joints).[2] The facet joints in the cervical spine are coronally oriented to enable flexion, extension, and rotation while resisting translation.[3] The ligamentum flavum is a ligament that attaches adjacent laminae, above to the front of the upper lamina and to the back of the lower lamina.[2] The ligamentum flavum blends medially from the facet joint capsule to the midline, where it partially fuses with the ligamentum flavum of the opposite side.[2] With increasing age, the ligamentum flavum becomes hypertrophied and can compress the cord posteriorly.[5] C3 to C7 also have a posterolateral lip (uncus or uncinate process) on the upper surface of the vertebral body.[2] This lip forms a joint with the vertebra above called the neurocentral (Luschka's) joint. With increasing age, the uncinate process enlarges, forming bone posterolaterally that may actually prevent disk herniation from this area.[5] Clinically, the anatomy of the cervical spine thus lends itself more to compression of the spinal cord (cervical myelopathy) compared with compression of nerve roots (cervical radiculopathy).

Biomechanics

The biomechanics of the cervical spine vary with the level. C1 holds the occiput, enabling nodding movements of the head.[7] The deep C1 superior facets receive the occipital condyles and prevent anterior, posterior, and lateral translation of the head on the spine while only permitting flexion and extension of 13 to 20 degrees.[7,8] C2 serves a weight-bearing function, with the weight of the head transferred to the cervical spine through the lateral atlantoaxial joints. C1 rotates around the odontoid process of C2 with a range of axial rotation in normal individuals of 43 to 50 degrees to each side. The inferior lateral facet of C1 is concave in nature, whereas the superior lateral facet of C2 is convex in nature such that the atlas moves in a direction opposite to the rest of the cervical spine.[8] The atlas extends when the cervical spine flexes and vice versa. The rest of the cervical spine generally is involved with flexion and extension movements. This results from the structure of the vertebral bodies. The anterior inferior border of the vertebral body hooks downward, whereas the superior surface of the vertebral body slopes downward and forward such that the intervertebral disk is in a plane that is oblique to the long axis of the vertebral bodies.[7] This flexion is limited by the PLL, ligamentum flavum, capsules of the facet joints, and the interspinous ligaments, whereas extension is limited by the ALL and the annulus fibrosus of the intervertebral disk. Flexion is initiated at C4 to C7, never at the midcervical levels, with C0-C2, C2-C3, and C3-C4 contributing maximally during the middle of the motion.[7,8] Extension is initiated and terminated between C4 and C7, with the middle of the movement involving the midcervical region. The total range of motion of the cervical spine is 80 to 90 degrees of flexion, 70 degrees of extension, 45 degrees of lateral flexion, and up to 90 degrees of rotation to one side.[8]

Clinical Presentation and Pathophysiology

Cervical spondylosis is a general term referring to degenerative diseases of the spine.[1,9] It encompasses several clinical presentations, including myelopathy (compression of the spinal cord), radiculopathy (compression of nerve roots), or both.[9] In general, radiculopathy can result in pain in the distribution of the affected nerve, weakness, numbness, or reduced reflexes. In comparison, myelopathy tends to produce nondermatomal/myotomal weakness or numbness and hyperreflexia.[9]

Cervical spondylotic myelopathy (CSM) is the most common cause of nontraumatic paraparesis or quadriparesis and is even cited as the most common cause of spinal cord impairment worldwide, although the exact incidence is unclear.[10-12] CSM affects more men than women, with an average age of diagnosis of 64 years and mostly at C5 and C6.[12] Both static and dynamic factors play a role in the pathophysiology of CSM (**Fig. 23.1**). Static changes as individuals age include degeneration of the intervertebral disk, resulting in increased mechanical stress on the adjacent vertebral body end plates.[5,10] This leads to the formation of the osteophytic bar, which acts to stabilize adjacent vertebrae, and to uncinate process hypertrophy, which can extend into the spinal canal and intervertebral foramen, respectively.[10] Disk degeneration and the resulting abnormality in spine biomechanics lead to thickening of the ligamentum flavum, which can also narrow the spinal canal.[5,10,13] Loss of disk height causes kyphosis of the cervical spine.[12] This is all exacerbated by dynamic flexion and extension of the neck, as flexion results in stretching of the spinal cord over ventral osteophytic bars and extension results in buckling of the ligamentum flavum and subsequent compression of the spinal cord.[10] At the molecular level, these stresses may mediate an ischemic response in addition to compromise of the blood–spinal cord barrier and apoptosis, which all mediate damage to the spinal cord.[11-13] Neuroinflammation secondary to slow and progressive compression of the spinal cord may exacerbate damage to the spinal cord, the exact mechanisms of which still remain elusive[12,13] (**Fig. 23.2**). Minimal evidence exists for specific risk factors for the development of CSM, which may include small spinal canals and larger vertebral bodies, while gender does not appear to be a risk factor.[14] There is conflicting evidence around increasing age as a risk factor for the development of CSM despite the fact that CSM is generally a disease of older individuals.[12,14]

Clinically, patients with degenerative myelopathy can present with a combination of gait disturbance, clumsiness, and long-tract signs. Classically, patients present with a history of gait unsteadiness and weakness of the legs.[9,10,12] They also present with neck stiffness because of spondylosis.[10] Patients complain of clumsiness with fine motor movements, such as buttoning shirts, handling zippers, or writing.[10,12] Urinary incontinence and loss of sphincter control are rare, although patients complain of urinary urgency, frequency, and hesitancy.[10,12]

Long-tract signs indicate an upper motor neuron lesion that reduces the usual inhibitory effect of these neurons on efferent signals from the spinal cord caudally.[9] The Babinski sign or plantar reflex is elicited by stroking the lateral aspect of the patient's foot with a blunt object, curving medially across the ball of the foot. A positive response is indicated by dorsiflexion of the big toe and fanning of the other toes. Similarly, Hoffman's sign can be elicited by forcibly flexing the distal phalanx of the third digit of the hand, resulting in flexion and adduction of the thumb and flexion of the index finger, which also indicate an upper motor neuron lesion. The pectoralis muscle reflex can be elicited by tapping the pectoralis tendon in the deltopectoral groove.[10] Adduction and internal rotation of the shoulder indicates hyperreflexia and compression between C2 and C4.[10] Severe cervical cord compression from stenosis or disk herniation may produce Lhermitte's sign, which results in electrical shock–like sensations down the spine with flexion of the neck, secondary to posterior column sensory dysfunction.[9,10] Patients also demonstrate ankle clonus and spasticity.[10]

In CSM, the motor examination usually reveals weakness. In the upper extremities, weakness is present in the triceps and hand intrinsic muscles; in the lower extremities, it is present in the iliopsoas and quadriceps femoris.[10,12] Wasting of the hand intrinsic muscles is classically seen.[10] Patients may exhibit clumsiness when asked to make and release a fist 20 times in 10 seconds.[10] Gait assessment may reveal a stiff or spastic gait.[10,12] The sensory examination may reveal numbness in the fingertips and hand in a nondermatomal distribution.[10] All of these clinical findings can be used to quantify disability secondary to CSM with the use of various scales, the most common of which are the Nurick Disability Scale (**Table 23.1**)[15] and the Japanese Orthopaedic Association Scale (**Table 23.2**).[16] More sensitive measurement scales are currently being developed, especially for milder cases of CSM.[12]

According to the Cervical Radiculopathy from Degenerative Disorders Work Group of the North American Spine Society Evidence-Based Clinical Guideline Development Committee, cervical radiculopathy is defined as pain in a radicular pattern related to compression or irritation of one or more cervical nerve roots, without evidence of spinal cord dysfunction.[17] It has an annual incidence of 1.79 per 1,000 person-years, according to a large military database study in the United States.[18] It results from pressure on the spinal nerve secondary to degenerative changes, including decreased disk height and disk herniation as well as degeneration of the uncovertebral joints and facet joints[19] (**Fig. 23.1a**). Mechanistically, this can result in hypoxia of the nerve root, and, similarly to CSM, inflammation plays an important role in radiculopathy as inflammatory mediators are released from herniated intervertebral disks.[19] There are currently limitations in the literature surrounding the natural history of cervical radiculopathy, although expert consensus suggests that in most patients signs and symptoms resolve spontaneously over a variable period of time.[17]

The presentation of cervical radiculopathy varies depending on the nerve root affected.[9,18] In C3 radiculopathy, patients generally complain of pain radiating to the occiput or upper neck or sensory loss, although this radiculopathy is rare, given the small size of the nerve and the relatively large C2-C3 intervertebral foramen. C4 radiculopathy generally presents with pain radiating to the posterior neck, trapezius, and anterior chest. C5 radiculopathy presents with pain radiating from the neck to the posterior shoulder and proximal lateral arm with weakness in the deltoid and bicep, sensory loss in the deltoid region, and diminished biceps and brachioradialis reflexes. Radiculopathy is most common in C6. It presents with neck pain radiating down the lateral arm into the radial forearm and thumb and index finger, weakness in the biceps and extensor carpi radialis (innervated solely by C6), numbness in the thumb and lateral index finger, and weak biceps and brachioradialis reflexes. C7 radiculopathy presents with neck pain radiating down into the interscapular region, the mid-arm, mid-forearm, and middle three fingers, with weakness in the triceps, sensory loss in the middle and index fingers, and a diminished triceps reflex. Finally, C8 radiculopathy presents with pain radiating down the medial arm and forearm into the medial two fingers, weakness in hand intrinsic muscles and finger flexion (the benediction sign demonstrates an inability to extend the fourth and fifth digits), and numbness in the medial two fingers. Special signs including the abduction relief sign and Spurling's sign can be used to determine if a radiculopathy is present. Relief of radicular symptoms by abducting the shoulder on the affected side suggests a positive abduction relief sign.[9,17] The placement of axial pressure on the patient's head while the patient extends and laterally bends the neck toward the affected side resulting in radicular pain is a positive Spurling's sign and indicates the presence of a radiculopathy.[9,17] The neck distraction test involves applying a gradual pulling force on the chin and occiput while the patient is supine, and the test is positive, suggesting radiculopathy, if symptoms are reduced or eliminated.[19] Analogous to CSM, outcome measures of

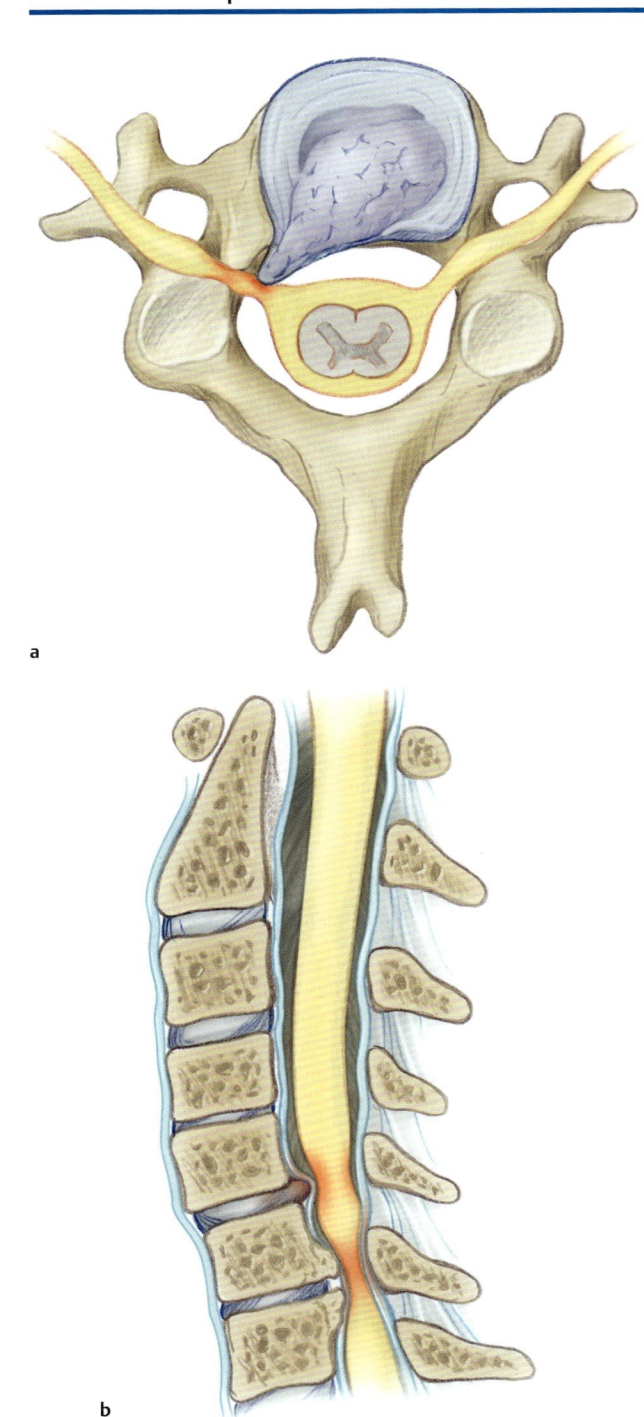

Fig. 23.1 Mechanisms of cervical radiculopathy and cervical spondylotic myelopathy in the cervical spine. **(a)** Cross-sectional view of a typical subaxial cervical vertebra. Cervical radiculopathy results from compression of the nerve root secondary to hypertrophy of the uncovertebral joint, hypertrophy of the facet joint, and herniation of the intervertebral disk. **(b)** Sagittal section through the cervical spine from C2 to C7. Disk degeneration results in loss of disk height, bulging of the intervertebral disk, osteophyte formation, and buckling of the ligamentum flavum which can compress the spinal cord. There is also associated kyphosis of the cervical spine. (Adapted from Carette S, Fehlings MG. Clinical practice. Cervical radiculopathy. N Engl J Med 2005;353:392–399. Reproduced with permission.)

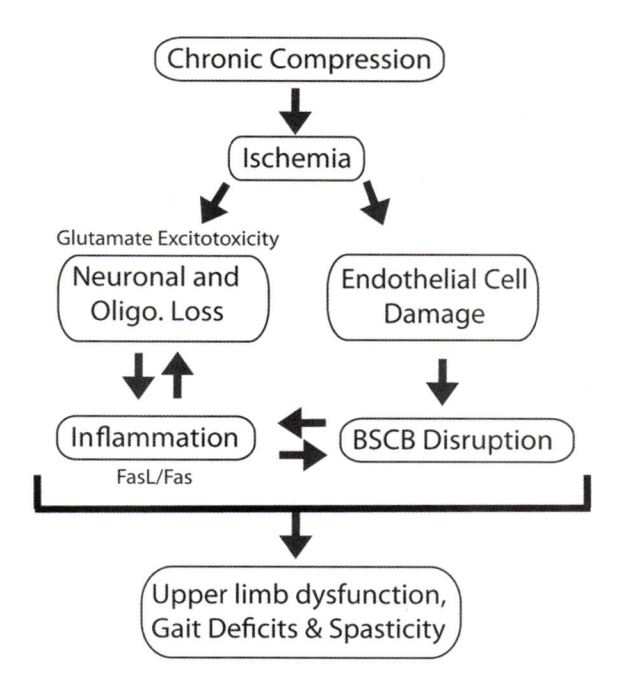

Fig. 23.2 At the cellular and molecular level, spinal cord compression results in ischemia that leads to oligodendrocyte, neuronal, and endothelial damage. The resulting inflammation further potentiates neuronal and oligodendrocyte loss in addition to exacerbating blood–spinal cord barrier (BSCB) disruption initiated by endothelial damage. BSCB disruption also potentiates further inflammation by allowing communication between the peripheral immune system and the spinal cord microenvironment. Inflammatory Fas ligand (FasL) signaling can also result in apoptosis of neurons and oligodendrocytes. This damage results in the neurologic deficits manifest in cervical myelopathy. (Adapted from Kalsi-Ryan S, Karadimas SK, Fehlings MG. Cervical spondylotic myelopathy: the clinical phenomenon and the current pathobiology of an increasingly prevalent and devastating disorder. Neuroscientist 2013;19:409–421.)

cord, and cord signal change indicate spinal cord damage.[12] More specifically, CSM appears as increased intramedullary signal intensity on T2-weighted imaging and decreased signal intensity on T1-weighted imaging. Cervical radiculopathy can demonstrate compression of an exiting nerve root by a herniated disk or osteophytic spur.[19] It is important to note that both CSM and cervical radiculopathy are not radiological diagnoses. Clinical examination with at least one symptom, one sign, and radiological confirmation of a compressive or irritating lesion can lead to a diagnosis of CSM or cervical radiculopathy. Indeed, reports in asymptomatic patients have demonstrated the presence of degeneration or narrowing of the disk on MRI.[20] This would lead to inappropriate diagnosis and treatment if only the radiological picture was used in these cases. Although incomplete, some research has attempted to define characteristics on MRI that can predict the outcome in CSM.[21] Patients with a high signal intensity on T2-weighted imaging, especially across a greater number of segments, may have a poorer prognosis, although more research into imaging characteristics that predict outcome needs to be performed.

Computed tomography (CT) can be used to supplement the MRI by providing more detail around the bony anatomy of the cervical spine and information about osteophyte formation, cervical lordosis, and vertebral body sclerosis.[10,12,17,19] CT can also be used as an initial study to correlate clinical findings with compressive lesions in cervical radiculopathy in patients with contraindications to MRI.[17] CT myelography may be an option in these patients.[10,17,19]

Other diagnostic tests including electromyography and nerve conduction studies are used on an individual basis. The use of electromyography is not generally recommended in the context of CSM, and insufficient evidence exists to make a recommendation for its use in the diagnosis of cervical radiculopathy.[10,17] Needle electromyography and nerve-conduction studies may help to distinguish cervical radiculopathy from other peripheral nerve lesions such as a brachial plexus injury.[19]

treatment for cervical radiculopathy that have been recommended include the Neck Disability Index, Short Form-36, Short Form-12, and Visual Analogue Scale.[17]

Evaluation and Imaging Studies

The evaluation of the patient with suspected cervical spondylotic disease begins with a careful physical examination. The physical examination should consist of a careful motor examination, sensory examination, and long-tract signs. Grading of muscle strength in the muscle groups innervated by the suspected affected nerves should be performed, and sensation including light touch, pin prick, and proprioception should be assessed. Reflexes should be graded appropriately. An assessment of gait should be performed. Testing of long-tract signs and other special tests, discussed earlier, can be performed to distinguish radiculopathy from myelopathy.

Radiographic evaluation is a hallmark of the full workup for cervical spondylosis (**Fig. 23.3**). Magnetic resonance imaging (MRI) is the study of choice in the initial evaluation of patients with cervical spondylosis,[10,12,17,19] because it provides excellent detail of the spinal cord and subarachnoid space in addition to disk pathology.[10,12] In CSM, such MRI findings as effacement of cerebrospinal fluid around the spinal cord, deformation of the

Table 23.1 Nurick Disability Scale

Grade	Signs and Symptoms
0	Signs or symptoms of root involvement but no evidence of spinal cord disease
1	Signs of spinal cord disease but no difficulty walking
2	Slight difficulty in walking that prevented full-time employment
3	Difficult in walking that prevented full-time employment or the ability to do all housework, but that was not so severe as to require someone else's help to walk
4	Able to walk only with someone else's help or with the aid of a frame
5	Chair-bound or bedridden

Source: Data from Nurick S. The natural history and the results of surgical treatment of the spinal cord disorder associated with cervical spondylosis. Brain 1972;95:101–108.

Table 23.2 Modified Japanese Orthopaedic Association Functional Scale

Dysfunction	Score
Motor Dysfunction of the Upper Extremities	
Inability to move hands	0
Inability to eat with a spoon but able to move hands	1
Inability to button shirt but able to eat with a spoon	2
Able to button shirt with great difficulty	3
Able to button shirt with slight difficulty	4
No dysfunction	5
Motor Dysfunction of the Lower Extremities	
Complete loss of motor and sensory function	0
Sensory preservation without ability to move legs	1
Able to move legs but unable to walk	2
Able to walk on flat floor with a walking aid (i.e., cane or crutch)	3
Able to walk up and/or down stairs with a hand rail	4
Moderate to significant lack of stability but able to walk up and/or down stairs without hand rail	5
Mild lack of stability but able to walk unaided with smooth reciprocation	6
No dysfunction	7
Sensation	
Complete loss of hand sensation	0
Severe sensory loss or pain	1
Mild sensory loss	2
No sensory loss	3
Sphincter Dysfunction	
Inability to micturate voluntarily	0
Marked difficulty with micturition	1
Mild to moderate difficulty with micturition	2
Normal micturition	3

Source: Data from Hirabayashi K, Miyakawa J, Satomi K, Maruyama T, Wakano K. Operative results and postoperative progression of ossification among patients with ossification of cervical posterior longitudinal ligament. Spine 1981;6:354–364.

Differential Diagnosis

The differential diagnosis of cervical radiculopathy and myelopathy is broad, and appropriate investigations should be undertaken to rule out these other possibilities, which include the following[10,19]:

- Amyotrophic lateral sclerosis: characterized by progressive degeneration of upper and lower motor neurons in the brain and spinal cord that ultimately leads to muscle weakness and death, usually from respiratory failure.[22] The diagnosis can be confirmed with electromyography, which can differentiate it from cervical spondylosis.
- Multiple sclerosis: a primary inflammatory disorder of the brain and spinal cord in which damage to myelin is mediated by focal lymphocytic infiltration.[23] The presentation of patients with multiple sclerosis is quite varied and can range from cognitive impairment to diplopia or vertigo; the diagnosis is supported by MRI, which can demonstrate lesions in the brain or spinal cord, and cerebrospinal fluid analysis (i.e., oligoclonal bands).
- Normal pressure hydrocephalus (NPH): a syndrome of gait disturbance, urinary dysfunction, and dementia in the absence of another cause.[24] MRI of the brain is usually performed to assess ventricular size, and lumbar punctures may be performed to assess opening pressures, the results of which determine whether NPH is less or more likely as a diagnosis.
- Spinal dural arteriovenous malformations: abnormal connections between a radicular artery into the spine and a venous plexus without an intervening capillary bed, leading to retrograde flow and intramedullary edema.[25] Patients present with progressive weakness and urinary and erectile dysfunction. MRI demonstrates cord edema on T2-weighted imaging with dilation of perimedullary vessels demonstrated as flow voids on the dorsal surface of the spinal cord. Spinal angiogram confirms the diagnosis.

The differential diagnosis also includes the following:

- Tumor
- Thoracic disk herniation
- Carpal tunnel syndrome
- Rotator cuff pathology causing shoulder pain
- Thoracic outlet syndrome
- Herpes zoster

Treatment Options

Treatment options vary for patients with cervical spondylosis. A recent narrative review by Karadimas et al[13] demonstrated that there is moderate evidence to suggest that 20 to 60% of patients with mild CSM deteriorate over time without surgical intervention, so patients should at least be counseled on the option of surgical decompression. This is supported by a recent systematic review demonstrating that there is little evidence that nonoper-

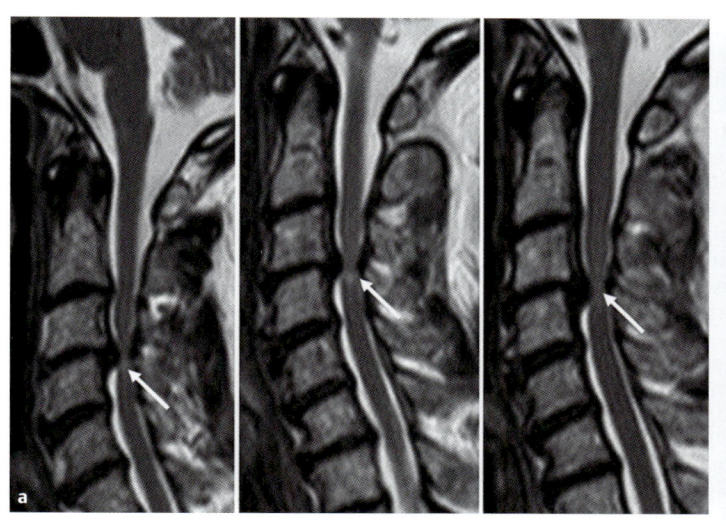

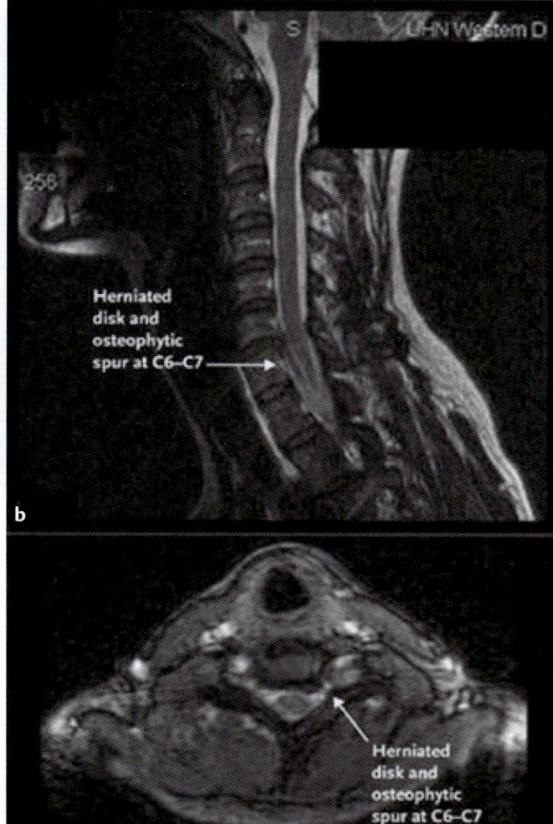

Fig. 23.3 Characteristic magnetic resonance imaging (MRI) sequence of a patient with **(a)** cervical radiculopathy and **(b,c)** cervical spondylotic myelopathy in the cervical spine. Cervical radiculopathy is characterized by compression of the exiting nerve root. Cervical spondylotic myelopathy demonstrates effacement of the cerebrospinal fluid around the spinal cord and compression of the spinal cord. This is associated with signal change seen on T2-weighted imaging *(arrows)*. (**a:** (Adapted from Kalsi-Ryan S, Karadimas SK, Fehlings MG. Cervical spondylotic myelopathy: the clinical phenomenon and the current pathobiology of an increasingly prevalent and devastating disorder. Neuroscientist 2013;19:409–421. **b,c:** Adapted from Carette S, Fehlings MG. Clinical practice. Cervical radiculopathy. N Engl J Med 2005;353: 392–399.)

ative treatment halts or reverses myelopathy, which tends to progress over time.[26] Fehlings et al[27] published a prospective multicenter cohort study that followed the effects of decompressive surgery on functional, quality-of-life, and disability-related outcomes at 1 year, in addition to complications. They found that there was a significant improved in the Modified Japanese Orthopaedic Association (mJOA) Scale, the Nurick Disability Scale, and the Neck Disability Index after surgery compared with the preoperative baseline status of patients enrolled in the study, with significant improvements in health-related quality of life demonstrated on the Short Form-36 version 2 scale. This study confirms that there is benefit to surgical decompression in symptomatic patients with CSM.

Another study attempted to create a clinical prediction model to determine surgical outcome in patients with CSM.[28] Based on a prospective cohort of 278 patients enrolled from multiple sites across North America between December 2005 and September 2007, a logistic regression model was created demonstrating that the odds of a successful outcome (defined as a mJOA ≥ 16) were greater when the patient had a higher preoperative mJOA score, did not smoke, did not have psychological comorbidities, did not have impaired gait, was younger, had a shorter duration of symptoms, and had a larger transverse spinal cord area. Certainly, these factors may help in determining who may benefit most from surgery, although future studies are needed to further validate this model.

After the decision to surgically treat CSM has been made, a decision to pursue an anterior or posterior approach also has to be made. A recent systematic review attempted to compare the effectiveness and safety of the anterior versus posterior approach, but the heterogeneity of the data and lack of well-designed studies prevented defining a superior approach.[29] Some factors to consider, including the location of the compression, the number of levels involved, and the overall cervical alignment, make individualizing the approach most appropriate. Even among anterior surgical approaches, there is debate about what type of operation to perform in the context of multilevel disease: multiple diskectomies versus multiple corpectomies versus diskectomy-corpectomy hybrid operations.[30] With minimal retrovertebral disease, a multiple diskectomy approach is favored over a corpectomy or diskectomy-corpectomy hybrid as it yields a better outcome and better sagittal alignment.[29] With significant retrovertebral disease, there is evidence to suggest a diskectomy-corpectomy hybrid is favored over multiple corpectomies.[30]

Similarly, the appropriate treatment of cervical radiculopathy also depends on various factors. Initial conservative management with the use of opioids and nonsteroidal anti-inflammatory drugs can be attempted.[19] Other nonsurgical interventions, such as short-term immobilization with a cervical collar to relieve pain, cervical traction, and exercise therapy may be attempted. A systematic review by the North American Spine Society found that no studies have adequately assessed the efficacy of pharmacological therapy, physical therapy, and chiropractic manipulation in the treatment of cervical radiculopathy.[17] Transforaminal epidural steroid injections may be considered with fluoroscopic or CT guidance, with the understanding that there is a risk of spinal cord injury and even death.

Surgical intervention is suggested for rapid relief of symptoms and is typically recommended with definite root compression on imaging, associated symptoms (neurologic or pain), and persistence of symptoms despite nonsurgical treatment for at least 6 to 12 weeks.[17,19] The type of surgical approach can vary widely, with comparable results for anterior decompression with and without fusion and with and without the addition of a cervical plate for single-level cervical radiculopathy.[17] There is a recommendation that an interbody graft for fusion and a cervical plate can improve sagittal alignment postprocedure.[17] Either anterior decompression and fusion or posterior foraminotomy can be used for single-level radiculopathy secondary to foraminal soft disk herniation, whereas an anterior approach is suggested for central or paracentral nerve root compression.[17]

Conclusion

The cervical spine is involved in a number of important functions include weight bearing, rotation, and flexion and extension of the head and neck. Over time, degenerative changes in the intervertebral disk, osteophyte formation, and thickening of the ligamentum flavum, collectively termed cervical spondylosis, can result in pain and neurologic deficit from compression of neural structures. Compression of nerve roots results in radiculopathy, whereas compression of the spinal cord results in myelopathy. A careful history, physical examination, and appropriate investigations to evaluate the spine while also ruling out other causes with similar presentations must be performed. Treatment with surgery may be indicated for symptomatic patients, and various surgical approaches may be employed with the intent to decompress neural elements and stabilize the spine.

References

1. Abbed KM, Coumans JVCE. Cervical radiculopathy: pathophysiology, presentation, and clinical evaluation. Neurosurgery 2007;60(1, Suppl 1):S28–S34
2. Sinnatamby CS. Head and neck and spine. In: Last's Anatomy: Regional and Applied. New York: Elsevier; 2006:438–451
3. Miele VJ, Panjabi MM, Benzel EC. Anatomy and biomechanics of the spinal column and cord. Handb Clin Neurol 2012;109:31–43
4. Xu R, Ebraheim NA, Nadaud MC, Yeasting RA, Stanescu S. The location of the cervical nerve roots on the posterior aspect of the cervical spine. Spine 1995;20:2267–2271
5. Bland JH, Boushey DR. Anatomy and physiology of the cervical spine. Semin Arthritis Rheum 1990;20:1–20
6. Tanaka N, Fujimoto Y, An HS, Ikuta Y, Yasuda M. The anatomic relation among the nerve roots, intervertebral foramina, and intervertebral discs of the cervical spine. Spine 2000;25:286–291
7. Bogduk N, Mercer S. Biomechanics of the cervical spine. I: Normal kinematics. Clin Biomech (Bristol, Avon) 2000;15:633–648
8. Swartz EE, Floyd RT, Cendoma M. Cervical spine functional anatomy and the biomechanics of injury due to compressive loading. J Athl Train 2005;40:155–161
9. Harrop JS, Hanna A, Silva MT, Sharan A. Neurological manifestations of cervical spondylosis: an overview of signs, symptoms, and pathophysiology. Neurosurgery 2007;60(1, Suppl 1):S14–S20
10. Baron EM, Young WF. Cervical spondylotic myelopathy: a brief review of its pathophysiology, clinical course, and diagnosis. Neurosurgery 2007;60(1, Suppl 1):S35–S41
11. Karadimas SK, Gatzounis G, Fehlings MG. Pathobiology of cervical spondylotic myelopathy. Eur Spine J 2015;24(Suppl 2):132–138
12. Kalsi-Ryan S, Karadimas SK, Fehlings MG. Cervical spondylotic myelopathy: the clinical phenomenon and the current pathobiology of an increasingly prevalent and devastating disorder. Neuroscientist 2013;19:409–421
13. Karadimas SK, Erwin WM, Ely CG, Dettori JR, Fehlings MG. Pathophysiology and natural history of cervical spondylotic myelopathy. Spine 2013;38(22, Suppl 1):s21–S36
14. Singh A, Tetreault L, Fehlings MG, Fischer DJ, Skelly AC. Risk factors for development of cervical spondylotic myelopathy: results of a systematic review. Evid Based Spine Care J 2012;3:35–42
15. Nurick S. The natural history and the results of surgical treatment of the spinal cord disorder associated with cervical spondylosis. Brain 1972;95:101–108
16. Hirabayashi K, Miyakawa J, Satomi K, Maruyama T, Wakano K. Operative results and postoperative progression of ossification among patients with ossification of cervical posterior longitudinal ligament. Spine 1981;6:354–364
17. Bono CM, Ghiselli G, Gilbert TJ, et al; North American Spine Society. An evidence-based clinical guideline for the diagnosis and treatment of cervical radiculopathy from degenerative disorders. Spine J 2011;11:64–72
18. Schoenfeld AJ, George AA, Bader JO, Caram PM Jr. Incidence and epidemiology of cervical radiculopathy in the United States military: 2000 to 2009. J Spinal Disord Tech 2012;25:17–22
19. Carette S, Fehlings MG. Clinical practice. Cervical radiculopathy. N Engl J Med 2005;353:392–399
20. Boden SD, McCowin PR, Davis DO, Dina TS, Mark AS, Wiesel S. Abnormal magnetic-resonance scans of the cervical spine in asymptomatic subjects. A prospective investigation. J Bone Joint Surg Am 1990;72:1178–1184
21. Tetreault LA, Dettori JR, Wilson JR, et al. Systematic review of magnetic resonance imaging characteristics that affect treatment decision making and predict clinical outcome in patients with cervical spondylotic myelopathy. Spine 2013;38(22, Suppl 1):S89–S110
22. Gordon PH. Amyotrophic lateral sclerosis: an update for 2013. Clinical features, pathophysiology, management and therapeutic trials. Aging Dis 2013;4:295–310
23. Compston A, Coles A. Multiple sclerosis. Lancet 2008;372:1502–1517
24. Shprecher D, Schwalb J, Kurlan R. Normal pressure hydrocephalus: diagnosis and treatment. Curr Neurol Neurosci Rep 2008;8:371–376
25. Krings T, Geibprasert S. Spinal dural arteriovenous fistulas. AJNR Am J Neuroradiol 2009;30:639–648
26. Rhee JM, Shamji MF, Erwin WM, et al. Nonoperative management of cervical myelopathy: a systematic review. Spine 2013;38(22, Suppl 1):S55–S67
27. Fehlings MG, Wilson JR, Kopjar B, et al. Efficacy and safety of surgical decompression in patients with cervical spondylotic myelopathy: results of the AOSpine North America prospective multi-center study. J Bone Joint Surg Am 2013;95:1651–1658
28. Tetreault LA, Kopjar B, Vaccaro A, et al. A clinical prediction model to determine outcomes in patients with cervical spondylotic myelopathy undergoing surgical treatment: data from the prospective, multi-center AOSpine North America study. J Bone Joint Surg Am 2013;95:1659–1666
29. Lawrence BD, Jacobs WB, Norvell DC, Hermsmeyer JT, Chapman JR, Brodke DS. Anterior versus posterior approach for treatment of cervical spondylotic myelopathy: a systematic review. Spine 2013;38(22, Suppl 1):S173–S182
30. Shamji MF, Massicotte EM, Traynelis VC, Norvell DC, Hermsmeyer JT, Fehlings MG. Comparison of anterior surgical options for the treatment of multilevel cervical spondylotic myelopathy: a systematic review. Spine 2013;38(22, Suppl 1):S195–S209

24 Intramedullary Tumors of the Spinal Cord

Paul C. McCormick

Spinal cord tumors account for 15% of central nervous system (CNS) neoplasms.[1] Most intradural tumors arise from the cellular constituents of the spinal cord and filum terminale, nerve roots, or meninges. Metastatic involvement of the spinal intradural compartment rarely manifests as a mass lesion. Intradural spinal cord tumors are broadly categorized according to their relationship to the spinal cord. Intramedullary tumors arise within the substance of the spinal cord, whereas extramedullary tumors are extrinsic to the spinal cord. A small number of neoplasms may have both intramedullary and extramedullary components that usually communicate either through a nerve root entry zone or the conus medullaris/filum terminale transition. Similarly, some intradural tumors may extend through the nerve root sleeve into the extradural compartment. This chapter discusses the incidence, epidemiology, pathology, clinical presentation, differential diagnosis, evaluation, and management considerations of patients with intramedullary tumors of the spinal cord.

Incidence

Intramedullary tumors are rare, accounting for only 5 to 10% of all spinal tumors.[2] In contrast, the benign encapsulated extramedullary tumors, such as meningiomas and neurofibromas, constitute between 55 and 65% of all primary spinal tumors. As a rule, intramedullary tumors are more common in children and extramedullary tumors are more common in adults. The histological characteristics of different types of primary and secondary spinal tumors are, to a large extent, similar to those of intracranial tumors.

A wide variety of pathological processes can arise from or secondarily involve the spinal cord as mass lesions. Primary glial tumors account for at least 80% of intramedullary tumors in most series[3-7] and include astrocytomas, ependymomas, and less common glial neoplasms such as gangliogliomas, oligodendrogliomas, and subependymomas. Hemangioblastomas account for 3 to 8% of intramedullary neoplasms.[8] Inclusion tumors and cysts, metastases, primitive neuroectodermal neoplasms, nerve sheath tumors, neurocytomas, and melanocytomas account for most of the remaining intramedullary mass lesions.[2,9] Metastatic involvement of the spinal cord accounts for fewer than 5% of intramedullary spinal cord tumors. Lung and breast are the most common primary tumor sites.[10]

Clinical Features

The clinical features of intramedullary spinal cord tumors are variable and usually reflect their indolent biology and slow growth. Early symptoms are usually nonspecific, and their progression may be subtle. Symptoms are often present for over a year before diagnosis.[3,7] The course of malignant or metastatic neoplasms is much briefer, in the range of several weeks to a few months.[3,7] Intratumoral hemorrhage can cause an abrupt deterioration, a presentation most often associated with ependymomas. In adults, pain and weakness are the most frequent presenting symptoms of intramedullary spinal cord tumors. The pain typically localizes to the level of the tumor and is rarely radicular. The distribution and progression of the symptoms are related to the tumor's location. Upper extremity symptoms predominate with cervical neoplasms. Thoracic tumors produce spasticity and sensory disturbances. Numbness is a common complaint and typically begins distally in the legs and progresses proximally. Tumors of the lumbar enlargement and conus medullaris often become symptomatic with back and leg pain. The leg pain may be radicular. Urogenital and anorectal dysfunction tend to occur early. In contrast to patients with medical myelopathies, such as multiple sclerosis and transverse myelitis, it is unusual for patients with benign intramedullary tumors to present with significant neurologic deficit. Often these tumors are quite sizable at the time of diagnosis, with little or no objective neurologic deficit. This reflects their slow growth rate and often serves to distinguish intramedullary benign tumors from inflammatory, infectious, or paraneoplastic processes that may involve the spinal cord.

Differential Diagnosis

The signs and symptoms of spinal tumors can resemble many other disorders affecting the spinal axis, including musculoskeletal pain syndromes (fibromyalgia), autoimmune disorders (transverse myelitis, multiple sclerosis), degenerative disease (ruptured intervertebral disks, spinal stenosis, synovial cysts), vascular lesions (cavernous malformations, arteriovenous malformations), infectious processes (epidural abscess, viral radiculitis, syphilis), traumatic lesions (syringomyelia, chronic dens fracture), congenital malformations of the spine and skull base (Klippel-Feil syndrome), motor neuron disease (amyotrophic lateral sclerosis [ALS]), and other miscellaneous disorders (arachnoiditis, hypertrophic arthritis, B_{12} deficiency). Information gathered from a careful medical history and a detailed neurologic examination can help to navigate through this extensive differential diagnosis. For example, a relapsing, remitting course compared with a slow, steady decline is much more typical of multiple sclerosis than of a spinal tumor. A patient with motor findings in the absence of any sensory disturbances hints at a motor neuron disease. The wide availability and heightened sensitivity of magnetic resonance imaging (MRI) has enabled accurate and timely identification of these neoplasms and differentiation from these other conditions.

Clinically and radiographically, nonneoplastic processes may present as intramedullary mass lesions. Examples include inflammatory conditions such as bacterial abscess, tuberculoma,

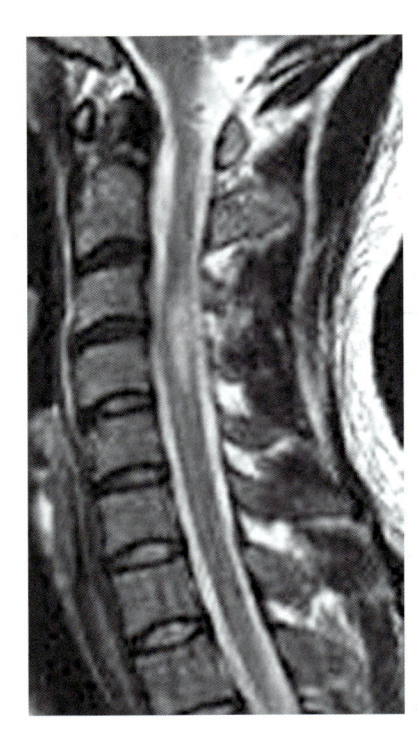

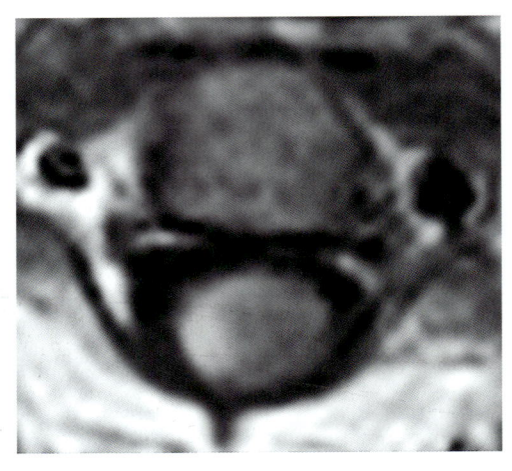

Fig. 24.1 T2-weighted sagittal (**a**) and axial (**b**) magnetic resonance imaging (MRI) scans of the cervical spine identify a focal area of increased signal abnormality localized to the lateral cervical cord white matter in a 24-year-old woman with acute onset of left-sided weakness. Note the lack of any spinal cord enlargement. This appearance and acute presentation are typical for demyelinating disease.

inflammatory pseudotumor, sarcoidosis, multiple sclerosis, viral or parainfectious myelitis, paraneoplastic involvement, or an intermediate entity between multiple sclerosis and acute disseminated encephalomyelitis.[11–14] An acute or subacute clinical course, characteristic of systemic involvement, further suggests the diagnosis. These conditions are associated with an acute or subacute myelopathy that advances rapidly over several hours to a few days but rarely longer. Indeed, an acute or subacute onset of a significant neurologic deficit with little or no spinal cord enlargement is nearly always associated with a medical myelopathy rather than an intramedullary tumor (**Fig. 24.1**). With demyelinating disease or sarcoidosis, the course occasionally is chronic and progressive or recurring with MRI features that may overlap with those of intramedullary tumors, and present difficulties with diagnosis (**Fig. 24.2**). Operative intervention in such patients should be undertaken with caution because tiny biopsy specimens tend to yield a nonspecific, inflammatory response and rarely provide the diagnosis or determine the medical treatment.

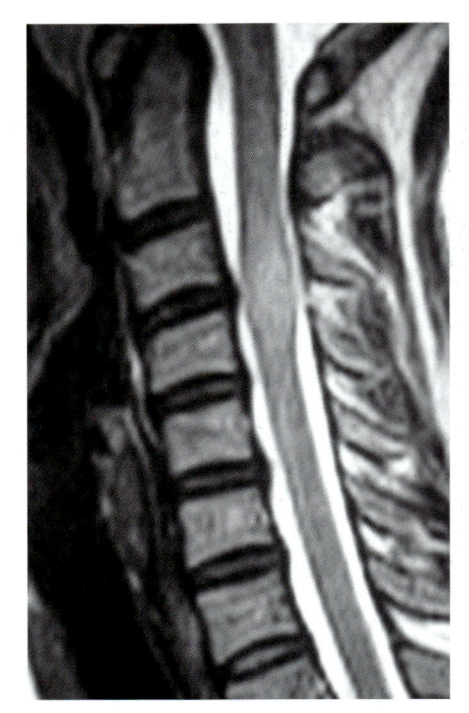

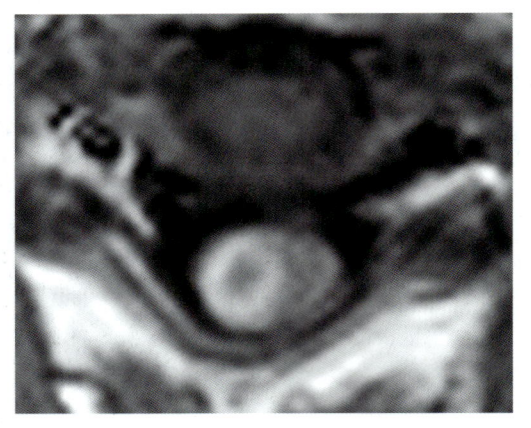

Fig. 24.2 T2-weighted sagittal (**a**) and axial (**b**) MRI scans of the cervical spine in 40-year-old woman with a more chronic progression of a neurologic deficit show abnormal increased signal in the spinal cord with a central hypointense area and modest spinal cord expansion caused by nonneoplastic undefined transverse myelitis.

Ependymomas

Ependymomas are usually slow-growing, benign lesions that are nonencapsulated but noninvasive. They are estimated to account for up to 60% of all intramedullary tumors in adults and 30% of those in children.[7] They most commonly present with axial pain, roughly arising from the level of the tumor or dysesthesias that are referred to limbs or dermatomes. Significant sensory changes and motor deficits may slowly develop over time if diagnosis is delayed. An acute neurologic deterioration may rarely occur due to intratumoral hemorrhage. Ependymomas tend to be hypointense to isointense to neural tissue on T1-weighted MRI and uniformly enhancing, although tumor cysts are fairly common (**Fig. 24.3**).[15] They can be associated with a syrinx, exhibiting a polar "capping" phenomenon. Although the typical ependymoma is centrally located within the spinal cord, it can occasionally exhibit some axial asymmetry on MRI, especially the subependymoma subtype. Subependymomas also often show limited or no contrast enhancement. A variety of histological ependymoma subtypes may be encountered. The classic cellular ependymoma is the most common and is considered a World Health Organization (WHO) grade II neoplasm. The classic ependymoma may have epithelial, tanycytic, or papillary features. Some ependymomas may exhibit a mixture of these histological patterns.

The presence of necrosis and intratumoral hemorrhage is frequent and is often related to factors unrelated to biological aggressiveness. These two features are often interpreted with caution in the grading of ependymomas. Most ependymomas may be rather well circumscribed and may present a relatively clear surgical plane for resection. In a small percentage, however, the tumor appears at least focally infiltrative or densely adherent to the spinal cord and presents a surgical challenge.

Astrocytomas

Astrocytomas are estimated to account for 36 to 45% of all intramedullary tumors in adults and 60% of those in children.[1,2,16] They most commonly present with pain and other sensory symptoms, with motor deficits occurring after disease progression. Like ependymomas, astrocytomas are hypointense to isointense on MRI, but, unlike ependymomas, they tend to enhance more heterogeneously with less well-defined margins (**Fig. 24.4**). They are more often to be eccentrically located within the spinal cord and are more likely than ependymomas to be cystic.[15] Histologically, the same WHO grading system governing intracranial lesions classifies them: grade I, pilocytic astrocytoma; grade II, fibrillary; grade III, anaplastic; and grade IV, glioblastoma. The vast majority of spinal astrocytomas are fibrillary, and indolent but invasive at their margins. There is more histological variability in children, where low-grade astrocytomas are usually fibrillary but can contain neural elements (gangliogliomas) or pilocytic features. Gangliogliomas and pilocytic astrocytomas tend to be more circumscribed and may carry a better prognosis.

Unlike their intracranial counterparts, grade III and IV lesions are rare, but when diagnosed carry a similarly dismal prognosis, with life expectancy ranging from a few months to 2 years after diagnosis.[17] High-grade spinal gliomas metastasize along cerebrospinal fluid (CSF) spaces in about half of reported cases, and extraneural metastases have been reported as well.[17,18] Surgical intervention is indicated for all astrocytomas if only for the limited goal of obtaining tissue. For high-grade lesions there is uncertain benefit of radical tumor resection with respect to preservation of neurologic function and tumor control. Irrespective of extent of resection, high-grade lesions are routinely irradiated after biopsy. For low-grade lesions, controversy exists regarding the roles of both radical resection and radiation. Some authors have found both a survival and a clinical benefit from aggressive surgical resection,[19] whereas others have not, neither in adults nor in children. Some studies cite a 5-year survival rate of 88% with maximal resection alone and see no advantage in adjuvant radiation.[19] Others point toward a modest benefit with radiation with 5-year survival rates of 50 to 90%, and recommend adjuvant radiation in cases of residual radiographic disease.[20-22] Various chemotherapy regimens, described in a few published reports, have been attempted for spinal gliomas. Still, no standard of care exists regarding chemotherapy.

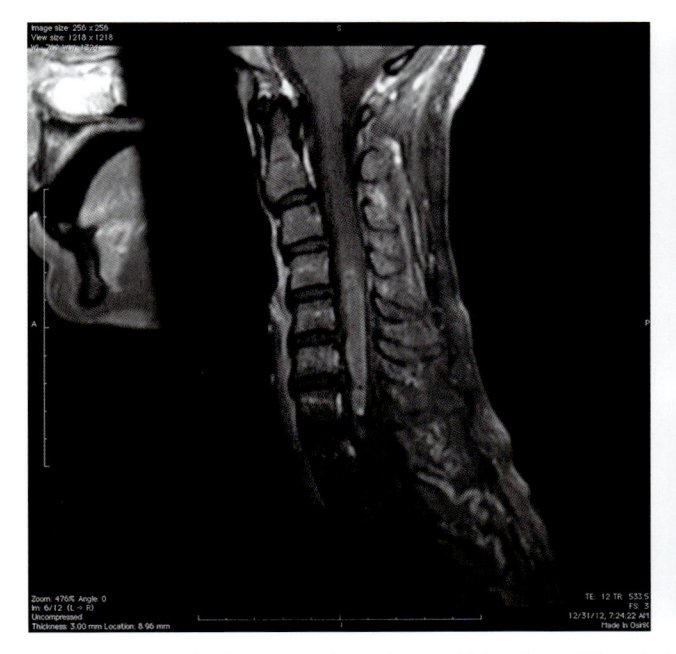

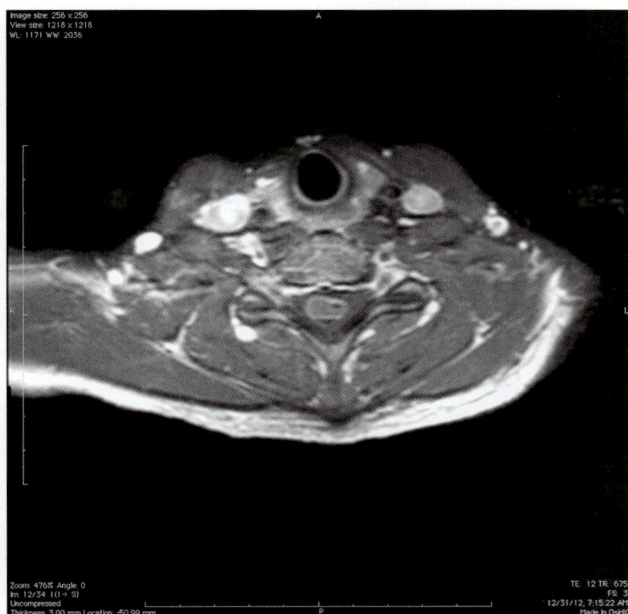

Fig. 24.3 T1-weighted contrast-enhanced sagittal (**a**) and axial (**b**) cervical MRI scans show a well-defined, uniformly enhancing, and centrally located expansile intramedullary mass in the cervical spine. This appearance is typical for an ependymoma.

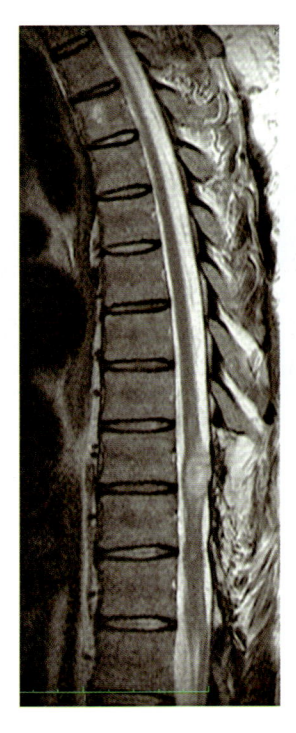

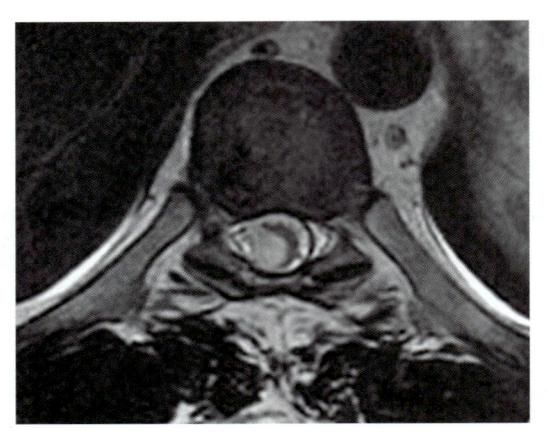

Fig. 24.4 T2-weighted sagittal (a) and axial (b) MRI scans of the thoracic spine show an eccentrically located mass with increased signal intensity that minimally enhanced following contrast administration. At surgery, a moderately well-defined astrocytoma was partially resected due to infiltration of the surrounding spinal cord.

Hemangioblastomas

In reported clinical series, 2 to 15% of primary intramedullary spinal cord tumors are hemangioblastomas. There is a male predominance for hemangioblastoma, with a reported male-to-female ratio of 1.6:1 to 5.5:1.[3,23–25] The majority of tumors occur in the cervical or thoracic spinal cord, but some can occur in the lumbosacral dorsal roots or filum terminale, which likely relates to the distribution and quantity of embryonic precursor cells.[26–28] The association of hemangioblastoma with von Hippel–Lindau (VHL) syndrome is strong: 20 to 45% of patients with spinal hemangioblastomas have VHL syndrome, 25 to 40% of VHL syndrome CNS tumors are spinal hemangioblastomas, and 60 to 80% of VHL syndrome patients have CNS hemangioblastomas.[25,27]

Microscopically, hemangioblastomas are histologically benign lesions that are composed of a dense vascular plexus surrounded by stromal cells, which have been identified as the neoplastic cell of origin.[28] The stromal cell has been further studied in VHL syndrome patients and seems to be an embryologically arrested hemangioblast derived from mesoderm that has the ability to form blood and endothelial cells.[28] This may explain some clinical patterns observed with hemangioblastomas. VHL syndrome–related hemangioblastomas usually appear in early adulthood, and circulating factors such as hormones that increase during and after puberty may promote the growth of these preexisting, dormant cells. In addition, the embryological distribution of this subset of hemangioblasts within the developing brain is also consistent with the observed locations of these tumors within the CNS. Therefore, the distribution of hemangioblastomas may result from developmental patterns rather than as a consequence of the migration of tumor cells.

Symptoms relate to the location of the tumor and the presence of edema, a cyst, or a syrinx; 80 to 90% of hemangioblastomas are associated with a tumor cyst or syrinx. A syrinx can result in a misleading clinical presentation because it can cause symptoms that localize to spinal cord segments remote from the tumor.[29,30] Symptoms may range from mild to severe, and include sensory or motor deficits, pain, dysesthesias, bowel dysfunction, urinary dysfunction, and occasionally bulbar symptoms from high cervical tumors or cervicomedullary syrinxes.

Contrast-enhanced MRI is the diagnostic modality of choice for spinal hemangioblastoma. Imaging characteristics often depend on tumor size.[24] Small tumors are usually located along the dorsal surface of the spinal cord. They are isointense on T1-weighted images, hyperintense on T2-weighted images, and homogeneously enhance with contrast (**Fig. 24.5**). Small symptomatic tumors are almost always associated with peritumoral edema and syrinxes. Larger hemangioblastomas have similar imaging patterns, but are more heterogeneous and often have flow voids consistent with the high vascularity of these tumors. Angiography can be useful for surgical planning to identify the feeding and draining vessels and to confirm the diagnosis. Embolization may be beneficial in some cases, but most surgeons do not believe that embolization should routinely performed.

Dermoids, Epidermoids, Lipomas, and Teratomas

Congenital spinal tumors are thought to result from embryological errors during neural tube closure between the third and fifth postconception week. Either as a result of the placement of cells with nonneural fates or the failure of properly positioned cells to receive appropriate differentiation signals, these rare lesions grow slowly in association with neural tissue and usually present in early childhood, often in conjunction with spinal dysraphisms such as dermal sinus tracts. Depending on the potentiality and fate of the ectopic cells, tumors form that mimic cutaneous and subcutaneous tissues. Epidermoids are growths of keratinized squamous epithelium, and some are thought to be seeded iatrogenically during lumbar puncture or surgical repair of myelomeningoceles. Dermoids contain sebaceous material and hair. Lipomas are ectopic fat deposits. Teratomas contain elements of all three embryological layers. The majority of congenital tumors occur in association with the conus medullaris and lumbar nerve roots.[31] Still, they may be entirely intramedullary and can

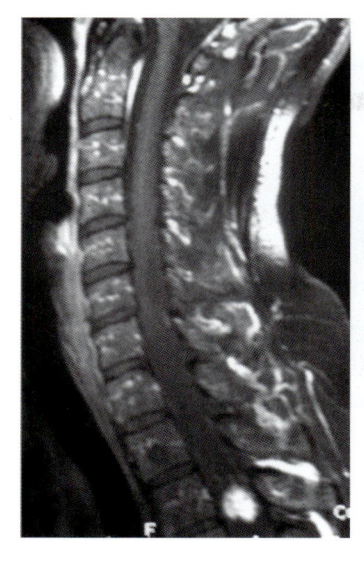

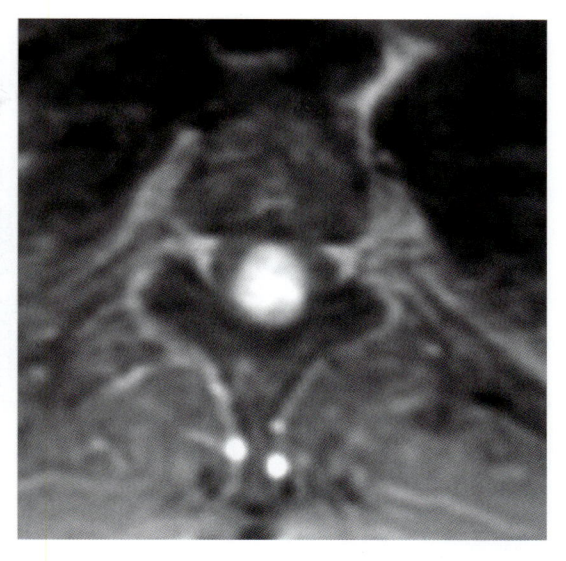

Fig. 24.5 T1-weighted contrast-enhanced sagittal (**a**) and axial (**b**) cervical and upper thoracic MRI scans show intensely enhancing mass arising from the dorsal aspect of the spinal cord at the T3-T4 level. At surgery, a hemangioblastoma arising from the dorsal pia was identified and resected.

occur throughout the neuraxis, although cervical lesions are exceedingly rare. When involving the conus medullaris, leg pain and urinary incontinence are common presenting symptoms, but many are diagnosed in asymptomatic patients after the discovery of a sacral skin abnormality leads to imaging studies.

On MRI, congenital tumors are generally nonenhancing. Epidermoids are homogeneously hypointense to neural tissue on T1-weighted images and hyperintense on T2-weighted images. Dermoids and lipomas reflect lipid content, which appears hyperintense on both T1 and contemporary fast spin echo T2 sequences (**Fig. 24.6**).[15]

When symptomatic, surgical resection is indicated, although total resection is usually limited by merging of the lesion margins into the surrounding neural elements. Because these are indolent lesions, disease control is often achieved, even with incomplete resection.

Intramedullary Spinal Cord Metastases

Although intracranial metastases and epidural metastases from systemic cancers are common, direct metastases to the spinal cord parenchyma are rare. Intramedullary spinal cord metastases (ISCMs) follow two patterns: direct invasion of a leptomeningeal metastasis across the pia, and intramedullary hematogenous spread from a pulmonary source. The latter appears to be exclusively from bronchogenic carcinomas, which are responsible for most cases of ISCM.[32] Other cancers known to metastasize to the spinal cord include breast, melanoma, and renal cell carcinoma. Although most patients develop ISCM in the setting of known metastatic disease, as many as 25% of patients present with ISCM as the initial manifestation of a systemic cancer. Some advocate surgical excision of ISCM in addition to radiation and histology-specific chemotherapy. Although life expectancy in patients with ISCM is usually less than a year, directed therapy can significantly extend this generalization.

Treatment Considerations

Accumulated experience with intramedullary tumors over the last few decades has clarified several observations regarding these lesions. First, the vast majority of intramedullary spinal cord tumors are histologically benign and biologically indolent. Second, surgery is the treatment of choice or the only effective treatment for these lesions. Conventional radiotherapy as a postsurgical adjuvant treatment is of some benefit in some patients with benign tumors, such as ependymomas, but the treatment response is neither uniform nor predictable. Finally, even successful tumor removal rarely results in neurologic improvement. In fact, most patients experience some loss of posterior column function following surgery due to the performance of the myelotomy

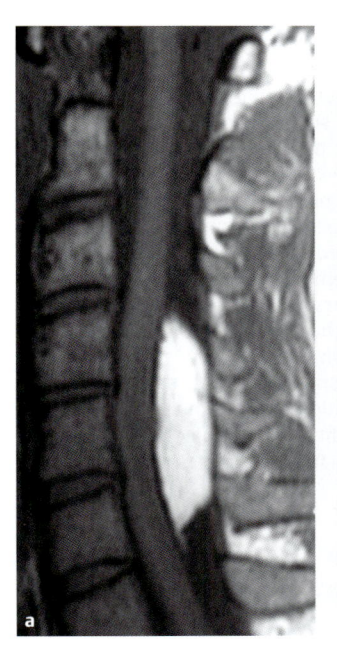

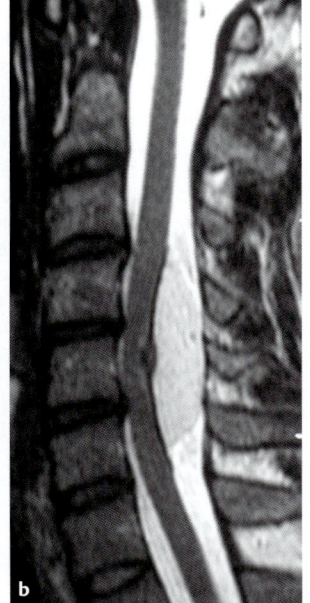

Fig. 24.6 T1-weighted noncontrast sagittal (**a**) and T2-weighted sagittal (**b**) MRI scans show a dorsal mass of increased signal intensity consistent with a subpial lipoma. At surgery, a radical subtotal resection was safely accomplished.

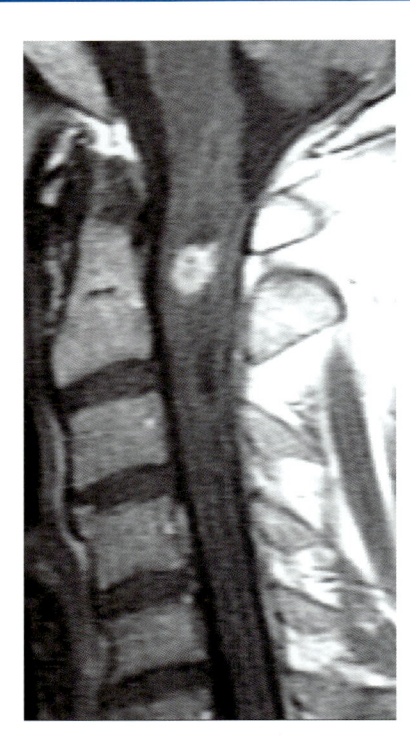

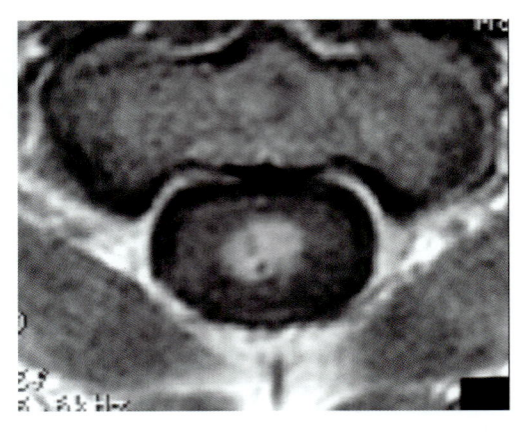

Fig. 24.7 T1-weighted contrast-enhanced sagittal (**a**) and axial (**b**) MRI scans of the cervical spine in an asymptomatic patient show a centrally located, nearly uniformly enhancing mass consistent with an intramedullary ependymoma.

through the posterior median septum. Thus, it is important to optimize both the timing and the performance of surgery in these patients. In this regard, the goals of surgical treatment are twofold: (1) preservation of neurologic function, and (2) optimization of surgical removal. These goals are generally compatible, but the first goal takes precedence because, in light of the biologically indolent behavior of most of these tumors, gross total resection is of little consolation in a patient with significant postoperative neurologic deficits.

A therapeutic dilemma is also presented by patients with no neurologic deficit and few or no symptoms. These patients are increasingly encountered because of the widespread use of MRI (**Fig. 24.7**). Serial imaging and clinical follow-up is more commonly recommended for patients with incidentally discovered intramedullary neoplasms. Once symptoms commence, then surgery is offered, before the onset of any significant neurologic deficit, because surgery is usually not effective in reversing neurologic deficits.

As always, the surgical strategy to accomplish the goals of safe resection of an intramedullary spinal cord tumor must be individualized. Although the vast majority of intramedullary ependymomas can be totally resected with preservation of neurologic function, there may be instances of more biologically aggressive tumors that are infiltrative at their margins, or even benign tumors whose adherence to the surrounding spinal cord prohibit safe total removal. Alternatively, astrocytomas, which are often reasonably well circumscribed, typically exhibit infiltration at their margin that precludes cytologically complete resection in most cases, although pilocytic astrocytomas often present with very well defined surgical margins. Hemangioblastomas are well circumscribed and encapsulated neoplasms, so gross total resection can be achieved in nearly all cases. However, clinical management differs between patients who have sporadic hemangioblastoma and patients with tumors as part of the VHL syndrome. Patients with sporadic tumors are usually symptomatic at diagnosis, and surgical resection is the primary treatment option. Incidental asymptomatic solitary lesions may be followed clinically with MRI surveillance at regular intervals. Hemangioblastomas are often multiple in patients with VHL syndrome and can be considered "symptoms" of a larger disease process that has no cure at the present time. Surgical resection, when medically feasible, is advocated for tumors that are clearly symptomatic or have developed significant radiographic progression of size, spinal cord edema, or syrinx.

In contrast, inclusion tumors and cysts often imperceptibly merge into the spinal cord at their margins to allow only subtotal removal to be safely accomplished in most patients (**Fig. 24.8**). As a general rule, assessment of the tumor–spinal cord interface under the operating microscope is the most important factor in determining the specific surgical objective for each patient with a benign intramedullary lesion, irrespective of tumor histology.

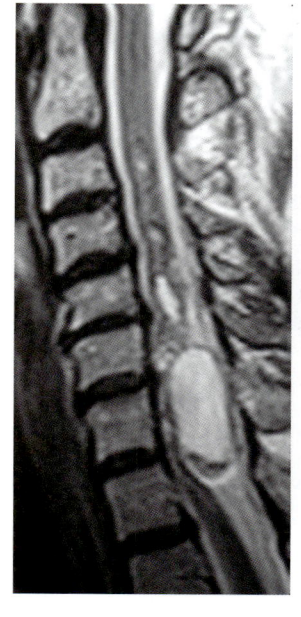

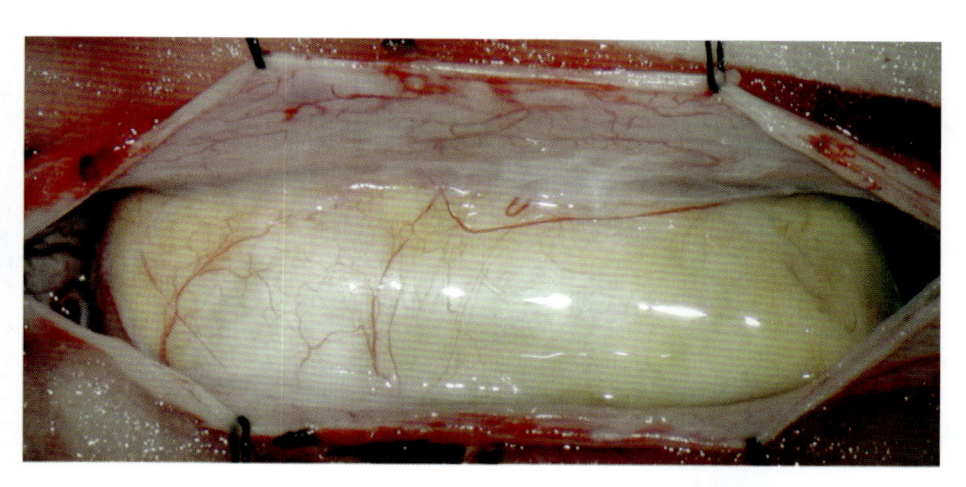

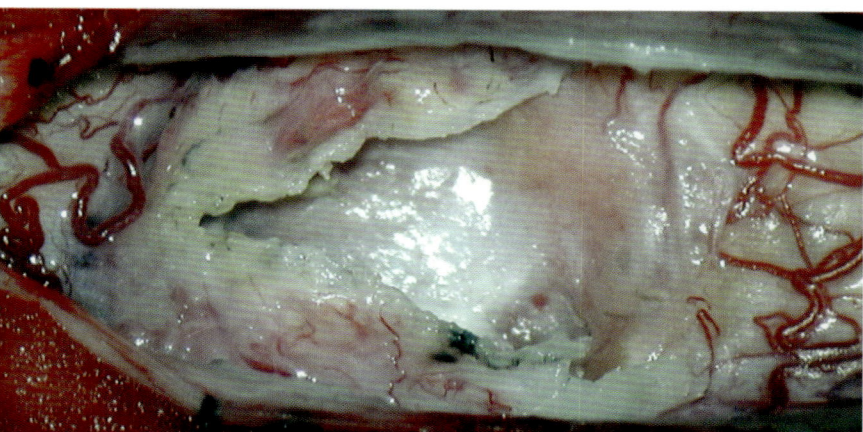

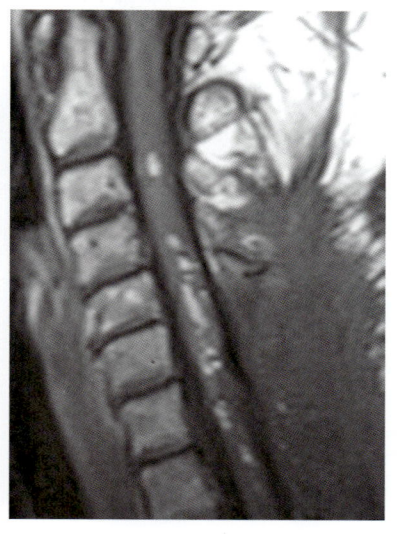

Fig. 24.8 (a) T2-weighted non–contrast-enhanced sagittal MRI scan of the cervical spine shows a predominantly intramedullary mass of mixed signal intensity with only minimal enhancement following contrast administration. (b) Intraoperative photo shows the exophytic portion of the dermoid tumor. (c) Intraoperative photograph following radical but subtotal resection due to infiltration of the lesion into the spinal cord. (d) Postoperative MRI scan document adequate decompression of the spinal cord but persistent intramedullary debris representing residual dermoid tissue.

References

1. Sloof JL, Kernohan JW, McCarthy CS. Primary Intramedullary Tumors of the Spinal Cord and Filum Terminale. Philadelphia: WB Saunders; 1964
2. Ogden AT, Schwartz TH, McCormick PC. Spinal cord tumors in adults. In Winn HR, ed. Youmans Textbook of Neurosurgery, 6th ed. New York: Elsevier; 2011:3131–3143
3. Cristante L, Herrmann HD. Surgical management of intramedullary spinal cord tumors: functional outcome and sources of morbidity. Neurosurgery 1994;35:69–74, discussion 74–76
4. Cooper PR. Outcome after operative treatment of intramedullary spinal cord tumors in adults: intermediate and long-term results in 51 patients. Neurosurgery 1989;25:855–859
5. Epstein FJ, Farmer JP, Freed D. Adult intramedullary astrocytomas of the spinal cord. J Neurosurg 1992;77:355–359
6. Epstein FJ, Farmer JP, Freed D. Adult intramedullary spinal cord ependymomas: the result of surgery in 38 patients. J Neurosurg 1993;79:204–209
7. McCormick PC, Stein BM. Intramedullary tumors in adults. Neurosurg Clin N Am 1990;1:609–630

8. Neumann HP, Eggert HR, Weigel K, Friedburg H, Wiestler OD, Schollmeyer P. Hemangioblastomas of the central nervous system. A 10-year study with special reference to von Hippel-Lindau syndrome. J Neurosurg 1989;70:24–30
9. Ellis JA, Rothrock RJ, Moise G, et al. Primitive neuroectodermal tumors of the spine: a comprehensive review with illustrative clinical cases. Neurosurg Focus 2011;30:E1
10. Costigan DA, Winkelman MD. Intramedullary spinal cord metastasis. A clinicopathological study of 13 cases. J Neurosurg 1985;62:227–233
11. McCormick PC, Stein BM. Miscellaneous intradural pathology. Neurosurg Clin N Am 1990;1:687–699
12. Jallo GI, Zagzag D, Lee M, Deletis V, Morota N, Epstein FJ. Intraspinal sarcoidosis: diagnosis and management. Surg Neurol 1997;48:514–520, discussion 521
13. Lee M, Epstein FJ, Rezai AR, Zagzag D. Nonneoplastic intramedullary spinal cord lesions mimicking tumors. Neurosurgery 1998;43:788–794, discussion 794–795
14. Kepes JJ. Large focal tumor-like demyelinating lesions of the brain: intermediate entity between multiple sclerosis and acute disseminated encephalomyelitis? A study of 31 patients. Ann Neurol 1993;33:18–27
15. Osborn AG. Diagnostic Neuroradiology. St. Louis: Mosby; 1994
16. Helseth A, Mørk SJ. Primary intraspinal neoplasms in Norway, 1955 to 1986. A population-based survey of 467 patients. J Neurosurg 1989;71:842–845
17. Santi M, Mena H, Wong K, Koeller K, Olsen C, Rushing EJ. Spinal cord malignant astrocytomas. Clinicopathologic features in 36 cases. Cancer 2003;98:554–561
18. Cohen AR, Wisoff JH, Allen JC, Epstein F. Malignant astrocytomas of the spinal cord. J Neurosurg 1989;70:50–54
19. Jallo GI, Danish S, Velasquez L, Epstein F. Intramedullary low-grade astrocytomas: long-term outcome following radical surgery. J Neurooncol 2001;53:61–66
20. Isaacson SR. Radiation therapy and the management of intramedullary spinal cord tumors. J Neurooncol 2000;47:231–238
21. Shirato H, Kamada T, Hida K, et al. The role of radiotherapy in the management of spinal cord glioma. Int J Radiat Oncol Biol Phys 1995;33:323–328
22. Linstadt DE, Wara WM, Leibel SA, Gutin PH, Wilson CB, Sheline GE. Postoperative radiotherapy of primary spinal cord tumors. Int J Radiat Oncol Biol Phys 1989;16:1397–1403
23. Mandigo C, Ogden AT, Angevine PD, McCormick PC. Intramedullary hemangioblastoma of the spinal cord. Operative Neurosurgery. 2009;65:1166–1177
24. Chu BC, Terae S, Hida K, Furukawa M, Abe S, Miyasaka K. MR findings in spinal hemangioblastoma: correlation with symptoms and with angiographic and surgical findings. AJNR Am J Neuroradiol 2001;22:206–217
25. Conway JE, Chou D, Clatterbuck RE, Brem H, Long DM, Rigamonti D. Hemangioblastomas of the central nervous system in von Hippel-Lindau syndrome and sporadic disease. Neurosurgery 2001;48:55–62, discussion 62–63
26. Lonser RR, Wait SD, Butman JA, et al. Surgical management of lumbosacral nerve root hemangioblastomas in von Hippel-Lindau syndrome. J Neurosurg 2003;99(1, Suppl):64–69
27. Lonser RR, Weil RJ, Wanebo JE, DeVroom HL, Oldfield EH. Surgical management of spinal cord hemangioblastomas in patients with von Hippel-Lindau disease. J Neurosurg 2003;98:106–116
28. Park DM, Zhuang Z, Chen L, et al. von Hippel-Lindau disease-associated hemangioblastomas are derived from embryologic multipotent cells. PLoS Med 2007;4:e60
29. Pai SB, Krishna KN. Secondary holocord syringomyelia with spinal hemangioblastoma: a report of two cases. Neurol India 2003;51:67–68
30. Wu TC, Guo WY, Lirng JF, et al. Spinal cord hemangioblastoma with extensive syringomyelia. J Chin Med Assoc 2005;68:40–44
31. Takeuchi J, Ohta T, Kajikawa H. Congenital tumors of the spinal cord. In: Vinken PJ, Bruyn GW, Myrianthopoulos NC, eds. Handbook of Clinical Neurology, vol. 32. New York: North-Holland; 1978:xii:588
32. Schiff D, O'Neill BP. Intramedullary spinal cord metastases: clinical features and treatment outcome. Neurology 1996;47:906–912

25 Extramedullary Tumors of the Spinal Cord

Paul C. McCormick

The majority of intradural spinal tumors arise outside of the spinal cord. With few exceptions these neoplasms are benign, well circumscribed, and amenable to complete surgical resection. As in the intracranial space, nerve sheath tumors and meningiomas account for most tumors that arise outside the substance of the central nervous system. Although spinal extramedullary tumors share many features with their intracranial counterparts, there are many distinctive aspects of these tumors that merit separate consideration. This chapter describes the incidence, epidemiology, pathology, clinical presentation, differential diagnosis, evaluation, and management considerations of patients with extramedullary tumors of the spinal cord.

Incidence

About two thirds of spinal cord tumors in adults are extramedullary. Nerve sheath tumors, meningiomas, and filum terminale ependymomas account for most extramedullary neoplasms.[1] Metastases, inclusion tumors and cysts, paragangliomas, and melanocytic neoplasms are rare. Most of these tumors occur in adults and, as such, present later in life than do intramedullary spinal tumors. The exception to this is filum terminale ependymomas, which are similar to intramedullary ependymomas in terms of occurrence.

Clinical Features

The clinical features of intramedullary tumors generally reflect their benign, slow-growing nature. Early symptoms are often quite mild, often intermittent, and of substantial duration. Nonspecific pain is an early symptom in most patients, but it is usually assumed to represent degenerative spine conditions, common in adult populations. In many cases tumors attain a large size prior to diagnosis, which reflects spinal cord and cauda equina accommodation to these slow-growing tumors. Early occurrence of radicular pain in the distribution of the root of origin of a nerve sheath tumor is a common but not universal complaint of patients with these tumors. Once symptoms/signs of spinal cord or cauda equina commence, they can often accelerate, indicating that there is a limit to the tolerance of the neural elements to slowly increasing pressure. Cervical tumors often present with proximal arm weakness and impairment of fine motor control with gait disturbance. Spasticity or an ataxic gait is common with thoracic cord compression, whereas pain and bowel/bladder dysfunction are common with cauda equina compression. Urinary retention, with or without overflow incontinence, is the most common form of bladder dysfunction.

Differential Diagnosis

From a clinical perspective, the differential diagnosis of intradural extramedullary tumors includes many conditions. Most commonly, these tumors present with mild, nonspecific, or intermittent pain that is usually interpreted as benign muscle strains or early osteoarthritic spine conditions or disk herniation/degeneration. Patients with cervical tumors who develop progressive myelopathy may overlap with patients with cervical spondylotic myelopathy, ossification of the posterior longitudinal ligament, or chronic disk herniation with spinal cord compression. Amyotrophic lateral sclerosis or other progressive or recurring medical myelopathies, such as multiple sclerosis, vitamin B_{12} deficiency, and Lyme disease, may have clinical profiles similar to these tumors. Thoracic tumors present either with radicular pain or myelopathy and include chronic thoracic disk herniation or stenosis as part of the differential diagnosis. It may be difficult to differentiate a densely calcified meningioma from a large calcified thoracic disk herniation, even with magnetic resonance imaging (MRI). Type I dural arteriovenous fistulas may also present with a slowly progressive myelopathy and must be considered in the differential diagnosis.

Tumors of the cauda equina most often overlap with much more common benign extradural spinal conditions, such as spinal stenosis, disk herniation, and degenerative spine conditions. Fortunately, MRI helps establish the correct diagnosis in the vast majority of patients.

Nerve Sheath Tumors

Nerve sheath tumors are categorized as schwannomas or neurofibromas. Although evidence from tissue culture, electron microscopy, and immunohistochemistry supports a common Schwann cell origin for neurofibromas and schwannomas, the morphological heterogeneity of neurofibromas suggests participation of additional cell types such as perineural cells and fibroblasts. Neurofibromas and schwannomas merit separate consideration because of their distinct demographic, histological, and biological characteristics.

The histological appearance of neurofibromas consists of an abundance of fibrous tissue and the conspicuous presence of nerve fibers within the tumor stroma.[2] Grossly, the tumor produces fusiform (plexiform) enlargement of the involved nerve, which makes it impossible to distinguish between tumor and nerve tissue. Multiple neurofibromas establish the diagnosis of neurofibromatosis (NF), but this syndrome should be considered even in patients with apparent solitary involvement. Both neurofibromatosis type 1 (NF1) and neurofibromatosis type 2 (NF2) are associated with nerve sheath tumors. Although neurofibromas predominate in NF1, schwannomas are more common in NF2.[3]

Schwannomas appear grossly as smooth globoid masses that do not enlarge the nerve but are suspended eccentrically from it with a discrete attachment. Their histological appearance consists of elongated bipolar cells with fusiform, darkly staining nuclei arranged in compact interlacing fascicles with a tendency toward palisade formation (Antoni A). A loosely arranged pattern of stellate-shaped cells (Antoni B) is less common.[4] Multiple schwannomas or "schwannomatosis" can occur in patients without NF, and these currently have no known genetic basis.[5,6]

Nerve sheath tumors account for ~ 25% of intradural spinal cord tumors in adults,[1,7] with an annual incidence of 0.3 to 0.4 per 100,000.[6] Most are solitary schwannomas that occur proportionally throughout the spinal canal. The fourth through sixth decades of life represent the peak incidence of occurrence. Men and women are affected equally.

Most nerve sheath tumors arise from a dorsal nerve root. Neurofibromas represent a higher proportion of ventral root tumors and often exhibit dumbbell growth.[8] Most nerve sheath tumors are entirely intradural, but 30% extend through the dural root sleeve as a dumbbell tumor with both intradural and extradural components.[6] About 10% of nerve sheath tumors are epidural or paraspinal in location. Transdural growth is common in cervical tumors because the intradural root segment is short.[6] One percent of nerve sheath tumors are intramedullary and are thought to arise from the perivascular nerve sheaths that accompany penetrating spinal cord vessels.[6] Centripetal growth of a nerve sheath tumor may also result in subpial extension, most often with plexiform neurofibromas. In these cases, both intra- and extramedullary tumor components are apparent. Brachial or lumbar plexus neurofibromas may extend centrally into the intradural space along multiple nerve roots. Conversely, retrograde intraspinal extension of a paraspinal schwannoma usually remains epidural.

About 2.5% of intradural spinal nerve sheath tumors are malignant.[9] At least half occur in patients with NF. Malignant nerve sheath tumors carry a poor prognosis; survival rarely extends beyond 1 year. These tumors must be distinguished from the rare cellular schwannoma that displays aggressive histological features but is associated with a favorable prognosis.

On MRI, nerve sheath tumors are isointense to neural tissue and usually enhance uniformly with contrast, although intratumoral cysts frequently confer a heterogeneous appearance (**Fig. 25.1**). Depending on the exact point of origin and the size of the tumor, nerve sheath tumors can be entirely intradural, extradural, or have both intradural and extradural components that evince a characteristic dumbbell shape. Because they often arise from the dorsal root, they typically lie dorsolateral to the spinal cord. Lesions with a significant extradural component often erode bone over time and can displace important local anatomic structures, although these will always lie outside the tumor margin if the tumor is benign (**Fig. 25.2**).

Meningiomas

Meningiomas are the second most common intradural extramedullary spinal tumor after schwannomas. The female preponderance seen in intracranial meningiomas is even more pronounced in the spine, with surgical series reporting female/male ratios of 4:1[10] to as high as 9:1.[11] Spinal meningiomas are thought to arise from cells within arachnoid villi, found at highest density around nerve root exit sites. This formulation likely influences the finding that the majority of spinal meningiomas are intradural, extramedullary, lie lateral to the cord, and are most prevalent in the segment of the spine with the most nerve roots, the thoracic spine.[10-13] The thoracic predilection, as high as 82%,[12] and the paucity of lumbar tumors, as low as 2%,[13] is perhaps not completely explained by the density of cell of origin, and some authors have found a more even distribution of thoracic and cervical meningiomas in men.[14] Meningiomas peak in late middle age, are uncommon in young adults, and are very rare in children.

The most common initial symptom is pain, but it is often mild or intermittent and usually does not lead to early investigation and diagnosis. Much more commonly patients present with a slowly progressive myelopathy. Conversely, due to the widespread use and availability of noninvasive imaging such as MRI, an increasing number of patients are diagnosed with incidental spinal meningiomas.[10,12,13]

On MRI, spinal meningiomas are isointense to neural tissue and homogeneously enhance with contrast administration (**Fig. 25.3**). Heavily calcified meningiomas may exhibit little or no contrast enhancement. They are often usually associated with the dura mater with the tumor mass compressing the spinal cord. Less than 10% of the time, spinal meningiomas exhibit significant extradural extension, although they may be entirely extradural.[10,12] Rarely have intramedullary meningiomas been reported.

Histologically, the vast majority of spinal meningiomas are benign and fall into the same subtypes as seen intracranially. The psammomatous subtype, however, is far more prevalent in the spine, and there is the suggestion in the literature that it is associated with less favorable neurologic outcomes after surgery. Younger patients are more likely to harbor the surgically recalcitrant angioblastic subtype, but true malignant meningiomas are exceedingly rare in the spine.

Filum Terminale Tumors

The vast majority of filum terminale tumors are myxopapillary ependymomas. Paragangliomas are less common, whereas astrocytomas, hemangioblastomas, and cavernous malformations are rare. About 40% of spinal canal ependymomas arise within the filum terminale,[15] most in its proximal intradural portion. Filum terminale ependymomas occur throughout life but are most common in the third to fifth decades. They occur in men slightly more often than in women. Filum ependymomas and cauda equina nerve sheath tumors occur with about equal frequency.

Myxopapillary ependymomas are by far the most common histological type encountered in the filum terminale. Their histological appearance consists of a papillary arrangement of cuboidal or columnar tumor cells surrounding a vascularized core of hyalinized and poorly cellular connective tissue.[4] Almost all are histologically benign.[16] These tumors, however, tend to be more biologically aggressive in younger age groups.[17] Due to the poor encapsulation of these tumors as well as their surface apposition to the cerebrospinal fluid (CSF) circulation, dissemination of these tumors, either rostrally or caudally, may result in tumor seeding through the spine and even the intracranial space. The MRI appearance usually shows an isointense mass that uniformly enhances following gadolinium administration (**Fig. 25.4**).

Paragangliomas

Paragangliomas are rare tumors that originate from the neural crest and may arise from the filum terminale or cauda equina.[18] They are benign, nonfunctioning tumors and resemble extra-

25 Extramedullary Tumors of the Spinal Cord

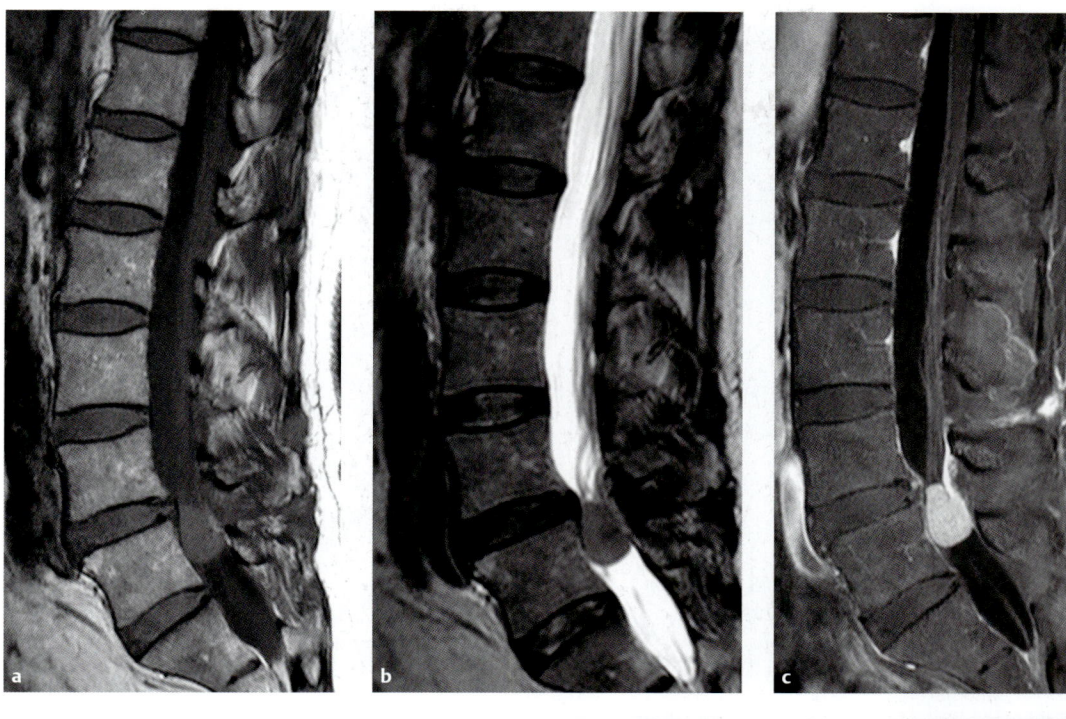

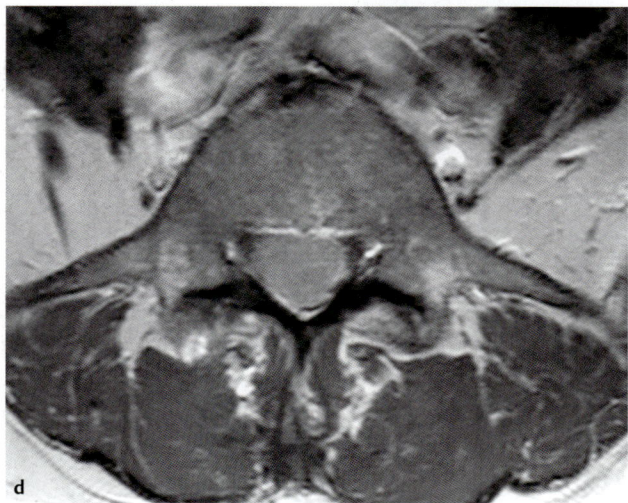

Fig. 25.1 (a) T1-weighted noncontrast sagittal magnetic resonance imaging (MRI) of the lumbar spine shows isointense intradural mass at the L5 level. (b) The lesion is hypointense on the T2-weighted sagittal image. T1-weighted contrast-enhanced sagittal (c) and axial (d) MRI shows uniform enhancement.

adrenal paraganglia (i.e., carotid body and glomus jugulare) histologically. Grossly, they appear as well-circumscribed vascular tumors that are indistinguishable clinically or radiographically from filum terminale ependymomas. Identification of dense core neurosecretory granules on electron microscopy establishes the diagnosis. Complete resection is usually possible except for large tumors that are tightly adherent to the cauda equina. CSF dissemination, either spontaneously or after surgical resection is more prevalent for these tumors than with myxopapillary ependymomas.

Diagnostic Imaging

Magnetic resonance imaging is the procedure of choice for the diagnosis and evaluation of intradural tumors. Most tumors are isointense or slightly hypointense on T1-weighted noncontrast MRI and nearly all exhibit some degree of enhancement following gadolinium administration. An exception is the densely calcified meningioma. Although most intradural tumors are identified on noncontrast MRI, small tumors may escape detection.

Myelography and postmyelography computed tomography (CT) are rarely used to evaluate intradural pathology except in patients who cannot undergo MRI, such as those who have a pacemaker. However, the spatial resolution of a myelography CT remains superior to that of MRI in certain instances. When a tumor is closely applied to the surface of the spinal cord and whether it is intra- or extramedullary is equivocal on MRI, its location can be better resolved on myelography CT. The intra- or extradural distribution of a paraspinal or dumbbell tumor also may be better resolved with myelography CT when MRI is unclear.

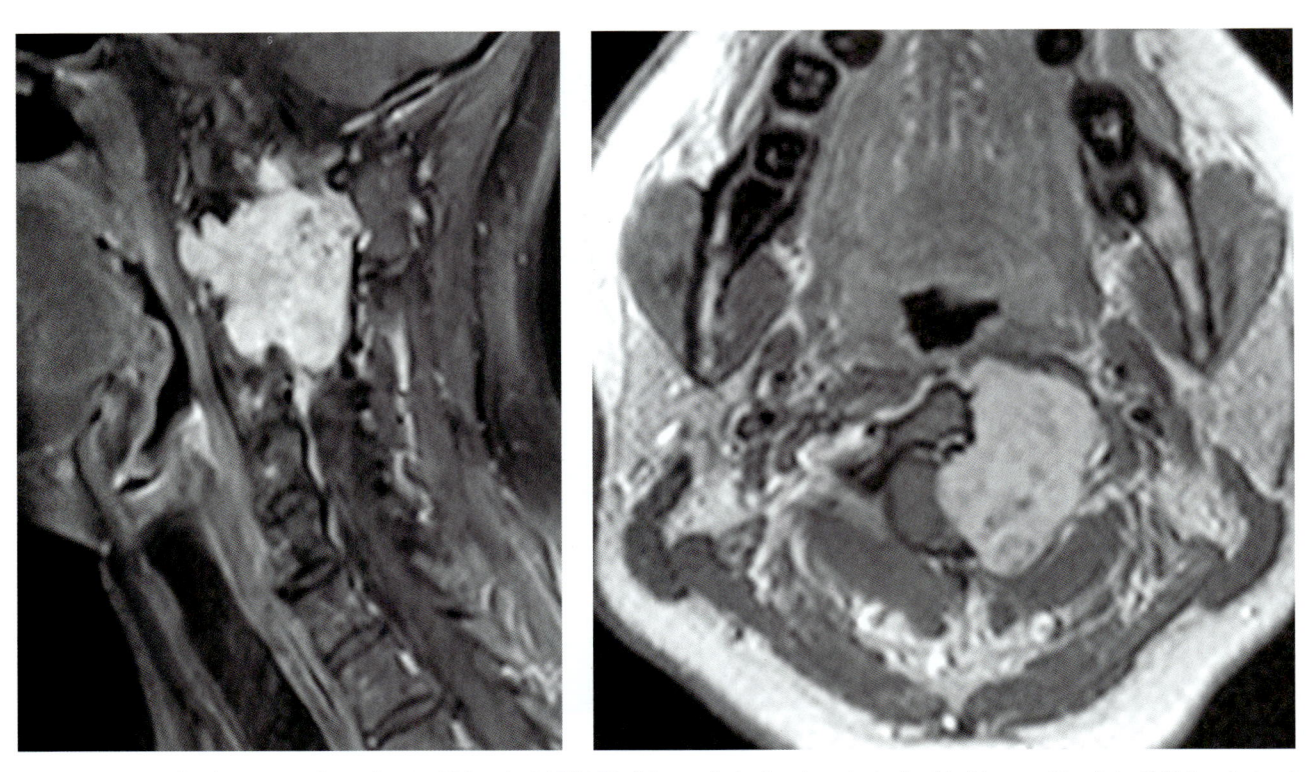

Fig. 25.2 T1-weighted contrast-enhanced sagittal **(a)** and axial **(b)** MRI of the cervical spine shows large dumbbell tumor with substantial intraspinal and paraspinal tumor components of a large dumbbell schwannoma. Note the degree of ventral bone erosion.

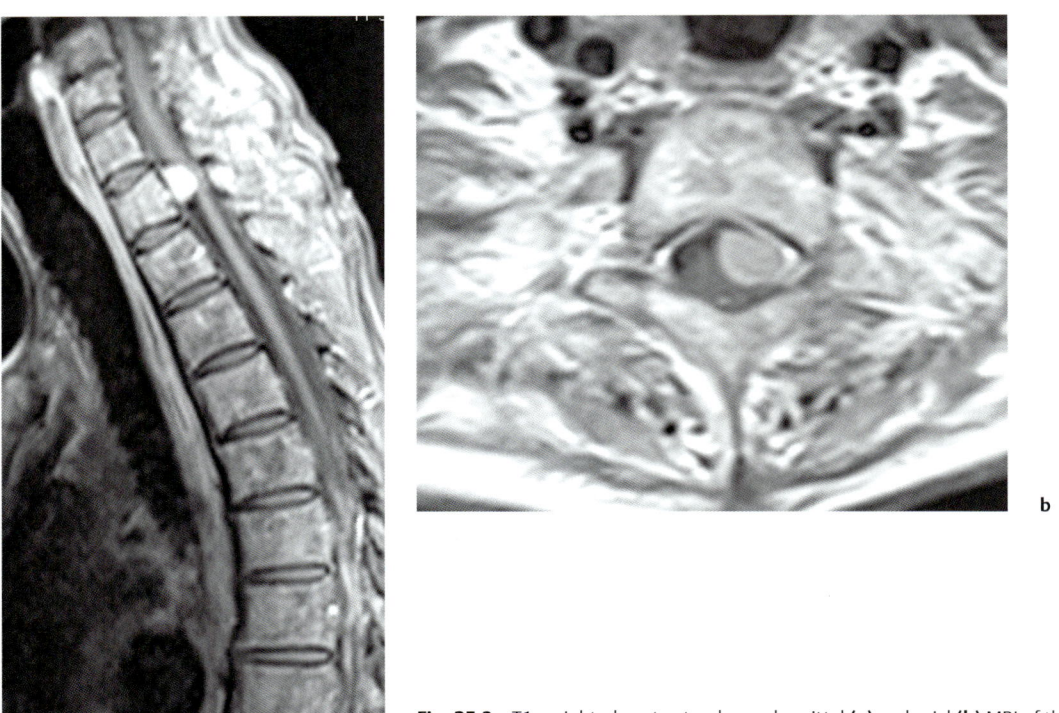

Fig. 25.3 T1-weighted contrast-enhanced sagittal **(a)** and axial **(b)** MRI of the thoracic spine shows a uniformly enhancing mass at the T2-T3 level with a broad-based ventrolateral dural attachment typical of a meningioma.

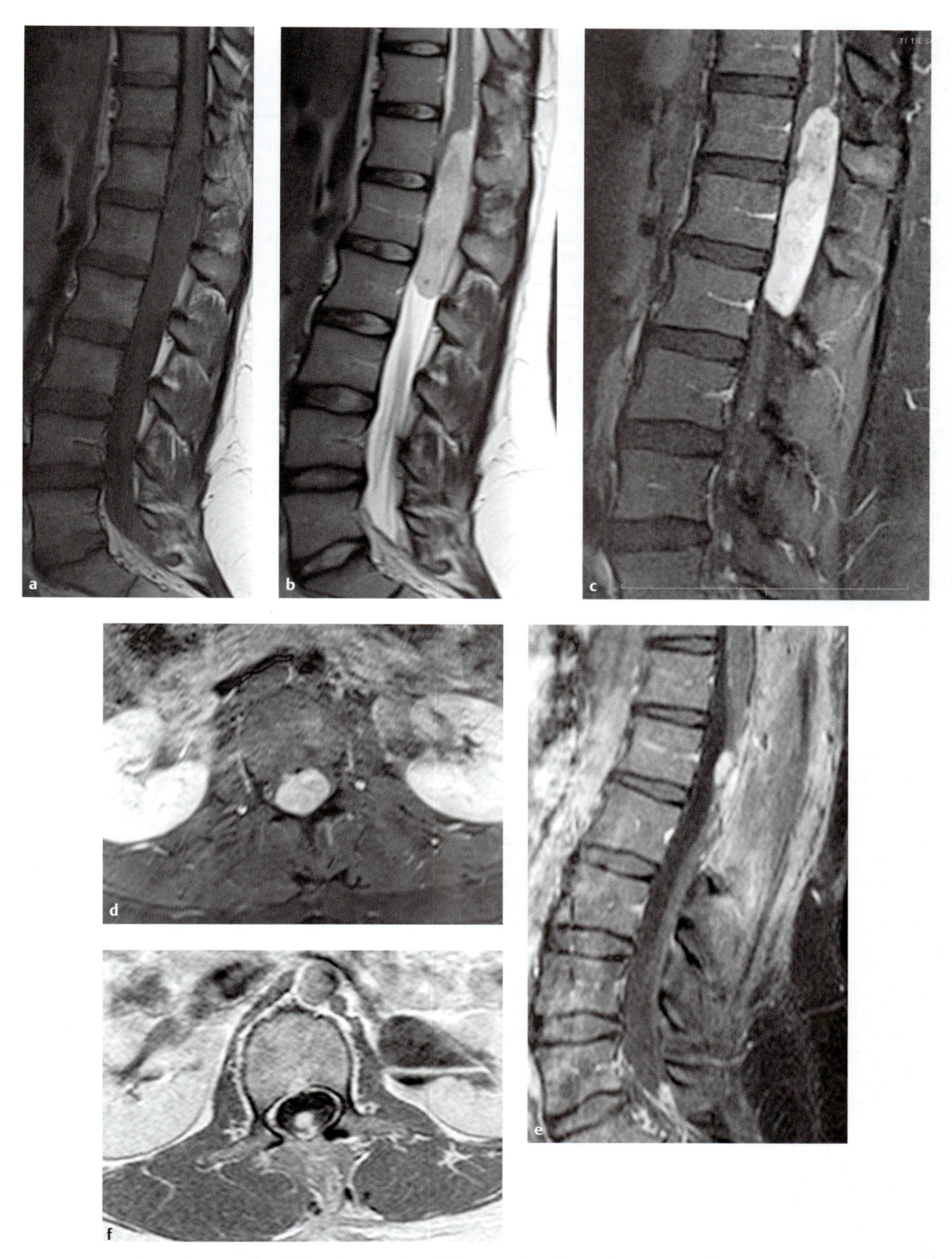

Fig. 25.4 Non–contrast-enhanced T1-weighted **(a)** and T2-weighted **(b)** sagittal MRI of the lumbar spine demonstrate a large intradural tumor extending from the T12 to L2 spinal level. The lesion is isointense on T1 and hyperintense on T2. T1-weighted contrast-enhanced sagittal **(c)** and axial **(d)** lumbar MRI shows uniform enhancement following contrast administration. The tumor occupies almost the entire cross-sectional area of the spinal canal on the axial image. Note the proximity and displacement of the distal conus medullaris along with the prominent draining veins on the spinal cord surface. The size of the tumor precluded safe en-bloc resection, so a subtotal piecemeal resection was accomplished. Due to residual tumor at the tip of the conus seen on postoperative contrast-enhanced sagittal **(e)** and axial **(f)** MRI, radiation therapy was administered.

Treatment Considerations

The fundamental goal of management for patients with extramedullary spinal cord tumors is either long-term tumor control or cure with preservation of neurologic function. Surgical resection of these tumors will accomplish either goal in the vast majority of patients. Surgery is clearly indicated in patients with symptomatic tumors, particularly those with large tumors producing significant compression of the spinal cord or cauda equina. For patients with smaller tumors or those with minimal subjective symptoms, it may be reasonable to follow them both clinically and radiographically over time. For small and asymptomatic tumors, interval radiographic surveillance can also be recommended. An exception for observation of asymptomatic tumors is the midline filum/cauda equina tumor. A substantial proportion of these tumors are filum terminale ependymomas that can exhibit spontaneous CSF dissemination. Early, en-bloc resection of these lesions is recommended in most instances.

There are several issues that must be considered in the planning of surgical resection of these tumors. The size, location (both in the axial and sagittal planes), spinal level, relationship of the tumor to the spinal cord, as well as tumor vascularity and consistency are relevant in this regard. The vast majority of intradural extramedullary tumors can be safely accessed and removed through a standard posterior laminectomy. Even most ventrally located tumors can be accessed posteriorly because lateral spinal cord displacement or rotation enables a safe corridor to debulk and remove most ventrally located tumors. However, pure ventral lesions may require a more lateral or ventral approach.[19] Dumbbell tumors usually require a unilateral facetectomy to allow access to foraminal and extraforaminal extension up to ~ 2.5 cm from the lateral dural margin. Whenever possible, it is preferable to remove the tumor through a single operative exposure to reduce morbidity and preserve surgical options. Instrumented fusion that extends one level above and below the facetectomy is usually performed.

Adjuvant therapy is typically not required following removal of these tumors. However, there may be instances where substantial tumor burden remains. Ventral meningiomas that encase the vertebral artery and lower cranial nerves at the foramen magnum–upper cervical region or large dumbbell extension into the upper cervical region may preclude safe surgical resection. Radiosurgery with either the linear accelerator (LINAC), in a single dose (e.g., 14 gray) or hypofractionated, or the gamma knife can be considered in these cases for long-term control of the residual tumor. Multifractionated radiation therapy is considered for patients following subtotal resection of myxopapillary ependymomas of the filum terminale (**Fig. 25.4e,f**).

References

1. Nittner K. Spinal meningiomas, neurinomas and neurofibromas, and hourglass tumours. In: Vinken PH, Bruyn GW, eds. Handbook of Clinical Neurology. New York: North Holland/America, Elsevier; 1976:177–322
2. Russell DS, Rubenstein LJ. Pathology of Tumors of the Nervous System. Baltimore: Williams & Wilkins; 1989
3. Halliday AL, Sobel RA, Martuza RL. Benign spinal nerve sheath tumors: their occurrence sporadically and in neurofibromatosis types 1 and 2. J Neurosurg 1991;74:248–253
4. Kernohan JW, Sayre GP. Tumors of the Central Nervous System, Fascicle 35. Washington, DC: Armed Forces Institute of Pathology; 1952
5. Purcell SM, Dixon SL. Schwannomatosis. An unusual variant of neurofibromatosis or a distinct clinical entity? Arch Dermatol 1989;125:390–393
6. Seppälä MT, Haltia MJ, Sankila RJ, Jääskeläinen JE, Heiskanen O. Long-term outcome after removal of spinal schwannoma: a clinicopathological study of 187 cases. J Neurosurg 1995;83:621–626
7. Levy WJ, Latchaw J, Hahn JF, Sawhny B, Bay J, Dohn DF. Spinal neurofibromas: a report of 66 cases and a comparison with meningiomas. Neurosurgery 1986;18:331–334
8. Seppälä MT, Haltia MJ, Sankila RJ, Jääskeläinen JE, Heiskanen O. Long-term outcome after removal of spinal neurofibroma. J Neurosurg 1995;82:572–577
9. Seppälä MT, Haltia MJ. Spinal malignant nerve-sheath tumor or cellular schwannoma? A striking difference in prognosis. J Neurosurg 1993;79:528–532
10. Klekamp J, Samii M. Surgical results for spinal meningiomas. Surg Neurol 1999;52:552–562
11. Levy WJ Jr, Bay J, Dohn D. Spinal cord meningioma. J Neurosurg 1982;57:804–812
12. Solero CL, Fornari M, Giombini S, et al. Spinal meningiomas: review of 174 operated cases. Neurosurgery 1989;25:153–160
13. King AT, Sharr MM, Gullan RW, Bartlett JR. Spinal meningiomas: a 20-year review. Br J Neurosurg 1998;12:521–526
14. Schiff D, O'Neill BP. Intramedullary spinal cord metastases: clinical features and treatment outcome. Neurology 1996;47:906–912
15. Sloof JL, Kernohan JW, McCarthy CS. Primary Intramedullary Tumors of the Spinal Cord and Filum Terminale. Philadelphia: WB Saunders; 1964
16. Sonneland PR, Scheithauer BW, Onofrio BM. Myxopapillary ependymoma. A clinicopathologic and immunocytochemical study of 77 cases. Cancer 1985;56:883–893
17. Davis C, Barnard RO. Malignant behavior of myxopapillary ependymoma. Report of three cases. J Neurosurg 1985;62:925–929
18. Reyes MG, Torres H. Intrathecal paraganglioma of the cauda equina. Neurosurgery 1984;15:578–582
19. Angevine PD, Kellner C, Haque RM, McCormick PC. Surgical management of ventral intradural spinal lesions. J Neurosurg Spine 2011;15:28–37

26 Vertebral Bone Tumors

Rakesh Ramakrishnan and William F. Lavelle

Bone tumors of the cervical spine are a rare entity. They may present as incidental findings on imaging studies or present with profound neurologic deficits. Symptoms vary greatly and may be as subtle as mild pain or as drastic as scoliosis with significant neurologic deficits. As with bone tumors in other areas, night pain is frequently associated with neoplasm. The common constitutional symptoms may also be present. Primary benign tumors generally occur in the younger population with a slightly higher prevalence in males. Malignant bone tumors are found primarily in the older population.[1,2]

Benign Tumors

Benign tumors of the cervical spine typically occur in the first two decades of life.[2,3] The most common symptom is neck pain or stiffness. There may be an associated torticollis or scoliosis. Although a neck mass may be palpable, this is not a sensitive physical examination finding and is definitely not the norm for tumors based in the vertebral body. Neurologic symptoms at initial presentation are generally uncommon. Diagnosis of these lesions is often delayed because imaging is not initially obtained due to the natural course of this type of pain. The most commonly reported benign subaxial vertebral body tumors are giant cell tumor, hemangioma, and eosinophilic granuloma.

Giant Cell Tumors

Giant cell tumors are generally slow-growing lesions that are locally aggressive and do not metastasize. When these lesions appear in the spine, they are typically located in the vertebral body but may expand to the surrounding cortical bone as the lesion grows. Radiographic findings include a lytic, expansile, well-circumscribed lesion without sclerosis. Complete excision is the treatment of choice because of the aggressive nature of these lesions. Due to the difficulty of obtaining a wide margin in the spine, these lesions have a high local recurrence rate. As a result, the routine use of computed tomography (CT) is recommended for postoperative follow-up care. Adjuvant radiation therapy has a 10% incidence of malignant transformation and should be avoided.[4] Recently, suppressive therapy with bisphosphonates for tumors that are either unresectable or incompletely removed has been used[5] (**Fig. 26.1**).

Hemangiomas

Hemangiomas in the vertebral body are common lesions. They are benign vascular tumors that are rarely symptomatic and are usually identified incidentally. Symptomatic individuals are typically older patients, and deformity associated with these lesions is rare in the cervical spine. Hemangiomas can generally be diagnosed on imaging. Prominent vertical striations are seen on plain films due to the abnormally thickened trabeculae of the vertebral body. Hemangiomas respond well to low-dose radiation therapy alone. If cord compression develops and surgical treatment is indicated, preoperative angiography should be considered.[1,6]

Eosinophilic Granuloma

Eosinophilic granuloma has generally been considered a self-limiting lesion, but its presentation and imaging studies refute this idea.[2] This process produces focal destruction of bone, and is difficult to distinguish radiographically from more malignant lesions or infection. Classically, this lesion is found in boys in the first decade of life. Laboratory tests are generally unremarkable, with the exception being the erythrocyte sedimentation rate, which is elevated in some cases. In the spine, the lytic lesion may cause the vertebral body to collapse, resulting in a common finding known as vertebral plana.[7] Surgical care is typically limited to biopsy to confirm the diagnosis.

Aneurysmal Bone Cysts

Aneurysmal bone cysts are uncommon bone pathology. Furthermore, those cases occurring in the spine are exceedingly rare. The most common clinical features are either pain or nerve root compression. The cysts are lytic, expansile lesions that are nonneoplastic. Although they are benign, their rapid enlargement can lead to neurologic compromise due to spinal instability or cord impingement. In their appearance in long bones, the cortex is typically markedly eroded. The cysts present more commonly in females and are generally found in patients under 20 years of age.[1] Although these lesions are almost always located in the posterior elements, they commonly extend into the vertebral body. Lesions in adjacent vertebrae are clues to this diagnosis. Magnetic resonance imaging (MRI) or CT is ideal for evaluation of the extension of the lesion and the internal contents of the cyst. Multiple fluid levels within the lesion, best seen on T2-weighted MRI, support the diagnosis. Often partial collapse of the body is identified. Surgical excision of the lesion is typically curative. Preoperative selective arterial embolization can be utilized to minimize bleeding during surgery.[8]

Malignant Tumors

Primary malignant tumors of the subaxial cervical spine also present with the primary complaint of pain. Night pain and spasms are common. Neurologic compromise can also be seen on initial presentation. In this region of the spine, plasmacytoma is the

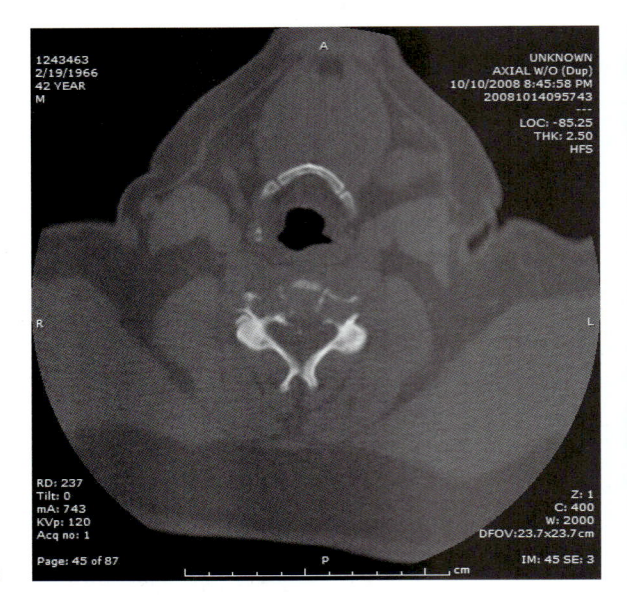

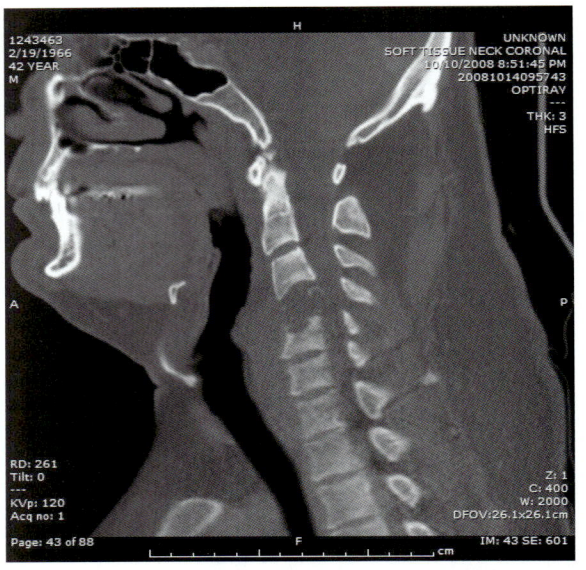

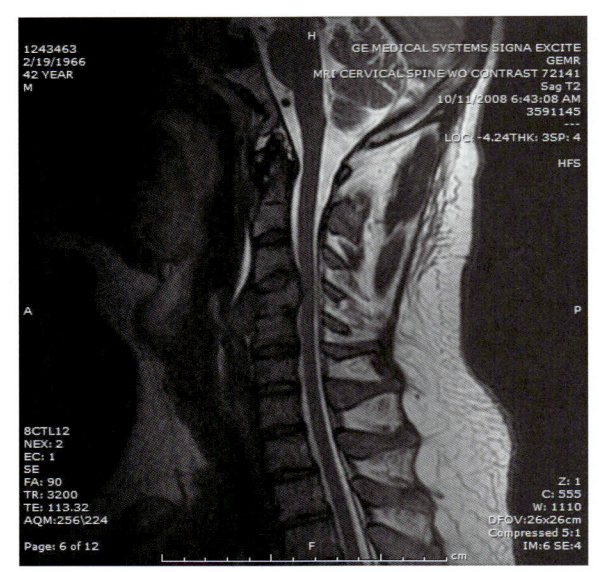

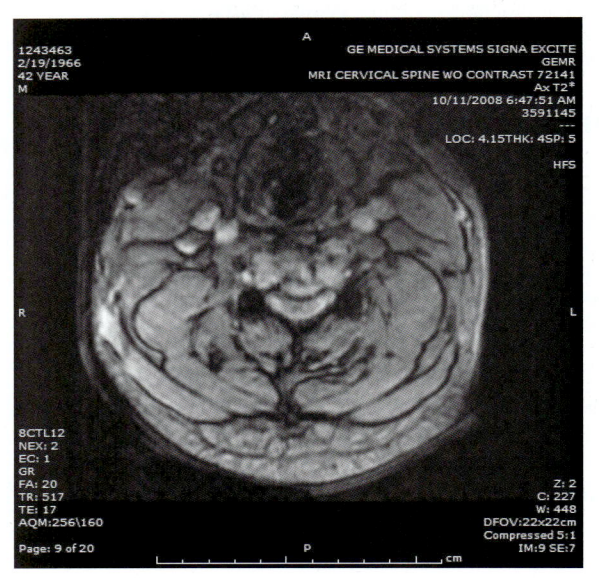

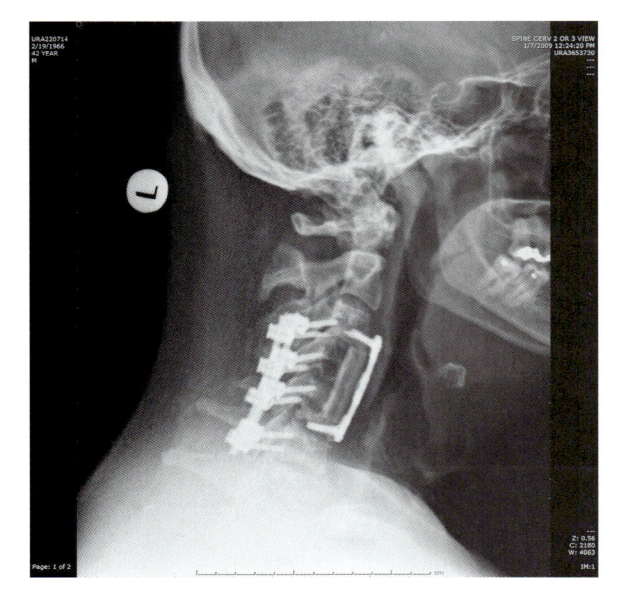

Fig. 26.1 A 42-year-old man presented to the hospital with progressive upper extremity weakness. The patient underwent an urgent decompression and fusion due to his progressive neurologic decline. He was treated with chronic bisphosphonate therapy, as his resection was interlesional due to the involvement of his vertebral arteries. **(a)** Axial and **(b)** sagittal CT showing a destructive bony lesion involving the vertebral body of C4. **(c)** Sagital T2 MRI demonstrating C4 Giant Cell Tumor with spinal cord compression. **(d)** Axial T2 MRI demonstrating C4 Giant Cell Tumor with spinal cord compression. **(e)** Lateral X-Ray demonstrating anterior and posterior decompression and fusion.

most common malignant tumor, followed by chordomas.[1] Malignant tumors in this region pose a particular problem because en-bloc resection in this region is more difficult than in the thoracic or lumbar regions due to the presence of the vertebral arteries as well as the involvement of the scalene muscles and cervical nerve roots.

Plasmacytoma

Plasmacytoma and multiple myeloma are both variations of B-cell neoplasms. True solitary plasmacytoma comprises ~ 3% of all plasma cell neoplasms.[1,9] As compared with patients with multiple myeloma, patients with solitary plasmacytoma tend to be younger and often have a significantly better prognosis. Radiation therapy is the treatment of choice. Surgery is only considered for neurologic deterioration or to ensure structural stability.[9,10] Some patients with solitary plasmacytoma may still develop generalized disease in the future even after adequate treatment (**Figs. 26.2 and 26.3**).

Chordoma

Chordoma is a rare malignancy that arises from remnants of the notochord. As a result, almost all the cases occur in the midline of the axial skeleton. About half of the cases occur in the sacrococcygeal area and a third at the base of skull. The cervical region is the most common area for the remaining cases. These are slow-growing lesions that cause clinical symptoms based on their location. In the cervical spine, they are usually centrally located within the vertebral body.[11] Anterior soft tissue extension can cause dysphasia, and posterior extension can lead to neurologic impairment. Systematic metastases occur in ~ 25% of cases. Wide resection can be curative, but local recurrence carries a very poor prognosis.

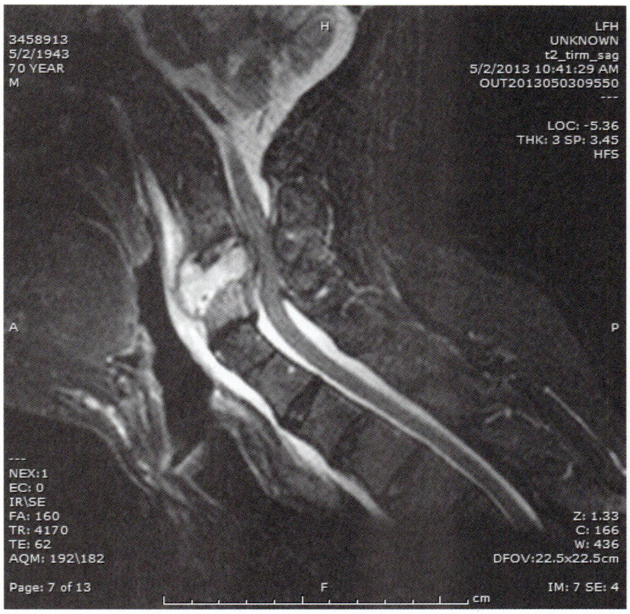

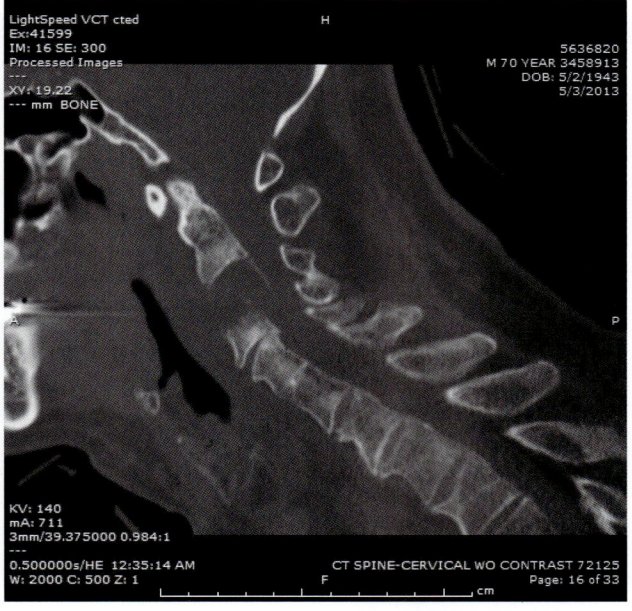

Fig. 26.2 A 70-year-old man presented to the hospital with severe neck pain and progressive arm weakness. He underwent an emergent anterior and posterior surgery based on his progressive deficit as well as the demonstrated bone loss on the computed tomography (CT) scan. Intraoperative pathology demonstrated a small round blue cell tumor that was later diagnosed as lymphoma. **(a)** Sagital T2 MRI demonstrating C3 tumor with spinal cord compression. **(b)** Sagital CT demonstrating lysis of C3 vertebra. **(c)** Lateral X-ray demonstrating anterior corpectomy with posterior stabilization.

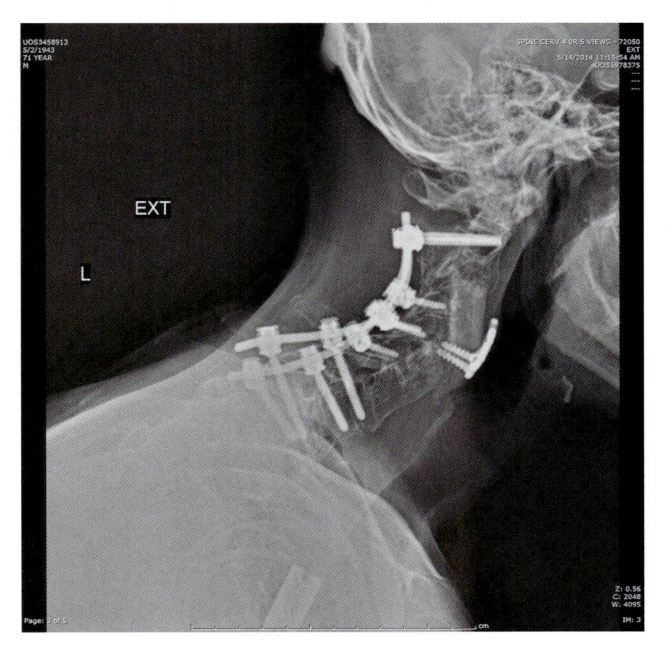

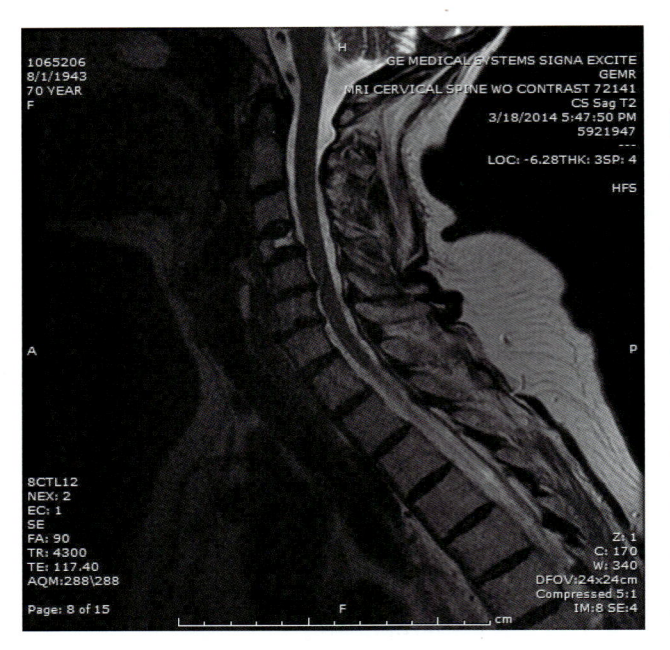

Fig. 26.3 A 70-year-old woman with a known history of multiple myeloma presented to the office with new-onset neck pain. A presumptive diagnosis of a multiple myeloma lesion was made, and the patient was treated with pain medication and radiation therapy.

Osteosarcoma

Osteosarcoma is the second most common primary malignant bone tumor, and ~ 2% arise in the spine.[2,12] As with other malignancies, pain is the primary symptom on presentation. More often than with other malignant tumors in the subaxial spine, osteosarcoma presents with neurologic compromise. Osteosarcoma appears as a lytic lesion that can have sclerotic areas. Cortical destruction and soft tissue calcification can also be seen. Prognosis for this lesion is very poor and treatment choices are limited. These include limited tumor resection and radiation therapy.

Chondrosarcoma

Chondrosarcoma is a malignant lesion that produces cartilage matrix, with up to 10% found in the spinal column. Generally, chondrosarcoma presents later in life because most are low grade and grow slowly.[1,3] Radiographically, there is a lytic area associated with a soft tissue mass with irregular calcifications. CT and MRI are recommended for full evaluation. These lesions are characteristically bright on T2-weighted MRI. They recur locally after incomplete excision, so negative margins are important.[13,14]

Metastatic Tumors

Metastatic tumors in the spine in general are common. The dominant symptom is neck pain in the majority of these patients. Many times this is the initial discovery of metastatic disease in this population. The metastatic spread to the cervical spine has been believed to be hematogenous.[15] Spinal metastases commonly involve the anterior and middle columns. The posterior column is much less susceptible and may be a function of not containing active red bone marrow throughout life. However, metastatic disease to the subaxial cervical spine is relatively uncommon.[16,17] Breast, lung, and prostate cancer account for most metastatic disease in the subaxial cervical spine. Given the low frequency of neurologic complications and less mechanical instability, this does not pose as much of a problem as metastases to the thoracic or lumbar spine. Nonoperative treatment is successful in many cases. Treatments include external immobilization, radiation therapy, or chemotherapy. The overall goals are stabilization of the cervical spine and the prevention of neurologic deterioration while resolving pain and maintaining the patient's mobility.[16,18] Surgical indications include instability, progressive neurologic compromise, and intractable pain.

Surgical intervention for metastatic disease in the subaxial cervical spine is palliative. Once the primary tumor is identified, the mechanical stability and the neurologic status must be assessed. Surgery is indicated to control pain and maximize stability and neurologic function. In the lower subaxial cervical spine, the risks of metastases are mainly neurologic secondary to compression of the spinal cord, requiring acute decompression and stabilization. The unknown preoperative variable is life expectancy. These vertebral body lesions are commonly approached anteriorly. Anterior decompression with stabilization is generally used to achieve the intended surgical goals. Polymethylmethacrylate (PMMA) can be used in patients with limited life expectancy. In those patients with prolonged life expectancy, bone graft rather than PMMA is indicated. Radiation therapy has been used in the immediate postoperative period; however, radiation is recommended either before surgery or 6 weeks postoperatively if bone graft is used.[16,17] Combined anterior and posterior stabilization should be considered in multilevel disease. C7-T1 is a transitional level that requires a specially adapted anterior surgical approach. Pain relief is obtained by adequate decompression and stabilization.

Postoperative survival can be dependent on the nature of the primary cancer. Several case studies in the literature point to a disparity in the length of survival. When the primary cancer was breast cancer or myeloma, the survival rate was double that of uterine or head and neck cancer[18] (**Fig. 26.4**).

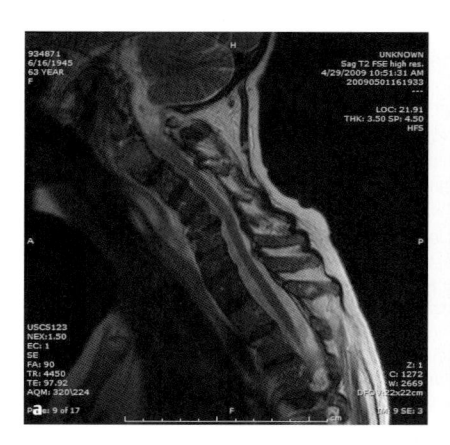

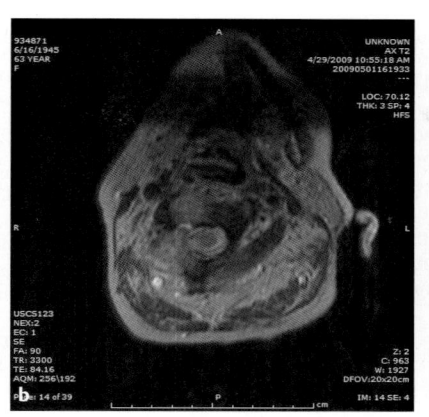

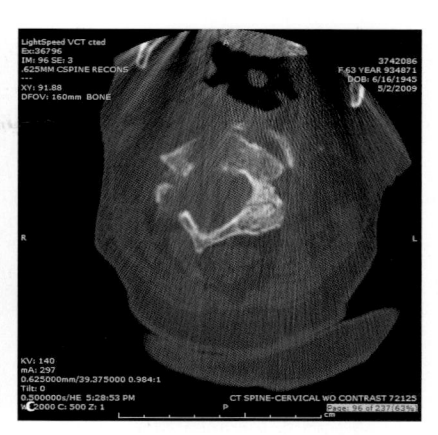

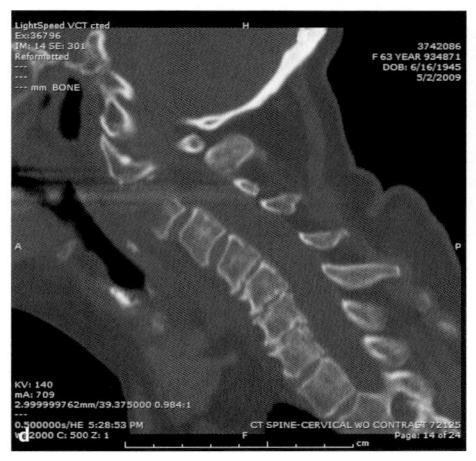

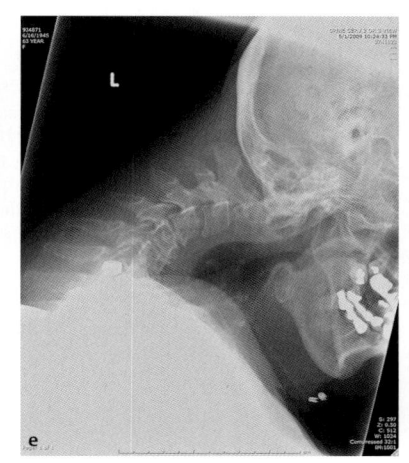

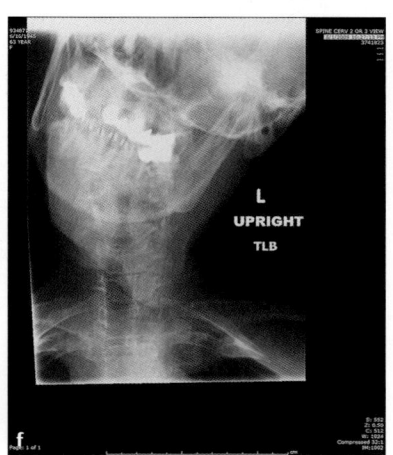

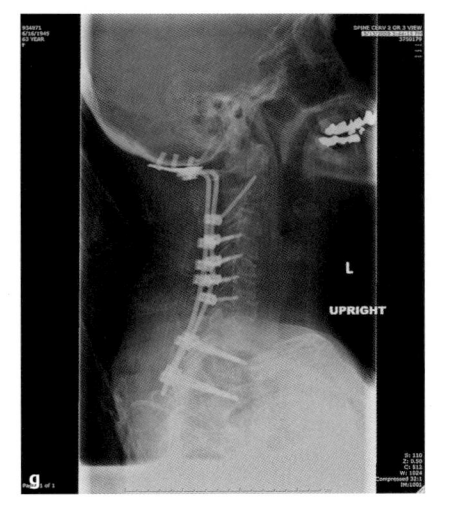

Fig. 26.4 A 65-year-old woman with a known history of small cell lung cancer presented to the hospital with severe and disabling neck pain. She was unable to raise or rotate her head. CT and magnetic resonance imaging (MRI) demonstrated an erosive C2 lesion that included the vertebral body and right lateral mass. She was offered the options of local fusion versus an extensive fusion to improve her cervical sagittal alignment. She underwent an occipital to thoracic spine fusion with posterolateral tumor debulking and bone grafting. **(a)** Sagital T2 MRI demonstrating C2 lytic tumor. **(b)** Axial T2 MRI demonstrating C2 lytic tumor. **(c)** Axial CT demonstrating C2 lytic tumor. **(d)** Sagital CT scan demonstrating C2 lytic tumor with kyphosis. **(e)** Lateral upright film demonstrating focal kyphosis. **(f)** AP plain film demonstrating head tilt. **(g)** Postoperative lateral X-ray demonstrating restoration an upright head and neck posture.

Conclusion

Bone tumors of the cervical spine are rare. They can be primary bone tumors or metastatic lesions. Regardless of the origin of the tumor, patient evaluation is paramount. The keys to treatment are determining the primary source of the lesion, tumor staging, mechanical and neurologic stability, prognosis, and quality of life. Surgical indications include (1) cord compression secondary to fracture or deformity, (2) instability, (3) progressive pain despite nonoperative treatment modalities, and (4) isolated spinal lesions unresponsive to nonoperative treatment.

References

1. Abdu WA, Provencher M. Primary bone and metastatic tumors of the cervical spine. Spine 1998;23:2767–2777
2. Weinstein JN, McLain RF. Primary tumors of the spine. Spine 1987;12:843–851
3. Dreghorn CR, Newman RJ, Hardy GJ, Dickson RA. Primary tumors of the axial skeleton. Experience of the Leeds Regional Bone Tumor Registry. Spine 1990;15:137–140
4. Hart RA, Boriani S, Biagini R, Currier B, Weinstein JN. A system for surgical staging and management of spine tumors. A clinical outcome study of giant cell tumors of the spine. Spine 1997;22:1773–1782, discussion 1783
5. Cornelis F, Truchetet ME, Amoretti N, et al. Bisphosphonate therapy for unresectable symptomatic benign bone tumors: a long-term prospective study of tolerance and efficacy. Bone 2014;58:11–16
6. Friedman DP. Symptomatic vertebral hemangiomas: MR findings. AJR Am J Roentgenol 1996;167:359–364
7. Bertram C, Madert J, Eggers C. Eosinophilic granuloma of the cervical spine. Spine 2002;27:1408–1413
8. Papagelopoulos PJ, Currier BL, Shaughnessy WJ, et al. Aneurysmal bone cyst of the spine. Management and outcome. Spine 1998;23:621–628
9. Valderrama JAF, Bullough PG. Solitary myeloma of the spine. J Bone Joint Surg Br 1968;50:82–90
10. McLain RF, Weinstein JN. Solitary plasmacytomas of the spine: a review of 84 cases. J Spinal Disord 1989;2:69–74
11. Boriani S, Chevalley F, Weinstein JN, et al. Chordoma of the spine above the sacrum. Treatment and outcome in 21 cases. Spine 1996;21:1569–1577
12. Shives TC, Dahlin DC, Sim FH, Pritchard DJ, Earle JD. Osteosarcoma of the spine. J Bone Joint Surg Am 1986;68:660–668
13. Shives TC, McLeod RA, Unni KK, Schray MF. Chondrosarcoma of the spine. J Bone Joint Surg Am 1989;71:1158–1165
14. Boriani S, De Iure F, Bandiera S, et al. Chondrosarcoma of the mobile spine: report on 22 cases. Spine 2000;25:804–812
15. Batson OV. The function of the vertebral veins and their role in the spread of metastases. Ann Surg 1940;112:138–149
16. Dunn EJ, Anas PP. The management of tumors of the upper cervical spine. Orthop Clin North Am 1978;9:1065–1080
17. Atanasiu JP, Badatcheff F, Pidhorz L. Metastatic lesions of the cervical spine. A retrospective analysis of 20 cases. Spine 1993;18:1279–1284
18. Rao S, Badani K, Schildhauer T, Borges M. Metastatic malignancy of the cervical spine. A nonoperative history. Spine 1992;17(10, Suppl):S407–S412

27 Trauma of the Mid- and Lower Cervical Spine

Daniel K. Resnick, Christopher D. Baggott, Bennie W. Chiles III, and Paul R. Cooper

The middle and lower segments of the cervical spine are the most common site of spinal injury. This area represents the most mobile portion of the spinal column and is thus particularly vulnerable to mechanical deformation and resultant structural damage when external forces are applied.

The general goals of management of patients with injuries of the middle and lower cervical spine are (1) preservation of function in patients who are neurologically intact, (2) prevention of additional loss of function and reduction of deficit in patients with neurologic compromise, and (3) restoration of spinal stability.

Initial Assessment and Stabilization

Management of patients with suspected cervical spine injuries begins at the scene of injury with strict immobilization of the neck during extrication from the scene and transport to the hospital. Rigid cervical collars, sandbags, and spine boards aid in protecting the patient with a potentially unstable cervical spine injury. Five percent of patients with severe systemic trauma have an unstable cervical spine, and two thirds of them have no initial neurologic deficit.[1,2] In recent years, the reported incidence of complete spinal cord injuries has decreased, likely due to wider recognition of the potential for secondary neurologic injury in the presence of an unstable spine.[3]

Proper airway management in spine-injured patients is vital to avoid hypoxemia, and clinicians should maintain a low threshold for early intubation and assisted ventilation. The technique used for intubation should take into account the potential for neurologic injury secondary to excessive neck manipulation. Hypotension may be present due to hemorrhagic shock or loss of systemic sympathetic vasomotor tone. The latter symptom generally responds to fluid resuscitation and, if necessary, pressors. An indwelling urinary catheter should be placed to prevent bladder distention and to monitor urine output.

Nasogastric tube insertion prevents aspiration of stomach contents and avoids abdominal distention, which may contribute to respiratory difficulties. A detailed, accurate initial neurologic evaluation is essential to specify areas for later imaging and to establish a baseline for the subsequent assessment of neurologic improvement or deterioration.

Radiological Evaluation

Patients with suspected cervical spine injury should undergo computed tomography (CT) imaging, if available. If CT is not immediately available, a three-view cervical spine series may be obtained with follow-up CT if there are suspicious or poorly visualized areas.[4,5] Depending on the results of the CT, further imaging may be considered including magnetic resonance imaging (MRI), often used to rule out ligamentous injury in obtunded patients but also useful in selected patients for demonstrating soft tissue compression of the spinal cord. The timing of MRI should be determined by the patient's clinical condition and imaging findings on CT. Patients with severe deficits and clear bony compression of the spinal cord may be better treated with prompt decompression prior to MRI, whereas patients without clear bony injury or with less severe injuries likely benefit from early MRI to define injury patterns and guide treatment.[4] For example, an awake patient with bilateral facet subluxation may be reduced using traction prior to MRI, whereas a patient with normal alignment and a significant deficit will require MRI to define the lesion. CT or MR angiography may be considered if there is concern regarding a vertebral artery injury, but the importance of imaging findings in the absence of symptoms may be questioned.[6]

Surgical Techniques

The goals of surgery in patients with injuries of the mid- and lower cervical spine include (1) decompression of the neural elements to facilitate maximal neurologic recovery; (2) immediate stabilization of injured and mechanically unstable spinal segments to enable early mobilization and avoid the wide variety of medical complications seen with prolonged recumbence; and (3) arthrodesis of these unstable spinal segments to prevent future deformity, pain, and neurologic injury. Decompression is accomplished anteriorly by diskectomy or vertebrectomy, and posteriorly by laminectomy, laminoplasty, or laminotomy. Immediate spinal stabilization is generally achieved with metallic implants. Anteriorly, this is almost universally done with screw-plate constructs. Posteriorly, lateral mass screw fixation has supplanted wiring as the stabilization technique of choice in the posterior cervical region. Arthrodesis can be performed utilizing a variety of bone-grafting techniques.

Anterior Versus Posterior Approach

The choice of an anterior or posterior approach for stabilizing the cervical spine after trauma depends on (1) the mechanism and type of spinal injury; (2) the presence of residual spinal cord compression; (3) the type of neurologic deficit, if any; and (4) the skills and preferences of the surgeon. Frequently, either approach is satisfactory to achieve immediate stability and prevent long-term deformity. The only absolute indication for anterior stabilization is the presence of anterior compression of the spinal cord in patients with preservation of some neurologic function below the level of the injury. An anterior approach enables restoration of the load-bearing structures of the spine and provides an advantage in resisting kyphosis.

There are no absolute indications for posterior stabilization except in the patient who has posterior spinal cord compression (e.g., a bilaminar fracture with anterior displacement). In general, though, it makes the most sense to use the posterior approach to treat instability resulting from injuries to the bony and ligamentous structures of the facet joints and injuries requiring multiple levels of fixation.

Circumferential techniques may be useful for highly unstable injuries or for limiting the length of fusion by providing anterior column support as well as a dorsal tension band.

Reduction, Positioning, and Anesthesia

All patients with acute, unstable injuries of the cervical spine require immobilization. Patients with malalignment of the spine, such as those with jumped facets, probably benefit from early decompression through reduction of the deformity. For positioning the patient, awake traction reduction with either Gardner-Wells cervical tongs or a halo ring is safe and usually effective.[7] Traction may be maintained to stabilize the spine during subsequent transfer to the operating room or for further imaging (if needed).

Ideally, intubation should be performed using an awake fiberoptic technique and the patient should be evaluated prior to the induction of general anesthesia to confirm that no new neurologic deficit has been incurred during intubation. If electrophysiological monitoring is to be performed, an appropriate combination of anesthetic agents is required, and baseline recordings should be obtained prior to positioning the patient on the operating table.

The use of intraoperative monitoring has been recommended by some as a means of detecting maneuvers during positioning or surgery that may result in increased neurologic deficit, enabling the surgeon to make appropriate technical adjustments.[8] The literature support for this hypothesis is very limited, however, and the choice to use monitoring should be made based on the condition of the patient, the procedure planned, and the preference of the surgeon. Monitoring is associated with increased complexity of the anesthesia, false alarms, and potential delays in decompression. Monitoring may be useful for the acutely unstable patient requiring intraoperative reduction of deformity if the surgeon has the ability and intent to "undo" the reduction if monitoring abnormalities are reported.[9]

Anterior procedures are generally performed with the patient in the supine position with the head on a horseshoe head support or donut and with the traction tongs left in place. Just before the induction of anesthesia and administration of muscle relaxants, the amount of traction weight should be reduced to 5 to 10 lb to avoid potential spinal cord injury from overdistraction.

Posterior procedures are generally performed with the patient in the prone position on chest rolls, and the head secured in a three-point skull fixation device or in traction. Intraoperative fluoroscopy is extremely useful for (1) confirming adequate positioning of the spine prior to the start of the procedure, (2) enabling rapid identification of the correct spinal levels intraoperatively, and (3) facilitating correct placement of metallic implants. To enable maximal radiological visualization intraoperatively, the patient's shoulders and arms should be pulled down and secured to the sides of the table with wide tape. Care should be taken to avoid excessive force in this maneuver, which can lead to a brachial plexus injury.

Anterior Stabilization

Anterior Decompression and Arthrodesis

Anterior decompression and arthrodesis are indicated for (1) traumatic disk herniation, with or without neurologic deficit; (2) extensive vertebral body injury, particularly if accompanied by significant loss of vertebral body height; and (3) anterior bony compression of the neural elements. Reduction of facet subluxation is possible via an anterior approach as well, although some authors prefer to approach such injuries with a posterior approach. When a three-column injury is present and a combined anterior/posterior procedure is planned, anterior approach is generally performed first.

The essence of the anterior approach to the cervical spine is dissection through a bloodless plane between the sternocleidomastoid muscle and carotid sheath laterally, and the trachea and esophagus medially (**Fig. 27.1**). The anterior approach to the cervical spine can be performed through a horizontal incision made in a skin crease in the anterior cervical triangle, or an oblique vertical incision made along the anterior border of the sternocleidomastoid muscle (**Fig. 27.2**). The former is appropriate for diskectomy and a one- or two-level vertebrectomy, and gives a better long-term cosmetic result. The latter is generally reserved for resection of more than two vertebral bodies when a greater amount of rostral-caudal exposure is required. The patient's body habitus also influences the incision, with shorter and heavier patients usually doing better with a horizontal incision.

The horizontal incision begins just off the midline and extends laterally to just beyond the medial border of the sternocleidomastoid muscle. Fluoroscopy can aid in proper localization of the skin incision, as can studying the preoperative images. Landmarks include the cricoid cartilage at approximately C5-C6 and the thyroid cartilage at approximately C4-C5. The right recurrent laryngeal nerve is aberrant in a small percentage of patients; the left recurrent laryngeal nerve is never aberrant, and a left-sided approach, therefore, may carry a lower risk of recurrent laryngeal nerve injury, particularly at lower cervical levels.[10] Recent findings, however, suggest a similar incidence of postoperative nerve injury regardless of the side of approach.

The skin, subcutaneous tissue, and platysma muscle are sharply divided and retracted with a blunt-toothed self-retaining retractor to expose the superficial cervical fascia. The superficial fascia is opened, and, using blunt dissection, the plane between the sternocleidomastoid muscle and carotid sheath laterally and the trachea and esophagus medially is developed. The carotid artery is identified and retracted laterally. The anterior cervical spine is rapidly palpated and identified. The prevertebral fascia is opened in the midline in a rostral-caudal direction. Proper identification of the midline is obtained by noting the medial attachments of both longus colli muscles, which lie on the anterolateral aspect of the cervical spine bilaterally. At this point, a spinal needle is placed in a disk space and the correct level is confirmed with an X-ray or a fluoroscopic image. With significant bony trauma, such as a burst fracture, one will also be able to visually appreciate other signs pointing to the correct level, such as a prevertebral hematoma or fracture of the affected vertebral body.

After adequate exposure and localization, the longus colli muscles are elevated bilaterally from medial to lateral. In the vertical direction, the length of longus colli mobilization must exceed the length of the necessary decompression. Various self-retaining anterior cervical retractor systems are available, the majority of which utilize curved blades whose teeth fit beneath the medial aspect of the longus colli muscles. Vertical retraction is accomplished using curved blades without teeth to minimize

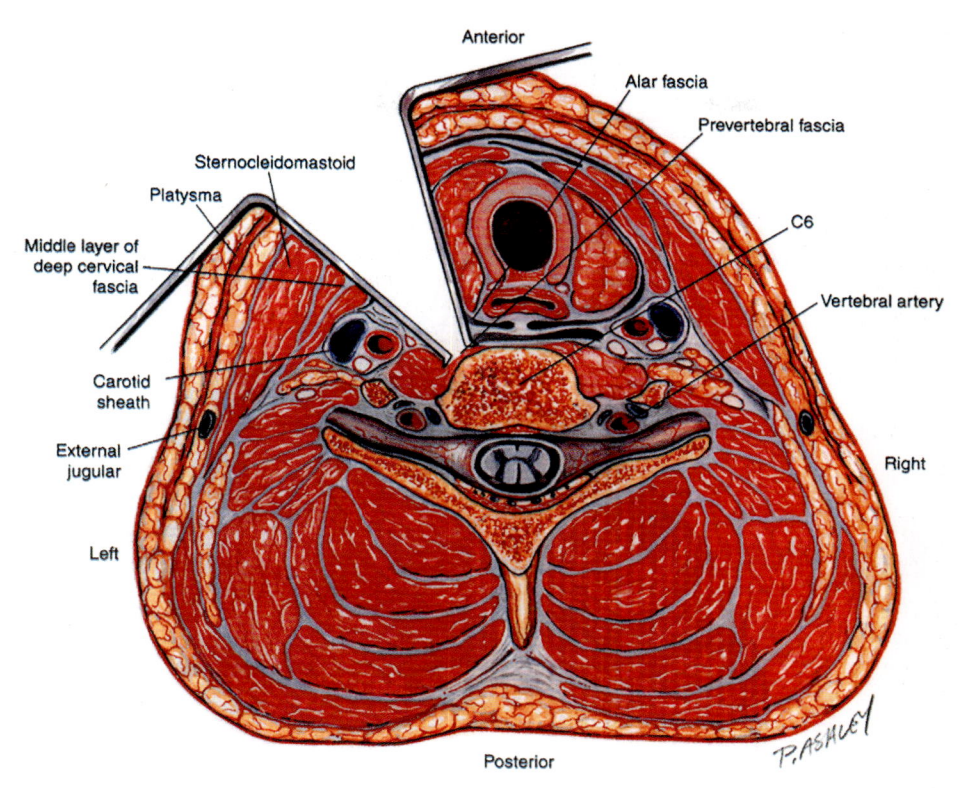

27 Trauma of the Mid- and Lower Cervical Spine 175

Fig. 27.1 Cross section through the C6 level demonstrating the correct anatomic plane through which the cervical spine is approached anteriorly. (Reproduced with permission of W.B. Saunders Company.)

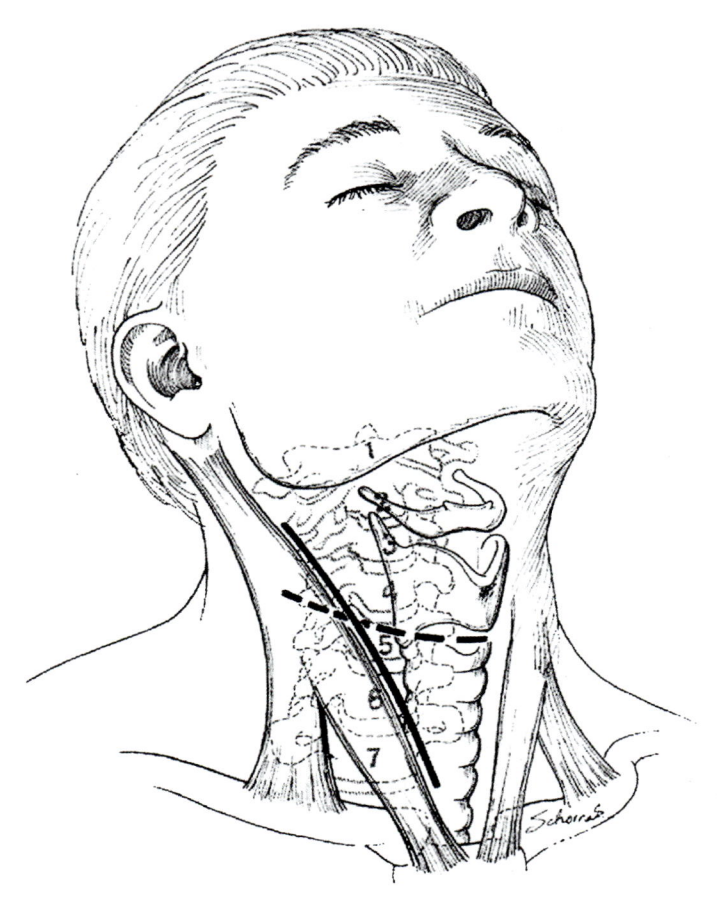

Fig. 27.2 Diskectomies at as many as three levels and single-level vertebrectomies can be performed through a horizontal incision. A vertical skin incision provides better exposure for multilevel vertebrectomies and anterior instrumentation. (Reproduced with permission of W.B. Saunders Company.)

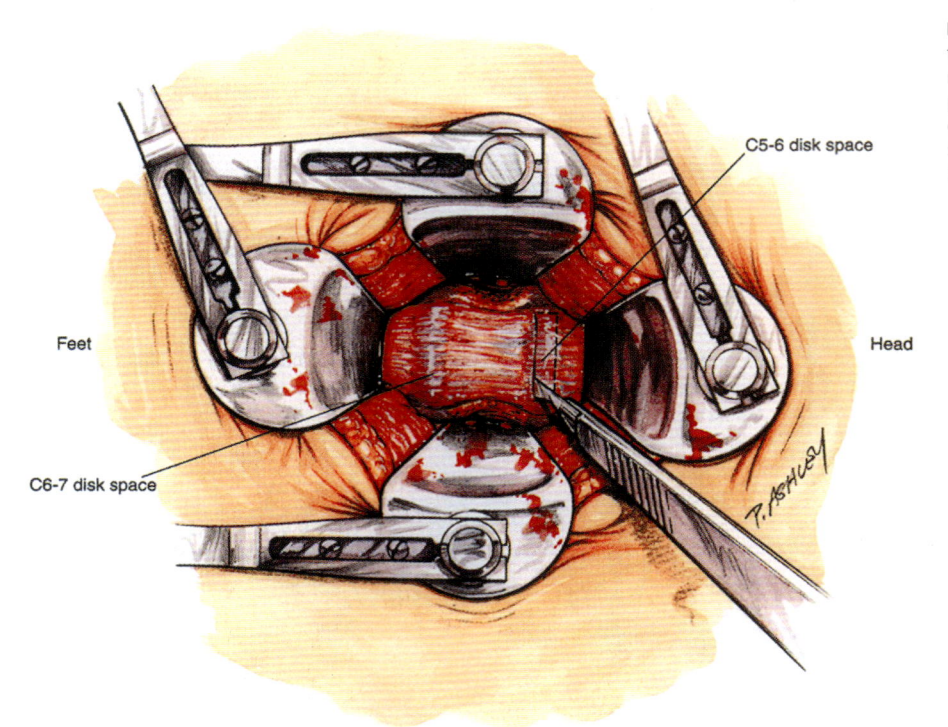

Fig. 27.3 Self-retaining retractors with teeth are placed under the longus colli muscles bilaterally. Smooth blades are placed in a vertical direction affording excellent exposure of the anterior cervical spine. (Reproduced with permission of W.B. Saunders Company.)

the possibility of retractor-associated damage to soft tissue structures (**Fig. 27.3**). Care should be taken to avoid dissection lateral to the longus colli muscles, which may injure the sympathetic chain and result in a postoperative Horner's syndrome.[11]

After retractor blades are inserted and the retractor mechanism opened, the cuff on the endotracheal tube is deflated and reinflated to just barely produce an airtight seal between the cuff and the trachea. This further minimizes the chances of recurrent laryngeal injury in the larynx by reducing the pressure between the retractor blade and the endotracheal tube.

After completion of the soft tissue exposure, the spinal portion of the procedure is performed. Occasionally, this consists of a diskectomy for a traumatic disk herniation. Removal of an entire vertebral body is often required if there is significant comminution, loss of height, or retropulsion of bone into the spinal canal. Reduction of a subluxation injury can be performed using either Caspar pins in adjacent vertebral bodies or a Cobb-type curette in the disk space.

We now describe the steps in performing a single-level vertebrectomy, probably the most common anterior operation performed in the setting of mid- and lower cervical spine trauma.

The disk spaces above and below the vertebral body to be resected are identified and incised with a fine-tipped knife blade. Partial diskectomies are then performed by mobilizing disk material with small curettes and removing it in a piecemeal fashion with pituitary forceps. The vertebral body can then rapidly be removed using a rongeur or high-speed drill to start, followed by continued use of the drill.

The decompression trough thus created should be shaped like a rectangle whose ends lie just at the vertebral end plates and whose sides are parallel to the sagittal plane (**Fig. 27.4a**). It is important to stay aware of the midline to avoid penetrating the lateral cortex and endangering the vertebral artery. An operating microscope is often useful to aid in visualizing the decompression.

As the ventral spinal canal is approached, the bone is "egg shelled" and micro-curettes and Kerrison punches are used to complete the decompression. Care must be taken to perform complete diskectomies and to adequately prepare the adjacent end plates for bone grafting. The trough should be at least 15 to 18 mm wide to ensure adequate bony decompression, but should not exceed 20 mm to avoid inadvertent injury to the vertebral arteries, which lie ~ 30 mm apart in the mid- and lower cervical spine (**Fig. 27.4b**).

After bone removal has been completed, the posterior longitudinal ligament (PLL) should be resected to ensure complete decompression of the epidural space. A small curette or nerve hook is initially used to lift and open the PLL, and its removal is then completed with small Kerrison punches, taking care not to compress the dura and underlying spinal cord.

Interbody arthrodesis is performed by placing a strut graft between the end plates of the vertebral bodies adjacent to the bony defect. We generally cut the graft a few millimeters longer than the measured rostral-caudal length of the defect and tamp it into place while the neck is distracted by the anesthesiologist (**Fig. 27.5**). This places the graft under compression, and enhances the likelihood of successful fusion. The graft should be countersunk 1 mm to prevent its extrusion, but should not exceed 13 mm in depth to prevent intrusion into the spinal canal. Iliac crest autograft and iliac crest, patella, or fibula allograft are all acceptable materials. Although autograft has a slightly higher fusion rate, allograft fusion rates are comparable, and the use of allograft eliminates donor-site morbidity.[12–14] Furthermore, current methods of obtaining and preparing allograft material virtually eliminate the possibility of infectious disease transmission.

Metallic, polymeric, or carbon fiber cages packed with morselized bone have become increasingly popular and are acceptable as an alternative to strut grafting, but are associated with substantially greater cost.

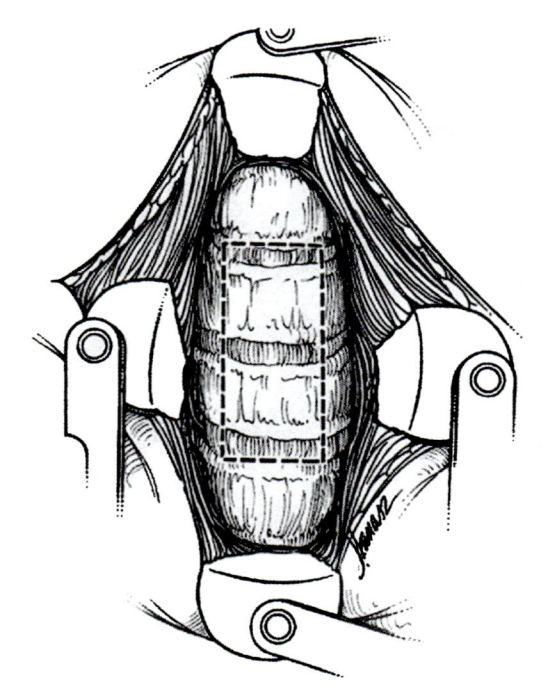

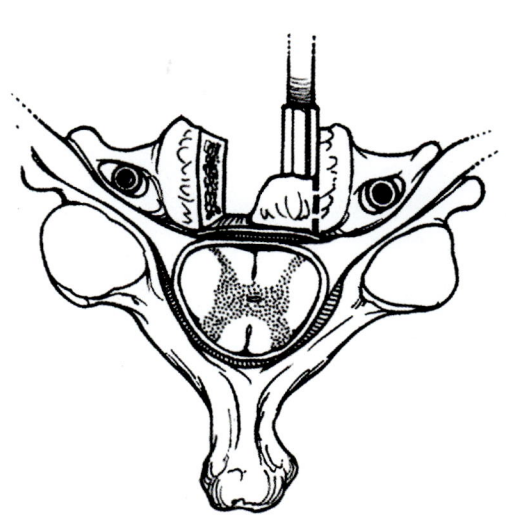

Fig. 27.4 (a) The extent of bone and disk removal for a two-level vertebrectomy *(dashed lines)*. (b) The width of the decompression should be adequate to ensure complete decompression of the spinal cord but should not exceed 20 mm to avoid vertebral artery injury. (Reproduced with permission of Lippincott, Williams and Wilkins.)

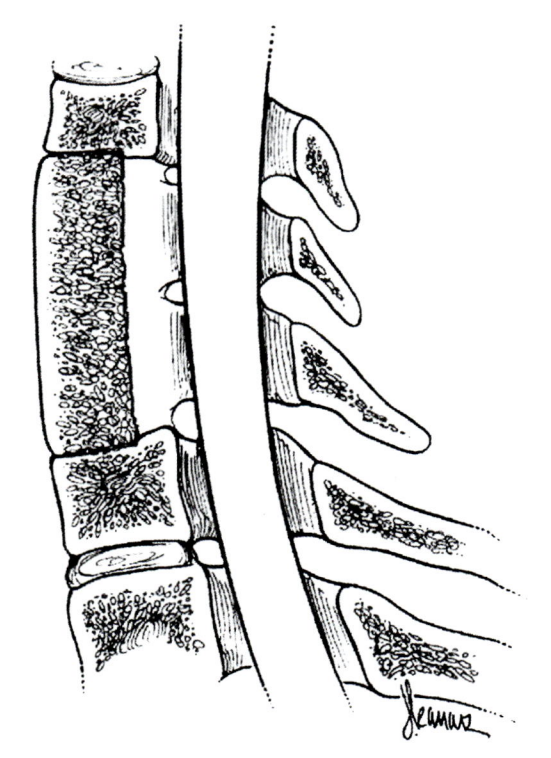

Fig. 27.5 Correct positioning of an interbody strut graft. The graft should be cut slightly longer than the decompression trough and placed while the neck is being distracted. Placement in this fashion will decrease the likelihood of graft dislodgment and will enhance the possibility of a successful fusion by putting the graft under compression. (Reproduced with permission of Lippincott, Williams and Wilkins.)

Anterior Cervical Plating

Screw-plate fixation of the anterior cervical spine has become increasingly popular to facilitate successful interbody fusion in a variety of pathological processes, particularly trauma. Anterior plates provide immediate rigid fixation, thus reducing the incidence of graft complications such as migration and pseudarthrosis, as well as obviating the need for postoperative halo-vest immobilization.[15-18] We routinely utilize cervical plating with single- and multilevel vertebrectomies performed for trauma.

Numerous cervical plating systems are available from a variety of manufacturers. A detailed discussion of the differences between the available systems is beyond the scope of this chapter, and the selection of any particular plate is largely a matter of the preference and experience of the surgeon. Plates made of titanium are generally used because they produce less artifact on postoperative MRI studies than stainless steel implants. The earliest available systems relied on bicortical screw placement, and, although they achieved excellent screw purchase, screws could penetrate the dura or cause spinal cord injury. Most current plating systems utilize unicortical screw placement, which is safer and technically easier to perform. To decrease the possibility of screw back-out, most systems have developed a mechanism to lock the screw head to the plate. The screw trajectory may be fixed, in which case the head of the screw is rigidly locked to the plate, or variable, in which the head of the screw is nonrigidly locked to the plate.

The ability to vary the angle of screw placement to achieve optimal screw placement provides surgeons with greater flexibility when confronted with abnormal anatomy or a thin, partially resected vertebral body. The variable trajectory systems may also be easier to use when working in the high cervical spine or near the cervicothoracic junction, where the jaw or the clavicle, respectively, may make standard instrument placement

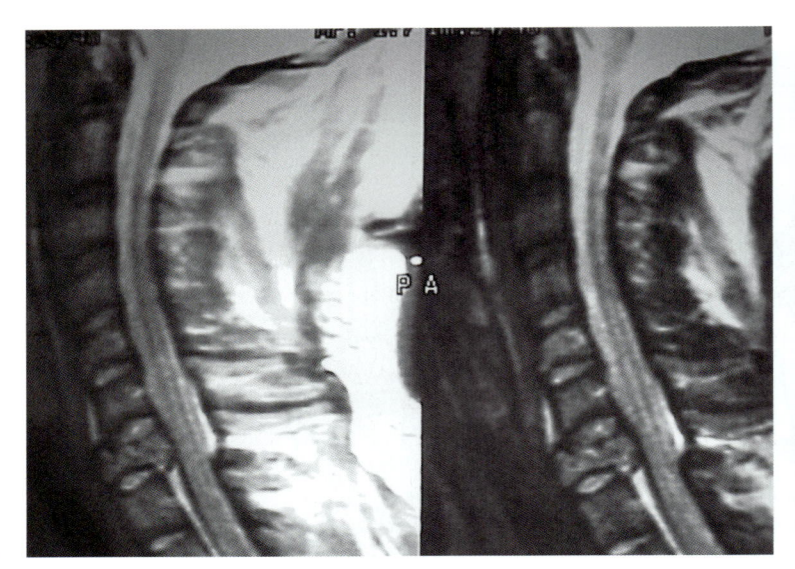

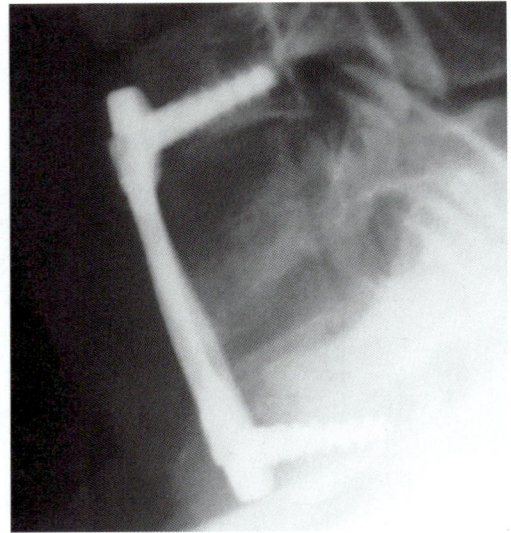

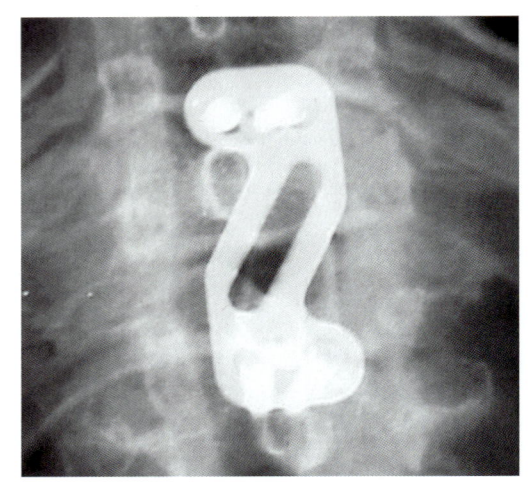

Fig. 27.6 A 17-year-old boy was involved in a high-speed motor vehicle accident. **(a)** Sagittal magnetic resonance imaging (MRI) scan demonstrates a burst fracture of C7 with bony retropulsion and spinal cord compression. **(b)** Lateral X-ray demonstrates interbody strut grafting from C6 to T1 and anterior cervical plating across the same segments using unicortical screws. **(c)** Anteroposterior view of the same construct seen in **a**, showing midline placement of the graft and plate.

more difficult. Variable trajectory systems are intrinsically less rigid than fixed trajectory systems and over time will demonstrate subsidence, which refers to a gradual load transfer from the implant to the bone graft. Theoretically, this facilitates the fusion process by placing the graft under greater compression, but it requires the screws to "windshield wiper" through the vertebral bodies, which may lead to loss of purchase.[12,19] For vertebrectomies, we now prefer to use translational plates that enable subsidence without requiring screw rotation within the bone. In the setting of trauma, any of the modern constrained four-screw (rigid screw–plate interface) plates may be used, and there is no evidence of the superiority of any particular design.

Regardless of which system is selected, the technical aspects of anterior cervical plating are similar. After completing the arthrodesis, osteophytes on the anterior aspect of the vertebral body, if present, are removed with a high-speed bur to enable the plate to sit flush on the ventral aspect of the spinal column.

Intraoperative fluoroscopy may aid direct inspection in selecting a plate of appropriate length. The plates are secured to the vertebral segments above and below the corpectomy defect with a pair of unicortical screws placed in the central portion of each body (**Fig. 27.6**). The screws should be turned with only finger-tightness to avoid "stripping" the hole. If this occurs, a larger diameter "rescue" screw can be inserted, or the plate can be repositioned and a new hole drilled. Care should be taken not to violate either the posterior cortex, which risks neural injury, or the vertebral end plate, which decreases the pullout strength of the screw. We do not recommend screw fixation of the plate to the bone graft because this may result in graft dislodgment if there is subsequent backout of the screw–plate construct and also weakens the graft.

Posterior Stabilization

Lateral Mass Plates and Screws

The use of lateral mass screws for the internal fixation of the cervical spine is an important advance in the management of patients with cervical instability and is now our preferred method for stabilizing fractures, dislocations, and ligamentous injuries to the posterior elements of the mid- and lower cervical spine. Application of either lateral mass plates and screws similar to those originally described and popularized by Roy-Camille or the new rod–screw systems are technically simple, produce immediate stability of the cervical spine, and are not dependent on the integrity of the laminae or spinous processes.[20–23]

Lateral mass screw fixation is ideal for facet dislocations caused by fractures or ligamentous injuries and is especially useful in patients with laminar and spinous process fractures when these structures cannot be wired.[23] Because the constructs are placed bilaterally at the locus of movement, they provide greater rotational stability than can be achieved with wiring of posterior midline structures.

There are few contraindications to the use of lateral screw fixation. However, this technique should be used with caution in patients with osteoporosis, metabolic bone disease, or conditions such as ankylosing spondylitis where the bone is soft; in these situations, screw pullout and loss of reduction are likely.[24] Additional points of fixation and alternative fixation techniques may be required to achieve adequate stability in these high-risk patients. Lateral mass screw fixation is also contraindicated in patients with residual neurologic function and persistent anterior compression of the spinal cord by bone, disk, or soft tissue. These situations should be addressed via an anterior approach.

Patients are brought to the operating room maintaining cervical precautions. After intubation, the patient is carefully turned to the prone position and is either placed in traction again or the head is fixed in a three-pin head holder. Intraoperative fluoroscopy is used to check alignment of the spine. A midline incision is made, and the posterior elements of the levels to be stabilized are exposed. It is important to remain in the avascular midline plane to avoid excessive bleeding and soft tissue injury. The muscles must be dissected off the bone laterally enough to expose the entire lateral mass at every location where a screw is to be placed. The levels are confirmed with fluoroscopy or a lateral X-ray.

If there is a facet dislocation that could not be reduced preoperatively, a curette or similar instrument may be wedged into the facet joint and the dislocation reduced. If this is not possible, a small bur is used to remove the superior facet of the inferior vertebra involved in the subluxation, and reduction is then performed.

The technical details of operative placement of lateral mass screws are straightforward and relatively simple and will be discussed subsequently. However, decision making regarding the number of motion segments requiring stabilization is frequently more complex; conceptual mistakes in the location of plate or rod placement probably account for more cases of inadequate fixation than technical failures.

The plates are always placed bilaterally and symmetrically (i.e., between the same vertebrae bilaterally). Two-hole plates are ideal for patients with single-level subluxations or facet dislocations (**Fig. 27.7**).

Three-level fixation is used for instability at two adjacent motion segments or when there is a fracture of the lateral mass or pedicle, precluding fixation of the lateral mass at that level. In

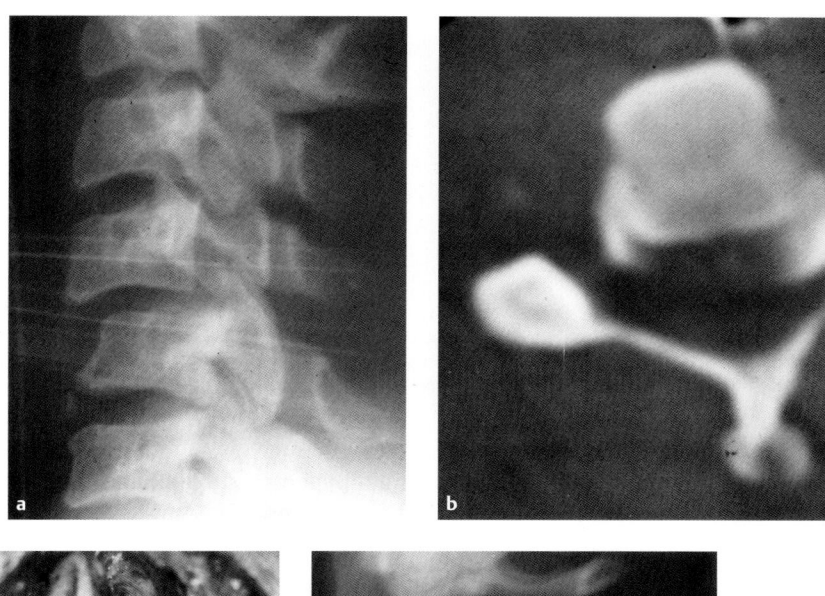

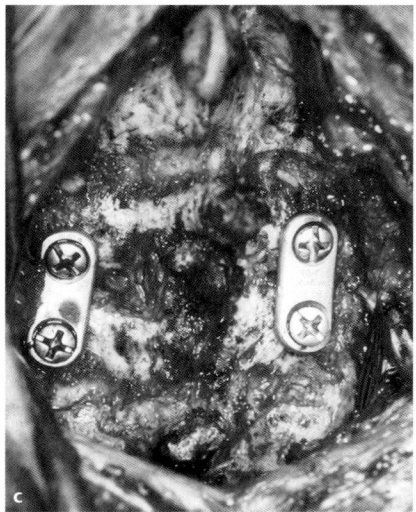

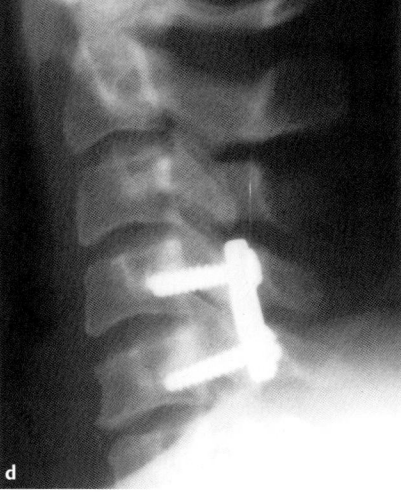

Fig. 27.7 **(a)** Lateral cervical spine X-ray showing C4-C5 subluxation. **(b)** Axial computed tomography (CT) scan at the level of subluxation demonstrates a jumped facet on the left. **(c)** Intraoperative photograph demonstrates plate placement. **(d)** Postoperative lateral X-ray demonstrates reduction of the subluxation and correct plate and screw placement at C4-C5.

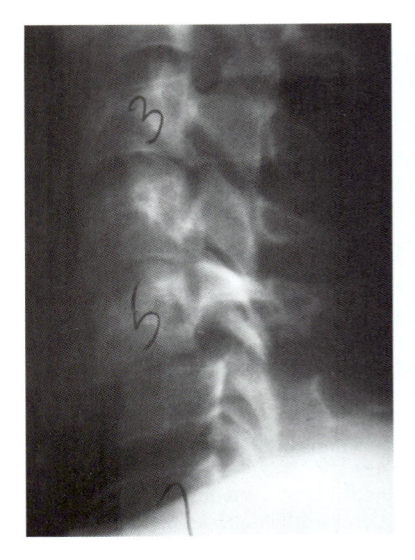

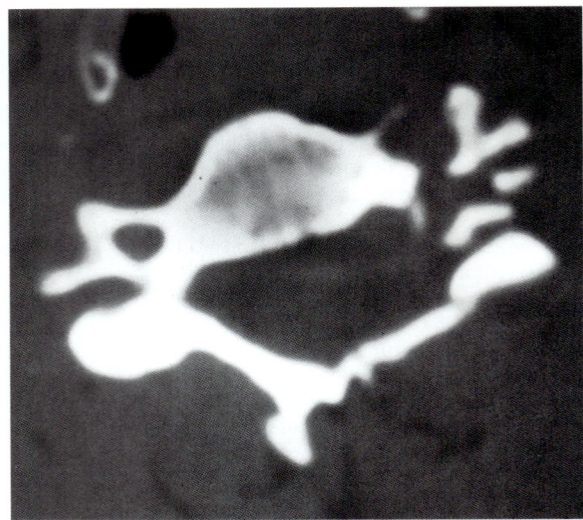

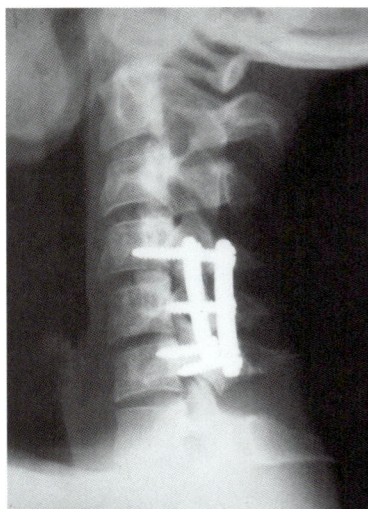

Fig. 27.8 (a) Lateral X-ray demonstrates a C5-C6 subluxation. (b) Axial CT at the C5 level demonstrates fracture of the C5 lateral mass and foramen transversarium on the left. (c) Postoperative lateral X-ray demonstrates excellent reduction of the C5-C6 subluxation. A screw could not be used to obtain fixation in the fractured left lateral mass of C5. Therefore, lateral mass plates were placed from C4 to C6. Note that there is only one screw at the C5 level.

this situation an additional adjacent motion segment must be incorporated into the construct. For example, if there is a subluxation at C4-C5 with an associated fracture of the lateral mass of C4, two-level fixation between C4 and C5 will immobilize this motion segment unilaterally only on the side of the intact lateral masses. Rotational stability will not be achieved and screw pullout and loss of alignment may occur. Application of three-level fixation from C3 to C5 is necessary in this situation (**Fig. 27.8**). The need to stabilize three or four motion segments using four- or five-level constructs is infrequent in traumatic situations, but if necessary, longer constructs will provide excellent posterior fixation.

The paraspinous muscles are reflected laterally to the most lateral aspect of the lateral mass. The lateral mass is defined by its four borders: (1) the superior facet, (2) the inferior facet, (3) the edge of the lateral mass laterally, and (4) the junction of the lateral mass and lamina medially. Two techniques have been described for screw-hole placement in the lateral mass (**Fig. 27.9**). Roy-Camille et al[23] place the hole in the exact center of the lateral mass and direct the hole 10 degrees laterally and directly anterior. Magerl et al[25] advocate hole placement 1 to 3 mm medial to the center of the lateral mass. The hole is directed 25 degrees cranially and 25 degrees laterally. Regardless of who described it, a trajectory must be selected to abut the screw tip in the "safe quadrant" of the lateral mass, which is the rostral lateral quadrant. Aiming rostrally directs the screw away from the neural foramen and nerve root, and aiming laterally directs the screw tip away from the vertebral artery. An easy technique to use when the midline structures are intact is to place the shaft of the drill guide against the subadjacent spinous process with the tip of the drill in a pilot hole just medial to the center of the lateral mass. This trajectory cannulates the longest dimension of the rhomboid-shaped lateral mass and directs the screw into the safe zone. Limiting screw length to 14 mm also decreases the likelihood of a neurovascular injury.

At C7, the lateral mass may or may not be suitable for lateral mass screw fixation. The C7 pedicle provides a strong fixation point. Placing C7 pedicle screws can be accomplished using a variety of techniques. We prefer to place the screws after performing a small laminotomy to palpate the medial, rostral, and caudal borders of the pedicle. The entrance point is generally located in the middle of (medial-lateral) and just caudal to the C6-C7 facet. The trajectory is "down and in" as opposed to "up and out" with lateral mass screws, and the drill is guided by direct palpation of the pedicle (**Fig. 27.10**). Image guidance and free-hand techniques have also been described. When incorporating a C7 pedicle screw

Magerl 25 to 30 degrees

25 degrees

Roy-Camille 10 degrees

10 degrees

25 degrees

10 degrees

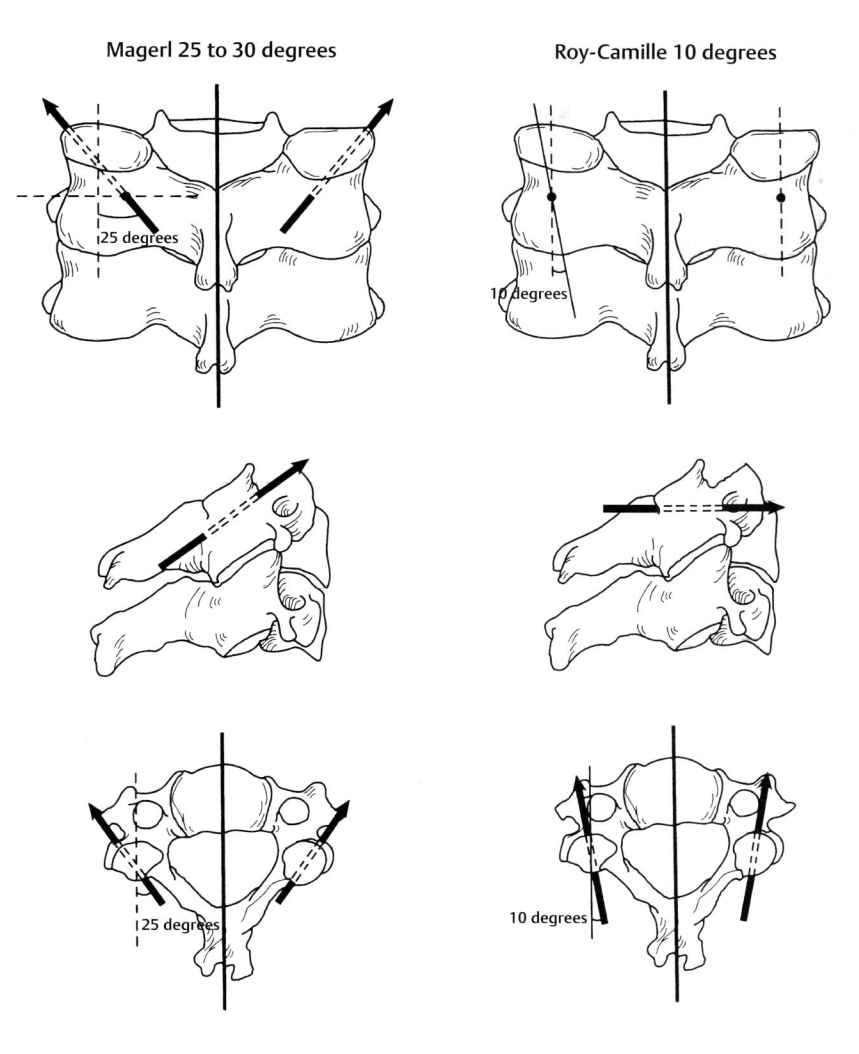

Fig. 27.9 Line drawings show two techniques for screw placement for lateral mass fixation as advocated by Magerl and Roy-Camille. See text for details. (From Montesano PX, Magerl F. Lower cervical spine arthrodesis: lateral mass plating. In: Clark C, ed. The Cervical Spine, 4th ed. Philadelphia: Lippincott-Raven; 1998:510. Reprinted with permission.)

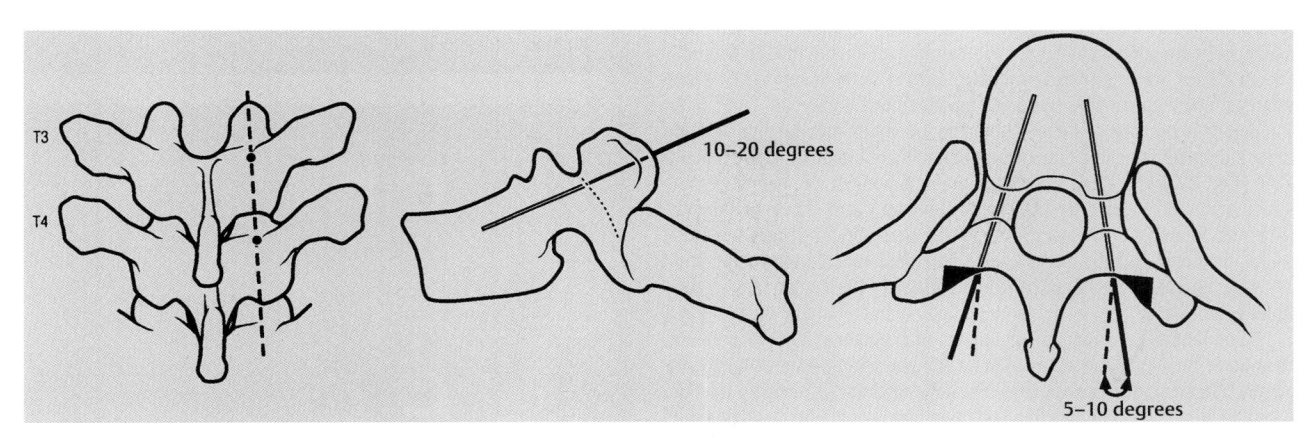

T3
T4

10–20 degrees

5–10 degrees

Fig. 27.10 Line drawing shows technique for pedicle screw placement in the upper thoracic spine. The screw hole is drilled in the midfacet line 1 to 2 mm below the superior edge of the facet. The hole is directed 10 to 20 degrees caudally and 5 to 10 degrees medially. (From Chapman JR, Anderson PA, Pepin C, Toomey S, Newell DW, Grady MS. Posterior instrumentation of the unstable cervicothoracic spine. J Neurosurg 1996;84:552–558. Reprinted with permission.)

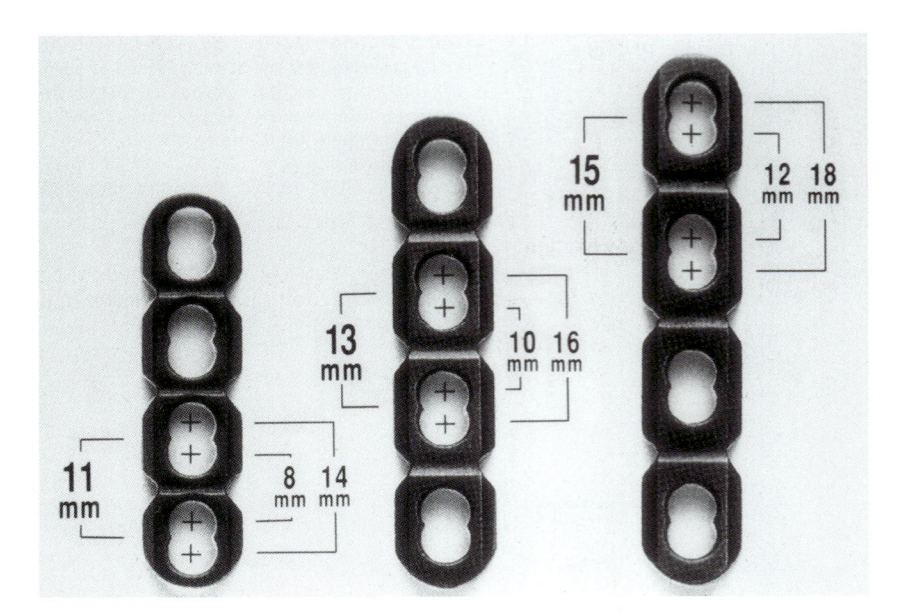

Fig. 27.11 Titanium bone plates (axis plates) manufactured by Sofamor-Danek. These are generic bone plates but are ideal for plating of the lateral mass. Plates are available in three sizes with interhole distances of 11, 13, and 15 mm.

into a cervical construct, it is important to recognize that the different trajectories of the C6 lateral mass and C7 pedicle screws result in an offset of the screw heads. This offset can usually be overcome using modern screw–rod systems, which allow for movement of the screw heads but may require sacrifice of the C6 screws in longer constructs.

Similarly, C2 does not have a lateral mass for screw fixation. Pars screws, pedicle screws, or translaminar screws may be used as points of fixation at C2. Although pars screws are easiest to incorporate into longer constructs, they do not resist flexion as well as other options. Both pars screws and pedicle screws carry the risk of vertebral artery injury, and careful study of preoperative studies is essential for safe application. C2 translaminar screws provide excellent resistance to flexion and can be placed under direct vision with no risk to the vertebral arteries. The main disadvantages of translaminar screw fixation are the requirement for intact posterior elements and some "fiddle factor" required for incorporation of the screws into screw–rod constructs. They cannot be used with older plate systems.

Several plating systems that may be used for stabilizing the cervical spine from a posterior approach are commercially available (**Fig. 27.11**). These systems perform well in the midcervical spine and reproduce the posterior tension band. They are more difficult to use at the craniocervical junction and cervicothoracic junction and do not provide intrinsic resistance to flexion or translation, necessitating extension of the construct if the facet is not intact.

The latest generation of screw–rod systems offers screws that have polyaxial heads into which a rod may be fitted and secured. These systems are quite versatile and are especially useful for multilevel fixation, where screws may not line up, making plate fixation difficult. Screw–rod systems also enable compression and distraction to be applied segmentally, which can be useful in helping to correct deformities and reduce subluxations (**Fig. 27.12**). However, these systems are significantly more expensive than plates, and are not generally necessary for straightforward one- or two-level stabilization procedures.

Once screws are placed (or immediately prior to screw placement if a plate system is used), the facet joints within the fusion are denuded with curettes and a high-speed drill with a matchstick bit. Small pieces of locally harvested autograft (spinous

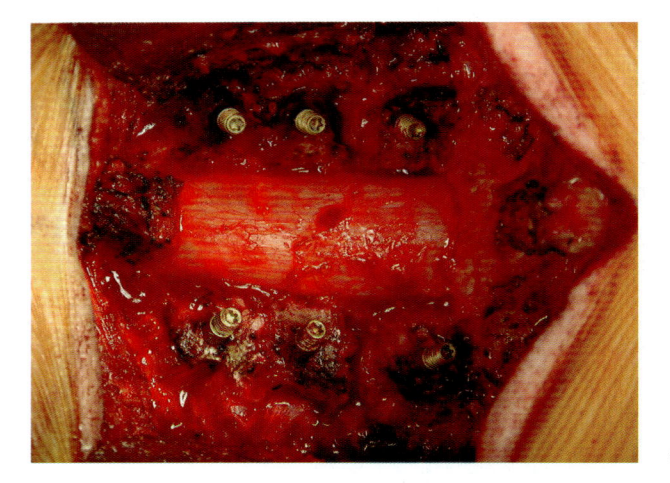

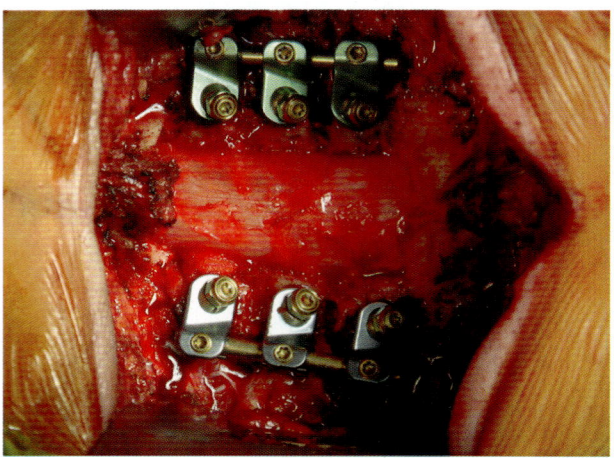

Fig. 27.12 An elderly man with central cord syndrome following a fall was brought to the operating room for laminectomy and fusion, and was found to have severe splaying of the facet joints at C5-C6. **(a,b)** Intraoperative photographs. The ability to compress across the rods facilitated reduction of the splaying, and the patient healed well postoperatively.

process) are packed into the joints to provide fusion. Extra bone graft may be placed laterally to enhance the fusion.

Patients are allowed out of bed the day after operation. The neck is immobilized for 6 weeks using a rigid collar. Lateral cervical spine films are taken once in the first week after operation and prior to collar removal. When the collar is removed, dynamic flexion and extension films of the cervical spine are taken to confirm stability.

Cervical Facet Wiring

Two types of cervical facet wiring have been reported. Callahan et al[26] have described a technique that entails drilling holes in the inferior facets of the vertebrae to be stabilized. Two strands of twisted 24-gauge wire are passed through each hole and tied around a corticocancellous iliac crest graft. The technique was originally described for the control of postlaminectomy instability and may also be used for patients with posttraumatic instability. Because it does not provide immediate internal fixation, it must be used with an orthotic device such as a halo vest until the bone graft fuses. This method of internal fixation is inferior to lateral mass plates and is now of historical interest only.

Cahill et al[27] have described bilateral wiring of the facet to the spinous process. They believe that this technique is particularly appropriate when one or both facet joints are disrupted by trauma, a situation where spinous process wiring may not provide sufficient rotational stability. Holes are drilled bilaterally in the inferior facet of the upper vertebra to be stabilized, and braided strands of 22- or 24-gauge wire are passed through the holes in the facets and tied around the inferior spinous process. Bilateral wiring is performed even if only one facet has been disrupted. After the wires are tightened, pieces of corticocancellous bone graft are placed over the posterior elements. The technique cannot be used if the posterior elements of the lower vertebra to be stabilized or the inferior facet of the upper vertebra has been fractured. Unfortunately, this precludes its use in a high percentage of patients with spinal fractures. Moreover, maintenance of stability depends on a thin piece of bone of the inferior facet; pullout of the wire through the facet may occur as the wire is tightened around the spinous process. This technique has also been largely supplanted by the use of lateral mass screw fixation.

Cervical Clamp and Hook Systems

Halifax clamps have historically been used to treat atlantoaxial instability but can also be used for stabilization of the subaxial spine. The device consists of two small hooks that engage the laminae of the vertebrae to be stabilized. The hooks are connected by a threaded screw, which is turned, resulting in progressive tightening of the clamps.[28–30] The more rounded hooks used at C1 are not employed, and only the square (more acutely angled) hooks are used to engage the cervical laminae to be stabilized. The hooks have several disadvantages in stabilizing the subaxial spine: (1) they cannot be applied if there are fractures of the posterior elements or pedicle; (2) the hooks hug the anterior aspect of the laminae and are located within the spinal canal, creating the potential for iatrogenic injury to the spinal cord; and (3) the hooks are poorly designed, with loss of fixation being not uncommon. For these reasons, they are not commonly used.

Interspinous Wiring

Interspinous wiring is the oldest method of posterior stabilization of the subaxial spine.[31] It is simple and easy to perform and requires no specialized equipment. However, it cannot be used when there are fractures of the spinous process, laminae, or facets of the vertebrae requiring stabilization. Because the wire is placed at the midline, it provides less rotational stability than bilaterally applied lateral mass fixation. Although this technique is less frequently employed since the advent of lateral mass screws, it is an effective means of stabilizing the subaxial cervical spine and is especially useful in patients with bone that is too soft to hold screws. It may also be used to supplement lateral mass plates and screws if there is concern about the adequacy of screw fixation.

Patients are managed preoperatively and positioned in the same manner described in the section Lateral Mass Plates and Screws, above. After exposure of the posterior elements to be stabilized, dislocated facets are reduced. If the level of instability is unclear at the time of exposure of the posterior elements, a lateral X-ray is taken. A right-angle drill or towel clip is used to make a hole in the base of the upper spinous process to be stabilized. It is essential that the hole be made at the most rostral portion of the spinous process and as close as possible to the base of the spinous process to minimize the chances of the wire cutting through the hole.

A 1.0- or 1.2-mm wire is passed through the hole and brought around the lower spinous process. Alternatively, a multi-stranded cable may be used to achieve fixation. The downward slope of the lower spinous processes usually prevents the wire from slipping off, but a small notch may be made at the base of the spinous process to provide a seat for the wire. The ends of the wire are brought around the lower spinous process and are tightened using a wire twister. Arthrodesis is then performed using pieces of cancellous and corticocancellous iliac crest autograft, which may be secured with the ends of the wire (**Fig. 27.13**). Closure is performed in the routine fashion without drains. Patients are kept in a rigid collar or halo for 3 months, after which flexion-extension X-rays of the cervical spine are obtained to assess stability.

Capen et al[32] have described a technique of interspinous wiring that is used in patients with fractures of the vertebral body, in which the spinous process of the injured vertebral body is skipped, and wiring is performed from the spinous process of the vertebra above to the spinous process of the vertebra below.

Inclusion of the vertebrae adjacent to the level of the injury is essential if the disk spaces adjacent to the vertebral body fracture have been injured. However, we prefer to include the spinous process of the injured vertebral body in the fusion construct.[31,33] Stabilization of two motion segments is also necessary when there is a fracture of the lamina, spinous process, or pedicle of a vertebra that was to be wired. In this case the fractured posterior element is skipped and wiring is performed to the spinous process above or below the fractured one.

The use of methylmethacrylate as an adjunct to posterior wiring has been advocated by Branch et al.[34] They contend that the technique avoids the necessity for bone grafting and results in immediate stability. Their reported results using the technique have been excellent. However, others have questioned the use of methylmethacrylate instead of bone grafting, and have reported a high incidence of failure of immobilization.[35] It is our opinion that methylmethacrylate is rarely, if ever, indicated for stabilization of the cervical spine following trauma. Methylmethacrylate poured over wire constructs adds little or no strength to the construct, it never fuses to bone, and forever remains a foreign body susceptible to infection. Bone grafts, on the other hand, are vascularized and are fused to adjacent posterior elements. They become stronger with time rather than weaker, and provide more strength over the long term than does methylmethacrylate.

The complications of posterior wiring techniques relate mostly to wire breakage or dislodgment. Failure of interspinous wiring may result if the wire cuts through the hole in the upper spinous process as a result of incorrect hole placement. Soft bone

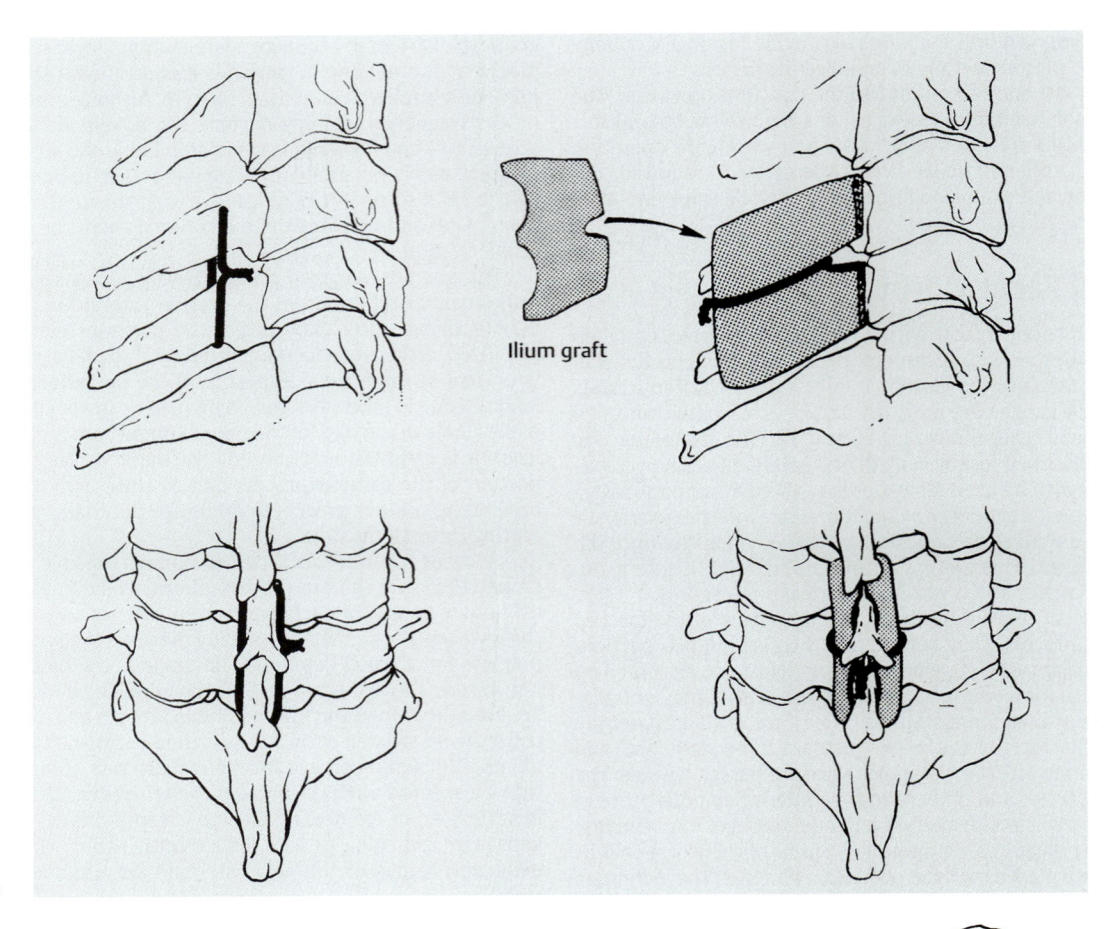

Fig. 27.13 **(a)** Line drawing shows technique of wiring two spinous processes. Stainless steel wire is passed through a hole at the base of the spinous process of the rostral vertebra and tightened around the base of the caudal vertebra. A piece of corticocancellous iliac crest graft is placed bilaterally against the spinous processes and secured with a second wire. **(b)** Technique for stabilizing three vertebrae with interspinous wires. The most rostral spinous process is wired to the middle spinous process, which is in turn wired to the caudal spinous process. Bone grafts may be placed as shown in **a**. (From Benzel EC, Kesterson L. Posterior cervical interspinous compression wiring and fusion for mid to low cervical spinal injuries. J Neurosurg 1989;70:893–899. Reprinted with permission.)

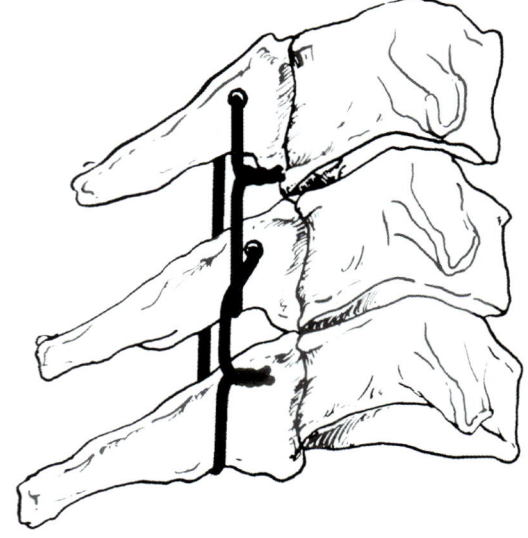

in patients with osteoporosis or metabolic bone disease may also result in wire pullout. Careful preoperative assessment with CT and intraoperative observation are essential to rule out fractures of the pedicle, spinous process, or facet of the vertebrae to be stabilized. Injury to any of these structures precludes wiring of the involved vertebra.

If the wire is insufficiently tightened or does not engage the lower spinous process at its base, the wire may slip off with loss of fixation. Because interspinous wiring provides less than optimal rotational stability, it is possible for facet dislocations to recur. In practice, however, this is infrequent.

Wire breakage is a distressing complication that may result in loss of reduction and necessitate reoperation. It occurs because of inadequate external mobilization or failure to use wires of sufficient diameter. Breakage of wires 1.0 to 1.2 mm in diameter is unusual.

Sublaminar Wiring

Sublaminar wiring is infrequently used in the subaxial cervical spine. Because the spinal canal in the lower cervical region is smaller than at C1-C2, sublaminar wiring techniques carry the risk of spinal cord injury and should be avoided.[36]

Combined Anterior and Posterior Stabilization

Combined anterior and posterior stabilization of the subaxial cervical spine is indicated when there is injury to both the anterior and posterior elements.[37] Such patients present with kyphosis, CT and plain film evidence of separation of the facets, and vertebral body fracture. If vertebrectomy must be performed to accomplish decompression of the spinal canal, bone grafting and anterior plating frequently do not provide sufficient fixation; plate loosening and graft extrusion are likely. In this situation we first perform anterior operation and then turn the patient and place posterior instrumentation to include two motion segments.

If the vertebral body is fractured but not retropulsed into the spinal canal and vertebrectomy is not necessary, posterior stabilization with wiring or lateral mass plates alone may be sufficient to stabilize the spine. However, compromise of anterior column support due to compression fracture and loss of height of the vertebral body may place considerable stress on the posterior instrumentation and predispose the construct to failure.

References

1. Marshall LF, Knowlton S, Garfin SR, et al. Deterioration following spinal cord injury. A multicenter study. J Neurosurg 1987;66:400–404
2. Wright SW, Robinson GG II, Wright MB. Cervical spine injuries in blunt trauma patients requiring emergent endotracheal intubation. Am J Emerg Med 1992;10:104–109
3. Gunby I. New focus on spinal cord injury. JAMA 1981;245:1201–1206
4. Ryken TC, Hadley MN, Walters BC, et al. Radiographic assessment. Neurosurgery 2013;72(Suppl 2):54–72
5. Walters BC, Hadley MN, Hurlbert RJ, et al; American Association of Neurological Surgeons; Congress of Neurological Surgeons. Guidelines for the management of acute cervical spine and spinal cord injuries: 2013 update. Neurosurgery 2013;60(Suppl 1):82–91
6. Harrigan MR, Hadley MN, Dhall SS, et al. Management of vertebral artery injuries following non-penetrating cervical trauma. Neurosurgery 2013;72(Suppl 2):234–243
7. Gelb DE, Hadley MN, Aarabi B, et al. Initial closed reduction of cervical spinal fracture-dislocation injuries. Neurosurgery 2013;72(Suppl 2):73–83
8. Epstein NE. Somatosensory evoked potential monitoring in cervical spine surgery. In: Cooper PR, ed. Neurosurgical Topics: Degenerative Diseases of the Cervical Spine. Park Ridge, IL: American Association of Neurological Surgeons; 1992:73–90
9. Resnick DK, Anderson PA, Kaiser MG, et al; Joint Section on Disorders of the Spine and Peripheral Nerves of the American Association of Neurological Surgeons and Congress of Neurological Surgeons. Electrophysiological monitoring during surgery for cervical degenerative myelopathy and radiculopathy. J Neurosurg Spine 2009;11:245–252
10. Bulger RF, Rejowski JE, Beatty RA. Vocal cord paralysis associated with anterior cervical fusion: considerations for prevention and treatment. J Neurosurg 1985;62:657–661
11. Graham JJ. Complications of cervical spine surgery. In: Cervical Spine Research Society, Editorial Committee, eds. The Cervical Spine. Philadelphia: Lippincott; 1989
12. Kaufman HH, Jones E. The principles of bony spinal fusion. Neurosurgery 1989;24:264–270
13. Prolo DJ. Biology of bone fusion. Clin Neurosurg 1990;36:135–146
14. Zdeblick TA, Ducker TB. The use of freeze-dried allograft bone for anterior cervical fusions. Spine 1991;16:726–729
15. Brown JA, Havel P, Ebraheim N, Greenblatt SH, Jackson WT. Cervical stabilization by plate and bone fusion. Spine 1988;13:236–240
16. Caspar W. Anterior stabilization with trapezoid osteosynthetic technique in cervical spine injuries. In: Kehr P, Weidner A, eds. Cervical Spine, vol. 1. New York: Springer; 1987:198–204
17. Kalfas IH. The anterior cervical spine locking plate: a technique for surgical decompression and stabilization. In: Fessler RG, Haid RW, eds. Techniques in Spinal Stabilization. New York: McGraw-Hill; 1996:25–33
18. Tippets RH, Apfelbaum RI. Anterior cervical fusion with the Caspar instrumentation system. Neurosurgery 1988;22(6 Pt 1):1008–1013
19. McAfee PC, Farey ID, Sutterlin CE, Gurr KR, Warden KE, Cunningham BW. 1989 Volvo Award in basic science. Device-related osteoporosis with spinal instrumentation. Spine 1989;14:919–926
20. Cooper PR, Cohen A, Rosiello A, Koslow M. Posterior stabilization of cervical spine fractures and subluxations using plates and screws. Neurosurgery 1988;23:300–306
21. Roy-Camille R, Saillant G, Berteaux D. Early management of spinal injuries. In: McKibbon B, ed. Recent Advances in Orthopedics. New York: Churchill Livingstone; 1979:57–87
22. Roy-Camille R, Saillant G, Judet T, Mammoudy P. [Recent injuries of the last 5 cervical vertebrae in the adult (with and without neurologic complications)]. Sem Hop 1983;59:1479–1488
23. Roy-Camille R, Saillant G, Laville C, Benazet JP. Treatment of lower cervical spinal injuries—C3 to C7. Spine 1992;17(10, Suppl):S442–S446
24. Eismont FJ, Bohlman HH. Posterior methylmethacrylate fixation for cervical trauma. Spine 1981;6:347–353
25. Magerl F, Grob D, Seemann D. Stable dorsal fusion of the cervical spine (C2-Th1) using hook plates. In: Kehr P, Weidner A, eds. Cervical Spine, vol. 1. New York: Springer-Verlag; 1987:217–221
26. Callahan RA, Johnson RM, Margolis RN, Keggi KJ, Albright JA, Southwick WO. Cervical facet fusion for control of instability following laminectomy. J Bone Joint Surg Am 1977;59:991–1002
27. Cahill DW, Bellegarrigue R, Ducker TB. Bilateral facet to spinous process fusion: a new technique for posterior spinal fusion after trauma. Neurosurgery 1983;13:1–4
28. Aldrich EF, Crow WN, Weber PB, Spagnolia TN. Use of MR imaging-compatible Halifax interlaminar clamps for posterior cervical fusion. J Neurosurg 1991;74:185–189
29. Aldrich EF, Weber PB, Crow WN. Halifax interlaminar clamp for posterior cervical fusion: a long-term follow-up review. J Neurosurg 1993;78:702–708
30. Holness RO, Huestis WS, Howes WJ, Langille RA. Posterior stabilization with an interlaminar clamp in cervical injuries: technical note and review of the long term experience with the method. Neurosurgery 1984;14:318–322
31. Benzel EC, Kesterson L. Posterior cervical interspinous compression wiring and fusion for mid to low cervical spinal injuries. J Neurosurg 1989;70:893–899
32. Capen DA, Garland DE, Waters RL. Surgical stabilization of the cervical spine. A comparative analysis of anterior and posterior spine fusions. Clin Orthop Relat Res 1985;196:229–237
33. White AA III, Panjabi MM. The role of stabilization in the treatment of cervical spine injuries. Spine 1984;9:512–522
34. Branch CL Jr, Kelly DL Jr, Davis CH Jr, McWhorter JM. Fixation of fractures of the lower cervical spine using methylmethacrylate and wire: technique and results in 99 patients. Neurosurgery 1989;25:503–512, discussion 512–513
35. Whitehill R, Cicoria AD, Hooper WE, Maggio WW, Jane JA. Posterior cervical reconstruction with methyl methacrylate cement and wire: a clinical review. J Neurosurg 1988;68:576–584
36. Geremia GK, Kim KS, Cerullo L, Calenoff L. Complications of sublaminar wiring. Surg Neurol 1985;23:629–635
37. Cybulski GR, Douglas RA, Meyer PR Jr, Rovin RA. Complications in three-column cervical spine injuries requiring anterior-posterior stabilization. Spine 1992;17:253–256

B. Anterior Approach

28 Cervical Spine: Anterior Approach, Diskectomy, and Corpectomy

Rueben Nair, Marco C. Mendoza, and Wellington K. Hsu

First introduced in the 1950s,[1] anterior cervical diskectomy and fusion (ACDF) is now widely used to treat cervical spondylotic radiculopathy and myelopathy with long-term clinical success.[2,3] ACDF enables removal of compressive lesions of the spinal cord, such as osteophytes, intervertebral disks, and ossified posterior longitudinal ligaments (OPLLs). Use of instrumentation (plating) has led to a further increase in fusion rates and a reduction of graft-related complications such as subsidence (see Video 28.1).[4]

Patient Selection

Patient selection is essential to achieving optimal results. Positive predictors of outcome include higher baseline Neck Disability Index scores, older age, and preoperative working status (if the patient had gainful employment prior to surgery). Conversely, negative predictors include ongoing litigation, workers' compensation, and dermatomal sensory loss.[5] Nonetheless, instrumented ACDF surgery has been shown to have clinical success rates of 97% and 94% for one- and two-level fusions, respectively, at a mean clinical follow-up ≥ 12 months.[6]

Corpectomy may be indicated when the extent of epidural compression extends beyond the level of the disk space, or if there is retrovertebral stenosis. Additionally, fusion rates for corpectomy with strut grafting are higher compared with diskectomy and interbody grafting in multilevel disease.[7,8]

Indications

- Radiculopathy/myelopathy from spondylosis or disk herniation
- Degenerative instability
- Kyphosis
- Trauma
- Tumor
- Infection

Relative Contraindications

- Multilevel congenital stenosis
- Severe ligamentum flavum hypertrophy
- Prior anterior neck infection/scarring
- Occupation dependent on voice
- Vocal cord dysfunction

Advantages

- Familiar, reproducible approach
- Successful outcomes in pain relief and resolution of neurologic symptoms
- Applicable to a variety of pathological conditions

Disadvantages

- Adjacent segment disease
- Neurologic/vascular injury
- Dysphagia, dysphonia
- Airway risks including reintubation
- Inability to address posterior spinal pathology

Preoperative Tests

- Upright plain radiographs to assess overall alignment and stability
- Magnetic resonance imaging (MRI) to evaluate neural compression
- Computed tomography (CT) myelogram if MRI contraindicated

Surgical Procedure

Anesthesia and Positioning

The patient is placed in the supine position on a standard operating room table. The head can be stabilized using a Mayfield horseshoe headrest (**Fig. 28.1**). A rolled towel is placed between the scapulae to increase accessibility to the anterior spine. Mechanical injury as a result of neck hyperextension during intubation must be avoided, especially in the setting of preexisting myelopathy. In an unstable cervical spine, the neck is kept in a neutral position and may require fiberoptic intubation. Gardner-Wells tongs may be utilized in situations where distraction is required (corpectomy). After adequate padding along the bony prominences, the arms are tucked to the sides. The shoulders are then pulled caudally and secured to the operating table with broad cloth tape, which facilitates optimal fluoroscopic visualization of the cervical spine, especially at C6-C7 and C7-T1 levels.

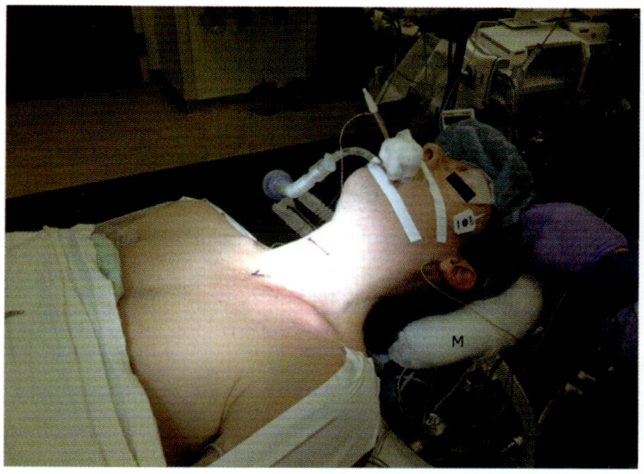

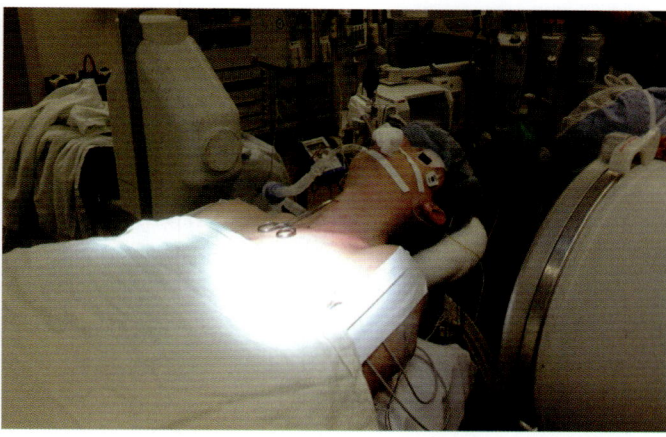

28 Cervical Spine: Anterior Approach, Diskectomy, and Corpectomy

Fig. 28.1 Positioning. **(a)** Supine position with head stabilized using Mayfield horseshoe headrest (M). Note the neck is in a neutral position. **(b)** Fluoroscope positioned to obtain lateral C-spine imaging. The shoulders are pulled in a caudal direction using cloth tape to facilitate adequate fluoroscopic visualization.

However, excessive shoulder traction could result in injury to the brachial plexus. Neuromonitoring with somatosensory evoked and motor evoked potentials may also be utilized depending on the surgical indication or surgeon preference.

Approach

Right Versus Left-Sided Approach

Multiple studies favor either a right- or left-sided approach.[9–12] Historical literature initially favored a left-sided approach based on the susceptibility of injury to the right recurrent laryngeal nerve (RLN) from more unpredictable anatomy. The right RLN makes a more oblique angle than the left RLN in the sagittal plane after looping around the subclavian artery traveling toward the midline. In addition, prior studies raised concern of its susceptibility to injury as it was thought to travel anterior and lateral to the tracheoesophageal groove[13] (**Fig. 28.2**). However, later anatomic studies have refuted this variation,[11,14] and clinical studies have demonstrated that the choice of operative side had no effect on the incidence of RLN palsy.[9,15] Additionally, there is some evidence suggesting that reduction in endotracheal cuff pressure during retractor placement decreases damage to the RLN.[16]

A right-sided approach does place the thoracic duct at risk. The thoracic duct is a conduit for the return of lymph to the bloodstream ascending dorsal to the aortic arch between the left side of the esophagus and pleura to the root of the neck dorsal to the left subclavian artery. Injury to this structure may result in chylothorax and severe metabolic derangements.[10]

Surgeon comfort can affect the choice of the approach, with right-handed surgeons being more comfortable with a right-sided approach and vice versa. Aberrant vasculature should also be noted on preoperative imaging studies, which may influence the choice of laterality. The carotid artery has been shown to be medial to its typical position (lateral to the foramen transversarium)

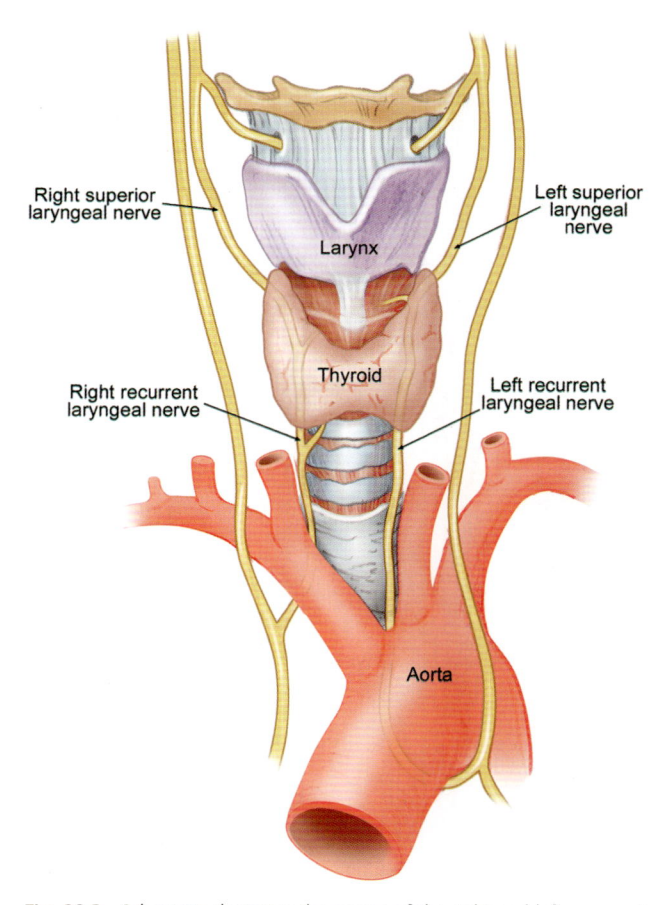

Fig. 28.2 Schematic depicting the course of the right and left recurrent laryngeal nerve (RLN). Note the corresponding vertebral levels.

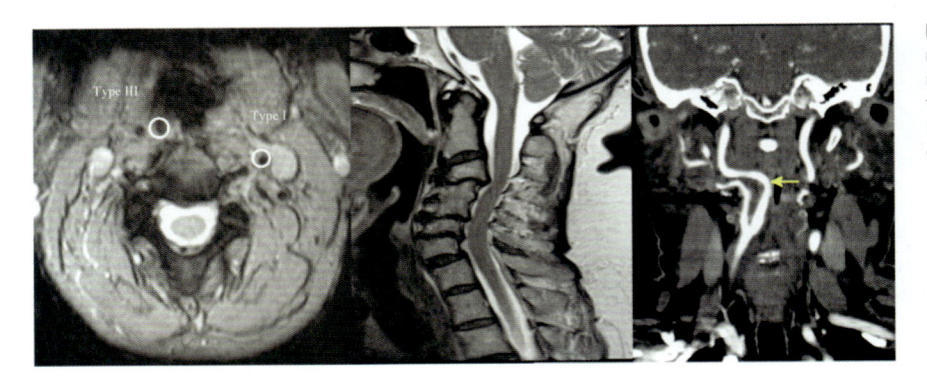

Fig. 28.3 Example of a right-sided retropharyngeal artery in a patient with spondylotic myelopathy. Note the retropharyngeal location of the right internal carotid artery (type III, *arrow*) compared with the normal position on the left (type I).

in as high as 12.3% of the population (**Fig. 28.3**).[17] We recommend critical analysis of the vasculature on preoperative MRI before the side of approach is chosen.

Illumination and Magnification

An operating microscope provides better illumination and visualization than do loupes and headlights. Additionally, the microscope affords the assistant the same view as the operating surgeon. It is necessary to continually adjust the viewing angle so that the line of sight remains parallel to the disk space to facilitate optimal visualization. Despite these marked benefits, the microscope does present another potential source of contamination into the field.[18] To maintain sterility, it is recommended that sterile members of the surgical team should change gloves after making adjustments to the optic eyepieces as well as avoid handling portions of the drape above the eyepieces.

Dissection

In one- to three-level diskectomies, a transverse incision is sufficient, but more extensile exposures may require either a longitudinal (vertical) incision or multiple transverse incisions. Lateral fluoroscopy or superficial landmarks (**Fig. 28.4**) are used to localize the level of the incision. Accuracy with incision placement can help prevent unnecessary dissection and exposure leading to adjacent segment disease. After completion of the skin incision, the platysma can be dissected in line with the skin incision using electrocautery. The sternocleidomastoid, enveloped by the deep cervical fascia, should now be identified, and blunt dissection is

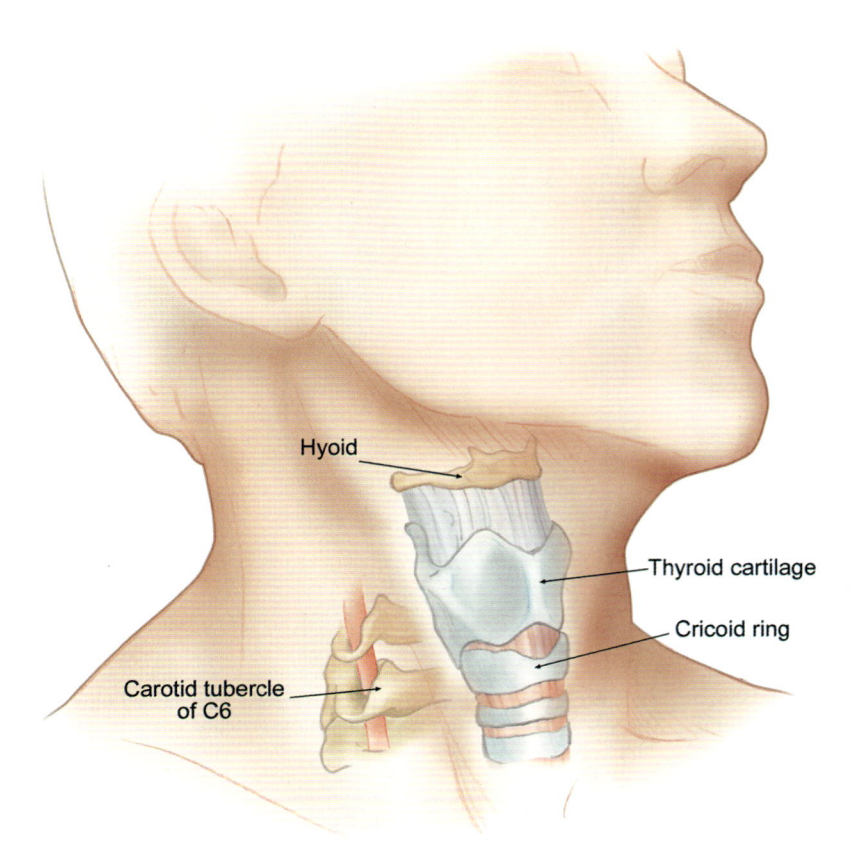

Fig. 28.4 Palpable structures in the neck may be used to determine the approximate level of the incision: hyoid bone C3, thyroid cartilage C4-C5, cricoid cartilage C6, carotid tubercle C6.

carried along its anteromedial aspect, retracting the strap muscles medially. Next, finger dissection is directed medially toward the anterior cervical spine, which proceeds between the carotid sheath laterally and the trachea and esophagus medially. The omohyoid muscle can be encountered during this step (usually at C5-C6), in which the surgeon can push either caudally or cranially depending on the location of the disk space. The prevertebral fascia, which directly lies over the cervical spine, can be bluntly stripped away with Kittner retractors to expose the medial edge of the longus colli muscles. These muscles can then be reflected laterally with electrocautery on the surface of the vertebral body, enabling subperiosteal placement of a self-retaining retractor beneath the longus colli. Sharp dissection should halt when the vertebral body begins to slope downward to the edge of the transversarium foramen. Straying lateral to the longus colli muscle places the sympathetic chain at risk, leading to a possible Horner's syndrome, which is a neurologic condition characterized by ptosis, miosis, and anhidrosis.

Diskectomy

After completion of adequate exposure, a spinal needle may be used to confirm proper operative levels. Because placement of a needle in an adjacent disk space can lead to a higher rate of degeneration,[19] one option may be to localize the operative level in a vertebral body. An anterior annulotomy is then performed sharply with a No. 15 blade scalpel with en-bloc resection and release of the disk space. Next, Caspar pins are placed in the vertebral bodies cranial and caudal to the corresponding disk (**Fig. 28.5**). The operating microscope can be introduced after this step with the retractors in place. After applying distraction, the diskectomy is completed with a combination of rongeurs and curettes. Uncinate processes are used as lateral borders of the decompression. Removing bone lateral to these structures places the vertebral artery at risk.[20] In spondylotic cases, there is commonly an anterior-inferior osteophyte from the cranial vertebra that should be removed to improve visualization of the posterior disk osteophytes. These bone spurs can be removed using an oscillating bur. There are different types of bur tips available. Our recommended approach is to use a side-cutting bur tip, which can protect the dura while applying direct pressure on the osteophyte. The side-cutting nature of the bur tip resects bone from the periphery rather than the tip where pressure can be applied onto neural structures. After adequate bony resection,

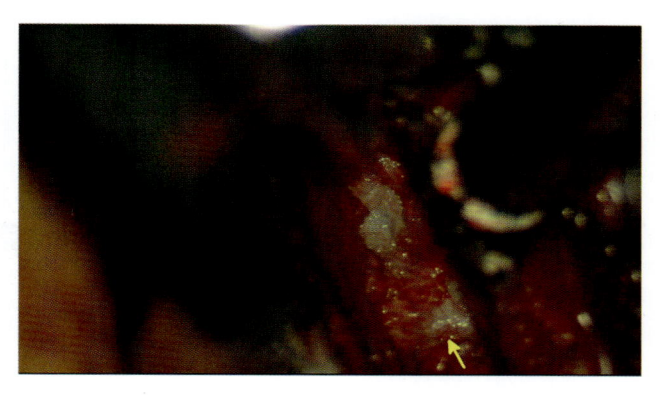

Fig. 28.6 Intraoperative view of the posterior longitudinal ligament (arrow) after removal of the annulus.

an angled Epstein curette may then be used to detach the posterior annulus fibers, exposing the posterior longitudinal ligament (PLL) either centrally or in the foramen (**Fig. 28.6**). A nerve hook can then be placed behind each vertebra and foramen to assess the adequacy of decompression. Complete resection of the PLL is not necessary except in the setting of central stenosis or a soft disk herniation beneath the PLL.

The final step before graft placement is the contouring of the end plates to accommodate the geometry of the implant. Depending on the graft used (lordotic or parallel), the end plates can be milled to facilitate a press-fit construct with either a cage or allograft spacer. Preliminary measurements can also be made from the preoperative MRI. Various commercially available graft sizers can be used. The trial rasps should have a secure interference fit under gentle Caspar pin distraction, thus ensuring an optimal fit after discontinuation of distraction. The graft should ideally fill as much space as possible without overdistraction or violation of the spinal canal.

Corpectomy

Diskectomy is first performed cranial and caudal to the vertebral body before bony resection. A Leksell rongeur can be utilized to remove the vertebral body for bone grafting, to be placed either in a cage or allograft spacer. A Penfield No. 4 instrument can then be used to palpate the foramen transversarium (where the vertebral body falls off) to identify the lateral borders of the corpectomy. A high-speed bur can then be used along the vertebral body to delineate the lateral borders of safe decompression for the corpectomy (medial edge of uncinate on each side). Understanding of relevant anatomy is critical to a successful corpectomy. The transverse foramina are ~20 mm apart; therefore, as a rule of thumb, only a 16- to 18-mm wide trough of bone centered at the midline should be resected to decompress the canal without inadvertent vertebral artery injury. The longus colli can also be used as landmarks to maintain orientation when performing the resection.

The residual posterior cortex is then removed with a curette or Kerrison rongeur to direct forces away from the canal to avoid potential neural injury. The residual PLL is then removed under direct visualization. A microcurette is used to disrupt the longitudinal fibers on the lateral aspect of the PLL to establish a dorsal plane to the PLL without inadvertent spinal cord damage. A 1-mm Kerrison rongeur can then be used to complete the PLL resection. The end plates should be appropriately decorticated and denuded of all cartilaginous material to facilitate bony union, but excessive end-plate removal must be avoided to prevent end-plate collapse or graft subsidence.

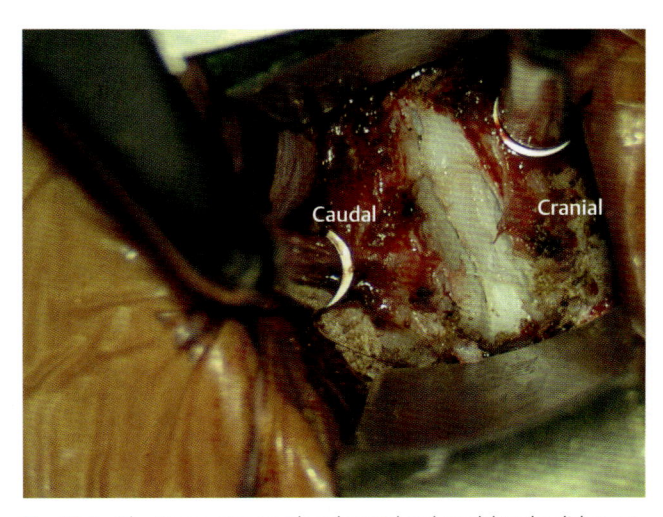

Fig. 28.5 The Caspar pins are placed cranial and caudal to the disk space, providing distraction and facilitating visualization for the decompression.

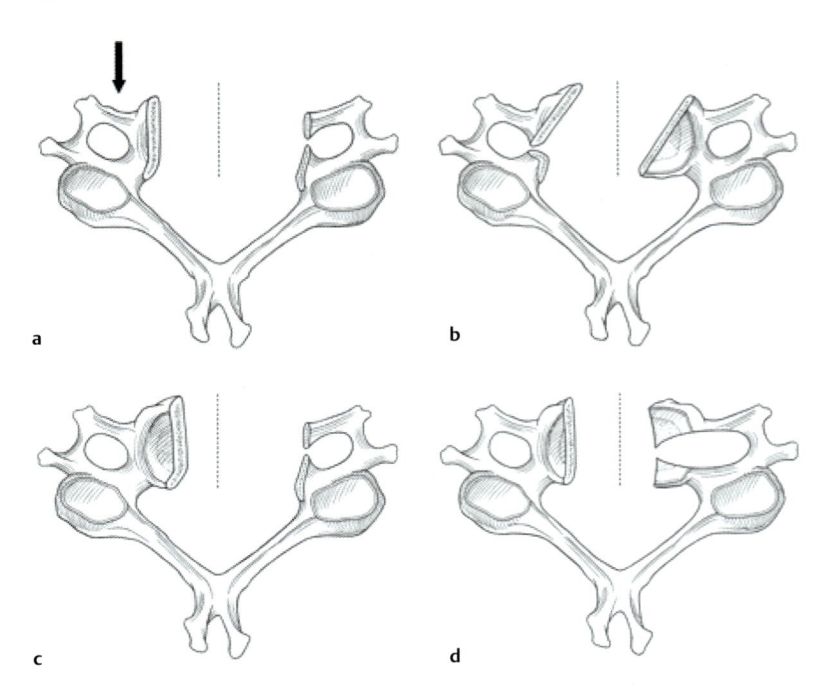

Fig. 28.7 Illustration demonstrating risk factors for vertebral artery injury. The *dashed line* indicates the midline. **(a)** Excessively wide corpectomy, with the costal process indicated by the *arrow*. **(b)** Oblique corpectomy caused by loss of the vertebral orientation landmarks. **(c)** Off-center corpectomy caused by loss of the vertebral orientation landmarks. **(d)** Tortuosity of the vertebral foramen, causing the vertebral artery to be located within the vertebral body.

One common mistake during a corpectomy is to lose the orientation of the bony resection and potentially violate the foramen transversarium (**Fig. 28.7**). This can occur if the line of sight in the operative field is inadvertently at an angle. Steps to avoid this include a complete visualization of the uncinate processes both above and below the vertebral body, identification of the center of the vertebral body with the Caspar pin, reorientation of the microscope to point directly perpendicular to the anterior border of the disk space, and the use of troughs along the lateral border of the corpectomy site to maintain line-of-sight during bur use.

Grafting Options

Anterior cervical diskectomy without fusion has recently fallen out of favor due to reported complications with postoperative kyphosis, worsening neck and contralateral arm pain, and poorer long-term outcomes compared with diskectomy with fusion.[21] The benefits of using an interbody graft include restoration of disk and neuroforaminal height, arrest of osteophyte formation in response to fusion, and reduced posterior compression as a result of unbuckling of the ligamentum flavum and the PLL.[22] Potential complications with use of an interbody graft include graft collapse, extrusion, pseudarthrosis, and donor-site morbidity.

Iliac crest autograft has historically been considered the gold standard for promoting fusion in ACDF,[23] but a significant drawback of this graft option is donor-site morbidity, including persistent pain, numbness, and impairment in ambulation.[24,25] There are numerous alternatives available that avoid these complications, including allogeneic bone graft, xenograft, and synthetic bone graft substitutes.[26] One-level instrumented ACDFs using allograft has fusion rates upward of 95%.[6,24,27]

A variety of anterior cervical cages are also available for use, including titanium and polyetheretherketone (PEEK) cages. These cages add structural stability and can be filled with local autograft from the decompression, allograft, or synthetic bone substitutes. Several studies show promising clinical results with the use of PEEK cages.[28,29]

Our preference is to use structural, machined corticocancellous allograft for both ACDF procedures. The surgeon must consider the pros and cons of various grafts when choosing which type of graft to use in anterior cervical spine surgery.

Instrumented Versus Noninstrumented Fusions

Anterior cervical plating in ACDF surgery offers many advantages compared with noninstrumented fusions, including improved fusion rates in multilevel ACDF,[30,31] increased stability, decreased rate of graft dislodgement,[32,33] and decreased segmental kyphosis.[27,34]

The size of the plate is determined once the graft has been placed. Optimal plate length enables the screws to be adjacent to the end plates. The shortest plate possible should be used to avoid encroachment on adjacent disk spaces. The plate should be centered in the coronal plane and should lie flush against the vertebral bodies (**Fig. 28.8**). Contouring of the anterior vertebral bodies with a high-speed bur can facilitate placement. Screws should be angled away from the graft, thus allowing longer screws than the ones directed parallel to the end plate. Although bicortical screw purchase has been described, we believe that screws should be unicortical to prevent potential spinal cord damage.

Various plating options are available, including constrained, semiconstrained, and dynamic plates. The evidence-based literature does not report significant differences in clinical outcomes with any of these plate designs.[35]

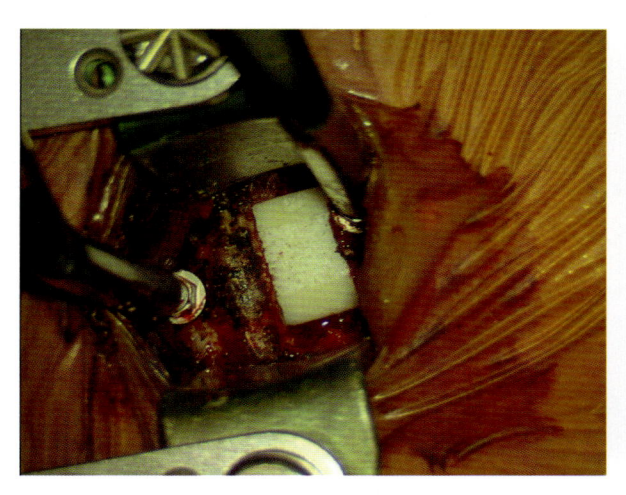

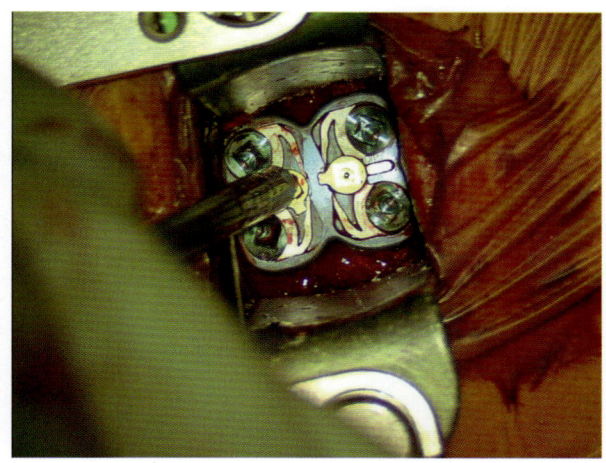

Fig. 28.8 (a) Intraoperative view of the structural corticocancellous allograft placement. (b) Final plate placement.

Postoperative Care

- Deep drain (Penrose) is left in the Smith-Robinson interval to prevent hematoma formation, typically removed on postoperative day 1.
- Soft cervical collar for comfort
- Diet is advanced as per nursing bedside swallowing evaluations.

Potential Complications and Precautions

- Vascular injury can be avoided by preoperative imaging assessment of potential aberrant carotid or vertebral arteries.
- Neurologic and visceral injury can be reduced with meticulous dissection and careful retraction.
- Pseudarthrosis rates can be reduced by the use of graft and instrumentation.
- Adjacent segment disease
- Dysphagia, dysphonia
- Durotomy

Conclusion

Since the description of the anterior approach for anterior cervical diskectomy and fusion by Smith and Robinson[36] in the 1950s, anterior cervical procedures have become one of the most common procedures performed by spine surgeons. Clinical success rates of this procedure are generally high, and adverse events are infrequent and manageable. Instrumentation and improved graft options have led to increased success rates and reduced morbidity. **Box 28-1** lists the key operative steps and the problems that can arise.

Box 28-1 Key Operative Steps and Potential Problems

Key Step	Problems
Positioning	- Inability to obtain lateral cervical radiographs due to inadequate shoulder retraction - Hyperextension of neck leading to increased risk of iatrogenic spinal cord injury
Dissection	- Carotid or vertebral artery injury due to aberrant anatomic course - Sympathetic chain injury due to excessive retraction of longus colli or extraperiosteal placement of retractor
Diskectomy	- Vertebral artery injury due to decompression lateral to uncinate processes - Spinal cord injury due to aggressive resection of PLL
Grafting	- Graft extrusion/subsidence secondary due to improper graft sizing
Instrumentation	- Encroachment of adjacent disk space due to improper plate positioning/sizing - Spinal cord injury due to screw malposition

References

1. Robinson RA. Fusions of the cervical spine. J Bone Joint Surg Am 1959;41-A:1–6
2. Bohlman HH, Emery SE, Goodfellow DB, Jones PK. Robinson anterior cervical discectomy and arthrodesis for cervical radiculopathy. Long-term follow-up of one hundred and twenty-two patients. J Bone Joint Surg Am 1993;75:1298–1307
3. Goffin J, Geusens E, Vantomme N, et al. Long-term follow-up after interbody fusion of the cervical spine. J Spinal Disord Tech 2004;17:79–85
4. Caspar W, Geisler FH, Pitzen T, Johnson TA. Anterior cervical plate stabilization in one- and two-level degenerative disease: overtreatment or benefit? J Spinal Disord 1998;11:1–11
5. Anderson PA, Subach BR, Riew KD. Predictors of outcome after anterior cervical discectomy and fusion: a multivariate analysis. Spine 2009;34:161–166
6. Fraser JF, Härtl R. Anterior approaches to fusion of the cervical spine: a metaanalysis of fusion rates. J Neurosurg Spine 2007;6:298–303
7. Hilibrand AS, Fye MA, Emery SE, Palumbo MA, Bohlman HH. Increased rate of arthrodesis with strut grafting after multilevel anterior cervical decompression. Spine 2002;27:146–151
8. Jiang SD, Jiang LS, Dai LY. Anterior cervical discectomy and fusion versus anterior cervical corpectomy and fusion for multilevel cervical spondylosis: a systematic review. Arch Orthop Trauma Surg 2012;132:155–161
9. Kilburg C, Sullivan HG, Mathiason MA. Effect of approach side during anterior cervical discectomy and fusion on the incidence of recurrent laryngeal nerve injury. J Neurosurg Spine 2006;4:273–277
10. Hart AK, Greinwald JH Jr, Shaffrey CI, Postma GN. Thoracic duct injury during anterior cervical discectomy: a rare complication. Case report. J Neurosurg 1998;88:151–154
11. Haller JM, Iwanik M, Shen FH. Clinically relevant anatomy of recurrent laryngeal nerve. Spine 2012;37:97–100
12. Cheung KM, Mak KC, Luk KD. Anterior approach to cervical spine. Spine 2012;37:E297–E302
13. Ebraheim NA, Lu J, Skie M, Heck BE, Yeasting RA. Vulnerability of the recurrent laryngeal nerve in the anterior approach to the lower cervical spine. Spine 1997;22:2664–2667
14. Monfared A, Kim D, Jaikumar S, Gorti G, Kam A. Microsurgical anatomy of the superior and recurrent laryngeal nerves. Neurosurgery 2001;49:925–932, discussion 932–933
15. Beutler WJ, Sweeney CA, Connolly PJ. Recurrent laryngeal nerve injury with anterior cervical spine surgery risk with laterality of surgical approach. Spine 2001;26:1337–1342
16. Jung A, Schramm J. How to reduce recurrent laryngeal nerve palsy in anterior cervical spine surgery: a prospective observational study. Neurosurgery 2010;67:10–15, discussion 15
17. Koreckij J, Alvi H, Gibly R, Pang E, Hsu WK. Incidence and risk factors of the retropharyngeal carotid artery on cervical magnetic resonance imaging. Spine 2013;38:E109–E112
18. Bible JE, O'Neill KR, Crosby CG, Schoenecker JG, McGirt MJ, Devin CJ. Microscope sterility during spine surgery. Spine 2012;37:623–627
19. Nassr A, Lee JY, Bashir RS, et al. Does incorrect level needle localization during anterior cervical discectomy and fusion lead to accelerated disc degeneration? Spine 2009;34:189–192
20. Schroeder GD, Hsu WK. Vertebral artery injuries in cervical spine surgery. Surg Neurol Int 2013;4(5, Suppl 5):S362–S367
21. Watters WC III, Levinthal R. Anterior cervical discectomy with and without fusion. Results, complications, and long-term follow-up. Spine 1994;19:2343–2347
22. Sonntag VK, Klara P. Controversy in spine care. Is fusion necessary after anterior cervical discectomy? Spine 1996;21:1111–1113
23. Epstein NE. Iliac crest autograft versus alternative constructs for anterior cervical spine surgery: pros, cons, and costs. Surg Neurol Int 2012;3(3, Suppl 3):S143–S156
24. Samartzis D, Shen FH, Goldberg EJ, An HS. Is autograft the gold standard in achieving radiographic fusion in one-level anterior cervical discectomy and fusion with rigid anterior plate fixation? Spine 2005;30:1756–1761
25. Silber JS, Anderson DG, Daffner SD, et al. Donor site morbidity after anterior iliac crest bone harvest for single-level anterior cervical discectomy and fusion. Spine 2003;28:134–139
26. Anderson DG, Albert TJ. Bone grafting, implants, and plating options for anterior cervical fusions. Orthop Clin North Am 2002;33:317–328
27. Zdeblick TA, Ducker TB. The use of freeze-dried allograft bone for anterior cervical fusions. Spine 1991;16:726–729
28. Kasliwal MK, O'Toole JE. Clinical experience using polyetheretherketone (PEEK) intervertebral structural cage for anterior cervical corpectomy and fusion. J Clin Neurosci 2014;21:217–220
29. Chen Y, Wang X, Lu X, et al. Comparison of titanium and polyetheretherketone (PEEK) cages in the surgical treatment of multilevel cervical spondylotic myelopathy: a prospective, randomized, control study with over 7-year follow-up. Eur Spine J 2013;22:1539–1546
30. Connolly PJ, Esses SI, Kostuik JP. Anterior cervical fusion: outcome analysis of patients fused with and without anterior cervical plates. J Spinal Disord 1996;9:202–206
31. Wang JC, McDonough PW, Endow K, Kanim LE, Delamarter RB. The effect of cervical plating on single-level anterior cervical discectomy and fusion. J Spinal Disord 1999;12:467–471
32. Geisler FH, Caspar W, Pitzen T, Johnson TA. Reoperation in patients after anterior cervical plate stabilization in degenerative disease. Spine 1998;23:911–920
33. Epstein NE. The value of anterior cervical plating in preventing vertebral fracture and graft extrusion after multilevel anterior cervical corpectomy with posterior wiring and fusion: indications, results, and complications. J Spinal Disord 2000;13:9–15
34. Wang JC, McDonough PW, Endow KK, Delamarter RB. Increased fusion rates with cervical plating for two-level anterior cervical discectomy and fusion. Spine 2000;25:41–45
35. Pitzen TR, Chrobok J, Stulik J, et al. Implant complications, fusion, loss of lordosis, and outcome after anterior cervical plating with dynamic or rigid plates: two-year results of a multi-centric, randomized, controlled study. Spine 2009;34:641–646
36. Smith GW, Robinson RA. The treatment of certain cervical-spine disorders by anterior removal of the intervertebral disc and interbody fusion. J Bone Joint Surg Am 1958;40-A:607–624

29 Cervical Arthroplasty

Manish K. Kasliwal and Zachary A. Smith

Spinal arthroplasty for the treatment of degenerative disorders of the cervical spine is becoming increasingly popular among spine surgeons. Anterior cervical diskectomy and fusion (ACDF) has been traditionally considered the definitive surgical treatment for symptomatic, single-level, cervical degenerative disk disease (DDD) for patients who have failed a trial of conservative management.[1] With increasing understanding of the biomechanics of the spine and with the fact that fusion alters the normal biomechanics, there has been growing concern about accelerated degeneration of the levels adjacent to cervical arthrodesis.[2-7] With its potential to maintain anatomic disk height, normal segmental lordosis, and physiological motion following surgery, cervical disk replacement (CDR) has emerged as an alternative to ACDF for degenerative disk disease.[8] The clinical effectiveness of cervical arthroplasty has been demonstrated in various randomized controlled trials, leading to the approval of several devices by the Food and Drug Administration (FDA). This includes both one-level and, in some instances, two-level applications. As a result, surgeons have multiple surgical options as well as several unique devices at their disposal.[9-13] This chapter discusses the surgical technique of, and specific indications for, cervical arthroplasty.

Patient Selection

The indications for cervical arthroplasty are not nearly as robust as those for cervical fusion, and this technique should not be assumed to be appropriate for all patients who may benefit from an ACDF.[14] The importance of careful patient selection cannot be overemphasized for the success of CDR. Symptomatic cervical disk pathology should be treated with a trial of nonoperative management before embarking on surgical treatment. Patients with cervical radiculopathy secondary to central or paracentral disk herniations and patients with minimal spondylosis at one or two levels are potential candidates for anterior cervical arthroplasty.[9-13] However, as cervical arthroplasty devices become available more widely outside clinical trials, the indications will continue to expand; in fact, CDR is performed outside of the United States for various indications in addition to the common single-level indication.[15]

Potential contraindications, including patient-specific anatomy, are important to consider. Cervical arthroplasty replaces only the disk and requires the posterior elements, such as the facets and ligaments, to be intact and functional.[16,17] As such, we suggest using computed tomography (CT) scans to assess the facet joints, to exclude patients with clinically significant facet degeneration. In addition, patients with cervical kyphosis, cervical spondylolisthesis with incompetent facets, severe multilevel cervical spondylosis (three or more levels), severe osteoporosis, or cervical trauma are typically excluded from this procedure.[9-11,18] Although patients with cervical kyphosis are at risk for migration of the arthroplasty because of abnormal local shear strains on the device, incompetent cervical facets with spondylolisthesis put patients at risk for early implant migration because of abnormal local shear strains.[9,14,16,17] Patients with severe multilevel spondylosis or ankylosis are unlikely to experience the benefits of arthroplasty because their baseline cervical range of motion is very limited. Patients with osteoporosis are at risk for pistoning of the implant through the weakened vertebral end plates. Trauma patients with ligamentous or facet injury are also at risk for device migration because of increased range of motion beyond normal anatomic constraints. The body habitus of the patient should be considered before beginning the procedure. Patients with large shoulders or short necks may present an added challenge to intraoperative fluoroscopic visualization of the appropriate cervical level, which makes precise implant placement difficult.

Indications[9-11,13,19]

The goals of cervical disk arthroplasty are to restore the intervertebral disk and foraminal height so as to prevent recurrence of nerve root compression along with preservation of motion. The indications are as follows:

- Radiculopathy caused by disk herniation
- Radiculopathy secondary to foraminal osteophytes
- Myelopathy due to a soft disk herniation
- Myelopathy due to large osteophytes: may not be ideal as it often requires too much vertebral bone resection

Contraindications[9-11,13,19]

- Cervical kyphosis
- Global deformity or segmental instability
- Cervical spondylosis with incompetent facets
- Three or more levels of cervical spondylosis
- Osteoporosis
- Cervical trauma with ligamentous or facet injury
- Recent history of infection or osteomyelitis
- Other relative contraindications include rheumatoid arthritis, renal failure, cancer, ankylosing spondylitis, ossification of the posterior longitudinal ligament, and diffuse idiopathic skeletal hyperostosis.

Advantages

- Familiar technique
- Preservation of motion
- Possible decreased risk of adjacent segment degeneration and disease
- No need for postoperative immobilization

Disadvantages

- Not suitable for multilevel disease
- Inadequate decompression may be more symptomatic.
- Arthroplasty may auto-fuse over time, obviating the potential advantages of motion preservation.
- The proposed benefit of CDR resulting in decreased incidence of adjacent segment disease still remains to be proved.[20–24]

Preoperative Tests

- Standing, neutral anteroposterior, and lateral plain radiographs to ensure normal sagittal and coronal alignment
- Lateral flexion and extension radiographs to rule out instability
- Magnetic resonance imaging (MRI) of the cervical spine
- Computed tomography (CT) myelogram (if MRI contraindicated)
- CT scan of the cervical spine (in patients whose X-rays and clinical exam are suspicious for facet disease/degeneration)

Surgical Anatomy

The surgical anatomy for cervical arthroplasty is similar to that for an ACDF, and is discussed in Chapter 28.

Surgical Procedure

The surgical technique for cervical artificial disk placement is very similar to that for ACDF, with some additional nuances.[25] The technique differs from device to device mainly in terms of achieving the fixation, but many of the surgical steps are shared and are important to optimize the overall outcome.[9–11,19,26] There is a greater need for surgical precision and proper alignment when performing arthroplasty as compared with arthrodesis. Although the surgical technique described in this chapter refers to that for ProDisc-C (DePuy Synthes, West Chester, PA) arthroplasty, we do not personally recommend any one device over the other. The ProDisc-C prosthesis consists of cobalt–chromium alloy end plates with a central keel for anchorage to the vertebral bodies and a locking core of ultra-high-molecular-weight polyethylene (UHMWPE) as a central polymer that provides a ball-and-socket articulation. The metal end plates have a keel design for enhanced primary stability and fixation, and the end plate coverage with titanium plasma spray coating enables bony ingrowth and long-term fixation (**Fig. 29.1**). Nevertheless, apart from the actual device implantation, most of the surgical steps including positioning and exposure do not differ much, irrespective of the devices used.

Patient Positioning

Intraoperative positioning of the patient is critical to the appropriate sizing and placement of a cervical arthroplasty. The arthroplasty device is designed to be placed in a neutral or mildly lordotic cervical spine.[12] The patient is placed in the supine position on a radiolucent table with the neck extended and supported dorsally with a roll to position the neck in a neutral or mildly lordotic position. The shoulders are caudally retracted to help with intraoperative fluoroscopic visualization. Patients are administered a dose of preoperative antibiotic. Intraoperative neuromonitoring with somatosensory evoked potentials and/or electromyography is optional. Intraoperative fluoroscopy is used to confirm and mark the level of surgery and to ensure that the vertebral level of interest can be visualized with lateral fluoroscopy.

Surgical Technique

Although either a right- or a left-sided approach may be selected depending on the surgeon's preference, we prefer to perform the standard anterior Smith-Robinson approach to the cervical spine through a transverse left-sided incision made through a preexisting skin crease if possible.[25] A scalpel is used to incise skin and subcutaneous tissue, followed by incising the platysmal muscle layer. A cephalad and caudad subplatysmal dissection is performed. The deep cervical fascia is then exposed and the

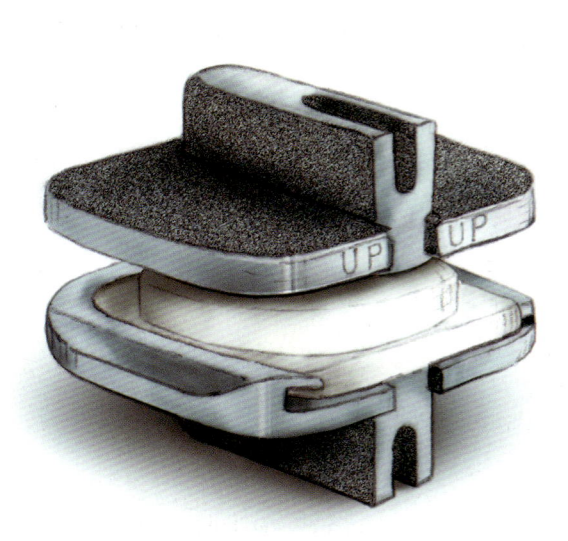

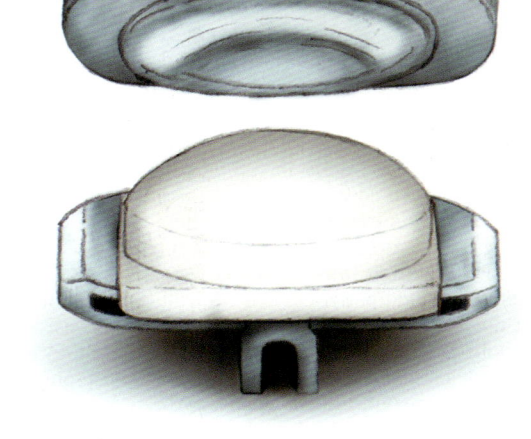

Fig. 29.1 Images demonstrating the ProDisc-C artificial cervical disk.

medial border of the sternocleidomastoid muscle (SCM) is identified. The deeper lateral carotid sheath is dissected from the medial tracheoesophageal bundle using a Kittner dissector. A localizing fluoroscopic X-ray is taken to identify and confirm the levels of intended arthroplasty.

Once the level is confirmed, handheld retractors are used to expose the longus colli muscles, which are mobilized subperiosteally with bipolar cautery and a Penfield elevator. A self-retaining anterior cervical retractor is placed under the elevated edges of the longus colli muscles. (Details and images of the dissection can be seen in Chapter 28.) An anteroposterior (AP) fluoroscopy is performed to mark the midline (**Fig. 29.2**). Instead of the regular Caspar distractor pins, the retainer screws are inserted exactly parallel to the end plates as far away from the disk space as possible. An awl should be used to initially perforate the cortex before placement of the retainer screws. These retainer screws should be long enough to engage the posterior cortex (**Fig. 29.3**). Fluoroscopy should be used to confirm the trajectory and depth of the retainer screws. The retainer is assembled and a light pretension is applied, avoiding the attempt to actually distract the disk space, which would be performed later with the use of actual distractor (**Fig. 29.4**). Standard diskectomy is performed using curettes and pituitary and Kerrison rongeurs, used with care to remove only the cartilaginous end plates. Although we personally prefer using an operating microscope beginning with this stage of the surgery, the whole procedure can be performed using loupe magnification.

The vertebral distractor is now placed, with the distractor tips placed up to the posterior margin of the vertebral bodies so as to avoid vertebral end-plate penetration under lateral fluoroscopy (**Fig. 29.5**). The distractor is manually distracted, and the retainer is adjusted to maintain the distraction achieved with the distractor. The distractor is then removed and the diskectomy is completed, removing all visible disks until the end plates and until the posterior longitudinal ligament is visualized, which is then removed. Posterior vertebral osteophytes are removed, and generous bilateral foraminotomies are performed, ensuring the removal of the uncovertebral joints bilaterally. Failure to adequately remove the uncovertebral joints may lead to new postoperative radiculopathy exacerbated during flexion of the implant. If the disk space has significant spondylotic changes, a power drill may be used to remove the disk and osteophytes. Nevertheless, drilling should strictly be kept to be a minimum,

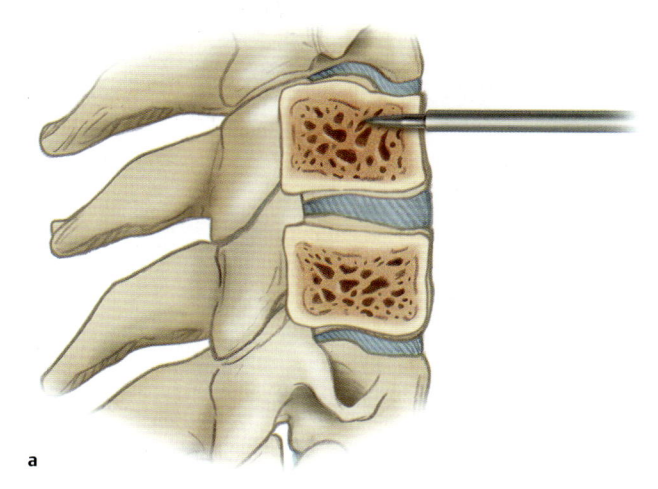

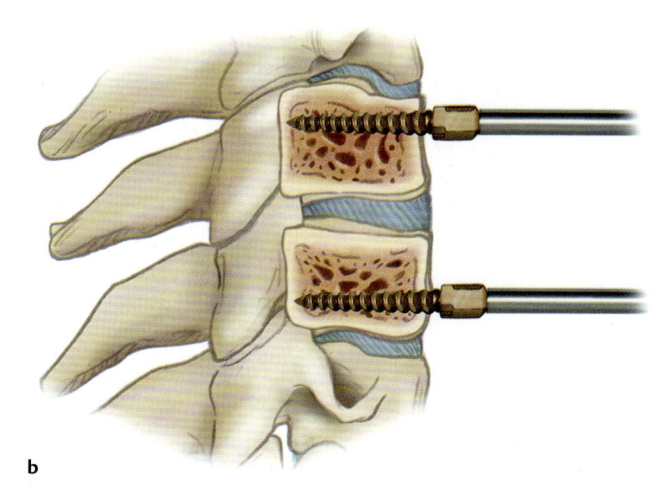

Fig. 29.3 (a) An awl should be used to initially perforate the cortex before placement of the retainer screws. (b) The retainer screws are inserted exactly parallel to the end plates as far away from the disk space as possible and should be long enough to engage the posterior cortex.

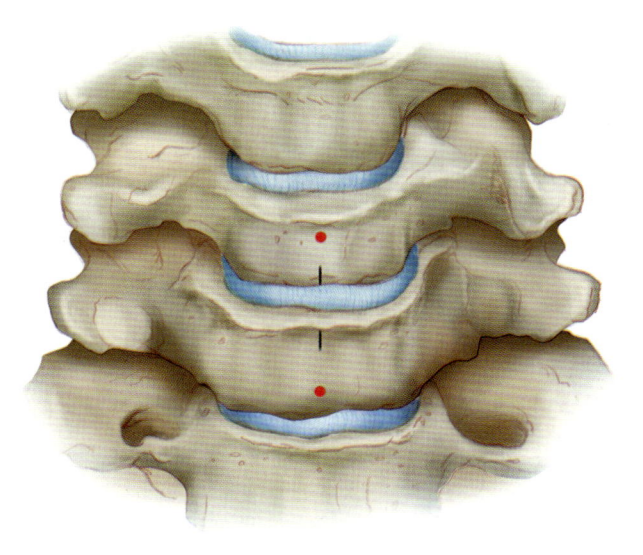

Fig. 29.2 Intraoperative anteroposterior (AP) image to mark the midline.

taking great care to avoid significant end-plate disruption, as it may lead to later implant subsidence into the vertebral body.

Implantation of the actual ProDisc-C device consists of three steps:

- Implant trial
- Keel preparation
- Insertion of the implant

The appropriate implant trial connected to the trial handle is placed snugly into the disk space, ensuring that the trial stop is fully seated by turning the handle clockwise until it does not advance any further (**Fig. 29.6**). The stop on the trial can be adjusted to allow the trial to advance more posteriorly until the optimal position is achieved. Lateral fluoroscopy should be used to confirm the optimal position of the trial implant, which should be at the posterior margin of the vertebral bodies and centered in the midline (**Fig. 29.7**). Although it is appropriate to aim for the largest implant footprint size and restoration of anatomic height, oversizing the trial should be avoided as it may limit the normal range of motion. The height of the normal adjacent disk is useful in selecting the smallest appropriate trial

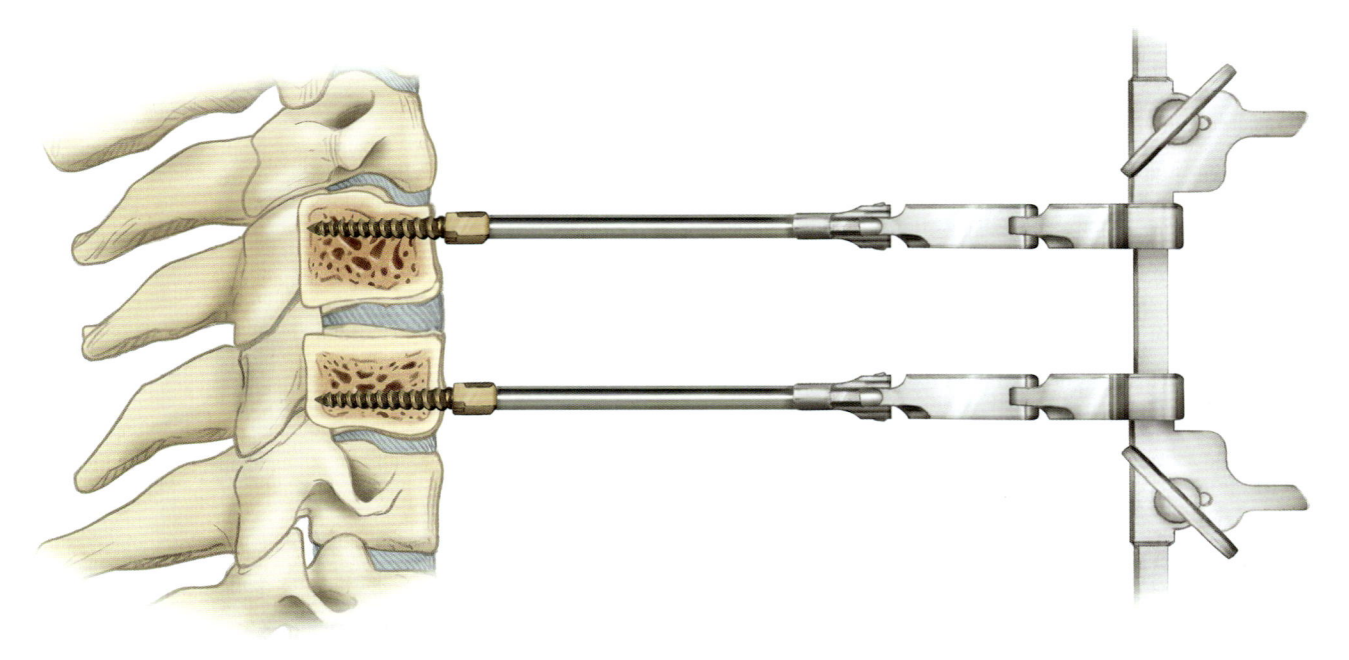

Fig. 29.4 Schematic diagram showing the retainer system that holds the distraction, which is applied with the help of an intervertebral distractor.

height. The distraction should be released while assessing the trial height, and once the trial is fully seated, distraction should be removed from the retainer with application of mild compression. The trial handle is then removed leaving the trial implant in place. Anteroposterior and lateral fluoroscopic images are obtained to ensure that the trial fits and is centered in the disk space. The surgeon should take the time to align the fluoroscope to obtain images without parallax.

The keel preparation is then performed using high-speed milling device. An appropriate size-milling guide is placed over the trial and the locking nut is tightened. AP fluoroscopy should be obtained to confirm the midline position (**Fig. 29.8**). A sharp temporary pin is placed through the inferior hole in the guide and manually driven into the bone. The milling device is inserted into the superior hole of the guide until the tip of the mill touches the anterior cortex, which should be confirmed by lateral fluoroscopy. The bit is advanced into the vertebral body under full power until it reaches the positive stop in the guide (**Fig. 29.9**). The bit is then swept toward the trial implant and then away from the trial to the full outer limit. The temporary pin is removed from the inferior hole and the milling procedure is performed in the inferior body just as it is performed superiorly. The trial implant and milling guide are removed and a keel

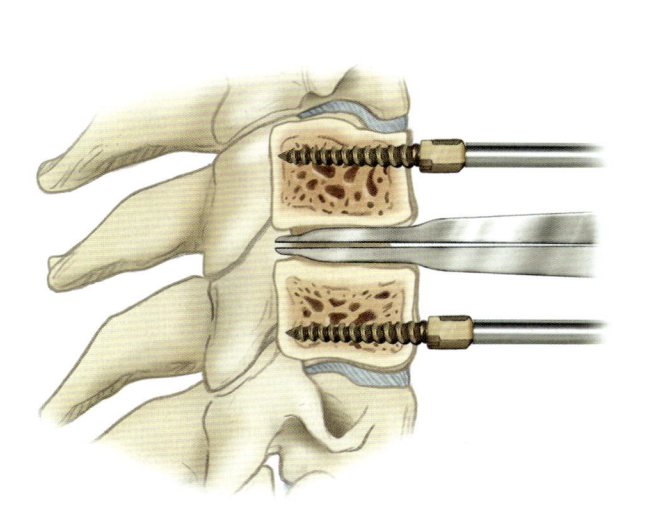

Fig. 29.5 Schematic diagram showing the vertebral distractor with its tips placed up to the posterior margin of the vertebral bodies, so as to avoid vertebral end-plate penetration under lateral fluoroscopy.

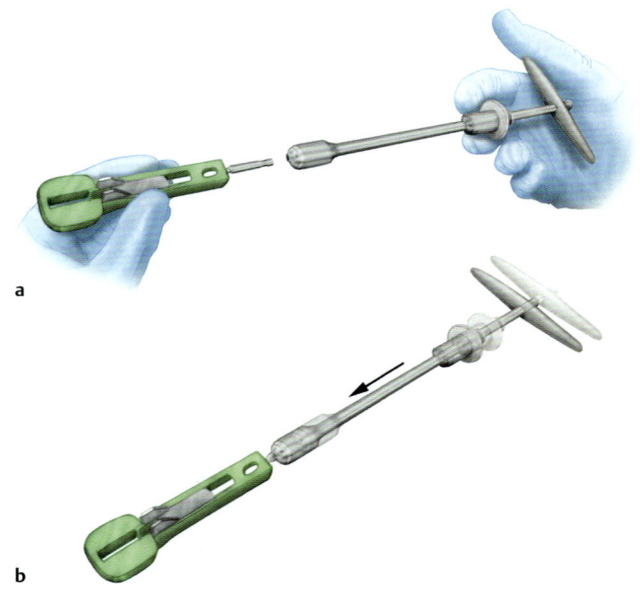

Fig. 29.6 (**a**) Schematic diagram showing the implant trial connected to the trial handle. (**b**) The trial implant can be advanced by turning the handle clockwise.

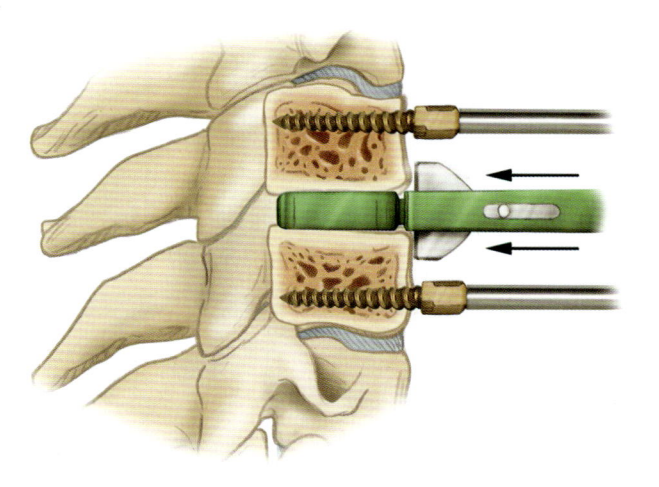

Fig. 29.7 Diagram showing the optimal position of the trial implant, which should be at the posterior margin of the vertebral bodies.

cut cleaner is inserted to verify the depth of the keel and to remove any bony debris from both the superior and inferior vertebral bodies, followed by extensive irrigation to clear any bony debris from the wound (**Fig. 29.10**).

The appropriate-size ProDisc-C implant is then loaded onto the implant inserter en bloc. Ensure that the "UP" indicator on the implant is attached to the UP side of the inserter. The implant is then aligned with the keel cuts already made and carefully advanced using lateral fluoroscopy, ensuring that the implant reaches the posterior margin of the vertebral body (**Fig. 29.11**). After confirming appropriate placement, the retainer system is removed and all screw holes and cancellous bone are waxed. A copious irrigation should be done to remove all the bony debris and other tissue. Final AP and lateral fluoroscopy should be performed to confirm the final implant position (**Fig. 29.12**). The platysma muscle layer is then closed, and the anterior cervical skin incision is closed with subcuticular suture followed by application of skin glue.

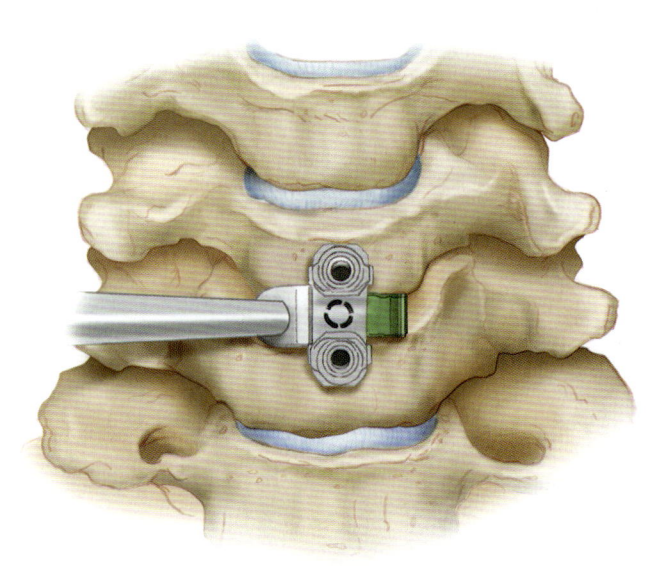

Fig. 29.8 Diagram showing a milling guide placed over the trial. AP fluoroscopy should be obtained to confirm the midline position.

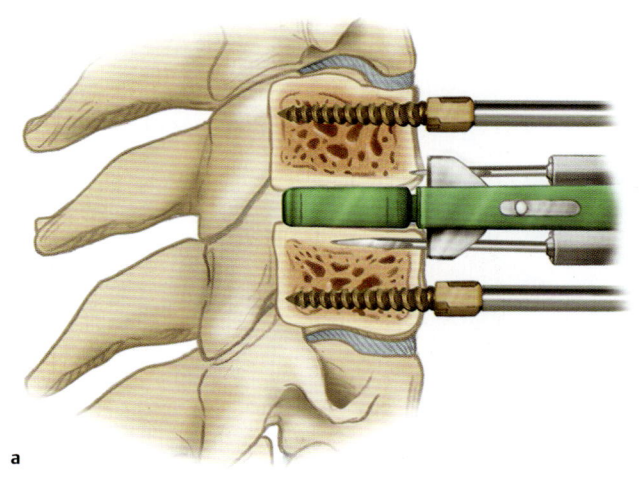

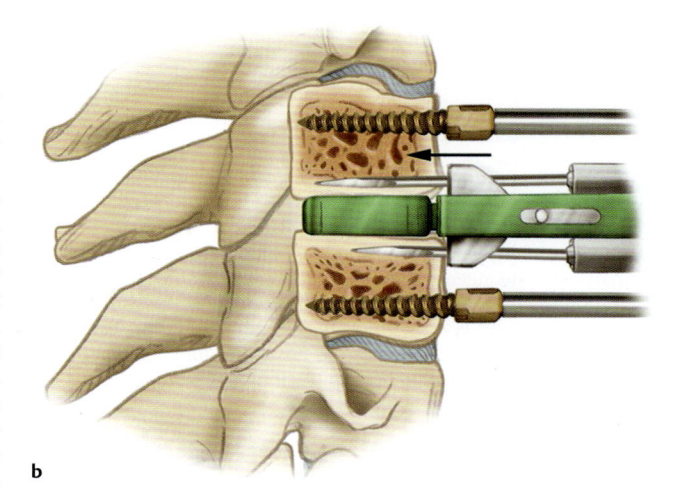

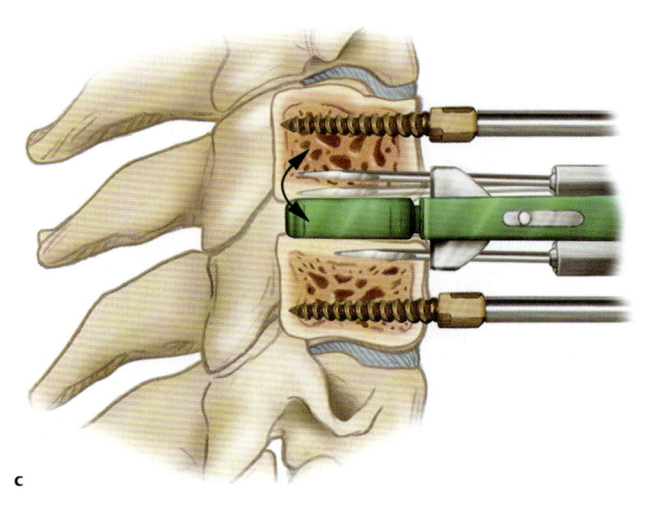

Fig. 29.9 Schematic diagram showing the milling process. (**a**) A sharp temporary pin is placed through the inferior hole in the guide and manually driven into the bone. (**b**) The milling device is inserted into the superior hole of the guide until the tip of the mill touches the anterior cortex, which should be confirmed by lateral fluoroscopy. The bit is advanced into the vertebral body under full power until it reaches the positive stop in the guide. (**c**) The bit is then swept toward the trial implant and then away from the trial to the full outer limit.

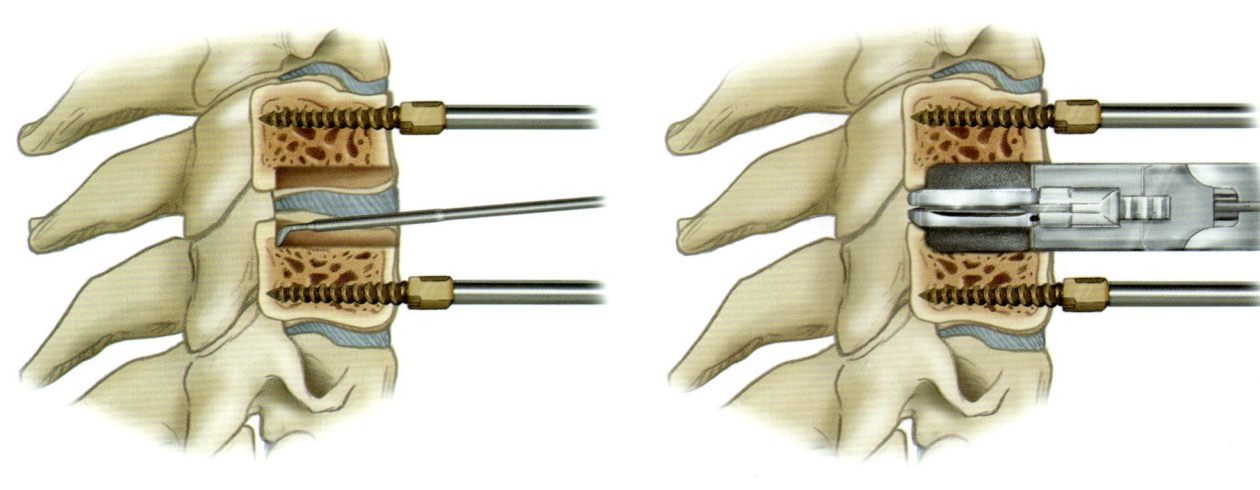

Fig. 29.10 Image demonstrating the use of a keel cut cleaner as it is inserted to verify the depth of the keel and to remove any bony debris from both the superior and inferior vertebral bodies.

Fig. 29.11 Schematic diagram showing the implant placement, ensuring that the implant reaches the posterior margin of the vertebral body.

Postoperative Care

The patient can be mobilized the day of surgery with no need for a collar, with resumption of activities as tolerated. Nonsteroidal anti-inflammatory drugs (NSAIDs) are prescribed for 2 weeks after surgery to minimize the risk of heterotopic ossification.[9,11,12,19] The need for physical therapy should be assessed based on the patient's preoperative neurologic status, and should be started in the weeks following surgery. Regular follow-up radiographs should be obtained to ensure proper functioning of the implant and detect any complications.

Potential Complications and Precautions

Patient positioning is critical. It is important to position the neck in the neutral position. Positioning the patient with the neck in kyphosis may not allow for selection of the appropriate arthroplasty size and fit. Complete bilateral decompression with uncinate resection should be performed, as persistent nerve root compression may not be well tolerated in the setting of preservation of motion. It is vital to ensure that all disk and cartilaginous material is removed from the end plates without completely violating the subchondral bone, to prevent improper fitting of the implant and subsidence. Fluoroscopy should be aligned so as to obtain images without parallax to help choose the appropriate implant size. If the sizing is too loose, the arthroplasty may migrate. Conversely, if the sizing is too large, it may restrict normal range of motion (ROM), as the facets and posterior ligaments will be over-distracted, thereby "stiffening" the segment. The lateral image should be carefully visualized to see if there are any radiographic gaps between the trial and the end plates or if there is splaying of the facet joints. AP and lateral fluoroscopic images after final implant positioning should be obtained to confirm that the CDR is implanted properly in both the coronal and the sagittal planes.

Complications following cervical arthroplasty can be approach or device related. Although the use of CDR can obviate complications such as pseudarthrosis and graft donor-site morbidity, it still may result in approach-related complications, including hoarseness of voice, dysphagia, and hematoma, and the risk of neurologic injury remains.[1,25] Complications specific to CDR may include heterotopic ossification (HO), postoperative kypho-

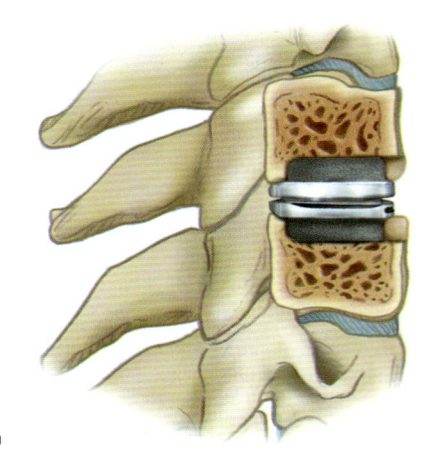

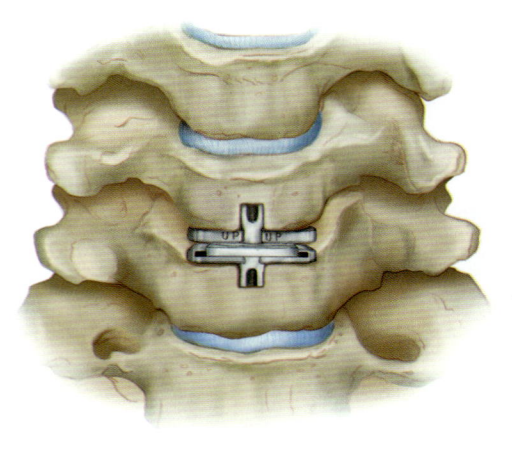

Fig. 29.12 Schematic diagram showing final AP **(a)** and lateral **(b)** images confirming the final implant position.

sis, device migration and subsidence, vertebral fracture, and hypersensitivity reaction. Overall, CDR has been very safe, as demonstrated in various randomized trials, with an excellent complication profile. HO is defined as formation of the bone outside the skeletal system and has been reported to occur in up to 70% of patients after cervical arthroplasty, depending on the definition of the term and the length of follow-up.[27-29] As HO potentially can result in loss of motion or fusion, negating the benefit of CDR, NSAIDs are often administered after surgery to minimize the incidence of HO. Most of the other device-related complications, such as postoperative kyphosis, device migration and subsidence, and vertebral fracture, can be prevented by careful patient selection and adherence to meticulous surgical technique.

Conclusion

Cervical arthroplasty has sustained the initial challenge of demonstrating equivalent clinical success as an anterior cervical fusion, at the same time preserving normal motion at the affected level. A large number of studies including multicenter randomized controlled trials have provided robust evidence showing the clinical success of CDR in the treatment of one- and two-level cervical degenerative disk disease. Short- and intermediate-term results with good clinical success and preserved range of motion favors the use of cervical spinal arthroplasty.[30-32] Careful patient selection and adherence to appropriate surgical technique are paramount to achieving a good clinical outcome following CDR and avoiding complications. Box 29-1 lists the key operative points and steps to take to avoid complications.

> **Box 29-1 Key Operative Points and Avoiding Complications**
>
> Patient positioning is critical. Position the neck in the neutral, slightly lordotic position.
>
> Perform complete bilateral decompression with uncinate resection to avoid postoperative nerve root impingement.
>
> Ensure removal of all disk and cartilaginous material from the end plates without completely violating the subchondral bone, to prevent improper fitting of the implant and subsidence.
>
> Fluoroscopy should be aligned to obtain images without parallax, so that an appropriate-sized implant can be chosen. Avoid both over- and under-sizing.
>
> Obtain anteroposterior and lateral fluoroscopic images after final implant positioning to ensure that the implant is seated properly in both the coronal and the sagittal planes.

References

1. Bohlman HH, Emery SE, Goodfellow DB, Jones PK. Robinson anterior cervical discectomy and arthrodesis for cervical radiculopathy. Long-term follow-up of one hundred and twenty-two patients. J Bone Joint Surg Am 1993;75:1298–1307
2. Bydon M, Xu R, Macki M, et al. Adjacent segment disease after anterior cervical discectomy and fusion in a large series. Neurosurgery 2014;74:139–146, discussion 146
3. Goffin J, Geusens E, Vantomme N, et al. Long-term follow-up after interbody fusion of the cervical spine. J Spinal Disord Tech 2004;17:79–85
4. Hilibrand AS, Carlson GD, Palumbo MA, Jones PK, Bohlman HH. Radiculopathy and myelopathy at segments adjacent to the site of a previous anterior cervical arthrodesis. J Bone Joint Surg Am 1999;81:519–528
5. Eck JC, Humphreys SC, Lim TH, et al. Biomechanical study on the effect of cervical spine fusion on adjacent-level intradiscal pressure and segmental motion. Spine 2002;27:2431–2434
6. Henderson CM, Hennessy RG, Shuey HM Jr, Shackelford EG. Posterior-lateral foraminotomy as an exclusive operative technique for cervical radiculopathy: a review of 846 consecutively operated cases. Neurosurgery 1983;13:504–512
7. Herkowitz HN, Kurz LT, Overholt DP. Surgical management of cervical soft disc herniation. A comparison between the anterior and posterior approach. Spine 1990;15:1026–1030
8. Chang UK, Kim DH, Lee MC, Willenberg R, Kim SH, Lim J. Range of motion change after cervical arthroplasty with ProDisc-C and prestige artificial discs compared with anterior cervical discectomy and fusion. J Neurosurg Spine 2007;7:40–46
9. Coric D, Nunley PD, Guyer RD, et al. Prospective, randomized, multicenter study of cervical arthroplasty: 269 patients from the Kineflex|C artificial disc investigational device exemption study with a minimum 2-year follow-up: clinical article. J Neurosurg Spine 2011;15:348–358
10. Davis RJ, Kim KD, Hisey MS, et al. Cervical total disc replacement with the Mobi-C cervical artificial disc compared with anterior discectomy and fusion for treatment of 2-level symptomatic degenerative disc disease: a prospective, randomized, controlled multicenter clinical trial: clinical article. J Neurosurg Spine 2013;19:532–545
11. Heller JG, Sasso RC, Papadopoulos SM, et al. Comparison of BRYAN cervical disc arthroplasty with anterior cervical decompression and fusion: clinical and radiographic results of a randomized, controlled, clinical trial. Spine 2009;34:101–107
12. Mummaneni PV, Robinson JC, Haid RW Jr. Cervical arthroplasty with the PRESTIGE LP cervical disc. Neurosurgery 2007;60(4, Suppl 2):310–314, discussion 314–315
13. Sasso RC, Kitchel SH, Dawson EG. A prospective, randomized controlled clinical trial of anterior lumbar interbody fusion using a titanium cylindrical threaded fusion device. Spine 2004;29:113–122, discussion 121–122
14. Kasliwal MK, Traynelis VC. Motion preservation in cervical spine: review. review J Neurosurg Sci 2012;56:13–25
15. Pimenta L, McAfee PC, Cappuccino A, Cunningham BW, Diaz R, Coutinho E. Superiority of multilevel cervical arthroplasty outcomes versus single-level outcomes: 229 consecutive PCM prostheses. Spine 2007;32:1337–1344
16. Acosta FL Jr, Ames CP. Cervical disc arthroplasty: general introduction. Neurosurg Clin N Am 2005;16:603–607, vi vi.
17. Durbhakula MM, Ghiselli G. Cervical total disc replacement, part I: rationale, biomechanics, and implant types. Orthop Clin North Am 2005;36:349–354
18. Puttlitz CM, Rousseau MA, Xu Z, Hu S, Tay BK, Lotz JC. Intervertebral disc replacement maintains cervical spine kinetics. Spine 2004;29:2809–2814
19. Mummaneni PV, Burkus JK, Haid RW, Traynelis VC, Zdeblick TA. Clinical and radiographic analysis of cervical disc arthroplasty compared with allograft fusion: a randomized controlled clinical trial. J Neurosurg Spine 2007;6:198–209
20. Bartels RH, Donk RD, Pavlov P, van Limbeek J. Comparison of biomechanical properties of cervical artificial disc prosthesis: a review. Clin Neurol Neurosurg 2008;110:963–967
21. Botelho RV, Moraes OJ, Fernandes GA, Buscariolli YdosS, Bernardo WM. A systematic review of randomized trials on the effect of cervical disc arthroplasty on reducing adjacent-level degeneration. Neurosurg Focus 2010;28:E5
22. Maldonado CV, Paz RD, Martin CB. Adjacent-level degeneration after cervical disc arthroplasty versus fusion. Eur Spine J 2011;20(Suppl 3):403–407
23. Nunley PD, Jawahar A, Kerr EJ III, et al. Factors affecting the incidence of symptomatic adjacent level disease in cervical spine after total disc arthroplasty: 2–4 years follow-up of 3 prospective randomized trials. Spine 2011
24. Yi S, Lee DY, Ahn PG, Kim KN, Yoon DH, Shin HC. Radiologically documented adjacent-segment degeneration after cervical arthroplasty: characteristics and review of cases. Surg Neurol 2009;72:325–329, discussion 329

25. Smith GW, Robinson RA. The treatment of certain cervical-spine disorders by anterior removal of the intervertebral disc and interbody fusion. J Bone Joint Surg Am 1958;40-A:607–624
26. Sasso RC, Smucker JD, Hacker RJ, Heller JG. Clinical outcomes of BRYAN cervical disc arthroplasty: a prospective, randomized, controlled, multicenter trial with 24-month follow-up. J Spinal Disord Tech 2007;20:481–491
27. Mehren C, Suchomel P, Grochulla F, et al. Heterotopic ossification in total cervical artificial disc replacement. Spine 2006;31:2802–2806
28. Parkinson JF, Sekhon LH. Cervical arthroplasty complicated by delayed spontaneous fusion. Case report. J Neurosurg Spine 2005;2:377–380
29. Tu TH, Wu JC, Huang WC, et al. Heterotopic ossification after cervical total disc replacement: determination by CT and effects on clinical outcomes. J Neurosurg Spine 2011;14:457–465
30. Burkus JK, Haid RW, Traynelis VC, Mummaneni PV. Long-term clinical and radiographic outcomes of cervical disc replacement with the Prestige disc: results from a prospective randomized controlled clinical trial. J Neurosurg Spine 2010;13:308–318
31. Goffin J, Van Calenbergh F, van Loon J, et al. Intermediate follow-up after treatment of degenerative disc disease with the Bryan Cervical Disc Prosthesis: single-level and bi-level. Spine 2003;28:2673–2678
32. Goffin J, van Loon J, Van Calenbergh F, Lipscomb B. A clinical analysis of 4- and 6-year follow-up results after cervical disc replacement surgery using the Bryan Cervical Disc Prosthesis. J Neurosurg Spine 2010;12:261–269

30 Transcorporeal Tunnel Approach for Unilateral Cervical Radiculopathy

Gun Choi and Alfonso Garcia Chávez

History

Minimally invasive spine surgery has addressed the entire spinal column from the cervical to lumbosacral segments, with the primary goal of achieving outcomes comparable to those of open surgery while minimizing healthy tissue damage and reducing recovery times and the length of hospital stays. The history of anterior microforaminotomy for cervical radiculopathy dates back to 1968,[1–3] when attempts were made to achieve decompression by partial removal of the offending disk material. Anterior cervical foraminotomy was described by Jho in 1996,[4] and the results of this technique were reported in 2002.[5] This approach was later modified by Saringer et al[6] in 2002, who recommended preserving a thin piece of lateral wall of the uncinate process, avoiding exposure of the vertebral artery but involving transverse resection of the longus coli muscle, therefore increasing the risk of injury to the cervical sympathetic chain and of Horner's syndrome. We have modified the technique of upper vertebral transcorporeal anterior foraminotomy for the treatment of cervical radiculopathy by avoiding breaching the medial wall of the transverse foramen and attempting to preserve the lower end plate.

The development and propagation of the anterior cervical approach, initially by Smith and Robinson,[7] and later by Cloward,[8] led to the development of today's anterior cervical diskectomy with or without fusion for patients suffering from cervical radiculopathy. Their principle was based on the simple idea of direct anterior decompression of the offending structure, but was associated with either loss of disk height (in patients without fusion) or loss of a mobile segment (in patients with interbody fusion). Furthermore, patients undergoing anterior decompression and fusion in the long run developed fusion-related complications, namely adjacent segment disease, pseudarthrosis, and other graft-related problems.[9] On the other hand, indirect decompression using minimally invasive posterior laminoforaminotomy fails to address the pathology anterior to the root, such as foraminal osteophytes and ruptured disks. Percutaneous endoscopic cervical diskectomy (PECD) is an excellent treatment modality for cervical radiculopathy, but its indications are grossly limited to soft central disk herniation. Also, the difficulty in maneuvering a scope in the narrow confines of the cervical foramen restricts its use to a few indicated cases. In an attempt to solve this problem, Choi et al[10,11] developed the transcorporeal tunnel approach for unilateral cervical spondylotic radiculopathy.

Anatomic Considerations

The lower five cervical levels (C3 to C7) are known as the *typical cervical vertebrae* and they are all alike in that they are small and their anterior body length is usually slightly less than the posterior length, whereas the cervical disks are wider anteriorly and narrower posteriorly. This unique disk shape contributes to cervical lordosis. The superior and inferior surfaces of the bodies are saddle shaped due to the laterally placed uncovertebral joints (a.k.a. the joints of Luschka). In the foramen, the cervical nerve root passes anterior to the facet joint and posterior to the uncovertebral joints, and this special joint arrangement frequently prevent a disk rupture from directly pressing on the nerve root. In contrast, osteophytes arising from these joints may cause compression on the nerve root,[12] and are a major etiologic factor in unilateral cervical radiculopathy.

Goals

- Direct anterior decompression
- Preservation of disk height
- Avoidance of complications related to anterior fusion surgery
- Avoidance of exposure and injury to vertebral artery and cervical sympathetic chain
- Minimally invasive option for cervical radiculopathy with less patient morbidity

Advantages

The anterior transcorporeal tunnel approach has the following advantages:

- Direct approach
- Motion preserving technique
- Faster recovery
- No need for postoperative rigid immobilization

Patient Selection

- A thorough physical examination with special attention on distribution of radicular pain
- A detailed history
- Correlation between clinical and radiological findings

Indications

- Unilateral cervical radiculopathy not responding to conservative treatment
- Acute radiculopathy responding to opioids
- Upper limb motor weakness secondary to herniated disk or foraminal stenosis
- Imaging studies corresponding to clinical features

Contraindications

- Dominant axial neck pain
- Cervical instability
- Cervical infections or tumors

Relative Contraindications

- Bilateral cervical radiculopathy
- Previous anterior cervical diskectomy and fusion (ACDF) surgery at, or one level above, the affected level
- Cervical stenosis
- High cervical levels (C3-C4 and above)

Surgical Options for Treating Cervical Radiculopathy

- PECD: the least invasive but for limited indications
- Transcorporeal tunnel approach
- Total cervical disk replacement
- ACDF

Preoperative Imaging

All patients undergoing surgery need to be assessed with X-rays (anteroposterior [AP], lateral, oblique, and flexion/extension views) and magnetic resonance imaging (MRI) of the cervical spine, axial and sagittal views, along with bilateral 45-degree foraminal views.

Computed tomography (CT) scans are especially useful in preoperative planning for measuring the depth and direction of the drill hole trajectory.

Anesthesia and Patient Positioning

After induction of intubated general anesthesia, the patient is placed in the supine position on a surgical table with a small roll below the neck to maintain cervical lordosis. All the pressure points are adequately padded.

After the operative area is scrubbed with povidone iodine, the patient is draped in such a way so as to allow free movement of the C-arm in both the AP and lateral views.

Surgical Technique

The surgeon stands on the symptomatic side of the patient, as the pathology needs to be approached from the ipsilateral side. The intended skin incision level is marked on the skin using a marker X-ray or fluoroscopy, and the standard Smith-Robinson approach is made from the affected side as in an anterior cervical diskectomy. The transverse skin incision, ~ 3 to 4 cm long, is made at one level higher than the ACDF (i.e., for a C6-C7 foraminal stenosis, the skin incision would be that for a C5-C6) (**Fig. 30.1**).

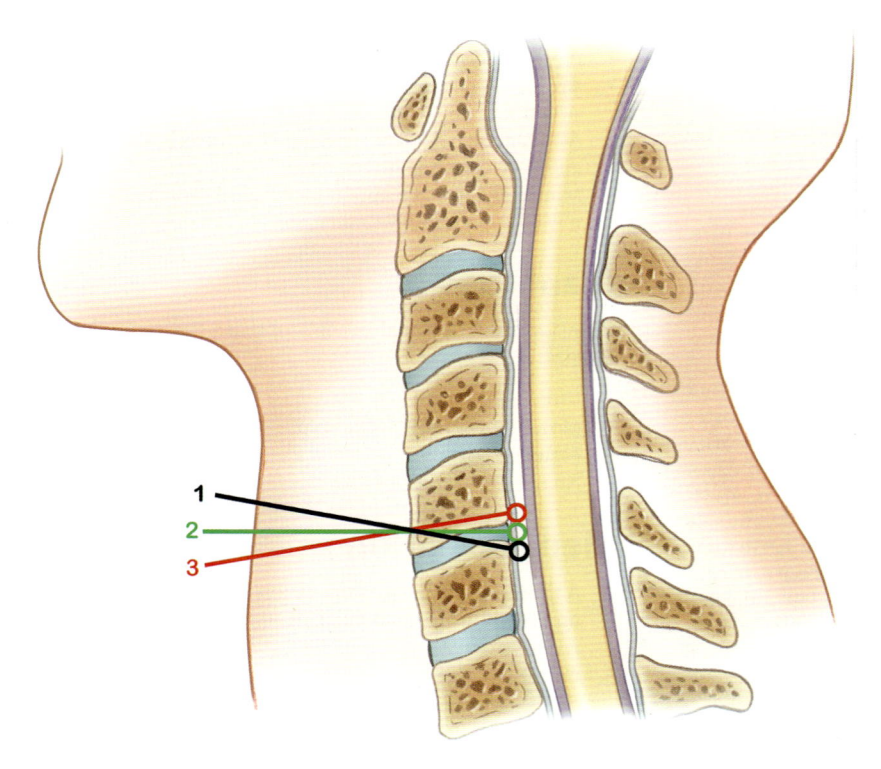

Fig. 30.1 The level of the skin incision depends on the location of the pathology. 1, steep cephalocaudad trajectory for target located at lower levels of disc space. 2, showing shallow trajectory in cephalocaudad direction for target located near to disc space level. 3, almost straight trajectory for the target located at retrovertebral level or above the disc space. *Note:* This diagrammatic representation is done for C5-6 level.

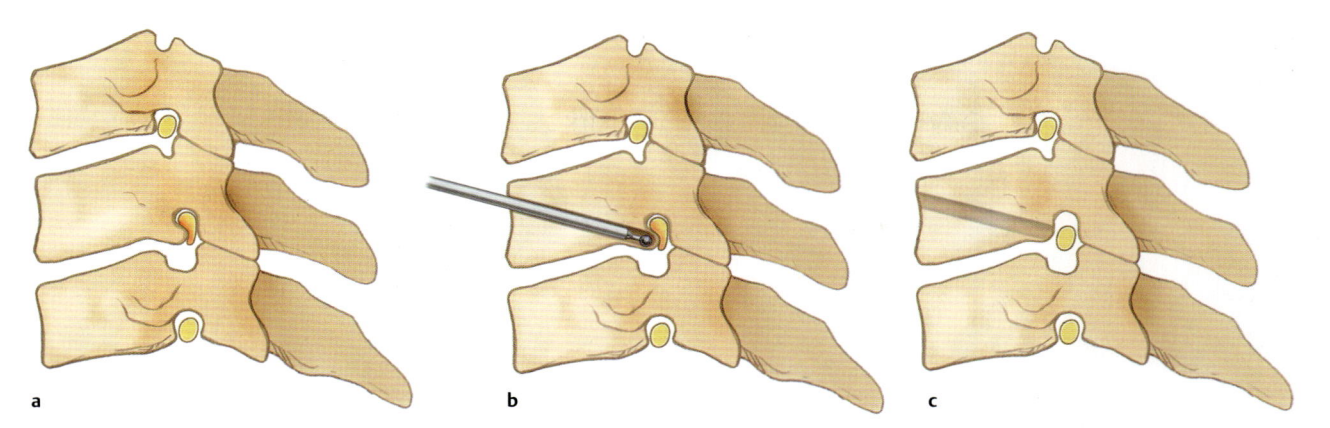

Fig. 30.2 Serial diagrams showing **(a)** a foraminal stenosis (bony spur), **(b)** the drilling trajectory, and **(c)** the decompressed foramen.

Dissection is continued down to the deep cervical fascia. Once the prevertebral fascia is opened, the midline is marked in relation to the two longus coli muscles, and the level is confirmed under fluoroscopy. The longus coli muscle is then lifted off its medial attachment subperiosteally, and self-retaining retractors are applied under the muscle.

One major difference between ACDF and the tunnel technique is that, in the latter, exposure of only the target disk and proximal vertebral body is required, without the exposure of the inferior vertebral body. This prevents unnecessary handling of the anterior longitudinal ligament and ultimately its ossification.

Level confirmation is done at this stage, and an operating microscope is brought in the field. Before the drilling is begun, indigo-carmine dye is injected in the affected disk to facilitate the orientation of the disk space while drilling. The position of the drill hole is 4 to 6 mm above the lower border of the proximal vertebra, at the level of the medial border of the longus coli muscle. The trajectory depends on the location of the target, which is determined preoperatively on the radiological imaging (**Fig. 30.2**). If needed, intraoperative fluoroscopy can be used to confirm the hole position and trajectory.

A 6 × 7 mm drill hole is made from medial to lateral, and because of the oblique trajectory of the cervical disk, this leads directly to the pathological site in the foramen. Drilling can be done using a 4-mm diamond bur initially and later with a 3-mm bur for better visualization and fine drilling. The length of the drill bit is tailored to each patient, as calculated preoperatively on the sagittal CT/MRI scan. It is useful to identify some bony landmark on the preoperative CT that helps orient the surgeon with the lateral margin of the vertebral body. At a one-third depth of the drilling, the bluish discoloration of the stained disk can be seen. Drilling can be safely continued, keeping the blue-stained material in the center of the hole so as to maintain the direction of the trajectory. After the desired depth is achieved, a blunt probe is used to palpate the base of the tunnel so that the thin ivory-white shell of the posterior vertebral wall can be carefully lifted with a fine bone punch or curette. The posterior longitudinal ligament still acts as a protective barrier between the instruments and the neural structures. Bone wax can be used to stop the bleeding from the spongy bone, and epidural bleeds can be managed with thrombin-soaked Gelfoam or FloSeal. The use of bipolar coagulation is strongly discouraged at this step.

After opening the posterior wall, the herniated disk stained blue with indigo-carmine and the hypertrophied uncovertebral region can be visualized. Small pituitary rongeurs can be used to remove the herniated disk. Foraminal decompression can be achieved by undercutting the bony prominences with a rongeur, taking care not to breach the medial foraminal wall (**Fig. 30.3**). Adequacy of the decompression can be confirmed by observing the bulging nerve root with cerebrospinal fluid (CSF) flow and palpating the superior and inferior pedicles along the course of the nerve root using a root probe.

Wound closure is the same as in ACDF, with a Hemovac drain for aspiration of postoperative hematoma (see Video 30.1).

Potential Complications and Precautions

- Meticulous preoperative planning for the location of the drill hole and the direction of the trajectory based on CT is crucial.
- Injury to the vertebral artery is one of the major complications. Dominance of the vertebral artery and the distance of the transverse foramen from the uncovertebral joint should be noted preoperatively.
- Subperiosteal retraction of the longus coli minimizes bleeding and protects the carotid artery.
- The use of indigo-carmine dye facilitates the approach by identifying the disk space as well as any herniated disk fragments.
- While using a long bur, wobbling may be encountered, so extra care should be taken to avoid untoward injury.
- The surgeon should attempt to follow the direction of the previously planned trajectory.

Postoperative Considerations

- Rigid immobilization is not required. A soft collar may be used if the patient complains of pain at the operative site.
- Patient can be mobilized on postoperative day 1.
- Routine physiotherapy is advised along with 3 days of intravenous antibiotics.

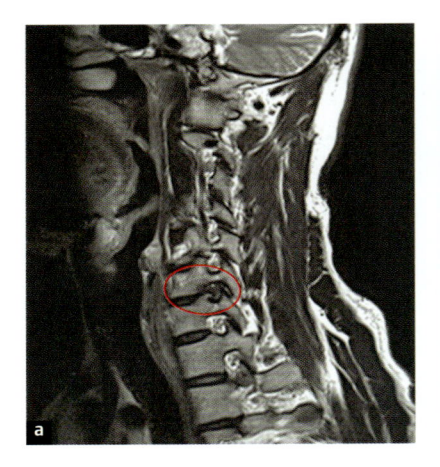

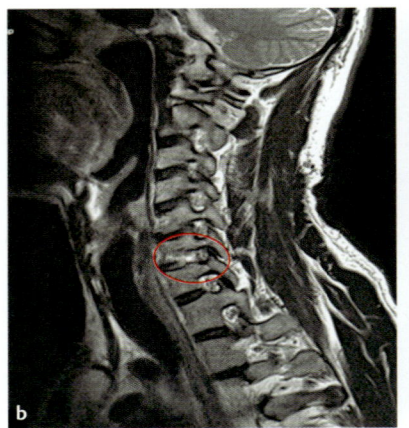

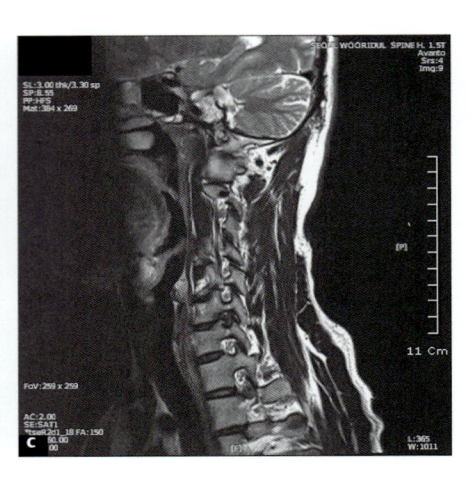

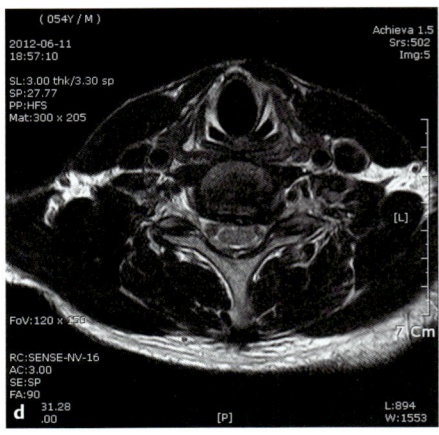

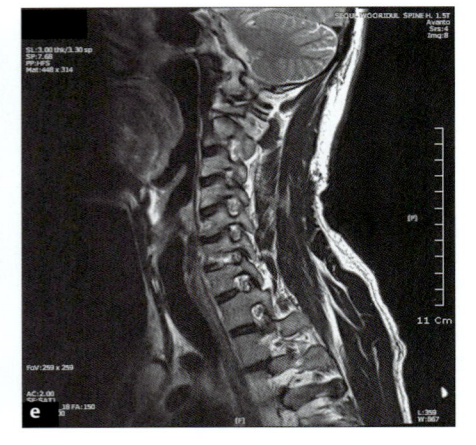

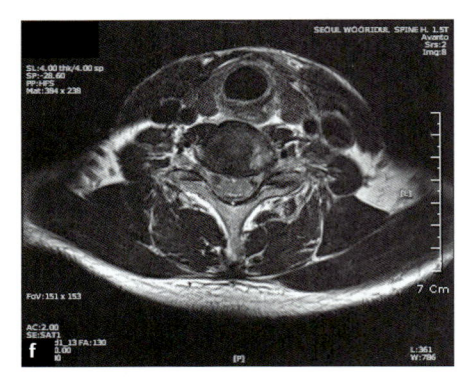

Fig. 30.3 Magnetic resonance imaging (MRI) of **(a)** the preoperative and **(b)** the postoperative foraminal view. **(c)** T2-weighted sagittal MRI showing the left C6-C7 foraminal stenosis with an osteophyte. **(d)** T2-weighted axial view at the C6-C7 foramen showing stenosis due to an osteophyte arising close to the left posterolateral uncovertebral margin. **(e)** Postoperative T2-weighted sagittal MRI of the same patient, after a transcorporeal approach was performed from the cephalad to the caudal direction, without damaging the C6-C7 disk. Successful removal of osteophyte and enlargement of foramen are demonstrated. **(f)** Postoperative T2-weighted axial view at C6. Note the narrow anterior window and the wider base posteriorly, which were done to decompress the left C6-C7 foramen.

Conclusion

The transcorporeal tunnel approach enables the surgeon to perform a direct anterior decompression without the need for interbody fusion. Meticulous planning and a cautious approach can provide an excellent surgical outcome.

References

1. Verbiest H. A lateral approach to the cervical spine: technique and indications. J Neurosurg 1968;28:191–203
2. Hakuba A. Trans-unco-discal approach. A combined anterior and lateral approach to cervical discs. J Neurosurg 1976;45:284–291
3. Lesoin F, Biondi A, Jomin M. Foraminal cervical herniated disc treated by anterior discoforaminotomy. Neurosurgery 1987;21:334–338
4. Jho HD: Microsurgical anterior cervical foraminotomy for radiculopathy: a new approach to cervical disc herniation. J Neuorsurg 1966;84:155–160.
5. Jho HD, Kim WK, Kim MH. Anterior microforaminotomy for treatment of cervical radiculopathy: part 1—disc-preserving "functional cervical disc surgery". Neurosurgery 2002;51(5, Suppl):S46–S53
6. Saringer W, Nöbauer I, Reddy M, Tschabitscher M, Horaczek A. Microsurgical anterior cervical foraminotomy (uncoforaminotomy) for unilateral radiculopathy: clinical results of a new technique. Acta Neurochir (Wien) 2002;144:685–694
7. Smith GW, Robinson RA. The treatment of certain cervical-spine disorders by anterior removal of the intervertebral disc and interbody fusion. J Bone Joint Surg Am 1958;40-A:607–624

8. Cloward RB. The anterior approach for removal of ruptured cervical disks. J Neurosurg 1958;15:602–617
9. Lopez-Espina CG, Amirouche F, Havalad V. Multilevel cervical fusion and its effect on disc degeneration and osteophyte formation. Spine 2006;31:972–978
10. Choi G, Lee SH, Bhanot A, Chae YS, Jung B, Lee S. Modified transcorporeal anterior cervical microforaminotomy for cervical radiculopathy: a technical note and early results. Eur Spine J 2007;16:1387–1393
11. Choi G, Arbatti NJ, Modi HN, et al. Transcorporeal tunnel approach for unilateral cervical radiculopathy: a 2-year follow-up review and results. Minim Invasive Neurosurg 2010;53:127–131
12. Goldstein B. Anatomic issues related to cervical and lumbosacral radiculopathy. Phys Med Rehabil Clin N Am 2002;13:423–437

C. Posterior Approach

31 Cervical Spine: Posterior Exposure

Sean Christie and Janet Martin

Historically, the initial operations on the cervical spine utilized a posterior approach. However, with the advent of anterior approaches and subsequent advancement of those techniques, the posterior exposure has lost some of its favor. Concerns about relatively more postoperative neck discomfort, longer hospital stays, and the development of postlaminectomy kyphosis have contributed to this trend. For many conditions, it is the surgeon's preference and patient characteristics that dictate whether an anterior or posterior approach is used. Nonetheless, the posterior approach is a familiar exposure to the cervical spine, and there are several pathological conditions that favor its use (**Table 31.1**).

Advantages

- Familiar to neurosurgeons
- Avoids risk to the anterior vascular and visceral structures

Disadvantages

- Potentially more postoperative discomfort and longer hospital stays
- Potential for postoperative kyphosis

Anatomy and Landmarks of the Posterior Spine

Although the regional anatomy of the anterior cervical spine was discussed in Chapter 28, several surface landmarks are of particular clinical utility with the posterior approach. Palpating downward from the base of the skull, the spinous process of the C2 vertebra may be identified as the most superior bony prominence encountered. Below C2, the vertebrae are frequently obscured by soft tissue to the level of C7, which is usually palpable in the midline of the base of the neck, and may be visible as an outward protuberance in nonobese patients. Placing the neck into flexion enables visualizing the ligamentum nuchae as a longitudinal ridge running between the spinous process of C7 and the external occipital protuberance, continuous inferiorly with the supraspinous ligament, and providing attachment to the trapezius and splenius capitis muscles. The musculature of the cervical spine is best visualized as three layers from superficial to deep (**Figs. 31.1 and 31.2**). The trapezius, running from the nuchal ligament to its scapular and clavicular attachments, lies immediately beneath the skin. Deep to the trapezius lies the splenius capitis, splenius cervicis, and levator scapulae. The deepest, or paraspinal layer, consists of the multifidus and long and short rotator muscles, including the semispinalis capitis, semispinalis cervicis, longissimus, and oblique capitis muscles. These areas are extensively vascularized, and good hemostatic control is of necessity for proper visualization; however, dissection through the ligamentum nuchae in the midline affords a plane of relative avascularity. The vertebral arteries run through the transverse foramen of the cervical vertebrae and are generally beyond the typical exposure from the posterior approach.

Morphologically, the cervical vertebrae are smaller, with bifid spinous processes, generally, to the level of C6 connected by the ligamentum flavum. As a rule, the cervical vertebrae display less shingling, enabling clear visualization of the interlaminar space. Clear distinction may be made between the lamina and the lateral mass/facet joints to the level of C6. At C7, this distinction becomes somewhat less apparent due to additional muscle attachments at this level. It should be noted that the lateral mass, also known as the zygapophyseal capsule, provides a readily visible landmark for the lateral extent of dissection in a majority of cases when instrumentation is not indicated.

Surgical Technique

Anesthesia

General endotracheal anesthesia is required for posterior cervical approaches. If there are concerns about cord compression during intubation or positioning, awake fiberoptic intubation may be used. Situations in which awake intubation should be considered include spinal trauma and pronounced spondylotic myelopathy in a cooperative patient[1]; if fiberoptic intubation is not available, intubation may be managed by maintaining the neck in a neutral position, with or without traction. In addition, several devices have been developed that utilize video assistance to safely intubate a patient without manipulating the neck. Real-time evoked potential monitoring may be extremely useful in monitoring the status of a patient during both the pre- and perioperative phases of surgery.[2] Preoperative assessment of patient positioning tolerance can be achieved by asking the patient to flex and extend the neck, while assessing for any neurologic symptoms.

Positioning

Although positioning of the neurosurgery patient can be challenging and must take multiple factors into account, the prone position is standard for this approach. In some cases, a seated position may be considered, but this position has been associated with hypotension, cord ischemia, and increased physical demand on the surgical team.[3] With the advent of microsurgical

Table 31.1 Choice of Surgical Approach Based on the Location of Pathology

Pathology	Anterior	Posterior	Both	Either
Midline "soft" disk herniation	++	–	–	–
Lateral "soft" disk herniation	+	++	–	++
Midline osteophyte	++	–	–	–
Lateral osteophyte	++	+	–	+
Spondylotic myelopathy with kyphosis	++	++	+	++
Spondylotic myelopathy without kyphosis	++	+	+	–
Ossified posterior longitudinal ligament—three levels	+	++	+	+
Ossified posterior longitudinal ligament—two levels	++	+	+	+
Vertebral artery decompression	++	+	–	–
Vertebral body osteomyelitis	++	–	–	–
Ventral epidural abscess	+	+	–	+
Posterior element osteomyelitis	–	++	–	–
Dorsal epidural abscess	–	++	–	–
Antero-posterolateral epidural abscess	–	+	–	–
Spinal arteriovenous dural fistula	–	++	–	–
Intracanalicular extradural neoplasia	+	++	–	+
Intracanalicular intradural neoplasia	–	++	–	–
Vertebral body fractures	++	+	–	+
Facet fracture-dislocation (reduced)	+	+	+	+
Facet fracture-dislocation (unreduced)	+	++	+	+
Occipitocervical fusion	–	++	–	–

+, accepted surgical option; ++ generally preferred surgical option; – generally not preferred surgical option.

techniques, its use has become vanishingly rare. The head should be positioned within a three- or four-pin fixation device, with the Mayfield three-pin head holder being the most common device used, due to its ability to fix both the head and the cervical spine while avoiding potentially damaging pressure to the optic nerve and face.[4,5] If an alternative means of fixation is used, such as a foam pillow, headrest, or horseshoe, care must be taken to avoid positional retinal ischemia. The cervical spine should be neutral or in slight flexion. Flexion will rotate the occiput away from the surgical field and tighten the skin and posterior musculature. However, it is important that flexion occur in the rostral cervical spine ("military tuck") and that the chin to chest distance is not less than two or three fingerbreadths (**Fig. 31.3**). Care should be taken to avoid overflexion, particularly if a fusion is being performed. In these cases, a neutral or slightly lordotic neck position will minimize fusion into a kyphotic position.[1] Difficulties in positioning may occur in obese patients, as well as those with short, wide necks.

The prone position, although enabling excellent access to the regional anatomy, is a logistically difficult position, due to the challenge of maintaining airway access, ventilation, perfusion, and hemodynamic stability. Designated frames (Wilson, Jackson, or similar) should be used wherever possible, with the use of additional chest rolls to support the chest wall and allow free movement of the abdominal wall, enabling improved diaphragmatic excursion, decreased abdominal pressure and surgical bleeding, and improved venous return from the lower extremities and pelvis.[6,7] The knees are flexed and bony protuberances should be well padded to avoid pressure ulcers, and care should be taken to avoid hyperextension in the abducted arms, to prevent incidental injury to the brachial plexus. Pneumatic compression devices should be used to minimize the risk of deep vein thrombosis.

Technique

Due to the multiple potential approaches to cervical spine pathology, as well as the potential adverse outcomes of the posterior approach, it is important to evaluate the patient's individual risk profile via a detailed history and imaging before finalizing a

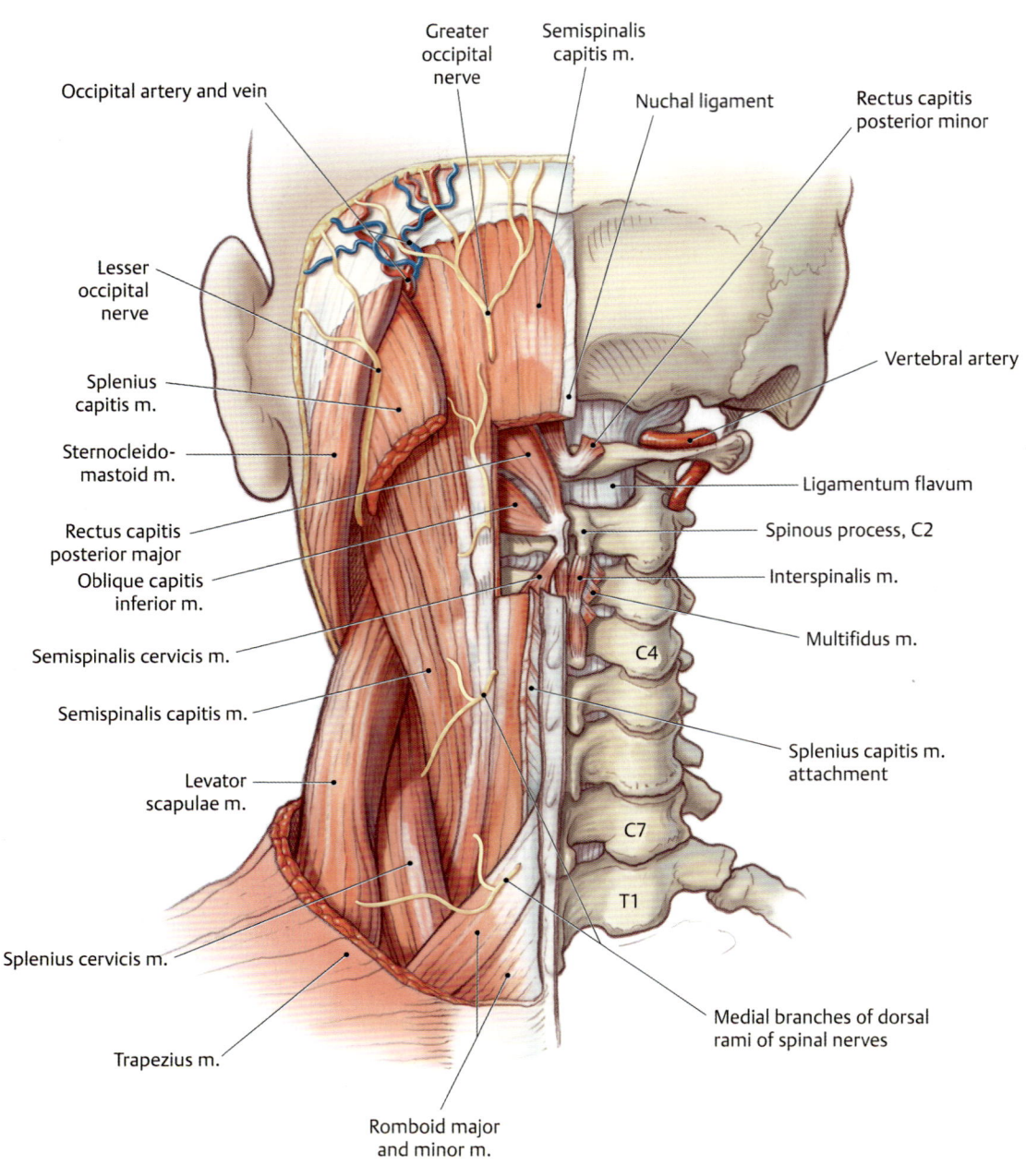

Fig. 31.1 Posterior cervical spine musculature.

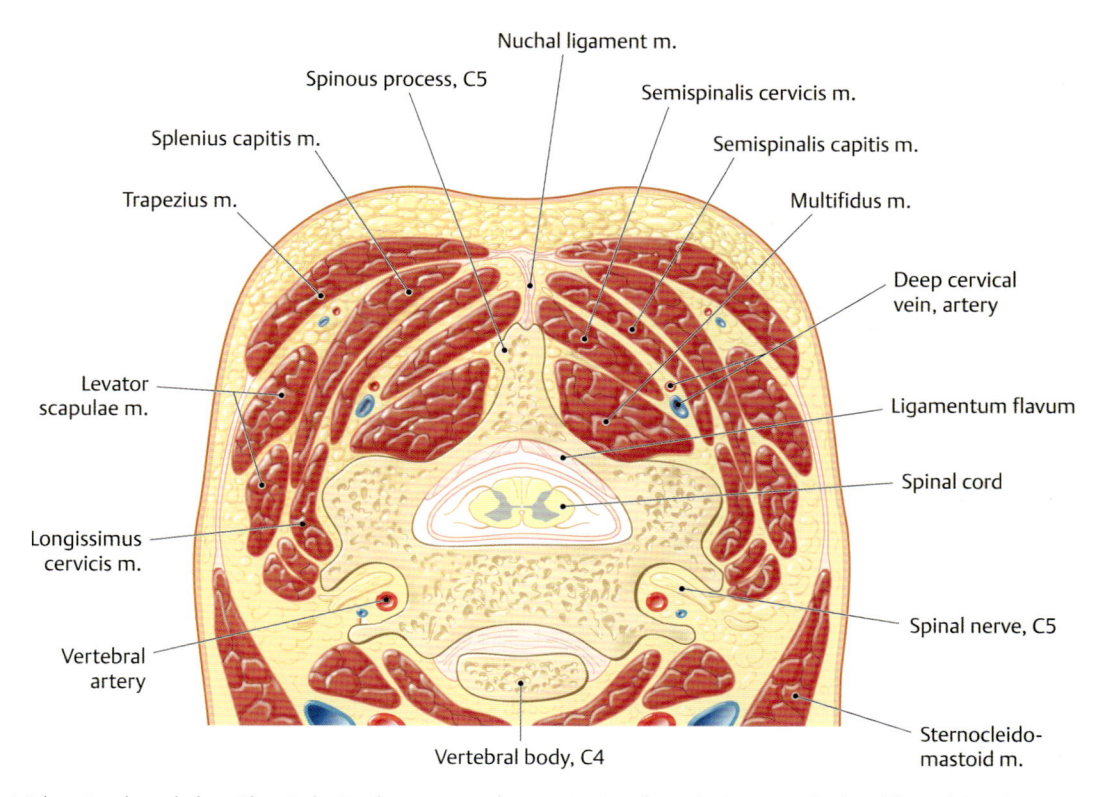

Fig. 31.2 Axial section through the midcervical spine demonstrates the organization of muscles into superficial, middle, and deep layers.

course of action. As with all surgical procedures, meticulous attention to detail and gentle tissue handling will yield the best results.

After obtaining informed consent and making arrangements for appropriate antibiotic prophylaxis, the patient is placed under general endotracheal anesthesia and positioned prone. Prior to incision, fluoroscopic imaging should be used to confirm spinal levels and alignment and to reduce the risk of cervical kyphosis, particularly in cases where laminectomy will be followed by fusion. The C-arm is then sterilely draped and left in position prior to commencement of the operation to minimize repositioning throughout the procedure.

Following marking of the incision line and infiltration of the skin with local anesthetic and epinephrine, a superficial incision is made with a scalpel, followed by monopolar electrocautery dissection to the level of the ligamentum nuchae (**Fig. 31.4**). The avascular plane of the ligamentum nuchae is followed, enabling lateral mobilization of the paraspinal musculature. Placement

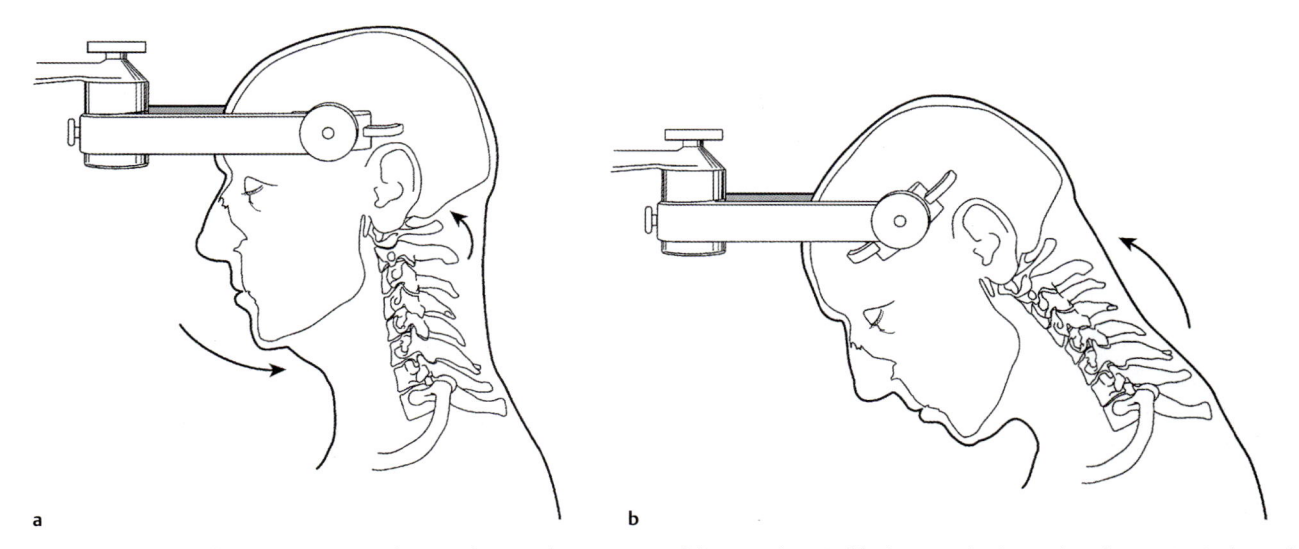

Fig. 31.3 Positioning for a posterior cervical approach. Note the conversion of the normal cervical lordosis into kyphosis when the position is changed from **(a)** flexion at the occiput-C1 level (military tuck position) to **(b)** flexion throughout the cervical spine.

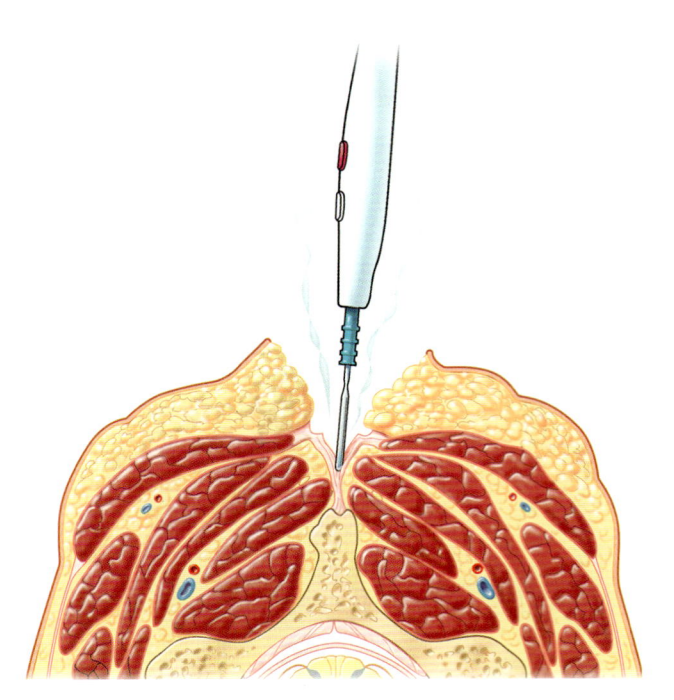

Fig. 31.4 Midline dissection along the ligamentum nuchae to expose the spinous processes.

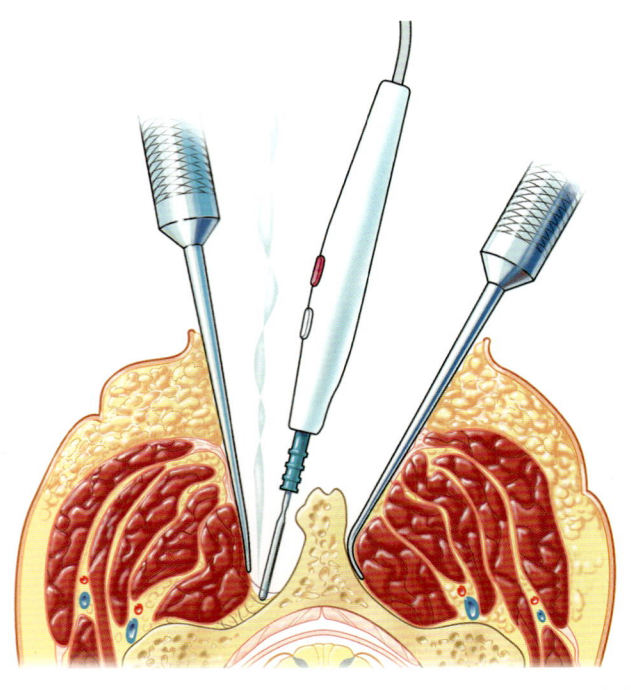

Fig. 31.5 Subperiosteal dissection with electrocautery. Straight or angled Cobb retractors can be used to expose the plane.

and frequent adjustment of a self-retaining retractor facilitates maintaining this plane. Once at the level of the spinous process and lamina, care should be taken to remain in the periosteal plane (**Figs. 31.5 and 31.6**), while also preserving structures associated with the adjacent zygapophyseal facet joints. Muscular attachments should be released perpendicular to the bone. Whether using electrocautery or curettage, the surgeon must be cautious while dissecting over the interlaminar space to avoid inadvertent injury to the spinal cord. Lateral dissection should extend to the medial border of the facet joints; to avoid destabilizing the spine and increasing the risk of subluxation or kyphosis, dissection of the lateral masses should only be undertaken if instrumentation, for the purpose of arthrodesis, is planned. The final exposure is maintained via two self-retaining retractors (**Fig. 31.7**).

Closure

Due to the highly vascular nature of the musculature of the cervical spine, some bleeding may occur upon removal of the retractors. This must be addressed prior to closure. Although drains may be placed in cases of severe bleeding, adequate hemostasis

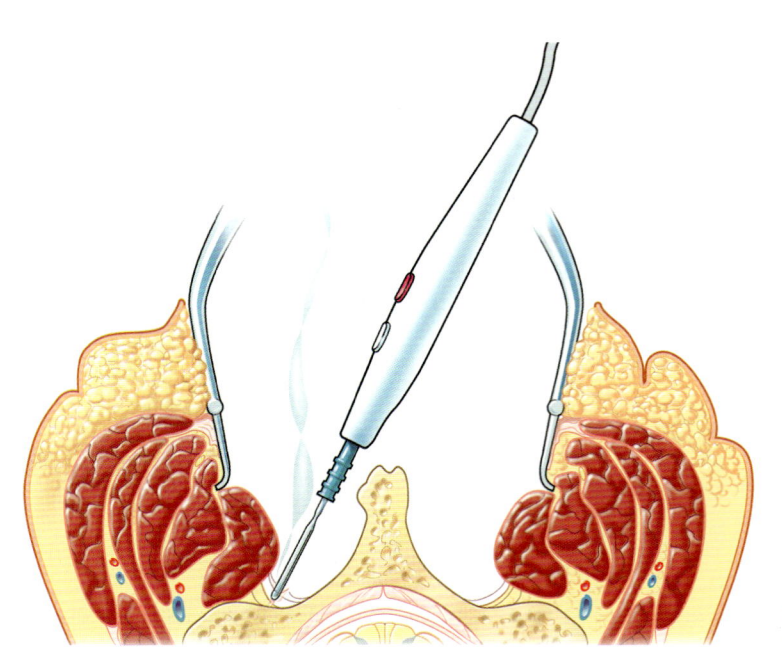

Fig. 31.6 The use of self-retaining retractors to provide sustained and uniform retraction.

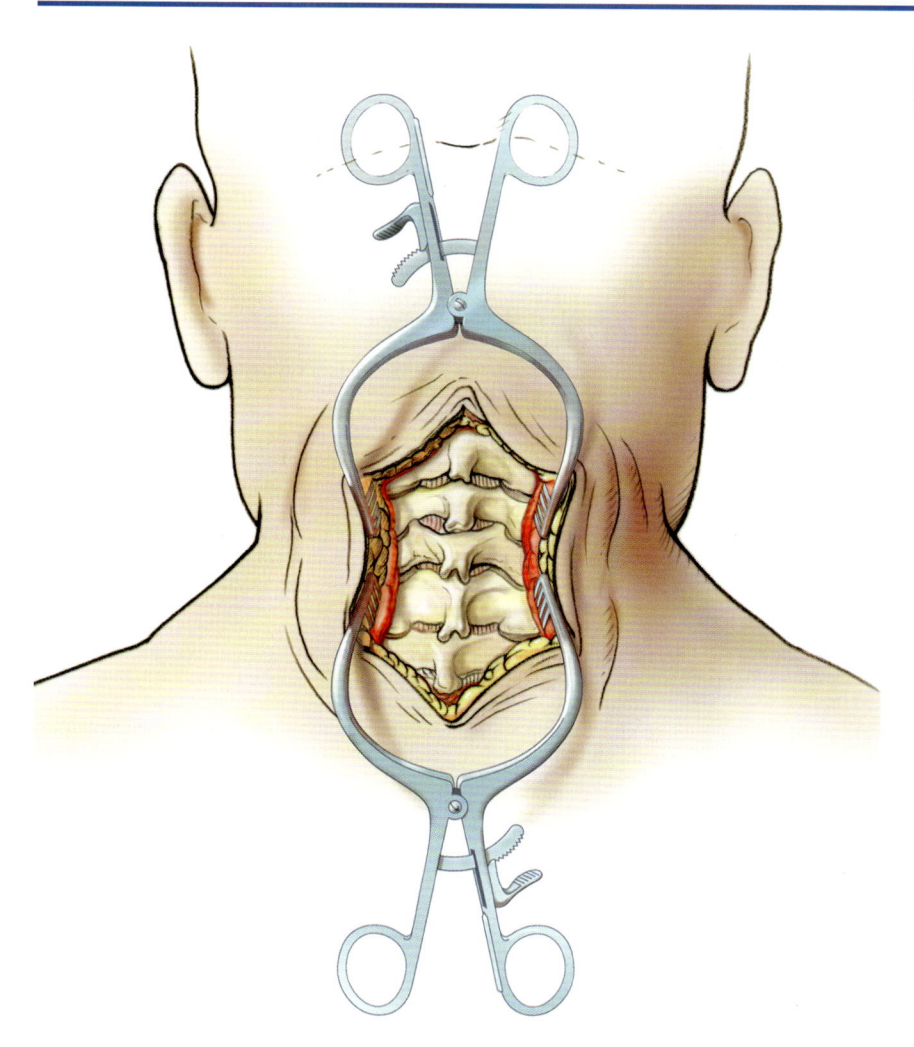

Fig. 31.7 Two angled, self-retaining retractors provide optimal exposure prior to commencing the decompression/laminectomy.

is associated with better patient outcomes.[6] Ischemia and necrosis are potential complications of reapproximation of the paraspinal muscles, which may be sutured with No. 0 polyglactin sutures, depending on surgeon preference. Due to the role of the muscles below C6 in shoulder girdle and upper limb movement, U-sutures should be used if repairing the musculature of the lower cervical spine, to allow for additional tensile strength. The fascia is then tightly closed with the same suture, and the subcutaneous tissues are reapproximated in layers with 2-0 or 3-0 inverted polyglactin sutures. The skin can be closed with staples or interrupted or subcuticular sutures. A sterile dressing is applied.

Complications of the Posterior Spine Approach

Complications associated with prone positioning include pressure sores, vascular compression or insufficiency, and brachial plexus injury, blindness, and, rarely, air embolism or quadriplegia.[7]

Along with the common operative risks of bleeding and infection, posterior cervical surgeries also carry a notable risk of postlaminectomy kyphosis, particularly in pediatric patients or patients with preoperative spinal instability or deformity.[8] Removal of more than 50% of one or more facet joints,[9,10] the associated capsule,[11] or extension of dissection over one or more levels[10,12] can be associated with segmental hypermobility. Spinal instability is a possible side effect of multiple procedures, although it appears to occur most commonly following laminectomy without fusion.[13] Pseudomeningocele is a rare complication resulting from intentional or incidental durotomy.[14]

Although vertebral artery injury is a rare complication of posterior spinal surgery, occurring in 0.07% of cases, it is more common with inexperienced surgeons and conveys a 10% risk of neurologic sequelae or death.[15] The risk of venous thromboembolism appears higher in patients undergoing posterior rather than anterior cervical fusion, but chemoprophylaxis is problematic due to the significant risk of postoperative epidural hematoma.[16]

Spinal surgery has long been associated with the risk of fifth nerve palsy.[17] This palsy is generally transient, presenting within the first week following surgery, at a rate ranging from 0 to 30%. Although putative causes include iatrogenic injury to the nerve root, tethering of the nerve root due to posteromedial shifting of the dural contents following surgery, segmental cord disorder, and ischemic/reperfusion injuries, there is no preponderance of clinical evidence in support of any particular option.[18] When conservatively managed, the majority of cases will resolve in under 6 months, and most patients will achieve full recovery within a year.[19]

Posterior cervical fusions, in particular, are associated with an increased risk of wrong-site surgery[20]; thus, we advocate the use of intraoperative radiological adjuncts to augment standard anatomic palpation.

Conclusion

The posterior approach to the cervical spine is a familiar and versatile approach for most neurosurgeons. However, the muscular dissection does yield more postoperative discomfort than most anterior approaches. Particular attention must be paid to hemostasis and avoiding facet joint disruption to reduce the risk of postoperative complications.

References

1. Tandon N, Vollmer DG. Midcervical spine: posterior approach. In: Fessler RG, Sekhar LN, eds. Atlas of Neurosurgical Techniques: Spine and Peripheral Nerves, 1st ed. New York: Thieme; 2006:233–238
2. Stecker MM. A review of intraoperative monitoring for spinal surgery. Surg Neurol Int 2012;3(Suppl 3):S174–S187
3. Porter JM, Pidgeon C, Cunningham AJ. The sitting position in neurosurgery: a critical appraisal. Br J Anaesth 1999;82:117–128
4. Schonauer C, Bocchetti A, Barbagallo G, Albanese V, Moraci A. Positioning on surgical table. Eur Spine J 2004;13(Suppl 1):S50–S55
5. American Society of Anesthesiologists Task Force on Perioperative Blindness. Practice advisory for perioperative visual loss associated with spine surgery: a report by the American Society of Anesthesiologists Task Force on Perioperative Blindness. Anesthesiology 2006;104:1319–1328
6. Wadsworth R, Anderton JM, Vohra A. The effect of four different surgical prone positions on cardiovascular parameters in healthy volunteers. Anaesthesia 1996;51:819–822
7. Rozet I, Vavilala MS. Risks and benefits of patient positioning during neurosurgical care. Anesthesiol Clin 2007;25:631–653, x
8. Deutsch H, Haid RW, Rodts GE, Mummaneni PV. Postlaminectomy cervical deformity. Neurosurg Focus 2003;15:E5
9. Zdeblick TA, Zou D, Warden KE, McCabe R, Kunz D, Vanderby R. Cervical stability after foraminotomy. A biomechanical in vitro analysis. J Bone Joint Surg Am 1992;74:22–27
10. Butler JC, Whitecloud TS III. Postlaminectomy kyphosis. Causes and surgical management. Orthop Clin North Am 1992;23:505–511
11. Zdeblick TA, Abitbol JJ, Kunz DN, McCabe RP, Garfin S. Cervical stability after sequential capsule resection. Spine 1993;18:2005–2008
12. Guigui P, Benoist M, Deburge A. Spinal deformity and instability after multilevel cervical laminectomy for spondylotic myelopathy. Spine 1998;23:440–447
13. Papadakis M, Aggeliki L, Papadopoulos EC, Girardi FP. Common surgical complications in degenerative spinal surgery. World J Orthop 2013;4:62–66
14. Morgan SL, Krishna V, Varma AK. Cervical pseudomeningocele as a cause of neurological decline after posterior cervical spine surgery. Neurol India 2012;60:256–257
15. Lunardini DJ, Eskander MS, Even JL, et al. Vertebral artery injuries in cervical spine surgery. Spine J 2014;14:1520–5
16. Schairer WW, Pedtke AC, Hu SS. Venous thromboembolism after spine surgery. Spine 2014;39:911–918
17. Scoville WB. Cervical spondylosis treated by bilateral facetectomy and laminectomy. J Neurosurg 1961;18:423–428
18. Sakaura H, Hosono N, Mukai Y, Ishii T, Yoshikawa H. C5 palsy after decompression surgery for cervical myelopathy: review of the literature. Spine 2003;28:2447–2451
19. Dai L, Ni B, Yuan W, Jia L. Radiculopathy after laminectomy for cervical compression myelopathy. J Bone Joint Surg Br 1998;80:846–849
20. Marquez-Lara A, Nandyala SV, Hassanzadeh H, Noureldin M, Sankaranarayanan S, Singh K. Sentinel events in cervical spine surgery. Spine 2014;39:715–720

32 Cervical Laminectomy

Sean Christie and Janet Martin

Despite the increased popularity of anterior approaches to cervical spine pathology, the posterior cervical laminectomy remains a commonly employed strategy to gain access to the spinal canal for decompressive purposes. It is crucial that the preoperative alignment be lordotic to minimize postoperative deformity. A list of indications can be found in Chapter 31, **Table 31.1**. In addition, cervical laminectomy remains the approach of choice for intradural tumors or vascular malformations and for continuous ossification of the posterior longitudinal ligament (OPLL). The primary advantage of the approach is its familiarity; in addition, it is an extensile technique, it easily accommodates multilevel decompressions, and it can be potentially motion preserving.

Indications

- Multilevel stenosis in patients with neutral or lordotic spinal alignment
- Compression or exposure of cord secondary to inflammation, infection, malignancy, fracture, or OPLL

Contraindications

- Kyphotic deformity of the spine

Advantages

- No risk of injury to anterior neck structures
- Ease of access; of particular use in multilevel disease
- Quickly performed and relatively undemanding

Disadvantages

- No direct access to anterior pathology
- Results may be less favorable than with anterior or anteroposterior approaches
- Potential destabilization
- Neck pain secondary to denervation of posterior musculature

Technique

The surgical anatomy, positioning, and exposure have been described in Chapter 31. Avoidance of hyperextension is critical in the context of cervical canal stenosis, as it will aggravate the narrowing through buckling of the ligamentum flavum. In addition, hyperflexion should be avoided when an arthrodesis is planned, to avoid an unnecessary kyphotic deformity. It is worth reiterating that the exposure should not extend beyond the beginning of the lateral masses unless an arthrodesis is planned, to minimize the risk of postoperative kyphosis.

Multiple techniques have been described to achieve the goal of cervical laminectomy, that is, to surgically remove any compressive structures (laminae and ligamentum flavum) while avoiding any trauma to the spinal cord or causing any instability. Common options include bony removal using a Leksell rongeur, a high-speed drill, or an en-bloc laminectomy.

During dissection, additional care must be taken to prevent iatrogenic injury to the stenotic spinal cord, and placement of instruments into the spinal canal should be avoided or performed with extreme caution and using a two-handed technique. In preparation for decompression, all soft tissue should be removed wherever possible to ease drilling, as residual tissue can bind the drill, cause it to skip, and potentially lead to inadvertent injury. Careful attention should be paid to hemostasis to provide optimal visualization. It should be noted that the ligamentum flavum is absent beneath the rostral aspect of the lamina and, as such, dura and spinal cord will be protected by minimal soft tissue.

Several techniques have been described to perform bony decompression. In the traditional approach, the spinous processes may be removed using a Horsley or Leksell rongeur to the level of the ligamentum flavum (**Fig. 32.1**). Following exposure of the ligaments, they may be gently "peeled away" from the laminar surface with a curette. The lamina may then be removed either manually or using a high-speed drill and bone punch (such as a Kerrison), and any residual ligamentum flavum trimmed back. It should be noted that this method enables the removal of the spinous processes without the drilling of laminotomy troughs, but also involves placement of a portion of the rongeur between the laminae and the dura. As such, care should be taken with this approach, particularly in cases of severe stenosis.

Alternatively, the laminae may be removed with the use of a high-speed drill. Two methods have been described to accomplish this, the first being en-bloc removal of the lamina via bilateral trough laminotomies (**Fig. 32.2**), using a procedure similar to a laminoplasty. The troughs may be created using a cutting bur attachment or by utilizing a footed attachment. The latter requires insertion of a thin footplate within the spinal canal and requires the same caution and care as mention above. With either en-bloc technique, it is critical that the cut lines angle medially and do not extend beyond the beginning of the lateral mass, to avoid injury to the exiting nerve roots. When elevating the en-bloc lamina (**Fig. 32.3**), care should be taken to remove it in a dorsal and caudal direction to avoid buckling and compression at the rostral extent. A 1- or 2-mm Kerrison rongeur can be used to release any remaining ligamentum flavum.

In the second method, the spinous processes may be removed using a Horsley or Leksell rongeur, bleeding surfaces waxed, and the entire lamina then thinned and removed along with its

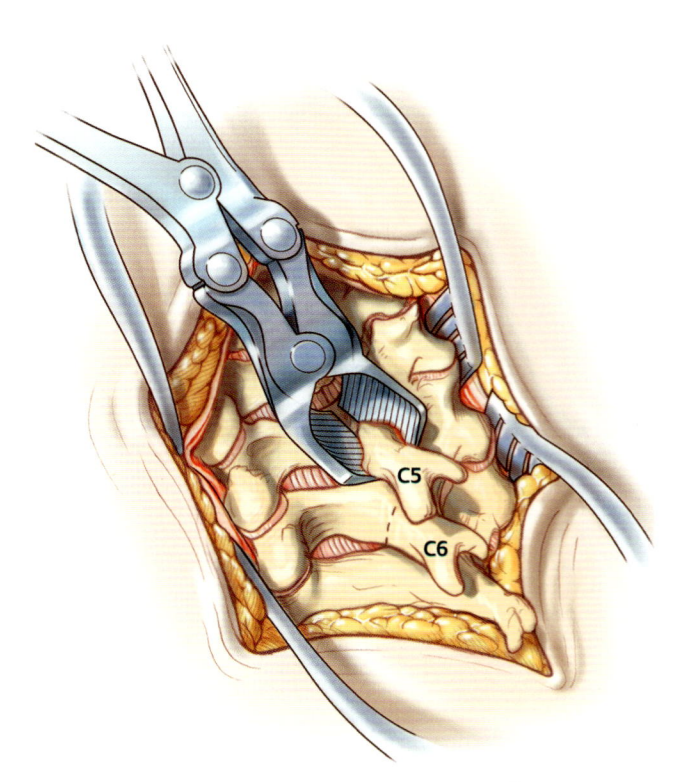

Fig. 32.1 Removal of the spinous processes using a Horsley rongeur.

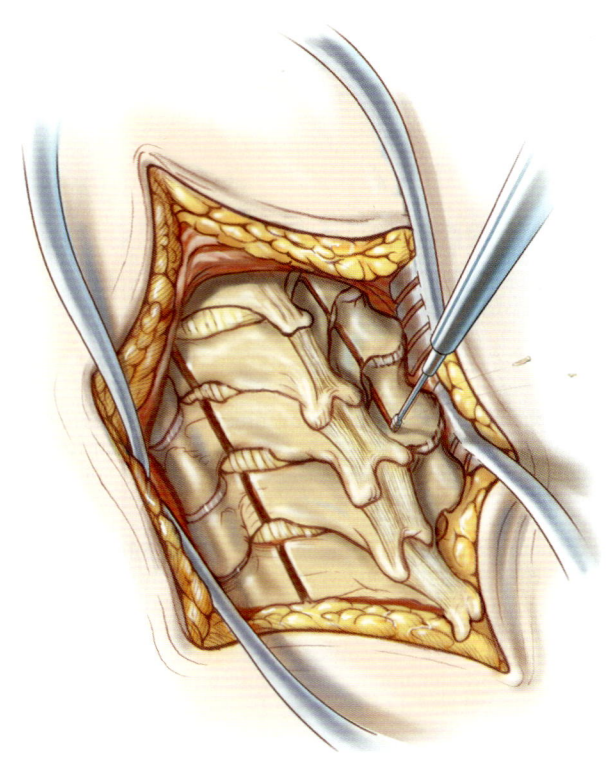

Fig. 32.2 En-bloc removal of spinous processes and laminae: drilling of troughs.

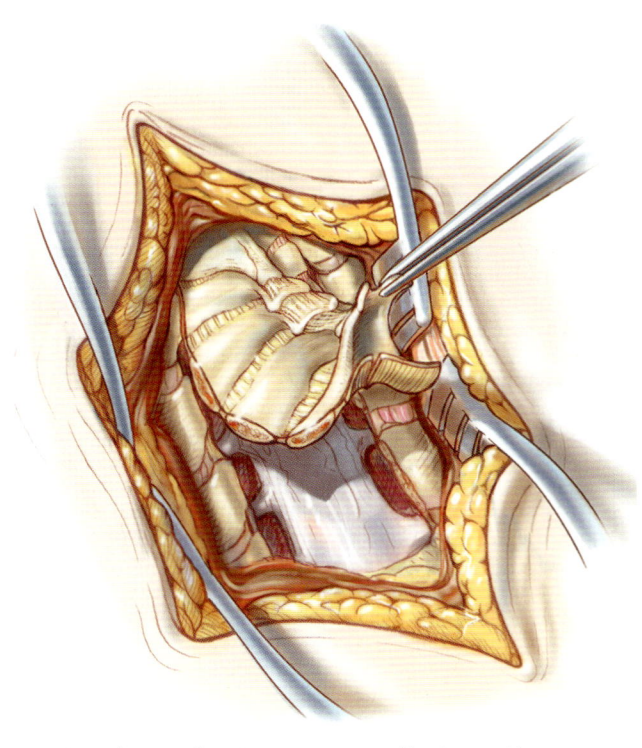

Fig. 32.3 Elevating the spinous processes and laminae en bloc.

attached ligaments using soft tissue instruments. A small cutting bur may be used to grind the bone down to a thin, inner cortical layer, which may then be further thinned using a precision drill if required (**Fig. 32.4**). During the drilling process, care should be taken to ensure proper irrigation and suction, both to improve visualization and to prevent thermal injury to the underlying bone and soft tissue.

The ventral aspect of the lamina requires deeper drilling to achieve total removal. As the lamina thins, the bone becomes increasingly pliant as it approximates the level of the ligamentum flavum (**Figs. 32.5 and 32.6**), changing in color from white-gray to reflect the yellowish coloration of the underlying dura, and becoming increasingly translucent. Suspected entry into the epidural space may be confirmed with gentle palpation using a nerve hook, or the drill bit itself.

Once the lamina is sufficiently thinned, the ligamentum flava may be elevated with fine-toothed forceps and gently split along the midline raphe prior to removal with rongeurs. The thinned lamina may be removed piecemeal (**Fig. 32.7**) using a No. 15 blade, surgical scissors, or Kerrison rongeurs. It should be noted that each individual vertebra does not exist in isolation; due to the shingling between adjacent vertebrae, full laminectomy of one vertebra often requires a partial laminectomy of the superior portion of the vertebra directly inferior to it.

Closure

Particular care should be taken in closure of the posterior cervical approach, due to the weight-bearing nature of the affected

32 Cervical Laminectomy

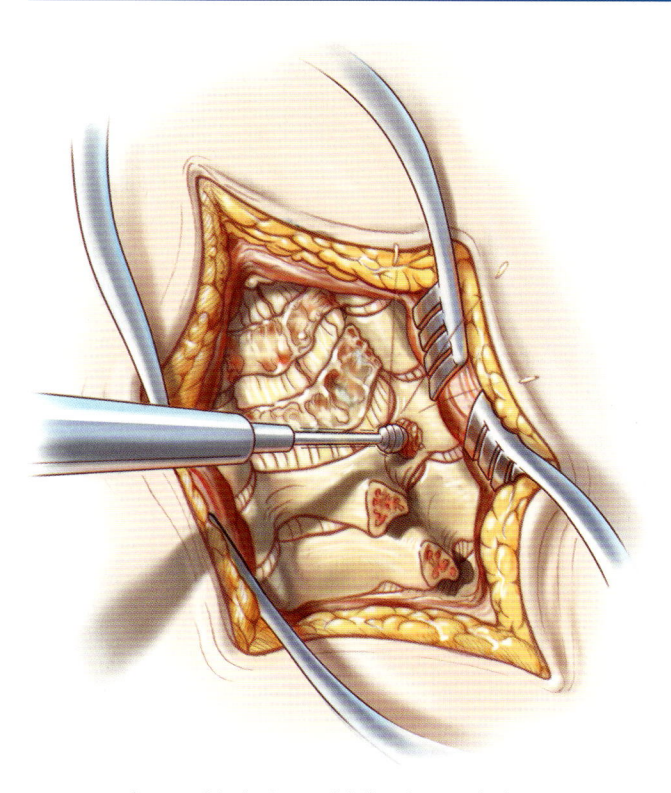

Fig. 32.4 The use of the high-speed drill to thin out the laminae.

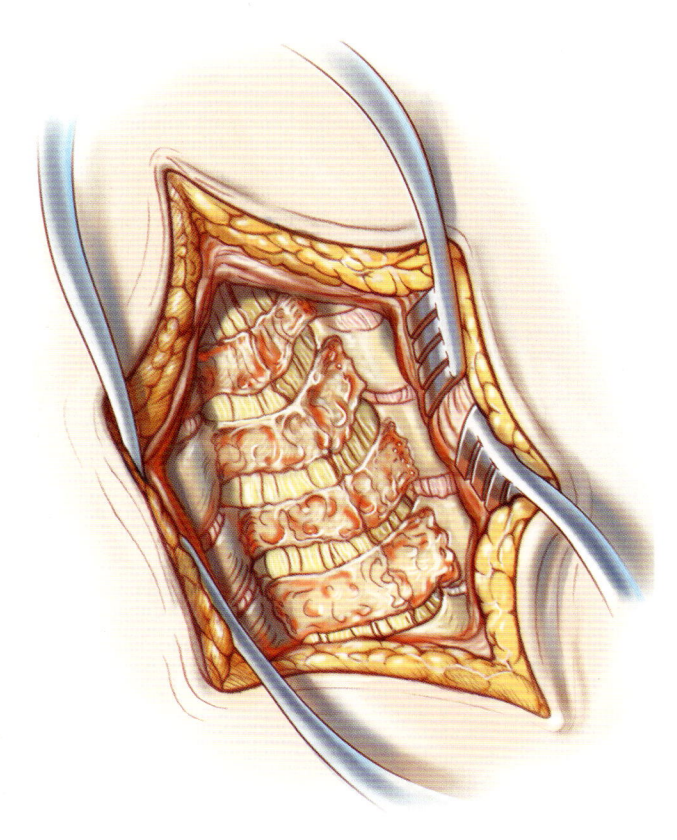

Fig. 32.5 Paper-thin laminae.

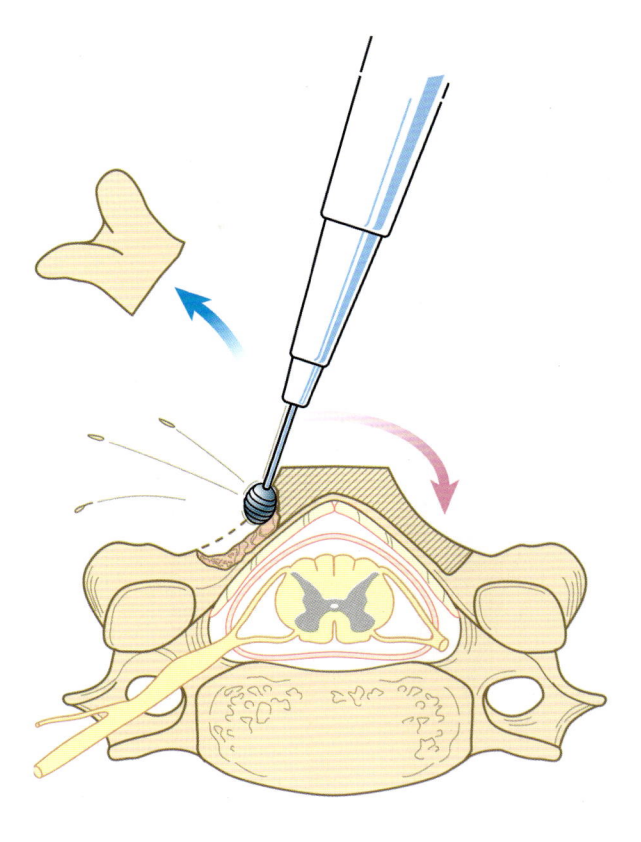

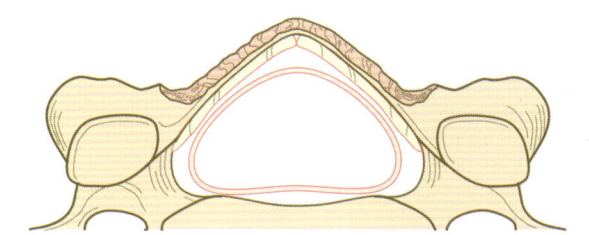

Fig. 32.6 Schematic representation in axial section of the process of thinning the laminae. Care is taken not to enter the joint capsule on either side.

musculature. Wherever possible, in segments adjacent to the laminectomy, transosseous reattachment of muscles to the spinous processes should be undertaken, followed by careful midline suturing of the fascial and dermal layers. There is some controversy with this approach, with some surgeons believing that muscle belly suturing leads to an increase in ischemia, muscle necrosis, and subsequent neck pain, and so they choose to suture only the subfascial and the dermis. A subfascial drain may be inserted, depending on surgeon preference.

Complications

Cervical laminectomy is subject to the general risks associated with major surgery, as well as those associated with the posterior approach to the spine discussed in Chapter 31, and specific complications related to the operation itself.

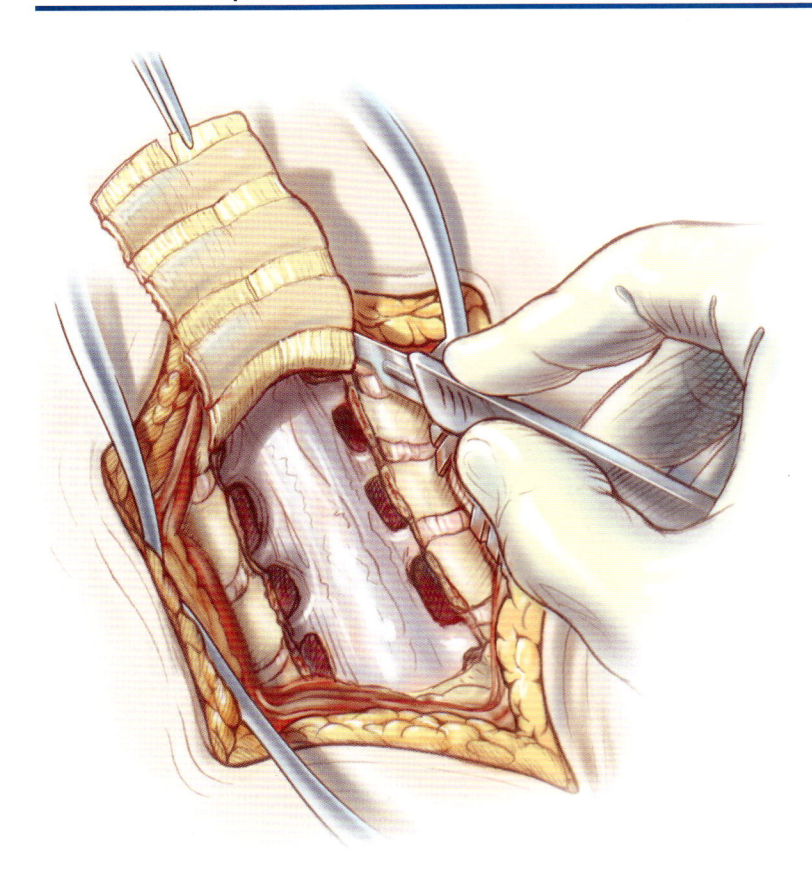

Fig. 32.7 Removal of the thinned laminae and the ligamentum flavum. This commonly occurs piecemeal as portions of laminae and ligament break off from their attachments.

Early complications involve the potential for intraoperative dural tear, which should be immediately sutured and sealed with a fibrin-based tissue glue.[1] Rates of spinal cord and nerve root injuries are surgeon and center dependent, but have been documented to occur in 5.5% of all cases.[2] Mechanisms of nonradicular injury are poorly characterized, with several factors, including cord ischemia, reperfusion injury, and syrinx development hypothesized to be causative.[3,4]

The most prominent late complication is the potential development of kyphosis, secondary to detachment of the paraspinous muscles from the spinous processes. Patient factors abetting the development of kyphosis or instability include advanced age, severe original myelopathy, and recent trauma.[1,5]

Although it is beyond the scope of this chapter, patients with implanted hardware including lateral mass screws will be subject to risks of screw malposition or loss, or, rarely, lateral mass fractures.[6,7]

Conclusion

Posterior laminectomy remains an important and extensile approach to cervical pathologies. It can be a stand-alone, motion-preserving, decompressive procedure, or performed in conjunction with an arthrodesis. Proper patient selection, including avoiding preoperative kyphotic spines, and meticulous surgical technique are keys to successful outcomes.

References

1. Epstein NE. Laminectomy for cervical myelopathy. Spinal Cord 2003;41: 317–327
2. Yonenobu K, Hosono N, Iwasaki M, Asano M, Ono K. Neurologic complications of surgery for cervical compression myelopathy. Spine 1991;16: 1277–1282
3. Tandon N, Vollmer DG. Midcervical spine: posterior approach. In: Fessler RG, Sekhar LN, eds. Atlas of Neurosurgical Techniques: Spine and Peripheral Nerves, 1st ed. New York: Thieme; 2006:233–238
4. Cybulski GR, D'Angelo CM. Neurological deterioration after laminectomy for spondylotic cervical myeloradiculopathy: the putative role of spinal cord ischaemia. J Neurol Neurosurg Psychiatry 1988l;51:717–718
5. Snow RB, Weiner H. Cervical laminectomy and foraminotomy as surgical treatment of cervical spondylosis: a follow-up study with analysis of failures. J Spinal Disord 1993;6:245–250, discussion 250–251
6. Aydogan M, Enercan M, Hamzaoglu A, Alanay A. Reconstruction of the subaxial cervical spine using lateral mass and facet screw instrumentation. Spine 2012;37:E335–E341
7. Katonis P, Papadakis SA, Galanakos S, et al. Lateral mass screw complications: analysis of 1662 screws. J Spinal Disord Tech 2011;24:415–420

33 Posterior Cervical Foraminotomy and Diskectomy

Sean Christie and Janet Martin

Cervical radiculopathy is commonly caused by compression of the cervical spinal nerve roots within the neural foramen. Although often associated with disk herniation, it can also occur secondary to spondylosis or ligamentous hypertrophy (**Fig. 33.1**). In these cases, the posterior approach to decompression offers a direct method for relief of foraminal compression causing radiculopathy.

Indications

- Cervical foraminal stenosis with symptoms correlating to affected nerve root documented on magnetic resonance imaging (MRI), computed tomography (CT), or CT myelogram
- Cervical osteophytic compression
- Symptoms refractory to medical management
- No myelopathy documented

Contraindications

- Symptoms not referable to the pathology seen on imaging
- Spinal cord compression visible on studies
- Significant herniation compressing the nerve root medial to the foramen
- Axial neck pain with no associated neurologic symptoms
- Significant kyphosis or mechanical instability at the cervical level of repair
- Any signs or symptoms associated with myelopathy, including upper motor neuron signs, pathological hyperreflexia, and preserved primitive reflexes
- Local skin infection

Advantages

- Does not destabilize the disk space
- Does not require fusion or device placement
- Avoids the risks of the anterior approach (carotid injury, esophageal or tracheal injury, recurrent laryngeal nerve injury, superior laryngeal nerve injury, thoracic duct injury, hoarseness after of the immediate postsurgical period)
- Direct approach and decompression; not technically complicated

Disadvantages

- More dissection of large erector spinae muscle mass, with a possible increase in postoperative neck pain
- Inability to deal with pathology affecting the central aspect of the canal
- Inability to deal with diseases of the ventral cord, such as ossification of the posterior longitudinal ligament (OPLL)

Surgical Technique

Anesthesia and Positioning

Under general anesthesia, the patient is placed in the prone or sitting position, but the sitting position may be associated with additional risks to the patient and fatigue for the surgeon. It is rarely used in uncomplicated cases of open posterior decompression but should be considered in cases where excessive bleeding, spinal cord hypotension, or respiratory complications are of concern, or when an endoscopic approach is planned (see Chapter 34). Positioning of the prone patient should be ensured by use of a Wilson frame or similar bolster under the torso, whereas the skull should be supported by a three-pin Mayfield skull clamp or well-padded horseshoe. The neck should not be hyperextended; a "military tuck" posture with the chin tucked aids in the approach to the posterior cervical disk space. The shoulders should be taped gently to facilitate a radiographic view of the neck, whereas the elbows should be padded to prevent nerve compression and taped to the patient's side. All other compression points should be checked and padded before commencement of the procedure.

After induction of general anesthesia and confirmation of appropriate intravenous access, a Foley catheter is placed, and a single dose of antibiotics (generally cephazolin or vancomycin) should be administered before the skin incision. Intravenous corticosteroids are generally not indicated for this procedure.

Somatosensory evoked potentials and myotomal electromyography (EMG) could be monitored throughout the procedure, with precordial Doppler available to monitor for air embolism, particularly with the patient in the sitting position. Use of neuromuscular paralytic agents should be minimized to enable intraoperative assessment of nerve root irritation.

Approach

A midline incision should be marked to a length of ~ 3 to 5 cm (1 to 1.5 inch) and infiltrated with local anesthesia (**Fig. 33.2**) Note that the length of the incision is a compromise between keeping the surgical aperture as small as possible and avoiding excessive muscle ischemia due to retraction. Before cutting, X-ray or fluoroscopy should be used to ensure good spine alignment, appropriate spinal level, and optimal incision placement.

Subperiosteal dissection (see Chapter 31) should be performed over the laminae of the vertebrae adjacent to the

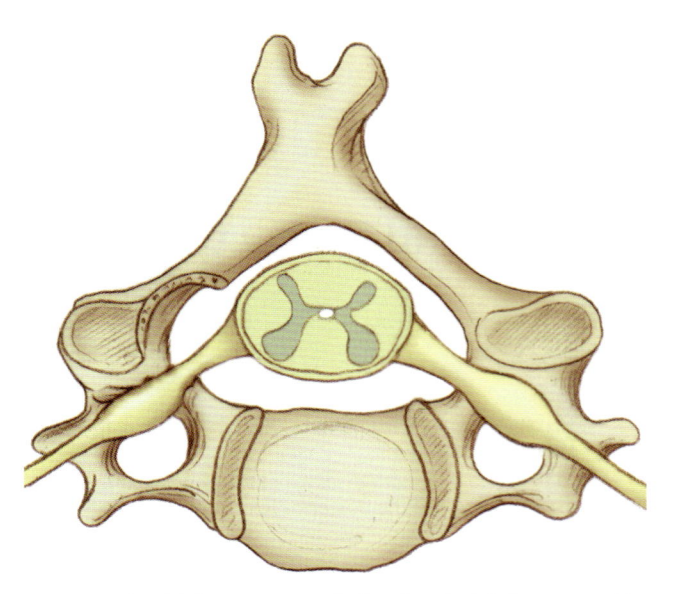

Fig. 33.1 The disk fragment is usually found on the inferior aspect of the root, coming up from the disk space.

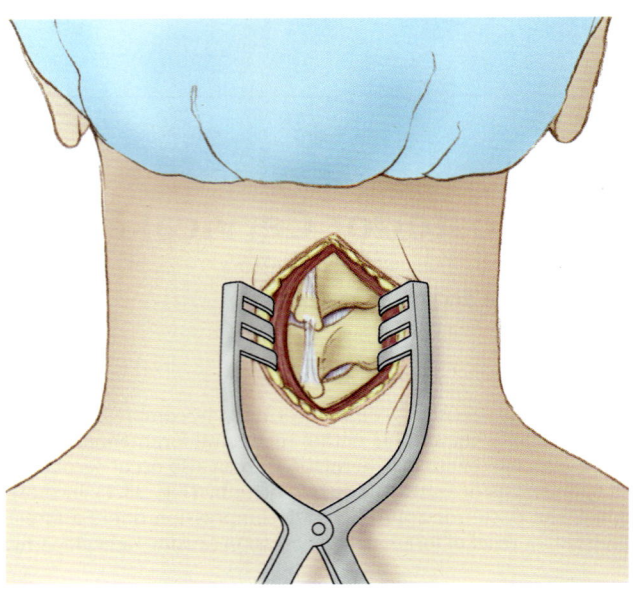

Fig. 33.2 The incision is made in the midline.

symptomatic foramen, strictly on the side of the pathology. The muscle should be dissected to expose the medial 50% of the facet joint (**Fig. 33.3**). Note that further medial or lateral dissection is not required to access the vertebral foramen and may destabilize the joint, leading to postoperative complications.

After the level is confirmed and adequate dissection achieved, the surgical exposure is maintained via placement of one or two self-retaining retractors.

Foraminotomy

The line marking the junction between the lamina and facet should be identified. Removal of bone should begin roughly medial to this point. Bone removal can be performed with a drill or thin-footed Kerrison rongeurs, according to the surgeon's preference.

The inferior aspect of the superior lamina should then be gently separated from the ligamentum flavum with small angled curettes or a dissector. As the very lateral aspect of the lamina is removed, the thecal sac should be visualized (**Fig. 33.4**).

If required, part of the superior aspect of the inferior lamina can also be removed to help identify the inferior pedicle.

Removal of the lateral lamina usually leads to spontaneous opening of the ligamentum flavum. If it remains intact after identification of the inferior pedicle, gently dissect with a small dissector or nerve hook, taking care to avoid puncturing the underlying dura. After dissection of the ligamentum flavum, the nerve root is visible, coursing laterally from the thecal sac into the vertebral foramen (**Fig. 33.5**). To aid in identification of the nerve root, the foramen can be palpated with a small nerve hook.

In cases where a large volume of bone remains dorsal to the nerve root, a small drill should be used to gently thin it as required, until only a shell remains. Note that the nerve can easily be injured at the foraminal junction; do not force instruments into a tight foramen. Instead, slowly continue to remove bone until the foramen becomes wide enough to allow free access. Bone fragments should be removed from the surgical site using 1- to 2-mm thin-footed Kerrisons.

As stated above, compression may be secondary to bony overgrowth, ligamentous hypertrophy, or both. To ensure proper decompression, all nonneural tissue dorsal to the nerve root should be carefully removed. Follow the nerve root laterally, removing tissue and palpating with a nerve hook as required, until the nerve is well decompressed. It is rare for more than 30 to 50% of the foramen to require unroofing.

Sites of compression may be visually identifiable at one or several areas within the foramen, where the nerve may appear discolored or thinned. In other cases, though, the nerve may appear undamaged, despite a high degree of compression. Although preoperative studies should be a guide to the extent of decompression required, by the end of the procedure, confirmatory

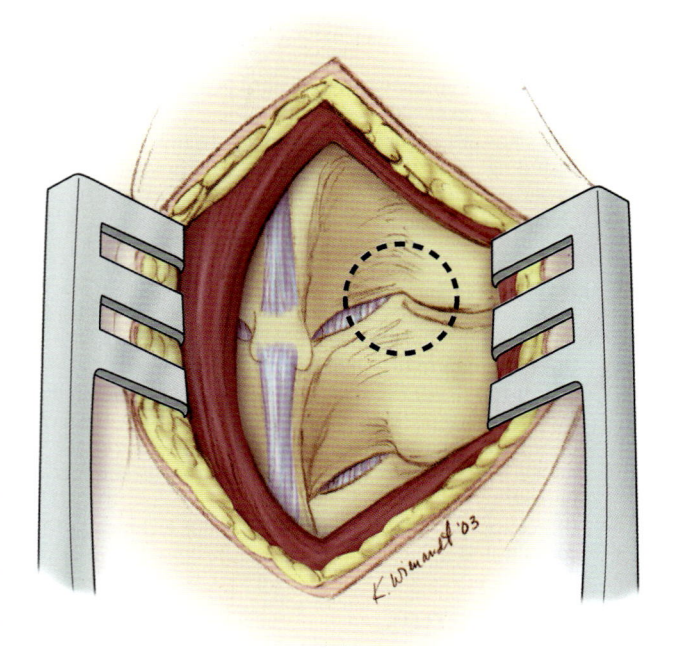

Fig. 33.3 The laminae are exposed only at the level of the pathology, taking care to leave the lateral 50% of the facet intact.

33 Posterior Cervical Foraminotomy and Diskectomy

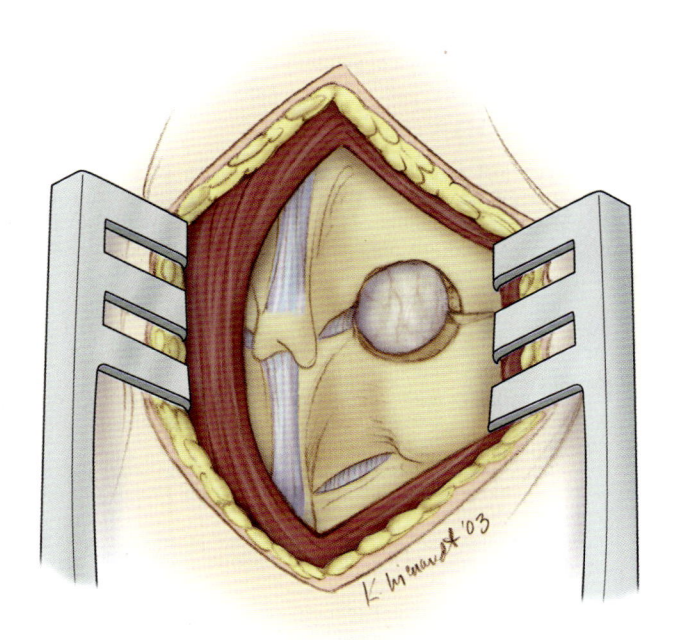

Fig. 33.4 The lateral lamina is removed to expose the central dura.

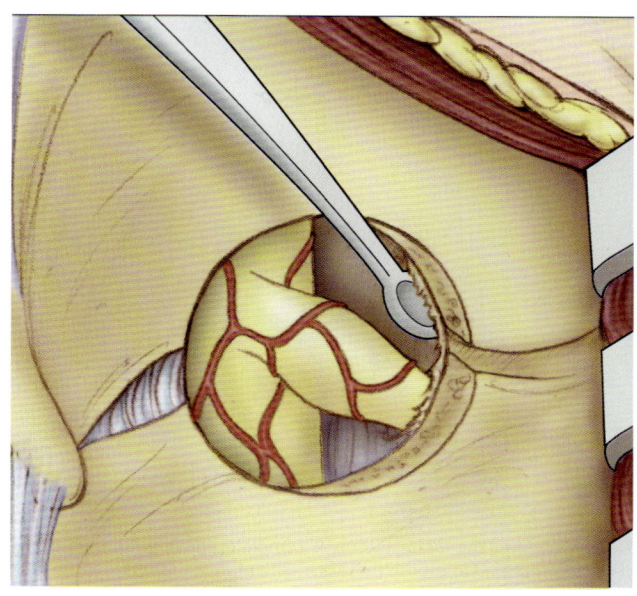

Fig. 33.5 The nerve root is exposed and followed out to the foramen.

palpation with a nerve hook should reveal a well-decompressed nerve root all the way out of the foramen. Decompression should be extended to the limits of the pedicles superiorly and inferiorly. Although some surgeons advocate drilling the pedicle itself, we believe that this is generally unnecessary and increases the risk of postoperative complications.

Diskectomy

If large anterior disk fragments are noted to be present, an additional diskectomy can be performed. After removal of dorsal compression, the superior portion of the inferior pedicle is removed with a drill. Note that this part of the procedure involves drilling in close proximity to the nerve root, and thus care must be taken to protect it. The perineural spaces are explored with fine, blunt dissecting instruments. Extruded fragments tend to migrate upward from the caudally located disk and are therefore typically found on the caudal side of the root (**Fig. 33.6**) Gentle superior retraction of the root gains access to the fragment (**Fig. 33.7**). Occasionally, the caudal portion of the superior pedicle requires some drilling to facilitate the retraction of the root and avoid undue compression. A small blunt nerve hook is used to palpate and deliver the fragment, which is then removed with a micropituitary rongeur (**Figs. 33.6 and 33.7**). Small anterior osteophytes can usually be ignored, but can be curetted with small curettes according to location and surgeon preference.

Significant bleeding can be a concern due to the prominent venous plexus surrounding the nerve root. Ensure hemostasis with bipolar coagulation or a synthetic hemostatic product, as available. Note that as much hemostatic material as possible should be removed prior to closure.

Closure

After irrigating the surgical field, a collagen sponge is placed over the root, the retractors are removed and the fascia is closed tightly with No. 0 or 00 polyglactin sutures. The subcutaneous tissues are reapproximated with No. 00 and 000 polyglactin sutures, and the skin closed with a dissolvable subcuticular running stitch. A sterile dressing is applied.

Complications

Major complications of posterior foraminotomy are both rare and fewer in number than those encountered with the anterior approach.[1] The most common complications reported are those implicit in the posterior approach, discussed in Chapter 31. Early complications directly related to the operation include direct or

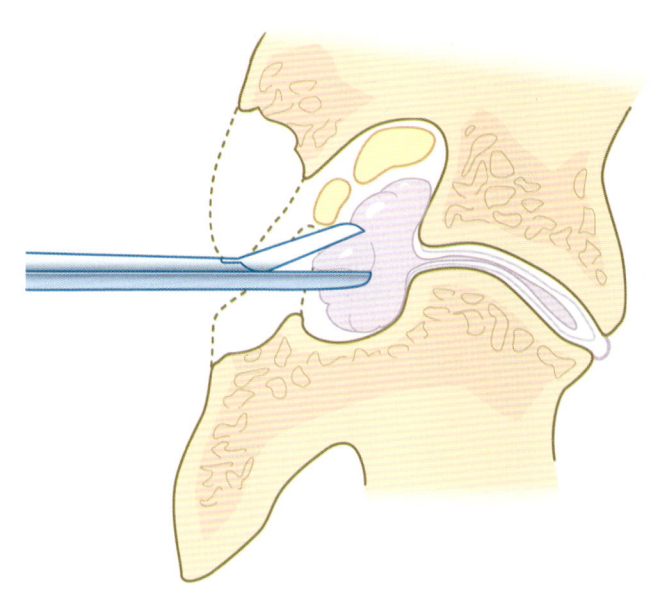

Fig. 33.6 Use of a pituitary rongeur to remove a "soft disk" from the axilla of the nerve root.

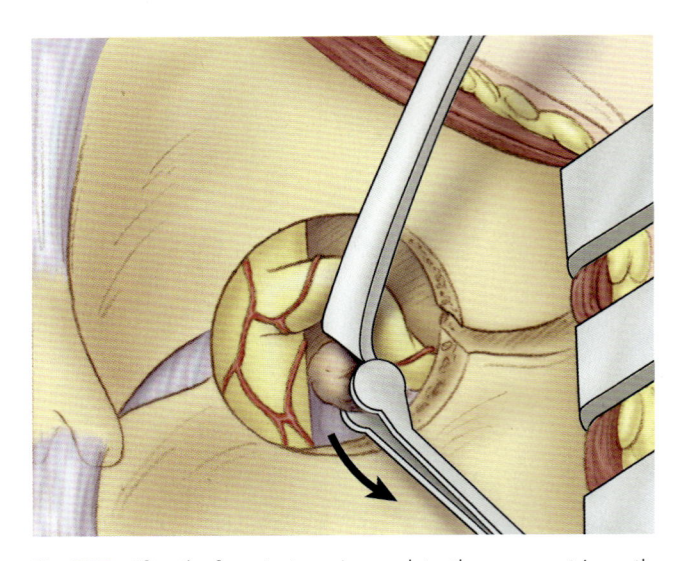

Fig. 33.7 After the foraminotomy is complete, the nerve root is gently deflected cephalad to expose the disk fragment.

indirect nerve root damage,[2] whereas the most prevalent late complication is recurrence of symptoms.[3,4]

Conclusion

Posterior cervical foraminotomy with or without diskectomy provides a straightforward and direct approach for root decompression in the management of radiculopathy. Although the procedure does not require an arthrodesis, it is limited to solely foraminal pathology.

References

1. Zdeblick TA, Zou D, Warden KE, McCabe R, Kunz D, Vanderby R. Cervical stability after foraminotomy. A biomechanical in vitro analysis. J Bone Joint Surg Am 1992;74:22–27
2. Davis RA. A long-term outcome study of 170 surgically treated patients with compressive cervical radiculopathy. Surg Neurol 1996;46:523–530, discussion 530–533
3. Galbraith JG, Butler JS, Dolan AM, O'Byrne JM. Operative outcomes for cervical myelopathy and radiculopathy. Adv Orthop 2012;2012: Article ID 919153
4. Zeidman SM, Ducker TB. Posterior cervical laminoforaminotomy for radiculopathy: review of 172 cases. Neurosurgery 1993;33:356–362

34 Minimally Invasive Posterior Cervical Diskectomy, Laminectomy, and Foraminotomy for Stenosis

Trent L. Tredway

Patients with symptoms secondary to compression of a cervical nerve root may present with radicular pain, dermatomal paresthesias, and/or motor weakness. The etiology of the nerve root compression is commonly associated with cervical stenosis secondary to neuroforaminal narrowing caused by degenerative changes. These degenerative changes occur as part of the normal aging process and include desiccation of the disk, hypertrophy of the ligamentum flavum, and advanced arthropathy of the facet complex. These alterations ultimately lead to narrowing of the spinal canal as well as the neuroforamen.

Compression of the nerve root can also be secondary to a lateral disk herniation that may occur acutely. Rarely, a cervical synovial cyst may also cause neural compression leading to radiculopathy. Despite the etiology, the clinical signs and symptoms are similar to those in patients with cervical foraminal stenosis. The first line of treatment usually consists of conservative management, and may include a regimen of physical therapy, nonsteroidal anti-inflammatory drug (NSAID) therapy, oral steroids, or epidural steroid injections. Overhead cervical traction may also help alleviate some of the symptoms as well.

Patient Selection

Patients presenting with a cervical radiculopathy from neural compression typically are diagnosed based on a clinical examination and imaging studies. Magnetic resonance imaging (MRI) is the preferred imaging modality to evaluate the anatomy of the spinal cord and exiting cervical nerve roots. T2-weighted images often demonstrate foraminal stenosis secondary to the degenerative changes described above (**Fig. 34.1**). The imaging may also demonstrate compression of the nerve root from a disk herniation or less commonly compression from a synovial cyst arising from the facet joint (**Fig. 34.2**). If a trial of conservative management utilizing the regimens cited above fails, then surgical intervention can be entertained.

Traditionally, cervical stenosis and laterally herniated disks were treated through standard open procedures that consisted of posterior laminoforaminotomies with or without diskectomy. There have been numerous reports documenting the excellent clinical outcomes and minimal complications associated with the procedure.[1-5] The posterior approach enables the surgeon to directly decompress the nerve root and does not require a fusion or subject the patient to the potential risks associated with an anterior cervical procedure.

Indications

- Cervical radiculopathy secondary to foraminal stenosis or lateral cervical disk herniation
- Failure of conservative therapy

Contraindications

- Medial disk herniations that would require retraction of the cervical cord (**Fig. 34.3**)
- Severe kyphotic deformity that may worsen if a posterior decompression is performed
- Instability of the operative level as identified on flexion/extension radiographs (> 3.5 mm)

Advantages and Disadvantages

One advantage of performing a posterior laminoforaminotomy is direct neural decompression without the need for fusion/stabilization, as typically performed via an anterior approach. Furthermore, the risks of performing an anterior approach, including injury to the recurrent laryngeal nerve, esophagus, ansa cervicalis, carotid artery, sympathetic chain, and thoracic duct, are obviated.

The advantages of performing a minimally invasive posterior cervical laminoforaminotomy compared with an open procedure include less soft tissue injury from retraction, less blood loss, less postoperative pain, and shorter hospital stays.[6] These minimally invasive procedures have also been reported to adequately decompress the neural elements in both cadaveric studies as well as in surgically treated patients.[7-9]

A disadvantage of performing a minimally invasive posterior cervical laminoforaminotomy is the additional time needed to place the patient in the sitting position. However, after performing these cases on a routine basis, the operative suite staff can help reduce the amount of time necessary for the setup of the procedure. It should also be noted that there is a learning curve in performing the minimally invasive procedures as well as an initial cost to obtain the specialized equipment. The initial investment includes the purchase of retractors, surgical instruments, endoscopes, light sources, and video display. However, the minimally invasive procedures are becoming more popular, and as our training programs incorporate this technology, more surgeons will be trained to perform the minimally invasive procedures. Finally, the patient-driven demand for less invasive procedures with quicker recovery times will most likely increase in the future.

Choice of Operative Approach

The surgeon chooses the approach based on the pathology. Patients harboring large midline disk herniations should be treated via an anterior cervical approach and may undergo either a fusion procedure or, if appropriate, an artificial disk procedure after the offending disk is removed. Patients with disk herniations

222   II   Midcervical Spine

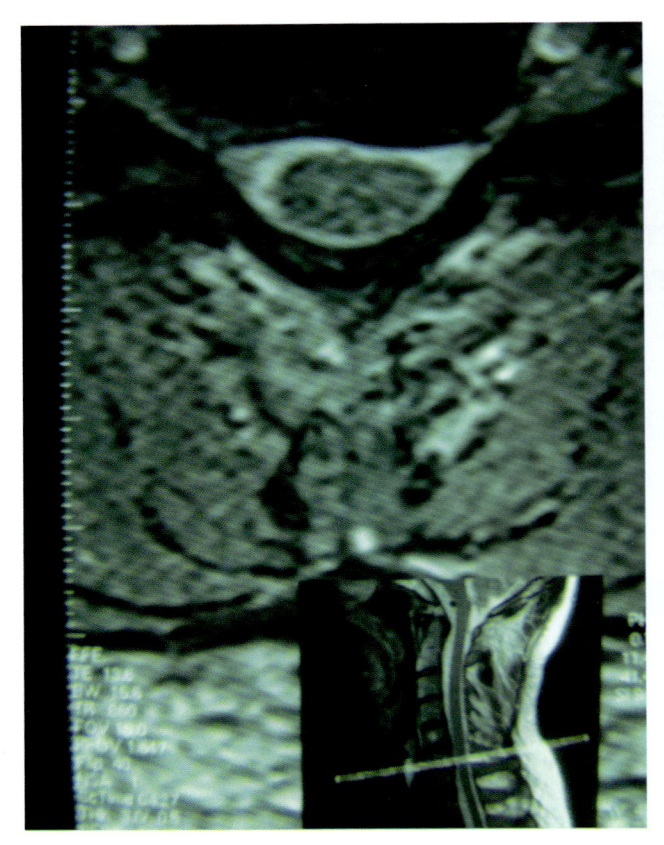

Fig. 34.1 T2-weighted axial magnetic resonance imaging (MRI) demonstrating left greater than right neuroforaminal stenosis.

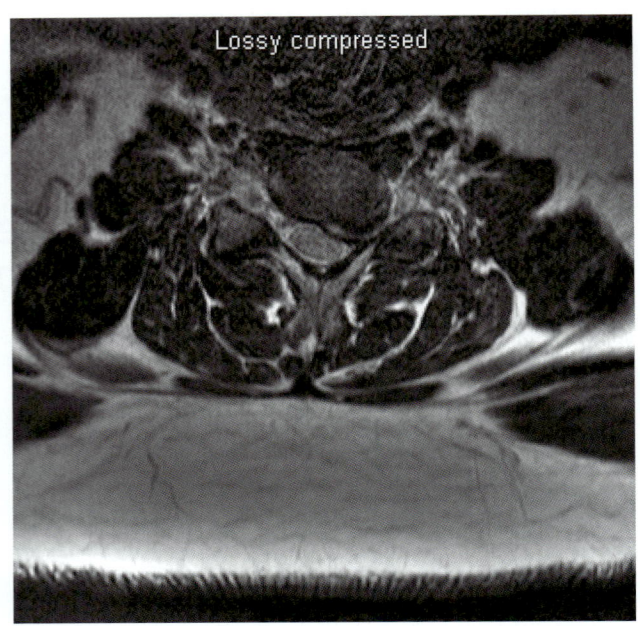

Fig. 34.2 T2-weighted axial MRI demonstrating nerve root compression secondary to a left lateral disk herniation.

and instability typically undergo an anterior decompression with fusion/stabilization to reduce the risk of cord and nerve root injury.

Unilateral neuroforaminal narrowing or unilateral disk herniations may best be treated with a posterior approach, and the

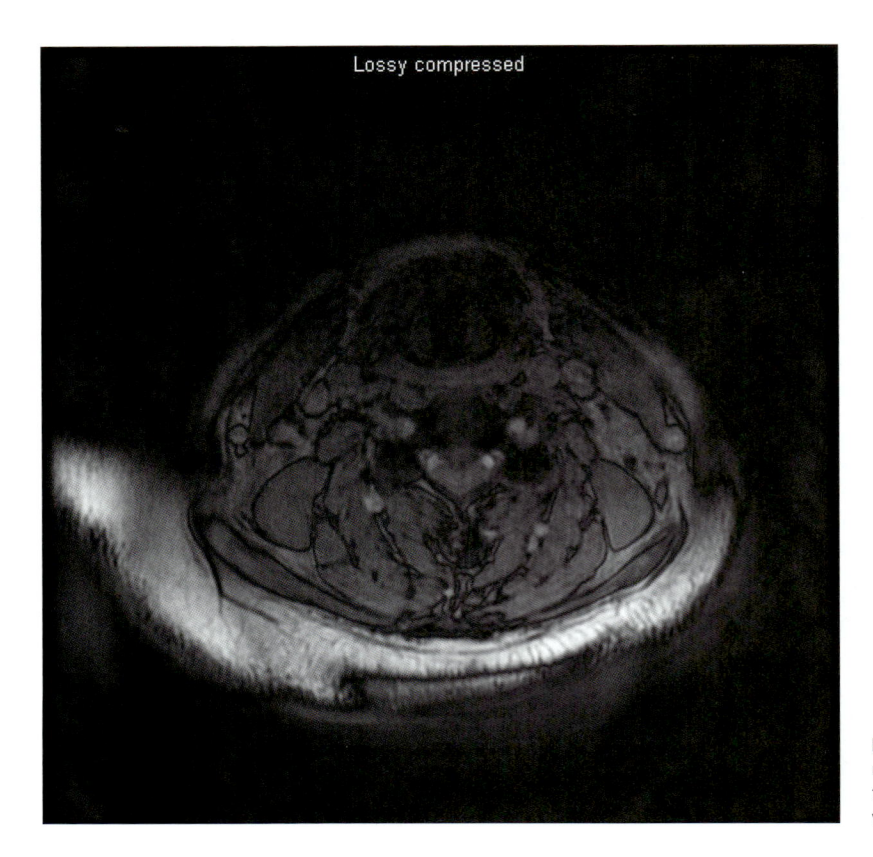

Fig. 34.3 T2-weighted axial MRI demonstrating a midline disk herniation causing severe compression of the spinal cord (a contraindication for a minimally invasive posterior laminoforaminotomy).

minimally invasive laminoforaminotomy with or without diskectomy enables the surgeon to treat the pathology directly without the risks described previously (see Video 34.1).

Preoperative Testing

The history and physical exam are paramount in making the correct diagnosis and determining the specific nerve root or nerve roots involved. The history should include detailed questioning regarding the onset, location, duration, and aggravating or relieving factors associated with the patient's complaints. Furthermore, a detailed physical exam concentrating on motor function, sensory exam, and increased or decreased reflexes will help determine the specific nerve root or roots that are affected.

On occasion, the history and physical exam may be perplexing and an electromyogram (EMG) may be necessary to rule out less common etiologies, including brachial plexopathies, median nerve compression (such as carpal tunnel syndrome [CTS]), ulnar neuropathy, radial nerve palsy, and the "double crush syndrome" that may occur secondary to both cervical radiculopathy (C6) and CTS. The EMG may also demonstrate an acute radiculopathy from a chronic problem as well as any form of reinnervation, suggesting that the healing process may have been initiated.

One of the most helpful preoperative tests is MRI of the cervical spine. However, some patients may not be able to undergo an MRI (e.g., patients with defibrillators), and therefore a computed tomography (CT) myelogram may be extremely helpful in solidifying the diagnosis.

Surgical Technique

Patient Position

The patient is brought to the operating room (OR), intubated, and placed in the prone or sitting position. I prefer placing the patient in the sitting position when performing the minimally invasive microendoscopic procedure because it entails less epidural bleeding. Epidural bleeding can cause a problem with visualization when using the endoscope, as the tubular retractor can fill up with blood and obscure the visual field. Also, this patient positioning is more comfortable for the surgeon. Cranial tongs are applied to the patient's skull. The OR setup includes a C-arm fluoroscopic unit to help verify the operative level as well as a monitor to facilitate visualization obtained through the endoscope (**Fig. 34.4**). Alternatively, the surgeon can utilize a microscope, but the operative position is somewhat more awkward and may require the surgeon to perform the procedure in a seated position to obtain the correct trajectory to the operative level.

Alternatively, the procedure may be performed by placing the patient in the prone position on a frame or chest rolls, and utilizing either the endoscope or microscope for visualization. An advantage of the prone position in performing a minimally invasive posterior cervical laminoforaminotomy is the familiarity of the setup for the OR staff and anesthesia team. As with the sitting position, cranial tongs are applied to the patient's skull. Care is taken to pad the bony prominences to decrease pressure-related complications. Another advantage of the prone position is that the patient's blood pressure is typically more normotensive in this position compared with the sitting position. However, the disadvantages to the prone position include difficulty in accurately determining the correct level, especially in the lower cervical spine, as well as the increased bleeding from the epidural space that may obscure visualization when using an endoscope.

Approach

The initial approach to the operative site is the most important step when performing minimally invasive procedures. To perform a safe approach to the posterior cervical spine, an incision is made ~ 1.5 cm to the side of the pathology. The incision is carried down through the posterior cervical fascia so that the sequential dilators may be used to gain access to the correct level. Several minimally invasive tubular retractor systems are available, and a few of the systems utilize a Kirschner wire (K-wire) to perform the initial approach. Due to the small caliber of the K-wire and the potential risk to the spinal cord and vertebral artery, some surgeons prefer to use the smallest blunt dilator tube instead of the K-wire. Next, a series of dilators are used, culminating in placing a tubular retractor, ~ 18 mm in diameter, over the laminofacet junction of the operative level (**Fig. 34.5**). This

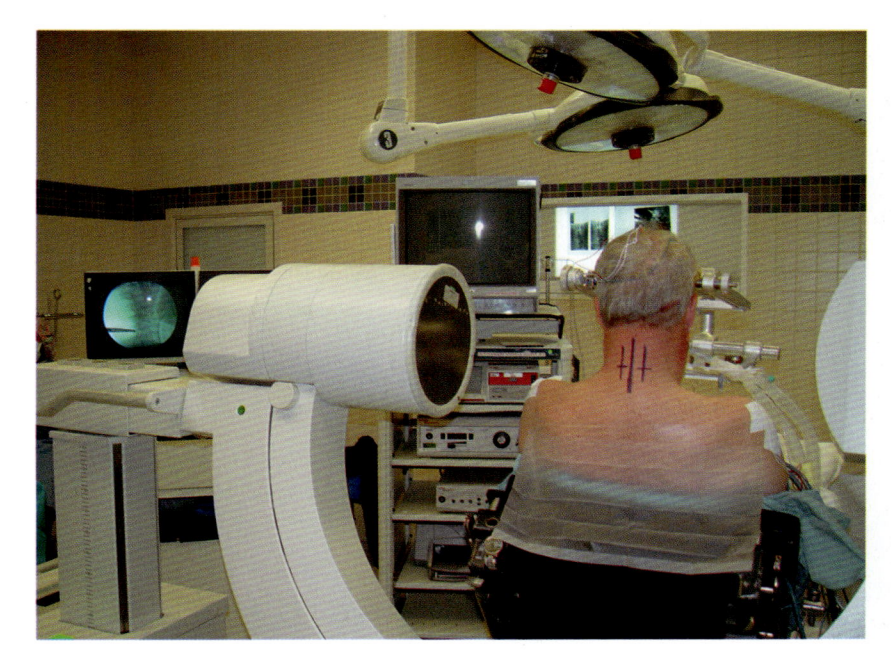

Fig. 34.4 Operating room setup for performing a minimally invasive posterior laminoforaminotomy. The patient is placed in the sitting position, with the C-arm fluoroscopic monitor and the endoscopic video monitor positioned so that the surgeon is able to visualize both easily.

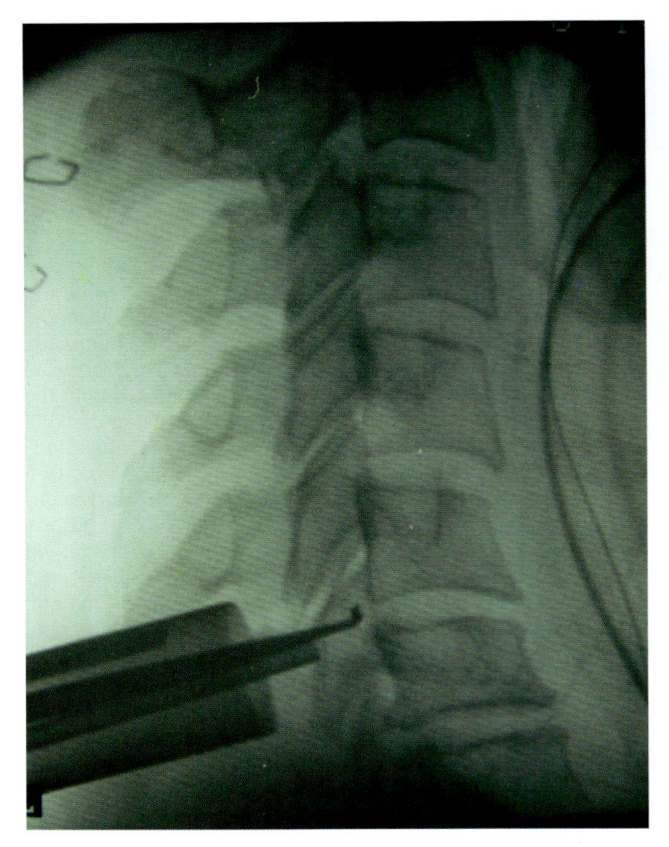

Fig. 34.5 Lateral C-arm fluoroscopic view of the tubular retractor and endoscope overlying the C5-C6 laminofacet junction and verification of the operative disk level.

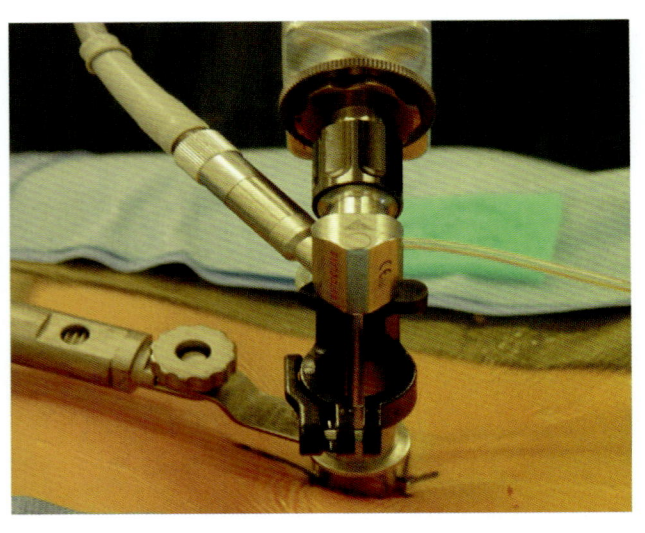

Fig. 34.6 The microendoscopic setup utilizes an 18-mm working channel with a 2.0-mm endoscope that attaches to the tubular retractor. An external light source is connected to the camera apparatus to provide excellent visualization down the tube.

retractor is locked into place with a flexible arm, and the endoscope is attached to the tubular retractor and centered to facilitate viewing in the anatomic position, with the most cranial level at the 12 o'clock position and the most inferior part of the surgical site at the 6 o'clock position (**Fig. 34.6**).

Dissection and Decompression

The soft tissue overlying the laminofacet junction of the operative index level is removed with a monopolar electrocautery. Next, the laminofacet junction is identified and verified prior to any bone removal (**Fig. 34.7**). A high-speed drill is used to remove the bone overlying the laminofacet junction. A small, angled curette is then used to dissect the cervical ligamentum flavum, and a 2-mm Kerrison rongeur is used to continue the bony removal overlying the lateral edge of the cervical dura and extending along the course of the nerve root into the medial facet complex. The decompression is carried laterally until the nerve root is free of compression, as can be verified with the use of a right-angled nerve root probe (**Fig. 34.8**). I typically try to maintain at least half of the facet complex, which can reduce the risk of postoperative instability. Furthermore, if the dissection is

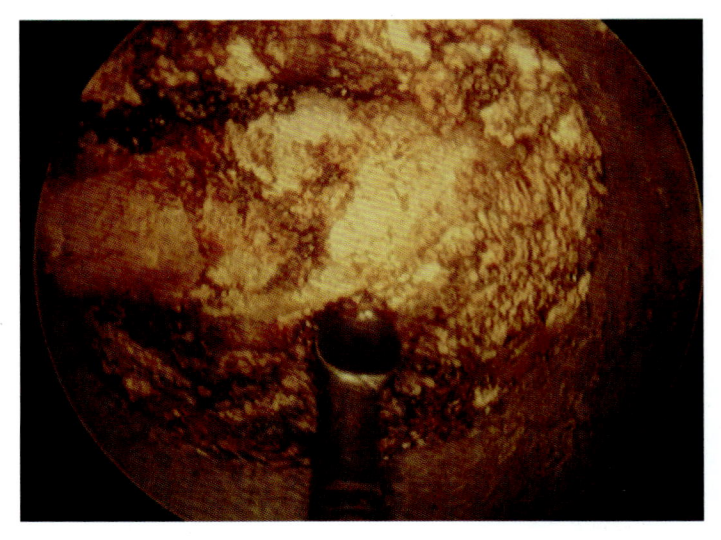

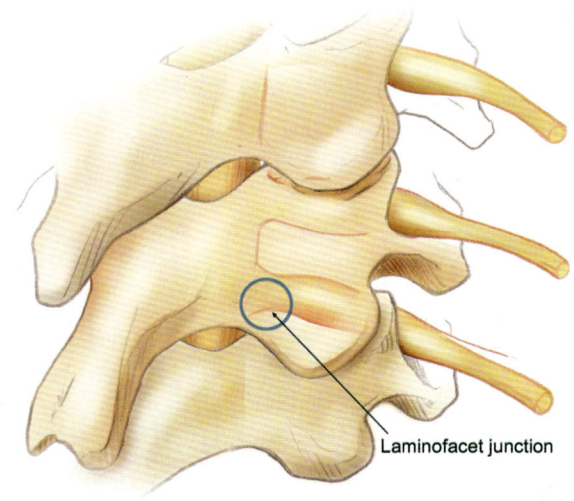

Fig. 34.7 (a) Intraoperative microendoscopic and (b) illustrative view of the laminofacet junction at the C5-C6 level.

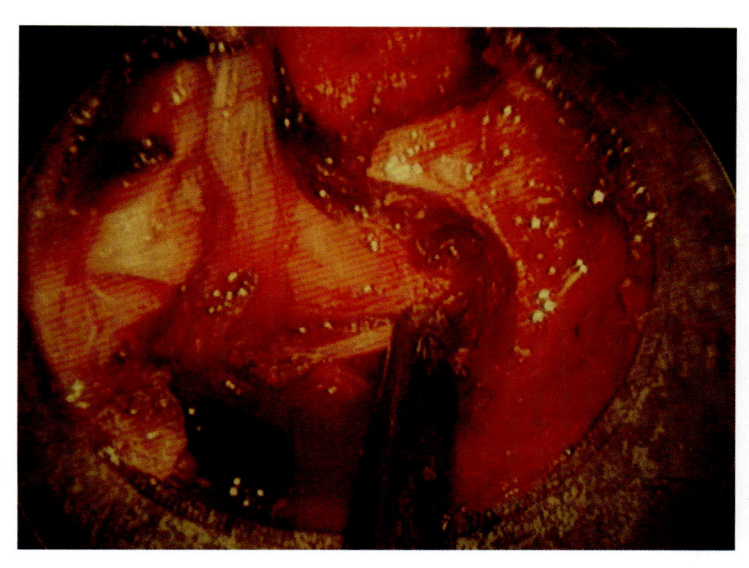

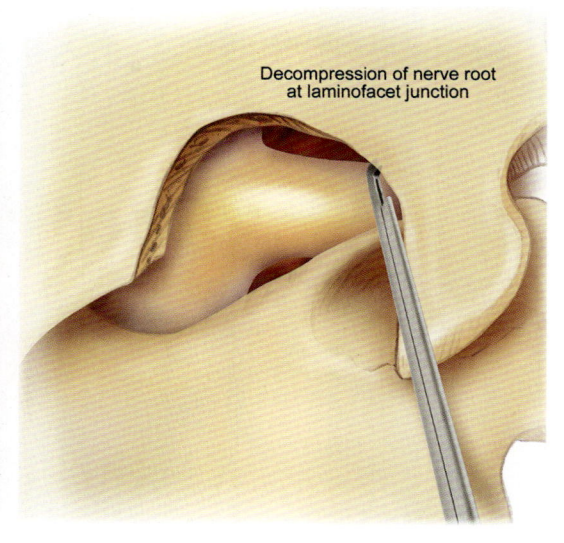

Fig. 34.8 (a) Intraoperative microendoscopic and (b) illustrative view of the lateral edge of the dura and exiting nerve root after performing a laminoforaminotomy.

carried too far lateral, the risk of vertebral artery injury is increased. Often, the surgeon may encounter some epidural bleeding after adequately decompressing the nerve root. This can be limited with the use of a bipolar electrocautery or hemostatic agents and gentle compression.

If the neural compression is secondary to bony foraminal stenosis, then a microendoscopic laminoforaminotomy is all that is performed to treat the symptoms. If there is a lateral disk herniation, then a diskectomy is recommended and the initial approach is the same as described for a laminoforaminotomy procedure; however, the disk may be visualized if herniated posterior, and it is usually inferior to the exiting nerve root. If the disk herniation is more osteophytic in nature, then drilling down the pedicle below the nerve root provides access to the disk space with minimal retraction on the nerve root[10] (**Fig. 34.9**). Once the disk is identified and verified using lateral fluoroscopic imaging, the disk is removed with a pituitary rongeur in a piecemeal fashion. The nerve root should be completely decompressed at the end of the procedure.

Closure

Once the nerve root is decompressed and the offending disk fragment/osteophyte is removed, attention is turned toward removal of the tubular retractor system and the endoscope. The muscle and fascia is cauterized with a bipolar electrocautery to decrease the risk of postoperative hematoma at the operative site. The area is cleansed with antibiotic irrigation, the fascia is closed with a running 2-0 absorbable suture, and the subdermal region is closed with a 3-0 absorbable suture in an interrupted fashion. The skin is closed with a 3-0 absorbable suture, and skin glue is applied to the suture line.

Postoperative Care

After the procedure, the patient is usually observed in the recovery room and treated with pain medications as well as agents to reduce muscle spasm. I typically perform these surgeries as an outpatient procedure, and the patient is discharged after the recovery from anesthesia is complete. The patient can expect some postsurgical pain at the operative site, but often the radicular pain component is significantly reduced. Careful instructions are given to the patient. If the patient has a new neurologic deficit, a postoperative hematoma or wound drainage is evaluated swiftly to decrease any risk of long-term neurologic deficits.

Potential Complications and Precautions

With posterior cervical spine surgery, care is taken to avoid injury to the spinal cord, nerve roots, and vertebral artery during the initial approach, and judicious use of fluoroscopy as well as gentle dissection of the fascia may reduce the risk significantly. To avoid becoming disoriented when using the minimally invasive procedures, the surgeon should identify the laminofacet junction on all approaches, to decrease the risk of injury to the spinal cord and nerve root. Once the laminofacet junction is identified, then the high-speed drill can be utilized to thin the lamina and medial facet to enable removal of the bony compression without disrupting the nerve root.

As stated earlier, care is taken to remove less than half of the facet complex, and if there is a durotomy noted at the time of surgical decompression, the durotomy is treated with a primary closure if possible, followed by a dural substitute and a dural sealant to help reduce the risk of postoperative pseudomeningocele formation. If there is a cerebrospinal fluid (CSF) leak noted, then it is recommended to keep the patient in an upright (90-degree) position in the immediate postoperative period (the first 12 hours). Direct neural injury is uncommon, but if it occurs, then steroids may be helpful in the immediate postoperative course.

Another complication of performing decompression of the cervical nerve root is a delayed nerve root palsy. The C5 nerve root is most commonly affected. This complication has been reported in ~ 5% of cervical decompression surgeries.[11] I typically treat delayed cervical nerve root palsies with a steroid dose pack, as most of these delayed palsies resolve.

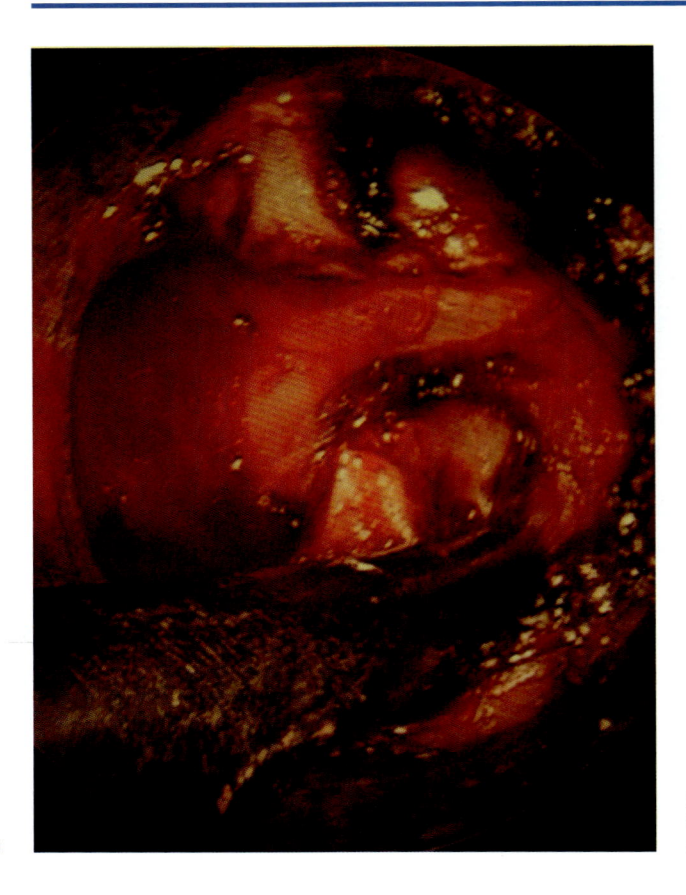

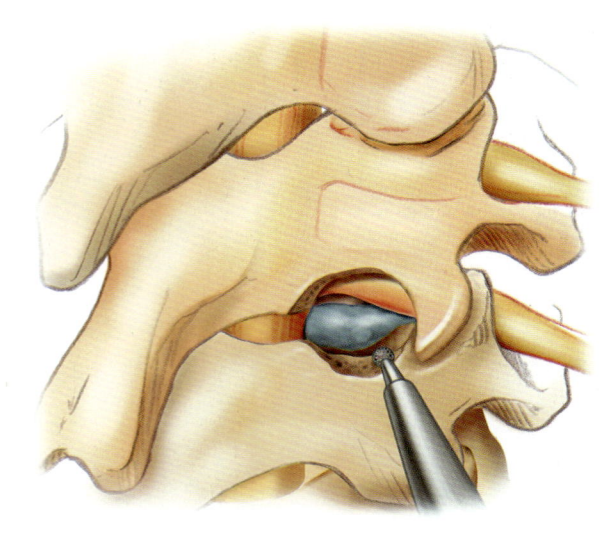

Fig. 34.9 (a) Intraoperative microendoscopic and (b) illustrative view of the exiting nerve root and disk space after performing a pediculotomy (often required to remove osteophytic disk complexes).

Conclusion

The minimally invasive posterior cervical laminoforaminotomy with or without diskectomy is an excellent surgical procedure for the treatment of cervical radiculopathy secondary to stenosis. The key operative steps are listed in **Box 34-1**. This procedure has been refined from the traditional open techniques and offers excellent relief of symptoms with good long-term outcomes. Recently, a systematic review comparing open versus minimally invasive percutaneous foraminotomies was performed that found that the latter technique required less OR time and resulted in less blood loss, reduced postoperative pain, and shorter hospital stays.[12] Moreover, a review of the microendoscopic procedure described in this chapter was recently published, with excellent long-term outcomes.[13] Finally, in regard to complications arising after a minimally invasive posterior cervical laminoforaminotomy, there is a low rate of reoperation at the index level (1.1% per index level per year).[14]

Box 34-1 Key Operative Steps

- The patient is placed in the sitting position with adequate visualization of the C-arm fluoroscopic monitor and the endoscopic viewing monitor.
- A 2-cm incision is made ~ 1.5 cm to the side of the pathology.
- The posterior cervical fascia is incised to allow the dilators of the tubular retractor to dock overlying the operative level.
- The 18-mm working channel and endoscopic unit is placed in the operative field, and the orientation is verified on the viewing monitor.
- The soft tissue is removed with a monopolar electrocautery.
- The laminofacet junction is identified, and a high-speed drill is used to perform a laminotomy and medial facetectomy to unroof the compressed nerve root.
- 1- and 2-mm Kerrison rongeurs are used to decompress the nerve root laterally.
- Extreme care is taken not to remove more than half of the facet and to remain cognizant of the course of the vertebral artery.
- If a diskectomy is required, then a pediculotomy can be performed underlying the nerve root to gain access to the disk/osteophyte complex.
- After decompression of the nerve root, the area is checked for hemostasis of the epidural veins, and the soft tissue is examined and cauterized after removal of the retractor.
- The incision is closed in a layered fashion culminating in closing the skin with a 3–0 absorbable suture using a subcuticular technique.

With the technological advancements in operative instrumentation and improved optics, there is a bright future for improving the minimally invasive techniques further. Recent reports utilizing smaller endoscopic approaches as well as three-dimensional visualization of the docking system may help reduce some of the complications that have been associated with approaching the posterior cervical spine through minimally invasive techniques.[15,16] It is hoped that these improvements will lead to even better clinical outcomes for patients with shorter, less painful procedures as well as decreased hospital stays.

References

1. Davis RA. A long-term outcome study of 170 surgically treated patients with compressive cervical radiculopathy. Surg Neurol 1996;46:523–530, discussion 530–533
2. Harrop JS, Silva MT, Sharan AD, Dante SJ, Simeone FA. Cervicothoracic radiculopathy treated using posterior cervical foraminotomy/discectomy. J Neurosurg 2003;98(2, Suppl):131–136
3. Kumar GR, Maurice-Williams RS, Bradford R. Cervical foraminotomy: an effective treatment for cervical spondylotic radiculopathy. Br J Neurosurg 1998;12:563–568
4. Silveri CP, Simpson JM, Simeone FA, Balderston RA. Cervical disk disease and the keyhole foraminotomy: proven efficacy at extended long-term follow up. Orthopedics 1997;20:687–692
5. Snow RB, Weiner H. Cervical laminectomy and foraminotomy as surgical treatment of cervical spondylosis: a follow-up study with analysis of failures. J Spinal Disord 1993;6:245–250, discussion 250–251
6. Burke TG, Caputy A. Microendoscopic posterior cervical foraminotomy: a cadaveric model and clinical application for cervical radiculopathy. J Neurosurg 2000;93(1, Suppl):126–129
7. Fessler RG, Khoo LT. Minimally invasive cervical microendoscopic foraminotomy: an initial clinical experience. Neurosurgery 2002;51(5, Suppl):S37–S45
8. Peng M, Qi C, Lv D, Cao X, Peng G, Ma X. [Efficacy of posterior microendoscopic foraminotomy for cervical radiculopathy]. Zhongguo Xiu Fu Chong Jian Wai Ke Za Zhi 2010;24:513–516
9. Roh SW, Kim DH, Cardoso AC, Fessler RG. Endoscopic foraminotomy using MED system in cadaveric specimens. Spine 2000;25:260–264
10. Webb KM, Kaptain G, Sheehan J, Jane JA Sr. Pediculotomy as an adjunct to posterior cervical hemilaminectomy, foraminotomy, and discectomy. Neurosurg Focus 2002;12:E10
11. Sakaura H, Hosono N, Mukai Y, Ishii T, Yoshikawa H. C5 palsy after decompression surgery for cervical myelopathy: review of the literature. Spine 2003;28:2447–2451
12. Clark JG, Abdullah KG, Steinmetz MP, Benzel EC, Mroz TE. Minimally invasive versus open cervical foraminotomy: a systematic review. Global Spine J 2011;1:9–14
13. Lawton CD, Smith ZA, Lam SK, Habib A, Wong RH, Fessler RG. Clinical outcomes of microendoscopic foraminotomy and decompression in the cervical spine. World Neurosurg 2014;81:422–427
14. Skovrlj B, Gologorsky Y, Haque R, Fessler RG, Qureshi SA. Complications, outcomes, and need for fusion after minimally invasive posterior cervical foraminotomy and microdiscectomy. Spine J 2014;14:2405–2411
15. Hilton DL Jr. Minimally invasive tubular access for posterior cervical foraminotomy with three-dimensional microscopic visualization and localization with anterior/posterior imaging. Spine J 2007;7:154–158
16. Ruetten S, Komp M, Merk H, Godolias G. A new full-endoscopic technique for cervical posterior foraminotomy in the treatment of lateral disc herniations using 6.9-mm endoscopes: prospective 2-year results of 87 patients. Minim Invasive Neurosurg 2007;50:219–226

35 Cervical Laminoplasty

Takashi Kaito and Kazuo Yonenobu

Until the 1970s, laminectomy was the only posterior decompression procedure for the cervical spine. However, postoperative neurologic deterioration supposedly due to the operative procedure (e.g., insertion of a rongeur or curette into the spinal canal) was not uncommon. The introduction of high-speed drills enabled delicate and safe decompression of the nerve tissue. Regardless, some cases exhibited postoperative neurologic deterioration believed to be due to the loss of mechanical stability, especially kyphotic deformity, caused by the excision of the posterior elements or scar tissue (i.e., laminectomy membrane) forming and occupying the void after the laminectomy. Accordingly, in 1973, Oyama and Hattori[1] invented the Z-plasty, which both secures the decompression of the spinal canal and preserves the posterior bony elements. After the first description of enlargement of the spinal canal without resecting the laminae, Hirabayashi et al[2,3] reported open-door laminoplasty and Kurokawa et al[4] reported double-door laminoplasty (i.e., spinous process-splitting laminoplasty, also called French door laminoplasty). Since then, many modified techniques based on these two laminoplasty techniques have been described,[5-10] aiming to secure the stability of enlarged spinal canal and minimizing invasiveness to the muscle and ligamentous structures. Although the preservation of posterior elements afforded by laminoplasty is thought to help reduce the incidence of postlaminectomy kyphosis and provide rigidity for the reconstructed spine, there is no conclusive evidence supporting this hypothesis.[11] This chapter describes the concept of cervical laminoplasty and the detailed techniques.

Patient Selection: Indications and Contraindications

The major indications for laminoplasty to be compressive cervical myelopathy due to developmental canal stenosis, multilevel spondylosis, and continuous or mixed-type ossification of the posterior longitudinal ligament (OPLL) requiring multilevel decompression is a reasonable treatment strategy. A retrospective comparative study between laminoplasty and multilevel anterior cervical decompression and fusion (ACDF) demonstrates that the incidence of complications is higher in ACDF than laminoplasty even though both procedures have similar clinical results.[12] ACDF is a standard procedure for one- or two-level cervical disk herniation.[13] Laminoplasty can also be performed in cases in which spontaneous involution is expected.[14] Laminoplasty is an alternative to ACDF, especially in young patients with concomitant developmental canal stenosis, and can help avoid adjacent segment disease.[15] In cases presenting with concomitant radiculopathy, foraminotomy can be easily combined. Neutral to lordotic alignment is advantageous for laminoplasty to allow indirect decompression of anterior factors by shifting the spinal cord posteriorly. In cases presenting with kyphotic alignment, neurologic recovery after laminoplasty is inferior to that in cases with neutral to lordotic alignment.[16] In addition, local severe spinal cord compression from the anterior (i.e., local OPLL) is a negative prognostic factor for neurologic recovery after laminoplasty.[17-19] Moreover, the addition of posterior fusion is recommended if local instability exists.

Advantages

- Enables simultaneous decompression for multilevel spinal cord compression
- Low incidence of serious complications as compared with ACDF
- Low incidence of adjacent segment disease as compared with ACDF
- Foraminotomy for radiculopathy can be performed if necessary.
- Reduced incidence of postlaminectomy kyphosis
- External fixation (i.e., collar use) can be omitted.
- Theoretically, cervical range of motion can be preserved as compared with multilevel ACDF.[20]

Disadvantages

- High incidence of axial pain (i.e., in the neck and shoulders)
- In cases with severe anterior compression or severe cervical kyphosis, laminoplasty may not provide sufficient indirect decompression.
- Segmental motor palsy (commonly C5 and rarely C6 and C7) occurs in ~ 5% of laminoplasties,[21,22] though the incidence is similar with multilevel ACDF.[23]
- Cervical alignment cannot be changed.

Choice of Operative Approach

Since the original report of laminoplasty, numerous modified procedures aiming to secure the enlarged spinal canal and minimize muscle detachment have been developed.[5-10] However, laminoplasty aims to preserve posterior bony elements while expanding the spinal canal. There are two main laminoplasty techniques: open-door and double open-door laminoplasty. Although two randomized controlled studies and three retrospective comparative studies report that these techniques are not significantly different with respect to neurologic recovery,[24-28] there is a lack of definitive evidence to conclude the superiority of either technique. This is partly because these techniques have been taught and developed in mentor–mentee relationships, meaning many surgeons are performing only one of these techniques.

Preoperative Tests

Physical Examination

The diagnosis of myelopathy should be based on meticulous evaluation of deep tendon reflexes, including the presence of pathological reflexes, motor and sensory loss, and bowel and bladder dysfunction.

Imaging Evaluation

Cervical alignment, canal diameter, and instability should be evaluated on plain radiographs. Computed tomography (CT) scan can help determine if spinal cord compression is due to ossified/calcified tissue or soft tissue. Knowing the precise dimensions and configuration of bone tissue is useful for selecting the location and depths of the troughs. Magnetic resonance imaging (MRI) can depict not only extrinsic compression of the spinal cord, especially soft tissue factors, but also the intrinsic changes of the spinal cord itself. Therefore, MRI is the most valuable tool for the diagnosis of cervical spondylotic myelopathy and exclusive diagnoses of tumors, infections, syrinx, and myelitis.

Surgical Procedure

Operative Position

The surgeon must avoid excessive cervical spine extension during the intubation process in the supine position. In cases of severe myelopathy, fiberscopic intubation is recommended. We routinely use the Mayfield head holder, which offers rigid immobilization of the cervical spine and places the patient on a Hall frame to decrease abdominal pressure when patient's position is changed to the prone position. The shoulders are taped down on both sides to provide traction, enabling better intraoperative radiographic visualization of the lower cervical spine. A slight flexed position of the neck makes the laminoplasty easier by diminishing the overlap of the laminae and facet joints; meanwhile, too much flex makes the exposure process difficult by increasing the tension of the paraspinal muscles. If spinal fusion techniques are to be applied, the position of the neck should be changed to a neutral position beforehand. The table is tilted into the reverse Trendelenburg position to make the incision site flat and avoid blood congestion in the operative field.

Incision and Exposure

The C2 and C7 spinous processes are usually easily palpable from the skin. After the dorsal midline skin incision from C2 to C7, the nuchal ligament between the right and left paraspinal muscles is in an avascular plane and is divided at the midline (Video 35.1). After the division of the nuchal ligament, all of the spinous processes are easily palpable. Laminoplasty originally involved exposure from C3 to C7. Laterally, the exposure of the inner half of the lateral mass is sufficient for the subsequent procedure. The semispinalis muscle attached to C2 should be maximally preserved to prevent the postoperative development and progression of kyphosis as well as mitigate postoperative axial pain. In cases in which there is overlap of the C2 and C3 laminae or compression of the cord at C2-C3, partial resection of the ventral portion of the semispinalis muscle enables dome-shaped laminoplasty of C2 and elevation of C3 lamina. The resection of muscles attached to the C7 spinous process (i.e., trapezium and rhomboideus minor muscles) is also reported to be associated with postoperative axial pain. Therefore, we usually implement laminoplasty from C3 to C6[29] (**Fig. 35.1**). In cases requiring de-

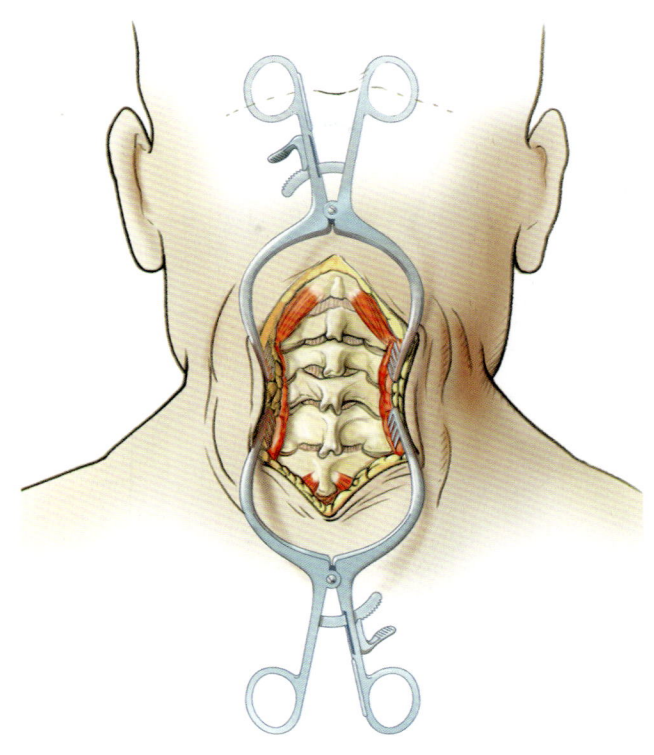

Fig. 35.1 Optimal exposure for laminoplasty from C3 to C6. Muscles attaching to C2 and C7 are completely preserved.

compression at the C6-C7 level, partial laminectomy of C7 (i.e., the cranial third) is added while keeping the muscles attached to C7 intact (Video 35.1).

Open-Door Laminoplasty

Following the exposure of the dorsal aspect of the cervical spine, the spinous processes of C3 through C7 (C6) are cut at the base with a Liston bone-cutting forceps and kept for use as bone grafts (**Fig. 35.2a**) (Video 35.1). Bone wax is used to stop bleeding from the cut surface of the bone. Bilateral troughs are made at the junction of lateral mass and lamina. To control the springiness of the elevated lamina, the open side of the "open door" is drilled first. A trough is made across each lamina using a high-speed drill with a 4-mm steel bur. Continuous irrigation is used to prevent thermal damage to the surrounding tissue and aid visualization of the bottom of the trough. After the inner cortex is exposed, the bur is replaced with a diamond bur. The drilling continues until the epidural venous plexus at the cranial half of the lamina and the yellow ligament at the caudal half of the lamina can be visualized through the thinned inner cortex (Video 35.1). Because of the inclination of the lamina and overlap of cranial lamina, the cranial portion of the lamina tends to be insufficiently thinned; surgeons must keep this in mind during the drilling process. After sufficiently thinning the inner cortex, an 8- to 10-mm raspatory is inserted into the trough and twisted. If the inner cortex is sufficiently thinned, the lamina makes a snapping sound when moved (**Fig. 35.2b**) (Video 35.1). Meanwhile, if there is a concomitant symptom of unilateral radiculopathy, opening the ipsilateral to the symptomatic side facilitates the concurrent foraminotomy. If the surgeon is right handed, the left side is chosen to be the open side. In cases of OPLL with severe laterality of the compressive factor, the compressive side is chosen

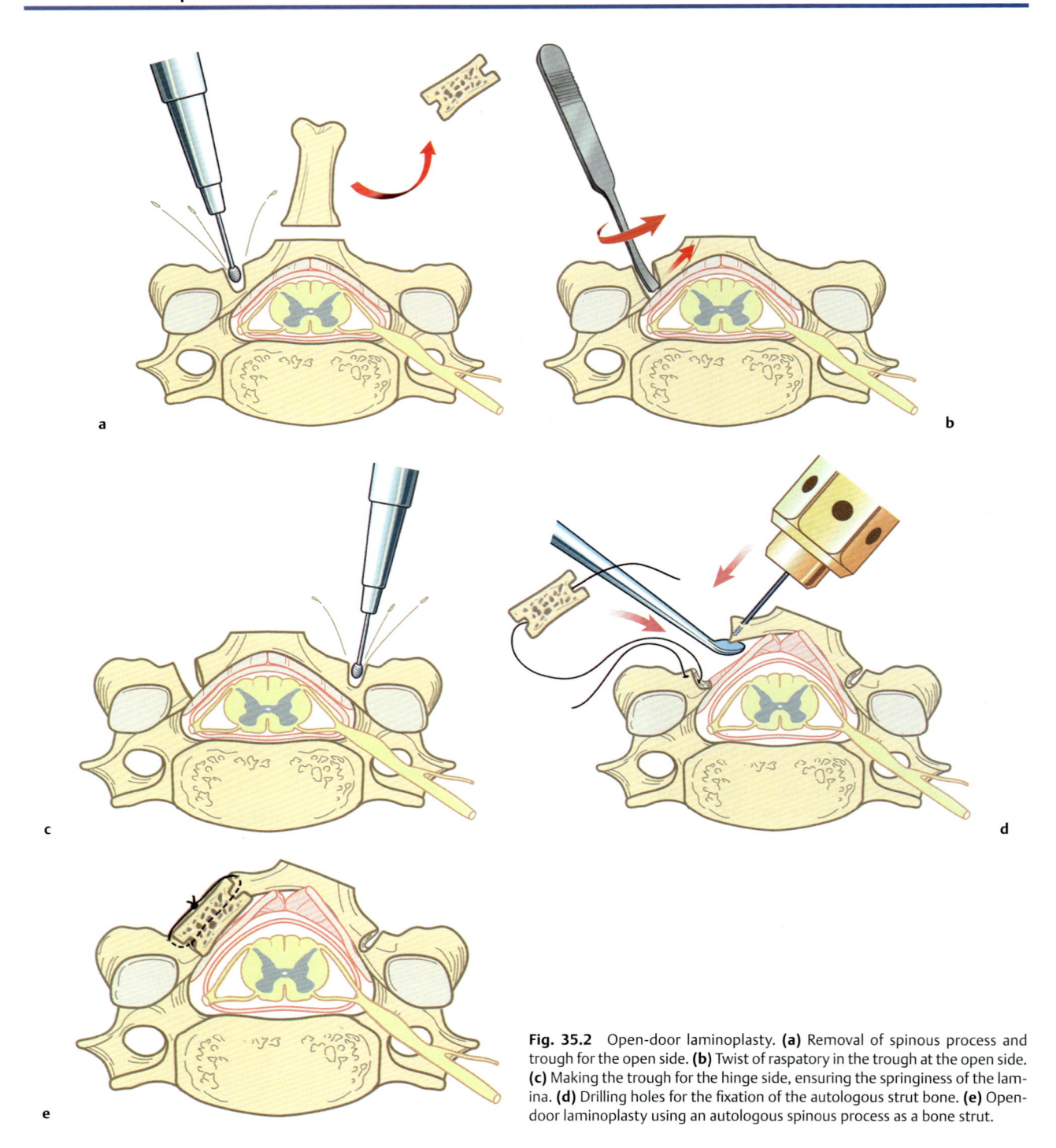

Fig. 35.2 Open-door laminoplasty. **(a)** Removal of spinous process and trough for the open side. **(b)** Twist of raspatory in the trough at the open side. **(c)** Making the trough for the hinge side, ensuring the springiness of the lamina. **(d)** Drilling holes for the fixation of the autologous strut bone. **(e)** Open-door laminoplasty using an autologous spinous process as a bone strut.

as the open side. The trough for the hinge side is subsequently made in the same manner (**Fig. 35.2c**).

When drilling down to the surface of the inner cortex of the lamina at the hinge side (2-mm trough depth for C4 and C5 where no cancellous bone exists in many cases), the springiness of the laminae should be checked frequently to prevent laminar fracture of the hinge side. The laminae are elevated starting from the caudal lamina to the cranial lamina (Video 35.1). The ligamentum flavum is cut under the trough and between the lamina at the cranial (C2-C3) and caudal (C6-C7 or C7-T1) ends, enabling the opening of the laminae over the extent of the laminoplasty. Hemostasis from the epidural venous plexus is achieved by bipolar cauterization. Collagen hemostatic agents may be used to gently tamponade bleeding sites. We use the autologous spinous processes from C6 and C7 (in case C7 spinous process is resected) as a supporting strut with a nonabsorbable 2-0 suture (**Fig. 35.2d,e**) (Video 35.1). In case the size and number of grafted materials are insufficient, hydroxyapatite spacers dedicated for open-door laminoplasty are placed instead (Video 35.1). A bone autograft or hydroxyapatite spacers are placed at C4 and C6 for C3 to C6 or

C3 to C7 laminoplasty. The placement of additional spacers can be considered if it is difficult to keep the nongrafted lamina elevated. The advantages of using autografts and hydroxyapatite spacers include low costs and the absence of radiographic artifacts.

Other Methods for Preventing Laminar Reclosure

1. From the hinge side: The original fixation method for laminae in open-door laminoplasty was suturing between the soft tissue at the hinge side and the spinous processes of the elevated laminae.[2] Two sutures are placed through the articular capsules and surrounding soft tissues on the hinge side, and both ends of the suture placed through the capsules are pulled out through the cranial and caudal interspinous ligaments to the open side. Then the threads are ligated at the open side of the spinous process to prevent the lifted laminae from closing.[30] The use of suture anchors was subsequently reported to ensure the elevation of the laminae. Nevertheless, the efficacy of suture anchors for preventing laminar reclosure remains controversial.[6,31]
2. From the open side: Titanium miniplates can be used to acquire further rigidity of the elevated laminae.[32] The miniplates are attached to the laminae and ipsilateral lateral mass with screws. Although some reports indicate miniplate fixation is effective for reducing postoperative neck pain or preventing other complications, there is a lack of strong evidence indicating the comparative benefits of using miniplates.[33]

Other Modifications to Preserve the Muscles Attached to C2 and C7

The preservation of the muscles attached to C2 and C7 is reported to reduce postoperative axial pain and kyphotic deformity progression.[34,35] Moreover, other modifications of laminoplasty procedures have been reported:

1. Laminectomy of C3 and laminoplasty from C4 to C7: In cases of degenerative cervical spine, the C2 and C3 laminae often overlap. In such cases, partial resection of the semispinalis muscle attached to C2 is required to elevate the C3 lamina. Laminectomy of C3 combined with laminoplasty at lower levels has been reported to minimize the resection of the semispinalis muscle.[36]
2. Laminoplasty from C3 to C6: The C7 spinous process, which is the largest spinous process of the cervical spine, is also the origin of the trapezium and rhomboideus minor muscles. Preservation of the muscle attached to C7 by performing laminoplasty from C3 to C6 with or without partial laminectomy of the cranial third of C7 lamina has been reported to reduce postoperative axial pain.[29]

Advantages

- Two troughs for the elevation of the laminae can shorten the operative time.
- In the original Hirabayashi procedure, no special implants are required to fix the elevated laminae. If the implants or autografts are placed as struts at the open side, the placement at every other lamina (i.e., skip placement) can provide satisfactory stability.
- Can be easily combined with foraminotomy
- The newly formed spinal canal is structurally stable compared with double open-door laminoplasty.[37]

Disadvantages

- Exposure of the epidural venous plexus at the open side can increase the risk of bleeding.
- Reclosure of the elevated laminae can occur if some kind of materials are not placed.

Double Open-Door Laminoplasty

After standard exposure of the laminae and medial aspects of the facet joints, the spinous processes from C4 to C7 (C6) are cut at the height of the C3 spinous process. A trough is made with a 2-mm diamond bur at the center of the spinous process until the inner cortex of the lamina is sufficiently thin. A raspatory is then inserted into the trough and twisted. The division of the spinous processes at the midline is confirmed by the movement of the lamina given sufficient thinning. Bilateral troughs are subsequently made with a 3-mm diamond bur at the junction of the laminae and lateral mass. After the springiness of the halved lamina is confirmed to be equivalent between the right and left sides, the bisected lamia is opened bilaterally. Bone grafts made from resected spinous processes or ceramic spacers are inserted between the opened laminae and secured in place with nonabsorbable sutures (**Fig. 35.3**).

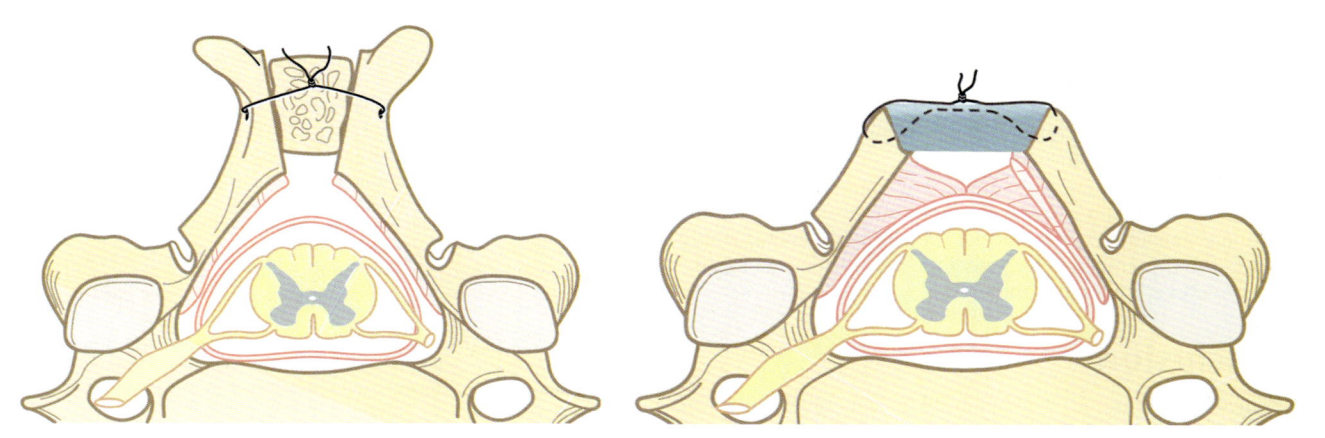

Fig. 35.3 Double open-door laminoplasty. **(a)** Double open-door laminoplasty using an iliac crest bone graft. **(b)** Double open-door laminoplasty using a hydroxyapatite spacer.

Advantages

- Bleeding from the epidural space is usually minimal because of the scarcity of venous plexus at the central portion.
- Midline division of the laminae enables symmetrical expansion of the canal, though the clinical significance is unclear.

Disadvantages

- Three troughs are required, which increases the time and complexity of the operation.
- In cases in which the divided spinous processes are thin, the ceramic spacers can migrate with the resorption of the tip of the spinous process.[37]
- Some kind of spacer must be inserted into each opened lamina, which can increase operative time and costs.

Postoperative Care

The drainage tube is removed 1 or 2 days after surgery. Sitting and walking are allowed from postoperative day 1. A neck collar is not used except for patients with severe neck pain. Cervical active range-of-motion exercises and isometric exercises are encouraged when pain is manageable.

Potential Complications and Precautions

The overall incidence of surgical complications in laminoplasty is reported to be lower than that in multilevel ACDF.[12] However, in addition to the common complications related to the cervical spine surgery (e.g., infection, hematoma, dural tear, nerve root injury, and spinal cord injury), there are several complications relatively characteristic of laminoplasty.

Axial neck pain is not specific to laminoplasty but common in cervical posterior surgery. The preservation of muscles attached to C2 or C7 may reduce the incidence and severity of this complication.[29,34,38] Furthermore, early mobilization of the neck may also mitigate symptoms.

Segmental motor palsy (commonly C5 and rarely C6 and C7) occurs in ~ 5% of laminoplasties.[21] Although segmental motor palsy usually shows favorable prognosis with full recovery within several months, some cases of severe palsy show incomplete recovery.[21,22] Because the etiology (i.e., nerve root injury including tethering phenomenon and thermal damage[39] or spinal cord disorder) has not been identified or may be multifactorial, several approaches have been attempted to decrease the incidence of this complication. The effect of prophylactic foraminotomy at bilateral C4-C5 for reducing the incidence of C5 palsy has been reported in a retrospective comparative study, but its effectiveness is inconclusive.[40]

Hinge-site fracture and subsequent laminar displacement can result in radiculopathy or myelopathy. The use of miniplate fixation when severe instability of the elevated laminae occurs secures the construct and may minimize the incidence of subsequent neurologic complications.

Conclusion

Cervical laminoplasty is well indicated for multilevel spinal cord compression without kyphotic alignment and severe anterior compression of the cord. The major advantages of laminoplasty are that the procedure is not technically difficult, multiple segments can be decompressed simultaneously, and the incidence of serious complications is lower than with the anterior approach. Although the problems of axial neck pain and segmental motor palsy remain, several modified techniques are expected to reduce their incidences. Nevertheless, additional well-designed randomized controlled studies are required to confirm the superiority of laminoplasty over laminectomy, anterior cervical decompression and fusion, and laminectomy and fusion. Surgeons must choose the optimal procedure depending on the etiology of each case while keeping in mind the benefits and drawback of each.

References

1. Oyama M, Hattori S. A new method of cervical laminectomy. The Central Japan Journal of Orthopaedic and Traumatic Surgery. 1973;16:792–794 [in Japanese]
2. Hirabayashi K, Watanabe K, Wakano K, Suzuki N, Satomi K, Ishii Y. Expansive open-door laminoplasty for cervical spinal stenotic myelopathy. Spine 1983;8:693–699
3. Hirabayashi K, Watanabe K, Wakano K, Suzuki N, Satomi K, Ishii Y. Expansive open-door laminoplasty for cervical spinal stenotic myelopathy. Spine 1983;8:693–699
4. Kurokawa T, Tsuyama N, Tanaka H, et al. Enlargement of spinal canal by the sagittal splitting of the spinous process. Bessatsu Seikeigeka 1982;2:234–240 [in Japanese]
5. Itoh T, Tsuji H. Technical improvements and results of laminoplasty for compressive myelopathy in the cervical spine. Spine 1985;10:729–736
6. Wang JM, Roh KJ, Kim DJ, Kim DW. A new method of stabilising the elevated laminae in open-door laminoplasty using an anchor system. J Bone Joint Surg Br 1998;80:1005–1008
7. Tsuzuki N, Abe R, Saiki K, Iizuka T. Tension-band laminoplasty of the cervical spine. Int Orthop 1996;20:275–284
8. Nakano K, Harata S, Suetsuna F, Araki T, Itoh J. Spinous process-splitting laminoplasty using hydroxyapatite spinous process spacer. Spine 1992;17(3, Suppl):S41–S43
9. Yoshida M, Otani K, Shibasaki K, Ueda S. Expansive laminoplasty with reattachment of spinous process and extensor musculature for cervical myelopathy. Spine 1992;17:491–497
10. Tomita K, Kawahara N, Toribatake Y, Heller JG. Expansive midline T-saw laminoplasty (modified spinous process-splitting) for the management of cervical myelopathy. Spine 1998;23:32–37
11. Ratliff JK, Cooper PR. Cervical laminoplasty: a critical review. J Neurosurg 2003;98(3, Suppl):230–238
12. Yonenobu K, Hosono N, Iwasaki M, Asano M, Ono K. Laminoplasty versus subtotal corpectomy. A comparative study of results in multisegmental cervical spondylotic myelopathy. Spine 1992;17:1281–1284
13. Yoshida M, Tamaki T, Kawakami M, Hayashi N, Ando M. Indication and clinical results of laminoplasty for cervical myelopathy caused by disc herniation with developmental canal stenosis. Spine 1998;23:2391–2397
14. Iwasaki M, Ebara S, Miyamoto S, Wada E, Yonenobu K. Expansive laminoplasty for cervical radiculomyelopathy due to soft disc herniation. Spine 1996;21:32–38
15. Hilibrand AS, Carlson GD, Palumbo MA, Jones PK, Bohlman HH. Radiculopathy and myelopathy at segments adjacent to the site of a previous anterior cervical arthrodesis. J Bone Joint Surg Am 1999;81:519–528
16. Suda K, Abumi K, Ito M, Shono Y, Kaneda K, Fujiya M. Local kyphosis reduces surgical outcomes of expansive open-door laminoplasty for cervical spondylotic myelopathy. Spine 2003;28:1258–1262
17. Iwasaki M, Okuda S, Miyauchi A, et al. Surgical strategy for cervical myelopathy due to ossification of the posterior longitudinal ligament: Part 1: Clinical results and limitations of laminoplasty. Spine 2007;32:647–653
18. Iwasaki M, Okuda S, Miyauchi A, et al. Surgical strategy for cervical myelopathy due to ossification of the posterior longitudinal ligament: Part 2: Advantages of anterior decompression and fusion over laminoplasty. Spine 2007;32:654–660
19. Fujiyoshi T, Yamazaki M, Kawabe J, et al. A new concept for making decisions regarding the surgical approach for cervical ossification of the posterior longitudinal ligament: the K-line. Spine 2008;33:E990–E993

20. Herkowitz HN. A comparison of anterior cervical fusion, cervical laminectomy, and cervical laminoplasty for the surgical management of multiple level spondylotic radiculopathy. Spine 1988;13:774–780
21. Sakaura H, Hosono N, Mukai Y, Ishii T, Yoshikawa H. C5 palsy after decompression surgery for cervical myelopathy: review of the literature. Spine 2003;28:2447–2451
22. Imagama S, Matsuyama Y, Yukawa Y, et al; Nagoya Spine Group. C5 palsy after cervical laminoplasty: a multicentre study. J Bone Joint Surg Br 2010;92:393–400
23. Lawrence BD, Jacobs WB, Norvell DC, Hermsmeyer JT, Chapman JR, Brodke DS. Anterior versus posterior approach for treatment of cervical spondylotic myelopathy: a systematic review. Spine 2013;38(22, Suppl 1):S173–S182
24. Okada M, Minamide A, Endo T, et al. A prospective randomized study of clinical outcomes in patients with cervical compressive myelopathy treated with open-door or French-door laminoplasty. Spine 2009;34: 1119–1126
25. Nakashima H, Kato F, Yukawa Y, et al. Comparative effectiveness of open-door laminoplasty versus French-door laminoplasty in cervical compressive myelopathy. Spine 2014;39:642–647
26. Yue WM, Tan CT, Tan SB, Tan SK, Tay BK. Results of cervical laminoplasty and a comparison between single and double trap-door techniques. J Spinal Disord 2000;13:329–335
27. Naito M, Ogata K, Kurose S, Oyama M. Canal-expansive laminoplasty in 83 patients with cervical myelopathy. A comparative study of three different procedures. Int Orthop 1994;18:347–351
28. Hirabayashi S, Yamada H, Motosuneya T, et al. Comparison of enlargement of the spinal canal after cervical laminoplasty: open-door type and double-door type. Eur Spine J 2010;19:1690–1694
29. Hosono N, Sakaura H, Mukai Y, Fujii R, Yoshikawa H. C3-6 laminoplasty takes over C3-7 laminoplasty with significantly lower incidence of axial neck pain. Eur Spine J 2006;15:1375–1379
30. Hirabayashi K. Expansive open door laminoplasty. In: Sherk HH, ed. The Cervical Spine: An Atlas of Surgical Procedures. Philadelphia: JB Lippincott; 1994:233–250
31. Matsumoto M, Watanabe K, Tsuji T, et al. Risk factors for closure of lamina after open-door laminoplasty. J Neurosurg Spine 2008;9:530–537
32. Frank E, Keenen TL. A technique for cervical laminoplasty using mini plates. Br J Neurosurg 1994;8:197–199
33. Heller JG, Raich AL, Dettori JR, Riew KD. Comparative effectiveness of different types of cervical laminoplasty. Evid Based Spine Care J 2013;4: 105–115
34. Riew KD, Raich AL, Dettori JR, Heller JG. Neck pain following cervical laminoplasty: Does preservation of the C2 muscle attachments and/or C7 matter? Evid Based Spine Care J 2013;4:42–53
35. Takeshita K, Seichi A, Akune T, Kawamura N, Kawaguchi H, Nakamura K. Can laminoplasty maintain the cervical alignment even when the C2 lamina is contained? Spine 2005;30:1294–1298
36. Takeuchi K, Yokoyama T, Aburakawa S, et al. Axial symptoms after cervical laminoplasty with C3 laminectomy compared with conventional C3-C7 laminoplasty: a modified laminoplasty preserving the semispinalis cervicis inserted into axis. Spine 2005;30:2544–2549
37. Kaito T, Hosono N, Makino T, Kaneko N, Namekata M, Fuji T. Postoperative displacement of hydroxyapatite spacers implanted during double-door laminoplasty. J Neurosurg Spine 2009;10:551–556
38. Hosono N, Yonenobu K, Ono K. Neck and shoulder pain after laminoplasty. A noticeable complication. Spine 1996;21:1969–1973
39. Hosono N, Miwa T, Mukai Y, Takenaka S, Makino T, Fuji T. Potential risk of thermal damage to cervical nerve roots by a high-speed drill. J Bone Joint Surg Br 2009;91:1541–1544
40. Ohashi M, Yamazaki A, Watanabe K, Katsumi K, Shoji H. Two-year clinical and radiological outcomes of open-door cervical laminoplasty with prophylactic bilateral C4-C5 foraminotomy in a prospective study. Spine 2014;39:721–727

36 Gardner-Wells Tong or Crown-Halo Reduction for Cervical Facet Dislocations

Joshua Bakhsheshian, Nader S. Dahdaleh, and Zachary A. Smith

The traumatic process of the inferior facet of the superior vertebrae moving anterior to the superior facet of the inferior vertebrae has been referred to as a dislocated, perched, jumped, or locked facet (**Fig. 36.1**).[1] For simplicity, we use *facet dislocation* as the umbrella term. Facet dislocations can be unilateral or bilateral, and are considered unstable. Bilateral facet dislocations occur when hyperflexion forces extend anteriorly, whereas unilateral facet dislocations often include an additional rotational force around one of the facet joints during flexion. Anterior displacement of the more cranial vertebral body exceeding 50% of the anteroposterior diameter of the caudal vertebral body usually results in bilateral facet dislocations. These injuries are commonly associated with significant neurologic deficits.

Cervical traction is frequently used and recommended to achieve reduction of dislocated facets, indirect decompression of the spinal cord and roots, and cervical spine stability.[2] A significant advantage of this approach is that patients are typically awake for the reduction process, and therefore are able to undergo interval neurologic examinations. Reduction in an alert patient is critical, as frequent patient examinations during reduction may provide early signs of impending neurologic injury. In these circumstances, traction conditions may be modified to prevent a permanent deficit. Closed cervical spine reduction can be accomplished through the application of traction using Gardner-Wells tongs or a crown halo.[3,4] The Gardner-Wells tongs entail a one-piece bow with two angled threaded pins (**Fig. 36.2**). The crown halo employs multiple pins that are inserted perpendicular to the cranium, and must be applied in a safe zone to avoid nerve injury (**Fig. 36.3**).

There is a high incidence of concurrent disk herniations with cervical spinal dislocations, but they may not always affect the neurologic outcomes following closed reduction.[2,5] Yet it is important to be aware of a traumatic disk herniation. In circumstances where a large traumatic herniation is present, closed reduction prior to operative decompression may precipitate a neurologic injury. In these circumstances, judicious decision making is critical. We recommend obtaining a magnetic resonance imaging (MRI) scan of the cervical spine to rule out traumatic disk herniation prior to the application of traction.

Patient Selection

This technique is appropriate in patients who require immediate reduction and can respond reliably to interval neurologic examinations.

Indications

- Bilateral/unilateral facet dislocations
- Other cervical traumatic indications (e.g., hangman's fracture type II)

Contraindications

- Adjacent fractures or rostral injury
- Skull defect or fracture at pin site
- Hangman's fracture type IIA or III
- Occipitocervical dislocation

Objective

- Craniocervical traction is used to restore anatomic alignment and stability, and preserve or improve neurologic function by indirect decompression.

Advantages

- Easy and rapid application
- May eliminate the need for a surgical procedure
- An awake patient responds to interval neurologic examinations
- May be supplemented with subsequent fixation if necessary (**Fig. 36.4**)

Disadvantages

- Does not allow investigation of the foramina and exiting nerve roots
- Does not allow direct manipulation of the joint
- Fails to reduce some facet dislocations
- Does not provide segmental fixation for unstable injuries

Preprocedural Imaging

- Lateral X-ray for fractures and dislocations
- Computed tomography (CT) for exact anatomy of fracture character/anatomy
- Cervical MRI is strongly advised if a consistent neurologic exam is not available.

36 Gardner-Wells Tong or Crown-Halo Reduction for Cervical Facet Dislocations

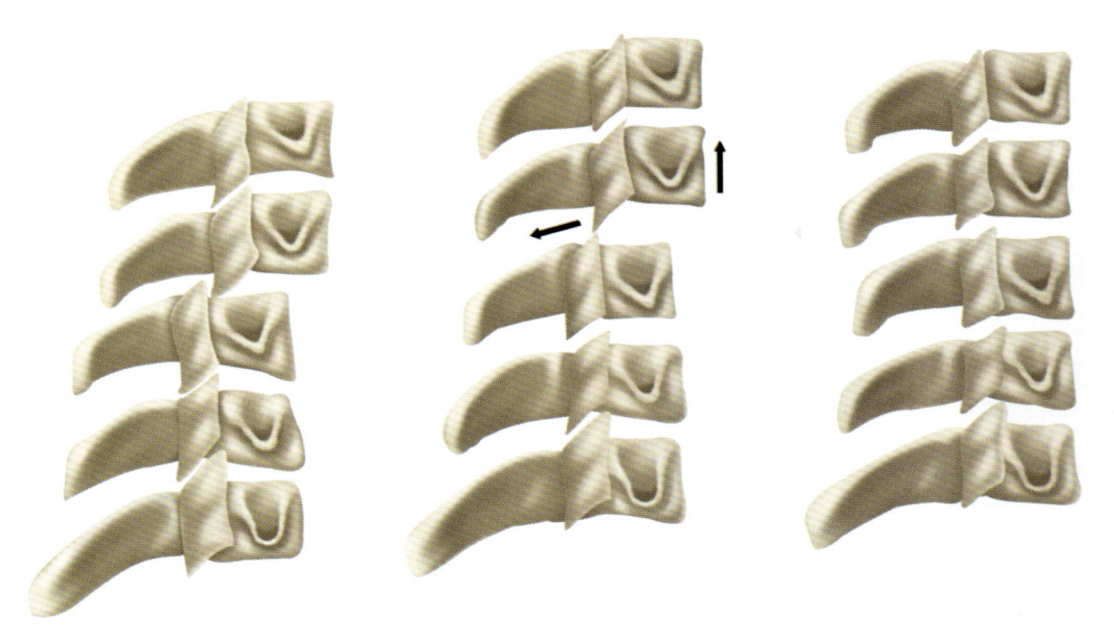

Fig. 36.1 Inferior lip of the C4 facet translated superiorly and anteriorly over the superior lip of C5 facet. With longitudinal traction the facets can be reduced to achieve anatomic alignment.

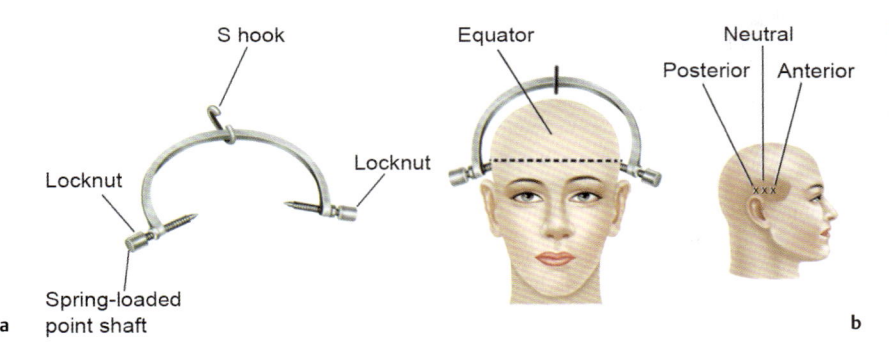

Fig. 36.2 The application of Gardner-Wells tongs. (a) Illustration of tongs with threaded angled pins on each side, and one spring-loaded point shaft. (b) The tongs should be placed below the greatest biparietal diameter of the skull. Changes in the vector of traction can be achieved by placing the pins more posterior, causing flexion, or more anterior, causing extension.

Fig. 36.3 The application of the halo skeletal fixator. (a) The safe zone for placement of the anterior pins is 1 cm superior and two-thirds lateral to the orbital rim. On the medial aspect of the orbital rim are the supraorbital and supratrochlear nerves and frontal sinus. (b) Schematic demonstration of the four-pin placement. The ring should provide 1 to 2 cm clearance of head circumference. (c) Illustration of the halo-vest orthosis with a rigid ring attached to the skull with pins.

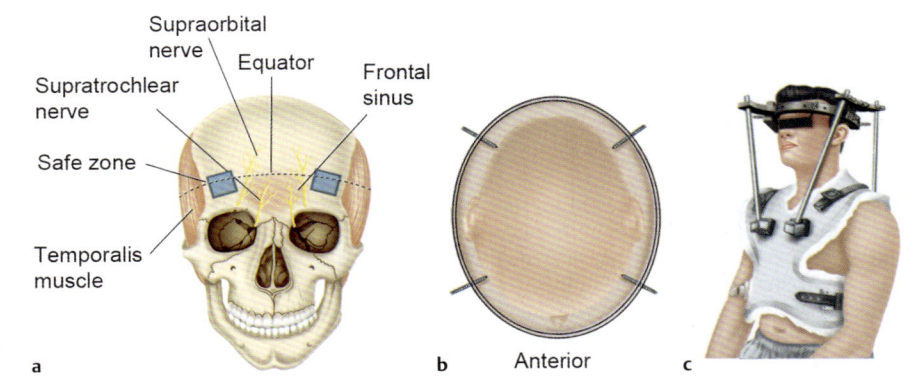

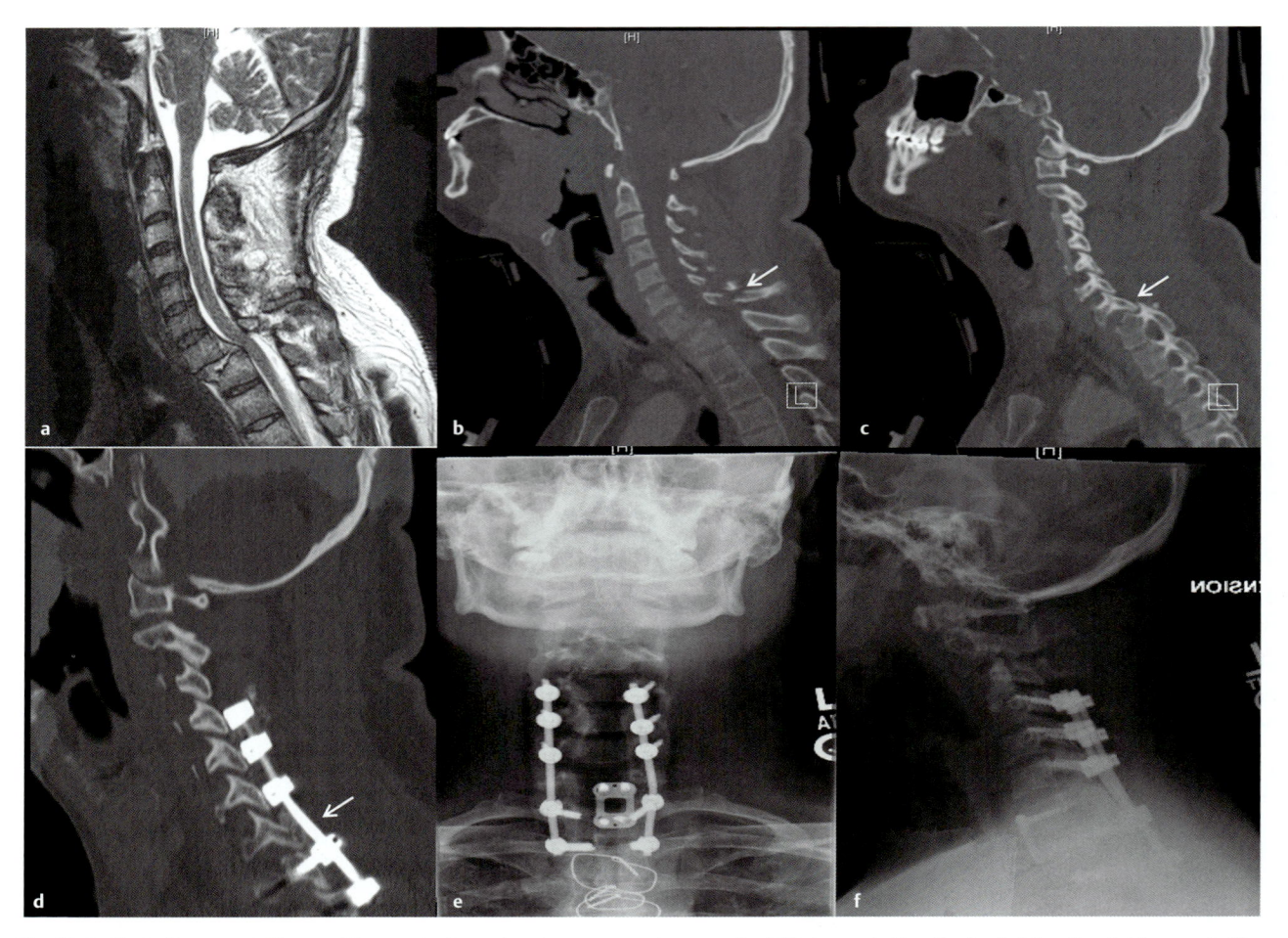

Fig. 36.4 Illustrative case. A 50-year-old man who is employed as a construction worker presented to the emergency room after a metal beam fell directly onto his head from a height of ~ 10 feet. Subsequent radiographic images demonstrated cervical facet dislocation at C7-T1. **(a)** Lateral magnetic resonance imaging (MRI) demonstrating a decreased anterior-posterior diameter of the spinal canal at the cervical dislocation site. **(b,c)** Computed tomography (CT) demonstrating the facet dislocation *(white arrow)*. After immediate closed reduction in the awake patient, general anesthesia was induced and the patient underwent combined anterior-posterior fixation. **(d–f)** Postoperative images demonstrate anatomic alignment of the prior facet dislocation on **(d)** lateral CT *(white arrow)*, **(e)** anterior-posterior X-ray, and **(f)** lateral X-ray.

Choice of Approach

Gardner-Wells tongs are indicated when longitudinal traction will be temporarily applied. They may provide a relatively rapid reduction of cervical dislocation. The tongs do not provide immobilization of the spine, and therefore the patient should be restricted to bed rest. The fixed size of the tongs can make it cumbersome for fitting larger or smaller heads. MRI compatible graphite tong and titanium pins are available but may be more prone to slippage when compared with stainless steel tongs and pins.[6]

The halo ring provides several advantages over the Gardner-Wells tongs. It enables optimum head control with circumferential pin fixation while decreasing the distribution of the pin load. Postreduction immobilization with the halo orthosis provides a rigid fixation of the cervical spine. Halo rings are available in a variety of sizes, making their use more compatible for varying head circumferences. The pullout strength of the halo ring has been shown to be double that of the Gardner-Wells tongs, thereby providing the opportunity of adding more weights for traction.[7,8] However, both devices provide the pullout strength required for safe cervical reduction.

Although the focus of this chapter is subaxial facet injuries, it should be noted that both Gardner-Wells traction and halo-vest orthosis have frequent applications in the treatment of spinal trauma. In many circumstances, fracture reduction can be obtained in both a closed and an open manner. When open fixation is elected after a closed reduction, it is our experience that a halo vest provides the stability for safe transportation to, and positioning in, the operating room. This is strongly aided by the use of halo-vest attachments on many modern Jackson tables. Furthermore, in situations where closed reduction is sufficient, the halo vest may be worn until fracture healing is confirmed.

Surgical Procedure

Closed Reduction

Patient Position and Sedation

The patient is placed in the supine position. A reverse Trendelenburg position or ankle weights may be used to counteract the pull from the traction weights. The hair is shaved, the skin is prepped in a sterile fashion, and the pin is inserted directly into the skin. Local anesthetic is injected into the skin to infiltrate the periosteum region.

Pin Placement

When using the Gardner-Wells tongs, pins should be placed below the greatest biparietal diameter of the skull, ~ 2 to 3 cm above the pinna, while avoiding the temporalis muscle and the superficial temporal artery and vein (**Fig. 36.2**). Avoid asymmetric pin placement, which may result in asymmetric forces to the cervical spine. For most cervical spine injuries, the pins can be placed superior to the external auditory meatus for neutral reduction. Small changes in the vector traction by placing the pins more posterior will cause flexion, and placing the pins more anterior will extension. In cases of jumped facets, the tong should be placed slightly more posterior because the flexion moment of the spine will assist in reducing the perched facets. Sterile pins are placed orthogonally while tightening the pins by alternating sides to maintain symmetry. A spring-loaded force indicator is contained in one of the pins. The pins should be tightened until the indicator demonstrates greater than 1 mm protrusion.

When using the halo ring, choose a ring size that provides 1 to 2 cm clearance of head circumference. The pins should be placed below the greatest circumference of the patient's skull. The halo ring can be stabilized with blunt position pins until the locations for the sharp pins are determined. The safe zone for placement of the anterior pins is 1 cm superior and two-thirds lateral to the orbital rim at the level of the equator (**Fig. 36.3**).[9] On the medial aspect of the orbital rim are the supraorbital and supratrochlear nerves and the frontal sinus. There is minimal risk with the placement of the posterior pins. Ask the patient to relax the forehead and keep the eyes closed when advancing the anterior pins to avoid tenting of the skin. Posterior pins are placed diagonal to the anterior pins, perpendicular to the cranium, and at ~ 1 cm above the pinna. Pins are sequentially tightened to "finger tightness." Using a calibrated torque wrench, pins are inserted at a torque of 8 inch-pounds (in-lb) for adults.[9] For pediatric patients, a major concern is the risk of pin penetration due to the immaturity of the skull. To avoid this complication, more pins are placed at a torque of 2 to 4 in-lb to further distribute the load.[10,11] A CT head scan is recommended in children younger than 6 years of age to locate the best pin sites. Lock nuts are placed to secure the pin to the halo ring.

Serial Reduction

After Gardner-Wells tongs or a halo ring is applied, an initial weight of 5 to 10 lb is added and a lateral X-ray is immediately taken to evaluate the alignment. The weight is increased in increments of 5 to 10 lb, waiting 10 to 15 minutes after each addition of weight to avoid overdistraction and allow tissue relaxation. After each weight is added, it is strongly suggested to continue interval lateral X-rays and neurologic examinations. The patient should be completely relaxed, and intravenous diazepam may be used for paraspinal muscle relaxation to assist in the reduction process. Doses of muscle relaxants should be limited by the ability to still acquire meaningful interval neurologic exams. One may need more weight traction for unilateral facet dislocations versus the bilateral facet dislocation due to the intact facet capsule on the contralateral side of the unilateral facet dislocation. When the facets are "perched" (tipping point of reduction), gentle cervical extension may be achieved by placing a small towel-roll between the shoulder blades to facilitate final reduction of the facets. After reduction is achieved, the patient is placed in a halo vest, and traction is reduced to 10 to 20 lb.

The maximal amount of weight safely applied for cervical traction remains controversial. Studies have shown that 50 to 140 lb have been used safely in patients with cervical trauma to obtain reduction of the spine.[7,12] However, the majority of patients do not need more than 50 lb. The patient's size, body weight, and body habitus should be considered when assessing the maximum cervical traction weight. In practice, we usually do not exceed 10 lb per vertebral level to avoid overdistraction. In addition, weight is added gradually when a consistent exam is possible. Reduction is discontinued if neurological status of patient deteriorates, greater distraction occurs at the site of injury, or when maximum weight is applied. Cervical traction can also be a temporary measure until a more permanent stabilization is performed intraoperatively (**Fig. 36.4**).

Postprocedural Care

The patient should be admitted to the intensive care unit or step-down unit, with interval neurologic examinations performed. The aspiration risk should be assessed to determine if a nasogastric tube is needed. The pins should be cleaned once a day with hydrogen peroxide. After 24 to 48 hours, the pins should be retightened; thereafter, additional retightening should be avoided to prevent penetration of skull. Early physical therapy should be encouraged.

Potential Complications and Precautions

- Loss of cervical reduction may require operative internal stabilization (see Chapter 37).
- Failed reduction may be due to anatomic obstacles including facet fractures and disk herniations. Preoperative imaging can assist the preprocedural planning.
- The risk of the pins penetrating the skull is low.[13] This can be guarded against by not applying pins too tightly or placing pins over thin bone.
- Pin migration may occur due to inadequate tightening or to overused tongs, which should be recalibrated or replaced.[8]
- Overdistraction can be avoided by increasing the weight in increments of 5 to 10 lb, and waiting 10 to 15 minutes after each addition of weight.
- Neurologic deterioration can occur (rarely due to pre-reduction herniated disks) and can be avoided with reduction in an alert patient with interval neurologic examinations. We recommend obtaining an MRI scan of the cervical spine to rule out traumatic disk herniation prior to the application of traction.
- Infection can be reduced with good pin care (e.g., hydrogen peroxide cleansing). An optimal strategy has not yet been identified.[14]

Conclusion

Craniocervical traction with a tong or halo is useful for closed reduction and stabilization of dislocated facets. Closed reduction may be safely used in an awake, alert, and cooperative patient with interval neurologic examinations and lateral radiographs. Caution should be exercised when applying additional weight due to the risk of overdistraction. **Box 36.1** summarizes the key steps and the problems that can arise.

Box 36.1 Key Steps and Potential Problems

Step	Problems
Pin placement	• Asymmetric pin placement • Skull penetration *Gardner-Wells:* • On temporalis muscle or superficial temporal vessels • Anterior to external auditory meatus, causing extension and difficulty in reduction *Halo ring:* • On supraorbital and supratrochlear nerves or frontal sinus • Tenting of the skin • Pediatrics with immature skull anatomy
Serial reduction	• Overdistraction • Pin migration • Neurologic deterioration

References

1. Andreshak JL, Dekutoski MB. Management of unilateral facet dislocations: a review of the literature. Orthopedics 1997;20:917–926
2. Gelb DE, Hadley MN, Aarabi B, et al. Initial closed reduction of cervical spinal fracture-dislocation injuries. Neurosurgery 2013;72(Suppl 2):73–83
3. Gardner WJ. The principle of spring-loaded points for cervical traction. Technical note. J Neurosurg 1973;39:543–544
4. Botte MJ, Garfin SR, Byrne TP, Woo SL, Nickel VL. The halo skeletal fixator. Principles of application and maintenance. Clin Orthop Relat Res 1989;239:12–18
5. Grant GA, Mirza SK, Chapman JR, et al. Risk of early closed reduction in cervical spine subluxation injuries. J Neurosurg 1999;90(1, Suppl):13–18
6. Blumberg KD, Catalano JB, Cotler JM, Balderston RA. The pullout strength of titanium alloy MRI-compatible and stainless steel MRI-incompatible Gardner-Wells tongs. Spine 1993;18:1895–1896
7. Cotler JM, Herbison GJ, Nasuti JF, Ditunno JF Jr, An H, Wolff BE. Closed reduction of traumatic cervical spine dislocation using traction weights up to 140 pounds. Spine 1993;18:386–390
8. Lerman JA, Haynes RJ, Koeneman EJ, Koeneman JB, Wong WB. A biomechanical comparison of Gardner-Wells tongs and halo device used for cervical spine traction. Spine 1994;19:2403–2406
9. Botte MJ, Byrne TP, Abrams RA, Garfin SR. Halo skeletal fixation: techniques of application and prevention of complications. J Am Acad Orthop Surg 1996;4:44–53
10. Lauweryns P. Role of conservative treatment of cervical spine injuries. Eur Spine J 2010;19(Suppl 1):S23–S26
11. Letts M, Girouard L, Yeadon A. Mechanical evaluation of four- versus eight-pin halo fixation. J Pediatr Orthop 1997;17:121–124
12. Cotler HB, Miller LS, DeLucia FA, Cotler JM, Davne SH. Closed reduction of cervical spine dislocations. Clin Orthop Relat Res 1987;214:185–199
13. Lerman JA, Dickman CA, Haynes RJ. Penetration of cranial inner table with Gardner-Wells tongs. J Spinal Disord 2001;14:211–213
14. Lethaby A, Temple J, Santy-Tomlinson J. Pin site care for preventing infections associated with external bone fixators and pins. Cochrane Database Syst Rev 2013;12:CD004551

37 Posterior Approach for the Treatment of Locked Cervical Facets

Ricardo B.V. Fontes, Manish K. Kasliwal, and Vincent C. Traynelis

So-called locked cervical facets are a widely recognized form of distractive-flexion cervical injury that may be present in up to 5% of cervical injuries with neurologic deficits.[1] The number of clinical series in the literature discussing its treatment, however, is deceptively small.[2] Hadra[3] first described spinous process wiring for cervical flexion-distraction injuries in 1891 and, 2 years later, Walton described this type of injury in greater detail. Although 125 years have elapsed since Hadra's publication, there is no consensus regarding the ideal management of these injuries.[4] Nonoperative therapies have been largely abandoned due to suboptimal results and the safety and efficacy of contemporary operative options. Traditionally treated with posterior wiring methods, application of anterior fusion in the 1960s and screw-based posterior cervical instrumentation in the 1980s for this type of injury have greatly improved fusion rates and decreased surgical morbidity.[2,5,6] Current operative strategies include anterior, posterior, or combined anterior-posterior (360-degree) approaches.

Perched or locked facets are a type of distraction-flexion injury as described by Allen et al[7] in 1982. Under more modern, treatment-oriented classification systems such as the Cervical Spine Injury Severity Score (CSISS) or the Subaxial Injury Classification (SLIC), these injuries are severe enough that they are usually grouped within the "surgical treatment" categories (CSISS > 7 points or SLIC > 5 points).[8,9] The posterior surfaces of the inferior articular process of the cranial vertebra lie snugly anterior to the superior articular process of the caudal vertebra or in a "perched" position (**Fig. 37.1**).

Closed reduction of unilateral or bilateral locked facets may be performed with traction, in a manner reproducing the mechanism of injury in the opposite sequence. Although closed reduction in obtunded patients has been described under neurophysiological monitoring, in our practice this is performed in awake and oriented patients to enable an immediate decrease in weights should the exam change. Gardner-Wells tongs or a halo are applied under local anesthesia. The traction bed is placed in a reverse Trendelenburg position at 30 degrees to avoid patient displacement with the use of heavy weights. Traction is started at 2.5 kg per level of injury and gradually increased by 5 kg every 10 to 15 minutes. Lateral radiographs are obtained at baseline and at every increase in weight. Nonsedating muscle relaxants and analgesics can be administered and are particularly useful for muscular individuals. No definitive upper weight limit exists, but we typically do not increase beyond 7.5 kg per level as it would be considered futile. Other end points for traction include failure of tongs/halo, cranial movement of the patient in bed, neurologic exam change, or signs of craniocervical or subaxial overdistraction (e.g., any disk space height > 10 mm on lateral radiographs). Slight flexion (e.g., with a rolled towel behind the occiput) can be utilized in the initial stages of traction to "unlock" the facets. When the facets are distracted, a small roll may be placed behind the shoulders to slightly extend the head, and then the traction is reduced by 2.5 kg. This should enable final reduction.

Closed reduction enables the fixation procedure to be performed in a nonemergent setting. Open reduction can also be performed immediately, if possible from a logistical standpoint or in the case of failure of closed reduction. It can be reliably achieved intraoperatively through either an anterior or posterior approach; the latter is described here.

Patient Selection

Patients with distractive-flexion injuries of the subaxial spine are potential candidates for posterior open reduction and internal fixation (ORIF).

Indications

- Subaxial distractive-flexion injuries

Contraindications

- Hemodynamic instability
- Concomitant compressive injury (e.g., cervical burst fracture) at same or adjacent level requiring anterior approach
- Herniated disk fragment with cord compression (relative)
- Articular process/lateral mass fractures (relative)

Advantages

The advantages of the posterior approach include direct repair of the posterior tension band, which is the primary structure that fails during distractive-flexion trauma, although bilateral facet dislocation or extreme instability also imply an injury of more anterior structures such as the posterior longitudinal ligament and intervertebral disk. Reduction maneuvers are easier to perform from a posterior approach because the articular processes are being directly manipulated, as opposed to the vertebral bodies in an anterior approach. If direct manipulation does not reduce the articular processes, then a portion of the superior articular processes of the caudal vertebra can be resected to facilitate reduction. Finally, posterior constructs may be biomechanically more stable than anterior grafting and plating, especially if pedicle screw fixation is utilized, although it is unclear whether the difference is clinically significant.[10]

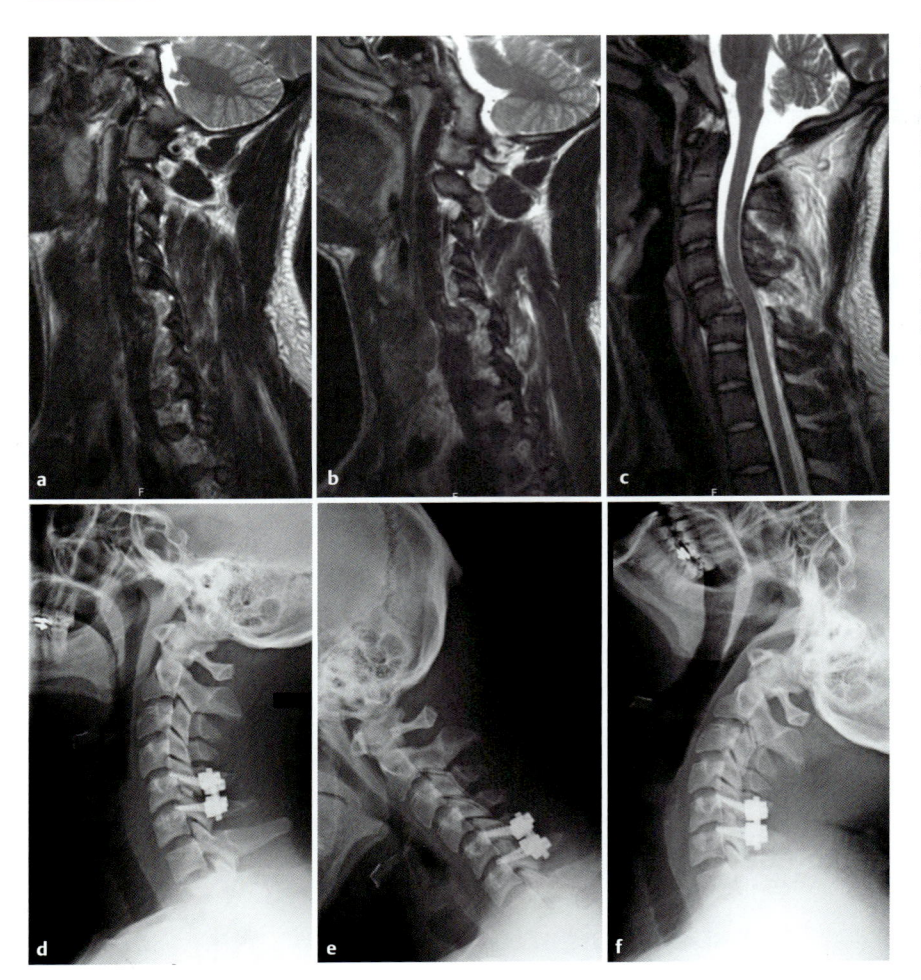

Fig. 37.1 Case example. A 19-year-old man dove into a shallow part of Lake Michigan while under the effect of alcohol. Neurologically intact, American Spinal Injury Association (ASIA) grade E. **(a)** Left perched and **(b)** right locked facets are demonstrated on magnetic resonance imaging. **(c)** A small disk fragment and subligamental hematoma are seen on the midsagittal view. **(d)** Closed reduction was unsuccessful and a posterior open reduction and internal fixation (ORIF) was performed with placement of intra-articular graft. **(e)** Flexion and **(f)** extension radiographs 1 year after surgery demonstrate solid fusion.

Disadvantages

The disadvantages of a posterior approach include the requirement for prone positioning with the need for strict cervical spine precautions while the patient is being positioned. This positioning may also complicate hemodynamic management in the case of patients with complete cord injuries. Compared with the standard anterior cervical approach, posterior exposures require more manipulation of muscle, which produces pain and tissue damage and creates dead space that may lead to increased infection rates and complicate the management of pseudomeningocele.

Choice of Operative Approach

Historically, the potential that a cervical disk herniation may occur concomitantly with cervical fracture-dislocation has been a concern, especially because disk disruptions may be detected in up to 90% of patients examined with computed tomography (CT) myelogram or magnetic resonance imaging (MRI).[11,12] The presence of a herniated fragment has been cited as a potential contraindication for closed reduction and indication for anterior repair of the bilateral dislocation and severely unstable injuries. Despite the elevated number of disk abnormalities detected via imaging, the risk of developing a new, permanent neurologic deficit during closed reduction is exceedingly small. Darsaut et al[11] demonstrated with MRI monitoring of closed reduction that the canal actually increases in size even when there is a fragment present. Nakashima et al[6] present a significant series of successful posterior ORIF with the presence of an anterior disk and no cases of deterioration. Many of the disk abnormalities seen on MRI are small or represent only the elevation of an intact posterior longitudinal ligament from the dorsal wall of the vertebral body. In such cases it is not unreasonable to reduce and fix a facet dislocation from a posterior route. In the setting of large disk herniations or when in doubt, it is best to choose an anterior approach.

Our group would avoid a posterior ORIF in the event the patient cannot be positioned prone or, due to surgeon's preference, a combined anterior-posterior fixation is planned to provide the best fixation from the biomechanical standpoint. In the latter case, the anterior approach is always performed first and is described in Chapter 28.

Preoperative Imaging

Every patient should have at minimum a CT of the cervical spine with sagittal and coronal reconstructions. If the locked facet(s) have been reduced with traction and the patient is intact, no further imaging is necessary. If the patient cannot be reduced with traction, an MRI scan should be considered, particularly if the patient is intact neurologically or has only minimal deficits. The presence of a large herniated disk fragment anterior to the cord would usually be handled with an anterior approach. Vascular imaging such as CT or MR angiography can be obtained in either case and is particularly useful if a neurologic deficit is asymmetric (as it may suggest a medullary infarction) or the patient is obtunded, although it is unclear how such information may impact the surgical procedure.

Surgical Procedure

The maintenance of adequate cord perfusion is of paramount importance during the entire procedure, particularly if the patient has an incomplete deficit. Invasive blood pressure monitoring is essential as is adequate intravenous (IV) access; a central venous line may be placed to ensure fluid replacement during surgery. A goal mean arterial pressure of 90 mm Hg is maintained throughout the procedure. The patient is intubated with cervical inline precautions. Prone positioning can be performed in two ways. If a Jackson table is available, the patient initially may be positioned supine with continuous traction and then turned with the table onto the open-frame attachment. Alternatively, the patient may be log-rolled onto a regular table with chest bolsters and the head secured in a Mayfield headholder, particularly if traction was unsuccessful. After applying the headholder, the surgeon holds the head at all times and traction is discontinued. The surgeon is responsible for maintaining alignment once the head frame is secured. If the prone position results in difficulty in maintaining adequate mean arterial pressure or compromises the ability to achieve appropriate ventilation, the patient is turned to the supine position and treated with an anterior operation.

Lateral fluoroscopy is utilized to localize the dislocation level, ensure proper alignment, and mark the skin incision. A midline longitudinal incision is made, and subperiosteal dissection is utilized to expose the lamina and bilateral lateral masses. Extensive damage to the ligamentous components of the posterior tension band is usually evident, with rupture of interspinous process and muscular hematoma. The initial step is to achieve reduction; a slight increase in head traction may facilitate this, but typically the patient who does not reduce with preoperative traction will require surgical manipulation of the segment. This may be performed in a variety of ways, all of which focus on focally distracting the segment or segments that are dislocated. This can be accomplished with dissectors; manipulation of the spinous processes of the cranial and caudal vertebra with clamps or towel clips sometimes may be helpful. As a last resort, the superior articular process may be resected. The presence of a concomitant lateral mass fracture not only can complicate the reduction but also impact the stabilization (purchase points, number of levels, etc.).

Once reduction is achieved, instrumentation is placed with lateral mass or pedicle screws as described in Chapters 40 and 41. Intra-articular grafting can be performed with autograft or allograft after denuding the facet of the cartilage. The incision is closed in the usual manner, and the patient is rolled into the supine position and transferred to the intensive care unit.

Postoperative Care

A rigid cervical collar is placed in the operating room if a posterior-only ORIF was performed. Mean arterial pressure precautions are maintained for a minimum of 24 hours postreduction if there was a preoperative deficit. Unless another traumatic injury is present or respiratory failure is a concern due to an injury above C4, there is no reason to maintain the patient sedated, and early extubation is advocated. Nutritional support is started as soon as possible through an enteral route, if possible. Mobilization and rehabilitation start on the first postoperative day. Ideally, deep venous thrombosis prophylaxis should be started with compression stockings even in the preoperative period; this is continued in the postoperative period, and appropriate prophylactic pharmacological therapy is instituted at the end of the first postoperative day if the patient is not ambulating. Transition to a regular hospital room and rehabilitation at a specialized spinal cord unit depending on the neurologic status can occur as early as the first postoperative day.

If a rostral injury is present, particularly above C4, respiratory function is assessed on the first postoperative day. When patients are unable to be weaned off the ventilator quickly, we have advocated early tracheostomy and percutaneous gastrostomy, as a means to decrease ventilator-associated pneumonia and start mobilization and enteral feeding as soon as possible. Lateral and anteroposterior cervical radiographs are obtained on the first postoperative day to serve as baseline controls. The rigid collar is worn continuously except when washing the neck, and at that time the patient should keep the neck in the neutral position. Six to eight weeks of immobilization is favored. Patients should be followed with serial radiographs to ensure maintenance of proper alignment and ultimately arthrodesis.

Potential Complications and Precautions

Complications inherent to any posterior cervical instrumented arthrodesis may occur, including, but not limited to, vertebral artery injury, incidental durotomy, neural element injury, and C5 palsy. The initial pathology being treated should not impact the management of such complications.

Complications specific to the treatment of facet dislocations include failure to reduce the dislocation, which should not happen when using the posterior approach, and failure to maintain alignment in the postoperative period. The latter is more likely to occur if there has been a significant disk injury or if the facets are completely incompetent, such as in the setting of a fracture or when the articular pillars have been resected to reduce the spine or decompress the root. Both scenarios diminish axial load support, and when this occurs it is wise to consider a 360-degree procedure or extend the number of instrumented segments if utilizing only posterior fixation.

Conclusion

Posterior reduction and internal fixation of distraction-flexion injuries is relatively easy to perform and results in a reliable correction. It is a safe technique, and treatment should not be delayed, even if closed reduction has been successful, so as to accelerate rehabilitation. **Box 37.1** lists the key operative points and steps to take to avoid complications.

Box 37.1 Key Operative Points and Ways to Avoid Complications

- Use of an arterial line and possibly a central line
- General anesthesia and intubation with the patient in the supine position; baseline neuromonitoring recordings with somatosensory evoked potentials (SSEPs) and motor evoked potentials (MEPs)
- Head in tongs under traction or Mayfield clamp
- Roll into prone position on regular table with gel bolsters or Jackson open frame.
- Lateral fluoroscopy confirmation and guidance throughout surgery
- Map midline posterior incision on the skin.
- Expose injured levels.
- Reduce fracture-dislocation; use a Penfield under inferior articular processes of the cranial vertebra, bilaterally.
- Distract and reduce; towel clamps attached to spinous processes may be helpful.
- Perform instrumented arthrodesis as usual.
- Close wound, roll patient into the supine position, and transfer to the intensive care unit.
- Maintain mean arterial pressure over 90 mm Hg if there is neurologic compromise.
- Compression stockings throughout procedure, subcutaneous heparin on postoperative day 1 (prophylactic dose).
- Early extubation, mobilization and rehabilitation
- If ventilator-dependent, early tracheostomy and gastrostomy

References

1. Maiman DJ, Barolat G, Larson SJ. Management of bilateral locked facets of the cervical spine. Neurosurgery 1986;18:542–547
2. Sonntag VK. Management of bilateral locked facets of the cervical spine. Neurosurgery 1981;8:150–152
3. Hadra BE. Wiring of the spinous process in injury and Pott's disease. Tran Am Orthop Assoc 1891;4:206
4. Aarabi B, Schweitzer K, Vaccaro AR. Subaxial injuries: distractive flexion injuries. In: Vaccaro AR, Anderson P, eds. Cervical Spine Trauma. Philadelphia: Rothman Institute; 2010:383–398
5. Cloward RB. Reduction of traumatic dislocation of the cervical spine with locked facets. Technical note. J Neurosurg 1973;38:527–531
6. Nakashima H, Yukawa Y, Ito K, Machino M, El Zahlawy H, Kato F. Posterior approach for cervical fracture-dislocations with traumatic disc herniation. Eur Spine J 2011;20:387–394
7. Allen BL Jr, Ferguson RL, Lehmann TR, O'Brien RP. A mechanistic classification of closed, indirect fractures and dislocations of the lower cervical spine. Spine 1982;7:1–27
8. Anderson PA, Moore TA, Davis KW, et al; Spinal Trauma Study Group. Cervical spine injury severity score. Assessment of reliability. J Bone Joint Surg Am 2007;89:1057–1065
9. Vaccaro AR, Hulbert RJ, Patel AA, et al; Spine Trauma Study Group. The subaxial cervical spine injury classification system: a novel approach to recognize the importance of morphology, neurology, and integrity of the disco-ligamentous complex. Spine 2007;32:2365–2374
10. Do Koh Y, Lim TH, Won You J, Eck J, An HS. A biomechanical comparison of modern anterior and posterior plate fixation of the cervical spine. Spine 2001;26:15–21
11. Darsaut TE, Ashforth R, Bhargava R, et al. A pilot study of magnetic resonance imaging-guided closed reduction of cervical spine fractures. Spine 2006;31:2085–2090
12. Harrington JF, Likavec MJ, Smith AS. Disc herniation in cervical fracture subluxation. Neurosurgery 1991;29:374–379

38 Subaxial Cervical Lateral Mass Screw Fixation

Joshua Bakhsheshian, Nader S. Dahdaleh, Richard G. Fessler, and Zachary A. Smith

Instrumentation and segmental fixation of the lateral masses is a widely accepted practice for fixation in the subaxial cervical spine (C3–C6). Following cervical lateral mass screw fixation, the fusion rate is high and carries a low risk of complications.[1] Modern polyaxial screw–rod constructs have evolved from lateral mass plating systems, and are more commonly used due to their versatility.[2] The angled-polyaxial constructs enable more rigid fixations while accommodating variations in cervical anatomy without compromising screw positioning.

Safe placement of lateral mass screws requires familiarity with the cervical anatomy. Multiple techniques have been described with different screw entry points and trajectory angles to prevent neurovascular injury.[3-7] The screw ideally travels lateral to the vertebral artery without violating the facet joint or neural injury. The length of the screw depends on the size of the lateral masses and should not be long enough to enter the foramen transversarium.

Patient Selection

Patients with subaxial cervical C3 to C6 lesions associated with instability are selected for lateral mass screw fixation based on careful evaluation of preoperative imaging. X-ray and computed tomography (CT) provide information on the type of fractures and dislocations involved. Further, CT demonstrates the size of the lateral masses and the position of the transverse foramen that encases the vertebral artery.

Indications

- Cervical instability due to trauma
- Reconstruction for degenerative and inflammatory diseases or neoplasms
- Cervical deformity or malformations
- Prevention of postlaminectomy kyphosis

Contraindications

- Metabolic bone disease
- Fracture or previous deformity of the lateral mass

Objective

- Obtain spinal stability by fixation and fusion while maintaining or improving neurologic function associated with the spinal pathology.

Advantages

- Can be utilized with spinous or laminar fractures
- Can be combined with decompression without compromising the fixation points
- Provides immediate rigid fixation

Disadvantages

- Lacks biomechanical stability of pedicle fixation
- Entails the risk of injury to the vertebral artery and neural structures (low risk)
- C7 lateral mass often has smaller anteroposterior dimension and may not accommodate instrumentation

Preoperative Imaging

- Anteroposterior and lateral X-rays
- CT
- Magnetic resonance imaging (MRI) may be useful in identifying ligamentous instability

Choice of Operative Approach

Roy-Camille et al[3] initially described the screw entry in the midpoint of the lateral mass with a 10-degree lateral trajectory. Magerl et al[4] described the screw entry 2 mm medial and caudal to the midpoint of the lateral mass with a 25-degree lateral and 40- to 60-degree cranial (parallel to facet joint) trajectory. When comparing both techniques, the cephalad projection provided by the Magerl technique decreased the risks of violating the facet joint.[8] This technique employs a screw entry 1 to 2 mm medial and superior to the midline, with a lateral 30-degree and a 40- to 60-degree cranial trajectory to avoid the above-mentioned complications (**Fig. 38.1**).[9] In general, safe screw placement can be achieved by maximal lateral angulation and sagittal angulation parallel to the facet joint. This chapter discusses the Magerl technique, focusing on C3–C6 lateral mass fixation.

Surgical Procedure

Positioning

In patients with cervical myelopathy, extra care should be taken to avoid neck motion during intubation. Ideally, fiberoptic intubation should be performed and the patient should be evaluated for any changes in neurologic status that may have occurred

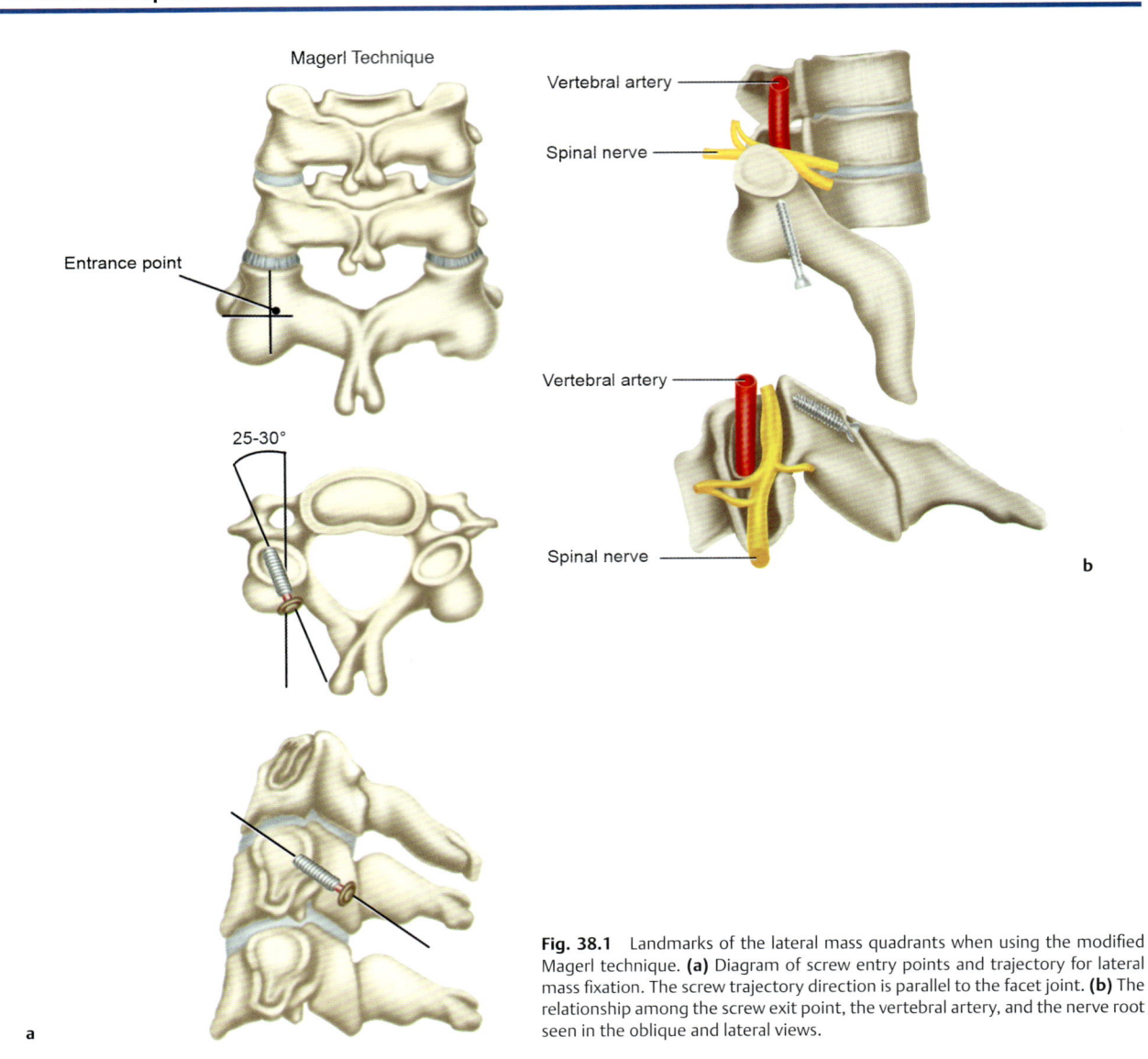

Fig. 38.1 Landmarks of the lateral mass quadrants when using the modified Magerl technique. **(a)** Diagram of screw entry points and trajectory for lateral mass fixation. The screw trajectory direction is parallel to the facet joint. **(b)** The relationship among the screw exit point, the vertebral artery, and the nerve root seen in the oblique and lateral views.

during intubation. General anesthesia appropriate for electrophysiological monitoring is used, and the patient is carefully placed in the prone position on chest rolls. Intraoperative neural monitoring (e.g., somatosensory evoked potentials, electromyogram, motor evoked potentials) is recommended to prevent intraoperative and perioperative neurologic deficits.[10,11] The neck is secured with a three-pin Mayfield headholder for immobilization during screw placement. A lateral fluoroscopy or X-ray may be utilized to ensure proper cervical spinal alignment and to help localize the pathology. The shoulders are taped down and the legs are flexed at the knees to enable maximal radiological visualization of the cervical spine. Bony prominences are padded, and then the patient is sterilely prepped in the standard fashion.

Incision

A midline incision is made over the levels to be stabilized. An electrocautery dissection is used to fully expose the facet joints and lateral borders of the lateral masses in a subperiosteal fashion. Dissecting more lateral than the lateral border of the lateral mass is often unnecessary. Bleeding from the venous plexus lateral to the lateral masses may occur and can be coagulated with electrocautery or an absorbable gelatin sponge. The facet joints adjacent to the level of fixation should be inspected for a possible ligamentous injury, which can be demonstrated on preoperative MRI. Great care should be taken not to disrupt the facet joints above and below the involved levels of fixation/stabilization to avoid late instability or fusion at those levels. The capsular ligaments and soft tissue from the involved facet can be removed with a small pituitary rongeur and by sweeping from medial to lateral with a curette.

Reduction

If reduction is needed and closed reduction was not successful, open reduction may be performed at this point. A curette or similar instrument may be wedged into the facet joint to facilitate reduction. If unsuccessful, a high-speed drill can be used to remove part of the superior articular process of the inferior vertebrae to facilitate realignment to the normal anatomic state. See Chapter 36 for more information on closed and open reduction.

Instrumentation

The center of the lateral mass can be located by defining the border between the lamina and the lateral mass. In many circumstances, a small up-going curette can be used to define the lamina–facet junction. The lateral mass can then be split into four quadrants, and the entry point is identified and marked. The technique focuses on projecting the screws to the upper lateral quadrant. The entry is 1 to 2 mm medial and superior to the midpoint (**Fig. 38.1**). A high-speed drill or awl is used to pierce the outer cortex of the bone at the entry point. This reduces the risk of the drill slipping over the lateral mass with screw placement, and provides entry through the superficial cortical bone.

After confirming that the joint capsule and soft tissue are removed from the involved facets, the joints can be decorticated with a high-speed drill with a small drill bit. Arthrodesis can be performed utilizing the patient's own bone from the laminectomy. In our clinical practice, we use a high-speed drill to partially drill into the superficial facet. This defines the borders of the lateral mass and also decorticates the facet margins for inter-facet fusion. Using a 4-0 Penfield, arthrodesis products can be placed into the superficial portion of the facet.

A high-speed electric drill can be used to create a path for the screws. The trajectory of the screws is 30 degrees laterally and 40 to 60 degrees cephalad (parallel to the facets) to avoid neurovascular injuries and unintended fixation of the superior facet of the next vertebra inferiorly. The lateral trajectory is best achieved from the contralateral side of the patient. One may lightly rest the drill on the spinous process (if present) for better control. If a self-tapping polyaxial screw is not available, the dorsal cortex can be tapped using a 3.5-mm cancellous tap.

Once the bone graft is in place and the facet is denuded, the lateral mass screws can be inserted with anatomic guidance (**Fig. 38.2**). The screws that are usually used have a 3.5-mm diameter and a length of 12 to 14 mm length for C3–C6. In specific circumstances (commonly traumatic fractures), 16-mm screws can be elected if the anatomy can accommodate these dimensions. Similarly, in certain patients, only a 12-mm screw can be used given the proximity of the vertebral artery. The final decision on length depends on the size of the lateral masses and the patient's specific anatomy, which can be assessed on prior CT imaging. The length should enable full penetration of the outer cortex. Lateral fluoroscopy can be used to assess the projection of the screws (**Fig. 38.3**). Although bicortical penetration is advocated for more unstable spines, these patients have a greater risk of nerve root injury without offering better purchase.[12,13]

Lateral mass screw can be placed in C7; however, the lateral mass is smaller and the pedicles are larger, so a pedicle screw may be more appropriate.[5,14] In circumstances that include cervicothoracic fixation, a C7 fixation point may be skipped to allow rod placement across the cervicothoracic junction.

If posterior decompression is indicated, it is our preference to mark, drill, and prepare the screw sites before performing a laminectomy. This protects the dura and spinal cord during the drilling process. After placing the screws, the appropriate-length rod is bent to conform to the lordosis of the cervical spine. Titanium rods 3 to 4 mm in diameter are most commonly used. The

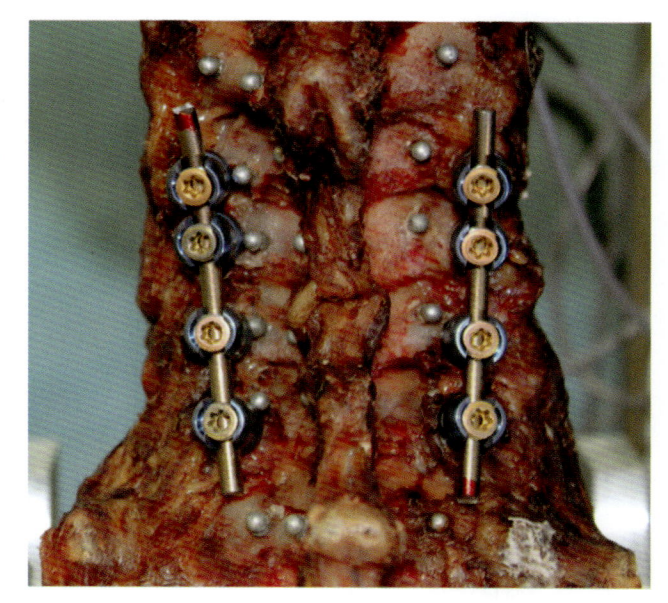

Fig. 38.2 Cadaveric model demonstrating posterior view of C3–C6 lateral mass screw–rod placement.

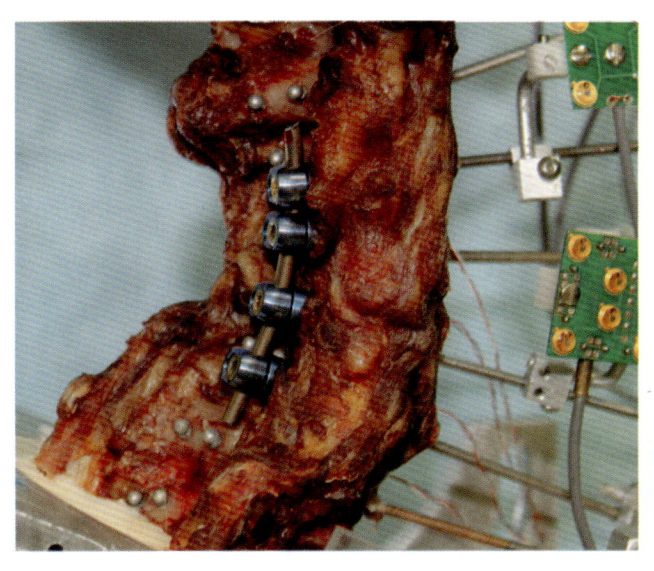

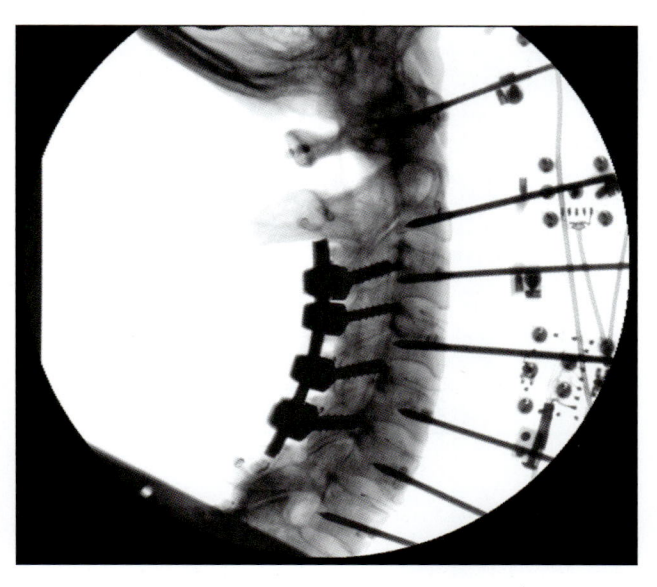

Fig. 38.3 C3–C6 lateral mass screw–rod placement demonstrated on (**a**) a cadaveric model and (**b**) a subsequent lateral fluoroscopic imaging.

use of cobalt chromium in spinal fusion-fixation instrumentation is relatively new, but may be preferred for deformity correction. Once the rods pass through the heads of all polyaxial screws, the rostral and caudal screws are secured with "set" screws and are tightened sequentially.

Closure

The wound is copiously irrigated with an antibiotic solution. Homeostasis is obtained with electrocautery, and a medium-sized Hemovac drain is placed below the fascia. The muscle and fascia are closed in their respective anatomic layers. The skin wound is reapproximated with staples, and adhesive dressing (Steri-Strips with Dermabond, Ethicon, Inc., Somerville, NJ) is applied.[15]

Postoperative Care

- The drain is typically removed 1 to 2 days after the surgery.
- No nonsteroidal anti-inflammatory drugs (NSAIDs) for 6 to 12 weeks.
- X-ray is performed the day after surgery to check the screw's positioning.
- The patient wears a rigid cervical collar for 2 to 3 months.
- Physiotherapy is recommended.

Potential Complications and Precautions

- Neurovascular injuries can be prevented with a proper drilling technique and screw size. Using intraoperative monitoring also decreases the risk of neural injury.[11]

Box 38.1 Key Operative Steps and Potential Problems

Step	Problems
Incision	• Dissecting muscular attachments superior to C2 • Disruption of facet joints above and below planned levels of fixation
Instrumentation	• Drill slipping over the lateral mass • Fixation of wrong cervical vertebrae • Violation of the facet joint • Vertebral artery injury • Nerve root injury • Screw placed too laterally (not enough bone laterally to hold it) • Violation of facet joint • Cerebrospinal fluid leak

- Loss of alignment due to hardware failure or screw pullout can occur if the screw is placed too laterally or if there is not enough bone lateral to the screw to hold it in place. Salvaging failed lateral mass screws can be accomplished with pedicle screw placements.

Conclusion

Lateral mass fixation is widely used for posterior cervical spinal stabilization, and is considered the standard of care in managing trauma, degenerative disease, and deformity. Lateral mass screw–rod fixation can be safely used for posterior cervical spinal stabilization. With extensive knowledge of the surrounding anatomy and understanding of techniques, there is minimal risk of injury to neurovascular elements. **Box 38.1** summarizes the key operative steps and the problems that can arise.

References

1. Coe JD, Vaccaro AR, Dailey AT, et al. Lateral mass screw fixation in the cervical spine: a systematic literature review. J Bone Joint Surg Am 2013; 95:2136–2143
2. Horgan MA, Kellogg JX, Chesnut RM. Posterior cervical arthrodesis and stabilization: an early report using a novel lateral mass screw and rod technique. Neurosurgery 1999;44:1267–1271, discussion 1271–1272
3. Roy-Camille R, Saillant G, Laville C, Benazet JP. Treatment of lower cervical spinal injuries—C3 to C7. Spine 1992;17(10, Suppl):S442–S446
4. Magerl F, Grob D, Seemann P. Stable dorsal fusion of the cervical spine (C2-Th1) using hook plates. In: Kehr P, Weidner A, eds. Cervical Spine I. New York: Springer; 1987:217–221
5. An HS, Gordin R, Renner K. Anatomic considerations for plate-screw fixation of the cervical spine. Spine 1991;16(10, Suppl):S548–S551
6. Anderson PA, Henley MB, Grady MS, Montesano PX, Winn HR. Posterior cervical arthrodesis with AO reconstruction plates and bone graft. Spine 1991;16(3, Suppl):S72–S79
7. Merola AA, Castro BA, Alongi PR, et al. Anatomic consideration for standard and modified techniques of cervical lateral mass screw placement. Spine J 2002;2:430–435
8. Heller JG, Carlson GD, Abitbol JJ, Garfin SR. Anatomic comparison of the Roy-Camille and Magerl techniques for screw placement in the lower cervical spine. Spine 1991;16(10, Suppl):S552–S557
9. Xu R, Ebraheim NA, Klausner T, Yeasting RA. Modified Magerl technique of lateral mass screw placement in the lower cervical spine: an anatomic study. J Spinal Disord 1998;11:237–240
10. Epstein NE. The need to add motor evoked potential monitoring to somatosensory and electromyographic monitoring in cervical spine surgery. Surg Neurol Int 2013;4(5, Suppl 5):S383–S391
11. Katonis P, Papadopoulos CA, Muffoletto A, Papagelopoulos PJ, Hadjipavlou AG. Factors associated with good outcome using lateral mass plate fixation. Orthopedics 2004;27:1080–1086
12. Heller JG, Estes BT, Zaouali M, Diop A. Biomechanical study of screws in the lateral masses: variables affecting pull-out resistance. J Bone Joint Surg Am 1996;78:1315–1321
13. Seybold EA, Baker JA, Criscitiello AA, Ordway NR, Park CK, Connolly PJ. Characteristics of unicortical and bicortical lateral mass screws in the cervical spine. Spine 1999;24:2397–2403
14. Ebraheim NA, Klausner T, Xu R, Yeasting RA. Safe lateral-mass screw lengths in the Roy-Camille and Magerl techniques. An anatomic study. Spine 1998;23:1739–1742
15. Hall LT, Bailes JE. Using Dermabond for wound closure in lumbar and cervical neurosurgical procedures. Neurosurgery 2005;56(1, Suppl):147–150, discussion 147–150

39 Subaxial Cervical Pedicle Screw Fixation

Alexander A. Theologis, Sang-Hun Lee, Justin K. Scheer, Shane Burch, and Christopher Pearson Ames

Cervical spine pedicle screws were first used in 1964 by Leconte et al to treat traumatic spondylolisthesis of the axis.[1] The use of these screws has since expanded to include stabilization of a variety of traumatic and atraumatic conditions of the axial and subaxial cervical spine because of their distinct clinical and biomechanical advantages compared with lateral mass screws, interspinous process wiring, posterior plate screws, and posterior hook plates.[2-6] They provide higher axial load to failure,[5] lower rate of loosening at the bone–screw interface,[4] and higher strength in fatigue[4] compared with lateral mass screws.

Cervical pedicle screws may be placed by free-hand techniques or image-assisted navigation. The accuracy of screw placement using a free-hand technique with or without fluoroscopy assistance is 12.5 to 93.3%.[7-11] This unpredictably is likely due to the extreme variability of the cervical pedicles' orientation and morphometry.[5,12,13] As image-assisted navigation systems enable a surgeon to visualize the anatomic variability in the cervical spine, they were initially promoted to increase the safety of cervical spine pedicle screw placement.[12,14-20] However, many of the original image-assisted navigation systems resulted in errors with registration and inaccurate screw placement because they relied on preoperative computed tomography (CT) scans and surface anatomy registration, which could not account for differences in spinal anatomy when the patient is in the supine position (preoperatively) or prone position (intraoperatively).[7,10,12,16] For example, compared with free-hand technique, Kast et al[7] found that image-guided navigation based on preoperative CT scans resulted in a higher rate of critical pedicle breaches (10% versus 5%) and lower overall accuracy rate (61% versus 77%).

The newest generation of image-assisted navigation, including the Iso-C³ᴰ system (Siremobil; Siemens, Erlangen, Germany) and the O-Arm and Stealth Navigation (Medtronic Inc., Louisville, CO), is based on intraoperative CT scans and three-dimensional (3D) image guidance.[17,18,20] As these systems enable immediate real-time image guidance, they have significantly increased the accuracy of cervical pedicle screw placement.[17,18,20] For example, Rajasekaran et al[18] placed 145 cervical pedicle screws in 33 patients assisted by the Iso-C³ᴰ system and found an 89.7% accuracy rate with no neurovascular injuries or critical breaches. Using O-arm imaging, Ishikawa et al[17] had an 88.9% accuracy rate for 108 cervical pedicle screws in 21 patients. They had no neurovascular injuries, and thus all the screws were considered "clinically safe." We have recently evaluated 21 patients with complex subaxial cervical and cervicothoracic spine pathology, including fixed cervicothoracic kyphosis and multilevel instability, necessitating rigid posterior-only or circumferential fixation, and found that 120 of 121 cervical pedicle screws were placed safely using the O-Arm and Stealth Navigation. This chapter presents the surgical techniques for free-hand and image-guided cervical pedicle screw placement.

Patient Selection

The aforementioned biomechanical advantages of cervical pedicle screws make them useful for patients requiring cervical fixation for reduction of translational deformities, and for fixed cervicothoracic kyphosis and multilevel cervical instability, which necessitate rigid posterior-only or circumferential fixation.[6,21] These screws should also be considered for patients with fragile or disrupted lateral masses or lamina,[2,3] which may been encountered in the settings of primary and metastatic tumors, spondylolysis, infectious spondylitis, facet fracture-dislocations, and spondyloarthropathy.[2,22-24]

Indications and Contraindications

Cervical pedicle screws are particularly valuable and advantageous in cervical deformity correction (translational deformities, cervical kyphosis, cervical sagittal malalignment), cervical reconstruction following tumor mass resections, and when lateral masses or lamina are disrupted, which may be encountered in the trauma setting. Caution should be taken when placing screws in pedicles with widths less than 3.5 mm.

Advantages and Disadvantages

Although the free-hand technique is relatively inexpensive to perform, it is associated with an extremely steep learning curve and the potential for significant neurovascular injury (i.e., nerve root, spinal cord, or vertebral artery injuries). Image-guided placement theoretically enables a more precise screw trajectory and fewer complications, as it allows one to assess the patient's anatomy in real time intraoperatively. However, the direct cost of obtaining image-guided technology is not insignificant, and there is also a steep learning curve associated with cervical pedicle screw insertion using image-guided technology.

Choice of Operative Approach

The posterior approach is the appropriate one for this technique.

Preoperative Testing

Safe and accurate cervical pedicle screw placement in the subaxial spine is challenging and is dependent on thorough preoperative surgical planning, a fundamental understanding of anatomic landmarks, and a firm working knowledge of navigation principles if using navigation. Preoperatively, a CT scan of the cervical spine may be obtained to evaluate the size and morphology of each subaxial cervical pedicle and transverse foramen (**Fig. 39.1**).

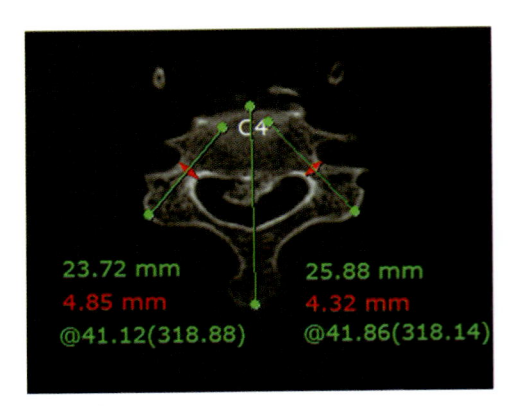

Fig. 39.1 Preoperative measurement of the pedicle diameter, medial convergence angle, and length of the screw on an axial computed tomography (CT) image.

Particular attention should be paid to the pedicle sizes of C3, C4, and C5, as the highest percentage of malpositioned cervical pedicle screws with free-hand and navigated techniques is reported to occur at these levels.[9,21] Yoshimoto et al[9] noted that of 134 cervical pedicle screws, all five complete pedicle perforations occurred at either C4 or C5. Of the 45 pedicle perforations observed by Abumi et al,[21] the highest perforation rate (10.6%) was at C4. Using image-assisted navigation, Richter et al[14] noted their only pedicle perforation (> 1 mm) occurred at C5.

Although C3 to C5 is the highest risk zone for inaccurate pedicle screw placement, the entire subaxial cervical spine is at risk during cervical pedicle screw placement and should be evaluated carefully. Pedicles with abnormal morphology and widths less than 3.5 mm should not be instrumented with cervical pedicle screws (**Fig. 39.2**). The last cervical vertebrae (C7) should also be assessed, as there is variability in the position of the vertebral artery at this level.[25] Kajimoto et al[25] demonstrated that 7.5% of vertebral arteries entered the C7 transverse foramen in a cadaveric model. Therefore, one may consider obtaining a CT angiogram preoperatively to determine the location of the vertebral artery relative to the C7 foramen, as neurovascular injury at C7 from a misplaced cervical pedicle screw is a true risk. Although a preoperative CT scan will help the surgeon determine which levels to instrument with cervical pedicle screws, it is not required if the plan is to use image-assisted navigation, because cervical pedicle anatomy may be characterized on intraoperative navigation images.

Surgical Procedures

The patient is brought to the operating room where intubation under general anesthesia is performed. Preoperative antibiotics are administered and a Mayfield frame is placed. The patient is placed in the prone position, the arms are tucked and well padded, and the shoulders are gently retracted with tape. A standard posterior-based midline incision is made over the posterior cervical spine extending to the most distal level of anticipated instrumentation. Standard subperiosteal dissection over the lateral masses is performed. If cervical deformity correction is a goal of the operation, cervical osteotomies (i.e., Smith-Petersen osteotomies) are subsequently performed and the cervical spine is realigned into the position of interest.

Free-Hand Technique[26,27]

To find the correct trajectory, the target of the virtual pedicle entrance point is identified, which is on the perpendicular line of the pedicle's axis (**Fig. 39.3a**). For the first step, a key slot–shaped entry is created on the medial half of the lateral mass with a 3-mm matchstick bur. The shape of entry is a rectangle in the coronal plane (**Fig. 39.3b**) and a triangle on the axial plane (**Fig. 39.3c**). The apex of the triangle is the virtual pedicle inlet, and the triangle's oblique side is the same as the pedicle's axis (**Fig. 39.3a,c**). In the sagittal plane, the depth of entry should be equivalent to two-thirds the thickness of the lateral mass (**Fig. 39.3d**). The detailed width, depth, and angle of the slot are adjusted according to the individual anatomy of each cervical vertebra on the preoperative CT images. When one first starts to use this technique, each screw's entry point and trajectory in the sagittal plane may be confirmed with a lateral fluoroscopic guide. After one becomes experienced in and comfortable with the technique, cervical pedicle screw placement is possible with a free-hand technique.

For the next step, the pedicle is cannulated as close to the medial wall as possible by gentle manual pressure using a 15-degree curved awl. After cannulating ~ 2 cm deep, pedicle wall integrity is confirmed using a ball-tip probe. If perforation is detected within the pedicle, the trajectory is changed or the segment is skipped for screw placement. Once a safe trajectory is determined, the pedicle is drilled and tapped, and then a screw is placed.

A screw with a head that is located on the lateral margin of lateral mass and a tip that is placed medial to the uncovertebral joint on plain radiographs are considered to be in the safest position. A tip positioned lateral to the uncovertebral joint area or a head located out of the lateral mass increases the risk of perforation (**Fig. 39.4**). This technique has been used safely and effectively to reconstruct an unstable subaxial cervical spine from trauma, perform a radical excision of tumor, and perform a one-stage correction of flexible or semi-rigid cervical kyphosis (**Fig. 39.5**).

Image-Guided Technique

Imaging and Navigation

Placing a passive reference array with reflective spheres is the first step of the navigation process, which is often the most important step. The reference array is placed on the spinous pro-

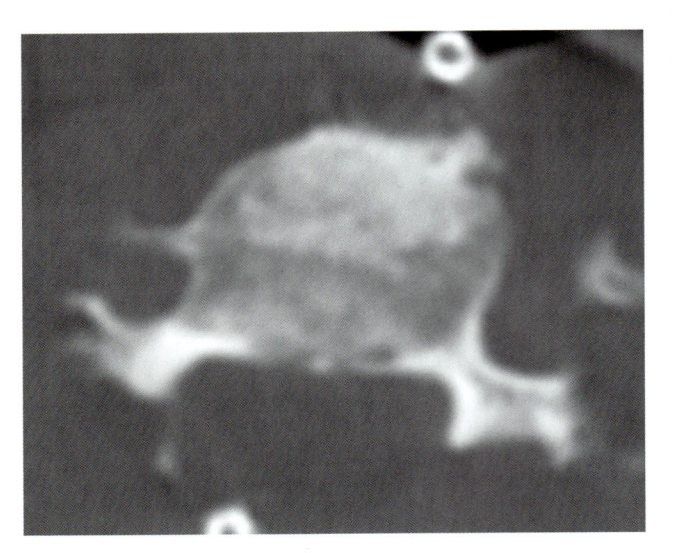

Fig. 39.2 Representative intraoperative axial O-Arm image of C4. The C4 pedicles were not instrumented, given their relatively small width and height (~ 3.5 cm).

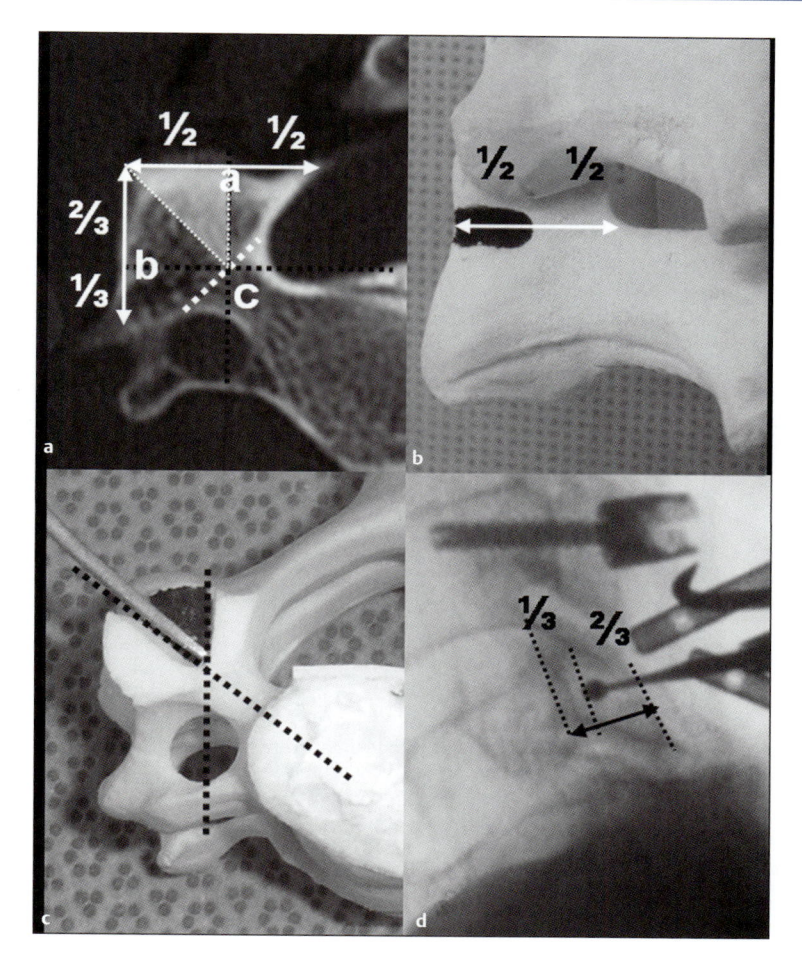

Fig. 39.3 **(a,b)** The key slot–shaped entry is created on the medial half of the lateral mass with a 3-mm cutting bur. The shape of entry is a rectangle in the coronal plane and a right-angled triangle in the axial plane with a being the width of the lateral mass, b being the anteroposterior width of the lateral mass. The apex of triangle is the virtual entry to the pedicle **(c)** and the oblique side is in the trajectory of the pedicle axis **(c)**. **(d)** Under fluoroscopic visualization, the bur is advanced to a depth that is two thirds of the lateral mass thickness in the sagittal plane.

cess of the vertebra one or two levels caudal to the most distal cervical pedicle screw to be placed by navigation. For example, if the last pedicle screw to be navigated is C7, the reference array may be placed on T2. The reference array should be firmly attached to the spinous process and be placed in a location that minimizes the risk that it will be moved by the surgeons and assistants, as movement of the reference array results in registration and navigation errors. Ideally, the optical camera (Stealth, Medtronic) is placed at the foot of the operating table at which the reference array is aimed. This arrangement provides an uninterrupted path between the optical camera and the reference array, as the working field is more cranial to each. An intraoperative 3D fluoroscopic scan is then obtained using the O-Arm with registration occurring automatically to identify and confirm each cervical level. The reference array and navigated instruments are then detected by the optical camera. The location of each instrument is subsequently projected onto a reconstruction of the spine based on the intraoperative imaging. On the projected image, each pedicle's morphology and size are evaluated, and the choice of which levels to instrument is made or confirmed. Again, caution should be taken in placing screws in pedicles with widths less than 3.5 mm.

If the planned procedure involves navigation of cervical pedicle screws and thoracic and lumbar pedicle screws, imaging and navigation should not be performed on a reference array placed in one location. For example, if a C2 to T10 posterior spinal fusion and instrumentation are to be performed, the cervical pedicle

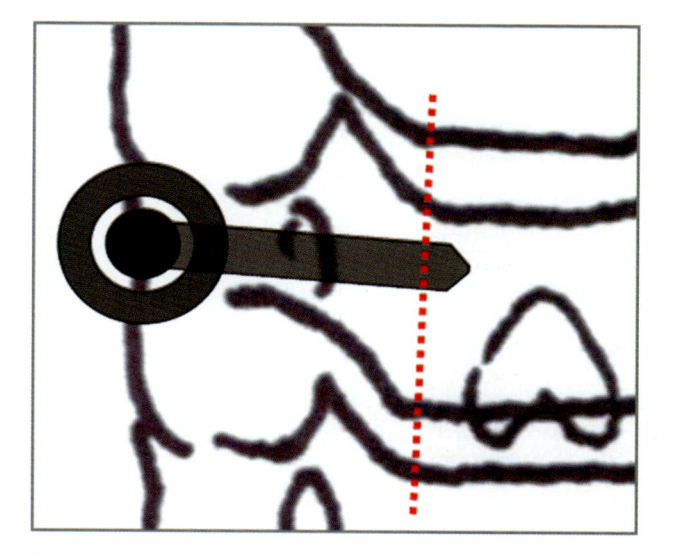

Fig. 39.4 A schematic drawing of an ideal cervical pedicle screw trajectory on an anteroposterior radiograph. A screw with a head that is located on the lateral margin of the lateral mass and a screw tip that is located medial to the uncovertebral joint *(dotted red line)* on plain radiographs is considered to be in a safe position. A screw tip positioned lateral to the uncovertebral joint area or a head located out of the lateral mass is expected to increase the risk of pedicle perforation.

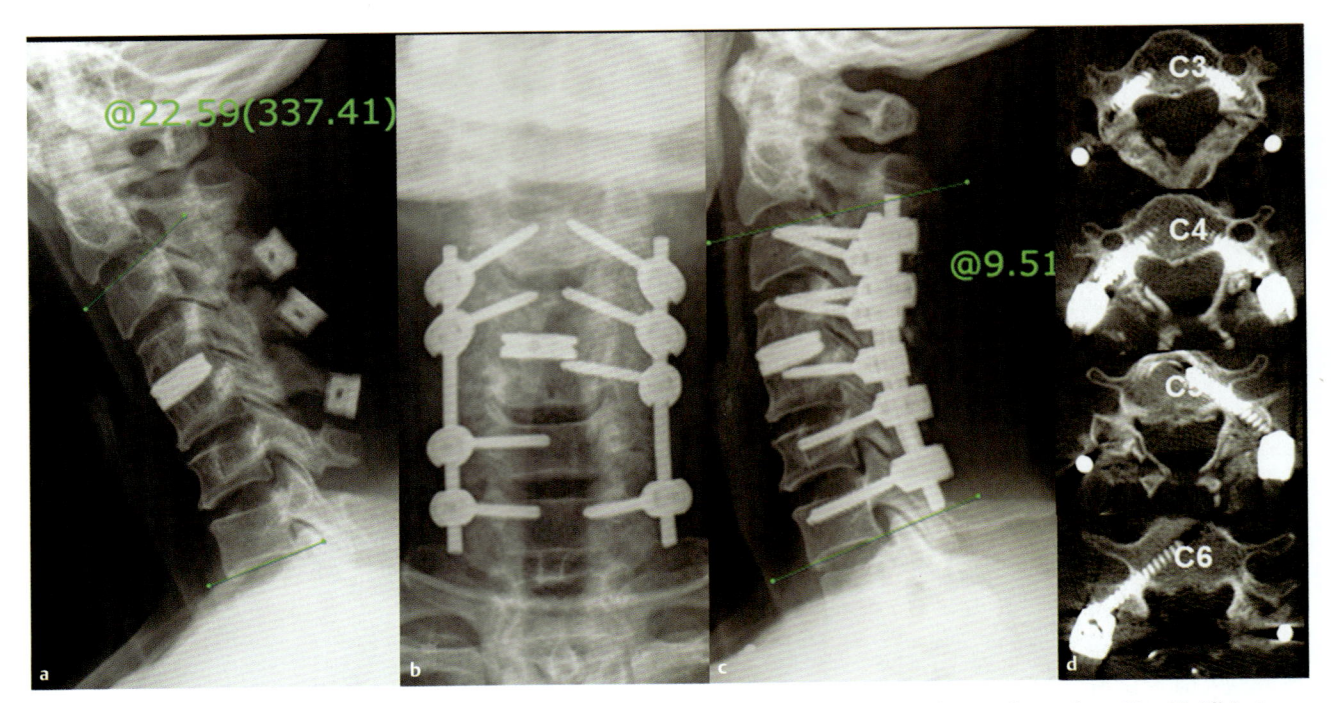

Fig. 39.5 (a) A preoperative cervical spine lateral radiograph of a 49-year-old woman with myelopathy and semi-rigid postlaminoplasty kyphosis. (b,c) Posterior decompression with one-stage correction of kyphosis was performed with subaxial pedicle screw fixation from C3 to C7. (d) Postoperative axial CT images demonstrate that all cervical pedicle screws are positioned accurately and safely without pedicle perforation.

screws should ideally be placed using imaging and navigation tools based on a reference array located close to the cervical spine (i.e., on the spinous process of T2), and the thoracic screws should be placed using imaging and navigation tools based on a reference array located in the lower thoracic spine (i.e., on the spinous process of T12). This may be accomplished by placing the reference array first on T2, obtaining an O-Arm scan, and then navigating the cervical pedicle screws. The reference array is then removed from T2 and secured on the spinous process of T12. A second O-Arm scan is obtained, and the thoracic screws are navigated. This is performed for two reasons. First, if the reference array is kept on T2 and thoracic pedicle screws are attempted to be inserted, the working field will be in between the reference array and optical cameras, which jeopardizes the accuracy of the navigated instruments. Second, if all screws are attempted to be placed based on a reference array that is initially placed on T12, the accuracy of the navigated cervical pedicle screws is at risk, as errors with registration increase as the distance from the reference array increases.

Pedicle Screw Placement

Each chosen cervical pedicle is cannulated using a navigated drill guide with 2.7-mm drill, followed by a 3.5-mm tap, and then an appropriate-sized screw. The trajectory of each of these steps is visualized on the axial and sagittal images on the Stealth Station (**Fig. 39.6**). Each pedicle is manually probed following cannulation and tapping of the pedicle. Of note, loss of registration may occur as one moves away from the passive frame. The rigidity of the cervical spine is critical to assess during the procedure. The more mobile the segments in the cervical spine, the less distance one is safely able to navigate away from the reference frame. It is important to consider cannulating the pedicle with a drill without downward and inward pressure to reduce the deformation of the spine in relation to the reference array to reduce error.

Therefore, with a reference array placed at T2, accuracy of C3 screws may be affected. Errors in registration may also be compounded by muscle retraction to achieve the lateral to medial pedicle trajectories and displacement of adjacent segments during pedicle screw placement. To evaluate pedicle screw location, a second intraoperative 3D CT scan may be obtained with the O-Arm after all screws are placed. On the basis of this second intraoperative O-Arm scan, the screws may be repositioned based on the surgeon's evaluation of their position or length within the pedicle.

Postoperative Care

Postoperatively, patients are immobilized with a hard collar. No unique postoperative care is required. However, postoperative signs and symptoms of a vertebral artery injury, a new radiculopathy, nerve root palsy, or spinal cord injury demand immediate attention. Symptoms suggestive of a vertebral artery injury include headache, difficulty speaking or swallowing, imbalance, visual loss, cranial nerve palsies, paraplegia, and Horner's syndrome. Angiogram is the study of choice to evaluate for a suspected vertebral artery injury, as there may be significant artifact with magnetic resonance angiography (MRA). Symptoms may develop acutely or several days after the operation due to a vertebral artery thrombosis.[28] For example, 3 days after undergoing bilateral pedicle screw placement at C4 and C5 using a free-hand technique, a patient developed a left facial nerve palsy and left hemiplegia (3/5 strength).[28] Complete perforation of the left C4 transverse foramen was detected by a CT scan, and a vertebral artery thrombus was detected by an angiogram. A CT scan is sufficient to evaluate screw position in patients with new radiculopathies or nerve root palsies. In the asymptomatic patient, routine postoperative CT scans may be ordered to assess pedicle screw accuracy if a second intraoperative O-Arm scan is not obtained to evaluate the final screw position. However, even

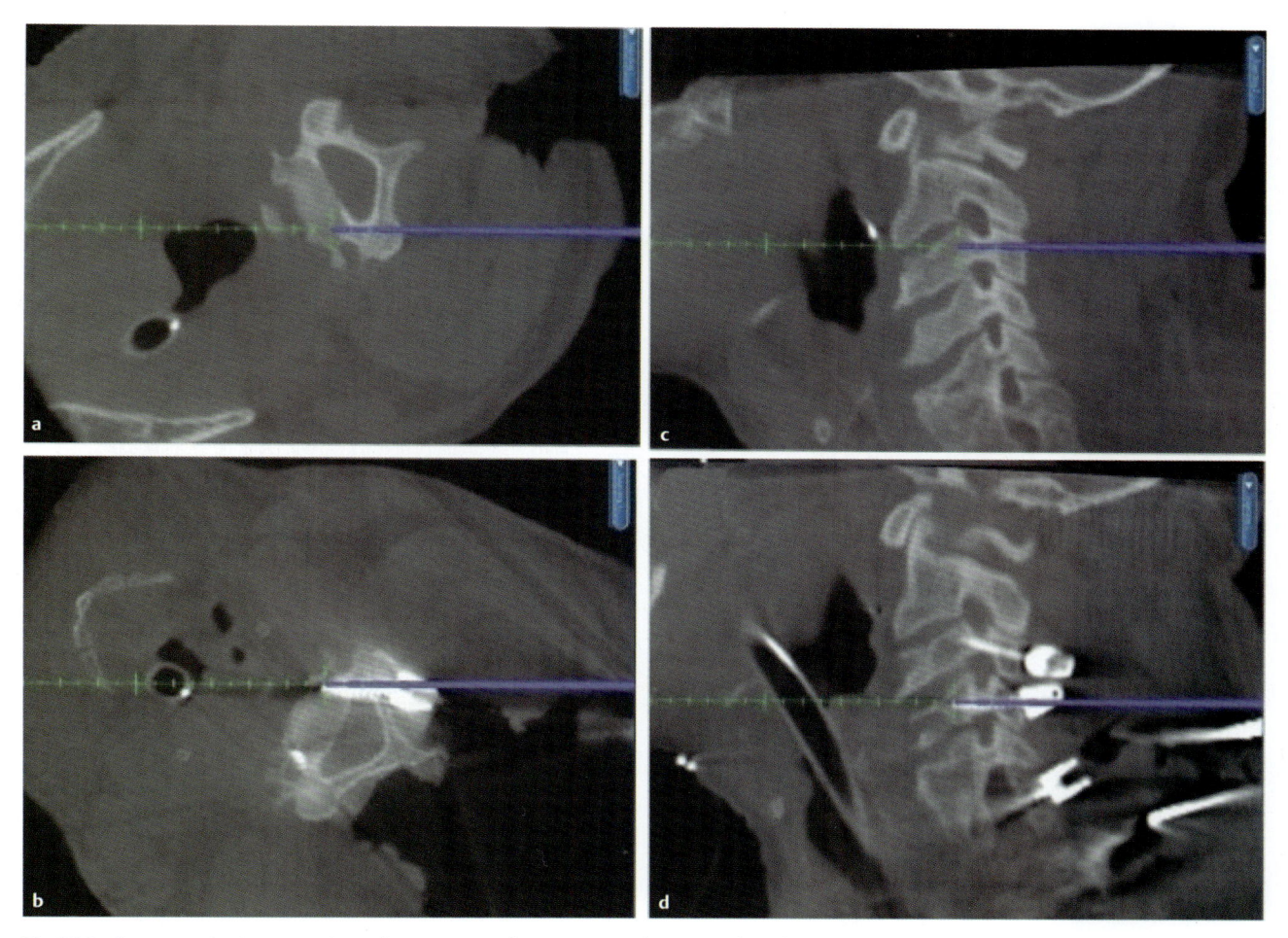

Fig. 39.6 Representative intraoperative real-time images of O-Arm acquired images and Stealth Navigation of cervical pedicle trajectory **(a,c)** and pedicle screw placement **(b,d)** in C3 and C4.

without a second intraoperative O-Arm scan, a "screening" postoperative CT scan after posterior cervical spine fusion in the asymptomatic patient is not required given concerns of radiation to the patient and costs.

Potential Complications and Precautions

The most dreaded complications associated with cervical pedicle screw placement are injuries to the vertebral artery, nerve root, or spinal cord. They are realistic risks associated with both the freehand and image-assisted techniques. Abumi et al[23] were the first to report on the accuracy and safety of subaxial cervical pedicle screw placement in clinical practice using their unique technique. Of 669 cervical pedicle screws, they noted 6.7% cortical penetrations, two of which caused a radiculopathy and one resulted in a vertebral artery injury without neurologic sequelae.[21] In a series of 100 patients treated with 419 cervical pedicles screws, Yukawa et al[8] reported an overall 14.3% breach rate and of those, 72% breached laterally with two intra-operative complications which were a vertebral artery injury and a transient radiculopathy. Avoiding a neurovascular injury is dependent on understanding the limitations of each technique and the steps at which errors may occur while establishing screw trajectories. For free-hand technique, a solid understanding of posterior cervical surface anatomy and radiographic criteria for a "safe" screw is paramount. Understanding how registration errors occur and how to avoid them when using image-guided technologies is key. Additionally, sound surgical technique in pedicle screw placement (i.e., palpating intact walls of the pedicle) remains a critical pillar in ensuring safe cervical pedicle screw placement for both techniques.

Conclusion

Placing pedicle screws in the subaxial cervical spine is technically challenging using free-hand and image-assisted navigation techniques. Surgeons attempting to place cervical pedicle screws with or without navigation must be well versed in anatomic landmarks of the cervical spine, and those using navigation technologies also need to be well versed in intraoperative navigation principles. Inaccuracy of the navigation systems can occur due to the hypermobility of the cervical spine. Therefore, loss of registration may occur as one moves further away from the passive frame. This is compounded by muscle retraction to achieve the lateral to medial cervical pedicle trajectories, which further compounds the displacement of adjacent segments and causes errors in registration. Although navigation systems appear accurate, fundamental knowledge of navigation principles is needed to perform this technique adequately and safely. **Box 39.1** lists the key operative steps and suggestions for each step.

Box 39.1 Key Operative Steps in the Placement of Cervical Pedicle Screws in the Subaxial Cervical Spine

Step	Tips and Tricks
Deformity correction	• Perform cervical osteotomies and realign the spine before proceeding with navigation imaging to minimize registration errors.
Reference array	• Place one or two levels caudal to the last instrumented level. • Firmly secure the frame to a spinous process, as movement of the reference frame will result in registration and navigation errors. • Aim at the optical camera (Stealth) situated at the foot of the operating table.
Imaging	• Assess the size and morphology of each subaxial cervical pedicle. • Subaxial cervical pedicles with widths < 3 cm are at high risk for breach and should not be instrumented.
Pedicle screw placement	• Loss of registration occurs as one moves away from the passive frame. • Muscle retraction to achieve the lateral to medial pedicle trajectories and subsequent displacement of adjacent segments may cause errors in registration. • To reduce error, consider cannulating the pedicle with a drill without downward and inward pressure to reduce the deformation of the spine in relation to the reference array.
Procedures involving the cervical and thoracic or lumbar spine	• Navigate/instrument cervical pedicle screws first, with the reference frame close to the cervical spine (i.e., T2 spinous process). • Move the reference array one or two levels caudal to the last thoracic/lumbar instrumented level. • Then obtain an O-Arm scan of the thoracic and lumbar levels and navigate or instrument the thoracic or lumbar screws.

References

1. Xu R, Ebraheim NA, Skie M. Pedicle screw fixation in the cervical spine. Am J Orthop 2008;37:403–408, discussion 408
2. Abumi K, Ito M, Sudo H. Reconstruction of the subaxial cervical spine using pedicle screw instrumentation. Spine 2012;37:E349–E356
3. Abumi K, Kaneda K, Shono Y, Fujiya M. One-stage posterior decompression and reconstruction of the cervical spine by using pedicle screw fixation systems. J Neurosurg 1999;90(1, Suppl):19–26
4. Johnston TL, Karaikovic EE, Lautenschlager EP, Marcu D. Cervical pedicle screws vs. lateral mass screws: uniplanar fatigue analysis and residual pullout strengths. Spine J 2006;6:667–672
5. Jones EL, Heller JG, Silcox DH, Hutton WC. Cervical pedicle screws versus lateral mass screws. Anatomic feasibility and biomechanical comparison. Spine 1997;22:977–982
6. Kotani Y, Cunningham BW, Abumi K, McAfee PC. Biomechanical analysis of cervical stabilization systems. An assessment of transpedicular screw fixation in the cervical spine. Spine 1994;19:2529–2539
7. Kast E, Mohr K, Richter HP, Börm W. Complications of transpedicular screw fixation in the cervical spine. Eur Spine J 2006;15:327–334
8. Yukawa Y, Kato F, Yoshihara H, Yanase M, Ito K. Cervical pedicle screw fixation in 100 cases of unstable cervical injuries: pedicle axis views obtained using fluoroscopy. J Neurosurg Spine 2006;5:488–493
9. Yoshimoto H, Sato S, Hyakumachi T, Yanagibashi Y, Masuda T. Spinal reconstruction using a cervical pedicle screw system. Clin Orthop Relat Res 2005;431:111–119
10. Ludwig SC, Kowalski JM, Edwards CC II, Heller JG. Cervical pedicle screws: comparative accuracy of two insertion techniques. Spine 2000;25:2675–2681
11. Abumi K, Shono Y, Kotani Y, Kaneda K. Indirect posterior reduction and fusion of the traumatic herniated disc by using a cervical pedicle screw system. J Neurosurg 2000;92(1, Suppl):30–37
12. Ludwig SC, Kramer DL, Balderston RA, Vaccaro AR, Foley KF, Albert TJ. Placement of pedicle screws in the human cadaveric cervical spine: comparative accuracy of three techniques. Spine 2000;25:1655–1667
13. Panjabi MM, Duranceau J, Goel V, Oxland T, Takata K. Cervical human vertebrae. Quantitative three-dimensional anatomy of the middle and lower regions. Spine 1991;16:861–869
14. Richter M, Cakir B, Schmidt R. Cervical pedicle screws: conventional versus computer-assisted placement of cannulated screws. Spine 2005;30:2280–2287
15. Takahashi J, Shono Y, Nakamura I, et al. Computer-assisted screw insertion for cervical disorders in rheumatoid arthritis. Eur Spine J 2007;16:485–494
16. Kotani Y, Abumi K, Ito M, Minami A. Improved accuracy of computer-assisted cervical pedicle screw insertion. J Neurosurg 2003;99(3, Suppl):257–263
17. Ishikawa Y, Kanemura T, Yoshida G, et al. Intraoperative, full-rotation, three-dimensional image (O-arm)-based navigation system for cervical pedicle screw insertion. J Neurosurg Spine 2011;15:472–478
18. Rajasekaran S, Kanna PR, Shetty TA. Intra-operative computer navigation guided cervical pedicle screw insertion in thirty-three complex cervical spine deformities. J Craniovertebr Junction Spine 2010;1:38–43
19. Ishikawa Y, Kanemura T, Yoshida G, Ito Z, Muramoto A, Ohno S. Clinical accuracy of three-dimensional fluoroscopy-based computer-assisted cervical pedicle screw placement: a retrospective comparative study of conventional versus computer-assisted cervical pedicle screw placement. J Neurosurg Spine 2010;13:606–611
20. Ito Y, Sugimoto Y, Tomioka M, Hasegawa Y, Nakago K, Yagata Y. Clinical accuracy of 3D fluoroscopy-assisted cervical pedicle screw insertion. J Neurosurg Spine 2008;9:450–453
21. Abumi K, Shono Y, Ito M, Taneichi H, Kotani Y, Kaneda K. Complications of pedicle screw fixation in reconstructive surgery of the cervical spine. Spine 2000;25:962–969
22. Abumi K, Ito M, Kaneda K. Surgical treatment of cervical destructive spondyloarthropathy (DSA). Spine 2000;25:2899–2905
23. Abumi K, Itoh H, Taneichi H, Kaneda K. Transpedicular screw fixation for traumatic lesions of the middle and lower cervical spine: description of the techniques and preliminary report. J Spinal Disord 1994;7:19–28
24. Abumi K, Kaneda K. Pedicle screw fixation for nontraumatic lesions of the cervical spine. Spine 1997;22:1853–1863
25. Kajimoto B, Addeo R, Campos D. Anatomical study of the vertebral artery path in human lower cervical spine. Acta Ortop Bras. 2007;15:84–86
26. Lee SH, Kim KT, Abumi K, Suk KS, Lee JH, Park KJ. Cervical pedicle screw placement using the "key slot technique": the feasibility and learning curve. J Spinal Disord Tech 2012;25:415–421
27. Lee SH, Kim KT, Suk KS, et al. Assessment of pedicle perforation by the cervical pedicle screw placement using plain radiographs: a comparison with computed tomography. Spine 2012;37:280–285
28. Onishi E, Sekimoto Y, Fukumitsu R, Yamagata S, Matsushita M. Cerebral infarction due to an embolism after cervical pedicle screw fixation. Spine 2010;35:E63–E66

40 C7 Pedicle Subtraction Osteotomy

Justin K. Scheer, Vedat Deviren, and Christopher Pearson Ames

Fixed sagittal malalignment at the cervicothoracic junction (CTJ) is very debilitating, resulting in severe pain, possible neurologic compromise, and loss of horizontal gaze.[1,2] Surgical correction of cervical deformity is technically demanding and poses potential high risks to the patient.[3-7] In general, the Smith-Petersen osteotomy with controlled fracture at C7 has been the standard to restore sagittal balance and horizontal gaze at the cervicothoracic junction, and has mostly been reported for cases of ankylosing spondylitis in which these controlled fractures are easier to accomplish compared with normal bone.[3-6,8-19] There are a few reports describing the pedicle subtraction osteotomy (PSO) at the cervicothoracic junction to correct severe flexion deformities,[20-24] which includes a wedge osteotomy of the vertebral body. Reported C7 PSO cases have been successful at correcting the deformity with beneficial outcomes, just as the lumbar PSO has been successful at correcting flexion deformities of the lumbar spine with positive clinical outcomes.[5,20,25-35] In addition, the cervicothoracic junction PSO may offer a more controlled closure,[21] greater biomechanical stability when compared with the Smith-Petersen osteotomy,[36] and no anterior open-wedge defect. This chapter discusses the C7 PSO technique.

Patient Selection

Patients with fixed cervicothoracic kyphosis requiring large sagittal correction who have good bone quality and few comorbidities are appropriate for this technique.

Indications and Contraindications

The indications include fixed sagittal malalignment of the cervical spine (mid- to low subaxial cervical spine) affecting horizontal gaze, persistent pain related to cervical sagittal imbalance despite conservative treatment, and high pelvic tilt causing low back pain driven by the cervical deformity following the failure of conservative management. Generally, an osteotomy is indicated when the deformity is irreducible (possibly following a trial of traction) and sufficient to result in severe pain and functional or neurologic impairment that cannot be relieved with a surgical decompression or stabilization procedure alone. This procedure is contraindicated in the presence of significant osteoporosis or debilitating comorbidities.

Advantages and Disadvantages

The CTJ PSO may be used to treat patients with fixed cervicothoracic kyphosis[20] because of the absence of the vertebral artery at this level. Once closed, there is bone contact in three columns, and the spinal canal is effectively shortened. Thus, the PSO procedure can provide excellent sagittal correction while simultaneously forming a stable construct and minimizing neural compression.

The PSO at the cervicothoracic junction has two key benefits compared with the traditional Smith-Petersen osteotomy. First, the PSO results in greater biomechanical stability (producing a mechanically stiffer result) than the Smith-Petersen osteotomy.[37,38] The Smith-Petersen osteotomy generally results in disk disruption or, in cases of ankylosing spondylitis, osteoclasis through a fused disk space or the anterior cortex of the vertebral body, causing a significant anterior gap in which the anterior longitudinal ligament is completely torn or the autofused anterior bridging osteophyte has been fractured. The PSO leaves the anterior longitudinal ligament intact. In addition, the PSO has a wedge component that cleaves the vertebral body, creating a larger bone-on-bone load-bearing interface even when compared with a Smith-Petersen osteotomy that is fully closed posteriorly. This greater bone-on-bone contact significantly increases stiffness, especially in compression, and may provide better fusion rates in patients who do not have ankylosing spondylitis, as the PSO provides a substantial load-bearing surface area in the uniting of the anterior, middle, and posterior columns upon closure.[37,38] No secondary anterior grafting is required. Second, the PSO results in a more controlled closure than the Smith-Petersen osteotomy because no sudden osteoclastic fracture is necessary.

Potential disadvantages are that this procedure is very complex, and it requires significant experience. Furthermore, this procedure results in a large osteotomy and increased blood loss compared with other cervical osteotomies.[20] The potential for neurologic compromise exists, as there is significant motion of a destabilized spine upon closure as well as identifying and mobilizing nerve roots.

Choice of Operative Approach

The posterior approach is the appropriate one for this technique.

Preoperative Testing

The deformity should be evaluated by anterior/posterior and lateral cervical radiographs along with dynamic lateral flexion/extension views. The deformity is then accurately measured (i.e., sagittal angle determination) and any other abnormalities noted (e.g., subluxation and pseudarthrosis).[39-41] It is important to obtain full-length posteroanterior and lateral 36-inch scoliosis radiographs to examine the overall sagittal and coronal alignment in these patients.[40-42] We assess cervical, thoracic, and lumbar sagittal alignment individually and globally, and define the effect of regional malalignment on cervical alignment and determine if it is a primary, secondary, or compensatory cervical deformity. The degree of required correction depends on the angle of the cervical deformity (the chin-brow to vertical angle), the C2 plumb line, and the desired final lordosis.[8,15,18,20,41] The goal of treatment is to obtain alignment, horizontal gaze, and cord decompression, and to normalize cord tension. Dynamic (i.e., flexion/extension) radiographs permit an assessment of the overall flexibility of the cervical spine, which is paramount when designing a treatment strategy. Computed tomography (CT) scans of the cervical spine are also useful in determining the presence of fusion or ankylosis of the facet joints and disks and in assessing fixation points such as C2 and the upper thoracic pedicles.

All patients should be evaluated with preoperative magnetic resonance imaging (MRI) or CT myelography. These image modalities help evaluate the compressive pathology. If significant ventral compressive pathology (disk, osteophyte) is present, a ventral decompressive procedure may first be performed before the correction of the deformity. In addition, patients should also have a CT angiography to determine the location of the vertebral artery and to verify that it enters at C6. This determination contributes to the safety of the procedure, because if the vertebral artery entered at C7, the procedure becomes exceedingly more complex and may have to be aborted in some cases.

Surgical Procedure

The patient is placed in the prone position in a halo ring, and transcranial motor evoked potential (TC-MEP), somatosensory evoked potential (SSEP), as well as electromyography (EMG) neuromonitoring are instituted. This setup is used to enable the correction to be adjusted if the monitoring system alerts the surgeon to the compression of the cervical roots, the buckling of the dura, or some other untoward event. A standard posterior surgical approach is made to the cervical spine creating an incision from C2 to T3/T5, depending on the location of the kyphotic apex and after the area had been shaved, prepped, and draped. The incision is taken sharply through the skin and down to the fascia. The paraspinous muscles are dissected in a subperiosteal fashion, exposing the spinous processes, laminar facets, and lateral processes of the cervical spine and transverse processes in the thoracic spine. After exposure, the spine is instrumented accordingly (C2 bicortical pedicle screws, cervical lateral mass screws, and thoracic pedicle screws). It is preferable to extend the fixation to C2 to obtain bicortical screw placement for a stronger fixation point than at the lateral masses of the inferior vertebrae. Furthermore, it is preferable to have the caudal extent of the fusion terminate at either T3 or T5, depending on the extent of thoracic kyphosis, to ensure the apex is within the fusion. Again, despite the fact that this is a cervical procedure, standing preoperative 36-inch radiographs are critical to analyze regional and global alignment patterns prior to the procedure. Cobalt-chrome rods are preferred to maintain alignment.

Following instrumentation, the osteotomies are performed (**Fig. 40.1**). Some patients may require laminectomies or resection of scar tissue from areas of prior surgery to prevent kinking of the dura on closure. Next, the Smith-Petersen osteotomy begins by performing facet release and removal of the facets of C6-C7 as well as C7-T1. The nerve roots at C7 and C8 are then identified and followed out the foramen. The dissection is then performed completely laterally, isolating the C7 pedicle. After the bilateral facetectomies and isolation of the C7 pedicle, the C7 pedicle is skeletonized and removed with Lempert rongeurs.

Sequential lumbar or custom wedge-shaped spinal taps are used to decancellate the C7 vertebral body combined with osteotomes and down-pushing curettes to create as wide a wedge as possible. The limiting factor is usually the proximity of the C7 and C8 roots. A 30-degree angle may be selected based on standard techniques used in the thoracolumbar spine and as a starting point intraoperatively.

The lateral wall of the C7 vertebral body is then dissected out with a Penfield No. 1 dissector and visualized (**Fig. 40.1**). The C7 lateral wall is removed with needle-nose rongeurs and osteotomes via the pedicle hole reamed out by the taps, followed by removal of the posterior vertebral body with a custom central impactor. After completion of the osteotomy, the head is then loosened from the table, and the halo ring is used to extend the head and close the osteotomy.

Postoperative Care

Standard postoperative care is instituted. Most patients may return to the surgical floor. For patients who sustain a complication or have significant comorbidities, the intensive care unit may be warranted.

Potential Complications and Precautions

Due to the recent advances in surgical technique, anesthesia, and intraoperative neuromonitoring, the cervicothoracic junction PSO is considered a safe, reproducible, and effective procedure for the management of cervicothoracic kyphotic deformities.[20] Cervicothoracic PSO has reported complications that include neurologic deficits, sudden subluxation, and even death.[15,42,43] However, in our reported series of 11 patients, eight of whom were over the age of 60 years, there were no perioperative neurologic deficits and there were perioperative medical complications in only two patients.[20] The lower medical complications rate and decreased incidence of dysphagia may be due to the all-posterior nature of this technique. Posterior-only deformity corrections have also been associated with lower complication rates in thoracolumbar surgery compared with staged anterior-posterior procedures.

Conclusion

The cervicothoracic junction PSO is a safe, reproducible, and effective procedure for the management of fixed cervicothoracic kyphotic deformities. It results in excellent correction of cervical kyphosis and chin-brow vertical angle with a controlled closure. Furthermore, it has greater biomechanical stability than the Smith-Petersen osteotomy by having a wedge component that cleaves the vertebral body, creating a larger bone-on-bone load-bearing interface by uniting of the anterior, middle, and posterior columns upon closure. This greater bone-on-bone contact significantly increases stiffness, especially in compression and may also provide better fusion rates in patients who do not have ankylosing spondylitis. Currently, we prefer the PSO at the cervicothoracic level for treatment of chin-on-chest deformity, especially for nonankylosing spondylitis patients with normal bone quality.

40 C7 Pedicle Subtraction Osteotomy

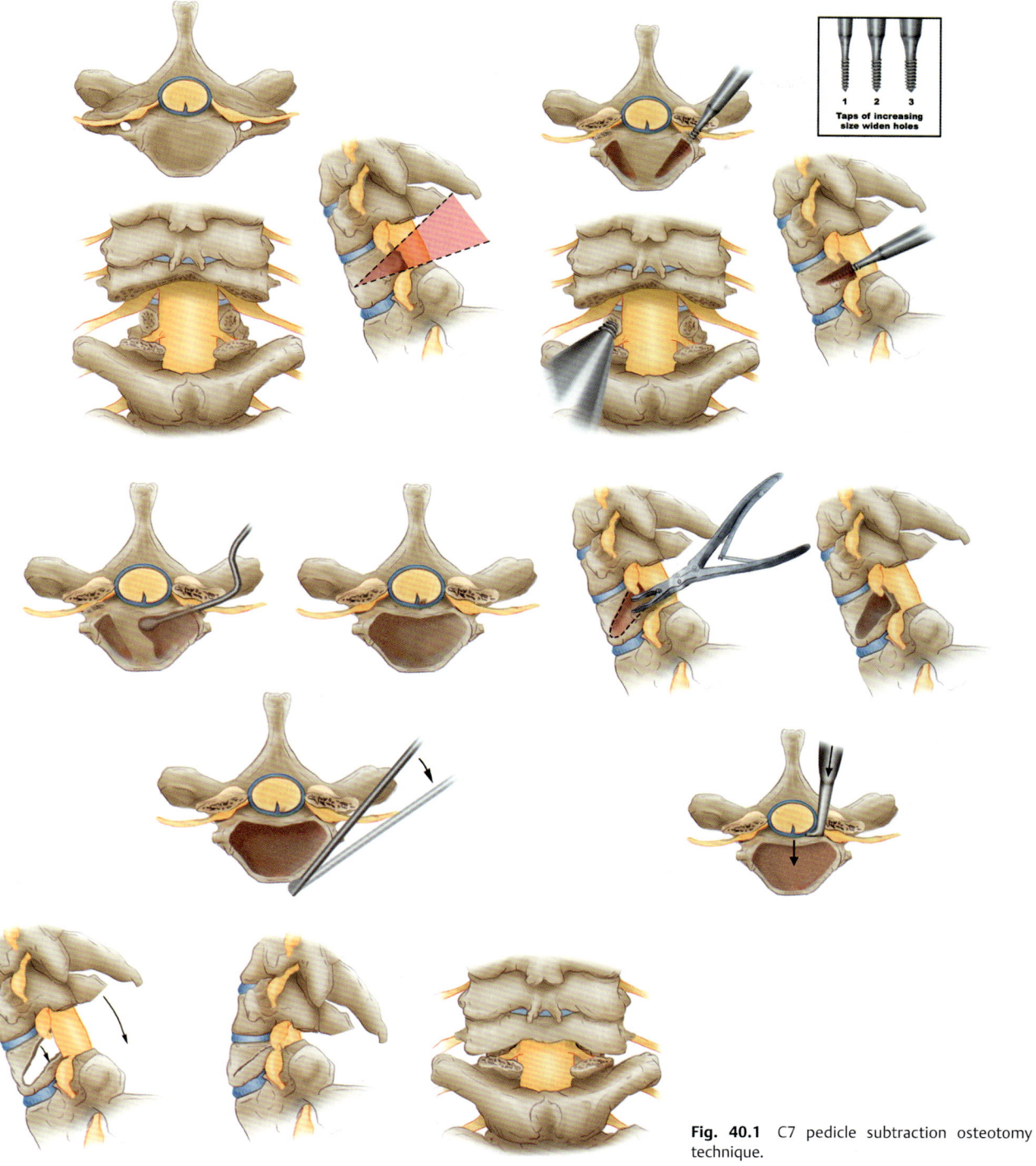

Fig. 40.1 C7 pedicle subtraction osteotomy technique.

References

1. Bradford DS, Tribus CB. Current concepts and management of patients with fixed decompensated spinal deformity. Clin Orthop Relat Res 1994; 306:64–72
2. Bridwell KH. Causes of sagittal spinal imbalance and assessment of the extent of needed correction. Instr Course Lect 2006;55:567–575
3. Etame AB, Than KD, Wang AC, La Marca F, Park P. Surgical management of symptomatic cervical or cervicothoracic kyphosis due to ankylosing spondylitis. Spine 2008;33:E559–E564
4. Etame AB, Wang AC, Than KD, La Marca F, Park P. Outcomes after surgery for cervical spine deformity: review of the literature. Neurosurg Focus 2010;28:E14
5. Gill JB, Levin A, Burd T, Longley M. Corrective osteotomies in spine surgery. J Bone Joint Surg Am 2008;90:2509–2520
6. Hoh DJ, Khoueir P, Wang MY. Management of cervical deformity in ankylosing spondylitis. Neurosurg Focus 2008;24:E9
7. Steinmetz MP, Stewart TJ, Kager CD, Benzel EC, Vaccaro AR. Cervical deformity correction. Neurosurgery 2007;60(1, Suppl 1):S90–S97
8. Belanger TA, Milam RA IV, Roh JS, Bohlman HH. Cervicothoracic extension osteotomy for chin-on-chest deformity in ankylosing spondylitis. J Bone Joint Surg Am 2005;87:1732–1738
9. Burton DC. Smith-Petersen osteotomy of the spine. Instr Course Lect 2006;55:577–582
10. Langeloo DD, Journee HL, Pavlov PW, de Kleuver M. Cervical osteotomy in ankylosing spondylitis: evaluation of new developments. Eur Spine J 2006;15:493–500
11. Law WA. Osteotomy of the cervical spine. J Bone Joint Surg Br 1959;41-B:640–641
12. McMaster MJ, Coventry MB. Spinal osteotomy in ankylosing spondylitis. Technique, complications, and long-term results. Mayo Clin Proc 1973;48:476–486
13. O'Shaughnessy BA, Liu JC, Hsieh PC, Koski TR, Ganju A, Ondra SL. Surgical treatment of fixed cervical kyphosis with myelopathy. Spine 2008;33:771–778
14. Savini R, Di Silvestre M, Gargiulo G. Cervical osteotomy by the Simmons method in the treatment of cervical kyphosis due to ankylosing spondylitis. Case report. Ital J Orthop Traumatol 1988;14:377–383
15. Simmons ED, DiStefano RJ, Zheng Y, Simmons EH. Thirty-six years experience of cervical extension osteotomy in ankylosing spondylitis: techniques and outcomes. Spine 2006;31:3006–3012
16. Simmons EH. The surgical correction of flexion deformity of the cervical spine in ankylosing spondylitis. Clin Orthop Relat Res 1972;86:132–143
17. Smith-Petersen MN, Larson CB, Aufranc OE. Osteotomy of the spine for correction of flexion deformity in rheumatoid arthritis. J Bone Joint Surg Am 1945;27:1–11
18. Suk KS, Kim KT, Lee SH, Kim JM. Significance of chin-brow vertical angle in correction of kyphotic deformity of ankylosing spondylitis patients. Spine 2003;28:2001–2005
19. Urist MR. Osteotomy of the cervical spine; report of a case of ankylosing rheumatoid spondylitis. J Bone Joint Surg Am 1958;40-A:833–843
20. Deviren V, Scheer JK, Ames CP. Technique of cervicothoracic junction pedicle subtraction osteotomy for cervical sagittal imbalance: report of 11 cases. J Neurosurg Spine 2011;15:174–181
21. Chin KR, Ahn J. Controlled cervical extension osteotomy for ankylosing spondylitis utilizing the Jackson operating table: technical note. Spine 2007;32:1926–1929
22. Pavlov PW. Correction and stabilisation in ankylosing spondylitis of the cervicothoracic spine. Eur Spine J 2009;18:1243–1244
23. Tokala DP, Lam KS, Freeman BJ, Webb JK. C7 decancellisation closing wedge osteotomy for the correction of fixed cervico-thoracic kyphosis. Eur Spine J 2007;16:1471–1478
24. Samudrala S, Vaynman S, Thiayananthan T, et al. Cervicothoracic junction kyphosis: surgical reconstruction with pedicle subtraction osteotomy and Smith-Petersen osteotomy. Presented at the 2009 Joint Spine Section Meeting. Clinical article. J Neurosurg Spine 2010;13:695–706
25. Berven SH, Deviren V, Smith JA, Emami A, Hu SS, Bradford DS. Management of fixed sagittal plane deformity: results of the transpedicular wedge resection osteotomy. Spine 2001;26:2036–2043
26. Booth KC, Bridwell KH, Lenke LG, Baldus CR, Blanke KM. Complications and predictive factors for the successful treatment of flatback deformity (fixed sagittal imbalance). Spine 1999;24:1712–1720
27. Bridwell KH, Lewis SJ, Edwards C, et al. Complications and outcomes of pedicle subtraction osteotomies for fixed sagittal imbalance. Spine 2003;28:2093–2101
28. Bridwell KH, Lewis SJ, Lenke LG, Baldus C, Blanke K. Pedicle subtraction osteotomy for the treatment of fixed sagittal imbalance. J Bone Joint Surg Am 2003;85-A:454–463
29. Dorward IG, Lenke LG. Osteotomies in the posterior-only treatment of complex adult spinal deformity: a comparative review. Neurosurg Focus 2010;28:E4
30. Hyun SJ, Rhim SC. Clinical outcomes and complications after pedicle subtraction osteotomy for fixed sagittal imbalance patients: a long-term follow-up data. J Korean Neurosurg Soc 2010;47:95–101
31. Ikenaga M, Shikata J, Takemoto M, Tanaka C. Clinical outcomes and complications after pedicle subtraction osteotomy for correction of thoracolumbar kyphosis. J Neurosurg Spine 2007;6:330–336
32. Kim KT, Suk KS, Cho YJ, Hong GP, Park BJ. Clinical outcome results of pedicle subtraction osteotomy in ankylosing spondylitis with kyphotic deformity. Spine 2002;27:612–618
33. Kim YJ, Bridwell KH, Lenke LG, Cheh G, Baldus C. Results of lumbar pedicle subtraction osteotomies for fixed sagittal imbalance: a minimum 5-year follow-up study. Spine 2007;32:2189–2197
34. Wang MY, Berven SH. Lumbar pedicle subtraction osteotomy. Neurosurgery 2007;60(2, Suppl 1):ONS140–ONS146, discussion ONS146
35. Wiggins GC, Ondra SL, Shaffrey CI. Management of iatrogenic flat-back syndrome. Neurosurg Focus 2003;15:E8
36. Scheer JK, Tang JA, Buckley JM, Pekmezci M, McClellan RT, Ames CP. Biomechanical analysis of osteotomy type (OWO, CWO) and rod diameter for treatment of cervicothoracic kyphosis. In: 17th Annual International Meeting on Advanced Spine Techniques. Toronto, Canada, 2010
37. Scheer JK, Tang JA, Buckley JM, et al. Biomechanical analysis of osteotomy type and rod diameter for treatment of cervicothoracic kyphosis. Spine 2011;36:E519–E523
38. Scheer JK, Tang JA, Deviren V, et al. Biomechanical analysis of cervicothoracic junction osteotomy in cadaveric model of ankylosing spondylitis: effect of rod material and diameter. J Neurosurg Spine 2011;14:330–335
39. Edwards CC II, Riew KD, Anderson PA, Hilibrand AS, Vaccaro AF. Cervical myelopathy. current diagnostic and treatment strategies. Spine J 2003;3:68–81
40. Chi JH, Tay B, Stahl D, Lee R. Complex deformities of the cervical spine. Neurosurg Clin N Am 2007;18:295–304
41. Mummaneni PV, Deutsch H, Mummaneni VP. Cervicothoracic kyphosis. Neurosurg Clin N Am 2006;17:277–287, vi
42. Mummaneni PV, Mummaneni VP, Haid RW Jr, Rodts GE Jr, Sasso RC. Cervical osteotomy for the correction of chin-on-chest deformity in ankylosing spondylitis. Technical note. Neurosurg Focus 2003;14:e9
43. McMaster MJ. Osteotomy of the cervical spine in ankylosing spondylitis. J Bone Joint Surg Br 1997;79:197–203

D. Combined Anterior-Posterior Approach

41 Combined Anterior-Posterior Approach for Complete Vertebral Resection in the Midcervical Spine

Mohamad Bydon, Rafael de la Garza-Ramos, Jean-Paul Wolinsky, and Ziya L. Gokaslan

Complete vertebral body resection, also known as spondylectomy, involves the removal of an entire spinal segment, most often to address oncological lesions or deformity.[1] This procedure entails removal of the vertebral body, pedicles, superior and inferior articulating processes, pars interarticularis, transverse processes, laminae, and the spinous process.[2] The term *spondylectomy* does not specify what the margins of resection were, nor does it specify that it was performed in an intralesional or en-bloc fashion. Rather, the term refers to a technique that has the objective of removing a specimen (tumor) in an en-bloc fashion with the intent of obtaining negative margins.

Spondylectomies are complex procedures with a high morbidity profile. They should be reserved for tumors that may oncologically benefit from resection, by being cured or by resulting in an increased long-term tumor-free survival, and for patients with neurologic deficits that may recover after neural decompression. They are usually indicated for the resection of primary malignant bone tumors, such as chordomas, chondrosarcomas, and osteosarcomas.[2] However, spondylectomies for spinal metastases have also been performed.[3] Some cases of spinal deformity (e.g., kyphoscoliosis) may also be treated with spondylectomy, sometimes in combination with spinal shortening techniques.[1,4]

There are several operative techniques for performing a spondylectomy. This chapter describes the combined anterior-posterior approach in the midcervical spine.

Patient Selection

There are several general indications to perform a spondylectomy. The risks and benefits of an invasive en-bloc resection must be thoroughly discussed with the patient, as well as the potential need for adjuvant chemotherapy or radiation therapy. Patients should undergo a complete medical evaluation prior to surgery.

Indications

- Resection of aggressive benign tumors[5]
- Resection of a primary malignant bone tumors (such as chordomas and chondrosarcomas)
- Resection of a solitary metastatic lesion of "biologically and prognostically favorable primary tumor (good prognostic scores)"[6]
- Severe deformity correction

Contraindications[6]

- Diffuse tumor spread of Tomita type 7
- Distant metastatic disease
- Biologically unfavorable tumors

Advantages and Disadvantages

The advantage of performing a spondylectomy is that it may result in a cure if the tumor is removed in its entirety. It also has the potential to increase disease-free survival and overall survival. The greatest disadvantage is the highly morbid profile, which includes potential injury to vascular structures, the spinal cord, and nerve roots.

Choice of Operative Approach and Surgical Planning

Surgery for spondylectomy can be divided into two stages: the preparatory stage and the tumor resection.[2] The preparatory stage can entail multiple procedures.

The goal of the first stage is to free the tumor from the surrounding tissues and structures so that the tumor can be removed with minimal damage to the spinal cord and critical nerves.[2] As a general rule of thumb, the preparatory stage occurs "on the side of the spinal cord, or thecal sac, opposite the tumor."[2] During this stage, vascular and neurologic structures may need to be sacrificed to adequately free the tumor, consequences that must be discussed in detail with the patient before surgery. The patient must understand, and agree to, the potential oncological benefits versus the potential loss of function.

Surgical Procedure

Midcervical Spine Spondylectomy

After the patient is appropriately selected, it is important to thoroughly review the radiological studies, including magnetic resonance imaging (MRI) and computed tomography (CT), to assess the tumor extent and infiltration (**Fig. 41.1**). A spondylectomy is only feasible in this region if at least one of the vertebral arteries is not infiltrated by the tumor.[2] Additionally, this non-infiltrated artery must be tested to determine whether it can provide adequate blood supply to the posterior fossa.[7] If the non-dominant artery is involved in the tumor, no further investigation is necessary. On the other hand, if the dominant artery is involved, additional investigation is required.

A cerebral angiogram can evaluate the patency of the circle of Willis to determine if the anterior circulation can provide enough blood supply to the posterior circulation.[2] A vertebral artery balloon occlusion test can also be performed to predict whether a patient will tolerate a vertebral artery sacrifice.

Another important consideration is the degree of nerve root involvement. The cervical spine nerves are involved in upper extremity function (via the brachial plexus), but also importantly

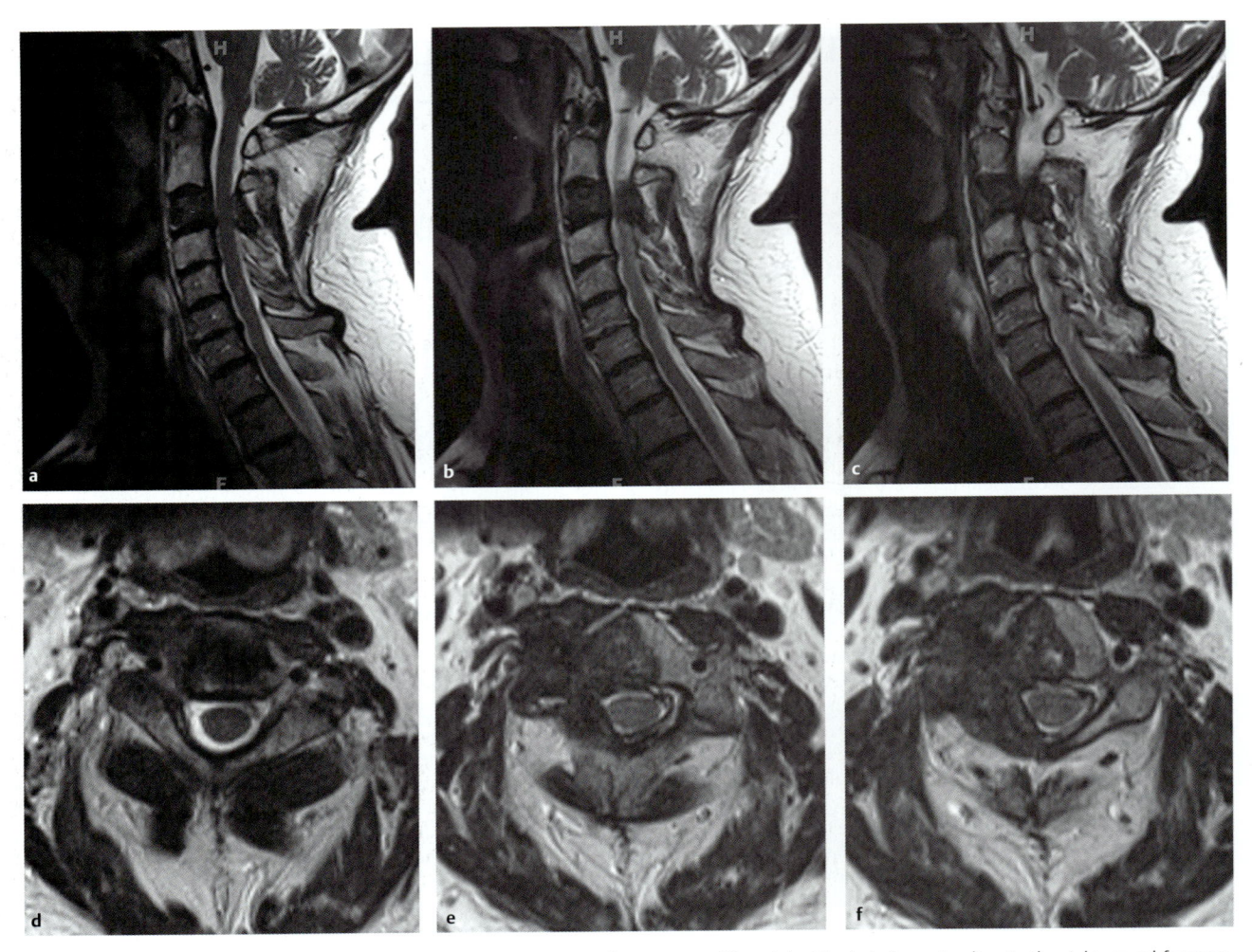

Fig. 41.1 A 72-year-old man with known renal cell carcinoma presented with progressive right upper extremity weakness and signs of myelopathy. **(a–c)** Serial sagittal T2-weighted magnetic resonance imaging (MRI) demonstrates a C3 vertebral body lesion extending to the right neural foramen. **(d–f)** Serial axial T2-weighted MRI demonstrates a C3 lesion involving the vertebral body, right pedicle, right lateral mass, and right lamina.

in innervation of the diaphragm (via the phrenic nerve in C3–C5). For this reason, careful planning and weighing of the risks and benefits must be done.

Preparatory Stage

The preparatory stage of a midcervical spondylectomy may require sacrifice of important vascular and neural structures. The vertebral artery spans from C6 to C1 in most patients, and may be either intentionally sacrificed or iatrogenically injured, both of which may result in ischemic posterior fossa stroke. The vertebral artery enters at the C6 level in 90% of patients, at C7 in 7%, and at C4 in 3%.[8] Sacrifice of nerve roots may result in significant loss of function (**Table 41.1**).[2] As mentioned earlier, the preparatory stage begins on the side of the spinal canal opposite the tumor. Thus, an anterior tumor may be first approached posteriorly, and in the second stage the tumor can be delivered anteriorly.

As in most posterior cervical approaches, a midline occipitocervical incision is made; the ligamentum nuchae can be separated by electrocautery. After a subperiosteal dissection, the laminae are removed, exposing the healthy thecal sac. If the anterior tumor extends laterally and involves a vertebral artery or nerve root, these structures may need to be sectioned. Based on a study by Simşek et al[9] of the anatomic parameters for subaxial cervical spondylectomy, it is recommended that three consecutive pedicles and two nerve roots be adequately visualized prior to spondylectomy.

Table 41.1 Neurologic Deficits from Specific Nerve Root Sacrifice in the Cervical Spine

Nerve	Deficit
C2	Loss of sensation on back of head
C3 and C4	Possible diaphragm weakness
C5	Deltoid, biceps weakness
C6	Bicep weakness
C7	Triceps weakness
C8 or T1	Hand intrinsic weakness

Once this is done, the nerve roots are identified, ligated, and sectioned proximal to the dorsal root ganglion.[2] However, as mentioned earlier, certain nerve roots are critical to upper extremity and diaphragm function, and sectioning of these roots may cause significant loss of function to the patient. Then the lateral masses cephalad and caudal to the tumor are resected with a high-speed diamond bur.[2] As the osseous elements are resected, the foramina for the nerve roots will be encountered, and ventral to the nerve roots lies the vertebral artery.[2]

Dissection of the vertebral artery must be done with care. A venous plexus surrounds this vessel, and if encountered, bleeding can be controlled with thrombin and powdered hemostatic gelatin (Gelfoam).[2] Prior to ligation, an aneurysmal clip can be put in place to test occlusion while monitoring the electroencephalogram and brainstem auditory evoked potentials.[2] If the test records any changes in potentials, the vertebral artery sacrifice should be aborted, unless a bypass can be performed.[2] Once the vertebral artery is identified cephalad and caudal to the tumor, it can be circumferentially ligated and sectioned.

After vertebral artery ligation, care must be taken to preserve the contralateral artery. The artery should be skeletonized with caution, as this step carries risk of vasospasm.[2] To diminish this risk, the vertebral artery should remain inside the foramen transversarium (if the tumor architecture permits it), and the sagittal osteotomies (lateral to the tumor) must be done medial to the artery and foramen transversarium. Once this is done, posterior instrumentation is placed with the addition of auto/allograft at the surgeon's discretion.

Tumor Resection

The second stage completes the preparatory stage, and it entails resecting the tumor. In the case of an initial posterior approach, the second stage involves an anterior cervical exposure.[2] Depending on the tumor, this can be achieved via a traditional Smith-Robinson approach,[10] a high cervical approach,[11] or a transoral transmandibular circumglossal approach (usually reserved for lesions in the upper cervical spine).[12] One drawback to the transmandibular approach is the increased risk of mandibular pseudarthrosis and pharyngeal dehiscence in patients scheduled to undergo adjuvant radiation therapy, and for this reason it is usually no longer an option.[2] Another approach used to treat low cervical spine and high thoracic lesions is the anterior transsternal approach,[13] although patients with a high-riding sternal notch may also require this approach. This operative technique may be challenging for the inexperienced surgeon, as it requires meticulous mobilization of the brachiocephalic vessels, superior vena cava, and aorta. Potential complications include (1) direct injury to the aforementioned structures, (2) hypotension for aortic retraction, and (3) increased airway resistance due to mobilization of the trachea.[13]

Once the approach is completed, osteotomies cephalad and caudal to the tumor should be performed. The osteotomies should be taken dorsally to the posterior longitudinal ligament.[2] Afterward, the specimen should be freed and removed en bloc.

Reconstruction

A spondylectomy results in destabilization of the spine. Biomechanically, the goal of an instrumented construct is to withstand the weight of the remaining cervical segments and head, and to bridge the spinal segments until a solid fusion is achieved.[2] Wolinsky et al[2] state, "In designing a specific construct after a spondylectomy procedure, an attempt to reconstruct all three columns should be made. Consideration should also be given to any postoperative adjuvant radiation therapy that may be given, and the implants should be designed to minimize interference with the therapy."

Posterior instrumentation is placed during the posterior approach, and usually involves a combination of midcervical lateral mass screws, C2 pedicle screws, C1 lateral mass screws, occipital fixation, or thoracic pedicle screws.[7,14,15] Anteriorly, reconstruction can be done utilizing mesh cages or allograft struts with anterior plating (**Fig. 41.2**).[16] Expandable cages, on the other hand, are usually avoided, as there is a limited amount of bone material that can be placed within the cage. Instrumentation usually involves two to three segments above and below the spondylectomy level.[16,17] Local autograft (such as the one obtained after a laminectomy) is usually avoided due to the increased risk of tumoral recurrence.

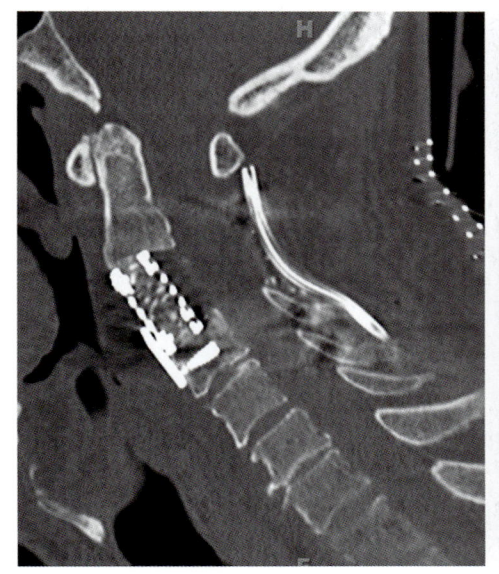

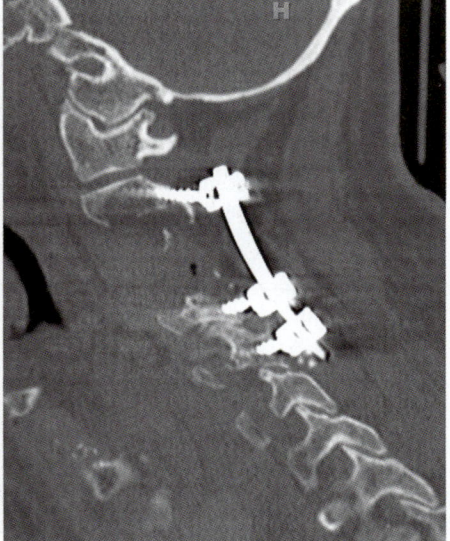

Fig. 41.2 The patient underwent a two-staged C3 spondylectomy with **(a)** anterior reconstruction using a mesh cage and plating and **(b)** posterior reconstruction using lateral mass screws and rods.

Complications

The extensive surgical wounds, blood loss, and prolonged operating time increases the risk of postoperative wound infection.[2] Special consideration must be given to antibiotic use and dosing and to the use of a complex plastic surgery flap.[2]

Postoperative cerebrospinal fluid (CSF) leak may be the result of an incidental durotomy or a fluid leak from a ligated nerve root. Fluid from the surgical drains may be sent to the lab for B-transferrin testing.[2] Once a diagnosis of CSF leak has been made, attempts at diversion such as a lumbar drain may be considered. If conservative measures fail, an operation to reexplore and close the leak may be necessary.

Instrumentation failure may result in anterior cage dislodgment or posterior instrumentation failure. Either of these complications may result in severe neurovascular injuries, and may require complex revision surgeries.[2] Other complications include vertebral artery injuries, esophageal perforation, and pseudarthrosis.

Vertebral artery injuries are estimated to occur in only 0.07% of all cervical spine cases, and ~ 23% of all injuries occur during anterior corpectomies.[18] Although 87% of patients may ultimately recover without any sequelae, ~ 5% may incur a cerebellar infarct.[18] Esophageal perforations are estimated to occur in 0.02 to 1.52% of cervical spine surgery cases,[19] with mortality as high as 19%.[20] Although some cases may be managed conservatively with nil per os, parenteral nutrition, and broad-spectrum antibiotics, the definitive treatment consists of using a sternocleidomastoid muscle flap.[21] Hsieh et al[7] reported both short- and long-term outcomes of five patients undergoing en-bloc excisions of chordomas; in three of the patients (60%) a pseudarthrosis required revision surgery. Hsieh et al concluded, "We also need to improve our ability for spinal reconstruction after aggressive tumor excision to provide patients with long-term fusion and stability of the spine."

Postoperative Care

Depending on each case, patients may require postoperative monitoring in the intensive care unit. Close monitoring of neurologic function is essential and should be done regularly. Patients should receive adequate fluid maintenance and be monitored for potential complications such as epidural hematoma. All patients should receive thromboprophylaxis and antibiotics as appropriate. Additionally, depending on the histology of the tumor, patients may require adjuvant chemo/radiotherapy.

Conclusion

The spondylectomy is a challenging procedure for the spine surgeon, with a high morbidity profile. The key to success is adequate preoperative planning and a thorough discussion with the patient about the risks and benefits of the procedure. Although most of these procedures are done to treat primary malignant tumors, other indications may include severe deformity.

Disclosures

Ziya L. Gokaslan is the recipient of research grants from Depuy Spine, AO Spine North America, Medtronic, Neurosurgery Research and Education Foundation (NREF), Integra Life Sciences, and K2M. He receives fellowship support from AO Spine North America. He holds stock in Spinal Kinetics and US Spine.

The other authors have no conflict of interests or funding sources to declare.

References

1. Barberá J. T12-L1 telescoped chronic dislocation treated by en bloc one-piece spondylectomy and spine shortening. J Spinal Disord Tech 2004;17:163–166
2. Wolinsky JP, Sciubba DM, Lastra-Power J, Gokaslan ZL. Spondylectomy for spinal tumors. In: Benzel EC, ed. Spine Surgery: Techniques, Complication Avoidance and Management. Philadelphia: Saunders; 2011
3. Yao KC, Boriani S, Gokaslan ZL, Sundaresan N. En bloc spondylectomy for spinal metastases: a review of techniques. Neurosurg Focus 2003;15:E6
4. Shimada Y, Abe E, Sato K. Total en-bloc spondylectomy for correcting congenital kyphosis. Spinal Cord 2000;38:382–385
5. Amendola L, Cappuccio M, De Iure F, Bandiera S, Gasbarrini A, Boriani S. En bloc resections for primary spinal tumors in 20 years of experience: effectiveness and safety. Spine J 2014;14:2608–2617
6. Druschel C, Disch AC, Melcher I, Luzzati A, Haas NP, Schaser KD. [Multisegmental en bloc spondylectomy. Indications, staging and surgical technique]. Oper Orthop Traumatol 2012;24:272–283
7. Hsieh PC, Gallia GL, Sciubba DM, et al. En bloc excisions of chordomas in the cervical spine: review of five consecutive cases with more than 4-year follow-up. Spine 2011;36:E1581–E1587
8. Civelek E, Kiris T, Hepgul K, Canbolat A, Ersoy G, Cansever T. Anterolateral approach to the cervical spine: major anatomical structures and landmarks. Technical note. J Neurosurg Spine 2007;7:669–678
9. Simşek S, Uz A, Er U, Apaydın N. Quantitative evaluation of the anatomical parameters for subaxial cervical spondylectomy: an anatomical study. J Neurosurg Spine 2013;18:568–574
10. Smith GW, Robinson RA. The treatment of certain cervical-spine disorders by anterior removal of the intervertebral disc and interbody fusion. J Bone Joint Surg Am 1958;40-A:607–624
11. Finn MA, Macdonald JD. C2-3 anterior cervical fusion: technical report. J Spinal Disord Tech 2013
12. DeMonte F, Diaz E Jr, Callender D, Suk I. Transmandibular, circumglossal, retropharyngeal approach for chordomas of the clivus and upper cervical spine. Technical note. Neurosurg Focus 2001;10:E10
13. Zengming X, Maolin H, Xinli Z, Qianfen C. Anterior transsternal approach for a lesion in the upper thoracic vertebral body. J Neurosurg Spine 2010;13:461–468
14. Chou D, Wang V. Two-level en bloc spondylectomy for osteosarcoma at the cervicothoracic junction. J Clin Neurosci 2009;16:698–700
15. Currier BL, Papagelopoulos PJ, Krauss WE, Unni KK, Yaszemski MJ. Total en bloc spondylectomy of C5 vertebra for chordoma. Spine 2007;32:E294–E299
16. Simsek S, Er U, Demir HA, Adabag A, Bavbek M. Two-stage multilevel cervical spondylectomy for aneurysmal bone cyst. Turk Neurosurg 2013;23:415–419
17. Wu W, Li F, Fang Z, et al. Total spondylectomy of C2 and circumferential reconstruction via combined anterior and posterior approach to cervical spine for axis tumor surgery. J Huazhong Univ Sci Technolog Med Sci 2013;33:126–132
18. Lunardini DJ, Eskander MS, Even JL, et al. Vertebral artery injuries in cervical spine surgery. Spine J 2013
19. Amhaz HH, Kuo R, Vaidya R, Orlewicz MS. Esophageal perforation following cervical spine surgery: A review with considerations in airway management. Int J Crit Illn Inj Sci 2013;3:276–278
20. Navarro R, Javahery R, Eismont F, et al. The role of the sternocleidomastoid muscle flap for esophageal fistula repair in anterior cervical spine surgery. Spine 2005;30:E617–E622
21. Ahn SH, Lee SH, Kim ES, Eoh W. Successful repair of esophageal perforation after anterior cervical fusion for cervical spine fracture. J Clin Neurosci 2011;18:1374–1380

Section III   Cervicothoracic Junction

A. Anterior Approach

42 Supraclavicular Approach to the Cervicothoracic Junction

Zachary A. Smith, Joshua Bakhsheshian, and Nader S. Dahdaleh

Surgical exposure of the anterior cervicothoracic junction (CTJ) can be challenging due to the major anatomic structures that are subject to abnormalities and pathology (**Fig. 42.1**). Disruptions to the CTJ can be caused by tumors or trauma or can be caused iatrogenically.[1] The major anatomic structures include the thyroid gland, the carotid sheath, and osseous structures such as the sternum and clavicle. When approaching the thoracic inlet, the surgeon must safely navigate through the trachea, esophagus, thoracic duct, and important nerves (e.g., vagus, recurrent laryngeal, phrenic, and sympathetics).[2] In cases of significant pathology, this can be complicated by poorly defined anatomic boundaries. For a successful outcome, a firm understanding of the neurovascular and bony anatomy is necessary.

The anterior cervical approach was initially described in the 1950s and subsequently modified to overcome the aforementioned challenges.[3,4] The anterior cervical region can be approached via the supraclavicular, transmanubrial-transclavicular, or transsternal route. The choice of the operative approach depends on the location of the pathological process and the surgeon's experience. This chapter focuses on the supraclavicular approach to expose the CTJ. This approach provides sufficient exposure up to T2 without disrupting the sternum or clavicle.[1] A transmanubrial approach is necessary to expose T3 and in patients with short necks; it is discussed in Chapter 43. The supraclavicular approach is essentially an oblique extension of the typical anteromedial approach. This technique can pose specific challenges in patients with prominent muscular development, short necks, or significant kyphosis. Furthermore, this approach can result in a deep operative field, thereby requiring an acute angle to place anterior instrumentation. When performed correctly, a successful outcome is attainable with this approach.

Patient Selection

The transmanubrial-transclavicular or transsternal approach may be employed to access the lower thoracic region of the CTJ. These approaches can also be used if a wider exposure to the CTJ region is needed in patients with a short neck or significant kyphosis.

Indications

- Tumor
- Infection
- Structural deformity

Contraindications

- Pathology below T2
- Limited exposure due to short neck, prominent musculature, or significant kyphosis
- Obstruction by anomalies of great vessels

Advantages

- Provides access to multiple levels of the anterior spinal column
- Enables simultaneous decompression and fixation

Disadvantages

- Limited access below the second thoracic vertebra
- No access to the posterior spinal column

Preoperative Imaging

- Anteroposterior and lateral X-ray
- Computed tomography (CT)
- Magnetic resonance imaging (MRI), especially with tumor pathology

Surgical Technique

Anesthesia and Positioning

General anesthesia appropriate for electrophysiological monitoring is used. Fiberoptic intubation is performed when there is evidence of cervical spinal cord myelopathy, compression, or instability. The patient should undergo a neurologic exam before and after intubation to evaluate any changes. A nasogastric tube can be placed to help localize the esophagus. Subsequently, the neck of the patient is slightly hyperextended and rotated away from the side of the operation. Straps are placed and the shoulders are pulled down. Lateral X-rays can then be used to localize the cervical pathology.

Incision

Developing a bloodless plane is critical to the surgical approach. Palpable anterior neck landmarks (mandibular angle at C2, hyoid

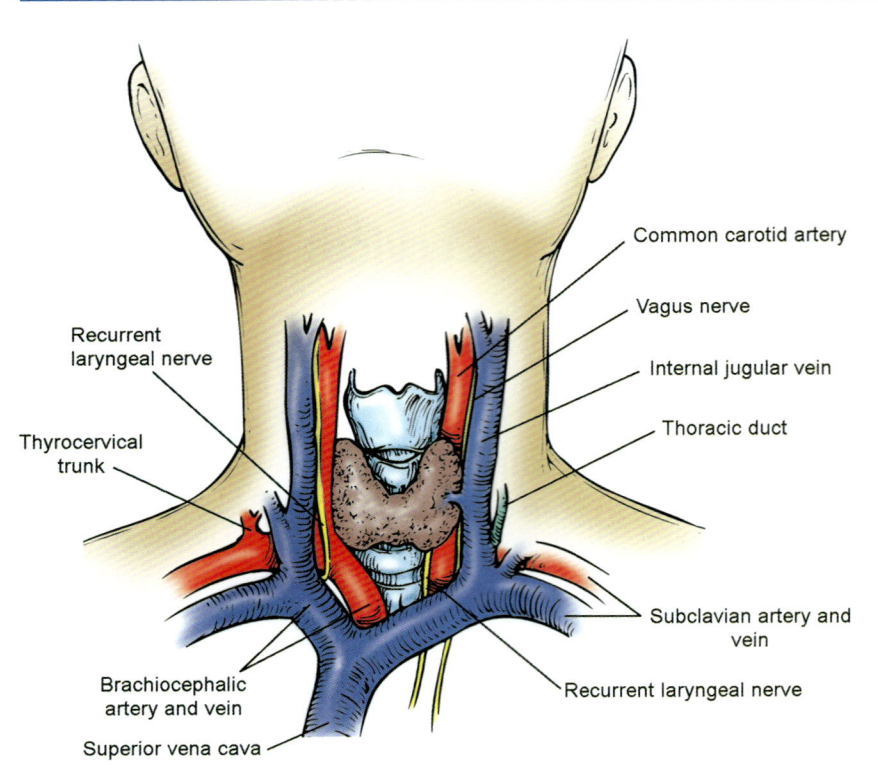

Fig. 42.1 Vascular anatomy at the base of the neck.

bone at C3, thyroid cartilage at C4-C5, and cricoid cartilage and carotid tubercle at C6) can help identify appropriate spinal levels (**Fig. 42.2**).[5] A transverse skin incision that is 2 cm above the clavicle is made, which extends from the midline to the lateral border of the sternocleidomastoid (SCM) muscle. As in many surgeries, a left-sided approach is employed due to the more consistent course of the left recurrent laryngeal nerve (**Fig. 42.3**).[6] However, a right-sided approach can be used if this nerve is suspected of having a potentially aberrant course.

The initial operative steps are similar to those employed with a traditional anterior cervical approach. Following careful dissection of more superficial structures (including the platysma), the first critical landmark is the SCM muscle. At the anterior border of this muscle, the superficial and deep cervical fascia should be dissected thoroughly, both cranially and caudally. The SCM muscle can be isolated with finger dissection, and its attachment to the sternal and clavicular heads identified. Subsequently, the muscular attachments can be transected in a subperiosteal manner and reflected superiorly (**Fig. 42.3**).

For complete surgical exposure, we suggest disarticulation of the clavicle from the manubrium. The free-floating portion of the clavicle can be removed. However, careful attention should be given to the undersurface of this bone fragment as the subclavian vein commonly underlies the clavicular head. In addition, the omohyoid and sternohyoid muscles can also be divided (**Fig. 42.4**). This facilitates visualization of the anterior scalene muscle and phrenic nerve.[7] The dome of the lung is also in close proximity to the anterior scalene muscle.

An equally important surgical landmark, the carotid sheath, should be given attention at this time. Located below the SCM muscle, the carotid artery and sheath should be laterally retracted, and dissection should occur in a plane medial to the carotid.[8] A potential pitfall during dissection of the caudal portion of this plane is injury to the recurrent laryngeal nerve that runs in the groove between the trachea and the esophagus (**Fig. 42.4**). If attention is not given to this structure, it can be damaged during the approach. Similarly, aggressive surgical dissection of the longus colli muscles laterally can lead to an injury of the sympathetic nerves and plexuses (**Fig. 42.5**). This may potentially result in a Horner's syndrome.[9]

At the most caudal portions of the exposure, there are additional structures that must be carefully identified and preserved.

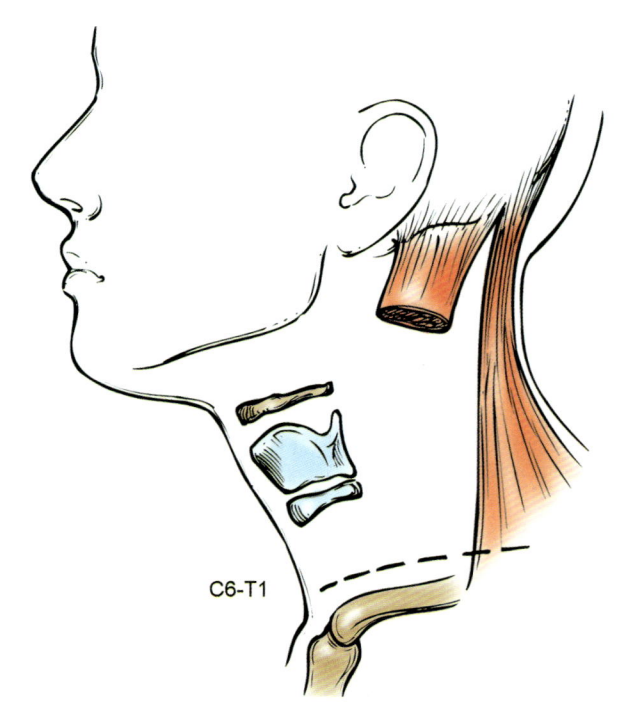

Fig. 42.2 Transverse skin incision of the supraclavicular approach.

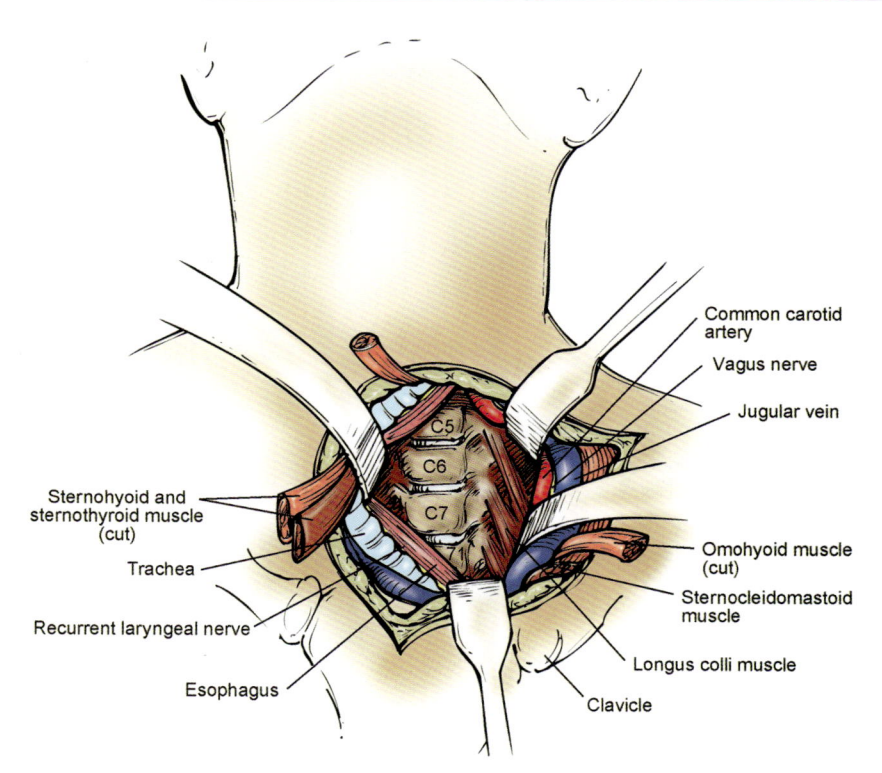

42 Supraclavicular Approach to the Cervicothoracic Junction 265

Fig. 42.3 The sternocleidomastoid (SCM) muscle is detached from the sternum and clavicle and reflected superiorly.

The thoracic duct is located laterally in the field, at the junction of the internal jugular and subclavian veins. If the dissection is focused medially from the carotid sheath, this structure is rarely injured. In addition, both the subclavian artery and the thyrocervical trunk are located inferiorly and can be injured with this approach.

When the level of pathology is reached, the prevertebral fascia must be incised in the midline to complete the exposure. The prevertebral fascia covers the vertebral bodies and encases the longus colli muscles. A bent spinal needle can be used to identify the surgical level with fluoroscopy, followed by development of longus colli "cuffs" to place permanent retractor

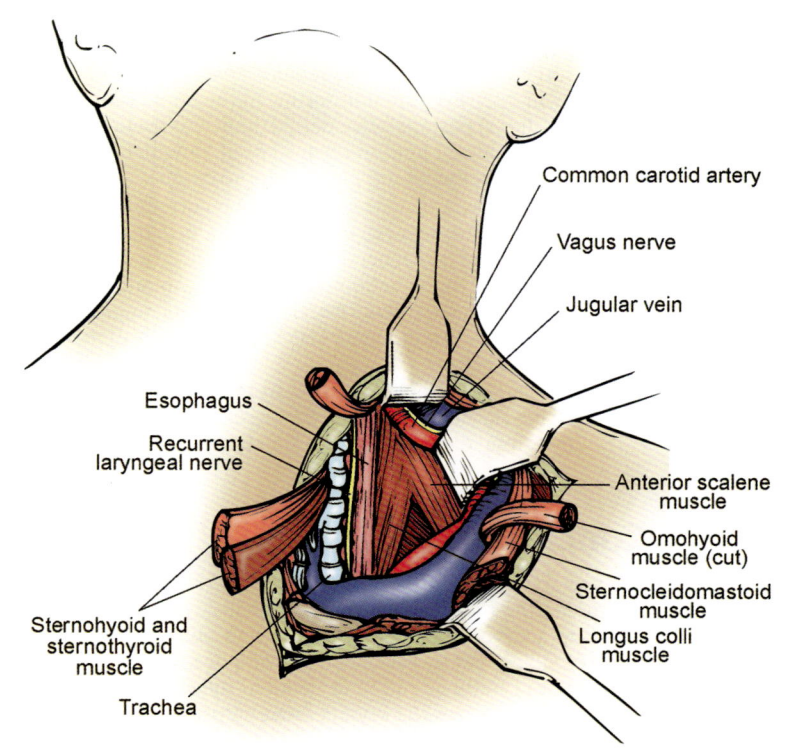

Fig. 42.4 Dissection should proceed along an anatomic plane between the carotid artery and sheath laterally and the trachea/esophagus medially.

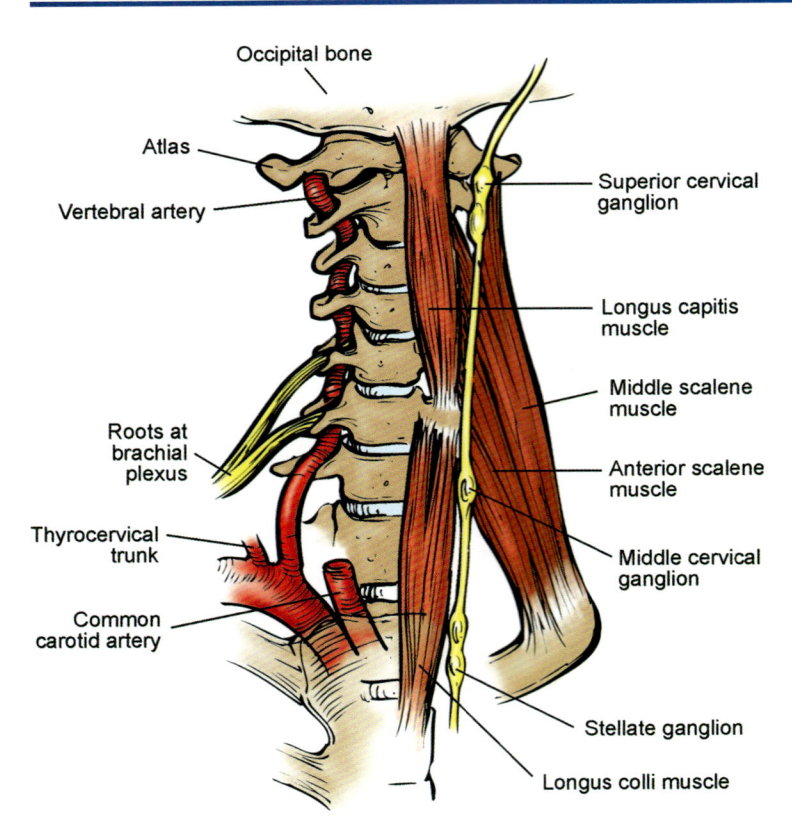

Fig. 42.5 Aggressive lateral dissection of the longus colli muscles can damage the sympathetic plexus or the vertebral artery.

blades. These muscular cuffs help to protect the midline esophagus and lateral carotid sheath from injury.[10] At this point of the procedure, the surgeon can address spinal column pathology in a fashion similar to that of other approaches in the spine (**Fig. 42.6**). However, because of the narrow opening of the thoracic inlet, wide surgical access is rarely possible. Therefore, if this is desired, splitting of the manubrium and sternum may be required (see Chapter 43).

Closing

After appropriate bone grafting and instrumentation, the area is irrigated copiously with antibiotic-impregnated saline. Hemostasis is obtained and fluoroscopy is used to confirm the placement of hardware or the bone grafting. We typically place a No. 7 Jackson-Pratt drain at the time of closure to prevent postoperative hematoma formation. Further, if there is any evidence of pleural violation, a chest tube can be inserted through a separate stab wound. Subcutaneous and skin tissue is closed in a routine fashion, and a cervical brace can be placed, according to surgeon preference.

Postoperative Care

- Jackson-Pratt drain in place for 2 to 3 days after the operation
- Intensive care unit monitoring for a minimum of 24 hours
- Monitor for respiratory difficulties
- Physiotherapy

Potential Complications and Precautions

- Soft tissue edema: Extra attention should be given to patients with extensive pathology or prolonged surgeries. These patients require close observation in an intensive care unit setting in the immediate (24-hour) postoperative period. Judicious evaluation for significant fluid shifts or signs of potential airway edema should be completed prior to extubation.
- Hoarseness: Due to traction on the recurrent laryngeal nerve, hoarseness can occur. In addition, damage to the superior laryngeal nerve can cause difficulty with clearing of the secretions and promote aspiration. Monitor these patients closely and promote rapid mobilization, pulmonary toilet, and the utilization of speech therapy.
- Horner's syndrome: Due to disruption of sympathetic chain, Horner's syndrome can occur. It can be avoided by careful dissection on the lateral border of the longus colli

Conclusion

The supraclavicular approach can be used to access the CTJ without disrupting the sternum or clavicle. This approach provides adequate access to several vertebral levels above T2 in a relatively bloodless plane. Perioperative complications can be prevented with careful attention to detail in the surgical anatomy. **Box 42.1** summarizes the key operative steps and the problems that can arise.

42 Supraclavicular Approach to the Cervicothoracic Junction

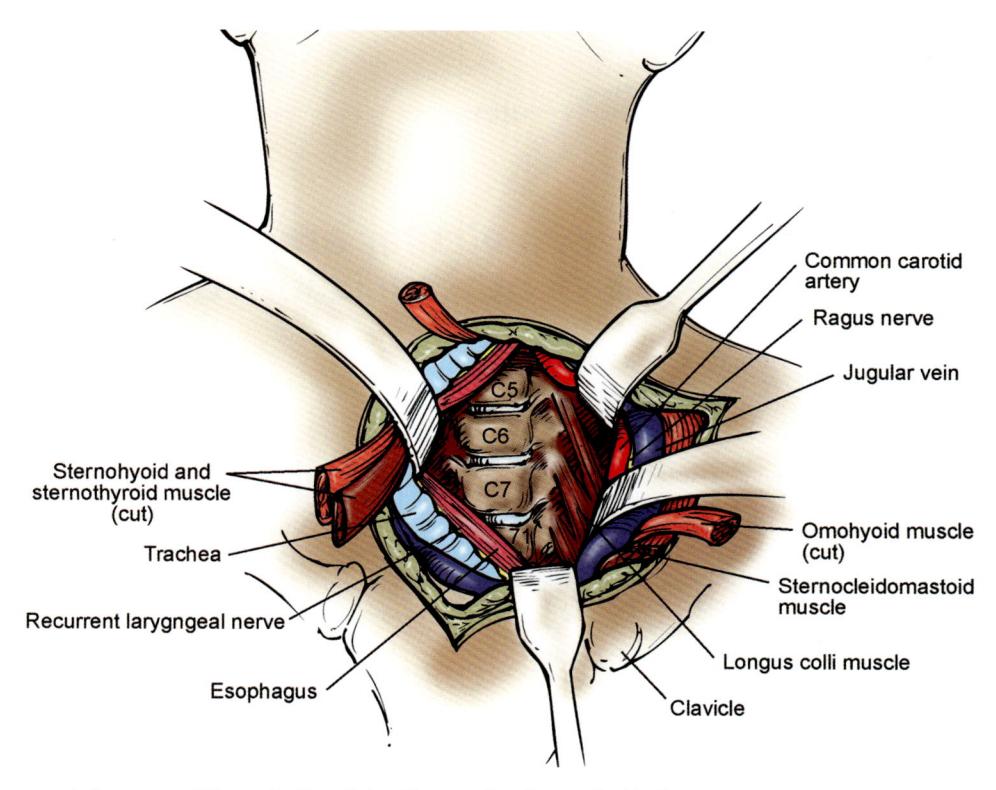

Fig. 42.6 Ultimate surgical exposure of the cervicothoracic junction revealing the vertebral bodies.

Box 42.1 Key Operative Steps and Potential Problems

Step	Problems
Left-side incision	Recurrent laryngeal nerve injury (low risk)
Dissection medial to the SCM	Dissection posterior to SCM can result in spinal accessory nerve injury
Disarticulation of the clavicle	Subclavian vein
Omohyoid and sternohyoid divided	Phrenic nerve injury
Carotid sheath retracted laterally	Recurrent laryngeal nerve injury. Dissection lateral to caudal portion of the carotid sheath can cause injury to thoracic duct, internal jugular and brachiocephalic vein, subclavian artery and vein, thyrocervical trunk, inferior thyroid artery
Dissection lateral to longus colli	Cervical sympathetic ganglion disruption causing unilateral Horner's syndrome

References

1. Wang VY, Chou D. The cervicothoracic junction. Neurosurg Clin N Am 2007;18:365–371
2. Lu J, Ebraheim NA, Nadim Y, Huntoon M. Anterior approach to the cervical spine: surgical anatomy. Orthopedics 2000;23:841–845
3. Choi S, Samudrala S. Supraclavicular approach to the cervicothoracic junction. In: Fessler R, Sekhar L, eds. Atlas of Neurosurgical Techniques. New York: Thieme; 2006:306–311
4. Watkins RG. Supraclavicular approach. In: Watkins RG, ed. Surgical Approaches to the Spine. New York: Springer; 2003:65–71
5. Auerbach JD, Weidner Z, Pill SG, Mehta S, Chin KR. The mandibular angle as a landmark for identification of cervical spinal level. Spine 2009;34:1006–1011
6. Sundaresan N, DiGiacinto GV. Surgical approaches to the cervicothoracic junction. In: Sundaresan N, Schmidek, HH, Schiller AL, Rosenthal DI, eds. Tumors of the Spine. Philadelphia: WB Saunders; 1990:358–368
7. McAfee P. Anterior surgical approaches to the lower and upper cervical spine. In: Sherk HH, ed. The Cervical Spine: An Atlas of Surgical Procedures. Philadelphia: Lippincott; 1994:37–69
8. Sundaresan N, Shah J, Foley KM, Rosen G. An anterior surgical approach to the upper thoracic vertebrae. J Neurosurg 1984;61:686–690
9. Civelek E, Karasu A, Cansever T, et al. Surgical anatomy of the cervical sympathetic trunk during anterolateral approach to cervical spine. Eur Spine J 2008;17:991–995
10. Albert T. Relevant cervical anatomy and anterior, middle, and lower cervical exposures. In: Albert T, Balderston RA, Northrup BE, eds. Surgical Approaches to the Spine. Philadelphia: WB Saunders; 1997

43 Transmanubrial-Transclavicular and Transsternal Approach to the Cervicothoracic Junction

Joshua Bakhsheshian, Nader S. Dahdaleh, and Zachary A. Smith

Lesions that occur in the anterior region of the cervicothoracic junction (CTJ) can result in significant vertebral kyphosis and spinal cord compression. The surgical exposure to pathological processes of the anterior CTJ can be challenging.[1,2] The CTJ can be defined as the region extending from C7 to T4, and it can be approached anteriorly via the supraclavicular, transmanubrial-transclavicular, or transsternal route. These approaches provide variable exposure to the upper thoracic region, and the choice of operative approach depends on the location of the pathological process.

The exposure provided by the supraclavicular approach is limited by the deep operative field. Further, the manubrium remains intact and shields T2 and the upper thoracic region. In contrast, the transmanubrial-transclavicular and transsternal approaches offer a perpendicular trajectory, thereby reducing the depth of the operative field (**Figs. 43.1** and **43.2**). The transmanubrial-transclavicular and transsternal approaches may be utilized for lesions extending to or below T2 or if a wider exposure is needed (e.g., obese patients and muscular patients with short necks). Depending on the location of the pathology, the focus and degree of sternal resection can be modified as needed. This chapter focuses on the transmanubrial-transclavicular and various transsternal approaches to expose the CTJ (see Chapter 42 for the supraclavicular approach).

With the transmanubrial-transclavicular approach, the medial third of the clavicle and a portion of the manubrium are removed.[3,4] This enables excellent exposure of the upper thoracic vertebrae and provides autologous bone for grafting. The exposure is limited by the amount of manubrium resected, as further resection can result in a larger manubrial defect and a higher risk of sternal nonunion. Multiple transsternal approaches that spare the sternoclavicular joint have been described, with a range in the extension of the sternotomy performed.[5-7] This also preserves the sternal and clavicular insertion of the sternocleidomastoid (SCM) muscle. Although these approaches are technically demanding, they can be both safe and effective when undertaken by an experienced surgeon.

Patient Selection

The transmanubrial-transclavicular and transsternal approaches may be employed to provide access to the lower thoracic region of the CTJ. These approaches can also be used if a wider exposure to the CTJ region is needed in patients with a short neck or significant kyphosis.

Indications

- Tumor
- Infection
- Structural deformity

Contraindications

- Obstruction by anomalies of great vessels
- Surgeon's lack of experience with regional anatomy
- Entail high surgical risks; therefore, benefits and life expectancy should be assessed

Objective

- To safely expose the targeted region in the CTJ while dissecting the sternum and clavicle only as necessary

Advantages

- Provides access to the anterior spinal column of the cervicothoracic region down to T3
- Enables simultaneous decompression and fixation
- Can preserve the SCM sternal insertion with the transsternal approach
- Can preserve the sternoclavicular joint with the transsternal approach

Disadvantages

- Anterior instrumentation at T4 is limited by the aortic arch.
- Posterior stabilization cannot be performed without repositioning the patient.
- The thecal sac is not visualized before performing a corpectomy.
- Risk of sternal nonunion and mediastinitis

Preoperative Imaging

- Anteroposterior and lateral X-rays
- Computed tomography (CT)
- Magnetic resonance imaging (MRI), especially with tumor pathology

Choice of Operative Approach

The anterior cervical region can be exposed with a supraclavicular, transmanubrial–transclavicular, or transsternal approach. Due to the steep surgical angle that is created with the supraclavicular method, the ability of anterior instrumentation along the T2 and T3 is limited. Therefore, the transmanubrial-transclavicular and transsternal approaches overcome this problem by

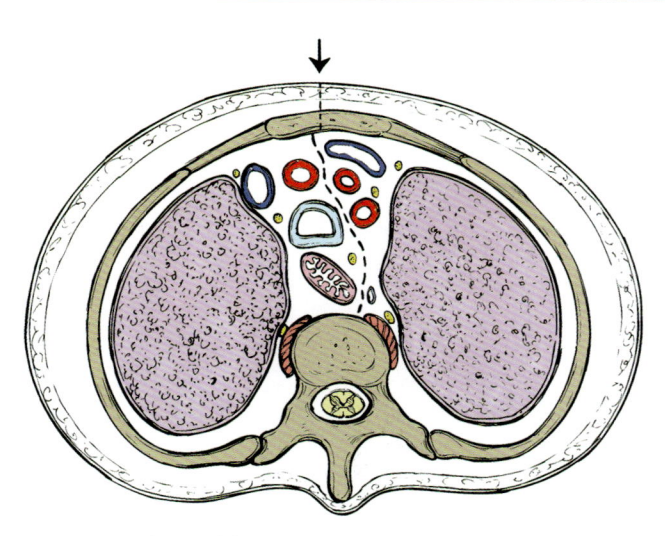

Fig. 43.1 Axial view of the anatomy at the second thoracic vertebrae. The *dashed line* represents the path taken from the manubrium to the vertebral body. The esophagus and trachea are dissected medially, whereas the contents of the carotid sheath are swept laterally.

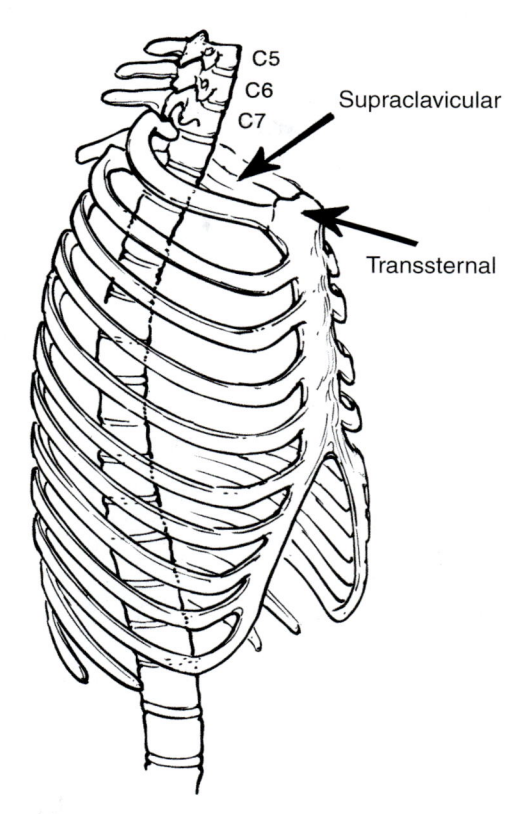

Fig. 43.2 The manubrium often shields the T1-2 intervertebral disk space. Consequently, the supraclavicular approach takes an acute angle over the sternal notch, making the placement of anterior plating difficult. The trajectory of the transsternal approach is perpendicular to the vertebral bodies. This reduces the depth of the operative field and facilitates anterior plating.

providing a perpendicular corridor. Preoperative CT and MRI help assess the need for a sternotomy. On CT, the lowest accessible disk space by the supraclavicular approach can be determined by drawing a straight line passing parallel through the disk space and above the manubrium.[8] On MRI, the location of the lesion relative to the cervicothoracic angle (angle formed between the axial plane of the suprasternal notch and the C7-T1 intervertebral disk) can be assessed to determine if a sternotomy is needed.[9]

The transmanubrial-transclavicular approach provides excellent exposure of the anterior vertebral bodies of the lower cervical vertebrae and T1-T3.[10] The vessels in the superior mediastinum are encountered when obtaining a more caudal exposure to T4, thereby limiting instrumentation in this region. A single- or double-sided clavicle resection can be employed depending on the exposure needed. Alternatively, the sternoclavicular joint can be spared by a partial manubriotomy.[11,12] Lesions found at the cervicothoracic region extending caudally to T5 may be resected with this approach. However, the resection of the clavicle significantly improves exposure and provides grafting material.

The transsternal approach spares the sternoclavicular attachments of the SCM muscle and sternoclavicular joint. This avoids compromising the function of the shoulder and potential cosmetic defects. A traditional sternotomy is limited by the aortic arch and great vessels, commonly located in the upper T5 region. The lower sternotomy does not significantly improve the exposure and carries higher operative mortality and morbidity. Although the vertebral level of the sternal angle varies between T2 and T7, it is most commonly at the T4 or T4-T5 intervertebral disk.[13] Therefore, the modified upper transsternal technique employs a sternotomy 2 cm distal to the sternal angle.[5–7] The final choice of the operative approach depends on the location of the pathological process and surgeon preference.

Surgical Technique

Anesthesia and Positioning

General anesthesia appropriate for electrophysiological monitoring is used. Fiberoptic intubation is performed when there is evidence of cervical spinal cord myelopathy, compression, or instability. The patient should undergo a neurologic exam before and after intubation to evaluate any changes. A nasogastric tube can be placed to help localize the esophagus. Subsequently, the neck of the patient is slightly hyperextended to facilitate exposure, and the head is turned contralateral to the approach. Straps are placed and the shoulders are pulled down. Lateral X-rays can then be used to localize the cervical pathology.

Transmanubrial-Transclavicular Approach

A curvilinear T-shaped incision is used for the transmanubrial approach.[14] This incision is usually 2 cm above the clavicle and extends to both sides of the SCM muscle (**Fig. 43.3**). The vertical portion of the incision extends down the midline and about halfway down the sternum. Subplatysmal flaps are created in a fashion similar to the classic anterior cervical approach. The supraclavicular nerves should be identified and protected. The external jugular veins and a portion of the jugular venous arch should be identified and mobilized. In some cases, these structures need to be sacrificed. A left-sided approach is preferred to limit the risk of damage to the recurrent laryngeal nerve.[15] However, a right-sided approach can be used if this nerve is suspected of having a potentially aberrant course.

The deep attachments of the SCM muscle are dissected, divided, and retracted laterally. In addition, the sternohyoid and sternothyroid muscles are dissected and reflected medially (**Fig. 43.4**). Careful attention must be given to the deep cervical fascia during the elevation of these muscles to minimize injury to the

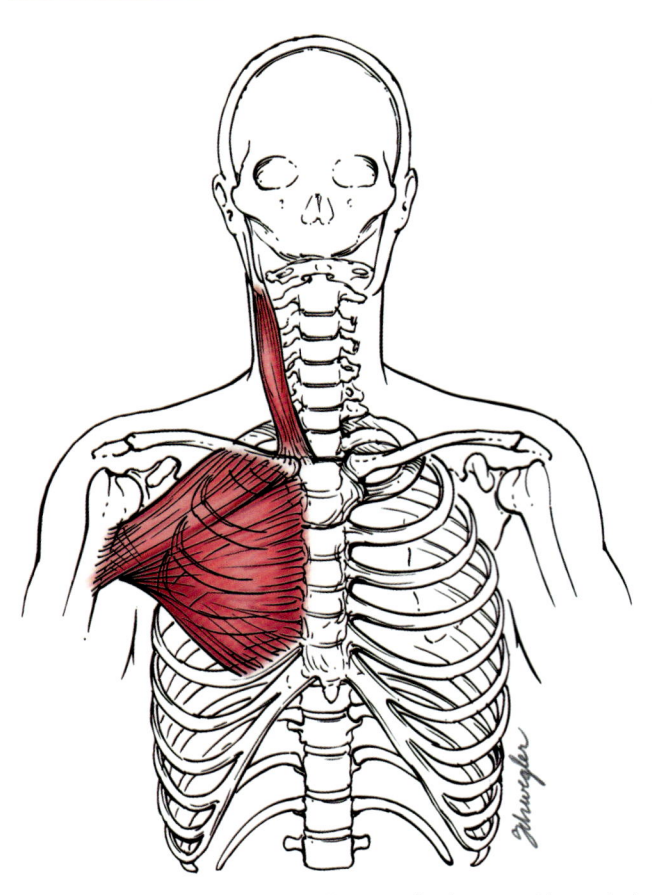

Fig. 43.3 The external landmarks relevant to the dissection. The cervical incision extends along the anterior border of the sternocleidomastoid muscle to the sternal notch. The thoracic incision extends to just past the junction of the manubrium and sternum.

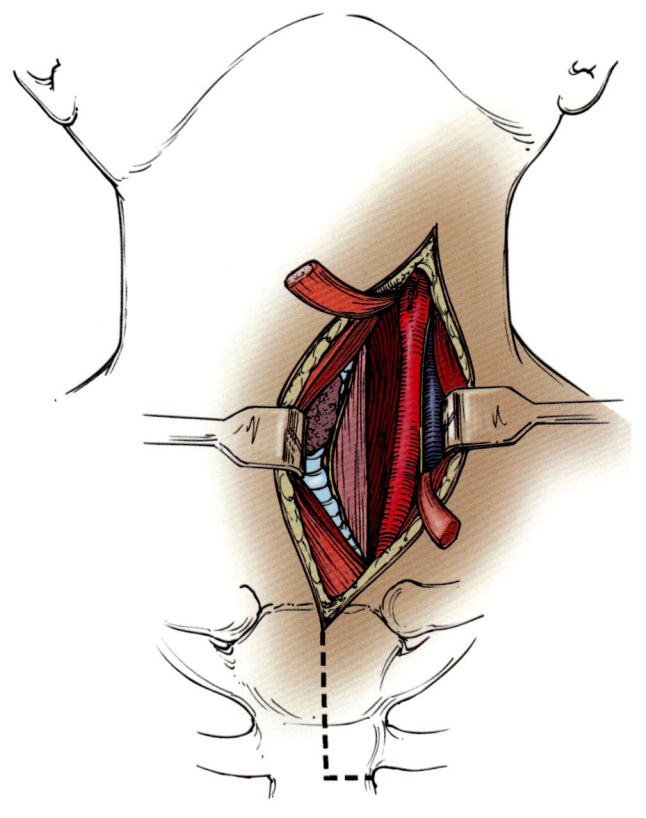

Fig. 43.4 The cervical dissection. The skin incision extends along the anterior border of the sternocleidomastoid muscle to the sternal notch. The platysma is divided. The omohyoid muscle is divided. The sternohyoid and sternothyroid muscles are identified at their sternal insertions. A plane is developed between the contents of the carotid sheath and the esophagus and trachea.

neurovascular bundles. The carotid plane is bluntly dissected, and the carotid sheath is retracted laterally. The suprasternal space is entered to complete the subperiosteal dissection. Once this is complete, the involved sternoclavicular attachment of the pectoralis major can be dissected.

Using a high-speed drill, resect the medial portion of the clavicle and then divide the first costal cartilage. The manubrium, sternoclavicular joint, and medial third of the clavicle can now be elevated with the SCM attached. One must exercise caution during this step to avoid injury to the underlying brachiocephalic and subclavian veins. Alternatively, the manubrium and medial clavicle can be resected with an osteotome and used for bone grafting (**Fig. 43.5**).

Deep dissection is continued until the greater vessels are identified and retracted caudally (**Fig. 43.6**). The inferior thyroid vessels can be ligated and divided if necessary. The pleural apices and Sibson's fascia (extension of transthoracic fascia) are also exposed. At this point, an avascular plane between the trachea and esophagus medially and the carotid sheath laterally is formed to enter the prevertebral space. Caudally, the surgical field is limited by the aortic arch and its branches at the T3 and T4 vertebrae. The prevertebral fascia is sharply dissected to expose the targeted vertebral bodies. A bent spinal needle can be used to identify the surgical level with fluoroscopy, followed by development of longus colli "cuffs" to place permanent retractor blades. These muscular cuffs help to protect the midline esophagus and lateral carotid sheath from injury.[16] The exposure can be further modified to the presenting pathology.

Transsternal Approach

A skin incision can be made along the anterior border of the left SCM muscle with a midline incision about halfway down the sternum. Subplatysmal dissection is performed, and the sternothyroid, sternohyoid, and omohyoid are identified. An avascular plane is created with the esophagus and trachea retracted medially, and the carotid sheath is retracted laterally, as described above.

The trans-upper-sternal approach is a partial sternotomy through the second intercostal space that can maximize exposure without being limited by the aorta and great vessels.[6,7] The sternotomy is extended transversely to the second intercostal space. This can be achieved with a unilateral (L-shaped) or bilateral (inverted T-shaped) dissection depending on the exposure needed. In performing a left unilateral transsternal approach, the left pectoralis major muscle is reflected to visualize the second intercostal space. Blunt finger dissection of the mediastinal contents from the inner table of the sternum is then performed.

After dissecting the upper anterior mediastinum, the sternum is then divided midline using a sternal saw. The dissection is carried caudally to a point 2 cm distal to the sternal angle. Gentle traction of the saw should be used, while being cautious

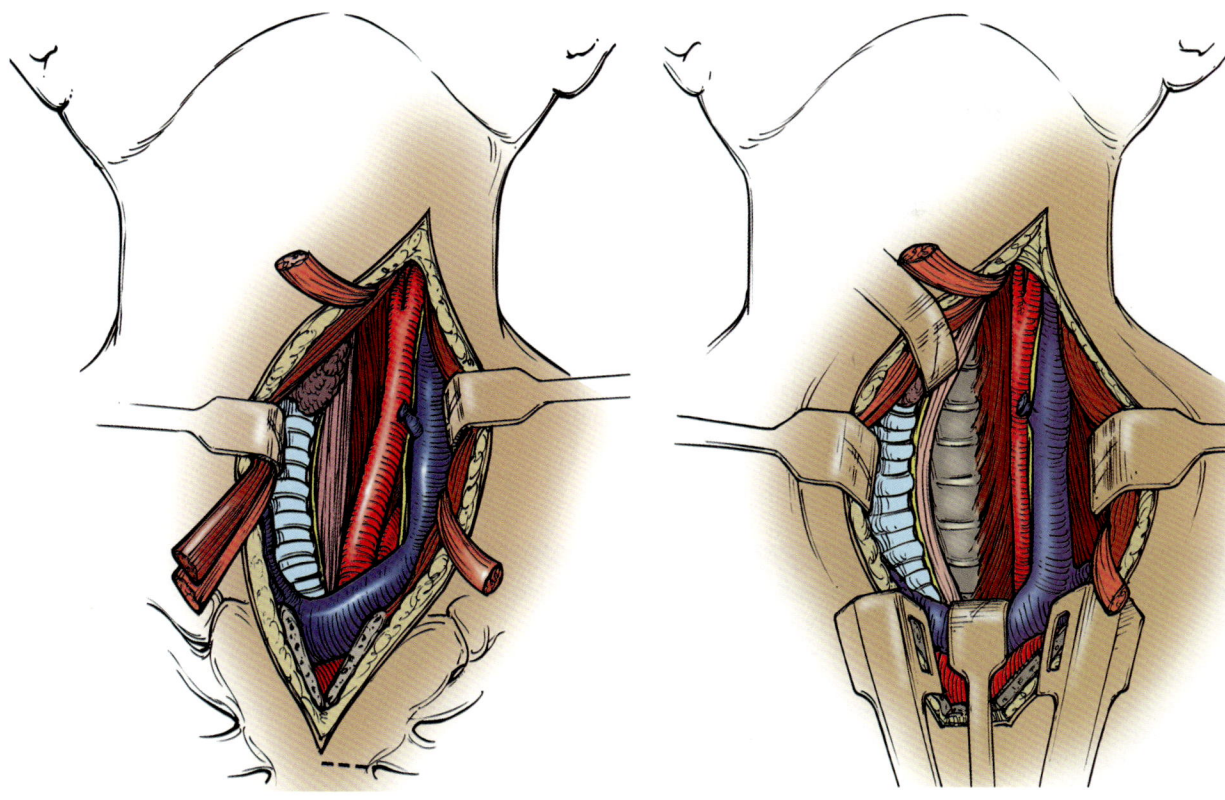

Fig. 43.5 A sternotomy is made just past the junction of the manubrium and sternum. The sternotomy is then extended to the left second intercostal space. Care must be taken to control the left internal mammary artery during this portion of the sternotomy. The sternohyoid and sternothyroid muscles are divided near their sternal insertions. The left innominate vein is identified. The left middle thyroid vein may be identified and ligated if the middle cervical spine is to be exposed. The prevertebral fascia and the longus colli muscles are identified.

Fig. 43.6 Gentle inferior retraction on the innominate vein reveals the third thoracic vertebra. Care must be taken to avoid overly vigorous caudal retraction on the innominate vein because the left recurrent laryngeal nerve travels from the aortic arch to the tracheoesophageal groove in this region.

of the underlying mediastinal structures and brachiocephalic vein. The left part of the sternum is then cut transversely in the second intercostal space, while being cautious of the internal mammary artery. Bleeding from the bone can be controlled with electrocautery, bone wax, and retractors. Excessive hemostatic methods may increase the risk for nonunion or pseudarthrosis.

At this point, the SCM is preserved while the sternothyroid and sternohyoid are dissected near the sternal region. This puts the cervical and thoracic regions in continuity. Retractors can be placed to provide access to the prevertebral fascia and sharply dissected as stated above. Extra care should be taken to avoid injury to the recurrent laryngeal nerve and subsequent injuries from vigorous retractions.

Closing

After appropriate bone grafting and instrumentation, the area is irrigated copiously with antibiotic-impregnated saline. Hemostasis is obtained, and fluoroscopy is used to confirm the placement of hardware or bone grafting. A Jackson-Pratt drain is placed at the time of closure to prevent postoperative hematoma formation. Further, if there is any evidence of pleural violation, a chest tube can be inserted through a separate stab wound. Subcutaneous and skin tissue is closed in a routine fashion and the manubrium can be reconstructed with mini-plates or sternal wires. A cervical brace can be placed, according to surgeon preference.

Postoperative Care

- Jackson-Pratt drain in place for 2 to 3 days after the operation
- Intensive care unit monitoring for a minimum of 24 hours
- Monitor for respiratory difficulties
- Physiotherapy

Potential Complications and Precautions

- Dissection of the manubrium and sternal splitting carries the risk of sternal nonunion and increases the risk for mediastinitis. The risk can be decreased by limiting the extension of the sternotomy and aggressive hemostasis.
- Shoulder-girdle weakness can occur with the transmanubrial-transclavicular approach. An isolated transmanubrial or modified transsternal approach may be employed to maintain the sternoclavicular joint.

- Soft tissue edema can occur with extensive pathology or prolonged surgeries. These patients require close observation in an intensive care unit setting in the immediate (24-hour) postoperative period.
- Hoarseness can occur due to traction on the recurrent laryngeal nerve. Monitor these patients closely and promote rapid mobilization, pulmonary toilet, and the utilization of speech therapy.
- Horner's syndrome can occur due to disruption of the sympathetic chain. This can be avoided by careful dissection on the lateral border of the longus colli.
- The thoracic duct is prone to potential injury with a left-sided approach. This should be identified at the junction with the internal jugular and subclavian veins.
- Internal mammary artery or intercostal neurovascular bundle injury can occur during resection or closure of the sternotomy. Keep the saw midline with gentle traction.
- Injury to the brachiocephalic vein can occur during instrumentation of the lower thoracic regions. This can be avoided by proper exposure and retraction techniques.

Conclusion

The challenges in the surgical exposure of the anterior CTJ can be overcome with the transmanubrial-transclavicular and transsternal approaches. They offer more exposure at the lower cervicothoracic regions down to T3-T4 while providing a perpendicular corridor. Perioperative complications can be prevented with careful attention to detail in the surgical anatomy. **Box 43.1** summarizes the key operative steps and the problems that can arise.

Box 43.1 Key Operative Steps and Potential Problems

Step	Problems
Transmanubrial-transclavicular	
Resection of the clavicle or disarticulation of the sternoclavicular joint	Injury to subclavian vessels
Resection of the manubrium for further exposure	Larger manubrial defect and higher risk for sternal nonunion The brachiocephalic and aortic vessels may be found higher (T2 instead of T3-T4) in patients with kyphosis
Transsternal	
Sternal saw midline and transversely to the second intercostal space	Injury to underlying mediastinal structures Injury to the internal mammary artery
Caudal retraction on the left brachiocephalic vein	Injury to the left recurrent laryngeal nerve that travels from the aortic arch to the tracheoesophageal groove
Both	
Left-side incision	Thoracic duct injury Recurrent laryngeal nerve injury (higher risk with right-sided approach)
Dissection medial to the SCM	Dissection posterior to the SCM can result in spinal accessory nerve injury
Disarticulation of the clavicle	Subclavian vein injury
Omohyoid and sternohyoid divided	Phrenic nerve injury
Carotid sheath retracted laterally	Recurrent laryngeal nerve injury Dissection lateral to caudal portion of the carotid sheath can cause injury to thoracic duct, internal jugular and brachiocephalic vein, subclavian artery and vein, thyrocervical trunk, and inferior thyroid artery
Dissection lateral to longus colli	Cervical sympathetic ganglion disruption causing unilateral Horner's syndrome

References

1. Wang VY, Chou D. The cervicothoracic junction. Neurosurg Clin N Am 2007;18:365–371
2. An HS, Vaccaro A, Cotler JM, Lin S. Spinal disorders at the cervicothoracic junction. Spine 1994;19:2557–2564
3. Sundaresan N, Shah J, Foley KM, Rosen G. An anterior surgical approach to the upper thoracic vertebrae. J Neurosurg 1984;61:686–690
4. Sundaresan N, Shah J, Feghali JG. A transsternal approach to the upper thoracic vertebrae. Am J Surg 1984;148:473–477
5. Darling GE, McBroom R, Perrin R. Modified anterior approach to the cervicothoracic junction. Spine 1995;20:1519–1521
6. Liu YL, Hao YJ, Li T, Song YM, Wang LM. Trans-upper-sternal approach to the cervicothoracic junction. Clin Orthop Relat Res 2009;467:2018–2024
7. Luk KD, Cheung KM, Leong JC. Anterior approach to the cervicothoracic junction by unilateral or bilateral manubriotomy. A report of five cases. J Bone Joint Surg Am 2002;84-A:1013–1017
8. Karikari IO, Powers CJ, Isaacs RE. Simple method for determining the need for sternotomy/manubriotomy with the anterior approach to the cervicothoracic junction. Neurosurgery 2009;65(6, Suppl):E165–E166, discussion E166
9. Teng H, Hsiang J, Wu C, et al. Surgery in the cervicothoracic junction with an anterior low suprasternal approach alone or combined with manubriotomy and sternotomy: an approach selection method based on the cervicothoracic angle. J Neurosurg Spine 2009;10:531–542
10. Kaya RA, Türkmenoğlu ON, Koç ON, et al. A perspective for the selection of surgical approaches in patients with upper thoracic and cervicothoracic junction instabilities. Surg Neurol 2006;65:454–463, discussion 463
11. Pointillart V, Aurouer N, Gangnet N, Vital JM. Anterior approach to the cervicothoracic junction without sternotomy: a report of 37 cases. Spine 2007;32:2875–2879
12. Lam FC, Groff MW. An anterior approach to spinal pathology of the upper thoracic spine through a partial manubriotomy. J Neurosurg Spine 2011;15:467–471
13. Mirjalili SA, Hale SJ, Buckenham T, Wilson B, Stringer MD. A reappraisal of adult thoracic surface anatomy. Clin Anat 2012;25:827–834
14. Khoo L, Samudrala S. Transmanubrial transclavicular approach to the cervicothoracic junction. In: Fessler R, Sekhar L, ed. Atlas of Neurosurgical Techniques: Spine and Peripheral Nerves. New York: Thieme; 2006
15. Sundaresan N, DiGiacinto GV. Surgical approaches to the cervicothoracic junction. In: Sundaresan N, Schmidek, HH, Schiller AL, Rosenthal DI, eds. Tumors of the Spine. Philadelphia: WB Saunders; 1990:358–368
16. Albert T. Relevant cervical anatomy and anterior, middle, and lower cervical exposures. In: Albert T, Balderston, RA, Northrup, BE, eds. Surgical Approaches to the Spine. Philadelphia: WB Saunders; 1997

44 Cervicothoracic Corpectomy

Robert F. Heary and John C. Quinn

Surgical treatment of cervicothoracic junction (CTJ) pathology poses several technical challenges due to the complex regional anatomy and unique biomechanical forces that exist in this region. Common pathologies encountered include primary or metastatic tumors, infections, or traumatic injuries. The majority of pathological processes occurring at the CTJ originate in the vertebral body. When these pathological processes result in compression of the spinal cord or significant junctional instability from loss of anterior column integrity, then frequently anterior decompression, stabilization, and fusion are indicated.

Ventral access to the CTJ enables simultaneously decompressing the neural elements and reconstructing the anterior column of the spine. At the CTJ, ventral access can be broadly divided into anterior and posterolateral exposures. A thorough discussion of the advantages and disadvantages of the various direct anterior and indirect posterolateral approaches are beyond the scope of this chapter. This chapter discusses the general techniques for performing a cervicothoracic corpectomy, including diskectomy, corpectomy, and end-plate preparation, as well as the specific techniques and technical considerations when performing a corpectomy following a direct anterior decompression and an indirect decompression following a posterolateral exposure.

Indications

- Vertebral body neoplasm: primary or metastasis
- Vertebral osteomyelitis or Pott's disease (tuberculosis)
- Vertebral body fracture with gross instability or spinal cord compression
- Fixed kyphotic deformity
- Ventrally situated extramedullary tumors
- Mediastinal tumor with contiguous vertebral body extension

Contraindications

- Poor medical condition
- Short life expectancy

Advantages

- Decompression of ventral compression (direct or indirect)
- Immediate reconstruction of anterior vertebral column
- Ventral release of fixed kyphotic deformity

Disadvantages

- Challenging exposures due to thoracic/mediastinal structures
- Potential need for additional posterior stabilization
- Risks injury to recurrent laryngeal nerve, thoracic duct, and sympathetic chain

Anterior Approach for Corpectomy

Anterior approaches to the CTJ require precise knowledge of the complex regional anatomy and careful preoperative planning. Despite modern tools and techniques, simultaneous exposure of the lower cervical and upper thoracic spine is technically difficult. Wide anterior exposure to this area is limited by the great vessels, clavicle, sternum, rib cage, thoracic duct, laryngeal nerves, sympathetic chain, esophagus, and trachea.[1,2] Complete descriptions of the techniques for anterior exposure to the cervicothoracic spine have been discussed in the previous chapters. In brief, the three main anterior approaches are (1) the modified low cervical supraclavicular approach, (2) the transmanubrial/transsternal/transclavicular approach, and (3) the transthoracic approach.[3,4]

In most patients, a standard low-cervical supraclavicular approach provides adequate exposure down to the T1 vertebral level. In patients with long necks, it may be possible to expose down to the T2 vertebral level. A significant limitation in using a supraclavicular approach to the proximal thoracic region is the steep working angle due to obstruction from the manubrium as well as the upper thoracic kyphosis. Furthermore, the great majority of pathologies treated surgically in this area are kyphogenic, which can make the working angles even more difficult than they would normally be. This difficult working angle impedes direct visualization and often makes decompression and instrumentation challenging. In general, with anterior exposures of the CTJ, the degree of upper thoracic exposure is limited by the size and position of the anterior bony thorax. Magnetic resonance imaging (MRI) studies have shown that while T3 was often cranial to the sternal notch, a straight trajectory was often limited to the T1-2 disk space in the vast majority of people.[5]

Limitations in visualization and surgical corridors caused by anterior chest wall structures may be addressed through the transmanubrial/transsternal approaches, which are greatly facilitated by the use of preoperative traction that can help to improve the kyphotic angulation and the working angle. These more extensive approaches provide a wide, direct exposure down to the T4 vertebral level through a surgical corridor that is relatively perpendicular to the vertebral bodies. This direct access is created by disruption or resection of bony anterior thoracic structures (sternum, manubrium, clavicle) and ligamentous structures. These approaches provide excellent visualization and improved surgical corridors, but can be associated significant morbidity. As a general rule, consideration should be given to enlisting assistance from cardiothoracic surgeons who routinely utilize this

44 Cervicothoracic Corpectomy

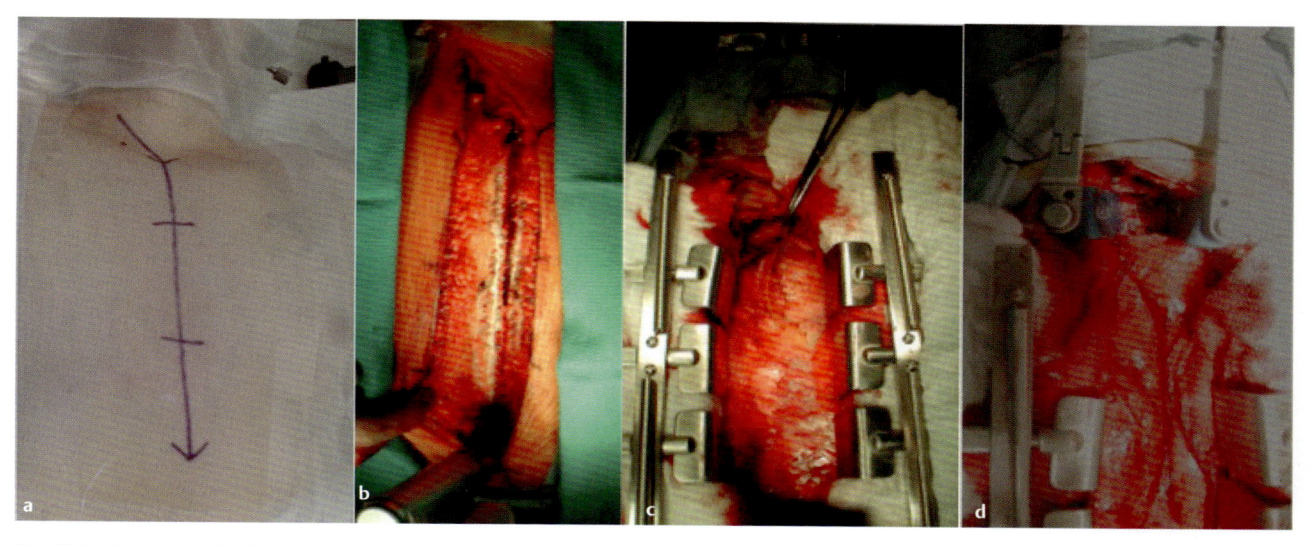

Fig. 44.1 Anterior cervicothoracic exposure: intraoperative photographs. **(a,b)** The positioning and incision for a transsternal approach for a T1 corpectomy. **(c,d)** Following a complete sternotomy, cervical and sternal retractors provide improved exposure to the ventral cervicothoracic junction (CTJ).

approach for coronary artery bypass surgeries. Other modifications such as the transmanubrial/transclavicular approach can provide visualization and access to the T3 vertebral level; however, this approach requires resection of the medial clavicle and sternoclavicular joint. In our experience, surgical disruption of the sternoclavicular joint is associated with greater morbidity than is a routine transsternal operative approach.[4] Similar exposure can be gained using a sternal-splitting approach when combined with the anteromedial approach through retraction of the great vessels. The posterior transthoracic approach enables reasonable access to the upper thoracic spine; however, this technique provides visualization that is often limited to the T1 vertebral body.

Anterior Thoracic Approach (Fig. 44.1)

Full descriptions of the various anterior approaches to the CTJ are discussed in Chapters 42, 43, and 45. This chapter discusses the steps in performing a corpectomy and preparing for anterior column reconstruction. It must be emphasized that an adequate, unobstructed exposure of the ventral vertebral bodies is essential prior to beginning the decompression and reconstruction.

Corpectomy Following Anterior Approach (Fig. 44.2)

Once the exposure has been completed, and the vertebral column visualized, a spinal needle should be placed in the most rostral structure exposed for a localizing radiograph. To avoid operating on the wrong level, the radiograph should extend superiorly into the lower cervical spine to count down from a known, radiographically confirmed, vertebral level. This ensures that the spinal needle will be well visualized for the localizing radiograph and not obscured by the shoulders.

Once the correct level has been identified, the disk spaces are marked with electrocautery. The prevertebral fascia and the

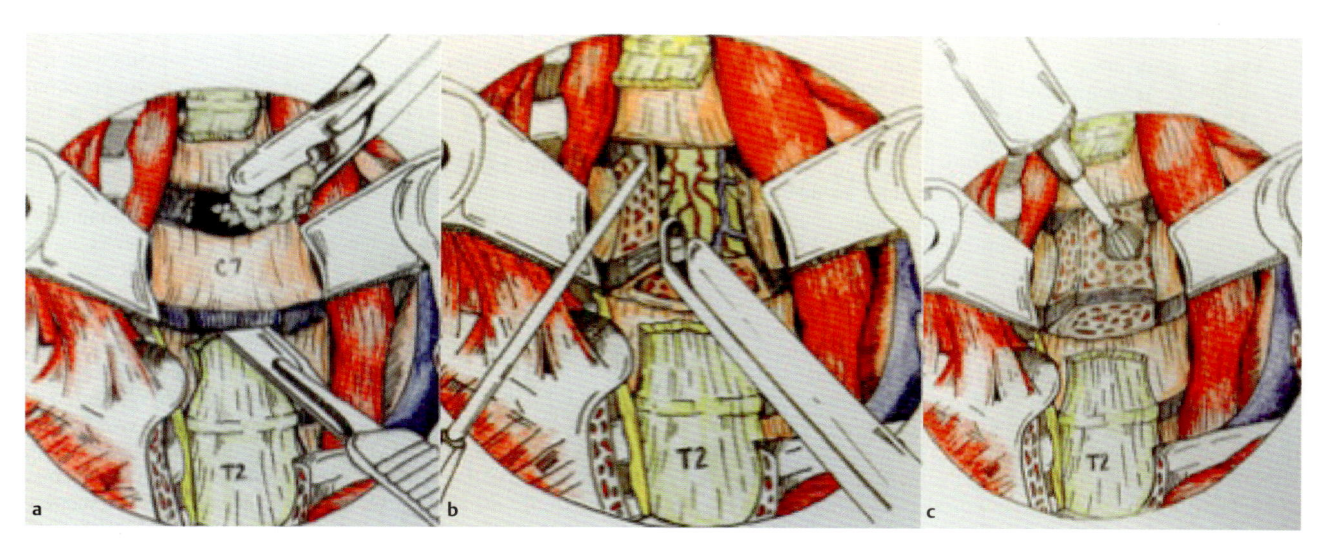

Fig. 44.2 Anterior cervicothoracic corpectomy. **(a)** Proximal and distal diskectomy using a high-speed drill. **(b,c)** The anterior cortical and cancellous bone are removed with either a drill or a rongeur, and the posterior cortex of the bone is routinely removed using the high-speed drill.

longus colli muscles are dissected away from the underlying bone and reflected laterally using both sharp dissection and bipolar cautery. Care must be taken to avoid injury to the esophagus medially and the carotid vessels laterally. Self-retaining retractors are placed after adequate lateral mobilization of the longus colli muscles in the manner that is familiar to most spine surgeons who perform the more common anterior cervical spine surgeries. Incomplete mobilization of the longus colli muscles may prevent secure anchoring of the retractor systems with the attendant risk of dislodgment or rotation of the retractor blades during surgery. Accidental dislodgment during surgery can damage critical structures in the operative field and must be avoided. The operating microscope may be introduced in the operative field at any time after the retractors are in place. We have found that a focal length of 500 mm is ideal for this approach to ensure that the surgical tools are able to be properly utilized. The operating microscope is useful in facilitating disk and vertebral body removal, as it provides excellent visualization of the spatial relationship between the instruments and the thecal sac, and 3D views of the surgical corridor.

Soft tissues remaining on the ventral aspect of the vertebral body of interest, and the vertebral bodies above and below, are cleared from end plate to end plate using a combination of monopolar cautery, curettage, and rongeurs. This exposes the position of the rostral and caudal vertebral bodies for eventual placement of a ventral stabilization plate. Performing this adjacent segment preparation, at this stage of the procedure, is easier than if it is done after the bony decompression is completed, as bleeding from the corpectomy site may obscure visualization during this process. Next, when technically feasible, distraction pins are inserted at the midpoint of the vertebral bodies above and below the planned corpectomy site. These pins should be placed as perpendicular to the vertebral body as possible. Gentle distraction across the corpectomy defect facilitates the decompression by opening the disk spaces while performing the diskectomies and aids in strut graft placement following the corpectomy. Slight distraction across the corpectomy enables placement of a slightly oversized strut graft by increasing the distance between the adjacent vertebral bodies, which upon release of the distraction will seat the anterior strut under compression. Either a structural bone graft or a cage filled with bone can be used as a strut in this location. Segmental distraction is also useful in cases of angular kyphotic deformity. Distraction following anterior release results in reduction of the kyphosis through improved alignment of the vertebral bodies in plane with the distraction.

Diskectomies are performed above and below the level of the planned corpectomy. Each disk space is incised with a scalpel and extended to the lateral border of the uncovertebral joints. Similarly to how this is performed in the cervical spine, these uncovertebral joints can be identified by the upward course of the end plates and will demarcate the lateral borders of the decompression. As the width of the spinal cord is routinely in the vicinity of 13 mm in this location, the decompression performed in this manner typically spans 17 to 18 mm to ensure that the spinal cord has been adequately decompressed. Removal of disk material is then performed using a combination of rongeurs, up-biting curettes, and pituitary rongeurs. A thorough diskectomy at the rostral and caudal disk spaces enables identifying the end plates above and below the area of planned resection and helps to prevent inadvertent violation of the end plates during the corpectomy. Removal of the disk is performed dorsally to the level of the posterior longitudinal ligament (PLL). Identification of the PLL prior to beginning the corpectomy facilitates an expeditious bony resection, as the depth of decompression is well visualized and appreciated.

Before starting the corpectomy, it is important to identify the borders of the planned bony resection. All remaining soft tissues overlying the vertebral body should be cleared to identify the lateral borders of the decompression to ensure a symmetric, rectangular decompression. Once the boundaries are identified, the vertebral body is resected using either rongeurs or a high-speed drill with a round cutting bur. We have found that utilization of a large, round bur (7 mm) improves the safety of the procedure by lessening the likelihood of an inadvertent slip. It may be appropriate to use a Leksell rongeur to initiate the corpectomy in order maintain a rectangular configuration of the region to be decompressed. Creating a rectangular decompression bed serves to ensure the adequacy of the decompression and creates an excellent graft recipient site.

After the anterior cortical and cancellous bone are removed, with either a drill or a rongeur, the posterior cortex of the bone is routinely removed using the high-speed drill. The posterior cortical bone should be drilled down to a very thin plate that can be easily removed using an upbiting curette or a thin Kerrison rongeur. The PLL is then lifted with a nerve hook and a small Kerrison is used to remove the PLL and bone fragments. The adequacy of decompression is judged by carefully sliding a blunt nerve hook under the superior and inferior vertebral bodies. After adequate bony resection, decompression, and removal of all devitalized bone and pathological tissue, the PLL is resected to expose the dura. Any tumor or bone impinging on the dural sac or nerve roots is carefully removed. In tumor cases, the goal of surgery should be a radical tumor resection and neural decompression. In patients who have previously received radiation therapy and in some sarcoma cases, the PLL may be adherent to the dura, making this part of the dissection particularly challenging. In these cases, it may be advisable to leave the PLL in place to avoid creating a dural tear. In most primary cases, the dissection plane between the tumor and the dura can be readily defined to assist in removal of the necessary structures.

End-Plate Preparation

Once an adequate decompression has been completed, the corpectomy defect is prepared for anterior column reconstruction. Commonly, this involves a structural strut graft along with fusion substrate. In cases of malignancy, where the life expectancy is less than 1 year, the goals of reconstruction are slightly different. In those instances, immediate, durable stability, and the ability to withstand the effects of radiation and or resist tumor invasion are paramount.

Whether or not a fusion is anticipated, the end plates of the vertebral bodies adjacent to the decompression site are prepared to accept a structural graft. The central portion of the end plates should be burred down to bleeding cancellous bone to promote fusion, if that is a goal. Care is taken to attempt to preserve the bony end plates around the periphery of the vertebral body in the area that will align with the cortical portion of a bone graft or with the edges of a cage. Flat surfaces should be developed to accept a graft with flat ends, thereby maximizing contact between the graft and host bone. A small posterior lip (2 or 3 mm) can be left in place to prevent graft intrusion into the spinal canal. Similarly, a small anterior lip may remain to prevent anterior graft extrusion. During end-plate drilling, the underlying cancellous bone should not be exposed by complete removal of the end plates. Destruction of the bony end plates will lead to reduction of the mechanical strength of the vertebral body and increase the risk that a loss of the strength of the vertebral body will occur. It will also increase the risk of the graft telescoping into or penetrating the weakened vertebral bodies. During end-plate preparation, it is important to keep in mind that the rostral and caudal end plates are of different shapes, and selective drilling must be used to ensure that the graft site has parallel surfaces with adequate cortical bone remaining to support the graft. One common mistake is the failure to remove sufficient ventral and dorsal end-plate lip, resulting in a central gap between the bone graft and the vertebral end plate. Another mistake that has more serious consequences is the "ramp effect," which occurs when excessive bone is removed from the ventral two thirds of the lower vertebral body. This excessive removal results in a graft site that is longer ventrally than dorsally, and this potentially predisposes to ventral dislocation of the graft.

Posterolateral Approach for Corpectomy (Fig. 44.3)

Direct anterior approaches to the CTJ can be challenging due to the complex anatomy of the bony thorax, great vessels, and mediastinal structures. As an alternative, posterolateral approaches have been developed to address CTJ pathology. Advantages of posterolateral approaches include the ability to decompress ventral pathology, to reconstruct the anterior column, and to place posterior instrumentation in a single stage. A major disadvantage of these techniques is the limited visualization of the neural elements during the decompression, relying instead on indirect decompression. Posterolateral approaches to the CTJ include the transpedicular approach, costotransversectomy, lateral extracavitary approach (LECA), and the lateral parascapular extrapleural approach.[2,6,7] Complete descriptions of the posterolateral approaches are found in Chapter 46. These techniques differ in the degree of lateral mobilization of parascapular musculature, and the removal of posterior spinal elements and costovertebral articulations. These approaches provide varying degrees of visualization, and the ease of vertebral body resection, reconstruction, and correction of kyphotic deformity also varies. Because of the limited viewing angle provided through these approaches, ventral decompression is often performed without direct visualization, which can increase the risk of neurologic injury. Anterior column lesions are often resected in a piecemeal fashion, through these approaches, and anterior column reconstruction may prove difficult.

The same basic principles and surgical techniques are applied when performing a corpectomy whether from an anterior or posterolateral approach. The major difference in the operative anatomy between the direct anterior approaches and the posterolateral approaches is the relationship of the vertebral body within the surgical corridor. In anterior approaches the decompression can be performed with a direct or slightly oblique view of the vertebral body and the neural elements. In posterolateral approaches this corridor is oblique, resulting in significantly limited direct anterior column visualization. Improved visualization of the lateral vertebral body can be attained by performing more extensive procedures including the LECA and the lateral parascapular approach. Bilateral exposures can also be used for improved circumferential anterior column access.

The different posterolateral approaches have unique anatomic constraints due to the complexity of the CTJ. One common anatomic constraint for posterolateral approaches is the presence of exiting spinal nerves within the surgical corridor. The presence of the spinal nerve root requires mobilization or sacrifice of thoracic spinal nerves in cases of en-bloc resection or extensive anterior reconstruction. Below T1, these nerve roots may be resected with limited clinical consequences, although care must be taken to cut the nerve proximal to the dorsal root ganglion to prevent the development of severe neuropathic pain.

Posterolateral Corpectomy (Fig. 44.4)

Following exposure, the intervertebral disks above and below the involved vertebral body are identified and incised initially by sharp dissection. Disk material is cleared with curettes and pituitary rongeurs. Removing the rib head enables identification of the ipsilateral pedicle and its continuation into the vertebral body. The pedicle is an important marker for the orientation and position of the spinal canal. Using sharp curettes, rongeurs, and a high-speed drill, the vertebral body is resected ventrally to dorsally, except for a rim of the ventral portion of the vertebral body. This rim protects the aorta and inferior vena cava from accidental trauma. Resection of the vertebral body can progress as far as the anatomic midline. For the entire dorsal aspect of the vertebral body to be removed, typically bilateral pedicle removal

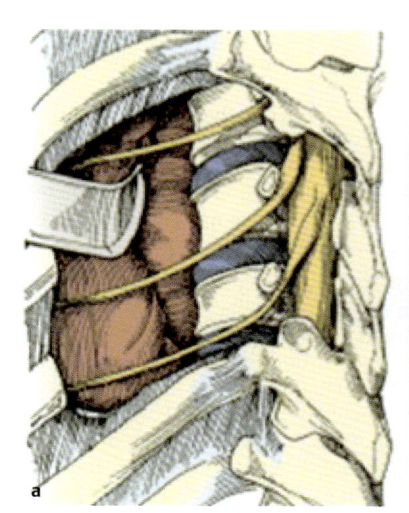

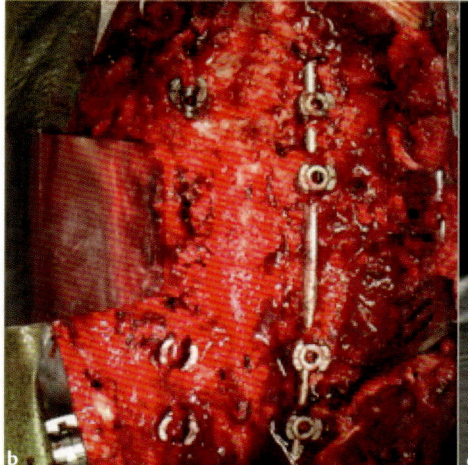

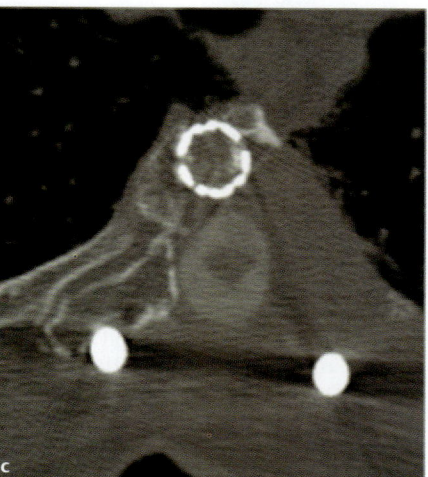

Fig. 44.3 Posterolateral cervicothoracic corpectomy: posterolateral approach to the CTJ. **(a)** Artist rendering demonstrating the operative exposure of a posterolateral approach for a thoracic corpectomy. **(b)** Intraoperative photograph demonstrating a multilevel posterolateral (lateral extracavitary) exposure for multilevel thoracic corpectomy. **(c)** An axial computed tomography (CT) scan following posterolateral corpectomy demonstrating the area of bone removed following a unilateral approach.

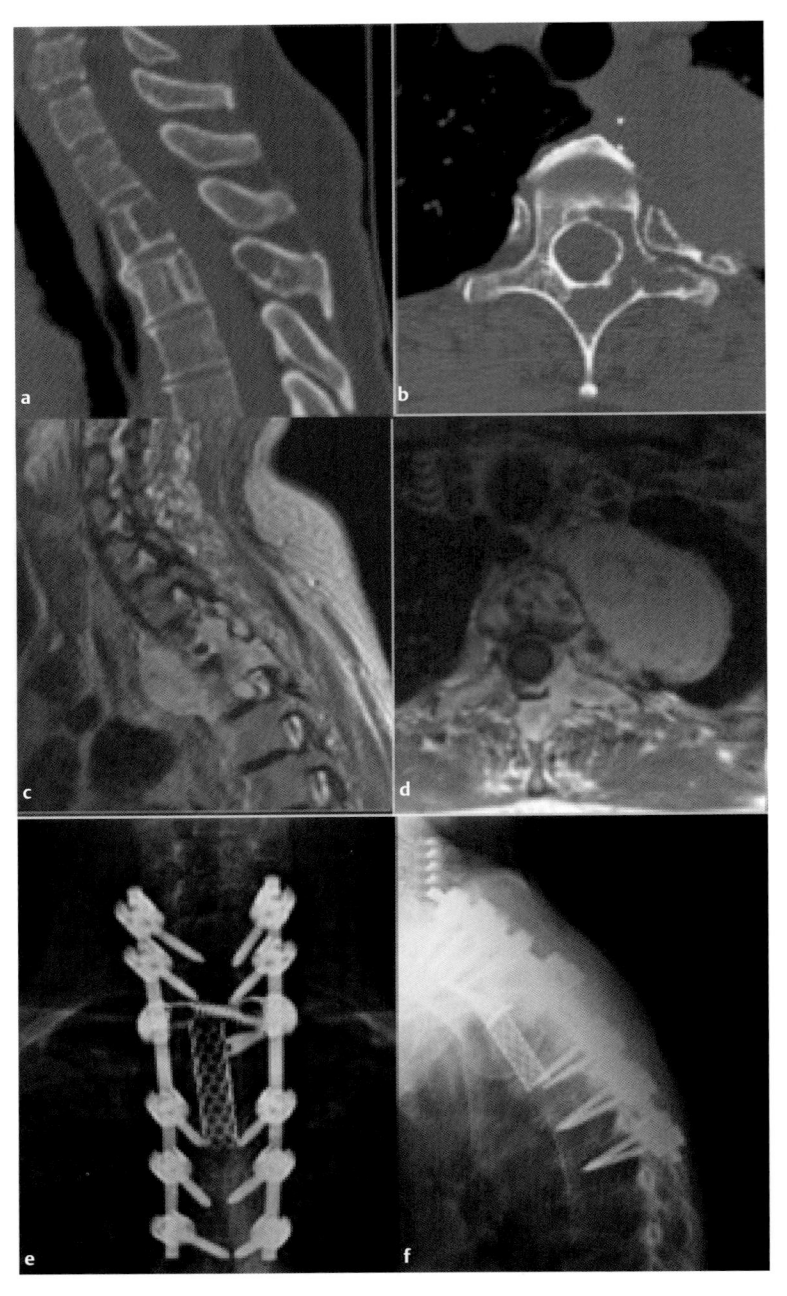

Fig. 44.4 Illustrative case of a 51-year-old woman with a capillary hemangioma involving the left thoracic apex, with extension into the ventral and dorsal elements of T2-T3. A sagittal and axial CT scan **(a,b)** and magnetic resonance imaging (MRI) with gadolinium **(c,d)** demonstrating an osteolytic, contrast-enhancing soft tissue mass involving the left thoracic apex with extension into the ventral and dorsal element of T2 and T3. The patient underwent a T2-T3 posterolateral corpectomy with posterior instrumentation of C7–T6. **(e,f)** Postoperative anteroposterior and lateral X-rays showing maintenance of sagittal and coronal balance.

is necessary. Sufficient bone needs to be removed to clear the PLL of any compression of the dura. The dissection can also be continued dorsolaterally to enable decompression of the spinal nerve roots. The tumor involvement and the quality of the residual bone for instrumentation determine the extent of bone removal.

Similar to anterior approaches, special care is afforded to the cartilaginous end plates and the central regions of cancellous bone of vertebral bodies adjacent to the corpectomy site. Removal is performed using a small high-speed bur or curette or osteotomes and rongeurs, depending on the bone consistency. This enables troughs to be created in the vertebral bodies above and below the corpectomy site to allow subsequent reconstruction with a bone graft, an implant, or an acrylic graft. Preparing the end plates to accommodate the construct requires special attention. In cases where bony fusion is the ultimate goal, the end plates require adequate vascular supply for achieving fusion, so aggressive decortication should be minimized. Posterior upper thoracic corpectomy for metastatic tumor resection is one of the few indications we have found for the use of expandable metallic cages. The cage can be delivered between the nerve roots into the ideal location and then expanded until it achieves adequate purchase on the adjacent vertebrae.

References

1. An HS, Wise JJ, Xu R. Anatomy of the cervicothoracic junction: a study of cadaveric dissection, cryomicrotomy, and magnetic resonance imaging. J Spinal Disord 1999;12:519–525
2. Mazel C, Hoffmann E, Antonietti P, Grunenwald D, Henry M, Williams J. Posterior cervicothoracic instrumentation in spine tumors. Spine 2004;29:1246–1253
3. Darling GE, McBroom R, Perrin R. Modified anterior approach to the cervicothoracic junction. Spine 1995;20:1519–1521
4. Sundaresan N, Shah J, Foley KM, Rosen G. An anterior surgical approach to the upper thoracic vertebrae. J Neurosurg 1984;61:686–690
5. Sharan AD, Przybylski GJ, Tartaglino L. Approaching the upper thoracic vertebrae without sternotomy or thoracotomy: a radiographic analysis with clinical application. Spine 2000;25:910–916
6. Fessler RG, Dietze DD Jr, Millan MM, Peace D. Lateral parascapular extrapleural approach to the upper thoracic spine. J Neurosurg 1991;75:349–355
7. Kraus DH, Huo J, Burt M. Surgical access to tumors of the cervicothoracic junction. Head Neck 1995;17:131–136

45 Anterior Reconstruction Following Cervicothoracic Corpectomy

Robert F. Heary and John C. Quinn

Cervicothoracic corpectomy for the treatment of tumor, infection, and traumatic fractures, or for deformity correction, can lead to significant instability. Although most causes of junctional instability can be managed with posterior instrumentation alone, anterior column reconstruction may be indicated after some anterior decompression procedures as well as traumatic or pathological processes that result in three-column instability.

Indications

- Anterior corpectomy for mass lesions
- Traumatic three-column instability
- Fixed kyphotic deformity

Goals of Reconstruction

Regardless of the primary pathological process, the primary goal of reconstruction is to achieve a stable spine that preserves neurologic integrity, is not painful, and maintains alignment without deformity. The ultimate goal of spinal column reconstruction depends on the nature of the lesion and the patient's life expectancy. In cases of trauma, benign lesions, or for patients with malignant tumors who have a relatively long life expectancy (> 2 years), the goal of anterior reconstruction is to provide three-column support, to correct or maintain appropriate alignment, and to promote bony fusion. In most cases where fusion is a primary goal, ventral instrumentation is utilized to promote graft incorporation by providing immediate stability at the bone–graft interface.

In patients with malignant processes (life expectancy < 1 year) a bony fusion would be inhibited by the use of adjunctive radiation or chemotherapy as well as the generally poor systemic health and nutritional status of these patients. In these patients, the primary goal of anterior reconstruction is to provide immediate structural support to alleviate pain and to prevent deformity or neurologic demise, without the expectation of achieving a bony fusion.

Reconstruction Considerations

Selection of Strut Graft (Fig. 45.1)

The appropriate type of material to use for spinal column reconstruction depends on the nature of the lesion and the patient's life expectancy. In cases of trauma or benign lesions, or for patients with malignant tumors who have a relatively long life expectancy, graft options for anterior column reconstruction include iliac crest autograft, allograft struts, or the use of an interbody cage filled with autogenous bone. Each graft alternative has unique advantages and disadvantages. Autogenous iliac crest bone graft is considered the gold standard against which all other graft options are measured. Iliac crest bone graft facilitates a faster biological incorporation and is less expensive; however, additional donor-site morbidity, including chronic pain and other complications, may occur.[1] A tricortical iliac crest bone graft can be used for up to a two-level corpectomy; however, multilevel corpectomy defects may necessitate fibular or other structural allografts. Although allograft struts may have greater immediate biomechanical strength than an autologous iliac crest, the high cortical bone content means that it may take up to a full year for the graft to incorporate. Supplemental local autograft including local bone from any vertebral body bone that is not involved in the pathological process may enhance the rate of fusion when using allografts.

In patients with malignant disease and a short life expectancy, autogenous bone grafts may have certain disadvantages. The use of radiation or chemotherapy will slow or prevent the bony fusion needed for stability, leading to graft failure. Additionally, incorporation of autogenous bone may serve as a site for local recurrence in cases of subtotal tumor resections. For patients with an expected survival of 18 months or less, a synthetic construct using polymethylmethacrylate (PMMA), with or without additional synthetic interbody cages or expandable cages, provides immediate structural stability.[2]

Interbody Cages

Use of prefabricated interbody cages has become a popular alternative to structural autograft or allograft for anterior column reconstructions. Interbody cages have been developed using a variety of materials including machined allograft, titanium, polyetheretherketone (PEEK), carbon fiber, and trabecular metal as well as expandable cages. A major advantage in the use of interbody cages is the ability to provide immediate structural stability irrespective of the patient's bone quality. Interbody cages are designed to prevent migration, and can simplify graft sizing and fitting. Titanium mesh cylindrical cages (Harms cages) are frequently used for anterior column reconstruction at the cervicothoracic junction. These mesh cages are implanted in a vertical orientation between the vertebral end plates of a corpectomy defect. In addition to overcoming issues of availability and morphology that constrain the application of structural autograft, the mesh cage is versatile with respect to diameter, length, and shape, and it enables the surgeon to make modifications to the inclination of its footplates to match the sagittal alignment of the adjacent vertebral end plates. Morselized, nonstructural autograft or allograft can be packed into and around the cage, and this promotes solid osseous union and eventually leads to long-term stability. The disadvantages of using prefabricated inter-

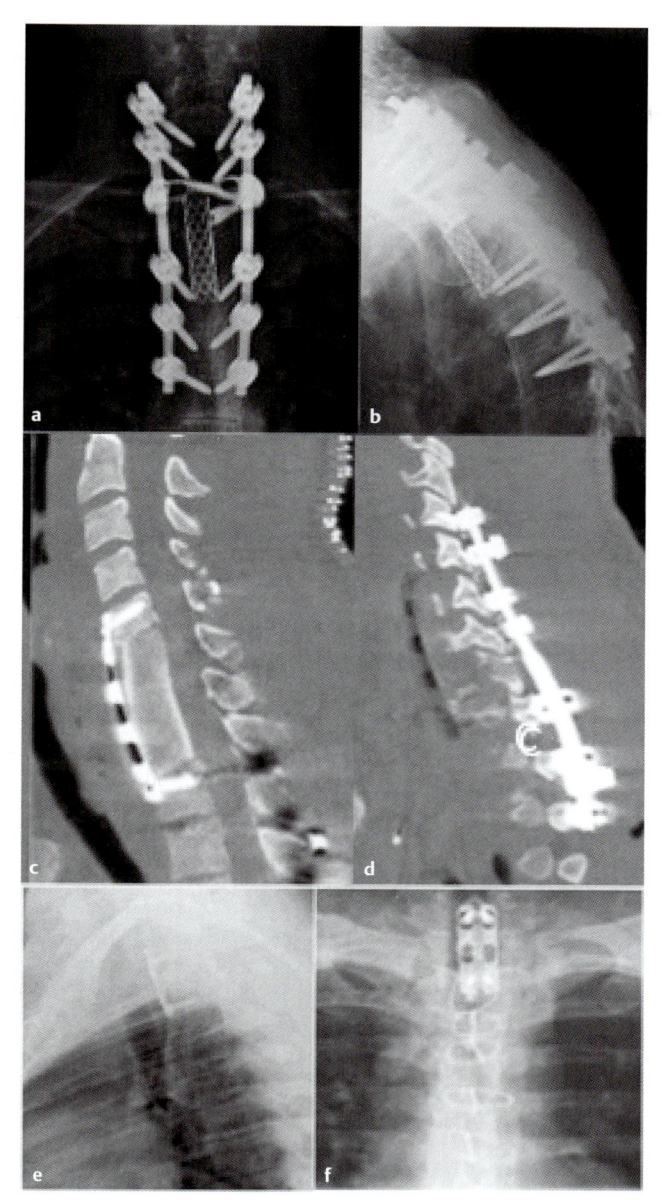

Fig. 45.1 Cervicothoracic junction anterior reconstruction alternatives. **(a,b)** Anteroposterior (AP) and lateral X-rays showing anterior column reconstruction using a titanium mesh cage following multilevel cervicothoracic junction (CTJ) corpectomy. **(c,d)** Sagittal computed tomography (CT) scan demonstrating the use of structural iliac crest autograft and an anterior plate for anterior column reconstruction along with posterior instrumentation spanning the CTJ. **(e,f)** AP and lateral X-rays showing anterior reconstruction following T1 corpectomy using a structural iliac crest without posterior instrumentation.

body cages are higher cost and the fact that these bulky devices can occupy space in the potential bone fusion bed.

Surgical Techniques

Graft-Site Preparation

After vertebral decompression through removal of the pathological lesion has been performed, the end plates of the vertebral bodies adjacent to the decompression site are prepared to accept a structural graft. As best as possible, flat, parallel surfaces should be created to maximize contact between the graft and host bone. A small posterior lip (2 to 3 mm) may remain to help prevent graft intrusion into the spinal canal. During end-plate preparation, it is important to keep in mind that the rostral and caudal end plates are of different shapes, and selective drilling must be used to ensure that the graft site has parallel surfaces with adequate cortical bone remaining to support the graft. One common mistake is the failure to remove sufficient ventral and dorsal end-plate lip, resulting in a central gap between the bone graft and vertebral end plate. Another mistake that has more serious consequences is the "ramp effect," which occurs when excessive bone is removed from the ventral two thirds of the lower vertebral body. This excessive removal results in a graft site that is longer ventrally than dorsally, predisposing to ventral dislocation of the graft.

Strut Graft Placement

The preoperative advanced imaging study, either computed tomography (CT) scan or magnetic resonance imaging (MRI), should be closely studied to identify the dimensions of the vertebra to be resected. A caliper and depth gauge should be used to measure the length and depth of the graft site accurately to determine the dimensions of the strut. The depth of the graft site is measured from the dorsal cortex to the ventral cortex along the midline of the vertebral body. The length of the graft site is measured with the vertebral bodies maximally distracted and is the distance between the end plates. Gentle distraction across the corpectomy defect, using pin distractors, facilitates the strut graft placement following the corpectomy. Slight distraction across the corpectomy enables placement of a slightly larger strut graft by increasing the size of the defect, which upon release of the distraction pins will seat the graft under compression. Segmental distraction is also useful in cases of angular kyphotic deformity. Distraction following anterior release results in a relative reduction of the kyphosis through realignment of the vertebral bodies in plane with the distraction. The width of the planned cage also needs to be properly planned to ensure that an optimal footprint is achieved. We have found that using a cotton patty of known size, typically a ¾" × 6" patty, is helpful to confirm that an adequate width of decompression has been achieved prior to placing a strut graft or a cage.

If an interbody cage is to be placed, prior to insertion, the cages are sized with a caliper and filled with iliac crest, local autograft, or morselized allograft. With the vertebral bodies distracted, the graft is gently placed into position and should fit without excessive force or hammering. Tactile inspection of the final position of the graft should be done using a blunt hook alongside the graft. Small pieces of cancellous bone can be gently impacted into the remaining gaps. However, care should be taken to avoid spinal canal compromise or compression of neural structures by these smaller pieces of bone.

If an expandable cage is to be used, the proper-sized footplates are attached to the cage. With the cage in place, the device is expanded to ensure a snug fit, taking care not to over-distract the disk space to preserve the integrity of the bony end plates. A concern with expandable cages has been the possibility of violating Wolff's law by unloading the graft material within the cage during the expansion process. Some authors attempt to pack additional bone into the cage after it is expanded; however, it is not clear whether this can be successfully accomplished to effectively "load" the graft material within the cage. As a result, we tend to reserve the use of expandable cages for cases where a fusion might not be absolutely necessary for the success of the surgical procedure (such as with malignant tumors).

Reconstruction Using Polymethylmethacrylate

In patients with a short life expectancy where fusion is not a primary end point, several reconstruction methods utilizing PMMA have been described.[2] One technique in which PMMA is injected into a Silastic tube that is fitted against the vertebral bodies above and below has been shown to provide adequate anterior column support. Silastic tubing is cut to span the corpectomy site. A 6-mm-diameter hole is made in the center of the tubing with a rongeur, and three small holes are made laterally, two at the rostral end and one at the caudal end. Small bites are also made at the ends of the tubing to allow extrusion of cement overflow. The side of the Silastic tubing facing the spinal cord is free of the central and lateral holes to avoid cement extrusion into the spinal canal. The Silastic tubing is passed into the space between two adjacent vertebral bodies at the corpectomy site and positioned so that there is no bending of the tubing that could obstruct cement flow. A low-viscosity PMMA preparation is mixed. When it has become semiliquid, the PMMA is injected through the center hold of the Silastic tubing, filling the tubing until PMMA can be seen passing out from the ends of the tube. While the PMMA is being injected, the tube must be observed carefully to avoid spilling the PMMA into the spinal canal. As the PMMA in the Silastic tubing solidifies, more PMMA is prepared and placed lateral to the Silastic tube until it is continuous with the borders of the upper and lower vertebrae. During polymerization and hardening of the PMMA, saline irrigation is used to dissipate the heat generated by the exothermic reaction.[2]

Anterior Instrumentation

Following placement of the interbody cage or graft in the cervicothoracic junction (CTJ), a screw–plate construct is routinely utilized. This plate is measured to span the corpectomy defect. The shortest plate possible is chosen that will avoid contact with the adjacent disk spaces. It is important to use a drill to remove any irregularities of the ventral surface of the vertebral bodies so that the plate can sit flush against them. A greater plate-to-bone contact provides increased structural stability for this construct. The length of the screws should be determined based on preoperative radiographs. Fixed-angle screws are placed to secure the inferior end of the plate to the inferior vertebral body. Care should be taken to avoid placing the screws into the graft or the adjacent disk space. Next, variable- or fixed-angle screws are placed to fixate the upper end of the plate to the superior body just above the end plate. The purpose of the variable screw placement above is to enable rotational subsidence of the variable-angle screws, which will load the graft and promote graft fusion. Once the vertebral body screws are in place, the screws are secured into position with the locking mechanism engaged to prevent screw backout. As a general rule, screw–plate systems are used in anterior cervical fusions for upper thoracic stabilization procedures.

Addition of an anterior plate to augment strut graft placement following cervical corpectomy has been shown to improve immediate stability and fusion rates compared with noninstrumented anterior cervical fusions.[3–5] Other benefits of plating include fewer complications from graft dislocation, end-plate fracture, and kyphotic collapse. Instrumentation at the CTJ employs techniques and plating systems similar to those used in anterior cervical fusions. Although many of the techniques are similar, the anatomic features of the CTJ make instrumentation in this region significantly more challenging. The thoracic inlet creates a difficult angle of approach for correct screw trajectory, especially at the more distal levels. Additionally, the natural kyphosis of the CTJ makes proper fitting of the cervical plates more difficult.

Posterior Stabilization

A particular area of concern in patients undergoing multilevel corpectomy is early construct failure leading to graft dislodgment. The early construct failure rate dramatically increases with multilevel constructs. Long strut grafts without points of intermediate fixation create significant stresses at the ends of long corpectomy constructs and are the likely mechanism underlying the relatively high complication rates and lower fusion rates seen in series utilizing multilevel corpectomies.[4] In the absence of posterior instrumentation, the large lever arm created in an anterior-only construct can lead to instability and graft dislodgment, even when an external fixator is used. The combination of anterior-posterior instrumentation has been shown to be an effective means of limiting motion with long constructs and decreasing graft migration and dislodgment.[6]

Some biomechanical and clinical studies suggest that anterior instrumentation and fusion techniques for CTJ pathology are inferior to techniques that use posterior-alone or combined anterior and posterior fixation.[7,8] At the CTJ, the indications for stand-alone anterior fixation are limited. Single-level anterior diskectomy and fusion at C7-T1 as well as single-level corpectomies at C7 or T1 can be successfully managed with anterior plating and a strut graft or cage, provided there is no posterior pathology or instability. When a corpectomy of two or more levels is performed at the CTJ level, supplemental posterior instrumentation is recommended. The goal of circumferential stabilization is to prevent subsequent spinal instability, spinal deformity, and excessive spinal movement that may predispose to loosening and dislodgment of the spinal construct at the corpectomy site. In general, the length of the posterior instrumentation is based on the bone quality and the overall alignment of the construct. Instrumentation should not be terminated in the midthoracic curve, to minimize the risk of pulling out the screws at the end of the instrumentation construct.

References

1. Heary RF, Schlenk RP, Sacchieri TA, Barone D, Brotea C. Persistent iliac crest donor site pain: independent outcome assessment. Neurosurgery 2002;50:510–516, discussion 516–517
2. Miller DJ, Lang FF, Walsh GL, Abi-Said D, Wildrick DM, Gokaslan ZL. Coaxial double-lumen methylmethacrylate reconstruction in the anterior cervical and upper thoracic spine after tumor resection. J Neurosurg 2000;92(2, Suppl):181–190
3. Fraser JF, Härtl R. Anterior approaches to fusion of the cervical spine: a metaanalysis of fusion rates. J Neurosurg Spine 2007;6:298–303
4. Singh K, Vaccaro AR, Kim J, Lorenz EP, Lim TH, An HS. Biomechanical comparison of cervical spine reconstructive techniques after a multilevel corpectomy of the cervical spine. Spine 2003;28:2352–2358, discussion 2358
5. Singh K, Vaccaro AR, Kim J, Lorenz EP, Lim TH, An HS. Enhancement of stability following anterior cervical corpectomy: a biomechanical study. Spine 2004;29:845–849
6. Sasso RC, Ruggiero RA Jr, Reilly TM, Hall PV. Early reconstruction failures after multilevel cervical corpectomy. Spine 2003;28:140–142
7. Bozkus H, Ames CP, Chamberlain RH, et al. Biomechanical analysis of rigid stabilization techniques for three-column injury in the lower cervical spine. Spine 2005;30:915–922
8. Prybis BG, Tortolani PJ, Hu N, Zorn CM, McAfee PC, Cunningham BW. A comparative biomechanical analysis of spinal instability and instrumentation of the cervicothoracic junction: an in vitro human cadaveric model. J Spinal Disord Tech 2007;20:233–238

B. Posterior Approach

46 Posterior Cervicothoracic Instrumentation and Fusion

Robert F. Heary and John C. Quinn

The goals of instrumentation and fusion for cervicothoracic instability are to restore and maintain anatomic alignment, preserve neurologic function, prevent progression of deformity, and alleviate pain. Several techniques have been described for the instrumentation of the cervicothoracic junction (CTJ), including anterior plating, posterior wiring, plating, and hook or screw-based rod constructs. Although frequently used in the subaxial cervical spine, anterior instrumentation and fusion is less commonly performed at the CTJ. Anterior fixation techniques require technically challenging approaches and are associated with significant complication rates. These techniques are generally reserved for cases requiring extensive anterior decompression or as part of the anterior-posterior procedures for treatment of three-column instability. Most causes of CTJ instability require only secure posterior stabilization.[1] Biomechanical and clinical studies have demonstrated the superiority of posterior-alone over anterior-alone stabilization techniques in this region, although combined anterior and posterior instrumentation provides the greatest stability.[1-3] Among posterior instrumentation techniques, screw-based systems (lateral mass screws in the cervical spine and pedicle screws in the thoracic spine) seem to provide the most robust fixation at the CTJ.[4]

Posterior stabilization of the cervicothoracic spine can be performed for numerous indications. An anterior pseudarthrosis at the CTJ, following either corpectomy or diskectomy, can often be treated by posterior fusion alone. Frequently, successful posterior fusion and instrumentation at this level posteriorly leads to eventual arthrodesis anteriorly as well. Traumatic injuries, such as facet fracture and dislocations at the CTJ, can often be treated posteriorly alone, following either a closed or open reduction.[5] Extensive anterior decompressions for cervical spondylotic myelopathy often require posterior stabilization, and if the decompression includes the lower cervical spine, posterior fixation is often extended distally to include the CTJ. Posterior cervical osteotomies for deformities due to ankylosing spondylitis are generally performed at the C7-T1 level.[6,7] Although these procedures can be performed without instrumentation, posterior instrumentation systems may increase the chance of successful fusion and, in selected cases, obviate the need for a halo brace. Finally, postlaminectomy kyphosis reconstruction of the cervical spine often involves both posterior and anterior procedures. Because of the extensive nature of this surgery, anterior and posterior fixation methods are often used, with the posterior instrumentation extending into the upper thoracic spine.

Indications

- Stabilization following decompression for tumor or infection
- Traumatic instability
- Proximal junctional kyphosis adjacent to thoracic instrumentation
- Stabilization following multilevel cervical fusion or three-column instability
- Kyphotic deformity correction

Biomechanical Considerations

The CTJ represents a transition zone from the mobile, lordotic cervical spine to the rigid, kyphotic thoracic spine. This dramatic transition is centered across a single motion segment creating significant biomechanical forces. With compromise of support structures as occurs with pathological processes or iatrogenic destabilization, the presence of these deformative forces can lead to progressive kyphosis with subsequent narrowing of the spinal canal and compression of the spinal cord. The transition from cervical lordosis to thoracic kyphosis at the CTJ results in transfer of weight from the posterior aspect to the anterior aspect of the spinal column, which results in significant translational stresses across the junction. In this region the anterior elements function to transfer compressive loads between adjacent vertebral levels, whereas the posterior elements provide stabilization through attachments to supporting paraspinal extensors muscles and ligamentous structures. Disruption of either component of this dynamic support structure can lead to progressive instability, deformity, and pain.[2]

Surgical Techniques
Anesthesia and Positioning

Patients with evidence of spinal cord compression are at risk for neurologic injury during intubation and induction of anesthesia. For these patients an awake, fiberoptic intubation is performed. Following induction, the patient is positioned prone on the operating room table and Gardner-Wells tongs are applied. Traction of 10 to 20 pounds is applied. Alternatively, a Mayfield head-holder may be used to rigidly fixate the skull and stabilize the neck in the prone position. The neck is positioned in a neutral or slightly lordotic position, but its position can be altered after decompression is performed to treat kyphotic deformities. Careful padding of the shoulders, elbows, and wrists in the neutral position is important to prevent peripheral nerve injury.

Care must be taken to fix the patient in an anatomic and neutral position to attain the best possible functionally normal position postoperatively. Fluoroscopy should be used to visualize cervical alignment before the surgery and during placement of instrumentation. In some instances following the decompression, the Mayfield device can be manipulated to improve the sagittal alignment of the CTJ prior to securing the fixation construct in place.

Radiological Evaluation

Prior to surgical intervention, anteroposterior (AP) and lateral radiographs of the region to be fused are required. Computed tomography (CT) scan should be obtained to evaluate the size and orientation of the osseous structures to be instrumented, and it enables preoperative calculation of screw lengths and angle of insertion. In general, the T1 pedicles tend to be larger with a more rounded cross section compared with the ovoid pedicles elsewhere in the thoracic spine.

Posterior Cervicothoracic Exposure

A standard midline approach is performed with the incision centered over the spinous processes. The length of the incision depends on the number of segments to be included in the construct. It is recommended that the incision extend one spinous process above and below the planned area of fixation to ensure adequate exposure and to attain proper, uninhibited working angles for accurate placement of the instrumentation. The paraspinal muscles are then elevated in a subperiosteal manner with the soft tissue exposure extended to the lateral edge of the lateral masses in the cervical spine and to the lateral edges of the transverse processes in the thoracic spine.

Instrumentation Alternatives

Many techniques that have been used in subaxial cervical fixation have been modified for use at the CTJ. Modified wire–rod constructs were the first to be developed; however, these have been largely supplanted by constructs incorporating rod–screw technologies. The development of methods for safe subaxial cervical spine instrumentation and pedicle screw fixation in the thoracic spine has significantly improved the ability to create stable, rigid internal constructs spanning the CTJ.[8]

Cervical Spine Lateral Mass Screw Placement

Lateral mass fixation has become the mainstay for stabilization of the subaxial cervical spine. Various techniques have been described including those of An, Magerl, Anderson, and Roy-Camille.[8,9] In the lower cervical spine, the proper screw starting point for lateral mass fixation is 1 mm medial to the center of the lateral mass. The medial boundary is defined by the inflection of the lamina and facet. The lateral boundary is the far edge of the articular mass. The superior and inferior boundaries are the respective facet joints. Preparation of the insertion site involves clear exposure of the boundaries of the lateral mass. After identification of the proper starting point, we recommend creating a small pilot hole with a 2-mm round bur or awl. This enables placement of the drill guide at the appropriate angle. The lateral mass screws should be directed 30 to 40 degrees rostrally and 20 degrees laterally. A fixed stop drill bit should be used and measured to the screw length as measured on the preoperative imaging. After drilling the hole, a fine, blunt-tipped probe is used to confirm the integrity of the walls of the hole and to verify that the cortex has not been penetrated. The pedicle finder is removed, and a pedicle probe is used to palpate five distinct bony borders, including a floor and four walls to ensure no bony breach. The appropriate length of the screw is determined by measuring the length of this probe using a clamp. The tract is then tapped 0.5 mm less than the diameter of the intended screw, which is inserted into the lateral mass in the same alignment as that of the probe removed just before screw placement. The length of the screw should not exceed the size of the drilled hole. Typically 3.5-mm screws with polyaxial heads can be used with a matching 4.0-mm rod. This can be connected to thoracic pedicle screws with a domino connection (side-to-side connector) or a tapered rod. Accurate placement is confirmed with fluoroscopy (**Fig. 46.1**).

Cervicothoracic Pedicle Screws

Pedicle screw fixation of C7 and the upper thoracic vertebrae is a good option in most cases of posterior instability, but it is technically challenging for several reasons: (1) The pedicles are narrow and routinely more tall than wide. (2) Intraoperative imaging of the pedicle can be difficult because of kyphotic alignment of the spinal column and obstruction from the shoulders. (3) The spinal canal is narrow, and violation of the medial pedicle can result in cord injury. (4) Vertebral arteries may occasionally be anomalous and enter the foramen transversarium of C7, or have a tortuous path and thus are at risk when the lateral cortical boarder is violated. (5) Starting points for the screws are not well defined and can be obscured by local pathology or degenerative changes.

Placement of pedicle screws at the CTJ can be performed either with the pedicles under direct visualization or through standard anatomic landmarks. With either technique, the preoperative imaging studies should be carefully examined to determine the medial angulation of the pedicle. Frequently, evaluation of the CT scan can also be very helpful in defining superficial landmarks. The relationships of the transverse processes to the pedicles should be noted and can often be useful when determining the starting point for the pedicle screws.

C7 Pedicle Screw Placement

C7 is a transitional vertebra that has characteristics common to both the cervical and the thoracic spine, with the lateral masses transitioning to the size and orientation of the thoracic transverse processes. The C7 lateral masses are often poor fixation points. They are the thinnest in the cervical spine and make traditional techniques for lateral mass screw placement more difficult and more likely to result in a fracture. In many cases, C7 pedicle screw placement offers a safer, more stable site of fixation than lateral mass screws. For safe and accurate placement of C7 pedicle screws, careful examination of the preoperative CT scan is essential for identification of the proper entry point, the pedicle diameters, and medial angulation. Techniques for placement based on bony landmarks that have been described recommend a pedicle entry point for the C7 pedicle 1 mm inferior to the midportion of the facet joint with 25 to 30 degrees medial angulation and perpendicular to the posterior arch. Alternatively, the pedicle may be identified by direct palpation with a cervical ball-tip probe if a laminotomy has already been performed. After determining the superior, medial, and inferior borders of the pedicle, the starting point is located, and a 2-mm bur or an awl is used to penetrate the posterior cortex. The pedicle can then be cannulated with a variety of devices. A pedicle probe or a power drill with an automatic stop on the guide may be used. Minimal force should be used when advancing the probe or the drill, to enable it to find its way in the confines of the pedicle. After advancing into the vertebral body, the walls of the pedicle can be palpated with a small, flexible ball-tip probe. Frequently, a portion of the pedicle will need to be tapped, due to the dense cortical bone. The screw can then be placed, with palpation of the borders of the pedicle, again with the ball-tip probe, to confirm

46 Posterior Cervicothoracic Instrumentation and Fusion

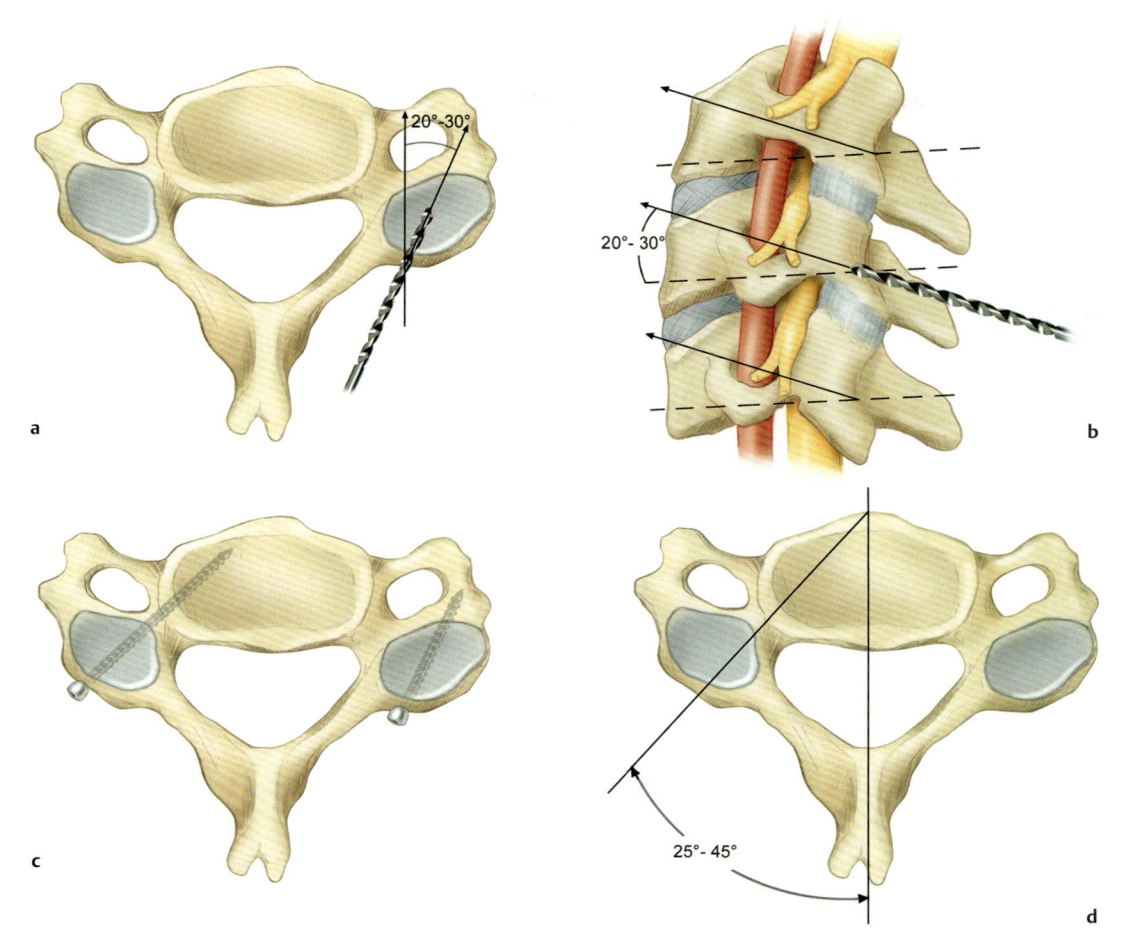

Fig. 46.1 Cervical instrumentation techniques. **(a,b)** Lateral mass screw placement. The starting point for lateral mass fixation is 1 mm medial to the center of the lateral mass. The medial boundary is the inflection of the lamina and facet, the lateral boundary is the edge of the articular mass, and the superior and inferior boundaries are the respective facet joints. The mass screws should be directed 30 to 40 degrees rostrally and 20 degrees laterally. **(c,d)** C7 pedicle screw placement. The starting point for the C7 pedicle is 1 mm inferior to the midportion of the facet joint with 25 to 30 degrees medial angulation and perpendicular to the posterior arch.

there has been no breach of the cortical walls of the pedicle. We most often utilize 24- to 26-mm screws in the C7 pedicles (**Fig. 46.1**).

Thoracic Pedicle Screw Placement

The same principles used for C7 pedicle screw placement apply for placement of upper thoracic spine pedicle screws. Wide exposure of the lamina and lateral mass (C7) and transverse processes (T1–T2) is performed with removal of the medial aspect of the transverse process of T1–T2 to enable the head of the pedicle screw to be seated. The starting point of the T1 to T2 pedicles is more lateral and more inferior than for the lower thoracic spine. Once a posterior cortical breach is made with a bur or an awl, a pedicle finder or a high-speed drill is placed into the base of the pedicle alternatively. The pedicle finder is advanced through the pedicle ~ 25 mm. Medial angulation is required for entry of the pedicle into the vertebral body, which averages ~ 30 degrees at the T1 level; subsequent inferior levels are more variable with T2 between 15 and 25 degrees and T3 and below in the 5-degree vicinity.

Translaminar Screw Placement

In cases with unfavorable upper thoracic pedicle anatomy, translaminar screws provide an effective alternative to pedicle screw fixation.[10] The translaminar screw insertion point is at the junction of the contralateral spinous process and lamina. The trajectory is approximately along the angle of the ipsilateral lamina, with the target being the intersection of the ipsilateral transverse process and superior facet. To place bilateral translaminar screws, the starting points have to be slightly different cephalad-caudal, and the lateral trajectories must be slightly divergent, to avoid collision of the screws. Furthermore, intact bony arches are needed, and as such this approach is used relatively infrequently (**Fig. 46.2**).

Rod Placement and Fusion Surface Preparation

After the screws are seated, a rod template is bent to the needed length. The rods, after being slightly bent to conform to the template, are placed onto the multiaxial screws and locked with

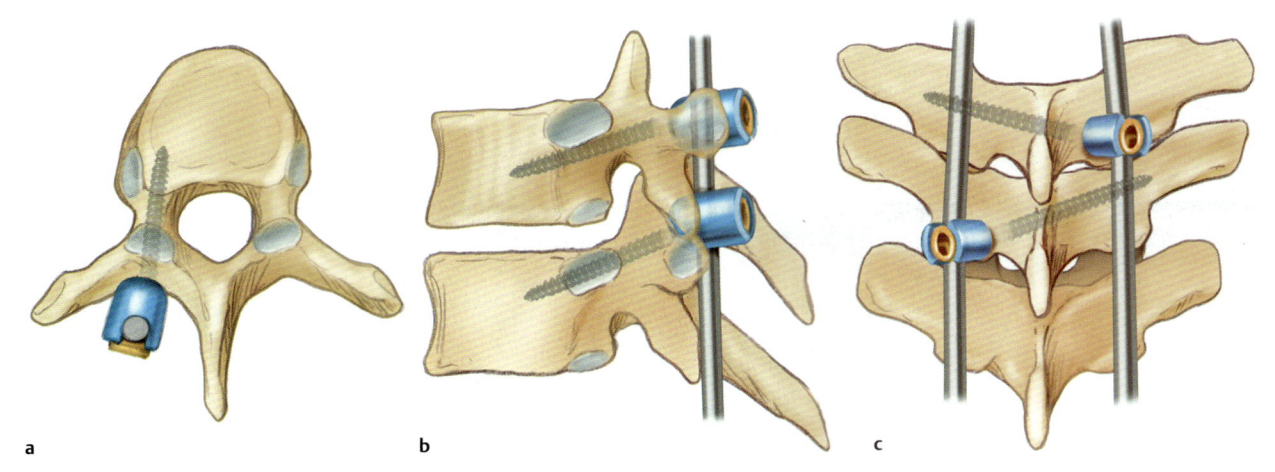

Fig. 46.2 Upper thoracic instrumentation. **(a,b)** Upper thoracic pedicle screw placement. The starting point is the midpoint of the transverse process (rostral-caudal) and the junction of the transverse process and lamina (medial-lateral). The medial angulation averages ~ 30 degrees at the T1 level; subsequent inferior levels are more variable, with T2 between 15 and 25 degrees and T3 and below in the 5-degree vicinity. **(c)** Thoracic translaminar screw placement. The starting point is the junction of the contralateral spinous process and lamina. The trajectory is along the angle of the ipsilateral lamina, aiming for the intersection of the ipsilateral transverse process and superior facet. To place bilateral translaminar screws, the starting points have to be slightly different cephalad-caudal, and the lateral trajectories must be slightly divergent, to avoid collision of the screws.

top-loading screws. If the rod does not drop easily onto the screw, a persuading device may be needed to pull the screw up to the rod. Caution is taken with these devices not to exert too much force because pullout and failure of the bone–screw interface can easily occur. Tapered rods are helpful in extending the construct into the thoracic spine. Typically, tapered rods vary from 3.5 mm in the cervical region to 5-mm diameter in the thoracic portion of the rod. Because of issues with rod fracture at their tapered portion, the rod is not bent at this site. Once the rods have been seated, the top-loading nuts are locked. Crosslinks are either rod-to-rod or screw-to-screw, depending on the available rod surface. If screw-to-screw fixation is desirable, this must be planned when the top-loading screws are placed.

An important component of any fusion surgery, regardless of the instrumentation technique chosen, is the preparation of the graft site and the type of graft used. In preparing a fusion bed, the posterior elements of the subaxial and proximal thoracic spine to be fused are decorticated with a cutting bur. The facet joints to be fused are opened sharply, the capsule removed, and a small curette is used to remove the joint cartilage and roughen the opposing surfaces of the facet joint. Cancellous bone graft is packed into the facet joint. Additional bone graft is laid around the screw–rod construct over the decorticated lateral masses, transverse processes, and any available laminae. Autograft remains the preferred material in most cervicothoracic fusions. Many sources of graft material are available for these techniques, including local autograft, iliac crest, and others.

Length of Construct

In terms of the numbers of levels fused, there are no specific guidelines. In cervicothoracic trauma, Chapman et al[5] fused all junctional motion segments. This usually involved two to three levels for a burst fracture but more if ligamentous injuries were present. In tumor cases, Mazel et al[11] recommended that the fusion be extended three levels above and three levels below if a vertebrectomy is performed. In general, the length of fusion depends on factors such as the age of the patient, underlying pathology, the length of decompression, and the bone quality. The degree of instability, specifically the number of columns involved, also plays an important role in the surgical treatment plan for pathology in this region. For a two-column instability at the CTJ, there is a trend toward increasing stiffness with extended thoracic fixation. Experimental models comparing constructs from C5–T1 to C6–T2 showed equivalent stability across the CTJ.[4,12] As such, most spine surgeons recommend C6–T2 fusion to save cervical fixation points. With three-column injuries, posterior fixation alone is often inadequate and results in excessive flexibility in flexion/extension, even with extension of instrumentation to T3. Supplementation with anterior column instrumentation leads to increased strength of the construct. Biomechanical models of three-column injury with corpectomy show similar results and suggest the requirement of both anterior and posterior instrumentation for adequate stabilization.[2]

Construct Design Challenges

In addition to significant biomechanical forces across an unstable CTJ, the transition in size and orientation of bony fixation points that occur when spanning this region make instrumentation across this region technically challenging.[9] Instrumentation must be strong enough to resist the forces of deformity correction yet flexible enough to be contoured to re-create the transition in curvature across the inflection point at the CTJ. In the past, cervical wiring and lateral mass plating were the mainstays for posterior cervical instrumentation. Especially with challenging long segment constructs spanning the CTJ, these systems had many design limitations and lacked the versatility for widespread application. Modern cervical spine rod–screw systems are versatile enough in design to enable integration into a thoracic spine instrumentation construct. These systems have improved flexibility with regard to correcting/accommodating deformity and achieving immediate rigid internal fixation and high rates of fusion. Rods may be contoured to the multiple points of cervical and thoracic fixation, including lateral mass screws, cervical pedicle screws, thoracic pedicle screws, and thoracic hooks.

Despite recent advances in instrumentation materials and technologies, assembling a cervicothoracic construct requires careful planning and execution, as there are several potential pitfalls that must be accounted for. In planning a long segment construct, one must take into account that the screw heads may

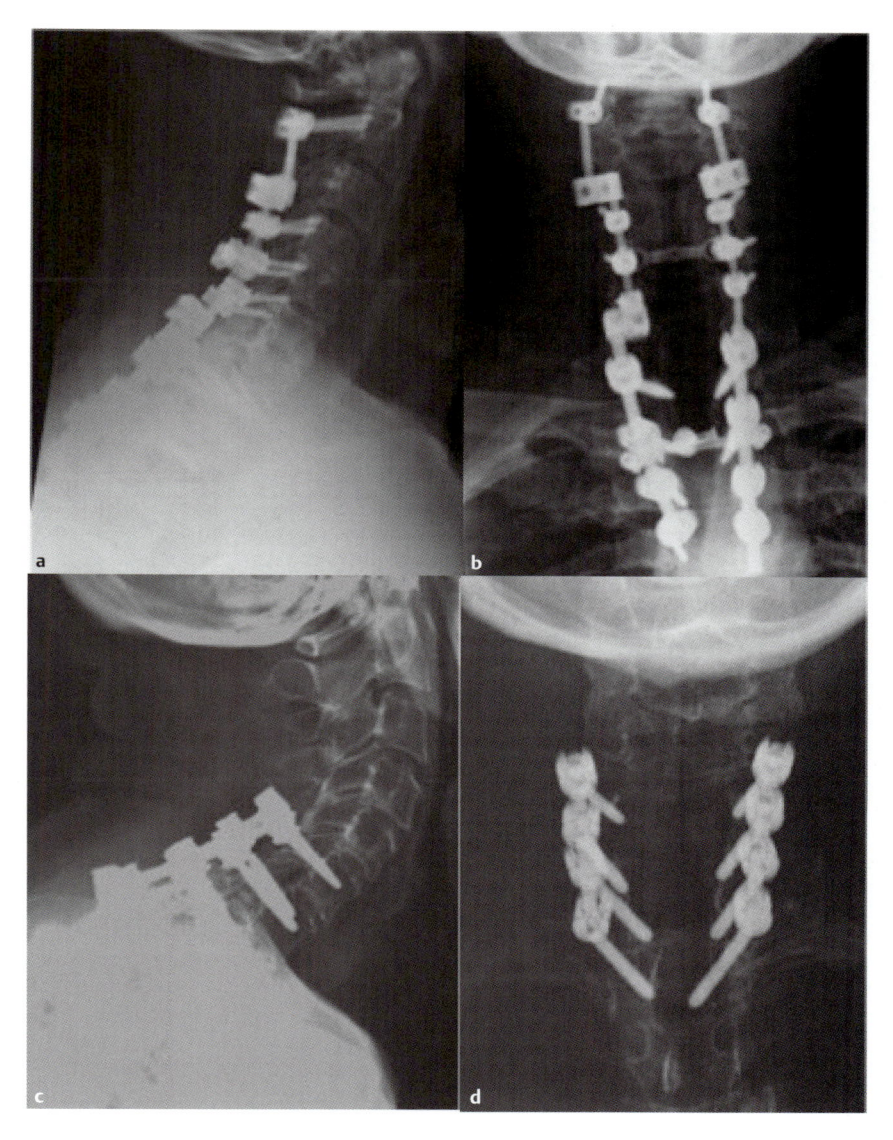

Fig. 46.3 Construct design challenges: anteroposterior (AP) and lateral radiographs. **(a,b)** A long segment cervicothoracic fusion (C2–T4) spanning the cervicothoracic junction (CTJ). This construct included C2 pars screws, C3–C6 lateral mass screws, and T1–T3 pedicle screws. The left side of the construct utilized a dual diameter 3.5- to 5.0-mm rod requiring an offset connector to link to the C2 pars screw. The right side required offset connectors to link the separate 3.5-mm rods between the C2 pars and lateral mass screws and a second offset connector to link up to a 5-mm rod in the thoracic spine. **(c,d)** AP and lateral radiographs demonstrating a short-segment CTJ fusion consisting of C6–T2 pedicle screws connected to a 5-mm rod.

interfere with each other. A C6 lateral mass screw will frequently interfere with that of a C7 pedicle screw. For this reason, C6 lateral mass screws may be left out if C7 pedicle screws are used. Alternatively, C7 screws may be left out if placement would offset the balance of a construct. In some instances where the cervical lateral masses are hypoplastic, such as with neurofibromatosis, extension of the rostral construct to the C2 pars level may be necessary to achieve satisfactory rostral fixation. Another difficult fixation problem crossing the CTJ is attaching a rod or plate to the lateral mass screw in C7 and a pedicle screw in T1. The lateral mass screw is angled up and out so that the head is inferior and medial while the pedicle screw is angled medial such that the head is lateral. Thus, over a very short distance, there exists a very significant lateral offset between the screw heads. This problem has been addressed by a polyaxial screw–rod system using an inner set screw and a lateral offset connector. Constructs may also take advantage of tapered rods, a domino connector, small thoracic pedicle screws that enable continuation of the small-diameter cervical rod into the thoracic region, or a rod-based end-to-end interconnect that enables the transition of one rod diameter to another at the CTJ (**Fig. 46.3**).

References

1. O'Brien JR, Dmitriev AE, Yu W, Gelb D, Ludwig S. Posterior-only stabilization of 2-column and 3-column injuries at the cervicothoracic junction: a biomechanical study. J Spinal Disord Tech 2009;22:340–346
2. Prybis BG, Tortolani PJ, Hu N, Zorn CM, McAfee PC, Cunningham BW. A comparative biomechanical analysis of spinal instability and instrumentation of the cervicothoracic junction: an in vitro human cadaveric model. J Spinal Disord Tech 2007;20:233–238
3. Kreshak JL, Kim DH, Lindsey DP, Kam AC, Panjabi MM, Yerby SA. Posterior stabilization at the cervicothoracic junction: a biomechanical study. Spine 2002;27:2763–2770
4. Rhee JM, Kraiwattanapong C, Hutton WC. A comparison of pedicle and lateral mass screw construct stiffnesses at the cervicothoracic junction: a biomechanical study. Spine 2005;30:E636–E640
5. Chapman JR, Anderson PA, Pepin C, Toomey S, Newell DW, Grady MS. Posterior instrumentation of the unstable cervicothoracic spine. J Neurosurg 1996;84:552–558
6. Mummaneni PV, Deutsch H, Mummaneni VP. Cervicothoracic kyphosis. Neurosurg Clin N Am 2006;17:277–287, vi
7. Belanger TA, Milam RA IV, Roh JS, Bohlman HH. Cervicothoracic extension osteotomy for chin-on-chest deformity in ankylosing spondylitis. J Bone Joint Surg Am 2005;87:1732–1738

8. Albert TJ, Klein GR, Joffe D, Vaccaro AR. Use of cervicothoracic junction pedicle screws for reconstruction of complex cervical spine pathology. Spine 1998;23:1596–1599

9. Pelton MA, Schwartz J, Singh K. Subaxial cervical and cervicothoracic fixation techniques—indications, techniques, and outcomes. Orthop Clin North Am 2012;43:19–28, vii

10. McGirt MJ, Sutter EG, Xu R, et al. Biomechanical comparison of translaminar versus pedicle screws at T1 and T2 in long subaxial cervical constructs. Neurosurgery 2009;65(6, Suppl):167–172, discussion 172

11. Mazel C, Hoffmann E, Antonietti P, Grunenwald D, Henry M, Williams J. Posterior cervicothoracic instrumentation in spine tumors. Spine 2004; 29:1246–1253

12. Bozkus H, Ames CP, Chamberlain RH, et al. Biomechanical analysis of rigid stabilization techniques for three-column injury in the lower cervical spine. Spine 2005;30:915–922

Section IV   Thoracic and Thoracolumbar Spine

A. Pathology

47 Congenital Abnormalities of the Thoracic and Thoracolumbar Spine

Sandi K. Lam, Jared Fridley, Christina N. Sayama, Bradley Daniels, and Andrew Jea

Congenital anomalies of the thoracic and thoracolumbar spine encompass a wide range of conditions that result from disorders in embryogenesis. This chapter provides an overview of these entities, describing the epidemiology, workup, diagnosis, and management of the more common congenital anomalies of the thoracic and thoracolumbar spine.

Radiological Evaluation

All patients with congenital abnormalities of the thoracolumbar spine should undergo imaging to determine the type and location of the vertebral anomaly, the presence of major and minor curvatures, the presence of spinal canal stenosis, and the association with important vascular structures, such as the artery of Adamkiewicz, and underlying central nervous system anomalies. This information is vital to predict the natural history of the abnormality and the optimal treatment approach if indicated.

In many cases, plain radiographs, computed tomography (CT), magnetic resonance imaging (MRI), and even spinal angiography should be performed concurrently. These imaging modalities should not be viewed as poor substitutions for one another; instead, they provide complementary data, such as movement of the spine with dynamic plain radiographs, delineation of bony anatomy with CT, definition of soft tissue structures with MRI, and localization of the artery of Adamkiewicz with spinal angiography.

Plain Radiographs

In general, plain radiographs are able to detect most osseous abnormalities of the cervical, thoracic, and lumbosacral spine in adults and children and provide an adequate global view of the spine.[1] Coronal and sagittal views performed with the patient in an upright position assess truncal balance. Serial radiographic measurements, performed over the same vertebral levels and showing a 10-degree increase to account for interobserver variability, indicate the progression of a spinal deformity. Flexion/extension X-rays of the cervical spine and lumbosacral spine are important to rule out subluxation or instability.[2] Side bending and traction views may be helpful in determining flexibility of the spinal deformity prior to surgery.

Computed Tomography

Axial CT of the spine may provide more detailed information regarding the bony anatomy of the spine, including the spinal canal. Sagittal and coronal reconstructions of the axial CT slices complete a three-dimensional analysis of the spine. High-quality CT scans are often most useful in identifying an occult, and possibly surgically correctable, vertebral abnormality.[2] Moreover, CT may suggest soft tissue abnormalities.

Although dynamic (flexion and extension) CT imaging is possible to perform, CT is performed in a static position in a majority of cases. If documentation about the motion of the spine is necessary, dynamic plain radiographs likely provide more clinically relevant information.

Magnetic Resonance Imaging

Magnetic resonance imaging has become the modality of choice in the assessment of soft tissue anatomy, such as the spinal cord, nerve roots, intervertebral disks, and ligaments. MRI is sensitive in detecting ligamentous aberrations and instability not seen on plain radiographs or CT.[3] MRI demonstrates the presence of damage to the spinal cord,[4] intradural pathology, and intrinsic anomalies of the spinal cord, such as split cord malformation. MRI has essentially almost replaced myelography in the evaluation of anatomy inside the spinal canal and intradurally.

Magnetic resonance imaging is useful in ruling out surgical lesions (i.e., those causing persistent cord compression).[5–7] It also helps in preoperative planning and evaluating the relationship of neural elements to the spinal anomaly.

Spinal Angiography

The artery of Adamkiewicz becomes an important additional consideration prior to surgery in the thoracolumbar region. The artery of Adamkiewicz is an intraforaminal structure that courses anterior to the spinal cord and most commonly arises between T9 and T12, although it has been documented to originate as high as T5 and as low as L5.[8,9]

Spinal angiography is the gold standard for imaging the artery of Adamkiewicz,[10,11] and is infrequently indicated as part of the preoperative workup. Complications associated with spinal angiography, including contrast reaction, paralysis, and retroperitoneal bleeding, have been reported in up to 4.6% of adults undergoing this procedure, depending on the number of vessels visualized and the underlying vessel pathology,[12,13] and thus temper its routine use. Other recent studies have examined the use of CT and MR angiography as alternative methods for identifying the artery of Adamkiewicz, with adequate visualization of the artery seen in 95% and 93% of patients, respectively.[11,14,15] CT angiography specifically was proven to be efficacious in depicting the artery of Adamkiewicz with a high degree of sensitivity in patients as young as 5 years of age.[11] However, one study compared CT angiography to traditional arteriogram and found that the arteriogram was superior to CT imaging in both identifying (94% versus 60%), and establishing continuity (87% versus 56%)

in, the artery of Adamkiewicz.[16] Thus, spinal angiography currently appears to be more accurate in identifying and tracing the artery of Adamkiewicz. Although the angiography procedure does carry risk, the reported rates of non–contrast-related risks are low, and, in our opinion, outweighed by the benefits of avoiding damage to critical vascular structures when surgery in the thoracolumbar region puts the segmental arteries at risk.

Embryology

Primitive Streak

In the human embryo, development of spinal elements begins around the 15th day of gestation. The embryo is a bilaminar disk whose two layers of primordial tissue are continuous above and below with the amnion and yolk sac. The layer continuous with the amnion is termed epiblast, considered to be primitive mesoderm and ectoderm, whereas the layer continuous with the yolk sac is termed hypoblast, considered to be primitive endoderm. The epiblast surface forms the primitive streak, a furrow extending toward the future caudal end of the organism from a depression (the primitive pit) at the midline. This establishes anterior-posterior directionality and left-right symmetry.[17]

Gastrulation

The bilaminar embryo becomes a three-layered structure as epiblast cells migrate caudally toward the primitive streak and delve in to populate the area between the epiblast and hypoblast. This gastrulation process results in a trilaminar disk composed of ectoderm, mesoderm, and endoderm.

A portion of epiblastic cells migrate beneath the primitive streak to form a line of mesoderm running cranially from the primitive pit along the midline, forming the notochord. Cells migrate from the epiblast embedding into the hypoblastic layer, and pinching off in the mesoderm. The structure that conveys these cells beneath the epiblast is the neurenteric canal. Pathology can result if the obliteration of this normally transient structure fails to happen[18] or if there is an anomalous persistent neurenteric canal that cleaves the future notochord,[19] which can precipitate neurenteric cysts and split cord malformations, respectively.

Primary Neurulation

The underlying notochord affects the region of ectoderm lying above it, making it thicken along the anteroposterior axis. By the end of gastrulation, a stripe of ectoderm (the neural plate) is along the middle aspect of the trilaminar disk. Lateral aspects (neural folds) stretch above the invaginating medial neural plate and fuse along the midline for neural tube closure, called primary neurulation. The anterior neuropore closes on about postovulatory day 24 and the posterior neuropore closes on about day 26. The superficial ectoderm separates from neural ectoderm in disjunction. Errors in primary neurulation result in neural tube defects, and abnormalities in disjunction result in spinal lipomatous lesions (or dorsal dermal sinus tracts in more focal failures of disjunction). If mesenchymal elements from surrounding mesoderm proliferate while the connection between cutaneous ectoderm and neural ectoderm is obliterated too early, intradural anomalies such as intramedullary lipomas and lipomyelomeningoceles[20] occur.

The molecular functional patterning of the developing neural tube is complex. The Sonic hedgehog (Shh) signaling molecule is important in ventral induction of the floor plate and motor cord (the basal plate),[21] whereas the transforming growth factor-β superfamily (bone morphogenic proteins) contributes to specialization of the dorsal aspects of the neural tube into sensory roles (the alar plate).[22]

Secondary Neurulation

A secondary neural tube forms caudally with mesenchymal-to-epithelial transition. The mesodermal caudal cell mass cavitates and re-differentiates into neural tissue of the sacral spine and distal sacral vertebrae. This secondary neural tube interfaces with the more rostral primary neural tube after closure of the caudal neuropore.[23,24] Errors in this secondary neurulation process result in sacral agenesis or caudal regression syndromes.

Somitogenesis: Formation of Vertebrae

Following gastrulation, several domains of mesoderm are fated to become various structures depending on their distance from the midline of the embryo. The paraxial mesoderm forms condensations (somites) flanking the neural tube bilaterally at approximately day 25 of gestation.[25] Somites differentiate to yield a dorsolateral dermomyotome and a ventromedial sclerotome. The sclerotome is compartmentalized into groups of mesenchyme destined to become bony structures supporting the future spinal cord. Medial aspects of each sclerotome migrate anteriorly, surrounding the notochord to become centra, vertebral disks, and bodies. Lateral portions of sclerotome migrate dorsally to surround the neural tube and become the posterior neural arch.[26]

The piecemeal nature of individual vertebrae formation can precipitate developmental abnormalities. These errors of formation most often include hemivertebrae, which can produce curvature in the vertebral column. Errors of formation affecting components of the neural arch in the lumbar spine can predispose toward dysplastic or developmental spondylolisthesis.

Resegmentation of the Vertebral Column

The distinct nature of each somite (or primary segment) as a developing unit changes. After resegmentation, each vertebra is composed of sclerotomic contributions from two adjacent somites: the caudal half of a cranial sclerotome and cranial half of the next-caudal sclerotome. Disks form at the midportion of each sclerotome, with the notochord around which centra organize contributing to the nucleus pulposus.[27] Remnants of the notochord may persist and form chordomas mostly in the cranial and sacrococcygeal regions.

Craniocaudal segmentation during somitogenesis is associated with a signaling cascade including receptors responding to the Notch transmembrane protein. Notch promotes an oscillating pattern of gene expression that alternates craniocaudally and drives resegmentation by specifying cranial and caudal halves of sclerotome.[27] Aberrances in Notch signaling yield errors of segmentation as adjacent somites fail to separate.[27] These resegmentation errors can manifest as congenital vertebral bars or block vertebrae as in Klippel-Feil syndrome.

Chondrification and Ossification

Sclerotomic mesenchyme starts to differentiate into cartilage at the sixth week of gestation, and by the tenth week ossification centers have been established and begin to convert cartilage into bone. Ossification of vertebral bodies follows a different temporal pattern than the ossification of neural arches. Studies using fetal CT scans and histological examination reveal that ossification of vertebral bodies commences around the notochord, beginning in the lower thoracic vertebrae and progressing both craniocaudally and caudocranially. Ossification of the neural arches progresses craniocaudally from the cervical column.[28]

Congenital Anomalies of Vertebral Bodies

Congenital Scoliosis

Congenital scoliosis is defined as scoliosis that occurs secondary to abnormal vertebral development (**Table 47.1**). These malformed vertebra lead to an abnormal curvature of the spine in the coronal plane, which can continue to worsen even after skeletal maturity. The true incidence of congenital scoliosis is unknown because minor deformities often go undetected. There is a female predominance among patients. There does not appear to be a genetic predisposition.[29,30] Nearly 20% of congenital scoliosis patients have associated intraspinal anomalies such as myelomeningocele, syringomyelia, occult spinal dysraphism, and diastematomyelia.[31] There are also a significant number of patients (30–60%) who have associated cardiac, genitourinary, and skeletal abnormalities.[32]

Embryologically, spinal deformities are secondary to a "failure of formation" or a "failure of segmentation" (**Fig. 47.1**, **Table 47.2**). Winter et al[33] developed a classification system for congenital spinal deformities based on the embryological development of the spine. This system divides the anomalies into (1) failures of formation, (2) failures of segmentation, and (3) mixed anomalies. Using this system, Winter et al were able to classify up to 80% of all abnormalities.

Table 47.1 Classification of Scoliosis

Type	Description
Congenital	Due to congenitally anomalous vertebral development
Idiopathic	A structural lateral spinal curvature for which no cause is established
Infantile	Spinal curvature that develops during the first 3 years of life (ages 0–3 years)
Juvenile	Spinal curvature that develops between age 3 and puberty (ages 3–10 years)
Adolescent	Spinal curvature that develops at or about the onset of puberty (10 years to maturity)
Neuromuscular	Due to a known abnormality of the central nervous system or of the muscles and nerves

Normal growth of the spine occurs at the end plates at the upper and lower surfaces of the vertebral bodies. Congenital vertebral anomalies can cause functional deficiency of the growth plates on one or both sides of the spine. A spine deformity occurs if there is asymmetric growth, which occurs as a functional deficiency on one side as compared with the other. The rate of angulation and the final severity of the congenital scoliosis are

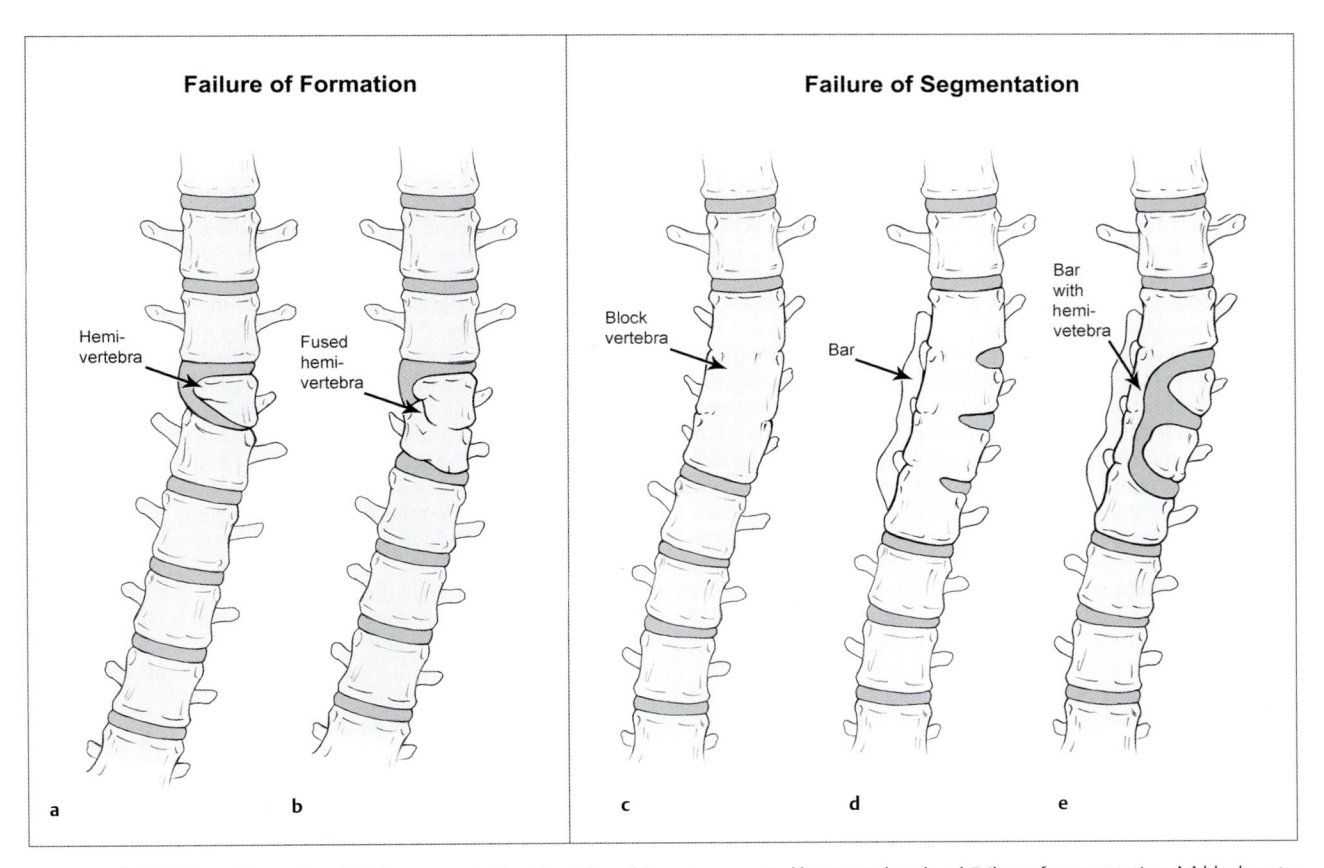

Fig. 47.1 (a,b) Failure of formation: (a) fully segmented hemivertebra; (b) semi-segmented hemivertebra. (c–e) Failure of segmentation: (c) block vertebra; (d) unilateral bar; (e) unilateral bar with hemivertebra.

Table 47.2 Congenital Spinal Deformity

Errors of Segmentation		
Congenital scoliosis (lateral)	Congenital lordosis (posterior)	Congenital kyphosis (anterior)
Unilateral bar		Winter type II
Block vertebrae		
Errors of Formation		
Congenital scoliosis	Spina bifida (posterior)	Congenital kyphosis (anterior)
Fully segmented hemivertebrae		Winter type I
Semi-segmented hemivertebrae		
Incarcerated hemivertebrae		
Nonsegmented hemivertebrae		
Combined Errors of Formation and Segmentation		
Congenital scoliosis (lateral)		Congenital kyphosis (anterior)
Unilateral bar with hemivertebrae		Winter type I

Failures of Formation: Hemivertebra

Hemivertebra results from a failure of formation of the vertebral body in which there is complete absence of half of the vertebral body, one pedicle, and one hemilamina. The hemivertebra is the most common cause of congenital scoliosis.[30,36] Hemivertebrae are usually diagnosed in infancy or childhood during periods of growth. There is no gender predilection. Many patients are asymptomatic, or they may present with abnormal spine curvature and undergo a scoliosis workup. Patients with significant scoliosis may develop neurologic deficits, developing pain or weakness. In cases of severe spinal deformity, pulmonary compromise may result from impeded chest wall movement.

X-rays show a sharply angulated, single curve or focal scoliosis, which serves as a significant diagnostic clue that there may be a hemivertebra. CT can show more detail and be a better test to delineate the hemivertebra or other bony abnormality. AP and lateral 36-inch scoliosis X-rays are a mainstay in the full evaluation of scoliosis and sagittal and coronal balance. MRI is helpful in evaluating the spinal cord, nerve roots, and any other associated spinal anomalies (such as lipoma, tethered cord, and diastematomyelia).

There are three types of hemivertebra (unsegmented, semi-segmented, and fully segmented), which are classified both by the relationship of the hemivertebra to the adjacent vertebrae and by whether the associated disks are morphologically normal (**Fig. 47.2**). An unsegmented hemivertebra is wedged between two bones without a growth plate. A semi-segmented hemivertebra is fused to either the lower or upper vertebra and has only one growth plate. A fully segmented hemivertebra has a full growth plate on either side and is the most common type of hemivertebra. The bone itself is of normal density and histology.[30,37]

The potential of a hemivertebra to cause significant scoliosis depends on its type, location, the number of hemivertebrae, their relationships (unilateral or bilateral), and the patient's age and growth potential. For example, paired bilateral hemivertebrae can result in a "balanced" scoliosis as the curves cancel out. However, one or more unilateral hemivertebra would result in an unbalanced and uncompensated scoliotic curve.

The fully segmented hemivertebra acts like an enlarging wedge and is located at the apex of the convexity of the scoliosis. The rate of progression for a single fully segmented hemivertebra depends on its location in the spine, with the worst prognosis for those located at the lower thoracic spine and the thoracolumbar junction. Earlier age at presentation usually portends a higher rate of curve progression. An incarcerated hemivertebra is a variant of the fully segmented hemivertebra in which the hemivertebra is set into defects in the vertebrae above and below it. The incarcerated hemivertebra is typically small and ovoid, with poorly formed disk spaces. The defects in the adjacent vertebrae tend to compensate for the hemivertebra, and the poor growth potential of the malformed growth plates results in less scoliotic deformity when compared with the standard fully segmented hemivertebra.[30]

A semi-segmented hemivertebra has mild to modest potential for scoliosis, as there are two active growth plates on each side. The nonsegmented hemivertebra has no associated growth plates and thus no potential for progression of scoliosis.

Failures of Segmentation

Segmentation failure causes a bony fusion between vertebrae. Defects of segmentation can be unilateral or bilateral. A block vertebra is a bilateral segmentation defect involving two or more vertebrae resulting in a loss of the growth plate bilaterally between the vertebrae. The spine is shortened but there is little propensity for progression because the disk spaces are either

proportional to the degree of growth imbalance produced by the vertebral anomalies. The portion of the vertebrae with deficient growth determines whether a pure scoliosis occurs or whether there will be a component of sagittal plane deformity with a component of kyphoscoliosis or lordoscoliosis. In general, 25% of all congenital scolioses do not progress, 50% progress slowly, and 25% progress rapidly.[33,34]

Although children are born with these vertebral anomalies, most patients may not develop noticeable spinal deformity until a growth spurt occurs later in childhood or adolescence.[30,33] Many patients reach adulthood without developing significant spinal deformity; only later is a vertebral anomaly discovered incidentally on radiographs performed for another reason such as trauma. Differences in number, location, and type of vertebral anomalies account for the wide range of clinical presentations seen in congenital scoliosis.[30,33,35] Patients may be asymptomatic or develop debilitating, progressive spinal deformity. Common presenting symptoms include pain, weakness, numbness, bowel or bladder problems, radiculopathy, or worsening cardiac/pulmonary function.

X-ray and CT are both done to evaluate bony abnormalities. Standing anteroposterior (AP) and lateral 36-inch scoliosis X-rays are a necessity to evaluate the extent of the scoliotic deformity. CT gives a more detailed view of the bone abnormalities and is helpful for preoperative planning when surgery is considered. MRI of the spine is performed to look for associated intraspinal anomalies. An echocardiogram and renal ultrasound should be performed in all patients to look for associated cardiac or genitourinary anomalies.

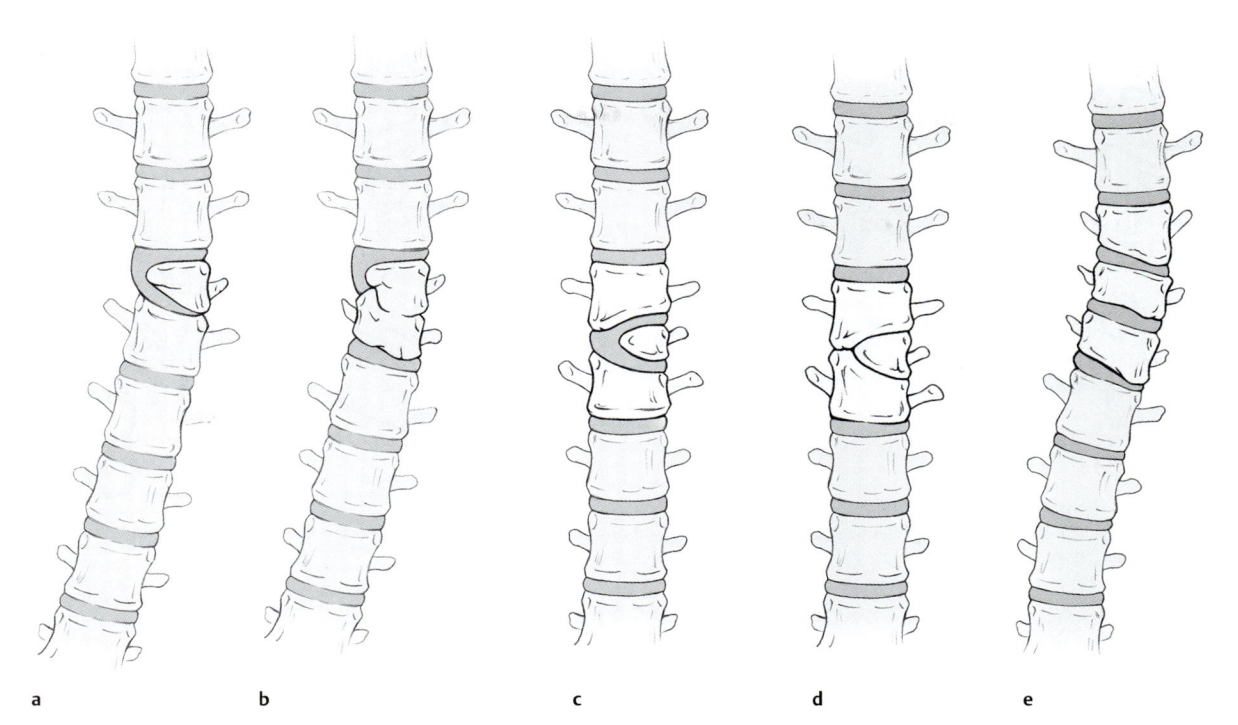

Fig. 47.2 Hemivertebra types: **(a)** fully segmented (unilateral complete failure of formation); **(b)** semi-segmented; **(c)** incarcerated; **(d)** nonsegmented; **(e)** wedge vertebra (unilateral partial failure of formation).

dysplastic or fused.[30,34,38] On the other hand, a unilateral unsegmented bar is a unilateral segmentation defect where one side of the spine is fused and the other side is left with normal active growth plates. This imbalance in growth results in scoliosis with the unsegmented bar in the concavity. Because growth potential exists on only half of the spine, the potential for deformity is significant. On average these curves deteriorate at a rate of 5 degrees per year and result in a significant deformity by puberty.[30] In a series of 43 patients with this specific anomaly, these deformities progressed at a rate of at least 6 degrees per year, with all exceeding 50 degrees by age 4.[36]

Children with congenital scoliosis must be closely observed over time for progression. Bracing in congenital scoliosis does not prevent curve progression as it does not correct the underlying pathology; thus, its use is controversial. Surgical correction for congenital scoliosis can be difficult and carry significant risk. Surgery is considered for symptomatic curves greater than 45 degrees, or progression of more than 10 degrees per year. The goals of surgery are to halt the progression of the deformity and, if possible to perform safely, correct the deformity. However, as these children often have multiple other comorbidities, all factors should be considered preoperatively to best optimize the situation to benefit the child's overall function and potential for growth.[32,34,36,39]

Congenital Kyphosis

Congenital kyphosis is an uncommon deformity in the sagittal plane and is even rarer than other forms of scoliotic deformity. Progression of kyphosis can lead to neurologic compromise; there is a high likelihood of neurologic deficit when left untreated. The cause of the kyphosis is failure of either formation or segmentation of a portion of the anterior column.[40–43]

The kyphosis is progressive and half of these patients present with some neurologic signs or symptoms. Symptoms are a result of compression of the spinal cord and nerve roots. The most common initial presentation is neurogenic bladder. Other symptoms include lower extremity abnormalities such as pain and weakness as well as orthopedic abnormalities such as equinocavovarus deformities of the feet.[44,45] The inherent instability of these kyphotic deformities places these patients at significant risk for catastrophic neurologic injury after minor falls or trivial trauma. Children can present with acute paraplegia and a "dislocated" spine.[44,45]

Imaging workup includes X-rays (AP and lateral as well as routine standing 36-inch scoliosis films), CT scan to fully delineate bony anatomy, and an MRI scan to evaluate the spinal cord and nerve root anatomy and to look for compression prior to any surgical correction.

Winter et al[46] classified congenital kyphosis into three patterns: type I, failure of vertebral body formation; type II, failure of anterior vertebral body segmentation, resulting in an anterior unsegmented bar; and type III, a mixed failure of formation and segmentation (**Fig. 47.3**). The type I kyphotic deformity is the most common and the most likely to progress rapidly and cause neurologic deterioration. The severity of the deformity is directly proportional to the amount of vertebral body that fails to form (**Fig. 47.4**). A variant of the type I error is a central and anterior failure of formation producing a "butterfly vertebra"[47] (**Fig. 47.5**). The type II kyphotic deformity is rarer and produces a less severe deformity that is less likely to progress to neurologic deficit. The etiology of the vertebral body aplasia or hypoplasia is not well defined. Initially, sclerotomal absence or malformation was proposed, but total disruption of the sclerotome would lead to posterior arch abnormalities, which are not typically seen in pure congenital kyphosis. One current theory proposes that there is a

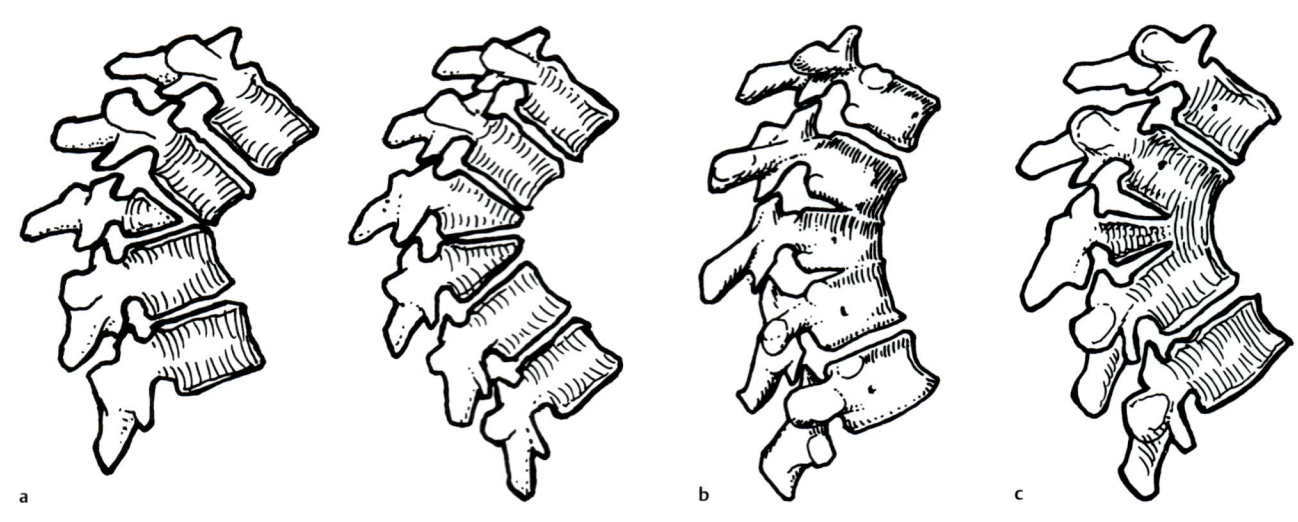

Fig. 47.3 Congenital kyphosis. Winter classification: **(a)** type I, failure of formation; **(b)** type II, failure of segmentation; **(c)** type III, mixed failure of formation and segmentation.

lack of vascularization of the developing centra of the vertebra during the end of chondrification or during ossification.

There is no clinical experience to support bracing or other nonoperative management for congenital kyphosis. For type I lesions, the ideal treatment is a simple posterior fusion without instrumentation, provided the child is between 1 and 5 years of age. For children older than 5 years, posterior fusion can be done if the angle of kyphosis is less than 55 degrees. If a posterior approach alone is employed in patients with greater than 55 degree of kyphosis, the pseudarthrosis rate may be as high as 54%. Therefore, for all adults and for children over 5 years of age whose kyphosis is greater than 55 degrees, a combined anterior/posterior approach is preferred.[43,44,48] The anterior surgery enables the release of tethering structures that prevent the correction of the kyphosis and enables the insertion of bone grafts to restore height and achieve solid union. For the less common type II kyphosis, treatment is posterior fusion one level above and below the segmentation defect. If the kyphotic deformity is advanced, then it may be necessary to perform an anterior osteotomy of the unsegmented bar followed by posterior stabilization.

Congenital Lordosis

Congenital lordosis is infrequently encountered, rarer than either congenital scoliosis or congenital kyphosis. This condition results from dorsal defects in segmentation accompanied by normal ventral growth. There may also be a deformity in the coronal plane with a lordoscoliosis when the location of the unsegmented bar is dorsolateral.[49,50] The most common complication of congenital lordosis is development of a severe impairment of pulmonary function, making it a potentially lethal deformity. Winter et al[35] report the case of a child with congenital thoracic

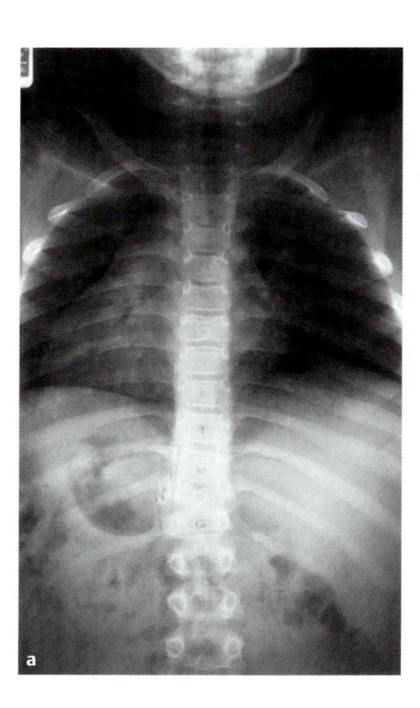

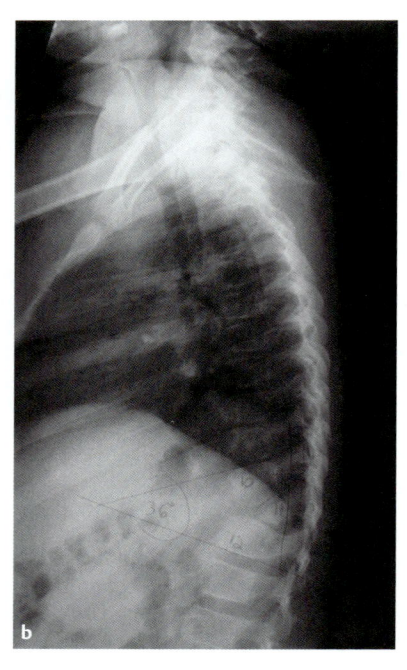

Fig. 47.4 Congenital kyphosis. Anteroposterior **(a)** and lateral **(b)** radiographs of a 6-year-old boy with an incidental abnormality found during an asthma evaluation. Winter type I congenital kyphosis with failure of formation of the anterior elements of T11.

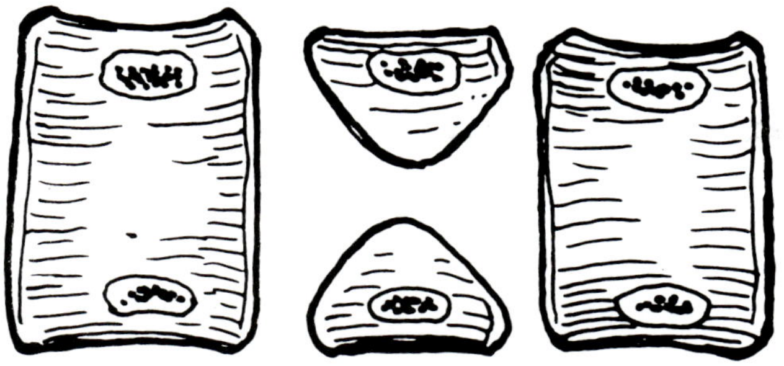

Fig. 47.5 Butterfly vertebra.

lordosis who died at age 9, whose autopsy revealed that the anterior aspect of the spine was only 8 mm from the posterior wall of the sternum.

Imaging should include X-rays (AP and lateral as well as routine standing 36-inch scoliosis films), a CT scan to clearly elucidate the bony abnormalities, and an MRI scan to evaluate for spinal cord or nerve root compromise. If pulmonary insufficiency is present, pulmonary function testing, medical optimization, and imaging should be done prior to surgery to ensure patient safety.

There is no role for conservative therapy once the diagnosis is made. The plan for surgical correction is either one of stabilization or one of correction depending on whether the patient has presented prior to the onset of major deformity. A preventive operation requires anterior arthrodesis of the involved segments and one or two vertebrae above and below the lesion. A corrective operation for major deformity requires a combined anterior/posterior approach.[50]

Dysplastic (Congenital) Spondylolisthesis

Spondylolisthesis is the slippage of all or part of one vertebral body on the vertebral body below. Spondylolisthesis is extremely rare during infancy.[51,52] A widely accepted classification of spondylolisthesis is by Wiltse et al.[53] They divided spondylolisthesis into five types: type I, dysplastic spondylolisthesis; type II, isthmic spondylolisthesis; type III, degenerative spondylolisthesis; type IV, traumatic spondylolisthesis; and type V, pathological spondylolisthesis. Wiltse and Rothman[54] later suggested a common congenital component in the etiology of dysplastic and isthmic spondylolisthesis and further refined classification of spondylolisthesis (**Fig. 47.6**).

Dysplastic spondylolisthesis accounts for 14 to 21% of the cases of spondylolisthesis, with a 2:1 female-to-male ratio.[51] It is characterized by structural anomalies of the lumbosacral junction, including dysplasia of the lamina and facet joints. The lack of the normal facet buttress provided by normal facet joints predisposes toward slippage of the superior vertebra on the inferior one. The dysplastic articular processes may be oriented in the axial or sagittal planes. In axial dysplasia, the articular processes have a horizontal orientation; this condition is often associated with spina bifida. In sagittal dysplasia, the facet joints are often asymmetric, and the neural arch is usually intact. Therefore, high-grade slippage seldom occurs.

Dysplastic spondylolisthesis can present with back or leg pain and neurologic deficit, such as paresthesia, weakness, or, rarely, incontinence of the bowel or bladder. Neurologic deficits are usually associated with high-grade slippage. Symptoms usually result from neural foramen stenosis secondary to the listhesis.

Several different etiologies have been identified with this condition. The role of upright posture contributing to development of dysplastic spondylolisthesis is recognized. The association of spondylosis with the onset of ambulation in early childhood has also been noted.[55,56] It has been suggested that spondylolisthesis results from a congenital defect or dysplasia that causes the development of a pars defect due to the stresses of upright posture and lumbar lordosis.

Diagnostic studies include X-ray, CT, and MRI. Upright X-ray is commonly the first imaging modality obtained and is useful for determining the grade of spondylolisthesis. Dynamic flexion and extension X-rays are important in evaluating the presence of instability. CT can better delineate bony structures, and is helpful for presurgical planning if surgery is indicated. MRI can also be helpful, especially in cases where there is neurologic compromise.

Initial treatment should be nonoperative unless progression is documented in the younger patients or slippage is greater than 50%. Fusion in situ is the most frequently performed surgical procedure, although some surgeons utilize reduction and fixation, especially in high-grade slips.[54,56]

Klippel-Feil Syndrome

Klippel-Feil syndrome (KFS) is a congenital spinal disorder characterized by multiple fused cervical vertebra due to a failure of cervical spine segmentation. Although most commonly associated with the classic clinical triad of a short neck, low posterior hairline, and decreased neck range of motion,[57] this trio of findings is seen in fewer than 50% of patients.[58] Commonly associated congenital abnormalities include scoliosis (> 50%), deafness, genitourinary abnormalities, Sprengel's deformity, cervical ribs, and cardiovascular abnormalities.[59] The incidence of KFS is not known.

Patients with KFS most often present with pain or neurologic compromise, usually secondary to spinal cord or nerve root dysfunction. High-quality radiographs or CT scans of the neck reveal multiple fused cervical vertebra. If neurologic deficits are present, MRI of the spine is recommended. On imaging workup, abnormalities of the craniocervical junction may be seen, and dynamic instability between fused segments may be present. There are three types of KFS as originally described[60]: type I, fusion of many cervical and upper thoracic vertebra; type II, fusion at one or two interspaces, which may be combined with other cervical spine abnormalities such as hemivertebrae; and type III, cervical fusions with thoracic or lumbar spine fusions. Of these, type II KFS has the lowest risk of developing significant scoliosis.[61] Workup of the KFS patient for abnormalities of the cardiac and renal organs typically includes an echocardiogram and renal ultrasound. Audiology testing is also done to identify a hearing loss.

Surgical treatment of KFS patients primarily occurs in the context of neurologic compromise due to stenosis, spinal instability, or spinal deformity. The heterogeneity of KFS spinal abnormalities necessitates that a spectrum of surgical solutions be available to address the problem to be corrected.

Spinal Dysraphism

Spinal dysraphism refers to congenital anomalies characterized by failure of fusion of midline structures of ectodermal and mesodermal origin. The failure of fusion of the bony posterior elements is termed spina bifida. Spina bifida ranges from mild, in the form of meningocele (meninges without neural elements protrude under the skin through an unfused cleft of malformed vertebral arch), to myelomeningocele (spinal cord and meninges protrude, not covered by normal skin), to severe, in the form of myeloschisis (neural folds did not close; neural plate is exposed, not covered by meninges or skin). These conditions are apparent at birth. In contrast, in spina bifida occulta, the unfused posterior

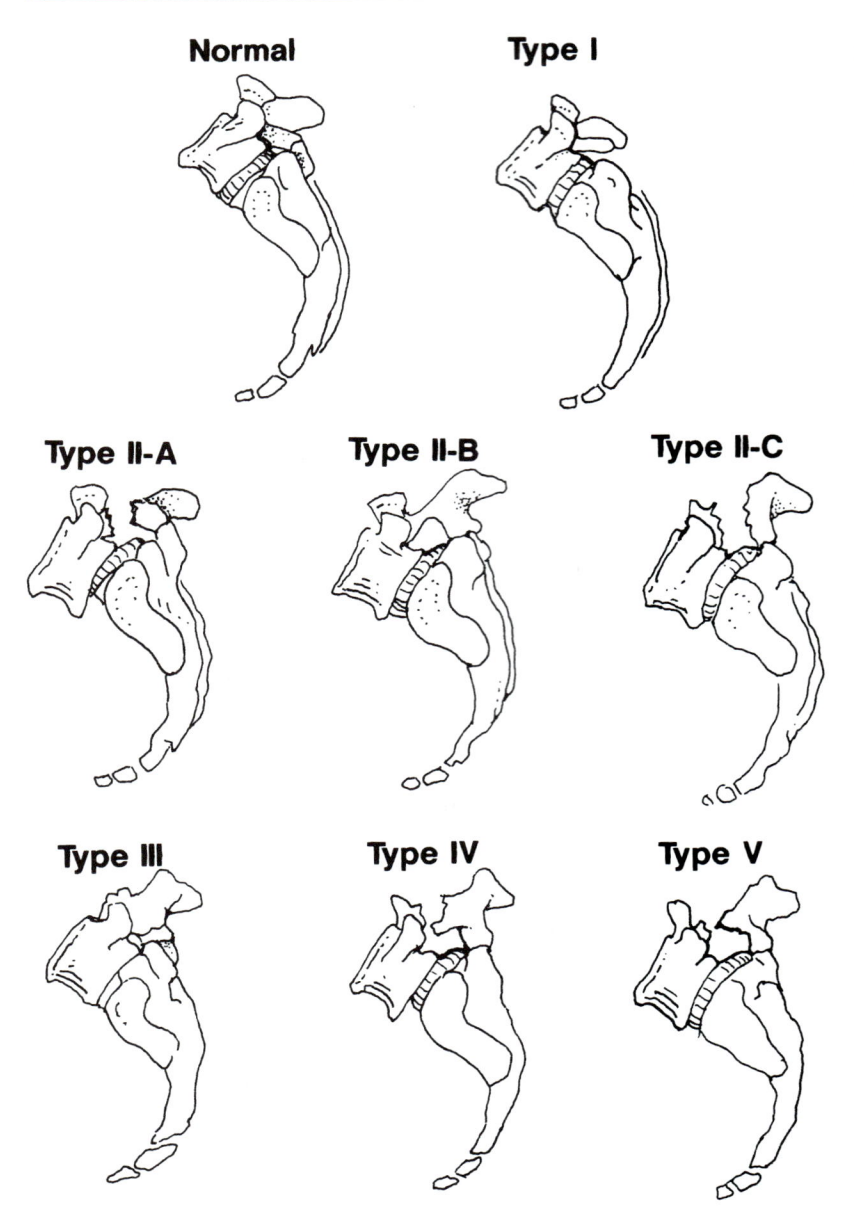

Fig. 47.6 Wiltse classification of spondylolisthesis. Type I: dysplastic congenital deficiency of the superior sacral and inferior fifth lumbar facets. Type II: isthmic; II-A lytic (fatigue fracture of the pars); II-B elongated but intact pars; II-C acute fracture of the pars. Type III: degenerative (facet joint degeneration allows translation, usually L4 on L5 in older patients). Type IV: traumatic (acute fracture in a region other than the pars). Type V: pathological attenuation of the pedicle secondary to structural weakness in the bone.

bony elements are typically detected only radiographically later in life. This finding may be seen in 10 to 20% of the population and are without neurologic consequence. A few studies suggest a higher incidence or more severe back pain with this finding, and even more studies have reported lack of association.[62]

There are other spinal dysraphism conditions, but unlike in open spinal bifida, the other spinal dysraphisms have no association with Chiari II malformation or hydrocephalus. Spinal dysraphism can encompass a variety of conditions including lipomyelomeningocele, lipoma of the filum terminale, tight filum terminale, diastematomyelia, and dermal sinus tracts (with or without intradural dermoid tumors) and neurenteric cysts. The defects are covered by skin; unlike myelomeningoceles, they are less readily apparent on clinical examination and may not be noted until later in life. The incidence of these conditions is not fully quantified as some remain undiagnosed.

Children may present with cutaneous stigmata, pain, orthopedic findings, neurologic changes, or radiographic abnormalities. The cutaneous stigmata include hairy patch, hemangioma, dermal sinus tract, subcutaneous mass, and rudimentary appendage.[63] Orthopedic examination may reveal scoliosis, leg length or size asymmetry, or cavovarus foot deformity. Neurologic changes include sensory and motor deficits typically in the lower extremities, as well as neurogenic bladder. Toddlers may present with delayed developmental motor milestones, whereas older children may present with a combination of both upper and lower motor neuron signs of one or more extremities. Bowel and bladder dysfunction are common; recurrent urinary tract infections in children should trigger workup for neurogenic bladder. The multidisciplinary care highlighted in the myelomeningocele section, below, may also apply to patients with other spinal dysraphisms depending on their degree of neurologic dysfunction.

Myelomeningocele

Myelomeningocele (MMC) is a neural tube defect (NTD) with potentially devastating presentations including paralysis, lifelong disability, and death. Since the implementation of folate supplementation and improved prenatal screening, the incidence of MMC in the United States has decreased 27% from 2.6 per 10,000 live births in 1995–1996 to 1.9 per 10,000 live births in 2003–2004.[64] Despite these efforts, the incidence of MMC has plateaued and continues to be prevalent in the U.S.[65] The incidence varies worldwide, with a rate as high as 8.7 per 1,000 live births in Belfast, Ireland, and almost similar in parts of India[66]; there are ethnic and racial variations, with a high a priori risk of NTD described in Irish and in Mexican-American populations. The overall incidence varies by socio-demography, race/ethnicity, genetics, geography, and environment. Risk factors include, but are not limited to, maternal folate deficiency, diet and vitamin intake, maternal glucose status, hyperthermia, maternal medication use (such as antiepileptics), and maternal substance use (alcohol, tobacco, illicit drugs). Epidemiological factors have also been implicated. No clear mode of inheritance for neural tube defects has been determined. First-degree relatives of an affected individual have a 3 to 5% risk, whereas second-degree relatives have a 1 to 2% risk of NTD.[67] Prenatal diagnosis is suggested by increased levels of maternal serum α-fetoprotein (AFP) or in amniotic fluid and by fetal imaging (such as ultrasound or MRI), most commonly fetal ultrasound.

Postnatal diagnosis of an open neural tube defect requires careful documentation of the anatomic level and the neurologic function, as well as assessment for hydrocephalus and Chiari II malformation symptoms. Evaluation for concomitant anomalies with cardiac and renal assessment is important preoperatively. Structural deformities such as kyphos as well as skin closure strategies should be actively considered during operative planning (**Fig. 47.7**).

The treatment rationale is to decrease the risk of central nervous system (CNS) infection from the open NTD, and to protect the exposed neural tissue from continuing additional trauma. Primary treatment of MMC is surgical closure of the defect following birth. Neurologic consequences of MMC include meningitis, hydrocephalus, and neurologic and functional deficits. Functional motor and sensory levels are typically consistent with the anatomic lesions at presentation. Associated Chiari II malformation and hydrocephalus with MMC contribute to the overall neurologic morbidity. Urologic sequelae arise from chronic neurogenic bladder dysfunction; proactive bladder management and bowel regimens are initiated early. Further urologic surgeries may be required. Orthopedic deformities and sequelae are from sensorimotor deficits or paralysis; patients also develop progressive spinal deformity over time. As well, patients need to be monitored for signs and symptoms of tethered cord over time, as up to 50% may require additional surgery for tethered cord release. Physical medicine and rehabilitation teams may help with bracing, assistive devices, and therapy to enhance independence. Long-term multidisciplinary care is needed for the life span of patients with myelomeningocele to prevent complications, maximize function, and optimize quality of life.

Alternatively, fetal surgery for in utero treatment of myelomeningocele was investigated through a multicenter randomized trial sponsored by the National Institutes of Health (Management of Myelomeningocele Study).[65] The rationale includes minimizing continued exposure of spinal tissue to amniotic fluid and closure of open cerebrospinal fluid (CSF) pathways at the lesion site. Long-term follow-up continues to be gathered, and early results show relative reduction in the number of children requiring CSF diversion for hydrocephalus and better motor function for the prenatal intervention cohort compared with the postnatal closure patients. Hindbrain herniation associated with Chiari II malformation also appears to resolve after some prenatal closures. There are risks to the fetus (including prematurity and death) and to the mother (including infection, massive hemorrhage, and fetal demise). A full treatment of this evolving topic is beyond the scope of this chapter.

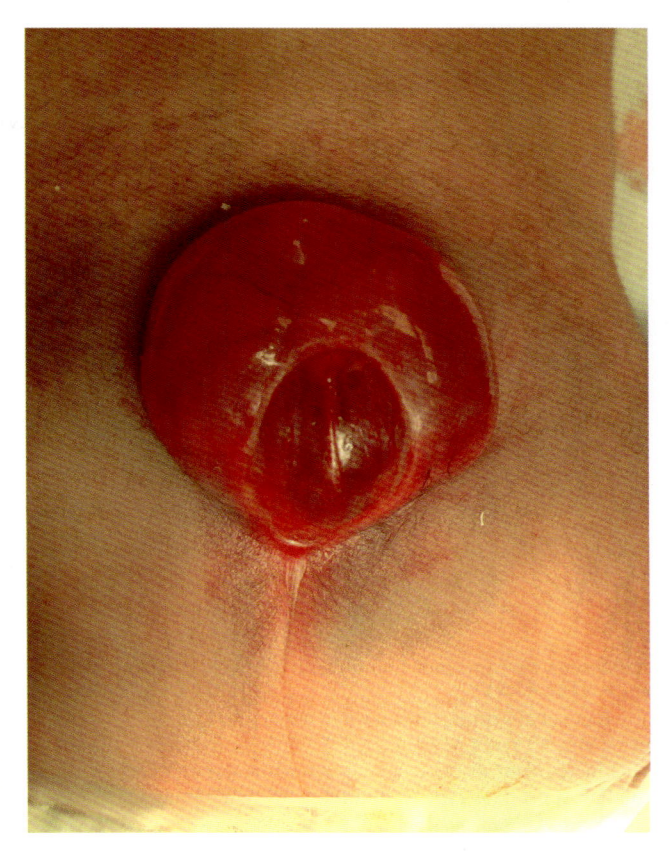

Fig. 47.7 Lumbar myelomeningocele.

Meningocele

Dorsal meningocele is a condition in which a sac of dura and arachnoid without neural elements protrude under the skin through an unfused cleft of malformed vertebral arch, typically with an underlying normal spinal cord and canal. Meningoceles are relatively rare, with one meningocele observed for every 10 to 20 myelomeningoceles. This entity likely represents a postneurulation disorder of dorsal mesenchymal development.

Meningoceles are usually covered with dysplastic or normal skin at birth, which is evident on clinical examination. The spinal cord is normal and remains in the spinal canal, and there are no neural elements in the herniated meningocele sac. The neurologic examination is normal. Association with Chiari malformation or hydrocephalus is uncommon. MRI delineates preoperative anatomy. Surgical repair of the meningocele is undertaken to correct the outward deformity and repair the protruded CSF sac. Prenatally, AFP levels in maternal serum and amniotic fluid are normal (**Fig. 47.8**).

Diastematomyelia (Split Cord Malformations)

There are two types of split spinal cord malformations (SCMs): diastematomyelia and diplomyelia. Diastematomyelia refers to a malformation with two hemicords contained in two separate dural sleeves, separated in the middle by a fibrocartilaginous or bony spur. This differs from diplomyelia, in which two separate

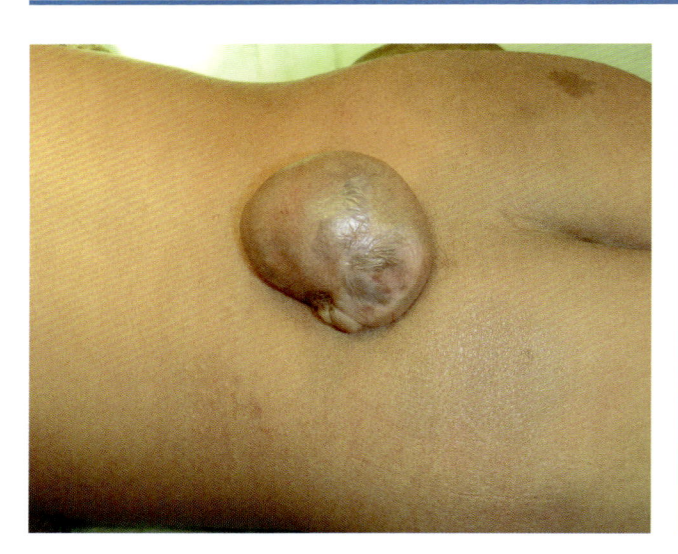

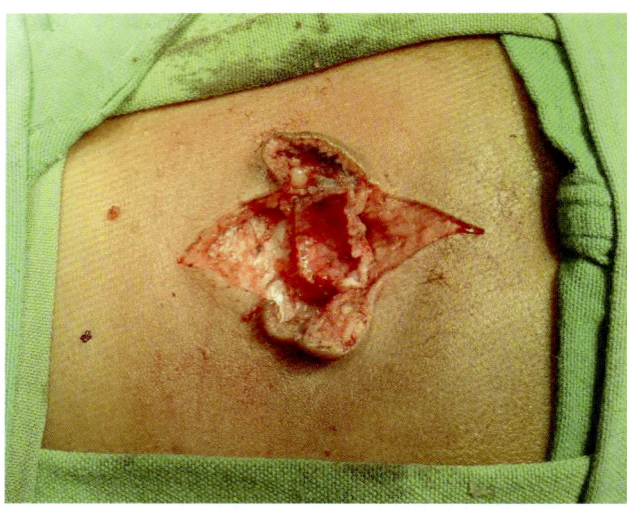

Fig. 47.8 **(a)** Late presentation of a lumbar meningocele in a child with no neurologic deficits. **(b)** Intraoperative photograph shows no neural elements within this dural sac.

hemicords are contained in one dural sac without an intervening spur[68] (**Fig. 47.9**).

Pang et al[19] proposed a unified theory for the embryogenesis of SCMs. A type I SCM refers to two hemicords each housed within its own dural tube separated by a osseocartilaginous median septum. A type II SCM refers to two hemicords within a single dural sheath (diplomyelia).

Both types of SCM are postulated to originate from one embryological error around the time of neural tube closure. The error occurs when an accessory neurenteric canal forms through the midline of the embryonic disk, maintaining a persistent communication between the endoderm and the ectoderm, which is normally only transient. Mesenchyme condenses around this tract, which splits the developing notochord and neural tube. The malformation phenotype depends on subsequent spinal development. An SCM results if the embryo is able to heal around the tract. If the tract is infiltrated with primitive cells from the mesenchyme destined to become the meninges, the two hemicords will each be invested in dura mater. The dura mater can stimulate bone growth that results in the midline spur in type I SCM. In Pang et al's[19] series of 39 patients, 19 patients had type I SCM and 18 patients had type II SCM, with two patients having composite lesions. Other authors have subsequently reported combinations of composite and tandem lesions. Although some advise inspecting for medial nerve roots from the split cords to help determine classification, medial nerve roots are also reported to be observed in 75% of both type I and type II SCMs.[19]

An SCM is typically observed from the high thoracic vertebra to the low lumbar vertebra, with a distribution of 50% in the thoracic and 50% in the lumbar regions. There is a female preponderance.[69] In one series, 79% had congenital scoliosis and 84% had neurologic manifestation in 43 patients with SCM.[70]

The presence of a cutaneous hairy patch is associated with underlying SCM. Plain X-rays of the spine may show a midline bony spur, widened interpedicular distance, scoliosis, or bony segmentation errors. MRI is helpful in delineating the pathological anatomy. CT with myelography is an imaging procedure of choice to study the overall bony architecture, to outline the anatomy of the hemicords, and to define the presence of a bony or fibrous tethering midline spur (**Fig. 47.10**).

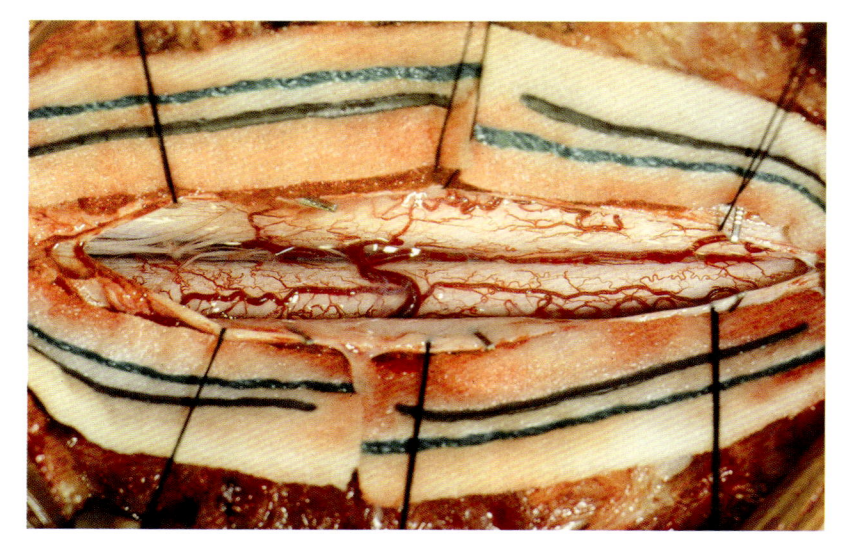

Fig. 47.9 Diplomyelia, intraoperative photograph.

47 Congenital Abnormalities

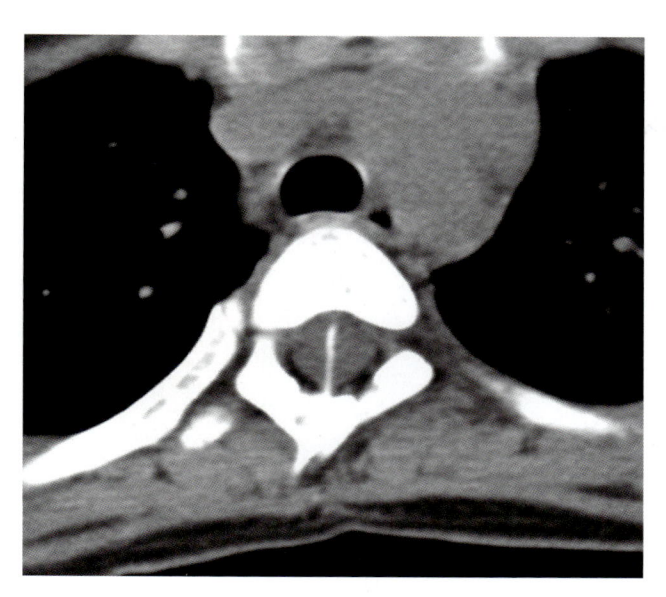

Fig. 47.10 Axial computed tomography (CT) scan showing a midline bony spur in a type 1 split cord malformation.

neurologic sensorimotor complaints are reported to respond well to surgical intervention.

Dermal Sinus Tracts

Dermal sinus tracts are estimated to have an incidence of 1 in 1,500 live births. They typically present as a small pit-like opening in the skin superior to the intergluteal crease. This is the entrance to a sinus tract lined by squamous epithelium that penetrates the thecal sac (anywhere along the lumbosacral spine to the occiput).[73] The position of the sinus tract opening above the gluteal crease helps to distinguish suspicion of the dermal sinus tract from a benign, blind-ended sacrococcygeal dimple or pilonidal pit.

Dermal sinus tracts are lined by stratified squamous epithelium. They may obliquely traverse several spinal levels compared with the external skin site before penetrating the dura and attaching to the filum or spinal cord. Intradurally, they may be associated with other dysraphic abnormalities.[74] About half of dermal sinus tracts end in an intradural dermoid or epidermoid lesion. Dermoids contain elements from two germ layers (such as hair, sweat glands, sebaceous glands), whereas epidermoids contain desquamated cells from the epidermal layer only. These tumors are also found in the subarachnoid space arising from isolated congenital rests of cells derived from the multipotential caudal cell mass.

Patients present with unexplained bouts of meningitis (typically *Staphylococcus aureus* or *Escherichia coli*) via dermal sinus tract communication with the CNS.[75] Patients may also present with signs and symptoms related to tethered spinal cord, neural compression, spinal abscess, or cutaneous infection of the sinus tract. MRI is the imaging modality of choice in further workup to delineate the lesion's anatomy for diagnosis and preoperative planning. MRI shows where the tract connects with the dura and reveals any associated intradural pathology[75] (**Fig. 47.11**). There is no role for conservative management, given the risk of recurrent CNS infection. Surgical intervention is recommended once

Split cord malformations may lead to tethering, neurologic deficits, and resulting orthopedic deformities. Patients diagnosed with SCM are recommended by some authors to undergo surgical exploration even in the absence of symptoms.[69,71] These authors note in their series that older patients at presentation tend to have more severe deficits. Others point out that there is no quality evidence in the literature supporting prophylactic surgical management.[72] Surgery for clinically symptomatic and neurologically deteriorating patients with SCM is less controversial. In cases with preoperative symptoms, preoperative pain and

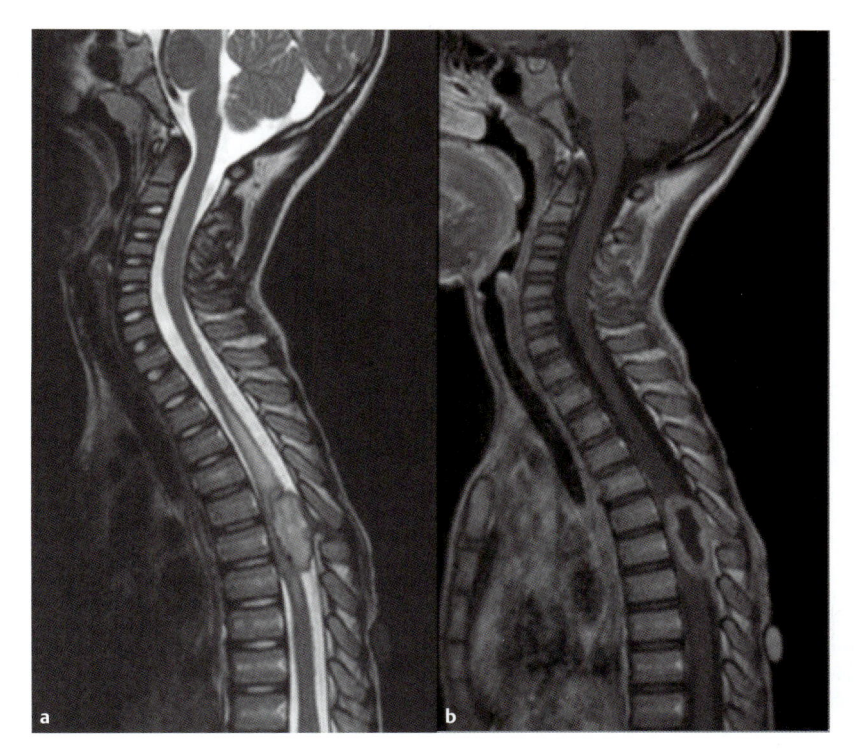

Fig. 47.11 Dermal sinus tract terminating in an infected intradural dermoid in the thoracic spine. Sagittal magnetic resonance imaging (MRI) of the thoracic spine: **(a)** T2-weighted sequence; **(b)** T1-weighted sequence with gadolinium.

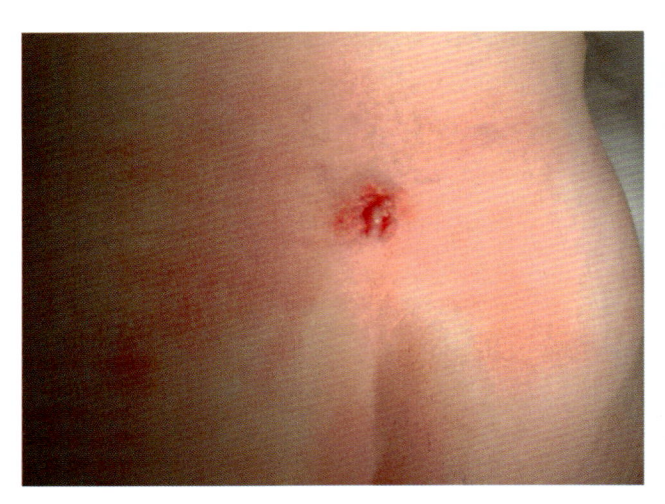

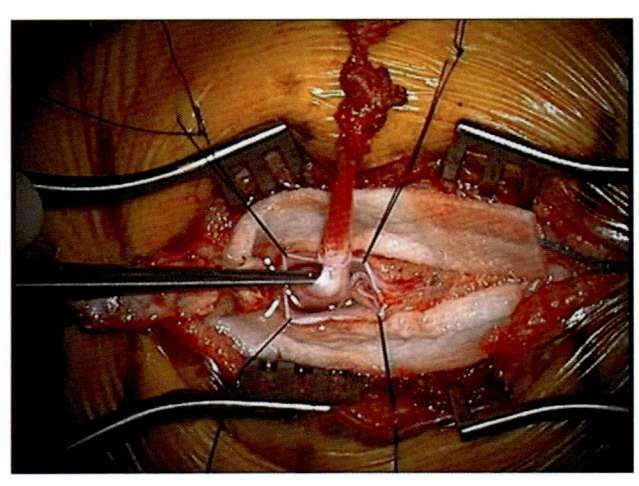

Fig. 47.12 (a) Lumbar skin lesion heralding occult spinal dysraphism. (b) Intraoperative picture of the associated spinal dermal sinus tract leading to a dermoid at the conus medullaris.

the diagnosis is made to completely excise the dermal sinus tract and any associated intradural pathology if present (**Fig. 47.12**).

Tethered Cord Syndrome

Tethered cord syndrome (TCS) signifies a clinical and pathological condition in which the conus medullaris is under tension, typically signified by an abnormally low position of the conus medullaris below the L1-2 disk space. Classically, TCS has been attributed to a thick filum terminale or fatty filum terminale. However, there are multiple etiologies that can lead to tethering of the spinal cord, including diastematomyelia, myelomeningocele, lipomyelomeningocele, lipoma, dermal sinus tract, and arachnoidal adhesions secondary to trauma, surgery, or infection.

The true incidence of TCS is unknown. Many patients with radiographic findings of possible tethered cord are clinically asymptomatic. The increasing use of high-resolution imaging such as MRI can lead to an incidentally found low-lying conus medullaris. Although most patients with TCS have a low-lying conus, some patients have a normally positioned conus with a "tight" filum.[76] Clinical symptoms of TCS include weakness, numbness, gait dysfunction, spasticity, urinary hesitancy/incontinence, and back/leg pain.[77] On examination, nearly 59% of patients have cutaneous stigmata such as a hairy patch, cutaneous hemangioma, lumbosacral appendage, or dermal sinus tract.[77] Many patients also present orthopedic findings, such as congenital vertebral abnormalities, leg length discrepancies, gluteal asymmetry, and foot/ankle deformities.

In patients with a history and physical examination suggestive of TCS, MRI constitutes an appropriate imaging workup. The location of the conus and any associated intradural pathology, such as a lipoma, is identified. When abnormalities of the bony spine are suspected, a CT scan is useful. If bladder dysfunction is suggested, urodynamic studies are performed. Urodynamic studies can help determine if there is true neurogenic bladder.

The treatment of TCS varies based on the underlying pathology. In patients with TCS secondary to a fatty filum or spinal dysraphism, surgical de-tethering of the spinal cord often results in significant pain and neurologic improvement.[78,79] Bladder dysfunction improvement is seen in 60 to 70% patients, particularly in those with primary TCS.[80,81] Patients who have surgery only with persistent signs and symptoms after medical management attain improvement of symptoms and favorable outcomes.[82] Clinical follow-up is mandatory, as patients can re-tether, requiring repeat operation.

Lipoma of the Terminal Filum

Lipoma of the terminal filum, otherwise known as a fatty filum, refers to a lipoma of the filum terminale that forms secondary to dysfunction during the process of secondary neurulation. The vast majority (> 90%) of patients with these lesions are asymptomatic, and increasingly these lesions are found incidentally on imaging.[83] In patients who have symptoms, it is usually due to tethering of the spinal cord, often becoming apparent during adolescent growth spurts. Common presenting symptoms include bladder dysfunction, low back pain, and leg pain. MRI is the imaging modality of choice for diagnosis, and usually reveals a T1 hyperintense, T2 hypointense fatty lesion within the filum terminale. An occult or asymptomatic fatty filum can be found in ~ 4% of the population.[84] Symptomatic patients with a fatty filum are typically expected to have an associated low-lying conus on imaging.[83]

Surgical treatment of this entity is controversial, especially in asymptomatic patients. Release of the filum terminale is associated with a low but present complication rate, and a reportedly low rate of re-tethering.[85] Prophylactic filum sectioning is advocated by some practitioners.[85,86] There is admittedly little evidence to support this practice of prophylactic surgery, and some data suggest the vast majority of lesions remain asymptomatic.[83] Many practitioners operate on only clinically symptomatic patients with a fatty filum and low-lying conus. The outcome in these patients is favorable, with an arrest in symptom progression or improvement in symptoms in nearly all patients.[86]

Lipomyelomeningoceles

Lipomyelomeningoceles are neural tube defects characterized by a union between spinal cord and fatty tissue, the interface of which is extraspinal. They occur in ~ 0.3 to 0.6 per 10,000 live births,[87] with a ~ 2:1 female-to-male ratio.[88] Tethered cord is nearly synonymous with lipomyelomeningocele due to the lipoma tethering down the spinal cord. There are also other associated conditions including genitourinary (GU) abnormalities, dermoids/epidermoids, diastomyelia, scoliosis, and syringomyelia. Most patient present with either a cosmetic defect or urinary incontinence, usually between the ages of 6 days and 18 years.[88]

Skin manifestations overlying the lipomyelomeningocele can include dimples, hemangiomas, hairy patches, tail-like appendages, and skin defects. Focal neurologic deficits are rare on initial presentation, but become much more common with age.

Lipomyelomeningoceles arise from failure of disjunction between the epithelial ectoderm and neural ectoderm during primary neurulation. This results in a union of neural tissue and fat forming mesenchymal tissue, manifested as a lipoma extending from the spinal cord, through the meninges and bony defects, and into the subcutaneous tissue. The extraspinal location of the neural placode lipoma interface differentiates this from lipomeningoceles, which have an intraspinal interface.

An MRI performed both prenatally and postnatally is useful for diagnosing lipomyelomeningoceles. There is expansion of the subarachnoid space with herniation of the neural tissue and meninges into the subcutaneous tissues. The fatty mass is best appreciated on T1-weighted sequences. Identification of the location of spinal cord, nerve roots, and lipoma is useful for minimizing injury during surgical planning. There are three types of lipomyelomeningoceles which describe the relative location of the lipoma and spinal cord: dorsal, transitional, and caudal. Dorsal lipomas attach to the spinal cord at the area of myeloschisis and are continuous with the subcutaneous tissue. Transitional lipomas further caudally down to the conus and are the most common type. Caudal lipomas arise mainly from the conus and may be covered by dura. Syringomyelia may be seen with tethering of the distal spinal cord (**Fig. 47.13**).

Goals for the treatment of lipomyelomeningocele are cord de-tethering, preservation of neural elements, and prevention of re-tethering of the spinal cord. The lipomatous tissue may or may not be possible to be excised. Due to the intimate association between the spinal cord and lipoma, various methods of lipoma resection have been devised to minimize the risk of neurologic injury including electrocautery, ultrasonic aspiration, and laser ablation. If the dura is not able to be closed primarily, duraplasty is performed.

Timing of surgery is controversial. Some practitioners advocate prophylactic surgery, whereas others offer surgery only with documented signs and symptoms of neurologic compromise such as neurogenic bladder or lower extremity dysfunction. Those that advocate early surgery (without neurologic compromise) point out that the surgical treatment of these patients carries a relatively low morbidity, with neurologic dysfunction recovery potential decreasing with age. Opponents point out that surgery carries the risk not only of neurologic injury and CSF leak, but also of scar tissue formation and spinal cord re-tethering, precipitating the need for more surgery in the future. Some patients may remain asymptomatic and not require surgery. Evidence in the literature supports the idea that clinical progression and deterioration are predictable based on the presenting anatomy of the lipomatous lesion, and surgery may not prevent progression over time.[85,89] Close multidisciplinary long-term monitoring is recommended to carefully track sensorimotor and urodynamic function as well as overall symptomatology to determine if and when surgery is clinically indicated.[72,90]

Neurenteric Cysts

Neurenteric cysts are congenital spinal cysts that account for 0.7 to 1.3% of all spinal axis lesions. These cysts originate from displaced endodermal tissue that has formed as a result of an abnormal connection between the endodermally derived foregut and the ectodermally derived spinal cord.[18,91] The mean age of presentation in the pediatric population is 6.4 years, and patients are predominantly male by a 2:1 ratio.[18,91] Most cysts occur in the thoracic or cervical spine and occur as solitary lesions located ventral to the spinal cord. Nearly 50% of patients with these lesions have other associated spinal abnormalities such as spinal dysraphism, split cord malformation, scoliosis, and Klippel-Feil syndrome.[18]

Presenting symptoms of neurenteric cysts vary by age. Most adolescent and adult patients present with back pain, leg pain, or neurologic deficits in the form of radiculopathy or myelopathy. Many children present only with cutaneous stigmata suggestive of an underlying dysraphic abnormality; the neurenteric cysts are then identified on imaging workup. There have been case reports of children presenting with aseptic meningitis, pyogenic meningitis, chronic pyrexia, incontinence, and paraplegia.[92]

Magnetic resonance imaging is the modality of choice to delineate the cyst and its relationship to neural structures; 90% are intradural and extramedullary. Neurenteric cysts are nonenhancing lesions that are isointense on T1-weighted imaging and hyperintense on T2-weighted imaging.[93] They are often intraspinal or dumbbell-shaped cystic lesions associated with an enteric/

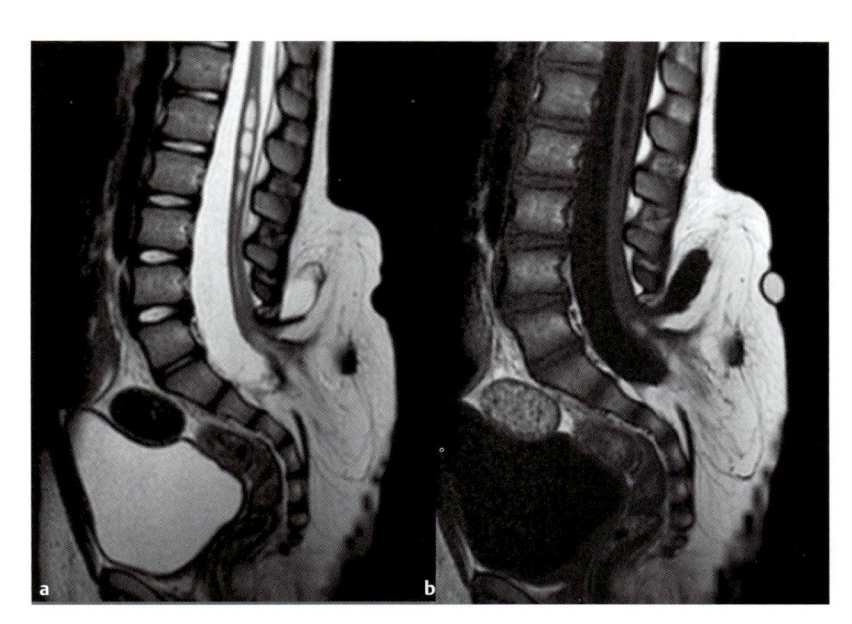

Fig. 47.13 Lipomyelomeningocele associated with syringomyelia. Sagittal T1-weighted **(a)** and sagittal T2-weighted **(b)** MRI of the lumbar spine.

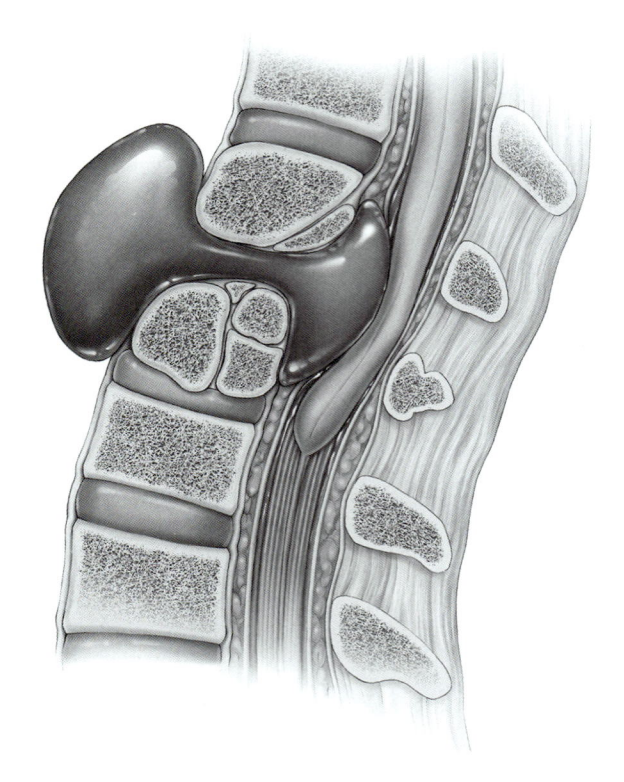

Fig. 47.14 Neurenteric cyst.

mediastinal cyst (**Fig. 47.14**). CT is used to identify any associated bony abnormalities.

On gross pathology, neurenteric cysts have a thickened outer membrane with a fluid-filled straw-colored center.[18,93] Histopathologically, they consist of mucin-producing, ciliated and nonciliated simple columnar and cuboidal epithelial goblet cells that surround a central cystic cavity.

Surgical resection is the first-line treatment for patients with neurologic deficits or significant debilitating pain. The goal of surgery is removal of the entire cyst. If remnant wall is left behind, there is a potential for cyst recurrence. Complete resection can be difficult and dangerous because of associated spinal vertebral abnormalities or adherence to nearby neural or vascular structures.[94] The selection of the approach for resection is entirely case dependent: anterior, posterior, or lateral approaches can be considered.

Cysts

Intraspinal Cysts

Intraspinal cysts, also known as congenital spinal meningeal cysts, are a heterogeneous group of congenital spinal cysts distinct from neurenteric cysts. They are commonly classified based on histopathology and on location within the spine. This is the basis for the Nabors classification system[95]:

- Type I: Extradural meningeal cyst without spinal nerve root fibers
    - Type Ia: Extradural meningeal cyst
    - Type Ib: Sacral meningocele
- Type II: Extradural meningeal cyst with spinal nerve root fibers
- Type III: Intradural spinal meningeal cysts

Type Ia: Extradural Meningeal Cyst

Extradural spinal meningeal cysts are outpouchings of arachnoid through a small dural defect that are contiguous with the spinal subarachnoid space.[96] They are thought to be related to transmitted hydrostatic pressure of CSF at areas of dural deficiency. These lesions are rare. Because many are found incidentally on imaging, the true incidence is unknown. They are most commonly found in the thoracic spine and are seen as enlargements of the subarachnoid space up to the level of the dorsal root ganglia.[95]

Patients typically present with radicular pain or paresthesias if they are symptomatic. These lesions may be difficult to visualize on MRI, as the cyst fluid appears the same as CSF. Adjacent bony changes on X-ray or CT, such as enlargement of a neural foramen or thinning of adjacent bone, can also consolidate the diagnosis.[96]

Asymptomatic incidental cysts can be observed. Surgical removal of an extradural spinal arachnoid cyst is the preferred option over simple aspiration for symptomatic patients with cysts. Surgery entails closure of the ostium between the cyst and the subarachnoid space, fenestration of the cyst, or shunting of the cyst.[96]

Type Ib: Sacral Meningocele

Sacral meningoceles are outpouchings of arachnoid from the caudal end of the thecal sac, adjacent to dorsal sacral or coccygeal nerve roots[95] (**Fig. 47.15**). The true prevalence is difficult to determine secondary to the rarity and the occult nature of this lesion. In symptomatic patients it does appear to have a male predominance.[97,98] Most patients are asymptomatic. When symptoms do occur, they commonly include pain and bowel or bladder dysfunction likely related to compression of adjacent dorsal

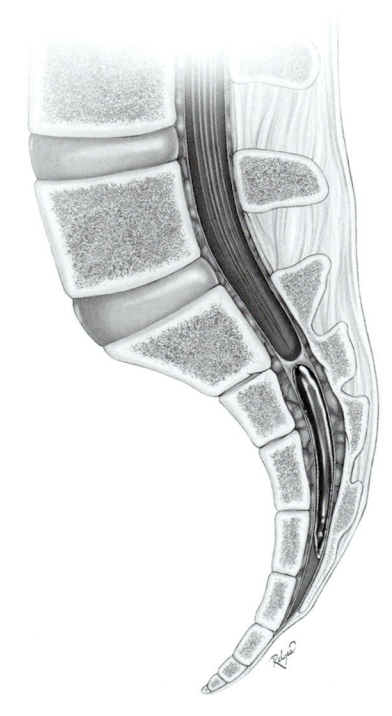

Fig. 47.15 Sacral meningocele.

sacral or coccygeal nerve roots. Pain can be described as a chronic, intermittent, deep tail bone pain.[98]

The imaging modality of choice is MRI, although the lesion, including the connection point, can be seen using CT myelography or myelography. The T1- and T2-weighted characteristics are the same as those of CSF on all sequences. CT often shows thinning of adjacent sacral lamina. Unlike a perineural cyst, the apex of the lesion usually appears midline.

On gross pathology there is a pedicle that connects the cyst to the thecal sac, which permits contiguous CSF flow. However, there are no meninges or neuronal elements surrounding or within the cyst. Histopathologically, the cyst is lined by fibrous connective tissue and has a single layer of simple cuboidal epithelium. The tissue is glial fibrillary acidic protein (GFAP) positive and consistent with the lining of the ependymal central canal wall.[98,99]

Asymptomatic lesions can be observed. Treatment for a growing symptomatic sacral meningocele is surgical ligation and obliteration of the cyst.[99]

Type II: Extradural Meningeal Cyst with Spinal Nerve Root Fibers

Commonly known as Tarlov's perineural cysts, these lesions typically occur in the sacral spine near the dorsal root ganglion; they contain nerve fibers, and can be isolated or come in multiples. They are located between the perineurium and endoneurium, hence the name perineural cyst. A perineural cyst appears as a dilatation of the arachnoid and dura of the spinal posterior nerve root sheath. Congenitally they are thought to arise from arachnoid proliferation within the root sleeve and subsequent obstruction of normal CSF flow.

Annual incidence is estimated to be around 5%, with a female predilection.[100] In over 80% of cases, patients are asymptomatic as these are usually incidental lesions. In the remaining 20% of cases, reported symptoms include back pain, sacral radiculopathy, urinary incontinence, bowel dysfunction, dyspareunia, and abdominal pain.[101] Cyst rupture has been reported to cause spontaneous intracranial hypotension.

Computed tomography and MRI are the most common modalities used to identify these lesions. On CT, the lesion appears hypodense and has similar characteristics of CSF. There is usually widening of the neural foramen due to chronic bone remodeling. On MRI sequences, the cyst is hypointense on T1-weighted imaging and hyperintense on T2-weighted imaging. On CT myelography, there is delayed opacification of the cyst with intrathecal contrast.

Grossly, the perineural cyst originates at the junction of the dorsal nerve root ganglion and has a clear to slightly cloudy cyst wall, with the nerve root traversing through or within the cyst wall. Histopathologically, the outer wall is epineurium lined by arachnoid and the inner wall is lined with pia mater.[101,102]

No treatment is needed for asymptomatic lesions. For patients with pain, conservative medical management with anti-inflammatory medications and physical therapy are appropriate. Surgical treatment, when indicated, includes microsurgical excision of the cyst with duraplasty or plication of the cyst wall.[102]

Type III: Intradural Spinal Meningeal Cysts

Intradural spinal arachnoid cysts are extra-axial cysts within the thecal sac that are thought to develop secondary to arachnoid proliferation. They rarely cause spinal cord pathology and thus the true incidence has not been reported. Most occur as solitary lesions posterior to the spinal cord, but are sometimes found in multiples or in association with other anomalies (such as syringomyelia, kyphoscoliosis, or spinal dysraphism). Because of their location, they can cause mass effect on adjacent spinal cord or nerve roots. Most symptomatic lesions are found within the thoracic spine. Patients can present with pain, paraparesis, hyperreflexia, paresthesias, and bowel or bladder incontinence. Symptoms may worsen with being upright[99,103] (**Fig. 47.16**).

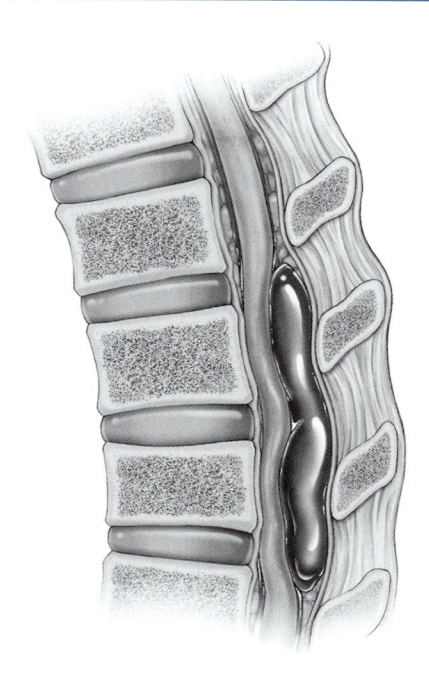

Fig. 47.16 Intradural spinal meningeal cyst.

Magnetic resonance imaging is the modality of choice. The lesion is hypointense on T1-weighted imaging and hyperintense on T2-weighted imaging. CT scan may show bony changes and enlargement of the spinal canal diameter. CT myelogram will show a filling defect at the location of the arachnoid cyst.

Grossly, the specimen appears as a cystic, well-circumscribed oval lesion. Histopathologically, the cyst wall is fibrous and lined with meningothelial cells.[96]

Surgery is indicated for symptomatic patients with symptoms attributable to the cyst. Unlike extradural spinal meningeal cysts, intradural spinal meningeal cysts are usually fenestrated rather than resected.

Neuroepithelial Cysts

Also known as ependymal cysts, these are extremely rare lesions, with only 18 intraspinal cases reported in the literature.[104,105] Neuroepithelial cysts are suspected to derive from ectopic ependymal fragments displaced from the central canal during embryological development and thus can occur anywhere along the spinal column. Clinical presentation has typically been reported as a slowly progressive myelopathy or a sudden deterioration following trauma.[104,105]

Imaging modalities of choice are MRI or CT myelography. On MRI, these cysts have variable appearances possibly secondary to the slight variation in protein and consistency compared with normal CSF. Typically, they are similar to CSF and are hypointense on T1-weighted images and hyperintense on T2-weighted images.[104] On CT myelography, the cysts appear as an intradural filling defect.

Grossly, the neuroepithelial cyst has been reported to have a glistening white wall with clear CSF-like fluid within. On histopathology the cyst wall consists of glial cells lined by a simple cuboidal to columnar epithelium. On immunohistochemical staining, the cells of the cyst wall are positive for S-100, GFAP, epithelial membrane antigen (EMA), and cytokeratin—all consistent with ependymal origin.[104,105]

Treatment is aimed at spinal decompression, which includes fenestration and decompression of the cyst. The goal is not usually total excision, as part of the cyst wall is commonly adherent to the spinal cord.[104] Alternatively, with failed cyst fenestration attempts, shunting is a possibility.

Syringomyelia

Syrinx cavities measure larger than 2 mm in axial diameter and tend to be eccentric. A syrinx cavity contains fluid similar to CSF in composition. Workup includes an investigation for the etiology of the syrinx, including Chiari malformations, tethered spinal cord, underlying enhancement suggestive of tumor, arachnoiditis/other CSF blockage, or posttraumatic history, as well as associated scoliosis. Asymptomatic dilated residual central canals can be visualized on MRI; these are typically round and located centrally. These dilated residual central canals are believed to have a stable nonprogressive natural history over time.[106] *Hydromyelia* is a term that refers to dilatations of the central canal that are at least partially lined by ependymal cells. Syringomyelia refers to cavities of the spinal cord parenchyma that may be lined by glial cells outside of the central canal.

Abnormality of CSF flow at the foramen magnum is commonly seen with syringomyelia. A majority of syrinx cavities associated with Chiari I malformations remain stable or resolve after Chiari decompression surgery. Recurrences are reported, and follow-up is thus recommended. Theories have evolved to explain the observed phenomena surrounding Chiari malformations and syringomyelia; proposals include the hydrodynamic theory, pressure differential theory, perivascular CSF dissection theory, venous hypertension and mechanical stress theory, and intramedullary pulse pressure theory.

Plain X-rays and CT aid in evaluation of bony abnormalities associated with Chiari malformations and syringomyelia, such as basilar impression, platybasia, assimilation of the atlas, canal abnormalities, congenital cervical fusions such as Klippel-Feil syndrome, scoliosis, or prior spinal trauma. CT is limited for evaluation of the posterior fossa and the foramen magnum area secondary to bony artifact. MRI is the diagnostic test of choice for evaluation of Chiari malformations and other etiologies of syringomyelia such as tethered cord, arachnoiditis or compression (sources of myelographic block), and spinal intraparenchymal tumor (**Fig. 47.17**). Although caudal displacement of cerebellar tonsils ≥ 5 mm below the level of the foramen magnum is the radiographic criteria for Chiari I malformation, this may not be clinically significant in isolation without symptoms. Other features that suggest CSF blockage at the foramen magnum may include peg-like cerebellar tonsils and effacement of subarachnoid spaces. Some groups suggest a possible clinical role for phase-contrast cine-MRI to evaluate flow at the level of the foramen magnum, although there is no consensus on its utility.[107] Twenty to 75% of patients with Chiari I malformation have concurrent syringomyelia. This concurrent diagnosis appears to be more common in clinically symptomatic patients.

Patients with Chiari II malformation may present with a variety of symptoms, including stridor/lower cranial nerve symptoms, brainstem symptoms, hydrocephalus symptoms, or spinal symptoms. Hydrocephalus/shunt failure is always suspected as the cause of symptoms first and foremost in this patient population with history of myelomeningocele, prior to workup of tethered cord, syringomyelia, and Chiari II pathologies.

Syringomyelia symptoms are related to the level, size, and location of the syrinx and affected spinal cord parenchyma. Clas-

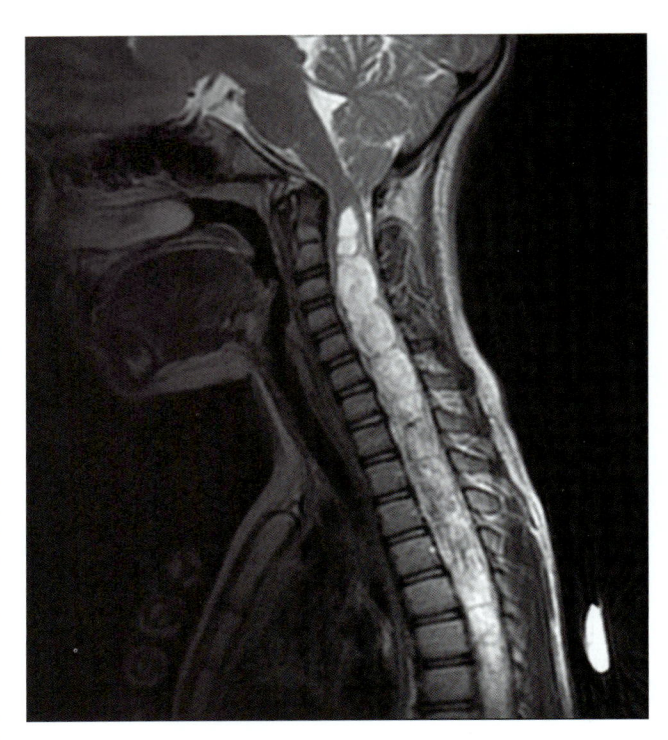

Fig. 47.17 Cervicothoracic syringomyelia associated with Chiari I malformation: sagittal T2-weighted MRI.

sically, dissociated sensory loss in a cape-like distribution is described (loss of pain and temperature sensation without loss of light touch and proprioception). Presentation is dependent on the anatomy of the individual syrinx itself, which may include asymmetry, variable pain involvement, Lhermitte's phenomenon, hand deformities, neurogenic arthropathy, autonomic symptoms, combined sensory loss, sensorimotor dysfunction, and musculoskeletal abnormalities.

Scoliosis in association with syringomyelia is thought to result from lateralized anterior horn compression manifesting as inequality in paravertebral muscle strength. Patients with underlying syringomyelia with scoliosis often present with scoliosis at a young age with an atypical curve, show rapid curve progression, and experience back pain symptoms.

There are no prospective randomized controlled studies or large-scale long-term prospective studies to date for syringomyelia. At present, a combination of clinical judgment and data from many case series are used for clinical decision support. Patients with asymptomatic Chiari I malformation do not necessarily require surgical intervention, whereas those with symptoms directly attributable to the Chiari I malformation have a favorable response to decompression. The presence of a syrinx in association with Chiari I malformation is typically surgically treated. The syrinx is thought to be likely to progress in size and in clinical symptoms if left untreated. Loss of neurologic function in syringomyelia is difficult to recover. In the setting of scoliosis, surgical management of scoliosis with an unrecognized syrinx is associated with the risk of neurologic complications. Intervention on syringomyelia with scoliotic curves less than 30 degrees has a more favorable prognosis in terms of avoiding future surgery and fusion.[108]

In this situation, surgical options range from posterior fossa decompression to drainage of the syrinx cavity, although direct drainage of the syrinx is not recommended as first-line treatment, as long-term outcomes are not favorable. The primary treatment of choice for Chiari I malformation with or without syringomyelia at a majority of pediatric centers is posterior fossa decompression. There is no consensus on optimal operative technique for posterior fossa decompression.[109] Posterior fossa decompression can be achieved by suboccipital bone decompression with or without C1 laminectomy. Bone-only decompressions in theory avoid the complications associated with opening the dura such as CSF leak, chemical meningitis, arachnoid scarring, vascular injury, and brainstem injury. There may be persistent blockage at the foramen magnum with bone-only decompression in a subset of patients, which would necessitate further surgery with intradural exploration. Dural opening, duraplasty, or cerebellar tonsillar shrinkage may be added at the initial surgery or at reexploration. The arachnoid may be left intact, or there may further intradural exploration with lysis of adhesions (such as arachnoid veils or webs at the foramen of Magendie). Use of intraoperative ultrasonography to ascertain adequate decompression and movement of the cerebellar tonsils with each cardiac cycle may aid in determining the type of decompression.[110,111] In general, the surgical goal is to establish CSF flow through patency of the subarachnoid space.[112] The choice of duraplasty material ranges from autologous tissue such as pericranium to synthetic dural substitutes; there is no consensus recommendation.

Management of symptomatic syringomyelia is approached by identifying and treating the etiology of the syrinx. Other important considerations include addressing hydrocephalus first, if present, prior to other corrective surgery for Chiari malformation or syringomyelia. In cases with concomitant craniocervical bony abnormalities or anterior compression of the brainstem, consideration is given to posterior occipital cervical fusion at the time of posterior fossa decompression, with or without anterior decompression, as neurologic compromise or progression has been reported in posterior fossa decompression alone. It is thought that these patients harbor chronic instability at the craniocervical junction.[113] Treatment strategies for such complex Chiari cases are tailored to the individual anatomy.

Spina bifida patients with Chiari II malformation with or without syringomyelia are a special population with intricate and challenging pathophysiology. Ventricular size may not change in the setting of shunt malfunction. Regardless of the presenting symptoms, treatment of hydrocephalus and patency of any existing shunt system need to be addressed first.[114] Tethered cord release and more rarely Chiari II decompression would be other considerations for a symptomatic spina bifida patient once hydrocephalus/shunt malfunction is ruled out.

If surgery is done for well-selected Chiari I malformation patients with appropriate targeting of the syrinx etiology, a majority of patients respond well symptomatically and demonstrate clinical and radiographic improvement or resolution of the syrinx.[112,115] In general, patients are more likely to have favorable outcomes if surgically treated for symptoms prior to the development of permanent deficits.

Persistent syringomyelia or persistent symptomatic Chiari I malformation is thought to be due to inadequate decompression or arachnoid scarring. Reoperation is advocated, especially if a syrinx does not resolve over time. Most syringes may show a trend toward resolution at the 3 month postoperative MRI, although there may be gradual improvement over a longer period of time. Drainage of the syrinx is considered a last resort. Shunting of the syrinx can be directed to the subarachnoid space or to more distant termini such as the pleural or peritoneal space. Syrinx shunting may be considered in patients with arachnoiditis who may fail lysis of adhesions, or in other carefully selected patients with low suspicion for CSF flow–related problems, although considerable morbidity from syrinx shunting is described.[116] Thecal shunting (from the subarachnoid space to a distant site) is an alternative to avoid morbidity of direct syrinx cavity shunting in this challenging population.[117]

Terminal Syringomyelia

A terminal syrinx is a cystic dilatation of the lower third of the spinal cord (cephalad to other manifestations of occult spinal dysraphism).[118] It is present in at least one third of occult spinal dysraphism cases evaluated by MRI; two thirds of these cases may be symptomatic with pain or neurologic deficit. The cause of this lesion is distinct from that of the cervical, Chiari-related syrinx,[119] or acquired syringes from tumor or trauma. A terminal syrinx is most frequently associated with tethered cord syndrome associated with low-lying filum, anorectal abnormality, meningocele manqué, diastematomyelia, or lipomyelomeningocele. MRI is the imaging study of choice. Syringomyelia is suspected if delayed deterioration in function occurs in a patient with occult spinal dysraphism. Relief of tension on the spinal cord is a surgical goal. Syringes may not resolve with surgical intervention or may persist and recur in the setting of re-tethering. In these cases, stenting or shunting of the syrinx cavity to the subarachnoid space may result in clinical and radiographic improvement.

Conclusion

Congenital anomalies of the thoracic and thoracolumbar spine encompass a wide range of disorders related to errors in embryological development, resulting in bony deformity to intradural pathology. Understanding the natural history is important. Prompt recognition, thoughtful management, and long-term follow-up are all necessary for successful treatment of this patient population.

References

1. Proctor MR. Spinal cord injury. Crit Care Med 2002;30(11, Suppl):S489–S499
2. Pang D, Wilberger JE Jr. Spinal cord injury without radiographic abnormalities in children. J Neurosurg 1982;57:114–129
3. Keiper MD, Zimmerman RA, Bilaniuk LT. MRI in the assessment of the supportive soft tissues of the cervical spine in acute trauma in children. Neuroradiology 1998;40:359–363
4. Grabb PA, Pang D. Magnetic resonance imaging in the evaluation of spinal cord injury without radiographic abnormality in children. Neurosurgery 1994;35:406–414, discussion 414
5. Davis PC, Reisner A, Hudgins PA, Davis WE, O'Brien MS. Spinal injuries in children: role of MR. AJNR Am J Neuroradiol 1993;14:607–617
6. Ahmann PA, Smith SA, Schwartz JF, Clark DB. Spinal cord infarction due to minor trauma in children. Neurology 1975;25:301–307
7. Walsh JW, Stevens DB, Young AB. Traumatic paraplegia in children without contiguous spinal fracture or dislocation. Neurosurgery 1983;12:439–445
8. Alleyne CH Jr, Cawley CM, Shengelaia GG, Barrow DL. Microsurgical anatomy of the artery of Adamkiewicz and its segmental artery. J Neurosurg 1998;89:791–795
9. Biglioli P, Spirito R, Roberto M, et al. The anterior spinal artery: the main arterial supply of the human spinal cord—a preliminary anatomic study. J Thorac Cardiovasc Surg 2000;119:376–379
10. Chen J, Gailloud P. Safety of spinal angiography: complication rate analysis in 302 diagnostic angiograms. Neurology 2011;77:1235–1240
11. Ou P, Schmit P, Layouss W, Sidi D, Bonnet D, Brunelle F. CT angiography of the artery of Adamkiewicz with 64-section technology: first experience in children. AJNR Am J Neuroradiol 2007;28:216–219
12. Savader SJ, Williams GM, Trerotola SO, et al. Preoperative spinal artery localization and its relationship to postoperative neurologic complications. Radiology 1993;189:165–171

13. Williams GM, Roseborough GS, Webb TH, Perler BA, Krosnick T. Preoperative selective intercostal angiography in patients undergoing thoracoabdominal aneurysm repair. J Vasc Surg 2004;39:314–321
14. Nijenhuis RJ, Mull M, Wilmink JT, Thron AK, Backes WH. MR angiography of the great anterior radiculomedullary artery (Adamkiewicz artery) validated by digital subtraction angiography. AJNR Am J Neuroradiol 2006;27:1565–1572
15. Muraki S, Tanaka A, Miyajima M, Harada R, Watanabe N, Hyodoh H. Adamkiewicz artery demonstrated by MRA for operated posterior mediastinal tumors. Ann Thorac Cardiovasc Surg 2006;12:270–272
16. Uotani K, Yamada N, Kono AK, et al. Preoperative visualization of the artery of Adamkiewicz by intra-arterial CT angiography. AJNR Am J Neuroradiol 2008;29:314–318
17. Schoenwolf G, Bleyl S, Brauer P, Francis-West P. Larsen's Human Embryology, 5th ed. Philadelphia: Churchill Livingstone; 2014
18. Savage JJ, Casey JN, McNeill IT, Sherman JH. Neurenteric cysts of the spine. J Craniovertebr Junction Spine 2010;1:58–63
19. Pang D, Dias MS, Ahab-Barmada M. Split cord malformation: Part I: A unified theory of embryogenesis for double spinal cord malformations. Neurosurgery 1992;31:451–480
20. Pang D, Zovickian J, Wong ST, Hou YJ, Moes GS. Surgical treatment of complex spinal cord lipomas. Childs Nerv Syst 2013;29:1485–1513
21. Echelard Y, Epstein DJ, St-Jacques B, et al. Sonic hedgehog, a member of a family of putative signaling molecules, is implicated in the regulation of CNS polarity. Cell 1993;75:1417–1430
22. Liem KF Jr, Tremml G, Roelink H, Jessell TM. Dorsal differentiation of neural plate cells induced by BMP-mediated signals from epidermal ectoderm. Cell 1995;82:969–979
23. Shimokita E, Takahashi Y. Secondary neurulation: Fate-mapping and gene manipulation of the neural tube in tail bud. Dev Growth Differ 2011;53:401–410
24. Yang HJ, Lee DH, Lee YJ, et al. Secondary neurulation of human embryos: morphological changes and the expression of neuronal antigens. Childs Nerv Syst 2014;30:73–82
25. O'Rahilly R, Müller F. Somites, spinal Ganglia, and centra. Enumeration and interrelationships in staged human embryos, and implications for neural tube defects. Cells Tissues Organs 2003;173:75–92
26. Monsoro-Burq AH, Duprez D, Watanabe Y, et al. The role of bone morphogenetic proteins in vertebral development. Development 1996;122:3607–3616
27. Dunwoodie SL. The role of Notch in patterning the human vertebral column. Curr Opin Genet Dev 2009;19:329–337
28. Skórzewska A, Grzymisławska M, Bruska M, Lupicka J, Woźniak W. Ossification of the vertebral column in human foetuses: histological and computed tomography studies. Folia Morphol (Warsz) 2013;72:230–238
29. Bernard TN Jr, Burke SW, Johnston CE III, Roberts JM. Congenital spine deformities. A review of 47 cases. Orthopedics 1985;8:777–783
30. McMaster MJ, Ohtsuka K. The natural history of congenital scoliosis. A study of two hundred and fifty-one patients. J Bone Joint Surg Am 1982;64:1128–1147
31. McMaster MJ. Occult intraspinal anomalies and congenital scoliosis. J Bone Joint Surg Am 1984;66:588–601
32. Jog S, Patole S, Whitehall J. Congenital scoliosis in a neonate: can a neonatologist ignore it? Postgrad Med J 2002;78:469–472
33. Winter R, Moe J, Eiler V. Congenital scoliosis: a study of 234 patients treated and untreated. J Bone Joint Surg Am 1968;50:1–47
34. Aslan Y, Erduran E, Mocan H, Yildiran A, Okten A, Gedik Y. Multiple vertebral segmentation defects. Brief report of three patients and nosological considerations. Genet Couns 1997;8:241–248
35. Winter RB, Lonstein JE, Boachie-Adjei O. Congenital spinal deformity. Instr Course Lect 1996;45:117–127
36. McMaster MJ. Congenital scoliosis caused by a unilateral failure of vertebral segmentation with contralateral hemivertebrae. Spine 1998;23:998–1005
37. McMaster MJ, David CV. Hemivertebra as a cause of scoliosis. A study of 104 patients. J Bone Joint Surg Br 1986;68:588–595
38. Morin B, Poitras B, Duhaime M, Rivard CH, Marton D. Congenital kyphosis by segmentation defect: etiologic and pathogenic studies. J Pediatr Orthop 1985;5:309–314
39. Chan G, Dormans JP. Update on congenital spinal deformities: preoperative evaluation. Spine 2009;34:1766–1774
40. Mayfield JK, Winter RB, Bradford DS, Moe JH. Congenital kyphosis due to defects of anterior segmentation. J Bone Joint Surg Am 1980;62:1291–1301
41. Montgomery SP, Hall JE. Congenital kyphosis. Spine 1982;7:360–364
42. Philips MF, Dormans J, Drummond D, Schut L, Sutton LN. Progressive congenital kyphosis: report of five cases and review of the literature. Pediatr Neurosurg 1997;26:130–143
43. Winter RB, Moe JH, Lonstein JE. The surgical treatment of congenital kyphosis. A review of 94 patients age 5 years or older, with 2 years or more follow-up in 77 patients. Spine 1985;10:224–231
44. Shapiro J, Herring J. Congenital vertebral displacement. J Bone Joint Surg Am 1993;75:656–662
45. Zeller RD, Ghanem I, Dubousset J. The congenital dislocated spine. Spine 1996;21:1235–1240
46. Winter RB, Moe JH, Wang JF. Congenital kyphosis. Its natural history and treatment as observed in a study of one hundred and thirty patients. J Bone Joint Surg Am 1973;55:223–256
47. Müller F, O'Rahilly R, Benson DR. The early origin of vertebral anomalies, as illustrated by a "butterfly vertebra." J Anat 1986;149:157–169
48. Kim YJ, Otsuka NY, Flynn JM, Hall JE, Emans JB, Hresko MT. Surgical treatment of congenital kyphosis. Spine 2001;26:2251–2257
49. Winter RB, Moe JH, Bradford DS. Congenital thoracic lordosis. J Bone Joint Surg Am 1978;60:806–810
50. Winter RB, Leonard AS. Surgical correction of congenital thoracic lordosis. J Pediatr Orthop 1990;10:805–808
51. Borkow SE, Kleiger B. Spondylolisthesis in the newborn. A case report. Clin Orthop Relat Res 1971;81:73–76
52. Boxall D, Bradford DS, Winter RB, Moe JH. Management of severe spondylolisthesis in children and adolescents. J Bone Joint Surg Am 1979;61:479–495
53. Wiltse LL, Newman PH, Macnab I. Classification of spondylolisis and spondylolisthesis. Clin Orthop Relat Res 1976;117:23–29
54. Wiltse L, Rothman S. Spondylolisthesis: classification, diagnosis, and natural history. Semin Spine Surg 1989;1:78–94
55. Newman PH, Stone KH. The etiology of spondylolisthesis. J Bone Joint Surg Br 1963;45:39–59
56. Rosenberg NJ, Bargar WL, Friedman B. The incidence of spondylolysis and spondylolisthesis in nonambulatory patients. Spine 1981;6:35–38
57. Klippel M, Feil A. The classic: a case of absence of cervical vertebrae with the thoracic cage rising to the base of the cranium (cervical thoracic cage). Clin Orthop Relat Res 1975;109:3–8
58. Hensinger RN, Lang JE, MacEwen GD. Klippel-Feil syndrome; a constellation of associated anomalies. J Bone Joint Surg Am 1974;56:1246–1253
59. Tracy MR, Dormans JP, Kusumi K. Klippel-Feil syndrome: clinical features and current understanding of etiology. Clin Orthop Relat Res 2004;424:183–190
60. Klippel M, Feil A. Un cas d'absence des vertebres cervicales, avec cage thoracique remontant jusqu'a la base du crane (cage thoracique cervicale) Nouv Incongr Salpet. 1912;25:223–250
61. Thomsen MN, Schneider U, Weber M, Johannisson R, Niethard FU. Scoliosis and congenital anomalies associated with Klippel-Feil syndrome types I-III. Spine 1997;22:396–401
62. van Tulder MW, Assendelft WJ, Koes BW, Bouter LM. Spinal radiographic findings and nonspecific low back pain. A systematic review of observational studies. Spine 1997;22:427–434
63. McAtee-Smith J, Hebert AA, Rapini RP, Goldberg NS. Skin lesions of the spinal axis and spinal dysraphism. Fifteen cases and a review of the literature. Arch Pediatr Adolesc Med 1994;148:740–748
64. Bowman RM, Boshnjaku V, McLone DG. The changing incidence of myelomeningocele and its impact on pediatric neurosurgery: a review from the Children's Memorial Hospital. Childs Nerv Syst 2009;25:801–806
65. Adzick NS, Thom EA, Spong CY, et al; MOMS Investigators. A randomized trial of prenatal versus postnatal repair of myelomeningocele. N Engl J Med 2011;364:993–1004
66. Cherian A, Seena S, Bullock RK, Antony AC. Incidence of neural tube defects in the least-developed area of India: a population-based study. Lancet 2005;366:930–931
67. Au KS, Northrup H. Genetic complexity of human myelomeningocele. Genetics 2013;2:116

68. Humphreys RP, Hendrick EB, Hoffman HJ. Diastematomyelia. Clin Neurosurg 1983;30:436–456
69. Erşahin Y. Split cord malformation types I and II: a personal series of 131 patients. Childs Nerv Syst 2013;29:1515–1526
70. Miller A, Guille JT, Bowen JR. Evaluation and treatment of diastematomyelia. J Bone Joint Surg Am 1993;75:1308–1317
71. Rauzzino MJ, Iskandar BJ, Oakes WJ. Occult spinal dysraphism. Contemp Neurosurg 1998;20:1–6
72. Drake JM. Surgical management of the tethered spinal cord—walking the fine line. Neurosurg Focus 2007;23:E4
73. Kanev PM, Park TS. Dermoids and dermal sinus tracts of the spine. Neurosurg Clin N Am 1995;6:359–366
74. Mete M, Umur AS, Duransoy YK, et al. Congenital dermal sinus tract of the spine: experience of 16 patients. J Child Neurol 2014;29:1277–1282
75. Vadivelu S, Desai SK, Illner A, Luerssen TG, Jea A. Infected lumbar dermoid cyst mimicking intramedullary spinal cord tumor: Observations and outcomes. J Pediatr Neurosci 2014;9:21–26
76. Warder DE, Oakes WJ. Tethered cord syndrome: the low-lying and normally positioned conus. Neurosurgery 1994;34:597–600, discussion 600 discussion
77. Bui CJ, Tubbs RS, Oakes WJ. Tethered cord syndrome in children: a review. Neurosurg Focus 2007;23:E2
78. Anderson FM. Occult spinal dysraphism: a series of 73 cases. Pediatrics 1975;55:826–835
79. Sarwark JF, Weber DT, Gabrieli AP, McLone DG, Dias L. Tethered cord syndrome in low motor level children with myelomeningocele. Pediatr Neurosurg 1996;25:295–301
80. Fone PD, Vapnek JM, Litwiller SE, et al. Urodynamic findings in the tethered spinal cord syndrome: does surgical release improve bladder function? J Urol 1997;157:604–609
81. Khoury AE, Hendrick EB, McLorie GA, Kulkarni A, Churchill BM. Occult spinal dysraphism: clinical and urodynamic outcome after division of the filum terminale. J Urol 1990;144(2 Pt 2):426–428, discussion 428–429, 443–444
82. Metcalfe PD, Luerssen TG, King SJ, et al. Treatment of the occult tethered spinal cord for neuropathic bladder: results of sectioning the filum terminale. J Urol 2006;176(4 Pt 2):1826–1829, discussion 1830
83. Cools MJ, Al-Holou WN, Stetler WR Jr, et al. Filum terminale lipomas: imaging prevalence, natural history, and conus position. J Neurosurg Pediatr 2014;13:559–567
84. Brown E, Matthes JC, Bazan C III, Jinkins JR. Prevalence of incidental intraspinal lipoma of the lumbosacral spine as determined by MRI. Spine 1994;19:833–836
85. Pierre-Kahn A, Zerah M, Renier D, et al. Congenital lumbosacral lipomas. Childs Nerv Syst 1997;13:298–334, discussion 335
86. La Marca F, Grant JA, Tomita T, McLone DG. Spinal lipomas in children: outcome of 270 procedures. Pediatr Neurosurg 1997;26:8–16
87. Sarris CE, Tomei KL, Carmel PW, Gandhi CD. Lipomyelomeningocele: pathology, treatment, and outcomes. Neurosurg Focus 2012;33:E3
88. Hoffman HJ, Taecholarn C, Hendrick EB, Humphreys RP. Management of lipomyelomeningoceles. Experience at the Hospital for Sick Children, Toronto. J Neurosurg 1985;62:1–8
89. Cochrane DD, Finley C, Kestle J, Steinbok P. The patterns of late deterioration in patients with transitional lipomyelomeningocele. Eur J Pediatr Surg 2000;10(Suppl 1):13–17
90. Drake JM. Occult tethered cord syndrome: not an indication for surgery. J Neurosurg 2006;104(5, Suppl):305–308
91. de Oliveira RS, Cinalli G, Roujeau T, Sainte-Rose C, Pierre-Kahn A, Zerah M. Neurenteric cysts in children: 16 consecutive cases and review of the literature. J Neurosurg 2005;103(6, Suppl):512–523
92. Shenoy SN, Raja A. Spinal neurenteric cyst. Report of 4 cases and review of the literature. Pediatr Neurosurg 2004;40:284–292
93. Cai C, Shen C, Yang W, Zhang Q, Hu X. Intraspinal neurenteric cysts in children. Can J Neurol Sci 2008;35:609–615
94. Kimura H, Nagatomi A, Ochi M, Kurisu K. Intracranial neurenteric cyst with recurrence and extensive craniospinal dissemination. Acta Neurochir (Wien) 2006;148:347–352, discussion 352
95. Nabors MW, Pait TG, Byrd EB, et al. Updated assessment and current classification of spinal meningeal cysts. J Neurosurg 1988;68:366–377
96. Hughes G, Ugokwe K, Benzel EC. A review of spinal arachnoid cysts. Cleve Clin J Med 2008;75:311–315
97. Azad R, Azad S, Shukla AK, Arora P. Role of screening of whole spine with sagittal MRI with MR myelography in early detection and management of occult intrasacral meningocele. Asian J Neurosurg 2013;8:174–178
98. Lohani S, Rodriguez DP, Lidov HG, Scott RM, Proctor MR. Intrasacral meningocele in the pediatric population. J Neurosurg Pediatr 2013;11:615–622
99. Bond AE, Zada G, Bowen I, McComb JG, Krieger MD. Spinal arachnoid cysts in the pediatric population: report of 31 cases and a review of the literature. J Neurosurg Pediatr 2012;9:432–441
100. Marino D, Carluccio MA, Di Donato I, et al. Tarlov cysts: clinical evaluation of an Italian cohort of patients. Neurol Sci 2013;34:1679–1682
101. Lucantoni C, Than KD, Wang AC, et al. Tarlov cysts: a controversial lesion of the sacral spine. Neurosurg Focus 2011;31:E14
102. Mummaneni PV, Pitts LH, McCormack BM, Corroo JM, Weinstein PR. Microsurgical treatment of symptomatic sacral Tarlov cysts. Neurosurgery 2000;47:74–78, discussion 78–79
103. Holly LT, Batzdorf U. Syringomyelia associated with intradural arachnoid cysts. J Neurosurg Spine 2006;5:111–116
104. Park CH, Hyun SJ, Kim KJ, Kim HJ. Spinal intramedullary ependymal cysts: a case report and review of the literature. J Korean Neurosurg Soc 2012;52:67–70
105. Findler G, Hadani M, Tadmor R, Bubis JJ, Shaked I, Sahar A. Spinal intradural ependymal cyst: a case report and review of the literature. Neurosurgery 1985;17:484–486
106. Yasui K, Hashizume Y, Yoshida M, Kameyama T, Sobue G. Age-related morphologic changes of the central canal of the human spinal cord. Acta Neuropathol 1999;97:253–259
107. Ellenbogen RG, Armonda RA, Shaw DW, Winn HR. Toward a rational treatment of Chiari I malformation and syringomyelia. Neurosurg Focus 2000;8:E6
108. Hwang SW, Samdani AF, Jea A, et al. Outcomes of Chiari I-associated scoliosis after intervention: a meta-analysis of the pediatric literature. Childs Nerv Syst 2012;28:1213–1219
109. Rocque BG, George TM, Kestle J, Iskandar BJ. Treatment practices for Chiari malformation type I with syringomyelia: results of a survey of the American Society of Pediatric Neurosurgeons. J Neurosurg Pediatr 2011;8:430–437
110. Milhorat TH, Bolognese PA. Tailored operative technique for Chiari type I malformation using intraoperative color Doppler ultrasonography. Neurosurgery 2003;53:899–905, discussion 905–906
111. Yeh DD, Koch B, Crone KR. Intraoperative ultrasonography used to determine the extent of surgery necessary during posterior fossa decompression in children with Chiari malformation type I. J Neurosurg 2006;105(1, Suppl):26–32
112. Batzdorf U, McArthur DL, Bentson JR. Surgical treatment of Chiari malformation with and without syringomyelia: experience with 177 adult patients. J Neurosurg 2013;118:232–242
113. Bollo RJ, Riva-Cambrin J, Brockmeyer MM, Brockmeyer DL. Complex Chiari malformations in children: an analysis of preoperative risk factors for occipitocervical fusion. J Neurosurg Pediatr 2012;10:134–141
114. Piatt JH Jr. Syringomyelia complicating myelomeningocele: review of the evidence. J Neurosurg 2004;100(2, Suppl Pediatrics):101–109
115. Tubbs RS, Beckman J, Naftel RP, et al. Institutional experience with 500 cases of surgically treated pediatric Chiari malformation type I. J Neurosurg Pediatr 2011;7:248–256
116. Batzdorf U, Klekamp J, Johnson JP. A critical appraisal of syrinx cavity shunting procedures. J Neurosurg 1998;89:382–388
117. Lam S, Batzdorf U, Bergsneider M. Thecal shunt placement for treatment of obstructive primary syringomyelia. J Neurosurg Spine 2008;9:581–588
118. Iskandar BJ, Oakes WJ, McLaughlin C, Osumi AK, Tien RD. Terminal syringohydromyelia and occult spinal dysraphism. J Neurosurg 1994;81:513–519
119. Strahle J, Muraszko KM, Garton HJ, et al. Syrinx location and size according to etiology: identification of Chiari-associated syrinx. J Neurosurg Pediatr 2015;16:21–29

48 Disk Disease of the Thoracic and Thoracolumbar Spine

Tobias A. Mattei, Alisson R. Teles, Kristin Huntoon, and Ehud Mendel

Thoracic disk herniation is an uncommon pathology that presents significant challenges for the spine surgeon in both its diagnosis as well as its treatment. In recent years, improvements in imaging techniques have resulted in the increased detection of thoracic disk disorders. The clinical presentation of thoracic disk herniations can be extremely varied, from no symptoms to axial or radicular pain, myelopathy, as well as symptoms mimicking those of other conditions such as lumbar disk herniation and cardiac, abdominal, or intrathoracic disorders. As a general rule, asymptomatic patients or those with only axial pain may be successfully managed conservatively. Thoracic diskectomy is indicated only for patients with refractory radicular pain or, more often, myelopathy.

The discrepancy between the small percentage of patients treated and the large number of described surgical techniques for this condition highlights the challenges faced by the spine surgeon when attempting to determine the best surgical approach to treat these patients. Historically, posterior approaches have been associated with high rates of neurologic morbidity (due to spinal cord retraction) and mortality. However, in recent decades, advanced surgical techniques and new approaches have led to a significant decrease in the associated surgical morbidity and mortality. The surgical decision-making process regarding the best surgical approach is based primarily on the location and characteristics of the herniated disk. Central calcified disks are better treated through an anterior or a far-lateral approach, whereas soft lateral disks can be successfully managed through posterolateral approaches. A deep understanding of the anatomy of the thoracic cavity, spinal canal, and associated neurologic structures, as well as a proper comprehension of the risks and benefits of the most common approaches are crucial for the safe application of the available surgical techniques for performance of thoracic diskectomies.

This chapter provides a general overview of the epidemiology, pathophysiology, clinical presentation, radiological evaluation, and clinical outcomes of contemporary published series reporting the results of the treatment of thoracic disk herniations through different surgical approaches.

Epidemiology

The prevalence of thoracic disk herniations in asymptomatic patients ranges from 5 to 37% in magnetic resonance studies[1-4] and from 7 to 15% in autopsy studies.[5-7] However, the estimated annual incidence of symptomatic thoracic disk herniations varies from 1 per 1,000 to 1 per 1,000,000 population,[8-13] and surgery for thoracic disks constitutes only 0.15 to 4% of the total number of surgical procedures for disk herniations.[14-18]

Despite being observed in all age groups, most symptomatic patients are in the 4th and 6th decades of life.[7-10,13,19] There is no significant difference in gender distribution.[6,8,15,20-22] A history of trauma is reported in 37% of symptomatic patients.[15] The association with Scheuermann's disease has also been reported by several authors,[23-29] but precise knowledge about the pathophysiology underlying the relationship between these two disorders is still unclear.

Most thoracic disk herniations are located in the lower thoracic spine,[13] with 75% of them occurring between T8 and T12.[13] A central or centrolateral location of the herniation is observed in the majority of the cases (70 to 90%).[13,15] Approximately 7% are intradural, and in 10 to 25% multiple-level disease is present.[15,30] Calcified thoracic herniations are observed in 22 to 65% of cases. Giant thoracic disk herniations (defined as those that occupy more than 40% of the spinal canal) can be found in up to 15% of patients.[30]

Pathophysiology

The decreased mobility of the thoracic spine in comparison to the cervical and lumbar spine suggests the existence of unique pathophysiological mechanisms underlying degenerative disk disease in the thoracic spine. In general, degenerative disk disease in the thoracic spine may be understood as a failure or breakdown in the underlying processes required to ensure a proper erect posture. Although some variations in the position of structures located outside of the spine (such as the head positioning and knee extension) may have a significant influence upon the overall body balance, the vast majority of stress attenuation and load-bearing capacity involved in the maintenance of the erect position is dependent on the spine. Specifically, the thoracic region is the only segment of the spine that displays connected surrounding structures (such as the thoracic cavities, the ribs, and the sternum) that may significantly aid in weight bearing.

The role of dehydration of the intervertebral disks in the pathophysiology of thoracic disk disease should also not be overlooked. Progressive changes in the biochemical composition of the intervertebral disk are responsible for a change in its water content, which has been demonstrated to be nearly 90% in early childhood and to decrease to less than 70% by the eighth decade.[31] Additionally, aging has been demonstrated to be associated with increased deposition of insoluble collagen within the intervertebral disk matrix, thus decreasing the gelatinous and elastic nature of the nucleus pulposus and annulus fibrosus, respectively.[32] Similarly, the nucleus pulposus has been shown to undergo a significant reduction of both cell clusters and physaliphorous cells during aging.[33] As the annulus becomes less elastic with age, the frequency of tears within its overall structure significantly increases, leading to a higher predisposition to disk herniation after minor traumatic events.

Disk degeneration is the final result of multiple eiological factors. All these underlying biochemical, anatomic, and biomechanical factors can be understood as ultimately leading to a critical point in which the combination of high pressures within the nucleus pulposus and the incapacity of the annulus fibrosus to counteract such radial forces lead to extravasation of the intranuclear material beyond the disk limits. As previously discussed, as the water content decreases, the ability of the nucleus pulposus to dissipate downward forces decreases, and the intradiskal pressure rises exponentially with increasing axial loading. Transmission of this biomechanical stress to the annulus fibrosus may lead to a disk bulge. The annulus fibrosus displays an eccentric structure, with its posterior portion being thinner. Thus, a breakdown in the integrity of the annulus fibrosus is more likely to occur in such posterior areas, where it is thinner and less reinforced. The posterior longitudinal ligament (PLL) is a band of connective tissue that travels segmentally along the posterior aspect of the vertebral bodies and spreads laterally at each disk–vertebra junction. The PLL is thicker at the midline and thinner toward the lateral aspects of the intervertebral disk. Consistently, many thoracic are "centrolateral" in their location,[15] occurring exactly at the segment where the PLL becomes thinner. Interestingly, a recent cadaveric study found that the PLL was stronger in the thoracic spine in comparison to the cervical and lumbar spine (average posterior distraction force to failure of 48.3 N in the cervical region, 61.3 N in the thoracic region, and 48.8 N in the lumbar region). Such inherent differences may account for the clinical observation that thoracic disk herniations are much rarer than their cervical or lumbar counterparts.

Clinical Evaluation

The most common symptom in patients with herniated thoracic disks is pain (76%).[15] The axial pain can be localized at the thoracic region (41% of the cases), or can radiate down the lumbar spine or paraspinal area (39%). Approximately 20% of patients may also present with thoracic radicular pain. Patients with thoracic disk also commonly present some sort of sensory impairment, ranging from dysesthesias/paresthesias (61%) to complete sensory loss. Bladder dysfunction has been reported in 24% of cases, with urgency being the most common complaint. Spasticity and hyperreflexia occur in 58% of patients, and a positive Babinski sign can observed in 55%. Interestingly, 24% of the patients motor impairment or hyperreflexia at presentation do not complain of pain or dysesthesias. An abnormal neurologic examination can be observed in 30% of the patients. Motor weakness in the lower extremity is found in 61% of patients: 72% of them presenting paraparesis, and the remaining 28% presenting monoparesis.[15]

The most characteristic chronological progression of symptoms of a thoracic disk herniation is pain followed by sensory disturbance, weakness, and, later, bowel and bladder dysfunction.[34] Acute myelopathy, defined as a variable degree of motor, sensory, and sphincter disturbances developing in less than 24 hours, is observed in approximately 4% of thoracic disk herniations.[35] Transitory or recurrent episodes of paraplegia have also been reported to occur in rare cases.[36]

The symptoms of disk herniations in the thoracolumbar junction may be slightly different, being specific to the affected level. Common findings in such patients are quadriceps and tibialis anterior weakness and atrophy, sensory disturbance, abnormal patellar tendon reflex and Babinski's sign, bladder dysfunction, lower extremity pain, and positive extension signs (i.e., straight leg raising test and femoral nerve stretch test).[37]

In addition to these classic symptoms, atypical presentations related to compression of extraspinal structures have also been reported in patients with thoracic disk herniations. These rarer symptoms include nausea, emesis, chest tightness, and chronic constipation.[38–41] Likewise, such unusual symptoms may include deep unilateral abdominal pain, further manifested by unilateral paresis of abdominal muscles.[42] The presence of acute chest pain in athletes (especially after traumatic injuries) should not be overlooked, as they may be a component of the clinical presentation of a thoracic disk herniation.[43] Positional headache and intracranial hypotension due to an intradural thoracic disk herniation have also been reported.[44] Familiarity with these atypical symptoms of thoracic disk herniations is essential to avoid potentially serious deleterious consequences related to a delay in the proper diagnosis.[41]

Differential Diagnosis

The differential diagnosis of thoracic axial pain includes primary and metastatic neoplasms, spondylodiskitis, fractures, ankylosing spondylitis, herpes zoster, costochondritis, and thoracic disk herniations.[38] As already mentioned, the pain symptoms associated with a herniated thoracic disk can mimic a variety of intrathoracic and abdominal disorders such as cardiac pain, renal colic, gallbladder colic, and colitis.[38–41] In patients presenting with myelopathy, the differential diagnosis includes central nervous system disorders (such as multiple sclerosis and amyotrophic lateral sclerosis), intraspinal tumors, spinal cord infarcts, spinal cord malformations,[45] vascular malformations, motor neuropathies,[46] and syringomyelia.

In patients who present with neurologic deficits and radiographic evidence of Scheuermann's disease, the differential diagnosis includes an extradural cyst or angular compression from the kyphotic deformity.[25,47]

Radiological Evaluation

Magnetic resonance imaging (MRI) is considered the most useful imaging tool for the diagnosis of a thoracic disk herniation.[48] Besides its high sensitivity, it is noninvasive and provides important additional information regarding the surrounding anatomic structures on the level of the disk herniation, such as its relationship with the thecal sac, the spinal cord, and the emerging nerve roots, as well as the presence of an intramedullary signal change.

However, it is important to emphasize that there are some reported pitfalls with the use of MRI for the diagnosis of thoracic disk herniations, such as exaggeration of the size of the herniation, difficulty in diagnosing calcified disk herniations, partial volume averaging (owing to the relatively large section thickness of the cuts), cerebrospinal fluid (CSF) flow void signs (i.e., regions of low signal intensity within the CSF related to its pulsatile motion), signal dropout from calcified disks, chemical shift artifacts from marrow fat, and mismapped signals from cardiac motion.[1,49–52] Finally, there have also been some reports of herniated thoracic disks mimicking calcified meningiomas[53] as well as intraspinal tumors.[54] The use of gadolinium contrast is usually helpful to differentiate herniated disks from such lesions.[55]

Additional information regarding the spinal anatomy and the intrinsic characteristics of thoracic disk herniations can be obtained with a computed tomography (CT) scan, especially regarding the presence of calcifications in the herniated disk. CT scan images may also enable proper visualization of posterior osteophytes, ossification of the posterior longitudinal ligament (OPLL) which is a common disease in Asians as well as the relationship of disk material to the dural sac.

Calcifications are found in 22 to 65% of thoracic herniations[15] and are associated with up to a 40% intraoperative incidence of dural tears.[28] Awwad et al[2,56] described a nuclear trail sign on axial CT slices, which represents a calcification that extends from the center of the intervertebral space to the calcified herniated disk. According to the authors, this sign is present in up to 45% of the herniated thoracic disks. Myelography CT may help to improve the accuracy of CT scan in detecting a possible intradural extension of the herniated disk, constituting an important diagnostic modality in those patients who cannot undergo MRI (such as those with cardiac pacemakers or implantable cardioverter defibrillators).[2,13,57]

The prevalence of multilevel thoracic disk herniations ranges from 10 to 25% of symptomatic patients.[15,30] In 30% of the patients such herniations are noncontiguous.[30] In such unique situations, care must be taken in order to identify the symptomatic disk that warrants treatment. Neurophysiological testing, such as motor evoked potentials (MEPs), somatosensory evoked potentials (SSEPs), and electromyography (EMG), may further aid in the proper identification of the likely source of symptoms in patients with multilevel herniated thoracic disks and myelopathy.[45,58]

Treatment

The natural history of asymptomatic thoracic disk herniations is relatively benign. Wood et al[59] observed 20 patients with 48 asymptomatic thoracic disk herniations. In a mean period of 26 months (range, 14 to 36 months), no patient developed symptoms. Of the 21 small thoracic disk herniations (defined as less than 10% of spinal canal compromise), 18 showed no significant change in size, whereas three showed a significant increase in size. Of the 20 medium-sized thoracic disk herniations (10 to 20% of canal compromise), 16 showed either a small or no change in size, one showed a significant increase in size, and three showed a significant decrease in size. Of the seven large thoracic disk herniations (defined as those with more than 20% of canal compromise), three demonstrated no change in size, and four demonstrated a significant decrease in size. In addition, five new disk herniations were detected in four patients during the follow-up period. Spontaneous regression of thoracic disk herniations has also been reported.[60,61]

The natural history of symptomatic calcified disk herniations is more controversial. Although there have been reports of reabsorption of calcified thoracic disks associated with resolution of the clinical symptoms,[53,62] some authors believe that this type of disk herniation does not usually regress and should be always treated surgically if symptomatic.[63]

The role of conservative treatment for symptomatic patients with thoracic disk herniations was first evaluated by Brown et al,[64] who retrospectively reviewed 55 patients with symptomatic thoracic disk herniations. Initially, only one patient underwent surgery due to an acute myelopathy with paraplegia. Initial treatment of the remaining 54 patients included bed rest, nonsteroidal anti-inflammatory drugs, and physical therapy. Of the 11 patients who initially presented with lower extremity symptoms (pain or weakness), nine ultimately required surgical decompression (82%). Five patients without preoperative lower extremity complaints failed conservative treatment and underwent surgery (11%). The majority of the 40 patients treated nonoperatively reported a good functional outcome, returning to their prior level of activity (78%).[64]

Although not standard in the clinical practice, there is anecdotal evidence in the literature of good clinical and radiological results without surgery for patients with acute myelopathy. Haro et al[65] reported on two cases of acute myelopathy due to thoracic disk herniations that resolved after clinical treatment with steroids and prostaglandin E_1. Both patients presented reabsorption of the disk herniations on follow-up imaging exams, with concomitant resolution of the symptoms. As a general rule, however, conservative treatment is reserved for patients with painful symptoms without signs of myelopathy. These conservative measures may include steroidal and nonsteroidal anti-inflammatories, bracing, modifications in the level of activity, physical therapy, and steroid injections.

In general, patients with lower extremity symptoms usually do not respond well to conservative measures and should be considered surgical candidates. Another reason to consider surgery in these patients is the potential risk of permanent damage to the spinal cord. The role of surgery as a means to control pain is controversial. It has been reported that radicular pain responds better to surgery than nonradiating axial thoracic pain.[21] In general, it is not unreasonable to offer surgical treatment to patients with thoracic disk herniations and refractory thoracic radicular pain who failed conservative treatment, even in the absence of myelopathy.

The surgical treatment of patients with symptomatic thoracic disk herniations can be challenging, and may be associated with variable degrees of risks depending on the unique morphological characteristics of each lesion, the location of the disk herniation, its adherence to the dura, the patient's age and comorbidities, and other anatomical and clinical factors. It is important to emphasize that preoperative MRI should include a general scout view of the spine which may allow the surgeon to determine the correct level of the herniated thoracic disk by counting both from the atlas down as well as from the sacrum up. In the operating room, fluoroscopy should be used to confirm the correct level, before skin incision and after the exposition of the bony landmarks. SSEPs and MEPs should be obtained before positioning to monitor any changes during the surgery. Intraoperatively, identification of the precise surgical level may be challenging in the thoracic spine, and it must be considered a crucial step during surgery for thoracic disk herniations.[66,67] Factors that make the thoracic spine challenging for proper target level localization include obesity, osteoporosis, shadows from the humerus or scapula, as well as anatomic variations in the number of thoracic ribs bearing vertebrae. Preoperative CT scan of the entire lumbar and thoracic spine may be helpful in identifying the relationship between the last thoracic rib to the herniated disk level as well as the presence of transitional lumbar vertebrae. As already mentioned, during the procedure, high-quality fluoroscopy may be of significant help, even in the presence of modern image-guidance systems, such as navigation.[67–74] It is usually easier to count the thoracic levels upward from the sacrum or using the ribs as a reference in the AP view, because the shoulders may obstruct the view of the cervical and upper thoracic spine.

A variety of surgical approaches can be used to treat thoracic disk herniations.[11,12,22,75–94] It is important for the spine surgeon to acquire familiarity not only with the indications and limitations of each surgical approach but also with the unique anatomic view provided by each one of them.

Basically, surgery can be performed through a posterior, posterolateral, lateral or anterior approach. The approach selection depends on the position, size, and consistency of the herniated thoracic disks as well as on the surgeon's expertise and comfort with each approach. The most important goal when choosing a surgical approach is to minimize manipulation of an already compromised thoracic spinal cord.[30]

In the past, simple thoracic laminectomy was proven to lead to high rates of morbidity and mortality, and thus it is not indicated.[82,95] Subsequent posterolateral and anterior approaches were developed with the goal of minimizing manipulation of the thoracic spinal cord. Posterolateral approaches (including the transfacetary, and the transpedicular routes, as well as the costotransversectomy technique) usually are appropriate for paracentral or lateral soft thoracic herniations. Lateral approaches, using the same avenue of the XLIF technique which has recently gained significant attention by spine surgeons, can also be used for such type of thoracic disc herniations. Anterior approaches (involving either an open thoracotomy or thoracoscopy) are more suitable to address large, midline, or calcified disk herniations. Recent reports have described a questionable posterior transdural diskectomy,[96,97] which, although feasible, raises several concerns related to dural violation and the increased incidence of postoperative CSF leaks and related complications.

The specific operative nuances of the several available surgical approaches for treatment of thoracic and thoracolumbar disk disease (such as posterolateral variations, the lateral and the anterior trans-thoracic approaches) are discussed in more detail in other chapters of this book.

References

1. Williams MP, Cherryman GR. Thoracic disk herniation: MR imaging. Radiology 1988;167:874–875
2. Awwad EE, Martin DS, Smith KR Jr, Baker BK. Asymptomatic versus symptomatic herniated thoracic discs: their frequency and characteristics as detected by computed tomography after myelography. Neurosurgery 1991;28:180–186
3. Wood KB, Garvey TA, Gundry C, Heithoff KB. Magnetic resonance imaging of the thoracic spine. Evaluation of asymptomatic individuals. J Bone Joint Surg Am 1995;77:1631–1638
4. Niemeläinen R, Battié MC, Gill K, Videman T. The prevalence and characteristics of thoracic magnetic resonance imaging findings in men. Spine 2008;33:2552–2559
5. Haley JC, Perry JH. Protrusions of intervertebral discs; study of their distribution, characteristics and effects on the nervous system. Am J Surg 1950;80:394–404
6. Abbott KH, Retter RH. Protrusions of thoracic intervertebral disks. Neurology 1956;6:1–10
7. Arseni C, Nash F. Thoracic intervertebral disc protrusion: a clinical study. J Neurosurg 1960;17:418–430
8. Love JG, Kiefer EJ. Root pain and paraplegia due to protrusions of thoracic intervertebral disks. J Neurosurg 1950;7:62–69, illust
9. Carson J, Gumpert J, Jefferson A. Diagnosis and treatment of thoracic intervertebral disc protrusions. J Neurol Neurosurg Psychiatry 1971;34:68–77
10. Benson MK, Byrnes DP. The clinical syndromes and surgical treatment of thoracic intervertebral disc prolapse. J Bone Joint Surg Br 1975;57:471–477
11. Sekhar LN, Jannetta PJ. Thoracic disc herniation: operative approaches and results. Neurosurgery 1983;12:303–305
12. Maiman DJ, Larson SJ, Luck E, El-Ghatit A. Lateral extracavitary approach to the spine for thoracic disc herniation: report of 23 cases. Neurosurgery 1984;14:178–182
13. Arce CA, Dohrmann GJ. Herniated thoracic disks. Neurol Clin 1985;3:383–392
14. Logue V. Thoracic intervertebral disc prolapse with spinal cord compression. J Neurol Neurosurg Psychiatry 1952;15:227–241
15. Stillerman CB, Chen TC, Couldwell WT, Zhang W, Weiss MH. Experience in the surgical management of 82 symptomatic herniated thoracic discs and review of the literature. J Neurosurg 1998;88:623–633
16. Chen CF, Chang MC, Liu CL, Chen TH. Acute noncontiguous multiple-level thoracic disc herniations with myelopathy: a case report. Spine 2004;29:E157–E160
17. Ohnishi K, Miyamoto K, Kanamori Y, Kodama H, Hosoe H, Shimizu K. Anterior decompression and fusion for multiple thoracic disc herniation. J Bone Joint Surg Br 2005;87:356–360
18. Whitmore RG, Williams BJ, Lega BC, Sanborn MR, Marcotte P. A patient with thoracic intradural disc herniation. J Clin Neurosci 2011;18:1730–1732
19. Brennan M, Perrin JC, Canady A, Wesolowski D. Paraparesis in a child with a herniated thoracic disc. Arch Phys Med Rehabil 1987;68:806–808
20. Albrand OW, Corkill G. Thoracic disc herniation. Treatment and prognosis. Spine 1979;4:41–46
21. Le Roux PD, Haglund MM, Harris AB. Thoracic disc disease: experience with the transpedicular approach in twenty consecutive patients. Neurosurgery 1993;33:58–66
22. Uribe JS, Smith WD, Pimenta L, et al. Minimally invasive lateral approach for symptomatic thoracic disc herniation: initial multicenter clinical experience. J Neurosurg Spine 2012;16:264–279
23. Van Landingham JH. Herniation of thoracic intervertebral discs with spinal cord compression in kyphosis dorsalis juvenilis (Scheuermann's disease); case report. J Neurosurg 1954;11:327–329
24. Bradford DS, Garica A. Neurological complications in Scheuermann's disease. A case report and review of the literature. J Bone Joint Surg Am 1969;51:567–572
25. Lesoin F, Leys D, Rousseaux M, et al. Thoracic disk herniation and Scheuermann's disease. Eur Neurol 1987;26:145–152
26. Currier BL, Eismont FJ, Green BA. Transthoracic disc excision and fusion for herniated thoracic discs. Spine 1994;19:323–328
27. Chiu KY, Luk KD. Cord compression caused by multiple disc herniations and intraspinal cyst in Scheuermann's disease. Spine 1995;20:1075–1079
28. Gille O, Soderlund C, Razafimahandri HJ, Mangione P, Vital JM. Analysis of hard thoracic herniated discs: review of 18 cases operated by thoracoscopy. Eur Spine J 2006;15:537–542
29. Kapetanos GA, Hantzidis PT, Anagnostidis KS, Kirkos JM. Thoracic cord compression caused by disk herniation in Scheuermann's disease: a case report and review of the literature. Eur Spine J 2006;15(Suppl 5):553–558
30. Oppenlander ME, Clark JC, Kalyvas J, Dickman CA. Surgical management and clinical outcomes of multiple-level symptomatic herniated thoracic discs. J Neurosurg Spine 2013;19:774–783
31. Adams P, Muir H. Qualitative changes with age of proteoglycans of human lumbar discs. Ann Rheum Dis 1976;35:289–296
32. Hunter CJ, Matyas JR, Duncan NA. The three-dimensional architecture of the notochordal nucleus pulposus: novel observations on cell structures in the canine intervertebral disc. J Anat 2003;202(Pt 3):279–291
33. Thompson RE, Pearcy MJ, Downing KJ, Manthey BA, Parkinson IH, Fazzalari NL. Disc lesions and the mechanics of the intervertebral joint complex. Spine 2000;25:3026–3035
34. Tovi D, Strang RR. Thoracic intervertebral disk protrusions. Acta Chir Scand Suppl 1960;Suppl 267:1–41
35. Cornips EM, Janssen ML, Beuls EA. Thoracic disc herniation and acute myelopathy: clinical presentation, neuroimaging findings, surgical considerations, and outcome. J Neurosurg Spine 2011;14:520–528
36. Lesoin F, Rousseaux M, Devos P, et al. [Transitory and recurrent paraplegia caused by a dorsal disk hernia. Physiopathological and therapeutic problems. Apropos of 3 cases]. Ann Chir 1985;39:367–370
37. Tokuhashi Y, Matsuzaki H, Uematsu Y, Oda H. Symptoms of thoracolumbar junction disc herniation. Spine 2001;26:E512–E518
38. Lyu RK, Chang HS, Tang LM, Chen ST. Thoracic disc herniation mimicking acute lumbar disc disease. Spine 1999;24:416–418
39. Xiong Y, Lachmann E, Marini S, Nagler W. Thoracic disk herniation presenting as abdominal and pelvic pain: a case report. Arch Phys Med Rehabil 2001;82:1142–1144
40. Rohde RS, Kang JD. Thoracic disc herniation presenting with chronic nausea and abdominal pain. A case report. J Bone Joint Surg Am 2004;86-A:379–381
41. Shirzadi A, Drazin D, Jeswani S, Lovely L, Liu J. Atypical presentation of thoracic disc herniation: case series and review of the literature. Case Rep Orthop 2013;2013:621476
42. Stetkarova I, Chrobok J, Ehler E, Kofler M. Segmental abdominal wall paresis caused by lateral low thoracic disc herniation. Spine 2007;32:E635–E639
43. Baranto A, Börjesson M, Danielsson B, Hellström M, Swärd L. Acute chest pain in a top soccer player due to thoracic disc herniation. Spine 2009;34:E359–E362
44. Rapport RL, Hillier D, Scearce T, Ferguson C. Spontaneous intracranial hypotension from intradural thoracic disc herniation. Case report. J Neurosurg 2003;98(3, Suppl):282–284
45. Kramer JL, Dvorak M, Curt A. Thoracic disc herniation in a patient with tethered cord and lumbar syringomyelia and diastematomyelia: magnetic resonance imaging and neurophysiological findings. Spine 2009;34:E484–E487
46. Hamilton MG, Thomas HG. Intradural herniation of a thoracic disc presenting as flaccid paraplegia: case report. Neurosurgery 1990;27:482–484
47. Ryan MD, Taylor TK. Acute spinal cord compression in Scheuermann's disease. J Bone Joint Surg Br 1982;64:409–412
48. Blumenkopf B. Thoracic intervertebral disc herniations: diagnostic value of magnetic resonance imaging. Neurosurgery 1988;23:36–40
49. Enzmann DR, Griffin C, Rubin JB. Potential false-negative MR images of the thoracic spine in disk disease with switching of phase- and frequency-encoding gradients. Radiology 1987;165:635–637

50. Ross JS, Perez-Reyes N, Masaryk TJ, Bohlman H, Modic MT. Thoracic disk herniation: MR imaging. Radiology 1987;165:511–515
51. Chambers AA. Thoracic disk herniation. Semin Roentgenol 1988;23:111–117
52. Williams MP, Cherryman GR, Husband JE. Significance of thoracic disc herniation demonstrated by MR imaging. J Comput Assist Tomogr 1989;13:211–214
53. Piccirilli M, Lapadula G, Caporlingua F, Martini S, Santoro A. Spontaneous regression of a thoracic calcified disc herniation in a young female: a case report and literature review. Clin Neurol Neurosurg 2012;114:779–781
54. Bose B. Thoracic extruded disc mimicking spinal cord tumor. Spine J 2003;3:82–86
55. Parizel PM, Rodesch G, Balériaux D, et al. Gd-DTPA-enhanced MR in thoracic disc herniations. Neuroradiology 1989;31:75–79
56. Awwad EE, Martin DS, Smith KR Jr. The nuclear trial sign in thoracic herniated disks. AJNR Am J Neuroradiol 1992;13:137–143
57. Epstein NE, Syrquin MS, Epstein JA, Decker RE. Intradural disc herniations in the cervical, thoracic, and lumbar spine: report of three cases and review of the literature. J Spinal Disord 1990;3:396–403
58. Taniguchi S, Tani T, Ushida T, Yamamoto H. Motor evoked potentials elicited from erector spinae muscles in patients with thoracic myelopathy. Spinal Cord 2002;40:567–573
59. Wood KB, Blair JM, Aepple DM, et al. The natural history of asymptomatic thoracic disc herniations. Spine 1997;22:525–529, discussion 529–530
60. Coevoet V, Benoudiba F, Lignières C, Saïd G, Doyon D. [Spontaneous and complete regression in MRI of thoracic disk herniation]. J Radiol 1997;78:149–151
61. Martínez-Quiñones JV, Aso-Escario J, Consolini F, Arregui-Calvo R. [Spontaneous regression from intervertebral disc herniation. Propos of a series of 37 cases]. Neurocirugia (Astur) 2010;21:108–117
62. Nicolau A, Diard F, Darrigade JM, Dorcier F, Vital JM. [Posterior hernia of a calcified disk in children. Apropos of 2 cases]. J Radiol 1985;66:683–688
63. Barbanera A, Serchi E, Fiorenza V, Nina P, Andreoli A. Giant calcified thoracic herniated disc: considerations aiming a proper surgical strategy. J Neurosurg Sci 2009;53:19–25, discussion 25–26
64. Brown CW, Deffer PA Jr, Akmakjian J, Donaldson DH, Brugman JL. The natural history of thoracic disc herniation. Spine 1992;17(6, Suppl):S97–S102
65. Haro H, Domoto T, Maekawa S, Horiuchi T, Komori H, Hamada Y. Resorption of thoracic disc herniation. Report of 2 cases. J Neurosurg Spine 2008;8:300–304
66. Mody MG, Nourbakhsh A, Stahl DL, Gibbs M, Alfawareh M, Garges KJ. The prevalence of wrong level surgery among spine surgeons. Spine 2008;33:194–198
67. Upadhyaya CD, Wu JC, Chin CT, Balamurali G, Mummaneni PV. Avoidance of wrong-level thoracic spine surgery: intraoperative localization with preoperative percutaneous fiducial screw placement. J Neurosurg Spine 2012;16:280–284
68. Rosahl SK, Gharabaghi A, Liebig T, Feste CD, Tatagiba M, Samii M. Skin markers for surgical planning for intradural lesions of the thoracic spine. Technical note. Surg Neurol 2002;58:346–348
69. Johnson JP, Stokes JK, Oskouian RJ, Choi WW, King WA. Image-guided thoracoscopic spinal surgery: a merging of 2 technologies. Spine 2005;30:E572–E578
70. Paolini S, Ciappetta P, Missori P, Raco A, Delfini R. Spinous process marking: a reliable method for preoperative surface localization of intradural lesions of the high thoracic spine. Br J Neurosurg 2005;19:74–76
71. Hsu W, Sciubba DM, Sasson AD, et al. Intraoperative localization of thoracic spine level with preoperative percutaneous placement of intravertebral polymethylmethacrylate. J Spinal Disord Tech 2008;21:72–75
72. Binning MJ, Schmidt MH. Percutaneous placement of radiopaque markers at the pedicle of interest for preoperative localization of thoracic spine level. Spine 2010;35:1821–1825
73. Sammon PM, Gibson R, Fouyas I, Hughes MA. Intra-operative localisation of spinal level using pre-operative CT-guided placement of a flexible hook-wire marker. Br J Neurosurg 2011;25:778–779
74. Thambiraj S, Quraishi NA. Intra-operative localisation of thoracic spine level: a simple "K-wire in pedicle" technique. Eur Spine J 2012;21:221–224
75. Garrido E. Modified costotransversectomy: a surgical approach to ventrally placed lesions in the thoracic spinal canal. Surg Neurol 1980;13:109–113
76. Lesoin F, Rousseaux M, Autricque A, et al. Thoracic disc herniations: evolution in the approach and indications. Acta Neurochir (Wien) 1986;80:30–34
77. Dietze DD Jr, Fessler RG. Thoracic disc herniations. Neurosurg Clin N Am 1993;4:75–90
78. Rossitti S. The extreme lateral approach to thoracic disc herniations: technique and preliminary results. Neurochirurgia (Stuttg) 1993;36:161–163
79. Simpson JM, Silveri CP, Simeone FA, Balderston RA, An HS. Thoracic disc herniation. Re-evaluation of the posterior approach using a modified costotransversectomy. Spine 1993;18:1872–1877
80. Levi N, Gjerris F, Dons K. Thoracic disc herniation. Unilateral transpedicular approach in 35 consecutive patients. J Neurosurg Sci 1999;43:37–42, discussion 42–43
81. Bilsky MH. Transpedicular approach for thoracic disc herniations. Neurosurg Focus 2000;9:e3
82. Chen TC. Surgical outcome for thoracic disc surgery in the postlaminectomy era. Neurosurg Focus 2000;9:e12
83. Vollmer DG, Simmons NE. Transthoracic approaches to thoracic disc herniations. Neurosurg Focus 2000;9:e8
84. Perez-Cruet MJ, Kim BS, Sandhu F, Samartzis D, Fessler RG. Thoracic microendoscopic discectomy. J Neurosurg Spine 2004;1:58–63
85. Eichholz KM, O'Toole JE, Fessler RG. Thoracic microendoscopic discectomy. Neurosurg Clin N Am 2006;17:441–446
86. Börm W, Bäzner U, König RW, Kretschmer T, Antoniadis G, Kandenwein J. Surgical treatment of thoracic disc herniations via tailored posterior approaches. Eur Spine J 2011;20:1684–1690
87. Kasliwal MK, Deutsch H. Minimally invasive retropleural approach for central thoracic disc herniation. Minim Invasive Neurosurg 2011;54:167–171
88. Quint U, Bordon G, Preissl I, Sanner C, Rosenthal D. Thoracoscopic treatment for single level symptomatic thoracic disc herniation: a prospective followed cohort study in a group of 167 consecutive cases. Eur Spine J 2012;21:637–645
89. Regev GJ, Salame K, Behrbalk E, Keynan O, Lidar Z. Minimally invasive transforaminal, thoracic microscopic discectomy: technical report and preliminary results and complications. Spine J 2012;12:570–576
90. Russo A, Balamurali G, Nowicki R, Boszczyk BM. Anterior thoracic foraminotomy through mini-thoracotomy for the treatment of giant thoracic disc herniations. Eur Spine J 2012;21(Suppl 2):S212–S220
91. Wait SD, Fox DJ Jr, Kenny KJ, Dickman CA. Thoracoscopic resection of symptomatic herniated thoracic discs: clinical results in 121 patients. Spine 2012;37:35–40
92. Falavigna A, Piccoli Conzatti L. Minimally invasive approaches for thoracic decompression from discectomy to corpectomy. J Neurosurg Sci 2013;57:175–192
93. Snyder LA, Smith ZA, Dahdaleh NS, Fessler RG. Minimally invasive treatment of thoracic disc herniations. Neurosurg Clin N Am 2014;25:271–277
94. Yoshihara H. Surgical treatment for thoracic disc herniation: an update. Spine 2014;39:E406–E412
95. Fessler RG, Sturgill M. Review: complications of surgery for thoracic disc disease. Surg Neurol 1998;49:609–618
96. Moon SJ, Lee JK, Jang JW, Hur H, Lee JH, Kim SH. The transdural approach for thoracic disc herniations: a technical note. Eur Spine J 2010;19:1206–1211
97. Coppes MH, Bakker NA, Metzemaekers JD, Groen RJ. Posterior transdural discectomy: a new approach for the removal of a central thoracic disc herniation. Eur Spine J 2012;21:623–628

49 Tumors of the Thoracolumbar Spine

Jonathan N. Sellin, Laurence D. Rhines, and Claudio E. Tatsui

Spinal neoplasia is a common problem for both patients and physicians. Metastatic disease is the most common form of spinal neoplasia, with an incidence of up to 20,000 new cases per year.[1] Up to 70% of spinal metastases arise in the thoracic spine or thoracolumbar junction, with a peak incidence in men during the fourth to sixth decades of life.[2] Hematogenous spread is the most common route of tumor dissemination, but direct extension of paravertebral tumors is also frequently seen.

Primary tumors of the spine are far more rare; they account for only 10% of spinal tumors[3] and can be either benign or malignant. Benign tumors tend to occur in young patients and involve the posterior elements, whereas malignant tumors affect older patients and tend to occur in the vertebral body.[4]

The management of spinal tumors is multidisciplinary and requires a variety of treatment modalities, with goals ranging from local disease control or cure to symptom palliation, prevention of neurologic deterioration, and spinal stabilization.

Symptoms

Thoracic spine tumors present in a variety of ways based on their location within the vertebra and the speed with which they grow. It is believed that tumor growth can lead to periosteal irritation, resulting in a deep, progressive, aching pain that is not related to movement, position, or effort. Classically, this pain is worse at night and is considered to be biological in nature. Bony or ligamentous destruction may cause spinal instability, which results in pain that is worse with movement and the upright position, improved with rest or the recumbent position, and considered to be mechanical in nature. Pathological fracture, progressive deformity, and tumor invasion may cause neural canal or foramen compromise, resulting in neurologic symptoms from root or cord compression. Thoracic radiculopathy is typically characterized by band-like radiating pain that originates in the posterior midline and wraps around the chest wall. Epidural extension may also cause epidural venous congestion and hypertension, resulting in spinal cord edema, frank hemorrhage, demyelination, or ischemia. In truth, most tumors cause symptoms through a combination of the above mechanisms.

Neurologic deficits may manifest themselves as frank lower extremity weakness if spinal cord compression occurs over a short period of time. In cases where epidural compression occurs more insidiously, neurologic symptoms may present subtly months or years after the onset of pain as thoracic myelopathy with spasticity, ataxia, loss of sensation, and paraparesis progressing to paraplegia. Autonomic symptoms may also develop, most commonly as bowel and bladder incontinence, but also with signs of orthostatic hypotension and impotence.

Thoracolumbar spine tumors may also cause symptoms via paravertebral extension with involvement of surrounding structures, such as the paravertebral muscles or the ventrally located mediastinum and great vessels. The constitutional symptoms of malignancy—fever, chills, fatigue, and cachexia—may also be present.

Radiological Evaluation

The specific imaging modalities best suited to evaluate spinal tumors depend on the underlying pathology. In general, any imaging should thoroughly evaluate all the segments involved. The appearance of tumor borders is often dependent on the rate of tumor growth. Clearly defined sclerotic margins usually occur in slow-growing tumors. Tumors that grow faster may lose their sclerotic rim and display mottled or ragged edges with a surround pseudocapsule. Rapidly growing tumors are more destructive and display a lytic pattern of bone destruction. Although particularly malignant tumors may prove an exception, tumor growth, in general, respects certain tissue planes, most notably the intervertebral disk, fascial planes, and spinal ligaments.

Tumor location within the spine is variable, but benign primary lesions tend to involve the posterior elements, whereas malignant lesions have a predilection for vertebral body and pedicles. Metastatic lesions, which spread hematogenously, tend to involve the vertebral body, but spread of these or any tumors through direct extension may involve any portion of the vertebra or the epidural space. Osteolysis and vertebral body collapse is common, but disk space height is usually maintained even with advanced vertebral destruction.

Radioisotope (99m-technetium) bone scanning is useful in detecting small osteoblastic lesions, although false positives may be seen with infection, fracture, or simple inflammation. False negatives may also occur in rapidly growing lesions with a relative paucity of reactive bone formation.

Computed tomography (CT) is highly sensitive to changes in bony anatomy and is excellent at capturing the extent of bony disease. Multiplanar image reconstruction aids in surgical staging and planning. CT is limited, however, in its visualization of neural elements. CT myelography does provide indirect visualization of the intradural contents, but this method entails procedural morbidity and requires unencumbered cerebrospinal fluid (CSF) flow in the caudal-cephalad direction, a process that may be limited by extensive epidural disease, neural element compression, and resultant obliteration of CSF channels.

Magnetic resonance imaging (MRI) is invaluable in identifying and characterizing tumors of the spine. It provides multiplanar images and is excellent at delineating soft tissue and neural elements, often obviating the need for CT myelography. MRI, however, is limited by poor visualization/delineation of bony anatomy.

Other miscellaneous studies may have a role in the workup of spinal tumors, depending on the suspected pathology. Angiography is useful in delineating spinal vascular anatomy—such as the artery of Adamkiewicz—and tumor vascularity, which may lead to concomitant therapeutic embolization prior to surgical intervention.

Medical Evaluation

Biopsy

In cases where the diagnosis is unknown, obtaining tissue for histological diagnosis is the first step in the management of any spinal tumor. Biopsies must be planned with care, to avoid tumor seeding along fascial planes or biopsy tracts, both of which increase the risk of recurrence. Areas of soft tissue extension or lytic destruction generally have the highest diagnostic yield.[5]

Biopsies can be divided into three categories: needle biopsy, open incisional biopsy, and open excisional biopsy. CT- or fluoroscopy-guided needle core biopsies are sufficient for tissue diagnosis in up to 86% of cases[6] and may be preferred over open biopsies due to their significantly lower morbidity. The most important shortcoming of needle biopsies is the limited tissue sampling, which can result in a nondiagnostic specimen, particularly in the case of densely blastic lesions, necrotic tumors, or vascular lesions.

If an open biopsy is decided upon, the biopsy incision should take into account an eventual excision during definitive surgical approach. Meticulous technique and homeostasis must be ensured, as hematomas can carry tumor cells along fascial planes. Bone windows must be small so as to avoid introducing instability or pathological fracture into a diseased spinal segment. Frozen section should be sent to the lab intraoperatively to ensure adequate tissue sampling. Culture should also be sent to rule out infectious pathology.

Medical Staging

The extent of surgical resection must be appropriate to achieve cure, local control, or palliation depending on the histology in question. Tokuhashi et al[7] developed a preoperative scoring system based on general condition (Karnofsky score), number of extraspinal bone metastases, number of metastases in the vertebral body, presence of and resectability of metastases to the major internal organs, primary site of disease (more aggressive histology yielding higher scores), and presence of neurologic deficit (Frankel score) to predict prognosis and lead to some general recommendations about the aggressiveness of treatment. Tomita et al[8] also developed a scoring system to guide and further characterize the degree of aggressive surgical resection, again using a prognostic scoring system. The validity of the Tokuhashi and Tomita scores, however, has yet to be established.

Differential Diagnosis

Benign Primary Tumors

Osteochondroma

Osteochondroma is the most common benign skeletal tumor.[9] It is a male-predominant, slow-growing lesion that is generally asymptomatic and incidentally found. When symptoms develop, they are usually exacerbated by degenerative changes secondary to the lesion, resulting in spinal canal or foraminal stenosis. These lesions usually cease growth at skeletal maturity, and progressive growth later in life should raise suspicion for possible degeneration into chondrosarcoma.[10] CT and MRI are the studies of choice for evaluating these lesions. Surgical treatment is generally recommended for symptomatic lesions or lesions that continue to grow after the onset of skeletal maturity. Osteochondroma are usually invested in a cartilaginous cap, which must be excised to prevent recurrence. Surgery for symptomatic cord or nerve root compression is quite effective, with improvement noted in up to 90% of patients.[11]

Osteoid Osteoma and Osteoblastoma

These benign tumors account for ~ 10% of primary spine tumors, have a male predominance (2–3:1), and occur in the second and third decades of life.[12] These osteoblastic lesions typically occur in the posterior elements of the lumbar spine. Mechanical pain is the most common presenting complaint. Aspirin, traditionally, is remarkably effective as an analgesic. Less commonly, radiculopathy or myelopathy can result from neural compression. On histological section, both tumor types are similar, as are findings on CT, which reveal a destructive nidus surround by osseous, expansile sclerosis with scalloped margins. On MRI, the nidus is T1 intermediately intense, T2 hypointense, with nidal enhancement on gadolinium imaging. The two tumor types are distinguished by size: tumors with a diameter > 2 cm are classified as osteoblastoma, and tumors with a diameter of 2 mm or more are classified as osteoid osteoma.[13]

Osteoblastoma, unlike osteoid osteoma, carries the risk of continued growth and malignant transformation. Traditional surgical treatment consists of intralesional, total excision that, when complete, results in resolution of symptoms. In cases where surgery is not possible, minimally invasive techniques such as percutaneous radiofrequency ablation have been proposed as alternative therapies.[14]

Aneurysmal Bone Cyst

These cystic, blood-filled lesions commonly occur in the posterior elements of the thoracolumbar spine in patients in the first to third decades of life, with a slight female predilection.[4,12] The most common complaint is mechanical back pain, although neural element compression, pathological fracture, or spinal deformity may be noted. CT imaging demonstrates a "soap bubble," lytic, multilobulated lesion, whereas MRI demonstrates fluid levels with variable T1 and T2 intensities consistent with blood of mixed chronicity and gadolinium enhancement (**Fig. 49.1**).

Angiography demonstrates blood-filled cavities within the lesion. Surgical excision is generally curative and may be coupled with preoperative embolization and low-dose radiation therapy. Successful treatment with stand-alone arterial embolization has also been reported.[15]

Hemangiomas

These benign lesions are rarely symptomatic despite their high prevalence in the general population, estimated at greater than 10% in autopsy studies.[16] They typically occur in the fourth to sixth decades, with a slight female predominance.[12] They are most often found incidentally in the vertebral bodies with a honeycomb pattern on radiographs, a "polka dot" appearance on CT, and a mottled, T1-isointense, T2-hyperintense, gadolinium-enhancing appearance on MRI. Angiography reveals contrast pooling within the lesion. These lesions, however, can become symptomatic during pregnancy, in particular, as pathological fractures, hematomas, or expansile vertebral body lesions. Surgery is typically reserved for lesions causing pathological fractures or significant neurologic deficit. Radiotherapy may be

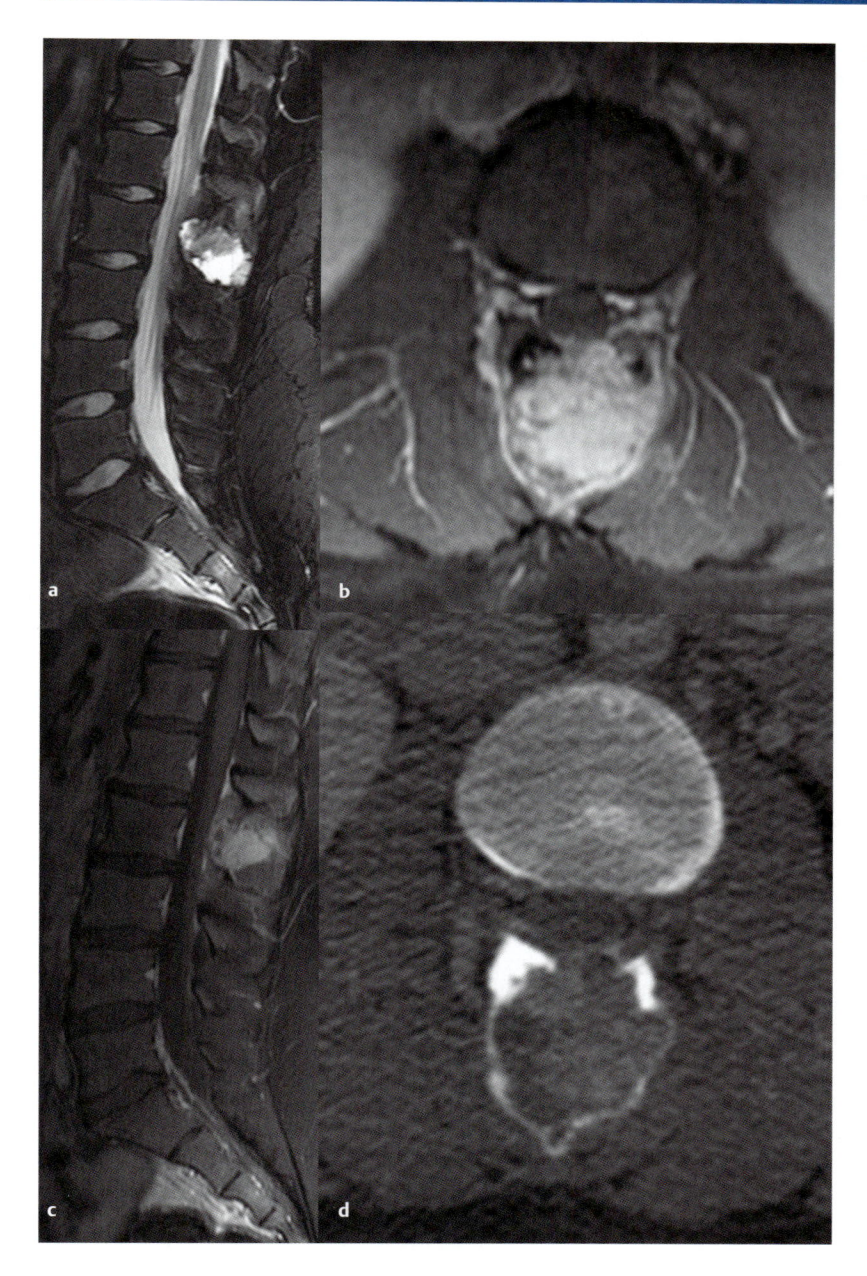

Fig. 49.1 Magnetic resonance imaging (MRI) and computed tomography (CT) imaging characteristics of an aneurysmal bone cyst (ABC). **(a)** Sagittal T2 sequence demonstrating a heterogeneous hyperintense lesion involving posterior elements of L2. Axial **(b)** and sagittal **(c)** T1 postcontrast sequences showing homogeneously enhancing lesion. **(d)** Noncontrast axial CT scan with characteristic "soap bubble" appearance.

recommended as a stand-alone therapy for back pain, whereas embolization is most commonly used as an adjuvant to surgery to reduce intraoperative bleeding.[5,17]

Eosinophilic Granuloma

This benign spinal lesion exists as one manifestation of a spectrum of disease, ranging from an isolated, self-limited process—Langerhans cell histiocytosis—to a single component of a multisystem disease process—Hand-Schüller-Christian disease and Letterer-Siwe disease. Spinal involvement is seen in up to 17% of children[18] with a male predominance (2–5:1), usually affecting the vertebral bodies of the thoracolumbar spine in children younger than 10 years of age.[12] These lesions cause lytic destruction of the vertebral bodies presenting as back pain, although pathological fracture may lead to deformity or neural element compression and deficit as well. CT imaging classically demonstrates a flattened vertebral body pancaked between two intact intervertebral disks, a finding known as vertebral plana, whereas MRI demonstrates a T1-isointense, T2-hyperintense ("flare reaction") image with soft tissue swelling and avid enhancement following contrast administration. Conservative therapy is the primary treatment, with surgery reserved for neural decompression or correction of progressive spinal deformity. Although observation is reasonable for asymptomatic lesions, bracing may be pursued in cases of a lesion-induced deformity that is not overtly unstable. Low-dose irradiation or corticosteroid injections can be pursued in advance of surgery, or in lesions not amenable to open treatment. Chemotherapy is reserved for cases of disseminated systemic disease. Generally, the disease regresses spontaneously with good prognosis and low recurrence rates.

Chondroma and Enchondroma

Chondromas are rare and benign cartilaginous tumors. These lesions are classified as chondromas when they originate in the hyaline cartilage and enchondromas when they arise in the medullary cavity. They occur more commonly in boys and young men in the second and third decades of life and occur throughout the mobile spine. Multiple enchondromas, also known as "enchondromatosis," is referred to as Ollier syndrome when isolated or the related Maffucci syndrome when hemangiomas are also present.[19] Growth typically resolves with skeletal maturity, but can cause neurologic deterioration in some cases. CT imaging demonstrates calcified, lytic lesions, whereas MRI demonstrates T1 hypointensity to intermediate signal intensity and T2 hyperintensity. Surgery with complete excision is recommended for tissue diagnosis and the prevention of neurologic deterioration; a small risk of sarcomatous degeneration has been described.[20]

Locally Aggressive (Malignant) Tumors

Giant Cell Tumor

Giant cell tumor (GCT) is most frequently encountered in women during the third and fourth decades of life.[12,21] The most common presenting symptom is pain, which may go unnoticed for months before the appropriate diagnosis is made. CT imaging demonstrates a lytic, cystic-appearing hypointense lesion, with areas of T1 and T2 hemorrhage and gadolinium enhancement on MRI. Associated soft tissue mass may be seen if cortical margins are violated. Although histologically benign, these tumors may be locally aggressive and cause significant morbidity and mortality. Wide surgical excision is the treatment of choice and is usually curative. Preoperative embolization is often employed.[22] Adjuvant radiotherapy has a role but may lead to an increased risk of sarcomatous degeneration.[23]

More recent investigation into the biology of GCT has identified a population of mononuclear stromal cells that express the receptor activator of nuclear factor kappa-β (RANK) ligand (RANKL), which has sparked interest in the use of denosumab, a monoclonal antibody against RANKL, as a therapeutic agent for recurrent or unresectable disease.[24] A phase 2 clinical study showed favorable radiographic or histological tumor response in 30 of 35 patients with an acceptable side-effect profile.

Chordoma

The most common primary locally aggressive tumor of the sacrum and mobile spine with an incidence of 0.08 per 100,000 individuals,[25] chordoma displays a male predominance (2:1) in the fifth to seventh decades of life, with an almost equal distribution among the sacrococcygeal region, the clivus, and the mobile spine.[26] These tumors arise from remnants of the notochord and are slow growing but locally aggressive lesions that may metastasize in around 30% of cases.[3,27] When affecting the mobile spine, the most common symptom is pain. On CT imaging, lesions appear lytic with mottled "calcific debris." MRI is useful for delineating soft tissue involvement, which is common, and demonstrates T1-hypointense and T2-hyperintense lesions with variable gadolinium enhancement. Metastatic imaging and workup is also necessary (**Fig. 49.2**).

Primary treatment involves surgery, and cure or a long-term disease-free interval may be achieved through en-bloc surgical resection. When en-bloc resection is not possible, aggressive tumor debulking with adjuvant radiotherapy may be the only treatment available, although external irradiation is of questionable value. In cases where biopsy is performed, the biopsy track must be excised to prevent seeding. Estimated 5- and 10-year survival rates of 84% and 64%, respectively, have been reported in patients following a combination of en-bloc or intralesional resection.[27] Bergh and colleagues[27] have noted that large tumor size, inadequate margins, tumor necrosis, and antecedent invasive diagnostic procedures outside a tumor center, thought to yield biopsy tract seeding and local recurrence, were adverse prognostic factors.

More recent technological advances in radiotherapy have enabled the delivery of significantly higher and more conformal radiation doses, with sparing of critical-adjacent structures, usually through the use of photon/proton beam therapy, hypofractionation, and radiosurgery. Data on proton beam therapy remains controversial. Chordoma are generally resistant to chemotherapy. Recently, progress has been made in the use of targeted molecular therapies. A study is currently underway in agents targeting the tyrosine kinase and angiogenesis pathways.[28]

Malignant Primary Tumors

Multiple Myeloma and Plasmacytoma

These neoplastic lymphoproliferative diseases, characterized by uncontrolled growth of plasma cells, are the most common type of primary tumor affecting the spine. They are most commonly found in the thoracic spine of men (2:1) over 50 years of age.[26] Plasmacytoma is a solitary soft tissue variant that progresses more indolently than multiple myeloma, but both can involve the spine, which may result in pathological fracture, deformity, instability, and neurologic deficit.

On CT, spinal lesions display lytic, "punched out" lesions of bone along the anterior column/vertebral bodies or pedicles and diffuse osteoporosis, which often culminates in vertebral body collapse.[5,12] This pronounced bony destruction may be linked to the ability of infiltrative plasma cells to cause bone resorption.[29] MRI, which is ideal for delineating the extent of bony involvement and paraspinal extension, demonstrates T1-hypointense, T2-hyperintense, gadolinium-enhancing lesions.

Because both plasmacytoma and myeloma lesions are fairly radiosensitive, conventional external beam radiotherapy is the primary treatment of choice. Surgical intervention has little effect on prognosis and is reserved for acute instability and neurologic compromise. Recent medical advances have improved multiple-myeloma therapy. Bisphosphonates have become a mainstay of therapy for the management of osteopenia and bone pain.[30] The use of thalidomide/dexamethasone and proteasome inhibitors like bortezomib now promise systemic disease control.[31,32] These new therapies have dramatically improved survival over the past two decades, with an improved overall survival from diagnosis of 44.8 month compared with 29.9 months in one large single institution retrospective.[31]

Osteosarcoma

Osteosarcoma is the most common malignancy of bone and the third most common primary spinal tumor, with a slight male predominance and predilection for the sacrum.[26] These lesions are bone-forming tumors that can occur as primary spine tumors, metastases from extraspinal primaries, or secondary lesions following spinal radiation in children or patients with preexisting Paget's disease, hereditary retinoblastoma, or fibrous dysplasia. Although lesions are commonly found in the long bones of young patients, the spine is the primary site of involvement in older

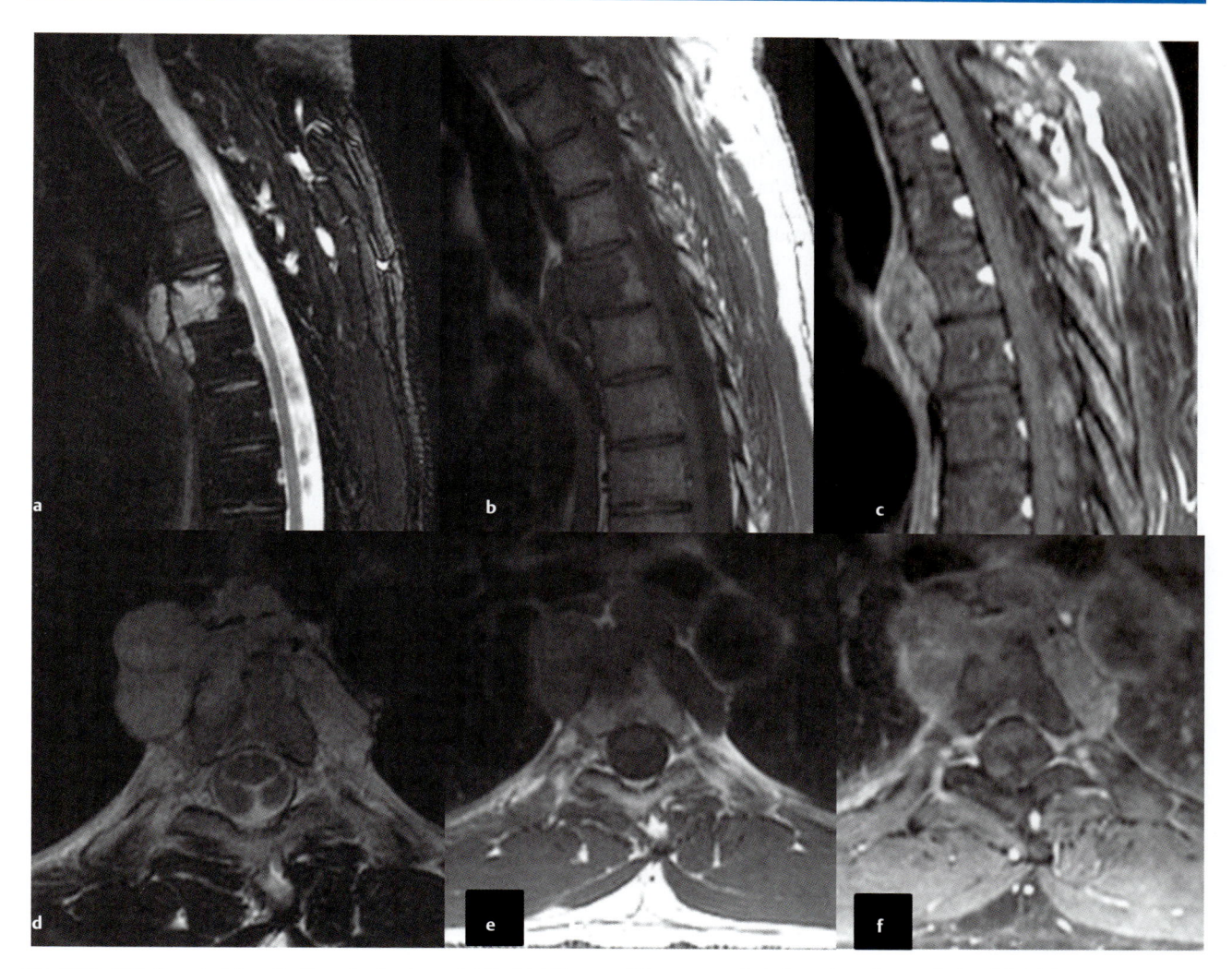

Fig. 49.2 MRI characteristics of a thoracic chordoma. **(a)** Sagittal T2 sequence demonstrating a hyperintense, lobulated, vertebral and prevertebral lesion. **(b)** Sagittal T1 precontrast sequence. **(c)** Sagittal T1 postcontrast sequence demonstrating heterogeneous enhancement pattern. **(d)** Axial T2 sequence displaying a hyperintense lesion. **(e)** Axial T1 precontrast sequence displaying a hypointense lesion. **(f)** Axial T1 postcontrast sequence displaying a heterogeneous enhancement pattern.

patients. Bony destruction results in pathological fractures, back pain, deformity, and neurologic compromise.

On CT imaging, osteoblastic and lytic lesion may be seen with matrix-mineralization. MRI better delineates soft tissue extension and reveals T1-hypotense, T2-hyperintense lesions without gadolinium enhancement, although signal intensity can vary with the extent of mineralization. Bone scans are useful in identifying multifocal disease. Chest imaging is important in excluding concomitant pulmonary metastases.

The ideal primary treatment for spinal lesions is aggressive surgical resection. However, achieving total resection can be difficult. Subtotal resection is associated with recurrence. Spinal involvement is associated with a poor prognosis; median survival times of up to 23 months have been reported, with metastatic disease, larger tumors, and sacral location harboring a worse prognosis.[33] Neoadjuvant chemotherapy may be employed to reduce tumor burden prior to surgery and subsequent adjuvant chemotherapy. Postoperative radiotherapy may be employed for palliation, but these tumors tend to be radioresistant, although studies have shown improved local control rates as high as 78% for patients undergoing gross total resection.[34]

Ewing's Sarcoma

This rare malignant tumor occurs in the first three decades of life with a slight male predominance and has a predilection for the sacrum, although posterior element involvement is commonly seen in the mobile spine.[12,17] Histologically, it is classified as a peripheral neuroectodermal tumor (PNET) and is characterized by small, round cells. Aberrant fusion proteins cause by translocations –t(11;22) are seen in all cases.[3] A common tumor of long bones and pelvis, vertebral involvement occurs in only 3.5 to 15% of cases.[35] Patients may complain of pain, neurologic deficit, or a sacral mass and fever. CT imaging demonstrates a lytic lesion with peripheral sclerosis, occasionally with vertebra plan. MRI demonstrates a T1-isointense, T2-hyperintense, gadolinium-enhancing lesion and aids in delineating soft tissue components. Intense tracer uptake is seen on technetium bone scan. Imaging for metastasis is required. Standard treatment involves upfront chemotherapy and radiotherapy. The role of surgery in achieving local control remains debated, with some authors advocating en-bloc resection in centers with this expertise because of the survival benefit conferred by superior local control.[3] Metastatic disease at onset and large primary tumor size remain the most significant biological factors. With newer chemotherapy regimens, 3-year survival rates approach 80% in patients with localized disease, although the prognosis in patients with metastatic disease remains grim.[36]

Chondrosarcoma

Chondrosarcoma is an indolent, cartilage-forming tumor with male predominance (2:1) that forms in the fourth decade of life, most commonly in the thoracic spine.[12] Pain and neurologic deficit are common presentations. These lesions can arise de novo as primary malignancies or as secondary sarcomatous transformations of osteochondromas, with primary chondrosarcomas tending to be lower grade. Lesions are typically classified as low, intermediate, or high grade. CT imaging varies depending on histological grade, with low-grade lesions causing cortical expansion and scalloping and high-grade lesions demonstrating frank lytic destruction of the vertebra. MRI demonstrates marked T2 hyperintensity and a "ring and arcs" gadolinium-enhancement pattern. Bone scan is helpful in identifying distant disease. These tumors, relatively resistant to traditional radiotherapy and chemotherapy, are treated with en-bloc surgical resection, when possible. More modern radiation therapies, however, are currently being investigated as a means to improve local disease control. A review of three studies with a total of 380 patients with chondrosarcoma of the skull base treated with proton beam therapy reported a 5-year progression-free survival of 95%, which was observed to be no different than the results of conventional therapy.[37] Prognosis depends primarily on histological grade and degree of tumor resection.

Metastasis

Spinal metastasis is by far the most common form of spinal tumor, with a slight male predominance, peak incidence in the fourth to sixth decades of life, and predilection for the thoracolumbar spine. Common symptoms are mechanical pain, radiculopathy, instability, and neurologic deficits from bony or epidural neural element compression. CT imaging delineates bony involvement, but MRI is the test of choice. Surgical treatment is generally palliative, reserved for intractable pain, acute neurologic deficit, or frank spinal instability. Radiotherapy has historically been considered the mainstay of therapy. Prostate, breast, and lymphoreticular metastases tend to be radiosensitive, whereas renal and gastrointestinal lesions tend to be radioresistant. Some radioresistant tumors may be addressed with surgical resection to improve local control. Life expectancy should be considered prior to performing surgical therapy. Preoperative embolization is a useful adjuvant to avoid blood loss. The evolution of spinal radiotherapy continues to change the treatment paradigm for these lesions.

Treatment
Medical Therapy

Chemotherapy, hormonal therapy, steroids, embolization, and external orthoses may play role to varying degrees in the management of spine tumors. In general, chemotherapy is best suited to treat the primary and systemic disease, but poorly suited to relieve acute neurologic symptoms or spinal instability. Hormonal therapy may be appropriate for hormone-dependent tumors as an adjuvant therapy. Steroids are useful in the acute phase of spinal cord compression as a bridge to surgical therapy.

Surgery
Staging and Classification

Enneking[38] described a staging system for tumors of the long bone that was subsequently applied to the spine.

In this system, benign tumors are divided into three stages: Stage 1 is asymptomatic tumors surrounded by a true capsule; these tumors display an indolent growth pattern and rarely require surgery. Stage 2 is tumors that grow actively, are symptomatic, and are surrounded by a thin capsule and a pseudocapsule of reactive tissue; these tumors require intralesional or en-bloc excision and recur infrequently. Stage 3 is tumors that are rapidly growing and, as a result are surrounded by a thin or incomplete capsule and by a hypervascular pseudocapsule; these tumors are locally aggressive and require en-bloc resection with the intent of doing a wide excision (**Fig. 49.3**).

Enneking's system classifies malignant tumors into three stages as well, each of which is further subdivided into type A

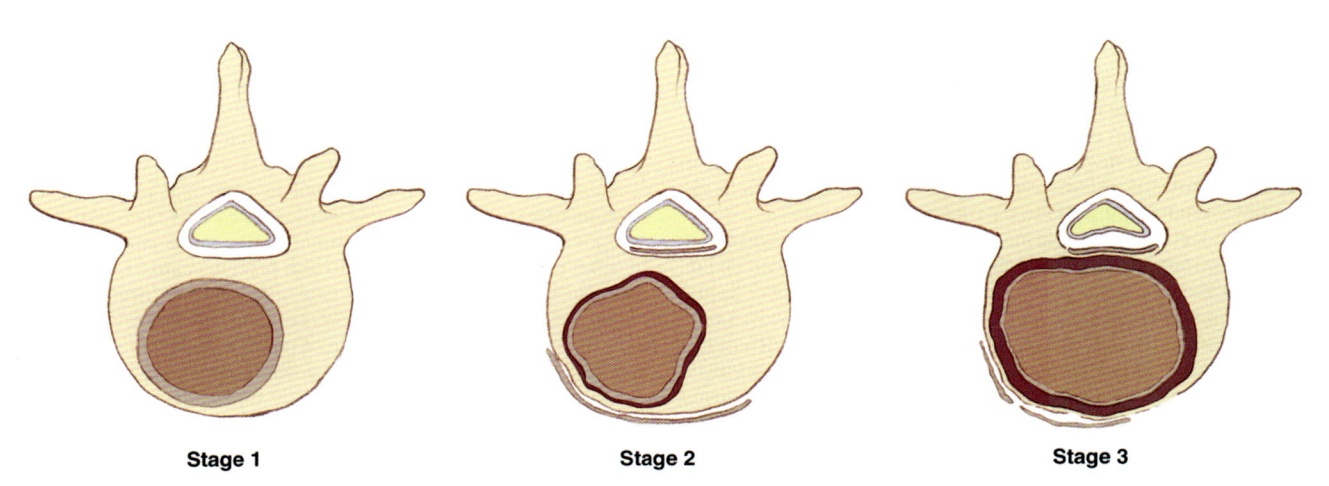

Fig. 49.3 Schematic for the Enneking staging system for benign tumors.

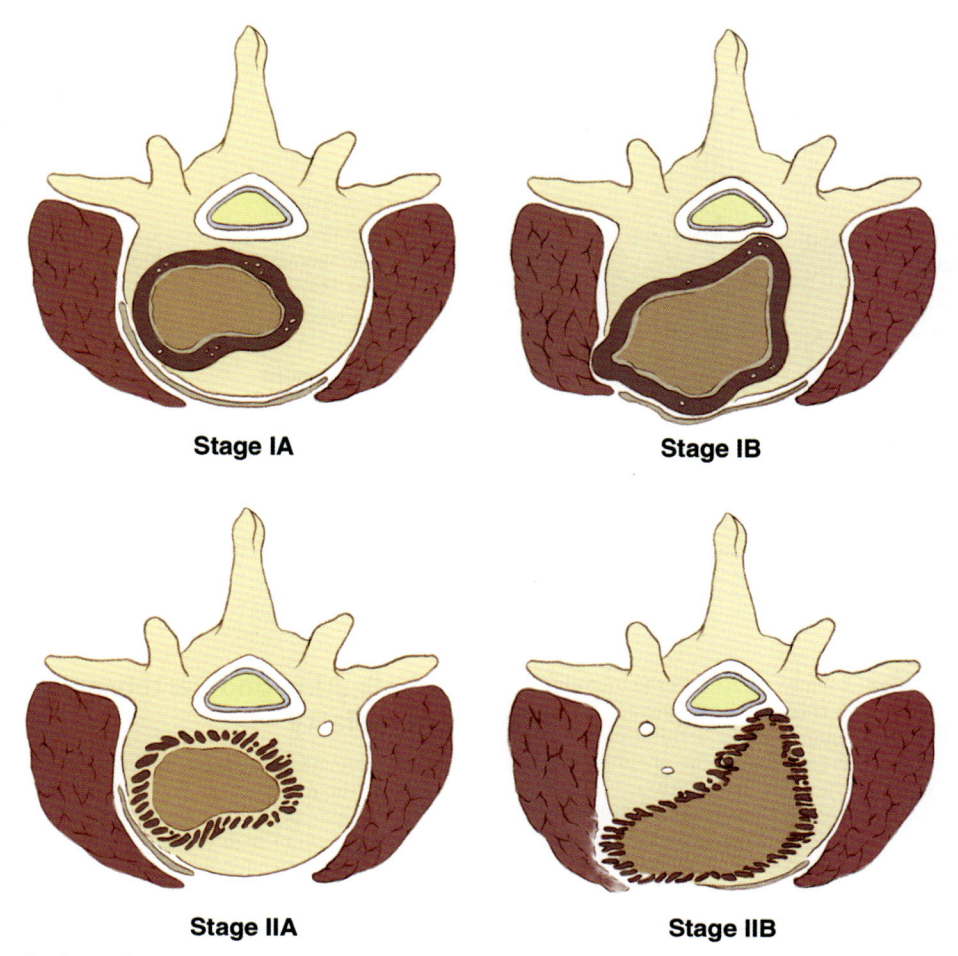

Fig. 49.4 Schematic for the Enneking staging system for malignant tumors. Stage III lesions (distant metastasis) are not represented.

lesions, in which tumor remains within the vertebra, and type B lesions, in which tumor extends beyond the bony confines of the spine. Stage I lesions are low grade, slow growing, and surrounded by a thick pseudocapsule, which contains microscopic rests of tumor tissue. Stage II tumors are high-grade, rapidly growing lesions whose rate of growth precludes formation of a reactive pseudocapsule and whose malignant pattern is characterized by continuous seeding of the surrounding tissue with satellite nodules, skip metastases, pathological fractures, and epidural invasion. Stage III lesions are similarly high-grade lesions that have metastasized to regional lymph nodes or distant organs (**Fig. 49.4**).

The adoption of the Enneking system in the management of spinal tumors has some limitations: it does not account for the continuous nature of the epidural compartment, does not acknowledge the devastating implication of sacrificing the spinal cord and roots when wide local excision is recommended, and does not address the need to maintain spinal stability following aggressive oncologic resection.

The Weinstein-Boriani-Biagini (WBB) surgical staging system was developed to recognize the unique anatomic complexity of the spine, and dictate operative technique, sparing the spinal cord without compromising surgical tumor margins.[39] This system divides the vertebrae into 12 radiating zones, progressing in clockwise fashion from the spinous process (zone I) at 12 o'clock, as well as five concentric layers (A to E) in the transverse plane, with A representing extraosseous soft tissue, B superficial intraosseous, C deep intraosseous, D epidural tumor extension, and E intradural tumor spread. The longitudinal extent of the tumor is based on the number of spine segments involved. The system provides a rational approach to surgical planning while taking into account the limitations of en-bloc excisions created by preservation of the cord (**Fig. 49.5**).

More recently, the Spinal Instability Neoplastic Score (SINS) has been developed to address the need for surgical stabilization in spine tumor surgery as a concern distinct from the ultimate degree of oncological resection.[40] The scoring system uses tumor location, patient pain, bone lesion quality, presence of preoperative spinal deformity, degree of vertebral body involvement/collapse, and posterolateral element involvement to stratify lesions into three categories based on their composite score: stable, potentially unstable, or unstable.

The terminology used in describing spine tumor surgery can be confusing. "Curettage" and "intralesional resection" refer to piecemeal removal of a tumor, whereas "en bloc" indicates removal of the whole tumor in one piece, with a layer of intact, surrounding healthy tissue. The specimen is submitted for histological study to further define the actual extent of resection. A specimen is labeled "intralesional" if the surgeon has cut within the tumor mass; "marginal" if the surgeon has dissected along the reactive pseudocapsule surrounding the tumor; and "wide" if the plane of surgical dissection is surrounded by a rim of

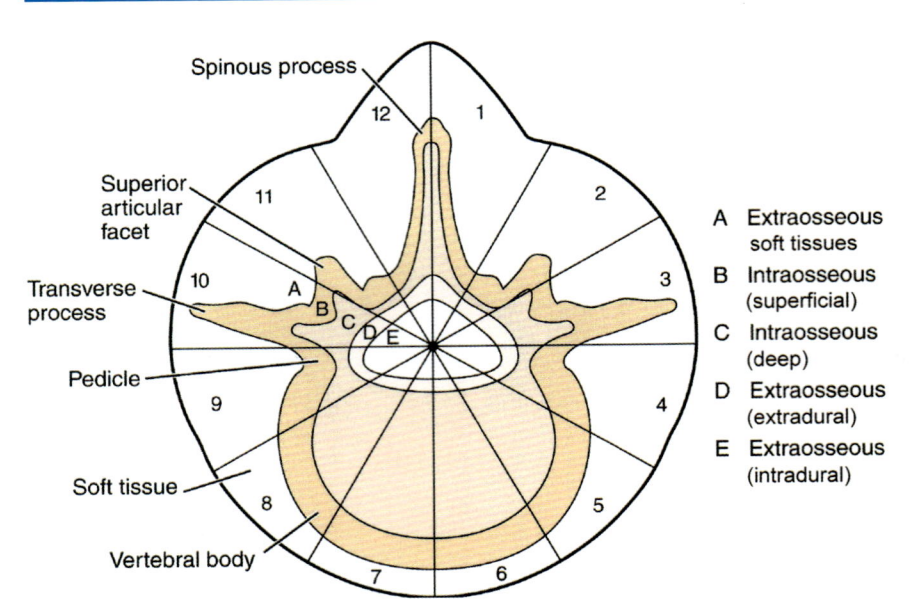

Fig. 49.5 Schematic for the Weinstein-Boriani-Biagini (WBB) staging system for spinal tumors.

A Extraosseous soft tissues
B Intraosseous (superficial)
C Intraosseous (deep)
D Extraosseous (extradural)
E Extraosseous (intradural)

continuous healthy tissue. A wide resection is the intended goal of an en-bloc procedure, but this goal is not always met. Intralesional resections provide symptom palliation but result in a high incidence of local recurrence due to the presumed spillage of residual tumor cells into the resection cavity.

The appropriate treatment for tumors of the thoracolumbar spine is dictated by the pathology in question and the patient's symptomatology. Instances of acute neurologic deficit, intractable pain, or progressive deformity usually require surgical intervention. Benign tumors that grow rapidly and are locally aggressive (stage 2 or 3 tumors in the Enneking classification) may prompt surgical resection—ideally en bloc—although the extent of resection is limited by the proximity of vital neural structures that cannot be sacrificed in an attempt to obtain surgical margins.

Posterior Decompression Versus Circumferential Decompression/Stabilization

Originally, a small randomized series and larger retrospective series called into question the value of the traditional surgical intervention of laminectomy plus radiotherapy, compared with radiotherapy alone, in the treatment of malignant—metastatic specifically spinal tumors causing high-grade epidural compression and neurologic deterioration.[41,42] After these studies, surgery for spinal metastases became less common. Laminectomy did little to address the ventral epidural and often bony compression from vertebral body infiltration and fracture. Moreover, it introduced further instability into an already pathological disease segment by removing the intact posterior column, a process that could result in further instability. Patchell et al[43] addressed this question by publishing a series advocating a more appropriate surgical intervention (circumferential decompression plus stabilization) than laminectomy alone, and showed such a significant improvement in symptom palliation with surgical intervention that their trial had to be halted prematurely for ethical concerns. After this landmark study, the pendulum of expert opinion swung back in the direction of aggressive surgical intervention for symptomatic metastatic epidural disease.

Embolization and Vertebroplasty/Kyphoplasty

Less invasive interventions have been developed to supplement or obviate the need for aggressive surgical resection in patients with multiple comorbidities or advanced disease. Blood loss during resection of highly vascular tumors can be significantly reduced when preceded by therapeutic embolization of vascular pedicles feeding such tumors.[44]

More recently, kyphoplasty and vertebroplasty have emerged as valuable interventions in the management of pathological fractures from spinal tumors. Fourney et al[45] reported 97 procedures performed in 56 patients, and found marked or complete pain relief in 84% that was significant for up to 1 year.

Radiotherapy

Radiotherapy has been used as an effective primary therapy for both primary and metastatic malignancies of the spine.[41,46] Subsequent evidence supporting aggressive surgical resection and stabilization in instances of cord compression has made radiotherapy an adjuvant therapy in these instances,[43] but external beam radiotherapy (EBRT) remains a staple of therapy in patients without neurologic symptoms or instability or with radiosensitive histologies. Traditionally, radiotherapy is indicated for the primary treatment of radiosensitive spinal tumors, axial or radiculopathic pain in the absence of neurologic deficits, widespread metastatic disease not amenable to surgical resection, limited life expectancy, or medical comorbidities that preclude operative intervention.

Response rates to EBRT vary depending on the relative radiosensitivity of the histology being treated. In general, prostate and lymphoreticular tumors are radiosensitive, breast and lung show moderate responses to radiation, and gastrointestinal, melanoma, and renal cell carcinoma are quite radioresistant.[47]

Spinal Stereotactic Radiosurgery and Separation Surgery

More recently, spinal stereotactic radiosurgery (SSRS) has emerged as a important tool in the management of spinal neo-

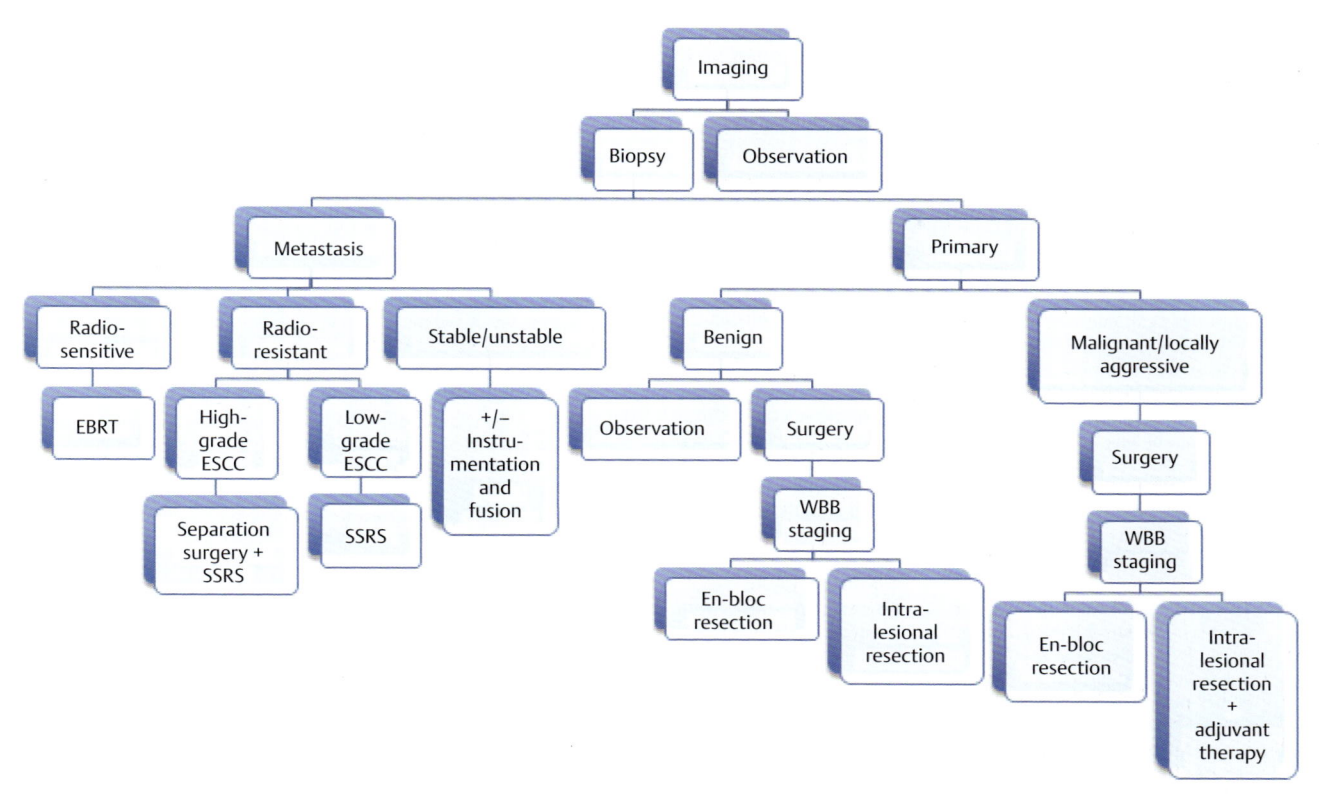

Fig. 49.6 Algorithm for diagnosis and management of tumors of the thoracolumbar spine. EBRT, external beam radiotherapy; ESCC, epidural spinal cord compression; SSRS, spinal stereotactic radiosurgery; WBB, Weinstein-Boriani-Biagini.

plasms, delivering higher conformal doses of radiation to smaller target volumes with decreased radiotoxicity to critical adjacent structures.[48] SSRS has also been effective in yielding pain relief and improving local control in the treatment of spinal metastases that were not causing significant neurologic deficits or structural instability.[49] Although SSRS has shown great promise, even with stereotactic conformal dosing, the delivery of radiation doses to the epidural space is limited due to concerns about regional neurotoxicity. Underdosed and undertreated epidural disease may be a future source of recurrent disease and neural element compression. Although effective, circumferential decompression and stabilization for such epidural disease carries with it significant morbidity and may not be suitable for all patients. More recent efforts have been made to use SSRS to control the bulk of nonepidural disease while employing more limited surgical resections with stabilization intended to remove epidural disease not amenable to appropriate radiation dosing by stereotactic methods—so-called separation surgery[50] (**Fig. 49.6**).

Conclusion

Tumors of the thoracolumbar spine are many and their treatment nuanced and complex. An overview of the field may provide a clinical framework for approaching patients with these tumors, but each patient should be evaluated on an individual basis, and clinical judgment, as always, remains paramount.

References

1. Ecker RD, Endo T, Wetjen NM, Krauss WE. Diagnosis and treatment of vertebral column metastases. Mayo Clin Proc 2005;80:1177–1186
2. Sciubba DM, Petteys RJ, Dekutoski MB, et al. Diagnosis and management of metastatic spine disease. A review. J Neurosurg Spine 2010;13:94–108
3. Sundaresan N, Rosen G, Boriani S. Primary malignant tumors of the spine. Orthop Clin North Am 2009;40:21–36, v.
4. Di Lorenzo N, Nardi P, Ciappetta P, Fortuna A. Benign tumors and tumor-like conditions of the spine. Radiological features, treatment, and results. Surg Neurol 1986;25:449–456
5. Levine AMCD. Treatment of primary malignant tumors of the spine and sac. In: Bridwell KH, DeWald RL, eds. The Textbook of Spinal Surgery, 2nd ed. Philadelphia: Lippincott-Raven; 1997
6. Ghelman B, Lospinuso MF, Levine DB, O'Leary PF, Burke SW. Percutaneous computed-tomography-guided biopsy of the thoracic and lumbar spine. Spine 1991;16:736–739
7. Tokuhashi Y, Matsuzaki H, Toriyama S, Kawano H, Ohsaka S. Scoring system for the preoperative evaluation of metastatic spine tumor prognosis. Spine 1990;15:1110–1113
8. Tomita K, Kawahara N, Kobayashi T, Yoshida A, Murakami H, Akamaru T. Surgical strategy for spinal metastases. Spine 2001;26:298–306
9. Malat J, Virapongse C, Levine A. Solitary osteochondroma of the spine. Spine 1986;11:625–628
10. Ahmed AR, Tan TS, Unni KK, Collins MS, Wenger DE, Sim FH. Secondary chondrosarcoma in osteochondroma: report of 107 patients. Clin Orthop Relat Res 2003;411:193–206
11. Albrecht S, Crutchfield JS, SeGall GK. On spinal osteochondromas. J Neurosurg 1992;77:247–252
12. Ropper AE, Cahill KS, Hanna JW, McCarthy EF, Gokaslan ZL, Chi JH. Primary vertebral tumors: a review of epidemiologic, histological, and imaging findings, Part I: benign tumors. Neurosurgery 2011;69:1171–1180
13. Atesok KI, Alman BA, Schemitsch EH, Peyser A, Mankin H. Osteoid osteoma and osteoblastoma. J Am Acad Orthop Surg 2011;19:678–689
14. Rosenthal DI, Hornicek FJ, Wolfe MW, Jennings LC, Gebhardt MC, Mankin HJ. Percutaneous radiofrequency coagulation of osteoid osteoma compared with operative treatment. J Bone Joint Surg Am 1998;80:815–821

15. Mohit AA, Eskridge J, Ellenbogen R, Shaffrey CI. Aneurysmal bone cyst of the atlas: successful treatment through selective arterial embolization: case report. Neurosurgery 2004;55:982
16. Barzin M, Maleki I. Incidence of vertebral hemangioma on spinal magnetic resonance imaging in Northern Iran. Pak J Biol Sci 2009;12:542–544
17. Boriani SW. Differential diagnosis and surgical treatment of primary benign and malignant neoplasms. In: Frymoyer JW, ed. The Adult Spine: Principles and Practice, 2nd ed. Philadelphia: Lippincott-Raven; 1997
18. Garg S, Mehta S, Dormans JP. Langerhans cell histiocytosis of the spine in children. Long-term follow-up. J Bone Joint Surg Am 2004;86-A:1740–1750
19. Pansuriya TC, Kroon HM, Bovée JV. Enchondromatosis: insights on the different subtypes. Int J Clin Exp Pathol 2010;3:557–569
20. McLoughlin GS, Sciubba DM, Wolinsky JP. Chondroma/Chondrosarcoma of the spine. Neurosurg Clin N Am 2008;19:57–63
21. Turcotte RE, Wunder JS, Isler MH, et al; Canadian Sarcoma Group. Giant cell tumor of long bone: a Canadian Sarcoma Group study. Clin Orthop Relat Res 2002;397:248–258
22. Hosalkar HS, Jones KJ, King JJ, Lackman RD. Serial arterial embolization for large sacral giant-cell tumors: mid- to long-term results. Spine 2007;32:1107–1115
23. Boriani S, Sudanese A, Baldini N, Picci P. Sarcomatous degeneration of giant cell tumours. Ital J Orthop Traumatol 1986;12:191–199
24. Thomas D, Henshaw R, Skubitz K, et al. Denosumab in patients with giant-cell tumour of bone: an open-label, phase 2 study. Lancet Oncol 2010;11:275–280
25. McMaster ML, Goldstein AM, Bromley CM, Ishibe N, Parry DM. Chordoma: incidence and survival patterns in the United States, 1973–1995. Cancer Causes Control 2001;12:1–11
26. Ropper AE, Cahill KS, Hanna JW, McCarthy EF, Gokaslan ZL, Chi JH. Primary vertebral tumors: a review of epidemiologic, histological and imaging findings, part II: locally aggressive and malignant tumors. Neurosurgery 2012;70:211–219, discussion 219
27. Bergh P, Kindblom LG, Gunterberg B, Remotti F, Ryd W, Meis-Kindblom JM. Prognostic factors in chordoma of the sacrum and mobile spine: a study of 39 patients. Cancer 2000;88:2122–2134
28. Casali PG, Stacchiotti S, Sangalli C, Olmi P, Gronchi A. Chordoma. Curr Opin Oncol 2007;19:367–370
29. Tricot G. New insights into role of microenvironment in multiple myeloma. Lancet 2000;355:248–250
30. Berenson JR, Hillner BE, Kyle RA, et al; American Society of Clinical Oncology Bisphosphonates Expert Panel. American Society of Clinical Oncology clinical practice guidelines: the role of bisphosphonates in multiple myeloma. J Clin Oncol 2002;20:3719–3736
31. Kumar SK, Rajkumar SV, Dispenzieri A, et al. Improved survival in multiple myeloma and the impact of novel therapies. Blood 2008;111:2516–2520
32. Utecht KN, Kolesar J. Bortezomib: a novel chemotherapeutic agent for hematologic malignancies. Am J Health Syst Pharm 2008;65:1221–1231
33. Ozaki T, Flege S, Liljenqvist U, et al. Osteosarcoma of the spine: experience of the Cooperative Osteosarcoma Study Group. Cancer 2002;94:1069–1077
34. DeLaney TF, Park L, Goldberg SI, et al. Radiotherapy for local control of osteosarcoma. Int J Radiat Oncol Biol Phys 2005;61:492–498
35. Ilaslan H, Sundaram M, Unni KK, Dekutoski MB. Primary Ewing's sarcoma of the vertebral column. Skeletal Radiol 2004;33:506–513
36. Grier HE, Krailo MD, Tarbell NJ, et al. Addition of ifosfamide and etoposide to standard chemotherapy for Ewing's sarcoma and primitive neuroectodermal tumor of bone. N Engl J Med 2003;348:694–701
37. Brada M, Pijls-Johannesma M, De Ruysscher D. Proton therapy in clinical practice: current clinical evidence. J Clin Oncol 2007;25:965–970
38. Enneking WF. A system of staging musculoskeletal neoplasms. Clin Orthop Relat Res 1986;204:9–24
39. Boriani S, Weinstein JN, Biagini R. Primary bone tumors of the spine. Terminology and surgical staging. Spine 1997;22:1036–1044
40. Fisher CG, DiPaola CP, Ryken TC, et al. A novel classification system for spinal instability in neoplastic disease: an evidence-based approach and expert consensus from the Spine Oncology Study Group. Spine 2010;35:E1221–E1229
41. Young RF, Post EM, King GA. Treatment of spinal epidural metastases. Randomized prospective comparison of laminectomy and radiotherapy. J Neurosurg 1980;53:741–748
42. Gilbert RW, Kim JH, Posner JB. Epidural spinal cord compression from metastatic tumor: diagnosis and treatment. Ann Neurol 1978;3:40–51
43. Patchell RA, Tibbs PA, Regine WF, et al. Direct decompressive surgical resection in the treatment of spinal cord compression caused by metastatic cancer: a randomised trial. Lancet 2005;366:643–648
44. Gellad FE, Sadato N, Numaguchi Y, Levine AM. Vascular metastatic lesions of the spine: preoperative embolization. Radiology 1990;176:683–686
45. Fourney DR, Schomer DF, Nader R, et al. Percutaneous vertebroplasty and kyphoplasty for painful vertebral body fractures in cancer patients. J Neurosurg 2003;98(1, Suppl):21–30
46. Maranzano E, Latini P. Effectiveness of radiation therapy without surgery in metastatic spinal cord compression: final results from a prospective trial. Int J Radiat Oncol Biol Phys 1995;32:959–967
47. Bilsky MH, Lis E, Raizer J, Lee H, Boland P. The diagnosis and treatment of metastatic spinal tumor. Oncologist 1999;4:459–469
48. Hamilton AJ, Lulu BA, Fosmire H, Stea B, Cassady JR. Preliminary clinical experience with linear accelerator-based spinal stereotactic radiosurgery. Neurosurgery 1995;36:311–319
49. Gerszten PC, Burton SA, Ozhasoglu C, Welch WC. Radiosurgery for spinal metastases: clinical experience in 500 cases from a single institution. Spine 2007;32:193–199
50. Laufer I, Iorgulescu JB, Chapman T, et al. Local disease control for spinal metastases following "separation surgery" and adjuvant hypofractionated or high-dose single-fraction stereotactic radiosurgery: outcome analysis in 186 patients. J Neurosurg Spine 2013;18:207–214

50 Trauma of the Thoracic and Thoracolumbar Spine

Nader S. Dahdaleh and Zachary A. Smith

A thorough understanding of current classification systems is crucial when managing thoracolumbar spine fractures. Most classification systems differentiate between fractures that are stable and those that are unstable and require instrumentation and internal fixation. Once the fracture is deemed unstable, the second step toward successful management is the selection of the appropriate approach and stabilization technique.

The immediate goals of treating a spinal fracture include the achievement of spinal stability, the restoration of anatomic alignment, and the ability to expedite patient mobilization. The long-term goals include healing of the fracture, maintenance of alignment, and avoidance of posttraumatic kyphosis.

Generally we make an effort, when possible, to spare motion at the segments above and below the fracture by minimizing the number of motion segments fused and utilizing short segment fixation.

Classification of Thoracolumbar Spine Fractures

In 1929 Boehler categorized thoracolumbar fractures into five entities: compression, flexion-distraction, extension, shear, and rotational fractures.[1] This was the first attempt to classify these fractures. In 1938, Watson-Jones[2] identified three thoracolumbar fracture patterns: simple wedge fractures, comminuted fractures, and fracture dislocations. Moreover, he introduced the concept of instability and was the first to associate the integrity of the posterior ligamentous complex (PLC) with spinal stability. Nicoll,[3] in 1949, categorized fractures as stable or unstable. He identified four structures that contribute to spinal stability: the vertebral body, the disk, the intervertebral joints, and the interspinous ligaments. Similarly, the integrity of the latter was an important determinant of stability. He then classified thoracolumbar spine fractures as anterior wedge, lateral wedge, fracture dislocation, and neural arch fractures.

The two-column theory of spinal stability was introduced by Holdsworth[4] in 1963. This classification recognized five mechanisms of injury: flexion, flexion-rotation, extension, compression, and shear forces. The fracture patterns identified by this classification were anterior compression, fracture dislocation, rotational fracture dislocation, and extension, shear, and burst fractures. According to this model, the spine was divided into anterior and posterior columns. The anterior column consisted of the vertebral body and the intervertebral disk, and the posterior column consisted of the neural arch, the facet joints, and the PLC (interspinal and supraspinal ligaments, and the ligamentum flavum). Fractures that included a posterior column injury were unstable.

In 1978, White and Panjabi[5] defined clinical instability as the inability of the spine under physiological loads to maintain relationships between vertebrae such that there is neither an acute nor subsequent neurologic injury, deformity, or pain.

One classification that stood the test of time is the three-column theory of the spine. This famous, simple, and reproducible system was introduced by Francis Denis[6] in 1983. It was based on reviewing radiographs of 412 fractures and 53 computed tomography (CT) images. According to Denis, the anterior column of the spine included the anterior longitudinal ligament and the anterior half of the vertebral body, annulus, and disk. The middle column included the posterior half of the vertebral body, annulus, and disk, in addition to the posterior longitudinal ligament. The posterior column included the neural arch, facets, and the PLC, consisting of the supra- and interspinal ligaments, ligamentum flavum, and facet capsules (**Fig. 50.1**). Stability was dependent on the integrity of two of the three columns. This classification identified four types of fractures: compression fractures resulting from failure of the anterior column under compression, burst fractures resulting from failure of the anterior and middle columns, flexion distraction injuries secondary to failure of the posterior and middle columns, and fracture-dislocations resulting from failure of all three columns. Flexion distraction injuries or seat-belt–type injuries were considered unstable in the first degree. Burst fractures with deficit were considered unstable in the second degree, and fracture dislocations were unstable in the third degree.

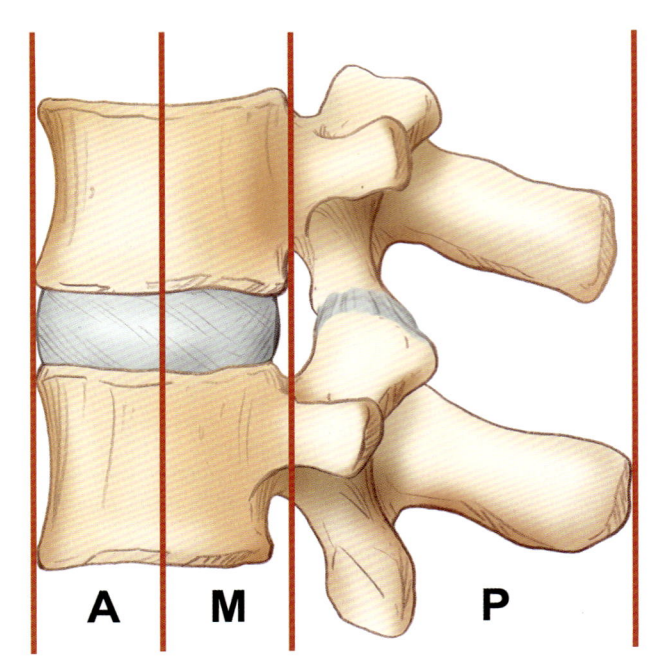

Fig. 50.1 Denis three-column spine model. A, anterior column; M, middle column; P, posterior column.

In 1983, McAfee et al[7] introduced a classification based on their review of the sagittal reconstruction of CT scans of 100 patients. They identified six fracture patterns: wedge compression, stable burst, unstable burst, Chance fracture, flexion distraction, and translational fractures. The stability of burst fractures was dependent on the integrity of the PLC.

In 1984, Ferguson and Allen[8] introduced the "mechanistic" classification, which consisted of seven fracture categories: compressive flexion, distractive flexion, lateral flexion, torsional flexion, translation, vertical compression, and distractive flexion.

The AO (Arbeitsgemeinschaft fur Osteosynthesefragen) classification system was introduced by Magerl et al[9] in 1989. This detailed system was based on a radiographic review of 1,445 thoracolumbar fractures. The classification recognized three main fracture types: A, compression; B, distraction; and C, fracture dislocation. Subdivisions and subcategories were created according to the severity of the fractures. This resulted in 53 fracture patterns with A1 being the least severe and C3 the most severe.

In 1994, McCormack et al[10] introduced the load sharing classification, which was based on the analysis of failures of thoracolumbar spine fractures managed with transpedicular short-segment fusion. The fractures were graded according to the degree of comminution of the body, the apposition of the fracture fragments, and the deformity. A point system was applied to each fracture from 1 to 3, with a higher number indicative of increased severity. Fractures with a score greater than 7 had a high risk of short–segment fixation failure. The main purpose of this classification was to guide surgeons in decision making when using short-segment fixation or anterior column graft support.

In 2005, the Spine Trauma Study Group led by Vaccaro introduced the Thoracolumbar Injury Severity Score (TLISS).[11,12] This classification was based on three injury characteristics: the mechanism of injury, the neurologic status, and the integrity of the PLC. Compression injuries were assigned 1 point, compression fractures with coronal plane deformity greater than 15 degrees and burst fractures were assigned 2 points, translational or rotational injuries were assigned 3 points, and distraction injuries were assigned 4 points.

Regarding neurologic injury, patients with an intact neurologic exam were assigned 0 points, patients with a nerve root injury or complete spinal cord injury were assigned 2 points, and patients with an incomplete spinal cord injury or cauda equina syndrome were assigned 3 points. In the original description, the integrity of the PLC could be assessed clinically by the presence of a palpable interspinous gap, radiographically by the presence of an interspinous gap on plane radiographs, or with the use of magnetic resonance imaging (MRI). Patients with an intact PLC were assigned 0 points, patients with a PLC of indeterminate integrity were assigned 2 points, and patients with a confirmed disruption were assigned 3 points.

The total TLISS score reflects the severity of the injury and aids in guiding the treatment. Patients with a score ≤ 3 are treated nonoperatively; patients with a score ≥ 5 are treated by surgical stabilization, and patients with score of 4 are deemed indeterminate and are treated according to the surgeon's preference. Later, the TLISS system, which emphasized the mechanism of injury, was modified into the Thoracolumbar Injury Classification and Severity Score (TLICS), which emphasized the morphology of fractures.[13] In contrast to the TLISS system, in the case of multiple mechanisms with one or more level involvement, this classification would only consider the most severe injury mechanism. In addition, the 1 point addition for coronal plane deformity was removed. The TLICS system included radiographic/mechanistic criteria, clinical criteria, and MRI based on the integrity of the PLC.

In 2006, Hitchon's group introduced the Iowa algorithm and classification scheme based on the management of 300 patients with thoracolumbar fractures who were prospectively followed.[14,15] This was the first classification that factored in the decision making the presence of persistent pain that precludes mobilization. The algorithm is based on three criteria: clinical, biomechanical, and radiographic. The clinical criteria evaluate the neurologic state and pain. The biomechanical criteria include the involvement of one, two, or three columns. The radiographic criteria address the degree of kyphosis, canal compromise, and the integrity of the PLC (**Fig. 50.2**).

Patients with a neurologic deficit and persistent pain that precludes mobilization are treated with operative intervention. In patients who are neurologically normal, the biomechanical criteria are addressed. Patients with a one-column injury are managed conservatively with or without bracing. Patients with a three-column injury are managed with operative stabilization. In intact patients with a two-column injury, the radiographic criteria are addressed. In this group patients with PLC disruption, kyphosis > 20 degrees, or a residual canal of less than 50% are managed with operative stabilization.

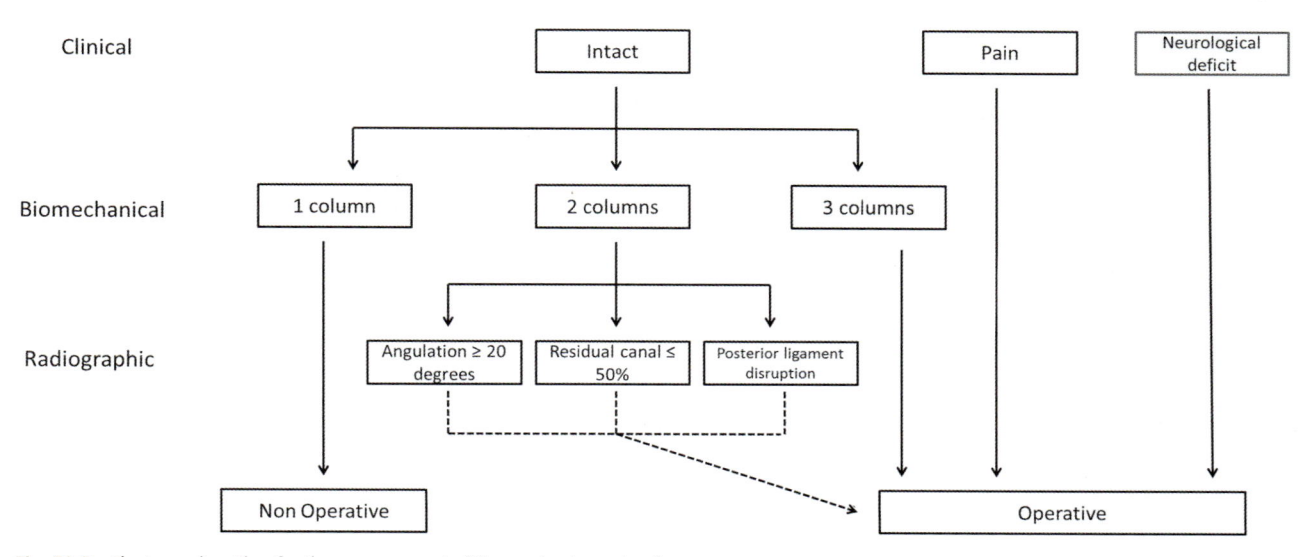

Fig. 50.2 The Iowa algorithm for the management of thoracolumbar spine fractures.

Fracture Types

For simplicity, we recognize four common fracture patterns identified and recognized by the most common classification schemes: compression fractures, burst fractures, distraction injuries, and fracture dislocations.

Compression Fractures

These fractures are also often called wedge compression fractures and are the most common fracture type. A compression fracture occurs when the anterior column fails under compression forces.[16] It often occurs in the thoracic spine due to the natural thoracic kyphosis. Axial loads in flexion are required for these fractures to occur in the straight thoracolumbar junction. These fractures spare the middle and posterior columns. The integrity of the PLC is often intact, and patients are neurologically normal. These fractures are considered stable and do not require internal fixation. Patients are usually treated with bracing and analgesia.

Burst Fractures

These fractures occur as a result of pure axial load application. The anterior and middle columns are involved. Bony retropulsion occurs to different extents, causing varying degrees of spinal canal compromise. The occurrence of associated neurologic injury is similarly variable, and its correlation with canal compromise is often controversial.[17,18] Operative intervention is necessary in the setting of neurologic injury for purposes of decompression and stabilization. Management of patients who are neurologically normal is controversial.[19,20] The presence of PLC injury, high load sharing scores, and persistent pain are drivers for surgical stabilization in these patients.

When surgical stabilization is deemed necessary, the choice of anterior column reconstruction or employment of long-segment fixation is dictated by the severity of the load sharing score. We usually reconstruct the anterior column when the load sharing score is > 6 (**Fig. 50.3**).

Distraction Injuries

Flexion Distraction Injuries

These injuries often involve the middle and posterior columns and sometimes all three columns. They were initially described by Chance.[21] They are often osseous injuries, but pure ligamentous forms do occur, making them hard to diagnose solely on plain X-rays, especially when a compression deformity is not detected. These fractures are unstable and are associated with neurologic injury if managed conservatively. The PLC is often disrupted. Posterior long or short pedicle screw fixation is often employed for stabilization. Percutaneous pedicle screw fixation has been increasingly used for these injuries, especially in the presence of an osseous fracture component (**Fig. 50.4**).[22]

Extension Injuries

These are three-column injuries that often occur in the setting of ankylosing spondylitis or diffuse idiopathic skeletal hyperostosis.[23]

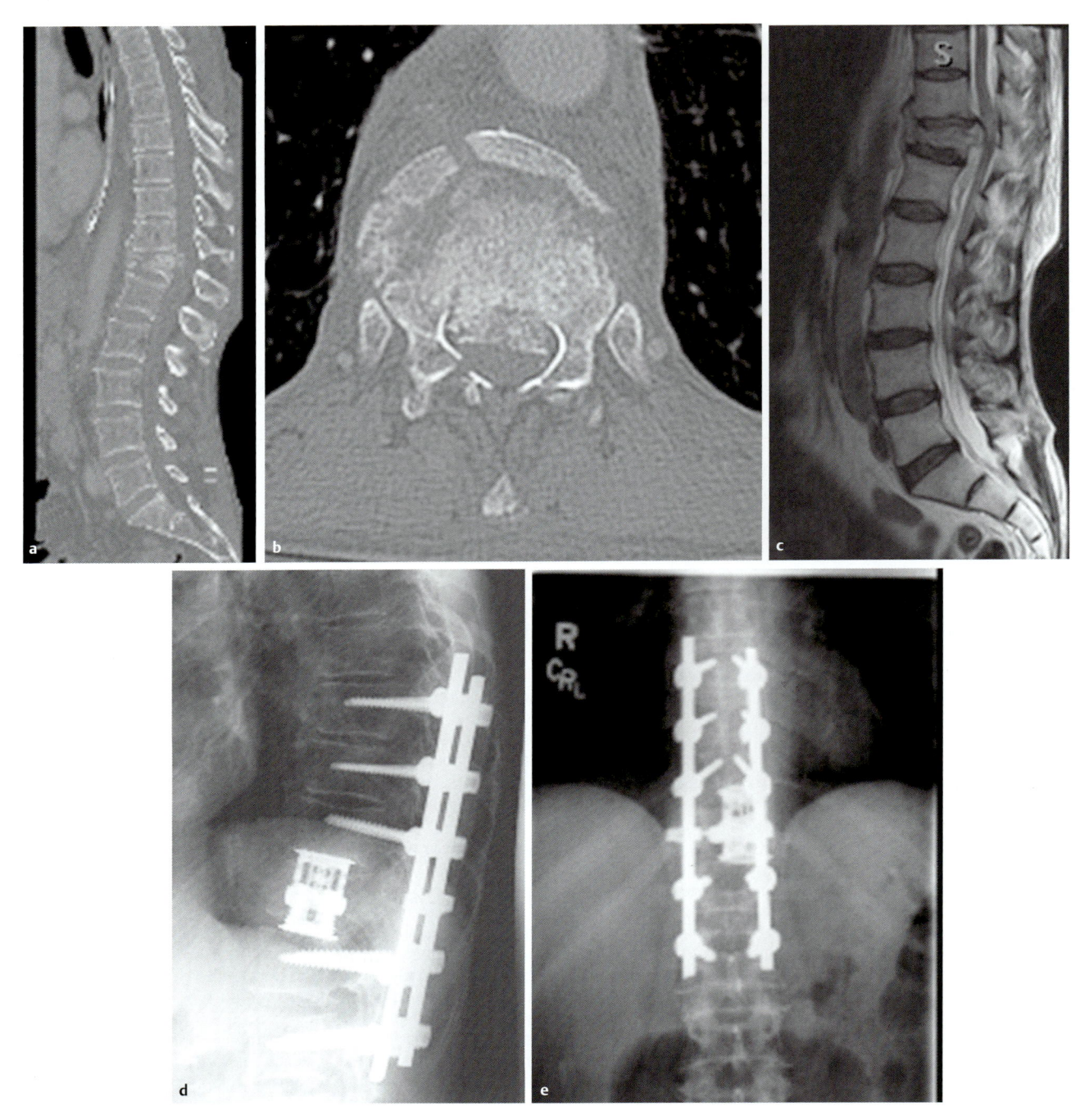

Fig. 50.3 A 56-year-old man suffered an injury at work when a wall fell on him and he was unable to move his legs. He was transferred to the emergency room, where an examination revealed 0/5 motor strength in the lower extremities. **(a,b)** He had a sensory level at T12 with reduced rectal tone. Computed tomography (CT) of the spine showed a T12 burst fracture with a 40% residual canal, with a load sharing score of 7. **(c)** A T2-weighted magnetic resonance imaging (MRI) sequence showed signal cord change at the level of the injury. The patient underwent an emergency transpedicular corpectomy and anterior column reconstruction with an expandable titanium cage as well as posterior long-segment pedicle screw fixation. By the 1-year follow-up [lateral **(d)** and anteroposterior **(e)** X-rays], the patient had regained motor strength and was ambulating with a walker, but he still had a neurogenic bladder.

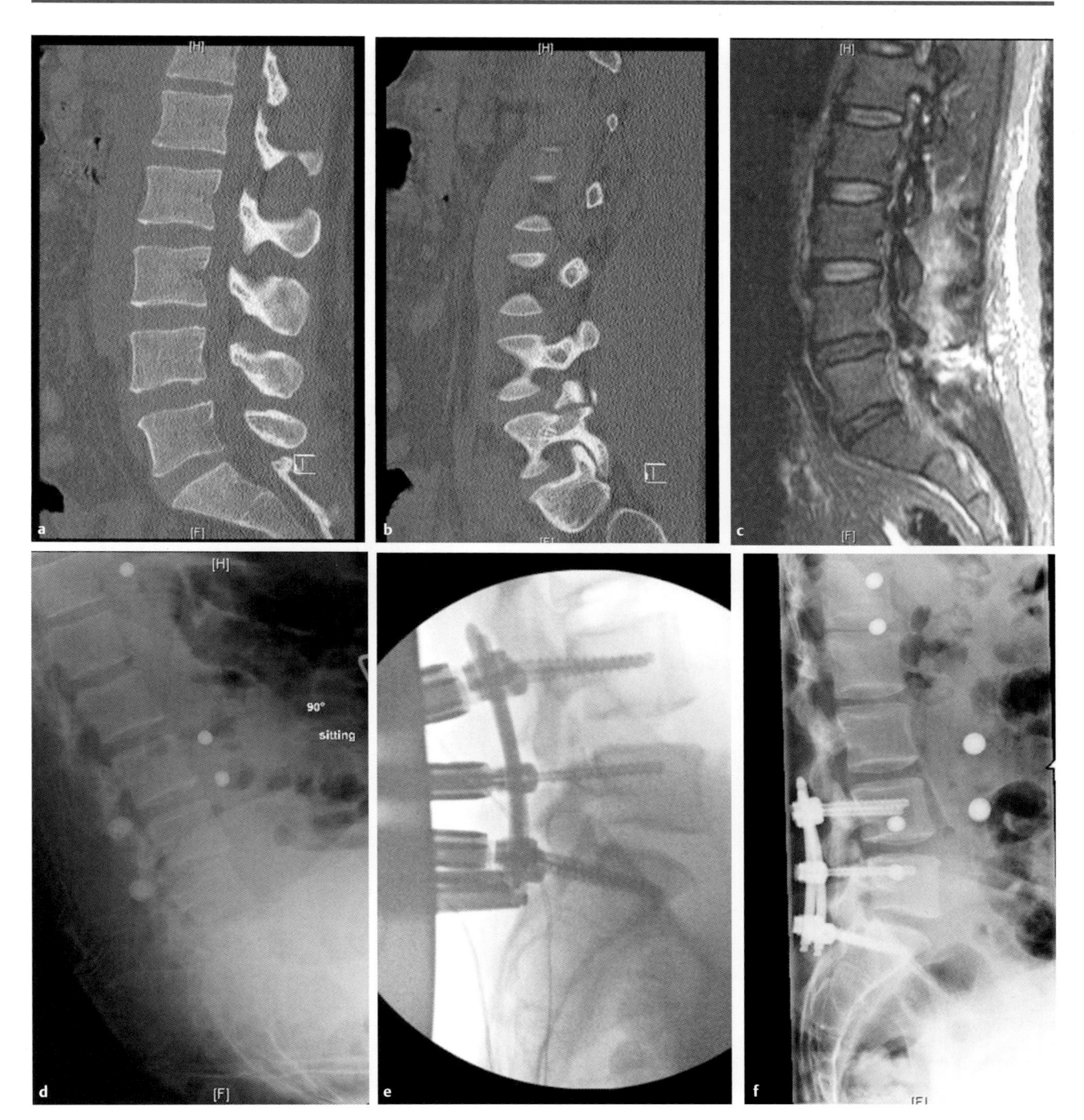

Fig. 50.4 A 29-year-old man was involved in a motor vehicle accident, in which he sustained multiple orthopedic lower extremity injuries. He underwent an emergency exploratory laparotomy and repair of a liver laceration. **(a,b)** CT of the lumbar spine showed fracture of the left superior articular process and pedicle of L4 but no subluxation. **(c)** MRI short tau inversion recovery (STIR) sequence revealed posterior ligamentous disruption. Because the patient had only a unilateral pedicle fracture, he was placed in a lumbosacral orthosis (LSO) brace. **(d)** However, 90-degree X-rays showed L4-L5 subluxation along with worsening lower back pain, indicating instability. The patient underwent percutaneous short-segment pedicle screw fixation. **(e)** X-ray at 3-month follow-up showed normal alignment. **(f)** The Visual Analogue Scale (VAS) rating of his back pain was zero.

These fractures are unstable and require posterior long-segment fixation. Because the levels above and below the fracture are autofused, forming a large level arm, multiple points of fixation above and below the fracture are recommended, to provide optimal biomechanical stability and to prevent failure and screw pullout (**Fig. 50.5**).

Fracture Dislocations

These are highly unstable three-column injuries that occur secondary to rotational shear forces, translational forces, or a combination of both. These fractures are highly associated with neurologic injury. Posterior reduction and pedicle screw fixation is often the treatment of choice (**Fig. 50.6**).

Conclusion

Most recent classification systems identify and differentiate stable and unstable fractures by assessing the fracture morphology, the neurologic state, the deformity, the integrity of the PLC, and the presence of persistent pain. These systems aid surgeons in deciding whether to operate or to use a brace. The second step in managing thoracolumbar fractures is the selection of the appropriate approach and technique for stabilization when the decision to operate is made. The surgeon should keep in mind that other important factors, such as the patient's age, bone health, and comorbidities, are not addressed by any classification system, thus necessitating that surgeon expertise and case-by-case individualization also be considered in determining how to treat the patient.

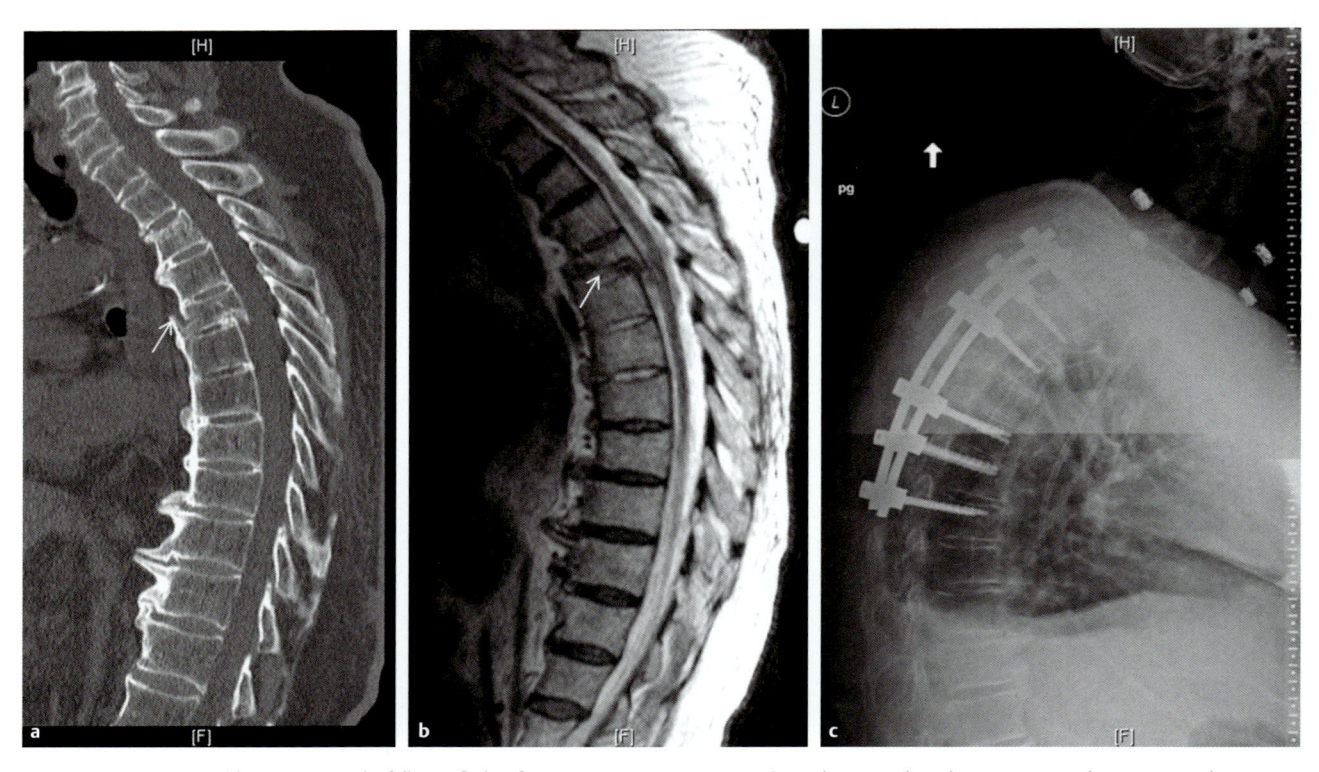

Fig. 50.5 An 86-year-old man sustained a fall on a flight of stairs. He presented to the emergency room with significant midthoracic pain. **(a)** CT of the spine showed an extension-type injury at T5, with posterior translation in the setting of diffuse idiopathic skeletal hyperostosis. **(b)** T2-weighted MRI sequence showed no spinal cord compression. The patient underwent an open posterior long-segment fixation. **(c)** X-ray at 6-month follow-up demonstrated adequate alignment and the patient's VAS rating of his back pain was zero.

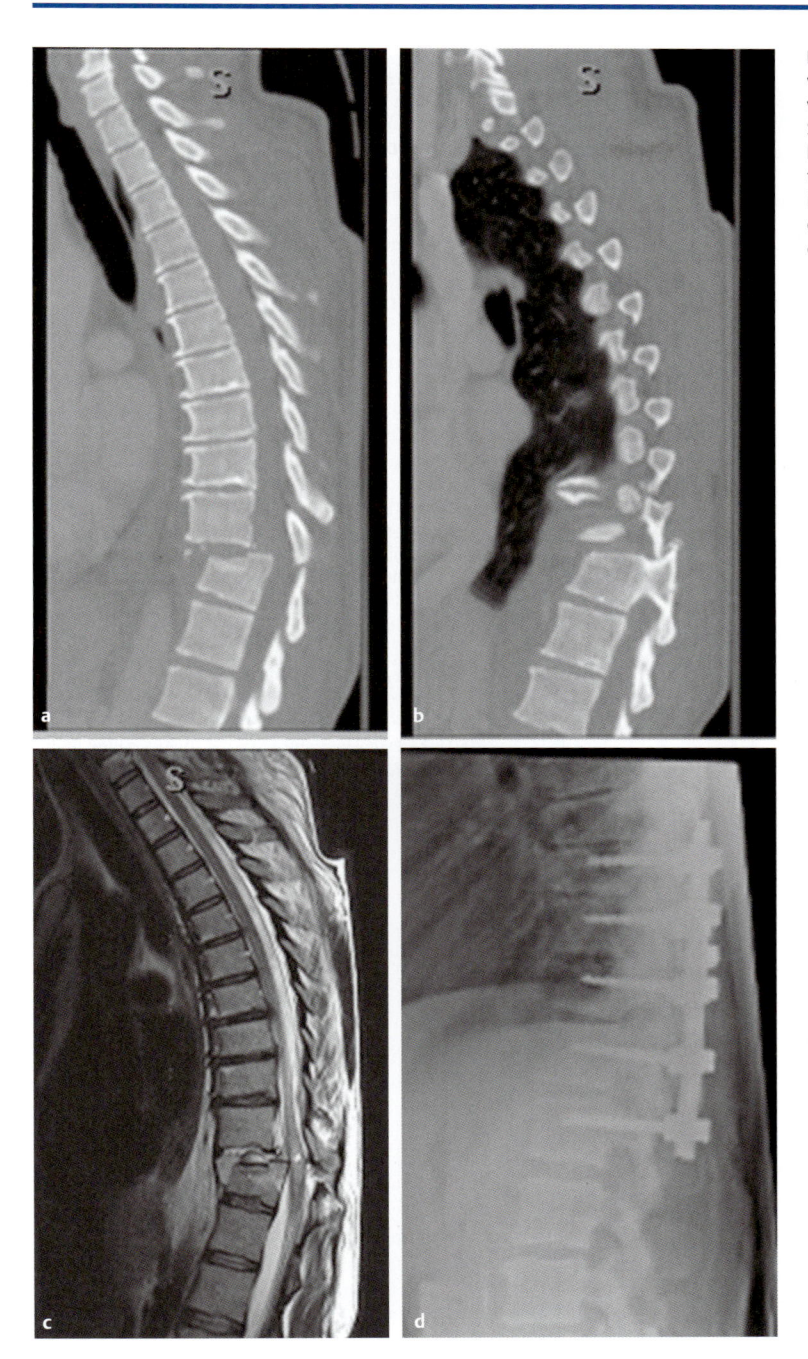

Fig. 50.6 A 47-year-old woman was involved in a motor vehicle accident. Upon arrival at the emergency room, she was found to have a complete spinal cord injury—American Spinal Injury Association (ASIA) grade A—with a sensory motor level at T10. **(a,b)** CT of the spine showed a fracture dislocation at T10-T11 with bilateral locked facets. **(c)** T2-weighted MRI sequence showed spinal signal cord change at the level of the injury. **(d)** The patient underwent posterior open reduction and long-segment pedicle screw fixation.

References

1. Sethi MK, Schoenfeld AJ, Bono CM, Harris MB. The evolution of thoracolumbar injury classification systems. Spine J 2009;9:780–788
2. Watson-Jones R. The results of postural reduction of fractures of the spine. J Bone Joint Surg Am 1938;20:567–586
3. Nicoll EA. Fractures of the dorso-lumbar spine. J Bone Joint Surg Br 1949;31B:376–394
4. Holdsworth F. Fractures, dislocations, and fracture-dislocations of the spine. J Bone Joint Surg Am 1970;52:1534–1551
5. White AA, Panjabi M. Clinical Biomechanics of the Spine. Philadelphia: JB Lippincott; 1978
6. Denis F. The three column spine and its significance in the classification of acute thoracolumbar spinal injuries. Spine 1983;8:817–831
7. McAfee PC, Yuan HA, Fredrickson BE, Lubicky JP. The value of computed tomography in thoracolumbar fractures. An analysis of one hundred consecutive cases and a new classification. J Bone Joint Surg Am 1983;65:461–473
8. Ferguson RL, Allen BL Jr. A mechanistic classification of thoracolumbar spine fractures. Clin Orthop Relat Res 1984;189:77–88
9. Magerl F, Aebi M, Gertzbein SD, Harms J, Nazarian S. A comprehensive classification of thoracic and lumbar injuries. Eur Spine J 1994;3:184–201
10. McCormack T, Karaikovic E, Gaines RW. The load sharing classification of spine fractures. Spine 1994;19:1741–1744
11. Vaccaro AR, Lehman RA Jr, Hurlbert RJ, et al. A new classification of thoracolumbar injuries: the importance of injury morphology, the integrity of the posterior ligamentous complex, and neurologic status. Spine 2005;30:2325–2333
12. Vaccaro AR, Zeiller SC, Hulbert RJ, et al. The thoracolumbar injury severity score: a proposed treatment algorithm. J Spinal Disord Tech 2005;18:209–215
13. Harrop JS, Vaccaro AR, Hurlbert RJ, et al; Spine Trauma Study Group. Intrarater and interrater reliability and validity in the assessment of the mechanism of injury and integrity of the posterior ligamentous complex: a novel injury severity scoring system for thoracolumbar injuries. Invited submission from the Joint Section Meeting On Disorders of the Spine and Peripheral Nerves, March 2005. J Neurosurg Spine 2006;4:118–122
14. Dahdaleh NS, Hitchon PW. Classification of thoracolumbar spine fractures. In: Benzel EC, Francis TB, eds. Spine Surgery: Techniques, Complication Avoidance, and Management. Philadelphia: Elsevier; 2012:593–599
15. Dahdaleh NS, Smith ZA, Hitchon PW. Percutaneous pedicle screw fixation for thoracolumbar fractures. Neurosurg Clin N Am 2014;25:337–346
16. Vollmer DG, Gegg C. Classification and acute management of thoracolumbar fractures. Neurosurg Clin N Am 1997;8:499–507
17. Meves R, Avanzi O. Correlation between neurological deficit and spinal canal compromise in 198 patients with thoracolumbar and lumbar fractures. Spine 2005;30:787–791
18. Mohanty SP, Venkatram N. Does neurological recovery in thoracolumbar and lumbar burst fractures depend on the extent of canal compromise? Spinal Cord 2002;40:295–299
19. Siebenga J, Leferink VJ, Segers MJ, et al. Treatment of traumatic thoracolumbar spine fractures: a multicenter prospective randomized study of operative versus nonsurgical treatment. Spine 2006;31:2881–2890
20. Wood K, Buttermann G, Mehbod A, Garvey T, Jhanjee R, Sechriest V. Operative compared with nonoperative treatment of a thoracolumbar burst fracture without neurological deficit. A prospective, randomized study. J Bone Joint Surg Am 2003;85-A:773–781
21. Chance GQ. Note on a type of flexion fracture of the spine. Br J Radiol 1948;21:452
22. Grossbach AJ, Dahdaleh NS, Abel TJ, Woods GD, Dlouhy BJ, Hitchon PW. Flexion-distraction injuries of the thoracolumbar spine: open fusion versus percutaneous pedicle screw fixation. Neurosurg Focus 2013;35:E2
23. Burkus JK, Denis F. Hyperextension injuries of the thoracic spine in diffuse idiopathic skeletal hyperostosis. Report of four cases. J Bone Joint Surg Am 1994;76:237–243

51 Thoracic Epidural Abscess and Vertebral Osteomyelitis

E. Emily Bennett and Edward C. Benzel

Since the time of its first characterization by Giovanni Battis Morgagni[1] in 1761, spinal epidural abscess (SEA) has remained a potentially neurologically morbid and fatal diagnosis.[2] The earliest surgical intervention for SEA was in 1901 by Barth.[3,4] Despite improved imaging techniques and management over the last century, morbidity has been reported in the range of 33 to 74% and mortality at ~ 5%.[2,5-8] Misdiagnosis or delayed diagnosis due to an often variable presentation is overshadowed by seemingly more acute medical illnesses; rapid onset of irreversible neurologic deficits may then ensue. Clinical outcomes are related to neurologic function at the time of presentation. The gold standard has been immediate surgical decompression and debridement. However, more recent evidence suggests that medical management with intravenous antibiotics alone in certain instances may produce similar outcomes.[4,7,9,10]

Epidemiology

The incidence of SEA has steadily increased over the last three decades. This increase, from 0.18 cases per 10,000 admissions to 2.8 cases per 10,000 admissions, could be a reflection of greater recognition and improved imaging.[11] Also, increased use of spinal instrumentation, intravenous drug abuse, immunodeficiency disorders, and an aging population may have contributed to this increase. SEA most commonly affects the thoracic spine, accounting for 25 to 50% of all spinal abscesses, followed by the lumbar region.[3,12] The relatively small epidural space in the thoracic region results in rapid and, at times, catastrophic development of neurologic deficits.

Etiology and Pathogenesis

An SEA results from purulent material collecting in the spinal canal between the dura and the ligamentous-vertebral structures. Bacteria can spread into the spinal canal via contiguous or hematogenous spread. Hematogenous spread accounts for half of the cases, contiguous spread accounts for one third, and no source is identified in the remaining cases.[8] In general, skin and soft tissue remain the major sources of infection, but urinary tract infections, dental procedures, traumas, spinal surgeries, and arteriovenous fistula infections can predispose to SEA formation as well.[13] The source of infection relates to the location of the SEA. For example, in intravenous drug users and upper extremity infections, the thoracic spine is most often involved.

Hematogenous spread occurs through the spinal epidural venous plexus (**Fig. 51.1**). SEA rarely forms from direct hematogenous spread without the presence of diskitis or osteomyelitis.[14] Vertebral osteomyelitis accounts for 5 to 45% of cases.[15] Thrombosis of these veins at the level of abscess and venous engorgement above and below the abscess are commonly seen.[16]

Staphylococcus aureus is the most common organism causing SEA. It accounts for almost two thirds of infections.[8] Furthermore, the proportion off SEA caused by methicillin-resistant *S. aureus* (MRSA) is on the rise and represents up to 40% of total infections at some institutions.[8] SEA caused by MRSA may develop more rapidly as well. Less common pathogens include coagulase-negative staphylococci (i.e., *Staphylococcus epidermidis*), streptococci, gram-negative organisms, fungi, parasites, anaerobic bacteria, and *Mycobacterium tuberculosis*.[8,17,18]

The location of an abscess in the epidural space is dictated by the anatomy of the spinal canal in the thoracic region and can be roughly divided into four groups (**Fig. 51.2**): (1) anterior symmetrical, (2) anterior asymmetrical, (3) posterior (dorsal), and (4) circumferential. It was often thought that the dorsal portion of the canal, due to its relatively larger volume and poorly vascularized epidural fat, was the most common site for infections to localize. However, dorsal predilection of SEA was challenged by a magnetic resonance imaging (MRI)-based study that found the ventral location to be the commonest (50%), then the circumferential (36%), and the dorsal (14%).[19] In contrast, a 2014 retrospective review of 128 patients who developed spontaneous SEA of the spine found the dorsal location to be the most common (41%), followed by the ventral (36%) and the circumferential (23%).[4] This review also noted that the location and extent of abscess did not significantly impact neurologic motor recovery.

The exact mechanisms by which thoracic epidural abscesses produce neurologic deficits remain unclear. Leading theories include a direct mechanical compression, an indirect vascular mechanism, or a combination of mechanical and vascular mechanisms.[8] Originally, microangiographic studies in rabbits showed that the initial neurologic deficits with experimental SEA were related primarily to mechanical compression.[18] Further, improvement after a laminectomy supports a mechanical pathophysiology.[8] But later studies utilizing animals showed that both mechanical compression and vascular ischemia have an additive effect on neurologic function.[8] Studies in a rabbit model and autopsied patients have shown the following vascular mechanisms: (1) venous compression and thrombosis, (2) thrombophlebitis of epidural space and spinal cord, (3) venous infarction and edema, (4) hypoxia secondary to rostral venous drainage obstruction and venous stasis, and (5) arterial thrombosis. This explains the rapidity of onset and often irreversibility of neurologic deficits. The pathophysiology of neurologic deficits may differ among patients, and it seems prudent to conclude that vascular and compressive factors likely act in combination to produce the full clinical picture.[8]

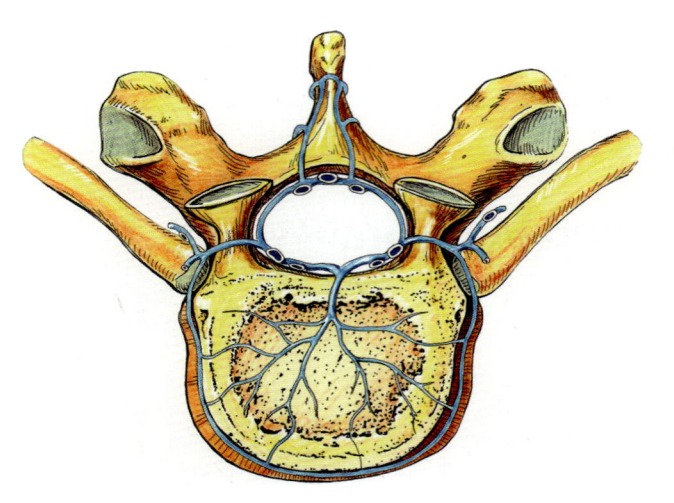

Fig. 51.1 The venous drainage of a typical thoracic vertebral segment.

Clinical Manifestations

Nearly 50% of patients are misdiagnosed at initial presentation.[4,20,21] High variability in the clinical picture often poses diagnostic difficulties. Fever and signs of systemic infection are common on initial presentation. Furthermore, patients often have more obvious and acute medical problems. Classic clinical evolution of SEA takes place through four clinical stages: (1) focal spinal pain and tenderness, (2) radicular pain, (3) weakness, and (4) paralysis.[8] A large meta-analysis by Reihsaus et al[6] found that up to 34% of patients presented with stage 4 or paralysis.

In Patel et al's[4] review, the most common presenting chief complaints were site-specific pain (100%), subjective fevers (50%), and extremity weakness (47%). Another retrospective study of 77 patients with spontaneous SEA found that axial pain was the most common presenting symptom, followed by focal weakness (55.8%), radiculopathy (29.9%), and myelopathy (5.2%).[2] The lumbar spine was most commonly affected in these two studies; however, presenting symptoms in these two larger reviews were similar to the four clinical stages as described above.

The latent period between onset of pain and neurologic deficit varies in each patient. Patients may be grouped into acute and chronic SEA based on time from progression of pain to weakness. Moreover, some investigators have classified patients with symptoms lasting less than 2 weeks as acute and those with symptoms lasting 2 weeks or longer as chronic. Acute patients generally display leukocytosis on evaluation. Chronic patients have less pain and slowly progressive paralysis. They have a better prognosis for neurologic recovery. Lastly, ascending neurologic deficits in a previously paraplegic patient could be a sign of developing SEA.

Laboratory and Radiographic Evaluations

Leukocytosis and elevated erythrocyte sedimentation rate are noted in the acute phase. Lumbar puncture is no longer necessary to make a diagnosis of thoracic epidural abscess. It carries the risks of neurologic deterioration, if performed below a block, and of traversing the abscess and transmitting the infection to the subarachnoid space. The possibility of isolating the infective organism from cerebrospinal fluid (CSF) is less than 25%.[8] On the other hand, blood cultures are positive for infective organisms in

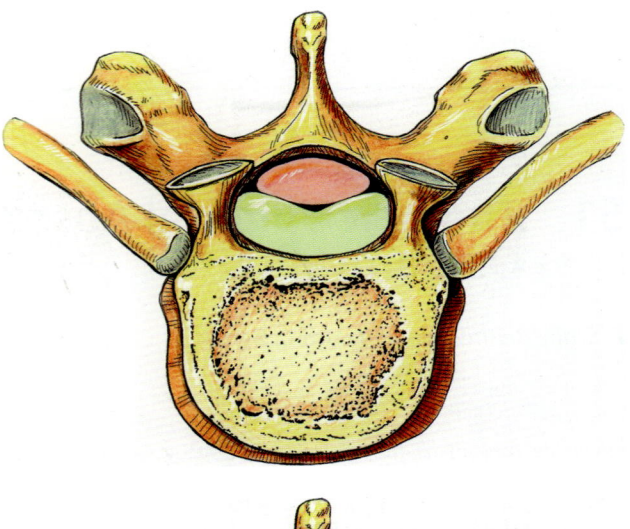

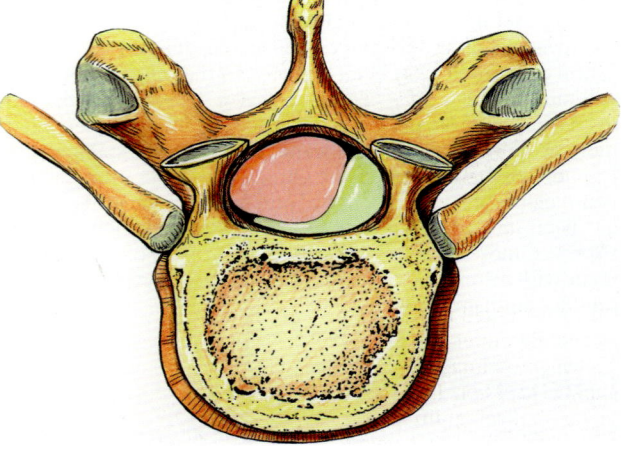

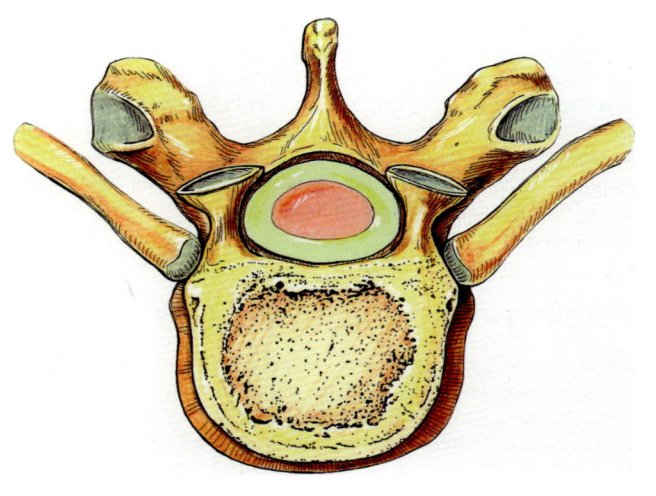

Fig. 51.2 Typical locations of epidural abscesses (dorsal not shown) **(a)** Ventral. **(b)** Ventrolateral. **(c)** Circumferential.

almost 60% of cases.[8] Still, the best yield is from the operative specimens.

Magnetic resonance imaging with intravenous administration of gadolinium is the investigation of choice in diagnosing SEA (**Fig. 51.3**). It shows the full extent of the abscess, bone, soft tissue, and spinal cord involvement. A spinal epidural abscess on T1-weighted images appears as an isointense extradural mass.

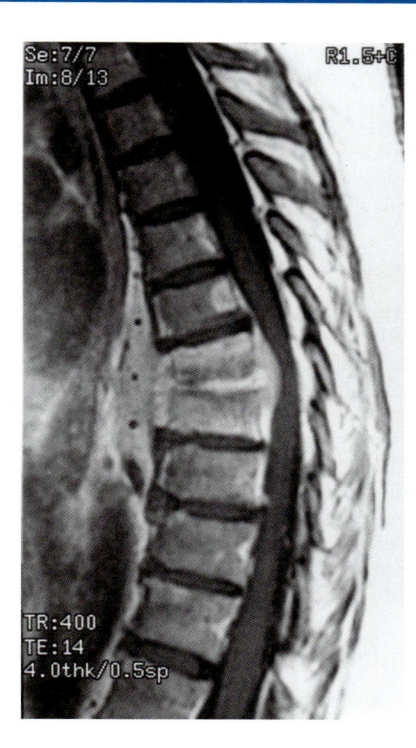

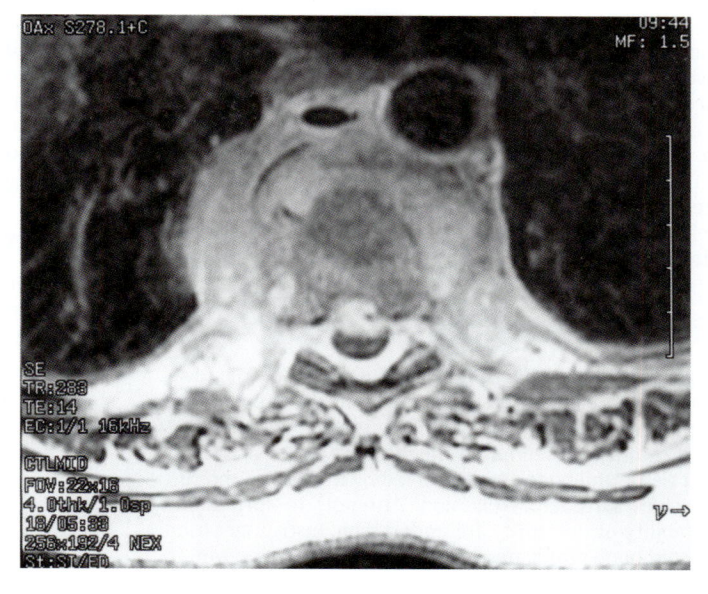

Fig. 51.3 Magnetic resonance image of spondylodiskitis. **(a)** Enhancement of the disk and symmetric destruction of the end plates are demonstrated. **(b)** Axial image demonstrating extent of ventral extension with thecal sac compression.

On T2-weighted images it appears to be completely silhouetted by the high intensities of the CSF. Gadolinium enhancement on T1-weighted images usually shows a homogeneous or capsule-enhancing lesion. If unable to obtain a MRI, computed tomography (CT) myelogram may be performed. Although sensitive in diagnosing SEA, CT myelogram is invasive and may not show the full extent of the lesion and status of the cord. Lastly, plain radiographs may show the bony destruction associated with spondylodiskitis.

Management

Traditionally, the gold standard treatment of thoracic SEA was emergency operative decompression for drainage and debridement. Randomized clinical trials remain difficult to perform due to the rarity of diagnosis and the ethical dilemma in randomizing patients.[8] Past retrospective studies support surgical decompression and intravenous antibiotics.[3,7,8,11,13,22] But a 2013 retrospective trial by Connor et al[2] found no statistical differences between operative and nonoperative cohorts with SEA. However, as with other retrospective studies finding similar outcomes, the operative group at presentation showed significantly greater focal weakness.[8] Generally surgery is indicated when patients with thoracic SEA have worsening neurologic deficits, spinal instability, or persistence of infection despite antibiotic treatment.[23]

As stated above, there is contradictory evidence in the literature regarding medical management alone. A 2014 study showed that > 41% of patients failed medical management alone and required surgical drainage.[4] Further, in these patients, who went on to surgical management, their ability to recover motor function was significantly impaired. The study found that diabetes, C-reactive protein > 115, white blood count > 12.5, and bacteremia predicted the failure of medical management. Moreover, MRSA infections have also been independent predictors of failed medical management (44% failure rate) as has age > 65 years.[23]

Generally, medical management alone is recommended only in patients with minimal or no neurologic deficits who can have frequent and vigilant neurologic assessment and rapid access to MRI. Some studies also recommend nonoperative therapy in patients who are poor surgical candidates because of multilevel extensive abscesses and profound neurologic deficits for more than 3 days or in those neurologically intact.[23] Many have noted that if complete paralysis persists longer than 24 to 36 hours, recovery is poor; paralysis may be a relative contraindication to surgical management.[8,10,13,22] Surgical management for these patients could be needed to treat epidural infection and control abscess but not to improve neurologic function.[8]

Medical management may be combined with CT-guided percutaneous needle drainage or biopsy for diagnosis or treatment. CT-guided percutaneous needle drainage has been utilized in selected patients with posterior SEA and no neurologic deficits. In a 2004 study, medical treatment alone or combined with CT-guided percutaneous needle drainage had comparable rates to the surgical arm regarding complete recovery and residual motor weakness outcome.[9] The results are limited, however, to only seven patients. Several other case reports have shown similar outcomes.[6,24,25] A risk of performing percutaneous needle drainage is transmitting the infectious material intradurally.[25] Still, in select patients this approach may be safe and effective. More studies are needed to support these findings.

Universally, antimicrobial therapy should be started immediately if the patient is septic and in all patients after the appropriate cultures are obtained. If biopsy or surgical results failure to grow microorganisms, tailoring antibiotics based on blood cultures results alone is generally feasible.[2] For this reason, withholding antibiotics prior to obtaining samples may not be supported by the evidence.[2] Empirical antibiotics should include first-line agents against staphylococci and gram-negative bacilli; synthetic penicillin and third- or fourth-generation cephalosporins are appropriate choices. Four to 6 weeks of intravenous antibiotics are usually recommended. A longer course is recommended in cases with poor clinical response, systemic infections, or infections caused by organisms such as tuberculosis, MRSA, or actinomycosis. Finally, patients who are immunosuppressed or of advanced age may need longer antibiotic courses.

It is recommended that affected patients remain immobile for at least 6 weeks during antibiotic therapy.[26] External bracing is helpful in relieving pain and promoting bony healing. It also minimizes spinal deformity. Orthoses are used for a minimum of 6 weeks. A thoracolumbosacral orthosis (TLSO) is used for mid- to lower thoracic spine stabilization.

Surgical Management

The surgical approach to the thoracic SEA depends on the location of the abscess. The basic principles of surgery remain the same despite the surgical approach. They include adequate exposure and complete resection of the infective material and involved soft tissue and bone. Healthy bleeding from bone and soft tissue indicates satisfactory excision. Attempts to correct the spinal instability or deformity are undertaken. Instrumentation and harvested bone grafts are used when indicated. The wound is primarily closed after thorough irrigation with antibiotic solution. An external drain usually helps evacuate some of the residual infection. Lastly, continuous irrigation using drainage tubes for inflow and outflow have been used at the time of surgery to improve debridement and removal of infected material.[27] These drains are inserted into the epidural space and provide continuous local administration of antibiotics directly to the wound as well. The closed irrigation suction system has several advantages, including avoiding secondary wound closure. It must be used carefully, though, due to the risk of congestion of irrigation flow and mismatching inflow and outflow.

Surgical Approaches

Surgical approaches to the thoracic spine can be categorized as ventral, dorsal, and dorsolateral. They can be used alone or in combination, and at the same time or in staged procedures. The surgical approach is determined by the pathological process, its location, evidence of spinal cord compression, instability, and the patient's medical condition. This chapter discusses dorsal and dorsolateral approaches. Dorsal surgical approaches to the thoracic spine include laminectomy (**Fig. 51.4a**) and the transpedicular approach. Dorsolateral approaches include costotransversectomy (**Fig. 51.4b**) and lateral extracavitary.

Laminectomy

Laminectomy (**Fig. 51.4a**), which is a midline surgical approach, is used exclusively for dorsally situated abscesses. It is not ideal for ventrally based abscesses due to inadequate exposure and the need for significant retraction of the dural sac. The stripping of paraspinal muscles exposes the laminae, which could be destroyed, and in turn exposing the thecal sac; thus, extra caution is called for. Removal of the lamina exposes the ligamentum flavum. Once the ligamentum flavum is removed, the dorsal thecal sac and overlying infected material are visualized. The purulent material and the granulation tissue are scraped off the dura, taking care not to perforate it. Healthy bleeding from the dural surface marks adequate debridement.

Transpedicular Approach

The transpedicular approach extends the laminectomy to provide more lateral and ventral exposure. As compared with the standard laminectomy, the extended exposure provides greater access with less retraction of the dural sac and spares the facet.

The exposure for the transpedicular approach is achieved through a standard midline incision (**Fig. 51.5**). The paraspinous muscles are reflected to expose the transverse process and facets at the affected levels. Laminectomy is optional but is often performed to increase exposure. The affected level foramen is exposed by drilling off the medial half of both the inferior facet of the superior vertebrae and superior facet and part of the pedicle of the inferior vertebrae. This exposes the lateral thecal sac and exiting nerve root. Bilateral transpedicular approaches can be performed for bilateral decompression.

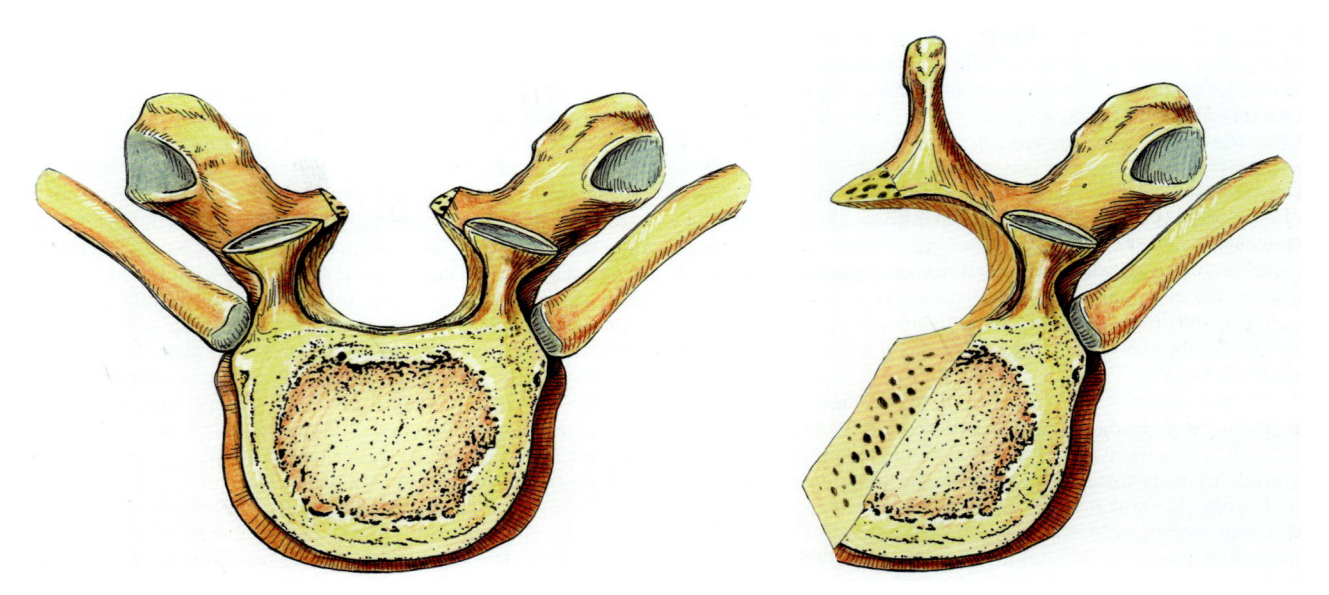

Fig. 51.4 Classic approaches to the thoracic spine showing degree of thecal sac exposure. **(a)** Laminectomy. **(b)** Transpedicular approach and costotransversectomy.

51 Thoracic Epidural Abscess and Vertebral Osteomyelitis 337

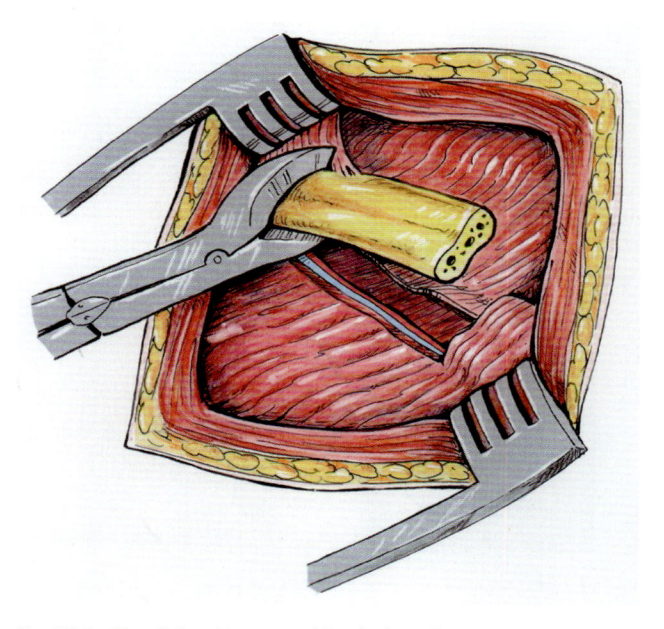

Fig. 51.6 The rib head is removed for the lateral extracavitary approach or the costotransversectomy. Care should be taken to protect the pleura during its removal. Note the neurovascular bundle, which can be used to find the neural foramen.

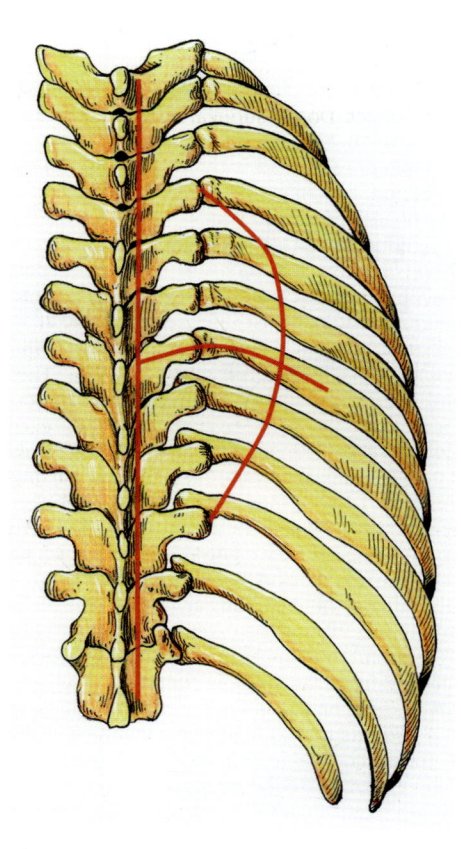

Fig. 51.5 Skin incisions for dorsal and dorsolateral exposures. The midline excision can be converted to a hockey-stick incision and will be used for midline pathology or in cases in which bilateral decompression is needed. The curved paramedian incision can be used for lateral extracavitary exposure or costotransversectomy. Neither incision precludes posterior instrumentation.

Costotransversectomy

Costotransversectomy and the other dorsolateral approaches are not facet sparing. This approach can be used at any thoracic level and provides further ventral exposure by removing the transverse process and proximal rib head (**Fig. 51.4b**).

Costotransversectomy is performed through a midline or curved paramedian incision (**Fig. 51.5**). The additional excision of a rib head (proximal 6 cm of the rib) and transverse process gives a wide lateral and ventrolateral access (**Fig. 51.6**). Partial vertebrectomy is technically more feasible and safer with this approach. Instrumented fusion is needed if there is instability due to extension of the infection into adjacent bone. Generally, two levels above and below the level of instability are fused with screws and rods.

Lateral Extracavitary Approach

The lateral extracavitary approach was first popularized in 1976 by Larson et al.[28] It provides even more lateral exposure than the costotransversectomy while at the same time enabling less retraction on the spinal cord. This approach does not violate the chest cavity and has less surgical morbidity than ventral approaches. Ventral vertebral body reconstruction and dorsal instrumentation can both be performed during this approach.

The patient is placed in the prone or three-quarter prone position and either a hockey-stick or paramedian incision can be used. A midline incision is also used when circumferential decompression is planned. The hockey-stick incision is a midline incision curved 45 degrees off midline for 6 to 8 cm in the lower portion. A paramedian incision centered over the lateral aspect of the paraspinal muscles can be used if midline exposure is not needed (**Fig. 51.5**).

A plane is then developed between the superficial and deep paraspinal muscles. A myocutaneous flap is thus lifted off to expose the lateral paraspinal muscle and rib cage. The paraspinal muscles are mobilized off medially to expose the underlying rib and transverse process. Now the midline structures dissection can be continuous with the lateral dissection beneath the paraspinal muscles. One or more ribs are then excised along with their ligamentous attachments without violating the pleura. The transverse process is also removed. The neurovascular bundle is isolated and used as a guide to the vertebral foramen. The pleura and the intercostal muscles are bluntly dissected away from the vertebral body (**Fig. 51.7**). The pedicle and the lateral vertebral body can then be drilled to expose the ventrolateral aspect of the thecal sac. The radicular artery is located in this region, and care is taken not to damage it. A thorough evacuation and debridement of infected material is done. Onlay and interbody bone grafts may be used for stabilization, which can further be reinforced by dorsal instrumentation. If pleural tears are encountered, they are repaired, and chest tubes may be necessary.

This approach can be performed on two sides to facilitate complete spondylectomy if necessary. Another option is to perform a lateral extracavitary approach on one side and either a transpedicular or costotransversectomy on the contralateral side.

Placement of bone graft and spinal instrumentation during the primary procedure is controversial. Placement of hardware in an infected surgical bed had been strongly discouraged in the past, and a small number of surgeons still defer to a staged procedure. In recent studies, however, no increases in complication rates were reported in instrumented fusion performed during

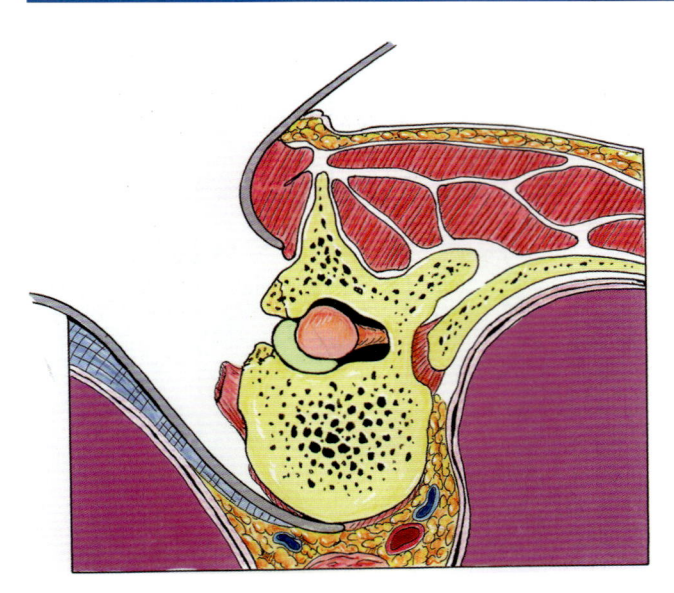

Fig. 51.7 Exposure afforded by the lateral extracavitary approach.

the primary procedure.[29–31] The autologous grafts are superior to nonvascularized grafts. Vascularized rib may be used due to its accessibility, high content of bone morphogenic protein, and vascularity.

Lastly, extensive SEA involving multiple and sometimes noncontiguous levels poses a unique challenge. Some authors have recommended less invasive methods for surgical SEA treatment.[25,32–34] In 2013, Safavi-Abbasi et al[25] described the successful management of noncontiguous thoracolumbar abscesses, using a tubular dilator system to perform hemilaminectomy, fenestration, and flavectomy for evacuation of SEA.

Outcome

The prognosis in patients with thoracic epidural abscesses has improved dramatically with the evolution of antibiotics and newer surgical approaches. The mortality rate, which was as high as 30 to 80% in older studies, has more recently been reported to be around 5%.[8] The neurologic outcome depends primarily on the degree of cord function and the duration of symptoms before drainage and decompression. Patients who are paralyzed for less than 36 hours are more likely to recovery neurologically after surgical decompression. The chance of recovery significantly decreases after this time frame. The degree of thecal sac compression and the age of the patient have a significant independent association in determining the outcome. In general, increased age and greater spinal canal compromise correlates with poor neurologic outcomes.

Vertebral Osteomyelitis

Although vertebral osteomyelitis is uncommon, it is associated with a high incidence of morbidity and mortality, especially in the elderly population. SEA is often associated with vertebral osteomyelitis as well as diskitis. When osteomyelitis occurs with discitis, it is referred to as spondylodiskitis. The vertebral osteomyelitis incidence is 1:250,000, and mortality rate ranges from 5 to 15% in the general population.[14,26] For reasons similar to those for SEA, its incidence is on the rise. The average age of presentation is in the fourth to fifth decades.[35] The lumbar spine is most commonly involved; thoracic involvement has been reported to occur in up to 35% of cases.[35,36]

Pathogenic microorganisms reach the vertebral osseous structures via direct inoculation or contiguous spread, or hematogenously through arteries or veins from similar sources to SEA.[35] Hematogenous spread is the most common mechanism of spine infection, but an estimated 37% of pyogenic spondylodiscitis have no identifiable source.[7,14,35,37] Osteomyelitis can then spread contiguously into the disk or into the epidural space. The most common organism is *S. aureus*. Streptococcus species, gram-negative bacilli, anaerobic bacteria, *Mycobacterium tuberculosis*, fungal infections, and parasitic infections are also observed.[35]

Similar to SEA, leukocytosis and acute phasic reactants may be elevated in acute infection but are nonspecific.[14] Contrastingly, blood cultures are more often negative, in up to 75% of patients.[14]

The gold standard for radiographic evaluation is MRI. T1-weighted imaging shows hypointensity within the marrow and disk space, and T2-weighted imaging shows hyperintensity within the marrow with active infection. The intervertebral disk is also hyperintense on T2-weighted imaging. With gadolinium intravenous infusion, the end plate–disc interface enhances, and usually this enhancement spreads away from the disk with progression of disease.[35] Once the extent of involvement is defined by MRI, CT is useful in defining related bony destruction.

Pain arising from the spine is the major presenting symptom.[14] Radicular leg or arm pain may be present as well in less than 10% of patients due to neurologic involvement.[14,35] Neurologic symptoms and progression of pain suggests formation of epidural abscess or vertebral collapse. Neurologic deficits are more common in patients with a delayed diagnosis.[30,35,36] Fever occurs in 20 to 50% of cases.[30,38]

It is generally recommended that tissue be obtained prior to antibiotic initiation. Biopsy is recommended for identification of the organism. Biopsy can be either closed or open, but a closed biopsy is recommended as the first-line treatment.[14] Closed needle biopsies, either percutaneous or fluoroscopy guided, have a 70% reported accuracy, whereas an open biopsy is diagnostic in over 80% of cases.[14,36] Once the pathogen is identified, it is generally recommended to treat with intravenous antibiotics for 2 to 6 weeks followed by a variable course of oral antibiotics.[14] Immobilization guidelines are similar to those described for SEA. Failure rates following conservative management range from 12 to 18%.[30] Five indications for surgery were described by Tay et al[14]: (1) obtaining a tissue diagnosis after failed closed needle biopsy or for tissue that is inaccessible by closed methods, (2) drainage of abscess causing sepsis or neurologic deficits, (3) treatment of neurologic deficits due to compression, (4) structural instability or deformity, or (5) failure of medical management.

For thoracic lesions, ventral decompression and fusion via a ventrolateral or dorsolateral approach is generally recommended.[14,29,40] Most commonly, the anterior elements are affected by infection, but some stability is still provided by the posterior elements. If a decompressive laminectomy is performed alone, the spine may be further destabilized.[40] The main goals of surgery are similar to those of SEA: debridement of infected tissue, decompression of neural elements, and spine stabilization when indicated.

Although 90% of patients may be managed nonsurgically, there remains a high rate of spinal dysfunction, up to 33%.[26,35] Many complications can occur from thoracic osteomyelitis, including mediastinitis; epidural or subdural abscess; meningitis; collapse of vertebral body and disk space, creating a pathological fracture and spinal instability; and neurologic impairment if infected bone or granulation tissue is retropulsed into the spinal canal.[14,30] Early diagnosis and antibiotic treatment remain the mainstays of management to decrease morbidity and mortality.

References

1. Morgagni G. De Sedibus, et causis morborum per anatomen indagatis: dissectiones, et animadversiones nunc primum et. Complectuntur propemodum innumeras, medicis, chirurgis, anatomicis profuturas. Venice, Italy: Ex Typographia Remondiniana, 1761
2. Connor DE Jr, Chittiboina P, Caldito G, Nanda A. Comparison of operative and nonoperative management of spinal epidural abscess: a retrospective review of clinical and laboratory predictors of neurological outcome. J Neurosurg Spine 2013;19:119–127
3. Baker AS, Ojemann RG, Swartz MN, Richardson EP Jr. Spinal epidural abscess. N Engl J Med 1975;293:463–468
4. Patel AR, Alton TB, Bransford RJ, Lee MJ, Bellabarba CB, Chapman JR. Spinal epidural abscesses: risk factors, medical versus surgical management, a retrospective review of 128 cases. Spine J 2014;14:326–330
5. Hadjipavlou AG, Mader JT, Necessary JT, Muffoletto AJ. Hematogenous pyogenic spinal infections and their surgical management. Spine 2000; 25:1668–1679
6. Reihsaus E, Waldbaur H, Seeling W. Spinal epidural abscess: a meta-analysis of 915 patients. Neurosurg Rev 2000;23:175–204, discussion 205
7. Curry WT Jr, Hoh BL, Amin-Hanjani S, Eskandar EN. Spinal epidural abscess: clinical presentation, management, and outcome. Surg Neurol 2005; 63:364–371, discussion 371
8. Darouiche RO. Spinal epidural abscess. N Engl J Med 2006;355:2012–2020
9. Siddiq F, Chowfin A, Tight R, Sahmoun AE, Smego RA Jr. Medical vs surgical management of spinal epidural abscess. Arch Intern Med 2004;164: 2409–2412
10. Savage K, Holtom PD, Zalavras CG. Spinal epidural abscess: early clinical outcome in patients treated medically. Clin Orthop Relat Res 2005;439: 56–60
11. Danner RL, Hartman BJ. Update on spinal epidural abscess: 35 cases and review of the literature. Rev Infect Dis 1987;9:265–274
12. Carey ME. Infection of the spine and the spinal cord. In: Youmans JR, ed. Neurological Surgery, 4th ed. Philadelphia: WB Saunders; 1996:3270–3304
13. Hlavin ML, Kaminski HJ, Ross JS, Ganz E. Spinal epidural abscess: a ten-year perspective. Neurosurgery 1990;27:177–184
14. Tay BK, Deckey J, Hu SS. Spinal infections. J Am Acad Orthop Surg 2002; 10:188–197
15. Carragee EJ. Pyogenic vertebral osteomyelitis. J Bone Joint Surg Am 1997; 79:874–880
16. Morikawa M, Sato S, Numaguchi Y, Mihara F, Rothman MI. Spinal epidural venous plexus: its MR enhancement patterns and their clinical significance. Radiat Med 1996;14:221–227
17. Heusner AP. Nontuberculous spinal epidural infections. N Engl J Med 1948;239:845–854
18. Feldenzer JA, McKeever PE, Schaberg DR, Campbell JA, Hoff JT. Experimental spinal epidural abscess: a pathophysiological model in the rabbit. Neurosurgery 1987;20:859–867
19. Eichbaum E, Martz P, McCormick B. Spinal infections. In: Benzel EC, Stillerman CB, eds. Thoracic Spine. St. Louis: Quality Medical Publishers; 1999:577–598
20. Tang HJ, Lin HJ, Liu YC, Li CM. Spinal epidural abscess—experience with 46 patients and evaluation of prognostic factors. J Infect 2002;45:76–81
21. Davis DP, Wold RM, Patel RJ, et al. The clinical presentation and impact of diagnostic delays on emergency department patients with spinal epidural abscess. J Emerg Med 2004;26:285–291
22. Rigamonti D, Liem L, Sampath P, et al. Spinal epidural abscess: contemporary trends in etiology, evaluation, and management. Surg Neurol 1999; 52:189–196, discussion 197
23. Kim SD, Melikian R, Ju KL, et al. Independent predictors of failure of nonoperative management of spinal epidural abscesses. Spine J 2014; 14:1673–1679
24. Lyu RK, Chen CJ, Tang LM, Chen ST. Spinal epidural abscess successfully treated with percutaneous, computed tomography-guided, needle aspiration and parenteral antibiotic therapy: case report and review of the literature. Neurosurgery 2002;51:509–512, discussion 512
25. Safavi-Abbasi S, Maurer AJ, Rabb CH. Minimally invasive treatment of multilevel spinal epidural abscess. J Neurosurg Spine 2013;18:32–35
26. Greenberg MS. Spine infections. In: Greenberg MS, ed. Handbook of Neurosurgery, 7th ed. New York: Thieme; 2010:376–383
27. Kim SH, Lee JK, Jang JW, Seo BR, Kim TS, Kim SH. Laminotomy with continuous irrigation in patients with pyogenic spondylitis in thoracic and lumbar spine. J Korean Neurosurg Soc 2011;50:332–340
28. Larson SJ, Holst RA, Hemmy DC, Sances A Jr. Lateral extracavitary approach to traumatic lesions of the thoracic and lumbar spine. J Neurosurg 1976;45:628–637
29. Si M, Yang ZP, Li ZF, Yang Q, Li JM. Anterior versus posterior fixation for the treatment of lumbar pyogenic vertebral osteomyelitis. Orthopedics 2013; 36:831–836
30. Shiban E, Janssen I, Wostrack M, et al. A retrospective study of 113 consecutive cases of surgically treated spondylodiscitis patients. A single-center experience. Acta Neurochir (Wien) 2014;156:1189–1196
31. Przybylski GJ, Sharan AD. Single-stage autogenous bone grafting and internal fixation in the surgical management of pyogenic discitis and vertebral osteomyelitis. J Neurosurg 2001;94(1, Suppl):1–7
32. Pradilla G, Nagahama Y, Spivak AM, Bydon A, Rigamonti D. Spinal epidural abscess: current diagnosis and management. Curr Infect Dis Rep 2010;12:484–491
33. Schultz KD Jr, Comey CH, Haid RW Jr. Technical note. Pyogenic spinal epidural abscess: a minimally invasive technique for multisegmental decompression. J Spinal Disord 2001;14:546–549
34. Tahir MZ, Hassan RU, Enam SA. Case report. Management of an extensive spinal epidural abscess from C-1 to the sacrum. J Neurosurg Spine 2010; 13:780–783
35. Skaf GS, Domloj NT, Fehlings MG, et al. Pyogenic spondylodiscitis: an overview. J Infect Public Health 2010;3:5–16
36. Sapico FL, Montgomerie JZ. Pyogenic vertebral osteomyelitis: report of nine cases and review of the literature. Rev Infect Dis 1979;1:754–776
37. Lestini WF, Bell GR. Spinal infections: patient evaluation. Semin Spine Surg 1990;2:244–256
38. Mylona E, Samarkos M, Kakalou E, Fanourgiakis P, Skoutelis A. Pyogenic vertebral osteomyelitis: a systematic review of clinical characteristics. Semin Arthritis Rheum 2009;39:10–17
39. Kornblum MB, Wesolowski DP, Fischgrund JS, Herkowitz HN. Computed tomography-guided biopsy of the spine. A review of 103 patients. Spine 1998;23:81–85
40. Rath SA, Neff U, Schneider O, Richter HP. Neurosurgical management of thoracic and lumbar vertebral osteomyelitis and discitis in adults: a review of 43 consecutive surgically treated patients. Neurosurgery 1996; 38:926–933

52 Vascular Malformations of the Spine

Bruno C. Flores, Daniel R. Klinger, Jonathan A. White, and H. Hunt Batjer

Vascular lesions that affect the spine are considerably less common than their intracranial counterparts, accounting for 5 to 9% of all vascular malformations of the central nervous system (CNS),[1] or 3 to 4% of all intradural spinal cord mass lesions.[2] Nonetheless, despite their pathological similarities with intracranial lesions, their clinical impact often has been comparatively worse. Spinal vascular malformations (SVMs) are a very heterogeneous group of vascular abnormalities that can cause acute, subacute, or chronic spinal cord dysfunction. The majority of the affected patients still present after a protracted course with severe neurologic dysfunction. Early reports from Aminoff and Logue,[3] published in 1974, showed that up to 48% of patients with untreated arteriovenous malformations (AVMs) of the spinal cord were confined to bed or wheelchair within 3 years of symptom onset, and complications of chronic paraplegia were directly responsible for a mortality rate of 15%. Early, correct recognition of the pathology and prompt intervention are mandatory to halt the progression of the disease, minimize permanent spinal cord injury, and improve long-term neurologic outcome.

This chapter describes the various types of vascular malformations of the spine, their pathophysiology, clinical presentation, and treatment strategies. The historical background, vascular anatomy, and its correlations to radiographic findings on pre- and postoperative evaluations of SVMs are briefly discussed. For the purposes of this chapter, the vascular malformations of the spine are categorized as arteriovenous fistulas (AVFs), arteriovenous malformations (AVMs), and cavernous malformations (CMs). The isolated occurrence of spinal cord aneurysms is extremely rare, and the majority of the lesions that come to the neurosurgeon's attention are concomitant with a spinal AVM.

History

The first clinical observation of an SVM was published in Germany in 1890. Berenbruch operated on a patient with a spinal abnormality, subsequently recognized as a vascular malformation at autopsy.[4] In 1910, Fedor Krause was the first to recognize a spinal lesion observed at laminectomy as a vascular abnormality.[4] In 1912, Charles Elsberg pioneered the first successful surgical intervention for a spinal cord vascular lesion, presumably a perimedullary AVF.[4,5] In his operative report, he described "a large mass of tortuous blood vessels.... Only part of the mass could be excised. No vessels appeared to come out of the cord itself, but there were a number of branches from the anterior surface of the cord."[6] Recovery from the operation was uneventful but without clinical improvement. In 1915, Cobb reported several cases of SVMs and outlined their variable clinical features. He was the first to report the combination of an SVM and vascular anomalies of the overlying skin, now known as Cobb syndrome.[5] The classic subacute necrotic myelopathy was described by Foix and Alajouanine in 1926, but the pathophysiology behind this eponymous syndrome was not further elaborated until the landmark studies of Wyburn-Mason[7] emphasized the role of thrombosis within the abnormal vessels of an SVM as a primary cause.[5]

The development of spinal angiography in the 1960s revolutionized the understanding of SVMs. Spinal aortography was introduced by Rene Djindjian and associates in France at the Lariboisière Hospital in 1962. Contemporary to that group, Doppman and DiChiro demonstrated the importance of subtraction angiography and selective catheterization techniques on their early studies on the topic at the National Institutes of Health (NIH) in the United States.[5]

Before the advent of modern anesthesia and microsurgical techniques, the few case reports on the surgical treatment of SVMs had overall discouraging results. Several of the performed operations focused on elevation and coagulation of the abnormal blood vessels from the dorsal aspect of the spinal cord, mainly due to the lack of an adequate comprehension of the pathophysiology of the disease. The so-called modern era in the treatment of SVMs began in 1969 with Krayenbühl and Yaşargil and the publication of their microsurgical technique, based heavily on the use of the operating microscope and bipolar cautery.[8,9] In 1977, Kendall and Logue[10] demonstrated that lesions on the surface of the spinal cord, formerly thought to be venous angiomas, were actually arterialized veins dilated by communication through a dural AVF.[4] Since then, a significant part of the current understanding of the different SVMs is a result of the combined effort from what Black[4] described as the American/English/French (ABF) connection. These contributions led to the development of the widely used classification of spinal AVMs, initially stratified into three types, I to III, but with a fourth type added later by Heros et al.[11] Over the last decade, other classifications have been introduced by different groups[12–14]; some of those are discussed later in this chapter.

Epidemiology

Spinal vascular malformations are rare lesions. Dural AVFs are more common than spinal cord AVMs, the latter of which have an incidence of ~ 10% that of brain AVMs.[15] Dural AVF is the most common of the vascular malformations; it accounts for 50 to 85% of all lesions.[16–19] Men are affected five times more often than women, and the mean age at the time of diagnosis is 50 to 60 years.[20,21] Patients younger than 30 years of age constitute less than 1% of patients with a DAVF. Most lesions are centered at the thoracolumbar spine, with up to 90% of those located between T4 and L3, according to Oldfield.[18,19] True intradural, perimedullary AVFs are significantly rarer, have no sex predilection, and tend to occur at the thoracolumbar region.[18,22] Most patients present at a relatively young age, typically within the second or third decades.[18,19]

The natural history of spinal AVMs is poorly understood. Most of the available literature consists of surgeon's personal experience and anecdotal case series. Spinal cord AVMs usually present in the third decade of life, but they can be diagnosed in the pediatric population.[12,15,18,19,23,24] In a recent meta-analysis analyzing spinal glomus AVMs, Gross and Du[24] reported no sex predilection. The majority of AVMs were thoracic (51%) and cervical (29%), and 29% had an associated aneurysm.

Previous surgical and autopsy studies have suggested that spinal cord CMs account for 5 to 12% of all spinal vascular abnormalities, or 3 to 5% of all CMs in the CNS.[25,26] There appears to be a slight female predominance. The mean age of presentation for symptomatic lesions is in the fifth decade. They appear to be more prevalent on the thoracic and cervical regions.[25]

Anatomy and Pathophysiology

A thorough understanding of the spine and spinal cord vascular anatomy is of paramount significance for the neurosurgeon treating SVMs. It facilitates adequate preoperative imaging interpretation, evaluation of the intrinsic pathophysiology, and the selection of the correct surgical technique.

The fetal spinal vascular anatomy develops in four stages: primitive segmental, initial, transitional, and terminal. The most likely stage of embryological development at which an AVM can arise is the second stage (3 to 6 weeks). Maldevelopment in this stage leads to persistence of thin-walled tortuous vessels that exhibit primitive capillary interconnections, arteriovenous shunts, and poorly developed elastic and medial layers that closely resemble intracranial angiomas.[27] The concept that intradural vascular malformations are congenital and are the result of fetal vascular maldevelopment is supported by the fact that 20% of patients with intradural AVMs have other associated congenital vascular anomalies.[27]

The anterior two thirds of the spinal cord are supplied by a single anterior spinal artery (ASA), running within the anterior median fissure. The ASA originates from the spinal branches of the vertebral arteries and is additionally supplied at multiple levels by spinal radicular branches of the segmental arteries. The majority of the radicular arteries regress during development, with an average number of six still present in adult life in an unpredictable pattern.[16] The artery of the cervical enlargement is a larger feeder often encountered between C4 and C8.[28] In the thoracolumbar region, two or three radicular arteries arise from the dorsal branches of either an intercostal or a lumbar artery. They follow the ventral nerve root through the intervertebral foramen until anastomosing with the ASA. After a short initial ascending course, the radicular artery follows a characteristic hairpin configuration at its junction with the ASA, with a smaller cephalad and a larger caudad branches arising from its apex. This classic configuration is very useful for angiographic identification of the anterior spinal artery. The most prominent is the artery of the lumbar enlargement or artery of Adamkiewicz (**Fig. 52.1**). It arises most commonly between T9 and T12, typically on the left side, seldom from the lumbar region or higher between T6 and T8. In the sacral region, the radicular branches may arise from the lateral sacral or iliolumbar arteries, which are branches of the internal iliac artery. In the conus, the anterior spinal artery terminates by anastomosing with the posterior spinal arteries, forming a basket-like configuration (rami cruciantes).[28]

The posterior third of the spinal cord is supplied by an extensive plexus with two dominant longitudinal systems, the posterior spinal arteries (PSAs), originating from the vertebral artery or the posterior inferior cerebellar artery. Surrounding the surface of the cord and connecting the anterior and posterior vessels is an extensive plexus (pial plexus). Numerous posterior radicular feeders arise from the extraspinal arteries and anastomose with the posterior inferior cerebellar arteries (PICAs), with a total of 11 to 16 posterior radicular arteries persisting through adulthood. As noted with the anterior spinal circulation, here also the posterior radicular arteries follow a classic ascending trajectory followed by a hairpin configuration and bifurcation into an ascending and descending branches, as they join the PSAs.[16]

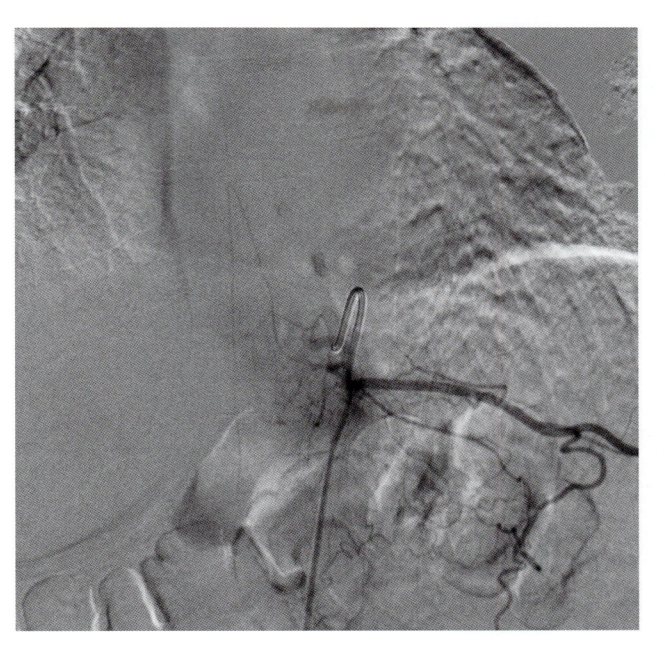

Fig. 52.1 Selective catheter spinal angiography, anteroposterior (AP) projection. Note the classic hairpin configuration of the artery of Adamkiewicz as it originates from the left radicular artery and anastomoses to the descending anterior spinal artery.

There is no definite parallel between the venous and arterial anatomy of the spinal cord. In fact, the variability of the venous system is even more pronounced. The intrinsic venous system consists of radial veins draining in a centrifugal manner toward the venous plexus of the pia mater. This complex anastomotic venous network drains toward the anterior and posterior median spinal veins. Both the anterior and posterior venous systems drain via medullary and radicular veins into the epidural venous plexus. The radicular veins, similar to their arterial counterparts, pierce the dura to follow the nerve roots. Although all of the mentioned veins are valveless, there is an anatomic narrowing at the dural penetration that some regard as a functional antireflux mechanism.[16] The epidural venous plexus, in turn, drains into the paravertebral veins, such as the vertebral vein in the neck, the azygous and hemiazygous veins in the thorax, the ascending lumbar vein, and the internal iliac vein.[28]

Kendall and Logue[10] were the first to understand the pivotal link between the intricate vascular anatomy and the pathophysiology of spinal cord vascular malformations. They correctly recognized a spinal cord AVF arteriovenous shunt site as dural, related to the nerve root sleeve. The arterialization of the coronal venous plexus caused by the fistulous connection resulted in venous hypertension and spinal cord ischemia and myelopathy. Since then, venous hypertension has been considered the major factor causing spinal cord ischemia in several types of SVMs. Direct intraoperative measurements of mean venous pressure as high as 74% of the systemic arterial pressure in patients with spinal dural AVFs helped consolidate this hypothesis.[29] Given that the spinal cord veins are valveless, the effects of gravity would also exacerbate the venous pressure gradients in the lower parts of the cord.[28]

Three other physiological mechanisms have been proposed to explain the neurologic deterioration in patients with SVMs: hemorrhage, vascular steal, and mass effect. Hemorrhage is most commonly seen with AVMs and CMs and can be subarachnoid, intraparenchymal, or both. Except for spinal dural AVFs in the cervical region, the risk of hemorrhage appears to be low in small or thoracolumbar AVFs. Vascular steal was first recognized in the late 1960s and 1970s.[5] It was then associated with high-flow, low-pressure AVMs and with large perimedullary AVFs fed by the ASA.[5,14,28] Vascular steal is a generally accepted mechanism, although it is contested by some authors.[30] Mass effect can occur with large AVFs with massively dilated venous structures and feeding vessels aneurysms. This phenomenon would explain, for example, some of the symptoms seen in extradural AVFs and conus medullaris AVMs.

Imaging

Historical Background

The initial descriptions of spinal vascular lesions predate the use of neuroimaging of the spine. Thus, these descriptions were largely derived from clinical investigation and postmortem pathological studies. Further autopsy studies cast light on the pathophysiology of subacute necrotizing myelopathy when Foix and Alajouanine noted regions of spinal cord necrosis associated with vascular abnormalities. However, it was not until the advent of lipoidal myelography in the 1920s that clinicians were able to identify spinal vascular lesions in the living patient.[5] Myelography then proved to be a viable diagnostic tool for identifying spinal vascular lesions but was limited by its inability to directly visualize the vascular anatomy itself. By the 1950s and 1960s, cerebral angiography became the gold standard for diagnosing and analyzing spinal vascular lesions, paving the way for the development of more anatomic classification schemes and targeted therapies. Currently, advances in computed tomography (CT) and magnetic resonance imaging (MRI) have proven useful adjunctive tools that may ultimately rival spinal angiography for the diagnosis and characterization of these lesions.

Magnetic Resonance Imaging

Magnetic resonance imaging has significant applications in the imaging of spinal vascular disease. Typically, MRI is the first imaging study ordered in the workup of these patients, who often present with some form of acute or subacute neurologic deterioration. The classic clinical presentation of progressive thoracic myelopathy associated with venous congestion, seen on cases of spinal dural AVFs, correlates with MRI findings of hyperintense T2 cord signal and cord edema over multiple spinal levels (**Fig. 52.2**). The swollen cord may demonstrate enhancement on postgadolinium sequences. In advanced disease, cord atrophy may be present. On T2-weighted sequences, dilated serpiginous perimedullary vessels can be seen as flow voids lining the dorsal or ventral surface of the cord usually over several spinal levels.[16] The T2 hyperintensity involves the conus in up to 90% of cases, and lack of T2 cord signal in the presence of an AVF is extremely rare. When there is a strong clinical suspicion of a symptomatic dural AVF, the sensitivity of MRI may be enhanced with gadolinium or myelographic sequences. Gadolinium administration may help identify enhancement within the cord itself or increase the visibility of the involved dilated perimedullary veins.

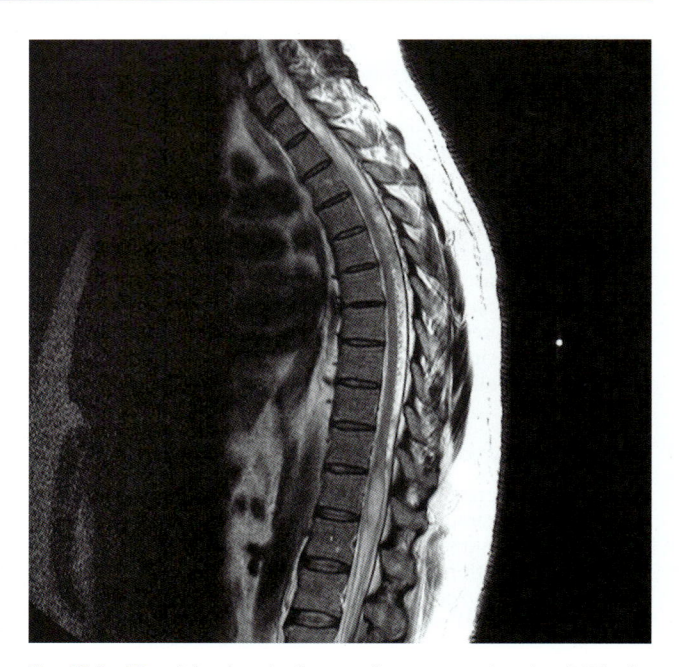

Fig. 52.2 T2-weighted sagittal magnetic resonance imaging (MRI) of a male patient diagnosed with an intradural dorsal arteriovenous fistula. Note the T2-hyperintense signal involving the enlarged thoracolumbar spinal cord, as well as the innumerous T2-hypointense flow void signals on the posterior thoracic subarachnoid space.

True spinal AVMs share some imaging features on MRI with intracranial AVMs. Typically, they form a mass of dilated peri- and intramedullary vessels visualized as flow voids on T2-weighted sequences (**Fig. 52.3**). As with dural AVFs, venous congestion may be present with hyperintense T2 cord signal and swelling. In AVMs with fistulous components, serpiginous flow voids extending several levels are common. AVMs that hemorrhage may demonstrate varying cord signal intensities consistent with acute or subacute blood products or subarachnoid hemorrhage.

Cavernomas are well-circumscribed intramedullary lesions that have a hypointense rim and hyperintense center on T2-weighted MRI sequences, the classic "popcorn" appearance well described intracranially (**Fig. 52.4**). Blood products in various stages of evolution may demonstrate varying signal intensities or blood-fluid levels. These lesions are angiographically negative and are less likely to be associated with significant vessel flow voids.

Magnetic Resonance Angiography

Recently advances in magnetic resonance angiography (MRA) imaging have improved the ability to confirm the diagnosis of spinal AVF or AVM and in many instances localize the lesion to a specific segment or spinal level. Although MRI alone may be helpful in making the diagnosis of an SVM, the findings of T2 cord hyperintensity, enhancement, or flow voids are not predictive of the level of the lesion; in the past, localization could only be confirmed through spinal angiography. Traditionally, the resolution of MRA to distinguish individual spinal arteries and veins and visualize fistulous connections was hampered by the trade-off between obtaining a large field of view to encompass the thoracolumbar spine while maintaining high spatial resolution. New protocols utilizing fast contrast-enhanced MRA enable more precise imaging of dilated perimedullary and radicular veins in dural AVFs or perimedullary fistulous AVMs from which

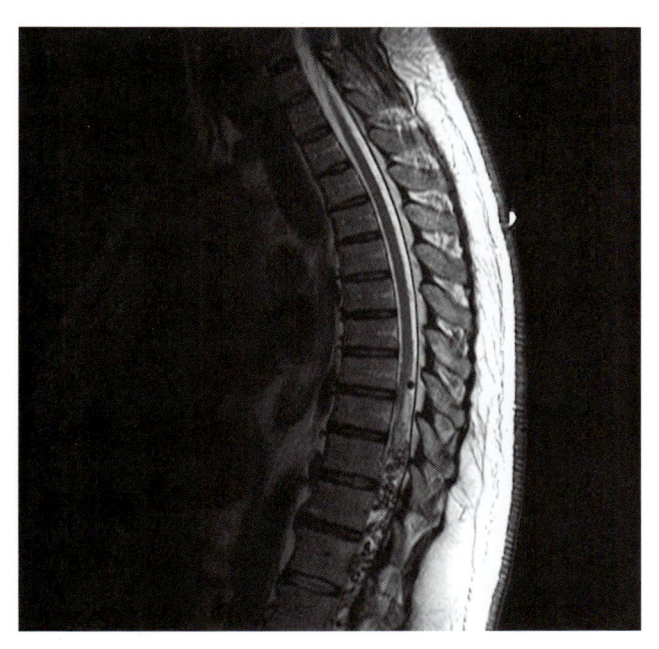

Fig. 52.3 T2-weighted sagittal MRI of a patient diagnosed with a large, diffuse thoracolumbar intradural intramedullary arteriovenous malformation (AVM). Note the innumerable flow void signals obscuring the anatomic margins of the normal thoracic spinal cord and conus medullaris. There is moderate cord compression caused by a large draining vein just cranial to the AVM nidus.

resonance angiography (CE-MRA) may at minimum enable a focused angiogram of the involved segments, potentially cutting down on procedure time, contrast load, time of fluoroscopic radiation exposure, and procedural complications.

Computed Tomography Angiography

Computed tomography angiography (CTA) and CT myelography remain options in the evaluation of spinal vascular disease. Many patients are unsuitable for MRI because they have incompatible implanted hardware such as cardiac pacemakers or defibrillators. A small series from China comparing CT spinal angiography to CE-MRA and spinal angiography found a 75% rate of detection of SVMs, which was comparable to that for CE-MRA.[32] CTA may suffer from impaired contrast resolution in the obese patient, and there is a potentially negative impact of the iodinated contrast use and ionizing radiation exposure.

Spinal Angiography

Spinal angiography remains the gold standard for diagnosis and characterization of spinal vascular lesions, particularly spinal dural AVFs and AVMs. Spinal angiography continues to be superior to MRI and CT in completely characterizing spinal vascular lesions because it enables a precise determination of the involved vessels and is a dynamic study that in many circumstances can pinpoint the exact fistulous component of a malformation and thus guide directed therapy. Many centers have developed specific protocols in the workup of spinal dural AVFs that include identifying the level of the artery of Adamkiewicz and any venous stasis suggestive of a fistulous connection followed by selective thoracic and lumbar intercostal injections. If these are unrevealing, further workup involves injecting the lateral sacral arteries, aorta and subsequently the arterial supply to the cervical cord and posterior fossa.[33] The subsequent addition of three-dimensional (3D) rotational spinal angiography has further

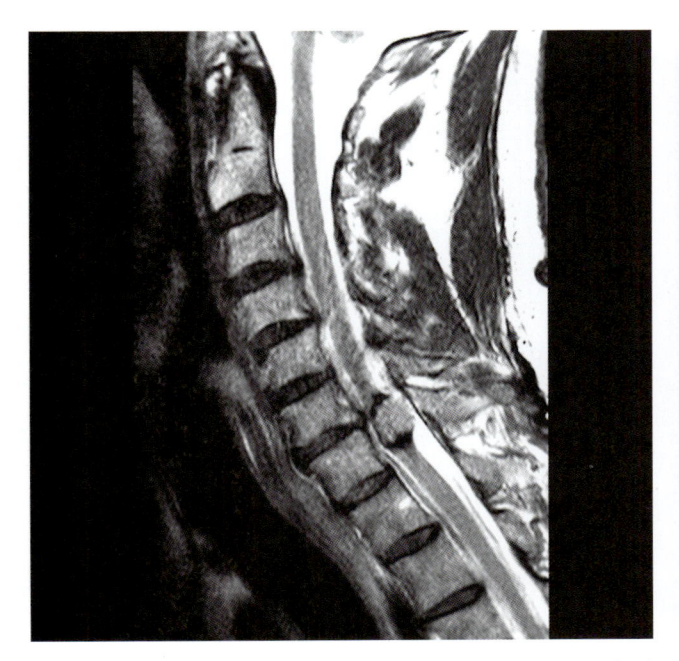

one could successfully infer the point (spinal level) of fistulous connection in up to 81% of cases.[31] The majority of these patients often require further spinal angiography for better characterization of the lesion, to initiate endovascular treatment or for microsurgical planning. Nevertheless, contrast-enhanced (CE) magnetic

Fig. 52.4 T2-weighted sagittal **(a)** and gadolinium-enhanced T1-weighted sagittal **(b)** MRI of a male patient with a cervical spinal cavernous malformation. Note the heterogeneous aspect with a T2-hypointense rim caused by hemosiderin deposits from previous hemorrhages. No significant contrast enhancement is seen.

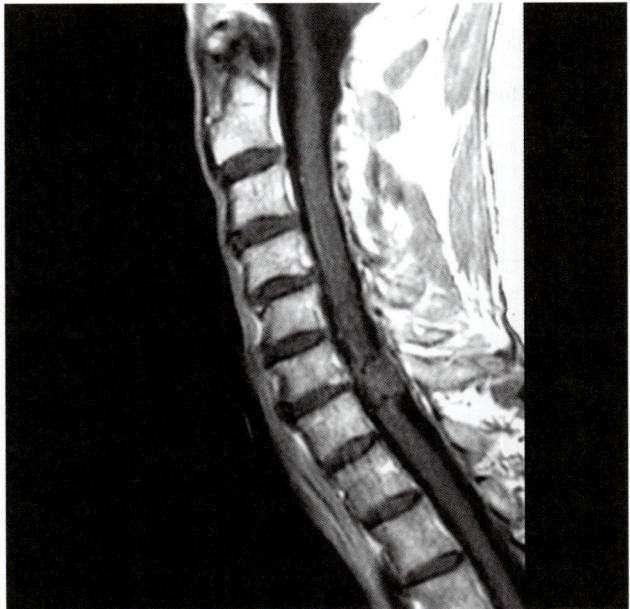

improved the imaging quality of spinal vascular lesions.[34] Despite these advances, conventional spinal angiography can require extended procedure times and multiple studies to define the offending pathology (particularly with dural AVFs). Conventional spinal angiography may require high iodinated-contrast loads and radiation doses to the patient and may continue to carry a small risk of procedural complication, including spinal cord ischemia and paraparesis. Spinal angiography also may be a means to treat spinal vascular lesions through direct embolization, as is discussed below.

Classification

The advent and development of modern spinal angiography and MRI revolutionized the understanding of the anatomy, pathophysiology, and treatment of SVMs. The continuous advancements in our knowledge of those lesions, however, also translated into a rapid proliferation of several different classification systems.[4,5,11–14] The heterogeneity of those classifications is multifactorial, certainly reflecting the contemporary understanding of SVMs at the time of publication, but also the lack of consensus on the utility of those different classification schemes.

The modern classification of the SVMs was first proposed by DiChiro, Doppman, and Ommaya in 1969.[4] They divided the SVMs into three types based on their landmark studies on spinal angiography. In 1986, Heros et al[11] reported a patient with an intradural perimedullary AVF and proposed that this SVM be classified as a distinct fourth type. The initial descriptions of a perimedullary AVF, not contemplated by the proposed classification above, are attributed to Djindjian et al in 1977.[5] The resultant classification, also known as the American/British/French (ABF) connection classification,[4] has had widespread acceptance and use in the neurosurgical literature since then (**Table 52.1**).

In 2002, Spetzler et al[13] proposed a modified classification system for SVMs based on specific anatomic and pathophysiological factors. This comprehensive classification incorporated into the ABF classification separate categories for spinal cord aneurysms and the so-called neoplastic vascular lesions (hemangioblastomas and CMs). The authors also described a newly proposed category of conus medullaris AVMs, characterized by their exclusive involvement of the conus medullaris and filum terminale, multiple feeding arteries, multiple niduses, and complex venous drainage (**Fig. 52.5**). They have multiple direct arteriovenous shunts that derive from the anterior and posterior spinal arteries and have glomus-type niduses that are usually extramedullary and pial based, but they may also have an intramedullary component (**Table 52.2**).

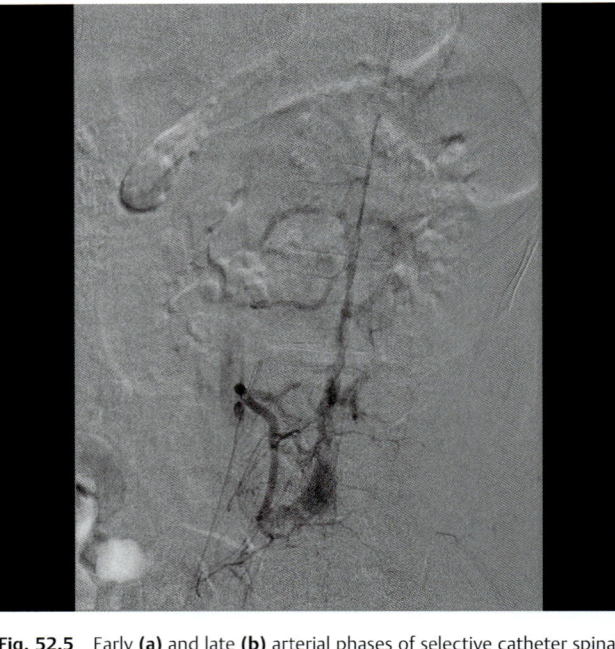

Fig. 52.5 Early (**a**) and late (**b**) arterial phases of selective catheter spinal angiography demonstrating a conus medullaris AVM. Note the presence of multiple feeding arteries, multiple diffuse niduses, and complex venous drainage.

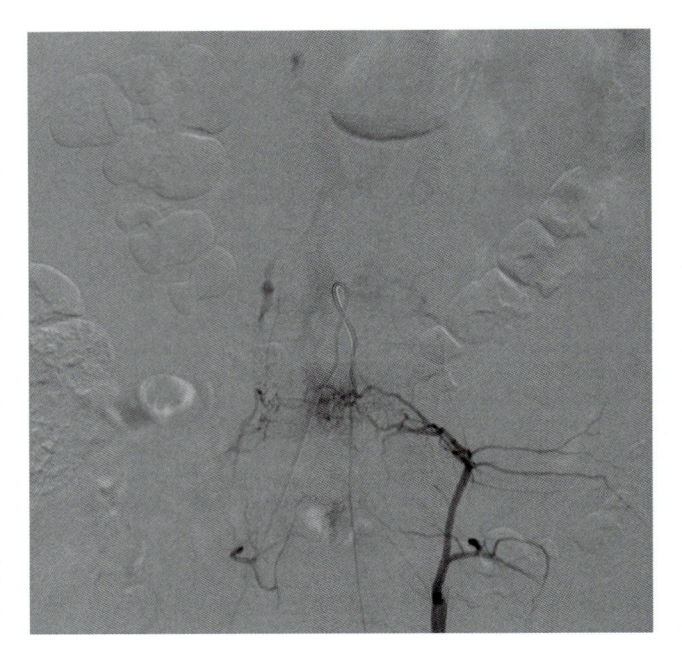

Table 52.1 American/English/French (ABF) Classification of Spinal Vascular Malformations

Type	Description
I	Spinal dural AVF (previous angioma racemosum venosum): located at the dural sleeve of a spinal root, associated with a single-coiled vessel on the dorsal pial surface of the spinal cord
II	Glomus AVM (previous angioma racemosum arteriovenosum): characterized by a true intramedullary nidus and with the arteriovenous shunting occurring deep into the pia
III	Metameric or juvenile AVM (previous Cobb syndrome): involvement of one or more metameres (and consequently of portions of the neural tissue, dura, bone, muscle and skin)
IV	Direct or perimedullary AVF: direct AVF, usually supplied by the anterior spinal artery, and drainage through the pial venous network, resulting in aneurysmal dilation of the draining veins

Abbreviations: AVF, arteriovenous fistula; AVM, arteriovenous malformation.

Table 52.2 Spetzler Classification of Spinal Vascular Malformations

Type	Examples
Neoplastic vascular lesions	Hemangioblastoma
	Cavernous malformation
Spinal cord aneurysms	
Arteriovenous fistulas	Extradural
	Intradural
	Ventral (type IV AVM)
Arteriovenous malformations	Extradural-intradural (type III AVM)
	Intradural
	Intramedullary (type II AVM)
	Conus medullaris

Abbreviations: AVM, arteriovenous malformation.

Clinical Presentation

The clinical presentation of vascular malformations of the spine is dependent on the lesion pathophysiology and classification. Two different categories can be roughly delineated: those with an acute presentation (associated with hematomyelia or subarachnoid hemorrhage) and those with a more protracted course with progressive neurologic deterioration (secondary to venous hypertension, cord ischemia, or mass effect). Acute presentation is usually seen in patients with spinal cord aneurysms, CMs, and intradural/intramedullary AVMs. Classic examples of the lesions with a protracted course include an AVF (extradural or intradural), conus medullaris, and juvenile AVM. Independent of the mode of presentation, untreated lesions tend to have a very poor neurologic outcome. By the time of diagnosis, the majority of patients already have a certain degree of motor and sensory deficits.[19] In their classic 1974 study on SVMs (mainly dural AVFs), Aminoff and Logue[3] defined the course of the disease as one of progressive neurologic decline and functional disability. One fifth of the 60 patients required crutches or were nonambulatory by 6 months after the onset of symptoms other than pain. Half of all patients were confined to a wheelchair or bed within 3 years of the onset of gait impairment, and 91% had restricted activity within 3 years of the onset of symptoms.[3,18]

Common to patients with AVMs and AVFs are symptoms of myelopathy, such as lower extremity weakness, loss of pain and temperature sensation, and bladder and bowel incontinence. Patients with spinal dural AVF often suffer from neurogenic claudication, with symptoms exacerbated by physical activities such as walking and standing, and relieved by sitting. Exercise or posture-induced symptoms are uncommon with AVMs. Subarachnoid hemorrhage is the presenting event in about one third of patients with AVMs of the spinal cord, but it is exceptionally rare with AVFs.[17] The presence of an associated nidal or feeding artery aneurysm has been reported in 16 to 48% of AVMs, and is often cited as a risk factor for hemorrhage.[19,24,35,36] Occasionally, a spinal bruit is associated with high-flow, juvenile AVMs, but this association has not been reported with AVFs. In a recent institutional review of 110 treated AVFs and AVMs, the most common presentation was paresis/paralysis (75.5%), paresthesias (60%), pain (51.8%), and bowel/bladder dysfunction (41.8%).[2] The distribution of frequencies of signs and symptoms was fairly similar between the two separate groups, except for a higher incidence of subarachnoid hemorrhage with AVMs (37.9%).

Despite the similarities, spinal dural AVFs are distinguished from intradural SVMs by several clinical features. They have a strong male predilection (> 80%) and present later in life (80% after the age of 40).[18,19] The majority of those lesions are located on the thoracolumbar region, which helps explain why upper extremity involvement is so unlikely.

In summary, the typical patient with a spinal dural AVF is an older (> 40 years) man with gradual onset of progressive lower extremities symptoms exacerbated by walking or standing. Differential diagnosis frequently involves spinal stenosis, demyelinating disease, spinal cord tumors, and, more rarely, conditions such as Guillain-Barré syndrome, amyotrophic lateral sclerosis, and peripheral vascular disease.[37] In contrast, the typical patient with a spinal AVM is a younger (< 30 years) man (if the pediatric population is included) with a greater risk of abrupt onset due to hematomyelia or subarachnoid hemorrhage, and more frequently with upper extremity symptoms, depending on the lesion location.[17] A distinct sensory level is present in most patients, and generally reflects the location of the vascular nidus along the spinal axis.[19]

Foix-Alajouanine syndrome is a classic but frequently misunderstood syndrome associated with spinal cord vascular malformations. Traditionally described as an acute or subacute myelopathy, it is attributed to a spinal cord venous thrombosis related to an AVM, resulting in venous infarction and necrosis. Spinal dural AVFs had not yet been described at the time of the original report in 1926.[38] In retrospect, it has been speculated that the patients in the original report by Foix and Alajouanine had type I AVFs. Pathological analysis of these initial cases did not show evidence of thrombosis, and symptoms may have been attributable to venous hypertension.[37,38]

Unlike other spinal arteriovenous lesions, conus medullaris AVMs frequently produce concomitant radiculopathy and myelopathy, and the radicular deficits are often prominent.[13] Wilson et al[39] described myeloradiculopathy as the initial presentation for 63% of patients. More than half of the study population had bladder or bowel dysfunction and 75% of the patients were ambulatory at presentation. Overall, 31% of their patients had a history of spinal hemorrhage.

Distinct clinical features are seen on SVMs in the pediatric population. In those patients, AVMs have been associated with inherited disorders such as hereditary hemorrhagic telangiectasia, familial cerebral cavernous hemangiomas, pulmonary AVMs, Klippel-Trenaunay-Weber syndrome, and Rendu-Osler-Weber syndrome.[35,40] In one of the largest studies on SVMs in a pediatric population, most of the patients presented with acute onset of symptoms.[35] Spinal cord AVMs (44.4%), perimedullary AVFs (23.6%), and Cobb syndrome (13.9%) were the most frequently diagnosed subtypes. No cases of spinal dural AVFs were found in that study. A bimodal incidence distribution was seen, with the first peak from birth to 2 years old, and the second peak and higher rate seen at the age of 12.[35] Other authors reported a spontaneous recovery rate without early treatment as high as 72% in pediatric patients.[30] Thus, the prognosis after hemorrhage may be better than initially thought, and early aggressive treatment would not be warranted.

Spinal cord CMs tend to closely resemble the course of spinal cord AVMs. Ogilvy et al[41] previously reported four types of clinical presentation in patients with CMs: (1) discrete episodes of neurologic decline with varying degrees of recovery between episodes; (2) slow progressive myelopathy; (3) rapid decline after acute onset of symptoms; and (4) gradual decline after acute onset of symptoms. As with their intracranial equivalents, repeated hemorrhage over several years with intervening periods of quiescence seems to be the rule. Acute neurologic deterioration can be caused by hemorrhage into eloquent spinal cord tissue. Although trauma, pregnancy, and strenuous activity have all been associated with acute deterioration from CMs, a causal link has not been established. Some authors have suggested that the neurotoxic effects from hemosiderin deposits or the mass effect secondary to repeat microhemorrhages may culminate in an episodic and stepwise neurologic deterioration, intercalated with periods of gradual but incomplete recovery.[25]

Treatment and Outcomes

Indications

Given the scarcity of spinal vascular lesions, there are limited data to support a specific treatment. Most studies are based on retrospective series that include less than 50 patients.[42,43] Spinal dural AVFs tend to produce venous hypertension, edema, and ischemia within the spinal cord itself, which manifests in a slowly progressive motor and sensory myelopathy over the course of months to years. Intervention through microsurgical or endovascular obliteration aims to halt or reverse this progression by eliminating flow through the abnormal fistulous connection and restoring normal spinal cord perfusion and intravascular pressures. Spinal AVMs, in particular those that are predominantly intramedullary as well as perimedullary fistulas, however, are more likely to present with an acute neurologic deficit secondary to intramedullary or subarachnoid hemorrhage. The goals of treatment in these lesions include preventing future hemorrhagic events, evacuating acute hemorrhage products, or selectively obliterating components of the malformation that are accessible to treatment and thought to be symptomatic (i.e., feeding artery aneurysms). Finally, with spinal cord cavernomas, the goal of treatment is gross total resection of the cavernoma to prevent a progressive neurologic decline from repetitive hemorrhage events.

Microvascular Treatment

Dural Arteriovenous Fistulas

The first successful surgical treatment of an SVM involved a thoracic laminectomy performed by Charles Elsberg at Mount Sinai Hospital (New York, NY) in 1914. He reportedly identified enlarged blood vessels adjacent to a thoracic nerve root, excising several centimeters of the abnormality where it penetrated the dura, and the patient recovered almost completely.[5] Subsequent efforts by other authors were less successful, as they often involved stripping the entire venous complex off the surface of the spinal cord, presumably incurring cord ischemia or worsening preexisting venous hypertension. Krayenbühl and Yaşargil brought modern microsurgical principles to the surgery of SVMs with the use of the operating microscope and bipolar cautery in 1969. However, it was not until Kendall and Logue identified the critical pathology of the dural AVF, later confirmed clinically by Symon and Oldfield, that microsurgery became an almost uniformly successful treatment modality.

Most commonly, dural AVFs involve one or several fistulous connections between a dural branch of a radicular artery and radicular vein located along the inner surface of the dura and laterally at the nerve root sleeve, most commonly in the thoracic or lumbar spine (**Fig. 52.6**). Once the level and side of the lesion is identified and the vascular anatomy is characterized by angiography, the exposure of the lesion typically is relatively straightforward. For classic lesions located at the nerve root sleeve, a laminectomy or laminoplasty is completed eccentric to the side of the lesion. The laminectomy may extend a level above and below the lesion to provide adequate access and to enable opening the dura rostral and caudal to the pathology, and it may extend laterally to the level of the pedicle above the involved neural foramen. The draining vein or veins are often abnormal appearing, enlarged, and arterialized. The fistulous connection is identified, and either a microsurgical clip is placed at the point of connection between the artery and the vein or the fistula is coagulated and subsequently cut.[44] Recently, the use of intraoperative indocyanine green (ICG) angiography has proven helpful in identifying the pathology and confirming the obliteration of the fistula.[12,45] Electrophysiological monitoring of motor evoked potentials (MEPs) and somatosensory evoked potentials (SSEPs) may be a useful adjunct during surgery to minimize the risk of cord injury and critical vessel sacrifice, as changes in MEPs or SSEPs after temporary vessel occlusion with microclips may potentially be reversible by clip removal.[22,46] Microscopically, once the fistula is obliterated, one may see the involved arterialized "red" draining vein develop stasis and a purple hue. Definitive confirmation of AVF resection requires a postoperative spinal angiogram. Once the lesion has been obliterated, closure proceeds in a standard fashion, with a watertight dural closure to prevent cerebrospinal fluid leak, infection, and pseudomeningocele formation. In cases requiring a significant bony removal of the ipsilateral facet complex and pedicle to access the lesion, an instrumented arthrodesis may be required to prevent postoperative instability.[42]

Outcomes of microsurgery for dural AVF are generally quite good (**Table 52.3**), but may vary based on the lesion complexity, the surgeon's experience, and perhaps most importantly, the preoperative neurologic status of the patient. Obliteration rates on postoperative angiography in several modern series are typically in the range of 94 to 100%, with recurrence rates typically less than 15%.[2,42,43] The vast majority of patients are either clinically improved or stable postoperatively. Complication rates have been reported to range from 5 to 15% in the modern era, and typically include pseudomeningocele, spinal instability, or worsened neurologic deficit.

Spinal Arteriovenous Malformations and Perimedullary Arteriovenous Fistulas

Spinal AVMs are, on the whole, less well defined vascular lesions than dural AVFs, and as such their surgical treatment is less well characterized. From a microsurgical standpoint, the anatomy of the individual lesion often dictates the role of surgery and the surgical approach. The location of the AVM within the spinal canal may determine the extent of bony removal and whether a posterior, posterolateral, or anterior approach is warranted.

52 Vascular Malformations of the Spine 347

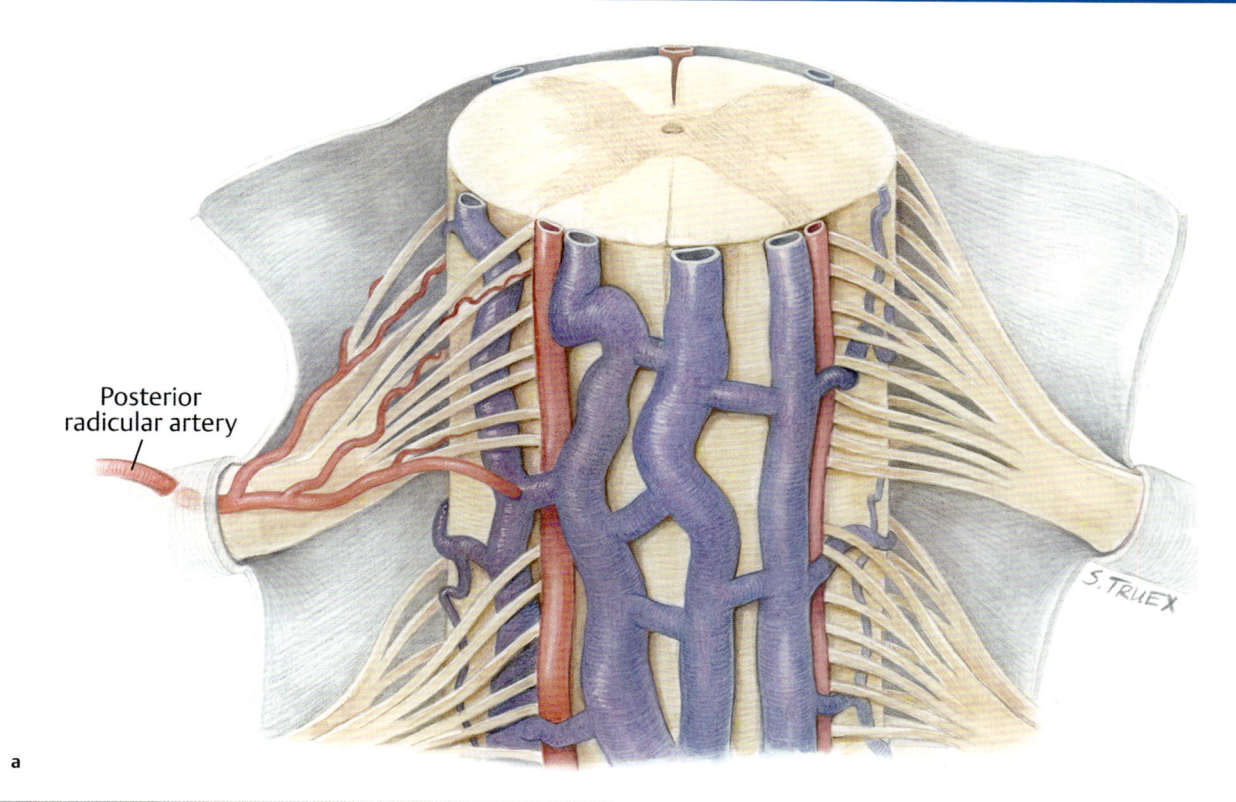

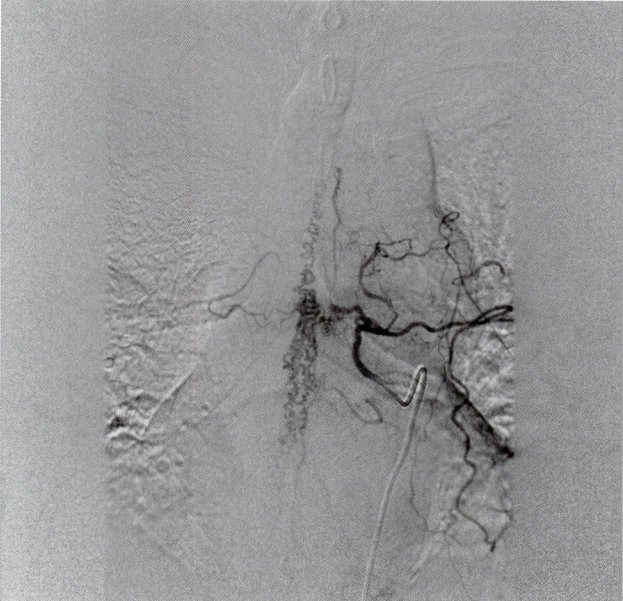

Fig. 52.6 (a) Schematic drawing of an intradural dorsal arteriovenous fistula. Note the fistulous connections between a dural branch of the posterior radicular artery and radicular vein, and the resultant engorgement and dilatation of the venous plexus. The fistula is usually located along the inner surface of the dura and laterally at the nerve root sleeve. (b) Selective catheter spinal angiography demonstrating a similar lesion with striking dilatation of the medullary venous plexus network.

Table 52.3 Case Series of Microsurgical Treatment of Spinal Arteriovenous Malformations

Authors	Patients (n)	Mean Age (yr)	Lesion Type	Treatment Modality (%)	Obliteration (%)	Mean Follow-Up	Outcome	Recurrence	Complication (%)	Mortality (%)
Rangel-Castilla et al (2014)[2]	110	42.3	AVF	S±E (86.4), E (12.7)	95.5	30.5 mos	Improved 71.4%, stable 26.3%	13.6	15.4	0
			AVM		75.5		Improved 43.6%, stable 42.8%	15		
Gross and Du (2014)*[36]	51	15	Juvenile AVM	E (44), E+S (24), S(9)	32	2.6 yrs	Improved 73%, stable 10%	—	—	—
Cho et al (2013)[43]	64	59	SDAVF	E (40), S(19), E+S (4)	94	20 mos	Improved 50%, stable 41%	0	23.4	0
		32	PMAVF		68	42 mos	Improved 58%, stable 37%			
		24	SAVM		50	56 mos	Improved 33%, stable 25%			
Gross and Du (2013)*[24]	293	29.1	Glomus AVM	S (68.2)	78	774.8 pt-yrs	Improved 57%, stable 31%	0.9/pt-yr	—	—
				E (31.7)	33		Improved 66%, stable 21%	11/pt-yr		
Velat et al (2012)[23]	20	30	Glomus AVM	S±E (100)	75	45.4 mos	Improved 55%, stable 45%	0	5	0

Study			Type	Treatment		Follow-up	Outcome			Mortality
Wilson et al (2012)[39]	16	34	Conus AVM	S±E (100)	88	70 mos	Improved 43%, stable 43%	19	7	0
Boström et al (2009)[60]	20	—	Glomus AVM	S (65), E+S (35)	78.5	55 mos	Improved 20%, stable 75%	15	15	0
Du et al (2009)[35]	72	9	AVF, AVM	S (14), E (54), E+S (28)	64	—	Improved 40%, stable 51.7%	—	—	0
Zozulya et al (2006)[61]	91	42.9	AVF	S (76.9), E (14.3), E+S (8.8)	100	—	Improved 82.4%, stable 11%	0	—	0
			AVM							
Steinmetz et al (2004)**[42]	19	60	SDAVF	S (100)	100	35 mos	Improved 55%, stable 34%	0	5	0
Connolly et al (1998)[62]	15	28	Glomus AVM	S±E (100)	94	8.5 yrs	Improved 40%, stable 53%	20	7	0
Rosenblum et al (1987)[19]	81	49	AVF	S (85)	100	3.7 yrs	Improved 72%, stable 28%	0	—	1.2
		27	AVM		59%		Improved 33%, stable 51%			

Abbreviations: AVF, arteriovenous fistula; AVM, arteriovenous malformation; E, embolization; S, surgery; SDAVF, spinal dural arteriovenous fistula.
*Pooled analysis.
**Single-institution series and meta-analysis.

Most lesions are accessible through a posterior laminectomy and partial facetectomy, however. Intradural AVMs that are ventral or ventrolateral to the spinal cord may warrant a generous arachnoid and dentate ligament opening to rotate the spinal cord medially. Similarly, nerve roots, particularly the thoracic ones, may need to be sacrificed intradurally for further exposure. Perimedullary AVFs (**Fig. 52.7**), also called fistulous AVMs, are fed by radiculomedullary arteries that drain to the superficial perimedullary veins, in contrast to dural AVFs. Their surgical treatment, as with dural AVFs, involves disconnecting the fistulous site or sites. Glomus AVMs (**Fig. 52.8**) contain a nidus that resembles that of a brain AVM and tend to be intramedullary. Depending on their location within the spinal cord, they may not be amenable to surgical resection or may carry an obligatory risk of postoperative neurologic deficit. Resection of the nidus may require a myelotomy, which traditionally can be dorsal midline, dorsal root entry zone, or lateral or anterior midline. These lesions are more likely to be associated with hematomyelia or subarachnoid hemorrhage, which may be evacuated intraoperatively. Pathological features such as feeding artery aneurysms or varices may also be targeted for resection in a focused manner in an attempt both to minimize the risk of incurring a postoperative deficit from resection and to prevent further lesional hemorrhages or edema.

Recently, for glomus AVMs with a significant intramedullary component, some surgeons have advocated subtotal resection of the extramedullary component of the lesion to minimize postoperative morbidity.[23] In this so-called pial resection technique, feeding arteries and draining veins along the surface of the spinal cord are coagulated and divided while minimizing subpial dissection. Myelotomies may be reserved for intramedullary hematoma evacuation and fenestration of associated intramedullary syringes. In a small number of patients, this strategy of subtotal resection of glomus AVMs has led to no increase in neurologic morbidity and even angiographic obliteration of the lesion. In general, complex spinal AVMs and AVFs increasingly require a multimodality approach that utilizes both microsurgery and endovascular embolization effectively. Outcomes for spinal AVMs (**Table 52.3**) may be worse than those for dural AVFs in regard to angiographic lesion obliteration, but may in general be better in regard to functional neurologic outcome, as many dural AVFs tend to present in older individuals at a significantly delayed interval from symptom onset.

Spinal Cord Cavernous Malformations

Microsurgical resection is the treatment of choice for symptomatic spinal cord cavernous malformations (SCCMs) to arrest the neurologic decline associated with episodic hemorrhages. As with dural AVFs and spinal AVMs, the location of the lesion determines the surgical approach and bony exposure. These lesions have a mixed signal intensity on T1-weighted MRI and may present to the pial surface. Posterior or posterolateral approaches predominate, and myelotomies to access the lesion are typically midline, dorsal root entry zone, or lateral. Intraoperative ultrasound may facilitate identification of the lesion and associated intramedullary hemorrhage. The dentate ligament may be sectioned and the spinal cord rotated medially for a more direct approach to more laterally located lesions. The resection is completed piecemeal, rather than en bloc, working within the sinusoidal hemorrhagic tissue of the malformation to minimize cord traction.[47] Unlike intracranial CMs in non-eloquent tissue, the yellow-stained and gliotic hemosiderin ring that surrounds an SCCM is generally not resected. Associated developmental venous

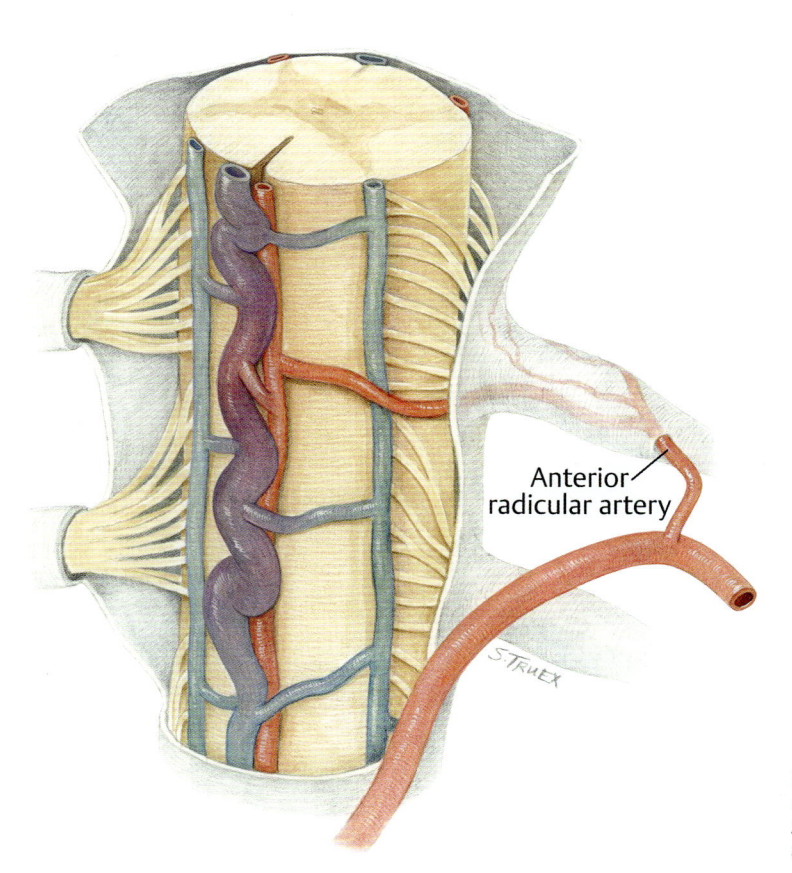

Fig. 52.7 Schematic drawing of an intradural ventral arteriovenous fistula (AVF) (i.e., type IV AVM or perimedullary AVF). Note the ventral fistulous connection between the anterior spinal artery and the venous plexus network.

Anterior radicular artery

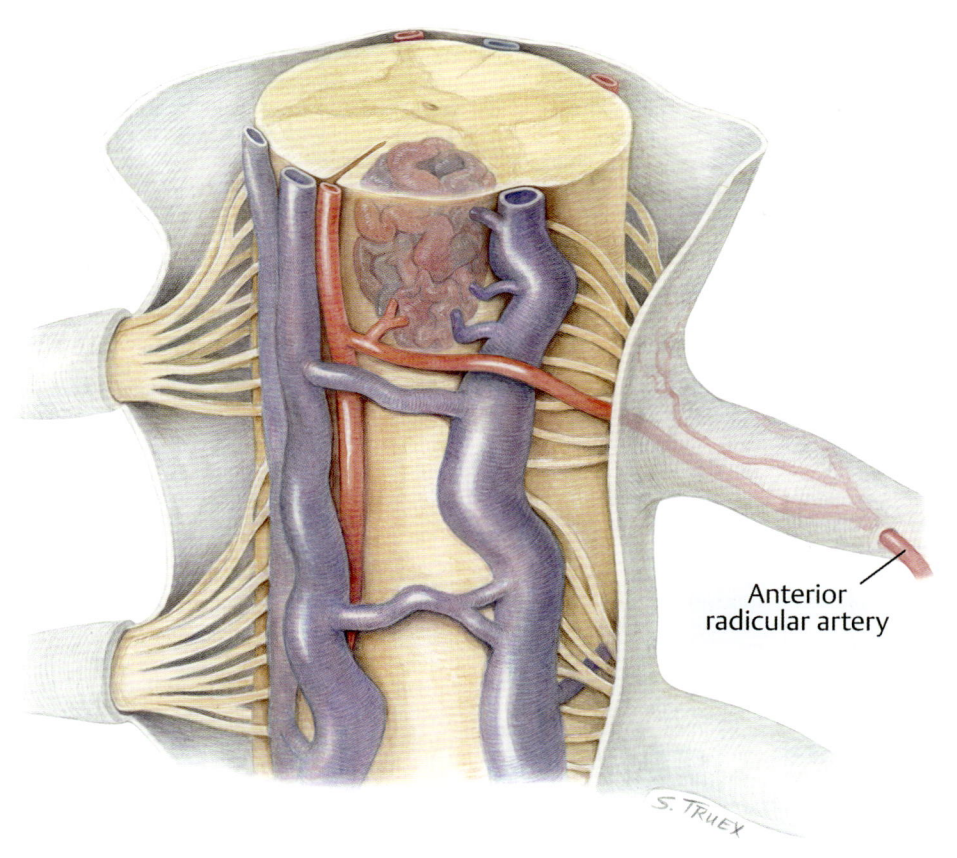

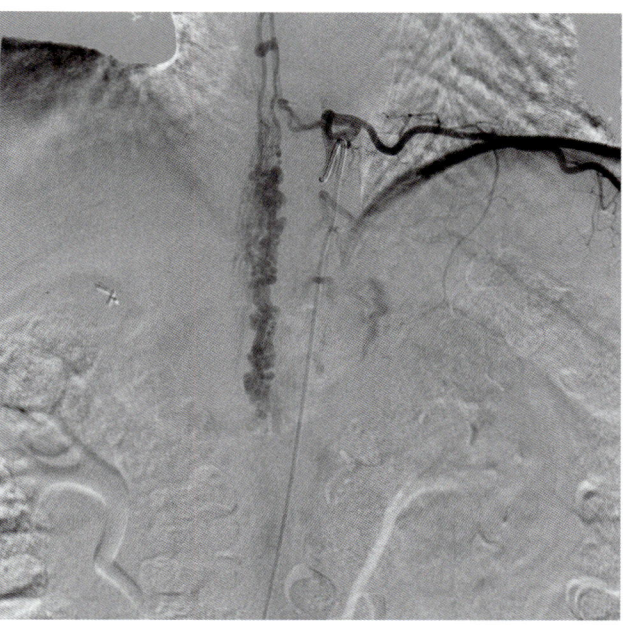

Fig. 52.8 **(a)** Schematic drawing of an intradural intramedullary arteriovenous malformation (i.e., glomus AVM). The AVM nidus can be compact, as shown here, or diffuse, but it is primarily parenchymal. **(b)** Selective catheter spinal angiography showing a large intradural intramedullary AVM with diffuse nidus. Note the enlarged anterior spinal artery and artery of Adamkiewicz with an associated flow-related aneurysm.

anomaly (DVA) should be preserved to avoid cord ischemia. Some surgeons advocate use of the CO_2 laser during resection to minimize trauma to adjacent spinal tracts.[47] Outcomes from microsurgical resection are generally favorable, with > 90% gross total resection in most series, and the majority of patients stable or improved postoperatively.[25,48–50]

Endovascular Treatment

Endovascular treatment of SVMs was initially described by Doppman et al in 1968.[5] Since then, the advent of modern spinal angiography, better microcatheter navigability, and liquid embolic agents such as *n*-butyl cyanoacrylate (nBCA) and Onyx have vastly expanded the role of embolization in the treatment of the various types of SVMs. For some of those lesions, surgery remains the treatment of choice, particularly when the malformation vascular supply is in intimal association with the ASA, posterior spinal artery (PSA) or artery of Adamkiewicz; in those cases, the risk of spinal cord ischemia and worse neurologic function with curative embolization may be prohibitive. Several reports have shown high rates of complete angiographic obliteration, and similar results on long-term neurologic outcome with minimal morbidity.[21,42,43,51,52]

Except for a few cases where preoperative embolization is the treatment goal, the use of particle embolization, such as with polyvinyl alcohol (PVA), Embosphere microspheres (Merit Medical Systems, South Jordan, UT), or Gelfoam, is not indicated and has been largely abandoned, due to its high recanalization rates.[21,30,52,53] The utility of endovascular treatment as monotherapy for SVMs is directly dependent on the lesion subtype, its angioarchitecture, and embolic agent selection. A detailed discussion of this topic is beyond the scope of this chapter. But the applicability of endovascular techniques for the treatment of the various SVMs is discussed below.

The endovascular literature is more focused on cases of AVFs. Higher rates of angiographic obliteration are described for spinal dural AVFs. In fact, several authors preconize embolization as the treatment of choice.[12,15,21,37,42,43] The goal of embolization is obliteration of the fistulous connection as well as the proximal aspect of the arterialized draining vein. Collateral supply must be ruled out at the time of treatment by injections at the correspondent levels on the contralateral side, as well as adjacent segmental arteries above and below the fistula. Initial obliteration rates vary from 25 to 100% (depending on the embolic agent used). Recurrence is much less frequent in the series treated with nBCA or Onyx (0–25%), compared with much higher numbers in the early PVA series (as high as 76%).[53] The analysis of the results for intradural AVFs is more complex, given the significant variability in the nomenclature (perimedullary AVFs, type IV, intradural ventral AVFs). The lesions with progressively larger shunts and marked dilated venous network appear to be the ones with better results, with initial obliteration rates of 67 to 100%.[53]

The role of embolization for the treatment of spinal cord AVMs has been studied by several authors.[43,54,55] In several institutions, it has become the treatment of choice.[15,51,52,54,55] There are fundamental differences in treatment concepts for spinal AVMs compared with brain AVMs. Similar to what occurs with ruptured cerebral AVMs, after a spinal AVM presents with hemorrhage, most authors would recommend a delay in treatment to promote hematoma reabsorption and to allow some improvement in neurologic function. However, in contrast to its intracranial equivalent, partial treatment or obliteration of spinal AVMs may be sufficient to dramatically improve prognosis, especially in patients in whom a complete resection or embolization would incur in neurologic deficits.[54] In unruptured spinal AVMs that have become symptomatic with venous congestion rather than hemorrhage, a reasonable goal of treatment would be to reduce the shunting volume (**Fig. 52.9**). The reported obliteration rates with liquid embolic agents varies from 33 to 100%, depending on the location and nidus size.[24,51–54] In a single-center experience with embolization of intramedullary AVMs with Onyx, 78% of patients had some history of spinal hemorrhage at the time of presentation.[51] After an average of 1.23 sessions per patient, total or subtotal obliteration was achieved in 68.75% of patients. Despite a relatively low rate of complete obliteration (37.5%), improvement in neurologic or functional status was seen in 82% of treated patients, with a permanent complication rate of 4.3%.[51] Partial obliteration of spinal AVMs may also be acceptable in patients with high-risk features, such as associated nidal or prenidal aneurysms or large venous varices. There appears to be a protective effect against hemorrhage even with partial obliteration of a spinal AVM. This has been studied on a recent pooled analysis of literature cases of glomus (type II) AVMs.[24] In this study, the overall annual hemorrhage rate was 4%, increasing to 10% in AVMs with previous hemorrhage. Despite a rate of complete endovascular obliteration of 33%, no postembolization AVM hemorrhages were reported over a total of 240.7 patient-years. The reduction in the annual hemorrhage risk was statistically significant even in the subgroup of partially embolized AVMs.

The modern treatment concept of SVMs necessarily entails a multidisciplinary approach to those lesions. Even in high-volume surgical centers, almost half of the SVMs are preoperatively embolized or treated with embolization alone.[2,13,14,17,18,22,23,39,40] The use of endovascular techniques to exclude high-risk features or obliterate deep arterial feeders otherwise not easily approached by microsurgery alone is of paramount importance to decrease the perioperative blood loss and to minimize spinal cord dissection injury and the incidence of postoperative new or worse neurologic deficits.

Radiosurgery

Radiosurgical treatment of SVMs has not been extensively studied and, thus, is not recommended. Over the last decade, a few reports have described the use of multisession CyberKnife radiosurgery for treatment of intramedullary spinal cord AVMs.[56,57] Overall, these results suggest a potential benefit of radiosurgery on hemorrhage risk; however, its effect on angiographic obliteration and long-term treatment results are yet to be determined.

Outcome

Several factors have significantly changed the treatment paradigm for spinal vascular malformations over the last three decades. The lower treatment morbidity has been coupled with improvements in long-term obliteration rates, making conservative management a distant third option for those lesions. Many SVMs can be safely treated with a multimodality approach that involves preoperative embolization and surgical resection. It remains true, though, that the treatment success rates depend directly on the lesion subtype and mode of presentation. Most of the treatment recommendations and outcomes published are based on case series or anecdotal experiences, and any generalization of clinical practice into guidelines is doomed to fail.

Of all the vascular lesions subtypes, spinal dural AVFs represent the most widely studied group. Their surgical obliteration rates approach 100%, and long-term functional improvement of 50% or greater is consistently reported on the case series.[2,12,17–19,21,43,44,52,58,59] The degree of preoperative neurologic function correlates strongly with the extent of postoperative recovery, independent of the treatment modality used.[17] Motor symptoms tend to respond better to treatment (66% overall improvement), whereas sensory symptoms such as numbness, dysesthesias, or burning pain tend to improve less frequently (12 to 45% of patients).[37] Recovery of sphincter dysfunction tends to be disappointing, with persisting symptoms in up to 73% of patients. Nevertheless, clinical recovery is possible even for patients with severe deficits, including paraplegia. Treatment should not be withheld from patients who are severely affected, because surgery may still be beneficial.[44,59] Although mild transient worsening of symptoms after surgery or embolization is common, it does not influence the short- or long-term outcome. Because many patients progress over a considerable period of time before a diagnosis is made, it can be argued that the delay in diagnosis rather than the degree of neurologic impairment is the major reason for incomplete recovery. Surgical intervention

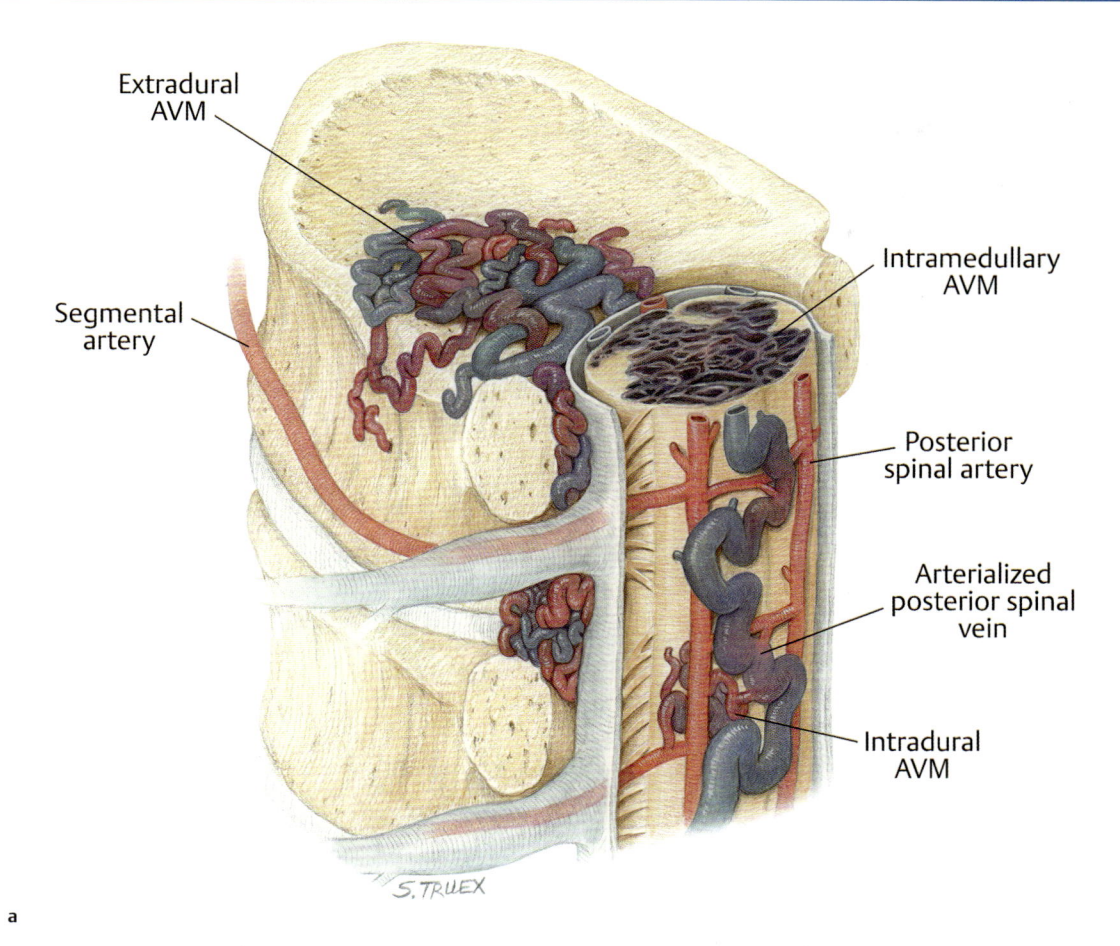

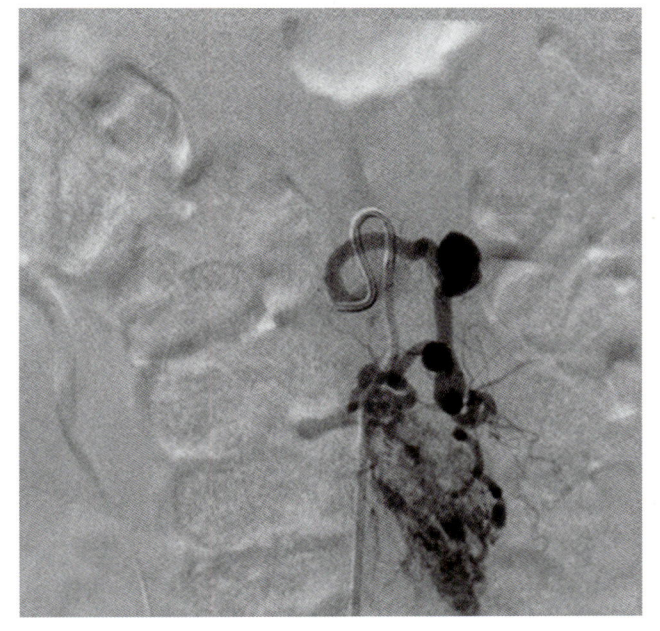

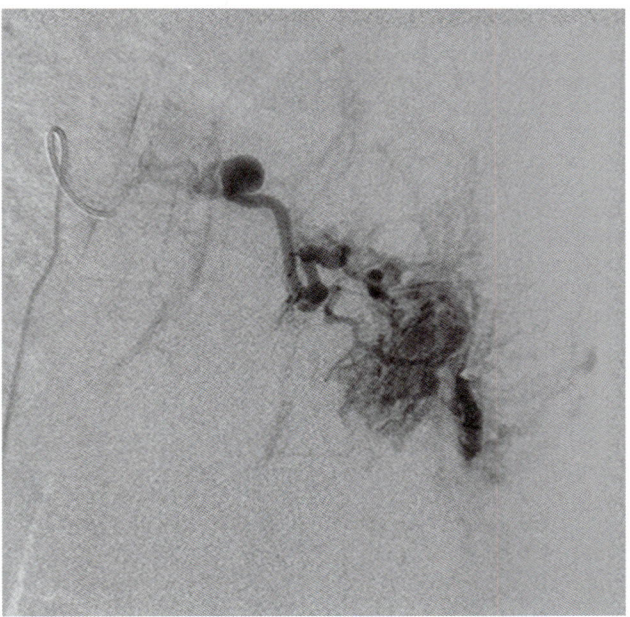

Fig. 52.9 **(a)** Schematic drawing of an extradural-intradural arteriovenous malformation (i.e., metameric AVM). Note the two distinct nidus components—intramedullary and extradural—involving the vertebral bodies and ventral epidural space. AP **(b)** and lateral **(c)** projections of a selective catheter spinal angiography, demonstrating a large metameric AVM. Note the enlarged radicular artery with flow-related and intranidal aneurysms.

historically has higher rates of obliteration, with lower rates of recurrence and comparable morbidity to endovascular treatment, and thus is the treatment of choice of several authors.[2,14,18,42,44] Radiological findings on MRI do not appear to be a reliable predictor of outcome, as neither the extent of preoperative nor the change in postoperative T2 signal abnormality correlate with postoperative clinical disability.[37]

Distinct from spinal dural AVFs, perimedullary or intradural ventral AVFs are rare; most of the case series with long-term follow-up and treatment results are relatively new. The preferred treatment modality differs by subtype (which takes into consideration the number and location of feeders and size of the fistulous component). Smaller lesions with single or few arterial feeders (types A and B) are better treated with surgery, whereas the larger lesions (type C) are usually managed with endovascular techniques. Using a multidisciplinary approach, Cho et al[43] reported the successful obliteration of 70% of perimedullary AVFs, with 95% favorable outcomes in long-term follow-up. The majority of lesions with complete obliteration were types A and B and were treated with surgery. Similar results have been recently published by other authors.[2]

Due to the heterogeneity of the patients and the complexity of the lesions, spinal AVMs represent the subgroup with the worst obliteration rates (32 to 94%), even in multimodality groups. Nevertheless, treatment is justifiable if one takes into consideration the high annual hemorrhage risk and the stepwise deterioration characteristic of those lesions. In two separate pooled analyses, Gross and Du[24,36] estimated an overall hemorrhage risk of 2.1% and 4% per year for glomus and juvenile AVMs, respectively. These numbers may underestimate the actual risk, because in their calculations the authors assumed that the AVMs were present since birth, which does not take into consideration the dynamic nature of some features of those lesions, such as the formation of associated aneurysms. The treating neurosurgeon might also keep in mind the substantial difference in treatment goals between spinal AVMs and the corresponding intracranial ones. As it has been noted by several authors, significant clinical recovery and functional improvement do not necessarily correlate with completeness of angiographic obliteration.[2,23,43,51] Targeted embolization of specific AVM angioarchitecture features (such as nidal aneurysms) may protect against future devastating events, such as intramedullary hemorrhage.[30,51,52]

Spinal cord cavernous malformations are associated with transient neurologic worsening in up to 40% of the patients, despite all the main series reporting stable or improved functional status in up to 90% of the cases.[48–50] Mitha et al[50] have found no correlation between long-term outcome and location of cavernous malformation, surgical approach, or preoperative neurologic status. Patients with pain as a presenting symptom appear to respond well to surgical intervention, with up to 56% of those patients experiencing an improvement in their preoperative pain levels. The degree of complete surgical resection reported in the literature appears to be higher than 90%, with a 5 to 6% complication rate reported on the main series. Gross surgical resection is associated with a significant decrease in the preoperative annual hemorrhage risk, previously reported to range from 1.4 to 4.5% per year.[48] Most patients who undergo resection of a spinal CM return at least to their preoperative neurologic level of function.[25] The prognosis and treatment recommendations for asymptomatic lesions are not well established, and treatment strategies vary significantly among treatment centers.

References

1. Chaloupka JC. Future directions in the evaluation and management of spinal cord vascular malformations. Semin Cerebrovasc Dis Stroke 2002; 2:245–256
2. Rangel-Castilla L, Russin JJ, Zaidi HA, et al. Contemporary management of spinal AVFs and AVMs: lessons learned from 110 cases. Neurosurg Focus 2014;37:E14
3. Aminoff MJ, Logue V. The prognosis of patients with spinal vascular malformations. Brain 1974;97:211–218
4. Black P. Spinal vascular malformations: an historical perspective. Neurosurg Focus 2006;21:E11
5. Akopov SE, Schievink WI. History of spinal cord vascular malformations and their treatment. Semin Cerebrovasc Dis Stroke 2002;2:178–185
6. Elsberg C. Diagnosis and Treatment of Surgical Diseases of the Spinal Cord and Its Membranes. Philadelphia: WB Saunders; 1916:194–204
7. Wyburn-Mason R. The Vascular Abnormalities and Tumours of the Spinal Cord and its Membranes. St. Louis: Mosby; 1943
8. Yaşargil MG. Surgery of vascular lesions of the spinal cord with the microsurgical technique. Clin Neurosurg 1970;17:257–265
9. Krayenbühl H, Yaşargil MG, McClintock HG. Treatment of spinal cord vascular malformations by surgical excision. J Neurosurg 1969;30:427–435
10. Kendall BE, Logue V. Spinal epidural angiomatous malformations draining into intrathecal veins. Neuroradiology 1977;13:181–189
11. Heros RC, Debrun GM, Ojemann RG, Lasjaunias PL, Naessens PJ. Direct spinal arteriovenous fistula: a new type of spinal AVM. Case report. J Neurosurg 1986;64:134–139
12. Rodesch G, Hurth M, Alvarez H, Tadié M, Lasjaunias P. Classification of spinal cord arteriovenous shunts: proposal for a reappraisal—the Bicêtre experience with 155 consecutive patients treated between 1981 and 1999. Neurosurgery 2002;51:374–379, discussion 379–380
13. Spetzler RF, Detwiler PW, Riina HA, Porter RW. Modified classification of spinal cord vascular lesions. J Neurosurg 2002;96(2, Suppl):145–156
14. Kim LJ, Spetzler RF. Classification and surgical management of spinal arteriovenous lesions: arteriovenous fistulae and arteriovenous malformations. Neurosurgery 2006;59(5, Suppl 3):S195–S201, discussion S3–S13
15. da Costa L, Dehdashti AR, terBrugge KG. Spinal cord vascular shunts: spinal cord vascular malformations and dural arteriovenous fistulas. Neurosurg Focus 2009;26:E6
16. Morris JM. Imaging of dural arteriovenous fistula. Radiol Clin North Am 2012;50:823–839
17. Watson JC, Oldfield EH. The surgical management of spinal dural vascular malformations. Neurosurg Clin N Am 1999;10:73–87
18. Oldfield E. Surgical treatment of spinal dural arteriovenous fistulas. Semin Cerebrovasc Dis Stroke 2002;2:209–226
19. Rosenblum B, Oldfield EH, Doppman JL, Di Chiro G. Spinal arteriovenous malformations: a comparison of dural arteriovenous fistulas and intradural AVM's in 81 patients. J Neurosurg 1987;67:795–802
20. Krings T, Mull M, Gilsbach JM, Thron A. Spinal vascular malformations. Eur Radiol 2005;15:267–278
21. Patsalides A, Santillan A, Knopman J, Tsiouris AJ, Riina HA, Gobin YP. Endovascular management of spinal dural arteriovenous fistulas. J Neurointerv Surg 2011;3:80–84
22. Atkinson J, Piepgras D. Surgical treatment of spinal cord arteriovenous malformations and arteriovenous fistulas. Semin Cerebrovasc Dis Stroke 2002;2:201–208
23. Velat GJ, Chang SW, Abla AA, Albuquerque FC, McDougall CG, Spetzler RF. Microsurgical management of glomus spinal arteriovenous malformations: pial resection technique: Clinical article. J Neurosurg Spine 2012; 16:523–531
24. Gross BA, Du R. Spinal glomus (type II) arteriovenous malformations: a pooled analysis of hemorrhage risk and results of intervention. Neurosurgery 2013;72:25–32, discussion 32
25. Lemole GM, Henn JS, Riina HA, Lanzino G, Kim LJ, Spetzler RF. Spinal cord cavernous malformations. Semin Cerebrovasc Dis Stroke 2002;2:227–235
26. McCormick PC, Michelsen WJ, Post KD, Carmel PW, Stein BM. Cavernous malformations of the spinal cord. Neurosurgery 1988;23:459–463
27. White JA, Kopitnik TA, Batjer HH. Spinal intradural vascular malformations. In: Benzel EC, ed. Spine Surgery: Techniques, Complication Avoidance, and Management, 3rd ed. Philadelphia: Saunders; 2012: 999–1004
28. Jahan R, Vinuela F. Vascular anatomy, pathophysiology, and classification of vascular malformations of the spinal cord. Semin Cerebrovasc Dis Stroke 2002;2:186–200

29. Hassler W, Thron A. Flow velocity and pressure measurements in spinal dural arteriovenous fistulas. Neurosurg Rev 1994;17:29–36
30. Rodesch G, Lasjaunias P. Spinal cord arteriovenous shunts: from imaging to management. Eur J Radiol 2003;46:221–232
31. Lindenholz A, TerBrugge KG, van Dijk JMC, Farb RI. The accuracy and utility of contrast-enhanced MR angiography for localization of spinal dural arteriovenous fistulas: the Toronto experience. Eur Radiol 2014;24:2885–2894
32. Si-jia G, Meng-wei Z, Xi-ping L, et al. The clinical application studies of CT spinal angiography with 64-detector row spiral CT in diagnosing spinal vascular malformations. Eur J Radiol 2009;71:22–28
33. Willinsky R, Lasjaunias P, Terbrugge K, Hurth M. Angiography in the investigation of spinal dural arteriovenous fistula. A protocol with application of the venous phase. Neuroradiology 1990;32:114–116
34. Prestigiacomo CJ, Niimi Y, Setton A, Berenstein A. Three-dimensional rotational spinal angiography in the evaluation and treatment of vascular malformations. AJNR Am J Neuroradiol 2003;24:1429–1435
35. Du J, Ling F, Chen M, Zhang H. Clinical characteristic of spinal vascular malformation in pediatric patients. Childs Nerv Syst 2009;25:473–478
36. Gross BA, Du R. Spinal juvenile (type III) extradural-intradural arteriovenous malformations. J Neurosurg Spine 2014;20:452–458
37. Fugate JE, Lanzino G, Rabinstein AA. Clinical presentation and prognostic factors of spinal dural arteriovenous fistulas: an overview. Neurosurg Focus 2012;32:E17
38. Foix C, Alajouanine T. Subacute necrotic myelitis, slowly progressive central myelitis with vascular hyperplasia, and slowly ascending, increasingly flaccid amyotrophic paraplegia accompanied by albuminocytologic dissociation. [in French] Rev Neurol 1926;33:1–42
39. Wilson DA, Abla AA, Uschold TD, McDougall CG, Albuquerque FC, Spetzler RF. Multimodality treatment of conus medullaris arteriovenous malformations: 2 decades of experience with combined endovascular and microsurgical treatments. Neurosurgery 2012;71:100–108
40. Kalani MYS, Ahmed AS, Martirosyan NL, et al. Surgical and endovascular treatment of pediatric spinal arteriovenous malformations. World Neurosurg 2012;78:348–354
41. Ogilvy CS, Louis DN, Ojemann RG. Intramedullary cavernous angiomas of the spinal cord: clinical presentation, pathological features, and surgical management. Neurosurgery 1992;31:219–229, discussion 229–230
42. Steinmetz MP, Chow MM, Krishnaney AA, et al. Outcome after the treatment of spinal dural arteriovenous fistulae: a contemporary single-institution series and meta-analysis. Neurosurgery 2004;55:77–87, discussion 87–88
43. Cho W-S, Kim K-J, Kwon O-K, et al. Clinical features and treatment outcomes of the spinal arteriovenous fistulas and malformation: clinical article. J Neurosurg Spine 2013;19:207–216
44. Narvid J, Hetts SW, Larsen D, et al. Spinal dural arteriovenous fistulae: clinical features and long-term results. Neurosurgery 2008;62:159–166, discussion 166–167
45. Walsh DC, Zebian B, Tolias CM, Gullan RW. Intraoperative indocyanine green video-angiography as an aid to the microsurgical treatment of spinal vascular malformations. Br J Neurosurg 2014;28:259–266
46. Niimi Y, Sala F, Deletis V, Setton A, de Camargo AB, Berenstein A. Neurophysiologic monitoring and pharmacologic provocative testing for embolization of spinal cord arteriovenous malformations. AJNR Am J Neuroradiol 2004;25:1131–1138
47. Mitha AP, Turner JD, Spetzler RF. Surgical approaches to intramedullary cavernous malformations of the spinal cord. Neurosurgery 2011;68(2, Suppl Operative):317–324, discussion 324
48. Gross BA, Du R, Popp AJ, Day AL. Intramedullary spinal cord cavernous malformations. Neurosurg Focus 2010;29:E14
49. Labauge P, Bouly S, Parker F, et al; French Study Group of Spinal Cord Cavernomas. Outcome in 53 patients with spinal cord cavernomas. Surg Neurol 2008;70:176–181, discussion 181
50. Mitha AP, Turner JD, Abla AA, Vishteh AG, Spetzler RF. Outcomes following resection of intramedullary spinal cord cavernous malformations: a 25-year experience. J Neurosurg Spine 2011;14:605–611
51. Corkill RA, Mitsos AP, Molyneux AJ. Embolization of spinal intramedullary arteriovenous malformations using the liquid embolic agent, Onyx: a single-center experience in a series of 17 patients. J Neurosurg Spine 2007;7:478–485
52. Rodesch G, Hurth M, Alvarez H, David P, Tadie M, Lasjaunias P. Embolization of spinal cord arteriovenous shunts: morphological and clinical follow-up and results—review of 69 consecutive cases. Neurosurgery 2003;53:40–49, discussion 49–50
53. Ducruet AF, Crowley RW, McDougall CG, Albuquerque FC. Endovascular management of spinal arteriovenous malformations. J Neurointerv Surg 2013;5:605–611
54. Krings T, Thron AK, Geibprasert S, et al. Endovascular management of spinal vascular malformations. Neurosurg Rev 2010;33:1–9
55. Veznedaroglu E, Nelson PK, Jabbour PM, Rosenwasser RH. Endovascular treatment of spinal cord arteriovenous malformations. Neurosurgery 2006;59(5, Suppl 3):S202–S209, discussion S3–S13
56. Potharaju M, John R, Venkataraman M, Gopalakrishna K, Subramanian B. Stereotactic radiosurgery results in three cases of intramedullary spinal cord arteriovenous malformations. Spine J 2014;14:2582–2588
57. Sinclair J, Chang SD, Gibbs IC, Adler JR Jr. Multisession CyberKnife radiosurgery for intramedullary spinal cord arteriovenous malformations. Neurosurgery 2006;58:1081–1089, discussion 1081–1089
58. Morgan MK. Outcome from treatment for spinal arteriovenous malformation. Neurosurg Clin N Am 1999;10:113–119
59. Tacconi L, Lopez Izquierdo BC, Symon L. Outcome and prognostic factors in the surgical treatment of spinal dural arteriovenous fistulas. A long-term study. Br J Neurosurg 1997;11:298–305
60. Boström A, Krings T, Hans FJ, Schramm J, Thron AK, Gilsbach JM. Spinal glomus-type arteriovenous malformations: microsurgical treatment in 20 cases. J Neurosurg Spine 2009;10:423–429
61. Zozulya YP, Slin'ko EI, Al-Qashqish II. Spinal arteriovenous malformations: new classification and surgical treatment. Neurosurg Focus 2006;20:E7
62. Connolly ES Jr, Zubay GP, McCormick PC, Stein BM. The posterior approach to a series of glomus (type II) intramedullary spinal cord arteriovenous malformations. Neurosurgery 1998;42:774–785, discussion 785–786

B. Antero/Anterolateral Approach

53 Open Lateral Transthoracic Approach

Tobias A. Mattei, Victoria Schunemann, and Ehud Mendel

This chapter addresses the standard lateral transthoracic/thoracotomy approach for anterior exposure of the thoracic spine. Other specialized approaches for anterior exposure of the cervicothoracic junction, upper thoracic spine (T1–T4), and thoracolumbar junction, namely the transclavicular, transmanubrial/transsternal, and combined transthoracic/retroperitoneal approaches, respectively, are addressed in other chapters. This chapter discusses the nuances of the lateral transthoracic approach, whereas the specific details of diskectomies and corpectomies performed through this approach are addressed in Chapter 54.

The first reported series of anterolateral transthoracic access to spine is from Hodgson and Stock[1] in 1960, who used this approach for the treatment of spinal tuberculosis (Pott's disease).

The transthoracic approach provides excellent access to the lateral and ventral aspect of the thoracic spine. Any level of the thoracic spine can be accessed by this approach; however, exposure of the most rostral levels (T1–T3) can be very challenging, requiring mobilization of the scapula, which, ultimately, limits the working space to the upper thoracic levels provided by this approach.

Patient Selection

Although the lateral transthoracic approach provides unique visualization of the anterolateral aspect of the thoracic spine, careful patient selection is crucial to avoid possible associated morbid events. Patients with previous lung pathologies (especially on the side of the approach), compromised cardiac function, or other major comorbidities that prevent selective ventilation through one lung may not be able to undergo such a complex procedure. In such cases the risk/benefits profile should be carefully evaluated, and other less invasive posterolateral approaches may present a more appropriate alternative to treat such patients without incurring high risks of perioperative complications.

Indications

The lateral transthoracic approach provides excellent visualization of the ventral aspect of the spine between the T4 and T12 levels, and may be considered for the treatment of the following pathologies:

- Thoracic disk herniations
- Anterior release and instrumentation for deformity correction
- Decompression, fusion, and instrumentation for spinal fractures
- Resection of metastatic tumors involving the thoracic vertebral bodies with subsequent reconstruction of the anterior column
- En-bloc resection of primary bone tumors involving the vertebral bodies
- Infections or osteomyelitis causing vertebral body collapse
- Abscesses or epidural empyemas with a significant collection located anterior to the spinal cord
- Biopsies (occasionally), as thoracoscopic approaches may consist in a minimally invasive alternative for such purposes

Choice of Operative Approach

The decision to perform a right-sided or left-sided approach may depend on several factors. Neoplastic lesions are usually approached through the side of greater tumor involvement. If neither side is predominantly involved by the lesion, the spine is generally approached from the left side in the lesions below T5 (as it is easier to dissect, mobilize, and manage eventual bleeding from the aorta than from the vena cava), and from the right side at or above T5 in order to avoid the aortic arch. Additionally, in the thoracolumbar junction (T10–L2), left-sided thoracotomy provides the advantage of avoiding liver retraction. Other factors such as a previous thoracotomy, pleurodesis, or infection/empyema should also be considered when choosing the side of the approach.

Advantages

- Provides access to the anterior column
- Enables decompression of the ventral portion of the spinal cord under direct visualization
- Enables reconstruction and stabilization of the anterior column without disruption of the posterior column
- Provides improved exposure of the anterior column in comparison to posterolateral approaches
- Preserves the paraspinal muscles

Disadvantages

- The contralateral pedicle and posterior elements are inaccessible through this approach.
- An access surgeon is usually required.
- Patients with a previous pneumonectomy or chronic obstructive pulmonary disease (COPD) may not tolerate single-lung ventilation.
- Specific morbidities related to this approach include great vessel injury, the need for a chest tube, and intercostal neuralgia.

Preoperative Testing

A careful physiological assessment of pulmonary and cardiac function should be performed before deciding on performing a lateral transthoracic approach. The pulmonary evaluation, which usually involve a pulmonary function test and, if necessary, even a ventilation/perfusion (V/Q) scan, is used to determine the patient's ability to tolerate prolonged single lung ventilation. Additionally, these preoperative tests may also assist in deciding from which side to approach the spine. The cardiac evaluation is performed if the patient demonstrates clinical signs of chronic heart failure, if the patient has multiple risk factors for coronary artery disease, or if there is a history of previous heart problems.

Surgical Procedure

Anesthesia

The patient is submitted to general anesthesia. A double-lumen tube should be used, as it is routine to deflate the ipsilateral lung to facilitate visualization of the spine. Other important anesthetic considerations, such as the necessity of large-caliber venous access for volume reposition as well as readily available type-and-crossed blood, are similar to those required for complex thoracic procedures that may eventually involve significant amount of blood loss.

Positioning and Monitoring

The operation is performed on a radiolucent table with the patient placed in the lateral decubitus position supported by either a beanbag or by foam supports in order to avoid undesirable movements in the anteroposterior direction (**Fig. 53.1**). It is important to emphasize that the top of the beanbag should not be higher than the level of the spinous process in order to enable unobstructed fluoroscopy. An axillary roll should be placed under the arm over which the patient is lying to protect the brachial plexus. The legs are slightly flexed, and all bony prominences are well padded. The desired spinal level can be placed in proximity to the break in the table in order to assist in the exposure by opening the disk spaces as well as to facilitate the anterior column reconstruction. The patient is secured to the table, and the spinal level is marked on the skin using anterior and lateral fluoroscopy.

The neurologic function is monitored throughout the whole procedure with somatosensory evoked potentials (SSEPs) and motor evoked potentials (MEPs). This is particularly important in cases with severe cord compression or spinal instability, where even subtle changes in position can result in neurologic deficits.

Incision, Dissection, and Exposure

The skin incision should be performed over the rib one or two levels above the vertebra to be addressed. It usually begins anteriorly at the mid-axillary line (although it can be extended until the costochondral junction). Overall, it should be noted that, in comparison with thoracotomies for other purposes, the thoracotomy incision for the lateral transthoracic approach should be more posterior than anterior.

Dissection is carried down through the subcutaneous tissues, and a retractor is placed. Then, the first layer of muscles (trapezius and latissimus dorsi) is identified and sectioned. In sequence, the second layer of muscles (rhomboids and serratus) is exposed and sectioned (**Fig. 53.2**). After exposing the rib, the periosteum is stripped off its surface with monopolar electrocautery. A curved periosteal elevator is then used to strip the intercostal muscles from the rib. Due to the directional nature of the intercostal muscle attachments, blood loss and tissue trauma can be reduced by stripping the tissue from posterior to anterior on the cephalad aspect of the rib, and from anterior to posterior on the caudal surface. At this point, it is important to carefully dissect the periosteum, neurovascular bundle, and parietal pleura from the undersurface of the rib so that they can be preserved.

In younger patients, entry into the thoracic cavity can be performed through the costal interspace after insertion and opening of a rib spreader, as the ribs are sufficiently mobile. Nevertheless, in adults it is usually necessary remove the rib with a rib cutter. It is advisable to cut the rib at the costochondral junction and as far posteriorly as possible, and then remove it. As most of the lateral transthoracic approaches to the spine involve some type of fusion, the rib can be saved to be used as a bone graft.

After resection of the rib, there are two options. One is to proceed through a transpleural approach, in which case the parietal pleura is sharply incised and the lung is carefully retracted to expose the spine. The other option is to proceed through a retropleural approach (**Fig. 53.3**). If the transpleural approach is chosen, the lung is gently retracted anteriorly and inferiorly and may be protected with a moist laparotomy sponge. It is important to remember that, in transpleural approaches, there is an additional layer of parietal pleura adjacent to the vertebral body that

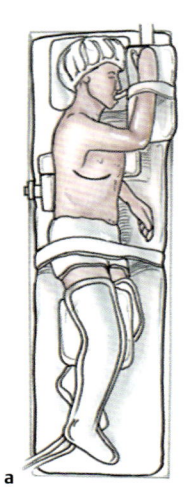

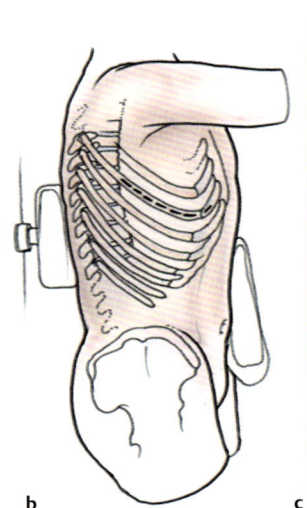

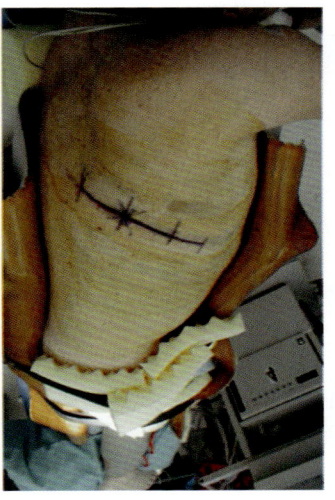

Fig. 53.1 **(a)** Patient positioning for the anterolateral transthoracic approach to the spine. Note the head support, the optional kidney rest, the airplane splint for the topside arm, the axillary roll to avoid compression of the brachial plexus, and the positioning of the patient's legs in a slightly bent fashion, with pillows under pressure points and with compression devices to prevent deep venous thrombosis. **(b)** The location of the planned incision, with an example of the pathology at the level of T8. Note that the incision is usually made along the course of the rib two interspaces above the vertebral level to be addressed. The incision is performed from the anterior border of the latissimus dorsi to the midaxillary line, although it can be extended anteriorly to the costochondral junction. **(c)** Surgical photograph of a patient positioned for an anterolateral transthoracic approach. In this case a beanbag with a suction system is used to provide anteroposterior support.

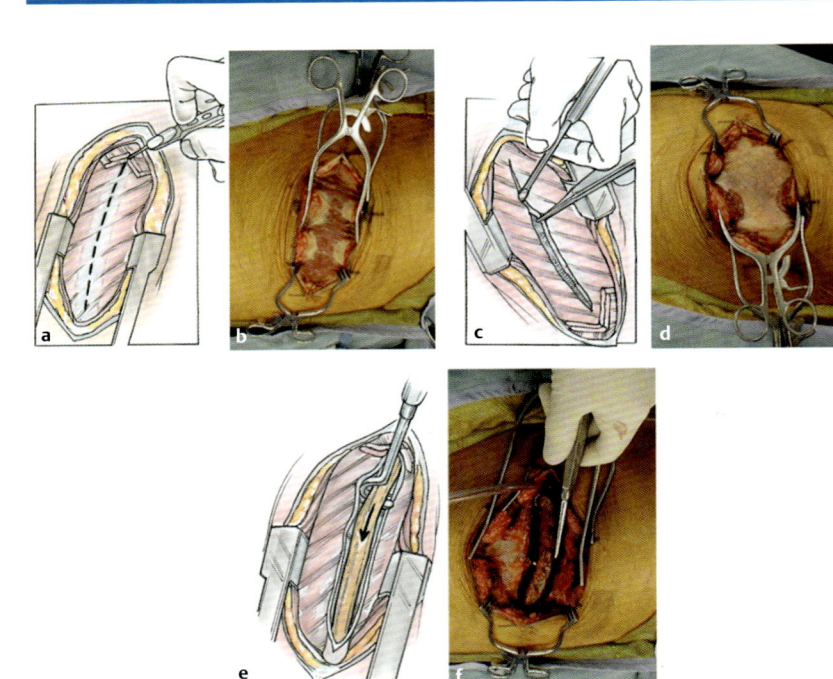

Fig. 53.2 Illustrative pictures **(a,c,e)** and surgical images **(b,d,f)** demonstrating the sequential steps of an anterolateral transthoracic approach. **(a,b)** After the initial skin and subcutaneous tissue incision, a retractor is placed and the first layer of muscles (trapezius and latissimus dorsi) is identified and sectioned. **(c,d)** In sequence, the second layer of muscles (rhomboids and serratus) is exposed and sectioned. **(e,f)** After exposition of the rib, the periosteum is stripped off its surface with monopolar electrocautery. A curved periosteal elevator is then used to strip the intercostal muscles from the rib. Finally, the rib is removed with a rib cutter while preserving the adjacent intercostal musculature and the neurovascular bundle on the pleural surface.

must be incised vertically along the lateral aspect of the anterior longitudinal ligament.

In the case of a retropleural approach, the pleura is carefully dissected from its attachment to the inner surface of the ribs with "sponge dissectors." This path is followed downward, until the head of the rib and spine are reached. Although the retropleural technique is significantly more challenging (because the parietal pleura is thin and frail), if successfully performed it avoids the necessity of a chest tube postoperatively.

When approaching lesions at the thoracolumbar transition it may be necessary to divide the diaphragm. In such cases it is important to place marking stitches in the divided portions of

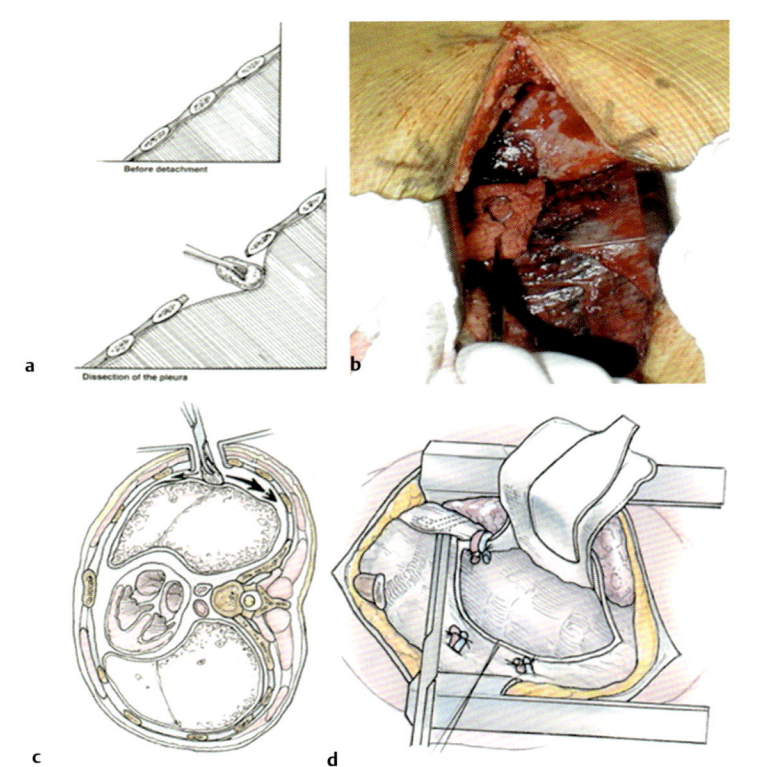

Fig. 53.3 After the initial thoracotomy, a retropleural or a transpleural approach can be performed. **(a,b)** In the retropleural approach, a cottonoid or a folded sponge is used to carefully detach the parietal pleura from the inner surface of the ribs. **(c)** The dissection proceeds posteriorly until the vertebral bodies are reached. **(d)** At this point the segmental vessels to those levels are ligated to enable full exposure of the vertebral bodies.

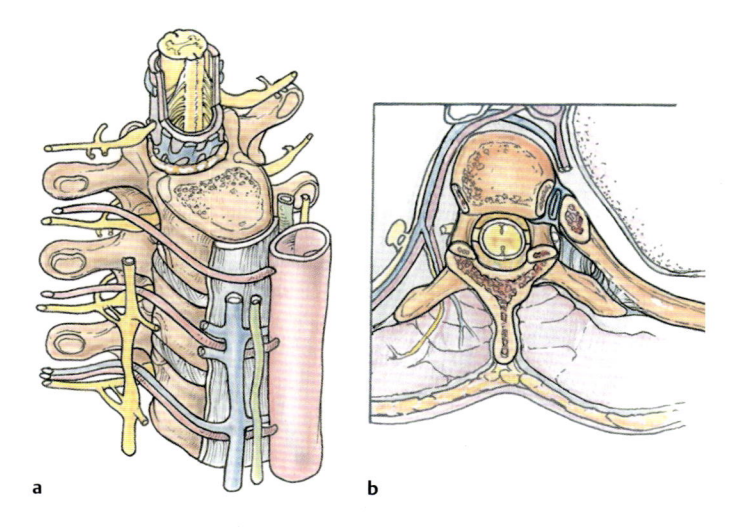

Fig. 53.4 (a) Illustration of the anatomy of the anterolateral vertebral column as it would be seen with all overlying periosteum and pleura stripped away. Note the anatomic relationships of the sympathetic chain, as well as the disk spaces and neural foramina relative to the segmental vessels. (b) Anatomy of the articulation and ligaments between the vertebra and rib. Note than in order for the surgeon to achieve full access to the neural foramen through an anterolateral approach, the head of the rib must be removed.

such muscle to enable proper identification of the corresponding portions that must be sutured back together during the closure step.

After identification of the rib head and the anterolateral portion of the vertebral body, intraoperative fluoroscopy is used to verify the appropriate level. Then, the segmental vessels of the level of interest (which course over the midportion of the vertebral body) are ligated in order to enable retraction of the great vessels from the anterior edge of the spine (**Fig. 53.4**). There is some consensus in the literature that up to three contiguous segmental vessels can be ligated at one side with minimal risk of neurologic deficit due to vascular compromise of the spinal cord.

During the anterolateral dissection of the vertebral body, a wrapped sponge in the form of a cylinder is used to progressively separate the great vessels from the spine. Conducting the dissection along the surface of the relatively avascular disk spaces helps to avoid bleeding. At this stage, care must be taken to preserve the structures running adjacent to the lateral aspect of the thoracic spine, such as the sympathetic chain and the thoracic duct.

If the normal anatomy is not altered by tumoral pathologies or fractures, the concave portions over the spine represent the vertebral bodies, and the disks appear as more prominent and elevated portions. Next, the head of the rib is identified and resected to expose the underlying pedicle, the key landmark point to the location of the neural foramen, which can be palpated with a small blunt dissector.

At this point the surgeon works on the vertebral bodies or disk spaces, depending on the pathology that is being addressed. Additional steps may include diskectomies or vertebrectomies, with the possibility of complete decompression of the anterolateral aspect of the spinal cord.

In the cases of vertebrectomies, the endplates above and below are freed from disk material, and the anterior column is reconstructed with either a bone graft strut or a cage (which can be either a carbon-fiber or an expandable cage) (**Fig. 53.5**). For single-level corpectomies, anterior segmental instrumentation can be placed using a lateral plate or a dual-rod construct to obviate the need of posterior instrumentation.

Closure

After completion of the spinal portion of the procedure, a chest tube must be placed if the parietal pleura has been violated. The chest tube should be tunneled subcutaneously and brought out through a separate small incision one interspace away from the operative incision. The chest tube must be externalized just above the rib to avoid the neurovascular bundle at its inferior surface. Additionally, after transpleural approaches, the parietal pleura overlying the spine is usually closed with interrupted absorbable sutures.

In retropleural approaches, usually a suction drain is left near the spine to prevent postoperative paraspinal hematomas. It is important to emphasize that if an unintended durotomy

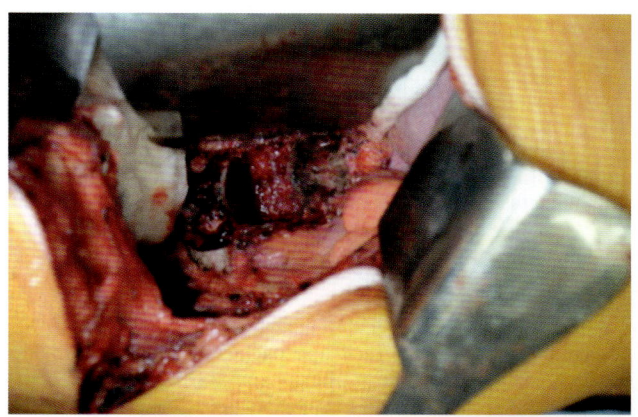

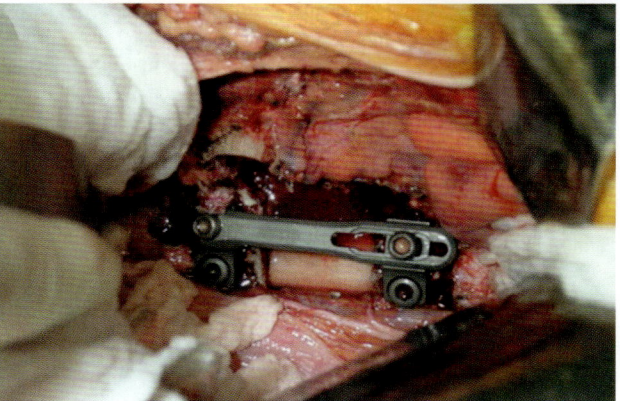

Fig. 53.5 Intraoperative photographs of a patient undergoing a thoracic vertebrectomy through a lateral transthoracic approach. After completion of the vertebrectomy and diskectomies at the level above and below (a), the anterior column is reconstructed with either a bone graft or a cage, and an anterolateral plating system is used for instrumentation (b).

occurred during the procedure, the chest tube should not be placed to suction. In such cases, primary closure of the durotomy is recommended, and a lumbar drain is usually left in place to prevent a cerebrospinal fluid (CSF) fistula to the pleural cavity. Such a situation may be very challenging, as the relatively negative intrathoracic pressure encourages the persistent flow of CSF from the intradural space to the pleural cavity.[2]

Finally, the chest wall retractor is removed and the lung is reinflated under direct visualization to confirm that all lobes appear well inflated. In the approaches to the thoracolumbar junction in which the diaphragm has been opened, this muscle is closed, with special care to match its correspondent portions in an attempt to restore, as best as possible, its normal contraction pattern.

If only one rib has been removed, it is usually possible to partially reapproximate the adjacent ribs with a few sturdy sutures around them. Finally, the latissimus dorsi is reapproximated, the subcutaneous tissue is closed, and the skin is closed with a subcuticular running stitch and steri-strips. The chest tube is secured to the skin and connected to 20 cm H_2O suction.

Postoperative Care

Besides the routine postoperative care regarding the hemodynamic status, wound care, deep venous thrombosis prophylaxis, gastrointestinal prophylaxis, and mobilization protocols typical of all spine patients, patients who have undergone surgery with a lateral transthoracic approach receive special attention in relation to the management of the chest tube (when used). In such cases, daily X-rays are usually obtained. Studies have shown that less than 200 mL of daily drainage can be used as a safe threshold to determine when to remove the chest tube.[3] However, before removing the chest tube, it is advisable to place a water seal (i.e., closed system without suction) for at least 6 hours and to obtain another chest X-ray to ensure that the patient will tolerate removal of the tube. Postoperative attention to pain management, pulmonary toilet, and ambulation (if possible) help prevent atelectasis and pneumonia.

Potential Complications and Precautions

Although lateral transthoracic approaches to the spine provide excellent visualization of the anterior spinal structures, they also entail unique risks related to possible lesions to the anterior great vessels, as well as other inherent complications related to transpleural approaches. Other reported complications are chronic radicular pain, Horner's syndrome, pleural effusion, pneumothorax, hemothorax, chylothorax, and lung herniation.[4,5]

In comparison to other approaches to the spine, lateral transthoracic approaches have been reported to incur higher morbidity rates.[6] In a series of 774 patients submitted to a variety of surgical approaches to the thoracic spine, the following complication rates were noted: lateral transthoracic approach, 39%; lateral extracavitary approach, 17%; costotransversectomy, 15%. In comparison to these last two approaches, the lateral transthoracic approach had also the highest rate of reoperation (3.5%) and the highest mortality rates (1.5%).

Despite such a morbidity profile, which includes a procedure-specific complication rate of 11.5%, other series have reported very low rates of mortality (around 0.3%) and of spinal cord infarction leading to paraplegia related to ligation of segmental vessels (0.2%).[7]

Finally, it has been reported that the addition of a posterior approach after a lateral transthoracic approach significantly increases the overall risk of complications to as high as 72%.[8]

Conclusion

The lateral transthoracic approach provides a unique exposure of the anterior elements of the thoracic and thoracolumbar spine for a broad range of degenerative, infectious, tumoral, and deformity pathologies.

Nevertheless, as such approach is less familiar to the general neurosurgeon than standard posterior approaches, several pre-, intra-, and postoperative nuances should be observed in order to avoid procedure-related complications.

Ultimately, despite its higher morbidity profile when compared with isolated posterior approaches, the lateral transthoracic approach constitutes a powerful tool in the armamentarium of the spine surgeon.

References

1. Hodgson AR, Stock FE. Anterior spine fusion for the treatment of tuberculosis of the spine: the operative findings and results of treatment in the first 100 cases. J Bone Joint Surg Am 1960;42:295–310
2. Raffa SJ, Benglis DM, Levi AD. Treatment of a persistent iatrogenic cerebrospinal fluid-pleural fistula with a cadaveric dural-pleural graft. Spine J 2009;9:e25–e29
3. Younes RN, Gross JL, Aguiar S, Haddad FJ, Deheinzelin D. When to remove a chest tube? A randomized study with subsequent prospective consecutive validation. J Am Coll Surg 2002;195:658–662
4. DiMarco AF, Oca O, Renston JP. Lung herniation. A cause of chronic chest pain following thoracotomy. Chest 1995;107:877–879
5. Rice TW, Kirsh JC, Schacter IB, Goldberg M. Simultaneous occurrence of chylothorax and subarachnoid pleural fistula after thoracotomy. Can J Surg 1987;30:256–258
6. Lubelski D, Abdullah KG, Steinmetz MP, et al. Lateral extracavitary, costotransversectomy, and transthoracic thoracotomy approaches to the thoracic spine: review of techniques and complications. J Spinal Disord Tech 2013;26:222–232
7. Faciszewski T, Winter RB, Lonstein JE, Denis F, Johnson L. The surgical and medical perioperative complications of anterior spinal fusion surgery in the thoracic and lumbar spine in adults. A review of 1223 procedures. Spine 1995;20:1592–1599
8. Campbell PG, Malone J, Yadla S, et al. Early complications related to approach in thoracic and lumbar spine surgery: a single center prospective study. World Neurosurg 2010;73:395–401

54 Open Lateral Transthoracic Diskectomy and Vertebrectomy

Tobias A. Mattei and Ehud Mendel

Open lateral transthoracic approaches provide several advantages for the treatment of lesions located at the anterior vertebral column and ventral to the spinal cord. Therefore, this approach is excellent for performing vertebrectomies as well as for thoracic diskectomies, especially in cases of central disk herniations.

Additionally, anterolateral access to the spine enables performing spinal decompression from pedicle to pedicle under direct visualization and reconstruction through a single approach, enabling anterior stabilization without the strict necessity of a posterior approach.

Crafoord et al[1] in 1958 and Perot and Munro[2] in 1969 pioneered the lateral transthoracic approach using a thoracotomy for the removal of herniated thoracic disks. The thoracotomy was an alternative to the pure posterior laminectomy, which entailed extreme morbidity, including high rates of paraplegia and death, and thus has been abandoned as an approach for thoracic herniated disks. Regarding thoracic disk herniations, the anterolateral transthoracic approach is best suited for centrally herniated disks.

The main disadvantage of anterolateral approaches is that they may entail the pulmonary complications of a thoracotomy, such as persistent pneumothorax, pulmonary contusion, pneumonia, pleural effusion, and empyema.

The specific details of the lateral transthoracic approach per se are presented in Chapter 53. In this chapter we focus on the operative nuances of performing diskectomies and vertebrectomies after a lateral transthoracic approach.

Indications

- Central or paracentral thoracic disk herniations causing neurologic symptoms (intractable radiculopathy or progressive myelopathy)[3]
- Diskitis
- Primary or metastatic vertebral neoplasms
- Unstable thoracic fractures
- Osteomyelitis or diskitis
- Spinal deformities and anterior release during scoliosis corrections
- Sequestered thoracic disk herniations causing neurologic symptoms

Contraindications

- Medical comorbidities, such as severe cardiopulmonary disease and acute respiratory distress syndrome (ARDS), which prevent safe access through the chest

Advantages

- Controlled exposure to the anterior portion of the dura
- Easier control of the radicular vessels
- Ability to reconstruct the anterior column (with either cages or bone strut grafts) and to place antero-lateral instrumentation

Disadvantages

- Increased incidence of pulmonary complications: atelectasis, pneumonia, pleural effusion, pulmonary contusion, chylothorax, persistent pneumothorax and bronchopulmonary fistula
- Possible increased incidence of medical complications as a result of a thoracotomy, such as thromboembolism and vascular injuries
- Increased postprocedural pain: postthoracotomy pain syndrome and intercostal neuralgia

Anesthesia and Positioning

Transthoracic diskectomies and vertebrectomies are performed using a standard lateral thoracotomy. For further details describing the approach, see Chapter 53. In addition to neurologic monitoring, adequate venous access and venous thrombosis prophylaxis, it is important to emphasize the necessity of the use of a double-lumen tube so that the lungs may be ventilated independently.

The transthoracic approach may be taken from either the right or the left side. The left side is typically favored by most surgeons for access to the lower thoracic spine due to the relative ease of mobilizing the aorta, as compared with the vena cava and azygous system found on the right side. Additionally, the orientation of the liver with respect to the spine also prompts most surgeons to favor the left-sided approach for operations around the thoracolumbar junction. In contrast, given the location of the great vessels, a right-sided posterolateral thoracotomy is usually the best choice to access the upper thoracic spine (from T2 to T6).

The patient is placed in the lateral decubitus position. Care is taken to ensure a 90-degree orientation to the floor. The lower leg is straightened, and the upper leg is bent to relax the ipsilateral psoas muscle and facilitate its dissection and mobilization away from the spine (**Fig. 54.1**).

Incision and Initial Dissection

X-rays are taken and the location for the skin incision is confirmed. The incision is made one to two levels above the level of interest, because the ribs tend to turn rostrally as they approach

362 IV Thoracic and Thoracolumbar Spine

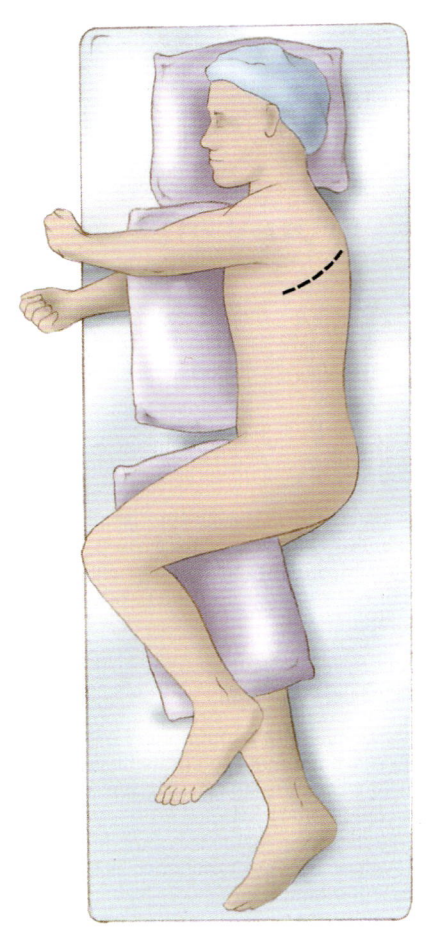

Fig. 54.1 Positioning and skin incision for an open lateral transthoracic approach to the upper thoracic spine. The location of the incision is based on the localization of the lesion according to the preoperative magnetic resonance imaging (MRI) and the fluoroscopic images. As a rule the incision should be placed one to two ribs higher than the disk space of interest.

the spine. Ultimately, the exact location of the incision should be based on the initial intraoperative image and should allow the surgeon a perpendicular access to the pathology.

After the skin is incised, the latissimus dorsi and serratus anterior muscles are incised. Subperiosteal dissection is used to expose the lateral aspect of the rib. The periosteum is then off of the medial aspect of the rib and a rib spreader is then placed.

Two standard approaches can be used to access the ventral thoracic spine, a retropleural or a transpleural route. The retropleural (or extrapleural) approach is performed within the space between the parietal pleura and the endothoracic fascia, a fascial layer tightly adherent to the periosteum of the rib and vertebral body. Blunt dissection is used to mobilize the pleura off the posterior chest wall and vertebral bodies.

In the transpleural approach, the ipsilateral lung is deflated and the parietal pleural between the ribs is incised. To expose the spinal structures, another layer of parietal pleura needs to be incised and flapped back with its base ventrally **(Fig. 54.2)**. This helps to expose the sympathetic chain, radicular vasculature, rib, and vertebral bodies.

As the first step to obtain full access to the neural foramen and intervertebral disk, it is necessary to first disarticulate the rib head and free it from its ligamentous (costotransverse and costovertebral) attachments using a down-going curette **(Fig. 54.3a)**. Then, the rib head is removed (with either an osteotome or a high-speed drill) and the anterior portion of the pedicle is drilled **(Fig. 54.3b)**.

The segmental vessels can be maintained when the goal is only removal of the disk (in the case of a thoracic disk herniation, for example), as these vessels lie midway between the disk spaces. By removing the rib, it is possible to identify the intercostal nerve from the undersurface of the rib and trace it back toward the neural foramen. This maneuver enables the surgeon to ascertain the location of the pedicle, the thecal sac, and the spinal cord. Then the diskectomies and vertebrectomies can be started.

Diskectomy

The disk is incised adjacent to the vertebral endplate using a No. 11 blade. Then a Freer elevator is used to dissect the disk

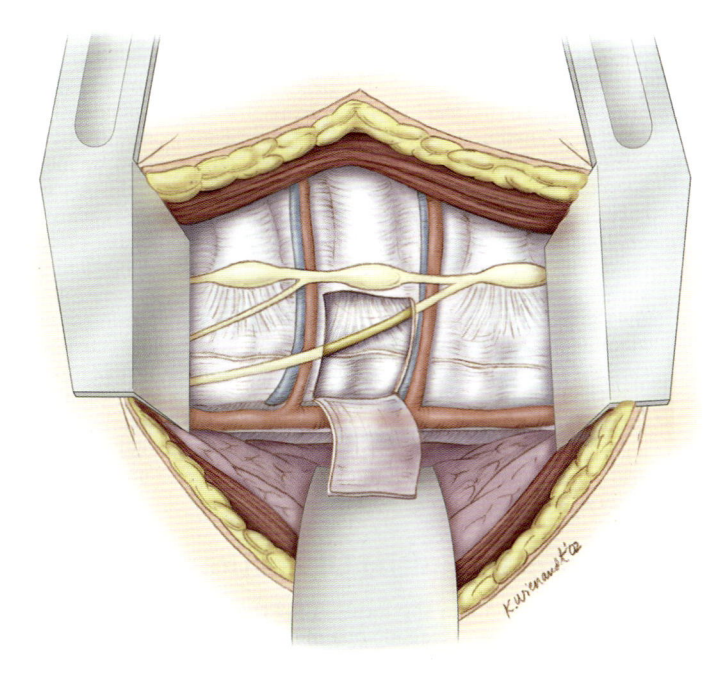

Fig. 54.2 After a lateral transthoracic approach, if a transpleural route is undertaken, the pleura is flapped back to expose the pathology. Here, the parietal pleural flap is based ventrally. At the end of the diskectomies and vertebrectomies, the pleura should be reapproximated.

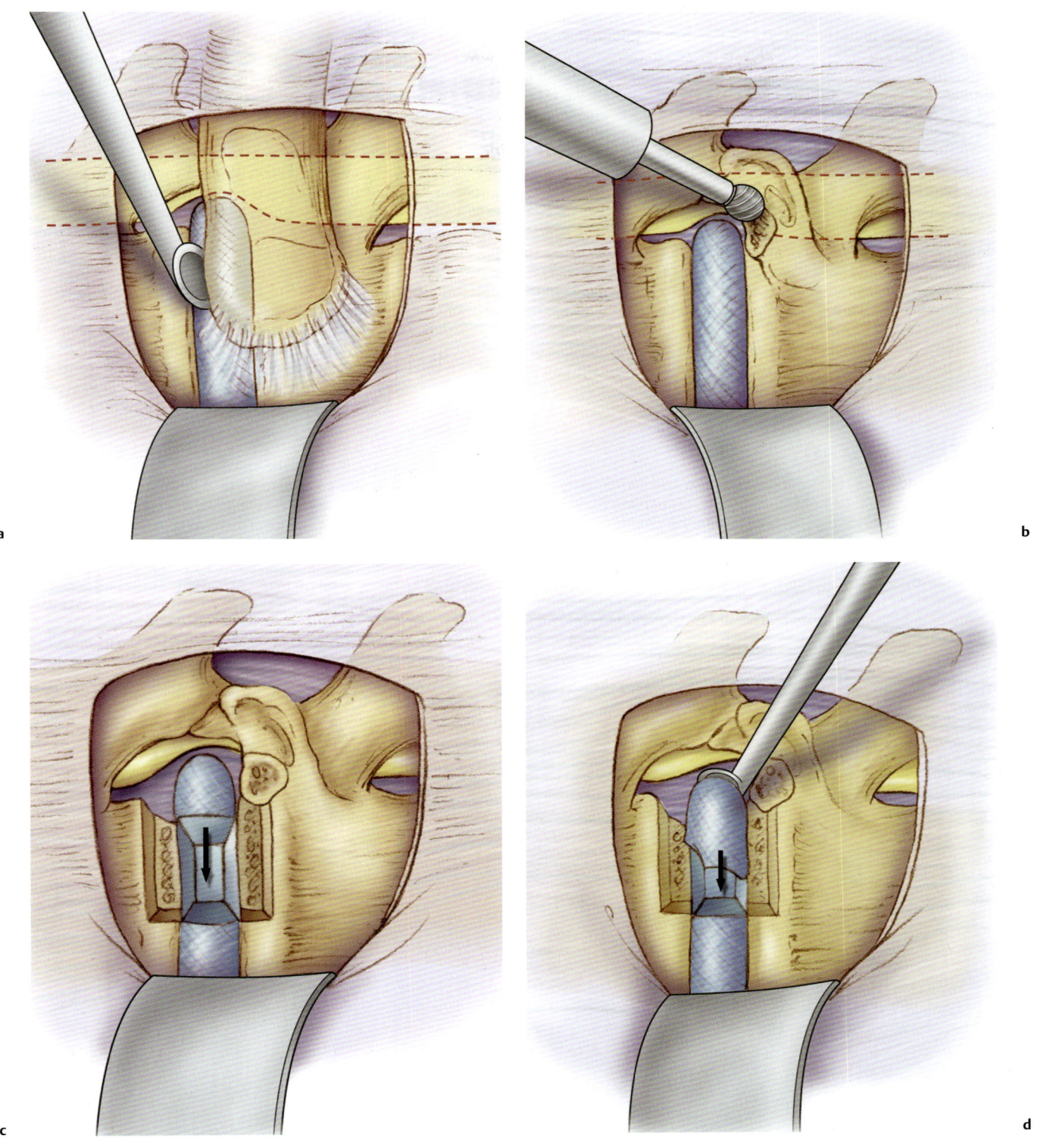

Fig. 54.3 Sequential steps of a thoracic diskectomy performed through a lateral transthoracic approach. **(a)** After exposing the head of the rib and the vertebral bodies, a down-going curette is used to free the rib head from its attachments to the vertebral body so that the disk space can be better visualized. At this point the head of the rib head is drilled to provide exposure of the neural foramen. **(b)** The drilling is extended to the upper portion of the pedicle, and a Kerrison rongeur is used to complete the exposure until the lateral aspect of the thecal sac is visualized. **(c)** The diskectomy should begin far from the thecal sac, creating a defect *(arrow)*. **(d)** Finally, a curette is used to push the remaining disk adjacent to the spinal cord toward the defect *(arrow)*, so that no pressure is exerted upon the spinal cord.

from the endplate in its whole extension. Then the diskectomy is performed. It is important to emphasize that, although the most posterior portion of the disk is closely related to the compression problem (in the case of thoracic disk herniations), the surgeon should first create a central cavity within the disk space (**Fig. 54.3c**). After that, the posterior portion of the disk adjacent to the thecal sac should be addressed. The correct maneuver is to push the disk fragments toward the cavity created in the center of the disk so that all forces are directed away from the spinal cord (**Fig. 54.3d**).

As it is common to observe calcifications and posterior osteophytes in the thoracic spine, it may be necessary to use down-going curettes to decompress the thecal sac. In order to minimize the epidural bleeding, the posterior longitudinal ligament should be kept intact throughout the diskectomy and, once this is completed, it may be cauterized and then removed as the last step.

At the end, a No. 4 Penfield or a Woodson can be used to inspect the whole anterolateral margin of the thecal sac from pedicle to pedicle to ensure that there are no hidden sequestered fragments left behind.

Vertebrectomy

Although there may be unique nuances to a vertebrectomy performed for a spinal tumor (**Fig. 54.4**) in comparison to one performed for a burst fracture, in general vertebrectomies performed through anterolateral approaches follow the same surgical principles of diskectomies. It is important to remember that, especially during vertebrectomies, positioning the patient with the spinal level of interest near the break of the table may significantly help obtaining proper exposure of the region (**Figs. 54.5 and 54.6**).

After resection of the head of the rib and identification of the neural foramen (**Fig. 54.7**), an empty shell should be created in the middle of the vertebral body, usually with a drill (**Fig. 54.8a**). In burst fractures, the bony fragments can be removed with a pituitary rongeur. When performing a vertebrectomy, diskectomies at the level above and below are required to enable reconstruction of the anterior column (either a cage or a bone graft strut) (**Fig. 54.8b**). In such cases we prefer to begin with the vertebrectomies, leaving the disks alone at the initial stage. One important caution that must be taken during the vertebrectomy is to avoid disruption of the endplates of the adjacent vertebrae, which may lead to late subsidence of the cage or bone graft used for anterior column reconstruction. In such cases, leaving the intervertebral disks intact at the initial portion of the vertebrectomy provides very useful landmarks for the limits of the vertebra which is intended to be resected.

After a large cavity is created in the middle of the vertebral body, the posterior portions of the body adjacent to the thecal sac can be removed by using curettes to push the fragments toward the empty cavity, making sure to direct all forces away from the thecal sac (**Fig. 54.9**). Finally, the posterior longitudinal ligament can be opened and the whole anterior aspect of the thecal sac can be inspected to ensure that there is no sequestrated fragment pushing on the spinal cord. After the diskectomies, the cartilaginous endplates are slightly drilled to enable bone contact with the cage or bone graft.

After the vertebrectomy and diskectomies, the anterior column must be reconstructed. The most common options are expandable titanium cages, carbon-fiber cages, and strut grafts, although cement can also be used (in such cases some surgeons prefer to inject the cement inside a chest tube to avoid cement extravasation toward the spinal canal). Each of these options has specific advantages and disadvantages. Expandable cages have the

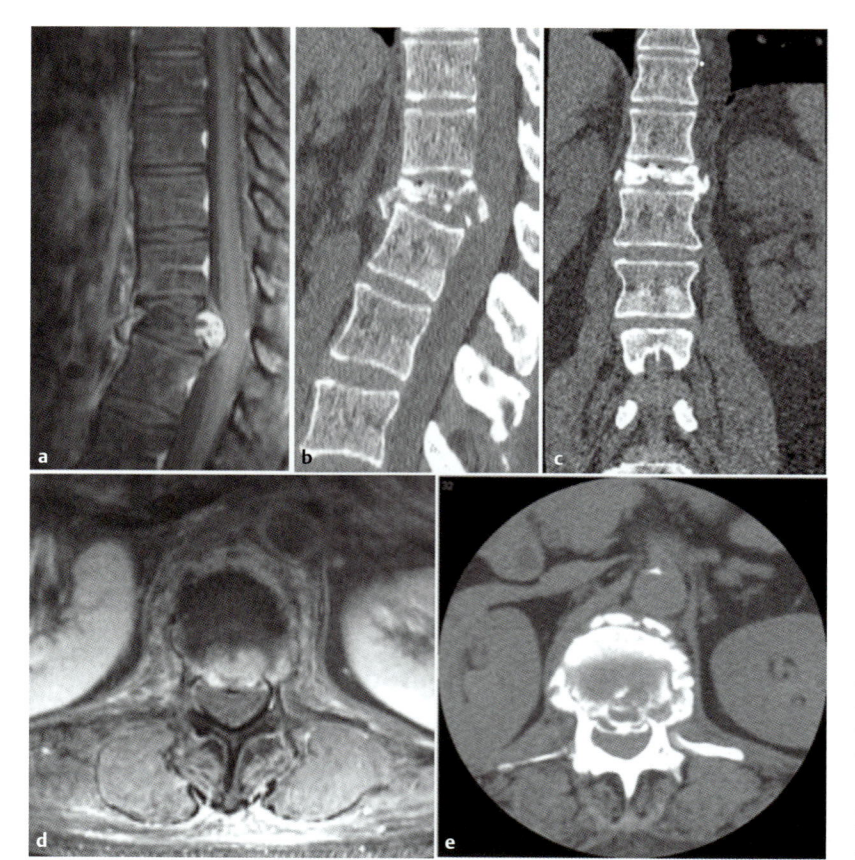

Fig. 54.4 Preoperative images of a 54-year-old patient with a history of metastatic breast carcinoma to the T12 vertebral body, leading to a compression fracture and moderate spinal cord compression. Sagittal **(a)** and axial **(d)** views of MRi with contrast. Sagittal **(a)**, coronal **(c)** and axial **(e)** slices of CT-scan. The patient was neurologically intact. The patient was submitted to a T12 vertebrectomy through a lateral transthoracic approach, as demonstrated in **Figs. 54.5 to 54.12**.

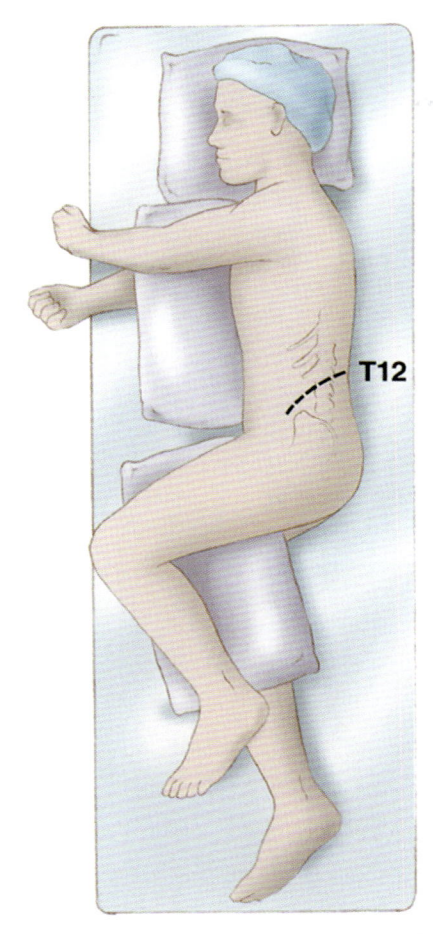

54 Open Lateral Transthoracic Diskectomy and Vertebrectomy

Fig. 54.5 The lateral decubitus position for a standard lateral thoracotomy for addressing the T12 vertebral body. The approach through the left side offers the advantage of avoiding liver retraction. Additionally, it is easier to deal with any eventual bleeding from the aorta than one from the vena cava.

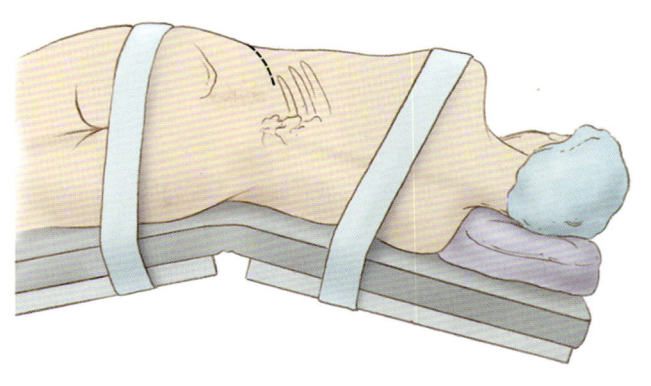

Fig. 54.6 The lateral view showing the incision for a T12 corpectomy. It is useful to position the region of interest at the level of the break of the table, so that the table can be flexed to increase the exposure to the pathological vertebrae.

capacity to be distracted and, therefore may enable further correction of local kyphosis. Additionally, by distracting the cage, it becomes more strongly impacted between the two vertebrae, reducing the chances of hardware extrusion. Carbon-fiber cages provide the unique advantage of being radiolucent, and therefore are ideal for anterior reconstructions after vertebrectomies performed for oncological reasons, enabling optimal follow-up images for surveilling of tumor recurrence, without the usual artifacts generated by titanium cages. Additionally, stackable carbon-fiber cages are significantly more robust than expandable titanium cages, enabling more bone to be compacted inside the cage (**Fig. 54.10**). Bone strut grafts have the best profile for bone growth and fusion in comparison to synthetic cages. Cement reconstruction with polymethylmethacrylate (PMMA), although being more laborious and not enabling bone fusion at the anterior column gap, is much less expensive than synthetic cages, and therefore may be a good option in limited-resources settings or during palliative surgery for patients with advanced stages of cancer.

Finally, after reconstruction of the anterior column, a lateral plate system is usually used to provide additional structural support to the construct. Some plate systems enable distraction between the lateral screws, enabling an optimal opening of the

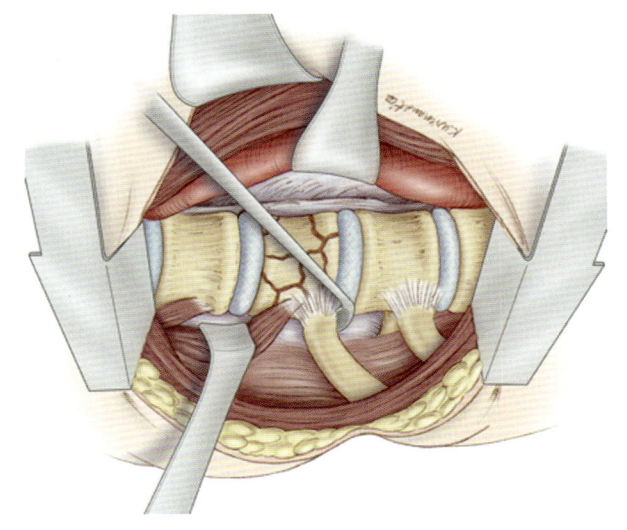

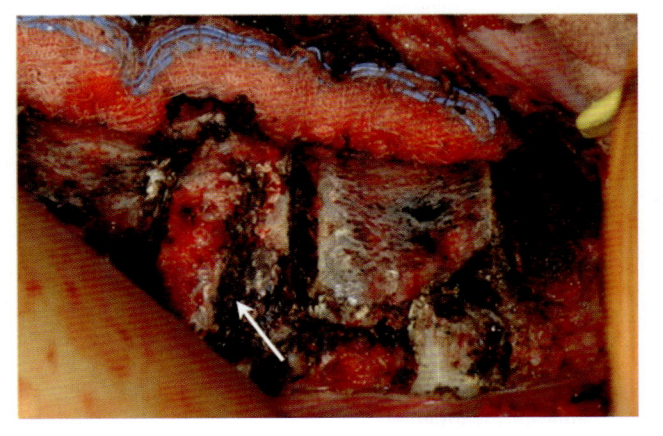

Fig. 54.7 To achieve access to the thoracolumbar transition, after a lateral transthoracic approach is performed (either trans- or retropleurally), it may be necessary to divide the diaphragm. **(a)** After exposure of the spinal structures, a curette is used to free the rib head from its attachments to the vertebral body so that the disk space located directly medial to the rib can be better visualized. **(b)** A folded sponge in a cylinder shape is used to dissect and separate the spinal structures from the great vessels.

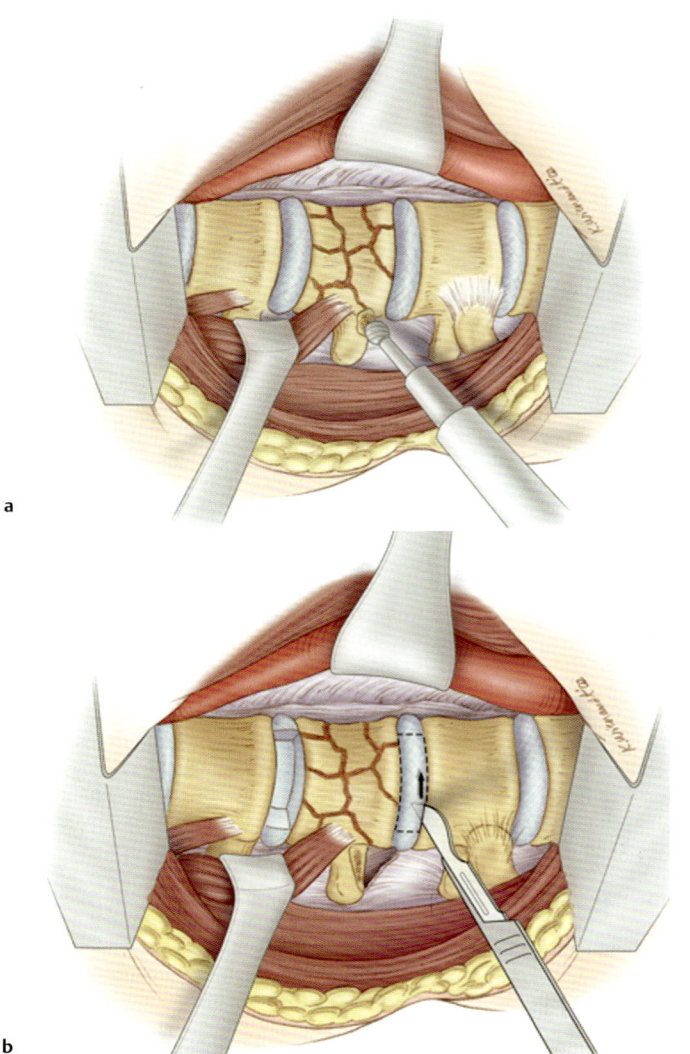

Fig. 54.8 (a) A high-speed drill is used to remove the head of the rib as well as the upper portion of the pedicle. A Kerrison rongeur can be used to complete the exposure of the neural foramen and the lateral aspect of the thecal sac. (b) During the diskectomies and the vertebrectomy, it is recommended to create an empty cavity at the central region so that it becomes possible to push the remaining bone and disk located adjacent to the thecal sac toward the defect (arrows). Proceeding in this fashion, all pressure is directed away from the spinal cord. (b) In the sequence, after completing the vertebrectomy, the diskectomies above and below the vertebrae of interest are performed.

Fig. 54.9 (a) During the diskectomies and the vertebrectomy, it is recommended to create an empty cavity at the central region so that it becomes possible to push the remaining bone and disk located adjacent to the thecal sac toward the defect *(arrows)*. Proceeding in this fashion, all pressure is directed away from the spinal cord. (b) After completion of the vertebrectomy and diskectomies, it is possible to achieve ample visualization of the anterolateral aspect of the thecal sac and the emerging nerve root.

space previously occupied by the vertebral body and the achievement of parallel endplates (**Fig. 54.11**). In dual-screw systems, the anterior screw should be oriented posteriorly and the posterior screw should be oriented anteriorly (**Fig. 54.12**).

Regarding the biomechanical strength of instrumentation following corpectomies, it has been shown that anterolateral plating stabilizes short posterior fixations but does not markedly affect long constructs stability.[4] In fact, following thoracolumbar en-bloc spondylectomy, it is the posterior fixation of more than one adjacent segment that determines stability. In contrast, short posterior fixation does not sufficiently restore stability, even with an anterolateral plate. Regarding to the method of anterior column reconstruction, the use of expandable versus nonexpandable cages does not seem to markedly affect stability.

In terms of clinical outcomes, surgical series have shown no difference in estimated intraoperative blood loss, performance status, pain outcomes (as measured on a Visual Analogue Scale [VAS]), or survival between anterior column reconstruction with expandable cages in comparison to PMMA, although there was a trend of better kyphotic reduction in the patients in whom expandable cages were used.[5]

Closure

If the diaphragm was incised for access to the spine near the thoracolumbar junction, it must be reattached at its lateral margin, with its crura being sewn directly to the anterior longitudinal ligament. Additionally, it is recommended to attempt to primarily

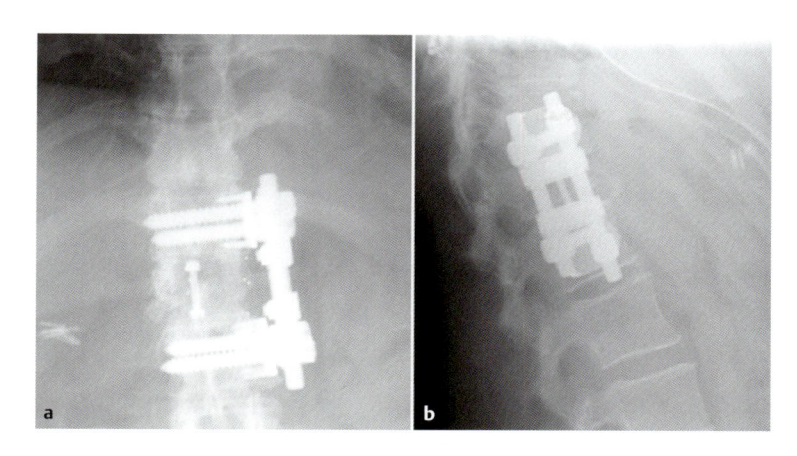

Fig. 54.10 Before implantation of the bone strut graft or interbody cage, it is important to make sure that the vertebral endplates are aligned. **(a)** The lateral plate (which can accommodate one or two screws in each vertebra, depending on the specific system) is positioned before the insertion of the screws. **(b)** After the insertion of the screws, it is possible to improve the alignment of the vertebral body endplates by retracting between the screws.

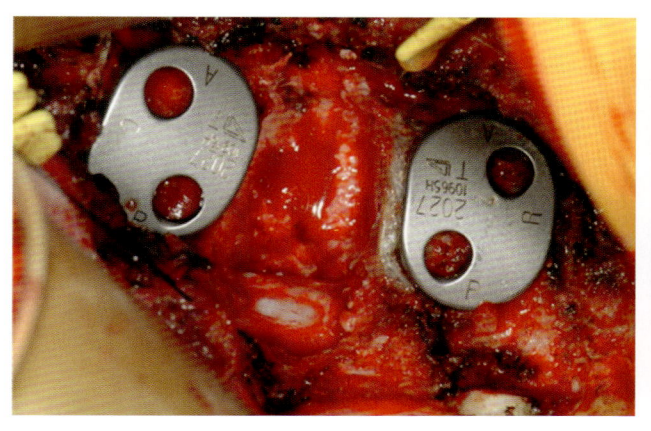

Fig. 54.11 **(a,b)** Postoperative X-rays after the T12 corpectomy through a lateral transthoracic approach and anterior column reconstruction with a carbon-fiber cage and anterolateral plating. Although not being expandable, the stackable carbon-fiber cage is advantageous in the setting of tumors as it is radiolucent and does not generate MRI artifacts as the titanium cages do.

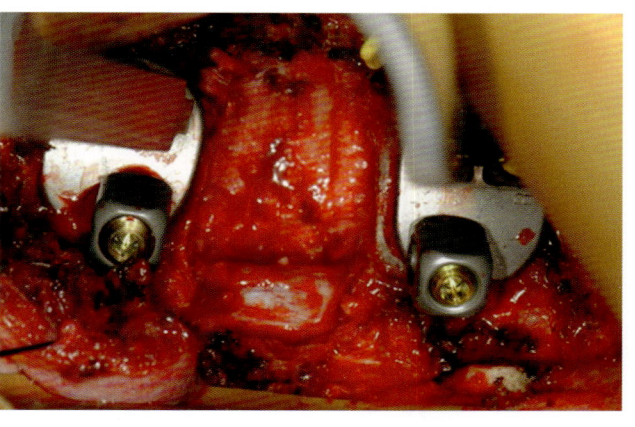

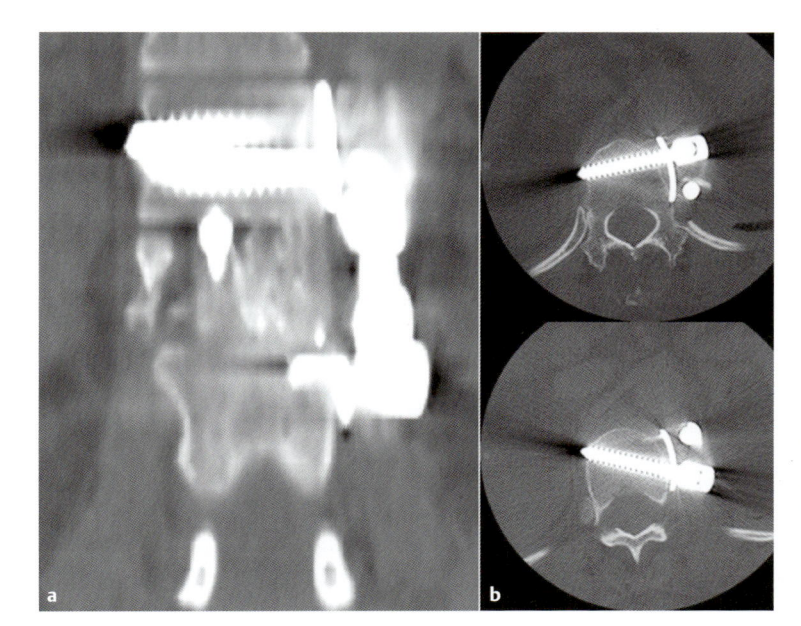

Fig. 54.12 Late postoperative computed tomography (CT) scan (**a**, sagittal; **b,c**, axial) after the T12 corpectomy demonstrating fusion between the bone inside the stackable carbon-fiber cage and the vertebrae above. Note that the lateral screws should be preferentially bicortical. Additionally, when using a dual-screw lateral plating system, the anterior screw should be oriented posteriorly **(b)**, whereas the posterior screw should be oriented anteriorly **(c)**.

close any occasional violations to the peritoneum. If this is not possible, the hole must be enlarged, as the main concern in such cases is bowel strangulation and secondary ischemia of bowel loops.

If the parietal pleura was entered, it is closed as well, overlying the operative site. If a retropleural exposure was performed, the wound should be filled with saline to confirm that no occult pleural laceration took place. If the pleura was entered, a chest tube is placed and tunneled out through a separate incision. After the wound is fully closed, the chest tube is placed on low wall suctioning and the lung is reinflated under direct visualization.

The intercostal musculature is closed using a running suture. The remaining tissue layers are closed with interrupted sutures. Subcuticular running suture can be used to close the skin. A sterile dressing is applied. Whether or not the pleura was entered, it is recommended to perform a chest X-ray in the recovery room or in the immediate postoperative period.

References

1. Crafoord C, Hiertonn T, Lindblom K, Olsson SE. Spinal cord compression caused by a protruded thoracic disc; report of a case treated with anterolateral fenestration of the disc. Acta Orthop Scand 1958;28:103–107
2. Perot PL Jr, Munro DD. Transthoracic removal of midline thoracic disc protrusions causing spinal cord compression. J Neurosurg 1969;31:452–458
3. Vollmer DG, Simmons NE. Transthoracic approaches to thoracic disc herniations. Neurosurg Focus 2000;9:e8
4. Disch AC, Schaser KD, Melcher I, Luzzati A, Feraboli F, Schmoelz W. En bloc spondylectomy reconstructions in a biomechanical in-vitro study. Eur Spine J 2008;17:715–725
5. Eleraky M, Papanastassiou I, Tran ND, Dakwar E, Vrionis FD. Comparison of polymethylmethacrylate versus expandable cage in anterior vertebral column reconstruction after posterior extracavitary corpectomy in lumbar and thoraco-lumbar metastatic spine tumors. Eur Spine J 2011;20:1363–1370

55 Endoscopic Lateral Transthoracic Approach

Justin C. Clark and Curtis A. Dickman

The surgical treatment of lesions affecting the anterior thoracic spine is challenging. Unlike mass lesions in the cervical and lumbar spine, the kyphotic curvature of the thoracic spine makes the posterior decompression of mass lesions compressing the anterior spinal cord untenable. The lessons about the difficulty of treatment were readily learned through cases of herniated thoracic disks treated with laminectomy, where posterior decompression led to unsatisfactory patient results.[1-4] From these experiences, it became clear that adequate surgical treatment of compressive thoracic lesions would require anterior approaches.

Surgical approaches to the anterior thoracic spine in the late 1950s were first described by Hodgson and Stock.[5] However, a desire to minimize the morbidity associated with this approach led surgeons to explore less invasive techniques.

Endoscopic approaches to the intrathoracic space were pioneered by cardiothoracic surgeons around 1990. Using new video-assisted thoracoscopic surgery (VATS) techniques, surgeons were able to accomplish via endoscopy many intrathoracic procedures that previously required an open thoracotomy. Soon after the development of VATS, the treatment of anterolateral thoracic spine pathology with endoscopic techniques was developed.[6,7]

The levels of the thoracic spine that can be accessed by the endoscopic lateral transthoracic approach (ELTA) vary with the type of surgery being performed. Certainly, the entirety of the thoracic spine from T1 through T12 can be visualized by this approach; consequently, endoscopy can be used to adequately treat paraspinal lesions from T1 through T12. However, because decompression of the anterior spinal cord requires that entry ports be placed parallel to the operative vertebral bodies or disk spaces, our experience has led us to believe that the ELTA should be used primarily to decompress the anterior thoracic spinal cord from T4 to T11.[8]

In the previous edition of this atlas, only a single chapter was devoted to anterior approaches to the thoracic spine. The pace at which minimally invasive surgical (MIS) techniques for the thoracic spine has evolved during the past decade is reflected in the fact that this edition devotes two of its three anterior thoracic spine approach chapters to MIS approaches (endoscopic and retropleural). As the popularity of these MIS techniques increases and demand rises, the breadth of surgical instruments available to the endoscopic spine surgeon will also increase. No doubt this resultant increase in technology will decrease the upfront learning curve and improve overall patient outcomes.

Patient Selection

Patients with pathologies involving the thoracic spine and paraspinal structures, along with the thoracic nerve roots and sympathetic chain, who have been considered for open thoracotomy may be candidates for the ELTA. For patients to be eligible for this procedure, they must be healthy enough to safely undergo single-lung ventilation. Morbidly obese patients often have excessive pleural fat, which makes visualization of the spine and paraspinal structures difficult from the endoscopic lateral thoracic approach; thus, this approach is usually not suitable for these patients.

Objective, Indications, and Contraindications

The objective of this chapter is to familiarize the surgeon with the basic steps involved in an ELTA to the spine, as well as the pertinent anatomy associated with the approach. Further illustration of the steps necessary to perform this surgery is provided in Video 55.1 Indications and contraindications for the ELTA are described in **Table 55.1**.

Advantages

- Less approach-related morbidity than with an open thoracotomy
- Shorter postoperative hospital stays than with an open thoracotomy
- Excellent visualization of the thoracic spine and its adjacent paraspinal anatomy
- Access to multiple thoracic spinal levels

Disadvantages

- Requires specialized endoscopic instruments
- Relatively steep learning curve
- Inadequate for dealing with complicated cerebrospinal fluid (CSF) leaks

Choice of Operative Approach

Many nuanced decisions must be made that are specific to each patient being considered for an ELTA to treat the patient's pathology. However, some general principles are discussed here. The most important variable to consider when choosing the ELTA for a patient is the surgeon's comfort level with the approach. It is recommended that the surgeon complete a significant number of proctored cases, as well as spend time in an endoscopic laboratory, before attempting this approach independently in patients. Next, it is important to determine whether the pathology is amenable to treatment with the ELTA. Our experience has taught us that certain lesions, such as giant ossified herniated thoracic disks, are poor candidates for this approach, because the ELTA does not enable the fine dissection movements required to deal with these formidable lesions, and the approach

Table 55.1 Endoscopic Lateral Transthoracic Approach

Indications	Contraindications
• Degenerative	• Prior thoracotomy on the side of access (high likelihood of dense pleural adhesions)
○ Herniated thoracic disk(s)	• Patient's inability to tolerate single-lung ventilation (e.g., poor pulmonary function)
○ Anterior release of scoliotic deformity	• Morbid obesity
• Trauma	• Surgeon's inability to access the surgical pathology because of proximity to the great vessels
○ Traumatic herniated thoracic disk	
• Infection	
○ Osteomyelitis/diskitis	
○ Abscess	
• Sympathectomy	
• Neoplasm	
○ Paraspinal neoplasm	
○ Spinal metastasis	
○ Primary spinal neoplasm	
○ Nerve sheath tumors	

does not enable the surgeon to deal with likely intraoperative complications, such as needing to repair a CSF leak. For these cases, a traditional open thoracotomy is preferred. That being said, the ELTA is well suited for treating pathologies that require a vast array of surgical maneuvers, including drilling, bimanual dissection, spinal cord decompression, sectioning of paraspinal vascular structures, and placement of spinal instrumentation.

Preoperative Testing

- Preoperative chest radiograph for rib count, to identify anomalous ribs
- Magnetic resonance imaging (MRI) or computed tomography (CT) from the clivus down to the level of the pathology
- Preoperative clearance from the internal medicine department
- Pulmonary function tests, if the patient has borderline pulmonary reserve

Surgical Procedure

Anesthesia

After being brought into the operating room, the patient is intubated by the anesthesiologist using a dual-lumen endotracheal tube (ETT), which allows for selective single-lung ventilation during the procedure. The proper placement of the ETT must be verified by the anesthesiologist via auscultation of breath sounds bilaterally, as well as maintenance of normal oxygenation parameters. Once the patient is intubated and under general anesthesia, invasive cardiac monitoring lines are placed to enable the precise measurement of systolic and diastolic blood pressure during the procedure. Large-bore intravenous access is achieved preoperatively to enable large-volume fluid replacement, in the event that one of the great vessels is damaged during surgery. Neuromonitoring leads are placed to record somatosensory, with or without motor, evoked potentials. A Foley catheter is placed for procedures lasting more than 1 hour.

Positioning

Upon completion of the steps noted above, the patient is then placed on the operating table in the lateral decubitus position with a deflatable beanbag underneath (**Fig. 55.1**). All pressure points are identified and well padded, which includes placing pillows between the legs at the levels of the knees and ankles. The head is supported with a pillow, and adequate access to the ETT is maintained throughout, so the anesthesiologist can troubleshoot airway issues during the procedure. An axillary roll is placed under the dependent arm, which is supported on an arm board. The nondependent arm is supported on an airplane splint and abducted up and out of the way of the surgical field. This provides wide surgical access to the lateral chest wall.

Before the beanbag is deflated, the patient is positioned in the manner required for the operation. For procedures requiring access to the upper thoracic spine and mobilization of the lung, the patient is positioned in a three-quarters prone position (**Fig. 55.2a**). Further passive lung mobilization can be achieved by placing the patient in the reverse Trendelenburg position and rotating the patient anteriorly. However, for procedures requiring access to the intervertebral disk spaces and placement of spinal instrumentation, the patient must be placed exactly perpendicular to the operative table (**Fig. 55.2b**). By keeping the patient perpendicular to the table, the surgeon can maintain proper orientation of hardware and facilitate perfect placement of screws in the spine. Upon proper positioning, the patient is well taped to the operating table to prevent movement during the procedure. The anesthesiologist and circuitry are positioned at the head of the bed and the endoscopic video monitors are positioned across from the spine surgeons (**Fig. 55.3**).

55 Endoscopic Lateral Transthoracic Approach

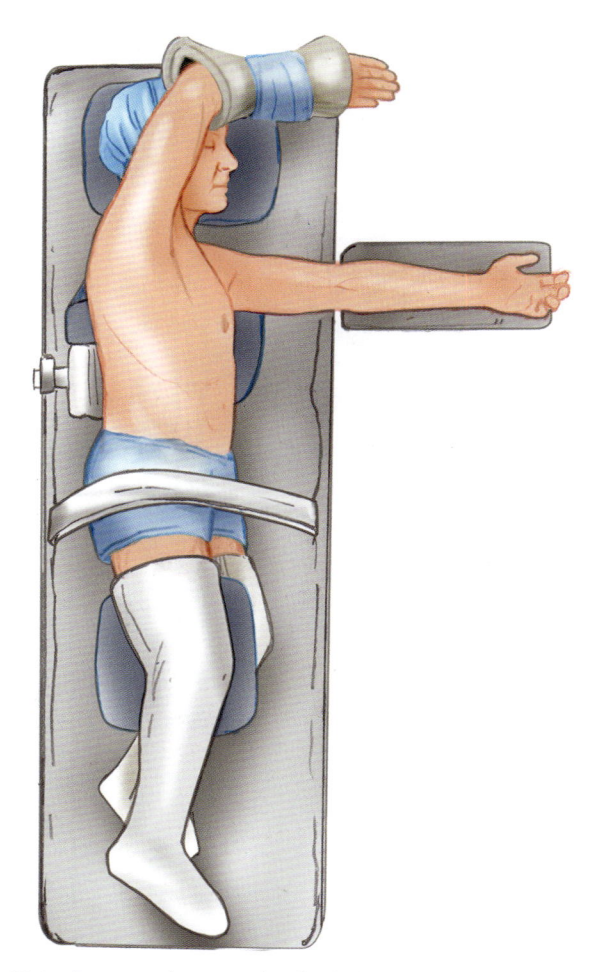

Fig. 55.1 Illustration of a patient placed in the left lateral decubitus position, in preparation for a right-sided endoscopic lateral transthoracic approach to the spine. The arm is supported in an airplane splint and abducted away from the surgical site. All pressure points are identified and well padded.

Localization

Correct localization of surgical levels in the thoracic spine is complicated, as compared with the cervical or lumbar spine. The presence of ribs and thoracic organs obscures the elements of the thoracic spine. The task is made even more challenging in patients who are obese or who have aberrant anatomy (e.g., anomalous ribs). Although the reported incidence of wrong-level surgeries in the thoracic spine is low, there is a concern that this problem is underreported in the literature.[9] However, wrong-level surgery can be avoided if the proper steps are followed. These steps include a preoperative chest radiograph for rib count, to identify any deviation from the normal number of ribs, as well as MRI or CT images that extend from the clivus down to the level of the pathology, and anterior-posterior fluoroscopy to count the ribs intraoperatively.

Incision Planning

Once the patient is positioned on the operating table, intraoperative fluoroscopy is used to count up from the lowest rib to the level of the pathology. Once the proper levels are identified, the vertebral bodies are marked on the patient using a surgical marker, and the incisions are planned directly lateral to the level of pathology (**Fig. 55.4a**). The number of incisions is dictated by the number of ports required during the case. In relatively simple cases, such as endoscopic sympathectomies, only two ports are required: one port for the endoscope and one port for the working instrument. A more complex case may require five or more ports to provide adequate access to the spinal pathology.

Port Selection

In keeping with the goal of minimizing patient morbidity, selected ports are expected to lead to minimal pain postoperatively. For this reason, either small rigid 5-mm ports or larger 1-cm flexible ports are used. Both types of ports attempt to put minimal compression on the intercostal nerve bundle running on the caudal aspect of each rib, thus decreasing postoperative intercostal pain.

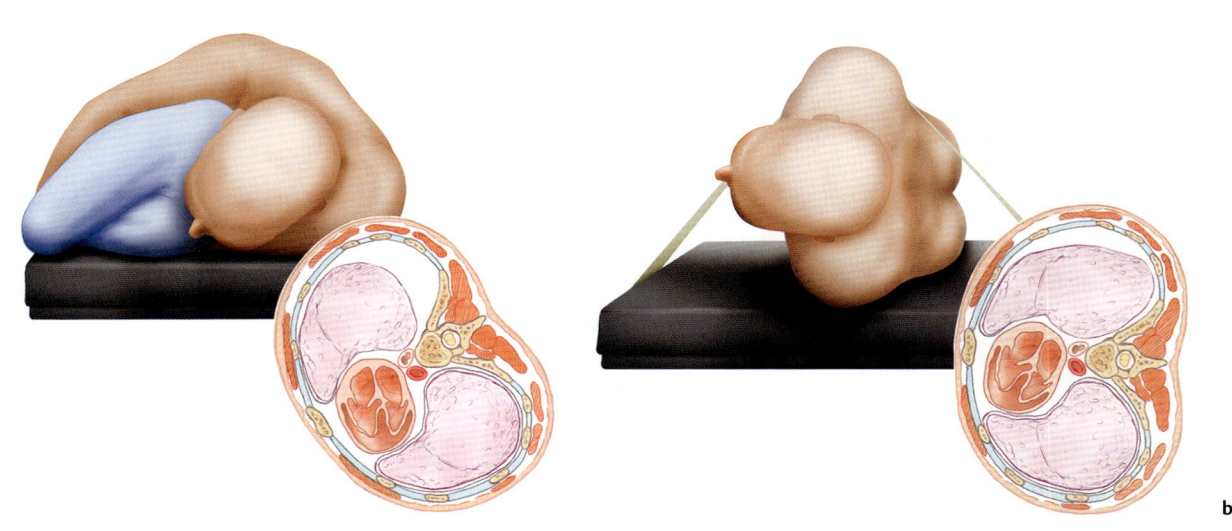

Fig. 55.2 A patient undergoing the endoscopic lateral transthoracic approach can be placed in either the three-quarters prone position **(a)**, to facilitate lung mobilization, or in the 90-degree position with the shoulders and hips perpendicular to the ground **(b)**, to facilitate the placement of spinal hardware.

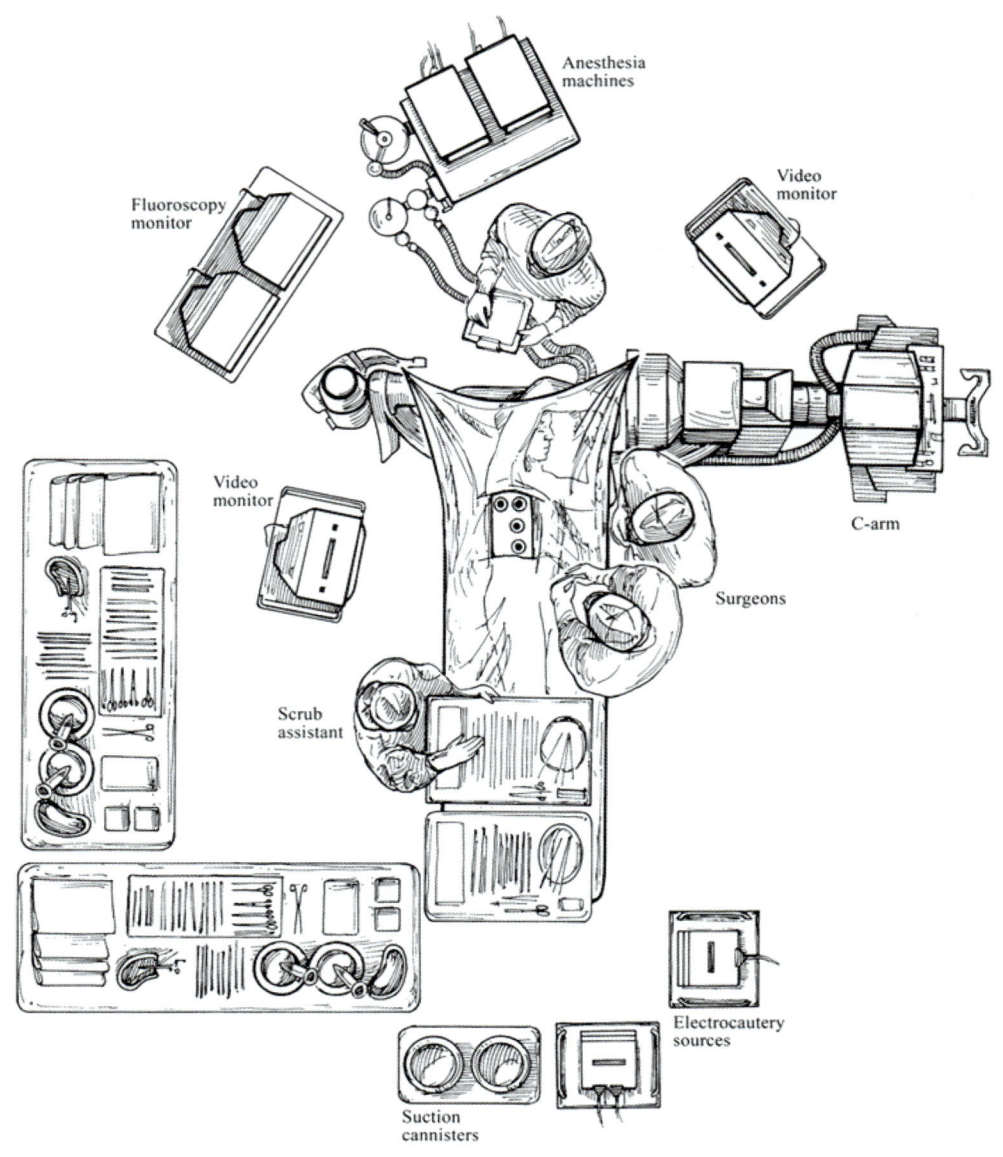

Fig. 55.3 The operating room is set up to provide the spine surgeons with full access to the patient and the surgical instruments, and with direct visualization of the endoscopic video screens and fluoroscopy screens. The anesthesiologist is positioned at the head of the bed to provide easy access for troubleshooting during the procedure. A fluoroscope can easily be maneuvered into position during the procedure, to assist with localization of pathology or placement of spinal instrumentation.

Port Placement

Incisions for the ports are placed in either the anterior axillary or posterior axillary line (**Fig. 55.4b**). The ports placed in the anterior axillary line are used for the working instruments and endoscope. The ports placed in the posterior axillary line are used for the endoscope and instruments for placing spinal hardware (**Fig. 55.5**).

Incision

Once the planned portal incisions have been mapped out, a potential thoracotomy incision that incorporates the portal incisions is drawn, which enables rapid conversion to an open thoracotomy if necessary during the surgery. If the surgeon is not credentialed by the hospital to perform open thoracotomy, then an approach surgeon needs to be available throughout the procedure, should emergent conversion to open thoracotomy be required. Next, the chest wall is prepped and draped using chlorhexidine and antimicrobial surgical drapes. Intercostal blocks are completed using 0.25% bupivacaine HCl with epinephrine, to assist with postoperative pain control. Incisions are made with a scalpel, and hemostasis is achieved with monopolar electrocautery. The anesthesiologist is then instructed to selectively ventilate only the dependent lung, allowing the ipsilateral lung to fall away from the chest wall. The thoracic cavity then is accessed using a hemostat, taking care not to damage the underlying lung parenchyma. The access point in the parietal pleura is then widened using the hemostat until it is large enough for the chosen port to be successfully positioned within it.

55 Endoscopic Lateral Transthoracic Approach

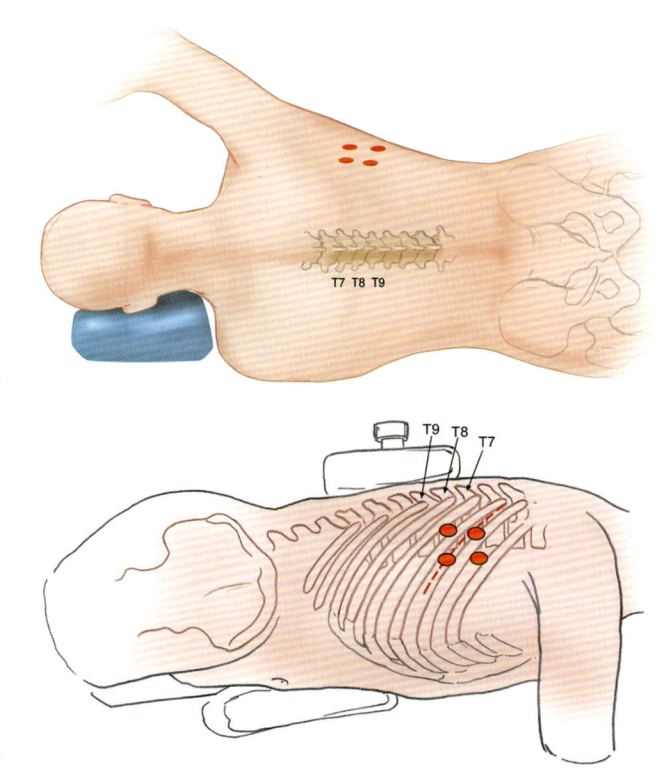

Fig. 55.4 (a) Fluoroscopy is used to identify the surgical levels, which are then marked on the patient's skin. (b) Once the surgical levels are identified, the incisions are planned perpendicular to the spine, in the anterior and posterior axillary lines.

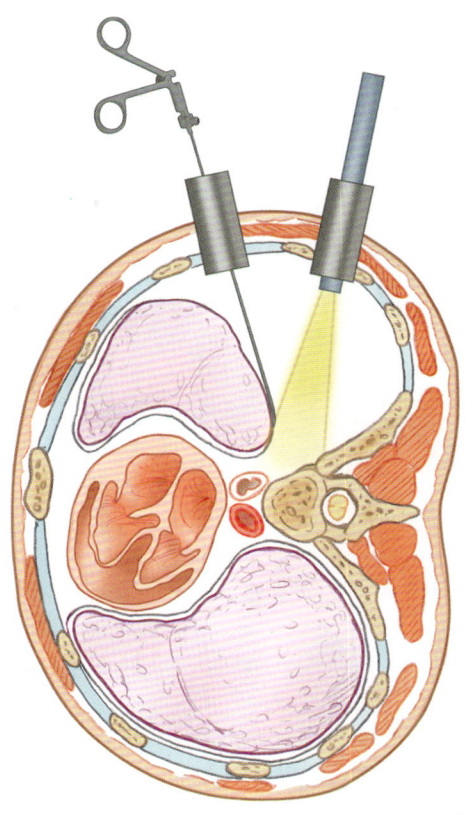

Fig. 55.5 Endoscopy ports are placed in the anterior and posterior axillary lines.

Introduction of Instruments

The endoscope is introduced into the thoracic cavity through the first access port to visualize the thoracic cavity. At this point, the lung should be partially deflated and should have fallen away from the chest wall. If the lung is still obstructing the operative site, several steps can be taken. The anesthesiologist can be asked to suction the lung, to actively deflate the lung. Once other ports have been placed, a fan retractor can be used to help retract the lung and keep it out of the way during surgery (**Fig. 55.6**). Care must be taken not to damage the lung during these maneuvers. Rotating the patient anteriorly can cause the lung to fall away from the spine, thus increasing the surgical space near the spine (**Fig. 55.2a**). In the same manner, placing the patient in the reverse Trendelenburg position when operating at the upper aspect of the thoracic spine can also help the lung to fall away from the surgical level. It is important to inspect the lung with the endoscope both at the beginning and end of the procedure to ensure that the lung parenchyma remains intact. Violation of the lung parenchyma can lead to an air leak and potentially increase patient morbidity. The endoscope is also used to look for lung adhesions. When minor adhesions are encountered, they can often be removed using endoscopic scissors through the same port as the endoscope (**Fig. 55.7**). If excessive adhesions are encountered, then it may be wise to abort the endoscopic approach and either convert to an open thoracotomy approach or reevaluate for a non-transthoracic approach to treat the lesion.

Once the surgeon is able to visualize that there is a safe distance between the lung and chest wall, then the subsequent ports can be introduced under direct visual guidance, using the endoscope (**Fig. 55.8**). This technique provides for safer introduction of ports, decreasing the risk of injury to the underlying lung. As mentioned earlier, it is imperative that ports be placed precisely, to provide adequate surgical access via the endoscopic technique. However, if upon entering the thoracic cavity, the surgeon discovers that the ports were placed in error in one of the four cardinal directions, extra ports can be placed without significant difficulty. This is in contrast to the open thoracotomy approach, for which making a new incision is very difficult to deal with cosmetically. The only real option in an open thoracotomy is to extend the incision in the anterior-posterior direction. Only through increased retraction on the adjacent ribs will extra cranial-caudal exposure be achieved in an open approach.

Procedure

After placing all of the ports necessary for the procedure, the surgeon can introduce the endoscopic instruments and begin the surgery. During the surgery, fluoroscopy can be easily brought into the surgical field whenever necessary (**Fig. 55.3**). Surgical aspects that are specific to various endoscopic thoracic cases are discussed in other chapters in this book.

Closure

After the surgical goals of the operation have been met, the closing portion of the procedure begins. Whenever possible, any parietal pleura that have been incised should be brought back together with Weck clips (**Fig. 55.9**). We believe that it is prudent

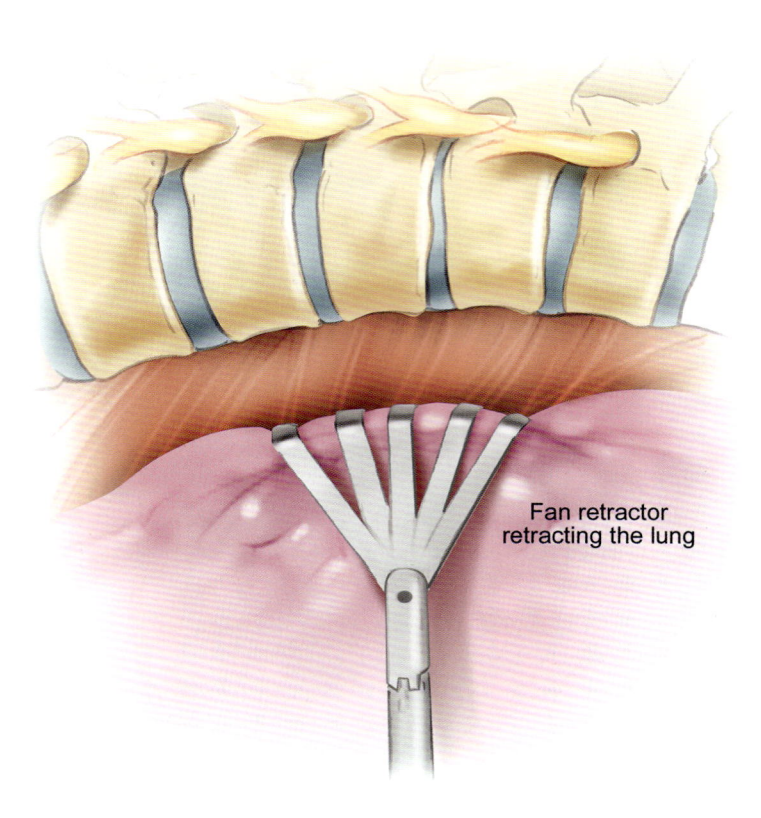

Fig. 55.6 If the lung is difficult to mobilize, a fan retractor can be used to help mobilize the lung out of the way.

to place a catheter of some kind at the end of every thoracic surgery, to evacuate as much air as possible from the thoracic cavity. This can be accomplished with either a traditional chest tube or a red rubber catheter. When a chest tube is placed, the surgeon has the option of removing it either at the end of the procedure or after the patient has recovered in the hospital during the postoperative period. Either way, the chest tube is tunneled out through one of the existing incisions from the placement of the ports. If the chest tube is kept in place overnight, then it is secured using a 2-0 nylon suture via a purse-string closure. A red rubber catheter is placed with the intention of removing it before the end of the procedure. The lung is then reinflated under direct endoscopic visualization, and the endoscopic ports are removed. The incisions are closed in layers. Absorbable 0-0 Vicryl

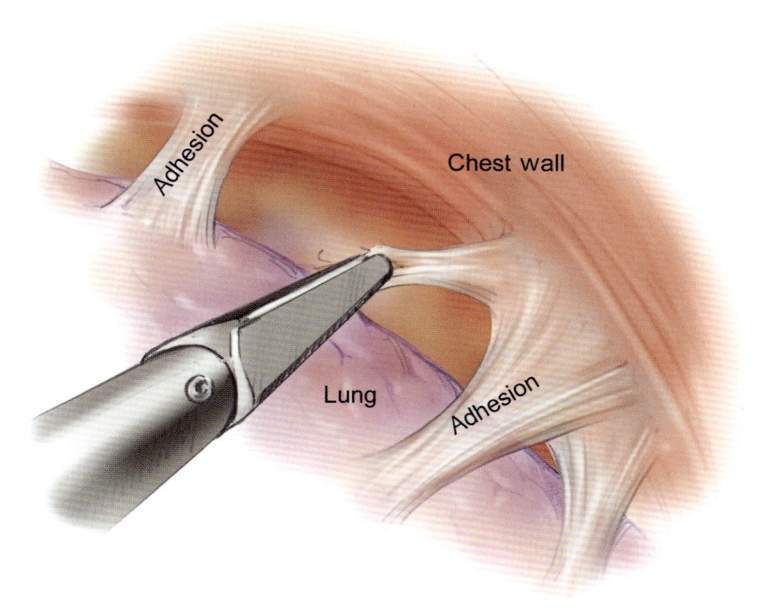

Fig. 55.7 When minor lung adhesions are encountered, they can be removed using endoscopic scissors.

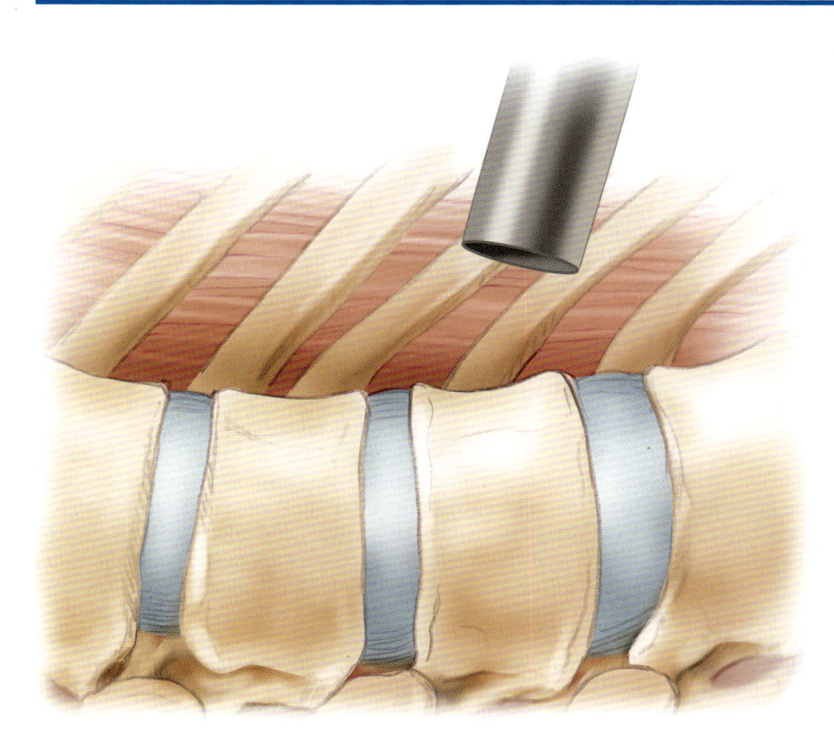

Fig. 55.8 Portals are placed under direct visualization, with the endoscope inserted in the first portal.

sutures (Ethicon, Inc., Somerville, NJ) are placed in an interrupted fashion to bring together the muscle layers. Smaller 3-0 Vicryl sutures are placed at the dermal-epidermal junction in an interrupted fashion to bring the skin together. A 4-0 Monocryl suture (Ethicon, Inc.) is placed in a subcuticular running fashion, followed by a layer of Dermabond (Ethicon, Inc.) to finalize the skin closure.

Postoperative Care

Most patients are extubated immediately at the end of the procedure. Surgeries of short duration that involve minimal pleural disruption, such as endoscopic thoracic sympathectomies, often allow the patient the option of being discharged later that same day. However, most other types of cases require the patient to remain in the hospital at least overnight for observation. All patients are given an incentive spirometer while in the hospital and upon discharge. They are instructed on how to use it and told to continue using it until their first postoperative visit at 10 to 14 days after the operation.

The postoperative period is highlighted by pain control, mobilization, and ensuring adequate pulmonary toilet (i.e., pulmonary hygiene). Adequate pain control should not be overlooked. If the patient's incisional pain is uncontrolled, then splinting can occur, which limits the patient's ability to inhale deeply, putting the patient at risk for atelectasis.

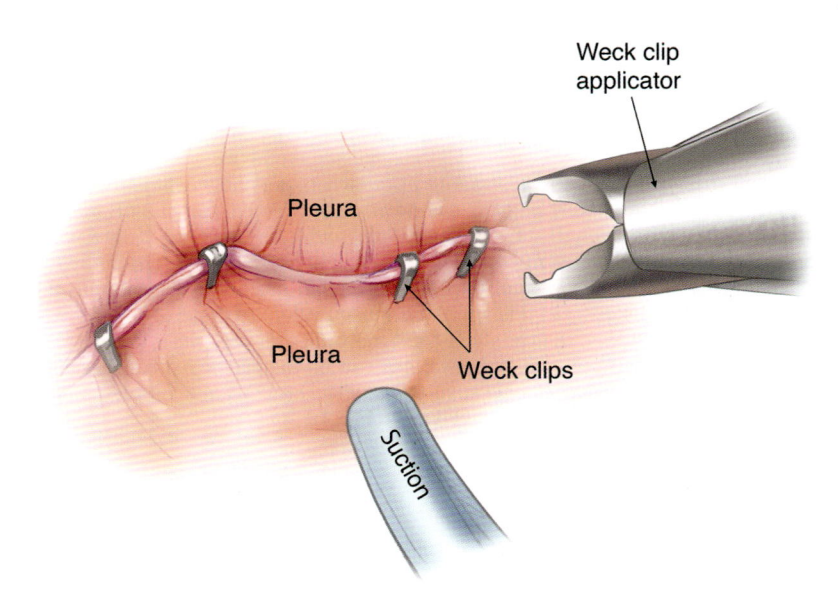

Fig. 55.9 During the closure portion of the procedure, any parietal pleura that have been incised should be brought back together with Weck clips, to promote pleural healing and decrease chest tube output.

Potential Complications and Precautions

The complications resulting from the ELTA can be categorized as immediate postoperative complications and long-term complications.

Immediate Postoperative Complications

Immediate postoperative complications can be subclassified into complications of the cardiopulmonary system and complications of the spine.

Cardiopulmonary Complications

Complications of the cardiopulmonary system include pneumonia, pleural effusions requiring drainage, respiratory distress requiring reintubation, and cardiovascular events. As stated above, all patients receive a postoperative chest radiograph to look for intrathoracic pathology. The most common postoperative clinical finding is a pneumothorax ipsilateral to the side of operation. This can usually be adequately treated with a chest tube as outlined above. Our practice is to leave a chest tube hooked up to wall suction at a pressure of −20 cm H_2O. The chest tube is left in place until the chest tube output decreases to less than 20 mL per 24 hours. The presence of a postoperative pneumothorax does not preclude immediately extubating the patient postoperatively. If a pneumothorax persists for more than 5 days, the patient may need to return to the operating room for a physical or chemical pleurodesis.

Other types of intrathoracic pathology that can complicate the immediate postoperative period are hemothorax, chylothorax, atelectasis, and tension pneumothorax. Similar to the treatment of a persistent pneumothorax, a persistent hemothorax or chylothorax requires reoperation; however, if the suspicion for these pathologies being present is high, return to the operating room usually occurs in a shorter period, such as by postoperative day 2 or 3, as these pathologies are less likely to resolve than a pneumothorax. Atelectasis requires extensive patient mobilization and pulmonary toilet to achieve resolution of the problem. Tension pneumothorax is an unusual complication, which results from inadequate closure of the chest walls. Treatment is emergent replacement of a chest tube.

Spine Complications

Complications of ELTA include all of the potential complications of any thoracic spine surgery, such as intraoperative spinal cord injury, intraoperative nerve root injury, incidental durotomy, incorrectly localized levels, and postoperative compressive syndromes such as epidural hematoma or epidural abscess. One possible complication of the ELTA that requires specific discussion is the intraoperative CSF leak. If a dural rent occurs during the operation, it is not easily repaired primarily through the endoscopic approach. Small leaks that occur can often be treated with Gelfoam and hydrogel (DuraSeal, Covidien, Mansfield, MA) being placed over the dura, followed by a lumbar drain being placed postoperatively while the patient is still in the operating room. In these cases, we keep the patient intubated for at least 1 day postoperatively and the chest tube is maintained at water seal to allow for positive pressure ventilation to occur, which discourages accumulation of CSF in the intrapleural space and decreases the risk of a CSF–pleural fistula forming. If a large dural rent is encountered intraoperatively, these same maneuvers can be attempted first; however, if they fail, then the surgeon may need to perform an open thoracotomy to primarily repair the dural rent and more definitively seal off the CSF from the pleural space.

Long-Term Postoperative Complications

Chronic postoperative complications usually involve pulmonary insufficiency or pain syndromes. Chronic atelectasis can cause long-term oxygenation issues. These issues are avoided by chest tube placement, early patient mobilization, good pulmonary toilet with incentive spirometry usage, and adequate pain control. Patients who have uncontrolled postoperative pain can suffer from splinting, which will make it impossible for them to achieve adequate insufflation of their lungs. Pain control via a combination of opiates and nonsteroidal anti-inflammatory drugs can allow the patient to achieve a state of adequate ventilation.

Pain syndromes resulting from the transthoracic approach are caused by one of two mechanisms. Chronic incisional pain is usually superficial pain that occurs specifically at the site of the incision. Although this pain usually resolves within a few weeks postoperatively for most patients, it can continue for some. Chronic intercostal neuralgia can result from damage to the subcostal nerves during the endoscopic approach, and it is characterized by a pain that wraps around the chest at the level of the incisions. Importantly, it does not extend dorsal to the incision. Chronic intercostal neuralgia can be difficult to differentiate from a painful radiculopathy; however, patients suffering from radiculopathy preoperatively can often differentiate between their preoperative radicular pain and their postoperative intercostal neuralgia. It is thought that this pressure on the neurovascular bundle can be avoided by using flexible endoscopic portals instead of the traditional rigid endoscopic portals. If the patient experiences chronic intercostal neuralgia despite these efforts, regular injections and gabapentin can help the patient manage these symptoms.

Chronic chest pain syndrome, which involves complaints of generalized chest pain, is thought to result from the disruption of the parietal pleura. This postoperative pain condition is uncommon and is very difficult to treat effectively when it occurs.

Conclusion

The ELTA is a versatile approach that enables the surgeon to adequately address a wide array of thoracic spinal pathologies. Its strengths are its ability to provide the surgeon with a wide field of vision within the thoracic cavity, as well as the ability to operate on multiple thoracic spinal segments. The long-term outcomes of this approach are equivalent to those of open thoracotomy, and the short-term morbidity for patients is lower. Most postoperative complications can be managed in a conservative manner. Key operative steps with the ELTA and problems that can arise are described in **Box 55.1**.

Box 55.1 Key Operative Steps and Potential Problems

Step	Problem
Intubation with dual-lumen endotracheal tube (ETT)	Poor ventilation from improperly placed ETT
Proper patient positioning	Movement that occurs when the operative bed is moved; it can be prevented by being certain the patient is well taped
Planning incision	Emergent thoracotomy; plan ahead
Incision	
Port placement	Damage to the neurovascular bundle on the caudal aspect of the ribs during introduction of ports
Introduction of endoscopic instruments	Pleural adhesions; remove them if necessary
Placement of chest tube(s) in the apex of the lung(s)	A chest tube placed in the caudal aspect of the lung allows for development of an apical pneumothorax
Closure of incisions	Inadequate closure; can lead to tension pneumothorax

References

1. Arseni C, Nash F. Thoracic intervertebral disc protrusion: a clinical study. J Neurosurg 1960;17:418–430
2. Hulme A. The surgical approach to thoracic intervertebral disc protrusions. J Neurol Neurosurg Psychiatry 1960;23:133–137
3. Logue V. Thoracic intervertebral disc prolapse with spinal cord compression. J Neurol Neurosurg Psychiatry 1952;15:227–241
4. Muller R. Protrusion of thoracic intervertebral disks with compression of the spinal cord. Acta Med Scand 1951;139:99–104
5. Hodgson AR, Stock FE. Anterior spine fusion for the treatment of tuberculosis of the spine: The operative findings and results of treatment in the first 100 cases. J Bone Joint Surg Am 1960;42:295–310
6. Mack MJ, Regan JJ, Bobechko WP, Acuff TE. Application of thoracoscopy for diseases of the spine. Ann Thorac Surg 1993;56:736–738
7. Rosenthal D, Rosenthal R, de Simone A. Removal of a protruded thoracic disc using microsurgical endoscopy. A new technique. Spine 1994;19:1087–1091
8. Wait SD, Fox DJ Jr, Kenny KJ, Dickman CA. Thoracoscopic resection of symptomatic herniated thoracic discs: clinical results in 121 patients. Spine 2012;37:35–40
9. Upadhyaya CD, Wu JC, Chin CT, Balamurali G, Mummaneni PV. Avoidance of wrong-level thoracic spine surgery: intraoperative localization with preoperative percutaneous fiducial screw placement. J Neurosurg Spine 2012;16:280–284

56 Endoscopic Thoracic Sympathectomy

Justin C. Clark and Curtis A. Dickman

Many clinical syndromes result from pathologically elevated sympathetic tone. Some of these conditions respond well to sectioning of the thoracic sympathetic chain ganglia, a procedure referred to as thoracic sympathectomy. Thoracic sympathectomy is an established surgical procedure that has been in use for more than 70 years.[1] Although it is indicated in the surgical treatment of many types of clinical pathologies, the majority of thoracic sympathectomies are performed to treat patients with medically refractory idiopathic (essential) palmar hyperhidrosis, which is characterized by excessive sweating of the hands.

The surgical approaches that can be used to perform the thoracic sympathectomy include the extrapleural or subpleural posterior approach, the transaxillary approach, the supraclavicular approach, and the anterior thoracotomy.[2–4] Like many surgical procedures, thoracic sympathectomy was initially performed as an open surgical procedure. As endoscopic techniques evolved, the open procedure for thoracic sympathectomy was superseded by the endoscopic approach. The clinical benefits of using the endoscope for thoracic sympathectomies include smaller incisions, shorter hospital stays, and overall lower patient morbidity.[5] As a result, the majority of thoracic sympathectomies today are performed via the endoscopic approach.

Patient Selection

Patients with debilitating symptoms despite optimal medical management are potential candidates for endoscopic thoracic sympathectomy. It is necessary for the patient to have enough shoulder mobility to enable adequate shoulder abduction during surgery.

Indications

- Hyperhidrosis
    - Craniofacial
    - Axillary
    - Palmar
- Upper extremity pain syndromes
    - Complex regional pain syndrome
    - Phantom pain
    - Cancer pain
- Cardiac arrhythmia

Contraindications

- Pleural inflammatory disease
- Cardiac or pulmonary disease precluding unilateral ventilation
- Extensive pleural adhesions/scarring

Relative Contraindications

- Prior ipsilateral thoracotomy or thoracoscopy
- Prior radiofrequency or alcohol sympathectomy
- Morbid obesity

Advantages

In comparison with an open approach, an endoscopic sympathectomy offers the following advantages:

- Decreased approach morbidity
- Decreased postoperative pain
- Decreased time to return to work
- Shorter hospital stay
- Clinical efficacy equivalent to that of an open procedure

Disadvantages

- Steep learning curve for thoracoscopic techniques
- Potential postoperative compensatory hyperhidrosis syndrome (CHS)
- Possibility of causing Horner's syndrome

Choice of Operative Approach

Patients who are debilitated by their condition and those for whom medical management has failed are candidates for thoracic sympathectomies. Patients who are free of the above-mentioned contraindications are candidates for endoscopic thoracic sympathectomy because of the extremely low morbidity associated with the procedure. If the patient is unable to undergo an anterior thoracic approach, a posterior approach or an axillary approach can also be offered. Patients who are not surgical candidates can be evaluated for percutaneous chemical sympathectomy.[6]

Preoperative Screening

Evaluating patients for hyperhidrosis requires ruling out endocrine (hyperthyroidism) and neoplastic causes for the patient's symptoms. If concern exists that these clinical entities are present, the patient should undergo screening evaluations for endocrinopathies or neoplastic conditions.

Surgical Procedure

The general details relevant to this approach are presented in Chapter 55 and will not be repeated here. A video demonstrating the surgical steps involved in this operation is available as part

> **Box 56.1 Instrumentation for Thoracoscopic Sympathectomy**
>
> Thoracoscope (5-mm diameter endoscope)
> Endoscopic harmonic scalpel
> Two 5-mm endoscope ports with trocars
> Three-chip endoscopic video system
> High-resolution monitor

of the supplemental material accompanying this text (Video 56.1). The instrumentation required for the operation is listed in **Box 56.1**.

Anesthesia

Before the procedure, surface temperature probes should be placed on the patient's forearms, to document a rise in temperature after the sympathectomy has been completed. The rise in temperature is expected to be at least 1 to 3°C and should occur within 10 to 20 minutes of the lesion being made (**Fig. 56.1**). If a rise in temperature is not seen, the sympathetic chain ganglia must be inspected for accessory connections that could be transmitting sympathetic tone to the arm.

In the case of bilateral sympathectomies performed during the same anesthesia session, the patient must be sterilely draped on one side, and then undraped, repositioned, and sterilely draped on the other side. During each half of the surgery, each lung must be selectively deflated and then re-inflated. It is of the utmost importance that the proper placement and functioning of the dual-lumen endotracheal tube is verified and re-verified during the procedure, to avoid difficulties with either ventilation or surgical exposure.

Whenever sympathetic lesions are being created, it is important to remember that the majority of the sympathetic tone provided to the heart is contributed by the left sympathetic chain. When the sympathetic ganglia on the left side are sectioned, most patients experience bradycardia for this reason.[7] This decrease in heart rate is usually minimal; however, the anesthesiologist should be prepared to treat lethal cardiac arrhythmias, as asystole has been reported.[8,9]

Positioning

Because the upper thoracic spine is slightly difficult to reach, patient positioning should be optimized to assist with access to this area. The patient is placed in a three-quarters prone position and then taped securely to the bed. Placing the patient in a three-quarters prone position on the operating bed and then maneuvering the patient into a reverse Trendelenburg position or rotating the bed anteriorly enables the patient's lung to fall away from the spine (**Fig. 56.2**). These maneuvers enable gravity to retract the lung away from the upper thoracic spine, thus exposing the upper thoracic sympathetic ganglia.

Incision Planning

In general, only two endoscopic portals are required for a unilateral endoscopic thoracic sympathectomy. The incision for the first portal, through which the endoscope will be inserted, is placed in the posterior axillary line of the fifth intercostal space. The second incision is for the working portal, and it is made in the third intercostal space of the anterior axillary line. Both planned incisions are 5 mm in length and are injected with 0.5% lidocaine with epinephrine before surgical incision (**Fig. 56.3**). A 5-mm trocar is inserted through each incision.

Procedure

Achieving adequate visualization of the upper thoracic spine enables the operation to proceed rapidly. The correct operative levels are located visually. The first rib is usually hidden behind the fat pad, making the second rib the first visible rib (**Fig. 56.4**). The stellate ganglion, sympathetic chain, and accessory sympathetic innervation can be visualized beneath the parietal pleura with the sympathetic chain being identified as it crosses over the rib heads. The stellate ganglion is located over the head of the first rib. It is typically surrounded by a fat pad within the thoracic outlet, adjacent to the subclavian vasculature.

The surgeon must take care not to injure the several large regional vessels. The second, third, and fourth intercostal veins merge to form the superior intercostal vein, before emptying into the azygos vein. The first intercostal vein is unique in that it drains directly into the brachiocephalic vein. Because it is positioned superficial to the segmental and intercostal vessels, the sympathetic chain can be transected without sacrificing any of these vessels.

Our preference for performing the endoscopic thoracic sympathectomy is to create a sympathectomy using either monopolar cauterization scissors or a harmonic scalpel. For palmar hyperhidrosis, we section the sympathetic chain as it passes across the second and third rib heads, effectively isolating the T2 ganglia (**Fig. 56.5**). The T3 and T4 ganglia are included for the treatment of axillary hyperhidrosis and bromhidrosis (axillary malodor).[10] Associated plantar hyperhidrosis resolves about 50%

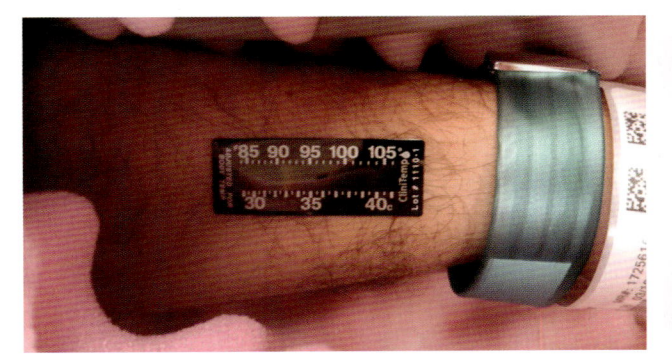

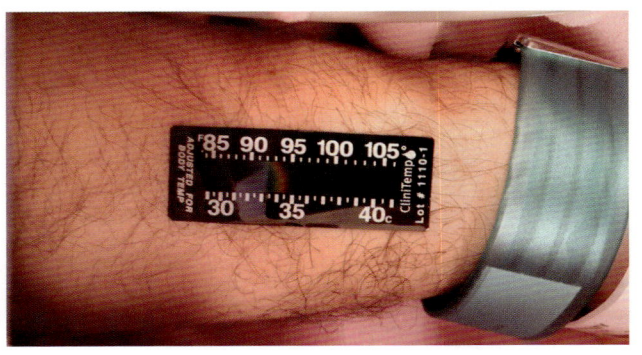

Fig. 56.1 When the sympathectomy has been successfully completed, the temperature probes on the patient's forearms will demonstrate an increase in temperature. Pictured here is an increase from a baseline of 33°C **(a)** to a final temperature of 34°C about 10 minutes after sympathectomy **(b)**. (Courtesy of Barrow Neurological Institute, Phoenix, Arizona.)

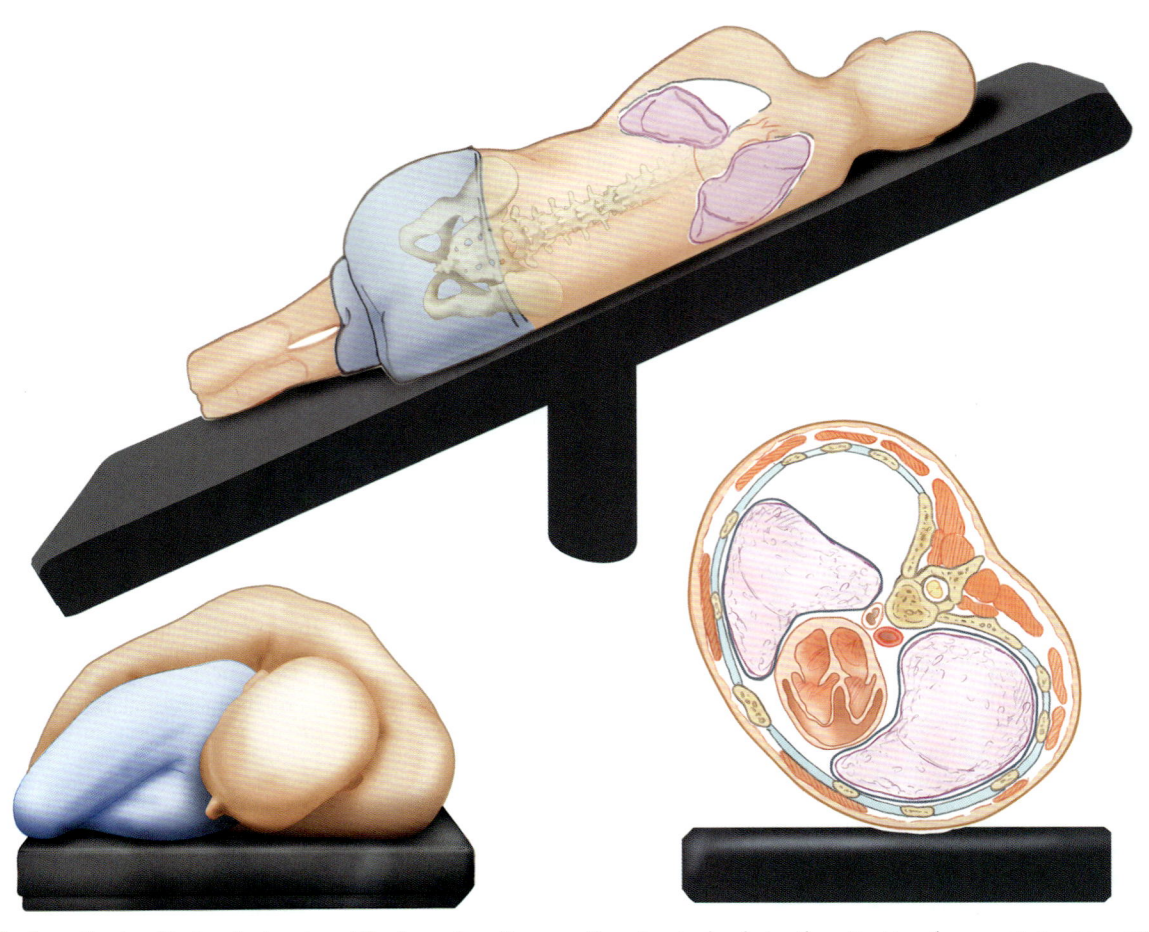

Fig. 56.2 For optimal positioning, the lung is mobilized away from the upper thoracic spine by placing the patient in a three-quarters prone position and placing the bed in a reverse Trendelenburg position.

of the time when hyperhidrosis of the upper extremities is relieved, and is referred to as a "dividend benefit" of the procedure because it is not an expected effect of transecting the upper thoracic sympathetic chain. Treatment of prolonged QT interval involves lesioning the ganglia on the left side from T1 through T4.[11] Sympathectomy can also be used to relieve pain related to pancreatic carcinoma.[12] This is done by lesioning the sympathetic ganglia on the left side from T5 through T9 to denervate the splanchnic nerve, and by lesioning the ganglia of T10 and T11 to denervate the lesser splanchnic nerve.

Once this is completed, a 20-Fr chest tube is placed through the anterior incision after removing the endoscopic portal. The chest tube is placed in the apex of the lung under direct visualization via the endoscope. The lung is then reinflated, which ensures adequate reexpansion and ventilation of the lung. The chest tube is then secured with a 3-0 nylon suture and connected

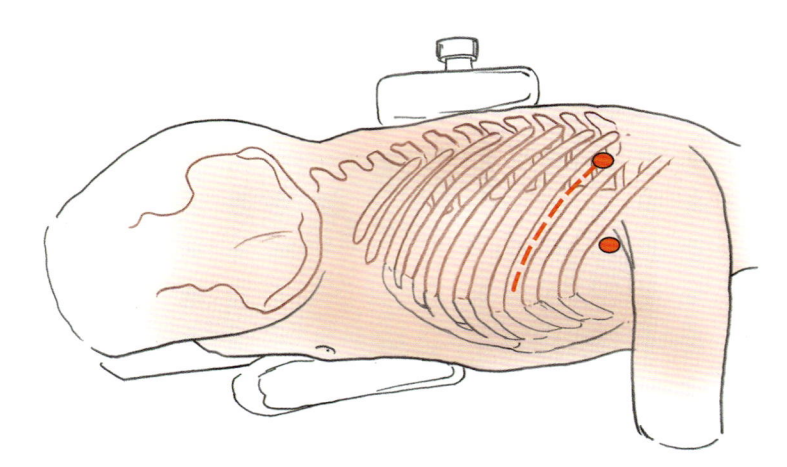

Fig. 56.3 The incisions for the portals are made in the posterior axillary line of the fifth intercostal space and the anterior axillary line of the third intercostal space. An incision for a thoracotomy is made incorporating the posterior incision, in case an emergent thoracotomy is required.

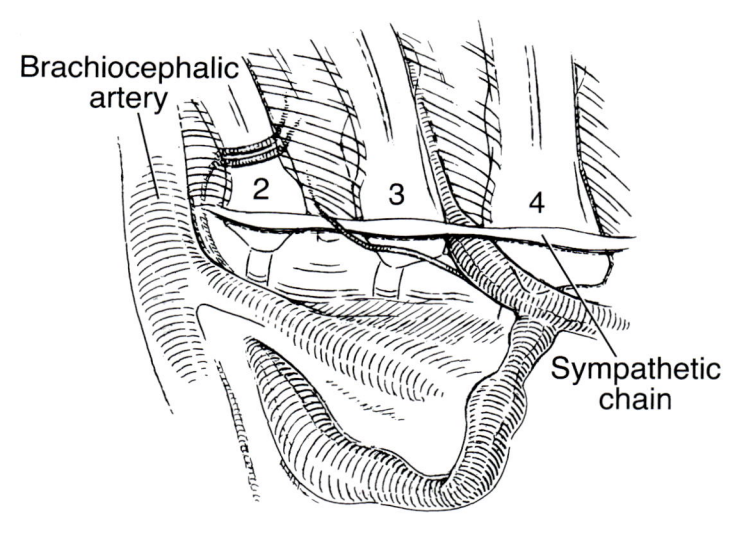

Fig. 56.4 The left pleural cavity is illustrated with the ipsilateral lung deflated, which exposes the vertebral column, rib heads (2, 3, and 4), and overlying sympathetic chain. (Courtesy of Barrow Neurological Institute, Phoenix, Arizona.)

to a chest drainage system. The posterior incision is closed in layers using 3-0 Vicryl sutures (Ethicon, Inc., Somerville, NJ) in the deep tissue followed by a 4-0 Monocryl subcuticular suture (Ethicon, Inc.). The chest wall then has a sterile dressing taped over it to keep the skin area around the chest tube sterile.

The sterile drapes are then removed and the patient is repositioned in the contralateral lateral decubitus position. An identical technique is used to perform the contralateral endoscopic thoracic sympathectomy. At the conclusion of the second-side operation, another 20-Fr chest tube is placed, as it was on the other side, and hooked up to a drainage system. The posterior incision is then closed using 3-0 Vicryl sutures for subcutaneous tissue closure. A 4-0 Monocryl suture is used for subcuticular closure. Once that posterior incision has been closed and suction has been applied to the chest tube for at least 5 minutes, a large insufflation of the lung is performed, to remove as much intrapleural air as possible. At the apex of insufflation, the chest tube is removed, and the skin incision is closed using 3-0 and 4-0 sutures, as mentioned above. The same steps for the removal of the chest tube are then performed on the side where the first chest tube was placed. After both chest tubes are removed and all incisions are closed, a chest radiograph is obtained while the patient is still intubated in the operating room to verify the absence of a pneumothorax (**Fig. 56.6**). It is important that the patient be placed in the sitting position during the radiograph, to facilitate identifying intrapleural air.

Postoperative Care

If the patient is hemodynamically stable and the chest radiograph demonstrates no intrathoracic pathology, then the patient can be extubated and taken to the postanesthesia recovery unit. Once the patient is fully awake, a thorough neurologic examination should be performed. Special attention should be paid to determining whether postoperative Horner's syndrome is present, indicating damage to the stellate ganglion. For patients who were severely affected by their palmar hyperhidrosis preoperatively,

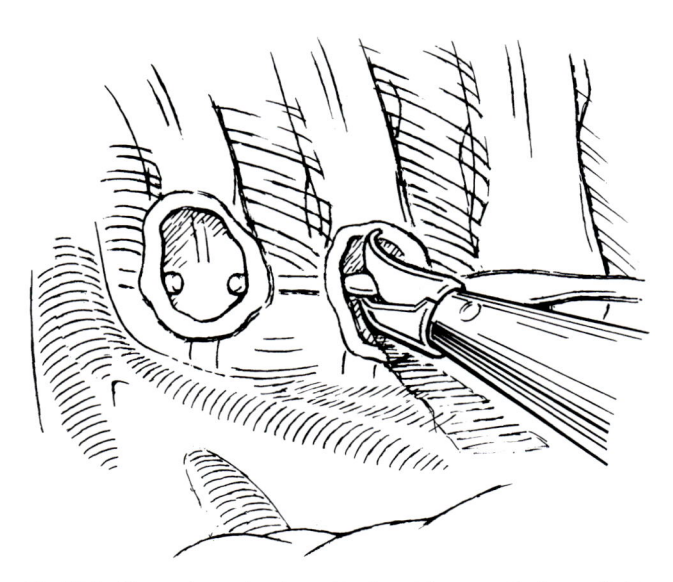

Fig. 56.5 Monopolar cautery is used to dissect the sympathetic ganglia laterally along the corresponding rib and then to transect the sympathetic chain completely. (Courtesy of Barrow Neurological Institute, Phoenix, Arizona.)

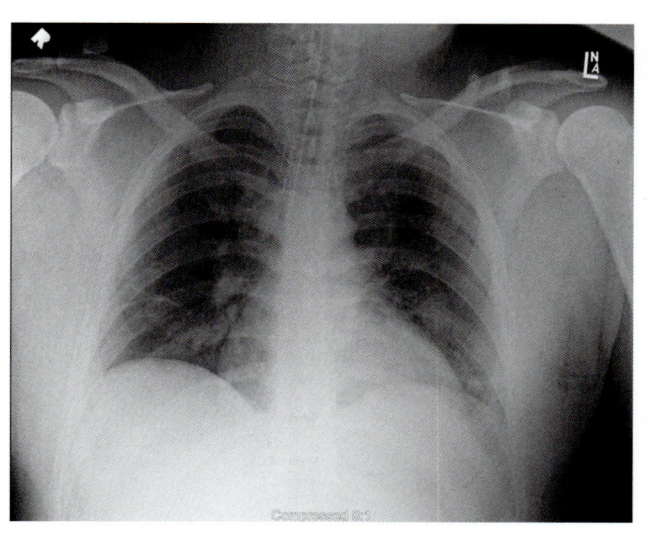

Fig. 56.6 Postoperative chest radiograph is performed at the end of the procedure to determine whether the patient has any cardiopulmonary complications that would preclude a discharge home later that day. (Courtesy of Barrow Neurological Institute, Phoenix, Arizona.)

Table 56.1 Thoracic Sympathectomy for Hyperhidrosis Syndromes*

Author, Year	No. of Patients	No. of Sympathectomies	Palmer Hyperhidrosis Relief, No. (%)	Plantar Hyperhidrosis Relief, No. (%)	Axillary Hyperhidrosis Relief, No. (%)	Compensatory Hyperhidrosis, No. (%)	Gustatory Sweating, No. (%)	Horner's Syndrome, No. (%)
Kux, 1978[18]	63	124	63 (100)	–	–	28 (44)	2 (3)	0
Lin, 1990[19]	21	42	21 (100)	3 (14)	–	1 (5)	–	0
Robertson et al, 1993[4]	22	–	22 (100)	–	–	3 (14)	0	1 (5) (transient)
Kao et al, 1994[3]	300	600	287 (96)	210 (70)	19/24 (79)	150 (50)	3 (1)	0
Lee and Hwang, 1996[20]	82	164	82 (100)	41 (50)	–	50 (61)	0	0
Johnson et al, 1999[15]	65	112	48/48 (100)	–	–	11 (17)	2 (3)	8 (12.3) (7 transient)
Lai et al, 1997[14]	72	144	67 (93)	–	–	71 (99)	12 (17)	5 (7)
Wait et al, 2010[9]	322	642	301/301 (100)	143/196 (73)	178/185 (96)	201/322 (62)	–	7/642 (1)
Baumgartner et al, 2009[21]	189	378	188 (99)	–	–	106 (56)	–	–

*The denominator used to calculate percentages is the total number of patients, unless otherwise indicated. The dash indicates that the series did not report data. The zero indicates that there were no results.

elimination of hand moisture should be appreciated immediately postoperatively. If no untoward events occurred intraoperatively, the patient can be discharged with a short course of oral pain medication and an incentive spirometer. The patient should be instructed on how to use the incentive spirometer prior to discharge. Clinical follow-up should occur within 2 weeks to evaluate incision healing, pulmonary function, and the relief of symptoms, as well as the presence of any complications.

Outcomes

The success rate of endoscopic sympathectomy for autonomic-mediated syndromes is highest for treating palmar hyperhidrosis. Multiple studies have reported success rates between 95% and 100% for the treatment of this disease in both North American and Asian populations (**Table 56.1**). In a report by the senior author (C.A.D.) about his use of the endoscopic thoracic sympathectomy, the clinical outcomes of 322 patients were analyzed. These patients presented with hyperhidrosis of the hands (13.4%), axillae (4.0%), craniofacial region (1.2%), or some combination of these three (81.4%). The results of this operation were excellent, with 99.7% of patients with palmar hyperhidrosis experiencing complete resolution of their symptoms. Results of axillary and craniofacial hyperhidrosis were also encouraging, with symptom resolution in 89.1% and improvement in 100% of these cases. The utility of this operation can be seen in the fact that 98.1% of patients who underwent treatment reported satisfaction and willingness to undergo the procedure again.[9] This treatment is effective not only in adults but also in adolescents.[13]

Potential Complications and Precautions

Potential complications of endoscopic sympathectomy are listed in **Box 56.2**. A significant number of patients treated with sympathectomy for hyperhidrosis experience CHS. A retrospective review of 104 patients in Taiwan treated with thoracoscopic sympathectomy reported CHS in 71 of the 72 patients available for follow-up.[14] CHS manifests as increased sweating of the chest, abdomen, legs, and/or back (non-denervated areas).[2,10,15,16] The severity of this response does not appear to be influenced by the extent of preoperative hyperhidrosis or by family history.[14] CHS symptoms typically improve or resolve within 6 months after surgery.[16] The incidence of CHS after sympathectomy in patients living in Israel, Austria, Ireland, and England ranges from 40 to 75%.[14] Most patients who develop CHS have mild or moderate sweating and are satisfied with the effects of their relief of palmar sweating. Only 5 to 10% of patients who develop CHS have severe sweating that drenches their clothing and bedsheets and creates a disabling problem.

Another complication associated with this surgical treatment is Horner's syndrome. This results from injury to the rostral stellate ganglion. In our experience, the incidence of Horner's syndrome in patients undergoing endoscopic thoracic sympathectomy was significantly reduced from 5% to 0.9% by changing the technique from excision of the sympathetic chain to in situ transection of the sympathetic chain at T2-T3.[9] We suspect that by cauterizing the sympathetic ganglia instead of putting traction on them and cutting them, we were able to decrease traction and subsequent injury on the rostral stellate ganglion and its ascending sympathetic fibers. Moreover, electrical or mechanical stimulation of the stellate ganglion is known to cause pupillary dilation that can be observed by the anesthesiologist. It has been reported as a useful test for identifying this condition.[17]

Vascular injury requiring conversion to an open procedure has not occurred in any of our cases and can be minimized by defining the regional anatomy with the thoracoscope before other endoscopic instruments are placed. Pneumothorax requiring replacement of a chest tube is rare, as long as the visceral pleura of the lung are not violated during the procedure. Intercostal neuralgia is avoided by minimizing dissection and traction against the intercostal bundle. In our experience, no procedures have required conversion to thoracotomy. Furthermore, no patients have required a second procedure because their preoperative complaints failed to improve or because they developed recurrent hyperhidrosis. Gustatory sweating, the result of aberrant synapses developing between sympathetic fibers and the vagus nerve, has been reported in 1 to 2% of patients.[14]

Conclusion

The endoscopic thoracic sympathectomy is a highly effective surgical technique for the treatment of diseases resulting from elevated sympathetic tone. By utilizing the sympathectomy technique, the incidence of Horner's syndrome can be greatly diminished. The morbidity associated with this procedure is low enough that it is commonly performed as an outpatient procedure with as little as 5 to 10 minutes of operative time per side. Key operative steps with the endoscopic thoracic sympathectomy and problems that can arise are listed in **Box 56.3**.

Box 56.2 Complications of Endoscopic Thoracic Sympathectomy

Intercostal neuralgia
Horner's syndrome
Compensatory hyperhidrosis syndrome
Gustatory sweating
Pneumothorax
Vascular injury

Box 56.3 Key Operative Steps and Potential Problems

Step	Problems and Precautions
Intubation with dual-lumen endotracheal tube (ETT)	Poor ventilation from improperly placed ETT
Proper patient positioning to encourage lung mobilizing away from the upper thoracic spine	Be certain the patient is well taped so no movement occurs when the operative bed is moved
Planning incision	Make certain that portals are placed as rostral as possible; be careful that the incisions do not encroach on the scapula
Sympathectomy, making sure that the forearm temperature increases at least 1°C	Identify the stellate ganglion and do not cauterize more than the lower third of it; look for accessory bundles of Kuntz
Removal of chest tube at the end of the procedure	Make certain the patient's chest is at maximum inflation when the chest tube is removed
Chest radiograph at the end of the procedure	Thoroughly inspect for any residual intrapleural air
Discharge later that day	Make certain the patient knows how to use the incentive spirometer and that the patient has enough pain medication so as not to experience "splinting" when trying to breathe deeply

References

1. Smithwick RH. The rationale and technic of sympathectomy for the relief of vascular spasm of the extremities. N Engl J Med 1940;222:699–703
2. Cloward RB. Hyperhydrosis. J Neurosurg 1969;30:545–551
3. Kao MC, Tsai JC, Lai DM, Hsiao YY, Lee YS, Chiu MJ. Autonomic activities in hyperhidrosis patients before, during, and after endoscopic laser sympathectomy. Neurosurgery 1994;34:262–268, discussion 268
4. Robertson DP, Simpson RK, Rose JE, Garza JS. Video-assisted endoscopic thoracic ganglionectomy. J Neurosurg 1993;79:238–240
5. Landreneau RJ, Hazelrigg SR, Mack MJ, et al. Postoperative pain-related morbidity: video-assisted thoracic surgery versus thoracotomy. Ann Thorac Surg 1993;56:1285–1289
6. Ebrahim KS. Percutaneous chemical dorsal sympathectomy for hyperhidrosis. Minim Invasive Neurosurg 2011;54:29–32
7. Cruz J, Sousa J, Oliveira AG, Silva-Carvalho L. Effects of endoscopic thoracic sympathectomy for primary hyperhidrosis on cardiac autonomic nervous activity. J Thorac Cardiovasc Surg 2009;137:664–669
8. Lin CC, Mo LR, Hwang MH. Intraoperative cardiac arrest: a rare complication of T2,3-sympathicotomy for treatment of hyperhidrosis palmaris. Two case reports. Eur J Surg Suppl 1994;572:43–45
9. Wait SD, Killory BD, Lekovic GP, Ponce FA, Kenny KJ, Dickman CA. Thoracoscopic sympathectomy for hyperhidrosis: analysis of 642 procedures with special attention to Horner's syndrome and compensatory hyperhidrosis. Neurosurgery 2010;67:652–656, discussion 656–657
10. Kao MC. Video endoscopic sympathectomy using a fiberoptic CO_2 laser to treat palmar hyperhidrosis. Neurosurgery 1992;30:131–135
11. Ouriel K, Moss AJ. Long QT syndrome: an indication for cervicothoracic sympathectomy. Cardiovasc Surg 1995;3:475–478
12. Worsey J, Ferson PF, Keenan RJ, Julian TB, Landreneau RJ. Thoracoscopic pancreatic denervation for pain control in irresectable pancreatic cancer. Br J Surg 1993;80:1051–1052
13. Wait SD, Killory BD, Lekovic GP, Dickman CA. Biportal thoracoscopic sympathectomy for palmar hyperhidrosis in adolescents. J Neurosurg Pediatr 2010;6:183–187
14. Lai YT, Yang LH, Chio CC, Chen HH. Complications in patients with palmar hyperhidrosis treated with transthoracic endoscopic sympathectomy. Neurosurgery 1997;41:110–113, discussion 113–115
15. Johnson JP, Obasi C, Hahn MS, Glatleider P. Endoscopic thoracic sympathectomy. J Neurosurg 1999;91(1, Suppl):90–97
16. Ray BS. Sympathectomy of the upper extremity; evaluation of surgical methods. J Neurosurg 1953;10:624–633
17. Segal R, Ferson PM, Nemoto E, Wolfson SK. Blood flow-monitored transthoracic endoscopic sympathectomy. In: Rengachary SS, Wilkins RH, eds. Neurosurgical Operative Atlas. Park Ridge, IL: American Association of Neurological Surgeons; 1998:163–171
18. Kux M. Thoracic endoscopic sympathectomy in palmar and axillary hyperhidrosis. Arch Surg 1978;113:264–266
19. Lin CC. A new method of thoracoscopic sympathectomy in hyperhidrosis palmaris. Surg Endosc 1990;4:224–226
20. Lee KH, Hwang PY. Video endoscopic sympathectomy for palmar hyperhidrosis. J Neurosurg 1996;84:484–486
21. Baumgartner FJ, Bertin S, Konecny J. Superiority of thoracoscopic sympathectomy over medical management for the palmoplantar subset of severe hyperhidrosis. Ann Vasc Surg 2009;23:1–7

57 Endoscopic Lateral Transthoracic Diskectomy and Vertebrectomy

Roque Fernandez, Inge Preissl, and Daniel Rosenthal

Thoracic disk disease presents a considerable therapeutic challenge because its symptomatology has not been determined, epidemiological studies are rare, and its natural evolution[1,2] has not been well studied. The disease cannot be characterized by its presentation pattern, and the therapeutic options range from conservative to surgical. Several surgical techniques have been reported in the last 30 years.[3] With this background, the surgeon has to decide if surgery will improve the patient's condition and, if so, which approach is the most optimal and the least risky for that patient.

Modern endoscopic procedures include the thoracoscopic and the endoscope-assisted trans- or retropleural minithoracotomy technique. Both procedures are suitable for diskectomy, vertebrectomy, and reconstruction procedures.

Anesthesia, Positioning, and Determining the Appropriate Level

Both techniques are performed under general anesthesia. Patients undergo double-lumen endotracheal intubation so that single-lung ventilation can be achieved, thus maximizing the surgical exposure. Regardless of the type of approach chosen, patients are placed in a strict lateral decubitus position (either left or right) for thoracoscopy or retropleural dissection. To prevent the position of the thorax from changing during surgical manipulations, the patient is secured with support aids at the pubis, at the sacrum, between the scapulae, and at the sternum, depending on the level that will be accessed (**Fig. 57.1**). In most cases, a table that has a break, which is used for the midlumbar region, is not necessary here.

The spinal level to be operated is determined and marked. Between T2 and T11 the ribs are the topographic landmarks. If the disk is situated between T6 and T7, the seventh rib will guide the surgeon to the disk space. The head of the rib always partially or completely covers the foramen, depending on the level of the dorsal spine to be treated. After removing the head of the rib, the surgeon gains access to the spinal canal, recognizing immediately its anterior border and spatial location.

The skin is sterilized and the surgeon places a needle above the rib that leads to the affected segment, perforating the pleura. By doing so when entering the thorax with the scope, the surgeon only has to find the tip of the needle, avoiding the need for intraoperative X-rays to locate the affected segment.

The positioning of the surgeon, assistant, instrumenting nurse, and equipment is shown in **Fig. 57.2**.

Approach

Thoracoscopy

The first portal is placed between the middle and posterior axillary line, slightly above the affected segment. The endoscope is inserted into the thoracic cavity and the lung is mobilized away from the anterior surface of the spine. If adhesions are present, they can be carefully detached using sharp dissection and coagulation until the lung is liberated completely. The ribs are recognized and counted up to the affected disk space, confirming the accuracy of the previously inserted needle, thus avoiding the need for intraoperative fluoroscopy. Further trocars are then inserted under direct vision.

The pleura is incised over the rib head and disk space and then mobilized. Its edges are folded laterally to expose the disk space and proximal rib over 2 to 3 cm. Any bleeding from the neurovascular bundle is controlled with bipolar cauterization. The proximal 2 cm of the rib is removed using the ultrasound blade, leaving a thin bony rim protecting the neurovascular bundle, which is always located at the lower distal edge of the rib. The costotransverse and costovertebral ligaments are detached from the rib head by using periosteal elevators, and after transecting it the bone is saved as graft material. The pedicle caudal to the disk space is then identified, leaving the entrance to the spinal canal free.

Mini-Open Trans- and Retropleural

Preoperative skin marking varies based on the shape of the thorax and the rib angulation, but the incision typically is two intercostal spaces above the targeted vertebral body or disk space.[1] The muscle layers are divided parallel to the skin incision until the underlying rib is exposed over a length of 8 to 10 cm. From this step onward, the transpleural technique splits the pleura parallel to the ribs. After the lung collapses, a rib spreader is brought in place to enlarge the intercostal space and open the chest cavity to expose the spine.

Entering and Working in the Spinal Canal

Regardless of the type of approach (thoracoscopy or retropleural), two important surgical steps are taken so that the surgeon can access the spinal canal safely.

First, the pedicle is partially removed at its base using a Kerrison rongeur, exposing the epidural space (**Fig. 57.3**). Epidural

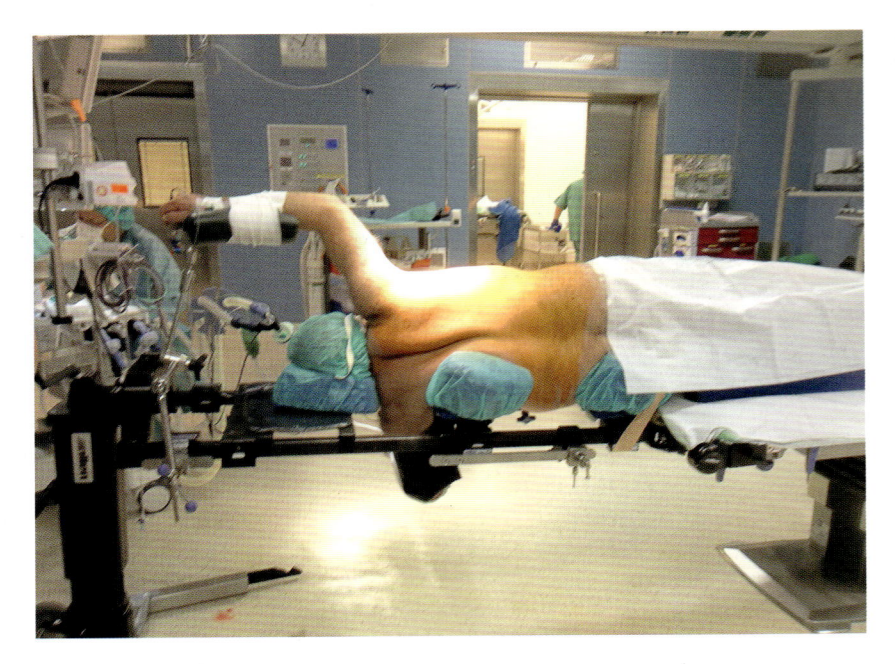

Fig. 57.1 Lateral decubitus position. Note that the table is in a horizontal position.

bleeding can occur, coming from the congested epidural plexus. Early identification of the dura enables the surgeon to visualize the anterolateral border of the spinal canal and gain visual control of the thecal sac during dissection (**Fig. 57.4**). Second, a cavity is created at the posterior edge of the disk space and adjacent vertebral bodies that provides enough room to move the disk material away (pulling it into the defect) from the epidural space.

Entering the compressed epidural space should be avoided before performing these two steps; the amount of bone resection that needs to be done is directly related to the size of the disk and the degree of compression. The cavity must be wide enough so that it extends cephalad and caudal to the disk herniation, enabling visualization of the dura at both ends of the compression. It should also be deep enough, up to the contralateral pedicle if needed, enabling the surgeon to resect the base of a calcified disk and expose the entire ventral surface of the dura across the spinal canal (**Fig. 57.5**). If the disk extends intradurally, a wider defect provides adequate exposure, enabling careful preparation of the arachnoid and pia mater with microdissectors. These two steps are of the utmost importance in order to decompress the spinal cord adequately and safely.

The retropleural approach is technically more demanding. After uncovering the rib, the periosteum is dissected, while the pleura and endopleural fascia are detached from the posterior surface of the rib, taking care not to harm these structures and carefully dissecting the neurovascular bundle at its lower border. A single or double (windowing) osteotomy of the rib is performed. The first option entails transecting the rib almost at the level of the posterior axillary line (in order to gain a better angle to enter the spinal canal), sliding the distal part of it up or down, depending on the surface the surgeon considers best to access the spine.[4] The second option entails cutting a piece of the rib, which can then be reinserted (fixing it with miniplates) or used as a bone graft to reconstruct the anterior column. Resection of two ribs is needed when a wider field of view or a multiple-level approach is planned (**Fig. 57.6**).

After displacing the rib cranially or caudally, the endopleural fascia is divided and the parietal pleura is then detached from the chest wall entering the retropleural space. Further dissection is performed using the fingers or instruments down to the head of the rib and vertebral body, taking care to avoid direct pressure against the pleura that, due to its fragility, can be easily disrupted. Once the surgical field is exposed, a self-retaining re-

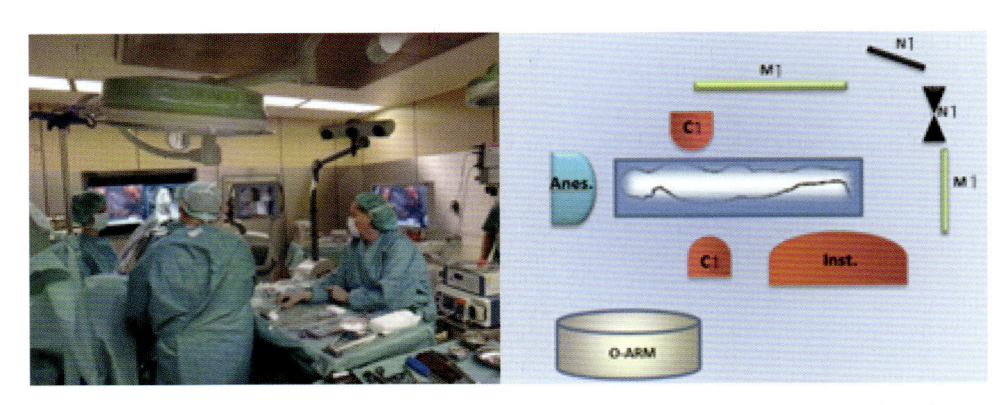

Fig. 57.2 Photograph **(a)** and diagram **(b)** of the positioning of the surgeon (C1), assistant (C2), instrumenting nurse, and anesthetist. M1, monitor 1; M2, monitor 2; N1, navigation monitor; N2, navigation tracking device. and a real image.

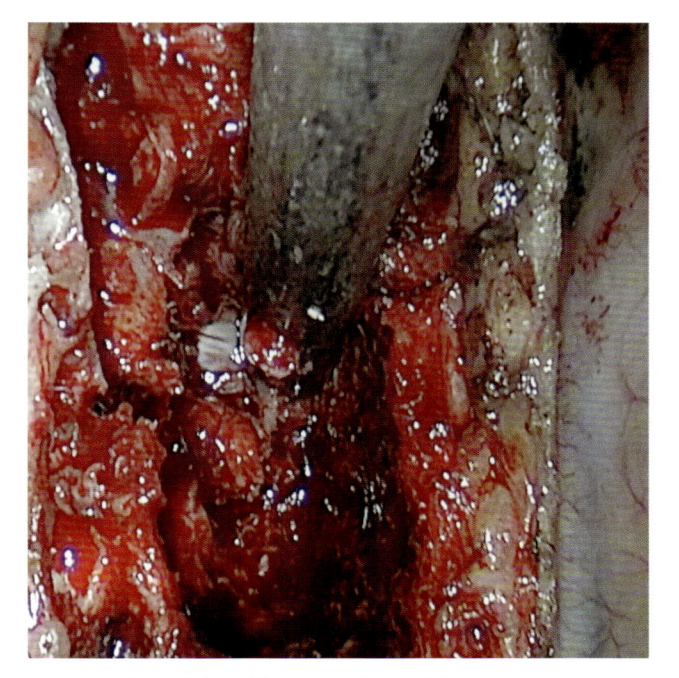

Fig. 57.3 The pedicle and foramen at the tip of the instrument.

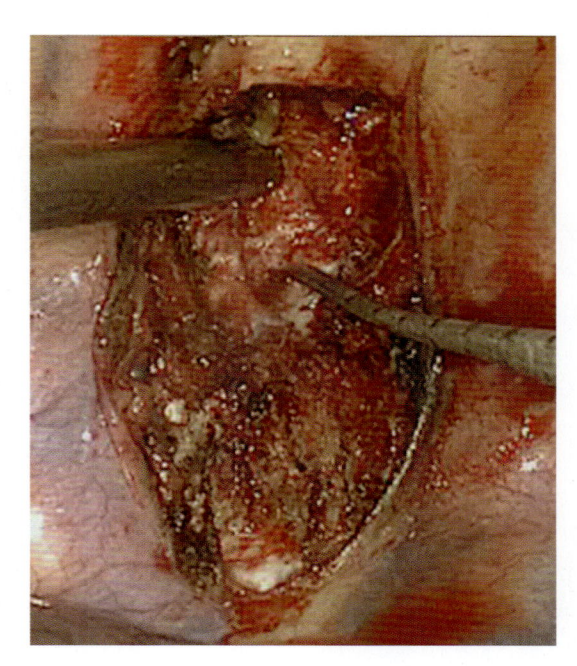

Fig 57.4 The pedicle partially removed, and the dura mater shines at the tip of the suction device.

tractor can be used. The detached pleura and the deflated lung are gently retracted anteriorly, enabling visualization of the spinal column and the affected segment.

Because the surgical field is relatively small, illumination and magnification are needed in order to visualize the surgical field properly. In addition to a light source, a surgical microscope or endoscope can be used for this task. One example is the Vitom[R] System (Karl Storz, Charlton, MA) that provides excellent magnification and illumination without needing to introduce the scope through the wound (**Fig. 57.7**).

Vertebrectomy

In cases where the vertebral body has to be removed totally or partially (such as for a fracture, tumor, or diskitis), both of the above-described approaches can be used to access the spine.

For exposure of the thoracic vertebral bodies and intervertebral disks, the surgeon proceed as discussed above (see Thoracoscopy section). The only difference is that for a vertebrectomy the segmental vessels are coagulated, clipped, and sectioned.

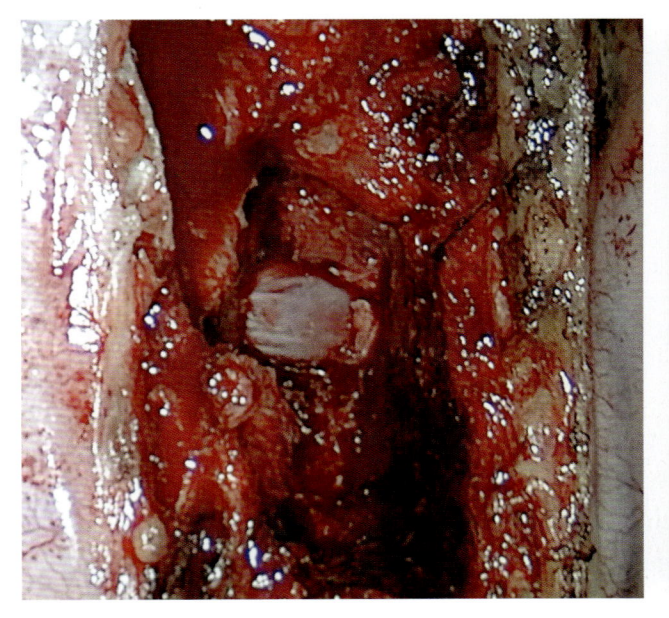

Fig. 57.5 The spinal canal and dural tube are completely decompressed.

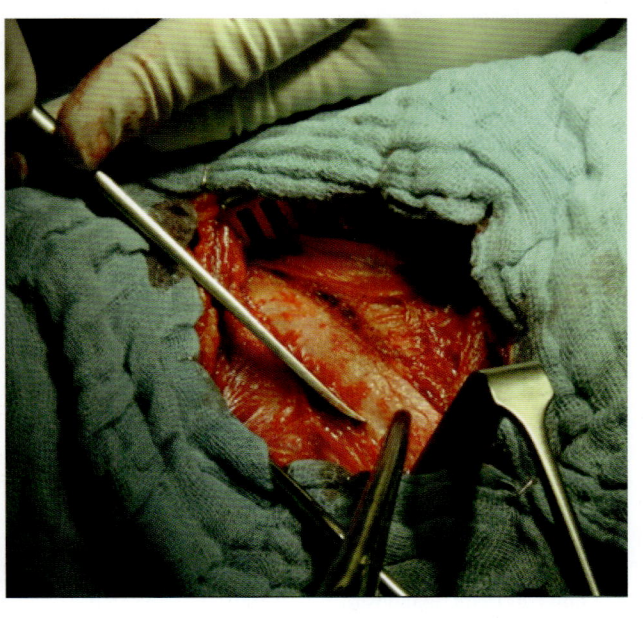

Fig. 57.6 After periosteal dissection, the pleura is detached from the rib.

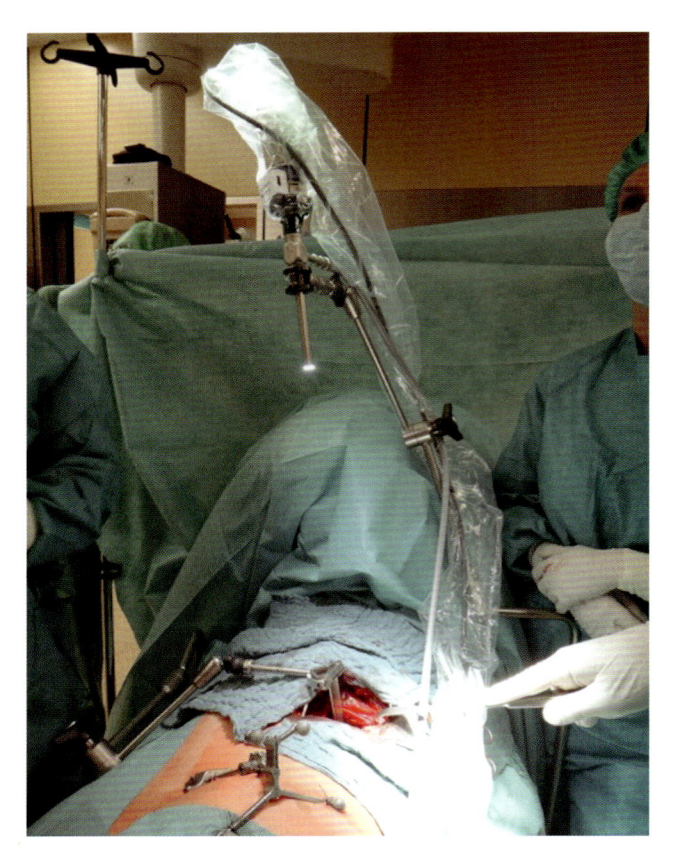

Fig. 57.7 The scope and retractors are in position.

Endoscopic diskectomy and corpectomy are performed in a manner similar to that described for open procedures. Disks adjacent to the diseased body are incised and removed. The intervening diseased vertebral body is removed by performing a median corpectomy using drills, osteotomes, or the bone scalpel. The depth of the corpectomy across the midline is verified either using fluoroscopy or tracking the instruments with the navigation system. Once the anterior defect has been created, the surgeon proceeds with the steps described above to enter and work in the spinal canal. Free bone fragments and epidural tumor are gently pushed into the central corpectomy cavity and removed. In cases of tumor removal, embolization (depending on the tumor type) is suggested in order to have complete control of the bleeding sources. Once decompression of the anterior spinal cord has been achieved, reconstruction of the vertebral body is performed.

Interbody Reconstruction and Endoscopic Stabilization

Anterior column reconstruction can be done with a variety of implants and materials, such as autologous bone, ceramics, polyetheretherketone (PEEK), or titanium. We prefer placing expandable cages for anterolateral thoracolumbar reconstruction because they can better adapt to the defect, the surgeon avoids the long and tedious tailoring of titanium mesh, and the stability of the construct is ensured. The proper-size implant is chosen; it is placed under fluoroscopic visualization and expanded until it sits press-fit in its final position. Allograft or bone can be packed around the cage to promote fusion. The construct can then be secured anteriorly using either screws and bars or plates systems, and brought into place using the usual techniques.

Closure and Postoperative Care

The thoracic cavity is rinsed and cleaned of debris, thus avoiding unnecessary adherences between the two pleural sheets. A small chest tube is placed in the chest cavity through one of the inferiormost ports under endoscopic visualization. Lung reinflation is visualized with the camera in place to ensure that no atelectatic lobes are overlooked. The chest tube is secured, and the ports are closed in a single-layer fashion and made airtight using methacrylate (Dermabond).

The chest tube is left without suction, especially in those cases where a cerebrospinal fluid (CSF) leak due to intradural disk extension has been confirmed. The chest tube is usually removed on the first postoperative day (or when the output is below 150 mL/d). A control chest radiography is obtained after removing the tube to confirm that no pneumothorax has occurred during tube removal. Patient are usually discharged on the fourth or fifth postoperative day.

Selection of the Surgical Approach

The selection of the surgical approach is based primarily on the location of the disk herniation (central or lateral), the nature of the herniation (hard or soft), the severity of symptoms, and the patient's ability to tolerate the procedure.[5]

Choosing the Right Approach

When approaching a thoracic disk, the surgeon considers the following factors:

- Pathophysiology of the illness
- Physical characteristics of the hernia (soft, calcified, size, and localization)
- Surgical expertise and experience
- Operating room setup and technical equipment required
- Clinical status of the patient

The combination of medullar compression at the narrowest section of the spinal canal in addition to the complex vascular anatomy of the spinal cord (watershed areas) may explain why the thoracic level is one of the most sensitive areas of the spinal cord.[6] The compensatory support provided in the lumbar and cervical regions does not exist in the thoracic region; consequently, compromise of these arteries results in regional ischemia.[7] In thoracic disk herniations, an increase in intradiskal pressures is transmitted to the neural elements, resulting in an increase in tissue interstitial pressures. The anterior approach enables the disk mass to be dissected away from the thecal sac, thus minimizing manipulation and compressive or tensile forces applied directly or indirectly to the spinal cord. For the same reason, bleeding control is of the utmost importance.[5]

Although most authors recommend anterior approaches for large calcified or medially located disks, there is no consensus on the approach when soft lateralized herniations need to be removed.[3] Posterior and posterolateral approaches achieve an indirect decompression of the spinal cord, requiring in some cases some degree of dural sac manipulation. If the integrity of the muscle–ligament and articular components of a spinal segment is important for spinal stability, modern and less aggressive anterior procedures should be a priority. Reports from large series using either thoracoscopy or retro- or transpleural techniques confirm this recommendation.[4,6,8–11]

The choice of the thoracoscopic or retropleural approach also depends on the quality of the physis and on whether or not the disk has an intradural component. Thoracoscopy is an excellent alternative for obese patients. In this case, we prefer a retropleural approach enabling the pleura to act as a second barrier against CSF leakage after covering the dura mater defect.

A complete discussion of the decision-making process is beyond the scope of this chapter, but the above is a sample of the points on which surgeons must focus when treating thoracic disks.

Why Choose an Anterior Approach to the Thoracic Spine?

Anatomic Basis

The spine and spinal cord have unique characteristics at the thoracic area. Due to the kyphotic curve of the spine, the spinal cord runs very close to the posterior wall of the vertebral bodies. The thoracic region is the narrowest of the spinal canal and the worst vascularized as well (watershed areas), making it very sensitive to ischemia.[6] In addition, the thoracic nerve roots and the dentate ligaments tether the cord, preventing it from drifting away from ventral mass-occupying lesions.

The working area that the surgeon creates using a ventral approach does not require retraction or sectioning of muscular structures. The dissection follows natural cavities (transthoracic) or unfolds them (retropleural).

Technical and Biomechanical Basis

Ever since laminectomy was largely abandoned for the operative treatment of thoracic disk herniation, due to the high degree of morbidity and mortality associated with the approach, a number of alternative surgical techniques have been developed to provide better access to the thoracic spine, such as costotransversectomy, lateral extra cavitary transpedicular, pedicle sparing, and thoracotomy.

Less disruptive procedures have marked the evolution of spine surgery during the last two decades, all of which aim to reduce unnecessary trauma on noble and functionally intact structures, thus achieving results that are equal to or better than those with conventional techniques. The term *minimally invasive spine surgery* (MISS) describes these procedures that divulse instead of detach muscle insertions, and unfold virtual cavities instead of widely opening them, reducing markedly the approach-related trauma. Of the techniques cited above, the anterior technique, with all its variations, is the only one that reaches the spine, sharply dissecting the skin and the pleura (in the transpleural varieties). All other structures strongly ligated to stability are kept intact (ligaments, capsule, articular surface, etc.).

Modern treatment of spinal pathologies is focused on optimizing, maintaining, or regaining stability. Thoracic stability is determined by the interaction of the vertebrae, disks, ribcage, and sternum.[12] Alterations in the integrity of these elements can lead to postoperative column insufficiency and mechanical instability. Although the approach technique varies between the anterior procedures (thoracotomy and its "mini" variations [trans- or retropleural] or thoracoscopy), the spinal step is identical for all the techniques and has been biomechanically tested in a report by Broc.[13] He concluded that although minimal biomechanical alterations of the operated segment occur, they do not lead to destabilization of the segment. One of the main advantages of approaching the spinal canal anteriorly is that the surgeon removes the mass-occupying lesion, pulling it away from the dural sac, rather than manipulating and holding it away during dissection.

Anterior instrumentation of the spine at the thoracic level is easier and safer as compared with a posterior instrumentation technique. The hardware needed can be brought into position through the same surgical corridor under direct visual control, and in the majority of the cases fewer pieces of equipment are needed compared with posterior or posterolateral techniques, thus reducing costs and radiation exposure. Finally, the bony surface available to achieve a stable bony fusion is larger at the anterior than at the posterior area of the vertebral body.[10]

Complications

The risk of life-threatening complications is cited by many authors as a reason not to use an anterior approach. However, the recent literature suggests that this risk is overstated. In publications with at least 100 cases performed endoscopically with a follow-up of at least 2 years, the overall complication rate varied between 15.6% and 21%.[9,10,12] The majority of the complications were pleural effusions and neuralgia. The mortality rate was 0%. No major vascular or pulmonary complications occurred. McAfee et al[14] found that the infection rate with MISS was extremely low, 0 to 0.2%, when compared with traditional open posterior approaches, which have an infection rate of 2 to 4%. This lower rate was also found with anterior thoracic approaches. In addition, no patient had either a wound infection or a deep-seated infection.

Steep Learning Curve

The majority of the authors favoring posterior or posterolateral approaches argue against anterior techniques because of the steep learning curve and because in some cases a thoracic surgeon must perform the thoracic part of the approach to the spine. But anterior approaches to the spine are not taught to spinal surgeons in training, so we do not know if the steep learning curve can be overcome. How easy and safe is the removal of a intramedullary tumor, or a lumbar radical resection of a sarcoma, or placing pedicle screws at the upper thoracic or lower cervical spine? Both the spinal cord and the vascular structures are in danger of presenting life-threatening complications, and the error margin at those levels is much higher than at the thoracic spine. But many centers worldwide perform these surgeries, with different degrees of expertise and surgical skills, varying amounts of equipment, and varying results, despite the steep learning curve.

We believe that the steep learning curve is used more as an excuse than as a real obstacle. New techniques always entail different anatomic and technical setups, and the learning process is not an obstacle for any of these approaches.

New Developments

Surgery is a dynamic specialty that fosters innovation and the never-ending search for less aggressive and more effective techniques or equipment to treat diseases. Endoscopy has certainly changed the balance among tissue damage, skill, and effectiveness. Percutaneous procedures are gaining a greater role in classic posterior instrumentation. Navigation will play a major role in the future, not only providing more accuracy in screws placement but also serving as a guide and aid in the anatomic approach. Our main goal as surgeons is to respect healthy and functional tissue as much as possible. Our therapeutic options for spinal disease seem unlimited, with new procedures continually being developed and our knowledge about the role or tissues, organs, muscles, ligaments, and bone, and the interrelations between them, continuing to increase, yielding improved results. Anterior spinal surgery is just starting to be applied for new approaches, in order to avoid unnecessary trauma on noble tissue.

References

1. Wood KB, Blair JM, Aepple DM, et al. The natural history of asymptomatic thoracic disc herniations. Spine 1997;22:525–529, discussion 529–530
2. Brown CW, Deffer PA Jr, Akmakjian J, Donaldson DH, Brugman JL. The natural history of thoracic disc herniation. Spine 1992;17(6, Suppl):S97–S102
3. Chen TC. Surgical outcome for thoracic disc surgery in the postlaminectomy era. Neurosurg Focus 2000;9:e12
4. Moran C, Ali Z, McEvoy L, Bolger C. Mini-open retropleural transthoracic approach for the treatment of giant thoracic disc herniation. Spine 2012;37:E1079–E1084
5. Ayhan S, Nelson C, Gok B, et al. Transthoracic surgical treatment for centrally located thoracic disc herniations presenting with myelopathy: a 5-year institutional experience. J Spinal Disord Tech 2010;23:79–88
6. Deviren V, Kuelling FA, Poulter G, Pekmezci M. Minimal invasive anterolateral transthoracic transpleural approach: a novel technique for thoracic disc herniation. A review of the literature, description of a new surgical technique and experience with first 12 consecutive patients. J Spinal Disord Tech 2011;24:E40–E48
7. Martirosyan NL, Feuerstein JS, Theodore N, Cavalcanti DD, Spetzler RF, Preul MC. Blood supply and vascular reactivity of the spinal cord under normal and pathological conditions. J Neurosurg Spine 2011;15:238–251
8. Rosenthal D, Dickman CA. Thoracoscopic microsurgical excision of herniated thoracic discs. J Neurosurg 1998;89:224–235
9. Anand N, Regan JJ. Video-assisted thoracoscopic surgery for thoracic disc disease: Classification and outcome study of 100 consecutive cases with a 2-year minimum follow-up period. Spine 2002;27:871–879
10. Quint U, Bordon G, Preissl I, Sanner C, Rosenthal D. Thoracoscopic treatment for single level symptomatic thoracic disc herniation: a prospective followed cohort study in a group of 167 consecutive cases. Eur Spine J 2012;21:637–645
11. Oskouian RJ, Johnson JP. Endoscopic thoracic microdiscectomy. J Neurosurg Spine 2005;3:459–464
12. Wait SD, Fox DJ Jr, Kenny KJ, Dickman CA. Thoracoscopic resection of symptomatic herniated thoracic discs: clinical results in 121 patients. Spine 2012;37:35–40
13. Broc GG, Crawford NR, Sonntag, VKH, Dickman CA. Biomechanical effects of transthoracic microdiscectomy. Spine 1997;22(6):605–612

58 Lateral Transthoracic and Retropleural MIS Approaches

Jason M. Paluzzi, Michael S. Park, and Juan S. Uribe

Surgical treatment for pathology of the thoracic spine has traditionally involved either an anterior or posterior approach, or a combination of them. These approaches include open thoracotomy, laminectomy, and costotransversectomy, as well as lateral extracavitary, thoracoscopic, and transpedicular approaches. However, they are associated with significant morbidity due to various anatomic considerations. The lateral retropleural thoracotomy was devised to permit a direct view of the neural elements while limiting injury to the intercostal nerve, aorta, vena cava, and sympathetic plexus, at the expense of a large incision and extensive rib resection. With the rise of expandable and tubular retractors, modified light sources, and specialized surgical instruments, minimally invasive surgery (MIS) variations of the lateral approach have been developed to circumvent these issues. The transthoracic and retropleural MIS approaches to the thoracic spine are technical variations that aim to achieve the same goals of the traditional approaches while minimizing associated morbidity.

Patient Selection

Patients with predominantly ventral or lateral thoracic spinal pathology have the greatest potential for benefit from these approaches. Additionally, patients with limited cardiopulmonary reserve who may not be able to tolerate longer procedures, extensive dissections, or single-lung ventilation may be preferentially selected for an MIS approach, in comparison with other approaches to the thoracic spine.

Objective

- To provide access to the ventral aspect of the vertebral column with a simultaneous view of the dura, neural elements, and anterior spinal pathology while minimizing complications associated with more extensive dissections

Indications

- Anterior compression of the neural elements or instability of the thoracic or thoracolumbar spine resulting from:
  - Unstable traumatic fracture
  - Infectious processes, including osteomyelitis, diskitis, and abscess
  - Primary or metastatic neoplasm involving the vertebrae or anterior/lateral meninges
  - Anterior degenerative disease such as thoracic disk herniation

Contraindications

- Pathology of the upper thoracic levels (T1–T4), as the presence of the mediastinum and axilla provides an anatomic constraint and limits access using these approaches
- Neoplastic processes involving predominantly the posterior elements with or without bilateral pedicle invasion, as a posterior or posterolateral approach is typically warranted
- Limited life expectancy, usually in the setting of metastatic tumors
- Previous ipsilateral thoracotomy, as dissection may be limited by significant pleural adhesions (relative contraindication)
- Medical comorbidities, such as advanced age, poor pulmonary function, and severe debilitation or medically frailty, were previously listed as contraindications, although these may be the patients who stand to gain the most from an MIS approach.

Advantages

- Offers direct visualization and concurrent control of the ventral thecal sac and anterior spinal pathology
- Smaller incisions result in fewer wound-related complications, decreased somatic pain, earlier mobilization, and shorter recovery
- Avoids extensive muscle dissection, rib resection, potential blood loss, and complications associated with single-lung ventilation seen in traditional anterior and posterior approaches
- Affords greater preservation of biomechanically important spinal anatomy such as the anterior and posterior longitudinal ligaments and the posterior ligamentous structures

Disadvantages

- There is a learning curve involved with MIS approaches due to a long working distance within a narrow space.
- Operative instruments may not be long enough for access in larger patients.
- Surgical planning requiring posterior instrumentation will necessitate a second incision.
- Chest tube drainage may be necessary postoperatively if sufficient air cannot be evacuated during closure (see below).

Choice of Operative Approach

As mentioned previously, the MIS lateral retropleural and transthoracic approaches are best suited for access to the ventrolateral thoracic spine from T4 to T12. If access to the upper thoracic spine is required, either an anterior transthoracic or a posterior approach may be more appropriate. For anterior approaches, with or without video endoscopy, the assistance of an access cardiothoracic surgeon is recommended. Posterior and posterolateral approaches are best suited for dorsal pathology; however, access to the ventral spine from a posterior corridor often requires a transpedicular approach, and although the lateral extracavitary approach can recapitulate the same ventrolateral exposure as the MIS approaches described here, it often requires greater muscle and soft tissue dissection.

Preoperative Imaging

Radiographic evaluation generally includes magnetic resonance imaging (MRI) of the affected region of the spine. This should include a contrasted sequence if a mass lesion such as a tumor or abscess is determined to be the primary pathology. If the patient cannot undergo an MRI, a computed tomography (CT) myelogram can delineate the lesion and assess the severity of neural compression. A noncontrasted CT scan should be obtained to evaluate vertebral integrity and for general surgical planning with respect to the bony anatomy. Standing scoliosis or flexion-extension radiographs may be indicated to determine the presence of a gross spinal deformity or instability, respectively. Angiography may be useful in the setting of hypervascular spinal tumors for potential preoperative embolization.

Surgical Procedure

Patient Positioning

The patient is placed and secured in a true lateral decubitus position on a radiolucent table (**Fig. 58.1**). The patient should be positioned with the table break under the mid-surgical level. An axillary roll is placed, and care is taken to pad all pressure points. Using fluoroscopy, the index level is identified and marked on the skin, as is the overlying rib. The side of the approach is dictated by the orientation of the pathology or, in some cases, the vertebral level.

Retropleural Approach

A 6-cm oblique incision is made directly over the rib overlying the index level in the midaxillary line. After dissecting through the soft tissue, latissimus dorsi, and intercostal muscles with monopolar electrocautery down to the rib periosteum, a 5-cm length of rib is exposed in a subperiosteal fashion. Using an Alexander or Doyen rib dissector, the underlying endothoracic fascia and neurovascular bundle are bluntly separated from the underside of the rib, with attention paid so as not to disrupt the latter. This length of rib is then removed and can be saved for use as autologous graft material. The rib resected typically correlates to two levels above the index vertebral level (e.g., the eighth rib for the tenth thoracic vertebra). Additional rib posteriorly may be removed with rongeurs to maximize exposure. The cut edges are waxed for hemostasis. The endothoracic fascia, which lies immediately underneath the rib and fuses with the periosteum, is identified and sharply cut to expose the parietal pleura. To stay in the retropleural space, the parietal pleura is swept anteriorly via blunt finger dissection to develop the appropriate plane.[1–3]

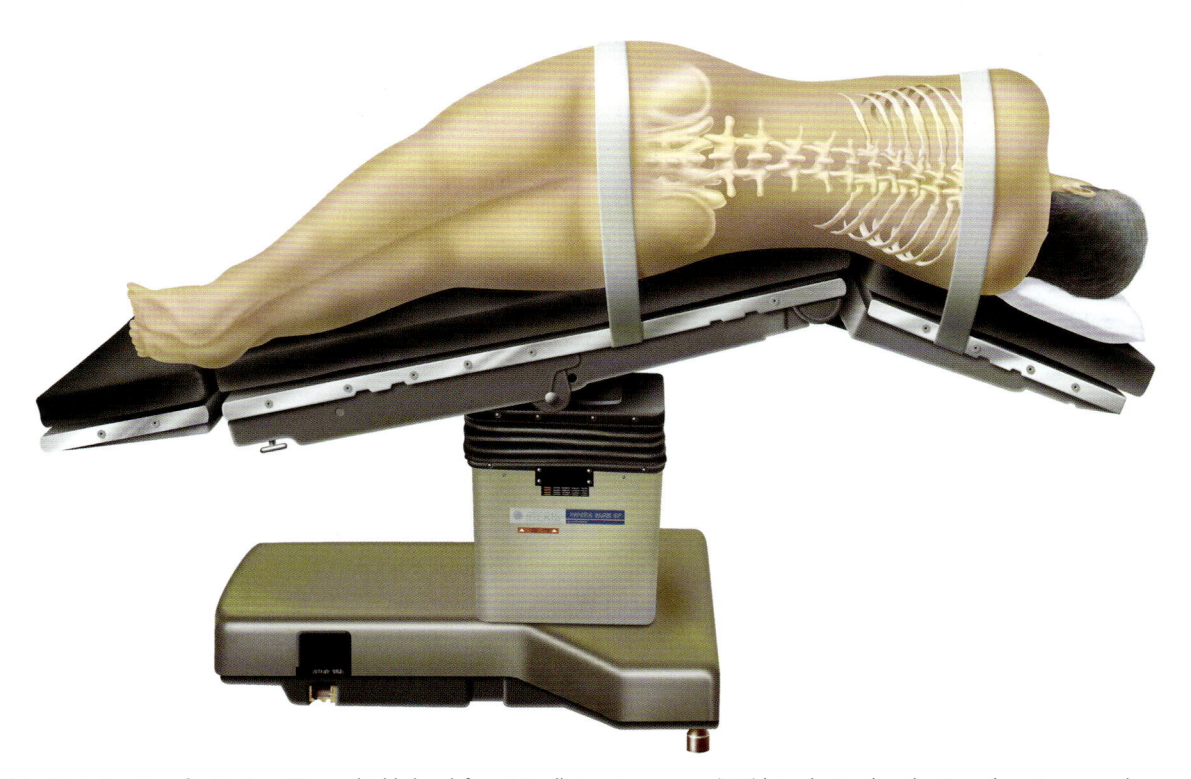

Fig. 58.1 Posterior view of patient position and table break for minimally invasive surgery (MIS) lateral retropleural or transthoracic approach.

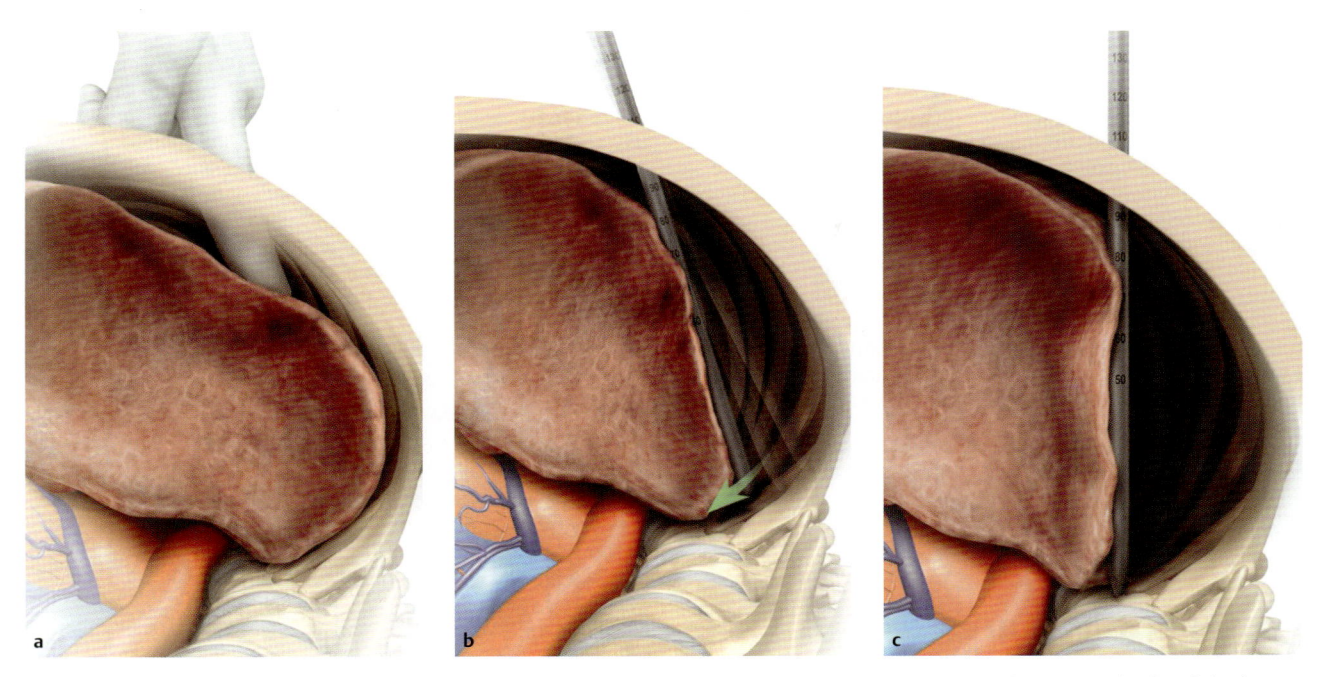

Fig. 58.2 (a) Digital access into the thoracic space with inflated-lung deflection. (b) The access dilator passing on the posterior border of the thoracic cavity (to prevent violation of the lung with the leading end of the dilator). (c) Accessing the lateral aspect of the disk space.

Transthoracic Approach

The positioning is identical to that for the retropleural approach. The incision for this approach is slightly shorter, 3 to 4 cm, parallel to and between the ribs. As with the retropleural approach, dissection through the subcutaneous tissue, latissimus dorsi, and intercostal muscles is performed with monopolar electrocautery. The endothoracic fascia and parietal pleura are incised to gain access to the thoracic cavity. For a transthoracic diskectomy, it is usually not necessary to perform rib resection, as the thorax can be entered directly between the ribs. However, for a vertebrectomy, rib resection is still necessary to obtain adequate exposure, with the skin incision made as for a retropleural approach.[1,3]

Dissection and Exposure

Regardless of whether a retropleural or transthoracic approach was used, the lung and parietal pleura (as well as the diaphragm, if performed at lower thoracic levels) are mobilized from the posterior thoracic wall with finger dissection or a sponge stick until the lateral vertebral body, pedicle, and intervertebral disks are visualized (**Fig. 58.2**). It is helpful to identify the ventral surface of the rib head and follow it back to the costovertebral junction; blunt dissection can then be performed with endoscopic Kittner dissectors. For access to the thoracolumbar junction, the posterior attachments of the diaphragm must be sharply dissected off the L1 transverse process, along with the attachment between the medial and lateral arcuate ligaments. The ipsilateral crus may be transected for more anterior exposure in this region.

For approaches from the left, the great vessels must be controlled as well. The aorta and hemiazygos vein are retracted anteriorly. Segmental vessels must be ligated as proximally as possible. Sequential tubular dilators are then inserted and docked on the index vertebral body. An expandable retractor system is then inserted over the last dilator, taking care to retract the aorta anteriorly if present (**Fig. 58.3**). This is secured in place using a flexible table-mounted arm, and expanded for the appropriate exposure.[1–3] From here, the desired operation can continue using MIS techniques, including decompression of neural elements, spinal stabilization, and resection of tumor.

Closure

After a transthoracic approach or in the event of injury to the parietal pleura, air must be removed from the pleural cavity to prevent a pneumothorax. This can be accomplished through placement of a chest tube intraoperatively. Alternatively, a red

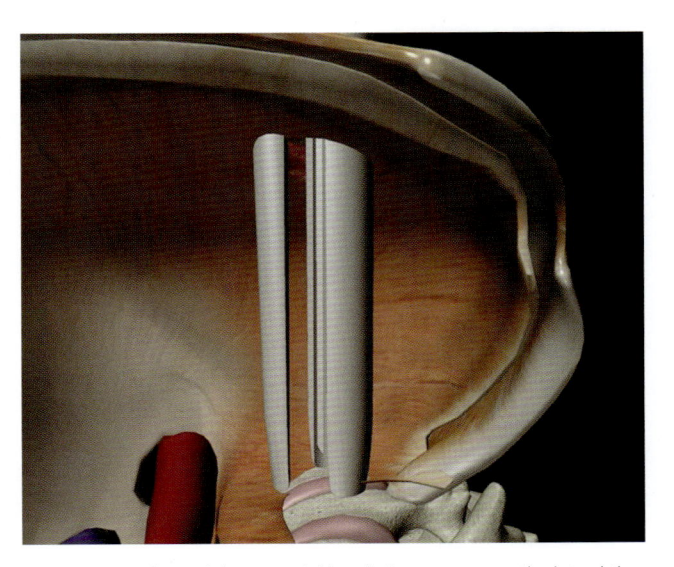

Fig. 58.3 Docking of the expandable tubular retractor on the lateral thoracic spine.

rubber catheter can be placed within the pleural space through the surgical wound. The distal end is submerged under water to prevent further ingress of air through the catheter. The surgical wound is then closed in a standard layered fashion. A purse-string stitch is placed around the catheter, and a Valsalva maneuver with end-inspiratory hold is performed until no more air is visualized within the water trap. At this point, the red rubber catheter is removed as the purse-string stitch is tied, obviating the need for a chest tube. In our experience, chest tube drainage is seldom necessary. It is also our practice to utilize this red rubber technique for retropleural approaches as well. If a drain is needed postoperatively, a Hemovac drain is placed in the wound, tunneled through a separate exit site, and connected to a suction canister under negative pressure. It can usually be removed the following day after inspection of the chest X-ray.[1]

Operative Video

An operative video of the MIS lateral transthoracic approach, as well as corpectomy and graft and plate reconstruction, is available online.[4]

Postoperative Care

A plain chest radiograph should be obtained immediately postoperatively and on postoperative day 1 to verify the absence of pneumothorax (if the red rubber catheter technique described above is used) or to verify the placement of an intraoperative chest tube. If placed, a chest tube is initially placed to low continuous wall suction and weaned to water-seal. Serial chest radiographs should be obtained to verify reexpansion of the lung prior to removal of the chest tube. Should a patient demonstrate respiratory distress or recurrence of a pneumothorax after removal, further evaluation and possible surgical reexploration may be warranted. It is our practice to obtain upright radiographs to confirm spinal stability and a postoperative CT scan to confirm hardware placement if any. Except in cases of diskectomy without interbody fusion, we mobilize our patients with a thoracolumbar orthosis.[5]

Potential Complications and Precautions

During removal of the expandable tubular retractor, the surgical field, bony surfaces, intercostal muscles, latissimus dorsi, and subcutaneous tissues can be inspected for any blood collection or ongoing bleeding. As mentioned previously, and as with any thoracic procedure, proper technique and vigilance is required to avoid the development of pneumothorax. Also, postthoracotomy pain syndromes, potentially leading to splinting and atelectasis, can occur; this can be addressed with local anesthetic infiltration at the time of closure or postoperative pain management consultation for intercostal nerve block.

Conclusion

The MIS lateral approach to the thoracic spine affords efficient visualization of the ventral and lateral spine with direct surgical access to the vertebral body and neural elements. It does so while avoiding the anatomy-related complications and significant morbidity associated with traditional anterior and posterior routes. The trajectory is modeled after the lateral retropleural thoracotomy while significantly reducing the extent of muscular and rib dissection. Although it requires experience with MIS techniques and may be technically demanding for those unfamiliar with the required instruments and practices, it may ultimately reduce complication rates that accompany other approaches to the ventral thoracic spine. **Box 58.1** summarizes the key operative steps and the problems that can arise.

Box 58.1 Key Operative Steps and Potential Problems

Step	Problems and Precautions
6-cm incision over the rib overlying the index level (retropleural approach) or parallel to and between the ribs (transthoracic approach)	Proper identification of the index vertebral level and the rib directly lateral to it
Exposure and removal of 5 cm of the overlying rib	Injury to the neurovascular bundle, violation of the parietal pleura
Blunt dissection along the pleural planes down to the vertebral body	Injury to the pleura or lung
Placement of sequential dilators and an expandable retractor system	Injury to the aorta, hemiazygos vein, or their segmental vessels

References

1. Uribe JS, Dakwar E, Le TV, Christian G, Serrano S, Smith WD. Minimally invasive surgery treatment for thoracic spine tumor removal: a mini-open, lateral approach. Spine 2010;35(26, Suppl):s347–S354
2. Uribe JS, Dakwar E, Cardona RF, Vale FL. Minimally invasive lateral retropleural thoracolumbar approach: cadaveric feasibility study and report of 4 clinical cases. Neurosurgery 2011;68(1, Suppl Operative):32–39, discussion 39
3. Kanter AS, Uribe JS, Bonfield CM, Mosley YI, Taylor WR. XLIF® Corpectomy: clinical experience and outcomes. In: Goodrich JA, Volcan IJ, eds. eXtreme Lateral Interbody Fusion (XLIF®), 2nd ed. St. Louis: Quality Medical Publishing; 2013:421–439
4. Ahmadian AA, Uribe JS. Mini-open retro-pleural thoracic corpectomy for osteomyelitis. J Neurosurg Multimedia, August 23, 2013; AANS Neurosurgery. https://www.youtube.com/watch?v=17Xo_u3WHNg&feature=youtube, accessed April 27, 2014
5. Park MS, Deukmedjian AR, Uribe JS. Minimally invasive anterolateral corpectomy for spinal tumors. Neurosurg Clin N Am 2014;25:317–325

59 Lateral Transthoracic MIS Diskectomy and Vertebrectomy

Michael S. Park and Juan S. Uribe

Historically, laminectomy was the surgical treatment for thoracic disk herniation and ventral spinal pathology. However, complications, most frequently ascribed to spinal cord injury secondary to intraoperative dural sac retraction, were common. In an early review of laminectomy for thoracic disk herniation, 44% of patients either failed to improve or deteriorated neurologically.[1] Transthoracic and dorsolateral (costotransversectomy) approaches were described in 1956[2] for the treatment of Pott's disease and in 1960,[3] respectively. More recently, endoscopic and mini-open lateral transthoracic and retropleural approaches, which were discussed in Chapter 58, have been reported in the neurosurgical literature. Thus, the history of surgery in the thoracic spine reiterates a basic neurosurgical tenet: whenever possible, compressive lesions in the nervous system should be removed directly.[4,5] In comparison to the early laminectomy reports, 80% of patients undergoing the mini-open lateral transthoracic approach for treatment of thoracic disk herniation achieved excellent or good outcomes.[6]

Thoracic disk herniations are much less prevalent than those seen in the lumbar or cervical spine, but despite their relative rarity, patients with symptomatic thoracic disk herniations present with significant neurologic sequelae, most frequently related to progressive myelopathy, and require aggressive treatment. The incidence of symptoms of myelopathy as presenting complaints is testament to the fact that these disk herniations tend to be central or paracentral, are relatively large, and tend to deform and compress the adjacent spinal cord. For these reasons, the natural history of this disorder is discouraging; without surgical intervention the majority of patients fail to regain their previous level of function.[4,5]

The benefits in using a thoracotomy for spine surgery are considerable. The surgeon's view of the anterior dura and posterior longitudinal ligament is unsurpassed when compared with the other routes to the thoracic spine. This fact is only reemphasized when one considers that the majority of pathology in the thoracic spine is ventral. Ventral spinal access affords the ability to perform a decompression (multilevel if necessary) and reconstruction (when required) through a single approach, enabling anterior stabilization with fusion under compression. The indications for transthoracic approaches have been broadened to include surgical treatment of spinal deformities, other forms of osteomyelitis, traumatic burst fracture, and tumors. The disadvantages include the medical complications related to the approach: persistent pneumothorax, pulmonary contusion, pleural effusion, and empyema. Furthermore, because the contralateral pedicle and posterior elements are not well visualized by this approach, a second operation is needed to address pathology of the posterior elements or for the placement of posterior instrumentation. But for centrally located thoracic disk herniations and pathology that lies anterior to the spinal cord, thoracotomy enables the surgeon to gain a pedicle-to-pedicle decompression under direct visualization, a luxury unobtainable through other approaches to the thoracic spine.[4,5]

Patient Selection

The incidence of thoracic disk herniation ranges from 7 to 37%, although only 0.25 to 0.5% of all disk herniations are symptomatic.[7] Therefore, identification of symptomatic patients who typically present with radiculopathy, in the form of pain or sensory loss, or with myelopathy, manifesting as bowel, bladder, or sexual dysfunction, paraparesis, or paraplegia, is important; symptoms and exam findings should correlate with radiographic data.[8] For vertebrectomy, patients with predominantly ventral or lateral thoracic spinal pathology have the greatest potential for benefit from this approach. Additionally, patients with limited cardiopulmonary reserve who may not be able to tolerate longer procedures, extensive dissections, or single lung ventilation may be preferentially selected for this minimally invasive surgery (MIS) approach.

Objective

For diskectomy, the objective is removal of the pathological disk fragment through a ventral approach. For vertebrectomy, the objective is removal of ventral thoracic vertebral pathology from a direct ventral and anterior approach. In both cases, decompression of the neural elements ventrally is the goal.

Indications

- Primary or metastatic vertebral neoplasm
- Osteomyelitis or diskitis
- Unstable thoracic fracture
- Scoliosis or spinal deformity
- Large sequestered thoracic disk herniation causing neurologic symptoms, including myelopathy, refractory radiculopathy, or both

Contraindications

- Medical comorbidity (severe cardiopulmonary disease, acute respiratory distress syndrome) preventing safe access through the chest or lateral positioning
- Limited life expectancy (a contraindication for vertebrectomy)

Advantages

- Controlled exposure to the anterior dura
- Procedure of choice for correction of scoliosis
- Ease in control of the radicular vasculature
- Ability to perform corpectomy and place ventral instrumentation (when indicated) from a single approach

Disadvantages

- Increased incidence of pulmonary complications (atelectasis, pneumonia, pleural effusion, chylothorax, persistent pneumothorax bronchopulmonary fistula)
- Increased postprocedural pain (postthoracotomy pain syndrome, intercostal neuralgia)
- Increased incidence of medical complications as a result of thoracotomy (thromboembolism, vascular injuries)
- May require a second operation to address posterior element pathology

Choice of Operative Approach

The choice of diskectomy versus vertebrectomy ultimately depends on the nature and extent of the underlying pathology, as well as the amount of spinal deformity and reconstruction needed. Naturally, for pathology limited to the intervertebral disk, such as central or paracentral disk herniations or diskitis, diskectomy will be sufficient, except in cases with a large sequestered fragment where vertebrectomy is necessary for adequate decompression. The side of approach is often dictated by the side and location of (i.e., ipsilateral to) the pathology.

Preoperative Imaging

Radiographic evaluation generally includes magnetic resonance imaging (MRI) of the affected region of the spine. This should include a contrasted sequence if a mass lesion such as a tumor or abscess is determined to be the primary pathology. If the patient cannot undergo an MRI, a computed tomography (CT) myelogram can delineate the lesion and assess the severity of neural compression. It should be noted that MRI and CT myelogram are both associated with a 14% false-positive rate for symptomatic thoracic disk herniation.[7] A noncontrasted CT scan should be obtained to evaluate the vertebral integrity and for general surgical planning with respect to the bony anatomy. Noncontrast CT may also be useful in demonstrating calcification of a herniated thoracic disk. Standing scoliosis or flexion-extension radiographs may be indicated to determine the presence of gross spinal deformity or instability, respectively. Angiography may be useful in the setting of hypervascular spinal tumors for potential preoperative embolization.

Surgical Procedure

Patient positioning and surgical approaches are discussed in Chapter 58. The importance of identifying the correct vertebral level(s) cannot be understated, given the lack of helpful identifying features to distinguish between adjacent vertebrae (e.g., C2, sacrum) and that wrong-level surgery occurs most commonly in the thoracic spine. It is our practice to obtain counting films (e.g., an overview MRI counting image) from C2 and especially from the sacrum, to enable us to count from the top and from the bottom in a redundant fashion at the time of surgery. As a reminder from Chapter 58, for a transthoracic diskectomy it is usually not necessary to remove the rib, aside from the rib head once the exposure is completed.

Once adequate exposure has been obtained, landmarks including the rib head are identified. For a diskectomy, the segmental vessel often can be maintained when operating on a thoracic disk, as these vessels usually lie essentially midway between disk spaces. Alternatively (or in the case of a vertebrectomy), they may be taken early in the procedure, on the vertebral body, to preserve the vascular structure more distally and to avoid ischemic cord complications. Ligation also helps to minimize blood loss later in the procedure.

The rib head (2–3 cm) is removed using an osteotome or high-speed drill (**Fig. 59.1**). The rib head is disarticulated by being freed from its ligamentous (costotransverse and costovertebral) attachments using a down-going curette). By removing the rib, it is possible to identify the intercostal nerve from the undersurface of the named rib and trace it back toward the neural foramen.[9] It is this maneuver that helps to ascertain the location of the pedicle as well and enables the surgeon to gain an early understanding of the location of the thecal sac.[4]

The upper portion of the pedicle can be drilled and then removed in part or completely using a Kerrison rongeur. Once removed, the lateral thecal sac is identified and can be visualized

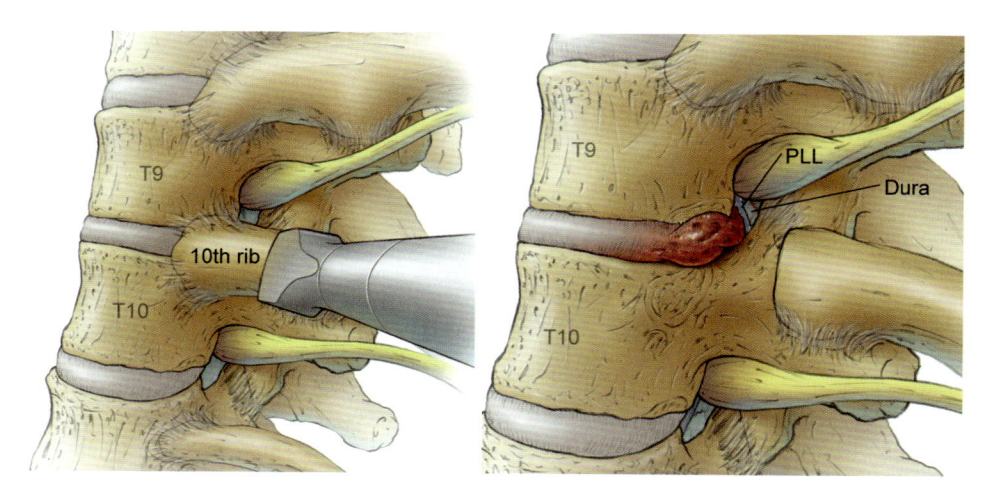

Fig. 59.1 The lateral disk space before (a) and after (b) rib head removal. PLL, posterior longitudinal ligament.

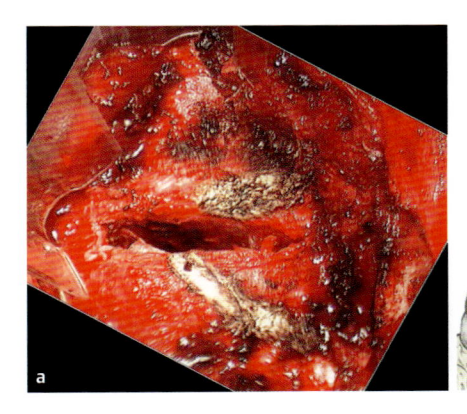

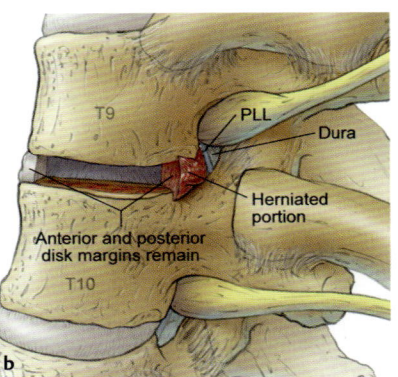

Fig. 59.2 Intraoperative photograph (**a**) and illustration (**b**), lateral view, demonstrating osteotomy of the posterior aspect of the adjacent vertebral bodies to facilitate complete canal decompression.

during the remainder of the procedure. Once the surgeon has determined the location of the spinal cord, it then becomes safe to begin the diskectomy.

Diskectomy

The disk is incised using a knife or the osteotome and removed anteriorly away from the thecal sac using pituitary rongeurs. Diskectomy is facilitated by removing a small section (~ 1 cm) of the neighboring vertebral bodies (**Fig. 59.2**). It may be necessary to widen this in the case of very calcified disks or those that have migrated behind the vertebral body. The initial diskectomy is performed by removing the disk material that clearly lies away from the ventral canal. The remaining disk can then be removed working from the thecal sac medially. Once a cavity is created (by performing the initial diskectomy and adjacent bone removal), the remaining disk can be reduced into this cavity, thereby directing all force away from the spine (**Fig. 59.3**). To minimize epidural bleeding, the posterior longitudinal ligament (PLL) is kept intact throughout the diskectomy. Once complete, it may be cauterized and then removed as a last step. A Woodsen or No. 4 Penfield can be used to ensure that no sequestered fragments lie hidden superior and inferior to the visualized area. The inspection should be undertaken from pedicle to pedicle, ensuring adequate decompression of the spinal canal and the complete removal of the offending pathology. If the contralateral pedicle cannot be felt, it is possible to take an anteroposterior film to confirm the extent of the decompression.[4]

Although not common, it is possible to destabilize a patient through this diskectomy (vertebrectomies are patently destabilizing and require anterior column reconstruction). In the case of extensive body removal (secondary to a large sequestered disk) the patient may require fusion. Although most authors do not believe that fusion is required for the majority of thoracic disk herniations,[4] it is our practice to place a polyetheretherketone (PEEK) interbody cage in the majority of cases, depending on the amount of disk removed.[6,8]

Vertebrectomy

For vertebrectomy, diskectomies at the adjacent levels above and below the pathological level are performed. Depending on the need for and the type of anterolateral plating system being used, additional rib head resections may need to be performed at the adjacent levels. For a vertebrectomy, the high-speed drill or osteotome is used to remove the majority of the anterior aspect of the vertebral body between the emptied disk spaces, helping to create a cavity anterior to and surrounding the area of neurologic compression. It is common to leave the anterior longitudinal ligament as well as the ventral and deep cortex intact to help secure the bone graft in place after the completion of the procedure (for more information, see Chapter 60). A more radical decompression can take place, especially in the case of tumor, but for the majority of cases this maneuver helps to create a barrier to prevent injury to the adjacent vascular and visceral structures.

The remaining disk and posterior cortex can be removed working from the thecal sac medially and ventrally. After a cavity is created (by performing the initial diskectomies and intervening bony removal), the remaining disk and bone can be reduced into this cavity, thereby directing all force away from the spine. The remainder of the diskectomies and vertebrectomy, including removal of the PLL and inspection of the decompression, is performed as described earlier for the diskectomy (**Fig. 59.4**). Anterolateral reconstruction is discussed in Chapter 60.[4,5]

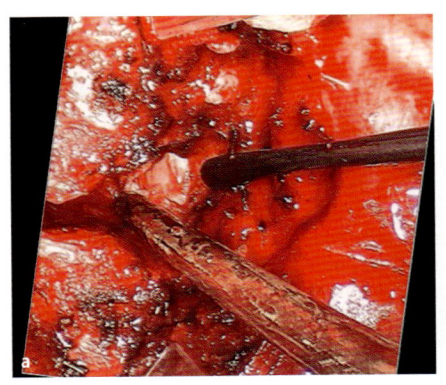

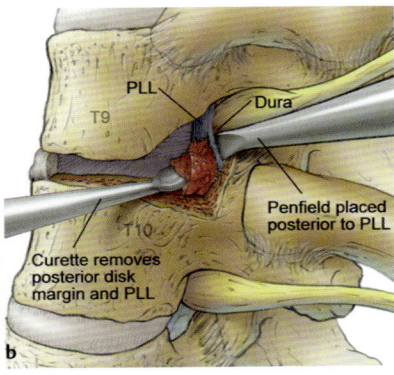

Fig. 59.3 Intraoperative photograph (**a**) and illustration (**b**), lateral view, showing completed thoracic herniated disk removal, demonstrating osteotomy of the posterior aspect of the adjacent vertebral bodies to facilitate complete canal decompression. PLL, posterior longitudinal ligament.

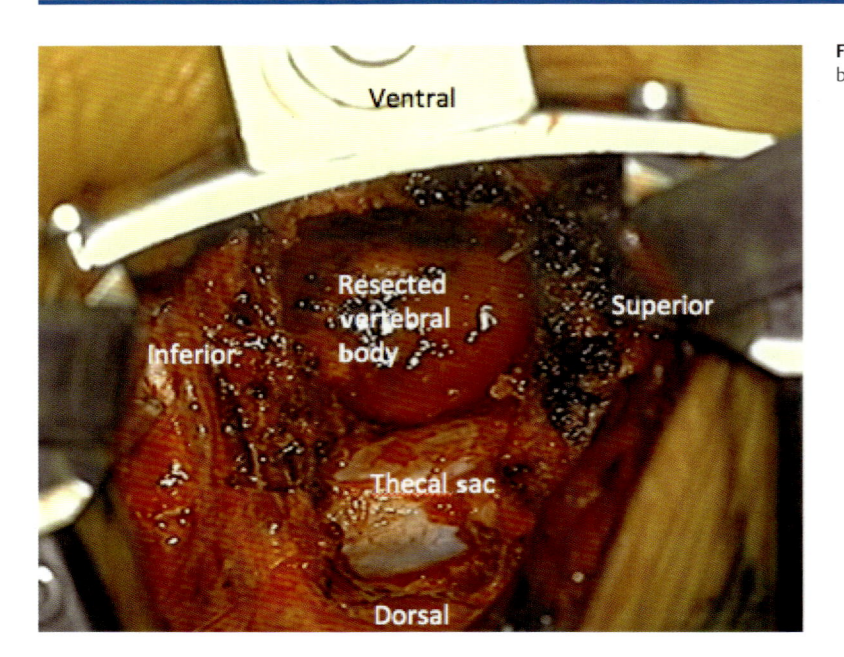

Fig. 59.4 Intraoperative photograph of the resection bed following corpectomy.

Closure

If completion of the diskectomy, with or without an interbody fusion, marks the end of the procedure proper, then the wound is irrigated with copious amounts of antibiotic-impregnated saline. Any durotomies, whether unintended or for resection of intradural tumor, should be closed primarily or with fibrin sealant; lumbar drainage may be necessary.[10] When incised for operations near the thoracolumbar junction, the diaphragm is reattached at its lateral margin, with the crura being sewn directly to the anterior longitudinal ligament. Any violations in the peritoneum should be closed primarily. When entered, the parietal pleura is closed as well, overlying the operative site. The red rubber technique described in Chapter 58 can be used to evacuate air from the wound, otherwise, a 28-French chest tube is placed and tunneled out through a separate incision, especially if the parietal pleura was entered. In our experience, however, it is seldom necessary to perform chest tube drainage. After the wound is fully closed, the chest tube is placed onto low wall suctioning. Alternatively, a Hemovac drain can be placed in the wound and tunneled through a separate incision (akin to a small diameter chest tube), and connected to a suction canister under negative pressure; it can usually be removed the following day after inspection of the chest X-ray. The lung is reinflated under direct visualization. The intercostal muscles, subcutaneous tissue, and skin are closed in standard fashion.

Operative Video

An operative video of the MIS lateral transthoracic corpectomy, as well as the approach and graft and plate reconstruction, is available online.[11]

Postoperative Care

A plain chest radiograph should be obtained immediately postoperatively and on postoperative day 1 to verify the absence of pneumothorax (if the red rubber catheter technique described in the previous chapter is used) or to verify the placement of an intraoperative chest tube. If placed, a chest tube is initially placed to low continuous wall suction and weaned to water-seal. Serial chest radiographs should be obtained to verify reexpansion of the lung prior to removal of the chest tube. Should a patient demonstrate respiratory distress or recurrence of a pneumothorax after removal, further evaluation and possible surgical reexploration may be warranted. It is our practice to obtain upright radiographs and a postoperative CT scan to confirm spinal stability and the degree of spinal decompression, respectively. We mobilize our patients with a thoracolumbar orthosis for 6 to 12 weeks, depending on whether their procedure was a diskectomy or vertebrectomy.[12]

Potential Complications and Precautions

Several authors recommend intraoperative neural monitoring for thoracic diskectomy and corpectomy.[4,5,13,14] During positioning, every effort should be made to place the patient in a truly orthogonal lateral decubitus position and to obtain true orthogonal anteroposterior and lateral intraoperative fluoroscopic views, to facilitate orientation in the surgical field. As with most cases of spinal cord compression, intraoperative hypotension should be avoided, to maintain spinal cord perfusion. Finally, it is suggested that surgical treatment of heavily calcified thoracic disk herniations is associated with a higher rate of intraoperative durotomy, which may be repaired primarily or with fibrin glue sealant.[13]

Conclusion

The MIS lateral transthoracic approach described in Chapter 58 can be used to perform thoracic diskectomy and vertebrectomy in a safe fashion with excellent results, with the advantages and disadvantages pertinent to the MIS nature of the approach and the surgical exposure afforded by this route of access to the thoracic spine. Experience with MIS techniques is recommended, if not required, as this surgery may be technically demanding for those unfamiliar with the required instruments and practices, but their application here has been demonstrated, at least preliminarily, to reduce complication rates that accompany other approaches to the ventral thoracic spine. **Box 59.1** summarizes the key operative steps and the problems that can arise.

Box 59.1 Key Operative Steps and Potential Problems

Step	Problems and Precautions
Resection of the rib head	Proper identification of the operative level
Identification of the intercostal nerve, neural foramen, pedicle, and thecal sac	Injury to the neurovascular bundle, violation of the parietal pleura
Partial pediculectomy and corpectomy	Unnecessary contact with dura
Diskectomy proper	Durotomy, especially with calcified disks
Vertebrectomy (if part of the procedure)	Vascular injuries

References

1. Perot PL Jr, Munro DD. Transthoracic removal of midline thoracic disc protrusions causing spinal cord compression. J Neurosurg 1969;31:452–458
2. Hodgson AR, Stock FE. Anterior spinal fusion a preliminary communication on the radical treatment of Pott's disease and Pott's paraplegia. Br J Surg 1956;44:266–275
3. Hulme A. The surgical approach to thoracic intervertebral disc protrusions. J Neurol Neurosurg Psychiatry 1960;23:133–137
4. Isaacs RE. Transthoracic diskectomy. In: Fessler LG, Sekhar LN, eds. Atlas of Neurosurgical Techniques: Spine and Peripheral Nerves. New York: Thieme; 2006:426–430
5. Isaacs RE. Transthoracic vertebrectomy. In: Fessler LG, Sekhar LN, eds. Atlas of Neurosurgical Techniques: Spine and Peripheral Nerves. New York: Thieme; 2006:431–435
6. Uribe JS, Smith WD, Pimenta L, et al. Minimally invasive lateral approach for symptomatic thoracic disc herniation: initial multicenter clinical experience. J Neurosurg Spine 2012;16:264–279
7. Ghostine S, Samudrala S, Johnson JP. Treatment of thoracic disk herniation. In: Winn HR, ed. Youmans Neurological Surgery, 6th ed. Philadelphia: Elsevier; 2011
8. Pekmezci M, Nacar OA, Deviren V. XLIF® for thoracic disc herniation: technique, outcomes, and comparison with conventional approaches. In: Goodrich JA, Volcan IJ, eds. eXtreme Lateral Interbody Fusion (XLIF®), 2nd ed. St. Louis: Quality Medical Publishing; 2013:283–300
9. Moro T, Kikuchi S, Konno S. Necessity of rib head resection for anterior discectomy in the thoracic spine. Spine 2004;29:1703–1705
10. Uribe JS, Dakwar E, Le TV, Christian G, Serrano S, Smith WD. Minimally invasive surgery treatment for thoracic spine tumor removal: a mini-open, lateral approach. Spine 2010;35(26, Suppl):s347–S354
11. Ahmadian AA, Uribe JS. Mini-open retro-pleural thoracic corpectomy for osteomyelitis. J Neurosurg Multimedia, August 23, 2013 AANSNeurosurgery. https://www.youtube.com/watch?v=17Xo_u3WHNg&feature=youtu.be, accessed April 27, 2014
12. Park MS, Deukmedjian AR, Uribe JS. Minimally invasive anterolateral corpectomy for spinal tumors. Neurosurg Clin N Am 2014;25:317–325
13. Huang RC, O'Leary PF, Taunk R. Open transthoracic discectomy. In: Vaccaro AR, Albert TJ, eds. Spine Surgery: Tricks of the Trade, 2nd ed. New York: Thieme; 2009:103–105
14. Kang JD, Khan MH. Open thoracic corpectomy via the transthoracic approach. In: Vaccaro AR, Albert TJ, eds. Spine Surgery: Tricks of the Trade, 2nd ed. New York: Thieme; 2009:106–109

60 Lateral Graft and Plate Reconstruction

Michael S. Park and Juan S. Uribe

After a corpectomy defect is created, anterior column support must be supplied. In general, the goal of any fusion is to produce a solid bony arthrodesis because no external hardware can confer long-term stability without this; in this sense all internal instrumented fixation can be thought of as a race between bony fusion and hardware failure. Previously, autologous or cadaveric bone grafts were used to reconstruct the anterior column[1]; in the case of metastatic disease, methylmethacrylate-filled Silastic tubing was described by Errico and Cooper[2] for this purpose. With the development of expandable cages, however, these techniques have been supplanted by this newer technology. We describe in this chapter the surgical technique for placement of an expandable cage and lateral plate instrumentation following corpectomy using a modular system; however, the reader is advised to remember that the choice of fixation (anterior or circumferential) is dependent on the amount of stability required, and must be tailored to each individual patient.

Patient Selection

Patients requiring lateral graft and plate reconstruction will have undergone corpectomy or vertebrectomy, as described in Chapter 59.

Objective

- Anterior column reconstruction and placement of internal fixation of the unstable thoracic spine from a minimally invasive surgery (MIS) lateral approach.

Indications

- Thoracic or thoracolumbar instability requiring anterior column reconstruction and internal stabilization resulting from the treatment of the following:
  - Primary or metastatic vertebral neoplasm
  - Osteomyelitis or diskitis
  - Unstable thoracic fracture
  - Large sequestered thoracic disk herniation
  - Scoliosis or other spinal deformity

Contraindications

- Medical comorbidity (severe cardiopulmonary disease, acute respiratory distress syndrome) preventing safe access through the chest
- As limited life expectancy is a contraindication to vertebrectomy, it will also preclude lateral graft and plate reconstruction.

Advantages

- Restores anterior column support
- Anterior construct forms a barrier to graft pullout
- Larger surface area for fusion
- May allow for shorter posterior constructs
- Anterior construct resists extension
- Ease in placement of the graft while the fusion takes place under compression

Disadvantages

- Increased incidence of pulmonary complications (atelectasis, pneumonia, pleural effusion, postthoracotomy pain syndromes, chylothorax, persistent pneumothorax bronchopulmonary fistula)
- Increased incidence of medical complications as a result of thoracotomy or placement of instrumentation (vascular injuries)
- May require a second-stage operation to address posterior element pathology or to complete circumferential fixation

Choice of Operative Approach

At the conclusion of an MIS lateral transthoracic or retropleural corpectomy, the expandable tubular retractor is maintained in its position, and the surgeon is prepared to proceed with lateral graft and plate reconstruction, after inspection of the surgical field to ensure adequacy of neural element decompression, resection of tumor (if applicable), and hemostasis.

Preoperative Imaging

For lateral graft and plate reconstruction, radiographic evaluation will have already taken place as for MIS lateral transthoracic or retropleural corpectomy. It may be helpful to measure the width of the cage footprint, the lengths of the lateral screws, and the height of the plate on preoperative imaging.

Surgical Procedure

Lateral graft and plate reconstruction is performed following decompression and corpectomy. The surgical approach is discussed in Chapter 58 and corpectomy is discussed in Chapter 59.

Regardless of whether decompression or the patient's primary pathology has caused destabilization, the goal of the anterior cage placement is to help restore normal anatomic alignment and promote stability. The reconstruction should be carefully

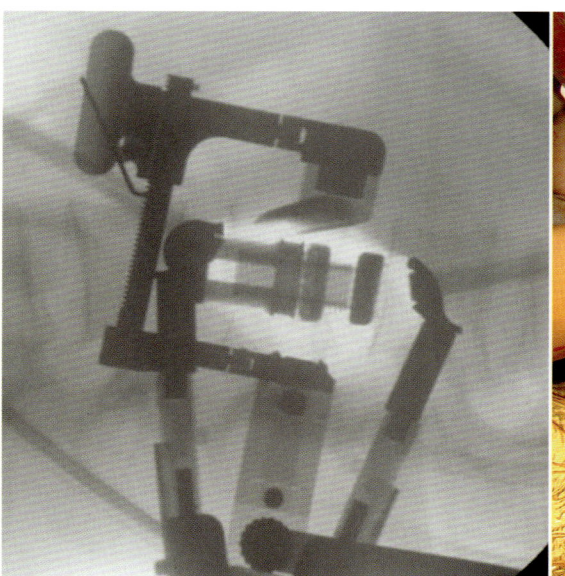

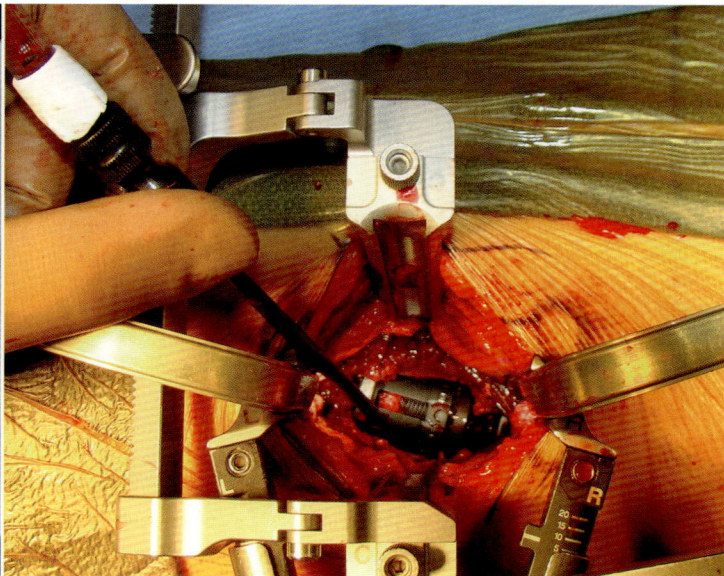

Fig. 60.1 Lateral fluoroscopic image **(a)** and intraoperative photograph **(b)** showing placement of a wide-footprint expandable cage for vertebral body replacement.

tailored to the defect to ensure proper seating of the implant, minimizing the risk of cage pullout while maximizing the patient's alignment and ability to form a solid fusion.

End-Plate Preparation

It is important that the disk material be fully removed to properly place the end caps of the expandable cage, which are designed to span the apophyseal ring of the vertebral body to provide maximum support.[3] Care must be taken not to violate the end plates of the adjacent vertebral bodies, as this will lead to cage subsidence. Once the end plates are prepared, the end caps and cage height are sized with trial devices and a distractor, respectively, and confirmed on fluoroscopy.

Expandable Cage Placement

The expandable cage is assembled from the modular system on a back table and packed with available autologous or allogeneic graft. The cage, which is compressed at this point, is placed using fluoroscopic guidance. Once proper positioning is confirmed, the cage can then be expanded until the intended amount of distraction is obtained (**Fig. 60.1**). At this point, the cage can be locked. If desired, additional graft can be placed surrounding the cage, although attention should be paid to avoid placement of graft material adjacent to the thecal sac.

Lateral Plating

Sizing for placement of a lateral plate can then be performed. If preparation of the lateral aspect of the vertebral bodies at the levels above and below the corpectomy have not yet been completed to this point, then this should be performed at this stage, to ensure proper and flush seating of the lateral plate.

An appropriately sized lateral plate is selected and placed through the expandable retractor in the desired location. In choosing the length of the lateral plate we generally avoid covering any more of the adjacent vertebral bodies than is necessary to span the corpectomy defect and ensure proper screw placement to reduce overhang. At the same time, undersizing the plate may reduce the biomechanical strength of the construct. Additional considerations when selecting an appropriate lateral plate length include the need for consecutive placement of lateral plating and the presence of pedicle screws. When lateral plating is applied to consecutive levels, staggering bolts that are placed within the same vertebral body in the anteroposterior plane may help to prevent potential stress risers and vertebral body fracture.[4] When lateral plating is used at a level that is cranial to preexisting pedicle screws at an adjacent level, either the screw's trajectory can be planned directly cranial to the screws and caudal to the end plate, or a longer plate may be chosen and the screw placed caudal to the pedicle screws. The former of these enables the screw to purchase more cortical bone, thereby increasing the biomechanical strength of the construct, but the latter is necessary if there is insufficient clearance between the pedicle screws and the end plate for the lateral screws.

An awl is used to pierce the cortex for each of the screws and then the screws are placed without prior tapping. Screws are most commonly placed parallel and ~ 2 to 3 mm off the end plates with bicortical purchase, which is desirable but not required. Screw placement can be confirmed with intraoperative fluoroscopy, taking care to maintain trajectories so as not to breach dorsally into the canal, ventrally into major vascular structures, or toward the end plate (**Fig. 60.2**). Slight craniocaudal angulation away from the expandable cage is acceptable, but excessively divergent trajectories should be used with caution as this may interfere with the screw locking mechanism (depending on the particular system) and increase the risk of construct failure. If a four-hole plate is selected, typically the anterior screws will be shorter than the posterior screws or bolts to minimize the risk of neurologic or vascular injury.[5]

Closure

The hardware is irrigated with copious amounts of antibiotic-impregnated saline. When incised for operations near the thora-

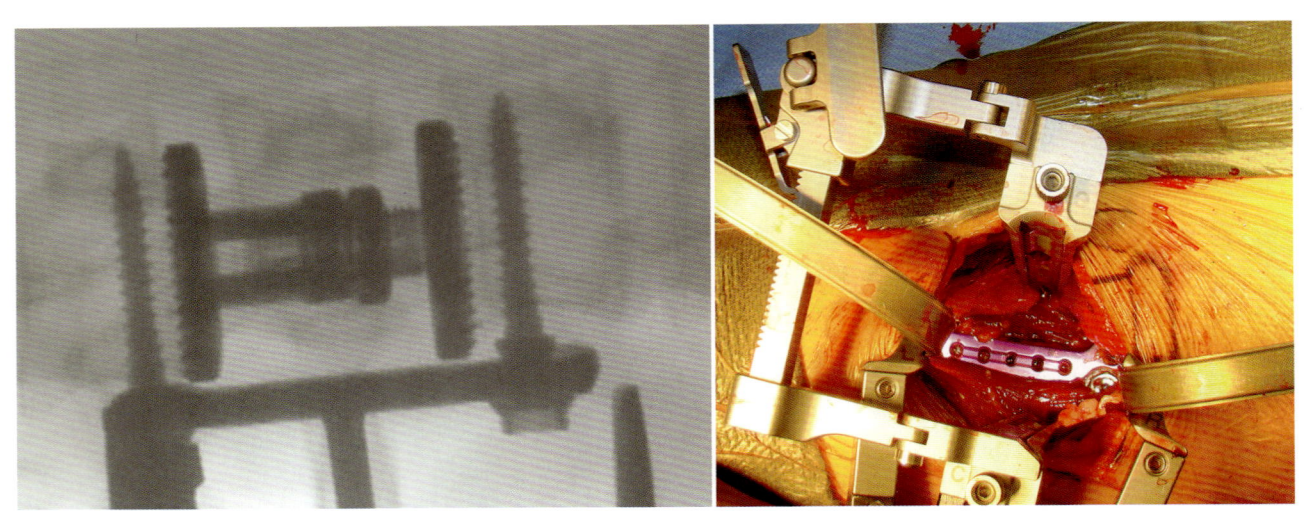

Fig. 60.2 Anterior fluoroscopic image (a) and intraoperative photograph (b) demonstrating the placement of the expandable cage and lateral plate.

columbar junction, the diaphragm is reattached at its lateral margin, with the crura being sewn directly to the anterior longitudinal ligament. Any violations in the peritoneum should be closed primarily. When entered, the parietal pleura is closed as well, overlying the operative site. The red rubber technique described in Chapter 58 can be used to evacuate air from the wound; otherwise, a 28-French chest tube is placed and tunneled out through a separate incision, especially if the parietal pleura was entered. In our experience, however, it is seldom necessary to perform chest tube drainage. After the wound is fully closed, the chest tube is placed onto low wall suctioning. Alternatively, a Hemovac drain can be placed in the wound and tunneled through a separate incision (akin to a small diameter chest tube), and connected to a suction canister under negative pressure; it usually can be removed the following day after inspection of the chest X-ray. The lung is reinflated under direct visualization. The intercostal muscles, subcutaneous tissue, and skin are closed in standard fashion.

Operative Video

An operative video of the lateral graft and plate reconstruction, as well as the MIS lateral transthoracic approach and corpectomy, is available online.[6]

Postoperative Care

A plain chest radiograph should be obtained immediately postoperatively and on postoperative day 1 to verify the absence of pneumothorax (if the red rubber catheter technique described in Chapter 58 is used) or to verify the placement of an intraoperative chest tube. If placed, a chest tube is initially placed to low continuous wall suction and weaned to water-seal. Serial chest radiographs should be obtained to verify reexpansion of the lung prior to removal of the chest tube. Should a patient demonstrate respiratory distress or recurrence of a pneumothorax after removal, further evaluation and possible surgical reexploration may be warranted. It is our practice to obtain upright radiographs and a postoperative computed tomography (CT) scan to confirm spinal stability and the degree of spinal decompression, respectively. We mobilize our patients with a thoracolumbar orthosis for 3 months.[7]

Potential Complications and Precautions

The wide footprint of the interbody cage distributes forces across a larger surface area of the end plate, reducing the risk of subsidence and increasing construct stability.[8] As mentioned previously, end-plate violation during preparation and diskectomy may lead to subsidence of the cage. Also, undersizing of the plate should be avoided, as this does not allow for complete body purchase when the bolts or screws are inserted. In some cases, a longer plate may be the better option, as this may help avoid pedicle screws. Finally, it is important to remember that in many cases, additional instrumentation (e.g., pedicle screw fixation) may be warranted, especially when the bone quality is suspect, or there is intraoperative evidence of either end-plate violation or adjacent vertebral fracture.

Conclusion

The development of expandable cages has contributed to the refinement of lateral graft and plate anterior column reconstruction from MIS lateral approaches to the thoracic spine. Use of large footprint end caps provides the largest contact surface area between the cage and the end plate, enabling the cage to rest on the apophyseal ring, and providing the highest resistance to subsidence. Lateral plating can be performed from this approach as well, although the choice of anterolateral versus circumferential instrumentation depends on several factors and must be tailored to each individual patient. **Box 60.1** summarizes the key operative steps and the problems that can arise.

Box 60.1 Key Operative Steps After Corpectomy Has Been Performed, and Potential Problems

Step	Problem
Adequate adjacent diskectomies and end-plate exposure	End-plate violation and decortication
Craniocaudal sizing of graft and footprint on end plates; packing and preparation of cage	Injury to the exposed spinal cord or thecal sac
Placement of cage	Not locking the expandable cage
Vertebral body preparation and placement of lateral plate	Inadequate vertebral body preparation for flush plate seating
Fixation of lateral plate with screws	Misdirection or cross-threading of screws

References

1. Isaacs RE. Anterolateral graft and plate reconstruction. In: Fessler LG, Sekhar LN, eds. Atlas of Neurosurgical Techniques: Spine and Peripheral Nerves. New York: Thieme; 2006:436–440
2. Errico TJ, Cooper PR. A new method of thoracic and lumbar body replacement for spinal tumors: technical note. Neurosurgery 1993;32:678–680, discussion 680–681
3. Pekmeczi M, Eastlick RK, Mundis GM Jr, Deviren V. XLIF® corpectomy: biomechanics. In: Goodrich JA, Volcan IJ, eds. eXtreme Lateral Interbody Fusion (XLIF®), 2nd ed. St. Louis: Quality Medical Publishing; 2013:223–232
4. Chou D, Lu DC, Weinstein P, Ames CP. Adjacent-level vertebral body fractures after expandable cage reconstruction. J Neurosurg Spine 2008;8:584–588
5. Tohmeh AG, Huntsman KT. XLIF® with lateral plating. In: Goodrich JA, Volcan IJ, eds. eXtreme Lateral Interbody Fusion (XLIF®), 2nd ed. St. Louis: Quality Medical Publishing; 2013:223–232
6. Ahmadian AA, Uribe JS. Mini-open retro-pleural thoracic corpectomy for osteomyelitis. J Neurosurg Multimedia, August 23, 2013. AANS Neurosurgery. https://www.youtube.com/watch?v=17Xo_u3WHNg&feature=youtu.be, accessed April 27, 2014.
7. Park MS, Deukmedjian AR, Uribe JS. Minimally invasive anterolateral corpectomy for spinal tumors. Neurosurg Clin N Am 2014;25:317–325
8. Reinhold M, Schmoelz W, Canto F, Krappinger D, Blauth M, Knop C. A new distractable implant for vertebral body replacement: biomechanical testing of four implants for the thoracolumbar spine. Arch Orthop Trauma Surg 2009;129:1375–1382

61 Open Thoracoabdominal Approach

Hasan R. Syed and Faheem A. Sandhu

Exposure of the anterior thoracoabdominal spine is often necessary for definitive treatment of various spinal disorders. The key features of this exposure are mobilization or partial mobilization of the diaphragm and entry into both the thorax and the retroperitoneum. The approach is versatile and provides good visualization of the anterior spine from T10 to L2. This chapter discusses the anatomic relationships encountered by the standard thoracoabdominal approach to the spine.

Indications

- Trauma: fracture-dislocation, compression fracture
- Tumors: primary tumor of vertebral body, metastatic disease
- Deformity correction: scoliosis, kyphosis
- Degenerative disk disease: herniation
- Pseudarthrosis
- Infection: osteomyelitis, ventral epidural abscess
- Spondylolisthesis
- Failed posterior fusion

Contraindications

- Medical illness that would preclude surgery
- Prior retroperitoneal surgery (relative contraindication)

Advantages

- Versatile approach
- Excellent visualization of and access to the anterior spine between T10 and L2
- Minimal disruption to intraperitoneal structures

Disadvantages

- Entry into the thorax and associated risks
- Complications of thoracotomy
- Potentially painful incision or postoperative neuralgia from damage to intercostal nerve
- Risk of injury to abdominal viscera
- Postoperative ileus common
- Risk of postoperative hernia via diaphragm or abdominal wall
- Risk of spinal cord infarction

Preoperative Imaging and Planning

Imaging studies of the thoracic and lumbar spine should be obtained to determine the level of surgery and confirm the number of ribs. Spinal alignment can also be observed using these images. A computed tomography (CT) scan provides better definition of bony anatomy, whereas magnetic resonance imaging (MRI) provides better visualization of spinal cord compression by tumor or soft tissue. Anesthesia considerations include the use of a central line in case there is unexpected blood loss, and double-lumen endotracheal intubation, which allows for collapse of the ipsilateral lung and enhanced exposure. A patient undergoing a thoracotomy must be hemodynamically stable enough to withstand single-lung intubation and possible significant blood loss.

Surgical Technique

Equipment

- Axillary roll
- Foam padding (for all pressure points)
- Fluoroscopy
- Rib dissector
- Rib spreader
- Rib cutter
- Chest tube

Approach

The thoracoabdominal approach is used to access T10–L2. The spine is usually approached from the patient's left side because arterial repair is easier than repair of the thin-walled vena cava. In addition, the liver is more difficult to mobilize when the approach is from the right. However, the location of the pathology and surgeon comfort often dictate the side of the approach. The use of a double-lumen endotracheal tube may aid in selective lung deflation.

Patient Positioning

The patient is placed in the right lateral decubitus position. Patient positioning is critical for adequate exposure of the spinal level of interest. The affected vertebral body should be positioned over the bend of the table to enhance exposure.

Incision and Dissection

The entire left side is prepped from the axilla to the iliac crest. The skin incision includes a simultaneous thoracic and retroperitoneal approach to the spine and is made over the 10th or 11th rib from the posterior axillary line extending to the lateral margin of the rectus sheath (**Fig. 61.1**). The dissection is carried down to the periosteum proximally and the oblique muscles and the transverses abdominus anteriorly. The cartilaginous rib tip is sharply dissected, and the rib is exposed. The intercostal muscles and neurovascular bundle are stripped subperiosteally from the rib (**Fig. 61.2**). The rib is harvested as far posterior to the costotransverse junction to provide adequate exposure and can be used as graft material. Care should be taken to avoid injury to the inferior neurovascular bundle.

The thoracic cavity is entered via the rib bend, and the diaphragmatic attachment to the ribs is identified. By blunt dissection, the retroperitoneum is entered and a plane established (**Fig. 61.3**). Once the diaphragm is free, it is incised at least 1 to 1.5 cm from its attachment to the rib cage. This muscular rim is denervated and must be tagged every 3 cm for later reattachment. Using a different-color suture for each side of the diaphragm can aid subsequent closure. The majority of the diaphragm remains innervated and fully functional because the phrenic nerve inserts centrally and radiates peripherally. The undersurface of the diaphragm is bluntly dissected from the retroperitoneum back to the crus. The pleura is then identified, incised, and dissected anteriorly, elevating it from the spine with the diaphragm. The crus of the diaphragm is also incised, leaving a small cuff on the spine for later approximation.

Following placement of retractors, T10 to L2 should be exposed. A radiograph is obtained to confirm the target level. The lung is deflated and packed, and a rib spreader is introduced to maximize the exposure. The vascular network of segmental vessels lies anterior to the vertebral bodies and these vessels are mobilized and ligated (**Fig. 61.4**). Two ligatures must be applied on the aortic stump, and ligation must be 1 cm from the vertebral foramen to avoid disruption of the anastomotic blood supply

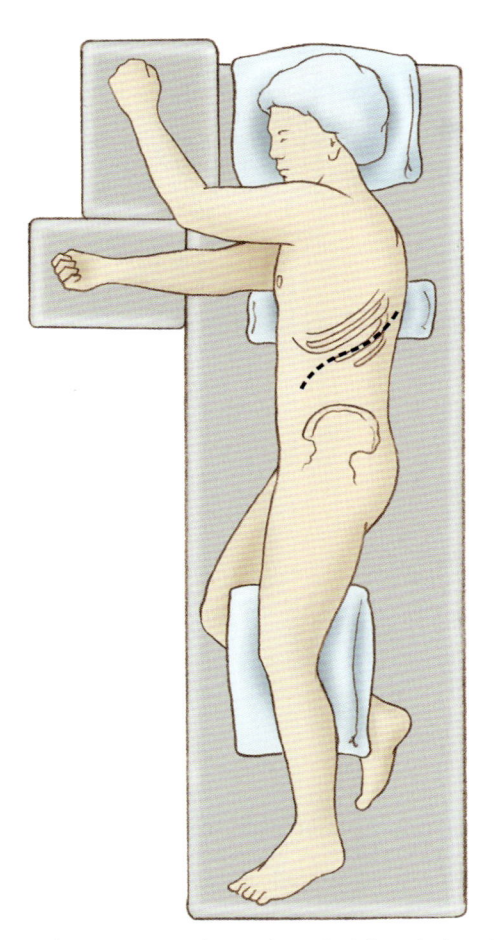

Fig. 61.1 A skin incision is made over the 10th rib from the lateral border of the paraspinous musculature to the costal cartilage. The incision is curved anteriorly to the edge of the rectus sheath.

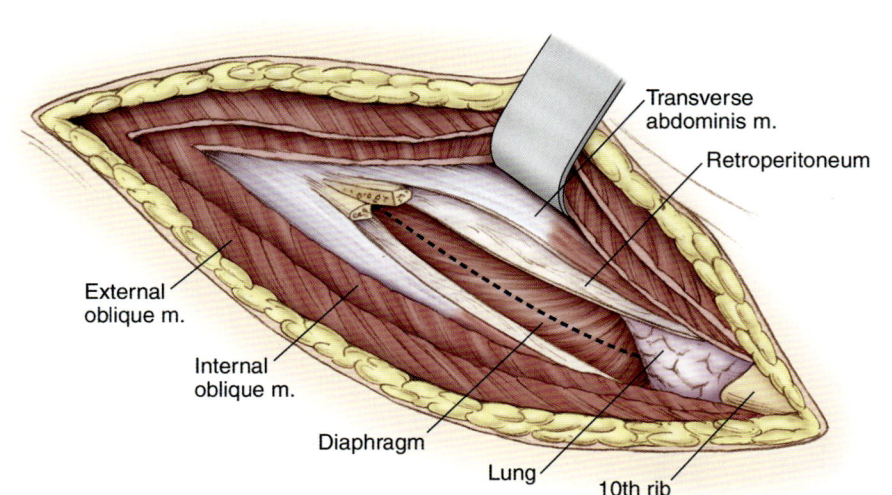

Fig. 61.2 The retroperitoneal space is entered by splitting the costal cartilage after removal of the 10th rib.

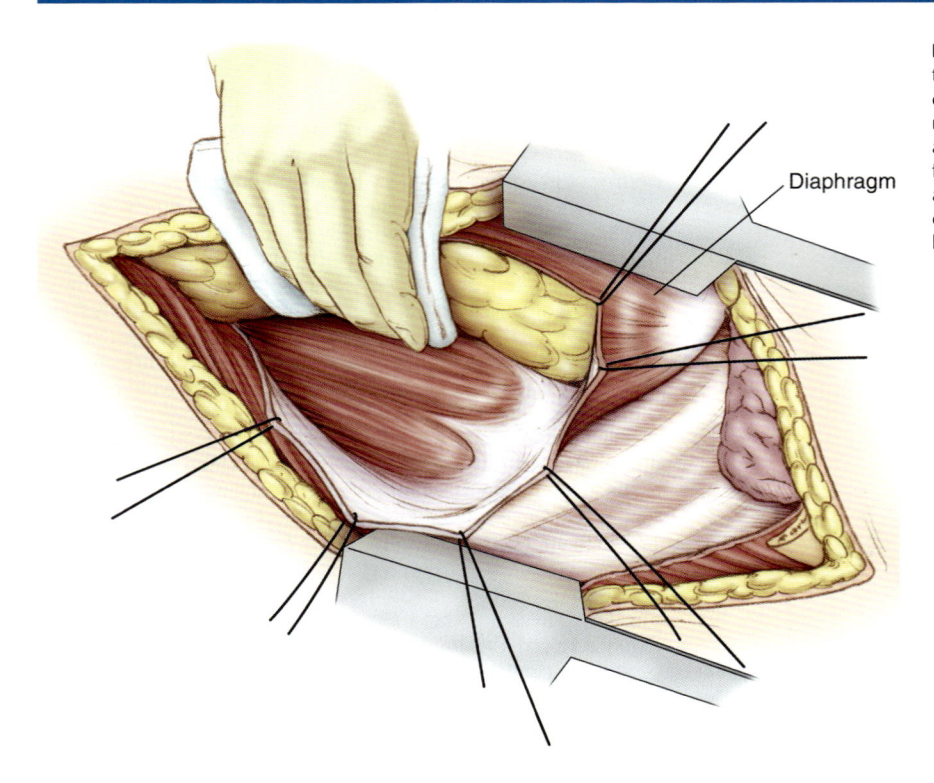

Fig. 61.3 The retroperitoneal space is identified by the light areolar tissue, and blunt dissection is performed to mobilize the peritoneum from the undersurface of the diaphragm and abdominal wall. The diaphragm is circumferentially incised 2.5 cm from the peripheral attachment to the chest wall. Marker stitches or clips are placed for resuturing the diaphragm later.

to the spinal cord. Care must be taken during the ligation process to avoid injury to the posterior sympathetic chain. To facilitate visualization of the spine, the proximal attachment of the psoas muscle may be incised and dissected posteriorly with a sharp elevator. At this point, the vertebrae are visualized and can be dissected to the neural foramina, pedicle, and anterior longitudinal ligament (**Fig. 61.5**). Once the surgeon has oriented the surgical working space within the anatomy, the diskectomy, decompression, and instrumentation can proceed. If indicated, the vertebral body can be removed after excision of the intervertebral disks above and below the operative level. For acute fractures, the vertebrectomy can be performed with a combination of rongeurs and curettes. A high-speed drill may facilitate removal of dense bone. After adequate decompression is achieved, strut grafting is required for reconstruction, and stabilization is achieved with an appropriate plating system.

Closure

Closure is initiated by approximating the diaphragmatic crus with nonabsorbable suture. The pleura is reapproximated with an absorbable suture. A running suture is used to approximate

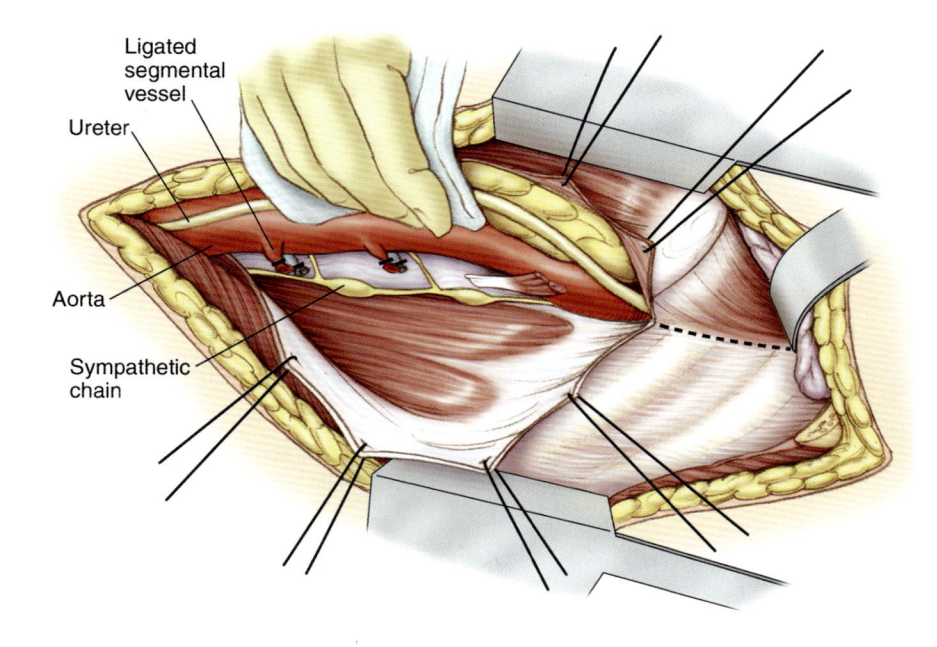

Fig. 61.4 The aorta is mobilized by ligating segmental vessels as necessary.

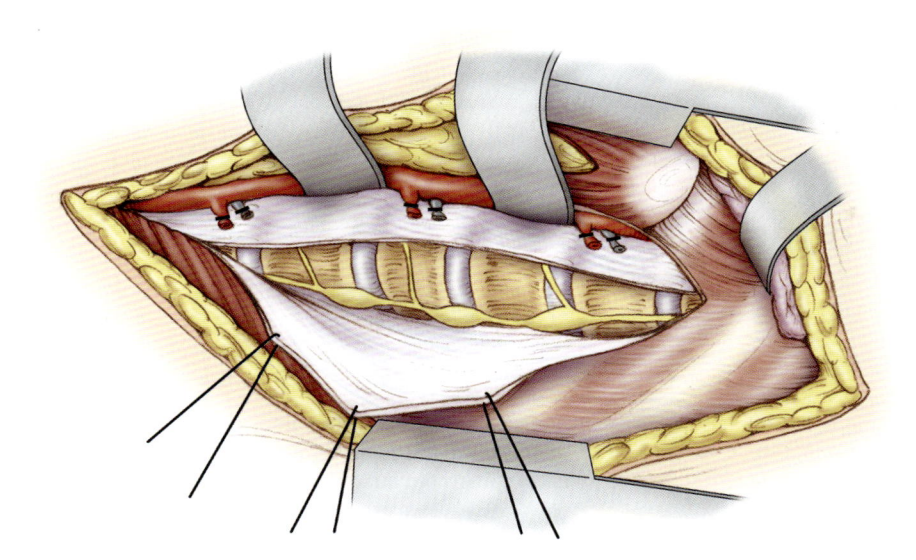

Fig. 61.5 The spine is exposed to the opposite cortex by mobilizing vessels and placing malleable retractors.

the diaphragm with supplemental interrupted sutures. A chest tube is placed through a separate stab incision under direct visualization through the thoracic portion of the exposure to evacuate blood and air. Two tubes may be necessary—one aimed superiorly to evacuate air and one aimed inferiorly to evacuate blood. The chest tube(s) are then secured with purse-string sutures. The lung is checked for air leaks by filling the thoracic cavity with saline. The ribs are approximated together with heavy suture. The periosteum and intercostal muscle layers are closed in airtight fashion with running suture. A drain in the retroperitoneal space may be placed but is not always required. The peritoneum is allowed to fall back into place. The transversalis fascia and aponeurosis of the transverses abdominus and oblique muscles are repaired to prevent hernia formation. The subcutaneous layers are closed with interrupted absorbable suture and the skin with staples.

Postoperative Care

Postoperative care is fairly routine in patients undergoing the standard open thoracoabdominal approach. It includes pain control, early ambulation, and physical therapy as the mainstay of recovery. A bowel regimen is useful, particularly for patients requiring a significant amount of narcotic medications. The chest tube(s) are placed under water-seal suction and removed when it is draining less than 100 mL in 24 hours. Daily chest radiographs enable the surgeon to monitor for pneumothorax and pleural effusions. Lumbar bracing is an option to facilitate arthrodesis if indicated. Routine imaging should be ordered to evaluate hardware placement if stabilization was performed.

Complications

The complication profile for the thoracoabdominal approach includes potential respiratory, vascular, and abdominal injury. Exposure of two body cavities adds significantly to the risks of surgery. Complications involving the abdomen may include injury to the stomach, colon, kidney, ureter, or spleen. Ileus may also be anticipated. Peritonitis may result from unrecognized intraperitoneal injury and should be suspected if prolonged ileus and abdominal pain are present. Iatrogenic sympathectomy may also be encountered with resultant limb warmth asymmetry. Inadequate closure of the diaphragm may result in herniation of abdominal viscera into the thorax. All complications of thoracic surgery may occur, including atelectasis, pneumonia, pleural effusion, pulmonary edema, and heart failure. Some patients suffer from postoperative thoracotomy or chest wall pain. Hemorrhage, delayed or immediate, is possible and may cause spinal cord compression if present in the epidural space. Finally, injury of the artery of Adamkiewicz with resultant spinal cord infarction is possible if intersegmental arteries are ligated too close to the neural foramen.

Conclusion

The standard open thoracoabdominal approach provides excellent exposure to pathology of the anterior spine from T10 to L2. Preoperative assessment, including anesthesia considerations, helps minimize the risk of intraoperative complications. An understanding of thoracoabdominal anatomy is critical, particularly in mobilizing the diaphragm from its attachments, and enables the proper exposure of the anterior spine.

62 MIS Thoracoabdominal Approach

Shane V. Abdunnur and Daniel H. Kim

Exposure of the anterior thoracolumbar spine is indicated for various pathologies. Although the relevant anatomy can be approached in an open fashion, minimally invasive surgery (MIS) techniques can enable the surgeon to approach T10 through L4 in a less morbid manner while still achieving the same clinical and radiographic results. Importantly, mastery of the open anatomy and surgical technique is a prerequisite to safely utilizing MIS techniques. This chapter discusses the anatomic relationships encountered in an MIS thoracoabdominal approach to the spine. Comparison with the open approach is made for further understanding of the similarities and differences between the techniques (**Table 62.1**). The chapter focuses on the minithoracotomy-transdiaphragmatic approach (mini-TTA) and the lateral retroperitoneal transpsoas approach to the lumbar spine.

Indications

- Trauma
- Tumors
- Deformity correction: kyphosis, scoliosis
- Degenerative disk disease
- Pseudarthrosis
- Osteomyelitis
- Spondylolisthesis
- Failed posterior fusion

Contraindications

- Medical illness that would preclude surgery
- Previous retroperitoneal or thoracoabdominal surgery

Advantages

- Versatile approach
- Good visualization of and access to the anterior spine between T10 and L4
- Minimal disruption to intraperitoneal structures
- Smaller skin incision (4–6 cm) compared with open techniques
- Less blood loss than with open techniques
- Shorter hospital stay compared with open techniques

Disadvantages

- Exposure limited by small incision (four to five disk levels)
- Requires mastery of open thoracoabdominal approach
- Entry into the thorax and associated risks
- Abdominal viscera at risk for injury
- Complications of thoracotomy
- Risk of spinal cord infarction

Surgical Technique

Approach

The mini-TTA is used to access T10 to L3. As the retroperitoneal anatomy is distinct at the L3-4 interspace and below, these interspaces are discussed elsewhere (Chapters 65 and 66). The spine is preferentially approached from the patient's left because mobilization and repair of the aorta, if needed, is far more straightforward than mobilization and repair of an injured inferior vena cava. In addition, the liver is more difficult to mobilize when the approach is from the right. It should be noted that dissection of the right side can be undertaken safely if the right-sided approach is indicated. Ultimately, the location of the pathology and surgeon comfort dictate the side of the approach. We routinely use a double-lumen endotracheal tube for selective lung deflation in transthoracic cases. If only L2-L3 and L3-L4 are being addressed, a double-lumen endotracheal tube is unnecessary, as the diaphragm will not be transgressed.

Patient Positioning

Patient positioning for the mini-TTA is the same as for the open thoracotomy and open direct lateral retroperitoneal transpsoas approaches. The operation is performed with the patient in the lateral decubitus position with an axillary roll under the dependent axilla. The patient should be positioned such that the spine's apex of curvature in the lateral view is maximized at the central level of the pathology. This is accomplished with the aid of a kidney rest and tilting of the operative table. The patient must remain in the true lateral position with the coronal axis perpendicular to the floor to maintain accurate surgeon orientation for spinal decompression and instrumentation. The hip is flexed to relax the psoas muscle for any operation below L1-2 and therefore to reduce tension on the lumbar plexus. The C-arm is brought into the field and used to confirm adequate positioning.

Incision and Dissection

The entire side is prepped from the axilla to the iliac crest such that conversion to the open technique is facilitated if required. Under direct fluoroscopic guidance, the target vertebra is projected onto the skin surface level and its borders are marked on the skin. The incision for the mini-TTA is typically centered over the T11 rib and extends posteriorly to the posterior axillary line and anteriorly to the costal cartilage. The average skin incision is 6 cm (**Fig. 62.1**). After the skin and subcutaneous tissues are

Table 62.1 Traditional Thoracoabdominal Approach vs Minithoracotomy-Transdiaphragmatic Approach (Mini-TTA)

	Traditional Thoracoabdominal Approach	Mini-TTA
Exposure	Extensive, access to seven to nine disk spaces	Limited, access from T10 to L3 vertebral bodies
Learning curve	Short: familiar technique	Moderate: extension of the traditional approach good requires working knowledge
Rib resection	More extensive	4–6 cm of T11 is split
Muscle dissection	Significant chest and abdominal wall dissection	No retroperitoneal muscle dissection
Operative time	Longer due to incision length and dissection	Shorter
Blood loss	Greater blood loss due to large incision, muscle splitting, and diaphragmatic incision	20–30% less blood loss
Pulmonary function	Transiently decreased due to rib resection and incisional pain	Transient decrease is less severe due to smaller incision and rib sparing
Chest tube duration	~ 3 postoperative days	~ 1–2 postoperative days
Hospital stay	4–6 days	2–3 days

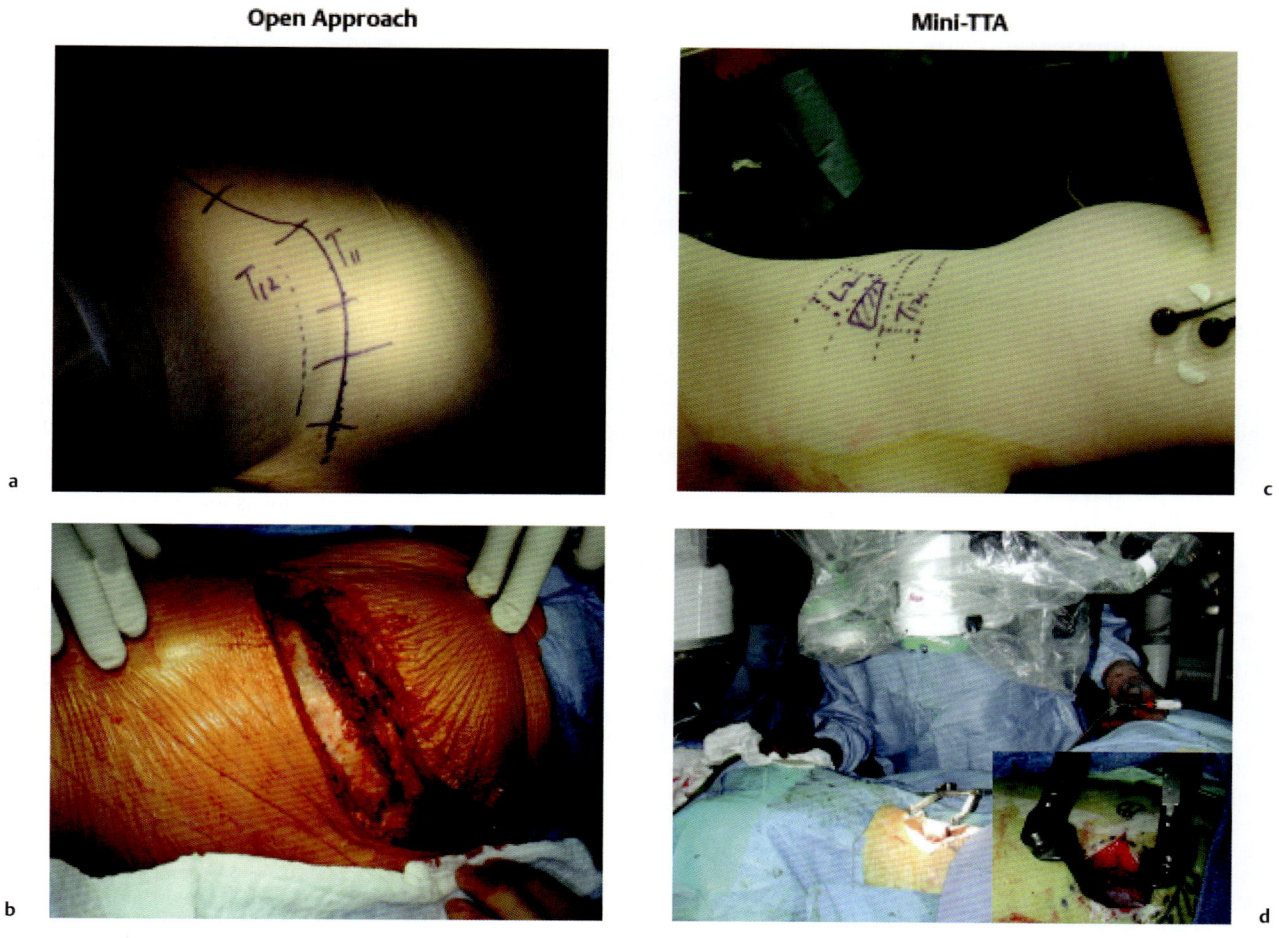

Fig. 62.1 Traditional open thoracoabdominal approach compared with the minithoracotomy-transdiaphragmatic approach (mini-TTA). The open exposure requires a large incision **(a)** with significant muscle dissection **(b)**. The mini-TTA incision is centered over the vertebral body of interest **(c)** and requires only a 6-cm incision **(d)**.

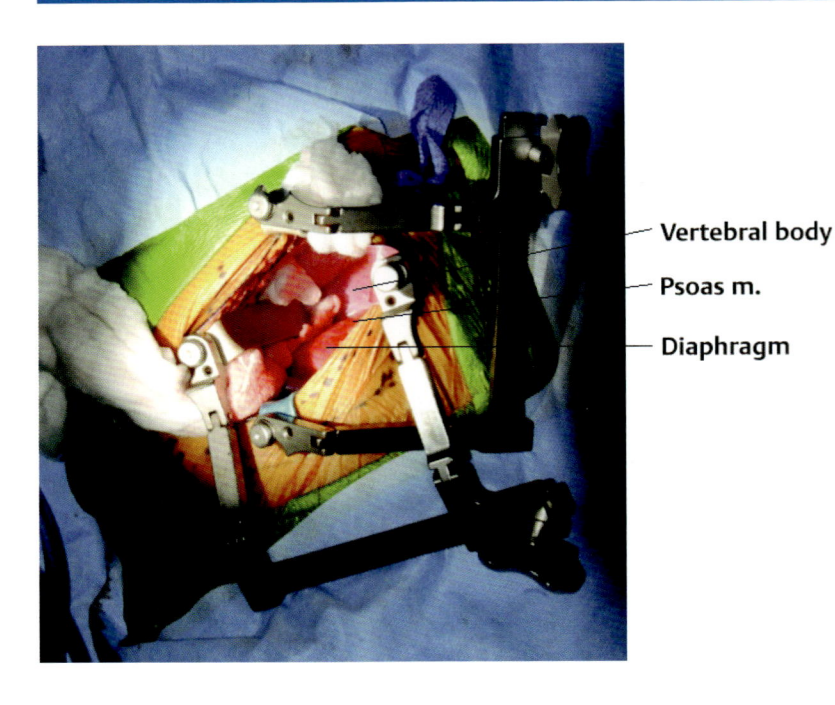

Fig. 62.2 Mini-TTA exposure. The superior aspect of the psoas muscle is noted under the margin of the diaphragm with the vertebral body and intervertebral disk medial. The diaphragm requires mobilization or retraction depending on the vertebral level needed for access.

incised, blunt muscle dissection and hemostasis should be obtained with bipolar electrocautery. The T11 rib is then dissected subperiosteally from the cartilaginous tip to the posterior margin of the skin incision, and the intercostal vein, artery, and nerve are gently dissected free from the rib. Single posterior osteotomy of the rib is completed so that the rib can be reflected inferiorly for preservation. The parietal pleura is visible just deep to the rib and is divided parallel to the direction of the rib. Selective ventilation is utilized, and the inferior lobe of the lung is retracted superiorly with a wet lap and blade retractors. Having completed this, the lateral recess convexity of the diaphragm becomes exposed and the diaphragm is visualized (**Fig. 62.2**).

The line of incision for diaphragmatic detachment is marked with monopolar cautery. The medial arcuate ligament should be retracted caudally to allow visualization of the lateral arcuate ligament of the diaphragm. The attachment of the medial and lateral arcuate ligaments to the transverse process is divided, which allows excellent inferior mobilization of the diaphragm. The crus of the diaphragm is incised such that a small cuff is left on the spine for later approximation. The retractor is now placed on the diaphragmatic opening and retracted inferiorly such that the superior end plate of L3 will be visualized. Retroperitoneal fat and the peritoneal sac are exposed and mobilized in an anterior-to-posterior direction along the psoas muscle at the L1 or L2 level to avoid injury to the lumbar spinal roots. The psoas muscle and its tendinous insertions into the vertebral bodies are carefully dissected from the bodies, avoiding damage to the segmental vessels. A 4- to 10-cm detachment of the diaphragm is required depending on the level approached. If access to the entire L2 vertebral body is needed, the diaphragmatic incision will be 8 to 10 cm in length. We prefer to use long cervical or narrow lumbar retractor blades. The surgeon may then expose the desired vertebral bodies and proceed with the indicated portion of the spinal procedure. The C-arm is utilized for intraoperative localization and instrumentation. The specific spinal techniques that can be utilized after securing this exposure are discussed in the previous chapters in this section.

For the direct lateral retroperitoneal transpsoas approach, a 3-cm incision is made vertically in the midaxillary line, centered over the disk space of interest. The three layers of abdominal wall musculature are split bluntly and the transversalis fascia, beneath the transversus abdominis, is incised sharply. Once that is completed, the retroperitoneal space is opened and the retroperitoneal contents are carefully mobilized from superior to inferior and posterior to anterior, thus deflecting the peritoneal contents anteriorly. This is completed with the surgeon's finger or a blunt instrument such as a sponge stick. The surgeon will feel the posterior lateral wall of the abdomen and the quadratus lumborum that leads directly to the psoas muscle.

The ipsilateral transverse processes can be palpated in the crevice that is formed from the medial border of the quadratus lumborum with the lateral boarder of the psoas muscle. Once this is palpated and the retroperitoneal space is clearly identified, the surgeon may place a blunt probe down onto the disk space or vertebral body of interest and confirm the location with lateral fluoroscopy. There are several systems available to the surgeon to complete the spinal portion of the procedure, and the specific steps that should be followed vary depending on which system the surgeon prefers. Generally, serial dilators are placed over a blunt probe after confirming adequate placement of the blunt probe. Retractors then take the place of the dilators, which allow direct visualization of the operative area.

Closure

For the mini-TTA, incisions less than 4 cm in the diaphragm are closed without any approximating sutures. In cases that require incisions larger than 4 cm, the cut edges of the diaphragmatic crus should be reapproximated with nonabsorbable suture. Both the medial and lateral arcuate ligaments should be reattached to the cuff that was left on the vertebral body at time the time of opening. The thoracic cavity is then irrigated and a single chest tube is placed through a separate stab incision under direct visualization. The chest tube is secured with a purse-string suture to the skin. Irrigant is used to assess the thoracic cavity for air leaks. The T11 rib is reapproximated with a No. 1 nylon suture after having drilled pilot holes on both sides of the cut edge. The transversalis fascia and aponeurosis of the transverses abdominis are oblique muscles are reapproximated with running suture to help prevent hernia formation. The subcutaneous layers are closed with interrupted absorbable suture and the skin with staples.

Closure is similar to that for the direct lateral retroperitoneal transpsoas approach but is less complicated because the diaphragm does not need to be addressed. After irrigating with the retractor system in place, the retractor can be removed slowly while it is still open. This enables the surgeon to assess and address any sites of bleeding in the psoas muscle. After the retractor is completely removed, a shallow self-retaining retractor is placed in the skin such that the transversalis fascia can be closed with several interrupted Vicryl sutures. The subcutaneous layer and dermis are then closed in a standard fashion.

Complications

Exposure of two body cavities adds significantly to the risks of surgery. Abdominal injuries may include injury to the stomach, colon, kidney, ureter, or spleen if the peritoneum is violated. Ileus may also be anticipated. Peritonitis may result from unrecognized intraperitoneal injury and should be suspected if prolonged ileus and abdominal pain are present. Iatrogenic sympathectomy may also be encountered with resultant limb warmth asymmetry. Inadequate closure of the diaphragm may result in herniation of abdominal viscera into the thorax. All complications of thoracic surgery may occur, including atelectasis, pneumonia, pleural effusion, pulmonary edema, and heart failure. Some patients suffer from postoperative thoracotomy or chest wall pain. Hemorrhage, delayed or immediate, is possible and may cause spinal cord compression if it occurs in the epidural space. Injury of the artery of Adamkiewicz with resultant spinal cord infarction is possible if intersegmental arteries are ligated too close to the neural foramen.

Several findings may be present after a direct lateral retroperitoneal transpsoas approach. These include hip flexor weakness from manipulation or injury to the psoas muscle and burning paresthesia in the groin or anterior thigh. The later findings are suggestive of nerve injury during the procedure. Lumbar plexus injuries during psoas muscle retraction can be avoided by minimizing the retraction time.

63 Open Retroperitoneal Approach

Hasan R. Syed and Faheem A. Sandhu

Anterior exposure of the upper lumbar spine is challenging due to the critical structures located in the abdominal cavity and thorax. However, numerous clinical situations dictate that an anterior approach be used to treat a pathological lesion. Access to the anterior lumbar spine can be readily accomplished by a retroperitoneal dissection. This approach poses less risk to the peritoneal organs and great vessels, while providing unilateral visualization of the vertebral body and intervertebral disk space. This chapter discusses the surgical technique required for a standard open retroperitoneal approach to the anterior lumbar spine from L1 to S1.

Indications

- Trauma: burst fractures
- Tumors: primary vertebral body tumors, metastatic disease
- Deformity corrections: scoliosis
- Infection: osteomyelitis
- Low-grade spondylolisthesis
- Anterior interbody fusion
  - Initial
  - After failed posterior fusion

Contraindications

- Medical illness that would preclude surgery
- Prior retroperitoneal surgery

Advantages

- Excellent unilateral visualization and exposure of the anterior lumbar spine between L1 and S1
- Minimal disruption to intraperitoneal structures
- Less risk to the peritoneal organs and great vessels

Disadvantages

- Larger incision with injury to abdominal wall musculature (versus minimally invasive approach)
- Risk of injury to vascular structures, especially with exposure of lower lumbar levels
- Risk of ureteral injury
- Risk of lumbosacral plexus injury

Preoperative Imaging and Planning

Preoperative considerations include imaging studies to assess the level of interest and the pathology relative to the iliac crest and ribs. A neuromonitoring plan should be established, with special attention to the lumbosacral plexus during approach. Typically, electromyography (EMG) is used to monitor the motor branches of the lumbosacral plexus, but sensory nerves cannot be monitored. Anesthesia must be compatible with neuromonitoring, as the patient must have muscle twitches during the surgery to enable EMG monitoring.

Surgical Technique

Equipment

- Axillary roll
- Foam padding (for all pressure points)
- Fluoroscopy
- Four-inch tape
- Cobb elevators
- Rongeurs
- Straight and angled curettes
- Cell Saver (Haemonetics, Braintree, MA)
- Neurophysiological monitoring (with EMG)

Patient Positioning

The patient is placed in the right lateral decubitus position, for several reasons. It is easier to mobilize and retract the aorta than the thin-walled vena cava, and if vessel injury occurs, repair of the thick-walled aorta is easier than repairing the vena cava. Also, retraction of the spleen is easier than retraction of the liver. Furthermore, the lateral decubitus position allows the peritoneal contents and the great vessels to fall away from the operative field. Support is applied to the shoulder, hips, and arms using tape, and the knees are flexed. Use of electrophysiological monitoring and the Cell Saver is recommended. The Cell Saver is an intraoperative salvage device that enables autotransfusion of red blood cells and thus reduces the need for donor blood transfusions.

Incision and Dissection

The incision is made at the midpoint between the lowest rib and the iliac crest from the midaxillary line to the edge of the rectus sheath. The level of the incision varies depending on the level operated. If upper lumbar exposure is desired, the skin incision is started over the 12th rib and extended transversely around to the anterior abdomen above the level of the umbilicus. To access lower levels, the incision is made one or two fingerbreadths below the costal margin and carried in an oblique fashion around the anterior abdomen below the level of the umbilicus (**Fig. 63.1**). The anterior portion of the 12th rib is dissected from the latissimus dorsi and serratus anterior. It is resected to facilitate an extensive exposure. The external oblique fibers are identified and split parallel to the incision. The fibers of the internal oblique and transversus abdominus muscles are cut in the same direction as the skin incision. The transversalis fascia is identified and the posterior portion is opened to access the retroperitoneal space (**Fig. 63.2**).

The peritoneum is identified and dissected medially from the transversalis fascia. Peritoneal injuries are more likely to occur lateral to the rectus sheath, and tears should be repaired primarily to avoid bowel herniation. In blunt fashion, the dissection is carried along the renal fascia posterior to the kidney in the plane between the quadratus lumborum, psoas, and renal fascia (**Fig. 63.3**). Mobilization of the peritoneum is carried medially from the inferior edge of the kidney down to the sacrum. The small-caliber genitofemoral nerve is identified on the belly of the psoas muscle. The cylindrical shape and peristaltic activity help identify the ureter, which is usually reflected medially with the peritoneal undersurface. If upper lumbar exposure is needed, the left diaphragmatic crus, which extends to the second vertebral body, can be taken down. Retractors are brought into the field to open the wound longitudinally. The concave shape, in contrast with the convex disk space, identifies the lumbar vertebral bodies. Radiograph or fluoroscopy is used to identify the desired level.

Vertebral body exposure requires lateral mobilization of the prevertebral structures. The lumbosacral plexus is located within the psoas muscle. Its ganglionic enlargements and yellow-white color traversing in the lateral aspect of the vertebral body distinguish the sympathetic trunk. In males, the first and second ganglia are involved in ejaculatory function. Arterial and venous anatomy must be considered during the exposure (**Fig. 63.4**). Segmental arteries are ligated and cut prior to their entry into the neural foramen to facilitate mobilization and retraction of the aorta. The ascending venous complex is located along the lateral aspect of the vertebral body; at the level of the neural foramen, segmental veins anastomose with the vena cava or common iliac if distal (fifth lumbar vein). These segmental vessels must be ligated midway between the neural foramen and the parent vessel to avoid avulsion injury. If exposure of L5-S1 is needed, the disk space is accessed between the common iliac vessels. The prevertebral structures (middle sacral vessels and hypogastric plexus) are bluntly dissected and swept to the opposite side, and the iliac vessels are retracted laterally. If extensive lumbosacral exposure is required or if arterial or venous anatomy prevents the interiliac approach, the common iliac vessels are reflected to the right. Mobilization of the iliac artery may require ligation of several branches, and the internal iliac vein also has many tributaries that should be identified and ligated. This exposure provides access to the lumbosacral spine and superior sacrum medial or lateral to the iliac vessels (**Fig. 63.5**).

Closure

After removal of the retractors, the peritoneum resumes its normal location. Placement of a suction drain is recommended. Each muscle layer is closed with running, nonabsorbable suture; the skin is closed with staples.

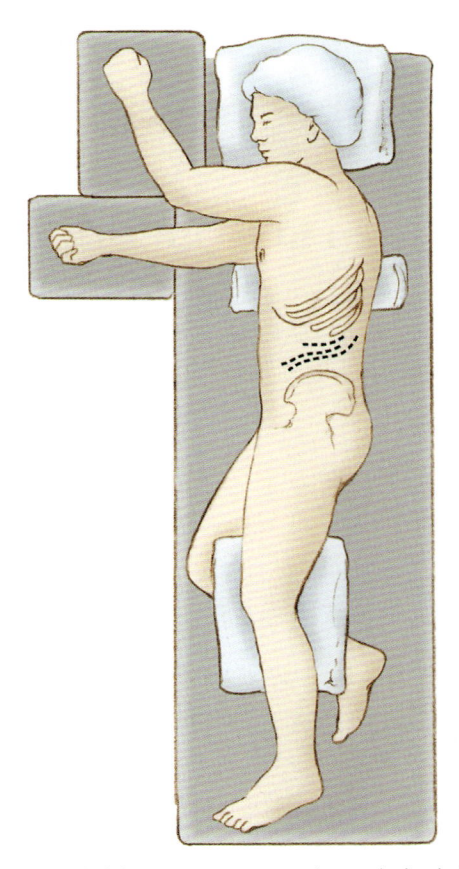

Fig. 63.1 The level of the incision varies according to the level of the spine approached. The patient is placed in the right lateral decubitus position with the left side up.

Postoperative Care

Postoperative care is fairly routine in patients undergoing the standard open retroperitoneal approach. It includes pain control, early ambulation, and physical therapy as the mainstay of recovery. Particular attention should be placed on assessing bowel function, due to the manipulation of the peritoneal cavity. A bowel regimen is useful, particularly for patients requiring a significant amount of narcotic medications. Lumbar bracing is an option to facilitate arthrodesis if indicated. Routine imaging should be ordered to evaluate hardware placement if stabilization was performed.

Complications

With the use of the retroperitoneal approach, injuries can occur to vascular structures and the bowel and ureter. Injury to a great vessel can result from congenital anomalies or adhesions. Tumors may be well vascularized, and a preoperative angiogram with embolization should be done if indicated. Injury to a great vessel must be addressed immediately with compression and primary repair to avoid potential massive hemorrhage. Peritoneal violation can occur in the setting of adhesions and scarring from prior surgery and radiation in oncology cases. Peritoneal laceration should be repaired primarily, and perforation of bowel requires the expertise of a general surgeon. To minimize postoperative

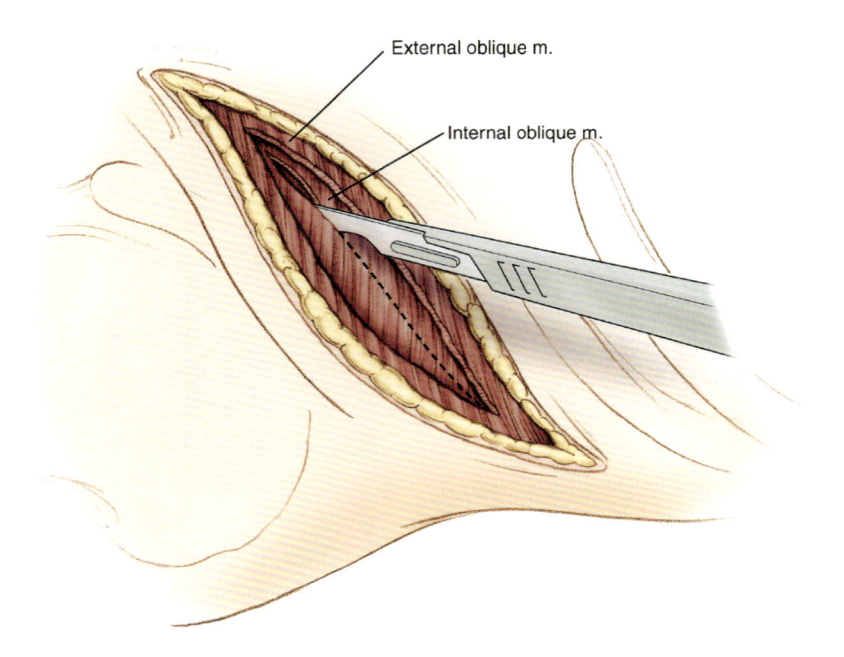

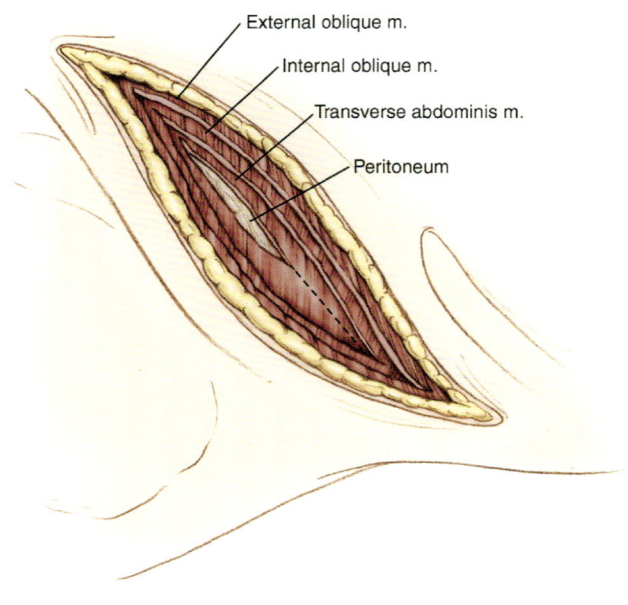

Fig. 63.2 (a) The skin incision extends from the midaxillary line to the edge of the rectus sheath. Dissection is through the external oblique, internal oblique, and transversus abdominis muscles. (b) The transversus abdominis muscle fascia is thin and very close to the peritoneum.

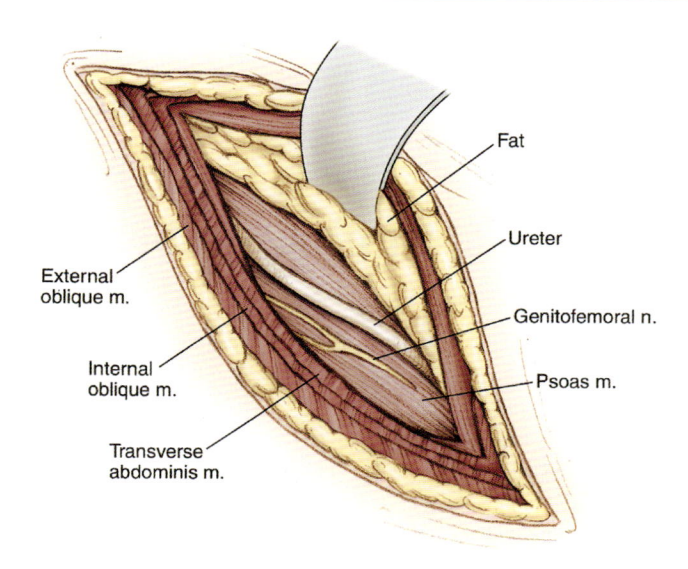

Fig. 63.3 Blunt dissection anterior to the psoas muscle and reflection of the peritoneum anteriorly should expose the spine. One should identify the genitofemoral nerve on the anterior surface of the psoas muscle, and the ureter along the undersurface of the peritoneum.

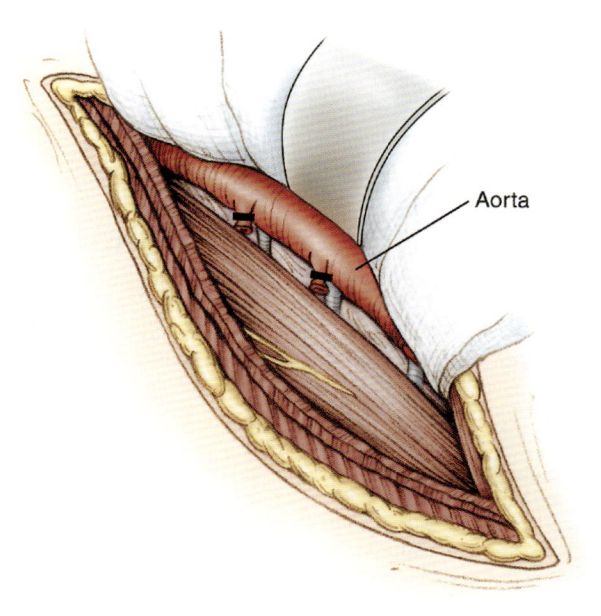

Fig. 63.4 The aorta is easily palpated, and the segmental vessels are ligated for mobilization.

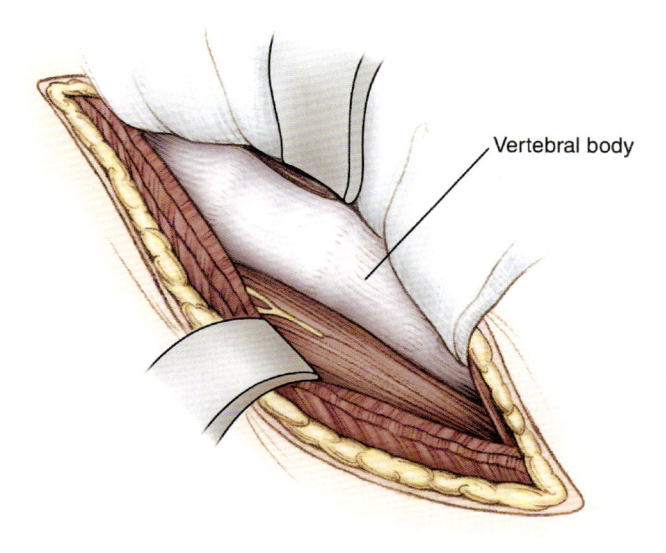

Fig. 63.5 Malleable retractors are positioned to expose the vertebral bodies.

ileus, the bowel and mesentery should be inspected for torsion prior to closure. Ureteral injuries can occur from retraction or manipulation. Renal anomalies can also preclude this surgical approach. Neurologic injuries largely comprise various nerve-related syndromes, as the lumbar contribution to the lumbosacral plexus lies within the substance of the psoas major muscle. Quadriceps weakness and leg dysesthesias can occur from stretch injury to femoral nerve. Wound infection and dehiscence are potential delayed complications. Use of preoperative antibiotics, meticulous skin preparation, and good surgical technique help avoid infections; proper closure of each muscular layer with strong suture material helps prevent dehiscence.

Conclusion

The standard open retroperitoneal approach provides excellent access to pathology of the anterior lumbar spine from L1 to S1. Compared with the traditional anterior approach, the retroperitoneal approach poses less risk to the peritoneal organs and great vessels. Although the risk of injury to the lumbosacral plexus exists, careful dissection of the psoas muscle, identification of the plexus, and the use of intraoperative monitoring help mitigate this risk.

64 Minimally Invasive Retroperitoneal Lateral Lumbar Interbody Fusion

Alexander Tuchman, Martin H. Pham, and John C. Liu

Interbody techniques allow a large surface area for bony fusion and are thus associated with low rates of pseudarthrosis. Unfortunately, accessing the intervertebral space can be technically difficult, and each approach has limitations. A posterior or posterolateral approach, such as posterior lumbar interbody fusion (PLIF) or transforaminal lumbar interbody fusion (TLIF), requires retraction on the thecal sac or nerve root when performing the diskectomy and placing the graft. This limits the graft size and places the patient at risk for complications such as nerve root injury or cerebrospinal fluid (CSF) leak. Traditional anterior approaches, such as anterior lumbar interbody fusion (ALIF), directly visualize a wide exposure of the disk space facilitating extensive disk removal, end-plate preparation, and larger graft placement. Approach-related risks include vascular complications, gastrointestinal complications, retrograde ejaculation, lymphocele, and sympathetic chain injury.

First described in 2001, the minimally invasive lateral lumbar interbody fusion has quickly gained popularity as a fusion technique because it enables large graft placement while avoiding some of the complications associated with anterior and posterior approaches.[1,2] Since its original description, the procedure has rapidly evolved thanks to advancements in our understanding of the regional anatomy, enabling variations in the technique. Originally described as a two-incision procedure that relied heavily on fluoroscopy and triggered electromyography to avoid nerve injury, recent variations include single incisions, oblique trajectories, retractor docking superficial to the psoas, and pre-psoas approaches. Indications have also expanded beyond degenerative disk disease; the procedure has been applied to many other lumbar pathologies, even being used in the correction of scoliotic deformities.[3] The lateral approach has a unique set of complications mostly associated with its proximity to the lumbar plexus as it travels through the psoas muscle.[4–6] Like all minimally invasive techniques it has a steep learning curve, but this is exacerbated by the relatively unfamiliar anatomy of the approach. Once mastered, this approach is a safe and effective method to achieve disk height restoration, segmental fusion, and deformity correction.

Indications

- Adjacent segment disease (ASD)
- Degenerative disk disease (DDD)
- Degenerative scoliosis
- Diskitis
- Foraminal stenosis (indirect decompression)
- Lumbar stenosis (indirect decompression)
- Postlaminectomy or posttraumatic kyphosis
- Pseudarthrosis
- Radiculopathy
- Spondylolisthesis
- Spondylolysis with instability
- Trauma

Contraindications

- Greater than grade 2 spondylolisthesis
- Vascular abnormalities
- Severe central canal stenosis (without complementary decompression surgery)

Relative Contraindications

- Previous surgery to the ipsilateral retroperitoneal space
- Previous radiation to the ipsilateral retroperitoneal space
- Severely collapsed disk space

Advantages

- No need for an access surgeon
- No increased rate of complications in obese patients[7]
- Safe and well tolerated in elderly patients[8]
- Lordotic grafts can assist with sagittal plane correction.
- Graft height and the trajectory of the implant enable powerful coronal deformity correction.
- Larger footprint compared with posterior interbody fusion procedures, which decreases the likelihood for graft subsidence in osteoporotic patients
- No retraction on the nerve root or thecal sac
- Leaves the anterior and posterior longitudinal ligament intact, maintaining anatomic structures for spinal stability

Disadvantages

- Reliance on indirect decompression of neural elements
- Often requires a separate approach for direct bony decompression and supplemental fixation
- Less visualization of abdominal and vascular structures compared with open procedures
- Less visualization of disk space and smaller graft size compared with open anterior approaches
- Risk of psoas pain and weakness postoperatively (usually transient)

- Requires reliable electrophysiological neuromonitoring to avoid the lumbar plexus and genitofemoral nerve injury

Objective

Minimally invasive techniques offer a variety of benefits when compared with their open counterparts, such as decreased blood loss, lower infection rates, less postoperative pain, and shorter hospital stays. Unfortunately, minimal access approaches can lead to less available surface area to achieve a solid bony fusion. The minimally invasive retroperitoneal lateral lumbar interbody fusion has the benefits of a small incision that follows natural planes to the spine and enabling a large surface area in the intervertebral space to achieve bony fusion. Beyond this, the intervertebral graft can be used to restore disk height, which can be helpful for indirect decompression and correction of sagittal or coronal deformities.[3] Lateral lumbar interbody fusions can be utilized as an anterior supplement for complex spinal reconstructions or as a stand-alone technique in the treatment of simple degenerative disk disease with an intact posterior tension band, no significant sagittal imbalance, and no requirement for direct decompression.[9]

Preoperative Planning and Imaging

Review the patient's history and preoperative imaging to determine the side of entry. Make sure to take note of a vascular or anatomic anomaly that precludes surgery on one side. A close examination of the patient's preoperative magnetic resonance imaging (MRI) can give helpful information about the bulk of the psoas muscle, the position of the lumbar plexus, and the presence of any vascular anomalies.[9] Review the patient's history for any previous unilateral retroperitoneal surgery to avoid dissection through postoperative adhesions. Note the coronal alignment of the lumbar spine. Approaching a deformity from the convex side can make the exposure and diskectomy easier, but positioning with the convexity up may put the psoas under greater stretch, increasing the risk for traction injury to the lumbar plexus. Entering on the concavity is often easier when addressing multiple levels or fusing L4-L5.

Surgical Technique

Anesthesia

The patient should be placed under general anesthesia for the procedure. Neuromonitoring is required to safely traverse the psoas muscle, so muscle relaxants and inhalational anesthetic agents must be minimized.

Patient Positioning

The patient is placed in a true lateral position on a breakable radiolucent bed. Care is taken to ensure that the iliac crest is below the break in the bed. An axillary role is placed and all pressure points are padded. The up knee and hip are flexed to decrease stretch on the psoas muscle, whereas the down leg can remain straight. The bed is then flexed no more than 20 degrees to increase the working space between the iliac crest and 12th rib. The patient is then firmly secured to the bed with tape around the hips, legs, and chest. Fluoroscopy is used to confirm a true lateral X-ray projection of the level of interest. If the image is not a true lateral projection, adjust the bed as needed while the fluoroscopy unit remains perpendicular to the floor. Anteroposterior (AP) fluoroscopy is then used to confirm that the spinous process is midline between the pedicles and that the pedicles project equally over the vertebral body. The fluoroscopy unit should be angled parallel to the end plates to provide a direct view of the disk space in question.

Incision, Dissection, and Exposure

Using fluoroscopy, the superior, inferior, anterior, and posterior boarders of the disk space or spaces of interest are marked out on the skin (**Fig. 64.1**). The incision is then made so that the surgeon can work directly perpendicular to the floor and access the disk space at a "safe zone" (**Fig. 64.2**). Safe zones for dilating through the psoas muscle and docking on the lateral intervertebral disk have been described in multiple anatomic and radiographic studies.[2-6,10,11] On a lateral X-ray, the vertebral bodies can be divided into four quartiles or zones. Zone 1 is the most anterior quartile of the disk space and zone 4 is the most posterior. Using these designations, the safe zones to traverse the psoas muscle while minimizing the risk for nerve or vascular injury have been defined as follows: L1-2 disk space, zones 2 and 3; L2-3 disk space, zone 3; L3-4 disk space, zone 3; and L4-5 disk space, zone 2[9] (**Fig. 64.3**). If a "shallow docking" (described below) technique is used to directly visualize and split the psoas muscle and genitofemoral nerve, rather than blindly placing sequential dilators, then the retractor should target zone 3. Using this technique, the surgeon can visualize and work around the genitofemoral nerve or work completely anterior to the belly of the psoas muscle.

A vertical incision can be easily lengthened if necessary when working at multiple levels. For a single-level interbody fusion, a 2- to 3-cm oblique incision parallel to the muscle fibers of the external oblique muscle is generally preferred. Scarpa's fascia is identified and opened to expose the muscle fibers of the external oblique muscle. The muscle fibers of the external oblique, internal oblique, and transversus abdominus are each split longitudinally to atraumatically dissect down to the transversalis fascia. The transversalis fascia is picked up and opened with scissors, taking care not to violate the peritoneum. Under

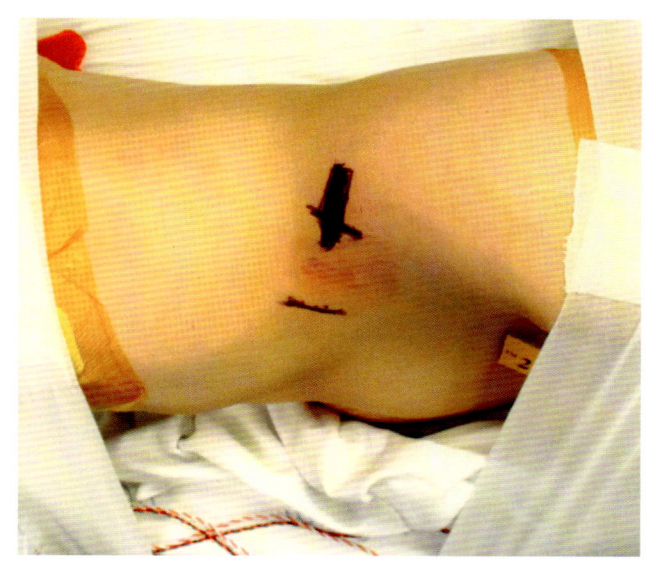

Fig. 64.1 Skin marking of the L3-4 disk space. The incision is marked out for a direct lateral approach directly over the disk space. The skin incision for an oblique approach is marked out further anteriorly.

418   IV   Thoracic and Thoracolumbar Spine

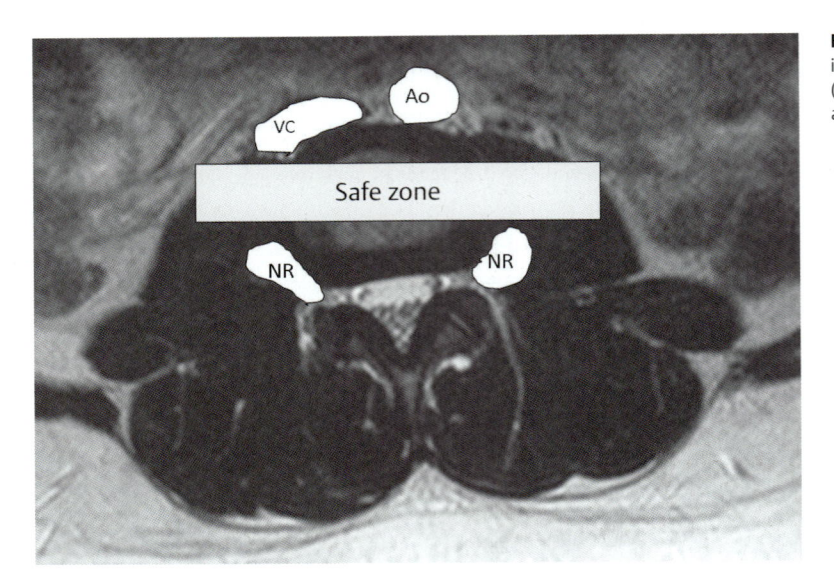

Fig. 64.2 Axial magnetic resonance imaging (MRI) showing the safe lateral working space between the nerve roots (NR) of the lumbar plexus and the vena cava (VC) and aorta (Ao).

direct visualization the peritoneum is swept anteriorly to create a corridor through the retroperitoneal space to the psoas muscle (**Fig. 64.4**).

At this point a neuromonitoring probe is slowly passed through the psoas muscle under direct fluoroscopic guidance to dock at the intervertebral disk within one of the previously mentioned safe zones.[11] Watch for a triggered electromyogram (EMG) response, and redirect the trajectory more anteriorly or posteriorly based on positioning on fluoroscopy to avoid lumbar plexus or genitofemoral nerve injury. Threshold values greater than 10 mA indicate sufficient space to proceed without major risk of nerve injury. Once the position on the lateral disk space is confirmed, the sequential dilators are passed through the psoas muscle until the retractor system can be inserted (**Fig. 64.5**). The superior and inferior retractor blades are then expanded so that the end plates of the vertebral body above and below can be visualized. To keep the blades in position, pins can be placed into the adjacent vertebral bodies.

Diskectomy

Once the annulus of the disk space is exposed, it is incised with a No. 15 blade. A combination of pituitary rongeur, curettes, and disk space shavers are used to perform the diskectomy and prepare the end plates under direct visualization. Confirming an appropriate trajectory with fluoroscopy and conservative utilization of the disk space shavers are key to preventing an end-plate violation at this step. The disk space shaver or a Cobb elevator can be gently malleted through the contralateral annulus to completely release the disk space. An AP radiograph is used to confirm passage of the instrument beyond the border of the contralateral annulus (**Fig. 64.6**).

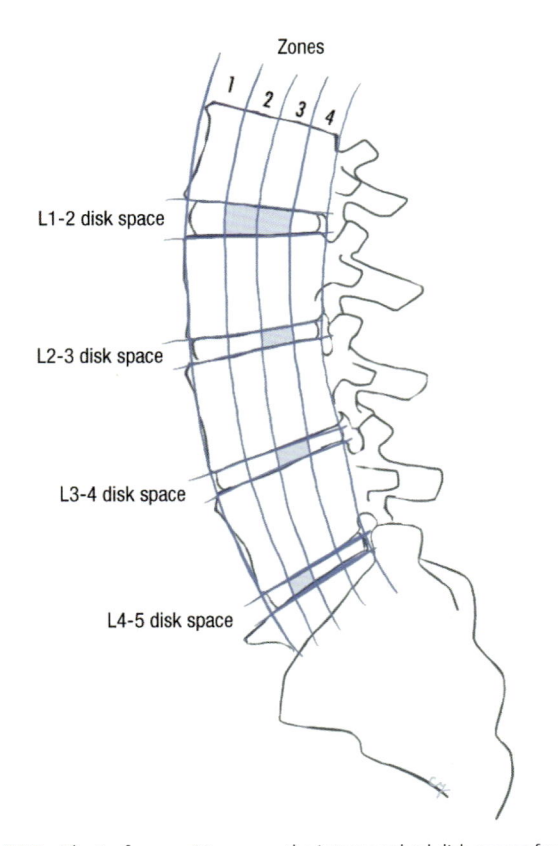

Fig. 64.3 The "safe zones" to access the intervertebral disk spaces from a lateral transpsoas approach. The preferred zones of entry are shaded at each level.

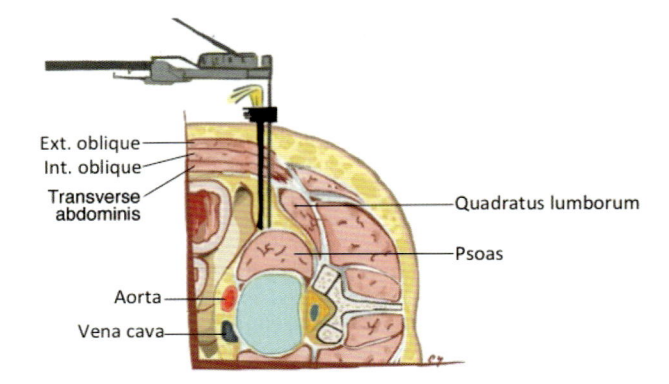

Fig. 64.4 The relevant axial anatomy en route to the L3-4 disk space via a lateral retroperitoneal approach.

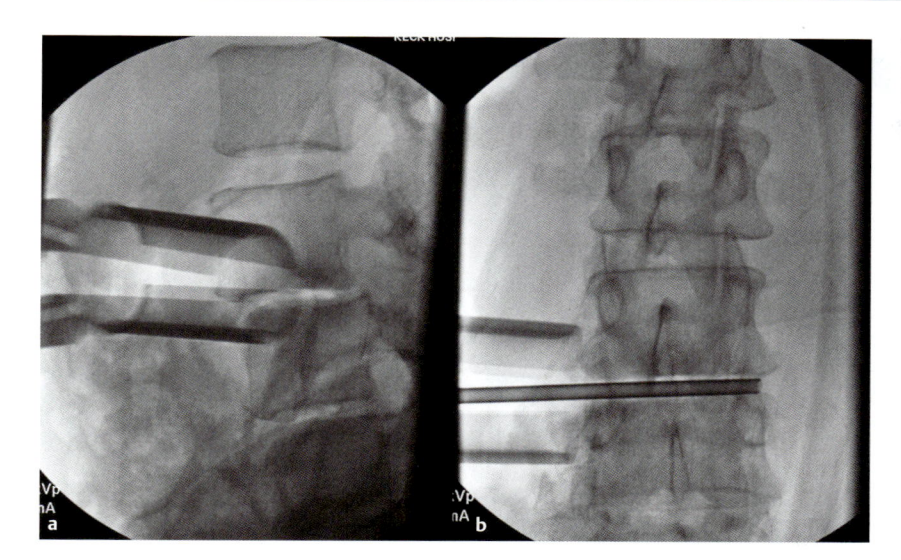

Fig. 64.5 Lateral **(a)** and anteroposterior (AP) **(b)** fluoroscopy of anterior oblique retractor placement for minimally invasive surgery (MIS) retroperitoneal lateral lumbar interbody fusion at L3-4.

Graft Placement

Sequential graft trials are then used to expand the disk space until a size with a snug fit and appropriate radiographic appearance is found (**Fig. 64.7**). Avoid over-distracting the disk space at this step, especially in osteoporotic patients, as it may lead to end-plate violation, putting the patient at increased risk for graft subsidence. The permanent interbody spacer is then filled with bone graft and placed in the intervertebral space. The ideal graft extends minimally beyond both lateral edges of the end plates. This ensures that the graft sits on the apophyseal ring bilaterally, thus engaging the strongest portion of the vertebral body. If the graft is too long, it can irritate the psoas muscle and cause mass effect on the lumbar plexus by sticking out to far.

Closure

Hemostasis is achieved and the retractor system is removed. The transversalis and Scarpa's fascia are closed with a braided absorbable stitch. Care is taken to perform a good closure at this step to avoid an incisional hernia. The subcutaneous tissues are closed with an inverted stitch and a subcuticular stitch is used to close the skin.

Alternatives

Rather than using sequential dilators to create a working space through the psoas muscle, we prefer a shallow docking technique (Video 64.1) such that the retractor system is docked above the psoas muscle and never advanced into the muscle itself.[12] Using this technique there is no need to blindly pass dilators through the retroperitoneal space and psoas muscle. The bladed retractor system can be docked over the psoas muscle with direct visualization. The position of the retractor is then confirmed with AP and lateral fluoroscopy. Care is taken to ensure that no unexpected structures, such as the peritoneum, ureter, or nerve, are adherent to outer surface. The superficial position of the retractor enhances visualization of these structures, enabling them to be dissected away prior to traversing the psoas muscle. Then, under direct visualization, the muscle fibers of the psoas are split, ensuring that no small nerves course through the track to the disk space. If a nerve is found to be running directly over

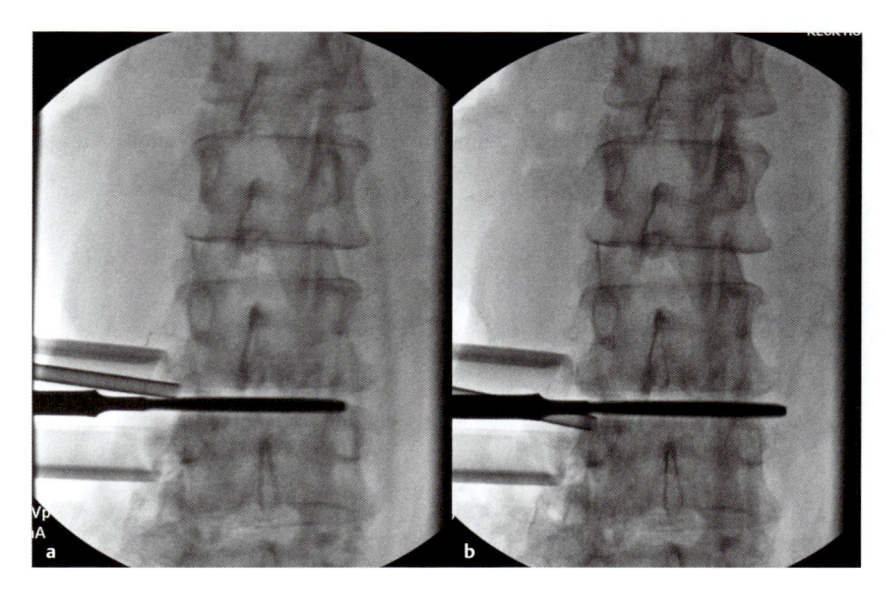

Fig. 64.6 AP fluoroscopy before **(a)** and after **(b)** the disk shaver is used to break through the contralateral annulus.

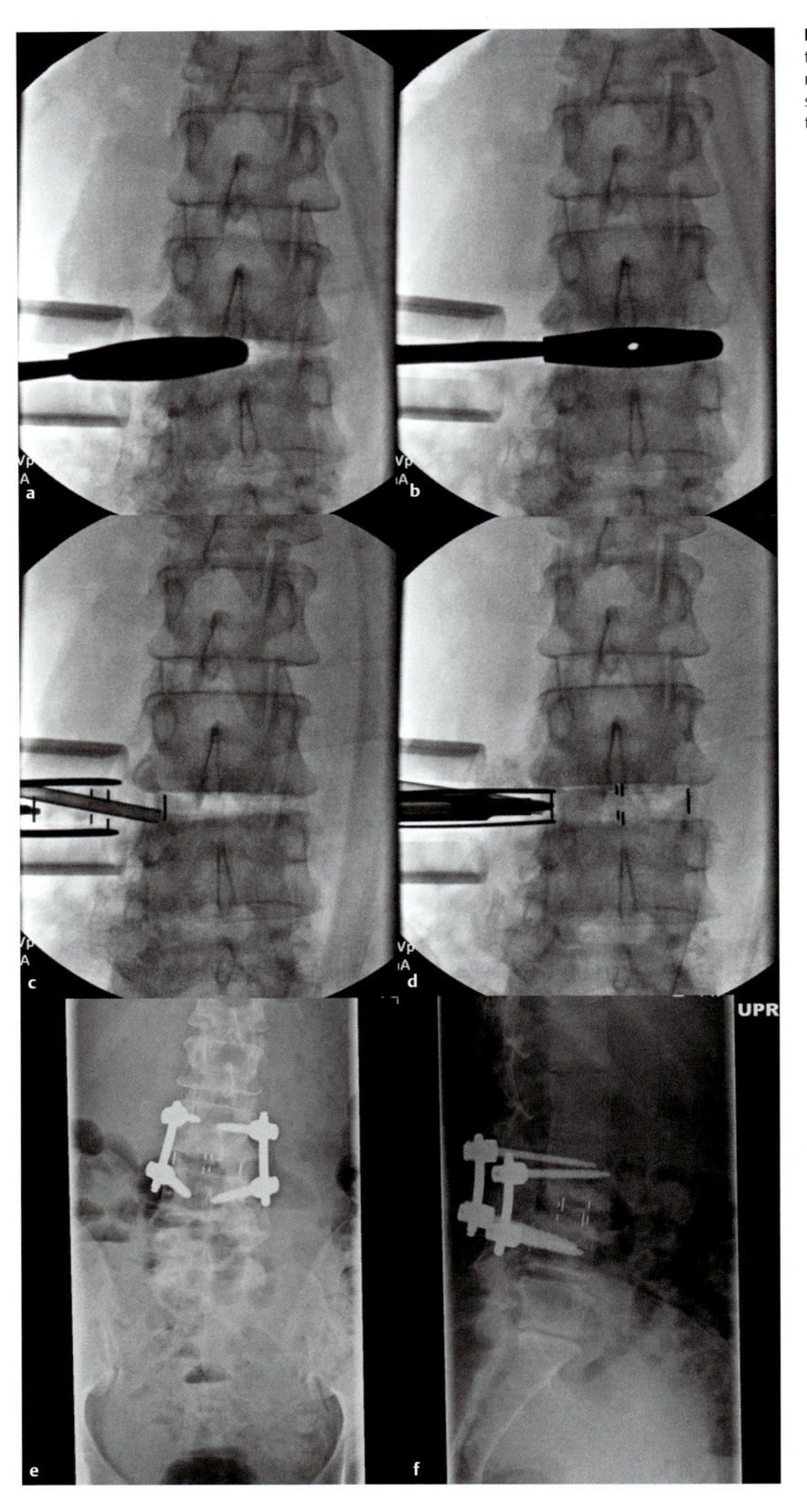

Fig. 64.7 **(a,b)** AP fluoroscopy placing a 10-mm trial at L3-4. **(c,d)** AP fluoroscopy placing the permanent graft at L3-4. Final AP **(e)** and lateral **(f)** standing X-rays of the lumbar spine following posterior fixation at L3-4 with MIS pedicle screws.

64 Retroperitoneal Lateral Lumbar Interbody Fusion

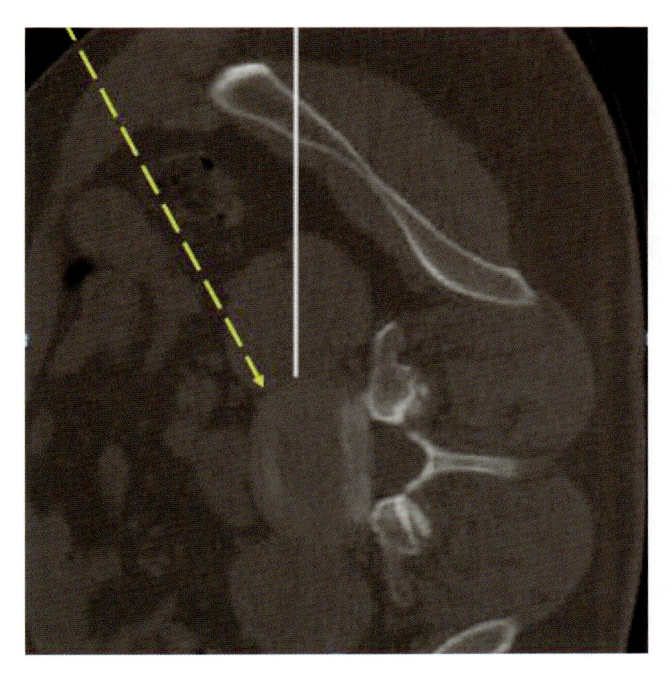

Fig. 64.8 Axial computed tomography (CT) scan showing the trajectory for oblique retroperitoneal *(yellow)* and a true lateral *(white)* approach to a lumbar disk space.

tem above the psoas muscle provides direct visualization of any nerves en route to the disk space, providing a third confirmation of safe trajectory. Persistent motor deficits have been correlated with four or more levels treated at once and the use of recombinant human bone morphogenetic protein-2 (rhBMP-2).[15]

Neurologic symptoms contralateral to the approach have also been reported and are thought to be caused by compression from fractured end plates or bone spurs, extruded disk material, or malposition of the interbody graft.[16] Avoid overzealous end-plate removal on the contralateral side, and confirm a lateral trajectory of the final graft without excessive graft overhang contralaterally to avoid this complication. Vertebral body fractures, graft subsidence, pseudarthrosis, adjacent segment disease, and hardware failure are always a risk, but can be minimized through good technique and patient selection.

When traversing the retroperitoneal space, it is important to recognize the anatomic relationships to avoid injury to the bowel, ureter, or vascular structures.[17,18] If any of these organs are injured, the key is to stabilize the patient and seek assistance as needed. A large vascular injury requires immediate action to control bleeding at the site, with compression above and below the injury. Do not hesitate to expand the incision to obtain better access. Vascular clamps may be necessary to gain temporary control of the bleeding. A bowel injury should be immediately repaired primarily. A ureteral violation requires primary repair or stenting, whereas compressive or vascular injuries to the ureter may lead to delayed fibrosis.[17]

the access to the disk, the retractor can be moved either more anteriorly or posteriorly to avoid putting undue retraction on the nerve. A thin-blade anterior-posterior retractor system can be used to keep this pathway open. The stimulator probe is used to confirm that the lumbar plexus is sufficiently remote from the entry point.

Often the height of the iliac crest prevents a direct lateral approach to the disk space, especially at the L4-L5 level. To overcome this limitation, an oblique approach can be used to gain access to the retroperitoneal space anterior to the iliac crest (**Fig. 64.8**). Using this approach, the skin incision and dissection through the abdominal wall musculature is done more anteriorly on the abdomen. Generally the incision is made 4 to 5 cm anterior to the direct lateral approach (**Fig. 64.1**). A good understanding of the retroperitoneal anatomy is critical for this approach to avoid ureter, vascular, or peritoneal violation. After the diskectomy is performed, the graft has to be angled back to a trajectory perpendicular to the floor to avoid compressing the contralateral nerve root. Another advantage of this approach is that, because of the oblique trajectory, the diskectomy often can be performed completely anterior to the psoas by retracting it posteriorly, thus avoiding the trauma associated with traversing the muscle.

Complications

A variety of complications unique to this approach have been described in the literature.[13,14] Transient neurologic symptoms (commonly ipsilateral proximal lower extremity pain, weakness, numbness, or dysesthesias) have an incidence of 1 to 60% in large reported series. This is likely related to psoas trauma, retraction on the lumbar plexus, and rarely from a nerve transection or crush injury. Using the anatomic safe zones for entry points to the disk space along with confirmatory EMG stimulation of the area can help avoid the lumbar plexus. Docking the retractor sys-

Key Points and Clinical Pearls

- The technique is in evolution.
- Patients generally do well with excellent fusion rates.
- The technique is a powerful tool for coronal deformity correction, but sagittal correction may require additional interventions (anterior longitudinal ligament release, facet resection).
- The safety data vary, but anterior thigh sensory or muscular changes are a concern though usually transient.
- Neuromonitoring is not all-protective.
- The risks and difficulty increase at L4-L5. The surgeon should have a backup plan if it is not possible to safely place a lateral interbody graft.
- Minimize retractor opening, and work efficiently to decrease retraction time on the psoas.
- Stay perpendicular during graft insertion to avoid injury to vessels or nerve structures.
- Do not overstuff the cage or exert excessive insertion force, to avoid end-plate injury.
- Remove the tube gradually and inspect the psoas and retroperitoneal space for bleeding.
- The technique entails a learning curve.

References

1. Pimenta L. Lateral endoscopic transpsoas retroperitoneal approach for lumbar spine. Proceedings of the 8th Brazilian Spine Society Meeting; May 2001; Belo Horizonte—Minas Gerais, Brazil
2. Ozgur BM, Aryan HE, Pimenta L, Taylor WR. Extreme lateral interbody fusion (XLIF): a novel surgical technique for anterior lumbar interbody fusion. Spine J 2006;6:435–443
3. Acosta FL, Liu J, Slimack N, Moller D, Fessler R, Koski T. Changes in coronal and sagittal plane alignment following minimally invasive direct lateral interbody fusion for the treatment of degenerative lumbar disease in adults: a radiographic study. J Neurosurg Spine 2011;15:92–96

4. Benglis DM, Vanni S, Levi AD. An anatomical study of the lumbosacral plexus as related to the minimally invasive transpsoas approach to the lumbar spine. J Neurosurg Spine 2009;10:139–144
5. Uribe JS, Arredondo N, Dakwar E, Vale FL. Defining the safe working zones using the minimally invasive lateral retroperitoneal transpsoas approach: an anatomical study. J Neurosurg Spine 2010;13:260–266
6. Moro T, Kikuchi S, Konno S, Yaginuma H. An anatomic study of the lumbar plexus with respect to retroperitoneal endoscopic surgery. Spine 2003; 28:423–428, discussion 427–428
7. Rodgers WB, Cox CS, Gerber EJ. Early complications of extreme lateral interbody fusion in the obese. J Spinal Disord Tech 2010;23:393–397
8. Karikari IO, Grossi PM, Nimjee SM, et al. Minimally invasive lumbar interbody fusion in patients older than 70 years of age: analysis of peri- and postoperative complications. Neurosurgery 2011;68:897–902, discussion 902
9. Nemani VM, Aichmair A, Taher F, et al. Rate of revision surgery after stand-alone lateral lumbar interbody fusion for lumbar spinal stenosis. Spine 2014;39:E326–E331
10. Guérin P, Obeid I, Gille O, et al. Safe working zones using the minimally invasive lateral retroperitoneal transpsoas approach: a morphometric study. Surg Radiol Anat 2011;33:665–671
11. Guérin P, Obeid I, Bourghli A, et al. The lumbosacral plexus: anatomic considerations for minimally invasive retroperitoneal transpsoas approach. Surg Radiol Anat 2012;34:151–157
12. Acosta FL Jr, Drazin D, Liu JC. Supra-psoas shallow docking in lateral interbody fusion. Neurosurgery 2013;73(1, Suppl Operative):ons48–ons51, discussion ons52
13. Patel VC, Park DK, Herkowitz HN. Lateral transpsoas fusion: indications and outcomes. ScientificWorldJournal 2012;2012:893608
14. Arnold PM, Anderson KK, McGuire RA Jr. The lateral transpsoas approach to the lumbar and thoracic spine: a review. Surg Neurol Int 2012;3(Suppl 3):S198–S215
15. Lykissas MG, Aichmair A, Hughes AP, et al. Nerve injury after lateral lumbar interbody fusion: a review of 919 treated levels with identification of risk factors. Spine J 2014;14:749–758
16. Papanastassiou ID, Eleraky M, Vrionis FD. Contralateral femoral nerve compression: an unrecognized complication after extreme lateral interbody fusion (XLIF). J Clin Neurosci 2011;18:149–151
17. Flouzat-Lachaniette CH, Delblond W, Poignard A, Allain J. Analysis of intraoperative difficulties and management of operative complications in revision anterior exposure of the lumbar spine: a report of 25 consecutive cases. Eur Spine J 2013;22:766–774
18. Czerwein JK Jr, Thakur N, Migliori SJ, Lucas P, Palumbo M. Complications of anterior lumbar surgery. J Am Acad Orthop Surg 2011;19:251–258

65 Minimally Invasive Retroperitoneal Vertebrectomy

Alexander Tuchman, Christina Yen, and John C. Liu

The anterior approach to the lumbar spine can be helpful in the treatment of a variety of pathological entities, including trauma, neoplasm, infection, and inflammatory lesions. This approach is particularly powerful in its ability to reconstruct the anterior and middle column through corpectomy and fusion. When compared with posterior-only constructs, anterior techniques have a more favorable durability for kyphosis correction.[1] The anterior approach affords visualization of ventral pathology, enabling direct decompression of the neural elements. A variety of approaches are used based on the levels required to be exposed. When treating pathology from L2 to L4 and sometimes L5, a lateral retroperitoneal approach in generally preferred for anterior exposure. The conventional retroperitoneal approach is associated with a large skin and abdominal muscle opening, long postoperative recovery, and significant blood loss.[2,3]

Recently, minimally invasive surgery (MIS) techniques have been applied to the retroperitoneal approach to the lumbar spine.[4–8] Several groups have demonstrated the feasibility of lumbar corpectomy using minimal access. Early reports found a low level of blood loss and fast postoperative recovery while achieving similar decompression and stability to classic open techniques.[6] When used in concert with an expandable cage and percutaneous pedicle screws, the MIS retroperitoneal corpectomy can be a powerful tool to decompress neural elements, correct deformity, and stabilize the lumbar spine. The MIS retroperitoneal vertebrectomy has evolved as a result of the increased proficiency with lateral approaches gained from the recent popularity of lateral interbody fusions. As such, the instrumentation requires further advancement from the large retractors required for vertebrectomy and the bulky instrumentation used during open corpectomy.

Indications

- Traumatic lumbar burst fracture
- Osteoporotic fracture with severe deformity or instability
- Osteomyelitis requiring corpectomy
- Metastatic tumors
- Scoliosis

Contraindications

- Previous retroperitoneal surgery with adhesions
- Vascular or anatomic abnormalities precluding minimally invasive approach
- Multilevel anterior corpectomy
- Primary bone tumor requiring en-bloc spondylectomy
- Medically unstable for surgery

Advantages

- Smaller incision
- Decreased postoperative pain and shorter recovery compared with open retroperitoneal approach
- Good exposure and visualization of anterior lumbar spine from L2 to L4
- Direct visualization of the anterior thecal sac
- Minimal disruption to organs in intraperitoneal compartment
- No need for an approach surgeon

Disadvantages

- Decreased visualization compared with traditional open retroperitoneal approach
- Pathology visualized from only one side
- Lateral plate can be cumbersome to place, with small working space usually requiring a separate posterior approach for stabilization and posterior decompression
- Temporary loss of visualization while passing the cage inserter, which has typically been designed for open corpectomy
- Risk of nerve injury to the lumbar plexus
- Risk of ureter injury
- Risk of injury to aorta and inferior vena cava
- High likelihood of transient postoperative iliopsoas pain or weakness related to trans-psoas approach
- Small working space
- Steep learning curve

Objectives

- Expose the pathological vertebral body from an anterior approach with the least "collateral damage" possible
- Decompress the neural elements
- Correct sagittal or coronal deformity
- Provide durable structural support to a compromised anterior and middle column
- Stabilize the spine
- Obtain good bony fusion

Surgical Technique

Anesthesia

The patient is placed under general anesthesia for the procedure. Neuromonitoring is preferred to safely traverse or retract the psoas muscle and while decompressing the thecal sac. Muscle relaxants and inhalational anesthetic agents must be minimized. Generally a short-acting paralysis agent is preferred. Nicotinic receptor agonists, such as succinylcholine, are contraindicated if the patient has concomitant paraplegia. These depolarizing agents have been associated with hyperkalemia and cardiac arrest in patients with denervated muscle.[9]

Positioning

On a radiolucent operating table, the patient is placed in a true lateral position with the back perpendicular to the floor. Either a left- or right-sided approach is selected, depending on the patient's anatomy and the pathology to be addressed. All things being equal, the left side is generally preferred because a right-sided approach can be complicated by the bulk of the liver and the proximity of the vena cava, which is more prone to injury and more difficult to repair than the aorta on the patient's left side. A gel roll is placed under the axilla to ensure that it is appropriately padded and that the patient's weight is distributed off of the down shoulder. The dependent arm is left straight and padded. A pillow is placed between the arms, and the up arm rests on the pillow with the elbow bent at 90 degrees. The dependent leg is left straight on the operating table. Pillows are placed between the legs, and the up leg is flexed at the hip and knee to relax the psoas muscle on the approach side. The patient is then secured to the operating table with tape over the hip, chest, and legs (**Fig. 65.1**).

To increase the opening between the 12th rib and the iliac crest, the operating bed can be flexed up to 20 degrees. During positioning, be sure that the iliac crest sits just below the break in the bed. Before the spine is instrumented, the patient must be returned to a neutral position to avoid fusing the patient with an iatrogenic coronal deformity.

The fluoroscopy unit is brought in to ensure that the spine is in a true lateral position. The bed, not the C-arm, should be rotated as needed to obtain a true lateral position. Anteroposterior (AP) fluoroscopy is then used to confirm that the spinous process is midline between the pedicles and that the pedicles project equally over the vertebral body. The fluoroscopy unit should be angled parallel to the end plates to get a direct view of each disk space in question. Working directly perpendicular to the floor is helpful for orienting the surgeon during the approach and

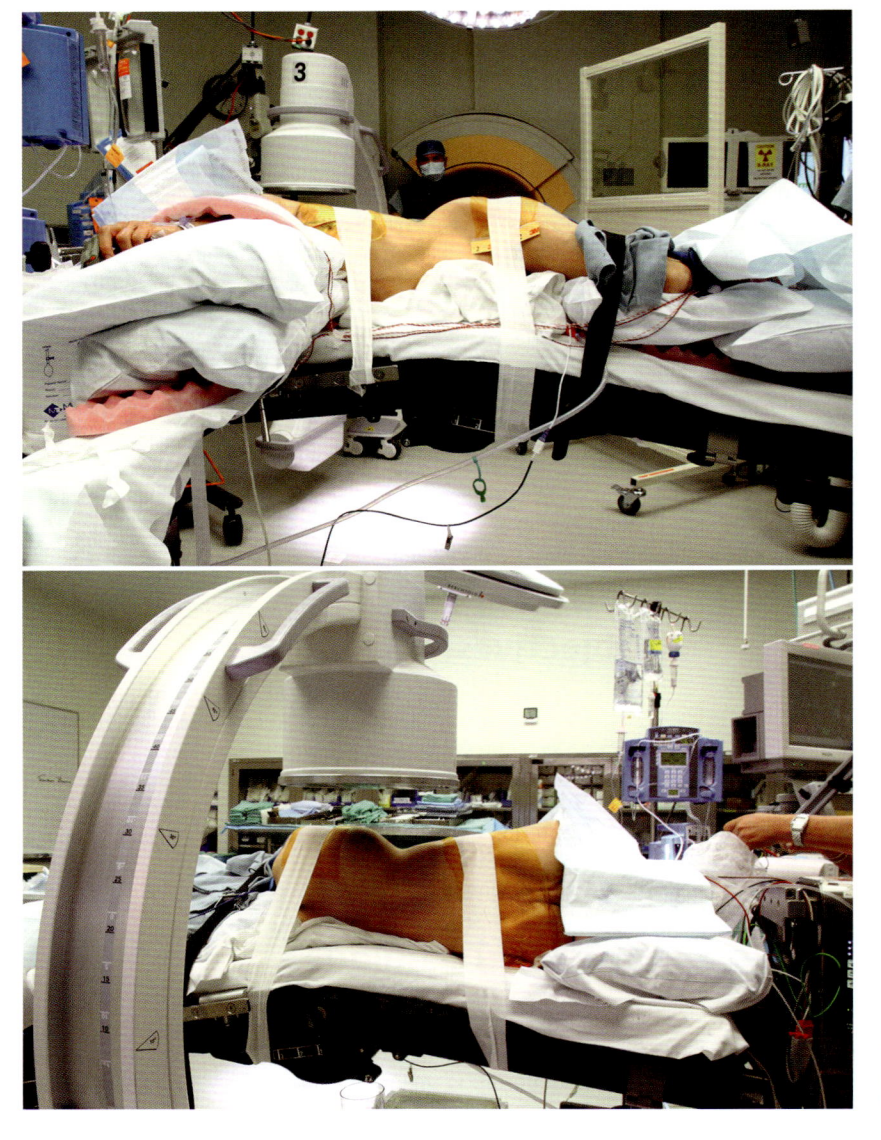

Fig. 65.1 Patient positioned lateral and slightly flexed on a radiolucent bed. **(a)** Anterior view. **(b)** Posterior view.

during placement of the instrumentation. Additionally, an intraoperative navigation system can be helpful to ensure adequate bone removal during the surgery. A reference probe can be inserted through the patient's posterior superior iliac spine from the lateral position after the patient has been prepped and draped.

Incision, Dissection, and Exposure

Using fluoroscopy, the superior, inferior, anterior, and posterior borders of the vertebral body of interest are marked out on the skin. The incision is planned so that the surgeon can work directly perpendicular to the floor and access just anterior to the anterior-posterior midpoint of the disk space above and below the corpectomy. A 3- to 5-inch incision is made parallel to the muscle fibers of the external oblique muscle (**Fig. 65.2**). If working at L2, a portion of the T12 rib will likely have to be removed. Scarpa's fascia is identified and opened to expose the muscle fibers of the external oblique muscle. The muscle fibers of the external oblique, internal oblique, and transversus abdominis are each split longitudinally to atraumatically dissect down to the transversalis fascia (**Fig. 65.3**). The transversalis fascia is picked up and opened with scissors, taking care not to violate the peritoneum.

Under direct visualization, the peritoneum is swept anteriorly to create a corridor through the retroperitoneal space (**Fig. 65.4**). A sponge stick can be helpful in gently freeing the peritoneum from the quadratus and psoas muscles. Along the superior portion of the dissection, the kidney may have to be retracted anteriorly to visualize the vertebral body. Avoid violating the renal fascia at this step.

At this point a neuromonitoring probe is slowly passed through the psoas muscle to dock on the lateral vertebral body. A safe entry point through the psoas should be chosen to avoid the lumbar plexus based on knowledge of its course through the psoas muscle.[10–12] Generally, an entry point anterior to the midpoint of the vertebral body should be safe in circumventing lumbar plexus injury. The genitofemoral nerve should be visible on the surface of the psoas muscle and avoided. If a response is noted on the electromyogram (EMG), the probe should be repositioned

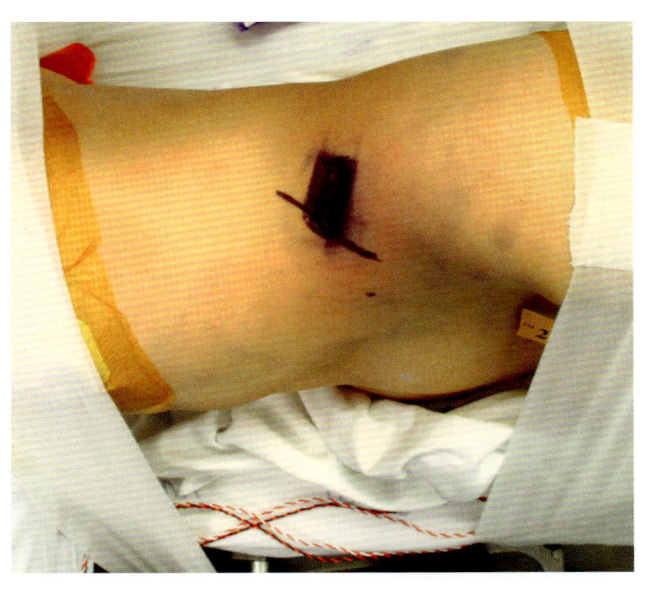

Fig. 65.2 Skin marking of the L3 vertebral body. A 6-cm incision marked out for a minimally invasive surgery (MIS) retroperitoneal vertebrectomy approach.

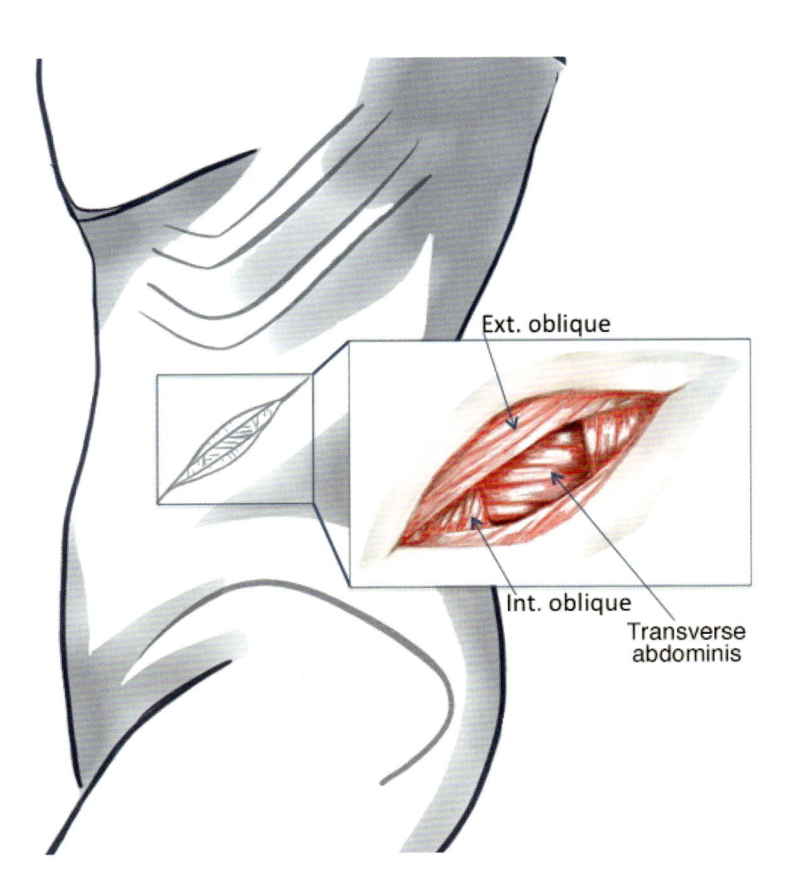

Fig. 65.3 Illustration of the opening of the abdominal wall musculature to access the retroperitoneal space, with the course of the muscle fibers at each muscle layer. The muscle fibers are retracted at each level rather than being transected.

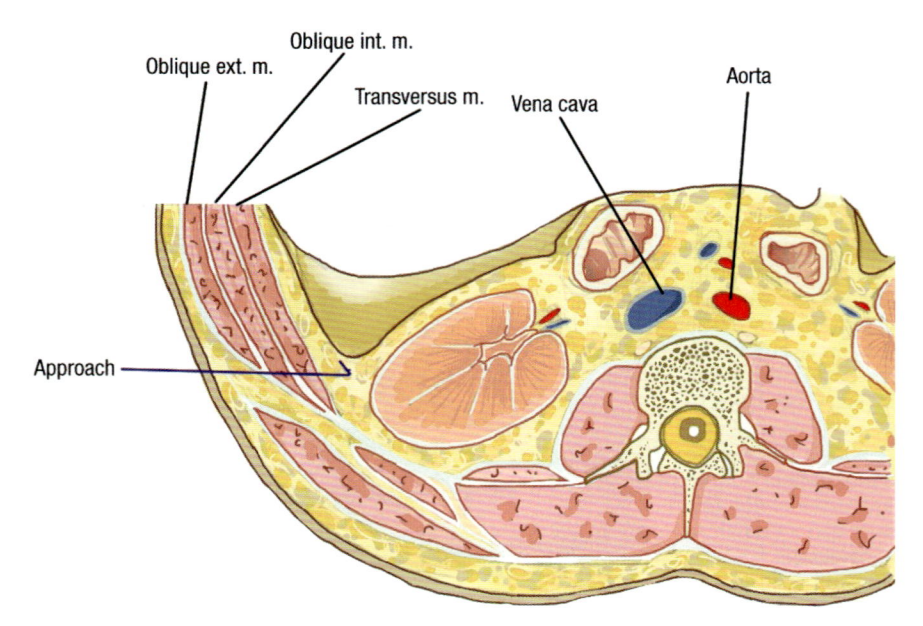

Fig. 65.4 Axial view of the relative anatomy en route to the lumbar spine from a lateral approach (modified image).

more anteriorly to avoid the plexus. Once the position on the lateral vertebral body is confirmed with fluoroscopy, the sequential dilators are used until the expandable retractor system can be placed. Alternatively, for patients with a smaller psoas muscle, a more anterior oblique trajectory can be used, keeping the entire retractor system anterior to the muscle and thereby circumventing the need for the dilators. The oblique approach also facilitates visualization of the anterior thecal sac if decompression is required.

The superior and inferior retractor blades are then expanded and advanced posteriorly such that they retract the psoas muscle and the end plates of the vertebral body above and below can be visualized (**Fig. 65.5**). To keep the blades in position, pins are placed into the adjacent vertebral bodies. When working at L2, the diaphragmatic crura will also have to be transected to visualize the L1-2 disk space. The anterior blade tip is then positioned in front of the pathological vertebral body. Care should be taken to ensure that the aorta and vena cava, which run just anterior to the vertebral body, are not injured while placing and opening the retractor. If possible, the retractor blade should be tucked just posterior to the anterior longitudinal ligament.

Diskectomies

Before bone removal, diskectomies at the level above and below the pathological vertebra are performed to clearly delineate the anatomy and avoid end-plate violation at the healthy segments. The annulus of the disk space is exposed, and it is incised with a No. 15 blade. A combination of pituitary rongeur, curette, and disk space shavers are used to perform the diskectomies and prepare the end plates under direct visualization. The disk space

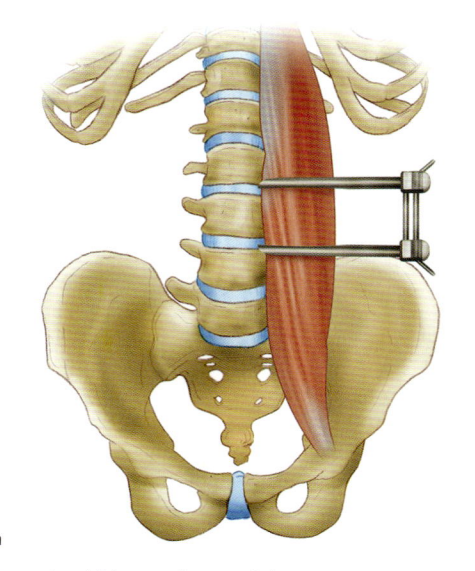

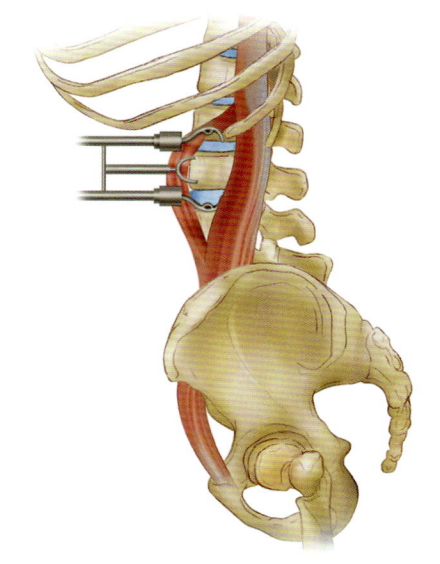

Fig. 65.5 (a) Coronal and (b) sagittal views of the retractor trajectory and blade positioning during an L3 MIS lateral retroperitoneal vertebrectomy.

shaver or a Cobb elevator can be gently malleted through the contralateral annulus to completely release the disk space.

Corpectomy

After the superior and inferior diskectomy have been completed and the end plates clearly identified, the corpectomy can commence. First the segmental vessels are identified and ligated. The segmental vessels are sacrificed proximally along their course, ensuring that there is a sufficient proximal vessel to hold the ligature without slipping off. Tearing the vessel or losing control at the proximal origin can lead to a hole in the side of the aorta or vena cava that is extremely difficult to control with a minimally invasive approach. The distal segmental artery is preserved as much as possible. In this region one of the segmental arteries may give rise to a low-lying dominant anterior radicular artery—the artery of Adamkiewicz. Taking a single segmental artery at the described location is normally safe and at extremely low risk for an anterior spinal stroke, as there is generally rich collateralization at the level of the neuroforamen.

The corpectomy is then performed within the space provided by the retractor with a combination of osteotomes, curettes, high-speed drill, pituitary rongeur, and Kerrison rongeur. Under direct microscopic visualization, the thecal sac is decompressed from pedicle to pedicle. A thin rim of bone is usually left in place along the ventral and lateral vertebral body to avoid injury to the great vessels and contralateral lumbar plexus, respectively. If indicated, as much bone as possible is saved during this step to use as autograft.

Graft Placement

Once the corpectomy has been completed, there are a variety of options in reconstructing the anterior column. Classically, this was achieved with allograft strut grafts such as of the femoral head, humerus, femoral shaft, or tibia. The outer cortical rim gives good structural support, and the hollow center can be filled with allo- or autograft to facilitate fusion. To insert a strut graft or any nonexpandable graft, the corpectomy defect is first measured with calipers. The graft is then cut to size and gently impacted into position under fluoroscopic guidance. Today, cages are more often used in the lumbar spine to circumvent issues with availability and size when using strut grafts. Titanium cages have also been demonstrated to be safe when instrumenting in the face of active infection.[13] Standard cage options include mesh and stackable cages.[14,15] Both can be packed with allograft or autograft and have high fusion rates, but they are sized externally, which can be time-consuming. Also, temporary distraction is recommended to achieve optimal compressive forces on the graft. This can be technically difficult to achieve through a minimally invasive approach.

Expandable cages have numerous advantages during a minimally invasive approach, including ease of insertion, in-situ expansion to allow for gentile distraction, and exact sizing to maximize engagement with the end plate.[16,17] When expanding the cage, care must be taken not to over-distract and place the end plates at risk for fracture.[18] Kyphosis correction should not be attempted by cage expansion alone. Adjunctive maneuvers, such as external pressure on the posterior spine at the level of the kyphosis or use of a vertebral body distractor system, are preferred to lessen the compressive forces on the end plate. Specific to the direct lateral trajectory, a wide footprint rectangular expandable cage can be used in place of a cylindrical cage to engage the apophyseal bilaterally.[8] Allograft or autograft is then packed around the cage while not exerting mass effect on the thecal sac.

Closure

Hemostasis is achieved, and the retractor system is removed. The transversalis and Scarpa's fascia are closed with a braided absorbable stitch. Care is taken to tightly approximate the fascial layers at this step to avoid incisional hernia. The subcutaneous tissues are closed with an inverted stitch, and a subcuticular stitch is used to close the skin.

Complications

Approach-related complications are rare but serious events. When traversing the retroperitoneal space, it is important to recognize the anatomic relationships to avoid injury to the bowel, ureter, or vascular structures.[19,20] Vascular injuries can be avoided by carefully inspecting preoperative films and modifying the approach if a vascular anatomic variant precludes lateral access on one side (**Fig. 65.6**). A large vascular injury requires immediate action to control bleeding at the site with compression above and below the injury. Do not hesitate to expand the incision to obtain better access. Vascular clamps should be available and may be necessary to gain temporary control of the bleeding. Assistance from a vascular surgeon may be required.

Bowel and ureter injuries can be harder to recognize, and a high clinical suspicion must be maintained to avoid much worse delayed complications. A bowel injury should be immediately repaired primarily. A ureteral violation requires intraoperative urology consultation for repair.[19] Be vigilant for compressive or vascular injuries to the ureter, which may lead to delayed fibrosis.

A durotomy obtained during decompression should be closed primarily if possible. If unable to get a watertight closure, a dural substitute and fibrin glue can be placed over the leak. A few days of lumbar drainage can promote healing of the leak postoperatively.[21]

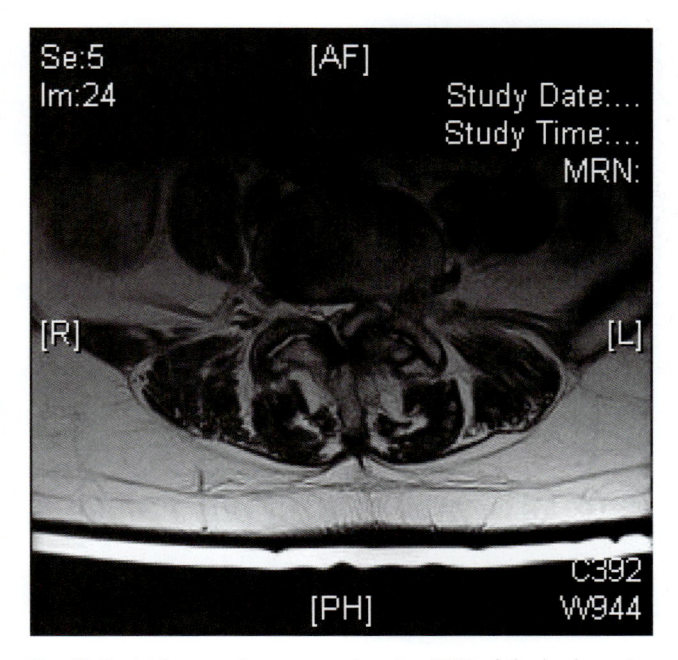

Fig. 65.6 Axial magnetic resonance imaging (MRI) of the lumbar spine demonstrating a vascular anomaly, making a right lateral approach unsafe.

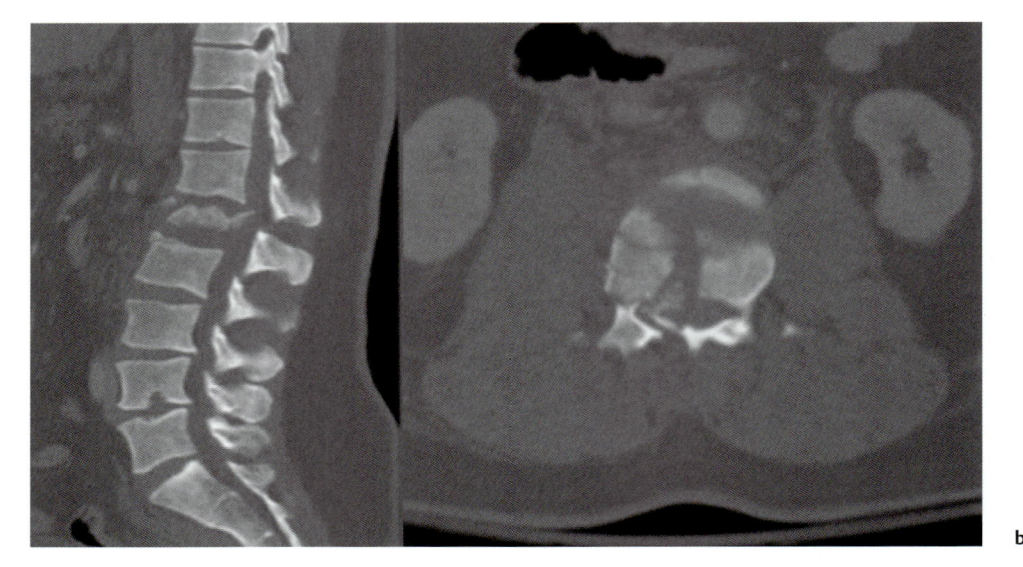

Fig. 65.7 Case example (see text). L2 burst fracture.

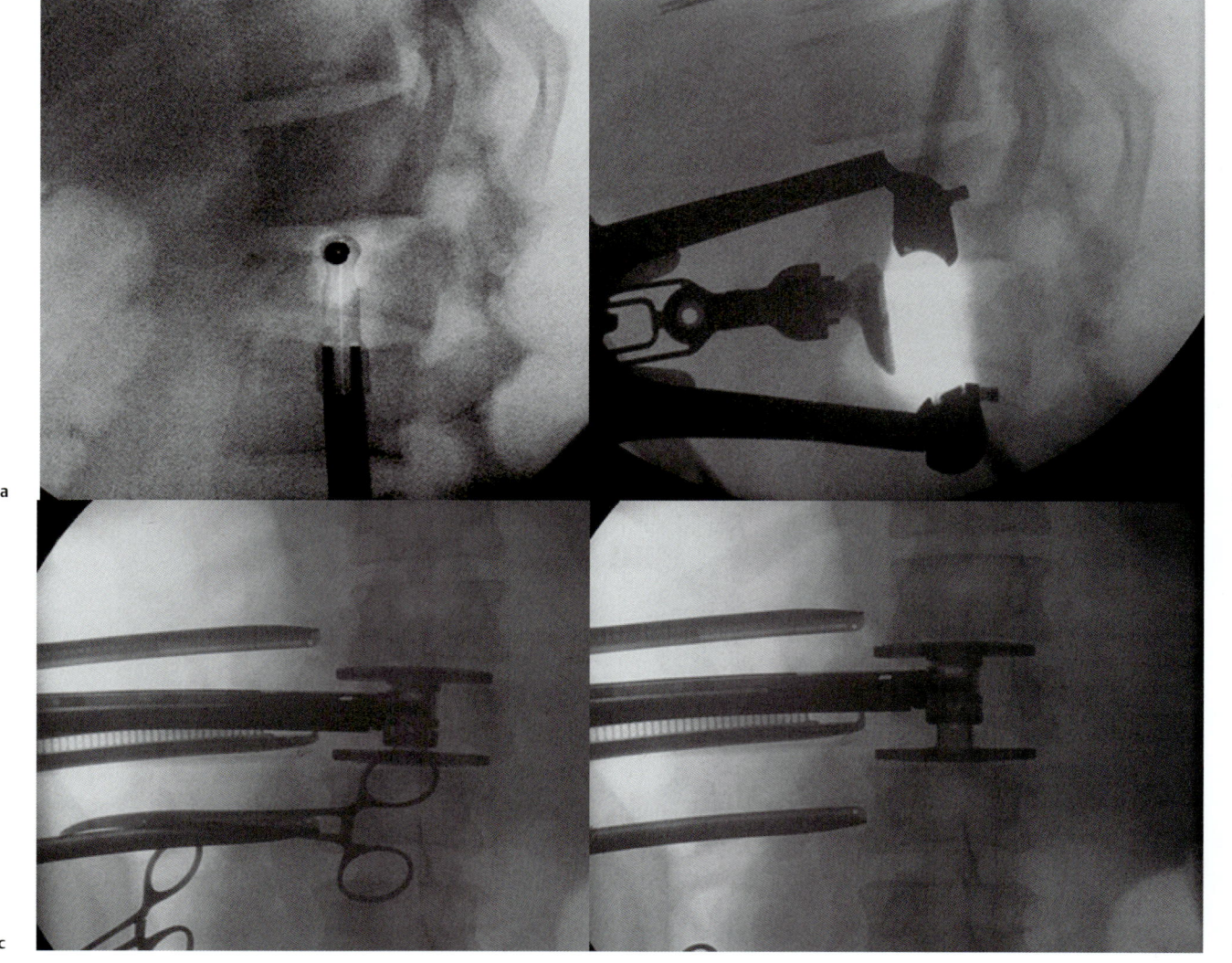

Fig. 65.8 Case example (continued). **(a)** Intraoperative fluoroscopy. **(b)** Expansion of the retractor system. Placement **(c)** and expansion **(d)** of a corpectomy cage with rectangular end caps.

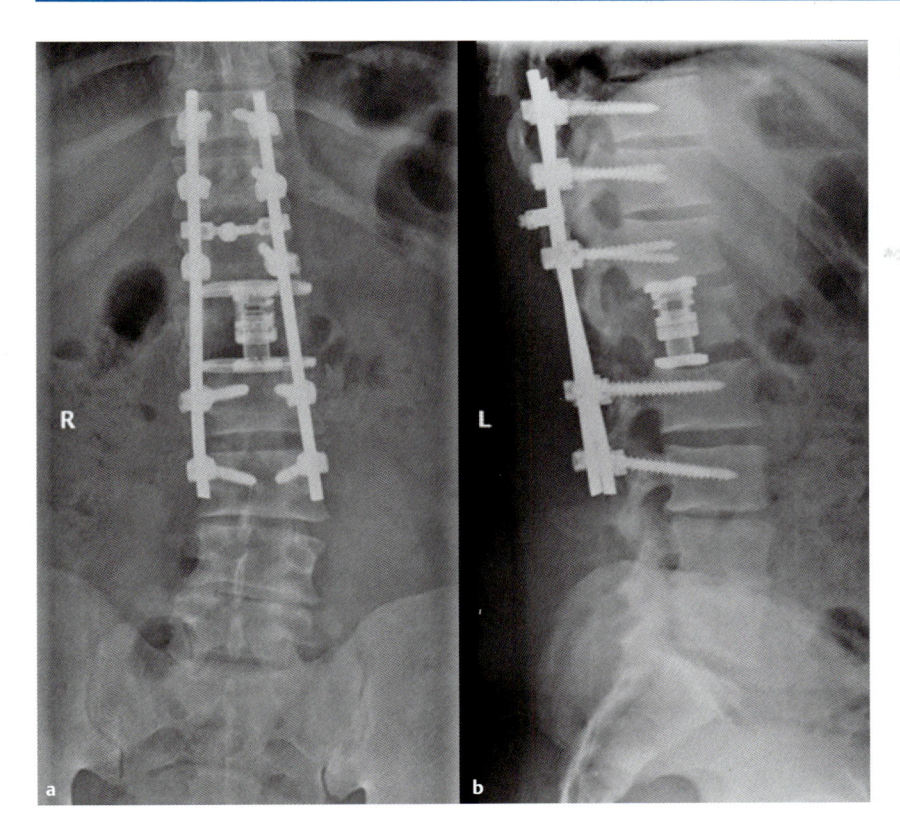

Fig. 65.9 (a, b) Case example (continued). Three-month follow-up.

Case Example of MIS Retroperitoneal Vertebrectomy

A 37-year-old man fell from a 40-foot-high bridge. In the emergency room he was found to be neurologically intact on initial evaluation. Imaging revealed a L2 burst fracture (the patient had an extra lumbar vertebra) (**Fig. 65.7**). Magnetic resonance imaging (MRI) confirmed a complete disruption of the posterior ligamentous complex, which has a Thoracolumbar Injury Classification and Severity *Score* (TLICS) of 5. The patient underwent a minimally invasive vertebrectomy with intraoperative fluoroscopy (**Fig. 65.8**). Because of the desire for posterior decompression along with multiple levels of posterior ligamentous injury at the thoracolumbar junction, we elected to supplement the anterior fusion with a long segment posterior spinal fusion during the same operation. The patient remained neurologically intact postoperatively and was doing well at 3-month follow-up (**Fig. 65.9**).

References

1. Sasso RC, Renkens K, Hanson D, Reilly T, McGuire RA Jr, Best NM. Unstable thoracolumbar burst fractures: anterior-only versus short-segment posterior fixation. J Spinal Disord Tech 2006;19:242–248
2. Harrington KD. Anterior decompression and stabilization of the spine as a treatment for vertebral collapse and spinal cord compression from metastatic malignancy. Clin Orthop Relat Res 1988;233:177–197
3. Lu DC, Lau D, Lee JG, Chou D. The transpedicular approach compared with the anterior approach: an analysis of 80 thoracolumbar corpectomies. J Neurosurg Spine 2010;12:583–591
4. Petteys RJ, Sandhu FA. Minimally invasive lateral retroperitoneal corpectomy for treatment of focal thoracolumbar kyphotic deformity: case report and review of the literature. J Neurol Surg A Cent Eur Neurosurg 2014;75:305–309
5. Tomycz L, Parker SL, McGirt MJ. Minimally invasive transpsoas L2 corpectomy and percutaneous pedicle screw fixation for osteoporotic burst fracture in the elderly: technical report. J Spinal Disord Tech 2015;28:53–60
6. Smith WD, Dakwar E, Le TV, Christian G, Serrano S, Uribe JS. Minimally invasive surgery for traumatic spinal pathologies: a mini-open, lateral approach in the thoracic and lumbar spine. Spine 2010;35(26, Suppl):S338–S346
7. Scheufler KM. Technique and clinical results of minimally invasive reconstruction and stabilization of the thoracic and thoracolumbar spine with expandable cages and ventrolateral plate fixation. Neurosurgery 2007;61:798–808, discussion 808–809
8. Amaral R, Marchi L, Oliveira L, Coutinho T, Pimenta L. Acute lumbar burst fracture treated by minimally invasive lateral corpectomy. Case Rep Orthop 2013;2013:953897
9. Brooke MM, Donovon WH, Stolov WC. Paraplegia: succinylcholine-induced hyperkalemia and cardiac arrest. Arch Phys Med Rehabil 1978;59:306–309
10. Benglis DM, Vanni S, Levi AD. An anatomical study of the lumbosacral plexus as related to the minimally invasive transpsoas approach to the lumbar spine. J Neurosurg Spine 2009;10:139–144
11. Uribe JS, Arredondo N, Dakwar E, Vale FL. Defining the safe working zones using the minimally invasive lateral retroperitoneal transpsoas approach: an anatomical study. J Neurosurg Spine 2010;13:260–266
12. Moro T, Kikuchi S, Konno S, Yaginuma H. An anatomic study of the lumbar plexus with respect to retroperitoneal endoscopic surgery. Spine 2003;28:423–428, discussion 427–428
13. Aryan HE, Lu DC, Acosta FL Jr, Ames CP. Corpectomy followed by the placement of instrumentation with titanium cages and recombinant human bone morphogenetic protein-2 for vertebral osteomyelitis. J Neurosurg Spine 2007;6:23–30
14. Eck KR, Bridwell KH, Ungacta FF, Lapp MA, Lenke LG, Riew KD. Analysis of titanium mesh cages in adults with minimum two-year follow-up. Spine 2000;25:2407–2415
15. Wang MY, Kim DH, Kim KA. Correction of late traumatic thoracic and thoracolumbar kyphotic spinal deformities using posteriorly placed intervertebral distraction cages. Neurosurgery 2008;62(3, Suppl 1):162–171, discussion 171–172

16. Eleraky MA, Duong HT, Esp E, Kim KD. Expandable versus nonexpandable cages for thoracolumbar burst fracture. World Neurosurg 2011;75:149–154
17. Snell BE, Nasr FF, Wolfla CE. Single-stage thoracolumbar vertebrectomy with circumferential reconstruction and arthrodesis: surgical technique and results in 15 patients. Neurosurgery 2006;58(4, Suppl 2):ONS-263–ONS-268, discussion ONS-269
18. Chou D, Lu DC, Weinstein P, Ames CP. Adjacent-level vertebral body fractures after expandable cage reconstruction. J Neurosurg Spine 2008;8:584–588
19. Flouzat-Lachaniette CH, Delblond W, Poignard A, Allain J. Analysis of intraoperative difficulties and management of operative complications in revision anterior exposure of the lumbar spine: a report of 25 consecutive cases. Eur Spine J 2013;22:766–774
20. Czerwein JK Jr, Thakur N, Migliori SJ, Lucas P, Palumbo M. Complications of anterior lumbar surgery. J Am Acad Orthop Surg 2011;19:251–258
21. Nairus JG, Richman JD, Douglas RA. Retroperitoneal pseudomeningocele complicated by meningitis following a lumbar burst fracture. A case report. Spine 1996;21:1090–1093

66 Thoracoabdominal/Retroperitoneal Graft and Lateral Plating

Shane V. Abdunnur and Daniel H. Kim

Exposure of the anterior thoracoabdominal spine is indicated for various pathologies and often requires an accompanying spinal reconstruction with grafting and instrumentation for the sake of arthrodesis. The most common procedure that necessitates a bone graft and lateral plating is a corpectomy for either tumor or trauma or a discectomy. Other indications are listed below. The type of construct utilized depends on the goals of the surgery itself. In general, the goal of any graft placement is to produce a solid bony arthrodesis, and restore normal anatomic alignment and structure. Although a comprehensive description of all the techniques and instrumentation systems is beyond the scope of this chapter, the discussion focuses on current overriding techniques and strategies for thoracoabdominal spine reconstruction with grafting and plating. Chapter 62 discusses the nuances of the approach.

Indications

- Vertebral body neoplasm (metastatic most common)
- Osteomyelitis/diskitis
- Unstable fracture
- Large sequestered thoracic disk herniation
- Degenerative scoliosis

Contraindications

- Medical illness that would preclude surgery
- Previous retroperitoneal or thoracoabdominal surgery

Advantages

- Ability to perform decompression and anterior instrumentation during a single approach
- Makes use of Wolff's law
- Resists compression and extension
- Restoration of anterior column support
- Large surface area for arthrodesis

Disadvantages

- Entry into the thorax entails associated risks.
- Abdominal viscera at risk for injury
- Complications of thoracotomy
- May require supplemental posterior instrumentation

Surgical Technique

Chapters 62 and 63 provide a complete description of the anatomic considerations for the thoracoabdominal and lateral retroperitoneal approach. Prior to performing a reconstruction with autograft or allograft, a decompression is first completed. Detailed descriptions of these procedures can be found in the preceding chapters in this section.

End-Plate Preparation

Because one of the main goals of anterior reconstruction is to restore normal anatomic alignment and promote stability during arthrodesis, end-plate preparation is the first key component that requires consideration. The inferior end plate of the superior-most level and the superior end plate of the inferior-most vertebral body being fused require preparation for acceptance of a graft that will provide stability and eventually arthrodesis. Removing all of the soft tissue, including disk material and cartilage, will enhance the surface area of bone-to-bone contact and facilitate fusion. Therefore, it is important to strip the bony end plate of its cartilage, leaving the cortical bone relatively intact. The cortical bone provides a firm foundation for fusion to take place. If its structure is compromised, the bone graft will be more likely to subside or telescope, possibly resulting in nonunion and instability.

Preparation of the end plate also requires shaping of the recipient end plates to accept flat surface graft, ensuring uniform compressive loads. If a lateral plate is eventually being placed, the lateral aspect of the vertebral bodies is shaved with a high-speed drill to enable flush seating of the plate.

Choice of Graft

Although it was once the autograft of choice, iliac crest has fallen out of favor during recent years due to the morbidity associated with the harvest as well as improvements in biologics and synthetic materials in promoting fusion. Still, autograft remains the most efficacious choice of material to promote fusion. At times during the exposure of the thoracoabdominal approach, the T11 rib is transgressed. Chapter 62 describes a technique of making a single posterior osteotomy and reflecting the T11 rib inferiorly. This can be easily converted into a T11 rib graft harvest with the addition of an anterior osteotomy and removal of a section of the floating T11 rib. In this manner, an 8- to 12-cm section of autograft can be obtained with little or no morbidity. If the initial approach does not transgress a rib, it is not recommended that

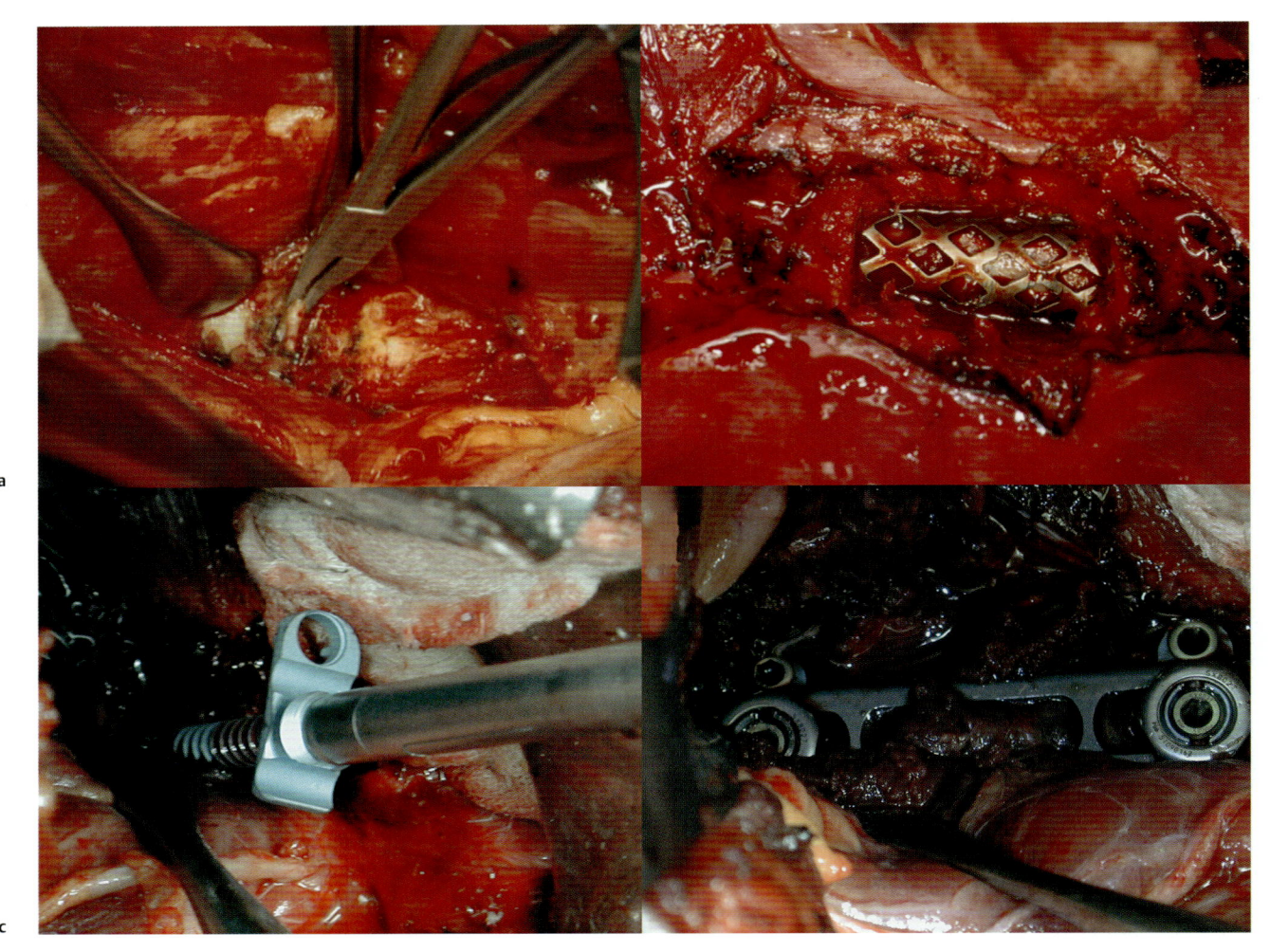

Fig. 66.1 Thoracoabdominal interbody cage and plate. After corpectomy has been completed **(a)**, a titanium strut filled with autologous bone graft is seated firmly in the corpectomy site under distraction of the vertebral bodies above and below **(b)**. **(c)** Bolts are placed in the vertebral bodies above and below the titanium cage, which are used to secure a lateral plate **(d)**.

the rib be harvested. When a corpectomy is being performed for a decompression, we recommend using a Leksell rongeur or similar instrument to remove the desired bone if it is acceptable as a graft. This is typically the case for traumatic fractures (**Fig. 66.1**). We do not take an autograft from the vertebral bodies if they are infiltrated with tumor or infection. There are numerous allografts available that range from cadaveric bone to osteoinductive and osteoconductive biologics. Numerous studies have been published regarding the characteristics of these various allografts, and their use is typically dictated by surgeon experience and preference.

If a simple diskectomy is performed, a small interbody cage can be place at each level, packed with either autograft or allograft. If, on the other hand, a corpectomy has been performed, there are numerous solutions that are currently available. Interbody devices that have been developed include stackable cages, fixed-length titanium mesh, and expandable titanium cages. Allogenic fibular strut grafting can also be utilized. Regardless of the scaffold used for reconstructing normal spinal alignment, the surgeon must ensure that the end plates of the vertebral bodies and the ends of the graft will seat together properly under physiological loading conditions. Graft should be packed into the cavity firmly but without undue force. Frequently, rib graft can be split longitudinally and placed anterior to the construct, thus placing it under direct axial load.

It is important to keep in mind that, depending on the length of the construct, arthrodesis may take 1 to 2 years to mature. In cases where patients are expected to live 1 year or less (some patients with metastatic cancer), the utility of grafting should be questioned. There are numerous reports of successful stabilization without grafting for arthrodesis. Alternatively, patients with pyogenic abscess should be treated on a case-by-case basis. Excellent results have been reported for patients who have a staged operation for decompression/stabilization and subsequent interbody fusion several weeks after corpectomy and intravenous antibiotics. There is no clear consensus regarding this last point, and the surgeon must consider the pros and cons of this strategy for each individual patient.

Reconstruction

The goal of reconstruction is generally to provide anterior support, resist axial loading, and restore normal alignment. In current practice, this typically takes the form of a titanium or polyetheretherketone (PEEK) cage, fibular strut graft, or polymethylmethacrylate (PMMA). The material used is at the discretion of

66 Thoracoabdominal/Retroperitoneal Graft and Lateral Plating

the surgeon and often dictated by the specific characteristics of the case. The thoracoabdominal and direct lateral retroperitoneal transpsoas approaches can be used to access T10 to L4, and as such, the typical goal of reconstruction is to provide a relatively straight construct. This transition zone of the thoracolumbar spine normally has slight lordosis at the L2-L3 level and 2 to 3 degrees of kyphosis at the T10-T11 level. Straight constructs will almost always provide excellent reconstruction in the thoracic spine. To avoid flat-back syndrome, 5 to 15 degrees of lordosis should be the goal per lumbar level being fused. This can be accomplished via interbody devices if necessary. Severe scoliosis can be one of the rare exceptions to this dictum.

Adequate reconstruction requires matching the diameter of the end plate to the diameter of the graft, as well as ensuring an appropriate length of graft. This is critical for both stability and eventual arthrodesis. As such, it is often advantageous to place the intervertebral construct while holding the superior and inferior vertebral bodies in distraction to facilitate placement of the graft. This can help ensure proper positioning, length, and diameter of the graft. There are several techniques that can be employed to attain the desired distraction. If a lateral plate is being used, it is often best to place the bolts in the vertebral bodies first and then employ a specialized distractor. Vertebral body spreaders can be utilized as well. Expandable cages can be placed in situ without distraction and subsequently expanded to properly seat the device in place. This is our preferred technique when it is suspected that there is poor bone quality at the level above or below.

Although there are a wide variety of techniques and materials currently available that help reconstruct the thoracolumbar junction, these are the guiding principles for the thoracoabdominal and direct lateral retroperitoneal approach. It is important for the surgeon to be familiar and comfortable with whichever system is used.

Plating

Plating for the thoracoabdominal retroperitoneal approach consists of a lateral support mechanism, typically a lateral plate that is secured to the vertebral body with two or more bolts. Again, there are numerous systems available, but the guiding principles are similar for each. Lateral plates primarily resist lateral bending. These systems also resist rotation and flexion/extension to some degree. The advantage of a lateral plate is that it can be placed during the same procedure. The nuances of one such system are discussed below (**Fig. 66.1**).

Prior to the interbody construct being placed, a depth gauge is used to measure the coronal diameter of the vertebral body above and below the corpectomy to determine the length of the bolts to be used. This distance can also be measured on preoperative computed tomography (CT) or magnetic resonance imaging (MRI). The single-bolt system is positioned in the coronal plane with bicortical fixation. A pilot hole is drilled in the anteroposterior (AP) center of the vertebral body. This should be placed in the inferior half, preferably the inferior third of the height of the vertebral body if posterior pedicle screws are planned, such that the trajectories of the posterior instrumentation will not be affected by the lateral bolt trajectory. After the pilot hole is drilled and its depth confirmed by blunt probe feel and fluoroscopy, it is tapped and then the bolt is inserted until it lies flush with the lateral surface of the vertebral body. These steps are completed at the level above and below the corpectomy. If desired, these bolts can be used for distraction and subsequent interbody device placement. The appropriate plate size can be measured by using the scale located on the distractor or by using a caliper. The plates have a fixed hole on one end and a slotted hole on the other end. The holes in the plate fit over the posts located on the bolts. It should be noted that the plate's lateral curvature should match the patient's physiological curvature. The nuts are placed over the posts and seated on the plate. Dynamic compression can then be added to the system as shown in **Fig. 66.1**. As the nuts are tightened, the compression becomes fixed and the final tightener with a countertorque handle is used to completely secure the system in place. Final alignment and hardware placement is confirmed by C-arm. **Fig. 66.2** illustrates an alternative system that utilizes two lateral rods connected to the bolts, in contrast to a plate. At the end of instrumentation, fluoroscopy confirms appropriate hardware placement and anatomic alignment (**Fig. 66.3**).

Closure

For the minithoracotomy-transdiaphragmatic approach (mini-TTA), incisions less than 4 cm in the diaphragm close without any approximating sutures. In cases that require incisions larger than 4 cm, the cut edges of the diaphragmatic crus should be

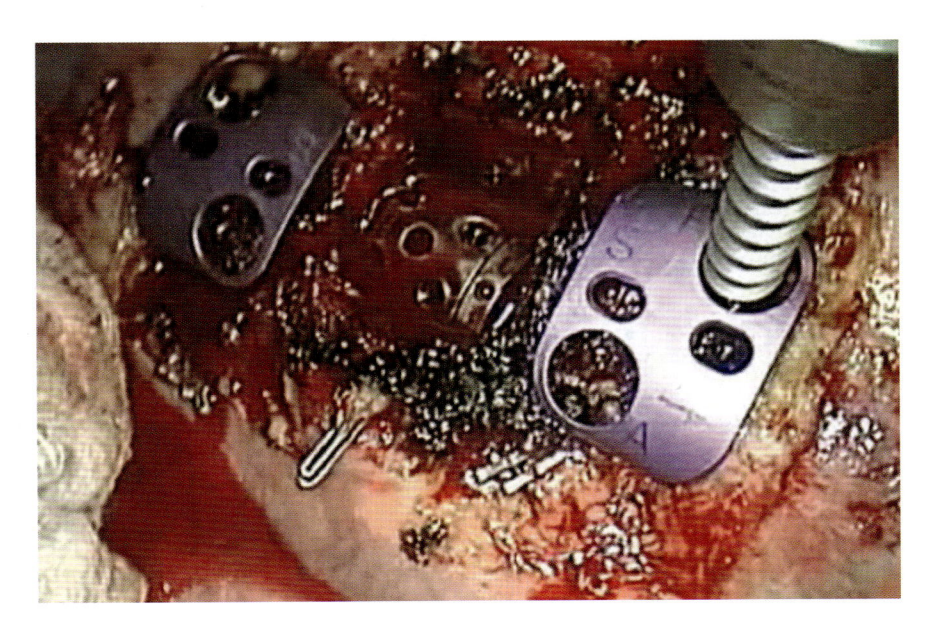

Fig. 66.2 Lateral rods are assembled under compression to aid arthrodesis and stability.

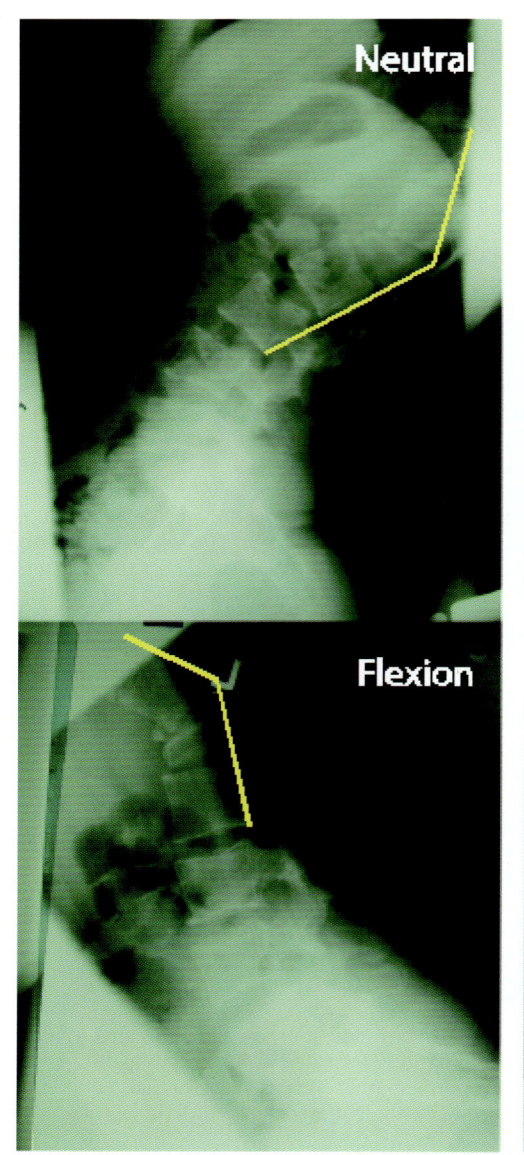

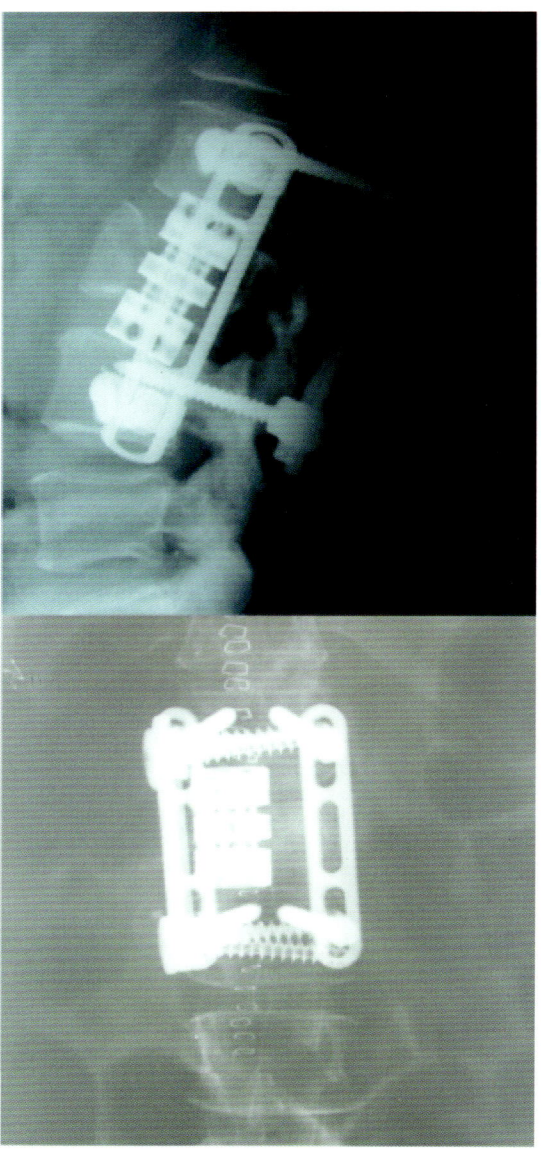

Fig. 66.3 L1 flexion/compression fracture. The thoracoabdominal/retroperitoneal approach is best suited for thoracolumbar junction pathology. **(a)** Preoperative lateral X-rays show a chronic unstable L1 fracture with increasing angulation in flexion. **(b)** Anterior cage with lateral plating, augmented by posterior spinal fusion (PSF) results in restoration of height and sagittal alignment.

reapproximated with nonabsorbable suture. Both the medial and lateral arcuate ligaments should be reattached to the cuff that was left on the vertebral body at the time of opening. The thoracic cavity is then irrigated, and a single chest tube is placed through a separate stab incision under direct visualization. The chest tube is secured with a purse-string suture to the skin. Irrigant is used to assess the thoracic cavity for air leaks. The T11 rib is reapproximated with a No. 1 nylon suture after having drilled pilot holes on both sides of the cut edge. The transversalis fascia and aponeurosis of the transverses abdominis are oblique muscles that are reapproximated with running suture to help prevent hernia formation. The subcutaneous layers are closed with interrupted absorbable suture and the skin with staples.

Closure is similar for the direct lateral retroperitoneal transpsoas approach, but it is less complicated because the diaphragm does not need to be addressed. After irrigating with the retractor system in place, the retractor can be removed slowly while it is still open. This enables the surgeon to assess and address any sites of bleeding in the psoas muscle. After the retractor is completely removed, a shallow self-retaining retractor is placed in the skin such that the transversalis fascia can be closed with several interrupted Vicryl sutures. The subcutaneous layer and dermis are then closed in a standard fashion.

Complications

- Pseudarthrosis
- Graft subsidence/telescoping
- Instability
- Hardware breakage/failure
- Neurologic or vascular injury from bolts or lateral screws

C. Posterolateral Approach

67 Open Costotransversectomy

Robert Andrew Rice, Rocky Felbaum, and Jean-Marc Voyadzis

Costotransversectomy is a far lateral posterior approach to pathologies of the thoracic spine. It involves resection of the rib and transverse process to provide greater exposure to the ventral aspect of the thecal sac than other posterior approaches to disk pathology. Menard first described the approach in 1894 in the treatment of Pott's disease to reach the vertebral body in an extracavitary manner. Hulme in 1958 was one of the first surgeons to report the use of costotransversectomy as an alternative management strategy for herniated thoracic disks, highlighting the lack of manipulation of the spinal cord otherwise necessitated by posterior procedures that had been employed previously.[1] The procedure has subsequently gained favor with many excellent results reported.[2-9] The typical surgical trajectory and planned bony removal are demonstrated in **Figs. 67.1 and 67.2**.

Indications, Contraindications, and Patient Selection

This technique is ideal for resection of soft or mildly calcified central and particularly lateral thoracic disk herniations. It is useful for sympathectomy, biopsy or resection of neoplasms, and removal of infectious processes, retropulsed bone fragments, or other anterolaterally oriented pathology compressing the spinal cord. It can be performed at multiple levels.[10] It is advantageous in its design by providing access to the lateral portion of the canal and the anterolateral portion of the thoracic vertebral body while avoiding violation of the pleural space and associated complications thereof. Costotransversectomy can be used to address pathology of the entire thoracic spine from T1 to T12, in contrast to anterior approaches that are limited by the thoracic inlet, mediastinum, and diaphragm. It can also be useful for patients whose clinical comorbidities would complicate a transthoracic approach. Finally, it obviates the need for the assistance of an approach surgeon for the thoracotomy. Conversely, its approach trajectory is less well suited than thoracotomy to address midline anterior pathology because of the limited view of the anterior spinal canal and dura that it affords.

Advantages

- Provides good exposure to the anterolateral aspect of the spinal canal and vertebral body
- Can be used to address pathologies of the entire thoracic spine
- Better tolerated by patients with complicated medical comorbidities
- Lower likelihood of pulmonary complications compared with thoracotomy

Disadvantage

- Midline anterior pathology difficult to visualize and address

Preoperative Testing and Imaging

Preoperative evaluation for costotransversectomy does not vary significantly from that for other thoracic spinal procedures. A detailed preoperative physical examination is paramount to delineate deficits and correlate them with imaging findings. Routine laboratory studies [complete blood count (CBC), basic metabolic panel (BMP), and prothrombin time (PT)/partial thromboplastin time (PTT)/international normalized ratio (INR)] should be performed for baseline values and predicting potential intraoperative intravenous (IV) volume needs. Packed red blood cells (RBCs) should be made available if significant blood loss is anticipated. Electrocardiogram (ECG) and chest X-ray are indicated for patients with known preexisting, or risk factors for, cardiopulmonary disease. Preoperative computed tomography (CT) can augment magnetic resonance imaging (MRI)-derived information to assess the degree of disk calcification. A "scout" sagittal MRI, including the lumbar or cervical spine, and anteroposterior (AP) and lateral radiographs to count lumbar vertebrae and ribs are helpful for localization. Fiducial markers can be placed at the index level prior to surgery to facilitate intraoperative localization. Alternatively, image guidance can augment the previously mentioned images.[11] A spinal angiogram can be performed when addressing pathology between T8 and L1, particularly on the left side, to visualize the artery of Adamkiewicz, as the approach puts the contents of the neural foramina at risk.[2,9,12]

Costotransversectomy for Thoracic Disk Herniations

Thoracic disk herniations account for only 0.15% of all spinal column disk herniations and 0.25 to 4% of all disk operations.[2,13] Most thoracic disk herniations that are symptomatic are found at or below T8[2,13] because of the increased mobility in the lower thoracic spine that results in a higher incidence of acute herniations associated with trauma as well as chronic spondylotic disease that presents more insidiously. These disks are generally central or paracentrally located, and their consistency varies from soft to heavily calcified.[9,14] Presenting symptoms may include any of the following: localized or radicular pain radiating along associated ribs and dermatomes, loss of sensation, lower extremity weakness, abnormal gait or difficulty ambulating, and bowel/bladder dysfunction.[2] Surgical indications include intractable pain refractory to conservative measures or progressive myelopathy.[13]

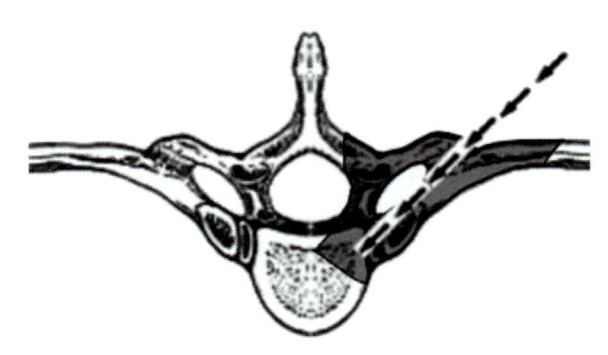

Fig. 67.1 Schematic of the surgical trajectory.

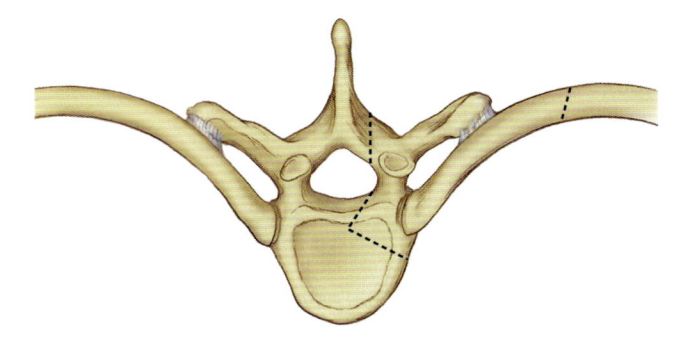

Fig. 67.2 Planned bony removal.

Surgical Technique

Preoperative antibiotics are administered within 30 minutes of the planned incision, and sequential compression devices are placed on the legs. General anesthesia is administered, and the patient is intubated in the standard fashion. Great care is taken to avoid hypotension in the setting of spinal cord compression, and arterial line monitoring is recommended. Neuromonitoring leads are then placed, and somatosensory evoked potentials (SSEPs) and motor evoked potentials (MEPs) are obtained throughout the procedure. The patient is positioned prone on gel rolls or a radiolucent Wilson frame to facilitate intraoperative fluoroscopic visualization, and all pressure points padded. This technique has also been performed in the three-quarter prone or modified lateral decubitus position. A C-arm machine is then maneuvered to localize the level of interest. Various incisions have been described and may be chosen based on surgeon preference. The most commonly used are a vertical midline, with or without a T-extension overlying the rib to be resected, or a straight paramedian incision along the lateral border of the erector spinae muscles, with or without a terminal curved "hockey-stick" extension (**Fig. 67.3**).

The laterality of the incision is chosen based on the eccentricity of the lesion and associated symptoms. In the absence of these considerations, some surgeons prefer an approach from the right side to avoid injuring the artery of Adamkiewicz, which usually emanates from the left side of the anterior spinal artery between T8 and L2.[2,12] The incision of choice is then marked, and the patient is prepped and draped in the usual sterile fashion.

Local anesthesia may then be injected. The incision is made and carried through the subcutaneous tissue and fascia with Bovie electrocautery. If the paramedian approach was chosen, these tissues are reflected medially. The superficial muscles and erector spinae muscles are then dissected and reflected toward the midline (or can be split transversely) to expose the angle of the ribs and ultimately costovertebral junction.

In the midline approach, standard subperiosteal dissection is performed laterally to the tips of the transverse processes, taking care to avoid disruption of the facet joints, to expose the costovertebral junction. Relevant muscular anatomy is shown in **Fig. 67.4**. Muscles encountered superficially in the upper thoracic spine include the trapezius and rhomboids, with the latissimus dorsi and serratus posterior found in the lower thoracic spine.[15] It is important to recall certain bony considerations. The medial scapula usually extends from approximately T2 to T7.[15] Access to a particular disk space necessitates exposure of the inferior rib and rib head (i.e., access to the T9-10 disk space necessitates exposure of the tenth rib). Additionally, the first, 11th, and 12th rib heads articulate only with their own vertebral body.[15] The ribs of interest are then exposed and skeletonized, including their articulations (superior, inferior, and transverse costal facets) and associated ligaments, as demonstrated in **Fig. 67.5**.

Care is taken to avoid unnecessary disruption of the intercostal neurovascular bundle along the inferior border of the exposed ribs. The dorsal pleura is gently freed from the ventral aspect of the ribs to be resected and ventrolaterally from the vertebral column and mobilized anteriorly. The skeletonized ribs and associated transverse processes are then resected to 3 to 6 cm from the costovertebral junction (**Fig. 67.6**). The fragments are typically saved to augment the fusion construct if applicable, although costotransversectomy does not in itself require fusion.

The relevant vertebral anatomy is seen in **Fig. 67.7**. The transverse processes and costovertebral ligaments are resected to enable disarticulation of the rib head(s) (**Fig. 67.8**). The neural foramina and associated pedicles are then identified, and subperiosteal dissection of the lateral aspect of their respective vertebral bodies is completed. Partial (or complete, if necessary) removal of the pertinent pedicles is then performed to visualize the ventrolateral dura and enable sufficient disk resection. Partial removal of the posterior portion of the inferior and superior aspects of the superior and inferior vertebral bodies, respectively,

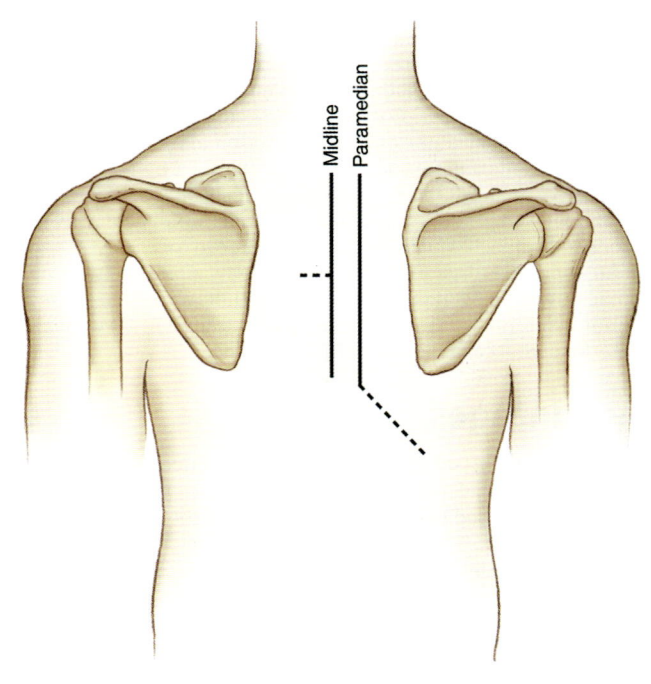

Fig. 67.3 Incision choices.

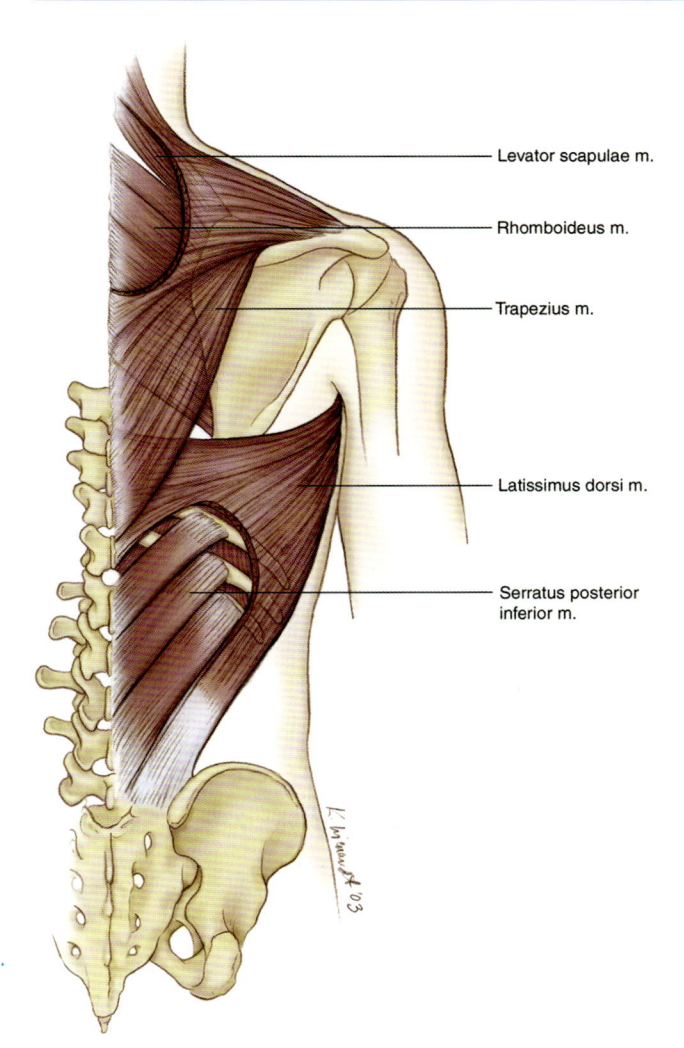

Fig. 67.4 Relevant muscular anatomy.

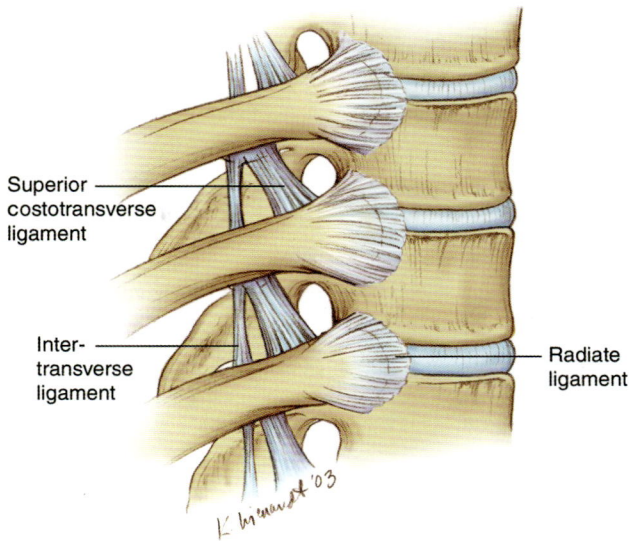

Fig. 67.5 Costovertebral ligamentous attachments.

The sympathetic nervous system (SNS) consists of bilateral chains of ganglia extending along the entire vertebral column oriented at the anterolateral aspect of each vertebral body. Sympathetic outflow arises from T1 to L2 in the intermediolateral nucleus of the spinal cord. The fibers leave the ventral roots via white rami communicantes and enter the sympathetic ganglia as preganglionic fibers. These fibers travel to the paravertebral or prevertebral ganglia. Postganglionic fibers then travel from these ganglia to innervate target organs via norepinephrine.[17]

Surgical Technique

Several approaches to the lower cervical and upper thoracic sympathetic chain have been described including the supraclavicular, transaxillary, and transpleural approaches. Using a posterior may also be required to avoid spinal cord manipulation. If a midline approach is used, a hemilaminectomy and facetectomy may also be performed if necessary.

Sufficient bony resection is crucial to avoid manipulation of the spinal cord. An operating microscope is commonly used to assist in bony removal near the thecal sac and of the lesion itself. After the lesion has been resected, attention can then be turned to instrumentation, if required. This can be done easily by exposing the contralateral lamina and transverse process if a midline approach was used, or it can also be performed percutaneously if a paramedian approach was used.

Costotransversectomy for Sympathectomy

The indications for surgical sympathectomy include causalgia, essential hyperhidrosis, Raynaud's disease, and various visceral pain syndromes refractory to nonsurgical management. The rationale for this procedure stems from theorized hyperactivity of or hypersensitivity to sympathetic outflow in these disease entities. Thus, disruption of this outflow has been shown to provide some relief for affected patients.[14] In addition, this technique can be used to alleviate the symptoms of Harlequin syndrome.[16]

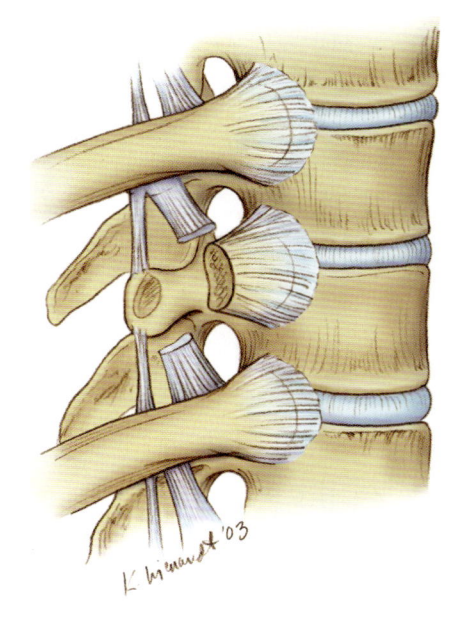

Fig. 67.6 View after the rib segment is resected.

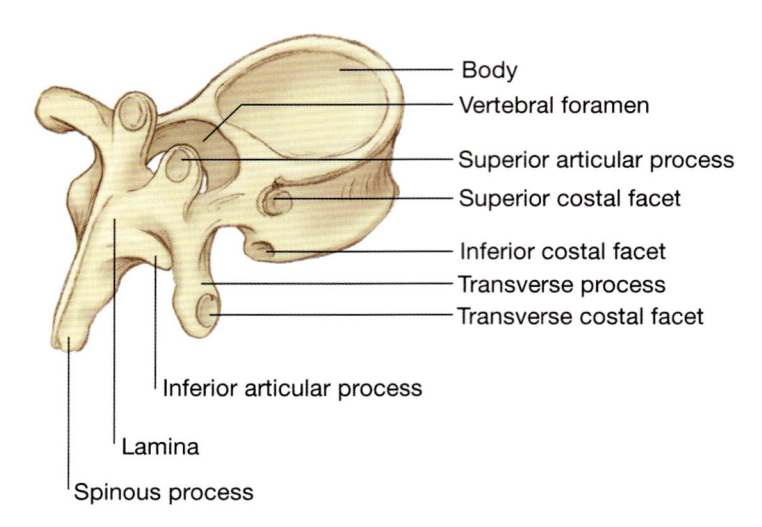

Fig. 67.7 Relevant vertebral anatomy.

midline incision, bilateral ganglionectomy can be achieved with the costotransversectomy approach. To achieve sympathetic denervation of the upper extremities, T2 is typically the only level requiring ganglionectomy.[14,18]

The patient may be placed in either a sitting or a prone position. A posterior midline incision is made over the spinous processes of T1 to T3 to provide sufficient exposure of anatomy surrounding T2. A C-arm X-ray device is used to confirm the identity of the T3 spinous process. Subperiosteal dissection of the musculature is then performed to the ipsilateral transverse process of T3, which is subsequently removed with a combination of Leksell and Kerrison rongeurs. The corresponding rib is then identified immediately deep to the previous location of the T3 transverse process. Careful dissection of the costovertebral junction is then performed as previously described, and the rib head is disarticulated from the vertebral body. Care is taken to protect the integrity of the pleura. The posterior mediastinum can be visualized by tilting the operating table while simultaneously elevating the ipsilateral side. Dissection is then carried anteriorly to expose the lateral aspect of the T3 vertebral body and the sympathetic chain, as well as superiorly to identify the T2 ganglion. The fibers of the rami communicantes connecting to the T2 intercostal nerve are divided. Surgical clips are then applied to the sympathetic chain adjacent to the ganglion superiorly and inferiorly, at which point the ganglion is removed (**Fig. 67.9**).[14,18] As similarly described above, the T3 costotransversectomy for T2 ganglionectomy is advantageous due to the low risk of pleural injury, coupled with a low risk of Horner's syndrome. Risks are also similar to those described above, including infection, empyema, radicular pain, and pneumothorax.

Wound Closure

The wound is then copiously irrigated, meticulous hemostasis is obtained, and the wound closed in anatomic layers (paraspinal muscles, lumbodorsal fascia, superficial muscles, skin) over a

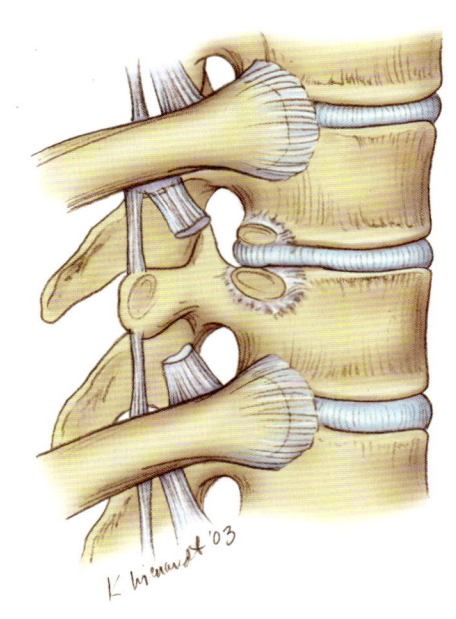

Fig. 67.8 View after the rib head is disarticulated.

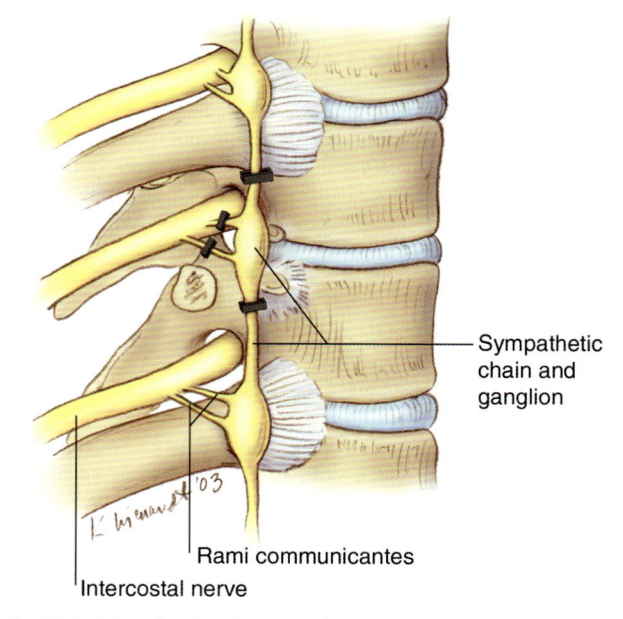

Fig. 67.9 View after the clips are applied to the sympathetic ganglion.

drain.[19] If the pleura was violated, it should be repaired primarily and a chest tube placed to avoid a postoperative pneumothorax.

Postoperative Care

A chest X-ray is obtained to assess the presence of pneumothorax after the patient is transported to recovery. Patients are ideally taken to a neurosurgical unit for close cardiopulmonary and neurologic monitoring. Routine chest tube care is instituted as necessary, as well as monitoring of surgical-site drain output.

Potential Complications and Precautions

Complications associated with costotransversectomy are intercostal neuralgia, pulmonary contusion/effusion, pneumothorax, atelectasis, and pneumonia or empyema. These are typically less common than in thoracotomy. The primary vascular complication, Although rare, is interruption of the major segmental arterial supply to the spinal cord (e.g., artery of Adamkiewicz), but this can be avoided by careful dissection and preoperative planning. Inadvertent durotomy can occur due to the limited anterior view of the thecal sac, especially in the setting of calcified or intradural disk. For small durotomies, postoperative lumbar drainage may be sufficient, but primary repair may be required for larger tears. Pleural injury and associated pneumothoraces are treated by chest tube placement. Spinal cord injury is rare owing to the far lateral nature of this technique that minimizes retraction of the thecal sac and its contents.[20]

Conclusion

Open costotransversectomy is an excellent option for accessing pathology of the anterolateral thoracic spine that minimizes potential complications and morbidity when compared with anterior transthoracic approaches. **Box 67.1** summarizes the key points.

Box 67.1 Key Points

- Use this technique for anterolaterally oriented pathology.
- Consider additional imaging or fiducials to confirm the level of interest.
- Avoid unnecessary ligamentous or neurovascular compromise (consider a right-sided approach).
- Expose the inferior rib/rib head to access the superior disk space.
- Fully mobilize the dorsal pleura from the rib and vertebral body.
- Resect the rib and transverse process, and then disarticulate the rib head.
- Remove enough bone to visualize the ventrolateral dura, avoid cord manipulation, and resect the lesion.
- Only T2 is typically needed for upper extremity denervation.
- Place a chest tube if the pleura is injured, or place a lumbar drain if a durotomy occurs.
- Assess the presence of pneumothorax postoperatively with a chest X-ray.

References

1. Burke TG, Caputy AJ. Treatment of thoracic disc herniation: evolution toward the minimally invasive thoracoscopic technique. Neurosurg Focus 2000;9:e9
2. el-Kalliny M, Tew JM Jr, van Loveren H, Dunsker S. Surgical approaches to thoracic disc herniations. Acta Neurochir (Wien) 1991;111:22–32
3. Fessler RG, Sekhar L. Atlas of Neurosurgical Techniques: Spine and Peripheral Nerves. New York: Thieme; 2006;441–447
4. Garrido E. Modified costotransversectomy: a surgical approach to ventrally placed lesions in the thoracic spinal canal. Surg Neurol 1980;13:109–113
5. Ghostine S, Samudrala S, Johnson J. Treatment of thoracic disc herniation. In: Winn RH, ed. Youmans Neurological Surgery. Philadelphia: Elsevier; 2011
6. Lubelski D, Abdullah KG, Mroz TE, et al. Lateral extracavitary vs. costotransversectomy approaches to the thoracic spine: reflections on lessons learned. Neurosurgery 2012;71:1096–1102
7. Otani K, Yoshida M, Fujii E, Nakai S, Shibasaki K. Thoracic disc herniation. Surgical treatment in 23 patients. Spine 1988;13:1262–1267
8. Wolfla C, Resnick D. Neurosurgical Operative Atlas: Spine and Peripheral Nerves, 2nd ed. New York: Thieme; 2007
9. Young S, Karr G, O'Laoire SA. Spinal cord compression due to thoracic disc herniation: results of microsurgical posterolateral costotransversectomy. Br J Neurosurg 1989;3:31–38
10. Lau D, Song Y, Guan Z, Sullivan S, La Marca F, Park P. Perioperative characteristics, complications, and outcomes of single-level versus multilevel thoracic corpectomies via modified costotransversectomy approach. Spine 2013;38:523–530
11. Kim KD, Babbitz JD, Mimbs J. Imaging-guided costotransversectomy for thoracic disc herniation. Neurosurg Focus 2000;9:e7
12. Stillerman CB, Chen TC, Couldwell WT, Zhang W, Weiss MH. Experience in the surgical management of 82 symptomatic herniated thoracic discs and review of the literature. J Neurosurg 1998;88:623–633
13. Stillerman CB, McCormick PC, Benzel EC. Thoracic discectomy. In: Benzel EC, eds. Spine Surgery: Techniques, Complication Avoidance and Management. New York: Churchill Livingstone; 1999:369–387
14. Bay JW, Dohn DF. Surgical sympathectomy. In: Wilkins RH, Rengachary SS, eds. Neurosurgery. New York: McGraw-Hill; 1996:3251–3256
15. Ahlgren BD, Herkowitz HN. A modified posterolateral approach to the thoracic spine. J Spinal Disord 1995;8:69–75
16. Sribnick EA, Boulis NM. Treatment of Harlequin syndrome by costotransversectomy and sympathectomy: case report. Neurosurgery 2011;69:E257–E259
17. Mallory B. Anatomy of the autonomic nervous system. In: Lin VW, et al. Spinal Cord Medicine: Principles and Practice. New York: Demos Medical Publishing; 2003. http://www.ncbi.nlm.nih.gov/books/NBK9506
18. Wilkinson HA. Surgery for hyperhidrosis and sympathetically mediated pain syndromes. In: Schmidek HH, Sweet WH, eds. Operative Neurosurgical Techniques: Indications, Methods, and Results. Philadelphia: WB Saunders; 1995:1573–1584
19. Johnson RM, Murphy MJ, Southwick WO. Surgical approaches to the thoracic spine. In: Herkowitz HN, Elsmont FJ, Garfin SR, et al, eds. The Spine. Philadelphia: Rothman-Simeone; 1999:1537–1557
20. Wiggins GC, Mirza S, Bellabarba C, West GA, Chapman JR, Shaffrey CI. Perioperative complications with costotransversectomy and anterior approaches to thoracic and thoracolumbar tumors. Neurosurg Focus 2001;11:e4

68 MIS Costotransversectomy

Justin K. Scheer, Nader S. Dahdaleh, and Zachary A. Smith

Through a posterolateral approach, the costotransversectomy provides access to the anterior and lateral portion of the vertebral canal and the anterior and middle columns of the thoracic spine. This approach provides the means by which the spinal canal may be directly decompressed and anterior column reconstruction and fusion may be performed. A costotransversectomy may be employed for decompression of traumatic or pathological fractured bone fragments, spinal osteomyelitis, rib pain, disk herniation, and biopsy or resection of neoplastic masses.[1,2] In general, the costotransversectomy is favored in patients who would poorly tolerate a traditional thoracotomy such as elderly patients or those with significant underlying pulmonary pathology. This approach has recently been modified to now include a minimally invasive option.

Minimally invasive surgery (MIS) has been shown to decrease hospitalization, decrease blood loss, and speed recovery in many spinal surgical techniques.[3–6] More surgeons are learning how to incorporate MIS approaches in common surgical spinal pathologies, and the field is only increasing.[5] The MIS costotransversectomy has been demonstrated to be safe and effective.[3,7–11] In addition to the advantages of a standard costotransversectomy, the advantages of the MIS costotransversectomy include clear visualization of thecal sac,[8,9] anterior stabilization,[7,9] and preservation of the posterior tension band.[9,10] However, it also increases radiation exposure and may limit complete bilateral decompression,[7,9] and a second incision may be needed for percutaneous stabilization.[9,10] This chapter discusses the technique of MIS costotransversectomy.

Patient Selection

Anyone requiring a costotransversectomy is appropriate for the MIS technique, especially the elderly who cannot tolerate transthoracic surgery.

Indications and Contraindications

The indications include decompression for traumatic or pathological fractured bone fragments, spinal osteomyelitis, rib pain, sympathectomy, disk herniation, and biopsy or resection of neoplastic masses.[1,2] Contraindications include cases in which rigid fusion is a concern, and there is poor bone quality as well as significant bilateral spinal canal compression. In these cases it is recommended to proceed with the open costotransversectomy instead of the MIS version.

Advantages and Disadvantages

The advantages of MIS costotransversectomy are numerous and include clear visualization of thecal sac,[8,9] anterior stabilization,[7,9] and preservation of posterior tension band.[9,10] Furthermore, costotransversectomy in general minimizes many of the complications related to thoracotomy, such as intercostal neuralgia, pneumothorax, pulmonary contusion, pneumonia, effusion, and atelectasis.[1] The lower incidence of pulmonary complications makes this procedure ideal for an elderly or high-risk patient. The disadvantages include significant blood loss and increased operating room time,[8,9] the decompression can only be unilateral,[7,9] a second incision is needed for percutaneous stabilization,[9,10] increased radiation exposure,[3] and the limited exposure of the anatomy.

Choice of Operative Approach

The posterolateral approach is used.

Preoperative Imaging

Imaging can be provided by anteroposterior (AP) and lateral plain film radiographs, 36-inch standing scoliosis radiographs, dedicated computed tomography (CT), or magnetic resonance imaging (MRI).

Surgical Procedure

After general endotracheal anesthesia is induced, the patient is turned prone onto a radiolucent four-poster or Jackson-type frame to ensure that the abdomen is free and not under pressure. This helps to reduce paraspinal and epidural venous congestion and hemorrhage during the procedure.[7] Prior to turning the patient prone, appropriate contact and pin leads for continuous neurophysiological monitoring with somatosensory evoked potentials or continuous electromyographic potentials are placed. Prior to draping the patient, the fluoroscopic C-arm is brought into the field to correctly identify the spinal level of interest.[7,11] If posterior fixation is indicated, such as with a corpectomy, AP views using fluoroscopic guidance are then obtained to plan for percutaneous pedicle fixation cranial and caudal to the level of interest.[11] Generally, pedicle screws are placed one or two levels above and below the level of the intended vertebrectomy. Following screw placement, the C-arm is rotated so that the disk space, facet complex, pedicle, and pars of the target level are clearly aligned, as the trajectory is such that the Kirschner wire (K-wire) and subsequent portal will glide down the rib angle toward the transverse process and pedicle of the body inferior to the target level of interest.[7]

The area is then prepared and draped in the usual fashion. Using fluoroscopic guidance, a paramedian skin incision ~ 3.5 to 4 cm is made 4 cm off midline, or two fingerbreadths.[7,8,10,11] A K-wire is then inserted through the posterior thoracic musculature and docked on the lateral facet at the level of the pathology. One may also mark the skin with a vertical 1.5- to 2-cm skin incision and then pass an 18-gauge spinal needle along the future surgical trajectory to ensure that it will dock at the appropriate spot and on bone.[7] Using this needle, a local anesthetic can then be infiltrated into the target area as the needle is withdrawn to the skin.[7] The 2-cm incision is then opened sharply through the fascia. A variant of the incision is to use a single midline incision and only open up to the fascia. Then in a suprafascial plane and laterally, the site for the dilators and retractor is opened.

Following either technique for the initial incision, sequential soft tissue tubular dilators are used to separate the posterior musculature and are placed along the oblique lateral trajectory up to a working portal of 22 to 24 mm.[7,8,11] The final tube is then secured to the flexible bed–mounted arm. Using the C-arm, biplanar fluoroscopic confirmation of the location of the docked working portal is obtained. In the lateral projection, the target lesion should lie essentially parallel to and in the center of the portal's working axis.[7] Once the final dilator tube is confirmed to be in the correct trajectory, retractor arms are opened to produce a minimal-access corridor.[8,11] Bipolar and unipolar cautery combined with pituitary rongeurs are used to free the inferior transverse process–facet complex. Any residual muscle or soft tissue attachments are then removed under microscopic guidance.[7,8,11]

The ipsilateral lamina, facet, transverse process, costovertebral joint, and proximal rib heads are exposed (**Fig. 68.1a**). A subperiosteal dissection is then performed to expose the rib heads at the level of interest and at the level below.[8,11] The lateral aspect of the lamina or pars interarticularis is identified and then removed from lateral to medial with the high-speed bur and Kerrison rongeurs. At this point, the ligamentum flavum becomes visible and is dissected free from the underlying nerve root and lateral aspect of the spinal cord using Kerrison rongeurs.[7,10,11] Next, the transverse process and facet joints are removed with a combination of Kerrison rongeurs, osteotomes, and a high-speed drill. For cases centered at T11 or T12, only the most peripheral fibers of the diaphragmatic attachment may be encountered. However, the surgeon will not need to mobilize or dissect this structure, given the approach angle in the prone position.[8,11] The pedicle and neural foramina are now exposed, and the rib head is then removed using a high-speed drill and Kerrison rongeurs.[8,10,11] The segmental nerve root is sutured or ligated. The underlying dura is then exposed following removal of the pedicle (**Fig. 68.1b**). At this point, the surgical correction of the interested pathology may then be completed.

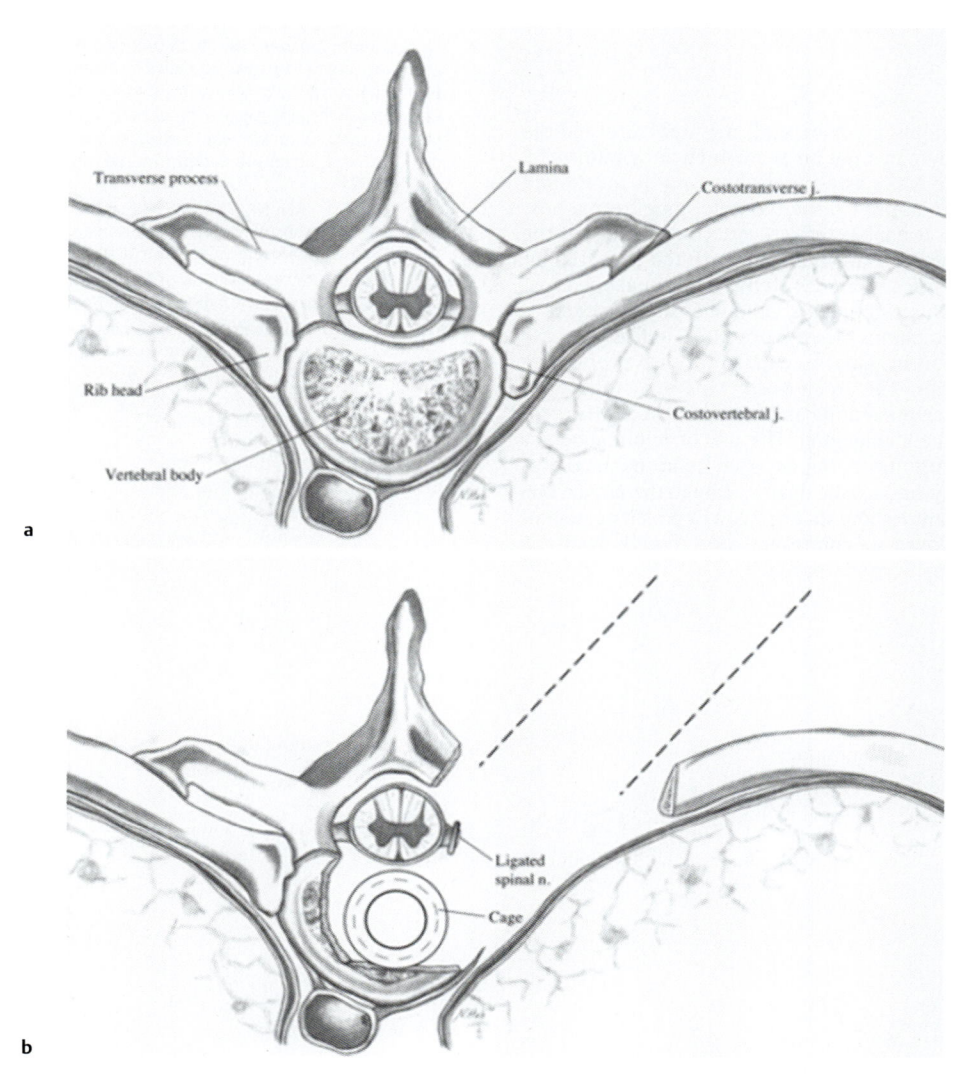

Fig. 68.1 Illustration of axial view for the costotransversectomy approach. **(a)** The normal preoperative anatomy. **(b)** The approach angle and correlative anatomy of bony removal and cage placement for a corpectomy.

Postoperative Care

Standard postoperative care is provided. Most patients may return to the surgical ward. But for those patients who sustain a complication or have significant comorbidities, the intensive care unit may be warranted.

Potential Complications and Precautions

Potential complications include pneumonia, wound infection, a dural tear, and neuralgia, with vascular complications being very rare.[1] One of the major disadvantages of the general costotransversectomy is that visualization of the contralateral central spinal canal is not as optimal as with other approaches. The exposure is even more limited in the MIS setting. If there is significant contralateral pathology, one may choose to dock a contralateral retractor. Another option for bilateral pathology is the use of the mini-open approach described by Chou et al.[12–14] This technique involves a midline incision and a trapdoor rib-head osteotomy.[14] Each side may be decompressed via this approach. However, regardless of the exact approach, very detailed knowledge of the anatomy in this region and careful patient selection are critical to avoid complications with this procedure.

Conclusion

The MIS spinal techniques are advancing at a rapid rate, and the costotransversectomy can now be performed in a minimally invasive fashion. The MIS costotransversectomy is a safe and effective technique to approach the thoracic spine from a posterolateral approach. It enables effective decompression of the spinal canal and anterior reconstruction, with the potential for decreased morbidity as compared with the traditional open costotransversectomy. This technique should decrease the complication rate that accompanies other procedures and may enable operative intervention in patients with otherwise prohibitive medical comorbidities. The open costotransversectomy is a technically demanding procedure, and the addition of MIS technology at first may be challenging. The use of minimal access techniques significantly limits the exposed anatomy, increases the use of fluoroscopy, and can be disorienting to the novice MIS surgeon. It is important to note that in cases in which persistent intraoperative challenges are confronted, one should always be prepared to convert to an open approach.

References

1. Lubelski D, Abdullah KG, Steinmetz MP, et al. Lateral extracavitary, costotransversectomy, and transthoracic thoracotomy approaches to the thoracic spine: review of techniques and complications. J Spinal Disord Tech 2013;26:222–232
2. Lubelski D, Abdullah KG, Mroz TE, et al. Lateral extracavitary vs. costotransversectomy approaches to the thoracic spine: reflections on lessons learned. Neurosurgery 2012;71:1096–1102
3. Falavigna A, Piccoli Conzatti L. Minimally invasive approaches for thoracic decompression from discectomy to corpectomy. J Neurosurg Sci 2013; 57:175–192
4. Massicotte E. The role of minimally invasive techniques in the management of spinal neoplastic disease: a review. J Neurosurg Sci 2013;57: 193–201
5. O'Toole JE. The future of minimally invasive spine surgery. Neurosurgery 2013;60(Suppl 1):13–19
6. Spoor AB, Öner FC. Minimally invasive spine surgery in chronic low back pain patients. J Neurosurg Sci 2013;57:203–218
7. Khoo LT, Smith ZA, Asgarzadie F, et al. Minimally invasive extracavitary approach for thoracic discectomy and interbody fusion: 1-year clinical and radiographic outcomes in 13 patients compared with a cohort of traditional anterior transthoracic approaches. J Neurosurg Spine 2011;14: 250–260
8. Kim DH, O'Toole JE, Ogden AT, et al. Minimally invasive posterolateral thoracic corpectomy: cadaveric feasibility study and report of four clinical cases. Neurosurgery 2009;64:746–752, discussion 752–753
9. Lall RR, Smith ZA, Wong AP, Miller D, Fessler RG. Minimally invasive thoracic corpectomy: surgical strategies for malignancy, trauma, and complex spinal pathologies. Minim Invasive Surg 2012;2012:213791
10. Musacchio M, Patel N, Bagan B, Deutsch H, Vaccaro AR, Ratliff J. Minimally invasive thoracolumbar costotransversectomy and corpectomy via a dual-tube technique: evaluation in a cadaver model. Surg Technol Int 2007;16:221–225
11. Smith ZA, Li Z, Chen NF, Raphael D, Khoo LT. Minimally invasive lateral extracavitary corpectomy: cadaveric evaluation model and report of 3 clinical cases. J Neurosurg Spine 2012;16:463–470
12. Chou D, Lau D, Roy E. Feasibility of the mini-open vertebral column resection for severe thoracic kyphosis. J Clin Neurosci 2014;21:841–845
13. Lu DC, Chou D, Mummaneni PV. A comparison of mini-open and open approaches for resection of thoracolumbar intradural spinal tumors. J Neurosurg Spine 2011;14:758–764
14. Chou D, Lu DC. Mini-open transpedicular corpectomies with expandable cage reconstruction. Technical note. J Neurosurg Spine 2011;14:71–77

D. Posterior Approach

69 Thoracic Laminectomy

Andrew James Grossbach, Stephanus Viljoen, Patrick W. Hitchon

Since it was first described by Smith in 1828, thoracic laminectomy has proven to be a mainstay in the treatment of several neurosurgical conditions of the thoracic spine. A contraindication for thoracic laminectomy is a large ventral compressive lesion, such as a herniated disk, the removal of which can result in a contusion of the cord, with worsening of the neurologic deficit.[1,2] Thoracic laminectomy remains the mainstay of treatment options for posterior pathologies of the thoracic spine, including epidural metastases (**Fig. 69.1**), infections (**Fig. 69.2**), and stenosis (**Fig. 69.3**), as well as providing exposure, as in implantation of epidural spinal cord stimulators. Results of thoracic laminectomy for appropriate indications depend on several factors, such as duration of symptoms, underlying pathology, age of the patient, and the presence of other risk factors.[3]

The anatomy of the thoracic spine differs from that of the cervical and lumbar spine. The spinal canal is smaller in the thoracic spine compared with the lumbar, and the pedicles are shorter, giving the surgeon less room to operate. Furthermore, care must be taken to preserve the blood supply to the thoracic cord, as it can be susceptible to infarction, most particularly between T4 and T9.[4] The main radicular artery supplying the lower thoracic cord is the artery of Adamkiewicz, which most commonly can be found on the left side between T9 and T11.

Recently, there has been growing interest in minimally invasive surgery (MIS) procedures. These procedures have the advantage of minimizing blood loss, tissue dissection, postoperative pain, and length of hospital stay.[5,6] MIS techniques can be used in the thoracic spine in cases of thoracic stenosis, or foraminal pathology such as lateral disk herniations or nerve sheath tumors. The limitation of MIS procedures is typically its smaller exposure as compared with open techniques.

This chapter discusses the common indications for thoracic laminectomy as well as the basic surgical technique for open and minimally invasive procedures.

Patient Selection

Thoracic laminectomy is appropriate for cases in which access to the spinal canal or thoracic nerve roots is needed.

Indications

- Posterior epidural tumor
- Epidural abscess
- Thoracic stenosis
- Bony tumor of the posterior arch
- Intradural extramedullary tumor
- Intradural intramedullary tumor
- Epidural hematoma
- Vascular malformation
- Exposure for placement of epidural spinal cord stimulator

Contraindications

- Central disk herniation
- Ventral epidural tumor
- Unstable spinal column due to trauma or bony destruction from neoplasm/infection

Advantages

- Familiar approach
- Less tissue disruption compared with posterolateral approaches
- Lower morbidity than with transthoracic approaches
- Lower risk for instability due to stabilization from rib cage

Disadvantages

- Limited access to ventral pathology
- Vascular "watershed" area at T4–T9
- When extensive, risk of kyphotic deformity

Choice of Operative Approach

Thoracic laminectomy should be considered for patients with dorsally located thoracic pathology. Other approach options for dorsally located pathology could include thoracic laminoplasty, which should be considered especially in the face of multilevel pathology when the posterior arch itself is not pathological. For ventrally located pathology, an anterior approach such as a thoracotomy/costotransversectomy should be considered, as this may improve access ventral to the cord.

Preoperative Testing and Imaging

Preoperative testing should include standard preoperative laboratories such as a complete blood count (CBC), basic metabolic panel (BMP), and coagulation factors. Preoperative imaging should be obtained, and varies based on the pathology encountered. For tumors and degenerative and infectious etiologies, a preoperative magnetic resonance imaging (MRI) is helpful. A computed tomography (CT) scan can help to identify calcified disks as well as other bony abnormalities. If instrumentation is anticipated, a CT scan also aids in preoperative planning. Plain anteroposterior (AP) and lateral radiographs should also be obtained, as they are useful in identifying the appropriate level intraoperatively,

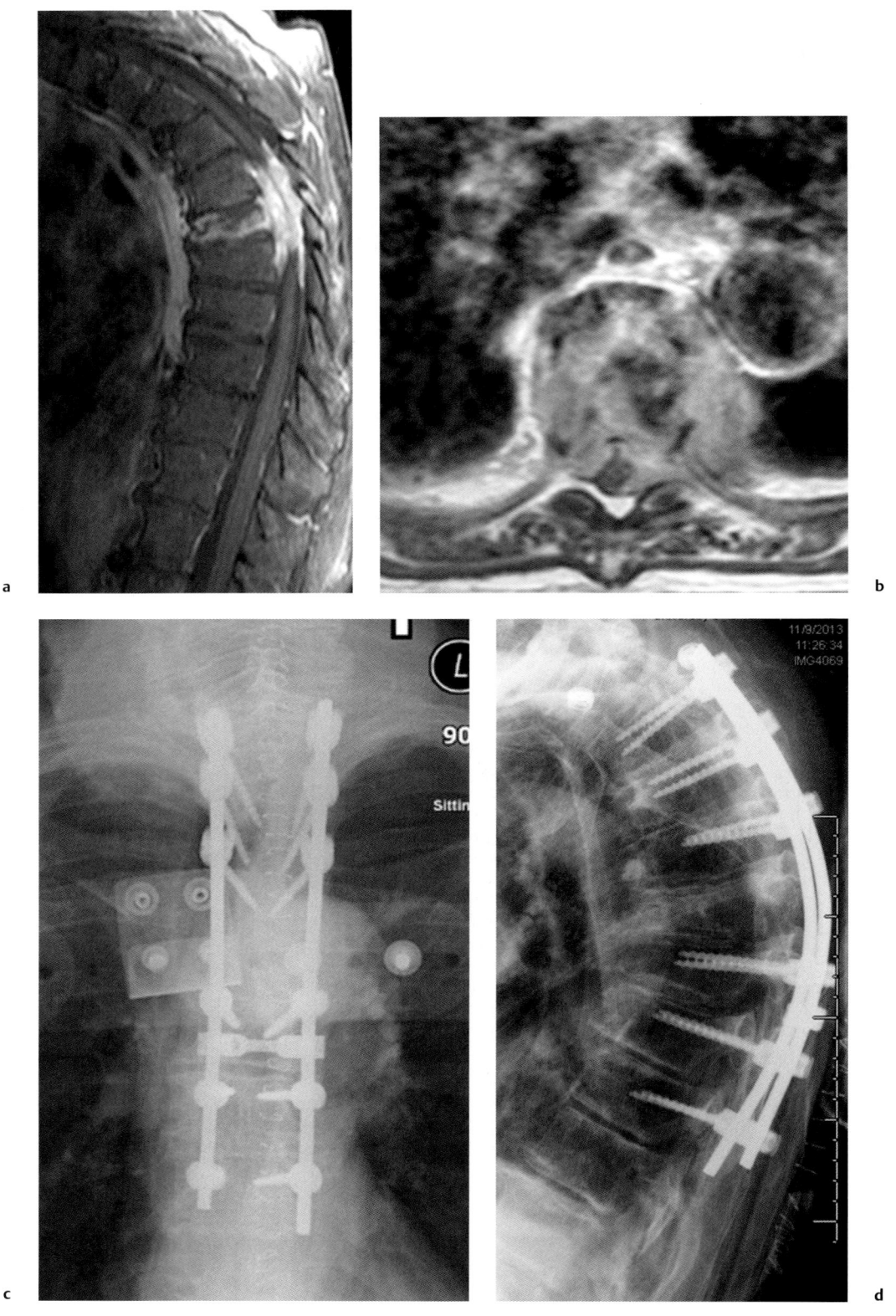

Fig. 69.1 An 82-year-old woman presented with a 4-week history of back pain and a 3-day history of numbness below the waist and weakness. The history included urothelial bladder cancer. On admission she had 3/5 motor strength in the legs with T6 sensory level. Sagittal **(a)** and axial **(b)** enhanced magnetic resonance imaging (MRI) scans show a T6 pathological fracture with enhancing tumor within the canal circumscribing and compressing the cord. The patient underwent a partial T6 laminectomy and partial laminectomy of T5 and T7 for decompression. Anteroposterior **(c)** and lateral **(d)** postoperative radiographs show pedicle screw fixation from T3 to T9. Postoperatively, motor strength in the legs was 4/5, and her pain was controlled. Pathology revealed metastatic urothelial carcinoma.

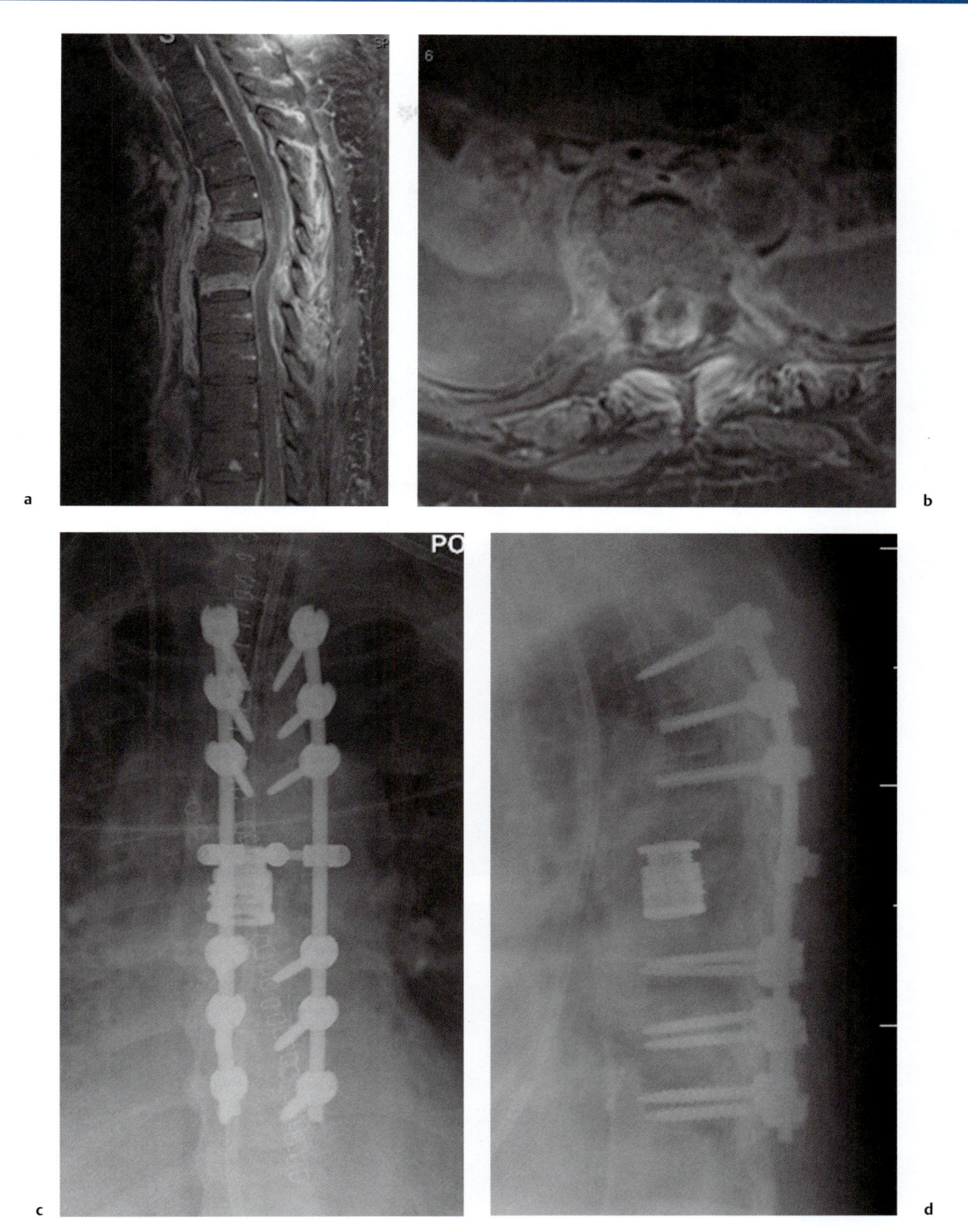

Fig. 69.2 A 73-year-old diabetic woman with obesity and atrial fibrillation was admitted with numbness in the legs and paraparesis. Sagittal **(a)** and axial **(b)** enhanced MRI scans show circumferential enhancement around the cord and in the paraspinal soft tissues compatible with a diagnosis of diskitis, spinal osteomyelitis, and epidural abscess. She underwent T6-T7 decompressive laminectomy, right-sided T6-T7 corpectomy with interbody grafting with an expandable cage, and pedicle screw fixation from T3 to T10. Anteroposterior **(c)** and lateral **(d)** radiographs show improved alignment with the hardware in place. Patient was unchanged neurologically and was discharged on meropenem for her *Escherichia coli* infection.

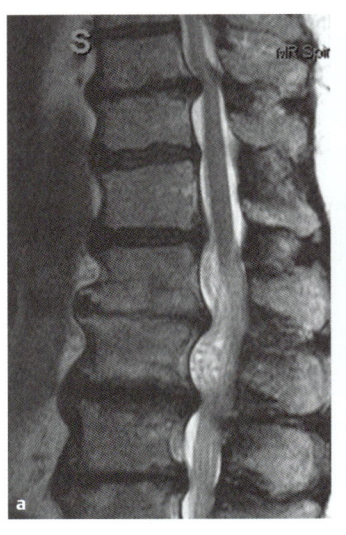

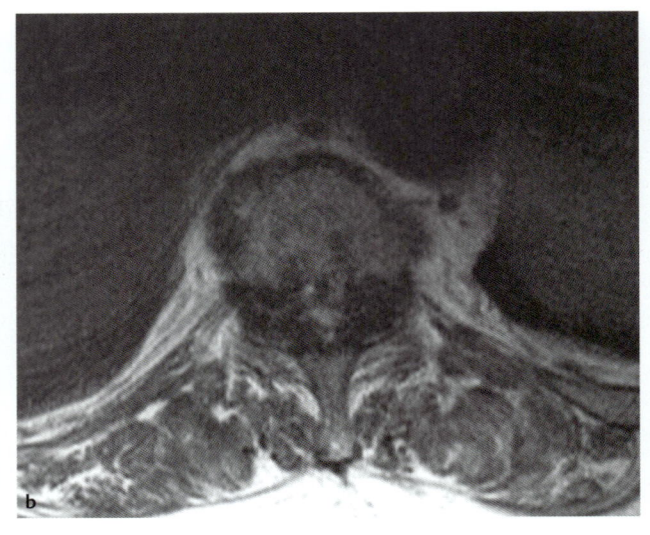

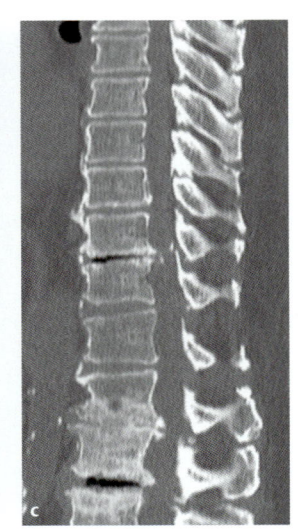

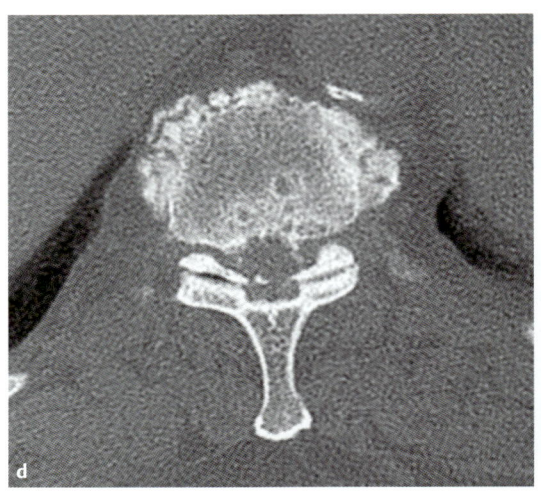

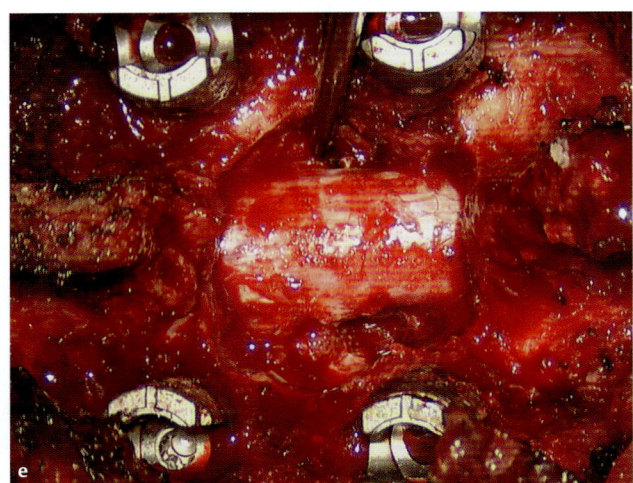

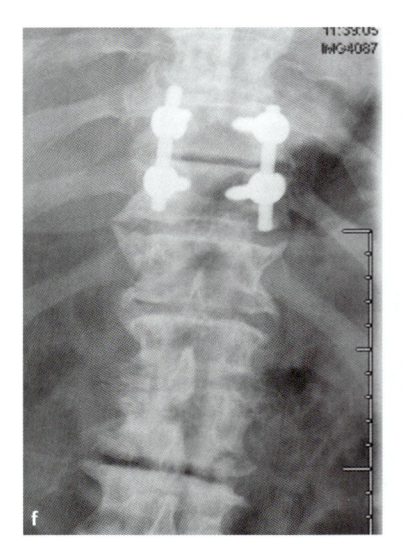

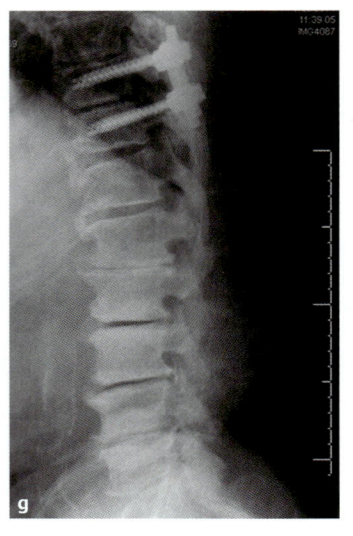

Fig. 69.3 A 72-year-old man with a long history of spinal degenerative disease of the cervical and lumbar spine, necessitating several operative procedures, presents now with numbness and weakness of the legs, necessitating the use of a walker. Examination shows paraparesis with 4/5 strength in both legs with hyperreflexia at the knees. Sagittal **(a)** and axial **(b)** MRI scans show circumferential stenosis at T10-T11 with increased signal from the cord. Axial **(c)** and sagittal **(d)** computed tomography (CT) scans confirm the bony nature of the stenosis at T10-T11. **(e)** Patient underwent T10-T11 laminectomy for decompression with pedicle screw fixation. Postoperative anteroposterior **(f)** and lateral **(g)** radiographs demonstrate the decompression and hardware in place.

which can be challenging in the thoracic spine. CT myelography may be necessary if the patient cannot tolerate MRI.

Surgical Procedure

The patient is placed in the prone position. We prefer to use the table from Mizuho OSI (Union City, CA), as it enable improved visualization with C-arm fluoroscopy. However, chest rolls may also be used. The OSI table also decreases intra-abdominal pressure, thus minimizing epidural venous bleeding during the procedure. All pressure points must be appropriately padded to minimize skin breakdown and neuropathies. C-arm fluoroscopy is mandatory to confirm the level of interest. In the surgeon's experience, this is best performed in the AP plane. As some patients may present with 11 or 13 ribs, it is recommended to count in both the rostral and caudal directions, so counting is confirmed from T1 caudally as well as from L5 rostrally. It is also recommended to compare the count with the preoperative images, as one of the most common complications with surgery on the thoracic spine is wrong-level surgery.

Once the appropriate level has been identified, the patient is then prepped and draped. A midline incision is made through the level of the deep fascia. The paraspinal musculature is dissected from the underlying lamina in a subperiosteal fashion using monopolar electrocautery or a Cobb periosteal elevator. Self-retaining retractors are used to maintain adequate visualization. Hemostasis in maintained using bipolar electrocautery. Dissection is performed laterally to expose the facet joints. Care should be taken not to violate the facet capsule. Care is also taken to avoid injury to the neurovascular bundle, which lies ventral to the facet joint and runs along the inferior aspect of the ribs.

The spinous processes are then removed using a Leksell rongeur, and the laminae thinned out with the same instrument. The neural arch can be quite unstable from tumor and needs to be removed carefully without inadvertent compression upon the cord. Once thinned out, the laminae can now be removed in one of three ways: using a 2-mm bone punch, a 2-mm power drill (**Fig. 69.4**), or a footplate (**Fig. 69.5**). If the craniotomy footplate is used, a small laminotomy needs to be performed at the caudal margin of the proposed laminectomy, large enough to allow insertion of the footplate. It is important to avoid infolding of the ligamentum flavum while performing the laminectomy to prevent inadvertent compression upon the cord. The lateral edge of the laminectomy coincides with the medial edge of the facet joint, which needs to be preserved for stability. After the ligamentum flavum is removed, the exposed dura is then visualized.

At this point, if the goal of surgery is spinal cord decompression, the procedure is complete. In cases of lateral epidural tumor or lateral thoracic herniated disk, a unilateral facetectomy may be performed to gain access to the neural foramen and disk space. In cases of pathological fracture and the need to decompress the canal with reversed curettes or a power drill, a pedicle or a portion thereof may have to be removed for access. Intraoperative ultrasound (**Fig. 69.6**) confirms the adequacy of decompression ventral to the cord.

Once decompression is complete, a subfascial vacuum drain may be used, which is brought out through a rostral exit wound, especially in cases involving multiple levels. Closure is performed using 2-0 absorbable sutures for the deep fascial layer, and 2-0 or

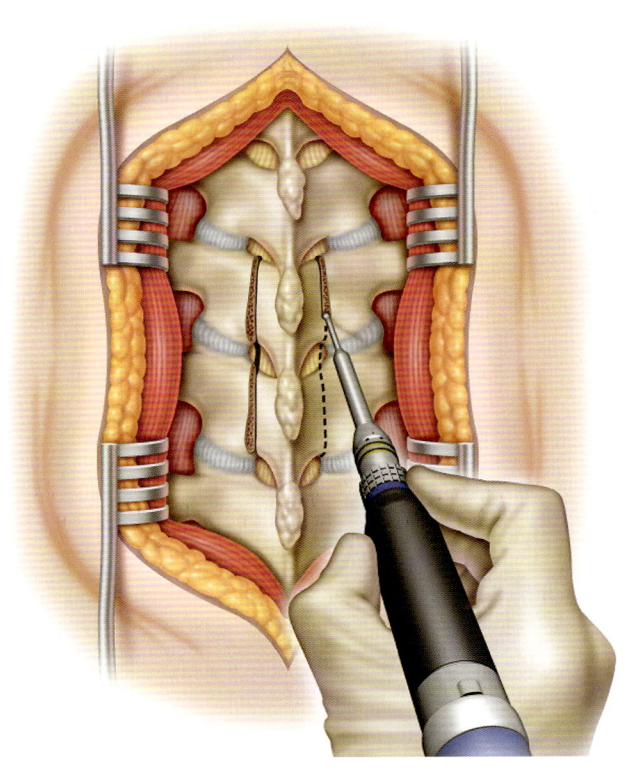

Fig. 69.4 Using a power drill with a 2- to 3-mm cutting bit, a trough is created on either side, without sacrificing the integrity of the facets. Care is taken to remain superficial to the ligamentum flavum with the bit.

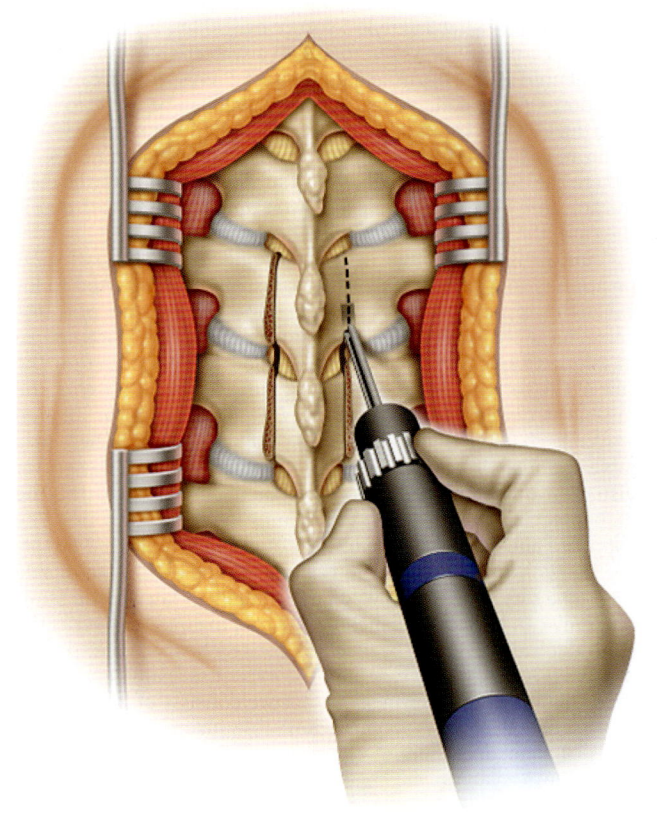

Fig. 69.5 Laminectomy can also be performed using a craniotome footplate. A small laminotomy of the caudal interlaminar space is necessary to introduce the footplate into the epidural space. The footplate is elevated for its entire course away from the dura.

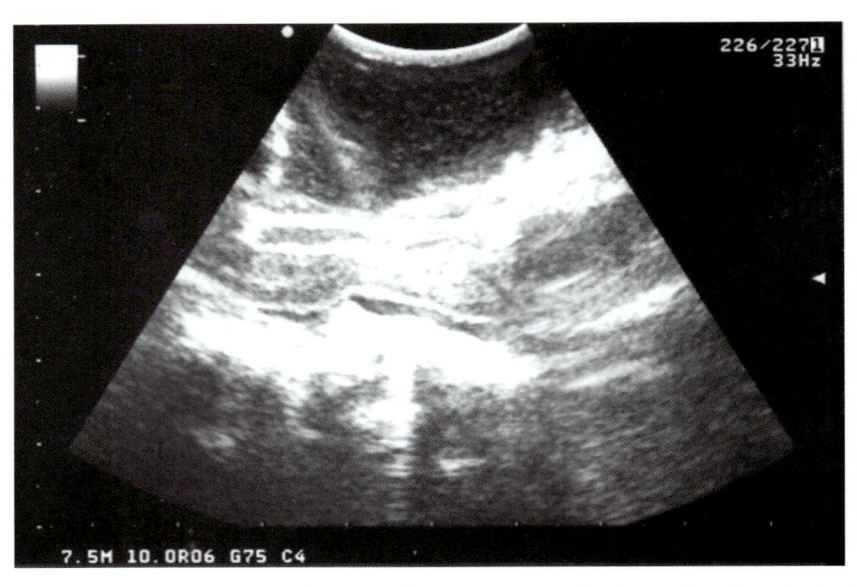

Fig. 69.6 Intraoperative ultrasonography demonstrates the adequacy of decompression, as well as the location of intradural pathology. This is particularly helpful in pathological fractures and ventral tumors.

3-0 absorbable suture for the subcutaneous layers. Skin is reapproximated using 3-0 nylon suture or staples. If the dura was entered, care must be taken to obtain a watertight dural closure and secured with a fibrin sealant (Tisseel, Baxter Healthcare Corporation, Deerfield, IL). A Valsalva maneuver can be used to check for a dural cerebrospinal fluid (CSF) leak. A lumbar subarachnoid drain may be used to aid in healing in the face of a CSF leak. Where the dura has been violated, a subfascial drain may be contraindicated, as it may keep the dural opening patent. If that is the case, the vacuum drain should be removed early.

For a minimally invasive hemilaminectomy, the patient is positioned in a similar fashion. Fluoroscopy is again used to localize the appropriate level, and a paramedian incision, or transverse incision in the obese patient, is used. The paramedian incision is typically 2 cm from the midline, depending on the size of the patient. Using a series of graduated blunt dilators, the muscle is dissected from the facets. Finally, an 18- or 22-mm working channel is docked on the lamina and attached to a table-mounted retractor. An operating microscope is used for visualization. Hemilaminectomy is then performed using the high-speed drill and 2-mm and 3-mm Kerrison rongeurs. The exposure and extent of the laminectomy can be enlarged by tilting the working channel from the ipsi- to the contralateral side (**Fig. 69.7**), as well as rostrally and caudally. A fairly wide laminectomy can be accomplished visualizing the ipsi- as well as the contralateral nerve root by working entirely beneath the spinous process (**Fig. 69.8**). The extent of the exposure again depends on the pathology being addressed. Closure consists of 2-0 absorbable sutures for the fascia, 3-0 absorbable sutures for the subcutaneous layer, and running 4-0 Monocryl for skin, followed by a skin adhesive.

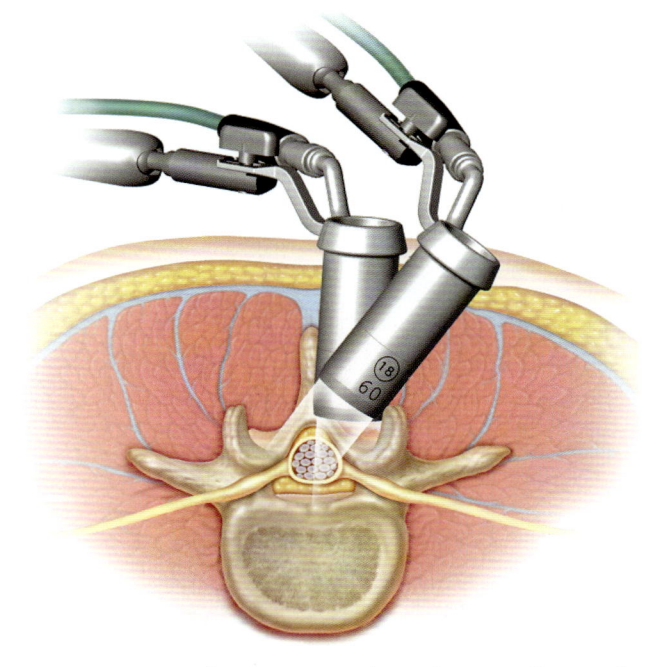

Fig. 69.7 For minimally invasive surgery (MIS), after tissue dilatation, the 18- or 21-mm working channel is used to visualize the base of the spinous process. The ipsilateral lamina is removed with bone punches or power drill. The working channel can be tilted to the contralateral side for further decompression and excision of the ligamentum flavum and inner table of the lamina.

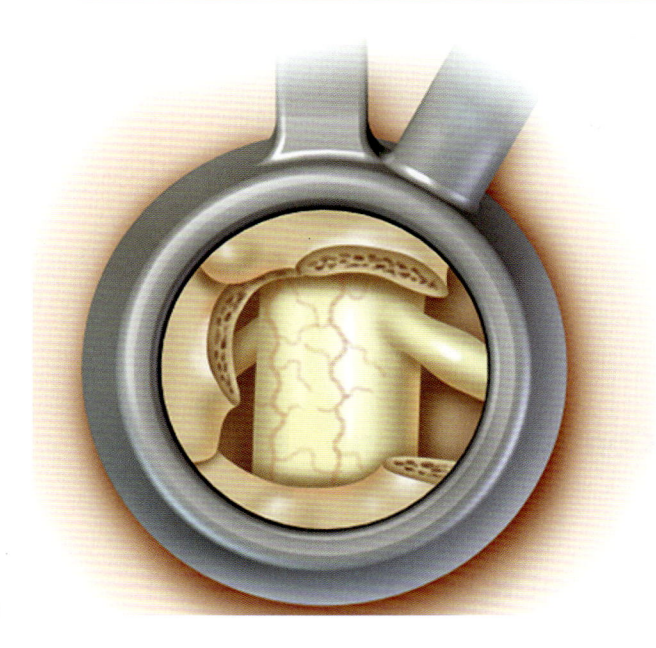

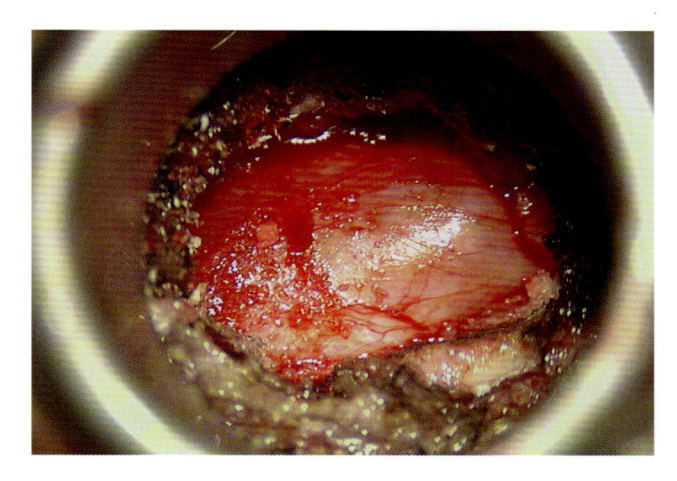

Fig. 69.8 Diagrammatic illustration (**a**) of the MIS laminectomy and the actual intraoperative view (**b**) of the decompressed dura.

Postoperative Care

Postoperatively, the patient should be mobilized as soon as possible. For intradural procedures, bed rest for 24 hours is recommended to minimize the risk of postoperative CSF leak or pseudomeningocele. Patients should be switched to oral pain medication as soon as possible. Wound dehiscence with postoperative radiation is a serious concern, and may warrant a dorsal figure-of-8 shoulder brace.

Potential Complications and Precautions

Common complications include wound infection and CSF leak. Adhering to strict guidelines can minimize wound infections. We instill topical vancomycin into the wound as well as cefazolin for perioperative antibiotics. Antibiosis should be continued for 24 hours postoperatively, or as long as a drain is in place. If there is an accidental durotomy, primary closure should be attempted. Likewise, if the dura must be entered for intradural pathology, a watertight closure should be achieved. A subarachnoid drain and flat bed rest may be useful in such situations. Another rare complication is cord infarction in the face of severe stenosis. Mean arterial pressure (MAP) should be kept elevated to help maintain cord perfusion. We prefer to maintain MAP > 80 mm Hg when there is cord compression from stenosis or mass lesions.

Conclusion

Thoracic laminectomy is a versatile procedure for dorsal access to the thoracic spinal canal, spinal cord, and nerve roots. However, for anteriorly located pathology, other approaches, such as thoracotomy or costotransversectomy, may provide better access and reduced complication rates. **Box 69.1** lists the key operative steps.

Box 69.1 Key Operative Steps

- Confirm the level beyond a doubt.
- A laminectomy for decompression must be performed with the utmost care to avoid a cord contusion.
- Ultrasonography at surgery confirms the adequacy of the decompression.
- Extensive laminectomy can lead to kyphosis.
- Laminectomy in the presence of vertebral body disease can lead to instability.
- In cases of preoperative kyphosis, vertebral body disease, or pathological fractures, instrumentation spanning the pathology is necessary.

References

1. Ridenour TR, Haddad SF, Hitchon PW, Piper J, Traynelis VC, VanGilder JC. Herniated thoracic disks: treatment and outcome. J Spinal Disord 1993;6:218–224
2. Lawrence FB. Surgical approaches to the thoracic and thoracolumbar spine for decompression and stabilization. In: Schmidek HH, Sweet WH, eds. Operative Neurosurgical Techniques, vol 2. Philadelphia: WB Saunders; 1995:1887–1893
3. Logue V. Thoracic intervertebral disc prolapse with spinal cord compression. J Neurol Neurosurg Psychiatry 1952;15:227–241
4. Chang UK, Choe WJ, Chung CK, Kim HJ. Surgical treatment for thoracic spinal stenosis. Spinal Cord 2001;39:362–369
5. Dommisse GF. The blood supply of the spinal cord. A critical vascular zone in spinal surgery. J Bone Joint Surg Br 1974;56:225–235
6. Grossbach AJ, Dahdaleh NS, Abel TJ, Woods GD, Dlouhy BJ, Hitchon PW. Flexion-distraction injuries of the thoracolumbar spine: open fusion versus percutaneous pedicle screw fixation. Neurosurg Focus 2013;35:E2

70 Thoracic Laminoplasty

Andrew James Grossbach, Sami Al-Nafi, and Patrick W. Hitchon

Laminectomy has been one of the main surgical tools for spinal surgeons. However, multilevel laminectomies serve to disrupt the posterior tension band and put the patient at risk for postlaminectomy kyphosis or kyphoscoliosis. Yasuoka et al[1] found that postlaminectomy deformity occurred in 46% of laminectomy patients under the age of 15 years and 6% of patients of ages 15 to 24 years. In the younger age group, four (36%) of the 11 patients who underwent thoracic laminectomies specifically developed deformity; however, the remaining seven did not undergo follow-up imaging.

Laminoplasty is the term now used to describe any technique in which the posterior elements are replaced. It is now widely used as a technique to gain access to the spinal canal while minimizing the risk of postsurgical kyphosis. This term has largely replaced such terms as *laminotomy* and *osteoplastic laminotomy* to describe these procedures.[2,3] The term *expansion laminoplasty* is used to describe techniques in which the spinal canal dimensions are enlarged, as is commonly performed in the cervical spine.[4] Titanium plating systems have improved the techniques to replace the bony posterior elements.[5]

This chapter discusses the technique of thoracic laminoplasty to access the thoracic spinal canal and nerve roots.

Patient Selection

Patients with dorsal pathology that does not involve the posterior bony arch are good candidates for thoracic laminoplasty.

Indications

- Intradural extramedullary tumors
- Intradural intramedullary tumors
- Epidural lipomatosis
- Vascular malformations
  - Spinal arteriovenous malformations
  - Dural arteriovenous fistulas
- Congenital spinal lesions
  - Arachnoid cyst
  - Syringomyelia
  - Diastematomyelia
  - Spinal cord herniation

Contraindications

- Pathology involving posterior bony elements
- Instability

Advantages

- Familiar approach
- Good access to posterior pathology
- Prevention of postoperative kyphosis or kyphoscoliosis

Disadvantages

- Increased operative time versus laminectomy
- Limited access to anterior pathology

Choice of Operative Approach

Patients with multilevel disease should be highly considered for laminoplasty, as compared with laminectomy, to minimize the risk of postoperative kyphosis with multilevel laminectomy. Patients with ventral pathology should be considered for an anterior approach, such as thoracotomy or costotransversectomy.

Preoperative Testing and Imaging

Preoperative testing should include standard preoperative laboratories such as a complete blood count (CBC), basic metabolic panel (BMP), and coagulation factors. Preoperative imaging should be obtained, and varies based on the pathology encountered. Plain anteroposterior (AP) and lateral radiographs should be obtained, as they are useful in identifying the appropriate level intraoperatively. For neoplastic, infectious, and degenerative pathology, magnetic resonance imaging (MRI) should be obtained. A computed tomography (CT) myelography may be necessary if the patient cannot tolerate MRI.

Surgical Procedure

The patient is positioned prone on the surgical frame from Mizuho OSI (Union City, CA) in a similar fashion as for a laminec-

70 Thoracic Laminoplasty   451

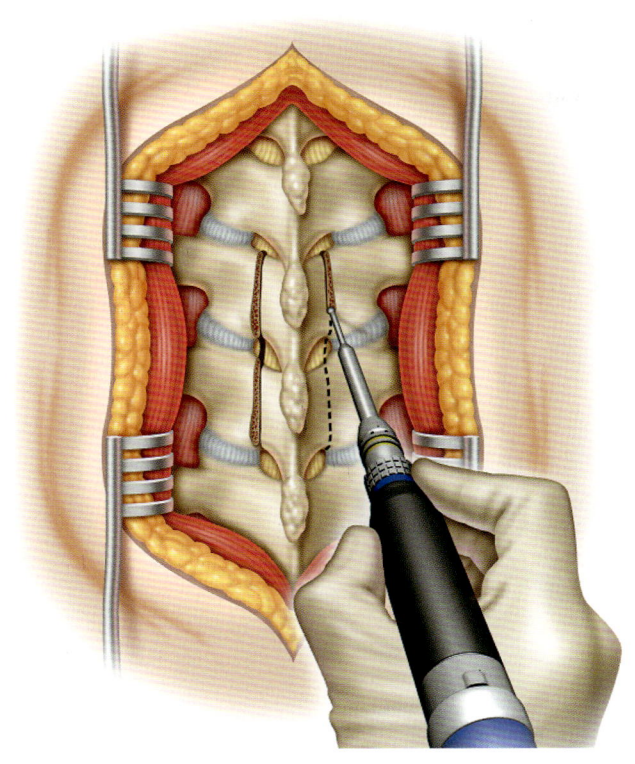

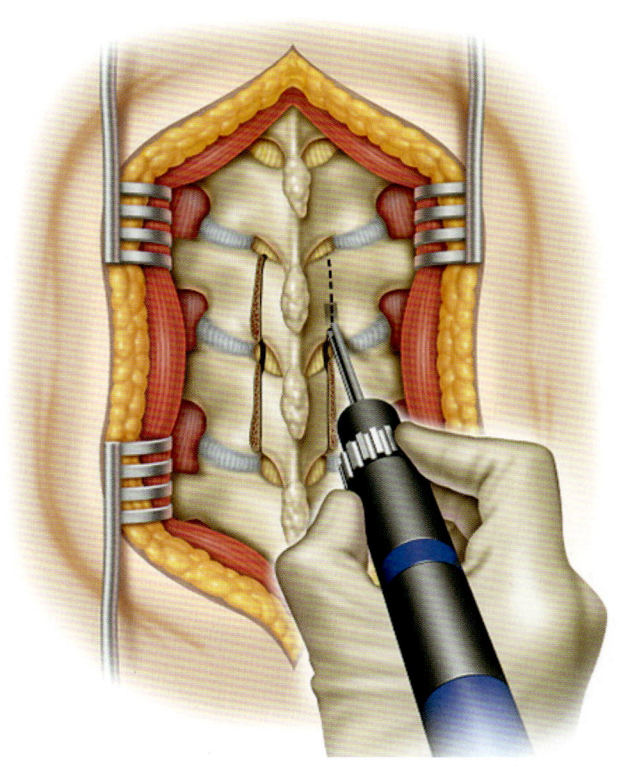

Fig. 70.1 A 2-mm bur is one option for cutting the lateral channels for the laminoplasty. The least amount of bone is removed to facilitate eventual bone fusion after the laminae are fixed.

Fig. 70.2 The use of the craniotome is the preferred method for the laminoplasty. In case of hypertrophied facets and severe scoliosis, this method may need to be abandoned in favor of using a bur or bone punch.

tomy. Pressure points are padded, and the appropriate levels are confirmed radiographically. Once the level of interest has been ascertained with intraoperative fluoroscopy, counting both from the top down and from the bottom up, the patient is prepped and draped. A midline incision is made through the level of the deep fascia. The paraspinal musculature is dissected from the underlying lamina in a subperiosteal fashion using monopolar electrocautery or a Cobb periosteal elevator. Self-retaining retractors are used to maintain adequate visualization. Hemostasis is maintained using bipolar electrocautery. Dissection is performed laterally to expose the facet joints, and care should be taken not to violate the facet capsule.

Laminoplasty in the thoracic spine entails not only obtaining adequate exposure to the pathology, but also replacing and fixing the laminae so that bony healing will eventually occur. This requires the creation of a narrow gutter at the lamina–facet interface, which is marked with a surgical pen. With the intent of replacing the laminae, bone is removed sparingly, such that the gap between the edges is minimized. This gutter or channel can be created using a 2-mm bone punch, a 2-mm matchstick bur (**Fig. 70.1**), or a craniotome footplate (**Fig. 70.2**). Although there is a slight learning curve for using the craniotome, we believe it is the best and most efficient technique. To insert the footplate at the caudal margin of the intended laminoplasty, a small laminotomy is made using a 2-mm punch. The ligamentum flavum is entered, and the footplate inserted between the dura and the ligamentum flavum. With the power on, the drill is gently advanced in a caudal to rostral direction while lightly pulling up on the footplate against the ventral surface of the lamina. Once the channel is completed on either side, the interspinous ligament is transected with heavy scissors, and the laminae lifted en bloc. Remnants of the ligamentum flavum still holding the laminae in place are sectioned with scissors or a 2-mm punch. Once the laminae are lifted, the dura is exposed, bleeding epidural veins are coagulated, and a hemostatic surgical agent (Ethicon, Johnson and Johnson, Somerville, NJ) is applied in the epidural space. The laminae are kept wrapped in bacitracin, and the epidural or intradural pathology is addressed.

Laminoplasty is appropriate where the laminae are healthy and uninvolved with tumor or infection. We believe that thoracic laminoplasty, like cervical laminoplasty, can avoid the postlaminectomy kyphosis that results from excision of the posterior tension band. This technique has worked well in the treatment of many spinal pathologies, including intradural tumors (**Fig. 70.3**), intradural arachnoid cysts (**Fig. 70.4**), and cord herniation (**Fig. 70.5**). Once the intradural pathology is dealt with, the

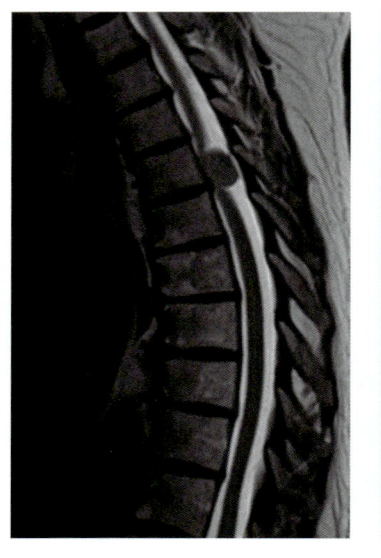

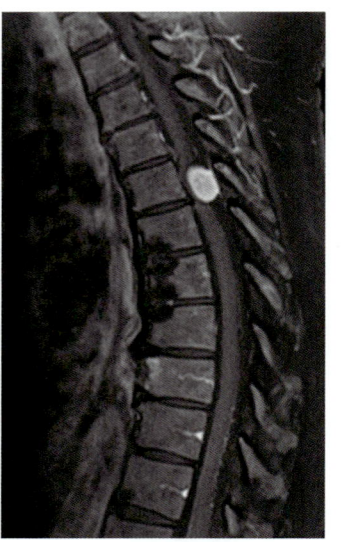

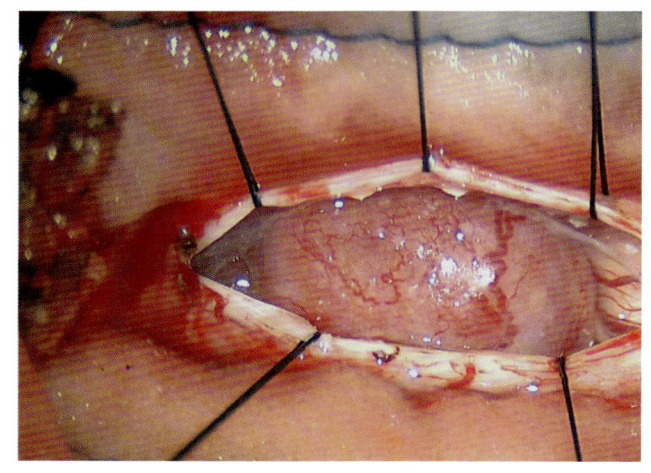

Fig. 70.3 A 50-year-old woman has a 2-year history of difficulty lifting her left leg, especially when walking, and this has gradually progressed to involve her right leg. On examination she has a T7 sensory level and hyperreflexia. T2-weighted **(a)** and enhanced **(b)** magnetic resonance imaging (MRI) scans show a T5 intradural extramedullary enhancing lesion with cord compression. Excision was approached with a two-level laminoplasty, and the tumor exposed and excised **(c)**. The laminae were affixed in position using cranial plates and screws.

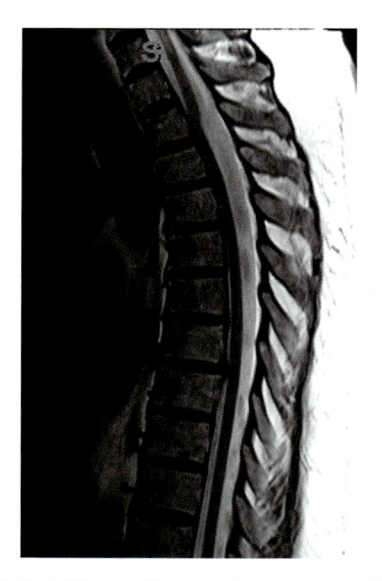

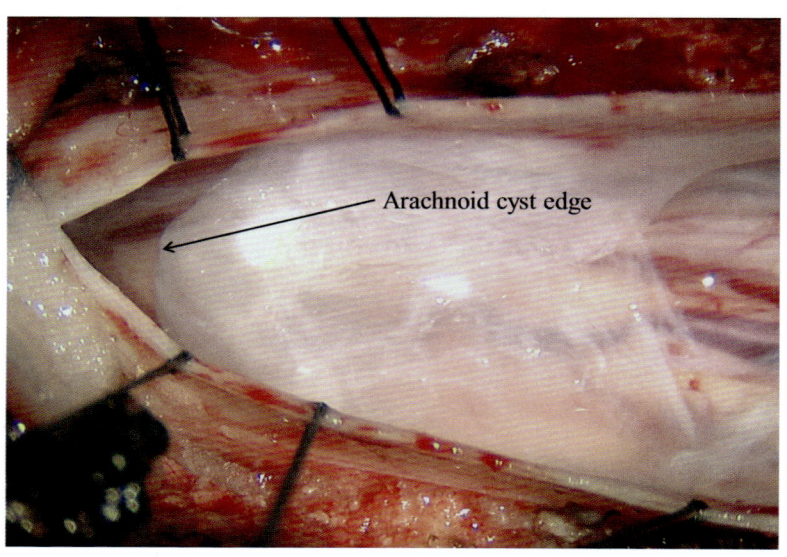

Fig. 70.4 A 56-year-old woman has experienced back pain and leg stiffness over the past year, eventually having to use a cane for her right leg weakness. **(a)** MRI of the thoracic spine shows anterior displacement of the cord from T2 to T5 with posterior flattening of the cord, suggestive of an arachnoid cyst. To excise the cyst, the selected approach was that of a four-level laminoplasty. **(b)** Intraoperative photograph shows the arachnoid cyst dorsal to the cord. Following excision of the cyst, the bone was affixed in place with cranial plates and screws.

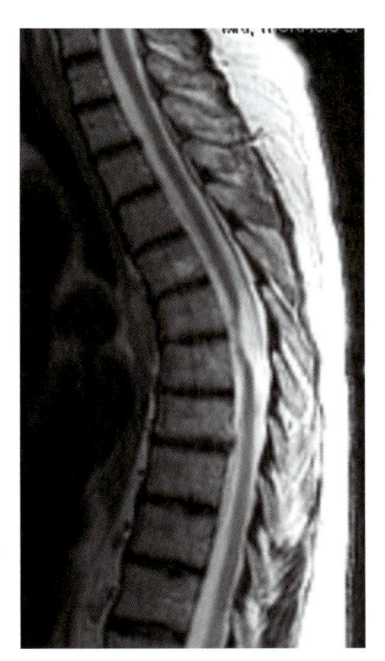

Fig. 70.5 A 59-year-old woman complains of low back and leg pain with burning in the feet. Examination shows a midthoracic sensory level with weakness in the right leg and footdrop. **(a,b)** Sagittal T2-weighted MRI scans show the cord displaced anteriorly with suspicion of either cord herniation or a dorsal arachnoid cyst. **(c)** Axial MRI slice above the lesion shows the cord in normal position. At the level of the lesion, the cord is displaced anteriorly and its borders ill-defined. **(d)** At surgery, a ventral dural defect is noted, with gliotic cord herniating through it.

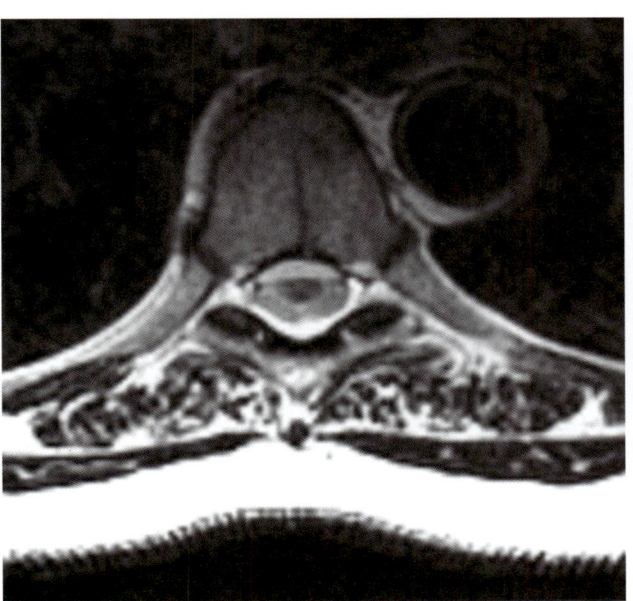

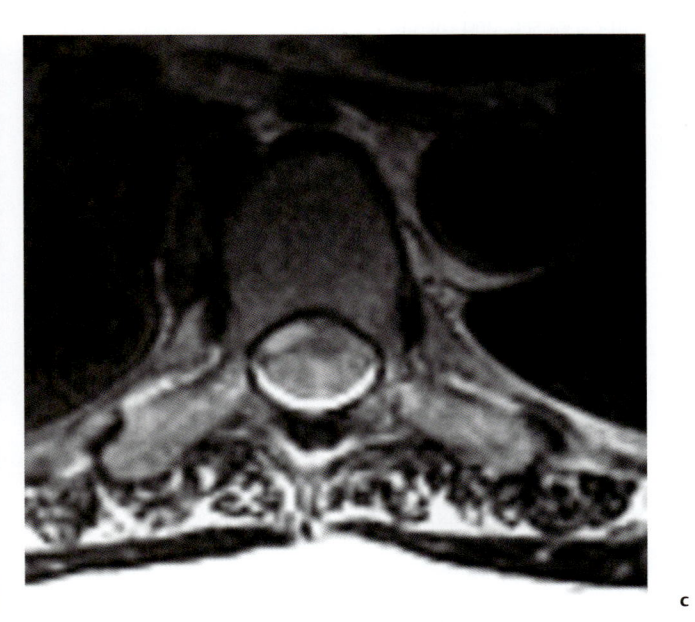

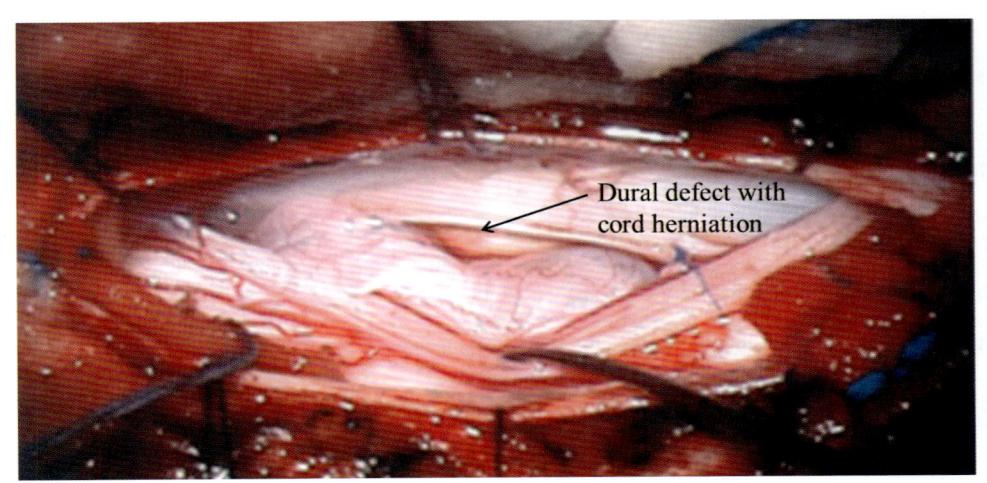

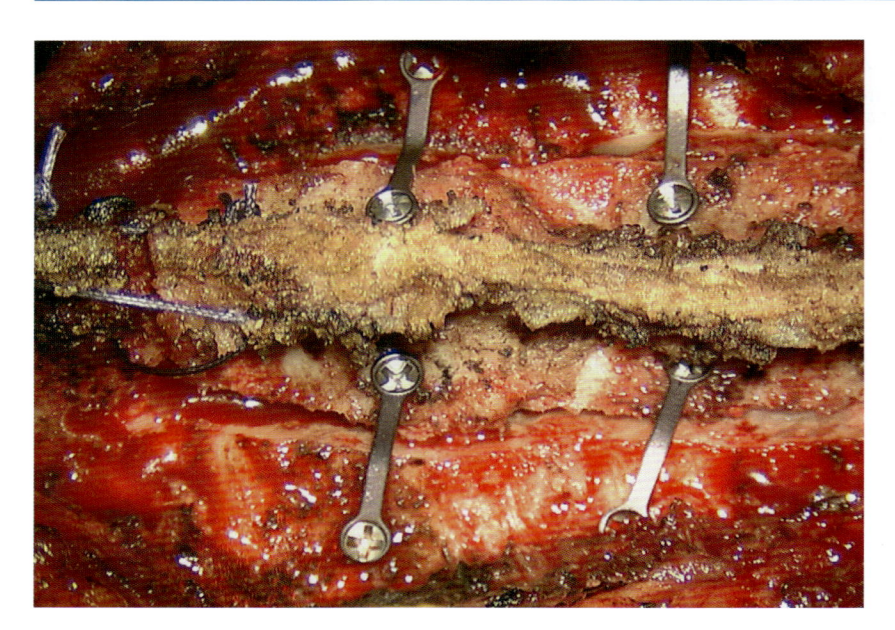

Fig. 70.6 The laminae are replaced and affixed in position using cranial plates and screws. One plate per lamina is sufficient. A 2-0 suture can also be used to reapproximate the supraspinous ligaments rostrally and caudally.

dura is closed, and the laminae are replaced and affixed. For fixation of the laminae, we have used nonabsorbable suture such as braided nylon. More recently, however, the preferred method is the use of cranial plates with 4- to 6-mm self-tapping screws (**Fig. 70.6**). One plate per lamina is generally sufficient. In addition to the cranial plates, a 2-0 suture is used to reapproximate the supraspinous ligament at both ends.

Postoperative Care

Postoperatively, the patient should be mobilized as soon as possible. No particular restrictions are necessary beyond those for any intradural exploration.

Potential Complications and Precautions

Common complications include wound infection and cerebrospinal fluid (CSF) leak. Adhering to strict perioperative guidelines regarding antibiotics, systemic as well as topical, can minimize wound infections. Topical vancomycin and perioperative systemic cefazolin for as long as the drains are in place are recommended. As with laminectomy, if there is an accidental durotomy, primary closure should be attempted. Likewise, if the dura must be entered for intradural pathology, a watertight closure should be achieved. A subarachnoid drain and flat bed rest may be useful in these situations.

Conclusion

Thoracic laminoplasty is an emerging tool for dorsal access to the thoracic spinal canal, spinal cord, and nerve roots. It has slightly more of a learning curve for surgeons compared with laminectomy; however, once mastered, it has the advantage of maintaining the posterior tension band and limiting postoperative kyphosis. **Box 70.1** lists the key operative steps.

Box 70.1 Key Operative Steps

- Confirm the level with radiographs. Do not compromise.
- Perform a laminoplasty using a craniotome. It must be wide enough to address the pathology.
- Make the dural closure watertight.
- Affix the laminae to the spine with plates. If the laminae are affected with tumor or infection, do not reimplant them.
- Avoid compromising the caliber of the canal.

References

1. Yasuoka S, Peterson HA, MacCarty CS. Incidence of spinal column deformity after multilevel laminectomy in children and adults. J Neurosurg 1982;57:441–445
2. Raimondi AJ, Gutierrez FA, Di Rocco C. Laminotomy and total reconstruction of the posterior spinal arch for spinal canal surgery in childhood. J Neurosurg 1976;45:555–560
3. Abbott R, Feldstein N, Wisoff JH, Epstein FJ. Osteoplastic laminotomy in children. Pediatr Neurosurg 1992;18:153–156
4. Shikata J, Yamamuro T, Shimizu K, Saito T. Combined laminoplasty and posterolateral fusion for spinal canal surgery in children and adolescents. Clin Orthop Relat Res 1990;259:92–99
5. Park AE, Heller JG. Cervical laminoplasty: use of a novel titanium plate to maintain canal expansion—surgical technique. J Spinal Disord Tech 2004;17:265–271

71 Transpedicular Thoracic Diskectomy

David M. Benglis, Jr., Richard G. Fessler, and Regis Haid, Jr.

Thoracic disk herniations (TDH) are a rare yet formidable problem encountered by spine surgeons, accounting for 0.15 to 4% of all disk herniations in the neuraxis.[1,2] Differential diagnosis includes extradural/intradural masses, syrinx, abscess, or vascular malformations.

Symptomatic patients may present with myelopathy, mono- or biparesis/paralysis, spasticity, sensory disturbances, bowel or bladder involvement, or back/radicular pain syndromes. The presence of any of these symptoms aside from pain is often an indication for surgical intervention. Severity and the time length of deficit often impacts the postoperative result. Causative mechanisms include traumatic (25%) versus degenerative (most common). These problems tend to arise in the fourth decade of life, and the majority of patients have disk herniations that occur below T8, with a few occurring at the thoracolumbar junction (T11-L1).[1,2]

Surgical management has evolved over the past 80 years to include such approaches as direct posterior, posterolateral, lateral, ventrolateral, and transthoracic (**Fig. 71.1**) More recently, minimally invasive surgery options have become available, such as ventral thoracoscopic and dorsolateral tubular retractor, and they are viable alternatives in specific cases, reducing intraoperative blood loss, surgery duration, postoperative pain, and the length of hospital stay.

This chapter discusses the transpedicular thoracic diskectomy approach for treatment of symptomatic disk herniations, including the clinical presentation and disease process, the history behind this approach, the imaging modalities available for diagnosis, and its advantages and disadvantages.

Historical Background

Era of the Posterior Midline Approach

In 1911, Middleton and Teachers described at autopsy a large lower thoracic disk herniation that had contributed to a patient's paraplegia.[3] The first report in the clinical literature of an antemortem diagnosis of a TDH was by Antoni in 1931.[3] Elsberg[4] and Adson around the same time were the first to operate on patients with such conditions.[5] Mixter and Barr,[6] who are often credited with ushering in the "dynasty of the disk," reported four cases of patients with TDH in 1934.[7] Early treatment, however, was from a midline posterior approach with intra- or extradural excision. Many of these patients were made worse following surgery (combined results from multiple series demonstrated that 28% of patients worsened and 11% showed no improvement), presumably from inadequate decompression of the ventral force, spinal cord retraction for those attempting to access a ventral disk, "watershed" blood supply, general smaller diameter of thoracic canal versus lumbar/cervical, and the absence of modern microsurgical instruments and techniques.[2]

The Search for a Better Approach

After reporting an initial complication of paralysis from a dorsal approach, Hulme[8] in 1960 was the first to adapt a version of the posterolateral technique (a version of the costotransversectomy originally described by Menard in 1900 for treatment of Pott's disease) through the foramina, with partial pedicle resection to access the TDH in a series of cases with good results. In 1969, Perot et al[9] and Ransohoff et al[10] described a ventrolateral or transthoracic approach for access and treatment of midline TDH, with admirable results. Carson and colleagues[11] reported on an alternate posterolateral approach with total removal of the facet complex accomplished through a T-shaped incision. An evolutionary trend followed for the posterolateral approach, whereby in 1978 Patterson and Arbit[12] went one step further: total facetectomy with total pedicle removal to gain access to the TDH. The transpedicular approach to TDH was born, and overall improvement in postoperative clinical results were noted.[1,2] Multiple subsequent studies followed, demonstrating its place in the treatment of TDH.[13,14]

Radiological Evaluation

Before the introduction of computed tomography (CT) following a spinal myelogram, diagnosis of this rare phenomenon was problematic, with the false-negative rate being reported at 8% and the incorrect initial diagnosis rate of 44%.[5,15] Magnetic resonance imaging (MRI) has essentially replaced CT and CT myelograms for the initial diagnosis, as it is excellent at demonstrating soft tissue features such as intrinsic spinal cord edema changes, extradural defects, and disk herniations on T2 sequences. Although calcification on MRI is often hypointense, CT myelogram and CT are superior in the determination of calcification content of the disk[16] (**Fig. 71.2**). Scout images from the sacrum or upper cervical region should be performed with any of these imaging modalities to determine the level. Plain X-ray findings may demonstrate disk space narrowing, wedging, or scoliosis.[16]

It is noted in some series that 15 to 20% of the population have TDHs that are found incidentally on MRI. The most common location of disk herniations are central to centrolateral, and some patients have multiple herniations.[1,2] Stillerman et al,[1] in their series of 71 patients with 82 herniated thoracic disks, found that 65% exhibited calcification on CT evaluation. Care should be taken to note where the spinal cord is displaced in relation to the disk herniation, and whether calcification, if present in the disk, extends to the contact point of the dura; if it does, the disk is likely adherent.[1] Intradural TDH may also occur, but is less common.[1,17] Level identification for transthoracic approaches may be aided by preoperative interventional radiology placement of cement in the thoracic body below the disk herniation.

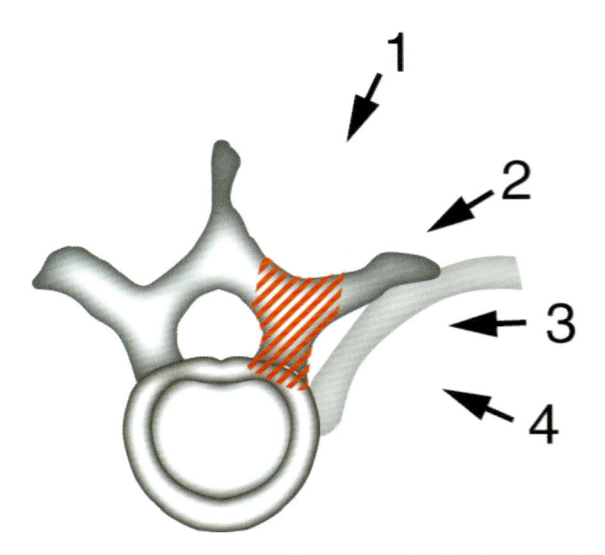

Fig. 71.1 Demonstration of the angle encountered with various approaches. *1*, transpedicular/transfacet (red stripes); *2*, costotransversectomy; *3*, lateral extracavitary; *4*, ventral transthoracic.

Overview of Approaches

Advantages

- Less invasive, no rib removal or chest tube required
- Identification of artery of Adamkiewicz not imperative preoperatively
- Reduced operative time
- Shorter hospital stay
- No need for the assistance of an access surgeon
- May perform at all spinal levels

Disadvantages

- Limited access to ventral disk herniations
- Less visualization of the decompression extent as compared with ventral and ventrolateral approaches
- Not ideal for calcified intradural disks
- May result in iatrogenic instability

Indication

- Transpedicular thoracic diskectomy is indicated for soft/partially calcified extradural lateral or centrolateral disk herniations.

Contraindication

- This approach is contraindicated for central fully calcified intra- or extradural thoracic disk herniations. These type of herniations can be accessed by the costotransversectomy or transthoracic approach.

Approach Options

Six broad options for the approach to TDH exist, each with respective advantages and disadvantages. Moving from dorsal to lateral, the approaches are the following: (1) dorsal midline (historical and not recommended due to reasons listed above); (2) dorsal lateral transfacet pedicle sparing; (3) dorsal lateral transfacet transpedicular; (4) costotransversectomy; (5) lateral extracavitary; (6) transthoracic (traditional open, retropleural, thoracoscopic)[18-20] (**Fig. 71.1**) Treatment algorithms have been developed to assist the surgeon in determining which approach may be the best for a particular situation[1,21] (**Table 71.1**).

In general, the posterolateral approaches including the transfacet and transpedicular are technically less challenging, require less operative time and entailing less blood loss and postoperative pain. They are ideal for removing both soft or partially calcified (nonadherent to the dura) centrolateral/lateral disks. Lateral and ventrolateral approaches (excluding thoracoscopic) include more extensive muscle dissection and trauma, or in the case of a thoracotomy deflation of the lung and placement of a chest tube postoperatively (unless the approach is retropleural). These lateral-anterolateral approaches also routinely require re-

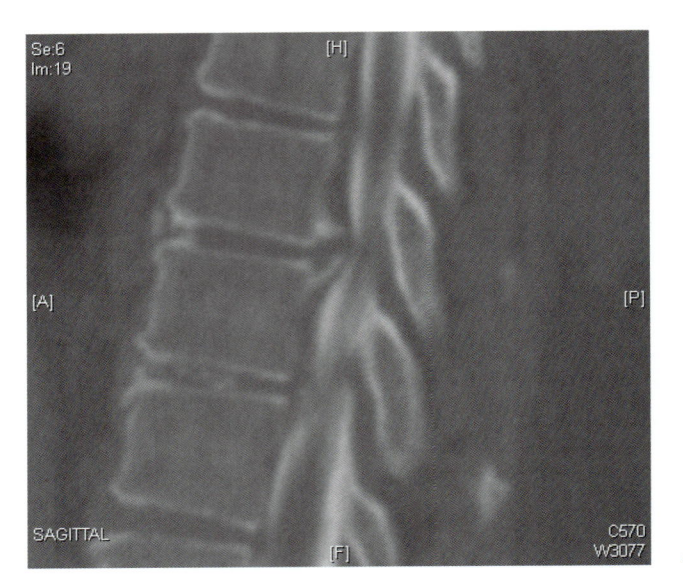

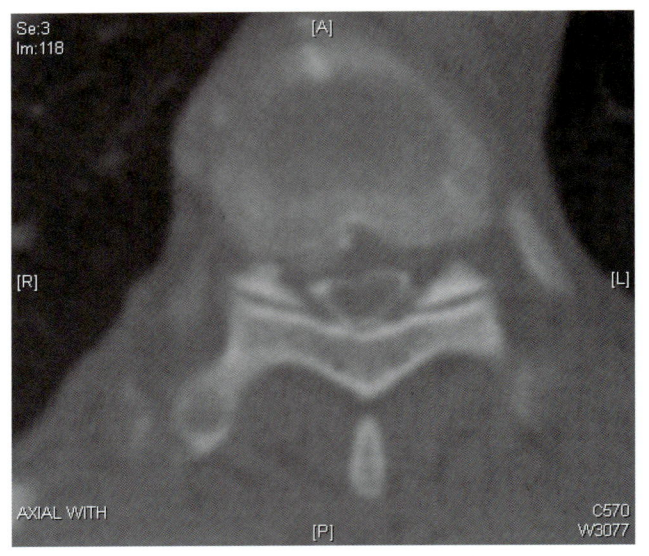

Fig. 71.2 Computed tomography (CT) thoracic myelogram sagittal (**a**) and axial (**b**) images of a centrolateral calcified extradural disk herniation at T10-T11.

Table 71.1 Location of Disk Herniation and Appropriate Spinal Approach

Location	Approach
Soft lateral disk: extradural	Transpedicular, costotransversectomy, transfacet pedicle sparing
Soft/hard lateral or centrolateral disk: extradural	Transpedicular, costotransversectomy, lateral extracavitary
Hard central disk: intra- or extradural	Costotransversectomy, lateral extracavitary

moval of at least a portion of a rib and often result in significant postoperative pain.

On the other hand, the lateral and ventrolateral approaches (costotransversectomy, lateral extracavitary, thoracotomy) enable greater ventral exposure. For example, a calcified, adherent, purely midline disk intra- or extradural with the thecal sac draped over, preventing a posterolateral safe working channel, would be better addressed through a thoracotomy or lateral extracavitary approach. The transpedicular approach with removal of the pedicle and facet may also contribute to postoperative iatrogenic instability.

For a lateral approach between T8 and L1, the artery of Adamkiewicz may be identified with a spinal angiogram preoperatively to avoid its injury. The opposite side or an alternate exposure is often recommended.[1] This is typically not a concern with the transpedicular approach.

Therapeutic Management/Surgical Technique

Open Technique

The patient is given a preoperative dose of steroids, and an arterial line is placed to maintain the mean arterial pressure (MAP) > 85 mm Hg for spinal cord perfusion. Continuous motor evoked potentials (MEPs) and somatosensory evoked potentials (SSEPs) are monitored throughout the case; therefore, only short-acting paralytics are used for the intubation. The patient is then turned prone after intubation and placement of a Foley catheter, and positioned on a Jackson table with a radiolucent Wilson frame, with padding of all pressure points, and with the arms either tucked (for disks T6 and above) or placed above the patient, not extending the shoulder beyond 90 degrees (for disks T7 and below). The patient is secured to the table with tape in case lateral rotation is needed; tilting the patient 15 to 20 degrees during disk removal maximizes visualization and minimizes manipulation of the spinal cord. Intraoperative fluoroscopy is brought in in the anteroposterior (AP) and lateral planes before a prep is performed. Preoperative X-ray or computed tomography (CT) verifies that the patient has 12 ribs. In the AP plane, a mark is made at the pedicle of interest and the patient is prepped and draped. If lateral fluoroscopy is used, a count is performed from the sacrum upward.

A midline incision is made ~ 5 to 8 cm over the disk space. Unilateral or bilateral subperiosteal muscle dissection is then performed, and the erector muscles are reflected laterally, exposing the facet complex and transverse process over the appropriate pedicle and disk space (**Fig. 71.3**). Williams self-retaining retractors (for unilateral muscle dissection) are placed. AP and lateral fluoroscopy is brought in again to reconfirm the correct level.

The lamina, facet, and pedicle located under the appropriate disk space are marked. The operating microscope is then brought into the field. The use of CT navigation may provide further anatomic guidance for surgeons who do not routinely perform this approach.

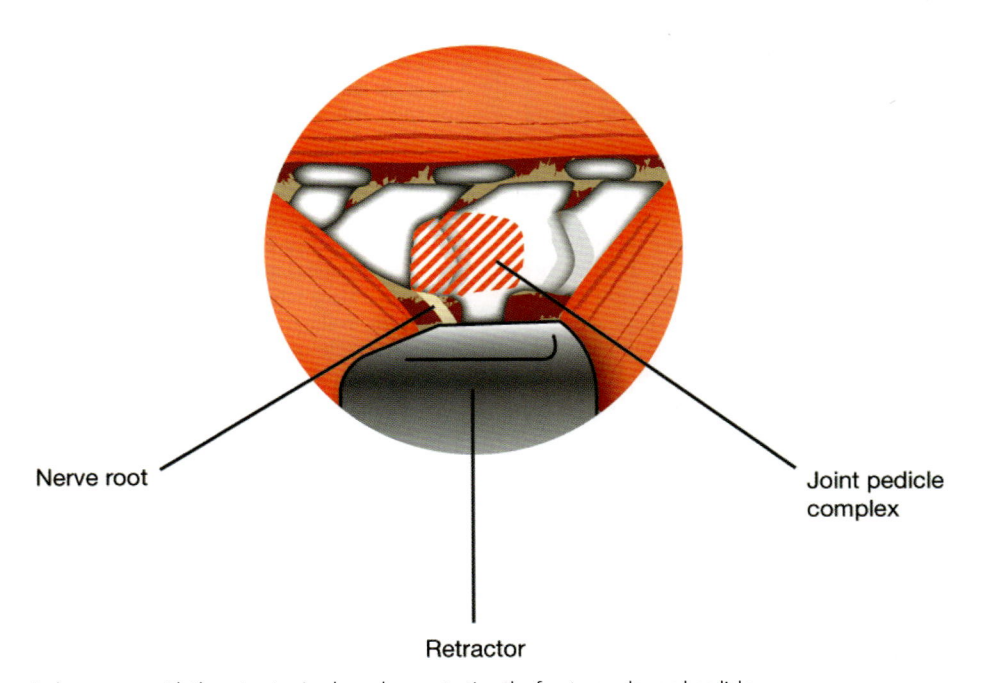

Fig. 71.3 Initial surgical exposure, with the retractor in place, demonstrating the facet complex and pedicle.

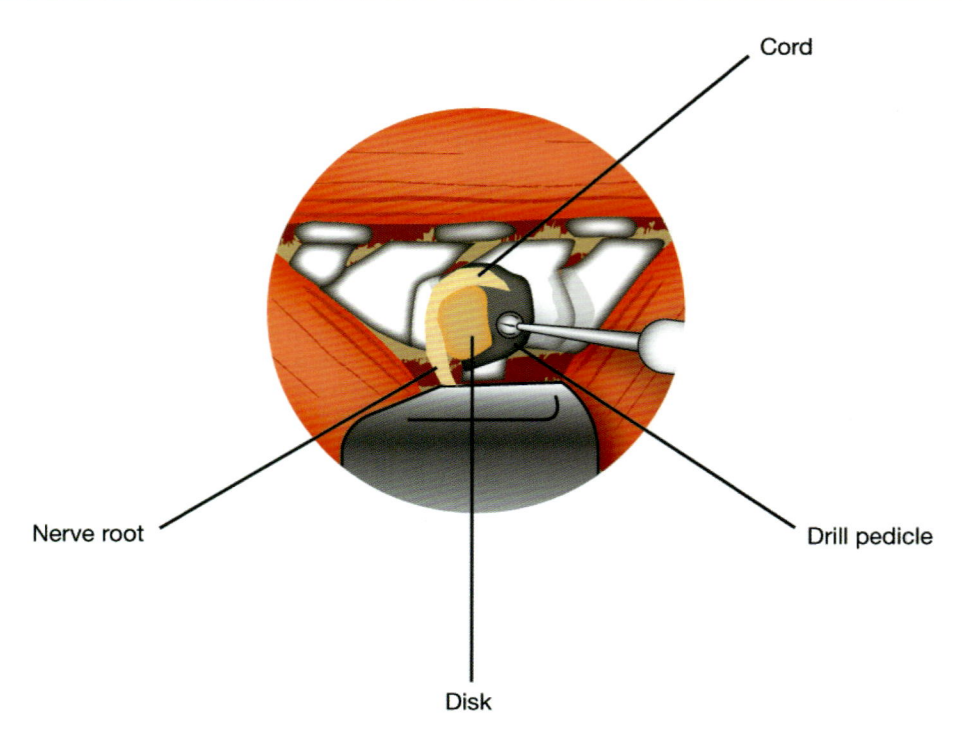

Fig. 71.4 The foramen including disk herniation, nerve root, and lateral thecal sac are viewed following drilling of the facet and pedicle.

The high-speed cutting bur is then utilized to enter the center of the pedicle through the facet. A laminotomy may also be performed for orientation purposes and may help to palpate with a microinstrument the medial wall of the pedicle. AP fluoroscopic imaging facilitates the pedicle removal and determining the orientation of the pedicle in relation to the disk space. Bone wax is used intermittently to achieve hemostasis.

The surgeon then transitions from a cutting to a diamond bur when cancellous pedicle bone changes to cortical and once the dura has been identified (**Fig. 71.4**). An attempt is made to preserve as much of the pedicle and facet as possible, but this should not compromise the exposure and the ability of the surgeon to accomplish the goal of complete decompression.

The disk space is entered superior to the pedicle and inferior to the neurovascular bundle, lateral to the thecal sac. A cavity trough is created where more medial disk abutting the ventral thecal sac may then be delivered into this empty space with down-biting curettes, microforceps, and Woodson instruments[16,21] (**Figs. 71.5 and 71.6**). This maneuver helps the surgeon to achieve decompression across the midline, and the thecal sac falls back into anatomic position (**Fig. 71.7**). If a calcified fragment is identified, then a larger trough is made extending into the vertebral body for its delivery. If a portion of the fragment is too adherent to the dura, it may be left, and, depending on recovery, reimaging may be necessary.

Minimally Invasive Thoracic Microendoscopic Diskectomy: Lateral Transforaminal Approach

This technique utilizes tubular muscular dilators/retractors via a posterolateral approach along with drilling of the lateral facet complex with or without resection of the pedicle. It is ideal for centrolateral or lateralized disk herniations causing myelopathy and radicular-type pain syndromes not responsive to conservative therapies.[22] Similar preoperative preparatory measures are induced as described above in the open approach.

Following the patient being positioned on a radiolucent Wilson frame, the fluoroscopy is brought into the field in a lateral position. A video monitor is placed across from the surgeon. After prepping and draping, a spinal needle is used to locate the herniated disk. The surgeon counts up from the sacrum to confirm the level. A Kirschner wire (K-wire) is placed at the medial aspect of the caudal transverse process at the level of the herniation. A 2-cm incision is made ~ 4 cm lateral to the midline, and a series of tubular muscle dilators are placed under fluoroscopic guidance. Following dilation, a tubular retractor is then affixed to a flexible arm secured to the operative table. An AP fluoroscopic image is then performed to confirm the medial/lateral position of the retractor. The proper level is then reconfirmed using lateral fluoroscopy.

The endoscope is then prepared and positioned properly (i.e., rostral-caudal anatomy, the same as the patient's position on the operative table). An alternative option at this step would be to bring in the microscope instead of the endoscope.

The muscle overlying the proximal transverse process and lateral facet complex is removed using an insulated Bovie cautery. Probing with a ball-tip probe helps define bony margins, and continued use of fluoroscopy throughout the procedure helps orient the surgeon. A high-speed long tapered drill facilitates removal of the transverse process, lateral facet joint, and pedicle.

The disk is identified and the epidural veins are coagulated and sectioned, the annulus is cut with a knife, and the diskectomy is performed. The advantage of the 30-degree endoscope is that it enables extensive disk removal under the thoracic spinal cord.[23]

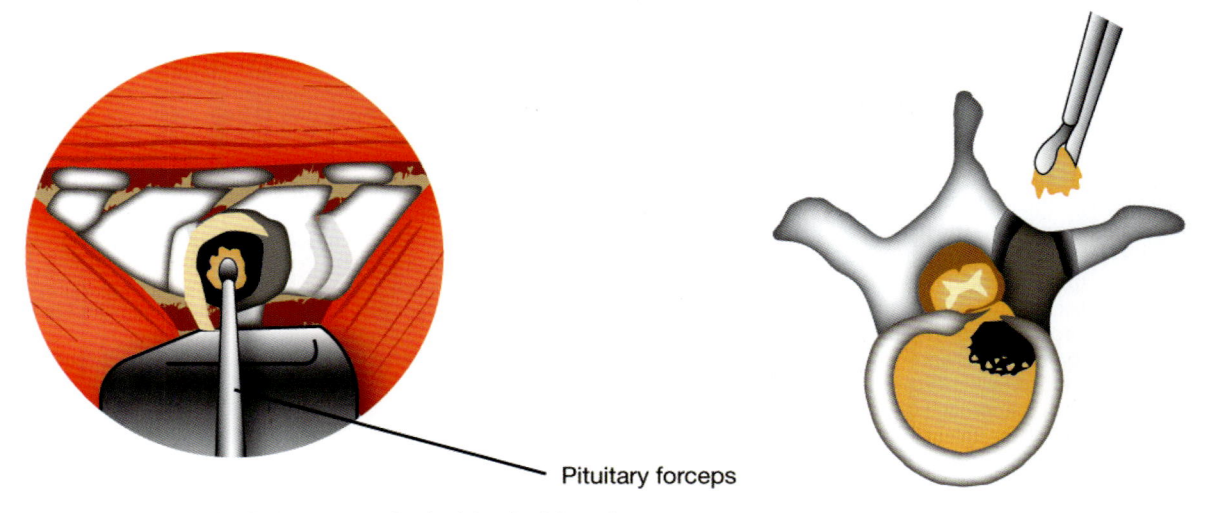

Fig. 71.5 A trough is created to facilitate a cavity for the disk to be delivered.

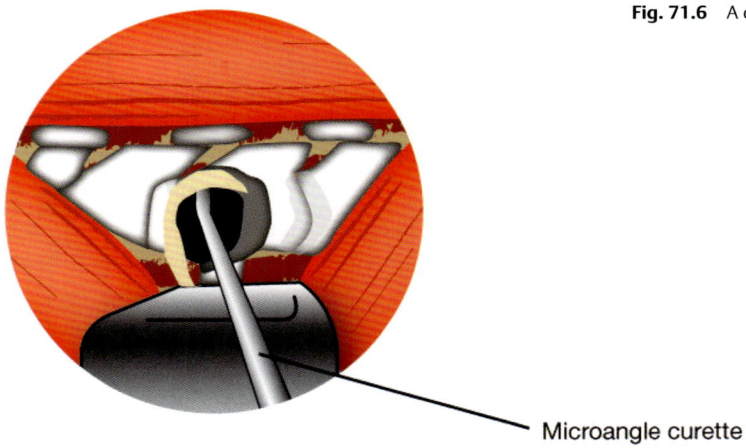

Fig. 71.6 A centrolateral disk is delivered down into the preformed cavity.

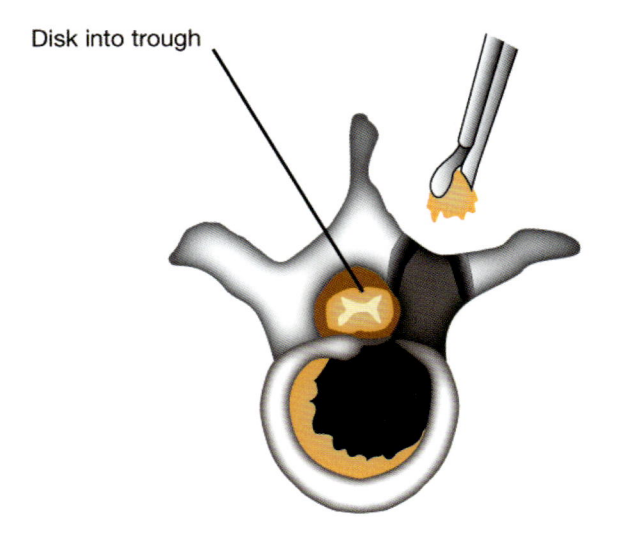

Fig. 71.7 Following decompression, the thecal sac falls back into anatomic position.

Outcomes and Complications

Due to the rarity of this condition and individual nuances favoring one approach over another, large series of TDH removal cases are not reported in the literature. Le Roux et al[16] performed a study of 20 patients who presented with symptoms related to thoracic disk herniation (pain and myelopathy most common), and had a transpedicular approach to address the problem. The authors noted significant improvement in all patients and no incidence of postoperative instability over a 12-month period. Most of the herniations were soft and centrolateral, and none were intradural. Other studies have reported good neurologic outcomes with the transpedicular approach, and in selected cases equivalence with more invasive anterior and lateral extracavitary approaches.[14,20,24–28] Nevertheless, removal of TDH remains one of the higher-risk surgeries in the spine. In a systematic review of complication rates from multiple approaches in the modern era of thoracic disk surgery (only a few cases of laminectomy reported), major complication rates ranged from 4.5 to 21.4% and they included permanent paralysis or worsened paraparesis, cerebrospinal fluid (CSF) leak, diskitis, creation of iatrogenic instability requiring later fusion, wrong level surgery (anterolateral approach), wrong diagnosis (arteriovenous malformation).[1]

Conclusion

The transpedicular approach utilizes a posterior and slightly lateral trajectory to address disk pathology. Patterson and Arbit,[12] in their original report on TDH removal, described the total removal of the facet and pedicle along with a laminectomy. Modifications to this approach include preserving some of the pedicle and facet complex, not performing a total laminectomy, and more recent incorporation of minimally invasive access techniques. Fusion is typically not necessary due to the stability provided by the ribs and anterior longitudinal ligament.

The transpedicular approach is ideal for soft or partially calcified, nonadherent, lateral/centrolateral disk herniations and can be used at any level in the spine. It is often a more familiar surgical approach that does not require rib removal or entry into the chest cavity, and it can be performed in much less time when compared with alternate procedures. In addition, minimally invasive tubular techniques have the potential of reducing incisional size, pain, blood loss, and hospital stays. The transthoracic and lateral extracavitary approaches, however, provide superior exposure for calcified central disk herniations.[9,14,20,25,27,29,30] **Box 71.1** lists the key points.

Box 71.1 Key Points

- Thoracic disk herniations are a rare (< 4% of all disk herniations) yet formidable problem encountered by spine surgeons.
- Patients who were treated via direct posterior midline approaches for thoracic disk herniation often had poor results.
- Thoracic MRI is essential in the diagnosis of TDH and can reveal T2 cord signal change.
- Thoracic CT myelogram, like MRI, can demonstrate cord compression and intra/extradural component, and is superior in demonstrating the calcium content of the disk.
- The transpedicular approach can be performed at all spinal levels and does not require the assistance of an access surgeon.
- The transpedicular approach is ideal for centrolateral to lateral disk herniations that are soft and extradural.
- Iatrogenic instability may occur if the entire pedicle and facet are removed.

References

1. Stillerman CB, Chen TC, Couldwell WT, Zhang W, Weiss MH. Experience in the surgical management of 82 symptomatic herniated thoracic discs and review of the literature. J Neurosurg 1998;88:623–633
2. Arce CA, Dohrmann GJ. Thoracic disc herniation. Improved diagnosis with computed tomographic scanning and a review of the literature. Surg Neurol 1985;23:356–361
3. Arseni C, Nash F. Thoracic intervertebral disc protrusion: a clinical study. J Neurosurg 1960;17:418–430
4. Elsberg CA. The extradural ventral chondromas (ecchondroses), their favorite sites, the spinal cord and root symptoms they produce, and their surgical treatment. Bull Neurol Inst NY 1931;1:350–388
5. Love JG, Schorn VG. Thoracic-disk protrusions. JAMA 1965;191:627–631
6. Mixter WJ, Barr JS. Rupture of the intervertebral disc with involvement of the spinal canal. N Engl J Med 1934;211:210–215
7. Parisien RC, Ball PA. William Jason Mixter (1880-1958). Ushering in the "dynasty of the disc". Spine 1998;23:2363–2366
8. Hulme A. The surgical approach to thoracic intervertebral disc protrusions. J Neurol Neurosurg Psychiatry 1960;23:133–137
9. Perot PL Jr, Munro DD. Transthoracic removal of midline thoracic disc protrusions causing spinal cord compression. J Neurosurg 1969;31:452–458
10. Ransohoff J, Spencer F, Siew F, Gage L Jr. Transthoracic removal of thoracic disc. Report of three cases. J Neurosurg 1969;31:459–461
11. Carson J, Gumpert J, Jefferson A. Diagnosis and treatment of thoracic intervertebral disc protrusions. J Neurol Neurosurg Psychiatry 1971;34:68–77
12. Patterson RH Jr, Arbit E. A surgical approach through the pedicle to protruded thoracic discs. J Neurosurg 1978;48:768–772
13. Ridenour TR, Haddad SF, Hitchon PW, Piper J, Traynelis VC, VanGilder JC. Herniated thoracic disks: treatment and outcome. J Spinal Disord 1993;6:218–224
14. el-Kalliny M, Tew JM Jr, van Loveren H, Dunsker S. Surgical approaches to thoracic disc herniations. Acta Neurochir (Wien) 1991;111:22–32
15. Baker HL Jr, Love G, Uihlein A. Roentgenologic features of protruded thoracic intervertebral disks. Radiology 1965;84:1059–1065
16. Le Roux PD, Haglund MM, Harris AB. Thoracic disc disease: experience with the transpedicular approach in twenty consecutive patients. Neurosurgery 1993;33:58–66
17. Fisher RG. Protrusions of thoracic disc. The factor of herniation through the dura mater. J Neurosurg 1965;22:591–593
18. Stillerman CB, Chen TC, Day JD, Couldwell WT, Weiss MH. The transfacet pedicle-sparing approach for thoracic disc removal: cadaveric morphometric analysis and preliminary clinical experience. J Neurosurg 1995;83:971–976
19. Simpson JM, Silveri CP, Simeone FA, Balderston RA, An HS. Thoracic disc herniation. Re-evaluation of the posterior approach using a modified costotransversectomy. Spine 1993;18:1872–1877
20. Otani K, Yoshida M, Fujii E, Nakai S, Shibasaki K. Thoracic disc herniation. Surgical treatment in 23 patients. Spine 1988;13:1262–1267
21. Mendel E, Guiot BH, Isaacs RE, Rhines LD, Fessler RG, Aaronson O. Diagnosis and management of thoracic disk herniation and the transpedicular decompression for thoracic disk herniation. In: Fessler RG, Sekhar L, eds. Atlas of Neurosurgical Techniques: Spine and Peripheral Nerves. New York: Thieme; 2006:469–477
22. Perez-Cruet MJ, Kim BS, Sandhu F, Samartzis D, Fessler RG. Thoracic microendoscopic discectomy. J Neurosurg Spine 2004;1:58–63
23. Perez-Cruet MJ, Samartzis D, Fessler RG. Microendoscopic thoracic discectomy. In: Perez-Cruet MJ, Khoo L, Fessler RG, eds. An Anatomic Approach to Minimally Invasive Spine Surgery. St. Louis: Quality Medical Publishing; 2006:431–447
24. Benson MK, Byrnes DP. The clinical syndromes and surgical treatment of thoracic intervertebral disc prolapse. J Bone Joint Surg Br 1975;57:471–477
25. Sekhar LN, Jannetta PJ. Thoracic disc herniation: operative approaches and results. Neurosurgery 1983;12:303–305
26. Bohlman HH, Zdeblick TA. Anterior excision of herniated thoracic discs. J Bone Joint Surg Am 1988;70:1038–1047
27. Russell T. Thoracic intervertebral disc protrusion: experience of 67 cases and review of the literature. Br J Neurosurg 1989;3:153–160
28. Lesoin F, Rousseaux M, Autricque A, et al. Thoracic disc herniations: evolution in the approach and indications. Acta Neurochir (Wien) 1986;80:30–34
29. Maiman DJ, Larson SJ, Luck E, El-Ghatit A. Lateral extracavitary approach to the spine for thoracic disc herniation: report of 23 cases. Neurosurgery 1984;14:178–182
30. Fessler RG, Dietze DD Jr, Millan MM, Peace D. Lateral parascapular extrapleural approach to the upper thoracic spine. J Neurosurg 1991;75:349–355

72 Intradural Extramedullary Tumor Resection

Paul C. McCormick

Tumors arising from the intradural extramedullary spinal canal reflect a wide variety of histopathologies. With few exceptions, however, these tumors are histologically benign and amenable to complete surgical resection. Long-term tumor control or cure with preservation or improvement in neurologic function can be achieved with surgery alone for most patients.[1-5] This chapter discusses direct surgical techniques and strategies for removal of these predominantly benign tumors.

Patient Selection

The main indication for surgery is the presence of an intradural extramedullary spinal tumor in a symptomatic patient. Symptoms vary based on the tumor location, type, and biology. Pain localized to the tumor level is common. The pain may worsen with activity, particularly in the case of lesions within the cauda equina. Classic night pain may also occur with these tumors, but this symptom may also occur with extradural primary or metastatic tumors of the spine. Alternatively, pain may be radicular in nature as a result of irritation or involvement of a local nerve root. Larger tumors ultimately cause local nerve root dysfunction and myelopathy or cauda equina syndrome.

Increasingly, however, these tumors are diagnosed in asymptomatic patients. This can present a management dilemma, because surgery must be considered prophylactic in these circumstances. These lesions are often biologically indolent and may exhibit only a very slow rate of growth. In these patients, a number of other issues need to be considered, such as patient age, comorbidity, and treatment preferences. Periodic surveillance with serial imaging may be an appropriate treatment option for many asymptomatic patients. One potential exception is the patient with a midline tumor of the cauda equina, because benign myxopapillary ependymomas can exhibit cerebrospinal fluid (CSF) dissemination. Early surgery to avoid this complication should be considered. Prophylactic surgery is rarely recommended in syndromic patients (e.g., neurofibromatosis, von Hippel–Lindau disease) with multiple lesions.

Choice of Operative Approach

Planning for resection of intradural spinal tumors includes numerous considerations such as tumor type, sagittal and axial location, and surgeon preference. Tumor-specific considerations, such as the presence of extradural tumor extension, the function of the root of origin for nerve sheath tumors, resection of the dural attachment in the case of meningiomas, or en-bloc resection for myxopapillary ependymomas, are also relevant. Despite these numerous factors, the vast majority of these lesions can be safely removed through a standard posterior exposure with a non-destabilizing laminectomy or osteoplastic laminoplasty. Modifications of the standard posterior exposures may be required to adequately access a ventral or paraspinal tumor extension.[6,7] More formalized posterolateral or even anterior exposures may occasionally need to be considered in some patients, particularly for midline ventral intradural tumors.[1] Minimally invasive exposures for resection of intradural extramedullary spinal tumors have also been described. In experienced hands, safe resection may be achieved by using these techniques.[8]

Preoperative Testing and Imaging

With few exceptions, surgical intervention is performed as an elective procedure. Optimization of the patient's medical condition is important and includes preoperative physical examination and appropriate age- and condition-specific radiographic imaging (e.g., chest X-ray), blood tests, and cardiac evaluation as determined by the patient's medical provider. If possible, platelet inhibiting anti-inflammatory medication should be discontinued 10 days prior to surgery.

Precise imaging of the surgical lesion is usually provided with a high-quality contrast-enhanced magnetic resonance imaging (MRI) **(Fig. 72.1)**. It is important, especially for thoracic lesions, that the correct level of the lesion be identified.

Surgical Procedure

General endotracheal anesthesia is induced. Inhalational anesthetics are typically avoided as they limit or prevent the recording of intraoperative electrophysiological monitoring. Instead, a total intravenous anesthesia (TIVA) technique is utilized. Perioperative intravenous antibiotics and steroids are administered. The leads for intraoperative somatosensory evoked potential (SSEP) and motor evoked potential (MEP) monitoring are placed, including sphincter electrodes for conus medullaris/cauda equina lesions as well as direct nerve root stimulation for lesions arising from the cervical or lumbosacral levels. In general, pre-positioning baseline recordings are not obtained for intradural lesions. The patient is turned into a prone position on a Wilson frame, with care taken to pad all bony prominences and subcutaneously coursing nerve trunks. For tumors below T6, a headrest is used and the arms are abducted not more than 90 degrees at the shoulders. For lesions above T6, a Mayfield head clamp is utilized and the arms are tucked at the side **(Fig. 72.2a)**.

Preoperative lateral and/or anteroposterior (AP) fluoroscopy is often used to localize the level of the incision. Intraoperative localization of the level of the lesion should be reconciled with the preoperative imaging localization. The operative field is prepped and draped in a sterile fashion. A midline skin incision and subperiosteal muscle dissection are performed **(Fig. 72.2b)**. A laminectomy **(Fig. 72.3)** or laminoplasty is performed. The degree of bone removal varies. A unilateral laminectomy may be performed for tumors that do not extend beyond the midline.

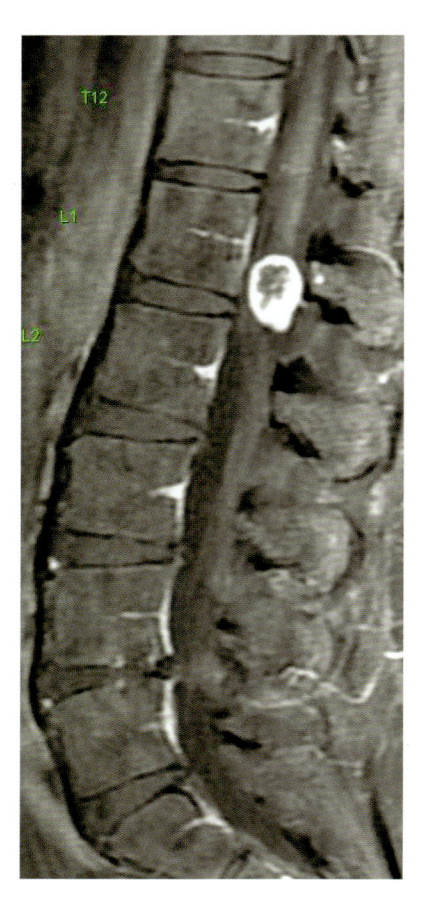

Fig. 72.1 (a) T1-weighted sagittal and (b) axial magnetic resonance imaging (MRI) of the lumbosacral spine demonstrates well-circumscribed heterogeneously enhancing intradural mass at the L1 spinal level. The appearance is typical for a spinal schwannoma.

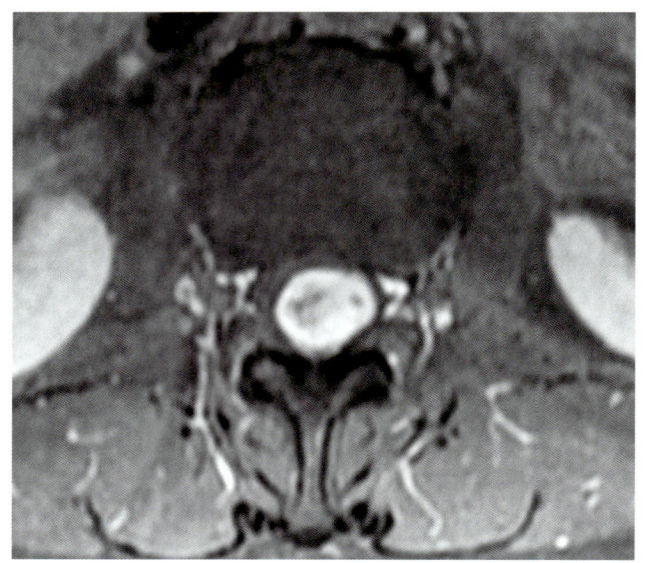

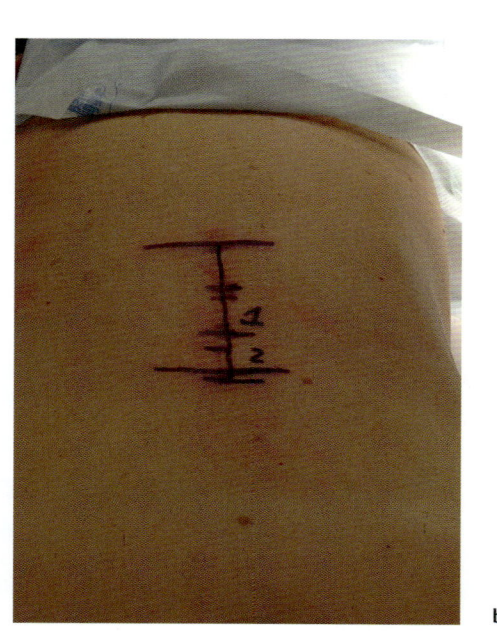

Fig. 72.2 (a) Intraoperative photograph of patient positioning for removal of a L1 spinal schwannoma. Note the use of a Wilson frame, which enables elevation of the surgical field and reduces lordosis. (b) Intraoperative photograph demonstrates the midline skin incision for bilateral L1 laminectomy.

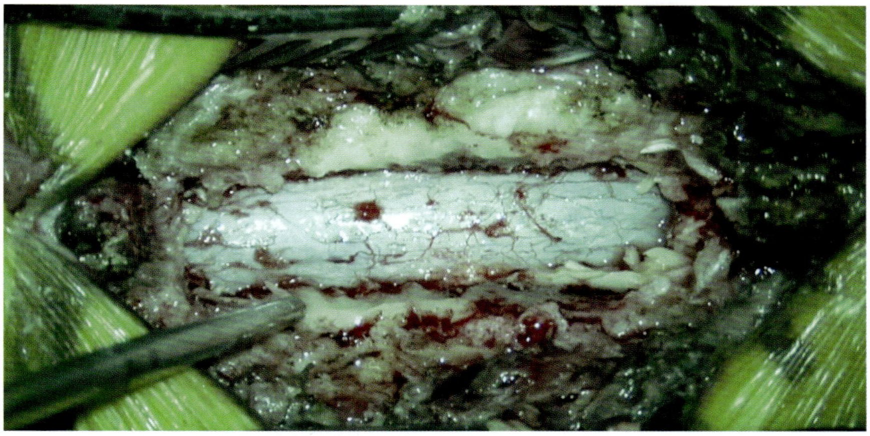

Fig. 72.3 Intraoperative photograph following completion of a bilateral L1 laminectomy. The majority of the facet joints are left intact to preserve spinal stability.

The facets are largely preserved, but a unilateral facetectomy may be required for a dumbbell tumor. The technique and strategies of tumor resection depend on the tumor type, location, and surgeon preference.

Nerve Sheath Tumors (See Video 72.1)

Most patients are approached through a standard laminectomy or osteoplastic laminoplasty that extends past the rostral and caudal tumor poles. The facet joints are completely preserved in most cases. A hemilaminectomy is performed if the tumor does not extend past the midline. With this exposure, the vast majority of intradural spinal schwannomas can be safely removed without compromise of spinal stability in adult patients. Some modification of this standard posterior approach may be needed for tumors located ventral to the dentate ligaments. Most ventral schwannomas occupy a unilaterally eccentric ventral location and produce some degree of spinal cord rotation and lateral displacement. In these circumstances, additional removal of portions of the facet joint and suture retraction of detached dentate ligaments usually provide adequate exposure for safe removal. Spinal stability may be compromised in some patients, particularly when significant removal of the lateral vertebral bone and joint components occurs. Pure ventral lesions without spinal cord rotation or lateral displacement may require a more formal anterior or anterolateral approach through a corpectomy or transforaminal exposure.

A midline or paramedian longitudinal dural opening is performed. The dural opening should extend just beyond the polar margins of the tumor to facilitate tumor removal and precise identification of the afferent and efferent nerve origin attachments. The dural edges are everted laterally and sutured to the paraspinal muscles to maximize intradural exposure and prevent the introduction of blood from the epidural space or paraspinal muscles into the dependent intradural surgical field. The intermediate arachnoid layer is sharply opened over the dorsal tumor surface. A second arachnoid layer is usually tightly applied to the tumor surface. This layer effectively compartmentalizes and ensheathes individual dorsal and ventral roots. Although the proximal portions of corresponding segmental dorsal and ventral nerve roots remain separate, they become compartmentalized within a common arachnoid sheath as they course toward the dural root sleeve.

Identification and opening of the arachnoid nerve sheath is important for two reasons. First, it enables the dissection to take place directly on the tumor surface. This layer is ultimately reflected off the tumor surface at its margins and can make mobilization and visualization of tumor margins difficult if the dissection is performed outside this layer. This is particularly important with regard to nonvisualized tumor margins that abut the spinal cord. Second, the corresponding nerve root is usually tightly applied to the tumor capsule within this arachnoid layer. Upon initial inspection, this nerve root may appear to be the nonfunctional nerve root of origin because of its tight attachment to the tumor surface. Upon opening this layer, however, it becomes clear that this root may be dissected off the tumor capsule and preserved. The same is not the case for the actual nerve of origin. Although a portion of the afferent and efferent components of the nerve of origin may be dissected and separated from the tumor capsule, eventually this dissection plane disappears as the nerve root becomes incorporated into the tumor capsule.

Once the tumor surface is identified, the polar margins are defined. Direct orthogonal visualization of both rostral and caudal tumor poles facilitates tumor removal. For large tumors, the dorsal tumor capsule is entered, and internal decompression with an ultrasonic aspirator or laser is performed. Sufficient internal decompression enable the progressive delivery of initially nonvisualized tumor into the resection bed. Division of the lateral dentate ligament attachment facilitates ventral access. Ultimately, the afferent and efferent tumor attachments need to be divided to achieve removal. Identification of these attachments depends on tumor size, origin, and location. In some cases, the afferent and efferent components may be immediately apparent on the dorsal surface of the tumor. Early division of these attachments facilitates removal of the tumor, particularly at the thoracic levels. More commonly, however, the afferent and efferent tumor attachments are not visualized on initial tumor exposure. The afferent root is often identified by its enlarged, congested, and hypervascular appearance. In contrast, the efferent root component usually appears normal.

Progressive internal decompression enables the delivery of the tumor margins into the resection bed until the attachments are visualized. The dorsal and ventral nerve roots may already be contained within a common arachnoid sheath at the proximal origin of cauda equina tumors. At these levels, the functional corresponding nerve root may appear to be part of the afferent root of origin. However, fascicles from the corresponding root will be reflected onto the tumor surface and can be dissected and preserved. Occasionally, some of the fascicles from the actual nerve root of origin may also be reflected onto the tumor surface and may be separable from the tumor capsule over much of, or occasionally the entirety of, the tumor surface. Unless these fascicles arise from critical cervical or lumbosacral levels and demonstrate intraoperative stimulation, they need not be preserved, as such futile dissection unnecessarily prolongs the resection. Tumors that arise from the very proximal portion of the nerve root may not have a definable afferent nerve root attachment. Instead, these tumors may abut and be adherent to the spinal cord at the root entry zone.

In some cases, proximal tumor growth may actually elevate the pia, where it is reflected at root entry zones, and occupy a subpial location. Great care must be taken to safely remove this subpial tumor component to avoid injury to the spinal cord or fragile epipial vascular network. In these cases, microsurgical dissection directly on the tumor surface usually enables safe and complete removal. This dissection can be difficult for removal of ventral root tumors, even with gentle retraction of a detached dentate ligament. Some portions of the pia may have to be incised to follow the subpial tumor component. If uncertainty regarding the margin of the tumor remains, then there should be no further dissection. Conversely, tumors arising more distally along the root of origin may have their distal margin near or just beyond the dural nerve root sleeve. In these cases, internal decompression, as well as early identification and division of the afferent attachment, provides adequate visualization and mobilization of the distal tumor component to enable preservation of a critical corresponding functional nerve root. Nerve root stimulation can be useful during this part of the dissection.

Following tumor resection, the subarachnoid space is irrigated with warm saline. The dura is closed with a running 4-0 silk or 5-0 Prolene suture (Ethicon, Inc., Somerville, NJ). A Valsalva maneuver to 35 mm Hg is then performed to verify watertight dural closure. DuraGen (Integra LifeSciences Corp., Plainsboro, NJ) may also be placed over the suture line. The paraspinal muscles, deep and superficial fascia, and skin are closed separately in a layered fashion (**Fig. 72.4**). A deep subfascial Hemovac drain is infrequently used. The patient is kept on bed rest until the morning of postoperative day 2 and then progressively mobilized.

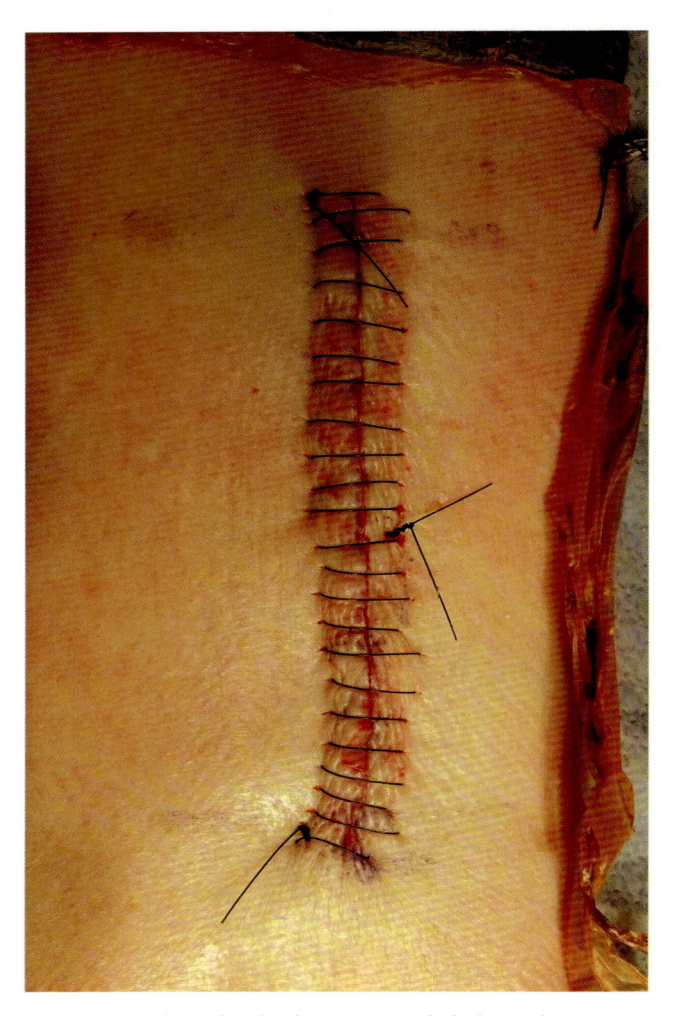

Fig. 72.4 The skin is closed with a running nonlocked 2-0 nylon suture to prevent cerebrospinal fluid (CSF) leakage.

Meningiomas

Most meningiomas of the spinal cord arise posterior, posterolateral, or lateral to the cord and therefore can be accessed by using a posterior approach. Patient positioning and the initial steps of intradural exposure are similar to those utilized for nerve sheath tumors. The exposed tumor surface should be visualized, including the rostral and caudal tumor poles. A small cottonoid is placed in each lateral gutter above and below the tumor margins. Division of one or more of the dentate ligament attachments to the lateral dura may improve access to ventral tumor extension. A well-defined arachnoid plane typically exists between the spinal cord and tumor capsule. Depending on the size and consistency of the tumor, internal debulking with an ultrasonic aspirator or laser facilitates visualization and development of the tumor margins. All traction on the tumor should be away from the spinal cord. The tumor surface may be quite friable and of variable vascularity. Cauterization of the dural base may reduce bleeding from highly vascular or friable lesions. Fortunately, due to a well-developed spinal epidural space, bony involvement does not typically occur. Management of the dural attachment depends on practical considerations. For dorsal tumors, resection of the dural origin facilitates resection. For more lateral and ventral tumors, cauterization of the tumor origin is preferred because of the difficulty of dural reconstruction in these locations. In either case, the rate of recurrence is quite low.

Filum Terminale Tumors

The basic principles of intradural surgical exposure also apply to filum terminale tumors. Ependymomas and paragangliomas should ideally be resected en bloc, as there is some evidence that piecemeal resection of these tumors increases the recurrence rates.[9] The tumor is carefully freed from adjacent nerve roots, and the filum is identified visually and tested with a neurostimulator. The filum terminale is cauterized above and below the tumor and divided, and the tumor is carefully rotated out of the canal (**Fig. 72.5**). It is often not possible to achieve en-bloc resec-

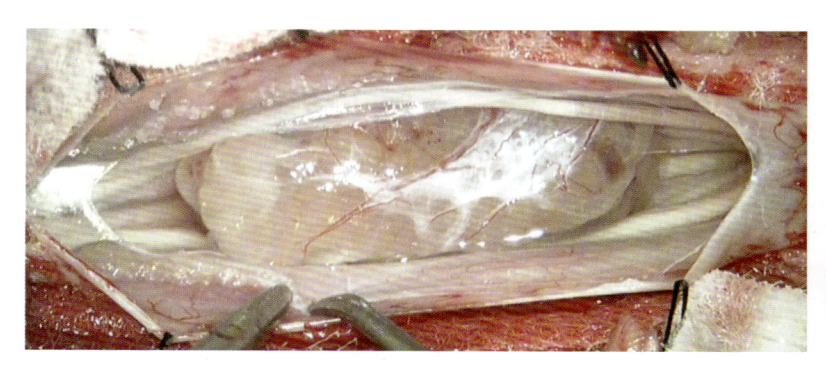

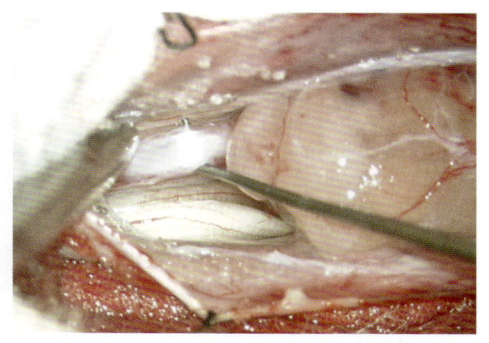

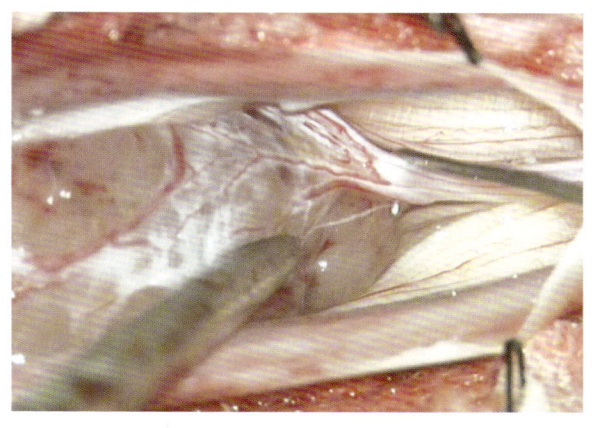

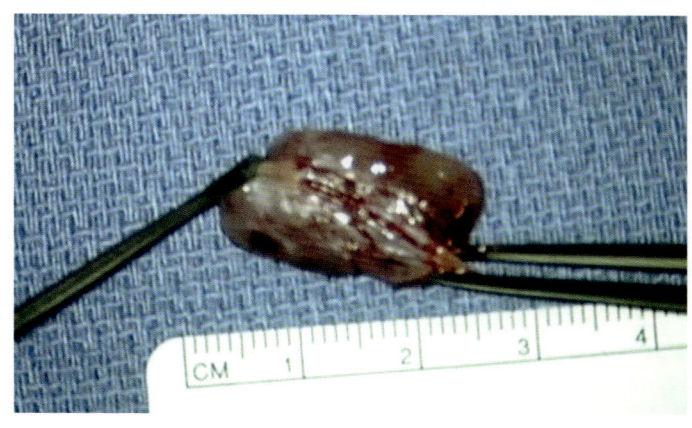

Fig. 72.5 (a) Initial intraoperative exposure of a cauda equina ependymoma. Note that both the rostral and caudal tumor poles are well visualized. (b) Magnified view of the rostral pole identifies the tumor origin from the filum terminale. The filum is differentiated from the surrounding cauda equina nerve roots by its white color and vascularity. (c) Magnified view of caudal pole demonstrates a distal filum terminale attachment to tumor. (d) Intraoperative photograph of tumor following en-bloc resection.

tion safely in larger tumors for various reasons. For example, the tumor may lack sufficient internal integrity and fall apart with even gentle manipulation. The tumor may also be too large to tease out without putting unacceptable amounts of traction on overlying nerve roots. Large tumors may exhibit sheet-like growth along arachnoid fenestrations. Functional roots may appear to course directly through the substance of the tumor. Safe resection can be impossible in these cases because the lack of supportive connective tissue matrix (i.e., epineurium) in the cauda equina nerve roots does not allow safe dissection of tumor off the involved roots. Only subtotal resection may be possible in these patients.

Postoperative Care

If a watertight dural closure is achieved, a subarachnoid lumbar spinal drain is unnecessary. The patient is kept flat in bed for 48 with sequential compression devices and a Foley catheter. If a spinal drain has been placed, it is generally clamped and removed prior to mobilizing the patient. Skin sutures are removed no earlier than 10 days following surgery. Early CSF leaks through the skin may be initially treated with recumbent and augmented skin sutures, but the patient is returned to the operating room for repair of persistent drainage. Delayed pseudomeningoceles are followed over time because many spontaneously resolve. Long-term clinical and radiographic follow-up is scheduled as needed.

Potential Complications and Precautions

Most complications relate to the wound and thromboembolic events. Meticulous wound closure will prevent most complications with CSF leaks, but if they do occur they should be treated promptly, especially if leakage through the skin is identified. Delayed pseudomeningoceles without skin drainage can be followed conservatively for many weeks in patients with no significant symptoms because they often spontaneously resolve. Persistent or symptomatic (e.g., postural headache) collections need to be drained via an open procedure. A small dural defect can usually be identified as the cause of the persistent leak and can be primarily repaired with suture and a small muscle graft.

Mechanical methods of deep vein thrombosis (DVT) prophylaxis are preferred in most patients due to the potential risks and consequences of delayed wound hematoma with pharmacological prophylaxis (e.g., low molecular weight heparins) but exceptions may be made in high-risk patients.

Conclusion

Intradural extramedullary tumors are overwhelming benign, well-circumscribed tumors that can be safely resected with good clinical results in the vast majority of patients. Timely diagnosis and early treatment in symptomatic patients utilizing contemporary neurosurgical techniques lead to favorable clinical outcomes for most patients. **Box 72.1** lists the key operative steps.

Box 72.1 Key Operative Steps

- Adequate bone and dural exposure to identify tumor poles
- Identification of tumor origin/attachment
- Internal decompression of large tumors to enable safe visualization/mobilization of tumor margins into the surgical field
- Attempt en-bloc resection of filum tumors if safely feasible
- Meticulous post-tumor resection subarachnoid space irrigation to prevent arachnoiditis
- Careful closure of all tissue layers to prevent postoperative CSF leak

References

1. Angevine PD, Kellner C, Haque RM, McCormick PC. Surgical management of ventral intradural spinal lesions. J Neurosurg Spine 2011;15:28–37
2. Cohen-Gadol AA, Zikel OM, Koch CA, Scheithauer BW, Krauss WE. Spinal meningiomas in patients younger than 50 years of age: a 21-year experience. J Neurosurg 2003;98(3, Suppl):258–263
3. Gottfried ON, Gluf W, Quiñones-Hinojosa A, Kan P, Schmidt MH. Spinal meningiomas: surgical management and outcome. Neurosurg Focus 2003;14:e2
4. Kim P, Ebersold MJ, Onofrio BM, Quast LM. Surgery of spinal nerve schwannoma. Risk of neurological deficit after resection of involved root. J Neurosurg 1989;71:810–814
5. Klekamp J, Samii M. Surgical results for spinal meningiomas. Surg Neurol 1999;52:552–562
6. McCormick PC. Surgical management of dumbbell and paraspinal tumors of the thoracic and lumbar spine. Neurosurgery 1996;38:67–74, discussion 74–75
7. O'Toole JE, McCormick PC. Midline ventral intradural schwannoma of the cervical spinal cord resected via anterior corpectomy with reconstruction: technical case report and review of the literature. Neurosurgery 2003;52:1482–1485, discussion 1485–1486
8. Nzokou A, Weil AG, Shedid D. Minimally invasive removal of thoracic and lumbar spinal tumors using a nonexpandable tubular retractor. J Neurosurg Spine 2013;19:708–715
9. Sonneland PR, Scheithauer BW, Onofrio BM. Myxopapillary ependymoma. A clinicopathologic and immunocytochemical study of 77 cases. Cancer 1985;56:883–893

73 Intramedullary Tumor Resection

Paul C. McCormick

Surgery represents the most effective treatment of benign well-circumscribed tumors, which constitute the majority of intramedullary neoplasms.[1–5] Long-term tumor control or cure, with preservation of neurologic function, can be achieved in most patients with microsurgical removal alone. The benign nature of most intramedullary neoplasms, the advances in microsurgical techniques, early clinical diagnosis with magnetic resonance imaging (MRI), and the ineffectual or inconsistent treatment provided by radiation therapy for most intramedullary tumors largely account for the expanded role of surgery in the management of these lesions.[6–10] This chapter describes the surgical techniques and strategies currently utilized to resect these neoplasms.

Patient Selection

The predominant benefit of surgery for an intramedullary tumor is prophylactic. Preservation, rather than restoration, of neurologic function is the most likely outcome after successful surgical treatment. In fact, significant improvement of a severe or long-standing preoperative neurologic deficit rarely occurs after a technically successful surgical excision. Surgical morbidity is also greater in patients with more significant preoperative deficits. This creates a therapeutic irony in which the risk of surgery is actually lower in patients with minimal or no objective neurologic deficit. Thus, early clinical diagnosis and, if possible, definitive initial treatment are critical to successful clinical management of most intramedullary tumors. A therapeutic dilemma arises, however, in the asymptomatic patient in whom an incidental intramedullary spinal cord lesion has been discovered. A posterior column deficit is a common consequence of a dorsal median myelotomy; thus, some degree of morbidity often accompanies even the most successful surgical removal. In completely asymptomatic patients, therefore, observation with serial clinical and radiological follow-up is an appropriate management strategy for most patients, especially those with conditions such as neurofibromatosis or von Hippel–Lindau disease.[11]

Indications and Contraindications

The primary surgical objective for intramedullary tumors is long-term tumor control or cure with preservation of neurologic function. The most important factor influencing the surgical objective is the nature of the tumor–spinal cord interface. This interface can be assessed accurately only through an adequate myelotomy, which extends over the entire rostrocaudal extent of the tumor. Benign tumors, such as ependymomas and hemangioblastomas, although unencapsulated, are noninfiltrative lesions that typically exhibit a distinct tumor–spinal cord interface. Gross total removal is the treatment of choice in these cases. Astrocytomas are more variable. Unlike the consistently benign histology, circumscribed nature, and natural history of ependymoma and hemangioblastoma, astrocytomas are much more variable with respect to histology, physical characteristics, and natural history. Although some benign astrocytomas are well circumscribed and are suitable for gross total resection, most exhibit variable infiltration into the surrounding spinal cord. This is often reflected in a gradual transition zone between the tumor and spinal cord. There is rarely a definitive dissection plane. Thus, whereas gross total resection may be achieved in some cases, the extent of removal is uncertain and poorly defined in most cases. Furthermore, more peripheral dissection beyond what is clearly tumor tissue risks loss of neurologic function from the resection of infiltrated, yet functionally viable, spinal cord parenchyma.

The surgical objective for spinal cord astrocytomas is unclear. Specifically, a correlation between the extent of resection and tumor control has not been definitively established.[12,13] Because preservation of neurologic function, rather than complete tumor resection, is the more prudent treatment objective in these cases, tumor removal is limited to tissue that is clearly distinguishable from the surrounding spinal cord. Therefore, the extent of tumor removal varies. Diffusely infiltrative tumors without a definite mass are biopsied, whereas gross total resection may be possible in well-circumscribed examples. Variable degrees of resection account for the remainder of the astrocytomas.

Choice of Operative Approach

The vast majority of intramedullary tumors are accessed through a standard laminectomy and midline myelotomy through the posterior median septum with the patient in the prone position. Minimally invasive techniques for intramedullary tumor removal have been described but are currently limited because the morbidity of these procedures resection is related to the intramedullary tumor resection, not the initial spinal exposure. More recently, lateral and ventral approaches have been described in selected patients with more ventrally located intramedullary tumors.[14,15]

Preoperative Imaging

Gadolinium-enhanced MRI is the procedure of choice for imaging and preoperative evaluation of an intramedullary tumor. Spinal cord enlargement and tumor enhancement are the characteristic findings (**Fig. 73.1**). Polar cysts are often present. Ependymomas are usually symmetrically located and exhibit uniform tumor enhancement, whereas astrocytomas are associated with a more variable appearance with respect to tumor margins and enhancement patterns. Prediction of these tumor types based on MRI appearance is often inaccurate, predominantly because of the variability of presentation on MRI scans, and is therefore avoided because it may unfairly influence the

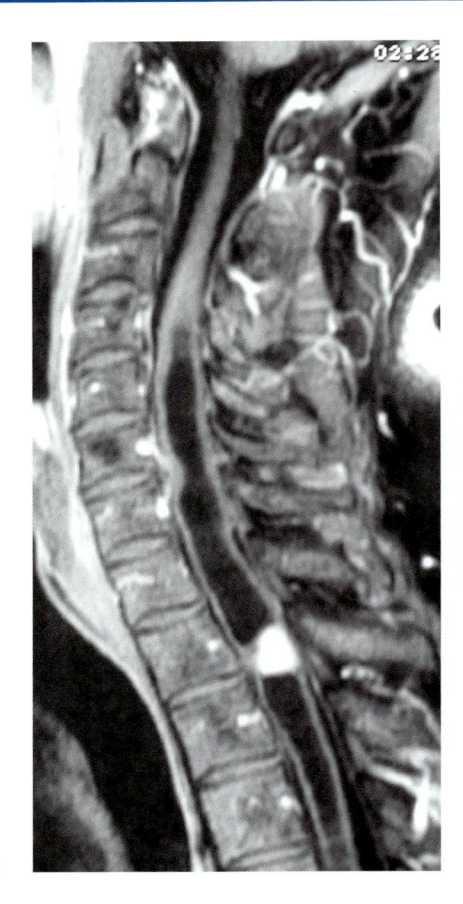

Fig. 73.1 T1-weighted contrast-enhanced sagittal (a) and axial (b) magnetic resonance imaging (MRI) of the cervicothoracic spine demonstrates an intramedullary ependymoma at the T2-T3 level with large rostral and caudal polar cysts.

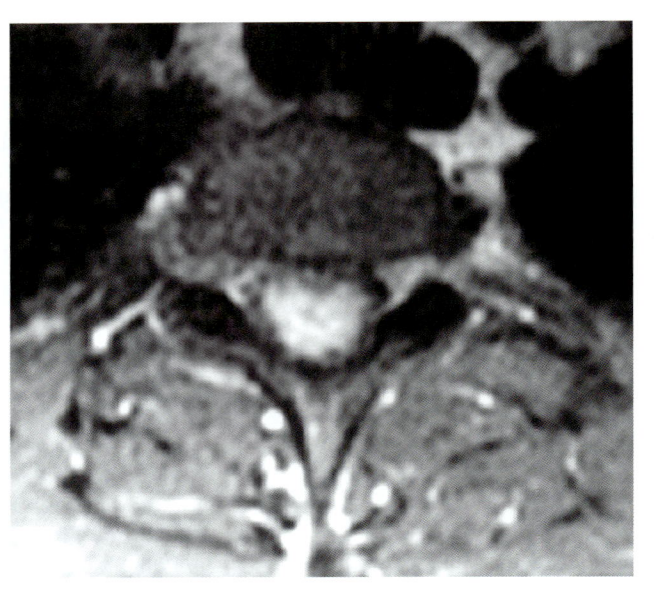

surgical objective. Hemangioblastomas usually appear as intensely enhancing eccentric masses or nodules. There is often diffuse spinal cord enlargement that may extend a considerable distance from the tumor. The cause of this tumor enlargement is most likely vasogenic edema.[16]

Surgical Procedure

Intramedullary Glial Tumors (Ependymomas, Astrocytomas)

After intubation and administration of perioperative steroids and antibiotics, the patient is turned to the prone position. A Mayfield skull clamp is used for cervical and upper thoracic lesions above the T6 level (**Fig. 73.2a**). Neck flexion and head elevation (i.e., military prone position) reduce the spinal curvature at these levels. Somatosensory evoked potential (SSEP) and motor evoked potential (MEP) monitoring may be used throughout the procedure. The acquired data, however, rarely influence the surgical technique or the surgical objective. The use of a total intravenous anesthesia (TIVA) technique has made intraoperative monitoring much more reliable.

A midline incision and subperiosteal bony dissection are made, and a standard laminectomy is performed (**Fig. 73.2b**). This should extend to at least one segment above and one segment below the solid tumor component. The facet joints are preserved, if possible. Delayed instability rarely occurs after laminectomy for intramedullary tumor removal in adults. Although laminoplasty may be a reasonable option, it is not required.[17] Concomitant spinal fusion is increasingly being performed, particularly following multilevel cervical or thoracic laminectomy and in high-risk pediatric and adolescent patients.[18]

Strict hemostasis must be secured before the dura is opened to prevent ongoing contamination into the dependent microsurgical field. Wide, moist, cottonoid "wall-offs" cover the exposed muscles. Oxidized cellulose (Surgicel) is generously spread over the lateral gutters to prevent contamination of the operative field with blood. The dura mater is opened in the midline and tented laterally to the muscles with sutures.

The arachnoid is opened separately, and the spinal cord is inspected for any surface abnormality. Most glial tumors appear with only localized spinal cord enlargement. The spinal cord may be rotated. Occasionally, the overlying spinal cord may be thinned or even transparent secondary to a large or eccentrically located tumor or polar cyst. Ultrasonography is useful for tumor localization and for ensuring adequate bony exposure.

Rarely, an exophytic component of a benign glial tumor may extend into the subarachnoid space through a nerve root entry zone. Malignant neoplasms may replace surface spinal cord tissue or fungate through the pia into the subarachnoid space. Most hemangioblastomas arise from the dorsal half of the spinal cord with a visible pial attachment.[19] The size of the pial attachment may bear no relationship to the underlying embedded portion of the tumor.

Exposure of most intramedullary glial neoplasms is through a dorsal midline myelotomy. Eccentrically located tumors that abut the pia may be exposed via an off-midline myelotomy that extends longitudinally from both ends of the visible tumor.

The dorsal midline septum is identified as the midpoint between corresponding dorsal root entry zones (**Fig. 73.3a**). Bipolar cautery marks the dorsal midline over the extent of the intended

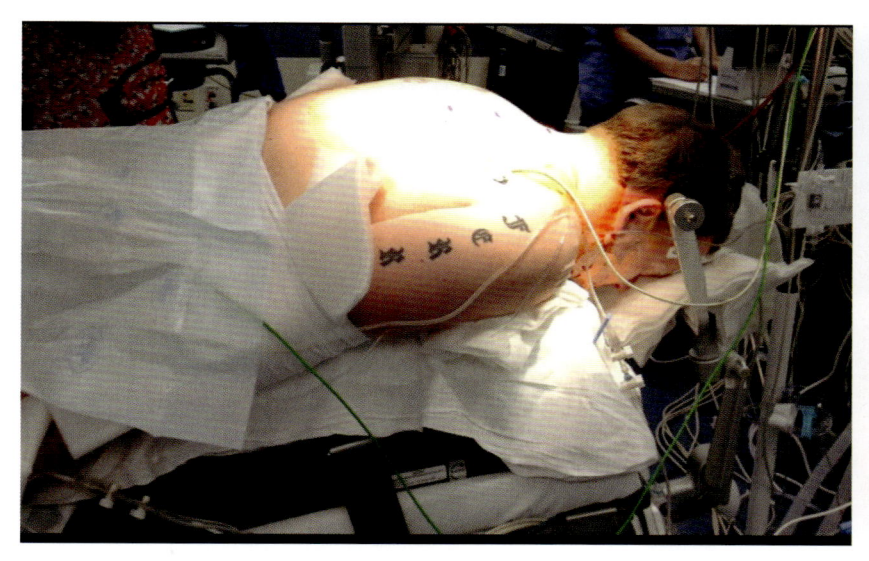

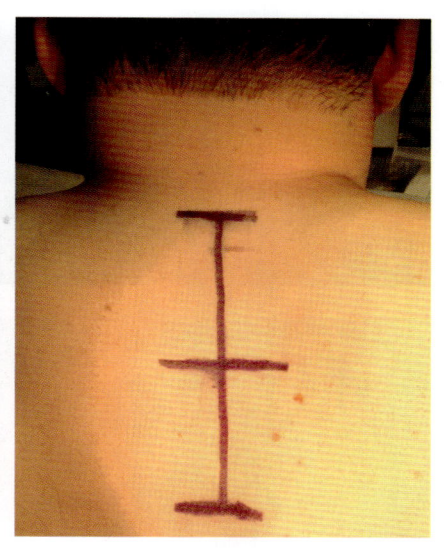

Fig. 73.2 (a) Patient placed in the prone position for removal of a T2-T3 intramedullary tumor. The neck is slightly flexed with the arms at the side and the head in a Mayfield head holder. (b) Intraoperative view of the skin incision for access to a T2-T3 intramedullary tumor.

myelotomy. The myelotomy is begun with a microknife in an avascular pial segment at the point of maximum spinal cord enlargement. The pia is a white, glistening fibrocartilaginous membrane that is tightly applied to the outer glial limiting membrane of the spinal cord. The pia is sharply incised over the entire extent of the tumor. Midline crossing epipial vessels are sequentially cauterized and divided. The myelotomy is deepened by gentle spreading with blunt microforceps and dissectors (**Fig. 73.3b**). Fibrous gliosis at the polar margins of the tumor may require sharp dissection with a microknife. The myelotomy continues until the entire rostrocaudal extent of the dorsal tumor surface has been identified. Although the myelotomy must extend a few millimeters beyond the solid portion of the tumor, it is not necessary to completely expose polar cysts. Size 6-0 pial sutures are placed and clipped laterally to the dura to maintain gentle traction (**Fig. 73.4**).

Evaluation of the tumor–spinal cord interface and frozen-section biopsy examination (to a lesser extent) determine the appropriate treatment objective. Ependymomas are usually characterized by a glistening reddish or brownish-red surface that may be slightly lobulated (**Fig. 73.4**). Blood vessels often course over the tumor surface. These tumors are clearly distinguishable from the surrounding spinal cord on the basis of color and texture. Although unencapsulated, these tumors do not infiltrate and can be easily distinguished and separated from the surrounding spinal cord. Astrocytomas are more heterogeneous with respect to physical characteristics, and they abut the spinal cord. Intratumoral cysts are quite common, but tumor color and consistency are variable. In adults, most astrocytomas appear as a definable

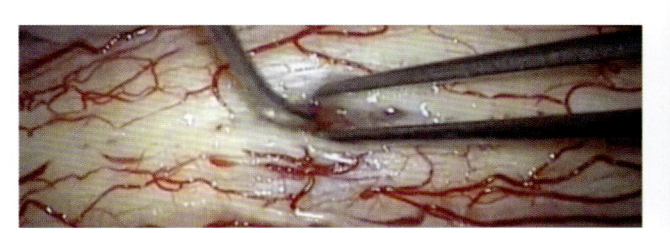

Fig. 73.3 (a) Identification of the posterior median septum by its midline vascular pattern and the midway point between dorsal root entry zones. (b) The posterior midline myelotomy is carefully developed with microforceps and microdissector.

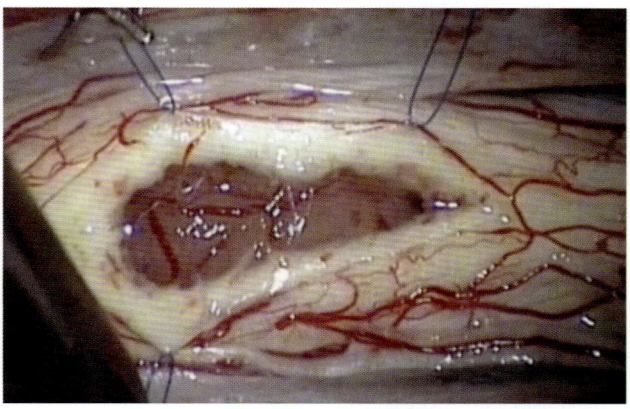

Fig. 73.4 The myelotomy is gently widened with pial sutures that are clipped to the dura. Note the well-defined tumor appearance that is characteristic of ependymomas.

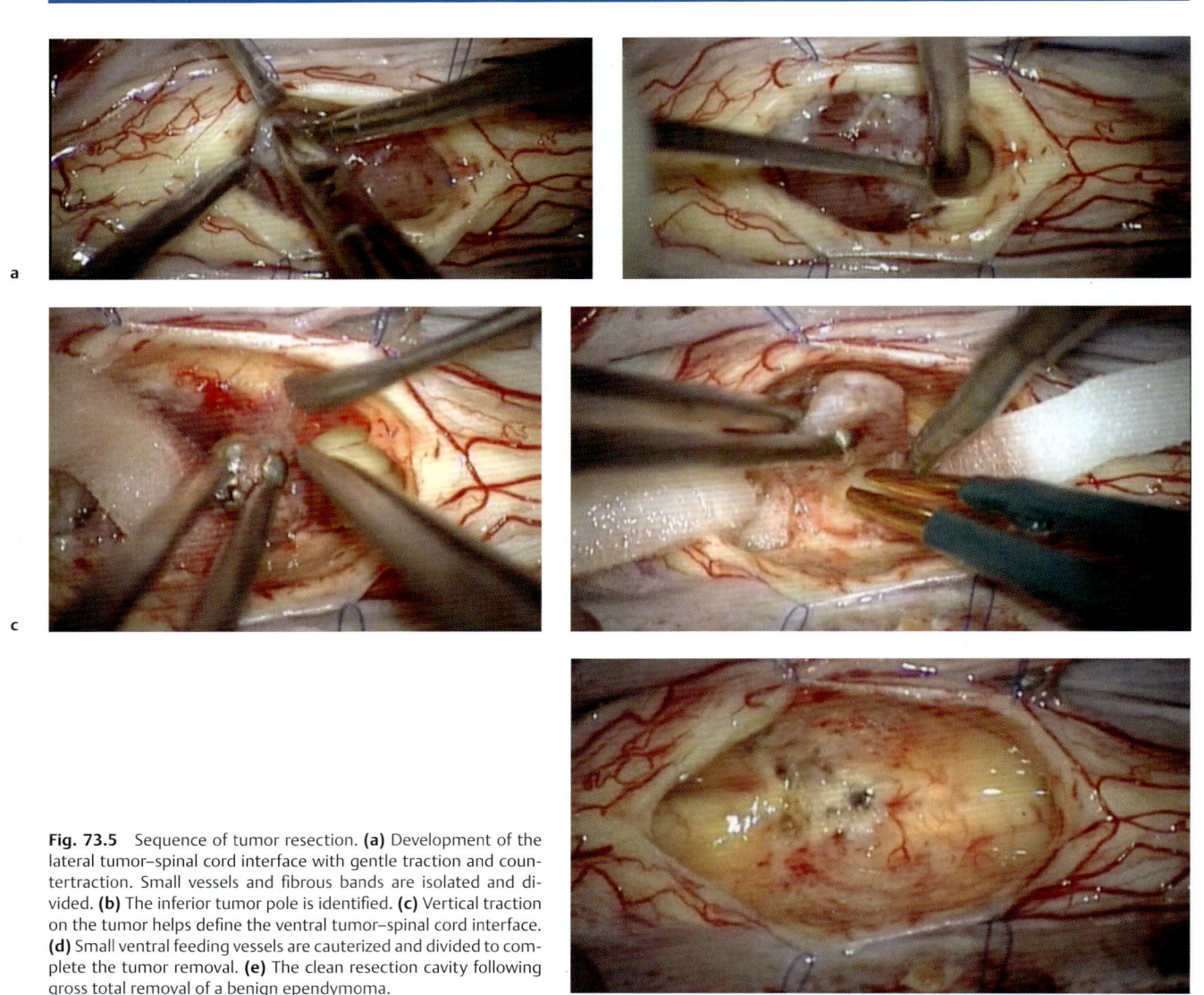

Fig. 73.5 Sequence of tumor resection. **(a)** Development of the lateral tumor–spinal cord interface with gentle traction and countertraction. Small vessels and fibrous bands are isolated and divided. **(b)** The inferior tumor pole is identified. **(c)** Vertical traction on the tumor helps define the ventral tumor–spinal cord interface. **(d)** Small ventral feeding vessels are cauterized and divided to complete the tumor removal. **(e)** The clean resection cavity following gross total removal of a benign ependymoma.

intramedullary mass with a gradual and indistinct transition between the tumor mass and surrounding spinal cord. This reflects the infiltrative nature of these neoplasms.

The technique of tumor removal depends on its juncture with the spinal cord and its size. Development of the tumor–spinal cord juncture is preferred for circumscribed tumors with a well-defined plane, as is the case with nearly all ependymomas and many astrocytomas. The dorsal tumor surface is exposed with pial sutures and gentle, blunt lateral displacement of the overlying dorsal hemicords with dissectors. Fibrous and vascular attachments that tether the spinal cord to the tumor surface are systematically cauterized and divided (**Fig. 73.5**). The development of the lateral and polar tumor margins is facilitated by forceps traction on the tumor and gentle pial suture and manual dissector countertraction on the spinal cord (**Fig. 73.5**). Larger tumors require internal decompression with an ultrasonic aspirator or laser to facilitate visualization and mobilization of the lateral and ventral tumor margins. Infiltrating tumors are removed using an "inside-out" technique. Internal decompression is continued peripherally until the clear distinction of the tumor and spinal cord is no longer obvious.

Following tumor removal, the resection cavity and subarachnoid space are copiously irrigated with a warm saline solution. Meticulous hemostasis is achieved. The dura is then reapproximated with a running locked 4–0 silk suture. A Valsalva maneuver to 35 cm H_2O is performed. Onlay dural substitutes, such as DuraGen (Integra LifeSciences Corp., Plainsboro, NJ), with or without a sealant such as DuraSeal (Confluent Surgical, Waltham, MA), can be used to cover the dura. The deep muscles are reapproximated with a running absorbable monofilament suture over a Hemovac drain. Absorbable braided suture is used to close the deep fascia and subcutaneous tissue, and a running nonlocked nylon suture is used for the skin closure. The patient is maintained on bed rest for 36 hours after surgery, and then mobilization is begun.

Hemangioblastoma

The techniques and principles of removal of spinal cord hemangioblastoma are distinct from those used for the resection of the much more commonly occurring glial tumors (astrocytomas and ependymomas).[11,19] Nearly all glial tumors occupy a completely intramedullary location and are surgically exposed via a dorsal midline myelotomy through the posterior median septum. Hemangioblastomas, however, are more accurately considered juxtamedullary tumors because they arise from the pia in the vast majority of cases. The surface presentation and pial origin of spinal cord hemangioblastomas provide the fundamental basis of the surgical resection strategy and technique. Circumferential release of the pial attachment at the interface of the tumor surface and spinal cord is performed to devascularize the tumor and to provide the exposure and mobility needed to access and safely remove the intramedullary component by detaching it from the adjacent neural structures (**Fig. 73.6a**). Variability in hemangioblastoma size and location, the relationship to the nerve roots, surface vascularity, edema and cyst, and surface-to-intramedullary tumor ratio, however, may necessitate some variation in surgical technique on a case-by-case basis.

After dural opening, inspection of the spinal cord under high magnification is performed to identify the surface component of the tumor. Most hemangioblastomas are located on the dorsal or dorsolateral surface of the spinal cord and are readily seen on initial inspection of the spinal cord under the microscope. The key to the initial dissection is identification of the surface component of the hemangioblastoma. The superficial tumor can be recognized by its characteristic sunset orange appearance (**Fig. 73.6b**). Large draining veins on the dorsal and dorsolateral spinal cord surface are typical and may partially or completely obscure visualization of the pial surface of the tumor. The tumor may be fairly small and superficially located. In some cases, there may be a significant exophytic tumor component ("snow cone" tumor), whereas in other cases, a very small surface tumor component belies a large underlying intramedullary extension ("iceberg" tumor) (**Fig. 73.7**). There is also variability in the degree and number of superficial draining veins.

Irrespective of these variations, the subsequent step after identification of the superficial pial tumor component is identification of the interface between the pial origin of the tumor and the surrounding normal pia. Draining veins that obscure visualization of the surface component of the tumor are systematically mobilized from their epipial attachment, cauterized, and divided. One or two major draining veins, usually at the polar margins of the tumor, are left intact until the end of the tumor resection. Dorsolateral tumors typically involve the dorsal root entry zone of at least one level. Often, this dorsal root partially obscures the surface of the tumor or the margin between the normal pia and

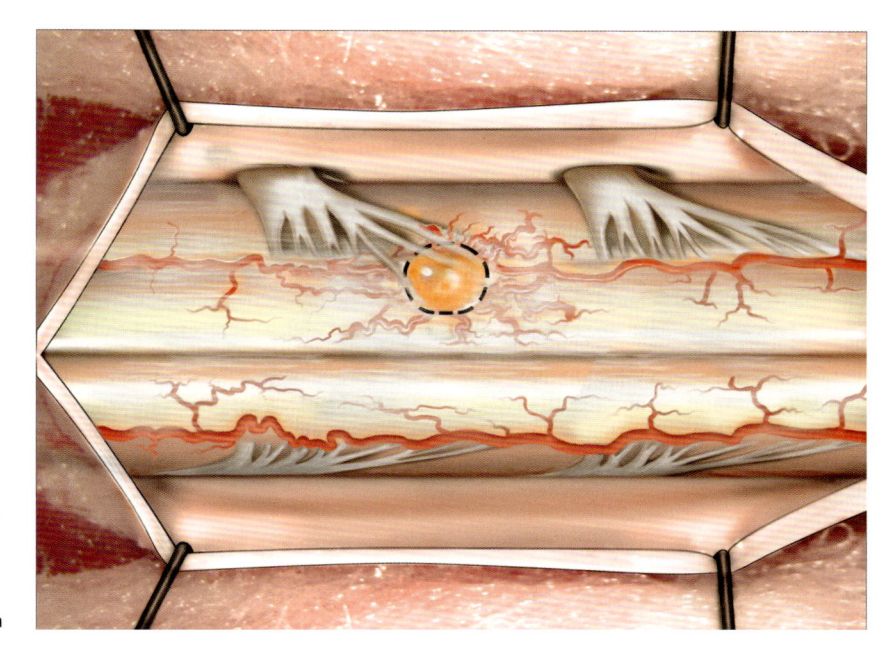

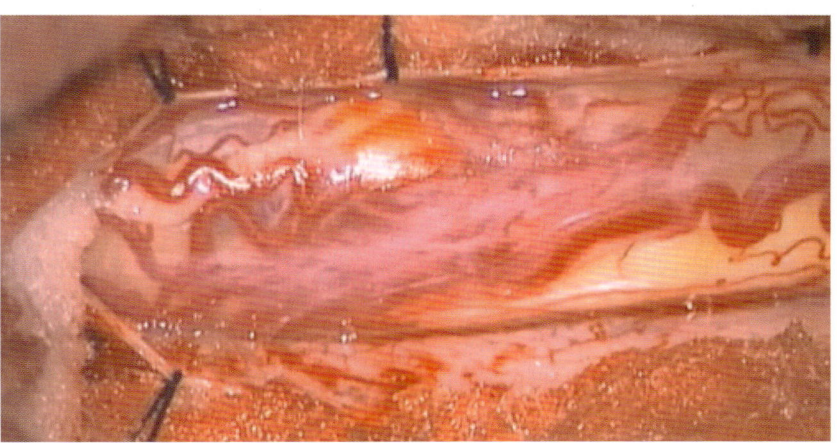

Fig. 73.6 (a) Artist's rendering of the circumferential detachment of the pial interface with a tumor capsule. (b) The characteristic dorsal lateral surface presentation of a sunset orange appearance of a hemangioblastoma that is partially obscured by large draining veins.

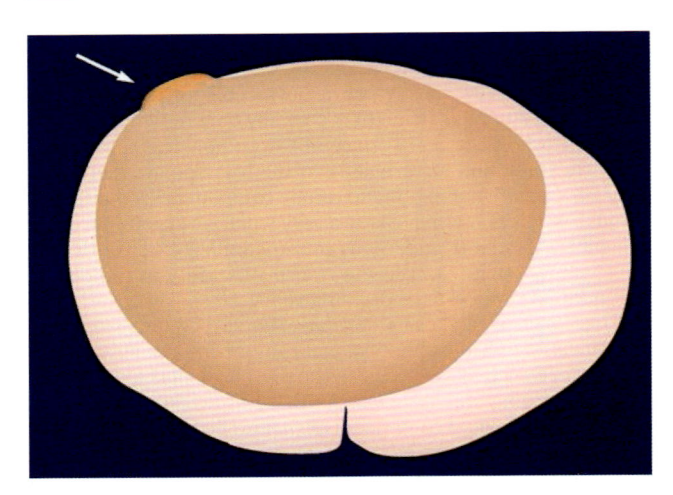

Fig. 73.7 Artist's rendering of an "iceberg" tumor with a small surface presentation *(arrow)* and a large intramedullary extension.

the pia overlying the tumor. These dorsal root fascicles must usually be mobilized and divided to facilitate tumor removal. Once the interface between the pia and the tumor is identified, it must be circumferentially detached. On its outer surface, an epipial matrix of arachnoid is loosely attached to the pia. The superficial vasculature of the spinal cord is loosely attached to the spinal cord surface within this epipial layer. Sharp dissection of the epipial arachnoid enables mobilization and isolation of surface draining veins to be cauterized and divided so that precise visualization of the interface between the tumor and the intima pia can be achieved.

Unlike the brainstem and cranial pia, the spinal intima pia is a robust membrane made up of longitudinally oriented fibers that have a characteristic glistening, white, striated appearance under the operating microscope. The intima pia is densely adherent to the underlying glial outer limiting membrane of the spinal cord. Detachment of this well-defined sturdy membrane requires sharp dissection with a microknife or scissors (**Fig. 73.8**). After the margin of the tumor has been circumferentially detached from the surrounding normal pia, removal of the intramedullary tumor component can begin. For tumors with limited or no intramedullary extension, the tumor is easily removed following the circumscribing pial incision. Tumors with larger intramedullary components, however, may require gentle traction on the tumor, with either tumor forceps or a suture through the pial origin, and progressive shrinkage of tumor volume through cauterization of the tumor surface with irrigating cautery on a low setting. This generally provides adequate exposure and visualization for safe resection of the intramedullary portion of the tumor. Tumors with very large intramedullary components, particularly those associated with a relatively small surface projection (i.e., "iceberg" tumors), may require the use of longitudinal polar myelotomies and pial traction sutures for safe removal (**Fig. 73.9**).

The intramedullary portion of these tumors is usually associated with a readily developed tumor plane whose dissection is further facilitated by the frequent presence of syringomyelia. The vast majority of arterial feeders and the venous drainage of these tumors are located at the pial surface. Very few deep feeding vessels or draining veins are encountered during the intramedullary dissection. Cauterization of the tumor surface can shrink the tumor volume to some degree and facilitate dissection, but this should be done under a low setting with somewhat broader tipped irrigating forceps because of the fragility of the hemangioblastoma vascular stroma. Internal decompression of the tumor or periodic compartmental tumor amputation can be used in some cases to facilitate deep exposure, but these maneuvers may be problematic because of tumor vascularity. Gentle traction on the tumor can be applied with a small traction suture in the pial surface of the tumor. The well-defined plane between the tumor and the spinal cord is progressively developed with traction on the tumor with a microdissector, tumor or microcautery forceps, or suction tip, and blunt gentle countertraction on the spinal cord with a microdissector (**Fig. 73.10**). Deep fibrous attachments and bridging vessels are systematically isolated, cauterized, and divided. Prolene pial traction 6-0 sutures may be used to provide gentle retraction to improve visualization and facilitate the intramedullary resection. Typically, at least one major draining vein is left patent at the polar margin of the tumor until dissection of the intramedullary tumor component is completed (**Fig. 73.11**). This vessel is then cauterized and divided. The pial traction sutures are removed and the wound is closed in layers.

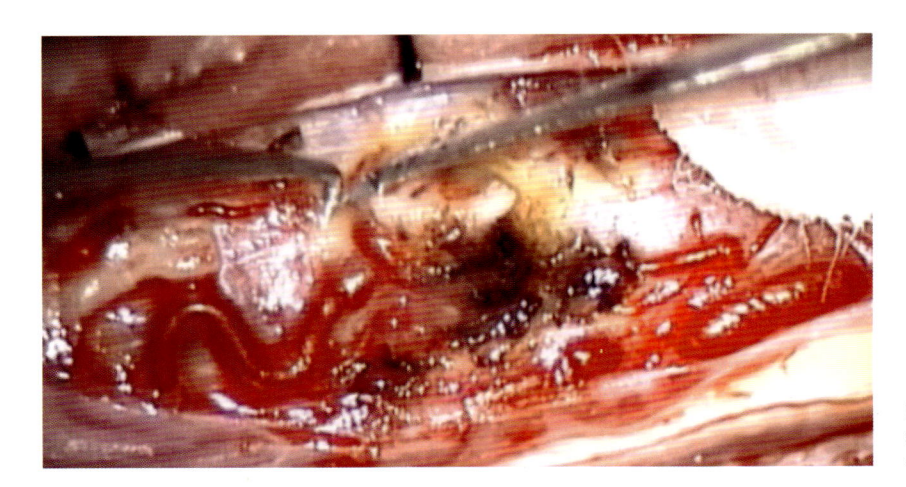

Fig. 73.8 Intraoperative photograph shows sharp dissection with a microknife at the tumor–spinal cord pial interface.

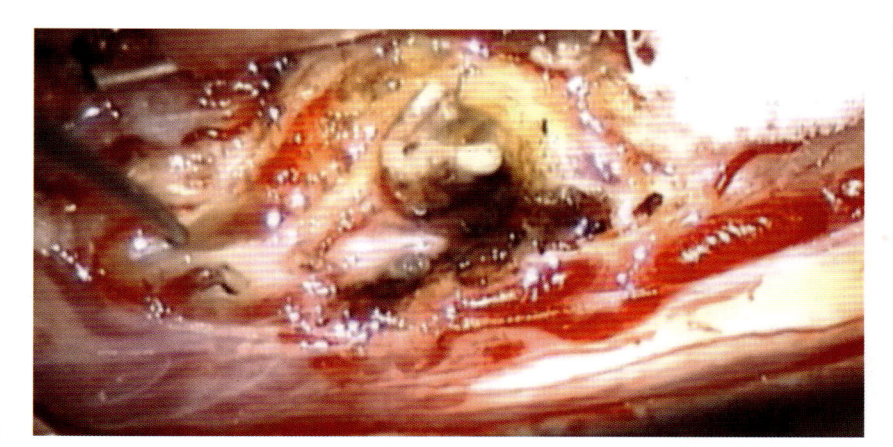

Fig. 73.9 (a) Due to a large intramedullary tumor component, a polar myelotomy is being performed at the rostral margin. (b) Artist's rendering of the technique of polar myelotomy.

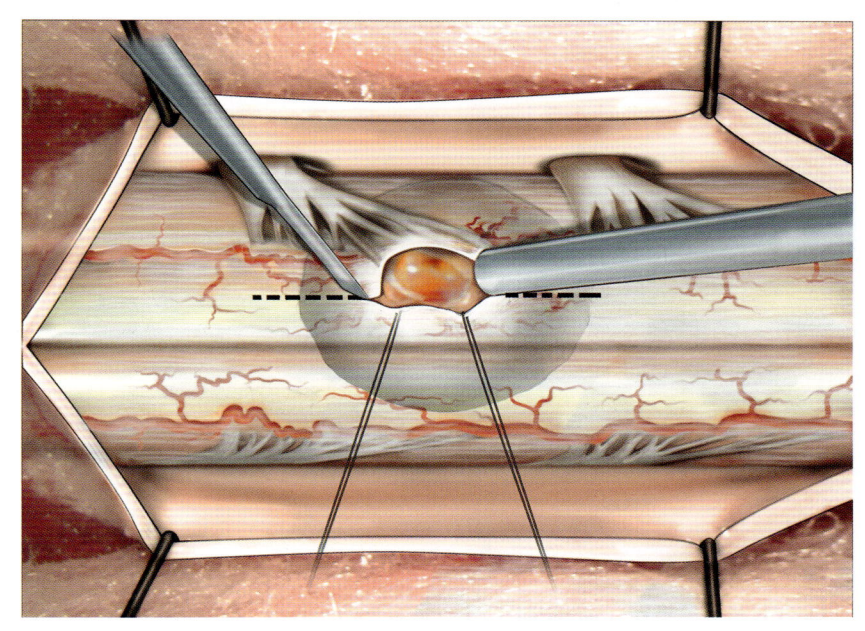

Postoperative Care

Postoperative management is standard. The benefits of early mobilization to avoid deep venous thrombosis or respiratory compromise must be balanced with safety and wound healing concerns, especially cerebrospinal fluid (CSF) leakage. The patient is usually kept in bed for 36 hours until mobilization is initiated. The Hemovac and urinary catheter are usually removed on postoperative day 3.

Potential Complications and Precautions

The most common complications relate to wound problems, infection, and thromboembolic events. Paretic patients are particularly vulnerable to thromboembolic complications. Sequential compression devices, initially placed immediately prior to surgery, are continued postoperatively until the patient is adequately mobilized. Subcutaneous heparin (5,000 units twice a day) or low molecular weight heparin (enoxaparin 40 mg every day) may also be considered on or about postoperative day 2, but may increase the risk of wound hematomas. CSF fistula can be problematic, especially with reoperations or previously radiated tumors. Delayed leaks may produce only contained pseudomeningoceles that usually spontaneously resolve over several weeks. Persistent collections, especially associated with postural headaches, may require reoperation for repair. CSF leakage through the skin must be aggressively managed to prevent infection. These patients are usually returned to the operating room for repair within 24 to 36 hours if the leakage persists.

Nearly all patients experience some degree of posterior column deficit following midline myelotomy. This is not so much a complication but a reality of the procedure. These deficits may improve but rarely completely resolve. This issue should be discussed with the patient as part of the preoperative preparation.

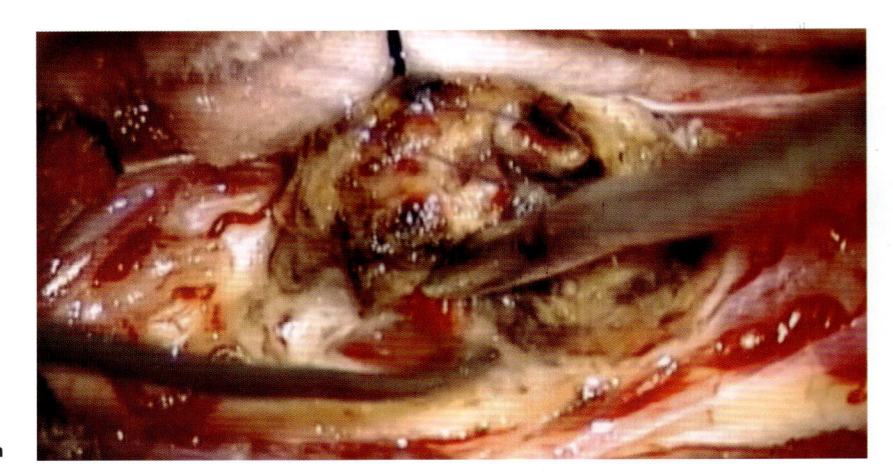

Fig. 73.10 (a,b) Intraoperative photographs illustrate the gradual deliverance of the tumor from out of the spinal cord once the circumferential pial attachment has been released.

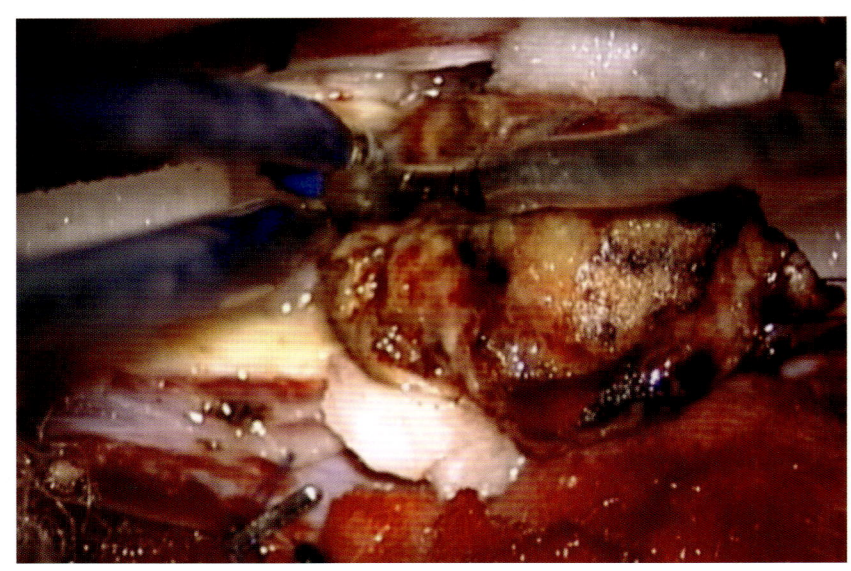

Fig. 73.11 Intraoperative photograph of a clean surgical cavity following gross total tumor resection.

Conclusion

Surgery represents the only established effective primary treatment modality for benign intramedullary neoplasms. Optimization of surgical outcome, therefore, is the most important treatment consideration. Aggressive initial management, appropriate judgment and technique, and adherence to strict microsurgical techniques are the most effective methods of avoiding complications and ensuring an optimal treatment outcome. **Box 73.1** lists the key operative steps.

Box 73.1 Key Operative Steps

- Adequate bone and dural exposure to identify tumor poles
- Identification of the posterior median septum for glial tumors
- Identification of the pial–tumor interface for hemangioblastomas
- Midline myelotomy over entire rostrocaudal extent of solid tumor
- Identify and develop plane between tumor and surrounding spinal cord
- Internal decompression of large glial tumors to facilitate resection
- Complete circumferential release of pial attachment of hemangioblastomas
- Careful closure of all tissue layers to prevent postoperative CSF leak

References

1. Aghakhani N, David P, Parker F, Lacroix C, Benoudiba F, Tadie M. Intramedullary spinal ependymomas: analysis of a consecutive series of 82 adult cases with particular attention to patients with no preoperative neurological deficit. Neurosurgery 2008;62:1279–1285, discussion 1285–1286
2. Lee J, Parsa AT, Ames CP, McCormick PC. Clinical management of intramedullary spinal ependymomas in adults. Neurosurg Clin N Am 2006;17:21–27
3. Raco A, Esposito V, Lenzi J, Piccirilli M, Delfini R, Cantore G. Long-term follow-up of intramedullary spinal cord tumors: a series of 202 cases. Neurosurgery 2005;56:972–981, discussion 972–981
4. Woodworth GF, Chaichana KL, McGirt MJ, et al. Predictors of ambulatory function after surgical resection of intramedullary spinal cord tumors. Neurosurgery 2007;61:99–105, discussion 105–106
5. McCormick PC, Torres R, Post KD, Stein BM. Intramedullary ependymoma of the spinal cord. J Neurosurg 1990;72:523–532
6. Sloof JL, Kernohan JW, MacCarthy CS. Primary Intramedullary Tumors of the Spinal Cord and Filum Terminale. Philadelphia: WB Saunders; 1964
7. Stein BM, McCormick PC. Intramedullary neoplasms and vascular malformations. Clin Neurosurg 1992;39:361–387
8. McCormick PC. Anatomic principles of intradural spinal surgery. Clin Neurosurg 1994;41:204–223
9. Gomez DR, Missett BT, Wara WM, et al. High failure rate in spinal ependymomas with long-term follow-up. Neuro-oncol 2005;7:254–259
10. Whitaker SJ, Bessell EM, Ashley SE, Bloom HJ, Bell BA, Brada M. Postoperative radiotherapy in the management of spinal cord ependymoma. J Neurosurg 1991;74:720–728
11. Lonser RR, Weil RJ, Wanebo JE, DeVroom HL, Oldfield EH. Surgical management of spinal cord hemangioblastomas in patients with von Hippel-Lindau disease. J Neurosurg 2003;98:106–116
12. Rossitch E Jr, Zeidman SM, Burger PC, et al. Clinical and pathological analysis of spinal cord astrocytomas in children. Neurosurgery 1990;27:193–196
13. Sandler HM, Papadopoulos SM, Thornton AF Jr, Ross DA. Spinal cord astrocytomas: results of therapy. Neurosurgery 1992;30:490–493
14. Ogden AT, Fessler RG, O'toole J, et al. Minimally invasive resection of intramedullary ependymoma: case report. Neurosurgery 2009;65:E1203–E1204, discussion E1204
15. Ogden AT, Feldstein NA, McCormick PC. Anterior approach to cervical intramedullary pilocytic astrocytoma. Case report. J Neurosurg Spine 2008;9:253–257
16. Lonser RR, Vortmeyer AO, Butman JA, et al. Edema is a precursor to central nervous system peritumoral cyst formation. Ann Neurol 2005;58:392–399
17. McGirt MJ, Garcés-Ambrossi GL, Parker SL, et al. Short-term progressive spinal deformity following laminoplasty versus laminectomy for resection of intradural spinal tumors: analysis of 238 patients. Neurosurgery 2010;66:1005–1012
18. Sciubba DM, Chaichana KL, Woodworth GF, McGirt MJ, Gokaslan ZL, Jallo GI. Factors associated with cervical instability requiring fusion after cervical laminectomy for intradural tumor resection. J Neurosurg Spine 2008;8:413–419
19. Mandigo C, Ogden FT, Angevine PD, McCormick PC. Intramedullary hemangioblastoma of the spinal cord. Operative Neurosurgery. 2009;65:1166–1177

74 Open Anterolateral Cordotomy

Joshua M. Rosenow

Open anterolateral cordotomy is predicated on the interruption of the spinothalamic and spinoreticular pathways in the anterolateral quadrant of the cord carrying pain inputs to the brain from the periphery. This procedure is intended to preserve the tracts carrying fine touch and proprioception through the dorsal columns. Within the spinothalamic tract, the sacral fibers are located more dorsolaterally and the cervical fibers more ventromedially. Moreover, at any spinal level, axons composing the spinothalamic tract are primarily projections from cells located in the contralateral cord beginning two or three spinal segments below the specific level. Therefore, a lesion should produce pain relief beginning two or three dermatomes below the level of the lesion.

Patient Selection

Patients selected for ablative neurosurgical procedures for the treatment of chronic pain should have significant pain that has failed to adequately respond to multiple other conservative nonsurgical treatments, such as rehabilitation, oral medications (antiinflammatories, narcotics, anticonvulsants, antidepressants), and injections. Typically these patients report an average Visual or Verbal Analogue Scale (VAS) score of greater than 5. Given the advances in neurostimulation and intrathecal drug delivery, it is also reasonable to conduct a trial of these therapies prior to considering ablative procedures. This is true both for patients with pain due to late-stage malignancies (due to their higher medical risk in undergoing surgery) and those with pain from nonmalignant causes (due to the risk of permanent neurologic morbidity from the procedures).

Once the patient is selected, it is just as important to carefully select the correct ablative procedure, considering both the etiology of the pain and its location within the nervous system, so as to maximize the potential pain relief.

Indications and Contraindications

Patients undergoing open cordotomy typically have intractable neuropathic pain of the lower body. Many already have significant motor or sensory deficits in the painful region.

Cordotomy is indicated more frequently for patients with extremity pain rather than pelvic pain. The latter is believed to respond better to midline myelotomy.

Advantages and Disadvantages

Cordotomy is relatively straightforward to perform and involves no device implants. However, its long-term efficacy is limited, especially for nonmalignant pain.[1] Most of the outcomes literature for cordotomy deals with cervical procedures.[2-5] However, of Nagaro et al's[6] series of 45 patients who underwent cordotomy, 33 experienced the development of new pain following cordotomy. In 28 patients, the new pain was in the mirror-image location of the original pain and could often be abolished by blockade of the nerves subserving the original pain.

Choice of Operative Approach

The procedure is typically performed via a laminectomy or hemilaminectomy and intradural exposure.

Preoperative Imaging

Preoperative spinal imaging with computed tomography (CT) or magnetic resonance imaging (MRI) is useful for understanding the patient's spinal anatomy and for determining if there is any baseline rotation or lateral shift in the cord location.

Surgical Procedure

In performing an open cordotomy, intradural exposure is first accomplished after laminectomy, followed by sectioning of the dentate ligament at the appropriate level. Grasping the free end of the dentate ligament enables the surgeon to gently rotate the cord away from the operative side and expose the ventral cord. A cordotomy hook with a 45-degree angle is inserted into the anterolateral quadrant and may be taken to the medial pia before sweeping ventrally. Closure is performed as is routine for any spinal intradural procedure.

Postoperative Care

The postoperative care is similar to that for patients who have undergone other intradural spinal procedures.

Potential Complications and Precautions

It is important to restrict the lesion to the region ventral to the dentate ligament to reduce the risk of inadvertent injury to the corticospinal tract, which is located more dorsally in the lateral spinal cord. Also, care must be taken not to violate the medial pia and risk injury to the anterior spinal vessels, which could cause spinal cord infarction. Attention should be paid to dural closure to avoid postoperative cerebrospinal fluid (CSF) leak.

Conclusion

Open anterolateral cordotomy plays a small role in the treatment of chronic neuropathic pain. Like many ablative procedures, it is probably best suited for those patients with a short life expectancy due to malignant pain, and is typically employed only after several other levels of invasive procedures have failed.

References

1. Jack TM, Lloyd JW. Long-term efficacy of surgical cordotomy in intractable non-malignant pain. Ann R Coll Surg Engl 1983;65:97–102
2. Tasker R. Percutaneous cordotomy for persistent pain. In: Gildenberg P, Tasker R, eds. Textbook of Stereotactic and Functional Neurosurgery, vol 1. New York: McGraw Hill; 1998:1491–1505
3. Kanpolat Y, Savas A, Ucar T, Torun F. CT-guided percutaneous selective cordotomy for treatment of intractable pain in patients with malignant pleural mesothelioma. Acta Neurochir (Wien) 2002;144:595–599, discussion 599
4. Fitzgibbon DR. Percutaneous CT-guided C1-2 cordotomy for intractable cancer pain. Curr Pain Headache Rep 2009;13:253–255
5. Kanpolat Y, Ugur HC, Ayten M, Elhan AH. Computed tomography-guided percutaneous cordotomy for intractable pain in malignancy. Neurosurgery 2009;64(3, Suppl):ons187–ons193, discussion ons193–ons194
6. Nagaro T, Adachi N, Tabo E, Kimura S, Arai T, Dote K. New pain following cordotomy: clinical features, mechanisms, and clinical importance. J Neurosurg 2001;95:425–431

75 Commissural Myelotomy

Joshua M. Rosenow

Commisural myelotomy involves severing the fibers of the spinothalamic tract where they cross the spinal cord in the anterior commissure. It is theorized that interrupting the flow of nociceptive information in this fashion produces analgesia at the spinal level of the myelotomy and just below. However, the extent of pain relief is often larger than would be predicted by the simple neuroanatomy and neurophysiology. This phenomenon is believed to be due to the presence of extralemniscal nociceptive pathways. Given that, even in the most talented of hands, commissural myelotomy does produce some damage to the dorsal columns due to the approach through these fibers and that the dorsal columns already carry multimodality sensory information, this is a leading contender for the location of this collateral pathway.[1-3]

Patient Selection

Myelotomy is considered primarily for patients with intractable pain in the lower body and pelvis that has failed to respond to numerous other medical and interventional techniques.

Indication

Myelotomy is considered primarily for patients with intractable pain in the lower body and pelvis.

Advantages and Disadvantages

Myelotomy, whether performed via an open or percutaneous approach, is a focused procedure that can usually be performed on even the most medically fragile patients. However, like most ablative procedures, the long-term efficacy is limited. Most patients are suffering from intractable malignant pain and have a limited life expectancy following the procedure. In Hirshberg et al's[1] series of eight patients, survival ranged from 3 to 11 months following myelotomy and all eight had significant pain relief up until death. One patient experienced new leg weakness following the procedure. Nauta et al's[2] group of six patients who underwent punctate midline myelotomy had similar results. However, in Kim and Kwon's[4] cohort of eight patients undergoing high thoracic myelotomy for visceral pain from gastric cancer, three developed new pain at other sites (with relief of the preoperative pain) and one developed proprioceptive deficits and paresthesias. Across the published series, the outcomes from punctate and traditional techniques do not differ much.[4-8]

Choice of Operative Approach

The procedure is typically performed via a laminectomy or hemilaminectomy and intradural exposure.

Preoperative Imaging Tests

Preoperative spinal imaging with computed tomography (CT) or magnetic resonance imaging (MRI) is useful for understanding the patient's spinal anatomy and for determining if there is any baseline rotation or lateral shift in the cord location.

Surgical Procedure

The spinal cord is exposed over the spinal neural level (rather than the bony spinal segment) corresponding to the pain. A small probe is inserted just lateral to the fibrous septum in the dorsal midline between the posterior columns (**Fig. 75.1**). Traditionally, this is then used to carefully section the midline crossing fibers until the anterior cleft of the cord is noted, taking care not to injure the ventrally located anterior spinal artery and other epidural veins. For lower body and pelvic pain, the cord is often exposed via a T9 or T10 laminectomy.

Nauta et al[2] started a trend of surgeons reducing the exposure and depth of dissection required for this procedure. In their technique, which may be performed either openly or stereotactically, a single punctate lesion is made in the dorsal midline of the cord. Given the theory that pain relief from this procedure is due to the lesioning of a dorsal column nociceptive pathway, some surgeons perform bilateral lesions of the paramedian dorsal columns without sectioning of the deeper midline crossing fibers.[9]

Closure is performed in the routine fashion for spinal intradural procedures.

Postoperative Care

The postoperative care is similar to that for patients who have undergone other intradural spinal procedures.

Potential Complications and Precautions

Care must be taken not to injure the anterior spinal vessels when crossing through the midline commissure. Moreover, because the lesion pathway traverses the dorsal columns, it is not unusual for patients to have at least temporary disturbances of dorsal column function.

Conclusion

Midline myelotomy plays a small role in the treatment of chronic neuropathic pain. Like many ablative procedures, it is probably best suited for those patients with a short life expectancy due to malignant pain and is typically employed only after several other levels of invasive procedures have failed.

References

1. Hirshberg RM, Al-Chaer ED, Lawand NB, Westlund KN, Willis WD. Is there a pathway in the posterior funiculus that signals visceral pain? Pain 1996;67:291–305
2. Nauta HJ, Soukup VM, Fabian RH, et al. Punctate midline myelotomy for the relief of visceral cancer pain. J Neurosurg 2000;92(2, Suppl):125–130
3. Vierck CJ Jr, Hamilton DM, Thornby JI. Pain reactivity of monkeys after lesions to the dorsal and lateral columns of the spinal cord. Exp Brain Res 1971;13:140–158
4. Kim YS, Kwon SJ. High thoracic midline dorsal column myelotomy for severe visceral pain due to advanced stomach cancer. Neurosurgery 2000;46:85–90, discussion 90–92
5. Fascendini A, Biroli F, Cassinari V. Critical evaluation of commissural myelotomy in the treatment of intractable pain. J Neurosurg Sci 1979;23:265–272
6. Gildenberg PL. Myelotomy and percutaneous cervical cordotomy for the treatment of cancer pain. Appl Neurophysiol 1984;47:208–215
7. Hwang SL, Lin CL, Lieu AS, et al. Punctate midline myelotomy for intractable visceral pain caused by hepatobiliary or pancreatic cancer. J Pain Symptom Manage 2004;27:79–84
8. Vilela Filho O, Araujo MR, Florencio RS, Silva MA, Silveira MT. CT-guided percutaneous punctate midline myelotomy for the treatment of intractable visceral pain: a technical note. Stereotact Funct Neurosurg 2001;77:177–182
9. Gildenberg PL, Hirshberg RM. Limited myelotomy for the treatment of intractable cancer pain. J Neurol Neurosurg Psychiatry 1984;47:94–96

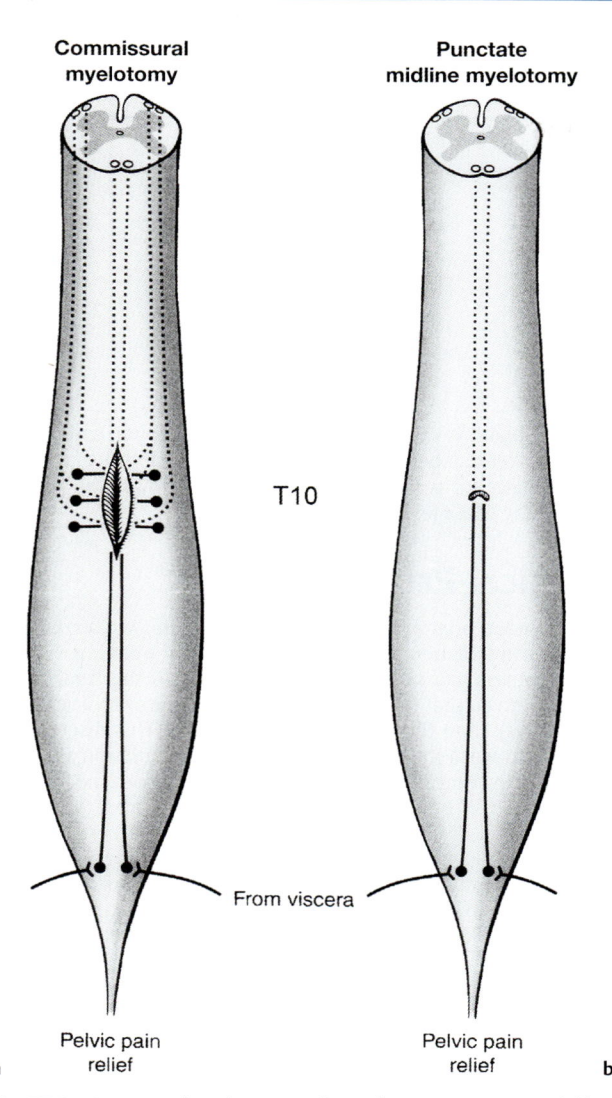

Fig. 75.1 Commisural myelotomy performed at various rostrocaudal levels. **(a)** In the past, commissural myelotomies were performed with the intent of eliminating crossing fibers of the spinothalamic tract segmentally for relief of pain. In addition to lesioning the portion of the spinothalamic tract crossing at the site of the lesion, the commissural myelotomy would also interrupt the pelvic pain pathway traveling in the midline. **(b)** Punctate midline myelotomy eliminates only the ascending pelvic visceral pain pathway, leaving the spinothalamic tract and most of the dorsal column intact.

76 Thoracic DREZ Operation

Joshua M. Rosenow

The dorsal horn of the spinal cord is an important relay center and integration site for sensory information. Sindou,[1,2] via coagulation in 1972, and Nashold,[3-8] via radiofrequency (RF) energy in 1974, lesioned the dorsal root entry zone (DREZ) of the spinal cord as a method of destroying the portions of the central nervous system involved in the central sensitization that perpetuates neuropathic pain following a peripheral lesion such as a nerve injury. The procedure is intended to destroy Lissauer's tract and preserve fibers subserving proprioception and certain aspects of touch that travel in the dorsal rootlets to the dorsal columns.

Larger series report reasonable rates of pain control. Dreval et al[9] published results of 124 patients with brachial plexus avulsion pain followed a mean of 47.5 months after DREZ and reported an 87% rate of good pain control. This has traditionally been the main indication for DREZ lesioning, and most series for this indication note good pain relief in a majority of patients (usually between 50% and 80% of the cohort). The limited series of results of DREZ lesioning for phantom limb pain show less favorable outcomes (14 to 67% good pain relief). The outcomes for DREZ lesioning when used for pain due to spinal cord injury and for truncal postherpetic pain are similar.[10]

Patient Selection

The DREZ lesioning is most commonly used in the cervical region for treatment of pain due to traumatic brachial plexus root avulsions. In the thoracic region, it may also be used for the treatment of pain due to sacral plexus avulsion, stump pain, or postherpetic neuralgia. A trial of spinal cord stimulation for this pain may be considered prior to performing an ablative procedure such as thoracic DREZ.

Indications

Thoracic DREZ is indicated for patients with intractable neuropathic pain in the thoracic region and lower extremities.

Advantages and Disadvantages

The DREZ procedure needs to be performed in an exacting fashion so as to only ablate the dorsal horn without creating a lesion that spreads to the adjacent spinal cord tracts, most significantly the lateral corticospinal tract located just ventral to the dorsal horn. Like other ablative procedures, the usefulness of DREZ lesioning for benign pain may be limited in the long term. Moreover, care must be taken to lesion the correct spinal segments. In the thoracic region, the dorsal rootlets converge to form the dorsal root, which exits one or two vertebral levels lower. This discrepancy increases toward the conus. DREZ does not involve an implanted device, so it may be a better choice for some individuals with thoracic radicular pain who are considered unsuitable for an implant. However, the ease of a trial of spinal cord stimulation, better risk benefit profile, and the reversibility of the procedure auger for consideration of a trial of stimulation prior to performing DREZ lesioning.

Surgical Procedure

The intended anatomic levels are exposed first via a complete laminectomy or hemilaminectomy and dural opening. As previously stated, consideration must be given to the levels to be lesioned, given that the dorsal root may exit one or two vertebral levels lower than the intended level of DREZ. This discrepancy increases toward the conus. Intraoperative stimulation and neuromonitoring may be used to identify rootlets from specific dermatomes to either include or exclude them from lesioning. Microsurgical dissection of the dorsal rootlets is performed to separate and isolate them from each other. After identifying the correct anatomic levels, either by electrical stimulation or by the presence of avulsed rootlets, lesions are created on the inferolateral aspect of the rootlet entry zone. The small lightly or unmyelinated fibers that carry pain signals to the dorsal horn enter from the lateral aspect of the DREZ, whereas the medial side contains primarily those fibers destined for the dorsal columns. Lesions are created either by coagulating and opening the pia on the lateral aspect of the dorsal rootlets followed by microbipolar coagulation of the DREZ (Sindou's method) or by using a DREZ RF needle (0.25-mm diameter) to make 1-mm spaced lesions at 75°C for 15 seconds (**Fig. 76.1**). Laser[11,12] and ultrasonically[9] created lesions have also been described.

Closure is performed in the routine fashion for spinal intradural procedures.

Postoperative Care

The postoperative care is the same as for patients who have undergone other intradural spinal procedures.

Potential Complications and Precautions

The most significant complication is the creation of a motor deficit. Great care must be exercised in targeting DREZ lesions due to the presence of the corticospinal tract just anterolateral to the dorsal horn. Moreover, the size and angulation of the DREZ and dorsal horn vary depending on the spinal level, being much thinner in the thoracic region. To minimize this risk, the location and depth of entry of the lesioning needle or the microbipolar must be carefully controlled. Moreover, the inherently tenuous vascular supply to the spinal cord must not be disrupted. Motor complications range from 0 to 69%.[10]

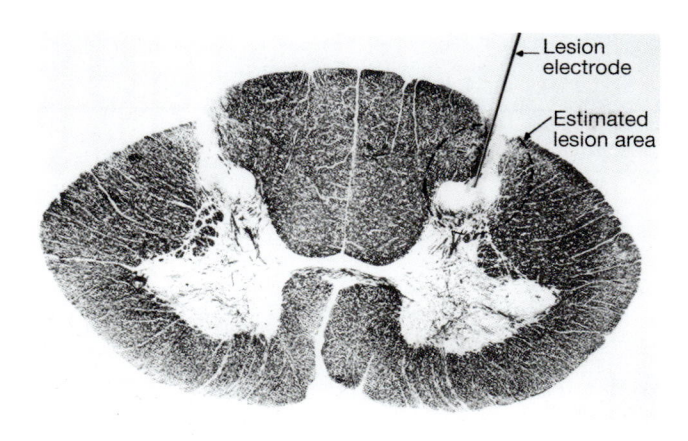

Fig. 76.1 Cross-section of the human cervical spinal cord. Note the dorsal root entry zone (DREZ) electrode tract and the estimated radiofrequency (RF) lesion size.

Closer to the conus, the risk of including unintended rootlets in the lesions increases due to the more tightly packed arrangement of the rootlets for the lower extremities and sacral nerves in this region. It may be difficult to lesion those rootlets from target regions in the legs and perineum without causing bladder or bowel dysfunction.

Conclusion

Thoracic DREZ maintains a small role in the treatment of chronic neuropathic pain. Like many ablative procedures, it is probably best suited for those patients with a short life expectancy due to malignant pain and is typically employed only after several other levels of invasive procedures have failed. For pain in the regions typically treated by thoracic DREZ, a trial of spinal cord stimulation should be considered prior to performing this procedure.

References

1. Sindou M. Drez lesions for brachial plexus injury. Neurosurgery 1988;23: 528
2. Sindou M, Jeanmonod D. Microsurgical DREZ-otomy for the treatment of spasticity and pain in the lower limbs. Neurosurgery 1989;24:655–670
3. Nashold BS Jr. Modification of DREZ lesion technique. J Neurosurg 1981;55:1012
4. Nashold BS Jr. Current status of the DREZ operation: 1984. Neurosurgery 1984;15:942–944
5. Nashold BS Jr. Neurosurgical technique of the dorsal root entry zone operation. Appl Neurophysiol 1988;51:136–145
6. Nashold BS Jr, Friedman A, Bullitt E. The status of dorsal root entry zone lesions in 1987. Clin Neurosurg 1989;35:422–428
7. Nashold BS Jr, Ostdahl RH. Dorsal root entry zone lesions for pain relief. J Neurosurg 1979;51:59–69
8. Nashold BS Jr, Ostdahl RH. Pain relief after dorsal root entry zone lesions. Acta Neurochir Suppl (Wien) 1980;30:383–389
9. Dreval ON. Ultrasonic DREZ-operations for treatment of pain due to brachial plexus avulsion. Acta Neurochir (Wien) 1993;122:76–81
10. Iskandar BJ, Nashold BS. Spinal and trigeminal DREZ lesions. In: Gildenberg P, Tasker R, eds. Textbook of Stereotactic and Functional Neurosurgery, vol 1. New York: McGraw Hill; 1998:1573–1583
11. Sindou M. Laser-induced DREZ lesions. J Neurosurg 1984;60:870–871
12. Young RF. Laser versus radiofrequency lesions of the DREZ. J Neurosurg 1986;64:341

77 Caudalis DREZ

Joshua M. Rosenow

For the treatment of facial pain, so-called caudalis dorsal root entry zone (DREZ) lesions may be made in the trigeminal nucleus caudalis. This is essentially a cranial continuation of the dorsal horn, extending from the brainstem down into the upper cervical spinal cord, and it receives much of the nociceptive signaling from the trigeminal system. As pioneered by Bernard et al,[1] these lesions are made from the upper rootlets of C2 to a point just above the obex. In the nucleus caudalis, the zones of the face are represented in an "onion skin" pattern of concentric circular dermatomes, with the most central facial regions represented most cranially toward the obex and the most peripheral regions of the face represented more caudally towards C1. The nucleus caudalis is wider (2 mm diameter) at the obex but only 1.5 mm wide at C2.

Caudalis DREZ procedure was initially associated with a high incidence of postoperative ataxia (up to 90%) due to the location of the nucleus caudalis approximately 1.2 mm deep to the surface of the cerebellum and just deep to the spinocerebellar tract. Nashold[2,3] developed angled, radiofrequency (RF) needles with a proximal insulated portion specifically for this procedure that protected this pathway from damage during lesioning of the nucleus caudalis, reducing the ataxia complication rate to 39%. In contrast to spinal DREZ, the best indication for caudalis DREZ is postherpetic facial pain (71% good to excellent relief in the Duke series). However, this procedure is rarely performed now.

Patient Selection

Patients considered candidates for caudalis DREZ procedures typically have neuropathic facial pain, such as that caused by trigeminal nerve injury/deafferentation, either unintentional or iatrogenic as part of the treatment of trigeminal neuralgia (including anesthesia dolorosa) or postherpetic neuralgia. Patients with deafferentation pain due to the resection of malignancy may also be considered candidates.[4]

Indications and Contraindications

Caudalis DREZ lesioning may be considered for those patients with neuropathic facial pain. Given the risks and outcomes from the procedure, patients should have failed multiple other interventional and medical treatments prior to undergoing caudalis DREZ lesioning. Patients who have a significant nociceptive component to their pain (such as many patients with malignancies) may not obtain as much relief from the procedure.

Advantages and Disadvantages

Like other central ablative procedures, the reported short- and long-term results of caudalis DREZ are highly variable, and the overall number of patients reported is small. Upper limb ataxia/dysmetria continues to be a significant risk, even though insulated electrodes have reduced the incidence of this complication.

Surgical Procedure

A small suboccipital craniectomy is performed, along with C1 and C2 laminectomies. After opening the dura, the nucleus caudalis is identified. The nucleus caudalis lies between the dorsolateral sulcus and the exiting accessory nerve rootlets (**Figs. 77.1 and 77.2**). The DREZ of C2 may be used as reference for line of lesions toward the obex, as the nucleus blends with the C2 DREZ. Using an angled, partially insulated caudalis DREZ needle (**Fig. 77.3**), lesions are made from the C2 DREZ cranially to the obex. They are most often created by lesioning at 75°C for 15 seconds each. Lesions are separated by 1 mm over a total distance of approximately 20 mm.

Potential Complications and Precautions

As previously indicated, the spinocerebellar tract lies superficial to the nucleus caudalis, especially in its more rostral portions. Lesions of the deeper nucleus caudalis often also affect this overlying tract as well, causing upper extremity dysmetria and ataxia. The introduction of electrodes with proximal insulation to selectively lesion the deeper structures has significantly reduced this problem. Care must be taken to avoid lesioning the exiting rootlets of cranial nerve XI as well.

77 Caudalis DREZ

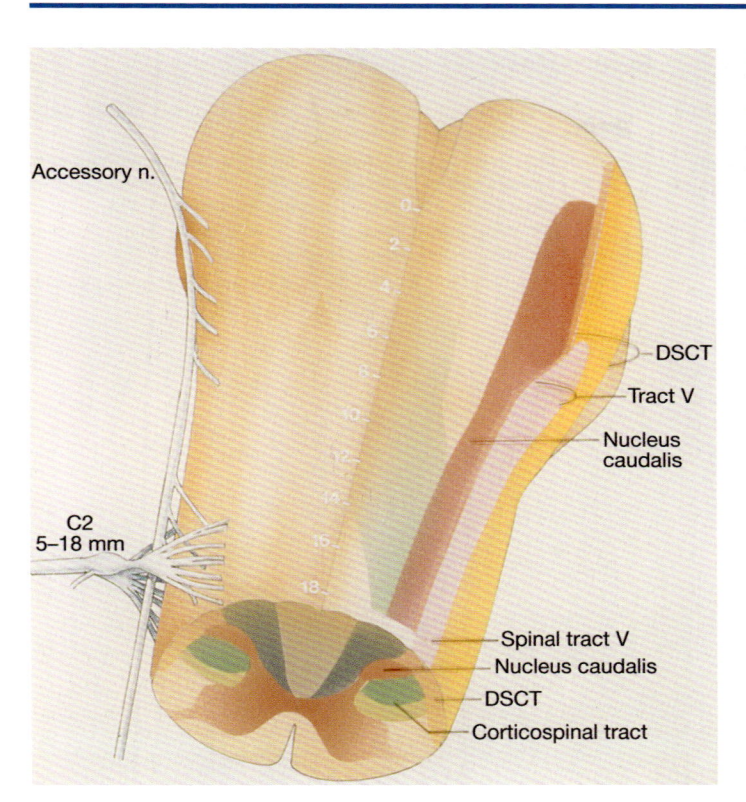

Fig. 77.1 The anatomy of the sensory and motor tracts at the cervicomedullary junction: dorsal view. Note the shape and size of the caudalis nucleus *(red)*. The nucleus is smaller in cross section at the level of the C2 dorsal root, and as it ascends rostrally to the region of the obex the caudalis nucleus doubles its cross-sectional diameter. This difference in size is the reason for using the two different types of caudalis DREZ electrodes to ensure that the nucleus is destroyed at the various spinal levels. Note the close proximity of the cortical spinal tract, which must be avoided in the lesioning. DSCT, dorsal spinocerebellar tract.

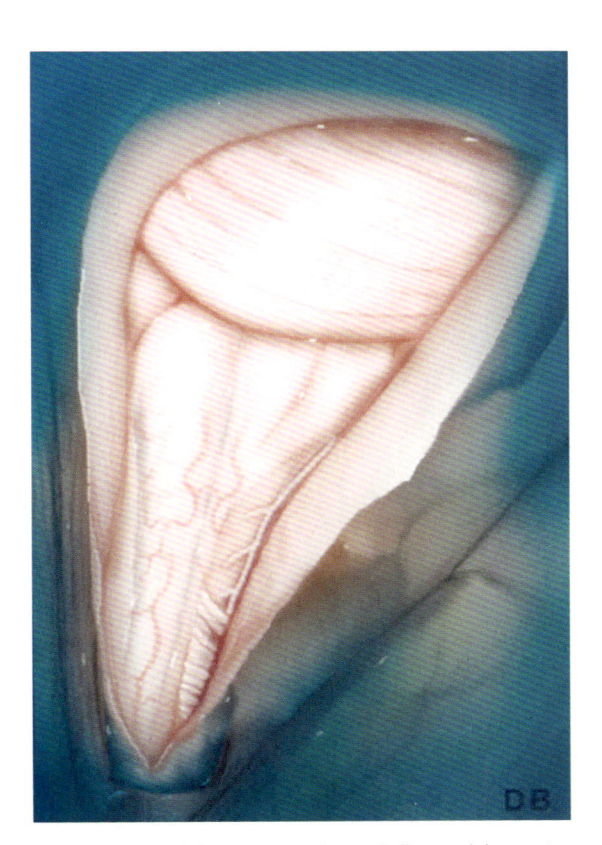

Fig. 77.2 The opened dura exposing the cerebellum and the cervicomedullary junction. Note the dorsal root of C2 and the spinal accessory nerve with its individual rootlets originating from the side of the cervical cord. The caudalis nucleus lies in the small zone between the C2 dorsal root and the origins of the spinal accessory rootlets.

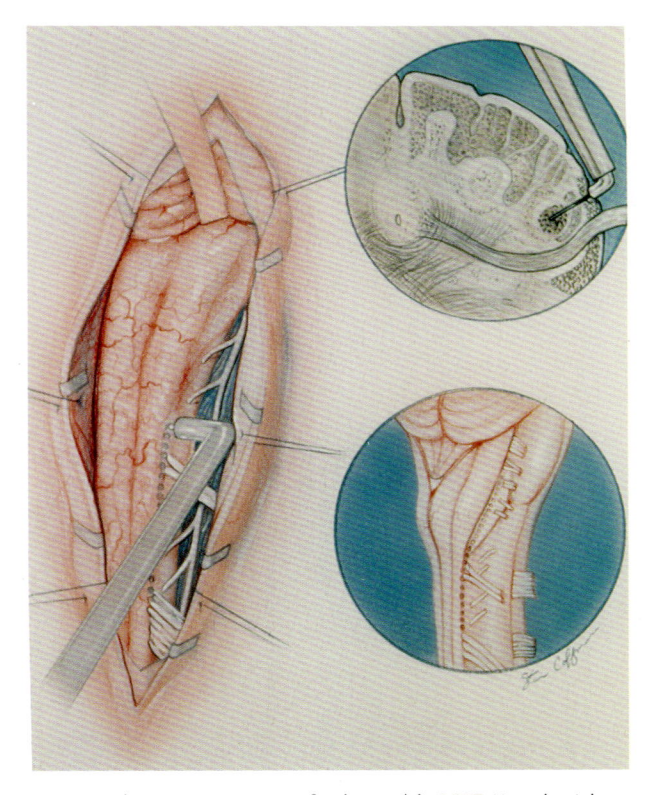

Fig. 77.3 The operative exposure for the caudalis DREZ. Note the right-angle DREZ electrode on the circular insert. Note the line of the lesions just below the caudalis DREZ electrode and its relationship to the cervical dorsal roots and the spinal accessory rootlets. In the *upper right circular inset,* the electrode can be seen as it is introduced into the spinal cord with the tip of the electrode in the caudalis nucleus.

Conclusion

Although not commonly used, certain ablative neurosurgical techniques continue to have a role in the management of medically intractable pain. Moreover, they have a role to play in our understanding of the pathophysiology behind the generation and maintenance of chronic pain states. With the rise in neurostimulation as a treatment of many types of neuropathic pain, there is significant concern that some of these valuable treatments will be lost forever. Physicians who treat chronic pain must continue to be trained in these procedures to ensure that they continue to be available for carefully selected patient populations. It is even more important for the neurosurgical community not to lose the experience in performing these procedures in an era of device implants for neurostimulation and intrathecal drug delivery.

References

1. Bernard EJ Jr, Nashold BS Jr, Caputi F, Moossy JJ. Nucleus caudalis DREZ lesions for facial pain. Br J Neurosurg 1987;1:81–91
2. Nashold BS Jr, el-Naggar AO, Ovelmen-Levitt J, Abdul-Hak M. A new design of radiofrequency lesion electrodes for use in the caudalis nucleus DREZ operation. Technical note. J Neurosurg 1994;80:1116–1120
3. Young JN, Nashold BS Jr, Cosman ER. A new insulated caudalis nucleus DREZ electrode. Technical note. J Neurosurg 1989;70:283–284
4. Nucleus caudalis DREZ for facial pain due to cancer. Br J Neurosurg 1990;4:81–82

78 Shunt Placement for Syringomyelia

Ulrich Batzdorf and Langston T. Holly

Aside from aspiration at surgery, shunting of syringomyelic cavities is the oldest technique employed for treating this disorder. The procedures were developed before our current level of understanding of the pathophysiology, aided particularly by magnetic resonance imaging. Although the shunt devices have been refined over the years, particularly shunt valves, and hemilaminectomy has supplanted laminectomy in many instances, the overall concepts of diverting accumulations of cerebrospinal fluid (CSF)-like fluid into a space from which the fluid can be absorbed into the body have not changed.

Syringomyelia is now believed to develop when there is a partial obstruction of the subarachnoid space in the spinal canal,[1] similar to that observed at the craniocervical junction. The pulsatile CSF, encountering this partial resistance to flow, more readily courses along the Virchow-Robin spaces[2] to enter the spinal cord, forming an intramedullary cavity. The possibility that persistence of the central canal in some individuals facilitates this fluid accumulation has been raised by Milhorat et al.[3] Differences in the timing and degree of involution of the central canal may explain why syringomyelia does not always develop in all individuals with spinal cord injury,[4] as is also true for patients with Chiari malformation.

> **Box 78.1 Focal Obstruction of CSF Flow**
>
> - Craniocervical junction
>   - Tonsillar ectopia, also called hindbrain descent (HBD) and Chiari malformation
>   - Membranous obstruction at the level of the foramen magnum, "Chiari 0 malformation," or obstruction at the outlet of the fourth ventricle
> - Primary spinal
>   - Arachnoid cyst
>   - Focal traumatic scar
>   - Tumor obstruction of the subarachnoid space
>
> **Diffuse Arachnoid Scarring with Obstruction of CSF Flow**
> - Primary spinal
>   - Postmeningitic
>   - Post–subarachnoid hemorrhage, including traumatic hemorrhage
>   - Postsurgical

Patient Selection

Shunting is recommended for patients with syringomyelia when an alternative procedure that would have the potential of restoring more normal physiological conditions is not feasible or when such a procedure has been performed and has failed. In planning treatment, it is important to consider the nature of the partial obstruction to CSF flow, whether it is focal or diffuse. Patients with syringomyelia may thus be considered under the categories listed in **Box 78.1**.

The extent and density of scar tissue formation varies with individuals, even under similar provocative circumstances, and may also have genetic determinants.

The distinction between focal and diffuse subarachnoid obstruction is important because it is now generally considered best to treat patients with focal obstruction of the subarachnoid space (SAS) with surgical procedures aimed at relieving this obstruction. This includes posterior fossa decompression (PFD) for tonsillar ectopia/hindbrain descent and resection of arachnoid membranes in the spine in primary spinal syringomyelia (PSS). In the great majority of such patients, the syrinx cavity does not re-form.

Diffuse arachnoid scarring poses a different challenge, and in many of these patients the interference with normal cerebrospinal fluid (CSF) flow extends over several vertebral levels and may also be nearly circumferential. Shunting would be considered for these patients and, as noted above, for patients in whom focal decompression has failed to arrest progression or achieve reduction of the syrinx cavity. Shunting may also be indicated when patient age or general health would make the less formidable shunting procedure preferable to PFD or a more complex spinal procedure.

Indications and Contraindications

Shunting of a syrinx cavity should be considered in the setting of progressive neurologic deficit, which may be inherent in the history as presented by the patient, or may be apparent to the physician on sequential examination of the patient over time. Unequivocal enlargement of the syrinx cavity over time on imaging studies should also be considered an indication for intervention, inasmuch as shunting might prevent or minimize more serious neurologic problems in these patients. As with any surgical procedure, the patient's expectations should be discussed and clarified by the surgeon. Limb atrophy, including hand atrophy, may stabilize but is very unlikely to improve. Likewise, sensory deficits may stabilize but not improve. Pain alone, particularly neuropathic pain, is not a good indication for shunting because it is not very likely to respond. The overall aim of shunting should be to stabilize the patient's neurologic condition. It is generally accepted that shunting will result in decreased filling of the syringomyelic cavity. In younger patients, collapse or near-collapse of the cavity may be seen on imaging after an appropriate time interval. In older patients, imaging may show only partial collapse of the cavity with widening of the SAS in the area of the syrinx. These differences presumably are the result of differences in tissue elasticity with age.

Hydromyelic cavities, which represent persistence of the central canal of the spinal cord, do not enlarge the cord and are not considered the source of clinical symptoms. Shunting is therefore not indicated when this is clearly the diagnosis.

Advantages and Disadvantages

The advantages and disadvantages of shunting can only be considered in relation to alternative strategies. As noted above, whenever a more physiological approach that would restore obstructed CSF circulation to normal is available, it is the preferable approach. The advantage of shunting is that it is relatively simple technically and may be performed through a hemilaminectomy, with minimal risk of spinal instability. Another advantage is that, following shunting, decompression of the syrinx cavity should be immediate, whereas reduction of the syrinx cavity following decompression procedures may take place over time (**Figs. 78.1 and 78.2**).

The greatest disadvantage of syrinx shunting is that shunts may fail. Shunts for syringomyelia have a failure rate that may approach 50% over 5 years following surgery. It is inherent in shunting that the syrinx cavity may collapse around the openings of the shunt tubing, thereby causing the shunt to obstruct. Shunt tubes are also subject to kinking, and shunts may become disconnected or dislodged, particularly with vigorous exercise. It must also be recognized that shunts are foreign object implants.

Choice of Operative Approach

Three general approaches are available for syrinx shunting. Placement of the shunt into the spinal cord is common to them all, but the approaches differ with respect to location of the distal end of the shunt, which may be placed to drain into

1. the spinal subarachnoid space (intrathecal),
2. the peritoneal cavity, or
3. the pleural cavity.

The advantages of intrathecal placement of the distal end of the tubing is that the entire procedure can be performed through a single incision, with the patient in the prone position on the operating table. It is not suitable for patients who have had very diffuse scarring of the SAS, such as one may see after meningitis or subarachnoid hemorrhage, because CSF may not be absorbed adequately in such situations. With this exception, it is our preferred approach.

Peritoneal placement of the distal shunt tube is relatively simple but requires that either the cord exposure be performed with the patient in the lateral position on the table, or that the patient be turned from prone to lateral during the procedure. The assistance of a general surgeon in placing the peritoneal end of the tubing may be helpful. Peritoneal shunt placement should not be performed in patients who have a past history of peritonitis or have a known tendency to form abdominal adhesions.

Pleural cavity placement of the distal end of the shunt, such as intrathecal placement, can be performed with the patient remaining in the prone position on the operating table. It requires temporary collapse of one lung and is therefore not recommended for patients with pulmonary problems.

Preoperative Imaging

Magnetic resonance imaging (MRI) is the generally accepted diagnostic technique for establishing the presence and extent of a syringomyelic cavity. It is important to establish the full extent of a syrinx cavity, that is, whether it is confined to the cervical

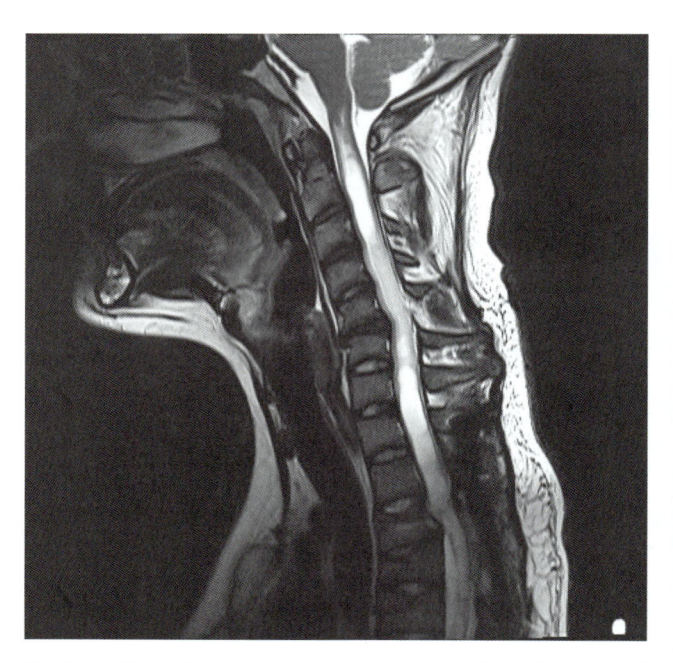

Fig. 78.1 T2-weighted magnetic resonance imaging (MRI) of the cervical spine showing a large syrinx cavity that developed following severe spine trauma at T3-T4. The syrinx cavity extended into the upper thoracic spinal cord.

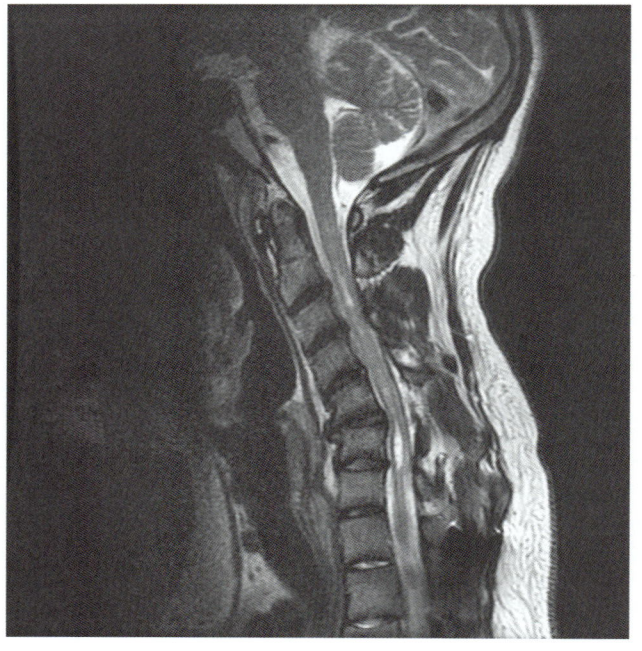

Fig. 78.2 Same patient as in **Fig. 78.1**. T2-weighted MRI of the cervical spine following thoracic laminectomy and placement of a syringoperitoneal shunt. Note the significant reduction in the size of the syrinx cavity.

78 Shunt Placement for Syringomyelia

usually near the site of trauma.[5] Because such shunts, in essence, drain the SAS by way of the syrinx cavity, a shunt valve is required to avoid intracranial hypotension. Another rare situation is a patient with a very high cervical cord obstructive syringomyelia, such as may be seen with high cervical cord injuries. Because of the risks to respiration with a high cervical cord myelotomy, valved shunting of the SAS rostral to the obstruction, instead of shunting the syrinx cavity itself, may be a safer alternative.[6] Shunting is not indicated for patients with a slit-like cavity of the cord, which really is a residual central canal.[7]

Techniques

Placement of the proximal (i.e., spinal) portion of the syrinx shunt catheter is independent of the location of distal shunt placement. A major consideration regarding the location of the myelotomy incision for placement of the shunt catheter is to minimize new or additional neurologic deficit and is discussed below. Broad-spectrum antibiotics are administered at the time of incision for all shunting procedures. Strict asepsis is essential.

Spinal Portion

Exposure of the Spinal Cord

Traditionally, shunts have been placed into the spinal cord exposed through a full laminectomy over the area intended for shunt placement. In many patients, however, it is possible to place the shunt through a hemilaminectomy, thereby leaving the spinous process and interspinous ligament, as well as the paraspinous muscles on the opposite side, intact.[8] These are important considerations in the effort to minimize spine deformity that may result from laminectomy in patients with syringomyelia. The level chosen for placement of the shunt tip is usually near the caudal end of the syrinx cavity. The spinal level, as determined on imaging studies, should be verified with an intraoperative radiograph. The choice of the entry point into the cord (discussed below) determines whether the midline of the cord needs to be exposed, or whether a lateral paramedian approach is selected. By drilling away some bone at the base of the spinous process from the hemilaminectomy approach, we have found it possible to expose the midline of the spinal cord through a unilateral approach. Some surgeons prefer to confirm the location of the syrinx cavity with intraoperative ultrasound, once the dura has been exposed.

Myelotomy

The myelotomy for shunt placement is most commonly performed through a midline incision near the lower end of the syrinx cavity, with two possible exceptions. If imaging studies show that the syrinx cavity is very eccentric and is of smaller size in the midline of the spinal cord, it may be well to take this into account and place the myelotomy incision over a wider portion of the syrinx. A second consideration pertains to patients who have profound long-standing sensory loss on one side in a distribution that corresponds anatomically to the level of the syrinx cavity intended for drainage. On the assumption that sensory recovery in this situation is very unlikely, myelotomies for shunt insertion have been placed in the dorsal root entry zone region on the side of sensory loss. The midline is often more difficult to identify in a cord with syringomyelia than would be true for a normal cord. The subtle dorsal raphe will be flattened by pressure from within the cord and can best be identified by noting the angulated course of blood vessels entering, or emanating from, the midline of the cord. The incision into the cord should

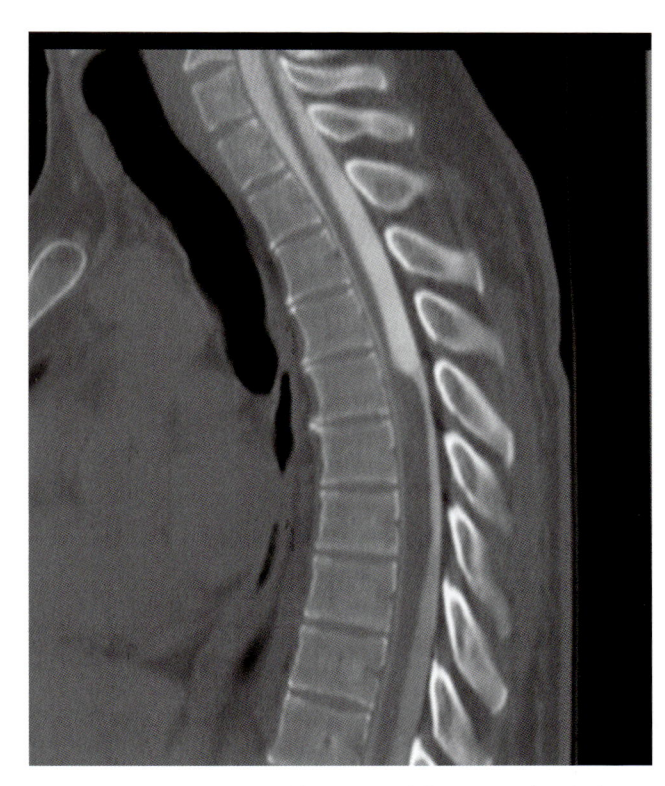

Fig. 78.3 Computed tomography (CT) scan following intrathecal administration of radiopaque contrast material via a C1-C2 puncture demonstrates a focal subarachnoid block at T5. The syrinx cavity was located just below this level.

region, or extends into the thoracic cord. In general, it is best to drain a syrinx cavity near the caudal end of the cavity. Axial MRI scans should also be checked for eccentric localization of the cavity and for evidence of longitudinal septation of the syrinx. When the syrinx cavity is compartmentalized in such a manner, separate shunting of separate cavities may be necessary. MRI may show the characteristic configuration of the SAS, pointing to the presence of an arachnoid cyst, and may also show evidence of diffuse arachnoid scarring. It is also essential in establishing the differential diagnosis between true syringomyelia and a tumor-related cyst as well as hydromyelia. High-resolution T2-weighted MRI scans have been helpful in defining the presence of septa in some instances. When there is doubt about the exact anatomic level of a subarachnoid obstruction or about the extent of an adhesive process, myelography followed by computed tomography (CT) of the region of interest may be extremely helpful (**Fig. 78.3**). Myelography with CT has also proven helpful in unclear cases to be certain that we are not dealing with a focal obstruction of the SAS, and, in rare cases, has established the diagnosis of idiopathic spinal cord herniation associated with a syrinx cavity.

Surgical Procedures

As detailed above, shunting is generally reserved for patients who have diffuse arachnoid scarring and patients who have syringomyelia in the absence of any documentable obstruction of the SAS, including those who failed decompressive surgery. Shunt systems for syringomyelia are generally without a valve because CSF pressure from the syrinx cavity is low. An exception is the rare posttraumatic syrinx cavity that has ruptured into the SAS, be small, so as to avoid CSF leakage around the tubing. The tubing should fit snugly into the opening. Use of a No. 11 scalpel blade, sometimes deepened with a No. 18 gauge spinal needle, will accomplish this. It is recognized the even the smallest incision, placed in the midline, may give rise to a small, usually segmental, sensory deficit.

Shunt Tube

A variety of biocompatible tubes have been used for syrinx shunts. The essential features of the shunt tubing are as follows:

- Small diameter, so as to minimize pressure on the adjacent cord tissue
- Multiple openings, to reduce the risk of shunt failure due to plugging of the drainage opening
- Ease of introduction, which requires either a certain degree of stiffness of the shunt material, or the ability to insert a temporary stiffener, such as nylon wire, during tip introduction

Ease of shunt tubing withdrawal might be another consideration, although it is recognized that if a shunt has stopped functioning as a result of glial ingrowth into the openings of the intracavitary portion of the tubing, it may be safer to amputate the shunt tube and insert a new one, rather than pulling too firmly on the shunt. The shunt tubing should be anchored to the pia and dura with a suture. In general, more complex shunt designs, such as T-shunts are to be avoided. T-shaped shunts have occasionally been shown to be able to twist around the exiting limb of the shunt, thereby occluding the drainage and causing cord trauma.[9] The dura needs to be well approximated, and a collagen sponge impregnated with fibrin glue is placed over the durotomy. Careful layer-by-layer soft tissue closure reduces the likelihood of wound complications.

A reduced tip lumbar drainage catheter with an outside diameter (OD) of 1.5 mm and a distal tube OD of 2.5 mm has worked well in our hands. Connectors used between segments of the shunt should be secured with a ligature placed around the tubing over the groove in the connector.

Distal Shunt Placement

Intrathecal

The distal end of the shunt tubing may be placed into the SAS, usually just caudal to the exit of the shunt tube from the cord (see Video 78.1). A single opening at the distal end of the tubing suffices. Placement of the tube anterior to the dentate ligament has proved most satisfactory[8] (**Figs. 78.4, 78.5, 78.6**). This approach should not be used when there is extensive obliteration of the SAS, such as may occur following meningitis or subarachnoid hemorrhage, because resorption of CSF from a scarred SAS may be problematic.

The advantage of this approach, when there are no contraindications, is that it requires only a single incision, placed in the dorsal midline.

Pleural

Placement of the distal shunt tube into the pleural cavity was described by Williams and Page[10] and is a useful technique. Repeated expansion of the chest cavity creates some negative pressure, which aids the flow of CSF. The fact that this procedure can be performed without moving the patient from the prone position for the laminectomy and the first step of the shunt placement is an advantage. The need to partially collapse the lung as the pleural space is entered is a disadvantage in patients with respiratory compromise. There also may be patients who had pleural or chest infections or other pulmonary problems in whom this procedure is contraindicated.

Technically, it is not a difficult procedure to perform. The shunt tube coming from the midline spinal incision is tied off and tunneled subcutaneously to a rib interspace over the posterior thorax. An incision is made ~ 8 to 10 cm from the midline and is carried down to the pleura with a muscle-splitting technique. The pleural cavity is entered while the anesthesiologist briefly holds the patient's respiration and the lung remains deflated. The shunt tube, of the usual 2.5-mm diameter with a single distal opening, is placed into the pleural cavity. To avoid an air lock, it is preferable to fill this tube with saline before connecting it to the syrinx drainage tube; 10 cm of tubing in the pleural cavity should suffice. The tube from the pleural cavity is attached to the tube from the spinal incision over a shunt connector, secured with silk ties. The system should be secured to the muscle or other soft tissue in the region of this second (i.e., thoracic) incision.

Peritoneal

Placement of the distal tube into the peritoneal cavity[11] requires that the laminectomy or hemilaminectomy be performed with the patient in the lateral position, so that the abdomen can be cleansed and draped simultaneously with the spinal and incision. The potentially greater risks of wound infection if the patient has to be turned during the procedure are obvious. A small (2–3 cm) flank incision, approximately in the axillary line, and located so it can be readily accessed even if the patient is turned, is used in either situation, and the shunt tubing is brought out

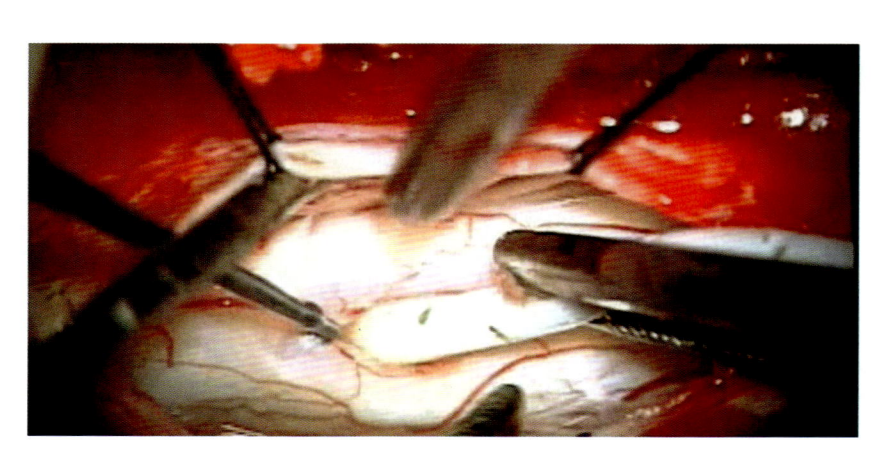

Fig. 78.4 Placement of a syringosubarachnoid shunt, with insertion of the reduced tip of the shunt into the syrinx cavity.

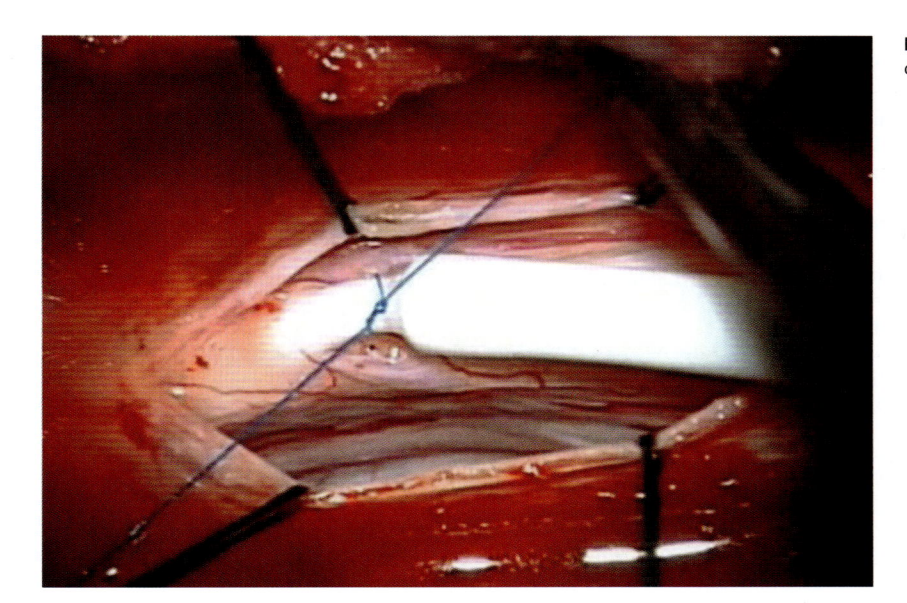

Fig. 78.5 The shunt has been inserted. An anchoring suture attaches the tubing to the pia mater.

from the spinal incision to the flank incision using a shunt passer. The distal end of the tubing should be tied off temporarily until it is ready to be inserted into the peritoneal cavity.

The abdominal incision (~ 10 cm in length) is generally made just below the level of the umbilicus, lateral to the rectus sheath. The external oblique muscle is divided sharply, parallel to its fibers, and the internal oblique and transverse abdominal muscles are spread bluntly, exposing the peritoneum. The peritoneum is incised sharply, making only a small incision. Using the shunt passer, the tubing is advanced from the flank incision to the abdominal incision and is then inserted into the peritoneal cavity for a distance of 15 to 20 cm, guiding the tubing toward the pelvis. Active flow of fluid through the tubing should be confirmed before it is inserted into the peritoneal cavity. The peritoneum is closed with an absorbable purse-string suture so that the tubing fits snugly but is not constricted. The transversus abdominis and internal oblique muscles are similarly approximated. The external oblique muscle, subcutaneous layer and skin are closed in layers.

Surgical treatment for syringomyelia that has developed in relation to a focal SAS block is directed toward removing this block to CSF circulation. In the case of HBD, posterior fossa decompression, preferably with an expansile duraplasty, is the preferred approach. In patients with PSS who have focal CSF obstructions, intradural exploration with resection of the arachnoid membrane is usually effective, and commonly is followed by partial or complete syrinx collapse.[12]

Postoperative Care

The broad aims of postoperative care of patients who have undergone syrinx shunting is to reduce the risks of postoperative complications. Foremost is minimizing the risk of CSF leakage from the spinal incision, a particular risk whenever the SAS has been opened and closed around a tube. To minimize the effect of gravity, many surgeons prefer to keep the patient lying on one side or the other rather than on the back, during the first 72 hours after surgery, or at least until the patient can sit up or walk. For the same reason, a firm dressing that can provide some counterpressure is helpful. Lumbar CSF drainage is not recommended unless the dural closure was problematic. Lumbar drainage, by producing a second entry to the SAS, theoretically increases the risk of infection at least slightly.

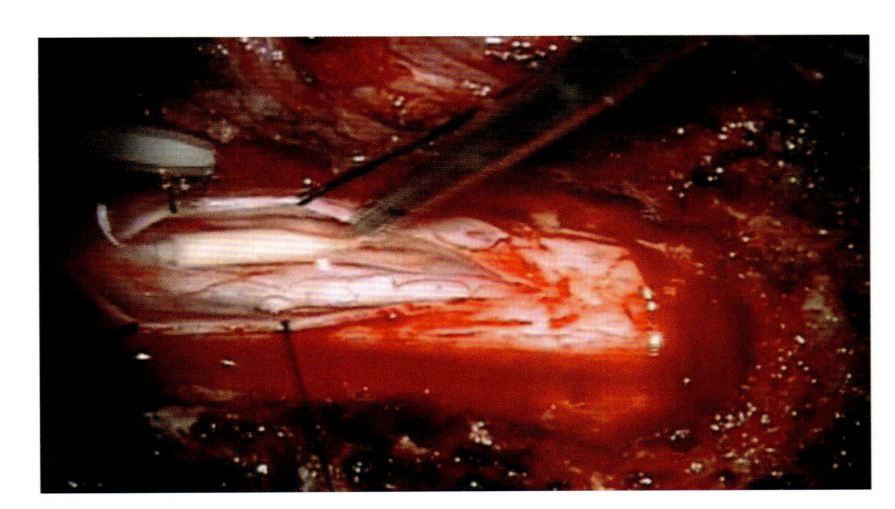

Fig. 78.6 The shunt is in place, with the distal portion of the shunt lying in the subarachnoid space, anterior to the dentate ligament.

Unless a patient is catheter dependent, an indwelling urinary catheter should be removed as early as possible after surgery. Stool softeners and appropriate laxative medication should be provided in the days and weeks after shunt surgery to reduce the likelihood of the patient straining. For similar reasons, coughing should be avoided if at all possible. If the patient develops an upper respiratory infection in the early postoperative period, it should be treated vigorously, if necessary with antibiotics, to reduce coughing and, thereby, straining.

Use of anti-embolism stockings and intermittent pressure devices is desirable, particularly in patients with impaired lower extremity mobility. Patients should be encouraged to be out of bed as early as possible.

Patients who underwent shunting into the peritoneal cavity should not be given food by mouth until bowel sounds have returned.

Potential Complications and Precautions

Acute or early complications must be considered separately from delayed complications.[13,14] The early postoperative complications include CSF leakage at the site of the laminectomy and dural opening, and acute wound infections. It is important to make only a small dural opening at the site of the planned myelotomy. Dural closure should be performed under magnification to minimize the risks of leakage. The spinal incision should be closed with care and in layers, apposing muscles and fascia tightly. Acute wound infection, as with all surgical procedures, can be avoided with meticulous attention to sterile technique and perioperative antibiotic administration.

Delayed complications are far more frequent and may be more difficult to avoid. Shunt obstruction is the most common problem and may result from collapse of the syrinx cavity around the perforations in the shunt tubing. Replacement of the proximal end of the system, if it can be safely withdrawn, is the best way to manage this complication. If the shunt tubing cannot be withdrawn, it should be amputated at the cord level and the proximal end of the shunt is replaced with a new tip. Obstruction of the distal end of the system, such as the peritoneal cavity, is rare. Separation of the shunt components at the site of a connector may occur, and would generally be evident as a subcutaneous fluid collection. Tethering of the shunt tube to the dura in such a way as to distort the cord and even impart motion to the cord with spine (particularly neck) movements may be seen in a few patients and generally relates to delayed changes in posture resulting from the innervation deficits caused by syringomyelia. It may benefit from maneuvers to restore more normal spinal alignment. Delayed infection of the shunt may occur in the course of septicemia from various sources, with microorganisms settling out on the shunt, an inert foreign body. Shunt replacement is generally necessary in this rare situation. Spine deformity at the level of shunt placement may also occur, and is thought to result from a combination of surgical muscle and bone dissection on a background of compromised innervations of the axial musculature resulting from syringomyelia.

Valve-less shunts placed in a situations of unrecognized communication of the syrinx with the SAS will lead to low CSF pressure symptoms, and must be corrected by placement of a valve into the shunting system. Failure to recognize longitudinal septation of a syrinx cavity may result in drainage of only one of two essentially parallel cavities and may require insertion of a second intraspinal shunt tube, which can be joined to the other outside of the spinal cord with an appropriate connector.

Conclusion

Shunting of syrinx cavities is a very useful technique for those patients whose imaging studies do not demonstrate a focal subarachnoid block that lends itself to local resection. When there is no reason to expect problems with resorption of CSF from the SAS, syrinx shunting into the SAS distal to the caudal end of the syrinx cavity may be preferable to shunting into an extraspinal location. Shunting into the peritoneal cavity is the more common site of extraspinal shunt placement. **Box 78.2** lists the key operative steps.

Box 78.2 Key Operative Steps

Laminectomy

- Verify the location with intraoperative radiographs.
- Verify the location of the syrinx cavity with intraoperative ultrasound.
- In a midline myelotomy, look for angulated vessels passing into the midline raphe.
- Dorsal root entry lesion just medial to rootlets attached to the cord
- Small myelotomy: No. 11 blade, No. 18 gauge needle
- Insert shunt with stiffener (nylon wire) to avoid kinking. Before insertion, identify the desired distance the tube is to be inserted into syrinx cavity.
- Anchor the shunt tubing to the dura; avoid kinking or obstructing the tubing with this suture.

Intrathecal Placement

- Identify the dentate ligament.
- Place an adequate length of tubing anterior to the dentate so it is less likely to dislodge.
- Avoid pulling on the shunt when placing the distal end to prevent dislodging tube from syrinx.
- Careful layer-by-layer wound closure

Peritoneal Placement

- Use a shunt passer to bring the tube out at the flank.
- Use a shunt passer to bring the tube from the flank incision to the abdominal incision.
- Abdominal incision just lateral to the rectus sheath; muscle splitting incision; small peritoneal opening
- Check that there is fluid flow from the catheter coming from the spinal incision.
- 10 cm of tubing into peritoneal cavity, directed inferiorly
- Purse-string closure of peritoneum snug but not occluding tubing; layered closure of abdomen

Pleural Placement

- Tunnel from midline to thoracic incision, ~ 10 cm from midline; use shunt passer
- Muscle splitting intercostals incision
- Anesthesia to hold breathing when lung is collapsed after pleura is opened
- Insert ~ 10 cm of tubing into the chest; make sure that there is fluid flow from the catheter coming from the spinal incision.
- Layered airtight wound closure

References

1. Heiss JD, Snyder K, Peterson MM, et al. Pathophysiology of primary spinal syringomyelia. J Neurosurg Spine 2012;17:367–380
2. Stoodley MA, Brown SA, Brown CJ, Jones NR. Arterial pulsation-dependent perivascular cerebrospinal fluid flow into the central canal in the sheep spinal cord. J Neurosurg 1997;86:686–693
3. Milhorat TH, Kotzen RM, Anzil AP. Stenosis of central canal of spinal cord in man: incidence and pathological findings in 232 autopsy cases. J Neurosurg 1994;80:716–722
4. Yasui K, Hashizume Y, Yoshida M, Kameyama T, Sobue G. Age-related morphologic changes of the central canal of the human spinal cord. Acta Neuropathol 1999;97:253–259
5. Milhorat TH, Capocelli AL Jr, Anzil AP, Kotzen RM, Milhorat RH. Pathological basis of spinal cord cavitation in syringomyelia: analysis of 105 autopsy cases. J Neurosurg 1995;82:802–812
6. Lam S, Batzdorf U, Bergsneider M. Thecal shunt placement for treatment of obstructive primary syringomyelia. J Neurosurg Spine 2008;9:581–588
7. Holly LT, Batzdorf U. Slitlike syrinx cavities: a persistent central canal. J Neurosurg 2002;97(2, Suppl):161–165
8. Iwasaki Y, Koyanagi I, Hida K, Abe H. Syringo-subarachnoid shunt for syringomyelia using partial hemilaminectomy. Br J Neurosurg 1999;13:41–45
9. Wester K, Pedersen P-H, Kråkenes J. Spinal cord damage caused by rotation of a T-drain in a patient with syringoperitoneal shunt. Surg Neurol 1989;31:224–227
10. Williams B, Page N. Surgical treatment of syringomyelia with syringopleural shunting. Br J Neurosurg 1987;1:63–80
11. Edgar RE. Surgical management of spinal cord cysts. Paraplegia 1976;14:21–27
12. Holly LT, Batzdorf U. Syringomyelia associated with intradural arachnoid cysts. J Neurosurg Spine 2006;5:111–116
13. Batzdorf U, Klekamp J, Johnson JP. A critical appraisal of syrinx cavity shunting procedures. J Neurosurg 1998;89:382–388
14. Sgouros S, Williams B. A critical appraisal of drainage in syringomyelia. J Neurosurg 1995;82:1–10

79 Posterior Approach and In-Situ Fusion of the Thoracic Spine

Hai Le, Rishi Wadhwa, and Praveen V. Mummaneni

Decompressive thoracic laminectomy (DTL) was once the universal approach performed for extradural spinal cord compression. Indications for this approach included compression secondary to neoplastic disease, hematoma, and abscess and canal or cord compromise secondary to traumatic fractures.[1]

This approach has been abandoned in recent years with the increasing popularity of the posterolateral approach. Moreover, the circumferential approaches are directed at the site of pathology and have been demonstrated to be safer when compared with DTL. However, DTL remains the standard approach for intradural pathology as well as dorsally located hematoma, abscess, tumor, and laminar fractures.

Removal of the posterior spinal elements, especially at the cervicothoracic or thoracolumbar junction, may compromise the stability of the spinal column. Therefore, in-situ fusion, or the use of bone graft to join adjacent vertebrae together, is often employed to stabilize the motion segments. Instrumentation with screws and rods can be subsequently utilized in selected cases to further strengthen the spinal column, correct spinal deformity, and facilitate spinal fusion.

This chapter describes the open posterior approach and in-situ fusion without instrumentation of the thoracic spine.

Patient Selection

Appropriate patient selection is essential for any successful surgery. A comprehensive history and physical examination should be done to identify the indications and contraindications to surgery as listed below. The patient with multiple medical comorbidities, especially cardiovascular and respiratory diseases, must be thoroughly evaluated and medically cleared for surgery. Although conservative measures should be carefully considered prior to surgery, we recommend that surgery, if indicated, should be done in a timely manner. Routine preoperative laboratory tests and imaging should be done. As with any surgery, the patient should be informed of the benefits, risks, and potential complications of the procedure, and should provide consent. If there is any concern about the possibility of poor fusion, the surgeon may consider spinal fusion with instrumentation to facilitate arthrodesis. The patient must also agree to partake in aggressive rehabilitation after surgery to promote and speed recovery.

Indications

- Dorsal epidural hemorrhage with incomplete cord injury or cauda equina syndrome
- Spinal cord tumors or arteriovenous malformations (AVMs) of the thoracic spine
- Spinal trauma leading to dorsal laminar fractures with neural compression
- Spinal osteomyelitis
- Degenerative disk disease
- Disk herniation

Contraindications

- Ventral neural compression
- Spinal trauma compromising integrity of the middle and anterior spinal columns
- Life expectancy less than 3 to 6 months
- Medical illness precluding major surgery

Advantages

- Familiar surgical approach
- Avoids the complications often associated with transthoracic approaches, such as complications from thoracotomy and risks of damaging vital neurovascular structures anterior to the thoracic spine
- Avoids the risks of placing instrumentation

Disadvantages

- Does not allow access to ventral compression
- Potentially lower fusion rates compared with instrumented cases
- Patient may need to wear orthosis postoperatively in contrast with instrumented cases

Objectives

- To obtain dorsal neural decompression and provide subsequent stabilization of the thoracic spine
- To obtain exposure to the dorsal thoracic spinal cord for resection of tumors or AVMs
- To obtain tissue biopsy of dorsally located pathology when previous less invasive attempts have failed, namely, computed tomography (CT)-guided biopsy

Choice of Operative Approach

Fusion of the thoracic spine can be performed by two main approaches—anterior and posterior. The choice should always be based on the location, size, and type of spinal pathology involved as well as the surgeon's experience and preference. The anterior approach usually involves fusion of fewer motion segments compared with the posterior approach, thus exerting less effect on the lumbar spine and lowering the risk for coronal imbalance and decompensation. However, access into the chest wall via thoracotomy or video-assisted thoracic surgery (VATS) is necessary. Therefore, there is a real risk of injuring vital neurovascular structures anterior to the thoracic spine. Pulmonary function may also be compromised. The posterior approach is a more familiar and straightforward approach for most surgeons, although more motion segments may need to be fused, and there may be prolonged postoperative back pain due to disruption of the paraspinal muscles.

Radiological Evaluation

Prior to surgery, anteroposterior (AP) and lateral radiographs of the spinal region to be fused should be obtained and carefully evaluated. Spinal deformity may require instrumentation for deformity correction and stabilization to facilitate fusion across motion segments. CT scan of the region should be obtained to better evaluate the anatomy of the thoracic spine and the extent of disease to precisely plan the surgery. If significant osteoporosis is suggested on imaging, bone densitometry may be performed to evaluate bone mineral density (BMD), because osteoporotic bone will lead to poor fusion rates. The use of alternative graft materials to local bone graft and spinal instrumentation may be needed for spinal fusion on osteoporotic spine. Of course, magnetic resonance imaging (MRI) should be obtained to carefully evaluate for sites of neural compression, keeping in mind that ventral compression cannot be directly decompressed via a posterior approach.

Surgical Techniques

Anesthesia and Positioning

Prior to surgery, type and screen or type and crossmatch should be performed if significant blood loss is anticipated. General endotracheal anesthesia and placement of a Foley catheter are performed with the patient in the supine position. The patient is then placed in the prone position on chest rolls with the arms tucked at the side. Care must be taken when positioning the arms so that all bony prominences and underlying neurovascular structures are protected. Adequate padding reduces the occurrence of postoperative pressure sores and nerve palsies. It is also imperative to allow the abdomen to hang freely to decrease the venous distention, especially in the lower thoracic/upper lumbar region. The anterior chest wall should also have adequate room for expansion during the procedure.

Incision and Musculocutaneous Flap

Prior to incision, appropriate prophylactic antibiotics should be administered if indicated. After adequate cleansing of the skin with antiseptic solution and sterile draping of the patient, an incision is made over the spinous processes of the levels involved. The localization of the incision may be facilitated with the use of fluoroscopy or with the use of radiopaque markers and plain radiographs. The incision is carried down to the fascia of the superficial muscular layer by blunt dissection. This layer consists of the trapezius muscle (C2–T12), the latissimus dorsi muscle (T6–lumbosacral fascia), and the rhomboid muscles (C7 and T1 insertion for the rhomboid minor and T2–T5 insertion for the rhomboid major) (**Fig. 79.1**). With the use of a Bovie electrocautery and a Cobb periosteal elevator, a subperiosteal dissection is performed through the superficial muscular layer. The intermediate layer, consisting of the serratus posterior muscle, is then dissected. The deep muscles are then encountered and dissected subperiosteally. The deep layer includes the sacrospinalis, semispinalis, multifidi, and rotator muscles (**Fig. 79.2**).[2] The use of self-retaining retractors facilitates the dissection and provides adequate visualization of the levels exposed. Furthermore, fluoroscopy or intraoperative radiographs help identify and verify the correct levels. The dissection needs to be performed laterally so that the transverse processes are generously exposed. This facilitates the decortication and placement of bone graft later in the procedure.

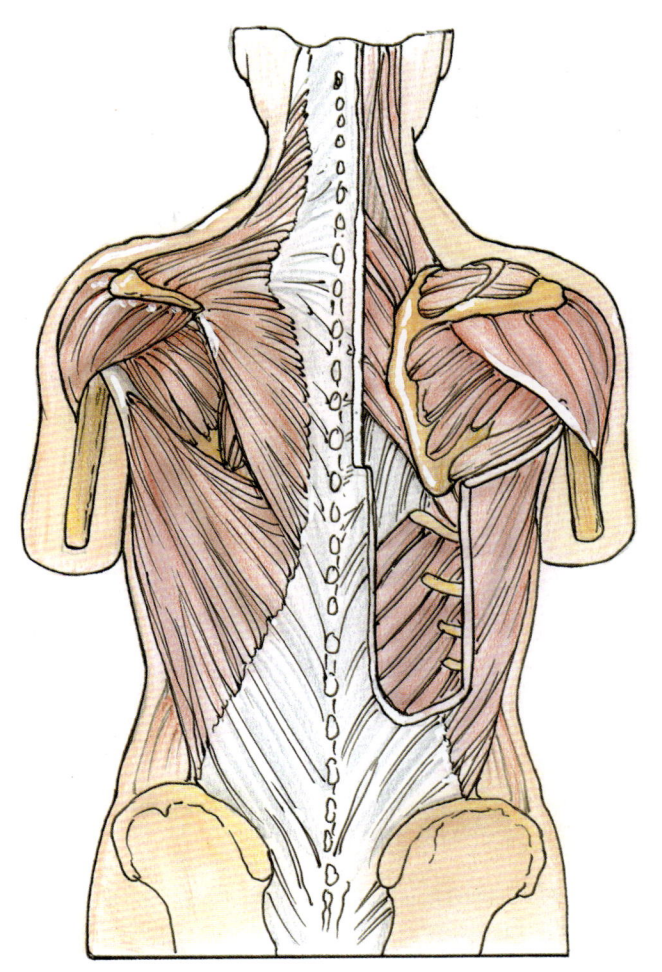

Fig. 79.1 Anatomy of the posterior thoracic spine.

Decompression

Once the posterior elements have been adequately exposed, a dorsal decompression is performed with removal of the spinous processes and laminae of the involved levels (**Fig. 79.3**). It is performed with a Kerrison rongeur or a high-speed drill with a cutting bur. An advantage of utilizing the Kerrison rongeur is that the bone may be used for subsequent grafting. One advantage of using the high-speed drill with a cutting bur is that it may decrease the operative time and thus the patient's exposure to anesthesia and wound contamination. However, risks associated with these instruments, including dural tears and injury to neural structures, should be taken into consideration. Then attention

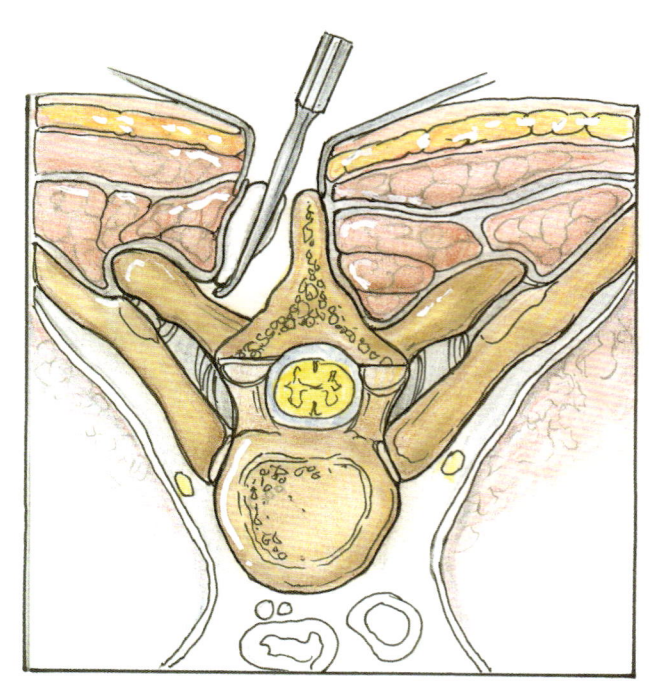

Fig. 79.2 Subperiosteal dissection of the thoracic spine musculature.

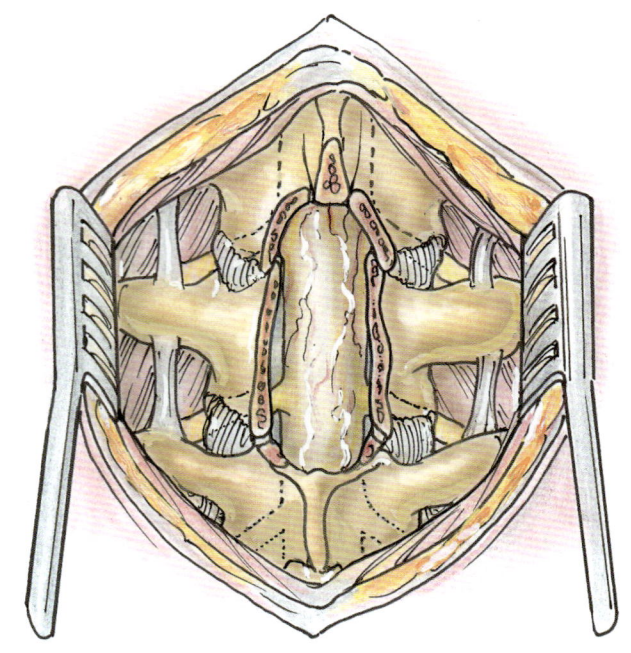

Fig. 79.3 Dorsal decompression with removal of the spinous processes and laminectomies.

is turned toward removing the extradural pathology, which may include tumor, abscess, hematoma, or bone fragments.

Decortication and Preparation for In-Situ Fusion

After adequate exposure and decompression have been performed, the transverse processes and facet joints are prepared for bone grafting. The transverse processes are decorticated with the use of sharp cupped curettes. A meticulous decortication enhances the fusion process. Next, facet joints should be resected and the cartilage removed. This process may also be performed with the use of a high-speed drill with a cutting bur (**Fig. 79.4**).

In-Situ Fusion

Once the transverse processes and the facet joints have been prepared, autologous bone graft is packed around the areas of decortication (**Fig. 79.5**). The graft may be composed of the local bone obtained during the dorsal decompression, but most often consists of autologous iliac bone graft.[3] For cases involving tumor or infection of the spine in which iliac bone grafting is anticipated, some surgeons may choose to harvest iliac bone graft first to avoid contamination. A skin incision over the iliac crest is made. Subsequently, the crest is harvested with a chisel and gouge. After adequate harvesting, the area is pulse-lavaged thoroughly. Adequate hemostasis should be achieved using bipolar cautery or Surgifoam. The iliac wound is closed in a layered fashion, and a drain can be tunneled out of the iliac crest.

Closure

Once hemostasis has been achieved and the bone graft has been carefully placed, the paraspinal muscles are returned to midline and the fascial layer is reapproximated with an absorbable suture (0 Vicryl). Some surgeons may choose to thoroughly irrigate the wound with antibiotic lavage prior to closure. The subcutaneous layer is then closed with a 2-0 Vicryl suture and the skin is closed with a 3-0 nylon suture. A 7-mm Jackson-Pratt drain may be placed overlying the fascial layer, which may reduce the formation of postoperative hematomas and seromas (**Fig. 79.6**).

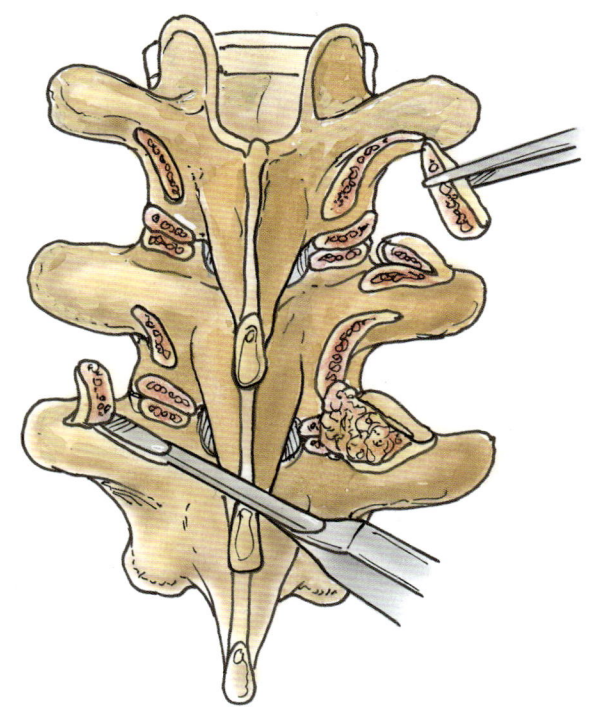

Fig. 79.4 Decortication of the transverse processes and removal of the facet joints.

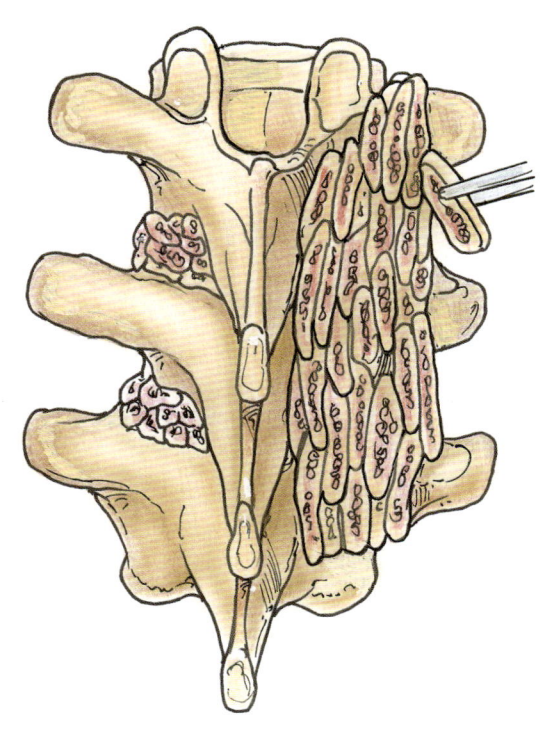

Fig. 79.5 Placement of bone graft on the transverse processes and facet joints.

If a cerebrospinal fluid leak occurs, the dura should be repaired primarily if possible. In the event that the dura cannot be repaired or the leak is not observable, placement of a lumbar drain is recommended.

Postoperative Care

Although the articulation with the rib cage provides some stability to the thoracic spine, an external orthosis (e.g., thoracolumbar brace) is recommended after a fusion without internal instrumentation is performed. Postoperative radiographs at 1-, 3-, and 6-month time intervals are used to assess any new deformity as well as a pseudarthrosis. Smoking cessation is recommended to the patient to improve the success of spinal fusion. The patient is also encouraged to be physically active, although heavy lifting, bending, or twisting should be discouraged until fusion is observed on radiograph. Pain should adequately be managed by oral pain medications, and new imaging studies, such as CT or MRI, are recommended to evaluate intractable postoperative pain.

Potential Complications and Precautions

Antibiotics may be given preoperatively and postoperatively to reduce the risk of deep infections. Prolonged antibiotic administration or reoperation may be needed should the wound become infected. Pseudarthrosis may require reoperation with spinal fusion and instrumentation for pain relief. Care must be taken during posterior decompression to avoid violation of the dura or posterior neural elements. Dural tears should be repaired primarily with placement of a subfascial drain.

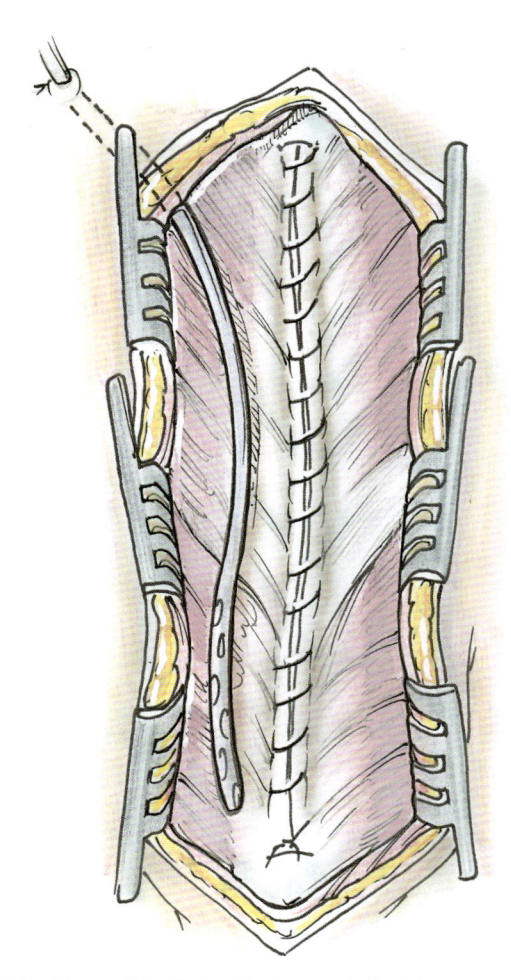

Fig. 79.6 Closure of the fascia with placement of a drain.

Conclusion

Decompressive thoracic laminectomy and fusion surgery are performed to relieve posterior spinal cord compression from various causes, including tumor, hematoma, abscess, and traumatic fractures. Generally, local or iliac crest autograft is used for in-situ fusion, although other bone graft options may be used. The direct posterior approach is more familiar to most surgeons and can be done safely without the complications associated with transthoracic approaches; however, its main drawback is that it does not enable direct ventral decompression. In selective cases, instrumentation with screws and rods can be subsequently performed to further strengthen the spinal column, correct spinal deformity, and facilitate spinal fusion.

References

1. Popovic EA. Decompressive thoracic laminectomy. In: Kaye AH, Black PM, eds. Operative Neurosurgery. London: Churchill Livingstone; 2000:1817–1826
2. Papadopolous SM, Fessler RG. The thoracic spine. In: Benzel EC, ed. Spine Surgery: Techniques, Complication Avoidance, and Management. New York: Churchill Livingstone; 1999:157–168
3. Simpson JM, An H. Posterior exposures of the thoracic spine. In: An HS, Riley LH, eds. An Atlas of Surgery of the Spine. New York: Lippincott-Raven; 1998:31–43

80 Pedicle Screw Instrumentation of the Thoracic Spine

Hai Le, Rishi Wadhwa, and Praveen V. Mummaneni

Traumatic or pathological fractures of the thoracic spine may compromise spinal alignment and stability, thus causing neurologic injury. Spinal deformity may also result from degenerative or iatrogenic conditions. Pedicle screw instrumentation and fusion are the mainstay of treatment.

Pedicle screw–rod instrumentation enables significant application of forces in multiple planes.[1] The pedicle screw fixation system offers many advantages over other options such as wire or hook–rod fixation. First, pedicle screws do not require that the dorsal elements be intact. Second, pedicle screw fixation avoids placement of instrumentation into the spinal canal. Hook systems and sublaminar wires occupy the spinal canal and pose more of a potential neurologic risk. Third, the fusion rates are reportedly higher with pedicle screw–rod fixation.[2]

The pedicle screw fixation system has disadvantages when compared with other systems, however. The primary disadvantage is the high cost.

Today, placement of thoracic pedicle screws can be performed either via an open approach or by minimally invasive surgery (MIS). Potential advantages of MIS fixation include muscle preservation, reduced blood loss, reduced operative time, lower risk of infection, and shorter hospital stay in comparison to standard open procedures.[3] Potential drawbacks of MIS fixation include increased exposure to fluoroscopy, inability to directly perform neurologic decompression, and limited space to place a bone graft.[3]

Sound knowledge of the anatomy of the thoracic spine is essential prior to performing thoracic pedicle screw fixation. The pedicle in most of the thoracic vertebrae is angulated by ~ 10 degrees from posterolaterally to anteromedially. The transverse pedicle angle decreases from T1 to T12.[4-6] The height of the thoracic pedicle is greater than its width, giving it a smaller transverse diameter compared with the lower lumbar pedicle.[5,7] Transverse pedicle width decreases from the upper thoracic vertebrae to the midthoracic vertebrae (smallest at T5-T6) and then increases again in the lower thoracic vertebrae. The length of the thoracic pedicle is shorter than the lumbar pedicle; thus, a greater segment of the screw is inserted in the thoracic vertebral body.[7]

Patient Selection

A comprehensive history and physical examination can identify the indications and contraindications to surgery as listed below. The patient with multiple medical comorbidities, especially cardiovascular and respiratory diseases, must be thoroughly evaluated and medically cleared for surgery. Although conservative measures should be carefully considered prior to surgery, we recommend that surgery, if indicated, should be done in a timely manner. Routine preoperative laboratory tests and imaging should be done. As with any surgery, the patient should be informed of the benefits, risks, and potential complications of the procedure and should provide consent. The patient must also agree to partake in aggressive rehabilitation after surgery to promote and speed recovery.

Indications

- Stabilization of the thoracic spine after neural decompression for tumor or infection
- Thoracic spinal column fractures
- Kyphotic deformities without significant osteoporosis
- Patients with deficient posterior spinal elements due to failed past surgeries
- Adolescent idiopathic scoliosis

Contraindications

- Significant osteoporosis (relative contraindication)
- Medical illness precluding major surgery
- Life expectancy less than 3 to 6 months
- Patients with thoracic pedicles too small for screw placement with screw diameter of at least 6 mm
- Compromised thoracic pedicles (e.g., fractured pedicles)

Advantages

- Does not require the dorsal elements to be intact
- Avoids placing instrumentation within the spinal canal
- Higher fusion rates
- Offers high stability with three-column involvement and three-dimensional correction forces
- Appropriate for cases that require only short-segment fixation and fusion

Disadvantages

- Smaller pedicles may result in higher incidence of durotomy or nerve injury
- Requires increased exposure to obtain necessary trajectory
- Medial screw misplacement can lead to iatrogenic neurologic injury

Objectives

- To relieve pain, preserve neurologic function, and maintain spinal alignment

- To obtain stabilization of the thoracic spine utilizing a three-column construct
- To provide posterior spinal stabilization to facilitate and augment anterior arthrodesis

Choice of Operative Approach

There are two main approaches to placement of thoracic pedicle screws—open and percutaneous. The choice of operative approach depends on the surgeon's experience and preference. Percutaneous screw insertion minimizes the skin incision and dissection of the paraspinal muscles. As with other MIS procedures, studies have found that percutaneous thoracic screw placement is associated with less postoperative pain, shorter hospital stay, lower blood loss, and decreased risk of infection. However, there is a high learning curve to be able to perform MIS safely and successfully.

Radiological Evaluation

Prior to surgical intervention, 36-inch anteroposterior (AP) and lateral X-rays of the regions to be stabilized and fused are required. Furthermore, a computed tomography (CT) scan examination of the region should be obtained to evaluate the size of the thoracic pedicles for appropriate preoperative planning. Magnetic resonance imaging (MRI) can be utilized to evaluate the integrity of the spinal cord and ligamentous structures. Note that MRI tends to underestimate pedicle dimensions.[8] If significant osteoporosis is suggested by the radiographs and CT scan, then bone densitometry may also be performed because osteoporotic bone will lead to poor fusion rates and increased instrumentation pullout.

Surgical Technique

Anesthesia and Positioning

General endotracheal intubation is performed, and the patient is then placed in the prone position on a radiolucent table. Care is taken to avoid pressure on the bony prominences and neurovascular structures by providing adequate padding. The anterior chest wall should have adequate room for expansion during the surgery.

Incision and Musculocutaneous Flap

The skin incision is made over the spinous processes of the levels involved. The construct should include three normal levels above the pathology and two normal levels below the pathology, and the incision should provide adequate exposure. The incision is carried down subperiosteally along the spinous processes and laminae, and should expose the transverse processes.

Placement of Thoracic Pedicle Screws

After adequate exposure of the dorsal thoracic spine has been achieved, the pathological process is addressed. Decompression, if indicated, removal of traumatic bone fragments, and biopsy or resection of tumor or abscess are performed prior to the stabilization and fusion.

The thoracic pedicle is oriented in a posterolateral to anteromedial direction by ~ 10 degrees along most of the thoracic spine (**Fig. 80.1**). There is a slight anterior and lateral angulation of the pedicle at T12.[9] It is recommended that fluoroscopy be available to assist in the proper trajectory. If the dorsal elements are intact, then a small laminotomy may be performed to enable direct palpation of the medial aspect of the pedicle. It is also important to note that the thoracic pedicle height is greater than the width and therefore smaller-diameter pedicle screws should be utilized in the thoracic region as compared with the lumbar spine (**Fig. 80.2**).

The entry point for a thoracic pedicle screw in the sagittal plane (using a straightforward trajectory) is at the midpoint of the thoracic transverse process (TP) at T1–T3 and at T10–T12. However, in the midthoracic spine (T4–T9), the entry point for the thoracic pedicle screw is superior to the TP (**Fig. 80.3**).[10] A high-speed drill with a cutting bur is used to remove the cortical surface overlying the entry point. Next, a pedicle probe is directed along the path of the pedicle screw. A sounding probe is then utilized to ensure that the path has cancellous bone in all directions. A Kirschner wire (K-wire) is then placed along the

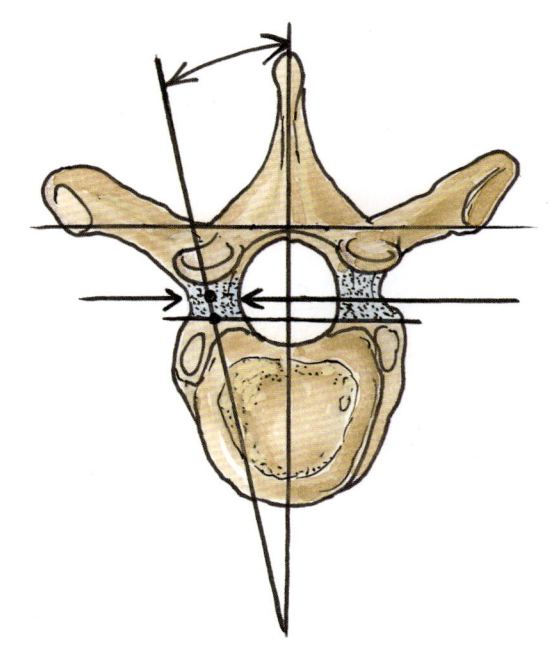

Fig. 80.1 Anatomy of thoracic pedicle.

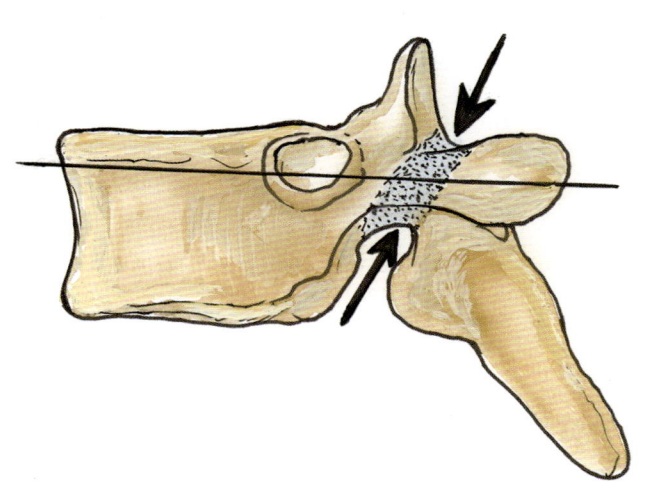

Fig. 80.2 The relationship of the pedicle height and width in the thoracic spine.

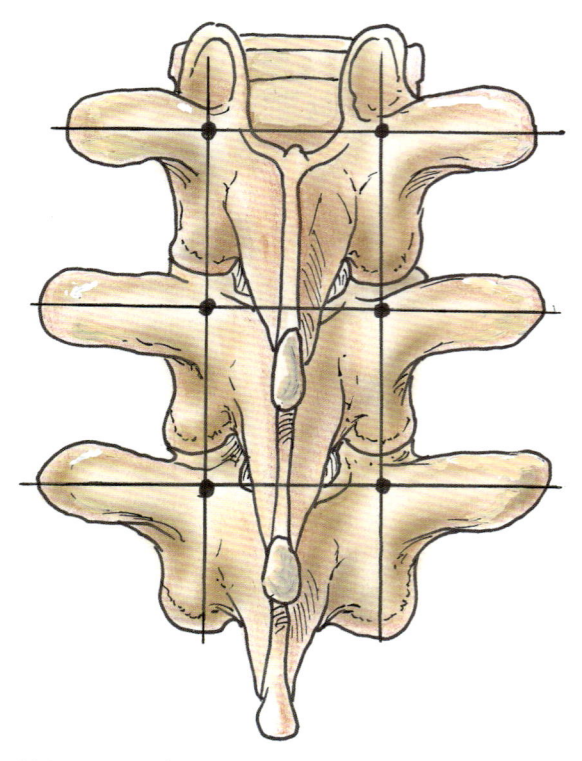

Fig. 80.3 Entry site for pedicle screw. For T1–T3 and T10–T12 pedicles, the entry point in the sagittal plane is at the midpoint of the thoracic transverse process (TP). For T4–T9 pedicles, the entry point is superior to the TP.

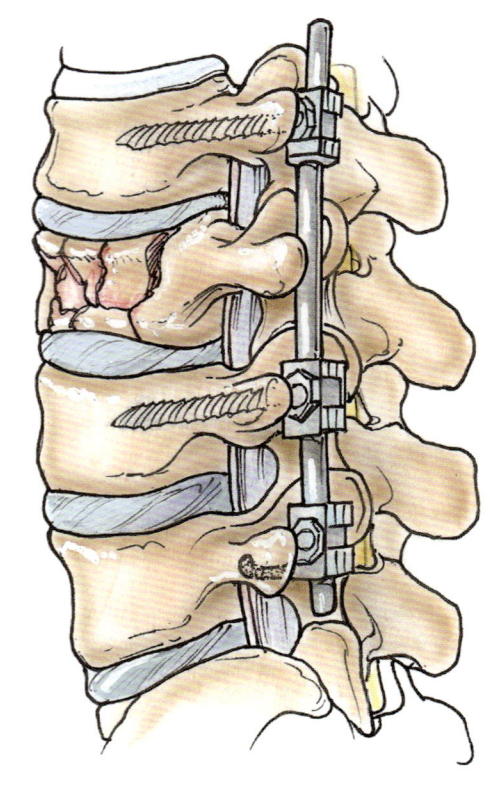

Fig. 80.4 Pedicle screws penetrating 50 to 80% of the vertebral body and connecting to a longitudinal member.

path, and the trajectory is assessed with fluoroscopy. After confirmation of the trajectory, a tap is used to prepare the bone for the pedicle screw. Newer systems use self-tapping screws, which reduce weakening of the cancellous bone when compared with the non–self-tapping screws. The length of the pedicle screw is determined by the K-wires, and should provide penetration of 50 to 80% of the vertebral body (**Fig. 80.4**). The screw strength is determined by the core diameter (minor), whereas the outside diameter (major) is an important factor in screw pullout.[1] Once the pedicle screw has been placed, the screws are connected to a longitudinal member (**Fig. 80.4**). The lateral aspect of the facet joint and the transverse processes are decorticated with a curette or bur, and bone graft is placed over the decorticated areas (**Fig. 80.5**).

Closure

The wound is treated with antibiotic irrigation, and hemostasis is obtained utilizing electrocautery. The deep fascia is closed with an absorbable suture (0 Vicryl), and the subcutaneous tissue is closed with a 3-0 absorbable suture. The skin is reapproximated and closed with a 3-0 nylon suture or with skin staples. A drain (7-mm Jackson-Pratt) may be placed overlying the deep fascial layer. The drain is brought through a percutaneous incision.

Postoperative Care

Anteroposterior and lateral X-rays should be obtained prior to discharge to evaluate the integrity of the construct and the degree of correction of the deformity. CT scan may also be obtained

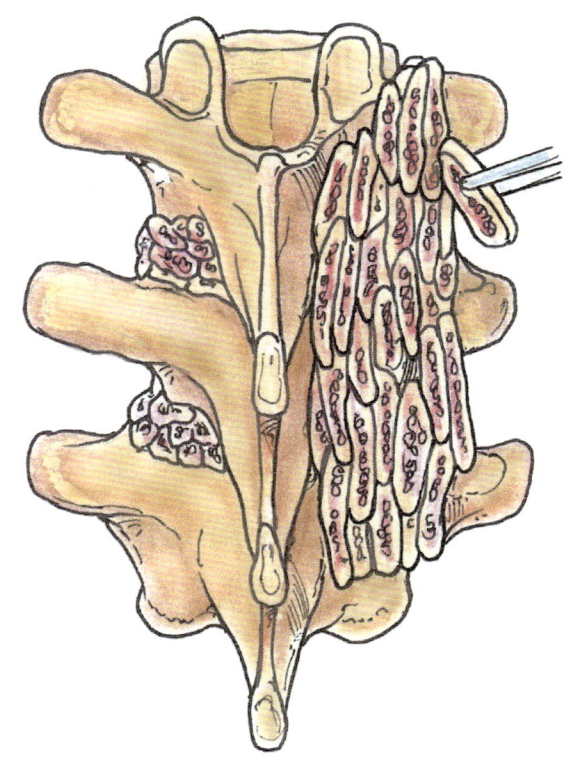

Fig. 80.5 Placement of bone graft along the transverse processes and facet joints after pedicle screw placement.

postoperatively if there is concern about pedicle breach. Patients may receive physical therapy for early mobilization during their hospitalization. Activity should be limited within the first 3 months to enable the fusion to solidify.[7]

Potential Complications and Precautions

Medial screw misplacement can lead to severe neurologic compromise. Laminotomies can be performed to enable direct palpation of the medial aspect of the pedicle, to facilitate identification of the entry point and screw pathway, thus lowering the risk of violating the medial pedicle wall.[4,5] If thoracic pedicle screw placement is performed by an MIS approach, there may be a need to convert to an open approach if there is any reasonable concern about screw breakout.[7] Intraoperative neurophysiological monitoring can be useful to assess the functional integrity of the neural elements.

Conclusion

Pedicle screw–rod instrumentation is widely considered the treatment of choice for fractures and deformity of the thoracic spine. Potential benefits of thoracic pedicle screw fixation include high fusion rates, good restoration of neurological function, and good maintenance of spinal alignment. It can be performed in combination with anterior procedures to provide posterior spinal stabilization to facilitate and augment anterior arthrodesis. Sound knowledge of the anatomy of the thoracic spine is essential to place thoracic pedicle screws safely and effectively. Great care must be taken to avoid violation of the medial wall during placement of these pedicle screws.

References

1. Halliday AL, Zileili M, Stillerman CB, Benzel E. Dorsal thoracic and lumbar screw fixation and pedicle fixation techniques. In: Benzel EC, ed. Spine Surgery: Techniques, Complication Avoidance, and Management. Philadelphia: Churchill Livingstone; 1999:1053–1064
2. Stillerman CB, Gruen JP, Roy R. Thoracic and lumbar fusion: techniques for posterior stabilization. In: Menezes A, Sonntag VKH, eds. Principles of Spinal Surgery. New York: McGraw-Hill; 1996:1199–1224
3. Court C, Vincent C. Percutaneous fixation of thoracolumbar fractures: current concepts. Orthop Traumatol Surg Res 2012;98:900–909
4. Fassett DR, Brodke DS. Percutaneous posterior insertion of thoracic pedicle screws. In: Vaccaro AR, Bono CM, eds. Minimally Invasive Spine Surgery. New York: Informa Healthcare; 2007
5. Tredway TL, Fessler RG. Pedicle screw instrumentation of the thoracic spine. In: Fessler RG, Sekhar L, eds. Atlas of Neurosurgical Techniques: Spine and Peripheral Nerves. New York: Thieme; 2006
6. Halpin RJ, Koski TR. Thoracic pedicle technique. In: Baaj A, Mummaneni P, Uribe J, Vaccaro A, Greenberg M, eds. Handbook of Spine Surgery. New York: Thieme; 2012
7. von Strempel AH. Thoracic pedicle screws: pedicular approach. In: Haher TR, Merola AA, eds. Surgical Techniques for the Spine. New York: Thieme; 2003
8. Lenke LG. Thoracic pedicle screw placement. In: Haid RW, Subach BR, Rodts GE, eds. Advances in Spinal Stabilization. New York: Karger; 2003
9. Papadopolous SM, Fessler RG. The thoracic spine. In: Benzel EC, ed. Spine Surgery: Techniques, Complication Avoidance, and Management. Philadelphia: Churchill Livingstone; 1999:157–168
10. Simpson JM, An H. Posterior exposures of the thoracic spine. In: An HS, Riley LH, eds. An Atlas of Surgery of the Spine. New York: Lippincott-Raven; 1998:31–43

81 Open Scoliosis Correction

Patrick A. Sugrue and Lawrence G. Lenke

The overall prevalence of scoliosis in the adult population has been reported to range from 1.4 to 20%,[1-4] but with a rapidly expanding elderly population, the incidence of adult scoliosis and adult spinal deformity is likely to increase significantly. The incidence of scoliosis in patients over 60 years of age with low back pain is 15%,[1,3] and thus, spine surgeons will certainly encounter varying degrees of spinal deformity that will require surgical intervention. Paulus et al[5] demonstrated the benefit of surgery compared with nonoperative treatment for symptomatic adult spinal deformity with significantly greater improvements in Scoliosis Research Society-22 (SRS-22), Oswestry Disability Index (ODI), and Short Form-12 (SF-12) outcome scores as compared with the scores for nonoperative intervention.[5]

In the pediatric population, the goals of intervention include the prevention of deformity progression and the optimization of cardiopulmonary development. The development of spinal deformity can influence lung compliance, lung volume, and alveolar growth.[6] Severe scoliosis leading to chest wall deformity can reduce lung compliance, leading to increased work of breathing and an elevated respiratory rate secondary to the inability to generate adequate tidal volumes during normal respiration.[6] Early-onset scoliosis has a high rate of progression in accelerated periods of growth and a high rate of cardiopulmonary complications, and untreated infantile and juvenile scoliosis leads to a high rate of pulmonary complications.[7] About 1% of idiopathic scoliosis cases occur in infants, 10 to 20% in children, and 80 to 90% in adolescents.[8,9]

The impact of surgical correction of spinal deformity can be significant in all age groups. However, there are multiple factors that the surgeon must consider when planning correction strategies in spinal deformity. This chapter discusses various correction techniques in the open treatment of scoliosis through an all-posterior approach. It cannot be overemphasized that deformity correction in all age groups is a technically and physiologically demanding task, and thus planning for such an operation begins when first meeting the patient. The use of multiple imaging modalities and a thorough medical evaluation help guide the correction strategy. Likewise, there are multiple steps that can be taken to optimize conditions for obtaining correction while minimizing patient risk.

Patient Selection

Planning surgical correction of spinal deformity at any age begins first with evaluation of the patient both clinically and radiographically. In the adult population, indications for surgical intervention include progression of deformity, neurologic deficit, and medically intractable pain impairing the patient's quality of life. By contrast, in the pediatric population, the indications for surgery focus on the magnitude of the deformity, cardiopulmonary development, cosmesis, and neurologic risk.

Radiographic Evaluation

The use of multiple radiographs is essential in the preoperative evaluation. In particular, the use of upright long-cassette 14 × 36 inch radiographs helps to evaluate the entire spine in a weight-bearing position. Likewise, the use of EOS imaging (EOS Imaging, Paris, France) (**Fig. 81.1**) can aid in assessing total body alignment and global sagittal and coronal balance. One of the most important factors in planning a correction strategy is assessing the flexibility of the deformity. Using multiple flexibility films such as supine, push-prone, side-bending, hyperextension, and traction films helps to determine the flexibility of the deformity and thus the extent of correction required. It can be helpful to categorize the rigidity of the curve based on these multiple films into groups such as flexible (type A) versus stiff (type B) versus stuck/fused (type C).[10] For example, type A deformity is passively flexible (≥ 50%) and does not require osteotomies to realign. Typically, this is a patient without prior spinal operations and without evidence of any autofusion. Although most of these patients do not require formal osteotomies, facet and ligamentous removal is helpful to increase the mobility of the deformity. Type B deformity is a stiff deformity with some movement on flexibility imaging (25–50%). Supine X-rays may not reestablish coronal or sagittal alignment, but the deformity certainly improves with positioning. These patients often require multiple posterior column osteotomies (PCOs) (**Figs. 81.2 and 81.3**) or a three-column osteotomy (3-CO) such as a pedicle subtraction osteotomy (PSO) or a vertebral column resection (VCR). Type C deformities show minimal or no flexibility and definitely require spinal osteotomies, often a PSO or a VCR to reestablish spinal alignment.

Classification

Aebi[11] first described three types of adult scoliosis: de novo adult scoliosis, progressive idiopathic scoliosis, and secondary degenerative scoliosis. Schwab et al[12] later developed a classification system for adult spinal deformity based on the radiographic findings that impact patient-reported outcomes, specifically addressing three important parameters: apical level, lumbar lordosis, and frontal and sagittal plane intervertebral subluxation. The authors concluded that in the adult population, coronal Cobb magnitude did not correlate with patient self-assessment but they found that thoracic, thoracolumbar, and lumbar curve patterns with a low apex and loss of lordosis led to a significant increase in patient disability as measured by the ODI and SRS scores. Likewise, the degree of intervertebral subluxation (> 7 mm) in the thoracolumbar and lumbar curves was found to significantly negatively impact patient reported outcomes. Later work by Schwab et al[12-16] added a global balance modifier, acknowledging the importance of overall spinal sagittal alignment by using the sagittal vertical axis (SVA). Finally, the Scoliosis Research

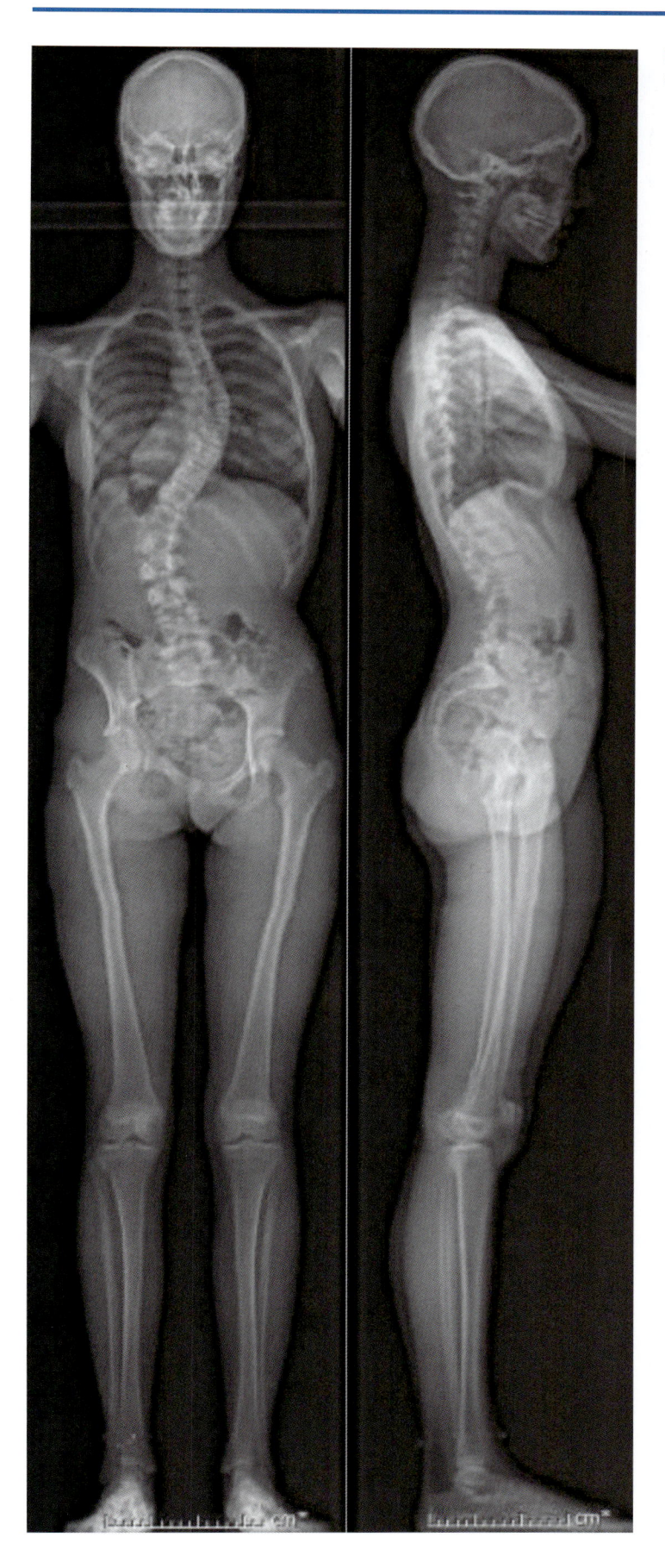

Fig. 81.1 EOS imaging demonstrating global body alignment in a patient with adolescent idiopathic scoliosis.

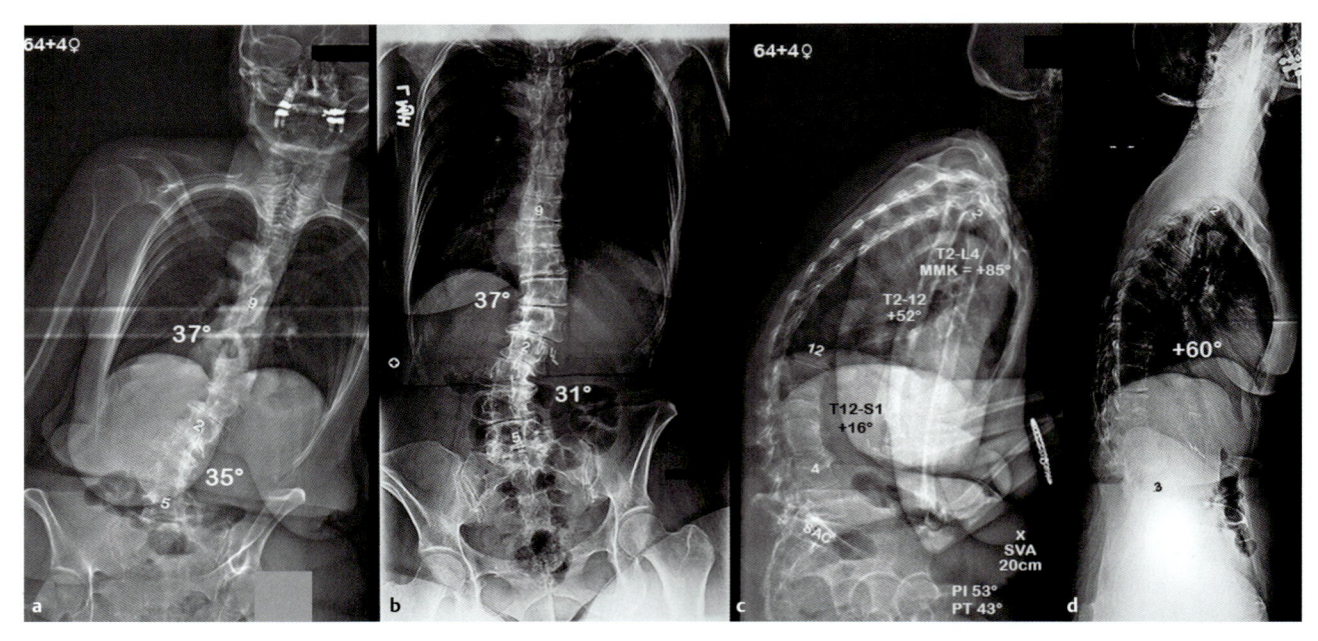

Fig. 81.2 Upright **(a,c)** and supine **(b,d)** radiographs demonstrating deformity correction in both the sagittal and coronal planes with supine positioning alone. Regional curve magnitudes are shown with additional radiographic parameters and labeled anatomic landmarks. SVA, sagittal vertical axis; PI, pelvic incidence; PT, pelvic tilt; MMK, maximum measured kyphosis; SAC, sacrum.

Society–Schwab classification system for adult spinal deformity **(Fig. 81.4)** emphasized the importance of the sagittal plane by first classifying a curve pattern in the coronal plane and then using three sagittal plane modifiers, thereby correlating specific radiographic measurable parameters with patient reported outcomes. By combining the three sagittal modifiers—pelvic incidence (PI)–lumbar lordosis (LL) mismatch, SVA, and pelvic tilt (PT)—the amount of correction required can be determined quantitatively.[16] Combining these data with the overall medical and physiological assessment of an individual patient enables the creation of a surgical plan that optimizes correction and patient safety. It is important to point out that the calculated correction required must be tempered by the age and medical condition of the patient. We do not yet fully understand the impact of neurodegenerative disorders such as Parkinson's disease on spinal alignment, and as all spines develop kyphosis over time, the amount of correction required is influenced by the patient's age.

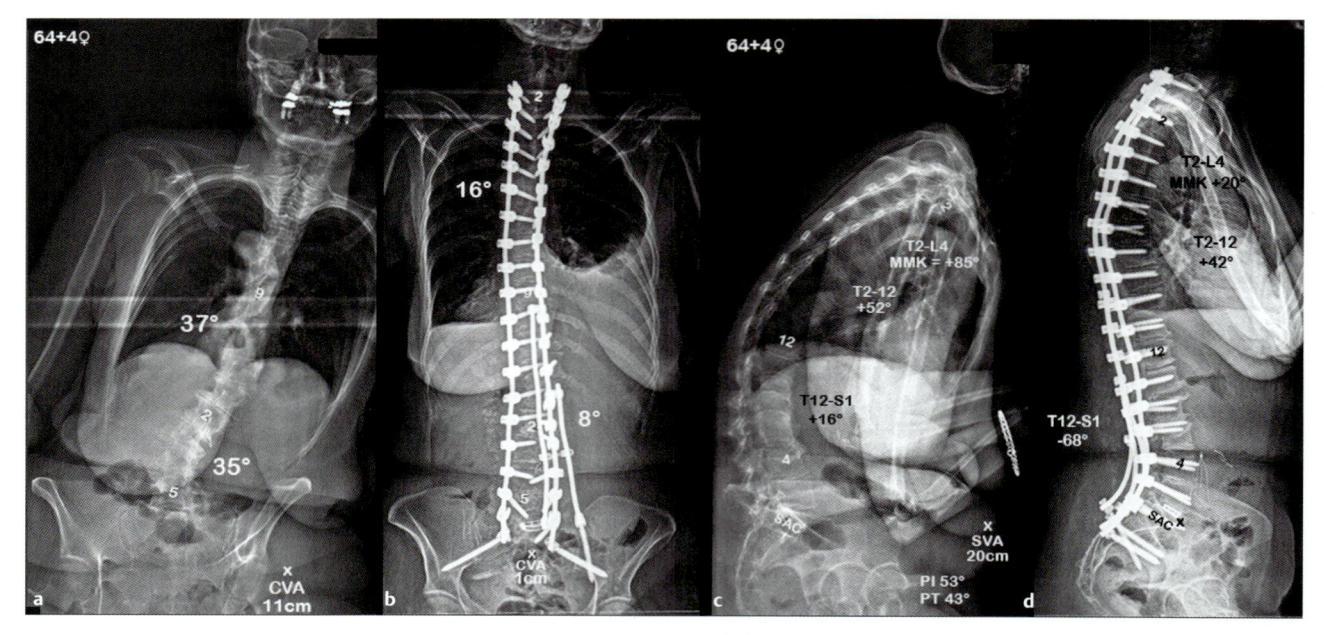

Fig. 81.3 Comparison of preoperative and postoperative standing upright radiographs in a 64-year-old woman with progressive back pain and adult degenerative lumbar kyphoscoliosis, with coronal and sagittal imbalance. She underwent C7-S1/ilium instrumented posterior spinal fusion using multiple posterior column osteotomies alone.

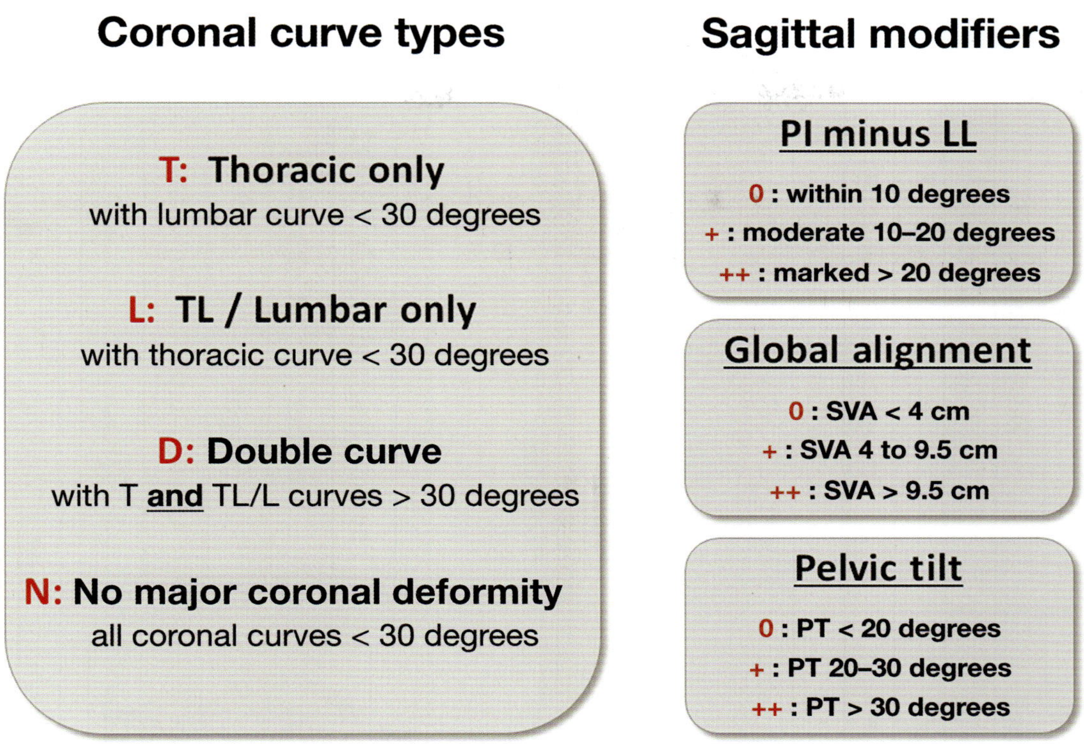

Coronal curve types

T: Thoracic only
with lumbar curve < 30 degrees

L: TL / Lumbar only
with thoracic curve < 30 degrees

D: Double curve
with T **and** TL/L curves > 30 degrees

N: No major coronal deformity
all coronal curves < 30 degrees

Sagittal modifiers

PI minus LL
0 : within 10 degrees
+ : moderate 10–20 degrees
++ : marked > 20 degrees

Global alignment
0 : SVA < 4 cm
+ : SVA 4 to 9.5 cm
++ : SVA > 9.5 cm

Pelvic tilt
0 : PT < 20 degrees
+ : PT 20–30 degrees
++ : PT > 30 degrees

Fig. 81.4 Scoliosis Research Society (SRS)–Schwab classification. L, lumbar; LL, lumbar lordosis; PI, pelvic incidence; PT, pelvic tilt; SVA, sagittal vertical axis; TL, thoracolumbar. (From Schwab F, Ungar B, Blondel B, et al. Scoliosis Research Society–Schwab adult spinal deformity classification: a validation study. Spine (Phila Pa 1976) 2012;37:1077–1082. Reprinted with permission.)

In the adolescent idiopathic population, the goals of correction are different, with a particular emphasis on preserving motion segments. The first classification system for adolescent idiopathic scoliosis (AIS) developed by King et al[17] was limited by its description of the coronal plane alone, its weak intra- and interobserver reliability, and its inclusion of only thoracic curves.[18] Lenke et al[19] later developed a classification system that accounted for both the coronal and sagittal planes and also addressed all potential AIS curve patterns. The Lenke classification also maintained high intra- and interobserver reliability and enabled the identification of structural curve patterns, facilitating more selective fusions, preventing postoperative decompensation, and preserving motion segments[18,20–22] (**Fig. 81.5**).

It is essential to point out the importance of addressing both the coronal and sagittal planes when evaluating spinal deformity. Although classification systems used for scoliosis are based on two-dimensional imaging, scoliosis is truly a three-dimensional deformity. The Scoliosis Research Society has formed a panel of experts to better understand and describe multiplanar scoliotic deformities and to help guide further treatment.[23]

In addition to using plain radiographs, advanced imaging such as magnetic resonance imaging (MRI), computed tomography (CT), and CT myelogram can provide valuable additional information about neurologic compression or three-dimensional anatomy. In cases of severe spinal deformity, especially in the revision setting, it may be helpful to have a three-dimensional model made to fully understand the anatomy of the deformity.

Evaluation of the patient's symptoms, physical exam findings, and ability to physiologically tolerate the proposed procedure must be taken into account along with the radiographic evaluation. Some institutions have utilized a high-risk spine protocol to provide a comprehensive medical evaluation of a patient prior to undergoing a spinal deformity operation; the protocol is carried through the patient's perioperative course.[24] The information obtained with such an evaluation may help guide the surgical planning in terms of weighing the risks and benefits of performing a potentially highly demanding and physiologically stressful procedure. Likewise, certain physical exam findings such as weakness or myelopathy may focus the surgical target and alter the timing, need, or degree of correction required. Particularly in the setting of myelopathy, the risk of further neurologic injury in the setting of an already diseased or injured spinal cord is much higher.

Deformities that require complex reconstruction should be undertaken only by experienced surgeons who are comfortable performing such operations and who have the anesthesia and critical care staff to support them. The complication rate for such long construct fusions in the adult population remains near 40%,[25,26] and one must have the appropriate preoperative, intraoperative, and postoperative support to minimize complications and optimize outcomes.

Spinal Alignment

It is important to fully understand the goals of correction before operating on a patient. Although there are many etiologies underlying different types of spinal deformity, the goals of correction focus on the need to reestablish balance and alignment. One of the most important factors in determining a patient's overall health status and surgical outcome is maintaining sagittal balance.[27,28] More specifically, true spinal balance is defined by the ability to maintain the head over the pelvis so as to enable energy-efficient physiological motion.[29] With this in mind, any

THE LENKE CLASSIFICATION SYSTEM FOR AIS

Curve Type	Proximal Thoracic	Main Thoracic	Thoracolumbar/Lumbar	Description
1	Nonstructural	Structural*	Nonstructural	Main Thoracic (MT)
2	Structural†	Structural*	Nonstructural	Double Thoracic (DT)
3	Nonstructural	Structural*	Structural†	Double Major (DM)
4	Structural†	Structural§	Structural§	Triple Major (TM)
5	Nonstructural	Nonstructural	Structural*	Thoracolumbar/Lumbar (TL/L)
6	Nonstructural	Structural†	Structural*	Thoracolumbar/Lumbar-Main Thoracic (TL/L-MT)

*Major curve: largest Cobb measurement, always structural; †Minor curve: remaining structural curves; §Type 4 - MT or TL/L can be the major curve

STRUCTURAL CRITERIA
(Minor Curves)

Proximal Thoracic — Side Bending Cobb ≥25°
  — T2-T5 Kyphosis ≥+20°

Main Thoracic — Side Bending Cobb ≥25°
  — T10-L2 Kyphosis ≥+20°

Thoracolumbar/Lumbar — Side Bending Cobb ≥25°
  — T10-L2 Kyphosis ≥+20°

LOCATION OF APEX
(SRS Definition)

CURVE	APEX
Thoracic	T2 to T11-12 Disc
Thoracolumbar	T12-L1
Lumbar	L1-2 Disc to L4

MODIFIERS

Lumbar Spine Modifier	Center Sacral Vertical Line to Lumbar Apex
A	Between pedicles
B	Touches apical body(ies)
C	Completely medial

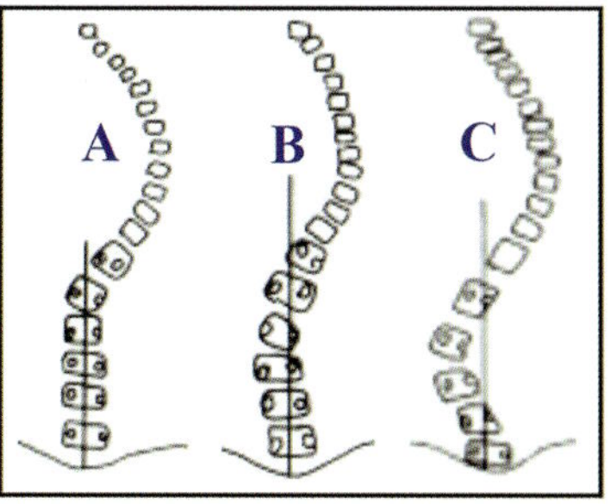

Thoracic Sagittal Profile T5-T12	
Modifier	Cobb Angle
− (Hypo)	<10°
N (Normal)	10° - 40°
+ (Hyper)	>40°

Curve Type (**1-6**) + Lumbar Spine Modifier (**A, B, C**) + Thoracic Sagittal Modifier (**−, N, +**) = Curve Classification (e.g. **1B+**): _____

Fig. 81.5 Lenke Adolescent Idiopathic Scoliosis Classification. (From Lenke LG, Betz RR, Harms J, et al. Adolescent idiopathic scoliosis: a new classification to determine extent of spinal arthrodesis. J Bone Joint Surg Am 2001;83A:1169–1181. Reprinted with permission.)

To compensate for spinal malalignment, patients often retrovert their pelvis, thus increasing pelvic tilt (PT). PT is the angle subtended by a vertical reference line from the center of the femoral heads to the midpoint of the sacral end plate (**Fig. 81.7**). Likewise, sacral slope (SS) is the angle subtended by a horizontal reference and the sacral end-plate line. Labele et al[34] have shown that PI = PT + SS. Together these parameters determine the alignment of the spine and ultimately the patient's ability to maintain the head over the pelvis and femoral heads. Glassman et al[28] have shown that there is a progressive decline in function with greater imbalance, and that relative lumbar kyphosis is poorly tolerated. Furthermore, Schwab et al[29] have described the need to maintain spinal alignment as part of the basic human need to preserve horizontal gaze and keep the head over the pelvis. Bridwell et al[35] have gone further to show that patients who have undergone operative correction of their deformity have experienced significantly greater improvements in ODI and SRS quality-of-life outcome scores compared with the scores for nonoperative management. Smith et al[36] confirmed these findings, and Schwab

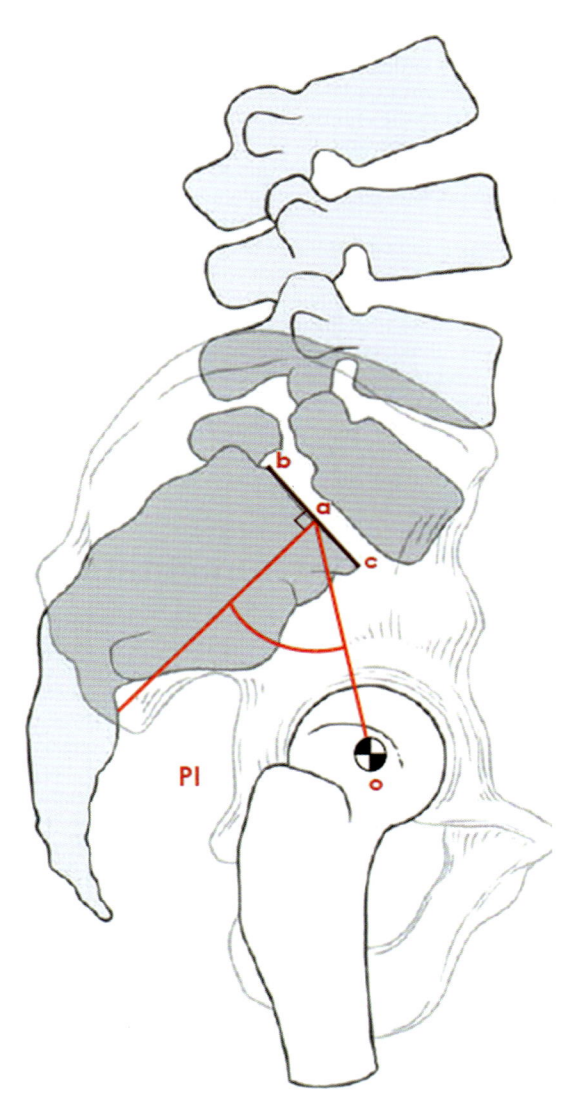

Fig. 81.6 Pelvic incidence (PI) is an angle subtended by a line that is drawn from the center of the femoral head to the midpoint of the sacral end plate and a line perpendicular to the center of the sacral end plate. (Courtesy of the Orthopaedic Research and Education Foundation [OREF]. From Legaye J, Duval-Beaupére G, Hecquet J, Marty C. Pelvic incidence: a fundamental pelvic parameter for three-dimensional regulation of spinal sagittal curves. Eur Spine J 1998;7:99–103. Reprinted with permission.)

corrective maneuvers must be directed at reestablishing global sagittal and coronal alignment. Dubousset[30] first introduced the idea of the "cone of economy," stating that to maintain an upright posture in an energy-efficient manner, one must position the head over the pelvis and femoral heads. The position of the pelvis in relation to the femoral heads is measured by the pelvic incidence (PI), which is the angle subtended by a line drawn from the center of the femoral heads to the midpoint of the sacral end plate and a line perpendicular to the sacral end plate (**Fig. 81.6**). The PI is a fixed value once a patient has reached skeletal maturity and defines the relationship of the spine to the pelvis.[31] The magnitude of PI determines how much lumbar lordosis (LL) is required, and the mismatch between PI and LL can lead to significant pain and disability.[32,33] Boulay et al[32,33] have determined that LL = PI ± 9 degrees. The amount of LL influences thoracic kyphosis, cervical lordosis, and ultimately the position of the head in space.

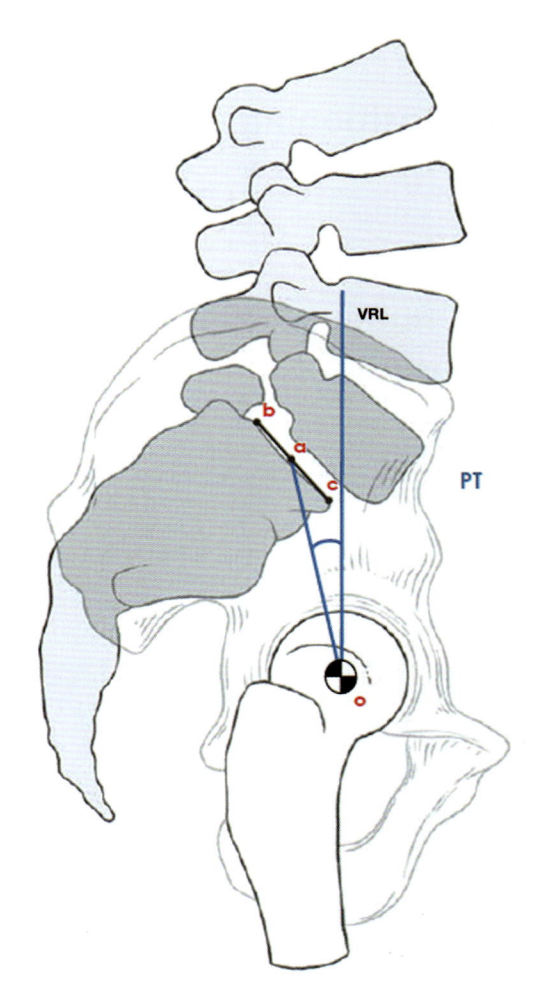

Fig. 81.7 Pelvic tilt (PT) is defined as the angle subtended by a vertical reference line (VRL) originating from the center of the femoral head (o) and the midpoint of the sacral end plate (a). The midpoint between the posterior aspect of sacral endplate (b) and anterior aspect of sacral endplate (c) is the midpoint of the sacral endpoint (a). (Courtesy of the Orthopaedic Research and Education Foundation [OREF]. Legaye J, Duval-Beaupére G, Hecquet J, Marty C. Pelvic incidence: a fundamental pelvic parameter for three-dimensional regulation of spinal sagittal curves. Eur Spine J 1998; 7:99–103. Reprinted with permission.)

et al[37] went on to determine that patients with a PI–LL mismatch > 11 degrees were more likely to have pelvic retroversion (PT > 22 degrees) and sagittal imbalance as well as a 3.9-fold greater risk of severe disability.

Preoperatively, the use of halo-gravity traction (HGTx) can be helpful in providing some curve correction. Sink et al[38] reported not only a 35% improvement in coronal Cobb angle but also improvement in trunk decompensation and trunk height in the pediatric population. Rinella et al[39] also demonstrated a 46% improvement in coronal Cobb angle, and Garabekyan et al[40] reported a similar 43% coronal Cobb correction and significant improvements in sagittal alignment (T5–T12), trunk height, and pulmonary function with preoperative HGTx. In a multicenter study, Sponseller et al[41] compared two groups of patients with severe scoliosis or kyphosis with and without preoperative HGTx. Following definitive spinal fusion, there was no significant difference in ultimate correction between the group that underwent HGTx and the group that did not, but the group with preoperative HGTx required significantly fewer vertebral column resections. The authors concluded that the use of HGTx enabled gradual deformity correction, and thus those patients did not require the more extensive procedure of a VCR with the associated neurologic risk and increased blood loss.[41]

Patient Positioning

Once the decision has been made to operate, and a surgical plan has been devised, the first step in obtaining correction is patient positioning. Using an open, radiolucent OSI Jackson table (Mizuho OSI, Union City, CA) with multiple posts/pads enables prone positioning in a physiological manner, optimizing the sagittal plane alignment. Multiple studies have addressed the impact of patient positioning on lumbar lordosis. Stephens et al[42] compared preoperative lumbar lordosis on standing radiographs with intraoperative radiographs obtained in the prone position on the OSI Jackson frame, and concluded that the OSI Jackson table does indeed duplicate physiological lordosis. Marsicano et al[43] also looked at the impact of the OSI Jackson table on lordosis and demonstrated an increase in the lordosis across the distal instrumented levels compared with preoperative radiographs in the AIS population. Furthermore, Harimaya et al[44] demonstrated that prone positioning in adult spinal deformity patients increases lordosis by 8.1 degrees compared with preoperative standing lateral radiographs, and patients with preoperative hyperlordosis (mean −25.9 degrees) experienced an even greater improvement in lordosis (mean 17.2 degrees) with positioning alone compared with upright radiographs. The hip pads should be placed distal to the anterior superior iliac spine to allow the abdomen to hang free and allow the lumbar spine to fall into lordosis. By paying careful attention to prone positioning, one can obtain improved sagittal plane alignment prior to making an incision.

With regard to positioning of the head, there are a variety of devices that can be utilized, each with advantages and disadvantages. In cases that require prolonged prone positioning, keeping the face free with the use of a halo, Gardner-Wells tongs, or Mayfield headholder can help reduce the risk of facial and airway edema. The use of a halo can be helpful in cases of severe upper thoracic kyphosis in particular. The halo helps keep the face free during the procedure and enables greater control of the cervicothoracic junction. The halo can rest on the prone headholder, and cervical traction can be applied when necessary via the halo (**Fig. 81.8**).

Exposure and Instrumentation

The dorsal exposure to the spine has been described in other chapters, but there are a few aspects worth pointing out. Correction techniques used in spinal deformity are dependent on the quality of fixation, and thus it is imperative to pay special attention to preparing the spine for the placement of instrumentation so that conditions are optimized for obtaining strong, reliable fixation. All dissection and exposure is done in the subperiosteal plane, and it must be wide enough to completely expose the lateral aspect of the transverse processes at every level. This ensures visualization of the complete segmental anatomy as well as exposing an appropriate bony bed for fusion. Also, all soft tissue must be completely removed from all aspects of the spine including the facet joints. Once the dorsal spine is completely exposed, denuded, and cleaned, it is time to prepare for the placement of instrumentation. In the thoracic spine, 3 to 5 mm of the inferior facet is removed using an osteotome, and the remaining cartilage should be removed with a curette or electrocautery to enhance conditions for intra-articular arthrodesis. Removal of the inferior facet has other advantages as well, namely exposing the superior facet so the starting point for pedicle screw placement can be easily visualized,[45] creating segmental mobility in the spine, and the harvested bone can then be utilized as

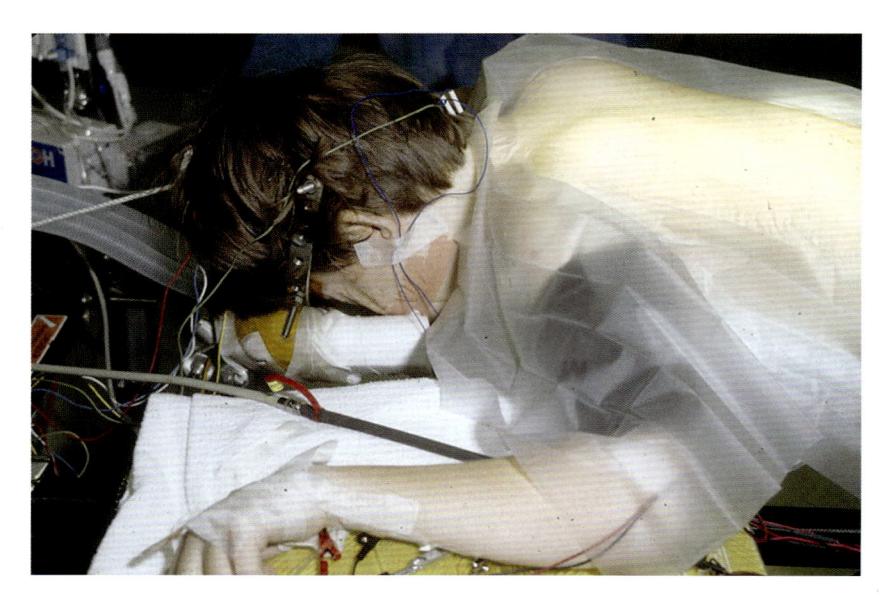

Fig. 81.8 The use of a halo traction intraoperatively can provide kyphosis correction and control of the cervicothoracic junction in cases of significant kyphosis, with constructs that extend to the proximal thoracic or distal cervical spine.

autograft for arthrodesis. Likewise, in the lumbar spine the inferior facet is also removed to expose the articular surface and properly identify the anatomy of the joint itself, particularly in the setting of common degenerative pathologies leading to facet hypertrophy. Freehand placement of thoracic and lumbar pedicle screws is then performed using the technique described by Kim et al.[46] The straightforward as opposed to the anatomic trajectory is utilized to maximize pullout strength and insertional torque.[47]

The use of hooks, sublaminar wires, pedicle screws, or other forms of segmental fixation is dependent on the surgeon's comfort with the various techniques, the goals of correction, and the patient's anatomy. Early segmental fixation methods involved the use of hooks and sublaminar wires.[48] Pedicle screws, however, provide three-column fixation and allow for greater correction force compared with hooks and wires.[49–52] The development of three-column fixation through pedicle screws has provided greater coronal and sagittal plane correction as well as enabled performing apical derotation. There are different types of pedicle screws that can be utilized throughout a construct, each with a specific purpose. For example, monaxial or uniplanar screws have been shown to be more effective in apical vertebral derotation compared with polyaxial screws.[53,54] However, the force required to secure the rod to uniplanar screws is greater than that for polyaxial screws,[55] and thus increases the force at the bone–screw interface.[56] Also, the use of reduction screws at the caudal aspect of a construct or at the concave apex may be helpful in bringing the rod to the screw head during correction. Often in the setting of severe deformity, many patients are malnourished, and thus soft tissue coverage over the implants can be an issue. At the cranial aspect of the incision, when possible, it is ideal to use as low profile a screw as possible. Closed multiaxial screws (CMASs) have a smaller screw head and a closed head, which can assist in correction with rod rotation and cantilever bending.

The size and material of the rod is also important in choosing the best construct for a specific patient. The most commonly used materials include stainless steel, titanium, and cobalt chrome alloy. Each has a specific stiffness and yield point, which is intrinsic to the rod material and diameter of the rod (**Fig. 81.9**). A detailed discussion of the memory and contourability of various rod systems is beyond the scope of this chapter, but suffice it to say that there many different options that should be matched to a patient's age, size, bone quality, and planned correction among other factors.

Osteotomy

There are many different types of osteotomies that can be used to obtain both sagittal and coronal correction. The decision to perform an osteotomy is based on many factors. The type of deformity—scoliosis, kyphosis, kyphoscoliosis, or lordosis—determines what type of correction is needed in both the coronal and sagittal planes. Likewise, the flexibility of the deformity determines how much of an osteotomy to perform. According to Schwab et al,[57] there are varying degrees of destabilization through an osteotomy based on the amount of bony resection, with six grades of potential destabilization:

Grade 1: partial facet release. Resection of the inferior facet and joint capsule creates little overall deformity correction but can provide some segmental flexibility, aid in arthrodesis, and generate autograft. A mobile intervertebral disk is required to provide any motion at that segment.

Grade 2: complete facetectomy. Removal of both the inferior and superior facets as well as the ligamentum flavum, lamina, and spinous process, also referred to as a posterior column osteotomy (PCO) (**Fig. 81.10**), creates an even greater degree of segmental mobility and is also dependent on a mobile anterior column. Smith-Petersen et al[58] first described performing a facetectomy for correction in a fixed deformity such as rheumatoid arthritis (**Fig. 81.11**). Ponte's group[59] also described performing a complete facetectomy for flexible deformity. The advantages of

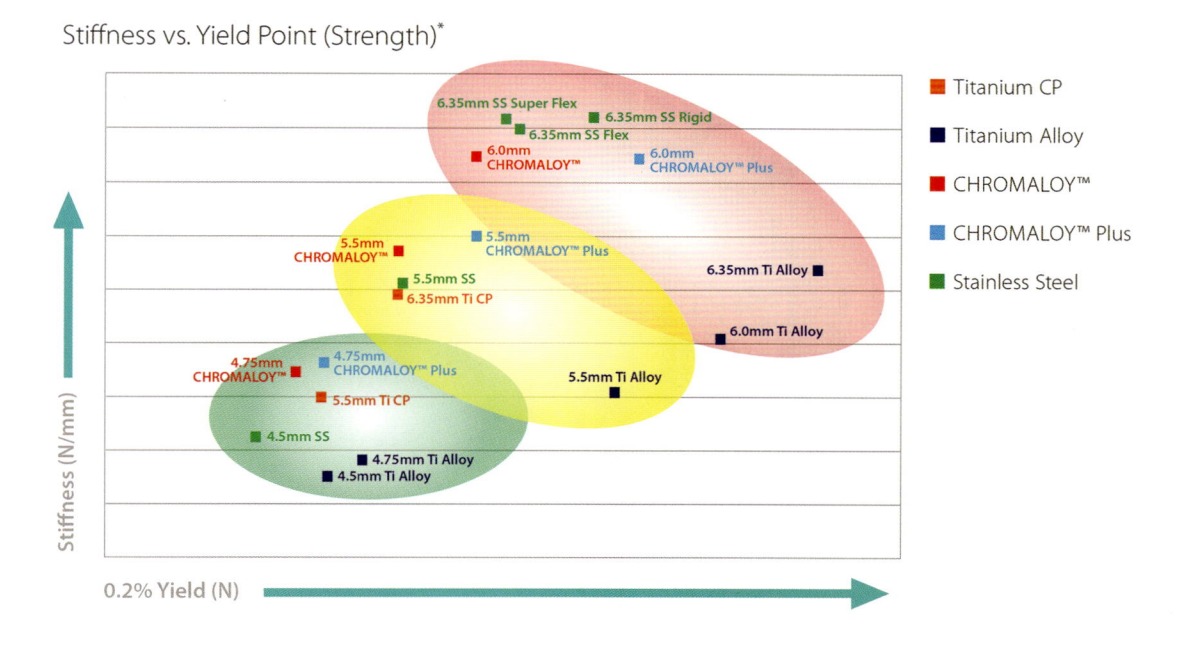

Fig. 81.9 Yield point versus stiffness for various types of rods. Chromaloy, cobalt chrome alloy; Ti, titanium alloy; SS, stainless steel.) (Courtesy of Medtronic, Inc. Reprinted with permission.)

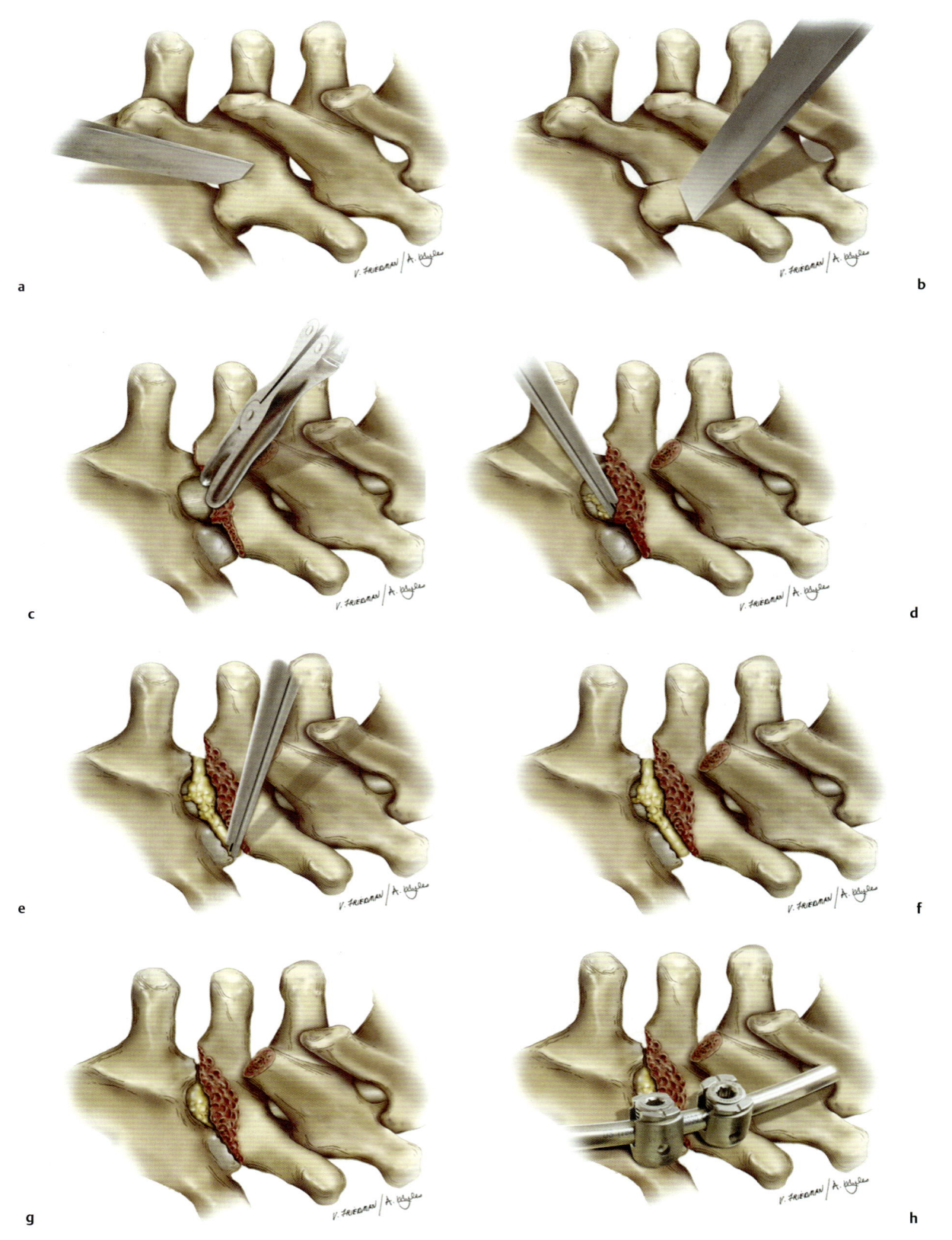

Fig. 81.10 Schematic demonstrating a posterior column osteotomy (PCO). **(a,b)** Using an osteotome, the inferior facet is removed, exposing the superior facet. The spinous process and lamina are removed, exposing the ligamentum flavum. **(d)** A Kerrison rongeur is then used to remove the ligamentum flavum and superior facet. **(e)** The osteotomy is performed to the lateral aspect of the joint and around the pedicle of the level below. **(f,g)** Once the osteotomy is complete, it is important to palpate cranially and caudally to ensure that there are no bony fragments that will compress the nerve root when the osteotomy is closed. **(h)** Compression using segmental fixation is used to close the osteotomy, providing focal lordosis.

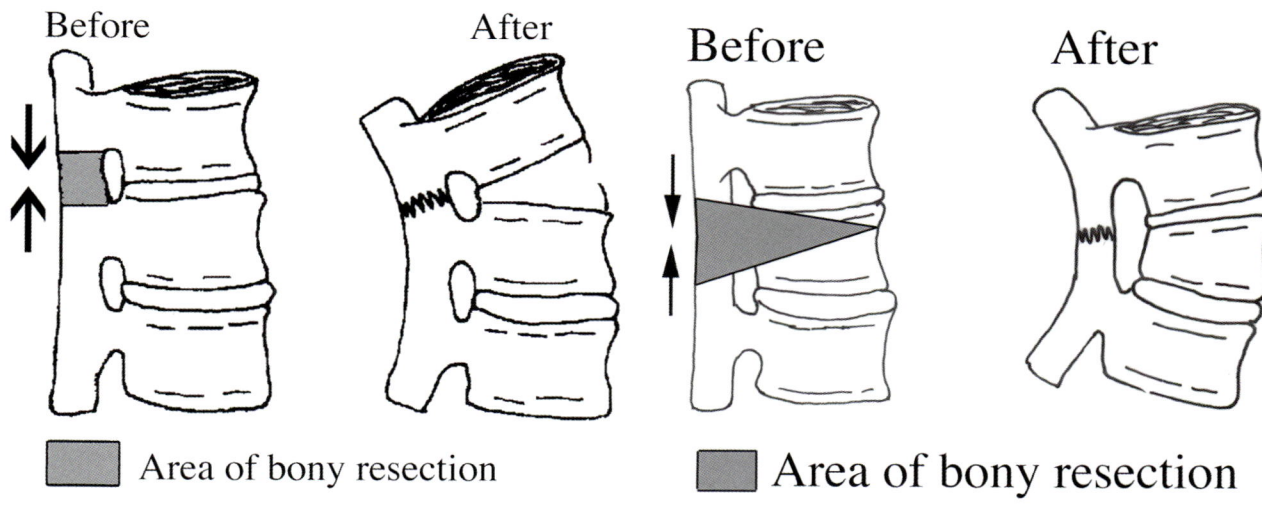

Fig. 81.11 Smith-Petersen osteotomy.

Fig. 81.12 Three-column pedicle subtraction osteotomy.

the use of multiple PCOs include relatively little blood loss and the ability to create smooth harmonious correction across multiple levels. On average, for each 1 mm of bone removed as part of a PCO, 1 degree of lordosis is generated.[60,61] Dorward et al[62] have shown an even greater impact of PCOs with an average of 8.8 ± 7.2 degrees of correction per level. Furthermore, they demonstrated regional differences in the amount of correction, with the greatest amount of correction obtained through PCOs in the lower thoracic and upper lumbar spine.

Grade 3: pedicle and partial vertebral body resection. A portion of the vertebral body and pedicles are resected along with the ligamentum flavum, lamina, and bilateral facets, creating a wedge-shaped osteotomy.[63] Most commonly known as a pedicle subtraction osteotomy (PSO)[63,64] **(Fig. 81.12)**, large, rigid deformities may require resection of a wedge of bone spanning the anterior, middle, and posterior columns to generate 25 to 35 degrees of correction.[60] The decancellation of the vertebral body can also generate a significant amount of autograft that can aid in arthrodesis. Although the primary application for a PSO is fixed sagittal imbalance, an asymmetric PSO can provide simultaneous sagittal and coronal correction. It is important to note that the use of a 3-CO is a *spine shortening* procedure. By shortening the spine, the cauda equine/spinal cord is taken off stretch into a much more relaxed position, thus reducing or minimizing the neurologic risk. Any maneuver that attempts to lengthen the spine puts the neural elements at significant risk. Thus, when placing distraction on the spine or in kyphosis correction without a 3-CO, caution must be taken to avoid stretching and potentially producing a neurologic deficit.

Grade 4: pedicle, partial vertebral body, and intervertebral disk resection. By extending the vertebral body resection to include the adjacent cranial intervertebral disk, the wedge created is thus enlarged and can increase the amount of correction. Ondra et al[65,66] have described the amount of posterior and middle column bony resection required to obtain a desired degree of correction by using a trigonometric calculation.

Grade 5: complete vertebral body and intervertebral disk resection. The vertebral column resection (VCR) involves complete resection of the vertebral body and adjoining ribs in the thoracic spine as well as the adjacent intervertebral disks. Resection of a complete vertebral body can be performed in the thoracic spine to generate 40 to 50 degrees of correction. The VCR includes resection of all posterior elements, facet joints and disks above and below, pedicles, and the entire vertebral body **(Fig. 81.13)** (Video 81.1). This technique enables a great deal of correction as the spine is disarticulated at the apex of the deformity and the proximal and distal limbs are slowly brought together. The entire spine is pushed slightly anterior with a VCR, and an anterior fusion is required using structural support (cage). It is important to point out that closure of the osteotomy is performed through segmental fixation. Cantilever force or compression can be used. By securing separate rods to multiple segments above and below the osteotomy and closing through a connector, construct-to-construct correction is utilized, which is much stronger and more able to withstand greater force during the closure **(Fig. 81.14)**.

Grade 6: multilevel adjacent vertebrae and intervertebral disk resection. The use of multiple VCRs allows for a tremendous amount of correction. However, a single-level VCR carries a significant neurologic and hemodynamic risk profile, and performing a multilevel VCR certainly adds to that risk. In fact, in a multicenter study of severe pediatric deformity, Lenke et al[67] have reported a 39% intraoperative complication rate, including a 27% rate of neurologic deficit with loss of intraoperative spinal cord monitoring, and a 15% rate of estimated blood loss greater than the patient's total blood volume.

Rod Rotation and Vertebral Body Derotation

There are a variety of techniques that can be used to correct the deformity once segmental fixation is in place. The flexibility of the spine can be increased significantly through facet releases and PCOs and dramatically by using a 3-CO. Ultimately, the final alignment is obtained through a combination of rod contouring, rod rotation, compression, distraction, direct vertebral derotation, in-situ translation, and cantilever bending. It cannot be overemphasized that the ability to perform these maneuvers is dependent on the flexibility of the spine, the strength of the implants, and the contour ability/memory of the rod material.

The techniques presented in this chapter are performed from an all-posterior approach. Prior to the use of pedicle screws and three-column fixation, vertebral body derotation required releasing the anterior column through a thoracotomy, thoracolumbar flank approach, or an anterior retroperitoneal approach. However, the use of multisegmental three-column pedicle screw fixation

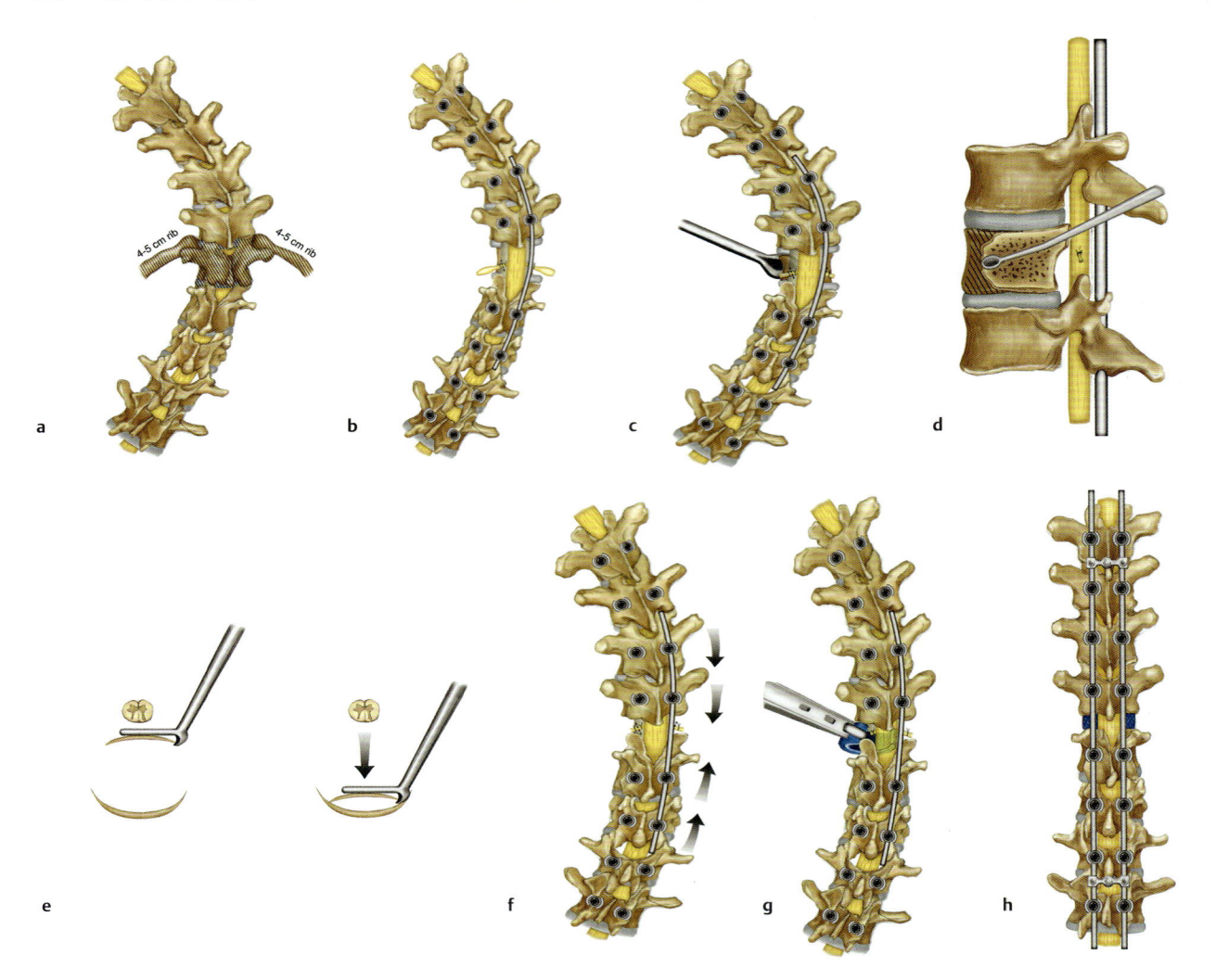

Fig. 81.13 Schematic demonstrating vertebral column resection (VCR). **(a)** The posterior elements including the lamina, facet, 4 to 5 cm of each rib, and ligamentum flavum are resected. **(b)** Once pedicle screw fixation is obtained at all levels, a temporary rod is secured in place, and the pedicles are resected until they are flush with the posterior vertebral body. **(c)** The lateral vertebral body is exposed, and a retractor is placed that reaches around the front of the vertebral body. **(d)** Decancellation of the vertebral body is performed, extending through the disk above and below. **(e)** The posterior body wall is impacted anteriorly into the defect created by removal of the vertebral body. **(f)** Compression is performed along the convexity creating coronal correction. **(g)** A structural anterior interbody cage is placed as a pivot point and to facilitate anterior fusion. **(h)** Final construct demonstrating coronal correction through a closed VCR.

has enabled surgeons to obtain improved sagittal and coronal correction through an all-posterior approach.[68–71] Furthermore, vertebral body derotation can provide significant reduction in the rib prominence as well as significant curve correction.[72–74] Cotrel and Dubousset introduced the technique of rod rotation to create sagittal and coronal plane correction; however this technique produced only a 9% apical rotational correction.[75–77]

One of the most common patient complaints in AIS is the cosmetic deformity associated with the rib prominence, which can be reduced using a thoracoplasty. However, thoracoplasty has been associated with a 23% reduction in pulmonary function testing 2 years after surgery.[77,78] By utilizing the strength and stability of three-column fixation with pedicle screws, the vertebral body itself can be derotated to reduce the chest wall rotational deformity. Moreover, fixed-angle screws provide even greater periapical derotation compared with polyaxial screws, as the torque through the screw is not dissipated in the multiaxial joint.[77,79] Derotation can be accomplished by pushing the concave

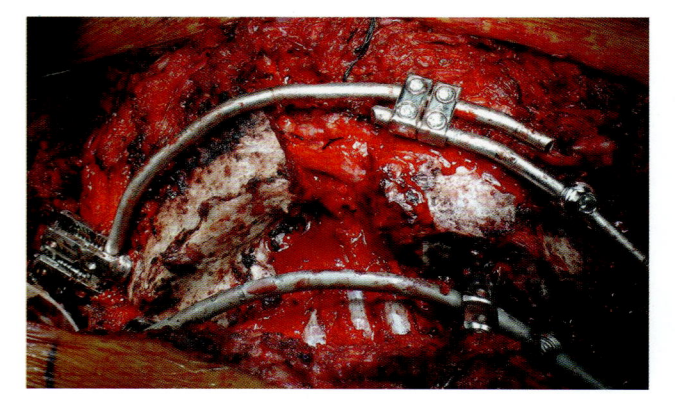

Fig. 81.14 Intraoperative photograph demonstrating construct-to-construct closure. Multiple fixation points both above and below the osteotomy are engaged with two separate rods connected through a domino connector.

apical screws laterally or pushing the convex periapical screws medially. Although the medial wall of the pedicle is stronger than the lateral wall, pushing the convex screws medially runs the risk of breaching the screw medially into the spinal canal. Likewise, forcing the concave screws laterally carries the risk of breaking the screw out laterally, potentially injuring major vasculature or simply losing fixation.

Lenke and Chang[77] describe the use of a vertebral column manipulator (VCM, Medtronic, Minneapolis, MN), a device that attaches to the heads of the periapical screws and triangulates the force of derotation to share the load across the convex and concave screws (**Fig. 81.15**). Connecting the two sides over multiple screws on each side creates a quadrilateral frame to distribute the force and share the stress[77,80] (**Fig. 81.16**). Prior to derotation with the VCM, the correcting rod is contoured to the desired sagittal profile. It is placed in the cranial two or three screws and blocked in place but not tightened. A rod rotation maneuver is then performed by rotating the rod counterclockwise to engage the caudal screws. Reduction screws at the caudal aspect of the construct can be helpful in capturing the rod. Once the rod rotation is complete, the caudal aspect is secured and the VCM is attached. When the quadrilateral frame is constructed, ventral manipulation of the convex handles produces a true derotation by medializing the apex. Translational forces can also be applied through the VCM by applying pressure on the convex apex and pulling up on the concavity. This helps push the apex medially up to the concave rod, creating correction in both the coronal and sagittal plane. The use of a reduction screw at the apex on the concavity can aid in capturing the concave apical rod. Once the correcting rod is fully seated and secured, the holding rod is then contoured to the desired sagittal profile and secured in place so that the VCM can be removed.

Performing a derotation maneuver, like many correction techniques, is dependent on the quality of segmental fixation. The fixation must be strong and the pedicle screws must be placed accurately. In the setting of thoracic hyperkyphosis (> 40 degrees), a derotation maneuver is not performed as it can place considerable force on the proximal screws. In the setting of a significant kyphotic component to the deformity, the convex rod is placed first and the coronal deformity and sagittal plane deformity are addressed simultaneously using a combination of rod rotation and cantilever bending.

The correction strategy is based on the pattern of the curve and the goals of correction. To demonstrate these points, we will use the Lenke classification[19] of AIS to illustrate various correction strategies from a posterior approach.

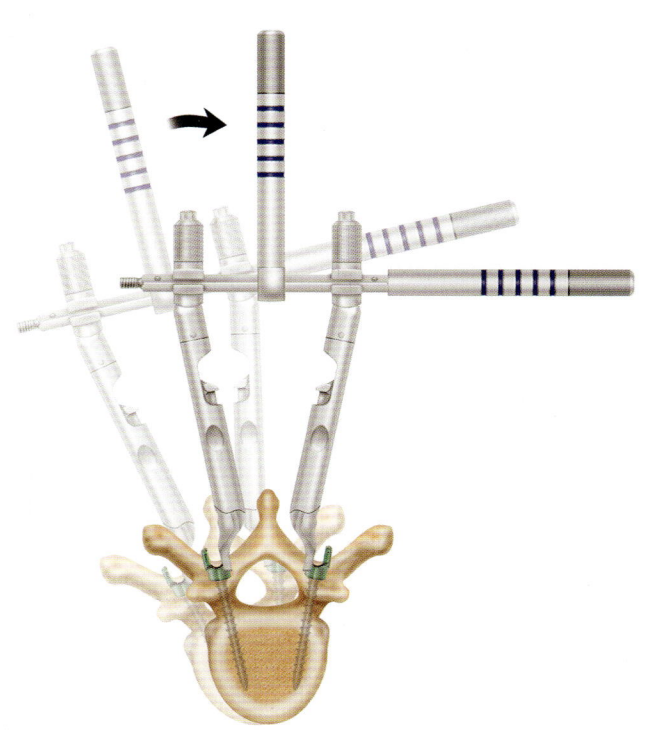

Fig. 81.15 Schematic demonstrating segmental direct vertebral derotation using VCM. (Courtesy of Medtronic, Inc. Reprinted with permission.)

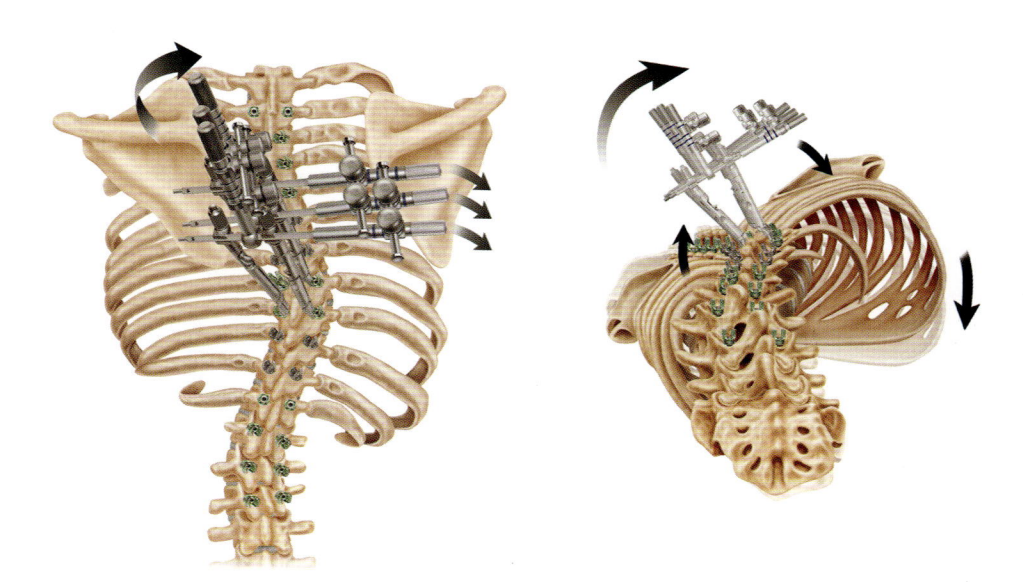

Fig. 81.16 Schematic demonstrating the use of VCM for direct vertebral body derotation through multiple levels using the quadrilateral frame. (Courtesy of by Medtronic, Inc. Reprinted with permission.)

Main Thoracic (Lenke Type 1)

The left/correcting rod is first contoured to the desired sagittal profile and inserted into all of the screws along the path of the right thoracic coronal curve without locking the rod in place. For large curves, the concave apical screws may not engage given the severity of the deformity. The rod is then rotated in the *counterclockwise* direction until the desired sagittal alignment is obtained. The caudal two or three set screws are then locked in place to hold the rod in the correct sagittal position. As with all corrective maneuvers, this should be performed in a controlled, cautious fashion, with close attention paid to the bone–screw interface, looking for pullout or loosening of the screws. Also, neuromonitoring with somatosensory evoked potentials (SSEPs) and motor evoked potentials (MEPs) should be followed closely during these maneuvers. Depending on the surgeon's preference and goals of correction, direct vertebral body derotation can then be performed as described above. Next, distraction is performed on the concavity. The apical screw is locked, and the upper screws are distracted cranially and the lower screws are distracted caudally. All the set screws are then locked in place and in-situ coronal benders are then used to fine-tune the correction while again paying attention to the bone–screw interface.

The right/holding rod is then contoured to a sagittal profile that is slightly less kyphotic. It is then attached to the most cranial screw in a kyphotic position and sequentially secured in place starting cranially and progressing caudally. Using cantilever force, the rod is secured in place, forcing the convex apex anteriorly and reducing the thoracic rib hump. The apical screw is then locked in place and compression is applied toward the apex, compressing the upper screws caudally and the lower screws cranially in an attempt to horizontalize the vertebral bodies and intervertebral disks. The amount of curve correction overall is determined by the selection of fusion levels and the magnitude and stiffness of the lumbar curve. By definition, the thoracolumbar/lumbar curve in a Lenke 1 scoliosis is nonstructural, and thus horizontalizing the lowest instrumented vertebra (LIV) is important and influenced by the extent of apical vertebral translation of the lumbar curve as graded by the Lenke lumbar modifier.[19]

Double Thoracic (Lenke Type 2)

The left/correcting rod is first contoured to the desired thoracic kyphosis (**Fig. 81.17a**), which is based on the flexibility of the curve, magnitude of the curve, quantity and quality of the fixation points, and size and material of the rod. The rod should first be secured but not locked to the cranial-most screws along the convexity of the proximal thoracic curve (**Fig. 81.17b**). A rod rotation maneuver is then performed to place the correcting rod in the appropriate sagittal orientation and then locked to the caudal screws to prevent it from rotating back (**Fig. 81.17c**). The apical screws on the main thoracic (MT) concavity may not engage the rod until more correction is obtained. The proximal thoracic curve is then corrected using compression toward the apex along the convexity (**Fig. 81.17d**). Once the proximal thoracic curve is reduced, the MT periapical vertebrae can be derotated using direct vertebral derotation, translating the concave apex dorsally and medially to engage the rod (**Fig. 81.17e**). While holding the spine in the derotated position, distraction is performed away from the apex on the MT concavity (**Fig. 81.17f**), and the rod is then secured to the MT concave screws. In-situ coronal benders can be used to adjust the alignment of the correcting rod (**Fig. 81.17g**).

The right/holding rod is then contoured in a hypokyphotic position and secured to the cranial one or two screws followed by sequential reduction to the caudal levels (**Fig. 81.17h**). In the event that there is a positive (+) sagittal modifier, cantilever

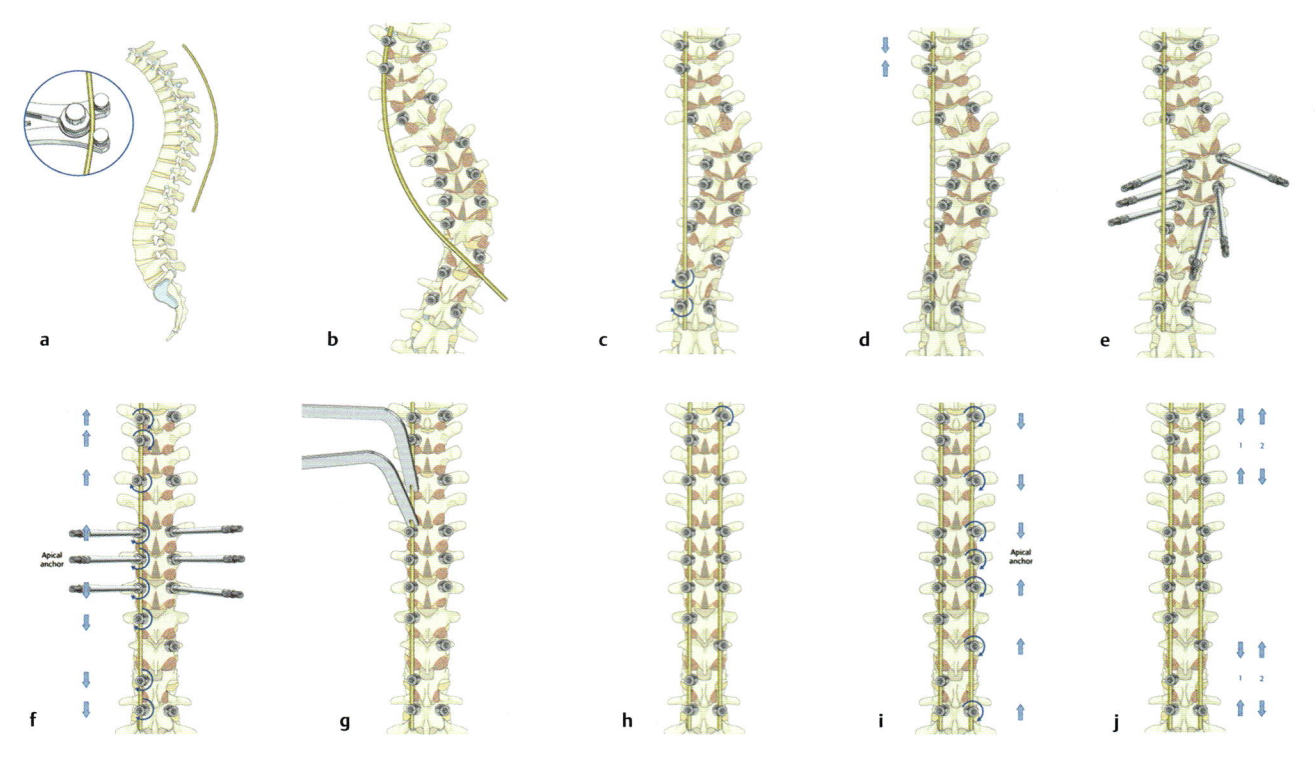

Fig. 81.17 Schematic demonstrating the sequence of techniques used for correction of a double thoracic idiopathic curve. (See text for a description of each panel.) (From AO Surgery Reference, www.aosurgery.org. Copyright by AO Foundation, Switzerland. Reprinted with permission.)

bending can be used to reduce the kyphosis. Finally, compression is performed toward the apex on the convexity (**Fig. 81.17i**). The most cranial and caudal segments can be adjusted using compression and distraction to make the shoulders level and/or to horizontalize the disk below the LIV (**Fig. 81.17j**).

Buchowski et al[81,82] have described the impact of temporary internal distraction for the correction of large deformities. Pedicle screws or a combination of an upgoing pedicle hook and downgoing laminar hook can be used on the concavity of large curves to augment distractive correction. However, posterior distraction creates kyphosis in the sagittal plane, and thus caution must be used in the amount of distraction that is applied. It must also be pointed out that distraction is a spine-lengthening maneuver that carries a higher neurologic risk than a spine-shortening maneuver such as compression.

Double Major (Lenke Type 3)

Similar to the Lenke types 1 and 2 curves, the double major curve is first addressed from the left. The left rod is contoured to the desired thoracic kyphosis and lumbar lordosis and secured, but not locked to the cranial one or two screws. The alignment should mimic the MT concavity and thoracolumbar/lumbar (TL/L) convexity. Rod rotation is then performed to establish the desired sagittal alignment by locking the caudal screws. Vertebral derotation is then performed both for the MT and TL/L curves in opposite directions. The MT curve is first derotated, pushing the thoracic apex medially and dorsally to engage the contoured rod. The TL/L curve is then derotated in the opposite direction to push the apical vertebra medially and ventrally to generate lumbar lordosis. In the derotated position, distraction is performed away from the apex on the concavity of the MT curve, compression is performed on the convexity of the TL/L curve, and the screws are then locked in place.

The right rod is contoured in the sagittal plane and sequentially secured to the screws using cantilever bending to reduce the convex thoracic apical rotational deformity. Compression can then be performed on the convexity of the MT curve and distraction on the concavity of the TL/L curve, and in-situ coronal bending can be used to fine-tune the correction.

Triple Major (Lenke Type 4)

The Lenke type 4 curve pattern or triple major curve by definition is composed of three structural curves. Thus, the correction strategy must address all three curves. The correcting rod is first contoured to the desired sagittal plane alignment, accounting for both the desired thoracic kyphosis and lumbar lordosis. The rod is placed in the cranial screws first and secured but not locked in place. A rod rotation maneuver is then performed until the desired sagittal alignment is reached and then locking the caudal screws. The proximal thoracic curve is first addressed using compression toward the apex on the convexity. Vertebral derotation of both the MT and TL/L curves is then performed. Then the MT curve is derotated, pushing the apex dorsally and medially to engage the rod on the concavity of the MT curve. Then the TL/L curve is derotated, pushing the apex ventrally and medially until the rod is engaged and locked in place. Distraction along the concavity of the MT curve is then performed, distracting away from the apex both above and below. Compression is utilized on the convexity of the TL/L curve to provide further coronal curve correction but also generate lordosis in the sagittal plane. In-situ coronal benders can then be used to horizontalize each vertebra and adjust the correction.

The right side is then addressed by first contouring the right rod to the desired sagittal profile and then securing it to the cranial screws. Cantilever force can then help reduce the thoracic rib hump and create the desire sagittal alignment. Distraction is then used on the concavity of the proximal thoracic and TL/L curves. Posterior distraction creates kyphosis in the sagittal plane; however, the correcting rod is locked in place holding the sagittal alignment. Compression can then be used on the convexity of the MT curve. In-situ benders can help to adjust the ultimate alignment of the construct.

Thoracolumbar/Lumbar (Lenke Type 5)

The Lenke 5 curve pattern, also known as the TL/L curve pattern, has a slightly different correction strategy, as the TL/L curve is the only structural curve, and typically it is convex on the left side. The left-sided rod is contoured to the desired sagittal profile, paying special attention to the amount of lordosis needed. The magnitude of lordosis is determined by the PI as well as by the thoracic kyphosis and magnitude of any nonstructural MT curve. The contoured rod is placed in the cranial-most screws and secured in place. The rod is then rotated to the desired lordosis and locked in place. Apical derotation is then performed, translating the apical vertebra ventrally and medially to provide coronal curve correction and generate lordosis.

The right rod is contoured with slightly less lordosis compared with the left side. The rod is secured to the cranial screws and then sequentially secured to the remaining caudal screws. Segmental sequential reducers can be utilized to translate the screws up to the rod dorsally to provide some apical derotation and curve correction. Compression toward the locked apical screw along the convexity on the left side is performed followed by distraction away from the locked apical screw on the concavity of the right side. Too much distraction reduces the amount of lordosis in the construct.

Depending on the surgeon's preference, there are anterior approaches that can be utilized for TL/L curves. The details of the anterior approach to the thoracic and lumbar spine are beyond the focus of this chapter, but it is worth mentioning that the anterior approach can be utilized in TL/L curves with either a neutral or negative sagittal profile.

Thoracolumbar/Lumbar–Main Thoracic (Lenke Type 6)

Similar to the Lenke type 3 double major curve, the Lenke type 6 pattern, by definition, consists of two structural curves—MT and TL/L. However, in the Lenke type 6 curve or TL/L–MT curve pattern, the TL/L curve is the major curve, but the overall correction strategy is very similar. The left rod is first contoured to the desired sagittal plane alignment, taking into account the amount of thoracic kyphosis and lumbar lordosis. The rod is then secured to the cranial screws and then rotated to the desired sagittal profile and locked at the caudal aspect. The MT curve is derotated first to translate the thoracic apex dorsally and restore the thoracic kyphosis. The TL/L curve can then be derotated in the opposite direction to push the TL/L apex ventrally to generate lordosis. Distraction on the concavity of the MT curve will correct the secondary curve, and compression toward the apex of the convexity of the TL/L curve is used to correct the major curve. In-situ benders can then be used once the screws are locked to adjust the alignment.

The right-sided rod is contoured to the desired sagittal profile and secured in place starting with the cranial screws. Cantilever bending from cranial to caudal can help reduce the thoracic rib hump on the apex of the MT curve, whereas sequential reduction through the lumbar screws will help to provide some apical derotation and TL/L curve correction. The use of some distal reduction screws can aid in sequentially engaging the rod in a controlled fashion. Compression toward the locked apical screw along the convexity of the MT curve is then performed, followed by distraction away from the apex of the concavity of the TL/L curve, being careful not to over-distract and lose lordosis. In-situ benders can then be used to fine-tune the construct.

Many of the same principles described for AIS curve correction apply to adult deformity as well. However, although coronal malalignment, risk of deformity progression, and cosmesis are the primary factors leading to surgical intervention in the pediatric population, most of the disability and symptomatology in adult deformity stems from sagittal plane malalignment and pain.[13,27,83,84] Furthermore, adults more often suffer from neurologic compression in the form of radiculopathy or neurogenic claudication, requiring decompression. Adults also more often require extension of the instrumented construct to the sacrum and pelvis, which adds an additional level of complexity and challenge in obtaining a solid fusion.

The principles discussed above with regard to patient clinical and radiographic evaluation apply to both the pediatric and adult population. The flexibility of the deformity is of the utmost importance and determines the amount or degree of an osteotomy required. Along with a thorough radiographic evaluation, other issues that need to be addressed include magnitude and angularity (sharp versus rounded) of the deformity, bone quality/density for screw purchase, goals of correction, and ultimately surgeon experience and ability to avoid and manage complications. Although O'Neill et al[25] have demonstrated the long-term benefit and durability of correction obtained through a 3-CO at a minimum 5 year follow-up, the literature also describes overall complication rates from 21 to 34%, an 11% neurologic complication rate, and a 59% complication rate for patients undergoing vertebral column resection specifically.[67,85–89] With that in mind, undertaking a PSO or a VCR should only be done in experienced centers.

The following example demonstrates the use of multiple correction techniques for a severe case of adult idiopathic scoliosis with a preserved sagittal profile in a patient with six lumbar vertebrae (**Fig. 81.18**). Using the freehand pedicle screw technique as described above, segmental fixation is first obtained at all levels. Next, transforaminal lumbar interbody fusions (TLIFs) are performed at the three most caudal segments (**Fig. 81.19a**). Because of the high biomechanical forces at the caudal aspect of a long construct to the sacrum and pelvis, the pseudarthrosis rate at the lumbosacral junction is high.[90,91] Interbody fusion providing anterior column support through an anterior or transforaminal approach has been advocated to decrease S1 screw strain[92] and increase fusion rates. Li et al[93] have described the use of TLIFs from a posterior approach in adult degenerative deformity correction. In this case, the TLIF approach is associated with a complete facetectomy and ligament resection, similar to a PCO, which provides not only deformity correction but also neural element decompression when necessary. Also, the use of pelvic fixation in long constructs to the sacrum is mandatory to reduce S1 screw strain and optimize conditions for fusion at the caudal segment.

In this example, posterior column osteotomies performed at the apical levels of the deformity increase curve flexibility and potential for correction (**Fig. 81.19b**). The concave (right) rod is then cut and contoured to the desired sagittal plane. Segmental realignment is then achieved using segmental compression on

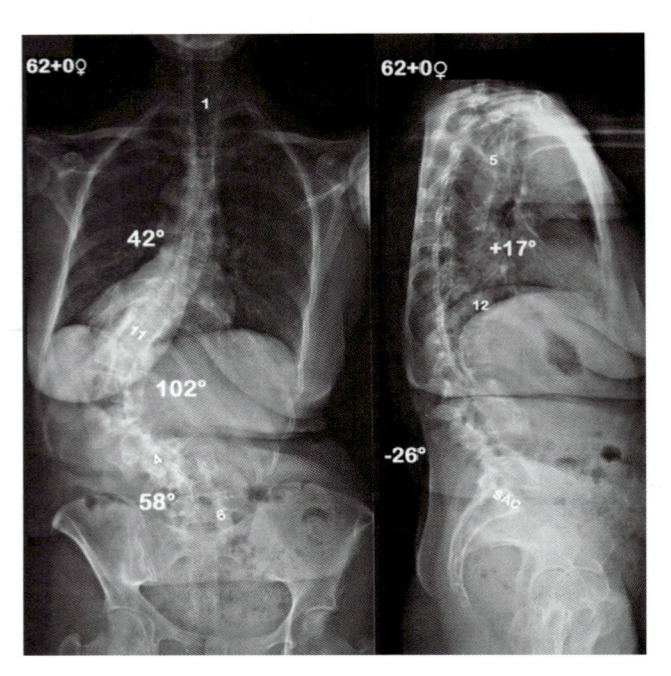

Fig. 81.18 Preoperative standing radiographs of a 62-year-old woman with severe adult idiopathic scoliosis with preserved sagittal alignment.

the convexity of the lumbosacral fractional curve (**Fig. 81.19c**). Further lumbosacral segmental realignment is achieved by distracting through the concavity of the fractional curve (**Fig. 81.19d**). Cantilever bending is then used with the left rod to generate lordosis through the mid-lumbar spine and push the convex apex ventrally (**Fig. 81.19e**). Sequential reduction with the right rod can also aid in pulling the concave apex dorsally. In-situ coronal contouring is then utilized to adjust the coronal alignment first through the left rod (**Fig. 81.19f**). Finally, in-situ translation is obtained through the right rod to achieve the final alignment (**Fig. 81.20**).

In cases of severe sagittal plane imbalance, multiple PCOs or a 3-CO may be required. The Schwab anatomic osteotomy classification[57] can help to determine what type of osteotomy is required, which is largely dependent on the flexibility of the curve.[10] Performing a 3-CO can be technically challenging and physiologically taxing to the patient. Thus, appropriate patient selection and thorough radiographic and medical evaluation is essential.

Conclusion

Both adult and pediatric deformities require significant preoperative planning to optimize outcomes and minimize risks. There are a variety of intraoperative techniques that can be utilized to obtain deformity correction including the use of osteotomies, vertebral derotation, and in-situ contouring, each with unique risk profiles. It is imperative to match the surgical plan with the appropriate patient, keeping in mind the goals of restoring spinal alignment to optimize outcomes.

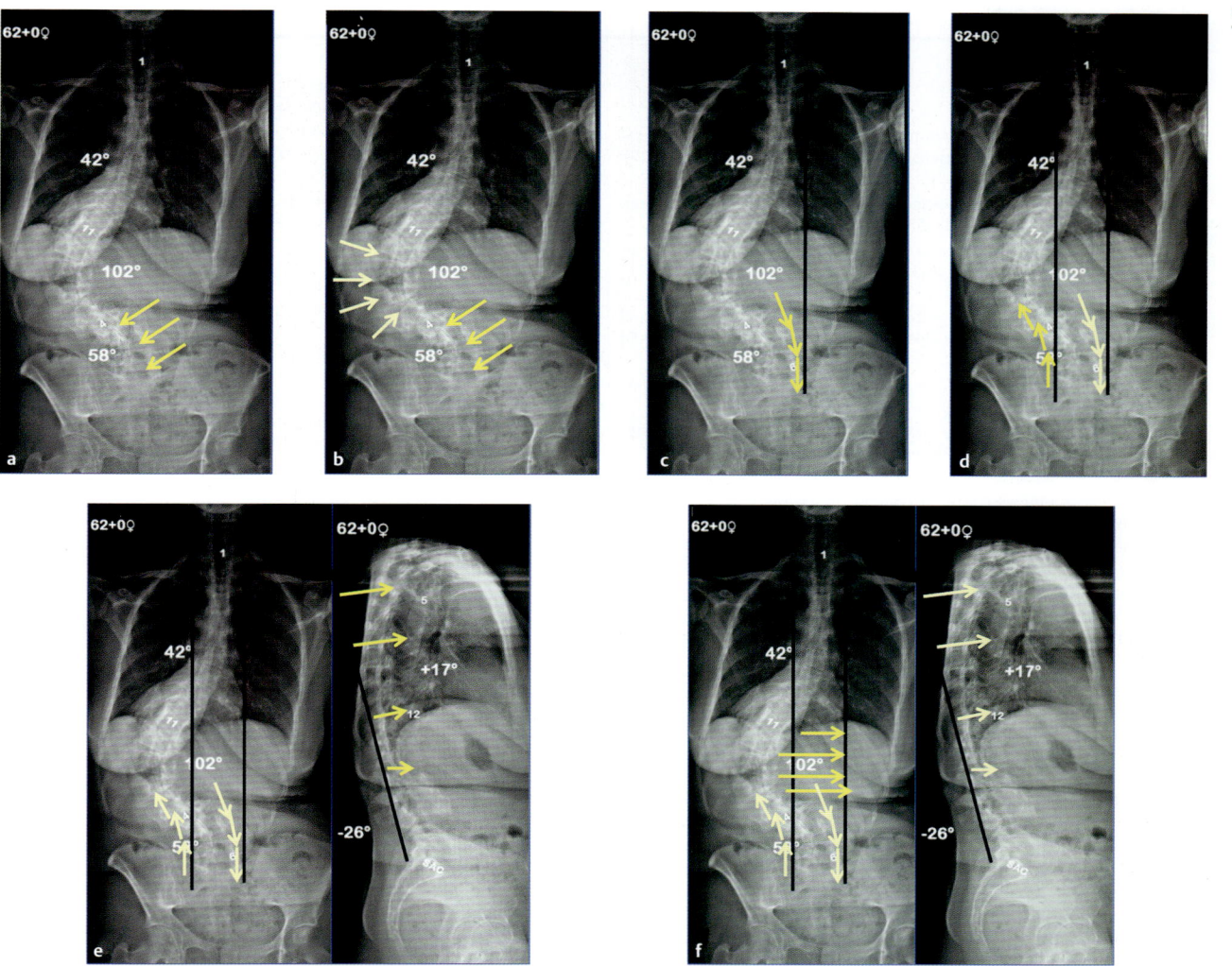

Fig. 81.19 Step-by-step schematic demonstration of final correction in a case of severe adult idiopathic scoliosis with posterior column osteotomies and transforaminal lumbar interbody fusions (TLIFs).

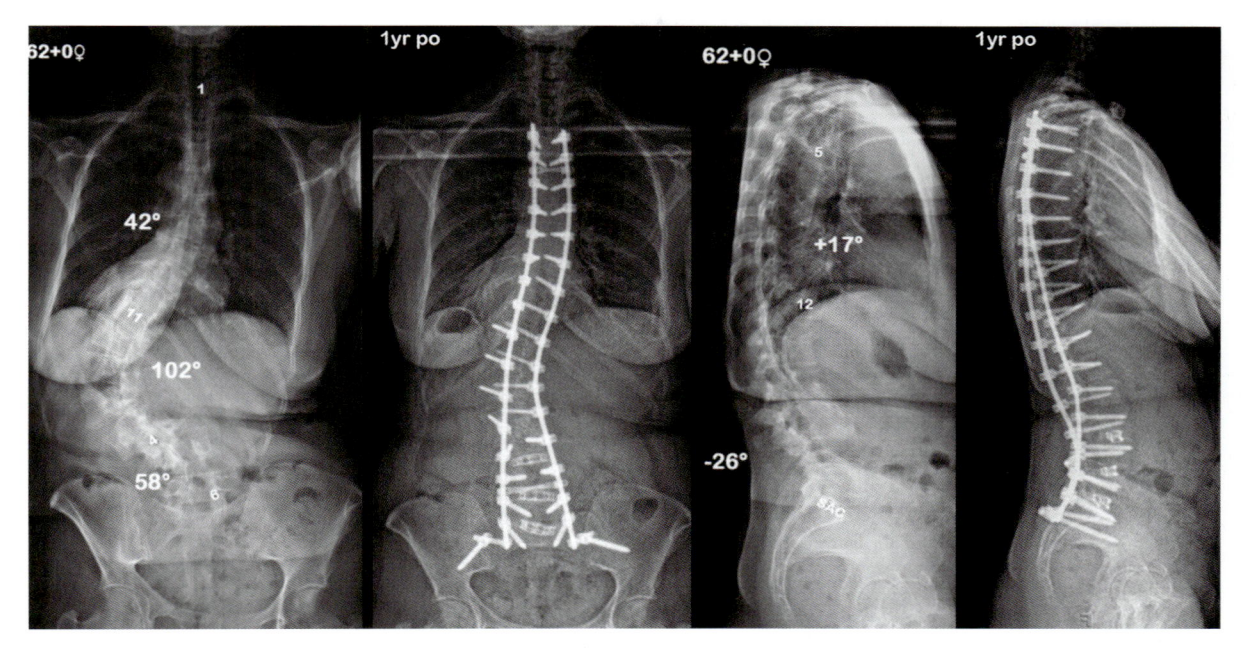

Fig. 81.20 Preoperative and 1-year postoperative standing radiographs of a 62-year-old woman with adult idiopathic scoliosis who underwent T4-S1/ilium instrumented posterior spinal fusion with five posterior column osteotomies and three TLIFs.

References

1. Bradford DS, Tay BK, Hu SS. Adult scoliosis: surgical indications, operative management, complications, and outcomes. Spine 1999;24:2617–2629
2. Kostuik JP, Bentivoglio J. The incidence of low back pain in adult scoliosis. Acta Orthop Belg 1981;47:548–559
3. Pérennou D, Marcelli C, Hérisson C, Simon L. Adult lumbar scoliosis. Epidemiologic aspects in a low-back pain population. Spine 1994;19:123–128
4. Schwab F, Dubey A, Gamez L, et al. Adult scoliosis: prevalence, SF-36, and nutritional parameters in an elderly volunteer population. Spine 2005;30:1082–1085
5. Paulus MC, Kalantar SB, Radcliff K. Cost and value of spinal deformity surgery. Spine 2014;39:388–393
6. Fletcher ND, Bruce RW. Early onset scoliosis: current concepts and controversies. Curr Rev Musculoskelet Med 2012;5:102–110
7. Pehrsson K, Larsson S, Oden A, Nachemson A. Long-term follow-up of patients with untreated scoliosis. A study of mortality, causes of death, and symptoms. Spine 1992;17:1091–1096
8. Bunnell WP. The natural history of idiopathic scoliosis before skeletal maturity. Spine 1986;11:773–776
9. Fernandes P, Weinstein SL. Natural history of early onset scoliosis. J Bone Joint Surg Am 2007;89(Suppl 1):21–33
10. Silva FE, Lenke LG. Adult degenerative scoliosis: evaluation and management. Neurosurg Focus 2010;28:E1
11. Aebi M. The adult scoliosis. Eur Spine J 2005;14:925–948
12. Schwab F, Farcy JP, Bridwell K, et al. A clinical impact classification of scoliosis in the adult. Spine 2006;31:2109–2114
13. Bess S, Schwab F, Lafage V, Shaffrey CI, Ames CP. Classifications for adult spinal deformity and use of the Scoliosis Research Society–Schwab Adult Spinal Deformity Classification. Neurosurg Clin N Am 2013;24:185–193
14. Schwab F, Lafage V, Farcy JP, et al. Surgical rates and operative outcome analysis in thoracolumbar and lumbar major adult scoliosis: application of the new adult deformity classification. Spine 2007;32:2723–2730
15. Schwab FJ, Lafage V, Farcy JP, Bridwell KH, Glassman S, Shainline MR. Predicting outcome and complications in the surgical treatment of adult scoliosis. Spine 2008;33:2243–2247
16. Schwab F, Ungar B, Blondel B, et al. Scoliosis Research Society–Schwab adult spinal deformity classification: a validation study. Spine 2012;37:1077–1082
17. King HA, Moe JH, Bradford DS, Winter RB. The selection of fusion levels in thoracic idiopathic scoliosis. J Bone Joint Surg Am 1983;65:1302–1313
18. Lenke LG, Betz RR, Bridwell KH, et al. Intraobserver and interobserver reliability of the classification of thoracic adolescent idiopathic scoliosis. J Bone Joint Surg Am 1998;80:1097–1106
19. Lenke LG, Betz RR, Harms J, et al. Adolescent idiopathic scoliosis: a new classification to determine extent of spinal arthrodesis. J Bone Joint Surg Am 2001;83-A:1169–1181
20. Edwards CC II, Lenke LG, Peelle M, Sides B, Rinella A, Bridwell KH. Selective thoracic fusion for adolescent idiopathic scoliosis with C modifier lumbar curves: 2- to 16-year radiographic and clinical results. Spine 2004;29:536–546
21. Lenke LG, Bridwell KH, Baldus C, Blanke K. Preventing decompensation in King type II curves treated with Cotrel-Dubousset instrumentation. Strict guidelines for selective thoracic fusion. Spine 1992;17(8, Suppl):S274–S281
22. Sanders AE, Baumann R, Brown H, Johnston CE II, Lenke LG, Sink E. Selective anterior fusion of thoracolumbar/lumbar curves in adolescents: when can the associated thoracic curve be left unfused? Spine 2003;28:706–713, discussion 714
23. Sangole A, Aubin CE, Labelle H, et al; Scoliosis Research Society 3D Scoliosis Committee. The central hip vertical axis: a reference axis for the Scoliosis Research Society three-dimensional classification of idiopathic scoliosis. Spine 2010;35:E530–E534
24. Halpin RJ, Sugrue PA, Gould RW, et al. Standardizing care for high-risk patients in spine surgery: the Northwestern high-risk spine protocol. Spine 2010;35:2232–2238
25. O'Neill KR, Lenke LG, Bridwell KH, et al. Clinical and radiographic outcomes after 3-column osteotomies with 5-year follow-up. Spine 2014;39:424–432
26. Yadla S, Maltenfort MG, Ratliff JK, Harrop JS. Adult scoliosis surgery outcomes: a systematic review. Neurosurg Focus 2010;28:E3
27. Glassman SD, Berven S, Bridwell K, Horton W, Dimar JR. Correlation of radiographic parameters and clinical symptoms in adult scoliosis. Spine 2005;30:682–688
28. Glassman SD, Bridwell K, Dimar JR, Horton W, Berven S, Schwab F. The impact of positive sagittal balance in adult spinal deformity. Spine 2005;30:2024–2029
29. Schwab F, Patel A, Ungar B, Farcy JP, Lafage V. Adult spinal deformity-postoperative standing imbalance: how much can you tolerate? An overview of key parameters in assessing alignment and planning corrective surgery. Spine 2010;35:2224–2231
30. Dubousset J. In: Weinstein SL, ed. The Pediatric Spine: Principles and Practice. New York: Raven Press; 1994;479–496
31. Legaye J, Duval-Beaupère G, Hecquet J, Marty C. Pelvic incidence: a fundamental pelvic parameter for three-dimensional regulation of spinal sagittal curves. Eur Spine J 1998;7:99–103
32. Boulay C, Tardieu C, Bénaim C, et al. Three-dimensional study of pelvic asymmetry on anatomical specimens and its clinical perspectives. J Anat 2006;208:21–33
33. Boulay C, Tardieu C, Hecquet J, et al. Sagittal alignment of spine and pelvis regulated by pelvic incidence: standard values and prediction of lordosis. Eur Spine J 2006;15:415–422
34. Labelle H, Roussouly P, Berthonnaud E, Dimnet J, O'Brien M. The importance of spino-pelvic balance in L5-S1 developmental spondylolisthesis: a review of pertinent radiologic measurements. Spine 2005;30(6, Suppl):S27–S34
35. Bridwell KH, Glassman S, Horton W, et al. Does treatment (nonoperative and operative) improve the two-year quality of life in patients with adult symptomatic lumbar scoliosis: a prospective multicenter evidence-based medicine study. Spine 2009;34:2171–2178
36. Smith JS, Shaffrey CI, Berven S, et al; Spinal Deformity Study Group. Improvement of back pain with operative and nonoperative treatment in adults with scoliosis. Neurosurgery 2009;65:86–93, discussion 93–94
37. Schwab FJ, Blondel B, Bess S, et al; International Spine Study Group (ISSG). Radiographical spinopelvic parameters and disability in the setting of adult spinal deformity: a prospective multicenter analysis. Spine 2013;38:E803–E812
38. Sink EL, Karol LA, Sanders J, Birch JG, Johnston CE, Herring JA. Efficacy of perioperative halo-gravity traction in the treatment of severe scoliosis in children. J Pediatr Orthop 2001;21:519–524
39. Rinella A, Lenke L, Whitaker C, et al. Perioperative halo-gravity traction in the treatment of severe scoliosis and kyphosis. Spine 2005;30:475–482
40. Garabekyan T, Hosseinzadeh P, Iwinski HJ, et al. The results of preoperative halo-gravity traction in children with severe spinal deformity. J Pediatr Orthop B 2014;23:1–5
41. Sponseller PD, Takenaga RK, Newton P, et al. The use of traction in the treatment of severe spinal deformity. Spine 2008;33:2305–2309
42. Stephens GC, Yoo JU, Wilbur G. Comparison of lumbar sagittal alignment produced by different operative positions. Spine 1996;21:1802–1806, discussion 1807
43. Marsicano JG, Lenke LG, Bridwell KH, Chapman M, Gupta P, Weston J. The lordotic effect of the OSI frame on operative adolescent idiopathic scoliosis patients. Spine 1998;23:1341–1348
44. Harimaya K, Lenke LG, Mishiro T, Bridwell KH, Koester LA, Sides BA. Increasing lumbar lordosis of adult spinal deformity patients via intraoperative prone positioning. Spine 2009;34:2406–2412
45. Lehman RA Jr, Kang DG, Lenke LG, Gaume RE, Paik H. The ventral lamina and superior facet rule: a morphometric analysis for an ideal thoracic pedicle screw starting point. Spine J 2014;14:137–144
46. Kim YJ, Lenke LG, Bridwell KH, Cho YS, Riew KD. Free hand pedicle screw placement in the thoracic spine: is it safe? Spine 2004;29:333–342, discussion 342
47. Lehman RA Jr, Polly DW Jr, Kuklo TR, Cunningham B, Kirk KL, Belmont PJ Jr. Straight-forward versus anatomic trajectory technique of thoracic pedicle screw fixation: a biomechanical analysis. Spine 2003;28:2058–2065
48. Cotrel Y, Dubousset J, Guillaumat M. New universal instrumentation in spinal surgery. Clin Orthop Relat Res 1988;227:10–23
49. Gaines RW Jr. The use of pedicle-screw internal fixation for the operative treatment of spinal disorders. J Bone Joint Surg Am 2000;82-A:1458–1476

50. Hamill CL, Lenke LG, Bridwell KH, Chapman MP, Blanke K, Baldus C. The use of pedicle screw fixation to improve correction in the lumbar spine of patients with idiopathic scoliosis. Is it warranted? Spine 1996;21:1241–1249
51. Kim YJ, Lenke LG, Cho SK, Bridwell KH, Sides B, Blanke K. Comparative analysis of pedicle screw versus hook instrumentation in posterior spinal fusion of adolescent idiopathic scoliosis. Spine 2004;29:2040–2048
52. Liljenqvist U, Hackenberg L, Link T, Halm H. Pullout strength of pedicle screws versus pedicle and laminar hooks in the thoracic spine. Acta Orthop Belg 2001;67:157–163
53. Dalal A, Upasani VV, Bastrom TP, et al. Apical vertebral rotation in adolescent idiopathic scoliosis: comparison of uniplanar and polyaxial pedicle screws. J Spinal Disord Tech 2011;24:251–257
54. Essig DA, Miller CP, Xiao M, et al. Biomechanical comparison of endplate forces generated by uniaxial screws and monoaxial pedicle screws. Orthopedics 2012;35:e1528–e1532
55. Wang X, Aubin CE, Labelle H, Parent S, Crandall D. Biomechanical analysis of corrective forces in spinal instrumentation for scoliosis treatment. Spine 2012;37:E1479–E1487
56. Wang X, Aubin CE, Crandall D, Parent S, Labelle H. Biomechanical analysis of 4 types of pedicle screws for scoliotic spine instrumentation. Spine 2012;37:E823–E835
57. Schwab F, Blondel B, Chay E, et al. The comprehensive anatomical spinal osteotomy classification. Neurosurgery 2014;74:112–120, discussion 120
58. Smith-Petersen MN, Larson CB, Aufranc OE. Osteotomy of the spine for correction of flexion deformity in rheumatoid arthritis. Clin Orthop Relat Res 1969;66:6–9
59. Geck MJ, Macagno A, Ponte A, Shufflebarger HL. The Ponte procedure: posterior only treatment of Scheuermann's kyphosis using segmental posterior shortening and pedicle screw instrumentation. J Spinal Disord Tech 2007;20:586–593
60. Bridwell KH. Decision making regarding Smith-Petersen vs. pedicle subtraction osteotomy vs. vertebral column resection for spinal deformity. Spine 2006;31(19, Suppl):S171–S178
61. Bridwell KH. Causes of sagittal spinal imbalance and assessment of the extent of needed correction. Instr Course Lect 2006;55:567–575
62. Dorward IG, Lenke LG, Stoker GE, Cho W, Koester LA, Sides BA. Radiographic and clinical outcomes of posterior column osteotomies in spinal deformity correction. Spine 2014
63. Bridwell KH, Lewis SJ, Rinella A, Lenke LG, Baldus C, Blanke K. Pedicle subtraction osteotomy for the treatment of fixed sagittal imbalance. Surgical technique. J Bone Joint Surg Am 2004;86-A(Suppl 1):44–50
64. Thomasen E. Vertebral osteotomy for correction of kyphosis in ankylosing spondylitis. Clin Orthop Relat Res 1985;194:142–152
65. Yang BP, Ondra SL. A method for calculating the exact angle required during pedicle subtraction osteotomy for fixed sagittal deformity: comparison with the trigonometric method. Neurosurgery 2006;59(4, Suppl 2):ONS458–ONS463, discussion ONS463
66. Ondra SL, Marzouk S, Koski T, Silva F, Salehi S. Mathematical calculation of pedicle subtraction osteotomy size to allow precision correction of fixed sagittal deformity. Spine 2006;31:E973–E979
67. Lenke LG, Newton PO, Sucato DJ, et al. Complications after 147 consecutive vertebral column resections for severe pediatric spinal deformity: a multicenter analysis. Spine 2013;38:119–132
68. Rhee JM, Bridwell KH, Won DS, Lenke LG, Chotigavanichaya C, Hanson DS. Sagittal plane analysis of adolescent idiopathic scoliosis: the effect of anterior versus posterior instrumentation. Spine 2002;27:2350–2356
69. Potter BK, Kuklo TR, Lenke LG. Radiographic outcomes of anterior spinal fusion versus posterior spinal fusion with thoracic pedicle screws for treatment of Lenke Type I adolescent idiopathic scoliosis curves. Spine 2005;30:1859–1866
70. Geck MJ, Rinella A, Hawthorne D, et al. Comparison of surgical treatment in Lenke 5C adolescent idiopathic scoliosis: anterior dual rod versus posterior pedicle fixation surgery: a comparison of two practices. Spine 2009;34:1942–1951
71. Luhmann SJ, Lenke LG, Kim YJ, Bridwell KH, Schootman M. Thoracic adolescent idiopathic scoliosis curves between 70 degrees and 100 degrees: is anterior release necessary? Spine 2005;30:2061–2067
72. Lee SM, Suk SI, Chung ER. Direct vertebral rotation: a new technique of three-dimensional deformity correction with segmental pedicle screw fixation in adolescent idiopathic scoliosis. Spine 2004;29:343–349
73. Hwang SW, Samdani AF, Lonner B, et al. Impact of direct vertebral body derotation on rib prominence: are preoperative factors predictive of changes in rib prominence? Spine 2012;37:E86–E89
74. Samdani AF, Hwang SW, Miyanji F, et al. Direct vertebral body derotation, thoracoplasty, or both: which is better with respect to inclinometer and scoliosis research society-22 scores? Spine 2012;37:E849–E853
75. Lenke LG, Bridwell KH, Baldus C, Blanke K. Analysis of pulmonary function and axis rotation in adolescent and young adult idiopathic scoliosis patients treated with Cotrel-Dubousset instrumentation. J Spinal Disord 1992;5:16–25
76. Wood KB, Transfeldt EE, Ogilvie JW, Schendel MJ, Bradford DS. Rotational changes of the vertebral-pelvic axis following Cotrel-Dubousset instrumentation. Spine 1991;16(8, Suppl):S404–S408
77. Lenke LG, Chang MS. Vertebral derotation in adolescent idiopathic scoliosis. Oper Tech Orthop 2009;19:19–23
78. Lenke LG, Bridwell KH, Blanke K, Baldus C. Analysis of pulmonary function and chest cage dimension changes after thoracoplasty in idiopathic scoliosis. Spine 1995;20:1343–1350
79. Kuklo TR, Potter BK, Polly DW Jr, Lenke LG. Monaxial versus multiaxial thoracic pedicle screws in the correction of adolescent idiopathic scoliosis. Spine 2005;30:2113–2120
80. Cheng I, Hay D, Iezza A, Lindsey D, Lenke LG. Biomechanical analysis of derotation of the thoracic spine using pedicle screws. Spine 2010;35:1039–1043
81. Buchowski JM, Bhatnagar R, Skaggs DL, Sponseller PD. Temporary internal distraction as an aid to correction of severe scoliosis. J Bone Joint Surg Am 2006;88:2035–2041
82. Buchowski JM, Skaggs DL, Sponseller PD. Temporary internal distraction as an aid to correction of severe scoliosis. Surgical technique. J Bone Joint Surg Am 2007;89(Suppl 2, Pt 2):297–309
83. Bess S, Boachie-Adjei O, Burton D, et al; International Spine Study Group. Pain and disability determine treatment modality for older patients with adult scoliosis, while deformity guides treatment for younger patients. Spine 2009;34:2186–2190
84. Schwab F, Dubey A, Pagala M, Gamez L, Farcy JP. Adult scoliosis: a health assessment analysis by SF-36. Spine 2003;28:602–606
85. Helenius I, Serlo J, Pajulo O. The incidence and outcomes of vertebral column resection in paediatric patients: a population-based, multicentre, follow-up study. J Bone Joint Surg Br 2012;94:950–955
86. Lenke LG, Sides BA, Koester LA, Hensley M, Blanke KM. Vertebral column resection for the treatment of severe spinal deformity. Clin Orthop Relat Res 2010;468:687–699
87. Sponseller PD, Jain A, Lenke LG, et al. Vertebral column resection in children with neuromuscular spine deformity. Spine 2012;37:E655–E661
88. Suk SI, Chung ER, Kim JH, Kim SS, Lee JS, Choi WK. Posterior vertebral column resection for severe rigid scoliosis. Spine 2005;30:1682–1687
89. Suk SI, Kim JH, Kim WJ, Lee SM, Chung ER, Nah KH. Posterior vertebral column resection for severe spinal deformities. Spine 2002;27:2374–2382
90. Dorward IG, Lenke LG, Bridwell KH, et al. Transforaminal versus anterior lumbar interbody fusion in long deformity constructs: a matched cohort analysis. Spine 2013
91. Kim YJ, Bridwell KH, Lenke LG, Cho KJ, Edwards CC II, Rinella AS. Pseudarthrosis in adult spinal deformity following multisegmental instrumentation and arthrodesis. J Bone Joint Surg Am 2006;88:721–728
92. Fleischer GD, Kim YJ, Ferrara LA, Freeman AL, Boachie-Adjei O. Biomechanical analysis of sacral screw strain and range of motion in long posterior spinal fixation constructs: effects of lumbosacral fixation strategies in reducing sacral screw strains. Spine 2012;37:E163–E169
93. Li F, Chen Q, Chen W, Xu K, Wu Q. Posterior-only approach with selective segmental TLIF for degenerative lumbar scoliosis. J Spinal Disord Tech 2011;24:308–312

82 Minimally Invasive Correction of Spinal Deformity

Nader S. Dahdaleh, Praveen V. Mummaneni, and Zachary A. Smith

The main premise of using minimally invasive surgery (MIS) in the spine is the avoidance of unnecessary muscle stripping, dissection, and devascularization through the utilization of direct portals and corridors while surgically addressing spinal disorders. The decrease in collateral damage during MIS has translated clinically into less postoperative blood loss, fewer infections, fewer cerebrospinal fluid leaks, shorter hospitalization, faster recovery, and greater cost-effectiveness without compromising long-term outcomes.[1]

The body of evidence demonstrating the efficacy of MIS has been increasing in the past two decades, especially in the degenerative spine literature. Surgeons have responded with enthusiasm after applying various minimally invasive techniques to the correction of spinal deformity and seeing first-hand that the potential benefits are more pronounced.[2]

The spectrum of spinal deformities in the adult population is wide, especially with an increasing elderly population and with revision surgeries. Generally, the indications for treating deformity include back or leg pain that is due to adult idiopathic scoliosis, iatrogenic deformity (flat back syndromes), and lumbar degenerative scoliosis. Curves can be (1) primarily scoliotic with normal sagittal balance, (2) kyphoscoliotic, or (3) primarily kyphotic resulting in positive sagittal balance. These curves can be flexible or rigid.

Open surgical techniques, including osteotomies of various kinds, effectively address the full spectrum of spinal deformities. However, these surgeries involve significant blood loss and long hospitalizations, and a considerable risk of morbidity and complications. Percutaneous techniques that obviate excessive blood loss and tissue disruption can effectively address primarily coronal curves in adult degenerative scoliosis. Moreover, newer advanced techniques have shown great promise in effectively treating kyphotic curves with positive sagittal balance.[3,4]

The Minimally Invasive Spine Deformity (MISDEF) Algorithm

Recently, the Minimally Invasive Surgery Section of the International Spine Study Group has proposed a treatment algorithm that guides spine surgeons in utilizing minimally invasive techniques for the correction of spinal deformity (**Fig. 82.1**).[5] The algorithm includes three general surgical approaches defined by three classes. Class I includes minimally invasive or mini-open muscle-sparing decompressions alone or single-level MIS fusions for a listhetic level. Class II includes MIS or mini-open techniques for interbody fusions that address curve apexes or the entire Cobb angle of the major curve. Class III entails traditional open surgical corrective techniques and osteotomies. According to the algorithm, percutaneous class II techniques can be applied to flexible curves with a sagittal vertical axis (SVA) > 6 cm as long as the lumbar lordosis (LL)–pelvic incidence (PI) mismatch is less than 30 degrees and the pelvic tilt (PT) is less than 25 degrees. In the setting of rigid curves with SVA > 6 cm and a PT > 25 degrees, open techniques with osteotomies are recommended.

This algorithm was validated by 11 fellowship-trained minimally invasive spine surgeons who applied the algorithm to a set of 20 published deformity cases. Two months later, the surgeons resurveyed the same cases. The initial interobserver kappa value was 0.58 and improved to 0.69 following the resurvey. The mean intraobserver kappa was 0.86.

Minimally Invasive Surgical Techniques for Deformity Correction

Lateral Transpsoas Lumbar Interbody Fusion (LLIF)

Since its introduction by McAffee and colleagues[6] in the late 1990s, lateral access surgery for interbody fusion has proved to be a powerful technique to address a wide variety of degenerative spinal disorders. It offers large surface areas for interbody fusion, effective indirect decompression of central canal and foraminal stenosis, and excellent clinical outcomes. Likewise, its application for coronal deformity correction has been gaining wide success. The average segmental correction ranges from 3 to 5.9 degrees in the coronal plan and 2.2 to 3.3 degrees in the sagittal plane[3] (**Fig. 82.2**).

Supplemental pedicle screw fixation is done percutaneously and has been shown to offer more stability, improved correction, and decreased risk of graft subsidence.[7-9]

Various reports have demonstrated the efficacy of lateral interbody fusion and posterior percutaneous pedicle screw fixation in the correction of scoliosis. The range of preoperative average coronal Cobb angles in these reports range from 18.9 to 38.5 degrees. Following correction, the postoperative average coronal Cobb angle improvement ranges from 6.1 to 14.0 degrees. In the sagittal plane, the correction is usually less than in the coronal plane. Some studies have even shown stability or a decrease in lumbar lordosis.[3]

Recently, to enhance sagittal plane correction during lateral lumbar interbody fusion, anterior longitudinal ligament release and placement of hyperlordotic cages have been pursued in a few cases with promising results.[4,10,11] One study compared nine patients who underwent 15 anterior column releases (ACRs) with 27 patients who did not undergo an ACR during LLIF. There was an improvement of 12 degrees in segmental lordosis, an improvement of 17 degrees in regional lordosis, and a correction of

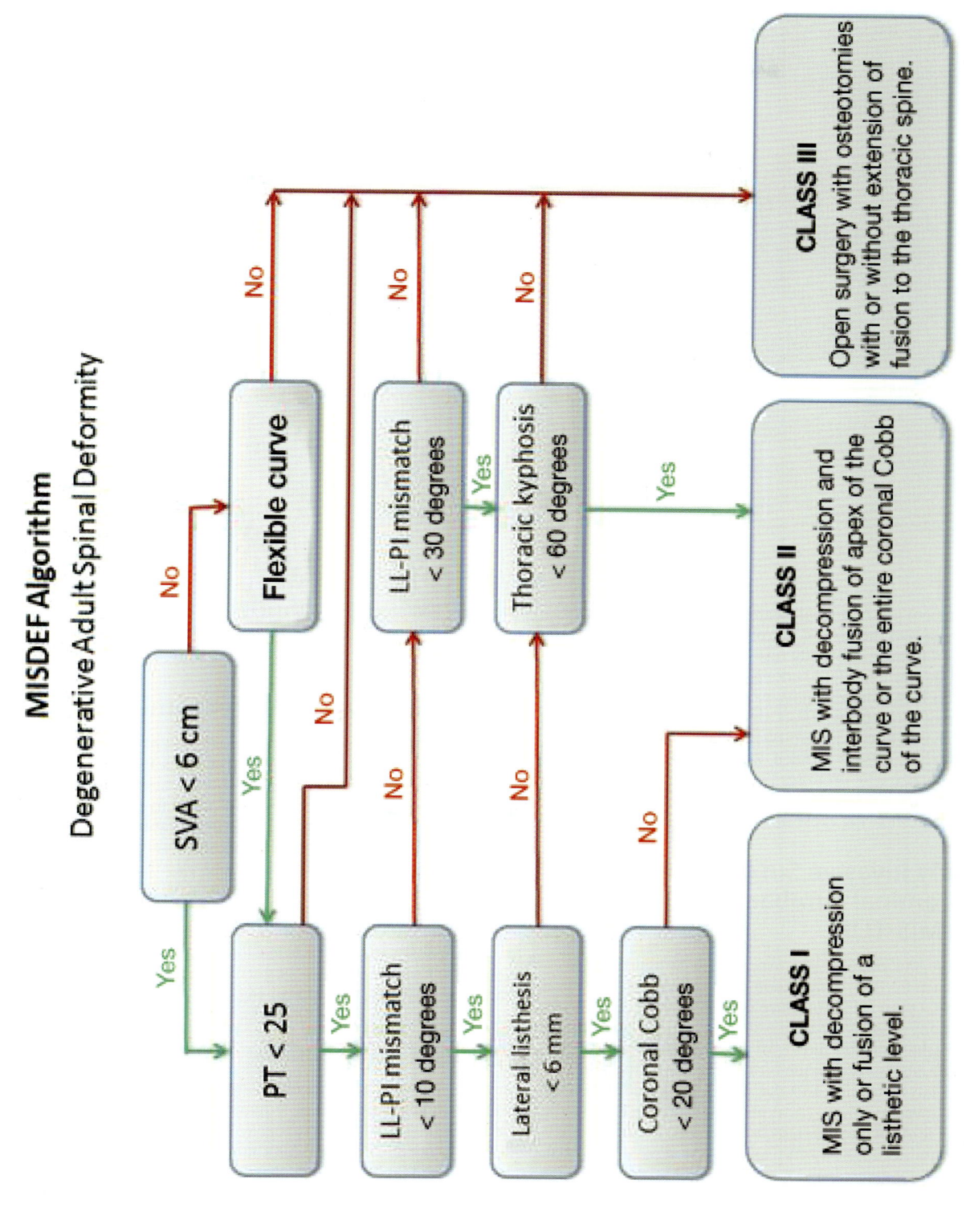

82 Minimally Invasive Correction of Spinal Deformity

Fig. 82.1 The Minimally Invasive Spine Deformity (MISDEF) algorithm. LL, lumbar lordosis; MIS, minimally invasive surgery; PI, pelvic incidence; PT, pelvic tilt; SVA, sagittal vertical axis. (Courtesy of the American Association of Neurological Surgeons. From Mummaneni PV, Shaffrey CI, Lenke LG, et al: Minimally Invasive Surgery Section of the International Spine Study Group. The minimally invasive spinal deformity surgery algorithm: a reproducible rational framework for decision making in minimally invasive spinal deformity surgery. Neurosurg Focus 2014;36:E6. Reprinted with permission.)

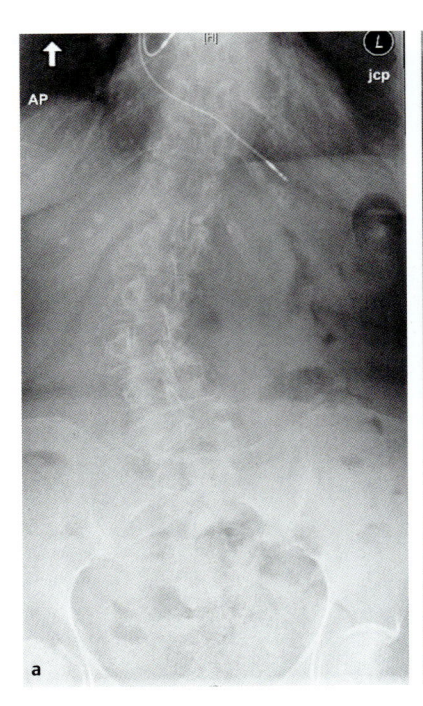

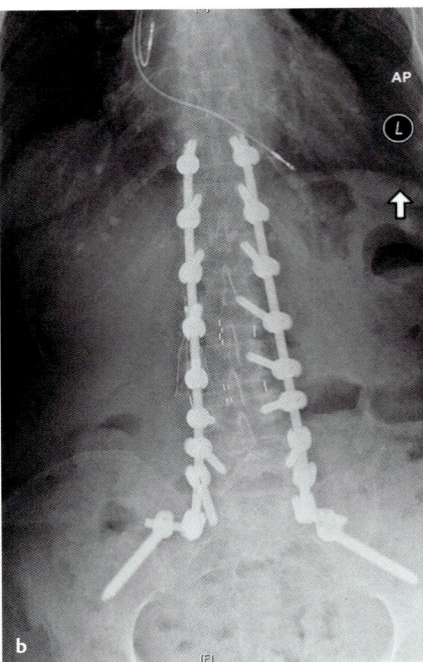

Fig. 82.2 (a) An 80-year-old woman presented with back pain and neurogenic claudications due to adult degenerative lumbar scoliosis. (b) After failing a period of conservative treatment, she underwent a two-stage purely minimally invasive correction of her deformity. The first stage consisted of lateral transpsoas lumbar interbody fusion (LLIF) at L2-3 and L3-4 and minimally invasive surgery for transforaminal lumbar interbody fusion (MIS-TLIF) at L4-5 and L5-S1 with bilateral decompression for stenosis at L4-5. The second stage consisted of percutaneous pedicle screw fixation spanning T11 through the sacrum/ilium as well as facet fusions at T11-12, L1-2, and L2-3.

the SVA of 3.1 cm per ACR level treated. There was no change in these parameters in the non-ACR group.[4]

The lateral lumbar interbody fusion technique was described in detail in Chapter 64. There is debate on whether to approach the correction from the concavity or the convexity. Proponents of the convexity approach report that it can address multiple levels through one or two incisions, and access to the L4-L5 level is easier if the iliac crest is avoided. Proponents of the concavity approach report that it provides better corrective forces with less stretch injury to the lumbar plexus. There have been no studies to date comparing these approaches in LLIF.

Minimally Invasive Surgery for Transforaminal Lumbar Interbody Fusion (MIS-TLIF)

This common and popular percutaneous technique enables a dorsal approach for interbody fusion with minimal or no thecal sac retraction. Often this procedure is used as an alternative to lateral interbody fusions for the correction of spondylolisthesis and lateral listhesis in the setting of coronal and sagittal deformity[12] (**Fig. 82.3**). This technique is described in Chapter 104.

Bilateral facetectomies and the use of steerable interbody cages (that allow the symmetrical placement of the cage in the anterior one third of the interspace) have been shown to improve segmental lordosis in MIS-TLIF.[13,14] One study found that, following bilateral facetectomies and steerable interbody cage placement segmental, lumbar lordosis improved by 8 degrees whereas there was no change in lordosis in patients undergoing unilateral facetectomy and bullet cage placement in MIS-TILF.[14]

Comparative studies evaluating clinical and radiographic outcomes in patients undergoing anterior lumbar interbody fusion during open deformity correction found similarly improved outcomes between both groups.[15,16] One study comparing anterior lumbar interbody fusion and transforaminal interbody fusion in long deformity constructs found that TLIFs require less operative time. Radiologically, anterior lumbar interbody fusions provided more segmental lordosis, whereas TLIFs provided better correction of scoliotic curves.[1]

Minimally Invasive Osteotomies

One main advantage of open surgical treatment for deformity is the ability to perform a variety of osteotomies as Smith-Petersen osteotomies, pedicle subtraction osteotomies, and vertebral column resections, which are powerful tools in correcting rigid coronal and sagittal deformities. We find that performing simple dorsal releases as Smith-Petersen osteotomies is feasible and relatively efficient using tubular retractors for the MIS technique. Currently, there are ceiling effects for the MIS technique in the reduction of large and rigid scoliotic and kyphotic curves, because of the difficulty of performing three-column osteotomies percutaneously, although it is feasible. Recently, pedicle subtraction osteotomies have been performed in minimally invasive or mini-open fashions with promising results.[17]

Percutaneous Pedicle Screw Fixation

Any long construct that involves lateral or transforaminal interbody fusions should be supplemented with percutaneous pedicle screw fixation. This Kirschner wire (K-wire)-based technique depends entirely on fluoroscopic guidance. Navigation that obviates the need for fluoroscopy also has been used in percutaneous pedicle screw placement with comparable accuracy.[18]

In long constructs, negotiating a long rod subfascially can be challenging. Patience and care must be taken while appropriately contouring the rod. Lateral fluoroscopic imaging is helpful to ensure appropriate seating of the rod through the tulips or extended tabs prior to the application of the set screws. Moreover, sequential and stepwise tightening of the set screws is recommended to avoid screw loosening and pullout. Newer technologies are evolving that aid in accurately contouring the

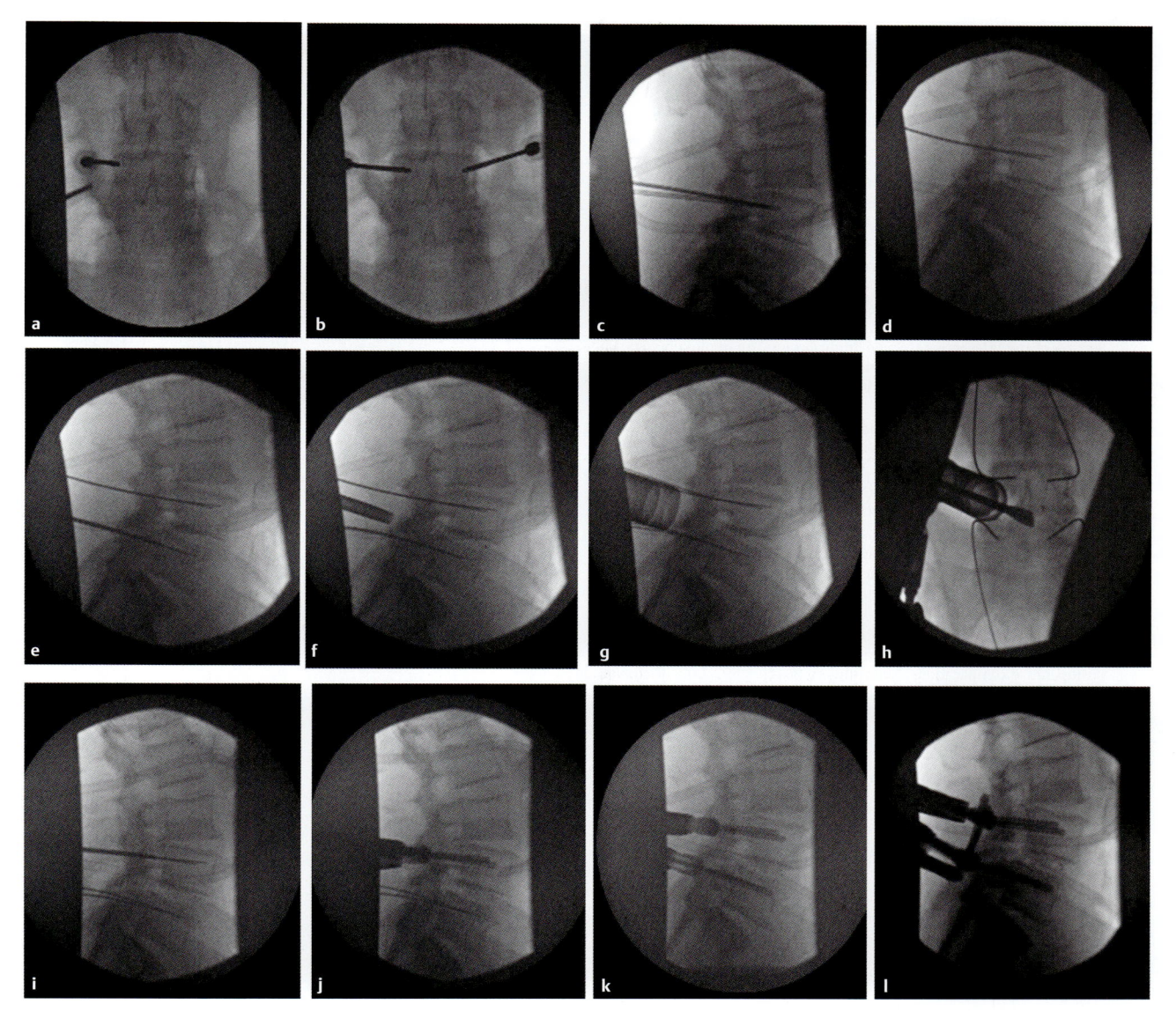

Fig. 82.3 Fluoroscopic based minimally invasive transforaminal lumbar interbody fusion (TLIF) and percutaneous pedicle screw fixation. **(a)** Under anteroposterior (AP) fluoroscopic view, the tip of the Jamshidi needle is docked at the lateral border of the pedicle. **(b)** The needle is advanced into the pedicle in a lateral-to-medial triangulated fashion such that it does not violate the medial border of the pedicle following 25 mm of advancement. The same procedure is done on the contralateral side. **(c)** Under lateral fluoroscopic view, Kirschner wires (K-wires) are placed through the Jamshidi needles into the vertebral body. **(d)** The Jamshidi needles are withdrawn leaving the K-wires in the vertebra. **(e)** The same procedure is repeated at the lower vertebra. **(f)** Sequential dilation is performed through the paraspinal muscles between the K-wires. **(g)** A working tubular table-mounted retractor is placed and docked usually at the level of the facet joint. **(h)** The TLIF is performed through the working tubular retractor, and an interbody fusion cage is placed. **(i)** A cannulated tap is placed, guided by the K-wire, to cannulate the pedicle (some surgeons place a cannulated awl prior to tapping). **(j)** Percutaneous pedicle screws with extended tabs or tulips are placed into the pedicle guided by the K-wire at the cranial vertebra. **(k)** Cannulated pedicle screws guided by the K-wires are placed in the caudal vertebra, following which the K-wires are withdrawn. **(l)** Using a rod introducer, a rod is placed subfascially engaging the pedicle screw heads. Set screws are then applied, and the extended tabs are removed or broken off the screw heads.

rod by utilizing intraoperative fiducials and navigation prior to rod placement.

Conclusion

With better understanding and appreciation of the impact of spinopelvic parameters on outcomes following spine surgery, there has been an increase in the number of deformity surgeries performed in the past two decades. These surgeries are often associated with a significant amount of blood loss, morbidity, and even mortality. Minimally invasive techniques that obviate muscle dissection and stripping have shown promise in the correction of spinal deformity while minimizing the morbidity in select patients.

References

1. Smith ZA, Fessler RG. Paradigm changes in spine surgery: evolution of minimally invasive techniques. Nat Rev Neurol 2012;8:443–450
2. Dangelmajer S, Zadnik PL, Rodriguez ST, Gokaslan ZL, Sciubba DM. Minimally invasive spine surgery for adult degenerative lumbar scoliosis. Neurosurg Focus 2014;36:E7
3. Dahdaleh NS, Smith ZA, Snyder LA, Graham RB, Fessler RG, Koski TR. Lateral transpsoas lumbar interbody fusion: outcomes and deformity correction. Neurosurg Clin N Am 2014;25:353–360
4. Manwaring JC, Bach K, Ahmadian AA, Deukmedjian AR, Smith DA, Uribe JS. Management of sagittal balance in adult spinal deformity with minimally invasive anterolateral lumbar interbody fusion: a preliminary radiographic study. J Neurosurg Spine 2014;20:515–522
5. Mummaneni PV, Shaffrey CI, Lenke LG, et al; Minimally Invasive Surgery Section of the International Spine Study Group. The minimally invasive spinal deformity surgery algorithm: a reproducible rational framework for decision making in minimally invasive spinal deformity surgery. Neurosurg Focus 2014;36:E6
6. McAfee PC, Regan JJ, Geis WP, Fedder IL. Minimally invasive anterior retroperitoneal approach to the lumbar spine. Emphasis on the lateral BAK. Spine 1998;23:1476–1484
7. Cappuccino A, Cornwall GB, Turner AW, et al. Biomechanical analysis and review of lateral lumbar fusion constructs. Spine 2010;35(26, Suppl):S361–S367
8. Nayak AN, Gutierrez S, Billys JB, Santoni BG, Castellvi AE. Biomechanics of lateral plate and pedicle screw constructs in lumbar spines instrumented at two levels with laterally placed interbody cages. Spine J 2013;13:1331–1338
9. Karikari IO, Grossi PM, Nimjee SM, et al. Minimally invasive lumbar interbody fusion in patients older than 70 years of age: analysis of peri- and postoperative complications. Neurosurgery 2011;68:897–902, discussion 902
10. Deukmedjian AR, Le TV, Baaj AA, Dakwar E, Smith DA, Uribe JS. Anterior longitudinal ligament release using the minimally invasive lateral retroperitoneal transpsoas approach: a cadaveric feasibility study and report of 4 clinical cases. J Neurosurg Spine 2012;17:530–539
11. Akbarnia BA, Mundis GM Jr, Moazzaz P, et al. Anterior column realignment (ACR) for focal kyphotic spinal deformity using a lateral transpsoas approach and ALL release. J Spinal Disord Tech 2014;27:29–39
12. Dahdaleh NS, Nixon AT, Lawton CD, Wong AP, Smith ZA, Fessler RG. Outcome following unilateral versus bilateral instrumentation in patients undergoing minimally invasive transforaminal lumbar interbody fusion: a single-center randomized prospective study. Neurosurg Focus 2013;35:E13
13. Yson SC, Santos ER, Sembrano JN, Polly DW Jr. Segmental lumbar sagittal correction after bilateral transforaminal lumbar interbody fusion. J Neurosurg Spine 2012;17:37–42
14. Lindley TE, Viljoen SV, Dahdaleh NS. Effect of steerable cage placement during minimally invasive transforaminal lumbar interbody fusion on lumbar lordosis. J Clin Neurosci 2014;21:441–444
15. Crandall DG, Revella J. Transforaminal lumbar interbody fusion versus anterior lumbar interbody fusion as an adjunct to posterior instrumented correction of degenerative lumbar scoliosis: three year clinical and radiographic outcomes. Spine 2009;34:2126–2133
16. Dorward IG, Lenke LG, Bridwell KH, et al. Transforaminal versus anterior lumbar interbody fusion in long deformity constructs: a matched cohort analysis. Spine 2013;Feb:25
17. Wang MY. Miniopen pedicle subtraction osteotomy: surgical technique and initial results. Neurosurg Clin N Am 2014;25:347–351
18. Stadler JA III, Dahdaleh NS, Smith ZA, Koski TR. Intraoperative navigation in minimally invasive transforaminal lumbar interbody fusion and lateral interbody fusion. Neurosurg Clin N Am 2014;25:377–382

83 Minimally Invasive Thoracic Decompression for Multilevel Thoracic Pathology

Cort D. Lawton, Nader S. Dahdaleh, Michael J. Harvey, Richard G. Fessler, and Zachary A. Smith

Compressive lesions in the thoracic spine often present with a gradual onset of symptoms and varied clinical manifestations, making the diagnosis and management challenging. Conservative therapy for thoracic myelopathy secondary to compressive lesions is often ineffective, as these patients invariably have progressive symptoms. In cases involving multiple levels, surgical approach–related morbidity and iatrogenic spinal instability become a concern.

Traditionally, the surgical intervention of choice involves multiple consecutive-level laminectomies with resection of the lesion through a large midline incision. This approach exposes the patient to extensive bilateral subperiosteal dissection of the paraspinal musculature and significant removal of the posterior spinal elements to expose the contents of the thoracic spinal canal. It is recognized that these large approaches predispose patients to significant postoperative pain and the potential for chronic pain. Additionally, extensive removal of the bony and ligamentous structures increases stress and loading on the facets of the surgical and adjacent levels. Biomechanical models have shown increased segmental instability following an open laminectomy procedure when compared with a unilateral minimally invasive hemilaminotomy procedure.[1,2] This increased instability identified when comparing the two procedures is likely magnified in cases requiring decompression at multiple consecutive levels. Furthermore, studies have suggested that the increased spinal instability resulting from multiple consecutive-level laminectomies may predispose patients to degenerative disease and iatrogenic spinal deformity, which is even more pronounced in the pediatric population.[3-6]

Tredway et al[7] described a unilateral minimally invasive approach for resection of intradural extramedullary neoplasms. The lesions resected were causing symptomatic neural compression spanning one or two levels in the cervical, thoracic, and lumbar spine. Smith et al[8] expanded upon this approach by describing a technique used for exposure and resection of extensive multilevel thoracic lesions through a minimally invasive thoracic decompression procedure. This procedure was performed through two small entry points at the cephalad and caudal ends of the pathology. Unilateral hemilaminotomies were performed through each entry point to enable resection of the lesions. The patients in this case series were experiencing myelopathy from lesions spanning five or six levels in the thoracic spine. Postoperative magnetic resonance imaging (MRI) studies demonstrated complete resection of the lesions, and the patients had complete resolution of symptoms, which was sustained at a mean long-term follow-up of 26.7 months.

In contrast to the traditional open procedure, the minimal access approach for multilevel decompression in the thoracic spine limits approach-related soft tissue injury, spares more of the posterior elements and bony anatomy, and decreases the alteration of spinal biomechanics and iatrogenic instability.[1-9] This chapter describes the minimally invasive multilevel thoracic decompression technique reported by Smith et al[8] for resection of multilevel thoracic pathology.

Patient Selection

Patients presenting with clinical myelopathy and radiographic evidence of structural thoracic spinal cord compression as a result of a dorsally located compressive pathology may be considered for this operation. An illustrative case is presented in **Fig. 83.1**.

Indications

- Thoracic myelopathy secondary to a dorsal compressive pathology
  - Epidural abscess
  - Epidural lipomatosis
  - Epidural hematoma
  - Epidural tumors (with the exception of lymphoma, multiple myeloma, and plasmacytoma)
  - Extramedullary hematopoiesis
  - Intradural arachnoid cyst
  - Intradural extramedullary tumors

Contraindications

- Spinal instability
- Ventral pathology

Objective

- To resect multilevel dorsal lesions causing symptomatic compression in the thoracic spine using a minimally invasive thoracic decompression technique

Advantages

- Less approach-related morbidity than with traditional open multilevel thoracic laminectomy techniques
- Lower risk of long-term spinal instability than with traditional open multilevel laminectomy technique
  - Less bony structure removal
  - Better preservation of ligamentous structures and posterior tension band

Disadvantages

- Difficult to access ventral pathology
- Steep learning curve
- Operating through limited working space
- Difficult to localize correct level intraoperatively

Preoperative Testing and Imaging

- Neurologic examination for evidence of thoracic myelopathy/radiculopathy
- MRI/computed tomography (CT)/X-ray of thoracic spine for characterization of lesion
- Somatosensory evoked potential (SSEP), motor evoked potential (MEP), electromyogram (EMG) monitoring if necessary

Surgical Procedure

Anesthesia and Positioning

Minimally invasive thoracic decompression is performed under general anesthesia with endotracheal intubation. For the prevention of intraoperative and perioperative neurologic deficits, intraoperative neural monitoring (SSEP, EMG, MEP) is recommended. It should be noted that the use of neurophysiological monitoring requires nonparalytic anesthetic agents at the appropriate stage of the procedure to assess MEPs.

The patient is placed in the prone position on chest rolls on a standard radiolucent operating table with the arms supported on arm rests or secured to the patient's side, depending on the levels of the pathology. The patient should be securely strapped to the operating table and all pressure points should be well padded. The head and neck is secured in a three-pin Mayfield headholder. Adequate positioning is essential to avoid pressure points and abdominal compression. Compression of the abdomen may lead to inadequate venous return and engorgement of the epidural venous plexus, leading to excessive intraoperative bleeding. The patient is then sterilely prepped in the standard fashion. Antibiotics are routinely given in the perioperative period.

Incision

It is essential to localize the appropriate level for the skin incision. Preoperative imaging should be utilized to determine the spinal level at the cephalad and caudal poles of the pathology (T3 and T8 in **Fig. 83.1a**). Surface landmarks may help to mark the incision by counting from the C7 spinous process; T3 is at the level of the scapular angle, and T7 is at the level of the inferior scapular tip. Additionally, lateral fluoroscopy with a marker

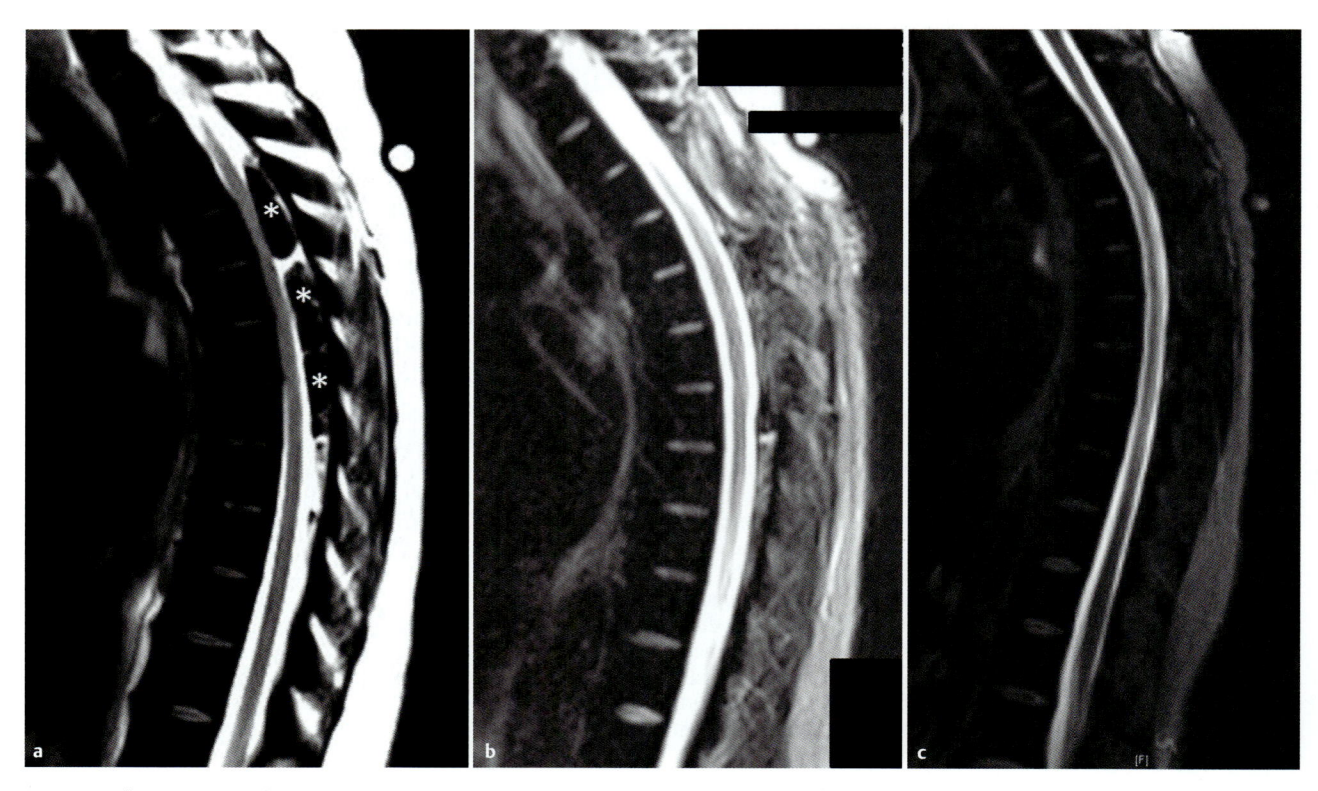

Fig. 83.1 Illustrative case of a patient undergoing minimally invasive multilevel thoracic decompression. A 45-year-old woman presented with a 2-year history of progressive thoracic radiculopathy, bilateral foot pain and numbness, and gait imbalance. Magnetic resonance imaging (MRI) of the thoracic spine demonstrated an extensive dorsal epidural lesion extending from T3 to T8 in the thoracic spine, with evidence of significant cord compression. **(a)** Preoperative T2-sagittal thoracic MRI demonstrating extensive dorsally compressive lesion *(asterisks)* from T3 to T8. The patient underwent minimally invasive left T3–T5 hemilaminotomies and right T6–T8 hemilaminotomies, via the described surgical technique. The lesion was resected and pathology was consistent with an extramedullary hematopoiesis. **(b)** T2-sagittal thoracic MRI demonstrating gross-total resection of the lesion with resolution of the spinal cord compression in the perioperative period. **(c)** T2-sagittal thoracic MRI at 1-year follow-up showing no recurrence or evidence of postoperative kyphosis. The patient's symptoms improved in the postoperative period, with complete resolution of symptoms sustained at 3-year follow-up.

should be utilized to localize the surgical levels by counting cephalad from the sacrum and confirming with anterior-posterior fluoroscopy by counting thoracic ribs. Due to the possibility for patient variation in the number of ribs, and because intraoperative radiographs may not cover all of the ribs, the surgeon should count both up from the bottom rib and down from the top rib to confirm the appropriate operative level. We often utilize preoperative CT to confirm placement of fiducials at the site of interest, which makes intraoperative localization accurate and less time-consuming.

With the appropriate operative levels confirmed, a skin incision should be marked 1.5 cm lateral to the midline and 3 to 4 cm long in a rostral-caudal direction at the cephalad pole of the lesion. A second skin incision should then be marked in a similar fashion on the contralateral side of the tension band at the caudal pole of the lesion. The skin incisions should then be made, followed by blunt dissection through the fascia. A series of muscle-splitting tubular dilators are docked onto the lamina one level below the cephalad end of the lesion (T4 in **Fig. 83.1a**). Lateral and anterior-posterior fluoroscopy should be used to confirm docking at the appropriate level. A Quadrant retractor tube (Medtronic Inc., Memphis, TN) is then placed over the dilators and the dilators are removed. The retractor is then secured to the operating table with a flexible arm and expanded in the rostral-caudal direction to expose the lamina of the superior and inferior surgical border (T3–T5 in **Fig. 83.1a**). The same steps should be used to position a second Quadrant retractor onto the lamina one level above the caudal end of the lesion (T7 in **Fig. 83.1a**). The Quadrant retractors should then be expanded in the rostral-caudal direction to expose the lamina of the superior and inferior surgical border (T6–T8 in **Fig. 83.1a**). **Fig. 83.2** demonstrates the intraoperative setup.

Electrocautery is then used to resect residual soft tissue that is obstructing visualization of the lamina. Bleeding from the venous plexus may occur and should be coagulated with electrocautery or absorbable gelatin sponge. Once adequate visualization and hemostasis is obtained, the same steps should be repeated at the contralateral caudal exposure.

Decompression

The laminar edges are defined using curettes. Multilevel hemilaminotomies are performed with Kerrison rongeurs and a high-speed drill at the cephalad segment (T3–T5 in **Fig. 83.1a**). Contralateral exposure is achieved using a shielded drill and drilling the ventral surface of the spinous process and contralateral lamina to the contralateral pedicle while being cautious not to create an accidental durotomy. The ventral surface of the contralateral lamina is removed. The same steps should be repeated to perform the hemilaminotomies on the contralateral side of the posterior tension band at the caudal multilevel segment (T6–T8 in **Fig. 83.1a**). Bipolar electrocautery, bone wax, and Surgifoam (Ethicon, Inc., Johnson & Johnson, Somerville, NJ) are used to achieve hemostasis. The ligamentum flavum can then be identified and removed to expose the dorsal epidural pathology.

For cases involving extradural pathology, the lesions can be resected with a combination of bipolar electrocautery, pituitary forceps, and microsurgical dissectors. Bipolar electrocautery and Gelfoam (Pharmacia & Upjohn Company, division of Pfizer Inc., New York, NY) can be used to achieve hemostasis during resection of the lesion.

For cases involving intradural pathology, the dura is opened at each exposure site and the pathology is resected throughout its rostral-caudal borders.

Closure

For cases involving intradural pathology in which a durotomy is performed, the dura is closed with 4-0 suture in a running fashion and sealed with fibrin glue (Duraseal, Covidien Company Inc., Mansfield, MA). If necessary, dural grafts can be sewn into place with similar techniques. In cases where the dura has been violated, a Valsalva maneuver and reverse Trendelenburg may be utilized to check for cerebrospinal fluid (CSF) leakage. Once hemostasis is obtained, the wound is copiously irrigated with an antibiotic solution. The retractors are then removed to allow the paraspinal muscles to reapproximate in normal anatomic alignment. The paraspinous fascia is closed using 1-0 Dexon suture. Proper closure of the dorsal fascia is essential due to the limited amount of tissue present above this layer in the event that a CSF leak were to become a problem. The subcutaneous layer is reapproximated with 3-0 Vicryl sutures, and the skin is closed using subcutaneous 4-0 sutures followed by Dermabond (Ethicon, Inc.) adhesive on the skin surface. Care should be taken to obliterate any potential dead space.

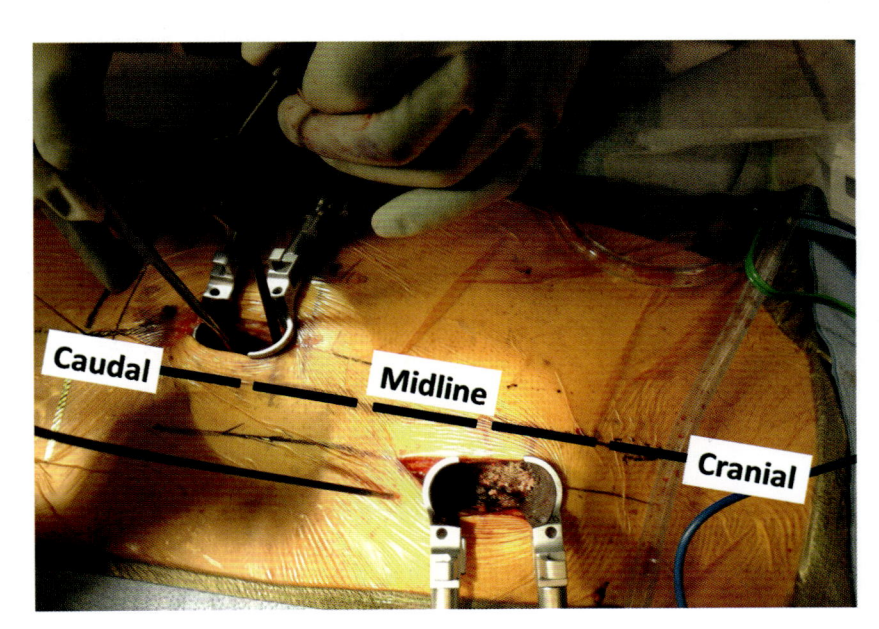

Fig. 83.2 Intraoperative image of operative setup and expanded Quadrant retractors.

Postoperative Care

- Routine neurologic examinations
- MRI of the thoracic spine
- Physical and occupational therapy

Potential Complications and Precautions

- A wrong-level starting point can be avoided by appropriate preoperative imaging and use of fluoroscopy for localization prior to skin incision.
- Nerve root and spinal cord injury can be avoided by proper drilling technique and intraoperative neural monitoring.
- Incomplete resection
- CSF leak can be avoided by proper drilling technique in cases of epidural pathology and by adequate dural closure in cases of intradural pathology.

Conclusion

The procedure described in this chapter is a minimal access technique using muscle-splitting tubular retractors that can be employed safely and effectively to treat various multilevel dorsally compressive pathologies of the thoracic spine. This technique may limit approach-related morbidity and long-term spinal instability when compared with the traditional multisegment decompression using open laminectomies. Performing the hemilaminotomies in this fashion helps to preserve the native musculoskeletal anatomy. **Box 83.1** lists the key operative steps and problems that can arise.

Box 83.1 Key Operative Steps and Potential Problems

Step	Problems
Anesthesia and positioning	Anesthesia not appropriate for MEP signaling
	Pressure points due to poor padding
	Abdominal compression
Incision	Wrong-level exposure due to poor localization
Decompression	Nerve root and spinal cord injury
	CSF leak
Closure	Creation of a potential space

References

1. Bresnahan L, Ogden AT, Natarajan RN, Fessler RG. A biomechanical evaluation of graded posterior element removal for treatment of lumbar stenosis: comparison of a minimally invasive approach with two standard laminectomy techniques. Spine 2009;34:17–23
2. Smith ZA, Vastardis GA, Carandang G, et al. Biomechanical effects of a unilateral approach to minimally invasive lumbar decompression. PLoS ONE 2014;9:e92611
3. Papagelopoulos PJ, Peterson HA, Ebersold MJ, Emmanuel PR, Choudhury SN, Quast LM. Spinal column deformity and instability after lumbar or thoracolumbar laminectomy for intraspinal tumors in children and young adults. Spine 1997;22:442–451
4. Duman I, Guzelkucuk U, Yilmaz B, Tan AK. Post-laminectomy rotokyphoscoliosis causing paraplegia in long term: case report. J Spinal Cord Med 2012;35:175–177
5. de Jonge T, Slullitel H, Dubousset J, Miladi L, Wicart P, Illés T. Late-onset spinal deformities in children treated by laminectomy and radiation therapy for malignant tumours. Eur Spine J 2005;14:765–771
6. Hsu W, Pradilla G, Constantini S, Jallo GI. Surgical considerations of spinal ependymomas in the pediatric population. Childs Nerv Syst 2009;25:1253–1259
7. Tredway TL, Santiago P, Hrubes MR, Song JK, Christie SD, Fessler RG. Minimally invasive resection of intradural-extramedullary spinal neoplasms. Neurosurgery 2006;58(1, Suppl):ONS52–ONS58, discussion ONS52–ONS58
8. Smith ZA, Lawton CD, Wong AP, et al. Minimally invasive thoracic decompression for multi-level thoracic pathologies. J Clin Neurosci 2014;21:467–472
9. Oktem IS, Akdemir H, Kurtsoy A, Koç RK, Menkü A, Tucer B. Hemilaminectomy for the removal of the spinal lesions. Spinal Cord 2000;38:92–96

Section V Lumbar and Lumbosacral Spine

A. Pathology

84 Spondylolysis and Spondylolisthesis in Children

Andrew J. Pugely and Stuart L. Weinstein

Spondylolysis and spondylolisthesis are frequent causes of low back pain among children. The term *spondylolysis* refers to a bony defect of the pars interarticularis without translation of adjacent vertebral bodies, whereas the term *spondylolisthesis* describes the anterior translation of adjacent vertebral bodies upon one another. Both the prefix "spondylo-" and the suffix "-olithesis" have Greek etymology and translate to "spine" and "to slip," respectively. In the pediatric patient, these conditions occur most commonly at the lumbosacral junction, involving the L5 pars followed by L4. Spondylolysis and spondylolisthesis encompass a spectrum of disease across which clinical presentation and treatment varies greatly. In most patients, symptoms resolve with nonoperative treatments, but in refractory cases and high-grade spondylolisthesis surgical intervention is often necessary. This chapter discusses the classification, epidemiology, clinical presentation, diagnostic evaluation, and treatment of spondylolysis and spondylolisthesis in children.

Classification

Although spondylolysis is defined as a defect in the pars interarticularis, it encompasses a spectrum of conditions. The term *isthmic spondylolysis* is applied to complete fractures with sclerotic margins. Incomplete disruption of the pars or adjacent elements carries the term *stress reaction*. Although not commonly used, the Tokushima classification grades spondylolysis defects as acute (early), progressive, or terminal (chronic) using axial computed tomography (CT).[1] The authors of the classification argue that spondylolysis grade may affect healing potential, although it has little effect on clinical outcome.

Spondylolisthesis refers to the anterior translation of the vertebral body upon the level below. The amount or degree spondylolisthesis was graded by Meyerding in 1941, and divided into five categories based on the percentage of anterior displacement of one vertebral body on another. Grades I (0 to 25%) and II (> 25% but < 50%) are considered low-grade spondylolisthesis (**Fig. 84.1**) and grades III (> 50% but < 75%) and IV (> 75% but < 100%) are high-grade spondylolisthesis, whereas spondyloptosis is defined as more than 100% translation. Like many pathologies of the spine, both spondylolysis and spondylolisthesis have multiple etiologies. In what has become the most common classification system, Wiltse and Newman characterized spondylolisthesis based on presumed etiology into five main groups: congenital, isthmic, degenerative, traumatic, and pathological.[2] Later modifications of the Wiltse-Newman system added a sixth category—iatrogenic.[3] Congenital (type I) and isthmic (type II) causes comprise the vast majority of cases in children, with isthmic being the most common. Degenerative spondylolisthesis (type III) occurs in adults and is the end-product of a multifactorial breakdown of the intervertebral disks and facet joints. In type III, translation rarely exceeds beyond Meyerding grade II.

Congenital or dysplastic spondylolisthesis (type I) describes a congenital bony abnormality of the posterior vertebral elements at the lumbosacral junction. Isthmic spondylolisthesis (type II) describes a deficit or elongation of the pars interarticularis, and has been subclassified into three types: IIA, IIB, and IIC. Type IIA is a disruption of the pars from a stress fracture typically induced secondary to repetitive loading (**Fig. 84.2**). High-impact activities in young athletes such as gymnastics, dancing, football, and wrestling have been associated with increased risk, as have motor vehicle accidents.[4] The bony defect does not typically heal but forms a fibrous union. Type IIB is a slip resulting from a chronic pars elongation caused by repeated bony callus formation. Type IIC is defined as an acute traumatic pars fracture; it is the least common subtype and usually unstable. This contrasts to a Wiltse-Newman type IV spondylolisthesis, seen in adults, which occurs from an acute fracture of posterior vertebral elements other than the pars.

Alternative classification systems such as the Marchetti-Bartolozzi,[5] Herman-Pizzutillo,[6] and Mac-Thiong/Labelle[7] classification have also been described. The former two systems attempt to clarify traumatic versus developmental causes in helping to guide nonoperative treatment. In the latter classification system by Labelle and colleagues, the spinopelvic relationship in spondylolisthesis is quantified and used to guide surgical treatment.[7] This classification scheme defines pelvic balance or imbalance, according to radiographic parameters such as pelvic incidence, sacral slope, and pelvic tilt (**Fig. 84.3**). The authors argue that the state of pelvic balance may aid in determining treatment for high-grade spondylolisthesis.[8] As the importance of global spinal balance has been appreciated more recently, many authors advocate making restoration of this balance a surgical goal in both adult and pediatric spinal deformity.[9,10]

Epidemiology

Although the exact prevalence of spondylolysis in the pediatric population has not been well defined, the reported incidence in adults ranges between 5%[11] and 11%.[12] Spondylolysis is more common among males but typically progresses more often in females.[13] Occurrence may follow genetic and ethnic lines, as demonstrated by a prevalence of 54% in the Alaskan Inuit, but only 2% in the African-American population.[14] Inherited predisposition among first-degree relatives may range between 22% and 26%.[15]

The natural history of spondylolysis and low-grade spondylolisthesis, Although not entirely understood, is generally benign. Given the close overlap of these conditions and heterogeneity of causes, the literature often does not precisely differentiate etiology. In general, successful clinical outcomes after nonoperative treatment of both conditions exceed 80% at 1 year, irrespective of bony healing.[16] Patients treated for spondylolysis probably have

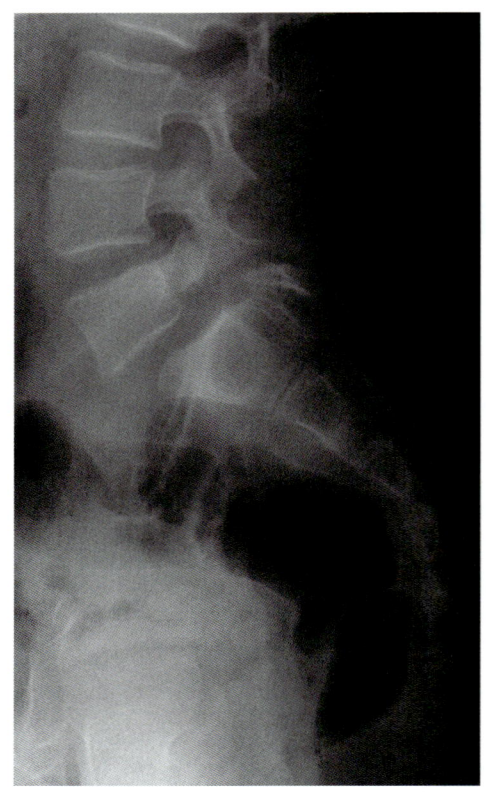

Fig. 84.1 Lateral radiograph of the lumbar spine showing spondylolysis at L4-L5 and a Meyerding grade I spondylolisthesis at L5-S1.

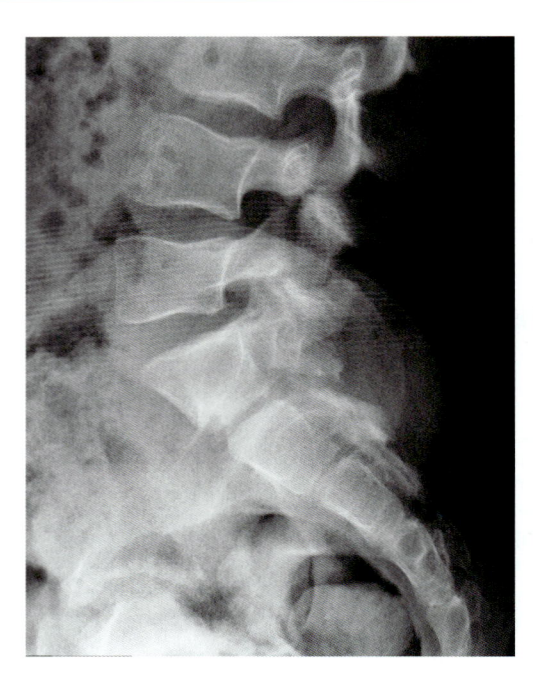

Fig. 84.2 Lateral radiograph of the lumbar spine showing a type 2a isthmic spondylolisthesis, Meyerding grade II at L5-S1.

slightly higher clinical success than those treated for low-grade spondylolisthesis.

In those with low-grade isthmic spondylolisthesis the risk of slip progression is considered quite low.[11,17] In spondylolisthesis, risk factors for slip progression in pediatric patients have not been consistent, but may include female gender, high-grade slips, and immaturity at presentation.[18] Risk of slip progression has been shown to be higher in dysplastic (type I) and high-grade (> 50% anterior translation) forms. In patients with low-grade dysplastic spondylolisthesis, however, the risk of slip progression and development of neurologic symptoms is higher because of abnormal sacral end-plate morphology and hypoplastic facets; the patients may experience a pincer effect of the posterior elements coming forward (contrasted to the posterior elements staying behind in isthmic slips). These patients, in particular, should be followed closely for any surgical treatment needs. Long-term follow-up studies of high-grade spondylolisthesis demonstrate that slip progression is high, but not inevitable, as 36% of patients were asymptomatic at 18-year follow, and progression to severe neurologic dysfunction was rare.[19] In patients

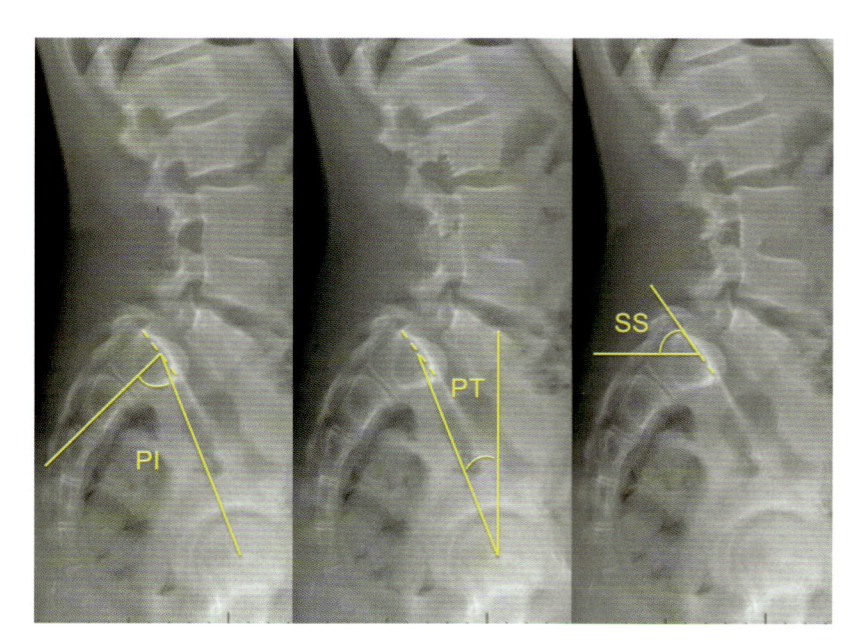

Fig. 84.3 Radiographic assessment of common pelvic parameters: pelvic incidence (PI), pelvic tilt (PT), and sacral slope (SS). The mathematical relationship between PI, PT, and SS is given by PI = PT + SS.

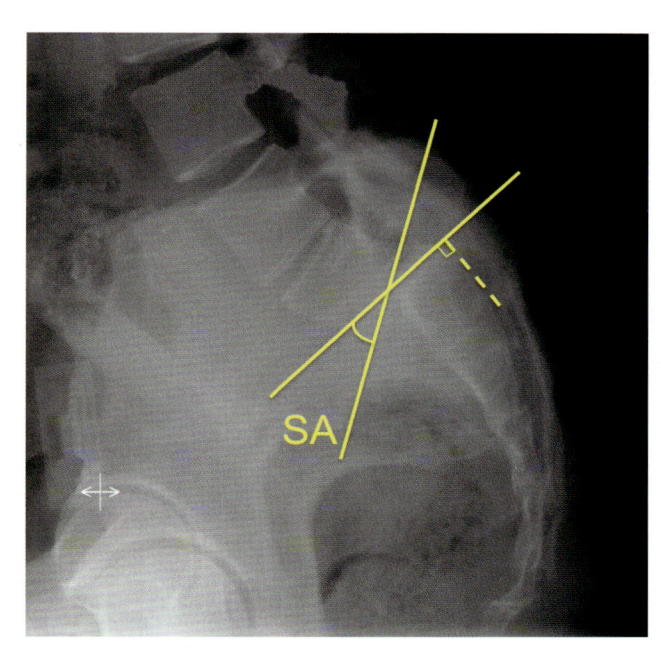

Fig. 84.4 Lateral radiograph of lumbar spine demonstrating a high slip angle (SA), indicating significant lumbosacral kyphosis.

with refractory neurogenic claudication or radicular symptoms, the long-term results of surgical intervention with fusion have proven superior to the results of nonoperative treatment.[20,21]

Radiographic spinopelvic parameters have been previously used to assess the likelihood of slip progression. The amount of lumbosacral (LS) kyphosis or verticality of the sacrum, measured as the angle between the superior end plates of slipped vertebra, has classically been quantified as the slip angle[18] (**Fig. 84.4**). Slip angles of greater than 50 degrees have been correlated with a significant risk of slip progression in children.[22] In addition, the relationship of the spinopelvic alignment has been recognized as important in guiding surgical treatment.[9,10] More recently, authors have argued that spinopelvic parameters should guide surgical treatment to maximize surgical success.[8]

Clinical Presentation

The most common complaint of children with spondylolysis is low back pain.

Unlike the more ubiquitous, self-limited back pain complaints in adults, back pain in children is often associated with underlying structural abnormalities and should be evaluated appropriately. Back pain from pediatric spondylolysis is typically mechanical in nature—activity related and relieved with rest. Children generally present with pain complaints that are more chronic in nature. In patients with spondylolysis, the musculoskeletal examination may reveal tenderness directly over the spine or in the lower lumbar flank region. Abnormalities in gait are uncommon. Neurologic complaints are also extremely rare in spondylolysis without spondylolisthesis.

Patients with low-grade spondylolisthesis commonly have similar presentations, with few abnormalities in gait or physical appearance of the back. With increasing degrees of spondylolisthesis, a palpable step between spinous processes may be felt at the level of the slip. In high-grade spondylolisthesis, an abnormal lumbosacral kyphosis may be present, associated with a compensatory thoracolumbar lordosis. In this circumstance, the child may have a shortened, waddling gait, known as the Phalen-Dickson sign. They have a tendency to flex at the knee and hip joints to maintain an erect posture. In advanced cases, a prolonged stooped posture is an effort to relocate the center of gravity shifted by the listhesis. Hamstring tightness may develop as a pelvic stabilizing mechanism, but the exact etiology remains unclear. A thorough neurologic examination in children with spondylolisthesis is mandatory. The exam is usually normal even when intermittent neurologic symptoms are reported. Special examination tests such as the straight-leg raise may be difficult to interpret, given concomitant hamstring tightness. Although true radiculopathy occurs infrequently, children may complain of radiation of pain into the buttock or legs. The presence of lower extremity weakness or bowel and bladder dysfunction is rare but has been reported and warrants appropriate urgent evaluation. A thorough history should also address previous trauma, athletics, and activity involvement. The rare neurologic deficit often involves the L5 nerve root, as spondylolisthesis of L5 over S1 is most common. The neural compromise resulting in neurologic dysfunction is typically due to both stretch and compression.

Diagnosis

Children who present with low back pain should have lumbar spine radiographs performed as an initial diagnostic step. Anteroposterior (AP) and lateral radiographs of the lumbar spine should be obtained with the child standing because the supine position may reduce any listhesis present. The lateral view is the most sensitive for detecting spondylolisthesis (**Fig. 84.1**), and a supine cross-table lateral with a bump underneath the LS junction can be used to assess mobility and reducibility of any lumbosacral kyphosis. The Ferguson-view posteroanterior (PA) radiograph is often helpful at further defining the lumbosacral bony morphology and robustness of the L5 transverse process. Although commonly ordered, the added utility of oblique spine views has been recently questioned.[23] Radiographs help identify and quantify the spondylolisthesis. The aforementioned Meyerding grading system is commonly used. A variety of spinopelvic measurements may aid in quantifying pelvic balance, predict progression, and potentially guide treatment (**Figs. 84.3 and 84.4**).

If radiographs are unrevealing but clinical history and exam are suggestive of spondylolysis, additional imaging may be warranted. Traditionally, a single photon emission computed tomography (SPECT) scan has been advocated, as it may add diagnostic precision in identifying spondylolysis (**Fig. 84.5**). The test is sensitive, while adding additional information about condition chronicity. High tracer uptake indicates an osteoblastic process, and implies a more acute process with greater healing potential than "cold" lesions. Relative decreases in signal uptake during the treatment process has also been correlated with clinical improvement.[24] More recently, however, the radiology literature has questioned the routine use SPECT for diagnosing lumbar spondylolysis.[25] These studies cite higher false positives,[26] such as infections, osteoid osteoma, and pars defects, which cannot be routinely differentiated. Additionally, the improved diagnostic precision of magnetic resonance imaging (MRI) as an alternative has increased the concerns about exposing children to ionizing radiation in SPECT.

In both spondylolysis and spondylolisthesis, modern, thin-section multidetector computed tomography (CT) is considered the best imaging modality for visualizing bony defects of the par interarticularis. CT offers additional details of the bony morphology and defect characteristics, and may aid in surgical planning. Sagittal reformatted CT images add additional precision, especially in incomplete pars fractures.[27] Well-defined sclerotic margins either on plain radiographs or on CT studies suggest a chronic pars defect, which may be less likely to heal. Healing, however, has low relevance to ultimate clinical outcome.[1]

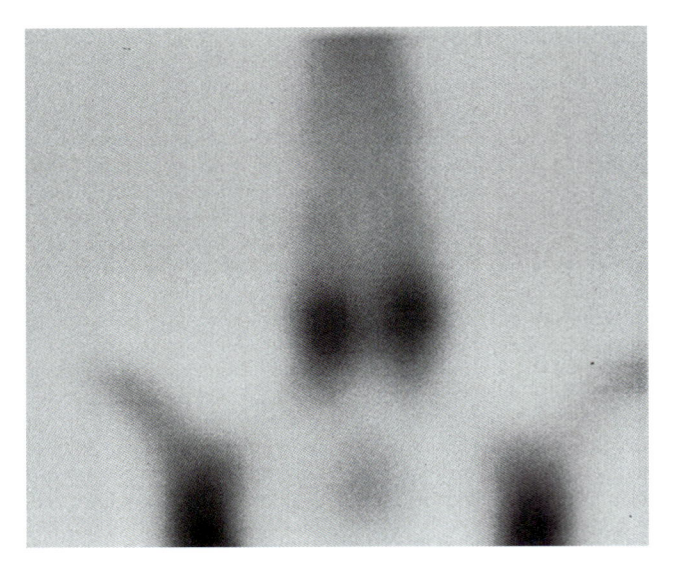

Fig. 84.5 Single photon emission computed tomography (SPECT) study showing increased uptake at the region of the pars interarticularis of L5.

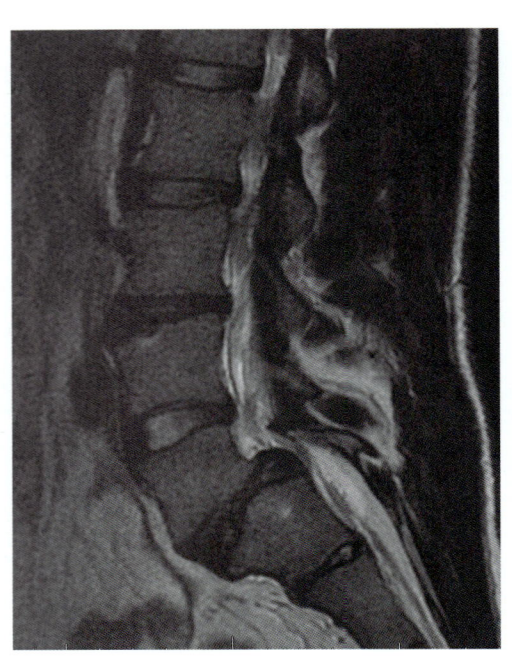

Fig. 84.6 Sagittal, T2-weighted magnetic resonance imaging of a child with spondylolisthesis.

Traditionally, MRI has been reserved for patients with neurologic complaints or findings (**Fig. 84.6**). The use of MRI as a primary diagnostic method for suspected spondylolysis, however, has not been well defined. Its use has been limited by high false-positive rates.[28] In spondylolysis, MRI also enables determination of injury acuity, as high T2-signal around the adjacent pedicle has been associated with a higher healing potential.[29] Healing, again, may have low clinical relevance. In cases of spondylolisthesis, MRI offers additional information about the intervertebral disks, neural tissues, and the presence of canal or foraminal stenosis. This may aid in surgical planning.

Management
Nonoperative

The initial treatment for spondylolysis is nonoperative. After appropriate workup, neurologically normal patients presenting with spondylolysis should be treated with various combinations of activity restriction, rest, rehabilitation, bracing, and anti-inflammatory medication, depending on symptom severity. Asymptomatic children with incidentally discovered spondylolysis should be allowed to continue activity without restriction. Although treatment may vary according to clinical presentation, chronicity, and etiology, offending activities, such as high-impact sports, should be limited for a 6- to 12-week duration. Thoracolumbar spinal orthosis (TLSO) bracing with or without a thigh extension should be considered for acute pars fractures. Our preference is to use a soft corset brace. Physical therapy may also be considered, to increase core muscle strength and to stretch an overly tight hamstring. Rehabilitation may improve spine biomechanics, maximizing the chances of recovery and reducing the potential for reinjury. After complete symptom resolution, gradual return to activity is permitted.

The goals of treatment should be carefully evaluated and explained to the patient. For most, especially those with chronic symptoms, symptom relief and formation of a stable fibrous union remain end points of treatment.[16] In patients with diagnostic evidence of an acute pars stress reaction or fracture, healing may be possible, but not necessarily the goal. In those treated conservatively for acute pars stress reactions or fractures, overall healing rates of less than 50%[30] have been reported, with L4 defects demonstrating greater healing potential than L5 defects (63% vs 9%).[1] Furthermore, unilateral pars defects are more likely to heal and not require surgery than bilateral defects.[31] In a meta-analysis, Klein et al[16] reviewed 665 pediatric patients from 15 studies of conservatively treated spondylolysis and low-grade spondylolisthesis and found that 83.9% had clinical success at 1 year. Additionally, subgroup analysis from this study failed to demonstrate a difference between bracing versus no bracing and outcome.

Patients with low-grade spondylolisthesis should undergo a similar course of nonoperative treatment as spondylolysis. Activity restriction, rest, bracing, and anti-inflammatory medication should remain the staples of treatment. Resolution of symptoms should remain the goal of treatment, as bony union has not been deemed relevant.[16] Although the outcomes after conservative treatment are generally excellent, the physician should be aware of a low likelihood of slip progression in the long term.[11,17] (Recall some of the clinical and radiographic risk factors for nonoperative failure that were discussed above; see Epidemiology section.) Regardless of treatment choice, children should be followed every 6 to 12 months until skeletal maturity with a standing spot lateral of the LS junction.

Operative

Indications for operative intervention include failure to relieve symptoms in spondylolysis and low-grade spondylolisthesis, progressive spondylolisthesis (anterior translation or LS kyphosis-slip angle), and asymptomatic high-grade spondylolisthesis in a skeletally immature patient. Although a variety of surgical treatment options exist, the indications and techniques for direct pars repair, in-situ fusion, and reduction with fusion remain controversial. In the following sections, we discuss the indications, methods, advantages, and drawbacks of these surgical options.

Pars Repair

In patients with spondylolysis and reducible low-grade spondylolisthesis who have failed nonoperative therapy, direct surgical repair of the pars interarticularis may be considered. Advocates cite the theoretical short- and long-term benefits of less invasive surgery, such as preserved lumbar motion with a lower likelihood of adjacent segment degeneration. Small, long-term follow-up series, however, fail to demonstrate a clear advantage, with no difference in clinical and radiographic outcomes between pars repair and uninstrumented posterolateral in-situ fusion at 14.8-year follow-up.[32]

Nevertheless, the ideal candidate has single-level defects above L5, with normal disk and facet soft tissues, no neurologic defects, and relief from local anesthetic injection around the pars.[16] Defects at the L5-S1 level should be considered for in-situ fusion, usually with instrumentation. Multiple surgical techniques have been described. Most techniques advocate fibrous nonunion debridement, decortication, bone grafting, and defect fixation. One of the first accounts of internal fixation was from Buck[33] in 1970. He used direct screw fixation of defects and achieved long-term clinical success. The Scott wiring technique utilizes a 20-gauge cerclage wire in a figure-of-8 format around the lamina and spinous process. Bradford and Iza[34] reported 80% good to excellent clinical results and a 90% fusion rate with the wiring technique. Although a variety of repair techniques have emerged over the last few decades, Kakiuchi[35] reported excellent results with the use of pedicle screw fixation and laminar hooks.[36] Another report advocated a U-shaped rod, anchored by pedicle screws and looped around the spinous process to compress across the defects.[37]

Low-Grade Spondylolisthesis and In-Situ Fusion

In patients with low-grade spondylolisthesis who have failed conservative care, in-situ fusion should be considered. For patients with < 50% anterolisthesis and a nonkyphotic lumbosacral angle, a single-level fusion is typically adequate. The gold-standard surgical treatment for low-grade spondylolisthesis, especially at the L5-S1 level, is considered in-situ, uninstrumented posterolateral fusion with postoperative cast or brace immobilization. Both a Wiltse paraspinal muscle splitting and a standard midline surgical approach to the lumbar spine have been advocated. Although the Wiltse approach has the advantage of sparing the posterior spinal elements from destabilization, it does not allow for central decompression (which is rarely needed).

Multiple authors have demonstrated durable, long-term results with uninstrumented posterolateral fusion for grades I and II spondylolisthesis.[13,38,39] With this technique, Lenke et al[38] reported > 80% clinical improvement, despite a 71% radiographic fusion rate. In those with neurologic symptoms (rare), wide decompression should accompany a spinal fusion to avoid further slip progression. Low-grade spondylolisthesis in patients with kyphosis at the lumbosacral junction is at higher risk of progression. In these cases, some have advocated use of a multilevel fusion, interbody fusion, or postural reduction techniques. In patients with deficient transverse processes, the addition of an interbody fusion may also be warranted. Despite the variety of available techniques, modern fixation for low-grade spondylolisthesis has shifted toward the use of single-level posterolateral spinal fusion, supported by pedicle screw fixation. This is the technique that we typically use. Transpedicular screw fixation in children has been proven safe with low complication rates.

High-Grade Spondylolisthesis

In-Situ Fusion vs Reduction and Fusion

In patients with high-grade spondylolisthesis (> 50% slip), surgical intervention should be considered, as long-term studies demonstrate high rates of slip progression and failure of symptom relief[17,19] (**Figs. 84.7 and 84.8**). Traditionally, an uninstrumented posterolateral fusion from L4 to S1 with postural reduction in a body cast has been the gold-standard treatment for high-grade spondylolisthesis in children in the pre-instrumentation era. Operative management has been superior to conservative care, but modern technique choices raise considerable controversy. In one of the largest series published, Pizzutillo et al[39] in 1986 found a pseudarthrosis and slip progression rate of only 5% with the aforementioned technique. Other studies, however, have reported less promising results.[13,19] Thus, for high-grade slips, in-situ posterolateral fusion without instrumentation has been questioned as an optimal treatment. Multiple studies have demonstrated higher rates of nonunion, slip progression, and bending of the fusion mass, with greater symptom progression and clinical failure.[13,19] In addition, surgery for high-grade spondylolisthesis poses a neurologic risk. Both nerve root compression and cauda equina syndrome have been reported.[40] These reports have tempered the enthusiasm for reduction techniques. Ultimately, elimination of pain and restoration of function remain important surgical goals, achievable with a stable fusion and restoration of spinopelvic balance.[8] Broad surgical options for high-grade spondylolisthesis include in-situ fusion versus reduction. The techniques of in-situ fusion also vary markedly; the use of instrumentation, the levels to fuse, anterior column support, and interbody fixation are debated. Likewise, a host of reduction techniques, from partial to complete reduction, have been described.

Given concerns about pseudarthrosis and failure following posterior fusion alone, multiple circumferential fusion techniques have been described. These anterior column stabilization procedures are used with both in-situ fusion and reduction/fusion approaches. Proponents argue the theoretical advances of circumferential fusion include a greater fusion bed, restoration of disk height, and indirect decompression of nerve roots in the foramina. Stabilization of the anterior column can also be achieved with transdiskal sacral pedicle screws that traverse the L5-S1 disks into the L5 vertebral body (**Fig. 84.9**). Proponents argue that this technique confers the clinical and biomechanical benefits of anterior stabilization with a single posterior approach.[41] Other techniques, including tunneling a fibular strut graft through the sacrum into the L5 vertebral body resection, have also been described.[42] In a long-term follow-up study, Lamberg et al[43] demonstrated that after 17 years, circumferential in-situ fusion provided slightly higher long-term results over isolated posterolateral or anterior in-situ fusion for high-grade spondylolisthesis.

The need for surgical reduction in high-grade pediatric spondylolisthesis remains controversial. Reduction of kyphosis and fusion may enhance fusion rates by diminishing shear forces across the lumbosacral junction, enable more instrumentation purchase, reduce nerve root traction and canal stenosis, and improve spinopelvic balance and cosmesis. Intraoperative reduction of high-grade slips, however, has been associated with a higher risk of injury to the nerve roots.[40] Other disadvantages include possible insufficiency fractures of the sacral dome, prolonged operative time, and increased blood loss. Multiple reduction

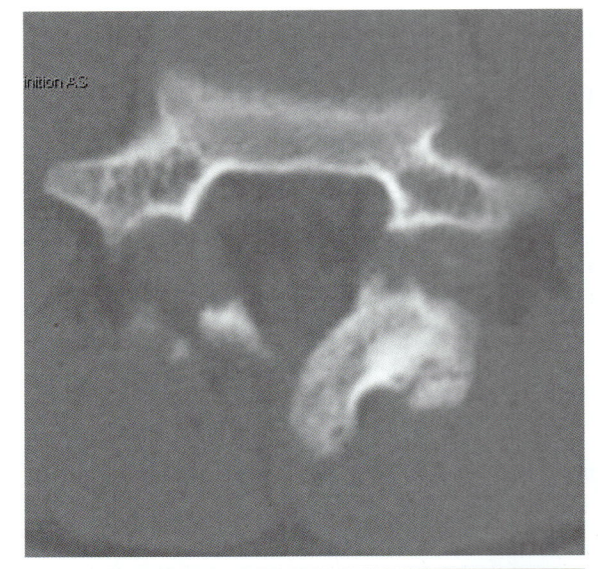

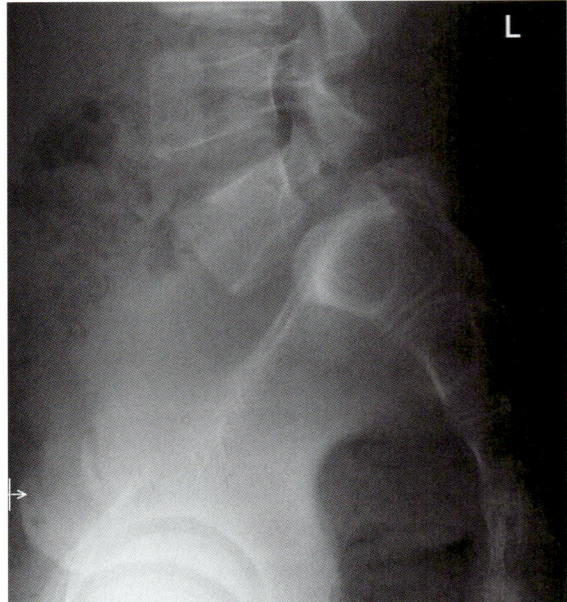

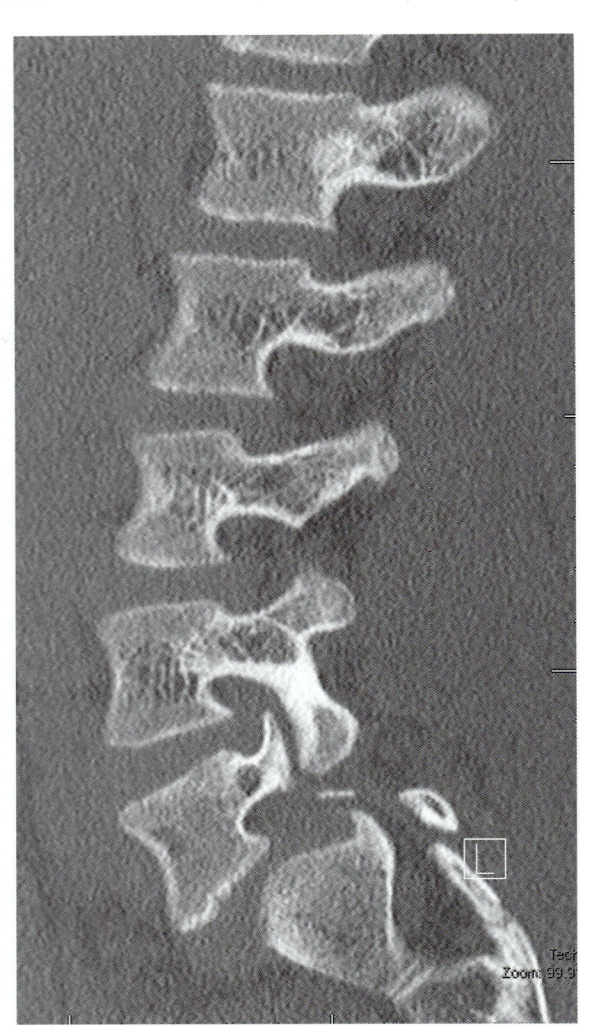

Fig. 84.7 A patient with grade II spondylolisthesis. **(a)** Axial computed tomography (CT). **(b)** Lateral CT. **(c)** Lateral standing radiograph.

techniques have been described, including halo-femoral traction, passive postural reduction,[44] anterior release with posterior instrumentation, and two-stage anterior–posterior surgery with vertebrectomy (Gaines procedure). The Gaines procedure has been used for spondyloptosis. In the passive postural reduction techniques, authors advocate hyperextension and compression of instrumentation **(Figs. 84.8 and 84.9)**. Extensive bony and soft tissue decompression should accompany many of these procedures, with wide laminectomies, foraminotomies, and diskectomies, to minimize iatrogenic neurologic injury if a clinical nerve root deficit exists.

In addition, intraoperative neurologic monitoring is considered the standard of care during surgical treatment of high-grade spondylolisthesis. Both transcranial motor evoked potentials (MEPs) and somatosensory evoked potentials (SSEPs) should be monitored throughout the procedure from L2 to S4. Triggered electromyograms may also help identify early nerve root irritation. An experienced anesthesia team may also help ensure maintenance of elevated mean arterial blood pressure and avoidance of anesthetics that interfere with neuromonitoring.

The outcomes for circumferential fusions and reduction techniques have not necessarily conferred clinical benefit over in-situ fusion for high-grade spondylolisthesis in the literature.

Muschik et al[45] compared an anterior procedure alone to a combined anterior-posterior procedure in children with severe spondylolisthesis. The radiographic results were better in the anterior-posterior group, but the authors could not demonstrate a difference in clinical outcome between the two groups. Molinari et al[46] described complications associated with three different approaches for the surgical treatment of high-grade isthmic spondylolisthesis in children. They concluded that the increased neurologic risks of circumferential fusion-reduction procedures

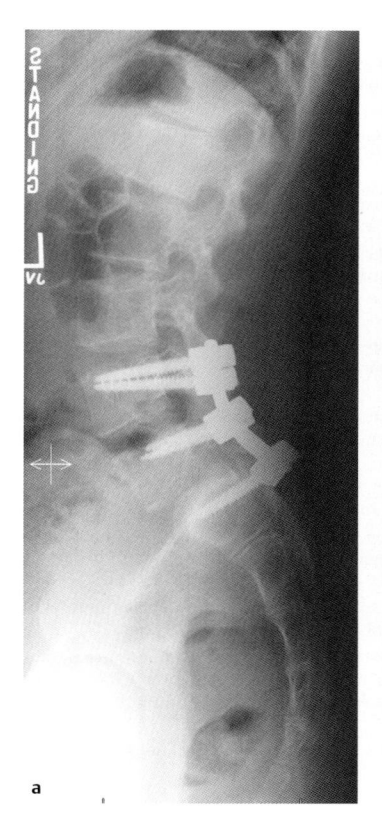

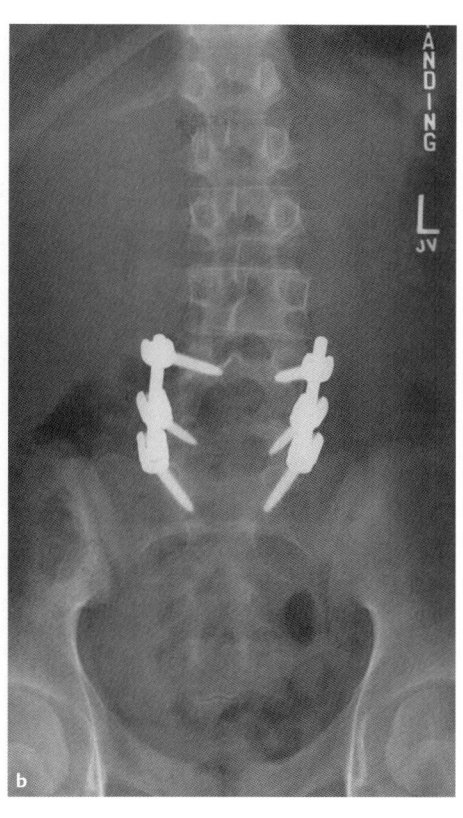

Fig. 84.8 **(a)** Lateral and **(b)** AP radiographs of patient in **Fig. 84.7** (grade II spondylolisthesis) treated with posterior spinal fusion and pedicle screw instrumentation of L4-S1. Note the partial reduction of the spondylolisthesis compared with preoperatively.

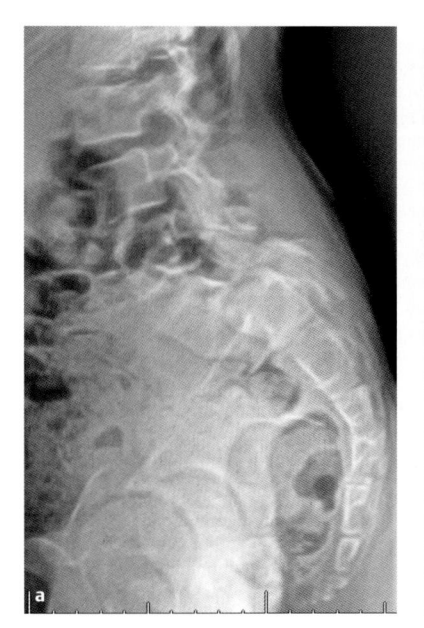

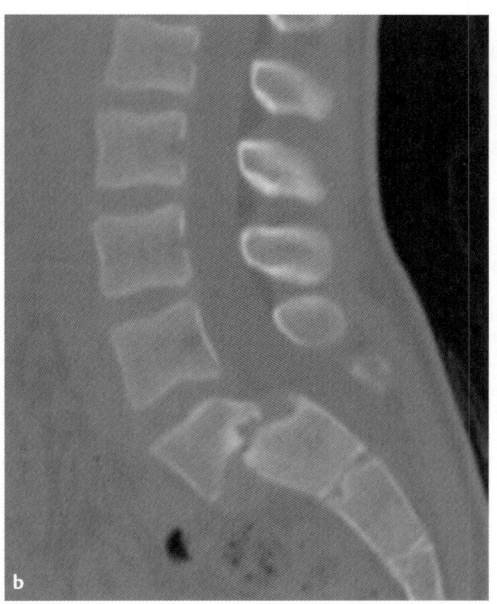

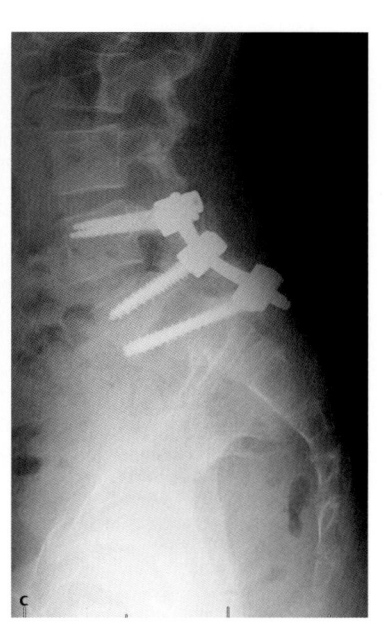

Fig. 84.9 **(a)** Lateral radiograph and **(b)** CT of the lumbar spine in a patient with high-grade spondylolisthesis with significant lumbosacral kyphosis, treated with postural reduction, posterior spinal fusion, pedicle screw instrumentation of L4-S1, and anterior column support **(c)**. Note the S1 screws traverse the L5-S1 disk space, ending in the L5 inferior end plate.

were acceptable given the fusion success rate, the degree of reduction achieved, and the improved patient outcomes with regard to pain and function. A literature review by Transfeldt and Mehbod[47] evaluated studies that compared reduction and fusion to in-situ fusion, and concluded that fusion rates may be higher with reduction even though clinical outcomes were similar between the groups. Poussa et al,[48] in a 15-year follow-up study, found that patients treated with in-situ fusion had a better outcome than those treated with reduction.

Conclusion

Given the mixed results reported in the literature, the surgical management of children with symptomatic high-grade spondylolisthesis remains controversial. Some basic concepts, however, can be summarized: (1) fusion alone carries a higher pseudarthrosis rate compared with instrumentation with fusion; (2) neural decompression should be accomplished when there is a preoperative neurologic deficit; (3) intraoperative attempts at reduction carry an increased risk of neurologic deficits; and (4) reduction of the spondylolisthesis, but particularly the lumbosacral kyphosis, may improve fusion rates and patient outcome.

References

1. Fujii K, Katoh S, Sairyo K, Ikata T, Yasui N. Union of defects in the pars interarticularis of the lumbar spine in children and adolescents. The radiological outcome after conservative treatment. J Bone Joint Surg Br 2004;86:225–231
2. Wiltse LL, Newman PH, Macnab I. Classification of spondylolisis and spondylolisthesis. Clin Orthop Relat Res 1976;117:23–29
3. Peter JC, Hoffman EB, Arens LJ. Spondylolysis and spondylolisthesis after five-level lumbosacral laminectomy for selective posterior rhizotomy in cerebral palsy. Childs Nerv Syst 1993;9:285–287, discussion 287–288
4. Rossi F, Dragoni S. Lumbar spondylolysis: occurrence in competitive athletes. Updated achievements in a series of 390 cases. J Sports Med Phys Fitness 1990;30:450–452
5. Hammerberg KW. New concepts on the pathogenesis and classification of spondylolisthesis. Spine 2005;30(6, Suppl):S4–S11
6. Herman MJ, Pizzutillo PD. Spondylolysis and spondylolisthesis in the child and adolescent: a new classification. Clin Orthop Relat Res 2005; 434:46–54
7. Mac-Thiong JM, Labelle H. A proposal for a surgical classification of pediatric lumbosacral spondylolisthesis based on current literature. Eur Spine J 2006;15:1425–1435
8. Hresko MT, Labelle H, Roussouly P, Berthonnaud E. Classification of high-grade spondylolistheses based on pelvic version and spine balance: possible rationale for reduction. Spine 2007;32:2208–2213
9. Dubousset J. Treatment of spondylolysis and spondylolisthesis in children and adolescents. Clin Orthop Relat Res 1997;337:77–85
10. Dubousset J. Three-dimensional analysis of the scoliotic deformity. In: Weinstein S, ed. The Pediatric Spine: Principles and Practice. New York: Raven Press; 1994:479–496
11. Fredrickson BE, Baker D, McHolick WJ, Yuan HA, Lubicky JP. The natural history of spondylolysis and spondylolisthesis. J Bone Joint Surg Am 1984;66:699–707
12. Kalichman L, Kim DH, Li L, Guermazi A, Berkin V, Hunter DJ. Spondylolysis and spondylolisthesis: prevalence and association with low back pain in the adult community-based population. Spine 2009;34:199–205
13. Seitsalo S, Osterman K, Hyvärinen H, Tallroth K, Schlenzka D, Poussa M. Progression of spondylolisthesis in children and adolescents. A long-term follow-up of 272 patients. Spine 1991;16:417–421
14. Simper LB. Spondylolysis in Eskimo skeletons. Acta Orthop Scand 1986; 57:78–80
15. Albanese M, Pizzutillo PD. Family study of spondylolysis and spondylolisthesis. J Pediatr Orthop 1982;2:496–499
16. Klein G, Mehlman CT, McCarty M. Nonoperative treatment of spondylolysis and grade I spondylolisthesis in children and young adults: a meta-analysis of observational studies. J Pediatr Orthop 2009;29:146–156
17. Beutler WJ, Fredrickson BE, Murtland A, Sweeney CA, Grant WD, Baker D. The natural history of spondylolysis and spondylolisthesis: 45-year follow-up evaluation. Spine 2003;28:1027–1035, discussion 1035
18. Boxall D, Bradford DS, Winter RB, Moe JH. Management of severe spondylolisthesis in children and adolescents. J Bone Joint Surg Am 1979;61: 479–495
19. Harris IE, Weinstein SL. Long-term follow-up of patients with grade-III and IV spondylolisthesis. Treatment with and without posterior fusion. J Bone Joint Surg Am 1987;69:960–969
20. Herkowitz HN, Kurz LT. Degenerative lumbar spondylolisthesis with spinal stenosis. A prospective study comparing decompression with decompression and intertransverse process arthrodesis. J Bone Joint Surg Am 1991;73:802–808
21. Weinstein JN, Lurie JD, Tosteson TD, et al. Surgical versus nonsurgical treatment for lumbar degenerative spondylolisthesis. N Engl J Med 2007; 356:2257–2270
22. Herman MJ, Pizzutillo PD, Cavalier R. Spondylolysis and spondylolisthesis in the child and adolescent athlete. Orthop Clin North Am 2003;34:461–467, vii
23. Beck NA, Miller R, Baldwin K, et al. Do oblique views add value in the diagnosis of spondylolysis in adolescents? J Bone Joint Surg Am 2013;95:e65
24. Anderson K, Sarwark JF, Conway JJ, Logue ES, Schafer MF. Quantitative assessment with SPECT imaging of stress injuries of the pars interarticularis and response to bracing. J Pediatr Orthop 2000;20:28–33
25. Leone A, Cianfoni A, Cerase A, Magarelli N, Bonomo L. Lumbar spondylolysis: a review. Skeletal Radiol 2011;40:683–700
26. Gregory PL, Batt ME, Kerslake RW, Webb JK. Single photon emission computerized tomography and reverse gantry computerized tomography findings in patients with back pain investigated for spondylolysis. Clin J Sport Med 2005;15:79–86
27. Dunn AJ, Campbell RS, Mayor PE, Rees D. Radiological findings and healing patterns of incomplete stress fractures of the pars interarticularis. Skeletal Radiol 2008;37:443–450
28. Saifuddin A, Burnett SJ. The value of lumbar spine MRI in the assessment of the pars interarticularis. Clin Radiol 1997;52:666–671
29. Sairyo K, Katoh S, Takata Y, et al. MRI signal changes of the pedicle as an indicator for early diagnosis of spondylolysis in children and adolescents: a clinical and biomechanical study. Spine 2006;31:206–211
30. Morita T, Ikata T, Katoh S, Miyake R. Lumbar spondylolysis in children and adolescents. J Bone Joint Surg Br 1995;77:620–625
31. Debnath UK, Freeman BJ, Grevitt MP, Sithole J, Scammell BE, Webb JK. Clinical outcome of symptomatic unilateral stress injuries of the lumbar pars interarticularis. Spine 2007;32:995–1000
32. Schlenzka D, Remes V, Helenius I, et al. Direct repair for treatment of symptomatic spondylolysis and low-grade isthmic spondylolisthesis in young patients: no benefit in comparison to segmental fusion after a mean follow-up of 14.8 years. Eur Spine J 2006;15:1437–1447
33. Buck JE. Direct repair of the defect in spondylolisthesis. Preliminary report. J Bone Joint Surg Br 1970;52:432–437
34. Bradford DS, Iza J. Repair of the defect in spondylolysis or minimal degrees of spondylolisthesis by segmental wire fixation and bone grafting. Spine 1985;10:673–679
35. Kakiuchi M. Repair of the defect in spondylolysis. Durable fixation with pedicle screws and laminar hooks. J Bone Joint Surg Am 1997;79:818–825
36. Patel RD, Rosas HG, Steinmetz MP, Anderson PA. Repair of pars interarticularis defect utilizing a pedicle and laminar screw construct: a new technique based on anatomical and biomechanical analysis. J Neurosurg Spine 2012;17:61–68
37. Gillet P, Petit M. Direct repair of spondylolysis without spondylolisthesis, using a rod-screw construct and bone grafting of the pars defect. Spine 1999;24:1252–1256
38. Lenke LG, Bridwell KH, Bullis D, Betz RR, Baldus C, Schoenecker PL. Results of in situ fusion for isthmic spondylolisthesis. J Spinal Disord 1992;5: 433–442
39. Pizzutillo PD, Mirenda W, MacEwen GD. Posterolateral fusion for spondylolisthesis in adolescence. J Pediatr Orthop 1986;6:311–316
40. Schoenecker PL, Cole HO, Herring JA, Capelli AM, Bradford DS. Cauda equina syndrome after in situ arthrodesis for severe spondylolisthesis at the lumbosacral junction. J Bone Joint Surg Am 1990;72:369–377
41. Abdu WA, Wilber RG, Emery SE. Pedicular transvertebral screw fixation of the lumbosacral spine in spondylolisthesis. A new technique for stabilization. Spine 1994;19:710–715

42. Bohlman HH, Cook SS. One-stage decompression and posterolateral and interbody fusion for lumbosacral spondyloptosis through a posterior approach. Report of two cases. J Bone Joint Surg Am 1982;64:415–418
43. Lamberg T, Remes V, Helenius I, Schlenzka D, Seitsalo S, Poussa M. Uninstrumented in situ fusion for high-grade childhood and adolescent isthmic spondylolisthesis: long-term outcome. J Bone Joint Surg Am 2007;89:512–518
44. Schwend RM, Waters PM, Hey LA, Hall JE, Emans JB. Treatment of severe spondylolisthesis in children by reduction and L4-S4 posterior segmental hyperextension fixation. J Pediatr Orthop 1992;12:703–711
45. Muschik M, Zippel H, Perka C. Surgical management of severe spondylolisthesis in children and adolescents. Anterior fusion in situ versus anterior spondylodesis with posterior transpedicular instrumentation and reduction. Spine 1997;22:2036–2042, discussion 2043
46. Molinari RW, Bridwell KH, Lenke LG, Ungacta FF, Riew KD. Complications in the surgical treatment of pediatric high-grade, isthmic dysplastic spondylolisthesis. A comparison of three surgical approaches. Spine 1999;24:1701–1711
47. Transfeldt EE, Mehbod AA. Evidence-based medicine analysis of isthmic spondylolisthesis treatment including reduction versus fusion in situ for high-grade slips. Spine 2007;32(19, Suppl):S126–S129
48. Poussa M, Remes V, Lamberg T, et al. Treatment of severe spondylolisthesis in adolescence with reduction or fusion in situ: long-term clinical, radiologic, and functional outcome. Spine 2006;31:583–590, discussion 591–592

85 Lumbar Degenerative Disk Disease

Ricardo B.V. Fontes, Josemberg S. Baptista, and John E. O'Toole

Intervertebral disks (IVDs) have been described in medical texts since ancient times, but it was Hubert von Luschka[1] who first devoted a medical manuscript exclusively to the IVD in 1858, describing its general organization, the vertebral end plates, and their cartilaginous nature. A slightly more detailed description of the human IVD as a two-part structure, consisting of a superficial, reinforced ring and a softer nucleus was widely found in anatomy textbooks at the beginning of the 20th century.[2,3] The first author to investigate patterns of normal and pathological aging of the IVD was Schmorl[4] in the late 1920s, followed by the seminal three-part work of Coventry et al,[5-7] who laid out the macro- and microscopic features of the lumbar IVD from early infancy into the ninth decade. They were also the first to formally postulate, and attempt to answer, the question of which degenerative features might be considered "normal" or "pathological"—a question that is still lacking a complete answer to this day.

This focused attention on the human IVD over the late 19th and early 20th century was not without reason. As health and sanitary conditions improved, so did life expectancy, and therefore the incidence of degenerative conditions increased. At the same time, development of neurology as a medical specialty, safer anesthesia, antiseptic conditions for surgery, and finally radiological techniques in the early 20th century enabled practitioners for the first time in history to advance beyond the natural history of disk pathology; they became able not only to alleviate pain with medications but also to diagnose clinically, support their hypothesis radiographically, and eventually perform surgery with acceptable results.

These new skills became useful for physicians, as low back pain (LBP) has emerged as one of the most common general medical complaints. Most men and women who reach late adulthood are expected to experience at least one clinically relevant episode of back pain, that is, an episode necessitating specialized medical attention. Different definitions and reporting methods may account for significant regional differences, but in a large literature review, Walker[8] reported figures of punctual prevalence in adults ranging between 12% to 33%, 1-year prevalence between 22% and 65%, and lifetime prevalence in the 11 to 84% range.[9] Although lifetime prevalence of LBP may be very high, in only a minority of these patients will the complaint last longer than 2 weeks, and in an even smaller number will this problem necessitate surgical intervention.[10]

Definitions

When describing morphological alterations in the IVD, widely different terms may be found even in the specialized literature. It is essential, however, to adopt and strictly adhere to a standard terminology to produce scientifically sound studies and comparisons. In 2001, a multidisciplinary task force from several North American subspecialty associations sought to standardize these terms. Recognizing the frequent lack of correlation between radiological features of the IVD and symptoms, this task force has arbitrarily established as a "normal" IVD the young disk without any alterations. The normal IVD is therefore virtual in the usual clinical practice because such disks are generally found only in very early childhood. Consequently, it was decided to group under the label "disk degeneration" all alterations at the cellular and macroscopic levels that IVDs undergo during their lifetime, thus avoiding a morphological distinction between "normal" and "pathological." Finally, it was decided to utilize the term *degenerative disk disease* (DDD) to designate only the clinical syndrome of LBP thought to derive from disk degeneration.[11] These definitions have been reaffirmed recently and should be utilized in all studies of this subject.[12]

Normal Anatomy and Embryology

The human IVD is a cartilaginous joint classified as an amphiarthrosis, given its roughly flat and slightly movable nature. Because the vast majority of disks are shown to persist throughout the entire life of the individual, it is further classified as a fibrocartilaginous symphysis. Although Luschka had initially identified the IVD as a synovial joint (and such theories persist until today), the fibrocartilaginous nature of the disk was proven as early as 1926, thus enabling Chiarugi[13] to accurately classify it.[1,14] This joint is composed of a superficial multilayered ring of connective tissue fibers known as the annulus fibrosus (AF) and a cell-poor, central core of loosely organized connective matrix known as the nucleus pulposus (NP). In the lumbar spine, this ring is complete but thinner in its posterior aspect; it is also wedge-shaped in the sagittal plane, thus accounting for the normal lumbar lordosis. The connective tissue fibers of the AF are organized in thick bundles that are displayed diagonally and alternately in the coronal plane in the anterior portion of the AF and insert themselves into the vertebral end plate in the form of Sharpey's fibers. Diagonal fibers exist in the posterior AF, but the primary orientation is longitudinal. In both the anterior and posterior sectors of the AF, there is no clear limit between the disk and the overlying longitudinal ligaments. In deeper areas of the lumbar IVD, there is also no clear limit between the AF and NP, though this limit is clearly seen at the vertebral interface because the NP does not have Sharpey-type insertions (**Fig. 85.1**). Although capillaries and venules may be found in the superficial layers of the AF, the deeper portions of the AF and NP are avascular. These characteristics play a dominant role in embryological development and in degeneration of the IVD.[15,16]

The notion that the human IVD may be embryologically derived from the notochord was based on early observations of Luschka and Kölliker of cells in the NP that morphologically resembled those from the notochord.[1,17] The development of the

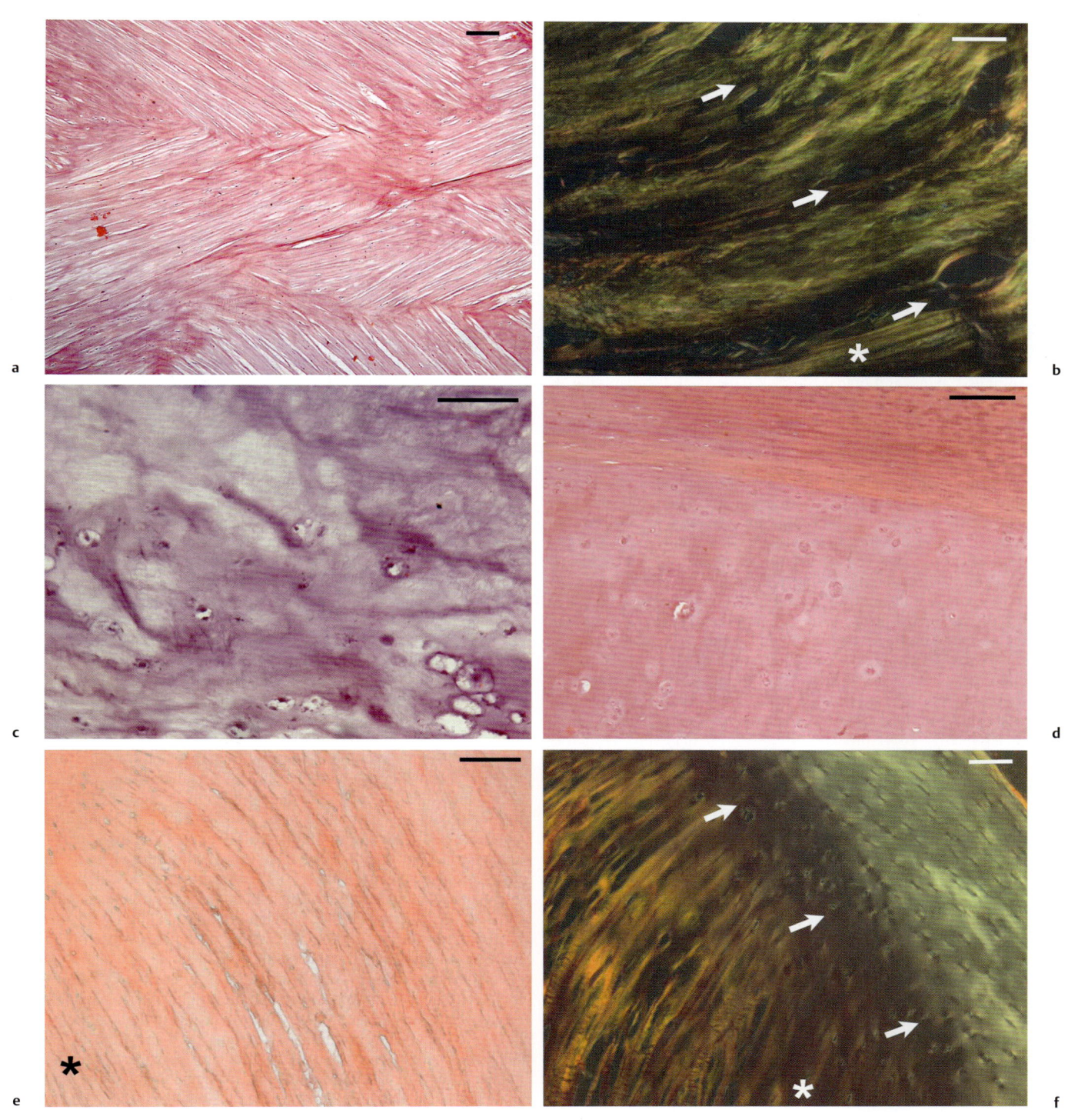

Fig. 85.1 Microscopy slides demonstrating the general histology of lumbar intervertebral disks (IVDs). *Arrows* mark the vertebral end plate, and *asterisks* indicate anterior direction in sagittal sections. **(a)** Coronal section of anterior annulus fibrosus (AF), demonstrating diagonally alternating fibrous lamellae. **(b)** Sharpey's fiber-type insertion of the anterior AF lamellae into the vertebral end plate. **(c)** Loose connective tissue composes most of the lumbar nucleus pulposus (NP), but in severely degenerated specimens **(d)** this is substituted by a much more compact matrix with chondrocyte clusters. **(e)** Sagittal section of the posterior AF with predominantly longitudinal bundles that also exhibit a Sharpey-type insertion into the end plate **(f)**. Scale bars = 100 μm.

embryonic spine may be divided into three phases: mesenchymal, cartilaginous, and osseous.[18,19] At approximately the fourth week of intrauterine life, axial sclerotome-derived mesenchymal cells migrate into a position around the notochord.[20] These mesenchymal cells are then grouped into an incompletely segmented column; this segmentation is complete only in its lateral aspect, where segmental arteries develop. Cells located next to the segmental arteries proliferate faster than those located farther away. In those areas with greater proliferation, mesenchymal cells from two adjacent somites are grouped together and form the primitive site or *anlage* of the vertebral body; this process was termed *resegmentation* by Remak,[19] and it occurs only in the central portion, so that the posterior elements are derived from a single somite. Due to the fast proliferation of mesenchymal cells in this location, notochord-derived cells disappear before the sixth gestational week. In contrast, those mesenchymal cells located farther away from the segmental arteries differentiate into fibroblasts and form the annulus fibrosus, adhering to the epiphysis above and below the disk. The AF and the epiphyseal ring, therefore, are derived from the same somite and may be considered a single structure from an embryological standpoint, comparable to the epiphyses of long bones.[18]

At 6 weeks of gestation, chondrogenesis centers appear within the vertebral bodies and the second stage of vertebral column formation begins. At 10 weeks, the fibers of the AF are well defined, and the differentiation between AF and NP becomes apparent. Notochord remnants eventually persist in the poorly vascularized central area of the disk; however, they do not simply die but rather differentiate into fibroblasts and adhere to the cranial and caudal end plates. These cells continue to proliferate during intrauterine life, albeit at a slower pace; there is more notochord-derived tissue in a single disk at birth than in the entire notochord at 4 weeks' intrauterine life.[18,20] These notochord cells also exert an important modulatory effect over the mesenchymal-derived cells: in organisms where the notochord was experimentally removed, the axial mesenchyma forms neural arches.[20,21] After birth, proliferation of disk cells is mainly along the fibrous and cartilaginous cell lines and derived from the vertebral end plates. This was correlated as early as 1932 with the gradual decrease and eventual disappearance of NP material during disk aging. In the second half of gestation, ossification centers appear in the vertebrae and initiate the last phase of vertebral column formation; this lasts until 8 to 9 years of age.[20]

Pathophysiology of Disk Degeneration

Based on the definitions of Fardon and Milette,[11] there is no clear boundary between normal disk development and degeneration. After the completion of the ossification phase of vertebral column formation, with the fusion of the epiphyseal ring to the rest of the vertebral body, the next dominant step in disk transformation is the closure of end-plate vascular channels, first described by Übermuth[22] in 1930. These channels typically disappear in the second decade of life and have not been demonstrated beyond 33 years of age in humans.[6] This event leads to a lower oxygen tension in the interior of the IVD, thus altering the biochemical pathway for proteoglycan synthesis. Proteoglycans are one of the two main macromolecule classes that make up most of the extracellular matrix of the IVD; the other is composed of proteins from the collagen family. Proteoglycans are glycoproteins with a central protein core and one or more lateral glycosaminoglycan (GAG) chains. The main glycosaminoglycans found in the human IVD are keratan sulfate, chondroitin sulfate, and hyaluronan.[23] The synthesis of chondroitin sulfate requires oxygen in its first step. It has been demonstrated experimentally that, in microenvironments with lower oxygen tension, the pathway is diverted into an anaerobic pathway that results in increased synthesis of keratan sulfate.[24] This explains not only the increased keratan sulfate/chondroitin sulfate ratio found in degenerated disks but also the phenomenon of disk dehydration, because water molecules are linked to GAGs inside the IVD and keratan sulfate has a much lower water-binding capability.[25] Furthermore, proteoglycans act as modulatory agents for the fibroblasts and chondrocytes of the IVD, particularly those from the small interstitial family of biglycan, decorin, fibromodulin, and lumican.[23,26]

Collagen content is also significantly decreased and modified during the degenerative process. Collagen turnover in the human IVD is known to be a very slow process, although estimates vary widely (from 9 months to 78 years).[23,27] It is known that overall collagen content is decreased in degenerated disks, but recent data suggest that turnover may actually be increased in these degenerated specimens.[27] More importantly, collagen profile is significantly altered in degenerated disks; whereas human lumbar disks show a 4:1 ratio between collagen II and IV at age 35, this ratio is decreased to almost 1:1 at age 65. Profile differences between collagen subtypes in the AF and NP (greater expression of collagens V, VI, and IX in the NP, greater expression of collagens II, III, and IV in the AF) disappear by the seventh decade (Ricardo Fontes et al, unpublished data) **(Fig. 85.2)**. Degradation of protein components (both PGs and collagens) of the disk extracellular matrix is performed by enzymes of the matrix metalloproteinase (MMP) family. MMPs are classified according to their protein target as *collagenases* (MMP-1, -8, -13, and -18, for example), *gelatinases* (MMP-2 and -9), and *stromelysins* (MMP-3, -10 and -11). These molecules are secreted into the extracellular medium as proenzymes and, once activated, they require the action of their inhibitors to be cleaved and inactivated; these inactivating enzymes are therefore grouped into a category termed *tissue inhibitors of matrix metalloproteinases* (TIMPs).[28-30] The actions of MMPs and TIMPs are in balance inside the normal disk and have been shown to be regulated by a large number of cytokines and growth factors both in vitro and in vivo. Tumor necrosis factor-α (TNF-α), transforming growth factor-β (TGF-β), vacular endothelial growth factor (VEGF), and interleukin-1 (IL-1) are examples of inflammatory molecules that have been shown to modulate MMP expression in vitro. For example, TNF-α and IL-1 were detected in increased levels in disks removed during surgery in symptomatic individuals.[31-33] Overexpression of MMPs, TIMPs, and modulatory enzymes, particularly VEGF, have also been demonstrated in highly degenerated disks from asymptomatic elderly individuals (Josemberg Baptista, unpublished data) **(Fig. 85.3)**.

These microscopic modifications of the disk microenvironment are translated into macroscopic alterations of disk morphology that are well known from autopsy and radiological study. Loss of AF-NP differentiation, loss of lamellar disposition of the AF, osteophyte formation, disk fissures, and peripheral neovascularization and herniations of disk material through the end plate (Schmorl's nodes) are typical features. Attempts have been made to classify these macroscopic alterations into normal and abnormal findings on the basis of frequency, severity, or chronology.[7,34] For example, Coventry et al,[7] on the basis of autopsy findings, determined that small or microscopic Schmorl's nodes were normal (present in 56 of 88 cadavers of varying ages), but large extrusions of disk material were not (present in 5/88 cadavers). Identification of so-called pathological morphology findings is complicated not only by the elevated prevalence of imaging findings in asymptomatic individuals but also by the demonstrated progression of such alterations without the development of symptoms.[35] Boden et al[36] demonstrated minor and significant degenerative changes in 57% and 28% of asymptomatic

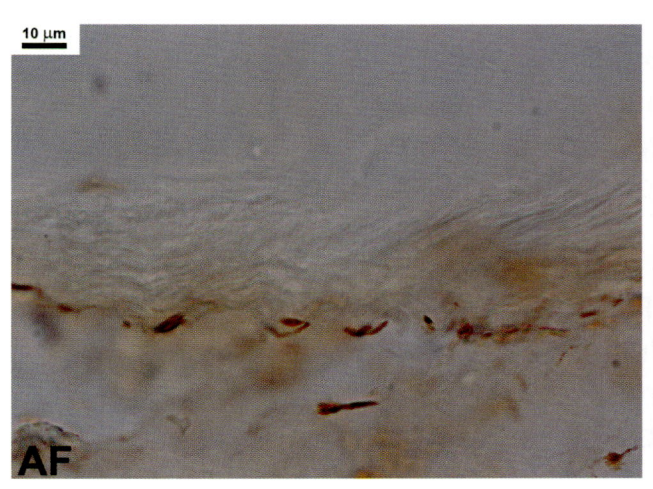

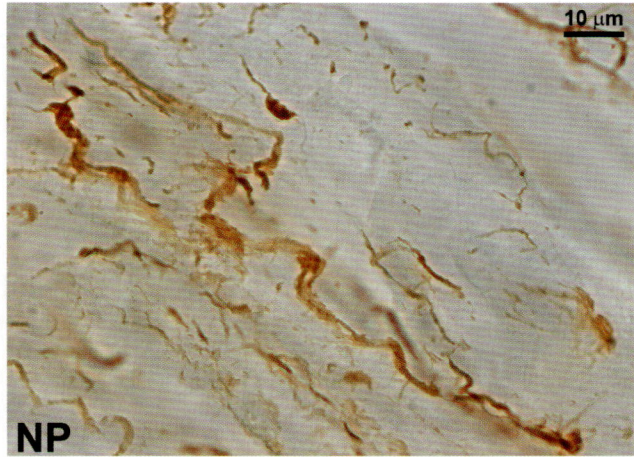

Fig. 85.2 Immunohistochemistry slides staining against **(a)** collagen II in the AF of an elderly (86-year-old) person and **(b)** collagen IX in the NP of a young (32-year-old) person. Collagen content is decreased by 80% during normal aging.

young (20 to 39 years of age) individuals, respectively. In asymptomatic subjects older than 60 years of age, 93% had major degenerative findings present in at least one lumbar disk[36] (**Fig. 85.4**). Several particular imaging findings have been identified over the years as pathological markers or at least significantly correlating with symptoms, such as underlying end-plate signal change (so-called Modic changes) and high-intensity zones in disk protrusions. Despite several studies correlating these findings with symptomatic or presymptomatic patient populations, other studies point out a significant percentage of the normal population with the same imaging findings.[35,37–39] In the particular case of Modic changes, even the underlying cause of these alterations is debatable, as recent publications have claimed them as manifestations of low-grade bacterial infection.[40]

Degenerative Disk Disease

As discussed above, the very definition of DDD is clinical: in individuals where other causes of nonradiated low back pain are excluded and disk degeneration is evident on imaging, the diagnosis of DDD is made. Despite the presence of degeneration, LBP is frequently multifactorial; inflammation of the joints in the spine from rheumatologic conditions is more common than once thought, and a myofascial component is almost always present in individuals with DDD.[41] It is, therefore, a complicated clinical exercise to identify the exact anatomic structure responsible for LBP. If muscles and ligaments that insert on the vertebrae are excluded, the two main pain generators found in the lumbar motion segment are the disk and the articular facets of zygapophysial joints. A basic requisite for any given anatomic structure to be considered a pain generator is the presence of nociceptive fibers and receptors. The synovial capsule and articular facets of the zygapophysial joints possess abundant Aδ and C nerve fibers. Free nerve endings are found in the superficial AF, which also exhibit the presence of substance P and calcitonin gene-related peptide (CGRP), which are neurotransmitters associated with nociception.[42–44] An increased density of nerve fibers in the more superficial aspects of the lumbar IVD, as well as their presence in the NP, was once thought to be a great insight into the pathophysiology of DDD and was published in high-impact, general medical journals. Over time, however, it was shown to be more common than previously thought, and a proprioceptive function for these nerves has also been proposed based on their association

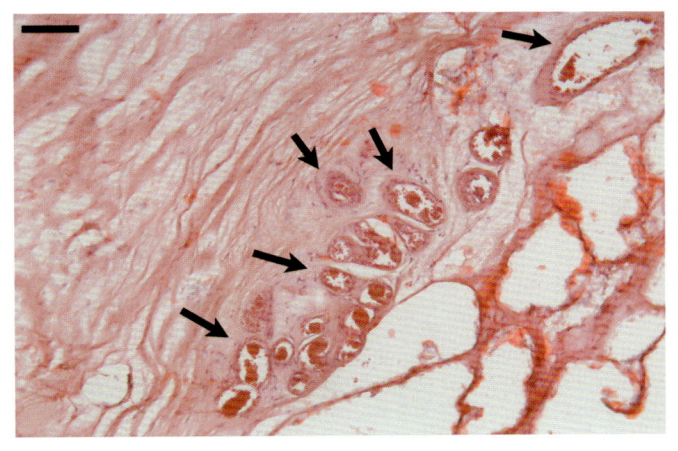

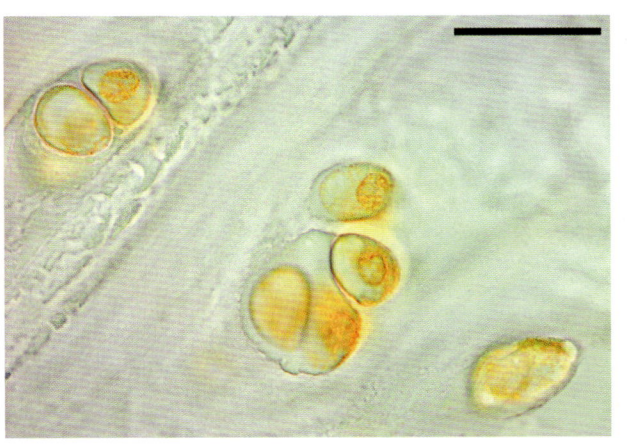

Fig. 85.3 **(a)** Hematoxylin and eosin (H&E) stain of the posterior AF of a lumbar IVD from an asymptomatic 71-year-old man. Prominent blood vessels are found within the superficial lamellae of the AF (*arrows*). **(b)** Chondrocytes from the interior of the same disk sample are positive for vascular endothelial growth factor (VEGF). Scale bars = 200 μm.

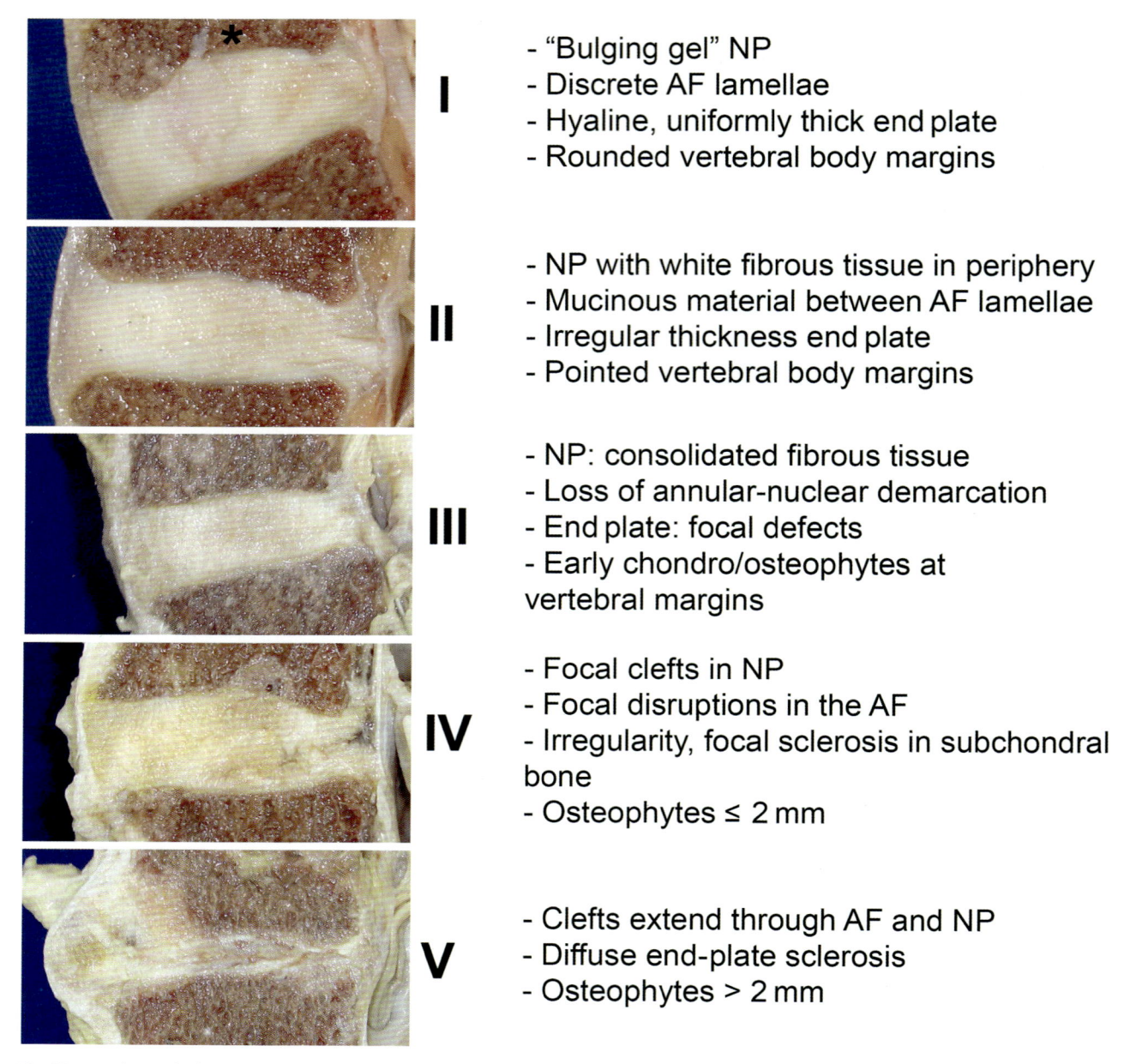

I
- "Bulging gel" NP
- Discrete AF lamellae
- Hyaline, uniformly thick end plate
- Rounded vertebral body margins

II
- NP with white fibrous tissue in periphery
- Mucinous material between AF lamellae
- Irregular thickness end plate
- Pointed vertebral body margins

III
- NP: consolidated fibrous tissue
- Loss of annular-nuclear demarcation
- End plate: focal defects
- Early chondro/osteophytes at vertebral margins

IV
- Focal clefts in NP
- Focal disruptions in the AF
- Irregularity, focal sclerosis in subchondral bone
- Osteophytes ≤ 2 mm

V
- Clefts extend through AF and NP
- Diffuse end-plate sclerosis
- Osteophytes > 2 mm

Fig. 85.4 Disk samples from the L4-L5 and L5-S1 levels from asymptomatic individuals demonstrating several macroscopic features of disk degeneration, grouped into the Thompson classification system.[53] *Asterisk* marks a small Schmorl node. AF, annulus fibrosus; NP, nucleus pulposus.

with type III mechanoreceptors.[43,45,46] It is likely that both the disk and zygapophysial joints contribute to nonradiated pain through nerve fibers that serve both nociception and proprioception.[44]

Whether the disk is intrinsically painful during a normally subthreshold stimulus for the generation of pain (*diskogenic pain*) or whether disk degeneration results in altered mechanical properties and overload of the zygapophysial joints may be ultimately irrelevant for the surgeon, as the initial degenerative locus is normally the disk. Kirkaldy-Willis et al[47] proposed the so-called three-joint complex in the 1970s to explain how disk degeneration would lead to facet hypertrophy and central or lateral recess stenosis. Since then, several imaging studies have demonstrated that in the overwhelming majority of cases, disk degeneration precedes facet degeneration.[48,49] Attempts to distinguish between diskogenic and "facetogenic" pain utilizing anesthetic blocks or diskography are fraught with problems.[44] Anesthetic blocks cannot be expected to act only upon the nerve fibers of the facet and synovial capsule.[50] A positive response on diskography is sometimes even cited as a diagnostic criterion for diskogenic pain. Although first performed by Luschka in 1929, there is still a lack of consensus on how to utilize this provocative maneuver.[51] It is generally agreed that patients fulfilling all of the International Association for the Study of Pain criteria for diskography have diskogenic pain (injection up to 50 psi provoking concordant pain, two negative control injections at adjacent levels, and compatible computed tomography findings including AF rupture), but these criteria are applicable only to a small minority of patients with localized LBP.[52] Therefore, identification of an effective diagnostic tool remains elusive, and the clinical definition persists as outlined by Fardon and Milette,[11] when consistent with imaging findings.

Conclusion

Despite the elevated prevalence of LBP and over 150 years of research focused on intervertebral disk biology, a complete understanding of the pathophysiology of degenerative disk disease is still lacking. We have been able, however, to understand several steps of the degenerative process and recognize today that morphological alterations are present in virtually every adult. Modern treatment of DDD still does not reflect all the advances that were made in the biology of the IVD. Although surgical innovations have made arthrodesis safer, easier to perform, and more available to sicker patients, it is essentially the same procedure performed 50 years ago for DDD and merely precipitates the "intended" end-result of degeneration. Arthroplasty as performed today is available for only a small subset of patients, and its efficacy in the lumbar spine remains debatable. Future advances in the treatment of DDD should lead to modulation therapies of the degenerative process in its mild and moderate stages through interactions with the mediating enzymes and cytokines. Given recent success with biological therapy for several diseases such as rheumatoid arthritis, there is reason to believe similar therapies may emerge for disk degeneration.

References

1. Luschka H. Die Halbgelenke des Menschlichen Körpers, 2nd ed. Berlin: Reimer; 1858
2. Poirier P, Charpy A, Cunéo B. Abrégé D'Anatomie, 1st ed. Paris: Masson; 1908
3. Testut L. Traité D'Anatomie Humaine, 1st ed. Paris: Octave Doin; 1905
4. Schmorl G. Über die an den Wirbelbandscheiben vorkommenden Ausdehnungs- und Zerreissungsvorgänge und die dadurch an ihnen und der Wirbelspongiosa hervorgerufenen Veränderungen. Verh Dtsch Ges Pathol 1927;22:250–262
5. Coventry MB, Ghormley RK, Kernohan JW. The intervertebral disc: its microscopic anatomy and pathology. Part I: Anatomy, development and pathology. J Bone Jt Surg Am. 1945;27:105–112
6. Coventry MB, Ghormley RK, Kernohan JW. The intervertebral disc: its microscopic anatomy and pathology. Part II: Changes in the intervertebral disc concomitant with age. J Bone Jt Surg Am. 1945;27:233–247
7. Coventry MB, Ghormley RK, Kernohan JW. The intervertebral disc: its microscopic anatomy and pathology. Part III: Pathological changes in the intervertebral. J Bone Jt Surg Am 1945;27:460–474
8. Walker BF. The prevalence of low back pain: a systematic review of the literature from 1966 to 1998. J Spinal Disord 2000;13:205–217
9. Cassidy JD, Côté P, Carroll LJ, Kristman V. Incidence and course of low back pain episodes in the general population. Spine 2005;30:2817–2823
10. Rubin DI. Epidemiology and risk factors for spine pain. Neurol Clin 2007; 25:353–371
11. Fardon DF, Milette PC; Combined Task Forces of the North American Spine Society, American Society of Spine Radiology, and American Society of Neuroradiology. Nomenclature and classification of lumbar disc pathology. Recommendations of the Combined task Forces of the North American Spine Society, American Society of Spine Radiology, and American Society of Neuroradiology. Spine 2001;26:E93–E113
12. Weinstein JN, Tosteson TD, Lurie JD, et al. Surgical vs nonoperative treatment for lumbar disk herniation: the Spine Patient Outcomes Research Trial (SPORT): a randomized trial. JAMA 2006;296:2441–2450
13. Chiarugi G. Istituzioni di Anatomia Dell'Uomo, 2nd ed. Milano: Società Editrice Libraria; 1926
14. Grignon B, Roland J. Can the human intervertebral disc be compared to a diarthrodial joint? Surg Radiol Anat 2000;22:101–105
15. Virchow R. Untersuchungen über die Entwicklung des Schädelgrundes im Gesunden un Krankhaften Zustanden und über den Einfluss derselben auf Schädelform, Gesichtsbildung und Gehirnbau. Berlin: G Reimer; 1857
16. Dursy E. Zur Entwicklungsgeschichte des Kopfes des Menschen und der Höheren Wirbeltiere. Tübingen: H Laupp; 1869
17. Kölliker A. Ueber die Beziehungen der Chorda Dorsalis zur Bildung der Wirbel der Selachier und Einiger Andern Fische. Verhandlungen Phys. Med Ges Wurzburg 1860;10:193–242
18. Keyes DC, Compere EL. The normal and pathological physiology of the nucleus pulposus of the intervertebral disc: an anatomical, clinical and experimental study. J Bone Jt Surg Am 1932;14:897–938
19. Remak R. Untersuchungen über die Entwickelung der Wirbelthiere. Berlin: G. Reimer; 1855
20. Christ B, Wilting J. From somites to vertebral column. Ann Anat 1992; 174:23–32
21. Bagnall KM, Higgins SJ, Sanders EJ. The contribution made by cells from a single somite to tissues within a body segment and assessment of their integration with similar cells from adjacent segments. Development 1989;107:931–943
22. Übermuth H. Altersveränderungen der menäschlichen Bandscheiben in der Wirbelsäule. Arch Klin Chir 1930;156:567–577
23. Singh K, Masuda K, Thonar EJ, An HS, Cs-Szabo G. Age-related changes in the extracellular matrix of nucleus pulposus and anulus fibrosus of human intervertebral disc. Spine 2009;34:10–16
24. Lyons H, Jones E, Quinn FE, Sprunt DH. Protein-polysaccharide complexes of normal and herniated human intervertebral discs. Proc Soc Exp Biol Med 1964;115:610–614
25. Taylor JR, Scott JE, Cribb AM, Bosworth TR. Human intervertebral disc acid glycosaminoglycans. J Anat 1992;180(Pt 1):137–141
26. Scott JE, Bosworth TR, Cribb AM, Gressner AM. The chemical morphology of extracellular matrix in experimental rat liver fibrosis resembles that of normal developing connective tissue. Virchows Arch 1994;424:89–98
27. Sivan SS, Hayes AJ, Wachtel E, et al. Biochemical composition and turnover of the extracellular matrix of the normal and degenerate intervertebral disc. Eur Spine J 2014;23(Suppl 3):S344–S353
28. Bachmeier BE, Nerlich AG, Weiler C, Paesold G, Jochum M, Boos N. Analysis of tissue distribution of TNF-alpha, TNF-alpha-receptors, and the activating TNF-alpha-converting enzyme suggests activation of the TNF-alpha system in the aging intervertebral disc. Ann N Y Acad Sci 2007; 1096:44–54
29. Bachmeier BE, Nerlich A, Mittermaier N, et al. Matrix metalloproteinase expression levels suggest distinct enzyme roles during lumbar disc herniation and degeneration. Eur Spine J 2009;18:1573–1586
30. Weiler C, Schietzsch M, Kirchner T, Nerlich AG, Boos N, Wuertz K. Age-related changes in human cervical, thoracal and lumbar intervertebral disc exhibit a strong intra-individual correlation. Eur Spine J 2012;21 (Suppl 6):S810–S818
31. Burke JG, Watson RWG, McCormack D, Dowling FE, Walsh MG, Fitzpatrick JM. Intervertebral discs which cause low back pain secrete high levels of proinflammatory mediators. J Bone Joint Surg Br 2002;84:196–201
32. Specchia N, Pagnotta A, Toesca A, Greco F. Cytokines and growth factors in the protruded intervertebral disc of the lumbar spine. Eur Spine J 2002;11:145–151
33. Nerlich AG, Bachmeier BE, Boos N. Expression of fibronectin and TGF-beta1 mRNA and protein suggest altered regulation of extracellular matrix in degenerated disc tissue. Eur Spine J 2005;14:17–26
34. Harris RI, Macnab I. Structural changes in the lumbar intervertebral discs; their relationship to low back pain and sciatica. J Bone Joint Surg Br 1954;36-B:304–322
35. Jensen MC, Brant-Zawadzki MN, Obuchowski N, Modic MT, Malkasian D, Ross JS. Magnetic resonance imaging of the lumbar spine in people without back pain. N Engl J Med 1994;331:69–73
36. Boden SD, McCowin PR, Davis DO, Dina TS, Mark AS, Wiesel S. Abnormal magnetic-resonance scans of the cervical spine in asymptomatic subjects. A prospective investigation. J Bone Joint Surg Am 1990;72:1178–1184
37. Modic MT, Ross JS. Lumbar degenerative disk disease. Radiology 2007; 245:43–61
38. Steffens D, Hancock MJ, Maher CG, Williams C, Jensen TS, Latimer J. Does magnetic resonance imaging predict future low back pain? A systematic review. Eur J Pain 2014;18:755–765
39. Takatalo J, Karppinen J, Niinimäki J, et al. Association of Modic changes, Schmorl's nodes, spondylolytic defects, high-intensity zone lesions, disc herniations, and radial tears with low back symptom severity among young Finnish adults. Spine 2012;37:1231–1239

40. Albert HB, Sorensen JS, Christensen BS, Manniche C. Antibiotic treatment in patients with chronic low back pain and vertebral bone edema (Modic type 1 changes): a double-blind randomized clinical controlled trial of efficacy. Eur Spine J 2013;22:697–707
41. Ahmad I, Tejada JG. Spinal gout: a great mimicker. A case report and literature review. Neuroradiol J 2012;25:621–625
42. Bogduk N, Tynan W, Wilson AS. The nerve supply to the human lumbar intervertebral discs. J Anat 1981;132(Pt 1):39–56
43. Edgar MA. The nerve supply of the lumbar intervertebral disc. J Bone Joint Surg Br 2007;89:1135–1139
44. Schwarzer AC, Aprill CN, Derby R, Fortin J, Kine G, Bogduk N. The relative contributions of the disc and zygapophyseal joint in chronic low back pain. Spine 1994;19:801–806
45. Freemont AJ, Peacock TE, Goupille P, Hoyland JA, O'Brien J, Jayson MI. Nerve ingrowth into diseased intervertebral disc in chronic back pain. Lancet 1997;350:178–181
46. Purmessur D, Freemont AJ, Hoyland JA. Expression and regulation of neurotrophins in the nondegenerate and degenerate human intervertebral disc. Arthritis Res Ther 2008;10:R99
47. Kirkaldy-Willis WH, Wedge JH, Yong-Hing K, Reilly J. Pathology and pathogenesis of lumbar spondylosis and stenosis. Spine 1978;3:319–328
48. Butler D, Trafimow JH, Andersson GB, McNeill TW, Huckman MS. Discs degenerate before facets. Spine 1990;15:111–113
49. Fujiwara A, Tamai K, Yamato M, et al. The relationship between facet joint osteoarthritis and disc degeneration of the lumbar spine: an MRI study. Eur Spine J 1999;8:396–401
50. Manchikanti L, Dunbar EE, Wargo BW, Shah RV, Derby R, Cohen SP. Systematic review of cervical discography as a diagnostic test for chronic spinal pain. Pain Physician 2009;12:305–321
51. Lindblom K. Diagnostic puncture of intervertebral disks in sciatica. Acta Orthop Scand 1948;17:231–239
52. Manchikanti L, Glaser SE, Wolfer L, Derby R, Cohen SP. Systematic review of lumbar discography as a diagnostic test for chronic low back pain. Pain Physician 2009;12:541–559
53. Thompson JP, Pearce RH, Schechter MT, Adams ME, Tsang IK, Bishop PB. Preliminary evaluation of a scheme for grading the gross morphology of the human intervertebral disc. Spine 1990;15:411–415

86 Tumors of the Lumbosacral Spine

Mohamad Bydon, Rafael De la Garza-Ramos, Jean-Paul Wolinsky, Ziya L. Gokaslan

Spinal vertebral tumors are rare lesions that can be broadly divided into metastatic tumors (90%) and primary tumors (10%).[1] Although vertebral tumors may occur throughout the spine, certain tumors have a predilection for the lumbosacral region, such as osteoid osteomas, chordomas, and Ewing's sarcoma.[2]

Primary benign and malignant vertebral tumors represent a heterogeneous group of lesions, and treatment often involves multidisciplinary approaches. Spine surgeons play a key role in evaluating, diagnosing, and managing patients with these lesions.

This chapter discusses the most common primary benign and malignant lumbosacral tumors, with special emphasis on the diagnosis and treatment of these lesions.

Evaluation and Initial Management

Although the most common presenting symptom of a vertebral tumor is pain, this finding is nonspecific, and a high index of suspicion is necessary to make an adequate diagnosis. Common red flags that prompt a more extensive evaluation include thoracic back pain, weight loss, point-tenderness over the posterior elements, and neurologic deficit (**Box 86.1**).

Plain radiographs are useful in the initial evaluation and may reveal a probable lesion. However, computed tomography (CT) and magnetic resonance imaging (MRI) are required for differential diagnosis and surgical planning.

> **Box 86.1 Patient Factors that Warrant More Extensive Evaluation in the Patient with Back Pain**
>
> Thoracic pain
> Pain duration > 5 weeks
> History of major trauma
> Unintentional weight loss
> History of malignancy
> History of immunosuppression
> History of intravenous drug abuse
> Intractable pain
> Fever and chills
> Spinous process tenderness
> Focal neurologic deficits
> Acute urinary, bowel, or sexual dysfunction

Primary Benign Tumors

Aneurysmal Bone Cyst

Aneurysmal bone cysts (ABCs) have an estimated incidence of 0.14 per 100,000 persons,[3] accounting for 10 to 20% of all primary spinal tumors.[4] These tumors occur most commonly in patients under the age of 30, and may arise de novo or as a secondary lesion from a primary hemangioma or osteoblastoma.[5,6] ABCs commonly arise from the posterior elements of the lumbar spine,[7] and presenting symptoms include back pain, neurologic deficits, or deformities such as scoliosis or kyphosis.[8–10]

The gross appearance of ABCs has been described as a "blood-filled sponge," which refers to blood-filled cavernous cysts separated by walls of osteoclasts and woven bone.[2]

The ABCs classically appear on CT imaging as "soap bubbles" that are "blown-out."[11] The large cystic lesions may compromise spinal stability, and ABCs may present with vertebral compression fractures.[12] MRI enhances the relationship of the lesion to neural tissues, and delineates fluid levels with a higher resolution than on a CT scan (**Fig. 86.1**). The cystic components show various degrees of intensity on MRI, and 96% of lesions show gadolinium enhancement.[13]

Although ABCs do not demonstrate histological features of malignancy, recurrence is very common irrespective of treatment.[8] If a lesion is suspected to be an ABC, the first recommended step in management is obtaining a biopsy, as sarcomas may be within the lesion.[14] The first recommended definitive treatment is arterial embolization, followed by complete curettage or en-bloc resection.[8] If the diagnosis is uncertain, an open biopsy is preferred, followed by curettage if the tissue sample is diagnostic. Spinal reconstructions via anterior or posterior approaches are recommended when bone removal is extensive (**Fig. 86.2**). Nevertheless, arterial embolization may be the definitive treatment in select cases.[15]

Radiation therapy may also play a role in the treatment of ABCs. Feigenberg et al[16] reported the use of radiotherapy (26 to 30 Gy) to treat nine patients with ABCs, three of whom had the tumor in the lumbosacral spine. The authors reported no secondary malignancies and no recurrences; all patients with significant preoperative pain had improvement.

Chondroma and Enchondroma

Chondromas are benign tumors that arise from cartilaginous tissue, and are called *enchondromas* when they arise in the medullary cavity.[2] They are most common in the second and third decades of life,[2] and account for less than 5% of all spinal bony tumors.[17]

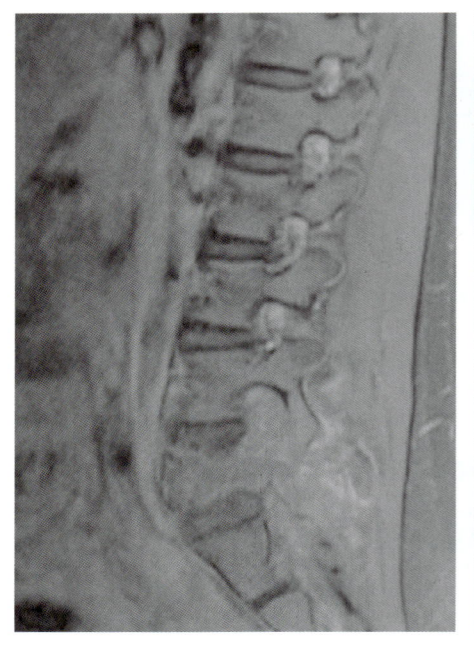

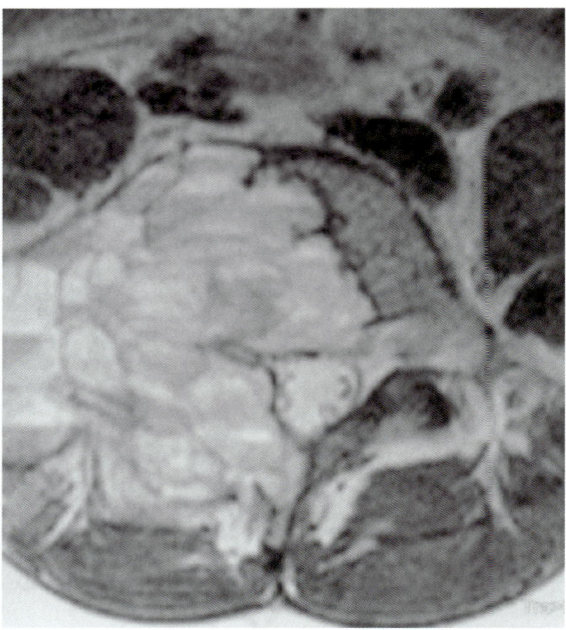

Fig. 86.1 A 12-year old girl presented with chronic low back pain and new-onset radiculopathy. **(a)** Sagittal T2-weighted magnetic resonance imaging (MRI) shows a large lesion in the L5 vertebrae, consistent with an aneurysmal bone cyst. **(b)** Axial T2-weighted MRI shows a large lesion infiltrating the right neural foramina.

Multiple enchondromas (i.e., "enchondromatosis") occur in Ollier syndrome or Maffucci syndrome (if hemangiomas are present). They typically appear as calcified lesions on CT scan and have intermediate to low signal intensity of T1-weighted and high intensity on T2-weighted MRI.[2]

However, definitive distinction between benign and malignant variant requires biopsy. The definitive treatment for these lesions is gross total resection, with the ultimate goal of maintaining spinal stability[17] and decreasing the risk of sarcomatous degeneration.[18]

Eosinophilic Granuloma

Eosinophilic granulomas are uncommon bone lesions that most commonly affect children under 15 years of age.[19] They are part of Langerhans cell histiocytosis, a proliferative disorder of dendritic antigen-presenting cells found in the skin. Eosinophilic granulomas are rare in the vertebral bodies, but may present as pathological fractures (vertebra plana) with back pain.[20]

Histologically, these lesions are characterized by Birbeck granules ("tennis racquet" shaped) in the cytoplasm.[2] On CT scan,

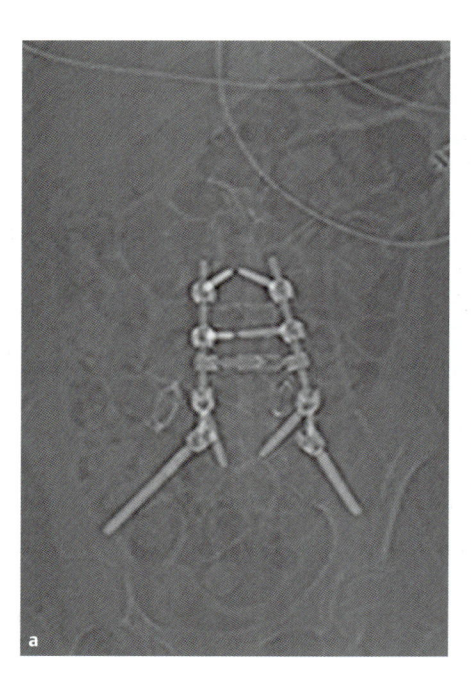

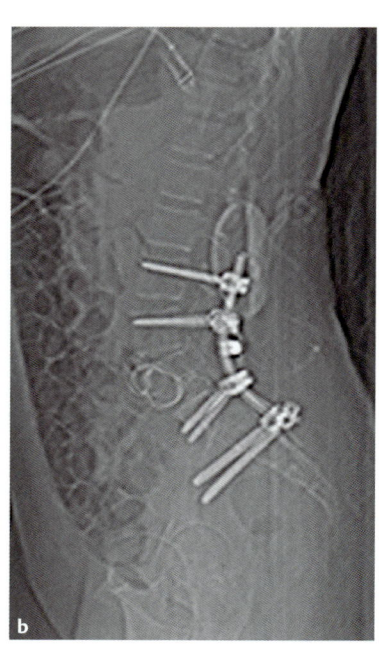

Fig. 86.2 The same patient as in **Fig. 86.1** underwent selective arterial embolization and extensive lumbopelvic reconstruction. **(a)** Anteroposterior and **(b)** lateral radiograph showing lumbopelvic instrumentation.

vertebral body collapse is often found with epidural or soft tissue extension.[21] On MRI, eosinophilic granulomas appear isointense on T1-weighted images and hyperintense on T2-weighted images.

Due to the extensive differential diagnosis of vertebra plana in children (including osteosarcoma, Ewing's sarcoma, and lymphoma), open or image-guided biopsy is recommended.[20] Patients without neurologic deficits may be treated conservatively with bed rest, bracing, and anti-inflammatory medications. Surgical treatment is usually reserved for patients with neurologic deficits or spinal instability,[22] and overall prognosis is excellent.[23]

Hemangiomas

Spinal hemangiomas are relatively common benign lesions, with 10% prevalence in autopsy studies.[24] The most common location is the vertebral body, but extension into the pedicles and spinous processes may occur. Most hemangiomas are asymptomatic, incidental findings on MRI. Nonetheless, these tumors may cause bone expansion, leading to back pain, or myeloradiculopathy.[25,26]

Microscopically, hemangiomas appear as multiple small vessels interspersed among bone trabeculae, which exhibit sclerotic changes due to the abnormal vessels.[2] They are subclassified as capillary or cavernous, depending on the associated vessels. Additionally, adipose tissue may be a component of hemangiomas, adding to the expansile nature of these lesions.

Radiographically, hemangiomas appear mottled on X-ray and CT scan, and may demonstrate a polka-dot pattern.[2] On MRI, hemangiomas appear as high signal intensity lesions on both T1- and T2-weighted imaging (**Fig. 86.3**).

Asymptomatic hemangiomas may be observed. Although uncommon, symptomatic hemangiomas may be treated with surgical decompression, resection and stabilization, vertebroplasty, radiation therapy, or transarterial embolization (**Fig. 86.4**).[25,27–29] Painful lesions without neurologic compression may be treated with embolization alone.[30]

Fibrous Dysplasia

Fibrous dysplasia refers to bony lesions composed of "curvilinear trabecular woven bone in a background of broken or retracted fibroblasts."[31] They are most common in children and adolescents, and may manifest as *monostotic* fibrous dysplasia or *polyostotic* fibrous dysplasia, depending on the number of bones affected. McCune-Albright syndrome is a form of polyostotic fibrous dysplasia with lesions throughout the skeleton accompanied by endocrine dysfunction and café-au-lait spots.

On CT imaging, fibrous dysplasia appears as an "expansile lesion with a blown-out cortical shell or a lytic lesion with a sclerotic rim."[31] MRI shows these lesions with varying degrees of intensity, with no specific features.

Patients with fibrous dysplasia require an endocrinologic workup to evaluate and treat vitamin D deficiencies, hyperparathyroidism, and phosphate wasting.[32] Patients with severe pain may be treated with oral bisphosphonates, and surgery is reserved for cases in which a diagnosis has not been established or for cases in which spinal stability is compromised. As with other spinal tumors, the ultimate goal of surgery is complete resection.[33]

Osteoid Osteoma and Osteoblastoma

Osteoid osteomas and osteoblastomas are both lesions that produce osteoid and woven bone. The former are smaller and self-limited; the latter are larger and may undergo malignant transformation.[2] Most osteoid osteomas occur in children and adolescents. These tumors are found in the spine in 10 to 20% of cases, most commonly in the posterior elements of the lumbar spine.[34,35]

The most common presentation is localized back pain of chronic duration, with nocturnal exacerbation and response to nonsteroidal anti-inflammatory medications.[2,36]

Histologically, these tumors appear as a "reddish nidus of osteoid and woven bone with interconnected trabeculae."[2] The

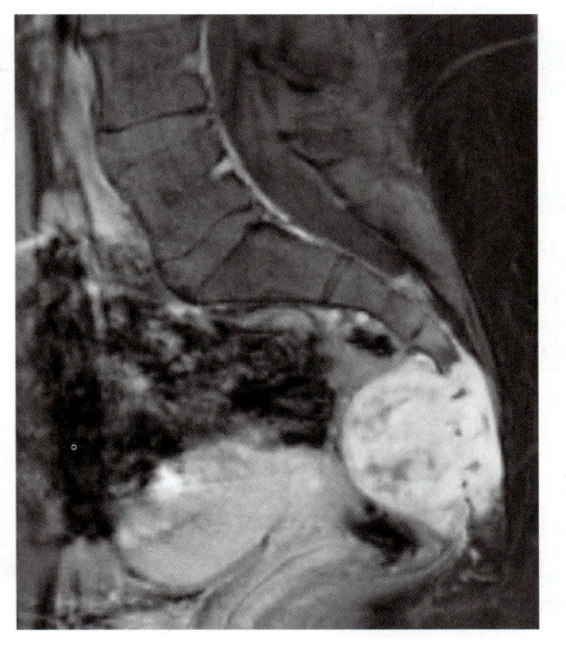

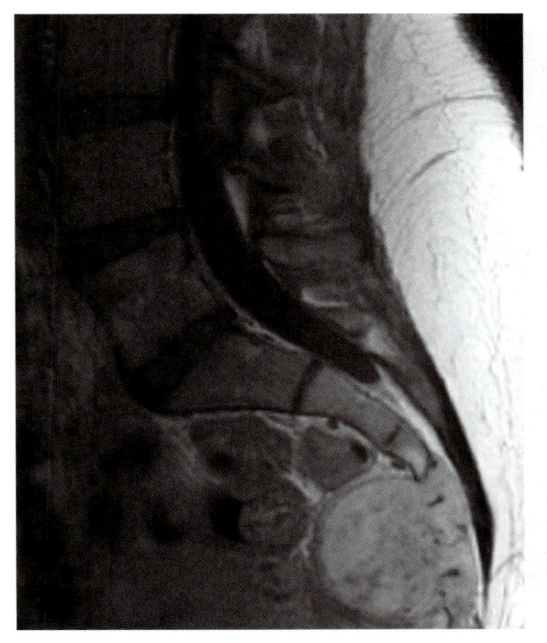

Fig. 86.3 A 24-year-old woman presented with a 7-week history of severe lower back pain. **(a)** Sagittal T1-weighted MRI shows a high signal intensity lesion on the presacral region (originating from S3–S5). **(b)** Postcontrast MRI shows a brightly enhancing lesion. Biopsy confirmed the diagnosis of hemangioma.

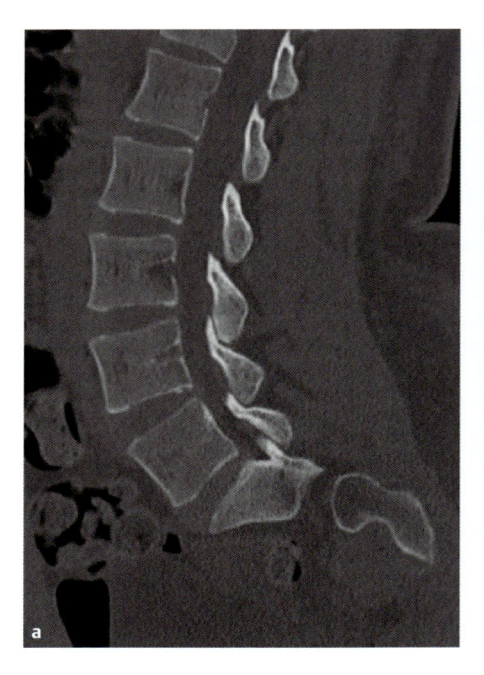

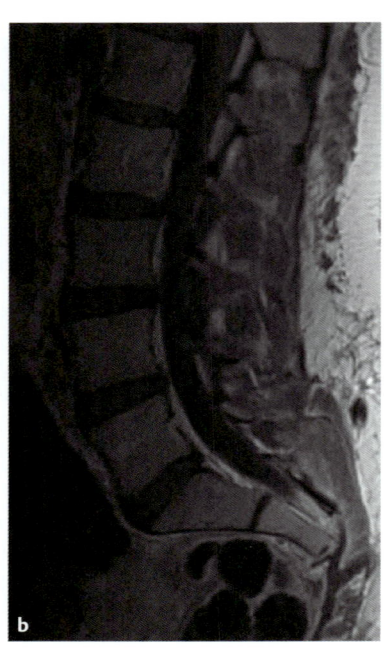

Fig. 86.4 The patient in **Fig. 86.3** underwent a midlevel sacral amputation with en-bloc resection of the hemangioma. **(a)** Postoperative sagittal computed tomography (CT) showing midsacral amputation. **(b)** Postoperative sagittal MRI.

lesions are well contained and may be surrounded by reactive bone; this has been referred to as "cloudlike appearance."[37]

On CT imaging, osteoid osteoma can be detected as an area of low attenuation accompanied by various degrees of peripheral sclerosis.[38] On MRI, the nidus appears hypointense on T2-weighted images, surrounded by marrow edema. On T1-weighted sequences, the nidus has an intermediate signal with areas of signal void due to calcifications.[39] The most sensitive diagnostic modality, however, is the technetium bone scan, which shows marked uptake of radionuclide activity within the nidus.[2] Osteoblastomas have a similar appearance on CT, but they are usually larger (> 1.5 cm)[40] and with less reactive sclerosis.[2] Additionally, osteoblastomas have been reported to undergo malignant transformation.[41]

Mild pain usually responds to medical treatment, but intractable pain or neural compression warrants complete surgical resection with instrumented stabilization.[36,42]

Primary Malignant Tumors
Chordoma

Chordomas are the most common primary malignant tumor of the mobile spine and sacrum. The estimated incidence is 0.08 cases per 100,000 persons per year.[43] These lesions arise from notochordal remnants and occur along the vertebral column; they account for 40% of all primary sacral tumors. In the mobile spine, the most common location is the cervical region.[44]

Although chordomas are considered slow-growing, they are locally aggressive and can metastasize in 5 to 40% of patients. Overall 5-year survival rates can reach 87%, and 10-year survival rates reach 64%.[43,45–47] Factors associated with more aggressive disease are Ki67-positive staining and tumoral necrosis.[46,48]

Histologically, chordomas consist of tumoral cells in a lobular arrangement with intervening fibrovascular septa.[31] These lesions have been described as "physaliphorous," owing to a large, round, and vacuolated cytoplasm.[46] Radiographically, chordomas appear as expansive, midline lytic lesions with irregular borders on CT scans.[49] Bone sclerosis and calcification is also common.

On MRI, chordomas exhibit hypointensity on T1-weighted images and hyperintensity of T2-weighted images. After gadolinium administration, enhancing patterns are variable, ranging from homogeneous enhancement to peripheral septal enhancement (**Fig. 86.5**).[50]

En-bloc surgical resection carries the best long-term prognosis,[51] but complex regional anatomy and widespread disease carries significant risks. A series of 36 patients with sacral tumors (30 chordomas) treated with en-bloc resection reported a 33% complication rate, with the most common being surgical wound infection.[52] The use of stereotactic radiosurgery is currently being explored for the treatment of sacral chordomas.[53]

Proton beam therapy is a type of particle therapy that relies on the use of high-energy protons to irradiate diseased tissue. Some of the advantages of proton beam therapy are in "dose deposition, including a sharp beam penumbra and the ability to define a stopping point for the radiation, beyond which normal tissues are completely spared from exit dose as would be seen with x-ray modalities."[54] Park et al[55] utilized high-dose proton beam therapy (mean dose of 71 Gy) to treat 21 sacral chordomas (14 primary and seven recurrent). Of these patients, 15 received proton therapy as adjuvant therapy and six as first-line treatment; overall survival at 10 years was 62.5%.

Giant Cell Tumor

Most spinal giant cell tumors (GCTs) involve the sacrum.[31] After chordomas, they are the most common primary bone tumor, occurring typically in patients 20 to 40 years of age.[56] These tumors are locally aggressive, with reports of malignant transformation and metastatic spread.[57]

Histologically, GCTs show multinucleated giant cells in a spindle-cell stroma. These giant cells have an osteoclastic nature and may contain over 100 nuclei.[31] On CT imaging, these lesions appear as expansive osteolytic lesions that destroy the adjacent bone cortex and may spread into surrounding structures.[51] On MRI, they appear to have low to intermediate signal intensity on both T1- and T2-weighted images and heterogeneously enhance with contrast. Occasionally, areas of hemorrhage appear hyperintense on T1 and T2.

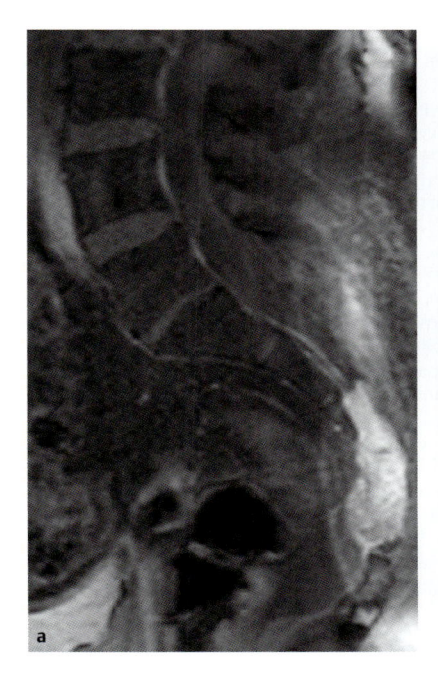

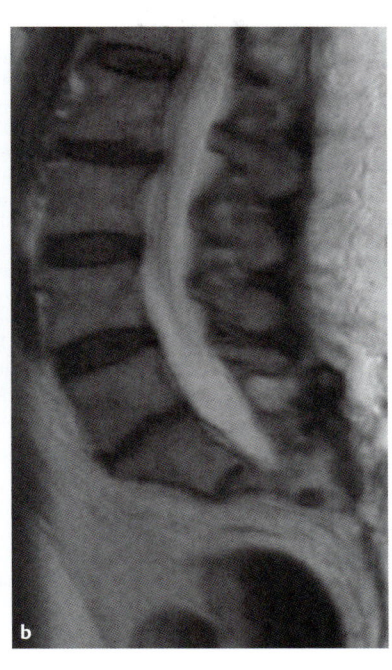

Fig. 86.5 A 67-year-old woman presented with a history of chronic intractable sacral pain. (a) Postcontrast sagittal T1-weighted MRI shows an enhancing lesion involving S2-S3. A CT-guided biopsy proved the diagnosis of chordoma. (b) The patient underwent en-bloc resection of the tumor, with a midsacral amputation and preservation of the S1 to S3 nerve roots bilaterally.

Intralesional excision with preoperative embolization is an alternative treatment method for these lesions, but with higher rates of recurrence.[58] A study by Li et al[59] reported outcomes of 32 patients with a sacral GCT who underwent wide resection (n = 2), marginal resection (n = 11), marginal resection plus curettage (n = 12), or curettage alone (n = 7). After a median follow-up of 42 months, 12 patients (37.5%) experienced local recurrence, including five of the seven patients who underwent curettage only. The authors reported an overall survival of 93.6%, and concluded that "curettage alone should not be used to treat GCT."

Another treatment modality for GCTs is intensity-modulated radiotherapy (IMRT). Roeder et al[60] reported five cases of GCTs (four sacral) treated with a median total dose of 64 Gy in conventional fractionation. After a median follow-up of 46 months, the authors reported local tumor control in four cases (80%) with significant improvement in symptoms. Nevertheless, there is also concern of malignant transformation of GCTs to sarcomas, which may occur in 5 to 15% of cases following radiation treatment.[4]

Denosumab, a monoclonal antibody that inhibits the receptor activator of nuclear factor kappa-B (RANK) ligand has proved useful in the treatment of a case of GCT of the cervical spine. Mattei et al[61] reported the use of this antibody as monotherapy, with the patient demonstrating complete remission and disappearance of the osteolytic process at 16 months of follow-up.

Ewing's Sarcoma

Ewing's sarcoma most often affects children and young adults in the second decade of life.[62] Although it most commonly occurs in the long bones and pelvis, up to 50% of cases may involve the sacrum.[63] Presentation often involves lower back pain and neurologic deficits.[64,65]

On histological examination, Ewing's sarcoma is composed of small, round cell with homogeneous-appearing nuclei[31]; the CD99 marker is sensitive but not specific.[66] Atypical histological features and necrosis are considered bad prognostic factors.[67]

Ewing's sarcoma appears as an osteolytic mass on CT scan, often involving the posterior elements.[63] On T1-weighted MRI, the tumor appears isointense, and on T2-weighted sequences it appears iso- to hyperintense. Contrast enhancement can also be seen, and intense tracer uptake is a characteristic of technetium bone scans.[31]

Treatment of these lesions relies primarily on chemotherapy, with the regimen developed by the Intergroup Ewing's Sarcoma Study consisting of cyclophosphamide, vincristine, dactinomycin, and doxorubicin.[40] Gross total or en-bloc resection may be considered in cases of severe epidural compression, nonresponsiveness to treatment, or spinal instability, but it is challenging to perform due to the complex anatomy involved in the lumbosacral region.[68] A study by Bacci et al[69] reviewed 43 patients with Ewing's sarcoma of the spine and sacrum treated with a combination of surgery, neoadjuvant chemotherapy (combination of vincristine, cyclophosphamide, Adriamycin, dactinomycin C, ifosfamide, and etoposide) and local radiotherapy (doses ranging from 44 to 60 Gy). The overall 5-year survival was 42% and the 10-year survival was 32%. The authors concluded that "regardless of the type of local treatment even when associated with neoadjuvant therapy, Ewing sarcoma in the spine and sacrum has a poor outcome and prognosis and is significantly worse than that of primary Ewing sarcoma in other sites."

Osteosarcoma

Osteosarcoma may occur anywhere in the spine, and it occurs frequently in the sacrum when it is associated with Paget's disease.[70] Similar to Ewing's sarcoma, the typical presentation may include pain and neurologic deficits.[71]

Histologically, osteosarcomas exhibit spindle cells with nuclear pleomorphism.[72] There are several subtypes, namely osteoblastic, cartilaginous, and fibroblastic, but most osteosarcomas have a mixture of these types.

Conventional X-rays demonstrate a dense and smooth appearance.[31] CT imaging demonstrates an osteolytic lesion with matrix mineralization.[37] MRI findings are nonspecific but typically show low signal intensity on T1-weighted images and high signal intensity on T2-weighted images.[73]

Optimal treatment for these tumors is en-bloc resection. A study by Bhatia et al[74] reported a 2-year survival of 44.1% for patients undergoing en-bloc resection, compared with 9.4% for patients only undergoing biopsy and debulking of the tumor. Chemotherapy and radiation therapy also play a role in these tumors. Typical oncological regimens include the use of caffeine-assisted intra-arterial chemotherapy with cisplatin[75]; neoadjuvant chemotherapy is usually given prior to en-bloc resection. Although osteosarcomas are generally considered radioresistant, the combination of intra-arterial chemotherapy and radiation (total fractionated dose of 41.6 Gy) has resulted in significant disease-free survival.[76] When treating osteosarcoma of the spine, radiation is usually given postoperatively; osteosarcoma in the upper or lower limbs may receive radiation preoperatively.[77]

Conclusion

Several primary benign and malignant tumors have a predilection for the lumbosacral spine. Although benign tumors have excellent prognoses, locally aggressive malignant tumors have poor prognoses and high recurrence rates. Surgical management of these lesions is a complex feat, and further research into less invasive and more effective treatment methods is necessary.

Disclosures

Ziya L. Gokaslan is the recipient of research grants from Depuy Spine, AO Spine North America, Medtronic, Neurosurgery Research and Education Foundation (NREF), Integra Life Sciences, and K2M. He receives fellowship support from AO Spine North America. He holds stock in Spinal Kinetics and US Spine.

The other authors have no conflict of interests or funding sources to declare.

\References

1. Hsu W, Kosztowski TA, Zaidi HA, Dorsi M, Gokaslan ZL, Wolinsky JP. Multidisciplinary management of primary tumors of the vertebral column. Curr Treat Options Oncol 2009;10:107–125
2. Ropper AE, Cahill KS, Hanna JW, McCarthy EF, Gokaslan ZL, Chi JH. Primary vertebral tumors: a review of epidemiologic, histological, and imaging findings, Part I: benign tumors. Neurosurgery 2011;69:1171–1180
3. Leithner A, Windhager R, Lang S, Haas OA, Kainberger F, Kotz R. Aneurysmal bone cyst. A population based epidemiologic study and literature review. Clin Orthop Relat Res 1999;363:176–179
4. Gasbarrini A, Cappuccio M, Donthineni R, Bandiera S, Boriani S. Management of benign tumors of the mobile spine. Orthop Clin North Am 2009;40:9–19, v
5. Bonakdarpour A, Levy WM, Aegerter E. Primary and secondary aneurysmal bone cyst: a radiological study of 75 cases. Radiology 1978;126:75–83
6. Martinez V, Sissons HA. Aneurysmal bone cyst. A review of 123 cases including primary lesions and those secondary to other bone pathology. Cancer 1988;61:2291–2304
7. Papagelopoulos PJ, Currier BL, Shaughnessy WJ, et al. Aneurysmal bone cyst of the spine. Management and outcome. Spine 1998;23:621–628
8. Boriani S, De Iure F, Campanacci L, et al. Aneurysmal bone cyst of the mobile spine: report on 41 cases. Spine 2001;26:27–35
9. Ozaki T, Halm H, Hillmann A, Blasius S, Winkelmann W. Aneurysmal bone cysts of the spine. Arch Orthop Trauma Surg 1999;119:159–162
10. Vergel De Dios AM, Bond JR, Shives TC, McLeod RA, Unni KK. Aneurysmal bone cyst. A clinicopathologic study of 238 cases. Cancer 1992;69:2921–2931
11. Burch S, Hu S, Berven S. Aneurysmal bone cysts of the spine. Neurosurg Clin N Am 2008;19:41–47
12. Codd PJ, Riesenburger RI, Klimo P Jr, Slotkin JR, Smith ER. Vertebra plana due to an aneurysmal bone cyst of the lumbar spine. Case report and review of the literature. J Neurosurg 2006;105(6, Suppl):490–495
13. Mahnken AH, Nolte-Ernsting CC, Wildberger JE, et al. Aneurysmal bone cyst: value of MR imaging and conventional radiography. Eur Radiol 2003;13:1118–1124
14. Bello Báez A, López Pino MA, Azorín Cuadrillero D, Sirvent Cerdá S. [Aneurysmatic bone cyst coexisting with osteosarcoma. Radiopathologic discussion]. Radiologia 2010;52:247–250
15. Amendola L, Simonetti L, Simoes CE, Bandiera S, De Iure F, Boriani S. Aneurysmal bone cyst of the mobile spine: the therapeutic role of embolization. Eur Spine J 2013;22:533–541
16. Feigenberg SJ, Marcus RB Jr, Zlotecki RA, Scarborough MT, Berrey BH, Enneking WF. Megavoltage radiotherapy for aneurysmal bone cysts. Int J Radiat Oncol Biol Phys 2001;49:1243–1247
17. Lozes G, Fawaz A, Perper H, et al. Chondroma of the cervical spine. Case report. J Neurosurg 1987;66:128–130
18. McLoughlin GS, Sciubba DM, Wolinsky JP. Chondroma/chondrosarcoma of the spine. Neurosurg Clin N Am 2008;19:57–63
19. Per H, Koç KR, Gümüş H, Canpolat M, Kumandaş S. Cervical eosinophilic granuloma and torticollis: a case report and review of the literature. J Emerg Med 2008;35:389–392
20. Garg S, Mehta S, Dormans JP. Langerhans cell histiocytosis of the spine in children. Long-term follow-up. J Bone Joint Surg Am 2004;86-A:1740–1750
21. Azouz EM, Saigal G, Rodriguez MM, Podda A. Langerhans' cell histiocytosis: pathology, imaging and treatment of skeletal involvement. Pediatr Radiol 2005;35:103–115
22. Bertram C, Madert J, Eggers C. Eosinophilic granuloma of the cervical spine. Spine 2002;27:1408–1413
23. Reddy PK, Vannemreddy PS, Nanda A. Eosinophilic granuloma of spine in adults: a case report and review of literature. Spinal Cord 2000;38:766–768
24. Barzin M, Maleki I. Incidence of vertebral hemangioma on spinal magnetic resonance imaging in Northern Iran. Pak J Biol Sci 2009;12:542–544
25. Acosta FL Jr, Sanai N, Chi JH, et al. Comprehensive management of symptomatic and aggressive vertebral hemangiomas. Neurosurg Clin N Am 2008;19:17–29
26. Templin CR, Stambough JB, Stambough JL. Acute spinal cord compression caused by vertebral hemangioma. Spine J 2004;4:595–600
27. Aich RK, Deb AR, Banerjee A, Karim R, Gupta P. Symptomatic vertebral hemangioma: treatment with radiotherapy. J Cancer Res Ther 2010;6:199–203
28. Fox MW, Onofrio BM. The natural history and management of symptomatic and asymptomatic vertebral hemangiomas. J Neurosurg 1993;78:36–45
29. Jayakumar PN, Vasudev MK, Srikanth SG. Symptomatic vertebral haemangioma: endovascular treatment of 12 patients. Spinal Cord 1997;35:624–628
30. Acosta FL Jr, Dowd CF, Chin C, Tihan T, Ames CP, Weinstein PR. Current treatment strategies and outcomes in the management of symptomatic vertebral hemangiomas. Neurosurgery 2006;58:287–295, discussion 287–295
31. Ropper AE, Cahill KS, Hanna JW, McCarthy EF, Gokaslan ZL, Chi JH. Primary vertebral tumors: a review of epidemiologic, histological and imaging findings, part II: locally aggressive and malignant tumors. Neurosurgery 2012;70:211–219, discussion 219
32. Kanter AS, Jagannathan J, Shaffrey CI, Ouellet JA, Mummaneni PV. Inflammatory and dysplastic lesions involving the spine. Neurosurg Clin N Am 2008;19:93–109
33. Medow JE, Agrawal BM, Resnick DK. Polyostotic fibrous dysplasia of the cervical spine: case report and review of the literature. Spine J 2007;7:712–715
34. Erlemann R. Imaging and differential diagnosis of primary bone tumors and tumor-like lesions of the spine. Eur J Radiol 2006;58:48–67
35. Kransdorf MJ, Stull MA, Gilkey FW, Moser RP Jr. Osteoid osteoma. Radiographics 1991;11:671–696
36. Zileli M, Cagli S, Basdemir G, Ersahin Y. Osteoid osteomas and osteoblastomas of the spine. Neurosurg Focus 2003;15:E5
37. Rodallec MH, Feydy A, Larousserie F, et al. Diagnostic imaging of solitary tumors of the spine: what to do and say. Radiographics 2008;28:1019–1041
38. Gamba JL, Martinez S, Apple J, Harrelson JM, Nunley JA. Computed tomography of axial skeletal osteoid osteomas. AJR Am J Roentgenol 1984;142:769–772

39. Harish S, Saifuddin A. Imaging features of spinal osteoid osteoma with emphasis on MRI findings. Eur Radiol 2005;15:2396–2403
40. Hitchon PW, Lindley T, Ebersold M. Primary bony spinal lesions. In: Benzel EC, ed. Spine Surgery. Philadelphia: Saunders; 2012:1023–1039
41. Woźniak AW, Nowaczyk MT, Osmola K, Golusinski W. Malignant transformation of an osteoblastoma of the mandible: case report and review of the literature. Eur Arch Otorhinolaryngol 2010;267:845–849
42. Burn SC, Ansorge O, Zeller R, Drake JM. Management of osteoblastoma and osteoid osteoma of the spine in childhood. J Neurosurg Pediatr 2009; 4:434–438
43. McMaster ML, Goldstein AM, Bromley CM, Ishibe N, Parry DM. Chordoma: incidence and survival patterns in the United States, 1973-1995. Cancer Causes Control 2001;12:1–11
44. Boriani S, Bandiera S, Biagini R, et al. Chordoma of the mobile spine: fifty years of experience. Spine 2006;31:493–503
45. Baratti D, Gronchi A, Pennacchioli E, et al. Chordoma: natural history and results in 28 patients treated at a single institution. Ann Surg Oncol 2003; 10:291–296
46. Bergh P, Kindblom LG, Gunterberg B, Remotti F, Ryd W, Meis-Kindblom JM. Prognostic factors in chordoma of the sacrum and mobile spine: a study of 39 patients. Cancer 2000;88:2122–2134
47. York JE, Kaczaraj A, Abi-Said D, et al. Sacral chordoma: 40-year experience at a major cancer center. Neurosurgery 1999;44:74–79, discussion 79–80
48. Pallini R, Maira G, Pierconti F, et al. Chordoma of the skull base: predictors of tumor recurrence. J Neurosurg 2003;98:812–822
49. Llauger J, Palmer J, Amores S, Bagué S, Camins A. Primary tumors of the sacrum: diagnostic imaging. AJR Am J Roentgenol 2000;174:417–424
50. Sung MS, Lee GK, Kang HS, et al. Sacrococcygeal chordoma: MR imaging in 30 patients. Skeletal Radiol 2005;34:87–94
51. Gerber S, Ollivier L, Leclère J, et al. Imaging of sacral tumours. Skeletal Radiol 2008;37:277–289
52. Clarke MJ, Dasenbrock H, Bydon A, et al. Posterior-only approach for en bloc sacrectomy: clinical outcomes in 36 consecutive patients. Neurosurgery 2012;71:357–364, discussion 364
53. Muacevic A, Drexler C, Kufeld M, Romanelli P, Duerr HJ, Wowra B. Fiducial-free real-time image-guided robotic radiosurgery for tumors of the sacrum/pelvis. Radiother Oncol 2009;93:37–44
54. McDonald MW, Linton OR, Shah MV. Proton therapy for reirradiation of progressive or recurrent chordoma. Int J Radiat Oncol Biol Phys 2013;87: 1107–1114
55. Park L, Delaney TF, Liebsch NJ, et al. Sacral chordomas: Impact of high-dose proton/photon-beam radiation therapy combined with or without surgery for primary versus recurrent tumor. Int J Radiat Oncol Biol Phys 2006;65:1514–1521
56. Randall RL. Giant cell tumor of the sacrum. Neurosurg Focus 2003;15:E13
57. Luther N, Bilsky MH, Härtl R. Giant cell tumor of the spine. Neurosurg Clin N Am 2008;19:49–55
58. Ming Z, Kangwu C, Huilin Y, et al. Analysis of risk factors for recurrence of giant cell tumor of the sacrum and mobile spine combined with preoperative embolization. Turk Neurosurg 2013;23:645–652
59. Li G, Fu D, Chen K, et al. Surgical strategy for the management of sacral giant cell tumors: a 32-case series. Spine J 2012;12:484–491
60. Roeder F, Timke C, Zwicker F, et al. Intensity modulated radiotherapy (IMRT) in benign giant cell tumors—a single institution case series and a short review of the literature. Radiat Oncol 2010;5:18
61. Mattei TA, Ramos E, Rehman AA, Shaw A, Patel SR, Mendel E. Sustained long-term complete regression of a giant cell tumor of the spine after treatment with denosumab. Spine J 2014;14:e15–e21
62. Sundaresan N, Rosen G, Boriani S. Primary malignant tumors of the spine. Orthop Clin North Am 2009;40:21–36, v
63. Ilaslan H, Sundaram M, Unni KK, Dekutoski MB. Primary Ewing's sarcoma of the vertebral column. Skeletal Radiol 2004;33:506–513
64. Marco RA, Gentry JB, Rhines LD, et al. Ewing's sarcoma of the mobile spine. Spine 2005;30:769–773
65. Sharafuddin MJ, Haddad FS, Hitchon PW, Haddad SF, el-Khoury GY. Treatment options in primary Ewing's sarcoma of the spine: report of seven cases and review of the literature. Neurosurgery 1992;30:610–618, discussion 618–619
66. Rocchi A, Manara MC, Sciandra M, et al. CD99 inhibits neural differentiation of human Ewing sarcoma cells and thereby contributes to oncogenesis. J Clin Invest 2010;120:668–680
67. Hartman KR, Triche TJ, Kinsella TJ, Miser JS. Prognostic value of histopathology in Ewing's sarcoma. Long-term follow-up of distal extremity primary tumors. Cancer 1991;67:163–171
68. Guo W, Tang X, Zang J, Ji T. One-stage total en bloc sacrectomy: a novel technique and report of 9 cases. Spine 2013;38:E626–E631
69. Bacci G, Boriani S, Balladelli A, et al. Treatment of nonmetastatic Ewing's sarcoma family tumors of the spine and sacrum: the experience from a single institution. Eur Spine J 2009;18:1091–1095
70. Sharma H, Mehdi SA, MacDuff E, Reece AT, Jane MJ, Reid R; Scottish Bone Tumor Registry. Paget sarcoma of the spine: Scottish Bone Tumor Registry experience. Spine 2006;31:1344–1350
71. Ilaslan H, Sundaram M, Unni KK, Shives TC. Primary vertebral osteosarcoma: imaging findings. Radiology 2004;230:697–702
72. Fletcher CDM. Diagnostic Histopathology of Tumors. New York: Churchill Livingstone; 1995
73. Greenspan A. Orthopedic Imaging: A practical Approach, 4th ed. Philadelphia: Lippincott Williams & Wilkins, 2004
74. Bhatia R, Beckles V, Fox Z, Tirabosco R, Rezajooi K, Casey AT. Osteosarcoma of the spine: dismal past, any hope for the future? Br J Neurosurg 2013
75. Tsuchiya H, Tomita K, Mori Y, Asada N, Yamamoto N. Marginal excision for osteosarcoma with caffeine assisted chemotherapy. Clin Orthop Relat Res 1999;358:27–35
76. Katagiri H, Sugiyama H, Takahashi M, et al. Osteosarcoma of the pelvis treated successfully with repetitive intra-arterial chemotherapy and radiation therapy: a report of a case with a 21-year follow-up. J Orthop Sci 2013
77. Dinçbaş FO, Koca S, Mandel NM, et al. The role of preoperative radiotherapy in nonmetastatic high-grade osteosarcoma of the extremities for limb-sparing surgery. Int J Radiat Oncol Biol Phys 2005;62:820–828

87 Trauma of the Lumbar Spine and Sacrum

Robert G. Kellogg

Lumbar trauma represents a significant portion of neurosurgical emergency consults. One estimate from a level 1 trauma center is that 6.3% of patients presenting with blunt trauma suffer thoracolumbar fractures. Thoracolumbar and lumbosacral trauma treatment requires an understanding of the anatomy, biomechanical limitations, and pathological forces affected by the injury. These traumas are challenging to treat, in part because no standard injury classification system has been established despite many attempts, beginning with Boehler in 1930. Additionally, the criteria for surgical intervention, and the subsequent timing and approaches of the surgery, continue to be debated.

Anatomy

The five lumbar vertebrae create a lordotic curve. Transitions in this curvature typically occur at L1-L2 from thoracic kyphosis to lumbar lordosis. Normal lordosis is 20 degrees at L4-L5.[1] Anatomic variations in the number of non–rib-bearing vertebrae make careful numbering important, especially in preoperative planning. A lumbarized first sacral vertebra or a sacralized fifth lumbar vertebra is a normal variant.

In the vertebral body, hard cortical bone encases the softer, trabeculated, and nutrient-rich inner cancellous bone. Cortical end-plate erosion is a degenerative condition contributing to pathological weakening of the body. Ankylosing spondylitis, diffuse idiopathic hyperostosis, and osteoporosis are other pathological states that can greatly affect the severity of a seemingly benign trauma. The posterior bony elements composed of the lamina, transverse process, and spinous process act as protection and conduit for the neural elements while providing strength and permitting motion.

The intervertebral lumbar disk is composed of an outer annulus fibrosus and an inner nucleus pulposus, with an acellular, avascular collagen and glycosaminoglycan meshwork. The disk ratio of nucleus to annulus is 2:1, which is greater than that of more cephalad disks, whose ratio is closer to 1:1. These elements distribute forces evenly over the inferior and superior vertebral body end plates. The average disk thickness is 9 mm, nearly two or three times as large as the cervical or thoracic intervertebral disks, respectively.[2]

Functionally considered as three groups, the anterior longitudinal ligament (ALL), posterior longitudinal ligament (PLL), and posterior ligamentous complex (PLC) support and regulate motion between the vertebrae. In general, ligaments resist dynamic loading forces better than do bony structures, thus necessitating significant force for a ligamentous rupture. Degenerative changes result in weakening of the PLL, predisposing the patient to intervertebral disk herniations. Similarly, ossification of the PLL can predispose the patient to trauma-induced myelopathy.[3]

The ALL and anterior annulus limit extension. In counterbalance, the PLL, posterior annulus, and ligamentum flavum limit flexion. This permits ~ 85 degrees of flexion and extension. Lateral bending averages 30 degrees. Limitation of axial rotation is divided between the intervertebral disk and facet complex (90%) and the interspinous and supraspinous ligaments (10%), allowing for ~ 10 degrees of movement.[4] Disk fiber strain has been shown to be greatest in extreme flexion and lateral rotations.[5]

The relative mobility of the lumbar spine reflects its lack of bony support. The thoracic spine is relatively rigid due to articulations with the rib cage, and the fused sacrum articulates with the pelvis. For these reasons, the thoracolumbar and lumbosacral junctions are most frequently the sites of traumatic pathology.

The clinician who is performing the trauma evaluation must appreciate the relationship of the spinal cord and cauda equina to the lumbar spine. The cord tapers to the conus between T12 and L2 before further dividing into the cauda equina. A higher injury may result in conus medullaris syndrome or paraplegia, whereas a lower lesion may cause cauda equina syndrome or even avoid neurologic injury altogether. The transverse diameter of the spinal canal increases by ~ 30% from the thoracolumbar junction to the sacrum, whereas sagittal diameter is preserved in descent.

Mechanisms

Injury occurs when external forces overwhelm the capacity of the bony, cartilaginous, or ligamentous structures. Most frequently, these forces are with axial loading or distraction forces. The AOSpine Spinal Cord Injury and Trauma Knowledge Forum proposes a three-category system with numerous subtypes to enable communication among clinicians and researchers. It has been shown to have reasonable reliability and accuracy.[6] Injuries are classified as compression, tension-band disruption, and displacement/translation.

Type A, compression, involves the anterior column and is typically due to failure under axial loading. This category may include injury to the transverse and spinous processes, but the integrity of the PLC is maintained. These injuries most commonly occur at the thoracolumbar junction secondary to the transition of curvature. They are uncommon in the lower lumbar spine. This type is further divided into five subtypes. The lowest grade of A0 designates clinically insignificant fractures isolated to the transverse or spinous process. The first significant fracture is synonymous with a "wedge" fracture—a fracture through the anterior body with preservation of the posterior vertebral height. The most severe subtype is a vertebral body burst fracture with preservation of the PLC (**Fig. 87.1**).

Type B, tension-band disruption, can occur in concert with type A fractures. These fractures are commonly associated with abdominal vascular and hollow viscus injuries. Type B has three subtypes. Type B1 is a monosegmental osseous fracture limited to a single level, extending from the posterior vertebral body

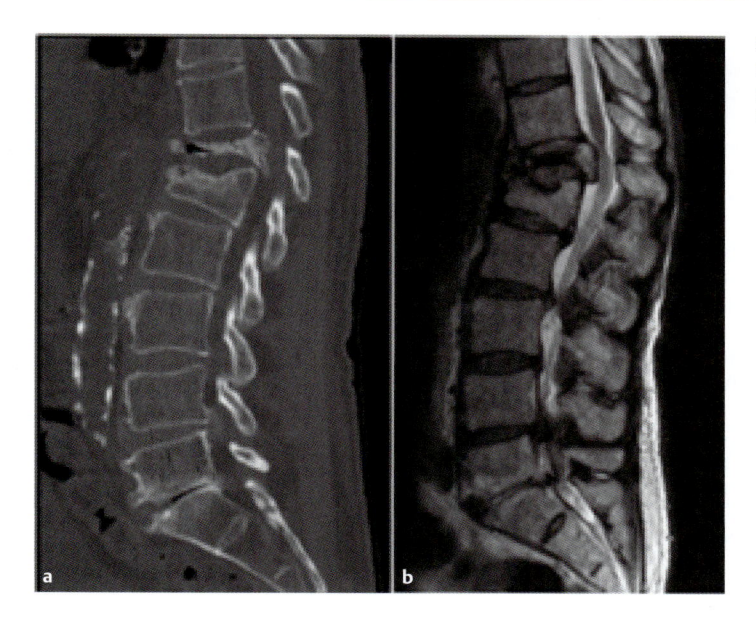

Fig. 87.1 Computed tomography (CT) scan **(a)** and T2-weighted magnetic resonance imaging (MRI) scan **(b)** of severe T12 and moderate L1 burst fractures with retropulsion of the body into the spinal canal.

through the pedicle and posterior bony structures. This is synonymous with the Chance fracture. Type B2 is another hyperflexion injury affecting an intravertebral level, and always affecting the PLC with or without bony injury. This type commonly occurs with type A burst fractures. Lateral radiographs or sagittal computed tomography (CT) images demonstrate longitudinal splaying of the spinous processes in these two subtypes. They are commonly referred to as seat-belt–type fractures, and their incidence has decreased with the addition of the shoulder strap to the lap belt in motor vehicles. Type B3 is a hyperextension/posterior-hinge injury resulting in disruption of the ALL, with or without bony injury.

Type C, displacement/translational, is the most severe type of injury. These injuries involve displacement of the cranial and caudal portions of an injured spinal column in any plane. This represents complete discontinuity of the bony and ligamentous complex. When occurring in shear forces in extension, there can be complete dissociation with the posterior elements. With rotational forces in flexion, it can be associated with multiple transverse process fractures. This type is most frequently associated with neural injury and dural tear. As with the other types, fractures pattern and ligamentous injury should be classified and noted in addition to the type C injury.

Classification

Although radiographic fracture pattern classification and inferred ligamentous assessment are paramount in guiding the clinician, they represent a portion of what decades of expert opinion has deemed necessary in classifying injuries. Several proposed models to conceptualize injury and assess stability have contributed in some way to the current understanding of lumbar trauma.

Regarded as the earliest publication on the matter, Boehler[7] described a purely anatomic classification system in 1930 in German. He identified five subtypes: compression fracture, flexion-distraction injury, extension injury, shear fracture, and rotational injury.

Holdsworth[8] in 1970 elaborated on the five fracture subtypes by describing their mechanisms in a two-column spine model. This model is predicated on an anterior load with a posterior tension band for support. The anterior column is composed of the vertebral body, intervertebral disk, ALL, and PLL. The posterior column is composed of the posterior neural elements and the PLC. Instability was inferred by disruption of both columns.

Denis[9] added a middle column to this model, which is composed of the posterior half of the vertebral body, the annulus fibrosis, and the PLL. Additionally, this model may have been the first to recognize that injuries can be considered biomechanically unstable, neurologically unstable, or neither or both. Wedge and compression fractures can be distinguished by involvement of the middle column. Denis also classified seat-belt injuries into two subtypes, distinguishing a single-level injury from one that traverses levels.[10] The Denis system perhaps has been oversimplified, as it is often reduced to a two-column failure that results in instability.

Panjabi and White[11] devised a system that includes clinical assessment in addition to the radiographic features of a fracture. The seven-item checklist assesses cauda equina damage, angulation deformity in the sagittal plane, destruction of the anterior or posterior elements, and predicted loading. A score of 5 or greater suggests instability. This system also has the benefit of being valid for nontrauma assessment, as it can evaluate stability in postoperative, neoplastic, and infectious pathological states.

Magerl et al[12] proposed an algorithm as a means of classification. Based on concepts originally applied to long bone fractures, injuries are classified into three types that are further divided into subtypes, subgroups, and subdivisions. In all, the algorithm generates 53 injury patterns, beginning with type A1 and ending with type C3. Perhaps due to its complexity, only moderate inter- and intraobserver reliability has been demonstrated in subsequent evaluation.[13]

The most recent thoracolumbar trauma classification is the Thoracolumbar Injury Classification and Severity Score (TLICS) proposed by the Spine Trauma Study Group.[14] The morphology of injury is determined by radiographic appearance, integrity of the PLC, and neurologic status of the patient. Assessment of these factors generates a score intended to guide the clinician in operative decision making. Compression injuries (type A) are assigned 1 point, tension-band disruptions (type B) are assigned 3 points, and displacement/translational injuries (type C) are assigned 4 points. A score of 3 or less warrants consideration of nonoperative treatment, whereas a score of 5 or more indicates a greater likelihood of requiring stabilization with or without decompression of neural elements. A score of 4 represents equipoise.

The integrity of the PLC can be evaluated through a variety of radiographic means. Morphological criteria as assessed with CT or plain film X-ray may be sufficient. Magnetic resonance imaging (MRI) has also been shown to be reliable in assessing PLC injury.[15] An intact PLC is assigned 0 points and a disrupted PLC is assigned 3 points. Indeterminate integrity is assigned 2 points. It bears noting that in the TLICS, as in other systems, a PLC injury alone is the criterion for surgical consideration.

The neurologic status of the patient's lower extremities places value on cases in which there is the potential to salvage function. An intact patient is assigned a score of 0. Injury isolated to a nerve root or a complete spinal cord injury is assigned 2 points, whereas an incomplete injury, conus medullaris, or cauda equina syndrome is assigned 3 points (**Table 87.1**).

Diagnosis

Forces required to generate lumbar spine pathology often are sufficient to damage other organ systems. Therefore, a classic airway, breathing, and circulation (ABC) trauma approach is paramount. One database review of trauma admissions in Canada found that 38% of traumatic spine fractures have an associated injury to an extremity, the spine, the head, the chest, or the abdomen, in descending order of frequency.[16] Securing an airway and ensuring oxygenation and hemodynamic stability must occur before attention can be diverted to a neurologic exam. Reviews have shown the co-occurrence of neurologic injury in 22% of thoracolumbar fractures.[12]

Assessment of consciousness and cranial nerve function must be done to assess the possibility of an intracranial injury. A spine-focused exam should include individual muscle group testing, sensation testing, deep-tendon reflexes, and long-tract signs. Pathological reflexes may provide important localizing information as to the level of the injury. Hoffman's sign indicates a lesion above C8, and Babinski's sign indicates an upper motor neuron injury. Testing of the sacral nerve roots provides insight into the completeness of the injury. A digital rectal exam to test the competence of the internal and external sphincters and sensation is of even greater importance in lumbar trauma. Absence of the bulbocavernous reflex in an acute spinal cord injury is indicative of spinal shock and can alter management significantly.

To amalgamate this plethora of data, Frankel et al[17] published their systematic evaluation of spinal cord injuries (**Table 87.2**). Each patient admitted to their National Spinal Injuries Centre in England received an "analysis pro forma" evaluation identifying injury causes and fracture morphologies, and an analysis of comprehensive spinal levels of motor and sensory function. This same evaluation was used to track recovery of function from admission to discharge. Five classes of neurologic status were identified, ranging from class A, complete injury, to class E, free of neurologic symptoms. This early work laid the foundation for future classifications as well as serving as a research metric by which intervention outcomes could be compared (**Table 87.3**). The current standard of neurologic status as devised by the American Spinal Injury Association (ASIA) draws heavily upon the work of Frankel and his United Kingdom colleagues.[18] The ASIA classification offers a well-defined evaluation of sensory and motor functions. Sensation is examined with light touch and pain for all 28 dermatomes bilaterally and classified as absent (0 pts), impaired (1 pt), normal (2 pts), or not testable. Motor function is tested through 10 paired myotomes on a 6-point scale: paralysis, palpable or visible contraction, active movement with gravity eliminated, full range of movement against gravity, full range of movement against gravity and moderate resistance, and normal movement. This evaluation is summarized in the five-class ASIA impairment scale as adapted from Frankel, in which class A is complete injury; classes B, C, and D are incomplete injuries; and class E is normal (**Table 87.3**).

A review of the 1-year outcomes in nearly 3,600 patients with traumatic spinal cord injury in the National Spinal Cord Injury Statistical Center Database found improvement of at least one ASIA grade in 16% of grade A patients, 60% of grade B patients, 70% of grade C patients, and 10% of grade D patients.[18] Sensory exam may be most helpful in localizing thoracic cord injury, as myotomes are not easily tested.

The array of imaging modalities available to the clinician may play a role in diagnosis and treatment.

Table 87.1 Thoracolumbar Injury Classification and Severity Score (TLICS)

Finding	Points
Injury Morphology	
Compression and burst	1
Translational/rotational	3
Distraction	4
Posterior Ligamentous Complex Integrity	
Intact	0
Suspect/indeterminate	2
Injured	3
Neurologic Status	
Intact	0
Nerve root, complete cord, complete conus medullaris injury	2
Incomplete cord, incomplete conus medullaris, incomplete cauda equina	3

Table 87.2 Frankel Injury Classification System

Grade	Motor Exam
0	Total paralysis
1	Palpable or visible contraction
2	Active movement, full range of motion with gravity eliminated
3	Active movement, full range of motion versus gravity ("antigravity")
4	Active movement, full range of motion versus moderate resistance
5	Active movement, full range of motion versus normally surmountable resistance (normal)

Table 87.3 American Spinal Injury Association (ASIA) Impairment Scale

Grade	Neurologic Progress	Expanded
A	Complete	No motor or sensory function is preserved in the sacral segments S4-S5.
B	Incomplete: sensory only	Sensory but not motor function is preserved below the neurologic level and includes the sacral segments S4-S5.
C	Incomplete: some motor	Motor function is preserved below the neurologic level, and more than half of the key muscles below the neurologic level have a muscle grade less than 3.
D	Incomplete: functional motor	Motor function is preserved below the neurologic level, and at least half of the key muscles below the neurologic level have a muscle grade of 3 or more.
E	Normal	Motor and sensory function is normal.

Computed tomography (CT) scan is ubiquitous in the trauma center. Frequently, areas of interest can be reconstructed from a CT chest/abdomen/pelvis obtained prior to consultation. CT offers the most information on bony and fracture anatomy and aids in surgical planning for hardware sizing and placement. Additionally, a CT aortogram, to ensure the health of the thoracoabdominal aorta, may be important in penetrating and high-impact injuries. CT myelogram may be useful in cases in which there is concern about posttraumatic cerebrospinal fluid (CSF) leaks. Additionally, this test may be required in evaluation of neural elements in patients with contraindications to MRI, such as those with foreign bodies (e.g., retained missiles) or medical devices (e.g., internal defibrillator).

Plain X-ray radiographs are less helpful than CT in diagnosis, but offer a relatively inexpensive option for following the patient pathology. In the acute setting, flexion-extension films can give dynamic views to establish ligamentous integrity. For certain nonoperative pathologies such as types of simple compression fractures, serial radiographs with and without bracing can be a cost-effective way to follow fracture healing or kyphotic deformity. Additionally, many clinicians choose to obtain baseline radiographs after instrumentation as a baseline for follow-up.

Magnetic resonance imaging (MRI) is the modality of choice for evaluating neural elements and ligamentous injury. T2-weighted images provide excellent imaging of the spinal cord and cauda equina, and demonstrates acute injury to these structures by traumatic pathology. T1-weighted, fat-suppressed imaging facilitates visualization of the exiting nerve roots in the neural foramen. Short tau inversion recovery (STIR) sequences are most sensitive for identifying ligamentous injury. Although MRI can reliably detect a PLC injury, there is a paucity of evidence that this information contributes to surgical decision making beyond what is determined by morphological criteria using plain radiographs and CT.[15] MR myelography is a second-line option to CT myelography for CSF leak identification in patients who are unable to undergo spinal puncture or who have certain dye allergies.

Treatment

Neurosurgical intervention begins after hemodynamic stability of the patient has been achieved. Securing an airway, oxygenating the blood, and perfusing the body are prerequisites to any neurosurgical procedure. Advance Trauma Life Support algorithms should be followed. Concomitant injuries that entail high mortality must be treated. Subsequently, the goals of the neurosurgeon are decompression of neural elements and stabilization to prevent secondary neurologic injury.

Indications for surgery include reversible neurologic deficit, gross or potential instability, and dural laceration/fistula formation. The mechanism of injury must be considered, as penetrating injuries from civilian gunshot wounds have a vastly different course than blunt trauma. In gunshot wounds, the only absolute indication for surgery is CSF fistula formation.[19] Given the focal nature of injury and the likely preservation of the ligamentous complexes with civilian ballistics, instability is unlikely to occur. Evidence of decompression of neural elements in an incomplete injury is mixed, but trends currently favor surgery in such cases.

Conservative management is generally accepted as first-line management in cases without neurologic injury or gross instability. Original research on the topic by Guttman et al[20] and Frankel et al[17] in the 1960s and 1970s demonstrated acceptable neurologic outcomes with immobilization. This entailed 6 to 12 weeks of bed rest and postural reduction; 60% of patients showed neurological improvement, but this population was at high risk for systemic complications. For this reason, modern methods focus on bracing to stabilize the affected levels and on early mobilization. Thoracolumbar spinal orthosis (TLSO), Jewett or hyperextension brace, and body casting have all been employed in this manner.[21] Given the paucity of head-to-head trials of bracing types, the decision currently relies on the clinician's access to and comfort with using these devices.

Thus, a significant proportion of injuries require surgical decompression and open stabilization. Decompression of neural elements varies based on the anatomy of the injury; retropulsion of vertebral body, neural foraminal compromise causing radiculopathy, epidural hematoma, or foreign objects can each dictate approach. Stabilization is performed to achieve immobilization to promote bony fusion. This must be coupled with restoration of sagittal balance, and minimizing the length of construct to maximize segment mobility.

Timing of surgery must be determined on a case-by-case basis. Risks of increased perioperative blood loss in hyperacute injury, intraoperative hypotension, as well as delay in treatment of concomitant injuries must be weighed against the benefits of stabilization and early mobilization after decompression and fusion. There is some evidence of decreased morbidity with interventions performed within 72 hours of injury.[22]

The surgical approach depends on the pathology type and ultimately surgeon comfort. As suggested by the TLICS guidelines, the two most important considerations for the surgical approach are neurologic status and integrity of the PLC. An incomplete neurologic injury generally requires an anterior decompression if anterior elements cause neural compression after postural or open reduction. Disruption of the PLC generally requires a posterior procedure. Therefore, a combined approach is necessary if an incomplete cord injury is coupled with anterior neural compression.

The anterior approach should utilize retroperitoneal access to the vertebral body to enable vertebrectomy and placement of a cage or strut graft. This approach is limited to the lower lumbar levels because of the intimate relationship of the abdominal aorta with the vertebral body prior to the bifurcation into the iliac arteries. In many centers this may require the assistance of an access surgeon.

The posterior approach enables lamina decompression along with pedicle screw fixation. Laminectomy is appropriate in cases of posterior compression, dural laceration, epidural hematoma, and radicular compression. This benefit must be considered along with the risk of disruption of the PLC, leading to further destabilization or long-term kyphosis. A measure of anterior decompression may be achieved through either retraction of the thecal sac and tamping of the vertebral body or ligamentotaxis. Pedicle screw fixation has largely replaced older fixation techniques, including rod or hook techniques. Biomechanical and clinical outcomes studies have shown that pedicle screw fixation enables high fusion rates with preservation of height and lordosis and lower rates of instrumentation failure and pseudarthrosis.[23,24]

Lateral extracavitary techniques were initially proposed by Capener in the 1950s and refined and applied to traumatic pathologies by Larson in the 1970s.[25] This approach offers simultaneous access to the ventrolateral and dorsal aspects of the spine. However, these open techniques frequently require the assistance of an access surgeon because of the neurosurgeon's unfamiliarity with costotransversectomy and retroperitoneal dissection at the thoracolumbar junction. Additionally, these procedures typically entail increased operative blood loss and increased incidence of gastrointestinal and pulmonary complications. These techniques lay the foundation for the minimally invasive lateral approaches that utilize muscle splitting instead of open dissection.

Minimally invasive and computer-assisted techniques are another advancement in the treatment of traumatic fractures. Although there is a paucity of high-level evidence in the trauma literature thus far, minimally invasive principles as supported in the degenerative spine literature should translate well to the trauma population[26] (**Fig. 87.2**). Minimizing blood loss and sparing of the paraspinal musculature may expedite functional recovery in posterior percutaneous segmental pedicle screw fixation. Anterior endoscopic techniques may decrease approach-related morbidity, but they entail a steep learning curve and require experience with the diaphragm and accompanying regional anatomy at the thoracolumbar junction.

For surgical treatment of isolated burst fractures, anterior and posterior approaches may have similar outcomes regarding kyphosis, pain, and function, although some studies have shown that posterior approaches entailed a higher incidence of adverse events.[27] With open techniques, limited evidence suggests that additional fusion and instrumentation may not be necessary in the treatment of burst fractures.[28] Data from randomized controlled trials comparing surgical techniques remain too limited to determine superiority of one approach over the other.[29]

Instrumentation constructs have seemingly limitless combinations and lengths. Some surgeons may advocate short fusion constructs spanning only two disk spaces in young patients with high fusion potential, or in lumbar fractures with anterior column integrity. Longer constructs (two above and two below) may be appropriate for patients with poor bone quality or low fusion potential, or in thoracic fractures and anterior column failure.[30] Additionally, instrumentation may be placed with the intention of removing it after fusion has occurred to preserve adjacent segment mobility and reduce iatrogenic disease at adjacent levels.

This patient population is at great risk for adverse events in the acute setting, including urinary tract infections, neuropathic pain, pneumonia, delirium, and ileus.[31] Several active preventive measures should be pursued. Early removal of indwelling urinary catheters in favor of clean intermittent catheterization should be performed. Sequential compression devices and thromboembolic deterrent (TED) stockings can be used, and chemoprophylaxis for deep venous thrombosis must be initiated early. Minimizing narcotic pain medicine and the use of adjuvant pain medication may prevent delirium and ileus. The pneumococcal vaccine should be administered. Aggressive bowel regimen via oral and rectal routes should be administered. Additionally, it

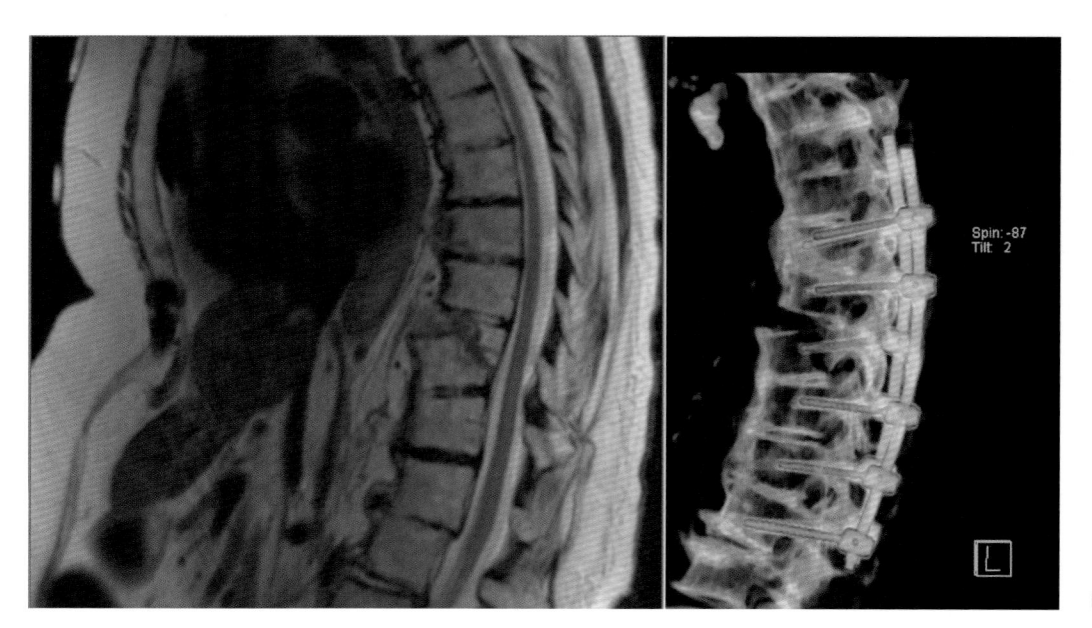

Fig. 87.2 An 87-year-old woman with osteoporosis presented after a fall backward. She was found to be neurologically intact and to have a T10 type B2 fracture **(a)**. She was treated via a minimally invasive technique. Percutaneous pedicle screws were placed bilaterally in T8 through L1, avoiding the left T10 pedicle because of the fracture pattern **(b)**.

is likely that all of these adverse events can be mitigated with early mobilization.

Ultimately, all conservative and surgical treatments are an effort to expedite rehabilitation and minimize the hospital stay.

Conclusion

The complex management of lumbar trauma is a reflection of the diversity of the pathology. Determination of the superiority of one method over the others has been difficult because of the lack of standard classification systems, despite the advancement in operative techniques for fusion. The most recent iteration of the TLICS has commendable inclusiveness, but it has yet to receive external validation. As supporting data continue to accumulate, conclusions will eventually be drawn to guide treatment decisions. As with all guidelines, focusing on the patient's pathological alterations in biomechanics and tailoring the treatment to the patient will remain paramount.

References

1. Bernhardt M, Bridwell KH. Segmental analysis of the sagittal plane alignment of the normal thoracic and lumbar spines and thoracolumbar junction. Spine 1989;14:717–721
2. Schafer RC. Clinical Biomechanics: Musculoskeletal Actions and Reactions. Baltimore: Williams & Wilkins; 1987
3. Saetia K, Cho D, Lee S, Kim DH, Kim SD. Ossification of the posterior longitudinal ligament: a review. Neurosurg Focus 2011;30:E1
4. Pintar FA, Yoganandan N, Myers T, Elhagediab A, Sances A Jr. Biomechanical properties of human lumbar spine ligaments. J Biomech 1992;25:1351–1356
5. Shirazi-Adl A. Biomechanics of the lumbar spine in sagittal/lateral moments. Spine 1994;19:2407–2414
6. Vaccaro AR, Oner C, Kepler CK, et al; AOSpine Spinal Cord Injury & Trauma Knowledge Forum. AOSpine thoracolumbar spine injury classification system: fracture description, neurological status, and key modifiers. Spine 2013;38:2028–2037
7. Boehler L. Die Techniek der Knochenbruchbehandlung im Grieden und im Kriege. Verlag von Wilheim Maudrich; 1930
8. Holdsworth F. Fractures, dislocations, and fracture-dislocations of the spine. J Bone Joint Surg Am 1970;52:1534–1551
9. Denis F. Spinal instability as defined by the three-column spine concept in acute spinal trauma. Clin Orthop Relat Res 1984;189:65–76
10. Denis F, Armstrong GW, Searls K, Matta L. Acute thoracolumbar burst fractures in the absence of neurologic deficit. A comparison between operative and nonoperative treatment. Clin Orthop Relat Res 1984;189:142–149
11. Panjabi MM, White AA III. Basic biomechanics of the spine. Neurosurgery 1980;7:76–93
12. Magerl F, Aebi M, Gertzbein SD, Harms J, Nazarian S. A comprehensive classification of thoracic and lumbar injuries. Eur Spine J 1994;3:184–201
13. Bono CM, Vaccaro AR, Hurlbert RJ, et al. Validating a newly proposed classification system for thoracolumbar spine trauma: looking to the future of the thoracolumbar injury classification and severity score. J Orthop Trauma 2006;20:567–572
14. Vaccaro AR, Lehman RA Jr, Hurlbert RJ, et al. A new classification of thoracolumbar injuries: the importance of injury morphology, the integrity of the posterior ligamentous complex, and neurologic status. Spine 2005;30:2325–2333
15. Oner FC, Wood KB, Smith JS, Shaffrey CI. Therapeutic decision making in thoracolumbar spine trauma. Spine 2010;35(21, Suppl):S235–S244
16. Hu R, Mustard CA, Burns C. Epidemiology of incident spinal fracture in a complete population. Spine 1996;21:492–499
17. Frankel HL, Hancock DO, Hyslop G, et al. The value of postural reduction in the initial management of closed injuries of the spine with paraplegia and tetraplegia. I. Paraplegia 1969;7:179–192
18. Maynard FM Jr, Bracken MB, Creasey G, et al; American Spinal Injury Association. International Standards for Neurological and Functional Classification of Spinal Cord Injury. Spinal Cord 1997;35:266–274
19. de Barros Filho TEP, Cristante AF, Marcon RM, Ono A, Bilhar R. Gunshot injuries in the spine. Spinal Cord 2014;52:504–510
20. Guttman L, Vinken PJ, Bruyn GW, eds. Handbook of Clinical Neurology, vol 26. New York: American Elsevier; 1976:285–306
21. Bakhsheshian J, Dahdaleh NS, Fakurnejad S, Scheer JK, Smith ZA. Evidence-based management of traumatic thoracolumbar burst fractures: a systematic review of nonoperative management. Neurosurg Focus 2014;37:E1
22. Bellabarba C, Fisher C, Chapman JR, Dettori JR, Norvell DC. Does early fracture fixation of thoracolumbar spine fractures decrease morbidity or mortality? Spine 2010;35(9, Suppl):S138–S145
23. Olerud S, Karlström G, Sjöström L. Transpedicular fixation of thoracolumbar vertebral fractures. Clin Orthop Relat Res 1988;227:44–51
24. Roy-Camille R, Saillant G, Mazel C. Plating of thoracic, thoracolumbar, and lumbar injuries with pedicle screw plates. Orthop Clin North Am 1986;17:147–159
25. Larson SJ, Holst RA, Hemmy DC, et al: Lateral extracavitary approach to traumatic lesions of the thoracic and lumbar spine. J Neurosurg 1976;45:628–637
26. Rampersaud YR, Annand N, Dekutoski MB. Use of minimally invasive surgical techniques in the management of thoracolumbar trauma: current concepts. Spine 2006;31(11, Suppl):S96–S102, discussion S104
27. Wood KB, Bohn D, Mehbod A. Anterior versus posterior treatment of stable thoracolumbar burst fractures without neurologic deficit: a prospective, randomized study. J Spinal Disord Tech 2005;18(Suppl):S15–S23
28. Chou P-H, Ma HL, Wang ST, Liu CL, Chang MC, Yu WK. Fusion may not be a necessary procedure for surgically treated burst fractures of the thoracolumbar and lumbar spines: a follow-up of at least ten years. J Bone Joint Surg Am 2014;96:1724–1731
29. Verlaan JJ, Diekerhof CH, Buskens E, et al. Surgical treatment of traumatic fractures of the thoracic and lumbar spine: a systematic review of the literature on techniques, complications, and outcome. Spine 2004;29:803–814
30. McLain RF. The biomechanics of long versus short fixation for thoracolumbar spine fractures. Spine 2006;31(11, Suppl):s70–S79, discussion S104
31. Glennie RA, Ailon T, Yang K, et al. Incidence, impact, and risk factors of adverse events in thoracic and lumbar spine fractures: an ambispective cohort analysis of 390 patients. Spine J 2015;15:629–637

B. Anterior Approach

88 Anterior Approach to the Lumbosacral Junction

Randall B. Graham, Nader S. Dahdaleh, and Tyler R. Koski

Anterior approaches to both the thoracic and lumbar spine have been utilized to treat a variety of spinal diseases since the early 20th century.[1,2] Dorsal and lateral approaches have recently proliferated, with a resultant movement away from anterior surgery. However, these approaches do not adequately solve all reconstructive issues. The anterior approach to the lumbosacral junction thus remains an essential and powerful tool not only for exposing the anterior and middle columns of the lumbosacral junction, but also for releasing rigid spinal deformities and achieving optimal lordosis restoration in the lumbar spine.

With an experienced access surgeon, straightforward anterior exposures can be performed efficiently and with minimal blood loss and relatively low morbidity through a reasonably small incision. Despite this, the fact remains that complications from this approach can be catastrophic. The inferior vena cava and iliac vessels are draped over the lumbar spine and lumbosacral junction. These vessels are typically mobilized during this operation, and can thus be injured or occluded by even the most seasoned access surgeon. Every access surgeon, therefore, should be comfortable with quickly triaging and repairing such damage with venous repair, arterial thrombectomy, or even vascular bypass techniques if necessary.

Patient Selection

Patients with either isolated lumbosacral pathology that is favorable to an anterior approach or multilevel thoracolumbar deformity with loss of lordosis through the lumbar spine and lumbosacral junction stand to benefit the most from an anterior approach.

Indications

- Severe degenerative facet or disk disease at the lumbosacral junction
- Postsurgical spinal instability or failed L5-S1 posterior fusion, L5-S1 spondylolisthesis, trauma/tumors/infections
- Multiplanar/ multisegmental deformity of the lumbar spine requiring caudal segment interbody support and lumbosacral lordosis restoration

Contraindications

- Morbid obesity or high sacral slope precluding adequate access
- Prior retroperitoneal/abdominal surgery or radiation therapy resulting in abundant fibrous scarring around the inferior vena cava and iliac vessels
- Severe aortoiliac disease or venous thromboembolism
- Poor bone quality in the setting of planned anterior lumbosacral interbody fusion (ALIF) surgery
- Males of reproductive age due to the risk of retrograde ejaculation (relative contraindication)

Advantages

- Extensive anatomic exposure of the anterior lumbosacral junction
- Aggressive treatment of pathological processes with lower injury to the neural elements than the dorsal approach in the setting of trauma/tumors/infections affecting the L5-S1 vertebral bodies
- Complete release of the anterior column, with subsequent ease in reduction and reconstruction for multiplanar deformities of the lumbosacral junction (i.e., spondylolisthesis)
- Correction of sagittal malalignment via lordosis restoration through the ALIF technique, particularly in the setting of large thoracolumbar constructs [3-6]

Disadvantages

- Assistance of an access surgeon
- Risk of vascular/visceral injury
- Venous thromboembolism
- Postoperative ileus
- Retrograde ejaculation

Choice of Operative Approach

The operative approach is anterior.

Preoperative Imaging and Testing

The choice of spinal imaging modality prior to performing an anterior approach to the lumbosacral spine depends on the pathology being treated. For most indications (e.g., trauma, tumor, infection, or degenerative disk disease), magnetic resonance imaging (MRI) through the lumbosacral spine is required, reserving gadolinium contrast-enhanced imaging for tumors, infections, or revision operations. Most indications also require computed tomography (CT) imaging to more fully evaluate bony anatomy. Coronal CT slices can identify and evaluate the transitional lumbosacral segments, which is crucial in preoperative planning. For older patients, it is often recommended to obtain preoperative bone-density testing, especially if instrumentation is planned.

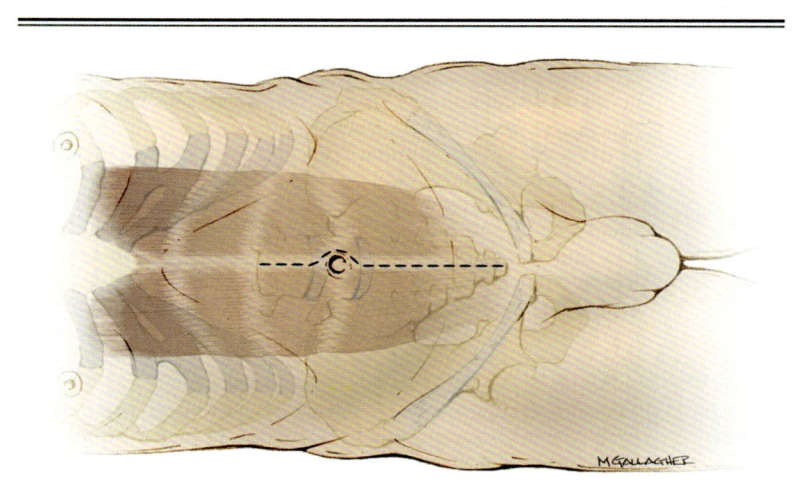

Fig. 88.1 Abdominal incision.

All patients should also have plain radiographs taken of the lumbosacral spine. If instrumentation is planned, standing anteroposterior (AP) and lateral views as well as flexion/extension lateral views should be included. Many surgeons (especially those who routinely use ALIF for deformity correction) also recommend obtaining full-length standing 36-inch cassette (scoliosis) radiographs to examine overall sagittal and coronal alignment. Before a deformity correction, spinal alignment is evaluated globally with measurements of the sagittal vertical axis (SVA), lumbar lordosis (LL), pelvic incidence (PI), and pelvic tilt (PT), with the goal of matching LL with PI while accounting for PT compensation.[7]

Patients with known vascular disease should be more thoroughly evaluated before undergoing an anterior approach. In the presence of known arterial disease or history of venous thromboembolism, preoperative ultrasound or angiographic studies can be useful for planning and avoidance of potential complications. Guidance from an experienced access surgeon is strongly recommended in these circumstances.

Surgical Procedure

The patient is placed supine on an AMSCO surgical table (Steris, Mentor, OH), configured in such a way as to allow fluoroscopic access. A gel-filled roll or foam axillary roll can be placed under the lumbosacral junction to generate a lordotic position if needed. A midline incision is made from just distal to about two thirds of the way to the pubic symphysis umbilicus. The umbilicus can be included depending on the number of levels (**Fig. 88.1**). The anterior abdominal fascia is then identified (**Fig. 88.2**) and incised vertically in the midline using monopolar electrocautery, and then elevated on the patient's left side with a handheld retractor. A dissection plane is then carried just deep to the left rectus muscle, allowing the endoabdominal fascia and peritoneum to fall away from the posterior rectus muscle. This dissection is carried as far laterally (toward the patient's left) as possible using a combination of electrocautery and blunt dissection, keeping the epigastric vessels superficially with the muscle layers.

The endoabdominal fascia is then incised vertically using tissue scissors, and blunt dissection is used to sweep the peritoneum medially until access to the left retroperitoneal space is gained (**Fig. 88.3**). This space is then carefully developed further, and the sacral promontory, left ureter, and iliac vessels are identified.

A fixed retractor system can then be deployed (we prefer the Omni system [Integra, Plainsboro, NJ]), with the appropriate blades positioned to hold the peritoneum in a rightward and cephalad direction. Direct pressure on the left ureter is avoided by placing the retractor superficial to it, so that the ureter can be visualized during the procedure on the right side of the field (anterior to the spine and attached to the peritoneum). The position and integrity of the major vessels, ureter, and spine are identified and verified. The vasculature is then carefully dissected, employing sharp technique for arteries and blunt dissection to the relatively thin-walled veins (**Fig. 88.4**).

For dissection around the lumbosacral junction, the peritoneum and ureter are mobilized together (as mentioned above),

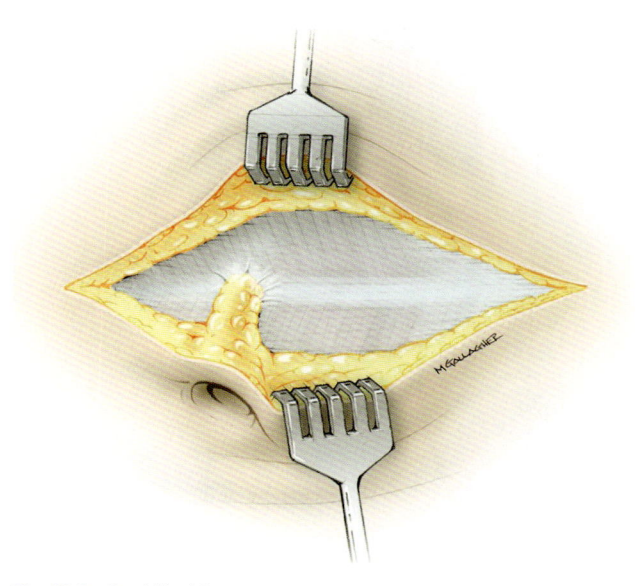

Fig. 88.2 Fascial incision.

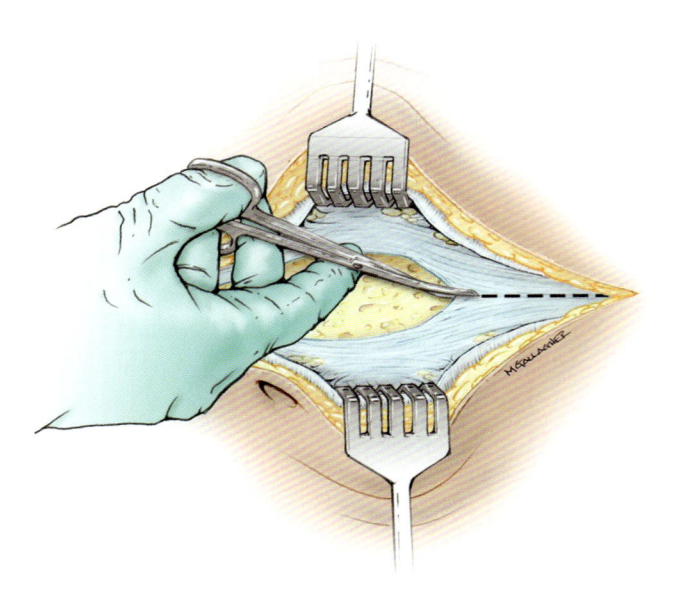

Fig. 88.3 Peritoneum division.

using long blunt sponge (or Kittner) dissectors toward the right side of the spine. The vessels are then carefully mobilized circumferentially, with small branches being carefully identified, ligated, and divided. The middle sacral vessels over the L5-S1 disk are identified, encircled with an angled clamp, and double clipped before being divided. There is typically one middle sacral artery with two veins, one of which branches off the left common iliac vein and courses toward the left border of the lumbar spine. This vessel is commonly missed and can cause significant blood loss if it is avulsed. Once they are identified and mobilized, the vessels can be gently retracted. The loose areolar tissue over the disk is then dissected free using a Kittner sponge. A spinal needle is then used to fluoroscopically confirm the L5-S1 level.

Once the L5-S1 disk is properly exposed and identified, a generous annulotomy is sharply performed, releasing enough disk at the anterolateral corners to prepare for lordotic distraction (**Fig. 88.5**). Large pituitary rongeurs are then used to remove the anterior annulus. A Cobb elevator and various curettes can then be used to remove further disk material and separate the cartilaginous end plates from the vertebral bodies (**Fig. 88.6**). It is important to remove and release enough disk to generate maximum mobilization for deformity correction and simultaneously achieve adequate arthrodesis of both end plates for fusion. Furthermore, great care must be taken to preserve the subchondral osseous structure of the end plates to prevent early graft subsidence. The prepared interspace is now filled with a structural lordotic interbody cage filled with graft material of the surgeon's choice. Screws are then introduced through the interbody device via manufactured screw holes to secure the cages and prevent dislodgment. Final AP and lateral radiographs are obtained upon completion of the construct.

Hemostasis is obtained via careful bipolar cautery and packing with topical hemostatic agents in the deeper spaces. The retractors are carefully removed, with thorough inspection to ensure adequate hemostasis. The peritoneum is gently swept back in place and inspected for rents, which are closed primarily with Vicryl suture. The abdominal fascia is then closed meticulously to prevent hernia formation, and the remainder of the wound is closed in anatomic layers.

Fig. 88.7 provides an example of an ALIF approach and its impact on lumbar lordosis.

Postoperative Care

Postoperative care after anterior approaches is centered mainly on careful diet advancement and prevention of venous thromboembolism. Patients are typically given nothing by mouth (NPO)

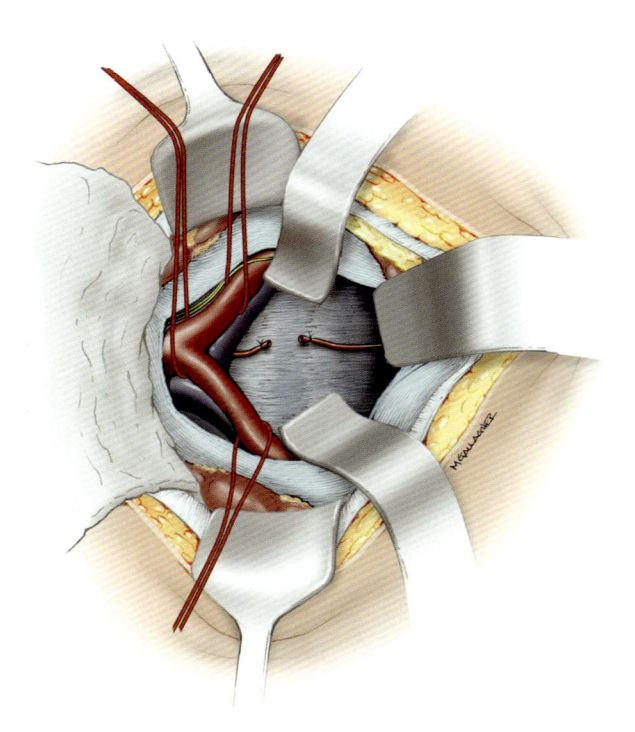

Fig. 88.4 Exposure.

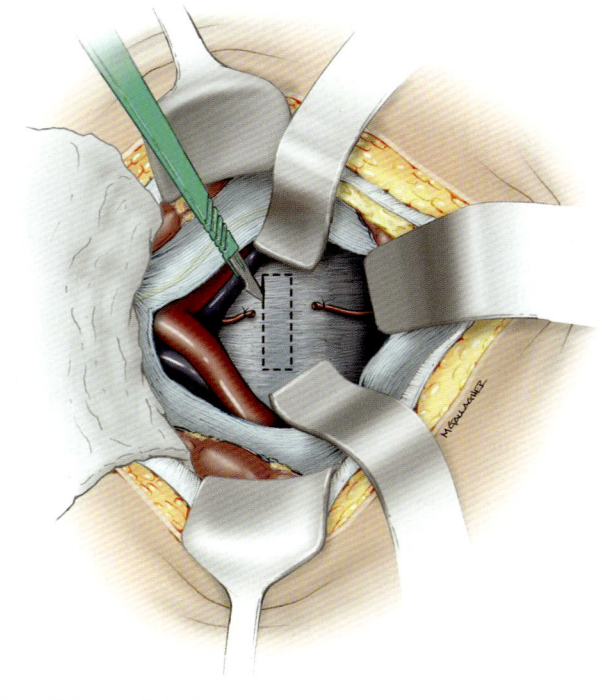

Fig. 88.5 Annular incision.

the first night after surgery, and then advanced slowly to sips of clear fluids the next day followed by a clear liquid diet after 24 to 48 hours, and then a regular diet once the patient begins passing flatus. A postoperative ileus is treated using an NPO status with intravenous fluids (potentially total parenteral nutrition, should the ileus persist) and frequent ambulation.

All patients are managed with sequential compression devices, frequent and early ambulation, and deep venous thrombosis (DVT) chemoprophylaxis (either fractionated or unfractionated heparin injected subcutaneously) starting the first postoperative day. If a second-stage posterior operation is planned within several days of the anterior approach (or if a DVT occurs), the patient is given an inferior vena cava filter.

Potential Complications and Precautions

The most common complications during anterior approaches to the lumbar spine are venous injuries. Circumferential exposure, control, and repair of the large venous structures can be exceedingly difficult due to their thin walls and the deep operative site with complex anatomy. Most small venous tears can be repaired with surgical clips deployed tangentially to the vein. Although oversewing these injuries can be dangerous (the slightest torque with a needle driver can exacerbate an injury due to the frail venous tissue) it is sometimes necessary to suture a longer tear. If this needs to be done, a delicate nonabsorbable monofilament

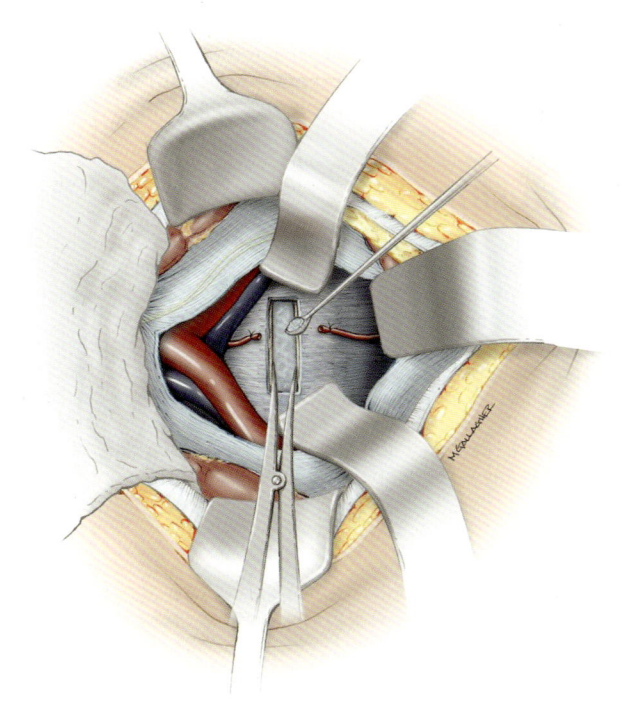

Fig. 88.6 Diskectomy.

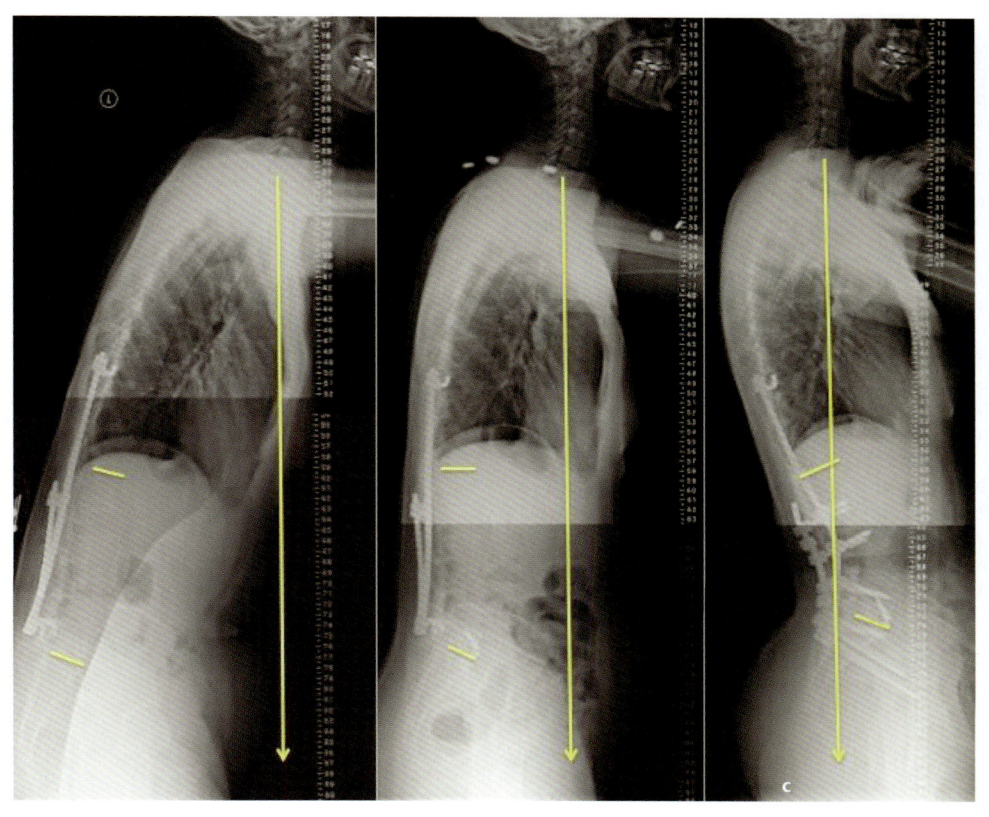

Fig. 88.7 The anterior approach to the lumbosacral junction can be a powerful tool for lordosis restoration via anterior lumbar interbody fusion (ALIF). **(a)** This patient previously underwent a thoracolumbar instrumented fusion for scoliosis, with resultant flat-back deformity and progressive sagittal imbalance due to severe degeneration at the lumbosacral junction. Note her grossly positive sagittal vertical axis (SVA; arrow) and lumbar lordosis measuring only 4 degrees (short bars). **(b)** Note the improvement in both lumbar lordosis (now 28 degrees) and SVA following L5-S1 ALIF. **(c)** The patient then underwent L2 to the sacrum/ilium instrumented posterior fusion with L4 pedicle subtraction osteotomy, with a final lumbar lordosis of 48 degrees and normal SVA.

suture on a tapered needle is recommended. Sometimes cotton pledgets need to be used to reinforce the tissue during repair.

Thrombosis of the iliac vessels can also occur due to prolonged retraction. Risk factors for vascular thrombosis (such as atherosclerosis, fibromuscular dysplasia, or venous thromboembolism) should be identified preoperatively. When operating on a patient with atherosclerotic iliac vessels, it is important to frequently check a distal left iliac pulse throughout the operation. A pulse oximeter can also be used on both lower extremities to monitor differential oxygen saturations. Furthermore, lower extremity somatosensory evoked potentials (SSEPs) can be monitored to detect decreased arterial blood flow. If a common iliac artery thrombosis occurs, 5,000 units of intravenous heparin is given immediately while circumferential proximal and distal control of the vessel is quickly obtained and an open thrombectomy is then performed.

Venous thromboembolism is typically seen in patients who sustained a venous injury during the exposure. If a patient develops leg swelling or pain in the perioperative period, an ultrasound is warranted to search for a DVT. It should be noted, however, that if the ultrasound is negative, a CT or MR venogram is warranted to evaluate the iliac veins, which cannot be evaluated via sonography.

Although rare, ureteral injuries can occur from intraoperative lacerations or ischemia due to direct pressure/stretching from retractor placement.[8] These injuries can result in immediate drainage of urine from the incision or delayed ureteral necrosis with "urinoma" formation or ureteral stricture leading to hydronephrosis. If a particularly difficult exposure is anticipated with a high risk of such an injury, ureteral stents can be placed to facilitate intraoperative identification of the ureters. Alternatively, a transperitoneal approach can be employed to avoid the more laterally located ureters. Ureteral injuries require urologic consultation for repair and long-term management.

Retrograde ejaculation occurs due to damage to the superior hypogastric nerve plexus, which courses over the left side of the sacral promontory. Disruption of these nerves causes dysregulation of the internal vesicular sphincters, resulting in ejaculation of sperm into the bladder rather than out of the penis. Retrograde ejaculation occurs in 0.42 to 10% of cases.[8–10] This injury results more commonly from thermal injury to the plexus through the use of monopolar cautery. Thus, blunt or bipolar dissection should be used when dissecting along the disk space, particularly in reproductive-age males. As mentioned earlier, many surgeons avoid the anterior approach if possible when performing elective lumbosacral spinal operations in reproductive-age males.

Bowel-related complications can range from a simple postoperative ileus to frank small-bowel injuries. Several days of postoperative ileus after this approach can be common, and are treated with NPO status, parenteral nutrition, frequent ambulation, and laxatives. Nasogastric decompression is reserved for patients who develop nausea and emesis. Patients' diets are generally advanced slowly in the postoperative period to prevent this. Frank bowel injuries are rare but serious complications that result from difficult intraperitoneal or retroperitoneal exposures or revision operations. Patients with bowel injuries can quickly become very ill and require complex repair and management by a qualified general surgeon.

Conclusion

The anterior approach to the lumbosacral junction is a technique with applications to traumatic, neoplastic, infectious, and degenerative diseases of the lumbar spine. It also provides direct access to the anterior column of the lumbosacral junction, and is thus one of the most powerful methods of adding lordosis and correcting sagittal plane deformity. Failure to understand the complex visceral and vascular anatomy of this region can result in potentially devastating complications, but in general this approach can be safely and efficiently performed when the regional anatomy is sequentially defined and controlled.

References

1. Hodgson AR, Stock FE. The Classic: Anterior spinal fusion: a preliminary communication on the radical treatment of Pott's disease and Pott's paraplegia. 1956. Clin Orthop Relat Res 2006;444:10–15
2. Hodgson AR, Wong SK. A description of a technic and evaluation of results in anterior spinal fusion for deranged intervertebral disk and spondylolisthesis. Clin Orthop Relat Res 1968;56:133–162
3. Hsieh PC, Koski TR, O'Shaughnessy BA, et al. Anterior lumbar interbody fusion in comparison with transforaminal lumbar interbody fusion: implications for the restoration of foraminal height, local disc angle, lumbar lordosis, and sagittal balance. J Neurosurg Spine 2007;7:379–386
4. Kim JS, Kang BU, Lee SH, et al. Mini-transforaminal lumbar interbody fusion versus anterior lumbar interbody fusion augmented by percutaneous pedicle screw fixation: a comparison of surgical outcomes in adult low-grade isthmic spondylolisthesis. J Spinal Disord Tech 2009;22:114–121
5. Dorward IG, et al. Transforaminal versus anterior lumbar interbody fusion in long deformity constructs: a matched cohort analysis. Spine 2013;38:E755–E762
6. Watkins RG IV, Hanna R, Chang D, Watkins RG III. Sagittal alignment after lumbar interbody fusion: comparing anterior, lateral, and transforaminal approaches. J Spinal Disord Tech 2014;27:253–256
7. Ames CP, Smith JS, Scheer JK, et al. Impact of spinopelvic alignment on decision making in deformity surgery in adults: A review. J Neurosurg Spine 2012;16:547–564
8. Rajaraman V, Vingan R, Roth P, Heary RF, Conklin L, Jacobs GB. Visceral and vascular complications resulting from anterior lumbar interbody fusion. J Neurosurg 1999;91(1, Suppl):60–64
9. Brau SA. Mini-open approach to the spine for anterior lumbar interbody fusion: description of the procedure, results and complications. Spine J 2002;2:216–223
10. Sasso RC, Kenneth Burkus J, LeHuec JC. Retrograde ejaculation after anterior lumbar interbody fusion: transperitoneal versus retroperitoneal exposure. Spine 2003;28:1023–1026

C. Anterolateral Approach

89 Anterolateral Retroperitoneal Approach to the Lumbosacral Spine

Jared J. Marks, H. Louis Harkey III, Timothy M. Wiebe, and Michael P. Schenk

In the current practice of spine surgery, there is an ever-increasing use of minimally invasive techniques to access the spine. However, the open anterolateral retroperitoneal approach still has its place in the armamentarium of the spine surgeon. This approach enables visualization of all lumbar vertebrae and access to the lumbar sympathetic chain (**Fig. 89.1**). It is practical for anterior pathology ranging from L2 to L4, whereas an approach to L5 or below may be complicated by the iliac vessels. Retroperitoneal dissection may avoid the complications of entering the pleural and peritoneal cavities.

In some cases an access surgeon, either a general surgeon of a vascular surgeon, may be needed to assist with the exposure, which requires mobilization of the great vessels and handling of the abdominal contents. The inclusion of an access surgeon on the surgical team can shorten the duration of the procedure and reduce the blood loss, and the access surgeon can repair vascular injuries as a result of surgical manipulation.

Indications

- Sympathectomy
- Decompression (tumor, trauma, and degenerative disease)
- Stabilization

Contraindications

- Morbid obesity (relative contraindication)
- Calcification of the great vessels
- Preclusive metastatic disease
- Prior abdominal surgery/infection (relative contraindication)
- Prior irradiation of the surgical path
- Retroperitoneal fibrosis

Advantages

- Enables visualization of all lumbar vertebrae
- Provides access to the lumbar sympathetic chain
- Enables ventral decompression
- Enables reconstruction and stabilization of lumbar spine pathology

Disadvantages

- Access to L5 obstructed by iliac vessels
- Right-sided approach limited by the liver
- Potential for complications to the abdominal viscera
- Rostral and caudal extent of the lumbar dissection may be limited
- Potential for vascular complications
- Potential for ureter damage
- Potential for damage to the genitofemoral nerve

Radiological Evaluation

Investigative studies are case specific. The delineation of soft tissues with magnetic resonance imaging (MRI) sequences is useful to visualize and characterize virtually all spinal pathology. Plain spinal radiographs may identify preclusive vascular calcification of the great vessels and delineate gross tumor, bone density, alignment, and stability, as well as landmarks to guide dissection. Plain spinal computed tomography (CT) clarifies the status of bone and ligamentous elements with regard to stability and thecal compression, and provides a template for measuring the screws and bolts to be used for instrumentation. Myelography delineates significant neural impingement and may complement CT and MRI. Selective spinal angiography may delineate tumor vascularity for preoperative embolization.

Intraoperative radiographs should be prearranged for non-instrumented cases, and a radiolucent operating table and C-arm fluoroscopy augment instrumentation procedures by enabling visualization of spinal levels and instrumentation. Similar information may be gained from image-guided surgical systems, which have the advantage of assisting in the selection of screw trajectory.

Preoperative Planning

Prior to elective spinal surgery, patients should be nutritionally optimized and counseled for smoking cessation. Autologous blood banking should be offered when available, whereas a red blood cell saver used intraoperatively may prevent exposure to blood products. For patients who will require an orthosis, it may be more convenient to have it prepared preoperatively. Ureteral stenting

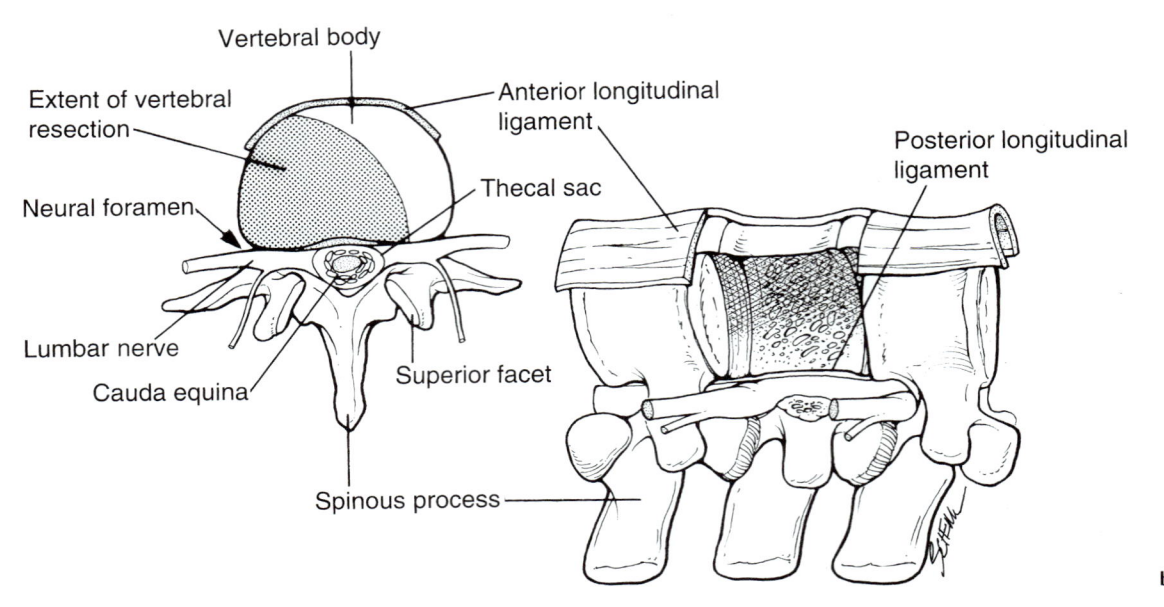

Fig. 89.1 Anatomic relationships in the anterolateral retroperitoneal approach. **(a)** Axial image. **(b)** Lateral view.

should be considered for ureteral identification in cases of related malignancy or fibrosis. Somatosensory evoked potential (SSEP) monitoring may be used to quantify the integrity of the central neuraxis and may indicate changes coincident or subsequent to surgical manipulation. Intraoperative microscopy can make thecal compression safer and more precise and should be considered based on the pathology.

Surgical Technique

Anesthesia and Positioning

Following induction, a nasogastric tube is placed for gastric decompression. Minimal vascular access includes peripheral venous and arterial catheterization, with case-selective central venous access for fluid administration and invasive monitoring. Antiembolus stockings and pneumatic compression devices are applied to the lower extremities. An indwelling urinary catheter will decompress the bladder and provide a measure of fluid status and renal perfusion.

Under general anesthesia, the patient is placed in the right lateral decubitus position, with the flank over the division in the operating table. A right axillary roll is positioned, after which the right arm is placed on an arm rest and padded at the cubital and carpal prominences. The left arm is supported by pillows parallel to the right arm. The hips are positioned on a deflatable beanbag. Pillows are placed between the legs to cover the medial tibial and malleolar prominences, and the right fibular and lateral malleolar prominences are also padded. The thighs are belted or taped to secure the patient to the table. A restraint may also be placed across the deltoid region.

In stable patients, slight table flexion at the flank reduces the angle of the costal margin with the iliac crest, and left hip flexion reduces tension of the psoas muscle. For many surgeons, anatomic orientation is enhanced by positioning the patient in an orthogonal anatomic plane. For the anterolateral approach, the patient should ultimately be positioned in the true lateral plane, which can be verified by the alignment of the pedicles and spinous processes on an anteroposterior radiograph view.

The anterolateral approach may be modified with the patient supine and the left flank elevated (paramedian approach), or, rarely, performed from the right side for sympathectomy and for cases with marked left-sided scoliosis. The left-sided approach avoids the liver and minimizes handling of the inferior vena cava.

The skin is shaved and draped from the left costal margin to a point below the left iliac crest, which may be taken for grafting. The intended incision is marked and hashed, followed with sterile preparation and draping, including the placement of an occlusive iodine-impregnated drape over the operative region.

In noninfected cases, administration of perioperative intravenous antibiotics for gram-positive coverage (cefazolin 1 g in patients weighing < 80 kg, and 2 g in patients weighing ≥ 80 kg) should commence 30 to 60 minutes prior to incision and continue 24 hours postoperatively. Consider vancomycin (1 g in patients weighing < 80 kg, and 1.5 g in patients weighing ≥ 80 kg) starting 2 hours before surgery and infused over 60 minutes for patients with allergic contraindications to cefazolin. Infected patients should begin antibiotics after cultures have been obtained.

Incision

The incision may be localized with fluoroscopy or image guidance. Empirically, the operating surgeon stands anterior to the patient and begins the flank incision at the posterior axillary line. To expose L1-L2, the incision begins above and two levels rostral to the desired level of exposure and terminates at the lateral border of the rectus sheath above the midpoint between the costal margin and the umbilicus. To expose L2–L5, an incision begins in the posterior axillary line equidistant between the costal margin and the superior iliac crest, and terminates at the lateral border of the rectus sheath. The incision for exposure of L2-L3 extends between the costal margin and the umbilicus; of L3-L4, toward the umbilicus; and of L4-L5, above the midpoint between the umbilicus and the pubic symphysis **(Fig. 89.2)**. To expose the lumbosacral junction, an incision begins slightly superolateral to the anterior superior iliac spine and continues

89 Anterolateral Retroperitoneal Approach to the Lumbosacral Spine

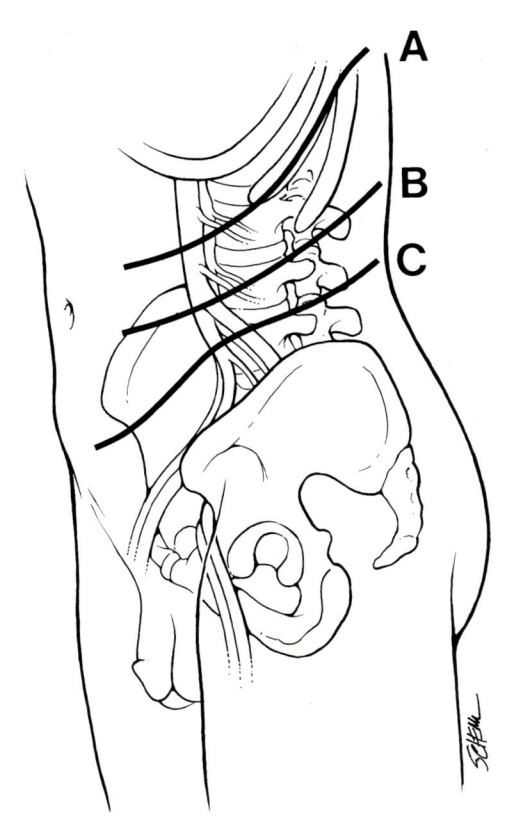

Fig. 89.2 Incisional considerations for the operative level. Incision A is for L2-L3 lesions, incision B is for L3-L4 lesions, and incision C is for L4-L5 lesions.

rostral and parallel to the iliac crest and inguinal ligament to a terminus at the lateral border of the rectus sheath.

Approach

A muscle-splitting approach involves division of the abdominal skeletal musculature along anatomic planes. Following skin incision, a Kelly clamp is used for dissection through the anatomic plane of the external and internal obliques and through the transversus abdominis muscles—the latter of which may be inapparent (**Fig. 89.3**). Anatomic dissection of the internal obliques limits exposure, rendering this approach most suitable for biopsy, drainage, and limited sympathectomy. Preservation of anatomic muscle planes reduces pain and promotes healing.

The flank approach involves linear electrocautery dissection through the anatomic planes of the external oblique and the transversus abdominis muscles (**Fig. 89.4**). In contrast to the muscle-splitting approach, the intervening internal obliques are transected against their anatomic plane to facilitate exposure.

The transversalis fascia should be opened laterally where the peritoneum is thickest and least likely to be adherent. The peritoneum is usually transparent gray, and if a peritoneal opening is encountered, it should be closed with absorbable suture prior to proceeding. Blunt dissection of the retroperitoneal plane between the renal fascia ventrally and the quadratus lumborum/psoas muscle group posteriorly leads to the vertebral column (**Fig. 89.5**). The inferior pole of the left kidney is retracted medially using a Deaver retractor padded with a lap sponge, and longitudinal retraction may be augmented with a Bookwalter retractor. The genitofemoral nerve exits the body of the psoas muscle medially near the level of L3 and should be protected during lateral retraction of the psoas muscle to avoid dysesthesia of the anterior thigh and inguinal region. Identification of the ureter may be confirmed by preoperative stenting and by Kelly's sign of visible ureteral peristalsis following application of gentle pressure. The ureter is gently elevated and retracted medially with the retroperitoneal fat pad when possible.

Exposure of the rostral lumbar spine may be augmented by costal resection two levels above the desired vertebral body. Resection of T11 and 12 ribs would expose the inferior body of L1. Division of the diaphragmatic crus from the anterior longitudinal ligament and subsequently of the arcuate ligament from the transverse process of L1 facilitates exposure of the caudal extent of T12. Diaphragmatic dissection should commence at the periphery, 2 cm from the lateral margin, to prevent injury to the phrenic nerve, which originates medially.

The lumbosacral junction lies below the iliac bifurcation. The hypogastric plexus overlies the middle sacral vessels in the interiliac space, and these structures may be mobilized by fascial dissection medial to the left common iliac vessels. Further exposure of the lumbosacral junction may require proximal ligation and division of branches of the internal iliac vessels for mobilization and distraction to the contralateral side over a vertebral body.

The subsequent steps are described in the following sections.

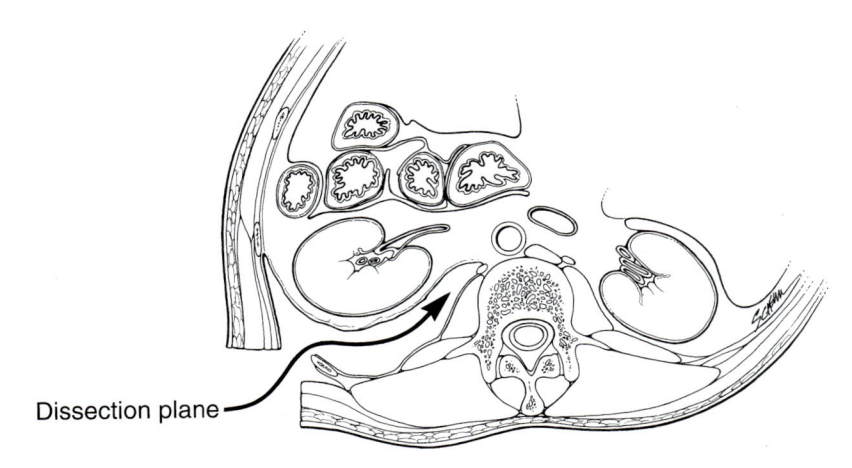

Fig. 89.3 Retroperitoneal approach utilizing a dissection plane for access to the anterolateral lumbar spine.

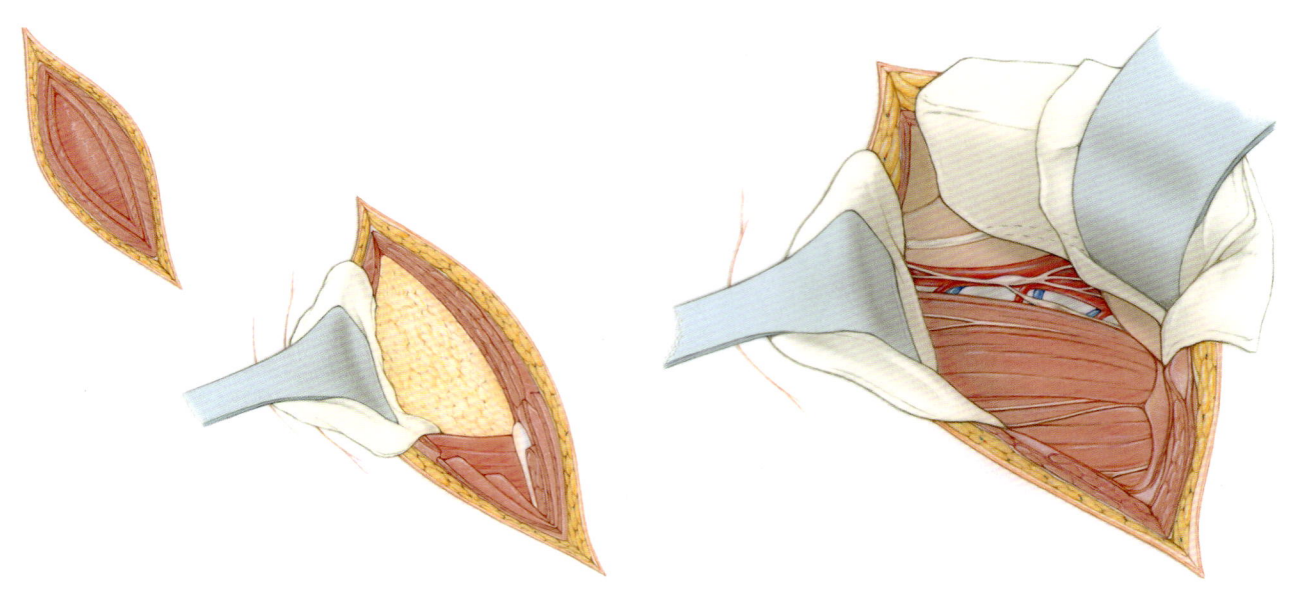

Fig. 89.4 Incision and dissection of musculature in the retroperitoneal approach.

Fig. 89.5 Retraction enables identification of relevant retroperitoneal structures.

Lumbar Sympathectomy

Indications

- Causalgia/reflex sympathetic dystrophy
- Pain—central and phantom hyperhidrosis
- Vascular insufficiency
- Post-frostbite syndrome

Approach

A muscle-splitting approach for focal exposure or a standard flank incision may be used. Alternatively, an oblique flank incision above the anterior superior iliac crest is continued toward the tip of the 12th rib. A right-sided approach may be indicated for right-sided pathology.

Following the standard approach, the sympathetic chain is identified along the lateral vertebral margin by its pale yellow hue and by its ganglionic swellings. The psoas muscle may be elevated bluntly from its attachments to the vertebral end plates and annulus using a Cobb periosteal elevator and bipolar cautery to facilitate exposure. Intervening lumbar veins may be divided, particularly on the right side, where the right sympathetic chain lies dorsal to the inferior vena cava.

For sympathectomy the chain is elevated with a blunt hook, clipped, and divided. Proximal lower extremity symptomatology may require sympathectomy as high as T12. Division at L1-L2 may lead to retrograde ejaculation. L2-L3 is divided for general lower extremity sympathectomy, and inclusion of L4 may yield a more complete result. Intervening rami communicantes should be divided to abolish communication from intermediate ganglia and contralateral circuits.

Diskectomy and Fusion

Approach

Following the standard approach the concave vertebral bodies may be discriminated visually and manually from the convex intervertebral disks. The prominence of the lumbosacral junction serves as a landmark. A 20-gauge spinal needle fashioned as a bayonet may safely mark the disk of interest for radiographic confirmation.

Disk exposure begins with psoas mobilization and retraction, which may occasionally require division of the psoas muscle. Segmental lumbar arterial branches arise at the midvertebral level. The radiculomedullary artery of Adamkiewicz (RA) is known to have a variable distribution and a tendency to arise from the left thoracolumbar region. As it nears the neural foramen, collateral vascular supply to the RA diminishes, and for that reason segmental lumbar arteries are divided in the midline. The anterior thoracolumbar spinal cord receives collateral vascular supply, and surgical division of a single segmental lumbar artery at the level of the neural foramen is not known to cause spinal cord infarction. Routine preoperative angiography to evaluate the RA is not indicated, nor should the occurrence of the RA in the surgical path warrant aborting an indicated thoracolumbar procedure.

The fifth lumbar vein occasionally enters the common iliac vein as the ascending iliolumbar vein, and it may be ligated and divided as it crosses the L4-L5 disk level on the left **(Fig. 89.6)**. The aorta is elevated medially.

The neural foramen is gently probed with a blunt right-angled nerve hook, and decompressed as necessary by removal of the anterior margin with an angled Kerrison rongeur. The anterior longitudinal ligament is dissected lateromedially from the anterior vertebral body and intervertebral disk with a Cobb

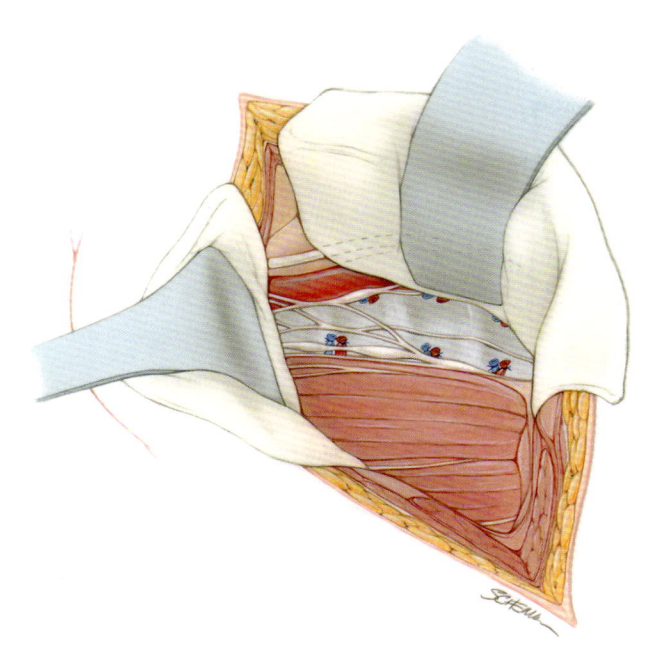

Fig. 89.6 Exposure and surgical intervention of the lumbosacral spine may require ligation of segmental vessels.

periosteal elevator. A window is sharply excised from the lateral annulus, and the diskectomy proceeds to the margins of the posterior longitudinal ligament with a pituitary rongeur. The posterior longitudinal ligament may be sharply incised and elevated with a blunt probe, then removed with angled Kerrison rongeurs for thecal decompression. The cartilaginous end plates of the disk space are sharply curetted and fashioned or slotted with a high-speed pneumatic drill bit for acceptance of a graft.

Vertebrectomy and Fusion

Approach

Vertebrectomy and instrumentation require vertebral exposure rostral and caudal to the level of pathology. The standard approach should be followed to anatomic levels flanking the level of interest and then proceed toward the region of pathology. The disks flanking the pathological vertebral level are grossly resected. Vertebrectomy proceeds from a lateral trajectory with an osteotome, followed by curettage to salvage bone for grafting. In cases where vertebral bone is unsuitable for graft, such as infection or malignancy, vertebrectomy is performed with a high-speed drill and a diamond bur. The anterior and contralateral margins of the vertebral body remain as barriers to the great vessels. Fine posterior bone dissection is performed with Kerrison rongeurs and curettage. The posterior longitudinal ligament may be excised for thecal decompression.

Flanking cartilaginous end plates are curetted and fashioned prior to fusion. Hemorrhage from bone surfaces along the fusion interface is stayed with thrombin-impregnated Gelfoam. Bone wax is deleterious to bone fusion and should be avoided. Physiological graft may include autologous costal struts and humeral or tibial allograft. Various cage systems can be fashioned to conform to end-plate margins and packed with autologous bone. Distraction pins may be used or the bend in the operating room table may be or adjusted to place the graft under compression. Caution should be used when distracting below calcified vessels, which may rupture.

Instrumented Stabilization

Approach

As an adjunct to interbody fusion, instrumented stabilization requires lateral exposure of vertebral bodies rostral and caudal to the level of pathology. Following the standard approach, segmental lumbar arterial branches are identified at the midvertebral levels of the vertebra to be plated and are ligated and divided in the midline. Division of segmental branches rostral and caudal to the level of fusion prevents vascular compression and avulsion during placement of instrumentation. Rarely, the psoas muscle may require incision for lateral exposure. Following lateromedial subperiosteal dissection, the lateral vertebral margins may be contoured with a high-speed drill and cutting bur to create flush apposition with the plates.

The nuances of cage, screw, and rod stabilizations vary with the system employed. Generally, lateral rods are affixed with screws in the midcoronal plane of the vertebrae rostral and caudal to the level of fusion. Accurate screw placement is vital to avoid neurovascular injury and should be confirmed with an intraoperative radiograph study.

Closure

Following irrigation with antibiotic solution, hemostasis is confirmed. Diaphragmatic openings may enlarge with time and predispose to diaphragmatic hernia, and for that reason they should be sutured closed. Peritoneal openings may be closed with a running suture. Drainage of the perivertebral space is usually not required. Muscles are closed in layers with interrupted resorbable sutures staggered through the aponeuroses. The dermis is closed with buried interrupted resorbable suture, and the skin is closed with the surgeon's choice of closure material.

Postoperative Care

In cases of fusion/instrumentation, biplanar radiographs are obtained while the patient is supine in the recovery room. Extubation proceeds in the early postoperative period. Patient-controlled anesthesia may augment early mobilization. Intravenous fluid maintenance continues until oral intake is advanced on the first postoperative day, coincident with returning signs of bowel function. Intermittent nasogastric suction may reduce nausea in the early postoperative period, but the nasogastric tube should be removed as soon as possible to prevent sinus infection. The urinary catheter should be removed by the first postoperative day, and signs of urinary retention should be sought and treated with intermittent urinary catheterization. Antibiotics can be continued for up to 24 hours.

External rigid orthosis is indicated for patients undergoing bone fusion of the lumbar spine. A thoracolumbosacral orthosis (TLSO) with a hip extension orthosis provides comfortable immobilization of the lumbar spine and augments lumbar bone fusion. The orthosis should be applied while the patient is supine, and subsequent lateral radiographs of the lumbar spine should be compared with the patient supine and standing. If there is no radiographic instability, the patient should be aggressively mobilized with assisted ambulation. Stability of the lumbar fusion segment is evaluated 3 months postoperatively with lateral flexion/extension radiographs of the lumbar spine or with a CT scan. If the spine appears stable, external orthoses may be discontinued or retained as necessary for patient comfort. Subsequent radiographs are attained at 6 months and 1 year postoperatively to evaluate bone fusion and to guide recommendations for progressive physical exertion.

Conclusion

Unlike some of the minimally invasive exposures to the lumbar spine, the anterolateral retroperitoneal exposure provides a large, open, and direct view of the lumbar spine. This approach can be applied to various types of surgical pathology and enables an anterior decompression of the thecal sac as well as reconstruction and stabilization of the lumbar spine.

Suggested Readings

Bauer R, Kerschbaumer F, Poisel S. Atlas of Spinal Operations. Stuttgart: Georg Thieme; 1993;64–66,270–302

Bauer R, Kerschbaumer F, Poisel S. Operative Approaches in Orthopedic Surgery and Traumatology. Stuttgart: Georg Thieme; 1987:41–63

Benzel EC. Biomechanics of Spine Stabilization. New York: McGraw-Hill; 1995

Bratzler DW, Dellinger EP, Olsen KM, et al. Clinical practice guidelines for antimicrobial prophylaxis in surgery. Am J Health Syst Pharm 2013;70:195–283. http://www.ajhp.org/content/70/3/195#sec-25

Colton CL, Hall AJ. Atlas of Orthopedic Surgical Approaches. Oxford: Heinemann; 1991:112–113

Hoppenfeld S, deBoer P. Surgical exposures in orthopedics. The Anatomic Approach. New York: Lippincott; 1994

Jagannathan J, Chankaew E, Urban P, et al. Cosmetic and functional outcomes following paramedian and anterolateral retroperitoneal access in anterior lumbar spine surgery. J Neurosurg Spine 2008;9:454–465

Orner GE, Spinner AL, Beek AL. Management of Peripheral Nerve Problems, 2nd ed. Philadelphia: Saunders; 1998

Spetzler RF. Op. Tech Neurosurg 1998;1:127–133

Wmter RB, Lonstein JW, Denis F, et al. Atlas of Spine Surgery. Philadelphia: Saunders; 1995:368–377

D. Posterior Approach

90 Open Posterior Lumbar Approach

Joseph S. Cheng and Scott L. Zuckerman

The open posterior lumbar approach for spinal surgery is a widely accepted technique to access the lumbar spine. The primarily muscular corridor to the osseous and neural anatomy of the spine avoids the more concerning complications and the surgical risks associated with anterior approaches, such as injury to the viscera and vascular anatomy, and obviates the need for the assistance of an approach surgeon.[1,2] Although there have been concerns regarding pain and damage to the lumbar muscles with the open posterior approach, understanding and respecting the tissues during dissection and retraction makes it possible to minimize the muscular damage and to limit the blood loss and postoperative pain.

The open posterior midline or paraspinal exposure of the lumbar spine remains one of the most widely utilized approaches in spinal surgery, and it is crucial that surgeons who perform lumbar spine surgery be intimately familiar with the practical surgical anatomy and techniques to perform a safe and efficient exposure of this area. This chapter reviews the anatomy of the lumbar spine and the techniques for the surgical exposure of the posterior lumbar spine.

Indications

- Lumbar decompression
  - Lumbar disk herniations
  - Lumbar stenosis
  - Facet synovial cysts
  - Lumbar spondylolisthesis
- Lumbar infections
  - Intervertebral diskitis
  - Vertebral body osteomyelitis
  - Spinal epidural abscess
- Lumbar trauma
- Lumbar tumors
  - Extradural neoplasms
  - Intradural neoplasms
- Spinal fusions
  - Correction of spinal deformity
  - Posterolateral intertransverse fusion
  - Pedicle screw fixation
  - Posterior lumbar interbody fusion
- Other indications
  - Iliac crest bone graft harvest

Advantages

- Common technique
- No major visceral or vascular structures at risk during approach
- Versatile for most pathology of the lumbar spine
- Cauda equina allowing retraction with low risk of spinal cord injury
- Easier localization of spinal level

Disadvantages

- Extensive muscle dissection needed
- Significant postoperative pain
- Higher risk of iatrogenic spinal instability
- Restricted access to anterior pathology

Anatomy

The anatomy and pathophysiology of the lumbar spine are important to understand when using these surgical techniques for exposure. The lordotic lumbar region bears 60 to 75% of the body's weight, and compromise of the muscles, tendon insertions, and ligamentous attachments during surgery affects the region's load-bearing abilities.

This region of the spine is made up of the vertebral body, the intervertebral disk, facet joints, paraspinal muscles, and ligamentous structures. The vertebral body is the main axial load-bearing structure of the spine, along with the disk, and typically 70% of the body weight is transmitted through it during neutral standing. The vertebral body is bounded by cortical bone peripherally and by a bony and cartilaginous end plate superiorly and inferiorly. The center of the vertebral body is composed of cancellous, spongy bone.[3] The cortical portions possess superior load-resisting properties, like a cylinder, with the cancellous center having less biomechanical strength in four main trabecular systems: the vertical system between the end plates, the horizontal system from posterior arch to transverse processes, and two oblique systems from end plates to the spinous process.[3] In patients with osteoporosis, it is the resistance of the spongy bone that varies, as it is dependent on mineral density, and, thus, osteoporosis results in weakness and decreased resistance.[4] This becomes more important in older patients, so it is important to assess their bone metabolism prior to surgery and for treatable problems such as vitamin D or Calcium deficiency. It is also important to assess their parathyroid hormone levels and bone mineral density before surgery. In patients with osteopenia or osteoporosis, as the width of the vertebral body increases as the spine descends, with an associated increase in pedicle width, it is important to choose a larger diameter pedicle screw to engage the inner cortical wall for purchase, as a mostly cancellous purchase may not be adequate for stability.

It is crucial to understand the anatomy of the lumbar intervertebral disk, given the frequency of disk degeneration and herniation, and to understand its importance in stabilizing each motion segment. Although the disk is a large avascular structure, it is biologically active with a hydrated core of proteoglycans in a loose collagen network in the nucleus pulposus surrounded by its fibrocartilaginous ring of the annulus fibrosus. The cellular function of the disk obtains its oxygenation and nutrition via diffusion from the end plates, and violation of the end plates through trauma or iatrogenically may lead to sclerosis, which prohibits diffusion, leading to cellular loss and degeneration. Lumbar disk degeneration is a situation of repetitive trauma to the disk space, as the load-carrying capacity of the disk increases 1 to 2.5 times during walking, and 10 times when lifting heavy objects. As the disk deteriorates, or "dehydrates" from the loss of diffusion of its nutrients and oxygenation, the load transfer properties are hindered.

The facet joints fulfill two basic movements: controlling the direction and amplitude of axial movement, and sharing the load-bearing of the vertebral body.[3,5] The facet joints increase in size and the orientation changes as the spine descends, and they accept typically 30% of the body weight in neutral position and up to 70% of the body weight in hyperlordotic positions.[3,6] The sagittal orientation of the lumbar facets provides significant resistance to rotation but not to flexion/extension or translation, and highlights the importance of the capsular ligament of the facet joint. The capsular ligament is one of the strongest ligaments in the region, due to its short length and proximity to the center of rotation of the lumbar spine, and it is frequently violated during an open posterior exposure. Minimizing the use of the monopolar cautery and of the subperiosteal technique helps preserve the ligament and prevents the high incidence of iatrogenic or postlaminectomy spondylolisthesis due the more sagittally oriented facets in this region.[7]

The extent of the exposure and degree of bone, joint, and ligament removal depend on the goal of the operation and the concern for spinal stability. For example, resection of a disk herniation can be performed via a small hemilaminotomy without destabilizing the facet joint or introducing iatrogenic spinal instability. However, a posterior lumbar interbody fusion with complete resection of bilateral facet joints requires a more extensive dissection, with resultant spinal instability to obtain adequate exposure of the intervertebral disk space with only minimal retraction of the nerve roots and dura to avoid significant neural injury. The optimal approach for each procedure is discussed in each section.

Pathophysiology

An older spine becomes rigid and stiff. As is expected, with the accumulation of facet joint osteoarthritis, dehydration of the intervertebral disk, and loss of normal spinal alignment, each segment of the spine undergoes characteristic degenerative changes. Central stenosis typically results from posterior bulging of the annulus, overgrowth and buckling of the ligamentum flavum, and hypertrophied facets with or without synovial cysts. Although the lumbar spinal canal is wide, stenosis can occurring during the fourth and fifth decades of life. Whereas the cervical region houses the upper cord, central stenosis in the lumbar region causes neurogenic claudication rather than myelopathy.

Proteoglycans of the nucleus pulposus have a high water content, and they enable the disk to sustain large axial forces in each subsequent vertebral body.[8] The disk degeneration process starts with loss of proteoglycans in the disk (i.e., loss of water), and substitution with dry, fibrotic tissue.[8] The fibrotic material behaves very differently from the hydrated gelatinous material, severely limiting the ability to absorb shock and trauma. Within the annulus, the arrangement of elastic fibers plays an important role in its mechanical strength.[9,10] In the degenerated annulus, shear stress, particularly anterior-posterior as seen in listhesis, causes the elastic fibers to become disorganized, which greatly alters the elasticity of the annulus. Permeability and annulus hydration also play a factor in its breakdown, similar to the nucleus pulposus.[8,11] An analogy for intervertebral disk degeneration is a car tire that loses height and bulges radially when compressed.[12,13] Any reduction in water content of the nucleus is like letting air out of a tire, so that an increasing load is applied to the annulus, rather than to the well-hydrated disk. Over time, nucleus pressure is reduced while compressive load-bearing by the annulus is increased.[12]

Facet hypertrophy and abnormal motion also play an important role in the degeneration cascade. The superior articulating process of one vertebra is separated from the inferior articulating process of the vertebra above by a synovium-lined articulation, which is called the zygapophyseal joint.[14] With changes to the articular cartilage, the facets and the zygapophyseal joint are at risk for damage and degeneration. As disks degenerate and lose height, greater stress is placed on the facet joint, with subsequent craniocaudal subluxation.[14] As the facet arthropathy progresses, the foramen is often encroached upon by the enlarging superior articular process. Pain can emanate from encroachment of the exiting or traversing nerve root, or directly from the pain fibers that innervate the synovial lining and joint capsule. Synovial cysts can also form from herniation of the synovium through the joint capsule.[15]

Preoperative Imaging and Testing

Preoperative imaging is needed for any surgical plan. An magnetic resonance imaging (MRI) scan is obtained to evaluate the neural elements if there is concern about neural compression, and computed tomography (CT) is needed to assess the bony elements. CT is most useful in revision surgery and deformities, where the surgeon can visualize the extent of the abnormal bone from the deformity or previous decompression. Standing X-rays are crucial to facilitate intraoperative localization of the spinal level, assess global alignment, and look for instability or spondylolisthesis that is not seen on supine CT or MRI scans. In addition to imaging, nuclear bone scans and tests for osteoporosis can provide further information. Obesity, smoking, and depression are three risk factors that have been shown to predict a worse outcome after spine surgery. A full discussion of these preoperative factors and how they should be considered in the surgical decision-making process is outside the scope of this chapter, but the surgeon should take these factors into account when planning the surgery.[16–19]

Anesthesia and Positioning

Most operations on the lumbar spine are performed under general endotracheal anesthesia. However, for relatively short procedures such as microdiskectomy, it has become more common to utilize regional anesthetic techniques such as a spinal epidural block or, in some instances, even local anesthesia supplemented with intravenous sedation. Just as proper positioning is central to safety and success for cranial procedures, such is also the case for operations on the spine. The posterior midline approach to the lumbar spine is most easily accomplished with the patient in the direct prone position. The patient may be positioned using a spinal frame or table in which the patient's legs are kept approximately in line with the spine, or using a knee-chest type of frame in which the hips and knees are flexed to 90 degrees and a major portion of the body weight is supported by the knees (**Fig. 90.1**). For ease and consistency, we prefer to use a Jackson-rail bed on which the patient is placed in the prone

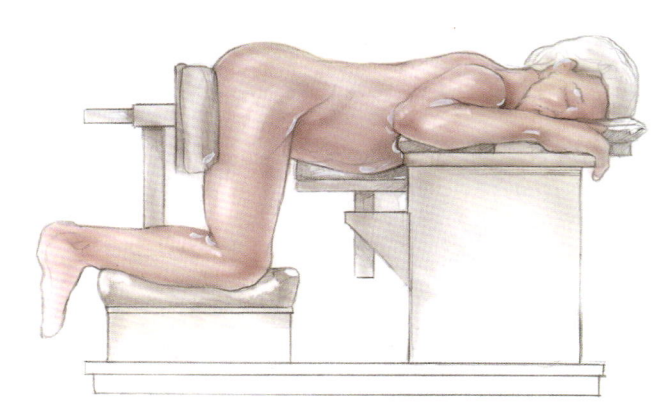

Fig. 90.1 The patient is positioned using a knee-chest frame, which enables the knees to support a significant portion of the body weight by keeping them flexed at 90 degrees.

position. The use of a sling enables the hips to flex, which decreases the lumbar lordosis and facilitates access for decompressions. In patients needing a fusion, a flat top is used to extend the hips and keep the legs parallel to the spine, which maintains the lumbar lordosis and prevents flat back deformities from the fusion. Improper positioning not only makes the surgical procedure more difficult, but also may result in additional morbidity unrelated to the procedure itself.

The Jackson rail system is commonly used to avoid any significant pressure on the abdomen that can produce elevated pressure in the epidural venous system and result in vexing bleeding during surgery. This system uses hip pads and chest pads, which need to be tempered by the patient's body habitus to avoid gravity effects, with pressure on the chin if the patient slips down, along with lateral femoral cutaneous nerve palsies. The chest should be properly supported to ensure adequate ventilation, and peak airway pressure should be checked, because with high peak airway pressures the patient can perform the Valsalva maneuver during the entire surgery. Proper positioning of the face requires collaboration between the surgeon and anesthesiologist, to make sure no additional pressure is placed on the eyes. We prefer the face to point straight toward the floor with the head supported on a large soft foam square. Alternatively, the head can be placed in a padded horseshoe headrest or immobilized in a Mayfield pin headholder. Regardless of the method, pressure on the orbits must be avoided to prevent corneal abrasions or visual loss. The neck should be maintained in a roughly neutral position and approximately parallel to the contour of the upper thoracic spine. The upper extremities should be positioned with the shoulder abducted and elbow flexed and supported by adequate foam padding. Excessive abduction or flexion of the shoulder should be avoided because this can result in a stretch injury of the brachial plexus. In addition, elbows not padded appropriately can lead to ulnar neuropathy, where the ulnar nerve passes between the olecranon and the medial epicondyle.[20,21]

As noted previously, the position of the legs is important in terms of ease of access to the spinal canal. Flexion of the hip reduces the amount of lordosis, increases the interspinous and interlaminar distances, and facilitates access to the spinal canal. However, one must remember that this position can give the surgeon a false sense of decompression, as this is not how the spine sits during ambulation, where more lordosis closes off the central canal and foramen. In contrast, depending on the goal of surgery, lordosis can be maintained by extending and elevating the hips. Flexion of the knee reduces the degree of stretch on the sciatic nerve. Although it is customary to place a safety strap across the buttock or upper thighs to stabilize the pelvis, a strap made too tight for a long procedure can result in a pressure palsy of the sciatic nerve. The feet should be elevated to facilitate venous drainage. Sequential compression devices should be worn for long cases, so as not to put pressure on the peroneal nerve. Pressure points such as the anterior iliac crest should be adequately padded to prevent a neurapraxia of the lateral femoral cutaneous nerve. Lastly, the genitals should be examined to ensure that they are free hanging and that the Foley catheter is still in place.

Radiological Evaluation

Accurate intraoperative localization begins with a careful preoperative review of the radiographic studies. In this regard, we routinely obtain an anteroposterior (AP) and lateral plain radiograph of the area of interest, to exclude aberrant anatomy such as an altered number of rib-bearing thoracic vertebra and lumbarized or sacralized segments caudally. Indeed, it is the responsibility of the surgeon to recognize any variations and operate on the correct level. In the lumbar spine (particularly for a single-level lumbar diskectomy), the level is initially approximated from the plain X-rays, realizing that the iliac crest usually passes through the L4-5 interspace (**Fig. 90.2**). Alternatively, after prepping the skin, a sterile 18-gauge spinal needle can be inserted and the position confirmed with a lateral X-ray. The tract can then be marked by injecting sterile methylene blue, although this is not our practice.

Once the superficial exposure is made, an intraoperative X-ray is obtained with a towel clip on the exposed spinous process or a Penfield probe under the lamina to confirm the operative level. Alternatively, one can use C-arm fluoroscopy, if available, for localization. However, regardless of the method utilized, the surgeon must always be confident that the level is correct. Any significant deviation from the expected pathological findings based on the preoperative imaging should prompt an immediate reassessment of the level. If there is any question, the surgeon should reexamine the imaging studies and obtain another confirmatory intraoperative X-ray. Wrong-level surgery is common, and every precaution, preoperatively and intraoperatively, should be taken to avoid this unwanted event.[22]

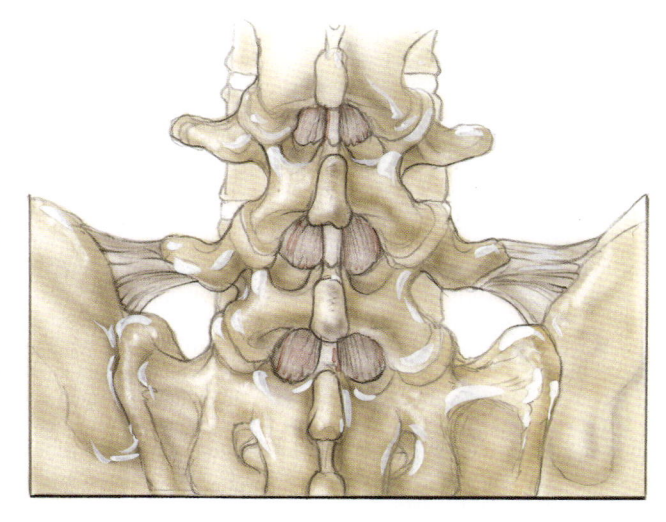

Fig. 90.2 The intercrestal line usually passes through the L4-5 interspace, which is approximated by careful preoperative review of the anteroposterior and lateral plain X-rays.

Operative Technique

Incision

The proposed skin incision and underlying subcutaneous tissues are infiltrated with a 50:50 mixture of 1% lidocaine with 1:200,000 epinephrine and 0.5% bupivacaine. Injection of local anesthetic with epinephrine reduces bleeding and limits the need for cautery in the subcutaneous tissues. The anesthesia team is always alerted prior to injection. The skin is sharply incised and extended into the subcutaneous tissues to the level of the fascia. Hemostasis is achieved at each step of the procedure as necessary using bipolar electrocautery, although excessive cauterization with charring of tissues should be avoided. Dissection of the subcutaneous tissues can be completed with either the scalpel or the monopolar electrocautery. The subcutaneous tissues are then retracted using a self-retaining Weitlaner retractor.

Fig. 90.3 Cross-sectional axial anatomy of the L5-S1 region.

Exposure

As one proceeds more caudally and encounters the segment overlying L5-S1, this becomes even more apparent and can be a helpful landmark in the very obese patient in whom precise localization can be problematic. The fascia is extremely robust in this region, being reinforced by the aponeuroses of the latissimus dorsi and posterior serratus inferior muscles (**Fig. 90.3**). The fascia is opened in the midline using either a fresh scalpel or the electrocautery. Alternatively, the fascia may be opened slightly off the midline. The latter technique may provide a slightly better cuff of fascia on either side to facilitate closure.

The next step in exposing the dorsal spine involves dissection of the paraspinous musculature using a subperiosteal technique. The lumbar paraspinous muscles are arranged into superficial and deep layers with specific attachments to the intraspinous region. In addition to the lumbodorsal fascia, which envelopes the underlying deep muscles, the superficial layer is primarily composed of the erector spinae muscles. The superficial layer consists of the spinalis, longissimus, and iliocostalis in a medial to lateral direction (**Fig. 90.4**). The deep layer of muscles includes the multifidus, rotatores, and intertransversarii. Although there are many techniques for performing a subperiosteal dissection of the paraspinous musculature, there are several themes that should be common to any technique, namely, safety, efficiency, and minimal blood loss. The fascial attachment to the spinous process is divided just off the midline to introduce a periosteal elevator at the most dorsal superior margin of the spinous process. The muscles are stripped from the spinous process superficial to deep using a periosteal elevator and can be continued over the laminar surface until the medial facet joint. This helps avoid muscle bleeding and injury, and insertion of a gauze sponge can facilitate the periosteal dissection, especially the medial to lateral dissection to expose the facets (**Fig. 90.5**).

We must emphasize the importance of the initial dissection technique. We perform the dissection sharply, with little to no use of cautery. The knife is taken down to the spinous process, where the lumbodorsal fascia is encountered. When accessing the bony elements, again, sharp dissection is continued. We use a combination of scraping the sharp end of the Cobb in a subperiosteal manner and heavy scissors to cut any remaining muscle or fascial attachments. The use of Ray-Tec sponges can help dissect the soft tissue in a subperiosteal manner. Although more bleeding is encountered, this sharp dissection preserves the muscle integrity and avoids excessive cautery. It has been our experience that excessive cautery in the muscle and the bony elements can cause thermal injury with irritation of the adjacent nerve roots. Complex regional pain syndromes and causalgia can ruin an otherwise well-performed operation if excessive cautery is used.[23,24]

Consider extending the incision if considerable force is being applied for dissection and retraction in obese or heavily muscled patients to accomplish the exposure. Excessive downward force should be avoided to prevent injury to the neural elements or creation of a dural tear and cerebrospinal fluid (CSF) leak. This can sometimes occur in patients with occult spinal dysraphism, and is also a potential pitfall in patients with posterior element fractures. Additionally, in some patients, the interlaminar space can be rather wide, in which case caution must be exercised to avoid inadvertent penetration into the spinal canal. The extent of the lateral dissection is determined by the operation, and is elaborated in subsequent chapters. For a simple hemilaminectomy and diskectomy, a unilateral exposure that extends just to the facet joint is customarily adequate. On the other hand, a posterolateral fusion requires a wide bilateral exposure that completely exposes the facet joint and the transverse processes, which lie more laterally and deep.

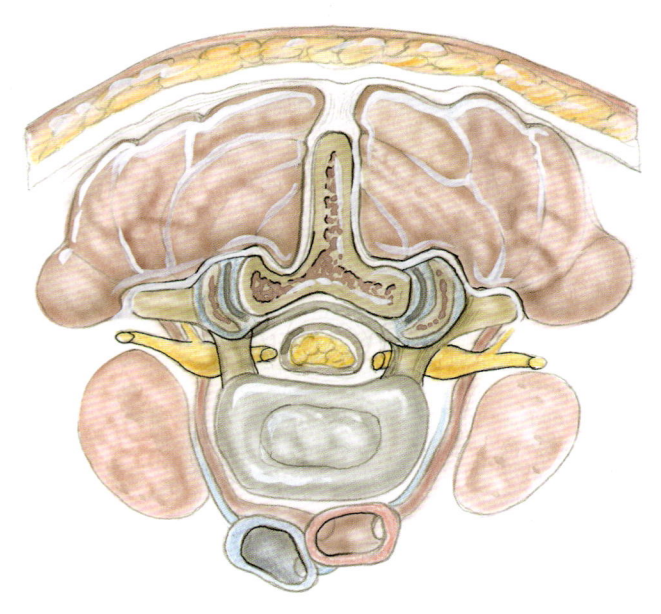

Fig. 90.4 Anatomic location of the deep paraspinal musculature in the L5-S1 region.

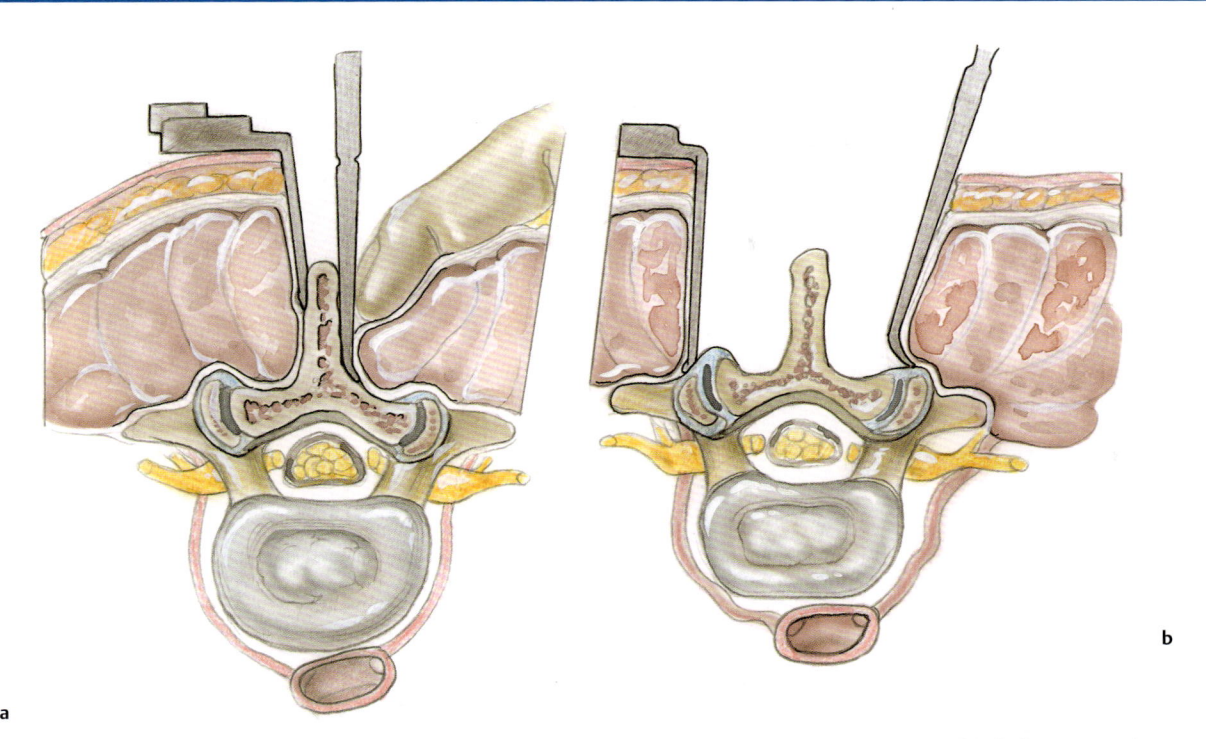

Fig. 90.5 **(a)** The paraspinal muscles are stripped superficial to deep from their attachment locations on the periosteum. **(b)** The laminar attachments are swept from medial to lateral to expose the facet.

There are numerous self-retaining retraction systems that can be utilized for maintaining the exposure. The ideal system is one that is simple to use, maintains a low profile so as to be unobtrusive and preserve lines of site to the surgical field, provides a variety of retractor blades, and is radiolucent so as not to interfere with the use of intraoperative imaging. Once dissection and retraction of paraspinous muscles are complete, the surgeon has a full view of the posterior spine (**Fig. 90.6**). The spinous processes become progressively larger in the lumbar spine. Although the spinous processes in the thoracic spine point inferiorly, this becomes less apparent in the lumbar spine. Indeed, at the lower lumbar levels, the spinous processes point directly posteriorly. Each vertebra articulates with its neighbor rostrally and caudally through the intervertebral disk and the facet joints (**Fig. 90.7**). Each facet consists of the inferior articular process of the vertebra above and the superior articular process of the vertebra below. The inferior process is situated medially with the superior process laterally. An important structure is the pars interarticularis, a portion of the lamina that provides the bony connection between the superior and inferior articular processes of an individual vertebra. The transverse processes project laterally from the level of the superior articular facet.

The important ligamentous structures include the supraspinous and interspinous ligaments, the ligamentum flavum, the facet capsule, and the intertransverse ligament. The iliolumbar ligaments run from the transverse processes of L5 to the iliac crests and help stabilize this area. The sacrum is composed of fused remnants of segmental bony elements. The dorsal surface is irregular owing to the presence of irregular crests overlying the fused spinous, articular, and transverse processes. On either side of the sacrum are four pairs of foramina for the passage of the dorsal rami of the sacral nerve roots. Caution must be exercised

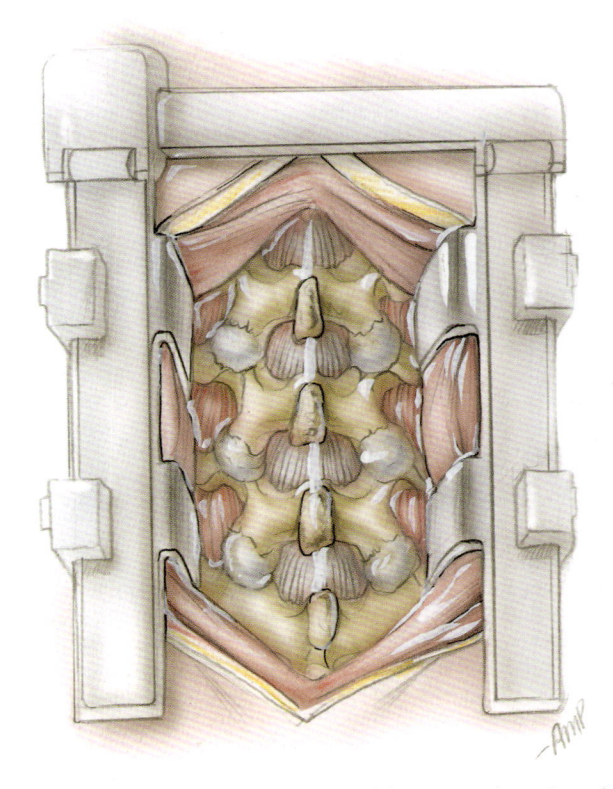

Fig. 90.6 After dissection and retraction of the paraspinal muscles, a full view of the dorsal aspect of the lumbar spine is available.

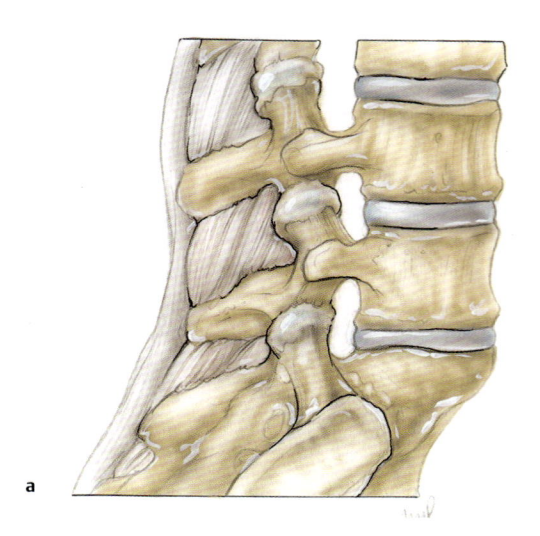

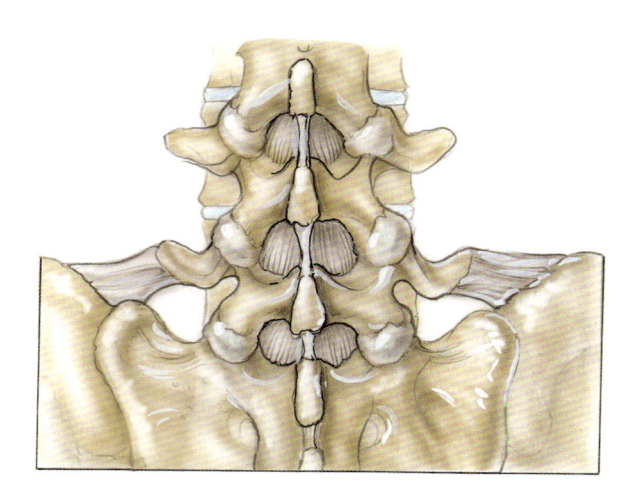

Fig. 90.7 (a) In the lower lumbar spine, each vertebra articulates with its neighbor rostrally and caudally through the disk and the facet joint. (b) Normal anatomy of the lumbosacral spine.

when exposing the sacrum, to avoid passage into these openings with resultant bleeding or CSF leakage. Lastly, during a decompression, parts of the dura often attach low down to the L5 and S1 lamina, and poor technique using the Kerrison rongeur can result in an unexpected CSF leak due to these dural attachments.

Closure

Prior to closure, the self-retaining retractors are loosened and meticulous hemostasis is performed. The surgeon may decide to leave a drain, largely based on the degree to which hemostasis can be achieved. It is our practice to favor placement of a drain for 24 to 48 hours if a dural transgression has not occurred. One should try to avoid an epidural drain if a dural tear and CSF leak have occurred, in an effort to avoid formation of a CSF fistula. The paraspinous muscles are then reapproximated with interrupted absorbable sutures such as 0 Vicryl, although tying the sutures excessively tight should be avoided. Rather, bleeding points should be controlled using bipolar cautery. The lumbodorsal fascia should be carefully and accurately closed with an absorbable suture. Interrupted or carefully secured continuous sutures of 0 Vicryl are preferred for the fascial closure. Sutures through the deep subcutaneous tissues can incorporate the fascia to eliminate any potential dead space. The skin is closed with a running absorbable suture (placed in traditional or subcuticular fashion) or can be reapproximated with surgical staples.

Postoperative Care

Postoperatively, patients are often monitored on the ward for one night. Length of stay depends on the extent of the procedure, but patients with single-level diskectomies, laminectomies, or foraminotomies are often kept for one night postoperatively. Adequate pain control is a must. Recent reports have recommend multimodal pain management, with multiple analgesic agents, in addition to narcotics, including gabapentin, Toradol, acetaminophen, and muscle relaxants.[25,26] Multimodal pain management helps avoid heavy dose narcotics, and patient-controlled analgesia (PCA) devices decrease the risk of respiratory depression and ileus, and shorten the hospital stay.[27] Prior to discharge, ambulation, urination, and tolerating oral liquids and solids must be achieved. Moreover, outpatient physical therapy is prescribed for all our postoperative spine patients.

Complications

Complications are elaborated in each individual procedure section. In terms of general complications with the posterior lumbar approach, extensive muscle dissection and lack of respect for tissue plans can lead to devascularization, atrophy, and complex regional pain syndromes. If hemostasis is not achieved, patients can require unnecessary transfusion and may go into shock.

Conclusion

Although the posterior midline approach to the lumbar spine seems simple, failure to understand variations in local anatomy and failure to adhere to meticulous surgical techniques can result in significant morbidity from the soft tissue exposure alone. However, the surgeon who has a grasp of the anatomy and adheres to strict principles of proper surgical technique will usually be rewarded with a successful outcome.

References

1. Canaud L, Hireche K, Joyeux F, et al. Endovascular repair of aorto-iliac artery injuries after lumbar-spine surgery. Eur J Vasc Endovasc Surg 2011; 42:167–171
2. van Zitteren M, Fan B, Lohle PN, et al. A shift toward endovascular repair for vascular complications in lumbar disc surgery during the last decade. Ann Vasc Surg 2013;27:810–819
3. Izzo R, Guarnieri G, Guglielmi G, Muto M. Biomechanics of the spine. Part I: spinal stability. Eur J Radiol 2013;82:118–126
4. Myers ER, Wilson SE. Biomechanics of osteoporosis and vertebral fracture. Spine 1997;22(24, Suppl):25S–31S
5. Jaumard NV, Welch WC, Winkelstein BA. Spinal facet joint biomechanics and mechanotransduction in normal, injury and degenerative conditions. J Biomech Eng 2011;133:071010
6. Dunlop RB, Adams MA, Hutton WC. Disc space narrowing and the lumbar facet joints. J Bone Joint Surg Br 1984;66:706–710
7. Yoganandan NHA, Dickman C, Benzel E. Practical anatomy and fundamental biomechanics. In: Benzel EC, ed, Spine Surgery: Techniques, Com-

plication Avoidance, and Management, 2nd ed. Philadelphia: Elsevier; 2005:109–134
8. Inoue N, Espinoza Orías AA. Biomechanics of intervertebral disk degeneration. Orthop Clin North Am 2011;42:487–499, vii
9. Smith LJ, Byers S, Costi JJ, Fazzalari NL. Elastic fibers enhance the mechanical integrity of the human lumbar anulus fibrosus in the radial direction. Ann Biomed Eng 2008;36:214–223
10. Smith LJ, Fazzalari NL. The elastic fibre network of the human lumbar anulus fibrosus: architecture, mechanical function and potential role in the progression of intervertebral disc degeneration. Eur Spine J 2009;18:439–448
11. Gu WY, Mao XG, Foster RJ, Weidenbaum M, Mow VC, Rawlins BA. The anisotropic hydraulic permeability of human lumbar anulus fibrosus. Influence of age, degeneration, direction, and water content. Spine 1999;24:2449–2455
12. Adams MA, Dolan P. Spine biomechanics. J Biomech 2005;38:1972–1983
13. Brinckmann P, Grootenboer H. Change of disc height, radial disc bulge, and intradiscal pressure from discectomy. An in vitro investigation on human lumbar discs. Spine 1991;16:641–646
14. Modic MT, Ross JS. Lumbar degenerative disk disease. Radiology 2007;245:43–61
15. Doyle AJ, Merrilees M. Synovial cysts of the lumbar facet joints in a symptomatic population: prevalence on magnetic resonance imaging. Spine 2004;29:874–878
16. Anderson JT, Haas AR, Percy R, Woods ST, Ahn UM, Ahn NU. Clinical depression is a strong predictor of poor lumbar fusion outcomes among workers' compensation subjects. Spine 2015;40:748–756
17. De la Garza-Ramos R, Bydon M, Abt NB, et al. The impact of obesity on short- and long-term outcomes after lumbar fusion. Spine 2015;40:56–61
18. Gulati S, Nordseth T, Nerland US, et al. Does daily tobacco smoking affect outcomes after microdecompression for degenerative central lumbar spinal stenosis?—A multicenter observational registry-based study. Acta Neurochir (Wien) 2015;157:1157–1164
19. Sekiguchi M, Yonemoto K, Kakuma T, et al. Relationship between lumbar spinal stenosis and psychosocial factors: a multicenter cross-sectional study (DISTO project). Eur Spine J 2015;24:2288–2294
20. DePasse JM, Palumbo MA, Haque M, Eberson CP, Daniels AH. Complications associated with prone positioning in elective spinal surgery. World J Orthop 2015;6:351–359
21. Kamel I, Barnette R. Positioning patients for spine surgery: avoiding uncommon position-related complications. World J Orthop 2014;5:425–443
22. Francis T, Benzel E. Wrong level spine surgery: a perspective. World Neurosurg 2013;79:451–452
23. Knoeller SM, Ehmer M, Kleinmann B, Wolter T. CRPS I following artificial disc surgery: case report and review of the literature. Eur Spine J 2011;20(Suppl 2):S278–S283
24. Wolter T, Knöller SM, Rommel O. Complex regional pain syndrome following spine surgery: clinical and prognostic implications. Eur Neurol 2012;68:52–58
25. Devin CJ, McGirt MJ. Best evidence in multimodal pain management in spine surgery and means of assessing postoperative pain and functional outcomes. J Clin Neurosci 2015;22:930–938
26. Garcia RM, Cassinelli EH, Messerschmitt PJ, Furey CG, Bohlman HH. A multimodal approach for postoperative pain management after lumbar decompression surgery: a prospective, randomized study. J Spinal Disord Tech 2013;26:291–297
27. Mathiesen O, Dahl B, Thomsen BA, et al. A comprehensive multimodal pain treatment reduces opioid consumption after multilevel spine surgery. Eur Spine J 2013;22:2089–2096

Recommended Readings

Kramer DL, Booth RE, Albert TJ, et al. Posterior lumbar approach. In: Albert TJ, Balderston RA, Northrup BE, eds. Surgical Approaches to the Spine. Philadelphia: WB Saunders; 1997:173–192

Long D, McAfee PC, eds. Atlas of Spinal Surgery. Baltimore: Williams & Wilkins; 1992:2–22

McLain R. Surgical approaches to the lumbar spine. In: Frymoyer JW, ed. The Adult Spine: Principles and Practice, 2nd ed. Philadelphia: Lippincott-Raven; 1997:1723–1744

Watkins RG. Posterior surgical approaches to the lumbar spine. In: Andersson G, McNeill TW, eds. Lumbar Spinal Stenosis. St. Louis: Mosby; 1992:31–45

91 Open Posterior Lumbar Foraminotomy

Joseph S. Cheng and Nikita Lakomkin

Indications

A foraminotomy is an important procedure for decompression of a symptomatic neural compression of the exiting nerve root by resecting portions of the ligamentum flavum or the superior and inferior articular process, which compose the medial facet joint. It is most commonly performed to treat foraminal stenosis with nerve root compression from the superior articular process and pedicle or from a foraminal disk herniation.[1-5] Less commonly, nerve root compression may result from an osteophyte that originates from the posterior aspect of the vertebral body (**Fig. 91.1**).

The primary goals of a foraminotomy are decompression of the exiting nerve root and preservation of segmental stability, which can typically be achieved by removing a portion of the undersurface of the articular process without violating the integrity of the facet joint proper. As the foramen is bounded by the facet joint, this differs from decompression of the central canal in lumbar stenosis, which does not enter the joint.

Advantages

- Directly addresses the causes of foraminal compression
- Preserves motion segment stability
    - Does not compromise the capsular ligament of the facet joint
    - Does not compromise the posterior tension band (spinous process and interspinous ligaments)
    - Preserves the majority of the facet joint

Disadvantages

- Restricted approach to neural foramen
    - Not applicable to more diffuse pathology
- Narrow operating field compared with larger approaches
- Potential onset of intraoperative epidural venous bleeding
- Potential to destabilize the facet joint

Anatomy

- Boundaries of the intervertebral foramen as noted in a prone position:
    - Superior: cephalad pedicle
    - Inferior: caudal pedicle
    - Roof: superior articular facet and ligamentum flavum
    - Floor: posterior vertebral body and intervertebral disk

The key to successfully performing a foraminotomy is having a thorough understanding of the anatomy of this region (**Fig. 91.2**). The superior boundary of the intervertebral foramen is the caudal surface of the superior pedicle, whereas the inferior boundary is formed by the cephalad surface of the inferior pedicle. The floor of the foramen consists of the posterior border of the cephalad vertebral body, the intervertebral disk, and the uppermost portion of the posterior aspect of the more caudal vertebral body. The roof is formed primarily by the superior articular process and pars interarticularis of the caudal segment, which is covered with the ligamentum flavum forming the anterior surface of the facet zygapophyseal joint capsule. In the lumbar spine, the exiting spinal nerve traverses the upper portion of the foramen, passing beneath its corresponding pedicle; in other words, the L5 nerve root passes beneath the L5 pedicle and exits through the L5-S1 foramen. The sinuvertebral nerve as well as its corresponding artery also passes through the foramen just inferior to the spinal nerve. Additionally, there are several veins that traverse the foramen. The dorsal root ganglion lies in the distal portion of the foramen.

Operative Technique

Positioning, the incision, and the initial exposure technique are discussed in Chapter 90. After proper exposure, a hemilaminotomy is performed centered over the medial facet line, and the ligamentum flavum is removed to enter the epidural space. Small Kerrison punches are used to remove the lateral portion of the ligamentum and extend the dissection as far laterally as possible, as the ligament extends laterally, forming the medial aspect of the facet joint. When gaining lateral exposure, the Kerrison punches should be placed with the footplate paralleling the dura and the mouth up against the ligament or bone to avoid injury to the nerve root. The traversing nerve root shoulder can be visualized, and concordant motion with the Kerrison punch may indicate grasping of the dura in the foramen. The exiting nerve root is typically hidden under the pars interarticularis, and not readily visualized. A Penfield No. 4 dissector is ideal for probing and verifying the plane between the lateral dura of the root sleeve and the lateral ligamentum that is to be removed. Once the ligamentum has been removed, it should be possible to visualize the nerve root winding around the pedicle and the site of compression within the foramen. The foramen can subsequently be probed to assess the extent of narrowing as well as root compression.

After the anatomy has been assessed, the undersurface of the superior articular facet can be removed along with the tip for decompression. This maneuver can be accomplished in several ways. Perhaps the simplest method is to use small angled Kerrison punches with a thin footplate. This footplate is inserted under the lip of the superior articular process and ligamentum flavum, and the portion of this structure is removed (**Fig. 91.2**). A second

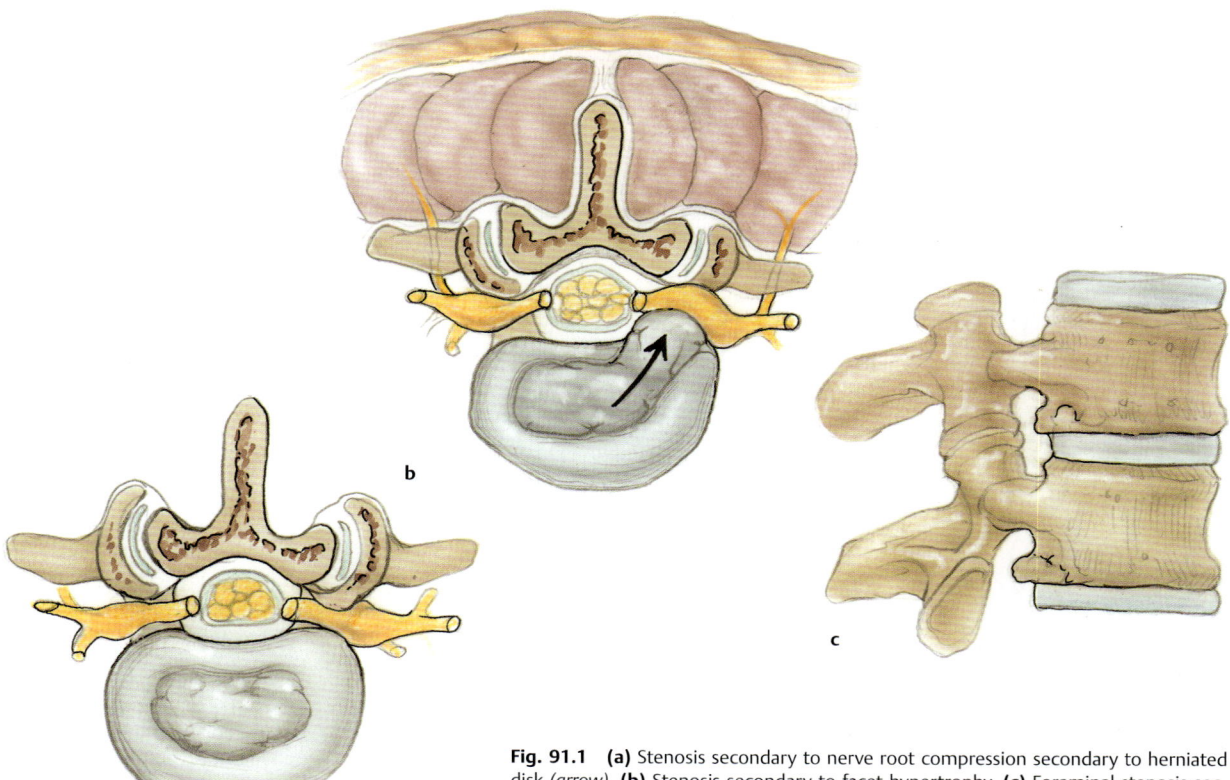

Fig. 91.1 **(a)** Stenosis secondary to nerve root compression secondary to herniated disk *(arrow)*. **(b)** Stenosis secondary to facet hypertrophy. **(c)** Foraminal stenosis secondary to foraminal osteophyte.

method for a foraminotomy is with the use of small osteotomes. This technique is similar to Ponte osteotomies with facet joint resection, but here, the osteotome is used instead of the drill to remove the medial portion of the articular process before grad-ually thinning the pedicle until the nerve root has been adequately decompressed (**Fig. 91.3a**). This technique involves removing thin slivers of bone; if one attempts to remove large portions, it becomes easy to fracture the zygapophyseal joint or the pedicle. It is important that fragments of bone not be driven into the nerve root or left in the foramen, which may cause residual compression. A third method of bone removal involves the use of a high-speed drill (**Fig. 91.3b**). This is the preferred method of many, including ourselves, and it is combined with the Kerrison rongeurs to complete the foraminotomy. If one elects to use a drill, it is critical that the nerve root and thecal sac be protected at all times either by leaving the ligamentum flavum until the bone work is completed, or with gentle retraction of the root medially. An appropriate cutting bur is then carefully used to complete the medial facetectomy, using a Kerrison to resect the superior articular processes tip to create sufficient space for the exiting nerve root. As bone is progressively removed and there becomes less compression on the nerve root, one may observe the root migrating laterally and the tension on the root lessening (**Fig. 91.3c**). Once decompression of the nerve root has been completed, the foramen is probed once more to assess the adequacy of the decompression (**Fig. 91.4**). If the foramen has been satisfactorily enlarged, the probe should pass easily, and it is used to palpate the region of the missing superior articular facet and ligamentum flavum. When the procedure has been completed, closure proceeds in a fashion identical to that described in Chapter 90.

Complications

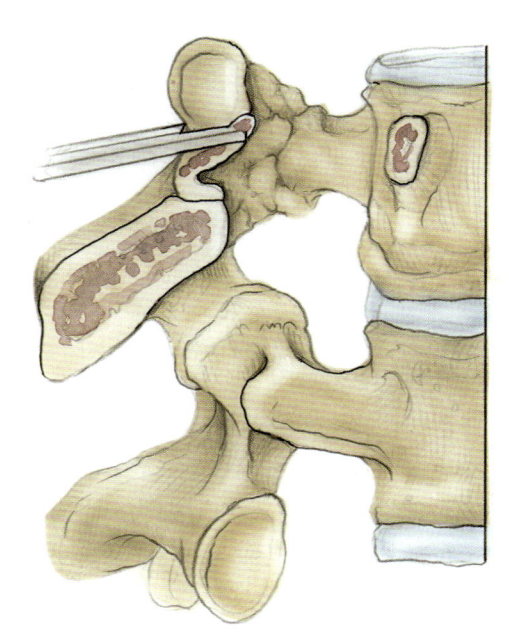

Fig. 91.2 Illustration depicting the anatomy of the foramen with a pathological process.

General complications that may arise after a lumbar foraminotomy are similar to those detailed for other types of spine surgeries.

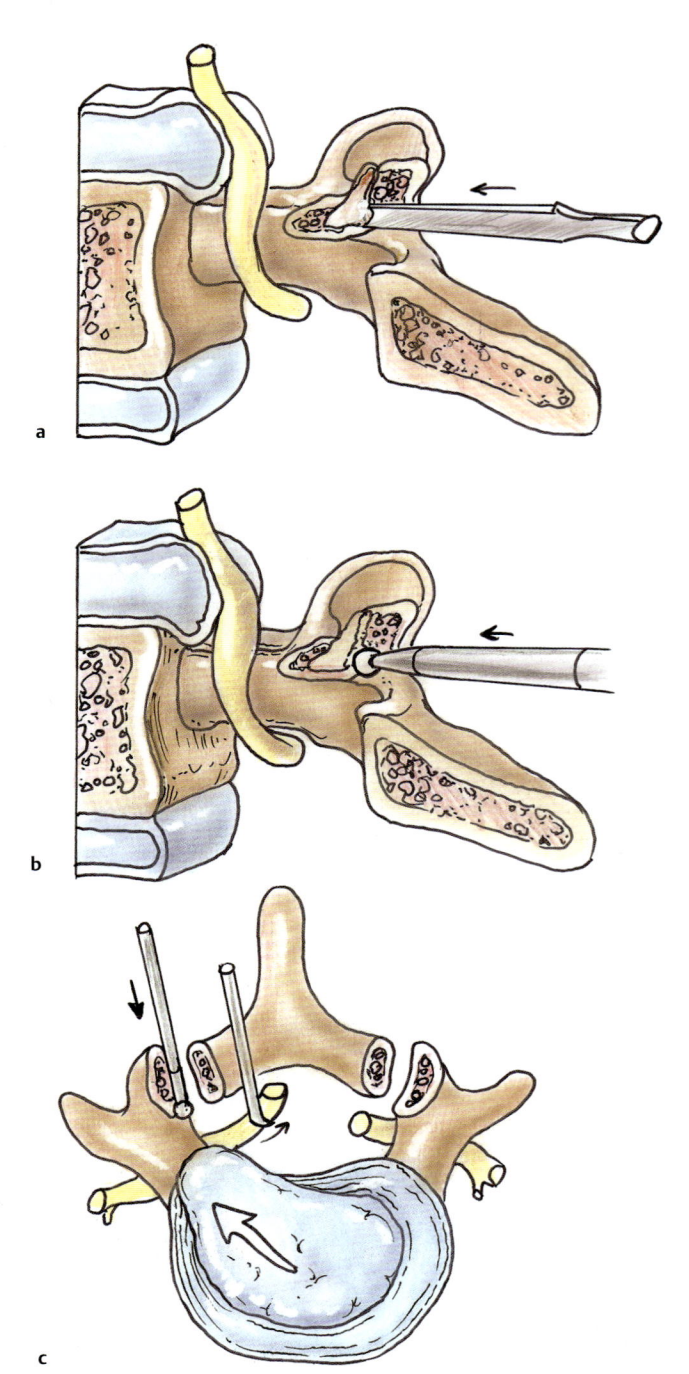

Fig. 91.3 **(a)** An osteotome is used to remove the inferior one half to two thirds of the superior articular process. **(b)** A high-speed drill can also be used to remove the bone. **(c)** As bone is progressively removed and compression on the nerve root lessens, one can actually observe the root migrate laterally and the tension on the root decrease.

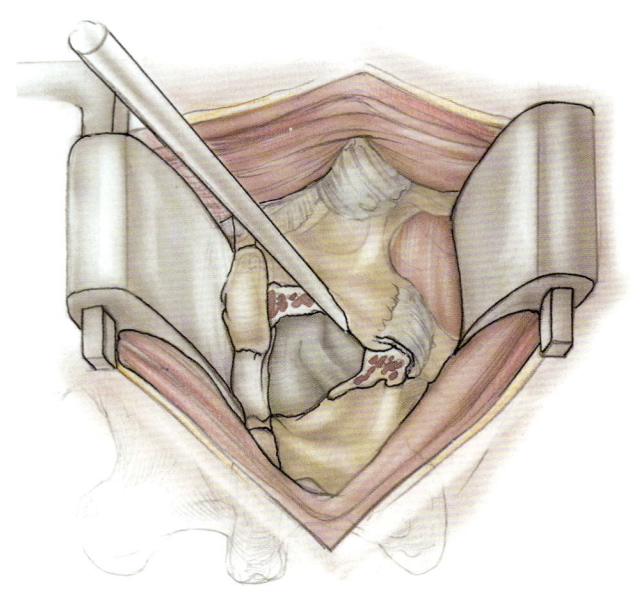

Fig. 91.4 After decompression of the foramen, the foramen is probed with a Penfield No. 4 instrument.

Infection, deep vein thrombosis (DVT), and damage to neural tissues may occur. The incidence of postoperative infection may be reduced via the use of prophylactic antibiotics, as described in Chapter 94, whereas nerve damage can almost always be avoided through meticulous attention to proper operative technique. The potential risks of developing DVT are typically mitigated through the implementation of early physical therapy (to reduce patient inactivity) as well as the use of anticoagulants. However, delayed complications should be noted if the resection thins the pars interarticularis too much, or there is too much resection of the facet joint, leading to the joint becoming unstable. The patient would present with mechanical back pain, and studies such as magnetic resonance imaging would show spondylolisthesis or fluid within the facet joint or facet diastasis, with the possible need for a fusion for stability.

References

1. Kramer DL, Booth RE, Albert TJ, et al. Posterior lumbar approach. In: Albert TJ, Balderston RA, Northrup BE, eds. Surgical Approaches to the Spine. Philadelphia: WB Saunders; 1997:173–192
2. Long D, McAfee PC, eds. Atlas of Spinal Surgery. Baltimore: Williams & Wilkins; 1992:2–22
3. Watkins RG. Posterior surgical approaches to the lumbar spine. In: Andersson G, McNeill TW, eds. Lumbar Spinal Stenosis. St. Louis: Mosby; 1992:31–45
4. McLain R. Surgical approaches to the lumbar spine. In: Frymoyer JW, ed. The Adult Spine: Principles and Practice, 2nd ed. Philadelphia: Lippincott-Raven; 1997:1723–1744
5. Torrens MJ. Lumbar laminectomy. In: Torrens MJ, Dickson RA, eds. Operative Spinal Surgery. Edinburgh: Churchill Livingstone; 1991:119–124

92 Open Posterior Lumbar Hemilaminectomy

Joseph S. Cheng and Peter Morone

Indications

Unilateral laminectomy, also referred to as a hemilaminectomy, is performed in a manner similar to that described for bilateral lumbar laminectomy.[1,2] The major difference is that the dissection is limited to one side of the interspinous ligament. Restricting the exposure to a single side facilitates limiting the size of the initial skin incision, muscle dissection, and bone removal. The primary reason for performing a hemilaminectomy is to create an exposure that enables completion of a foraminotomy, a microdiscectomy, or both. Indications for completing these procedures include foraminal stenosis, unilateral lower extremity weakness, and radiculopathy that does not improve with conservative treatment.

Advantages

- Small skin incision
- Unilateral muscle dissection
- Minimal bone removal

Disadvantages

- Decreased exposure, limiting the operative corridor
- Unable to visualize the complete lamina anatomy
- Increased risk of facet damage secondary to decreased visualization

Operative Technique

Positioning, the incision, and the initial exposure technique are discussed in Chapter 90. The patient is placed in the standard prone position, supported on a standard spinal frame or chest rolls (**Figs. 92.1, 92.2, 92.3**). The abdomen should hang free to avoid increased pressure in the epidural veins, which can lead to increased bleeding during the procedure. Alternatively, some surgeons prefer the lateral decubitus position. This position avoids pressure on the abdomen but can make visualizing the midline anatomy more challenging. Once the patient is properly positioned, prepped, and draped, lateral fluoroscopy is used to locate the appropriate lumbar level to minimize the length of the incision required.

The interlaminar space is now clearly defined along with the inferior edge of the rostral lamina and the inferior edge of the caudal lamina. The ligamentum superior flavum is detached from the inferior surface of the lamina above using a fine curette (**Fig. 92.4**). In some patients, the lamina may overlap significantly and there is essentially no interlaminar space. In these cases, a portion of the inferior lamina may need to be removed with a high-speed drill to gain access to the ligamentum flavum. The most inferior edge of the hemilamina is easily removed with a Leksell rongeur. The ligamentum flavum is detached more cephalad as necessary, and the hemilaminectomy is completed with 45-degree angled Kerrison punches (**Fig. 92.5**). The rostral extent of bone removal required to expose the disk varies from one individual to another and from one spinal level to another.

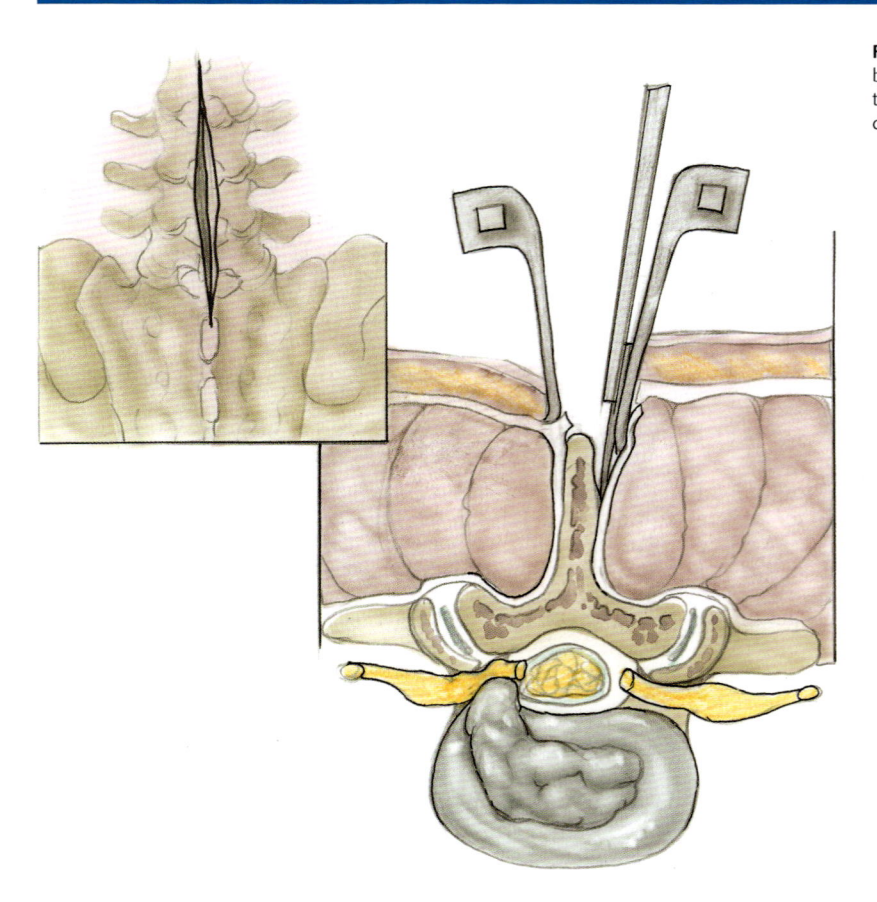

Fig. 92.1 A midline incision *(inset)* over the distance between the spinous process directly above and below the level of pathology is made to retract the lumbodorsal fascia.

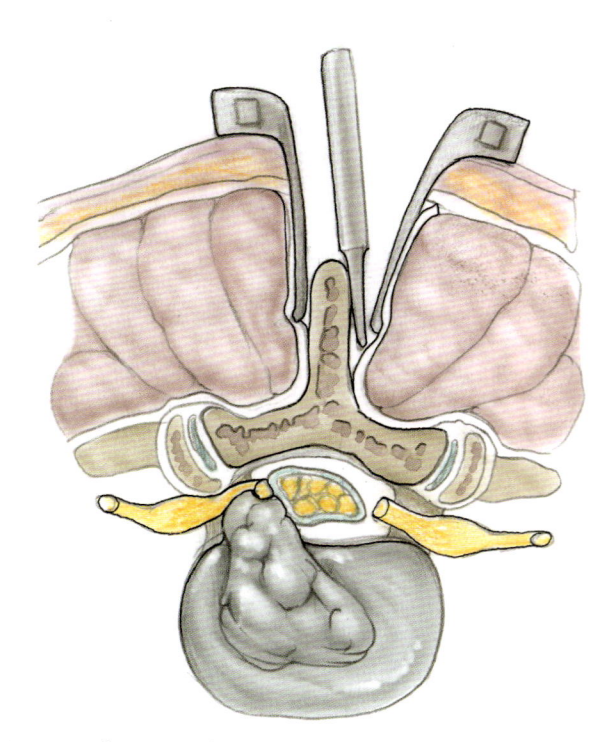

Fig. 92.2 The paraspinal muscles are detached from the spinous process to expose the laminae overlying the herniated disk.

For example, the L5-S1 disk space lies approximately at the level of the interlaminar space. Indeed, some individuals have an extremely large L5-S1 interlaminar space, making bone removal either unnecessary or minimal. However, as one progresses cephalad, the disk space becomes more cephalad in relation to the interlaminar space, and, therefore, exposure requires proportionately more bone removal. Some bone from the medial aspect of the facet or the pars interarticularis may need to be removed to achieve adequate lateral exposure. This is especially important with a large disk herniation to mobilize and retract the nerve root without undue pressure. Although the facet can be undercut to improve lateral exposure, the facet capsule should be preserved. Once the bone removal is complete, a small amount of bone wax applied with a Penfield instrument will easily control bleeding from the bone.

To expose the nerve root and underlying disk, the ligamentum flavum must be removed. This task can be accomplished in several ways; we perform it in the following manner. Using loupe magnification and a headlight (the operating microscope can also be used), the ligamentum flavum is grasped with a fine-toothed forceps and incised longitudinally using a No. 15 blade on a long handle (**Fig. 92.6**). The opening is made at an angle to avoid incising the ligament obliquely. A Penfield No. 4 is then used to further separate the fibers and gently "pop" into the epidural space. At this point, the fibers of the ligamentum flavum can be rather easily split longitudinally to enlarge the opening. A small cottonoid is inserted into the epidural space to protect the dura, and a generous window of ligament is excised. Additional ligament can then be removed using Kerrison rongeurs.

Fig. 92.3 (a) The paraspinal muscles are retracted laterally (b) using a Gelpi-Meyerding retractor that is anchored in the interspinous ligament.

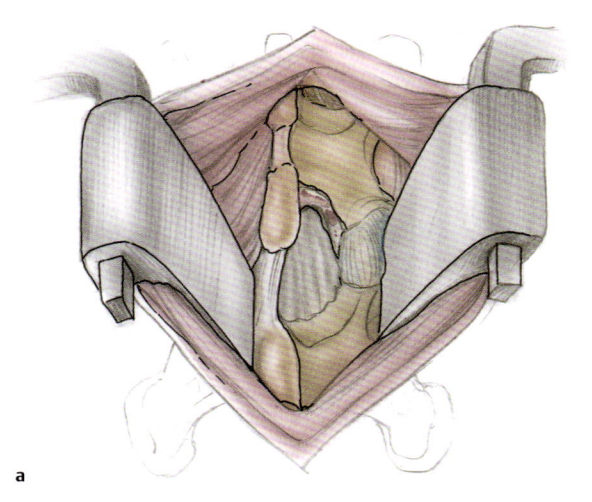

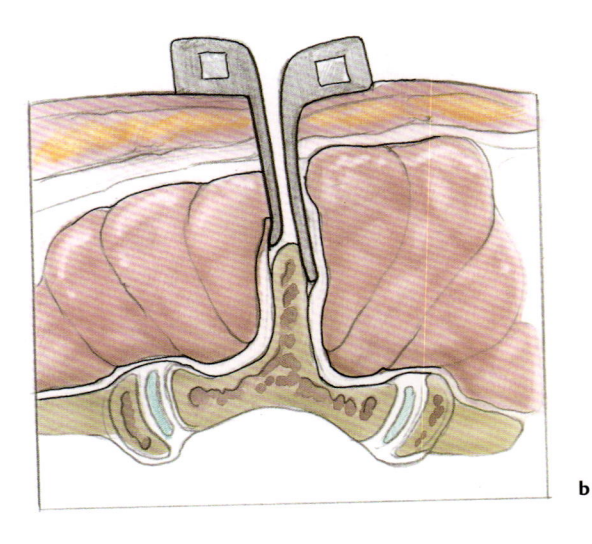

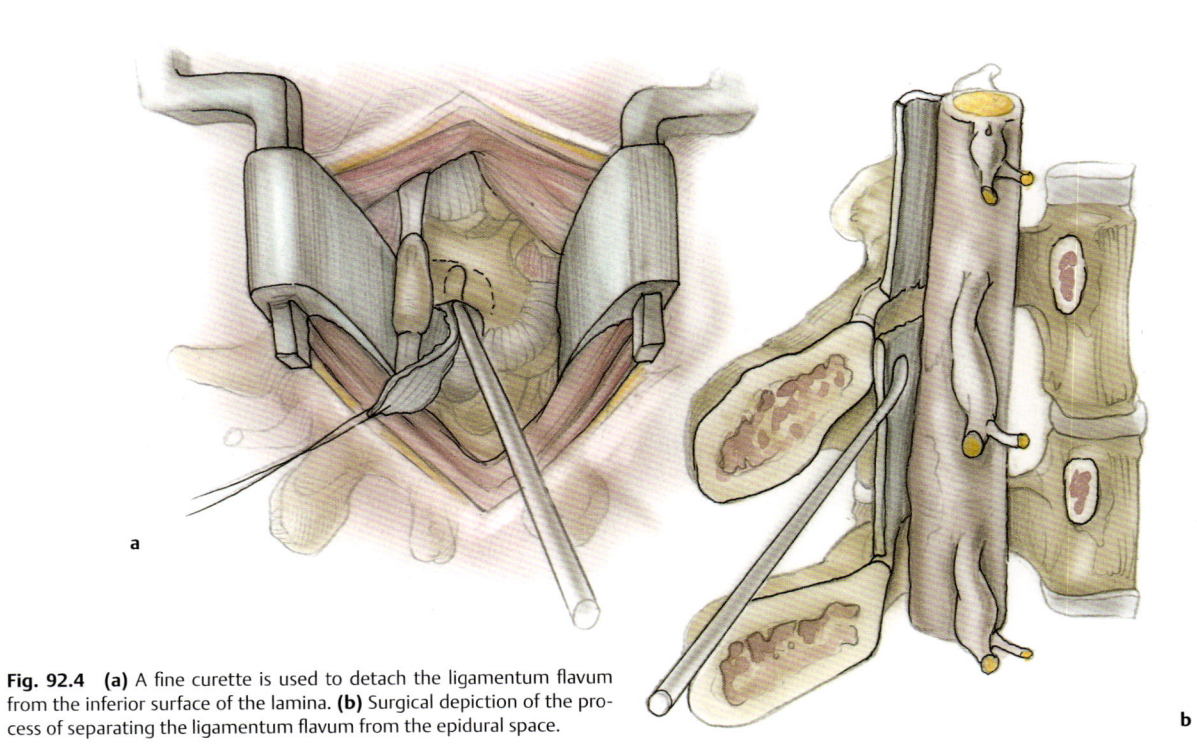

Fig. 92.4 (a) A fine curette is used to detach the ligamentum flavum from the inferior surface of the lamina. (b) Surgical depiction of the process of separating the ligamentum flavum from the epidural space.

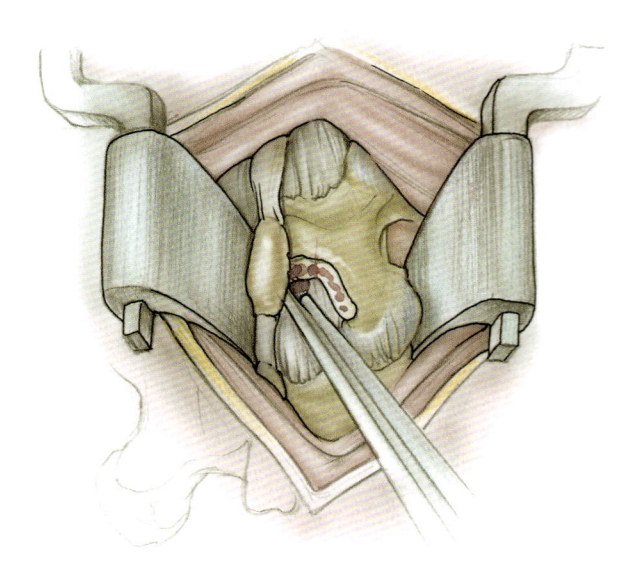

Fig. 92.5 A Kerrison punch is used at a 45-degree angle to complete the hemilaminectomy.

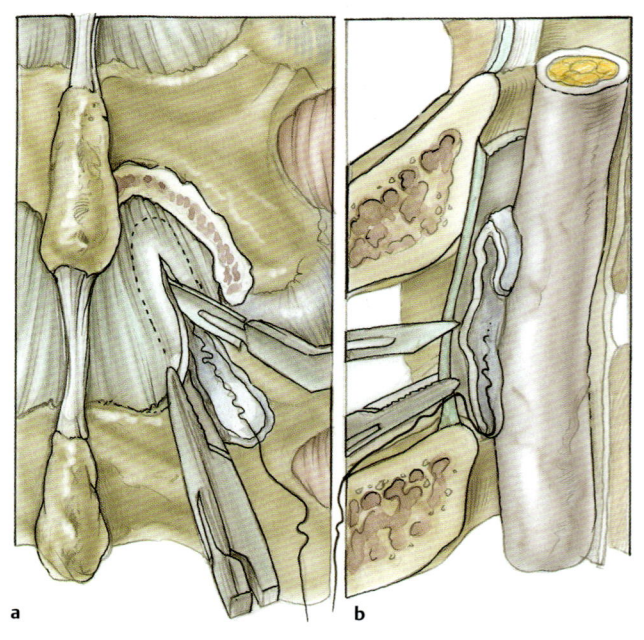

Fig. 92.6 The ligamentum flavum is secured with a toothed forceps **(a)** and the ligamentum flavum is incised longitudinally using a No. 15 blade **(b)**.

Complications

- Skin stretching and contusion secondary to a combination of a small incision and ample retraction
- When removing ligamentum flavum, extreme medial removal of ligament is not advised because placement of the footplate of the Kerrison medially has been known to produce dural tears outside the extent of the bony opening. This type of durotomy may go unnoticed at surgery and only become apparent when the patient returns postoperatively with cerebrospinal fluid (CSF) drainage from the incision or complaining of postural headaches and is discovered to have a pseudomeningocele.
- During lateral bony removal, disruption of the facet capsule can lead to significant, sometimes disabling, postoperative back pain. If the facet capsule and facet joint are damaged, it is often better to perform a complete medial facetectomy because this is less likely to cause significant postoperative back pain than is leaving a damaged unstable joint. As long as the contralateral facet is intact, unilateral facetectomy theoretically should not result in spinal instability.
- During rostral bony removal, ensure that the pars interarticularis is not violated. This structure must be preserved to maintain the stability of the motion segment.

References

1. Kempe L. Lumbar radiculoneuropathy: herniated intervertebral disk. In: Kempe L, ed. Operative Neurosurgery, vol 2. Berlin: Springer-Verlag; 1970:266–276
2. Hitchon P, Traynelis V. Lumbar hemilaminectomy for excision of a herniated disk. In: Rengechary SS, Wilkins RH, eds. Neurosurgical Operative Atlas, vol 1. Baltimore: Williams& Wilkins; 1991:135–140

93 Open Posterior Lumbar Microdiskectomy

Joseph S. Cheng and Scott L. Zuckerman

Indications

A lumbar diskectomy remains one of the most common procedures performed by neurosurgeons for nerve root compression and radiculopathy. Although the goals of the procedure remain the same, that is, performing either a diskectomy or fragmentectomy for decompression or removal of the offending disk herniation, the techniques have significantly evolved and include the use of minimally invasive techniques. Larger incisions and exposures for removal of a disk herniation have largely been supplanted by smaller, less invasive procedures. Lumbar microdiskectomy has become the norm rather than the exception.[1–3] As well, more minimally invasive techniques, such as percutaneous automated diskectomy and endoscopic diskectomy, are gaining more popularity and being presented as alternative options to the standard open microdiskectomy. However, open lumbar microdiskectomy still remains the gold standard, with its excellent outcomes against which other techniques must be compared, as the newer techniques accomplish the same goal with different techniques for access to the pathology.

Given the varying nomenclature used for lumbar diskectomies, clarification of the terminology is needed. For purposes of Current Procedural Terminology (CPT) coding, the definition of the procedure is based on the approach and visualization. That is, the primary approach and visualization defines the service, and a lumbar microdiskectomy is typically considered open unless otherwise specified. The following terms are used:

- Percutaneous: image-guided procedures (e.g., computed tomography [CT] or fluoroscopy) performed with indirect visualization of the spine without the use of a device that enables visualization through a surgical incision
- Endoscopic: spinal procedures performed with continuous direct visualization of the spine through an endoscope
- Open: spinal procedures performed with continuous direct visualization of the spine through a surgical opening
- Indirect visualization: image-guided (e.g., CT or fluoroscopy), not light-based visualization
- Direct visualization: light-based visualization; can be seen by the naked eye, or with surgical loupes, a microscope, or an endoscope

Even an open procedure such as a microdiskectomy can use microsurgical techniques and instrumentation for removal of a lumbar disk or a specific technique designated as microlumbar diskectomy (MLD), as introduced in 1977 by Williams.[3] Although microdiskectomy using the operating microscope and microsurgical instrumentation for removal of a lumbar disk imposes specific restraints on the technique, MLD is noted as an exact microsurgical technique specifically for initial "soft" disk herniations in patients with otherwise normal lumbar spinal canal, as depicted on CT or magnetic resonance imaging (MRI), to eliminate the most common tissue morbidities that are observed in patients following failed back surgery (**Box 93.1**). It should be acknowledged that most neurosurgeons do not perform a true MLD.

Box 93.1 Technical Parameters to Eliminate Tissue Morbidities of Failed Back Surgery

- Minimal radiographically localized midline skin incision
- No muscle incision or muscle suturing
- Absolute minimal removal of lamina and ligamentum flavum
- Complete preservation of epidural fat
- Constant visualization of the nerve root
- No annular incision
- No curettage of intervertebral disk
- No electrocoagulation in epidural space
- No foreign substances left in the spinal canal

Advantages

- Common procedure
- Minimal tissue disruption
- More familiar anatomy
- Wider exposure
- Avoid fusion

Disadvantages

- Limited application
- Potential for nerve root injury
- Potential for facet damage
- Small operating window than full laminectomy

Operative Technique

Preoperative Assessment

Understanding the anatomy of the disk helps determine the goal of the surgery to be performed. The surgical approach for a microdiskectomy for a free fragment of nucleus pulposus (NP) with associated inflammatory response as a cause of low back pain and radiculopathy may be much different than the surgical approach for a microdiskectomy for a protruding annulus fibrosus (AF) causing nerve root compression. As well, indications for a microdiskectomy alone without surgical stabilization depend on the expected natural history after surgery. The stability of the AF and its 10 to 20 densely packed concentric rings of collagen, and the state of the cartilaginous end plate and whether it enables continued passive diffusion of nutrients to the disk will factor into the iatrogenic changes and instability introduced to the desiccated disk.[4] The natural history is important for surgical planning, as when we age, pathological movement occurs, and the end plates become sclerosed, inhibiting diffusion to the disk. The NP loses its growth factors and nutrition, and loses its water content in place of fibrous material. This fibrous transformation places undue pressure on the AF, causing the thick cartilaginous rings to tear, as this was not their original function. As the AF tears, disk prolapse occurs. Disks can either bulge (where the annulus is intact), herniate (where the annulus tears and the disk protrudes), or become sequestered (the herniation is completely separate from the disk). In terms of classification, several gross pathological and radiographic grading scales exist. The Thompson classification[5] assesses gross disk appearance, the Pfirrmann classification[6] assesses disk appearance on magnetic resonance imaging (MRI), and the Modic classification[7] determines endplate changes associated with disk herniation.

The way to assess a possible symptomatic disk herniation is with an MRI. The T2 sequence can be used to determine the thecal sac and nerve root effacement, and the T1 sequence assesses the amount of epidural fat in the foramen; a disk compressing the foramen will have little to no fat in the foramen. On physical exam, a positive straight leg test is sensitive, whereas a contralateral straight leg test is more specific for a disk herniation. The type of disk herniation is crucial to successful operative treatment, and there are several types. Disks can be central, paracentral, foraminal, or lateral.[3] Foraminal herniations often present with intractable pain due to pressure on the dorsal root ganglion (DRG) and may require a far lateral approach rather than the open microdiskectomy technique. Furthermore, coronal location of the disk must be assessed.[3] Does the disk travel upward or downward, and is a pediculotomy needed for access to the disk? Intradural risks are rare, but should always be in the differential, as they often cannot be seen on imaging and can be verified only during the operation.[2]

Positioning

The lumbar microdiskectomy is typically performed with the patient prone and supported by a standard spinal frame. Frames that lessen the lumbar lordosis, such as the Wilson frame, will open up the interlaminar space and facilitate access. With any prone spinal position, one must be cautious about eye pressure and the rare incidence of blindness, which can be catastrophic.[8-10] The frames allow the abdomen to hang free to reduce the intraabdominal pressure, and thus the pressure within the epidural venous plexus and the associated bleeding in the surgical field. Along with standard sterile prep of the lumbar spine, localization of the spinal level for placement of the incision is performed typically with C-arm fluoroscopy or intraoperative X-rays. The lateral view of the spine with counting of the spine from the sacrum is recommended to mark the correct level, which highlights the importance of preoperative plain films to compare with for level localization. You need to be aware of congenital findings such as lumbarization of the sacrum or sacralization of the lumbar spine, in addition to anomalous ribs that may lead to misinterpreting the correct spinal level.

Operation

Positioning, the incision, and the initial exposure technique are discussed in Chapter 90. The interlaminar space and adjacent laminae should now be readily visible. Before proceeding with any bone removal, the level is again confirmed with fluoroscopy. The ligamentum flavum is detached from the surface of the inferior lamina, as it attaches at the edge unlike the superior lamina, using a fine curette. A hemilaminotomy is performed with Kerrison rongeurs taking the ligamentum flavum as it turns into the medial facet joint capsule. If a drill is preferred for the hemilaminotomy, this may be done before the ligamentum flavum is violated to help protect the dura underneath. The extent of the bone removal for the hemilaminotomy is determined by the location of the disk fragment or the level of the disk herniation. Depending on the cranial/caudal location, more of the superior lamina or inferior lamina is taken off to access the herniated elements. The rostral extent of the hemilaminectomy required varies from one spinal level to another. For example, the L5-S1 disk space lies approximately at the level of the interlaminar space. However, as one progresses cephalad, the disk space becomes more cephalad in relation to the interlaminar space and, therefore, exposure requires proportionally more bone removal. Some bone from the medial aspect of the facet or the pars interarticularis may need to be removed to achieve adequate lateral exposure of the underlying disk. This is especially important with large disk herniations to mobilize and retract the nerve root without undue pressure. However, it is important to watch the amount of pars remaining to avoid an iatrogenic or delayed pars fracture and subsequent spondylolysis.

From here on, magnification and additional illumination are utilized. This can be accomplished with the operating microscope or using surgical loupes and a headlight. Next, the ligamentum flavum is further removed to access to the epidural space. Although the ligamentum flavum can be incised longitudinally at the L5-S1 level, the sharp curette is typically used to separate out the insertion of the ligament and bone. Keeping the pressure of the curette against the bone decreases the risk of a durotomy. A Penfield No. 4 dissector can also be employed using a gentle sliding motion to further separate the fibers and gently "pop" into the epidural space. At this point, the fibers of the ligamentum flavum can be rather easily split longitudinally to enlarge the opening. It is now possible to insert a small cottonoid or pledget of Gelfoam into the epidural space to displace the thecal sac and protect the dura. In cases in which there is an extremely large disk protrusion that pushes the neural elements dorsally against the ligamentum flavum, this step may not be feasible. A generous window of ligament is excised. Additional ligament can then be removed laterally using Kerrison rongeurs to get lateral to the nerve root. It should be remembered that the ligamentum constitutes a portion of the medial wall of the facet joint capsule, and therefore as the ligamentum is removed, caution must be exercised not to open the facet capsule. Removal of only the needed ligament for decompression and access is recommended, as placement of the footplate of the Kerrison has been known to produce dural tears outside the extent of the bony opening. Indeed, these may sometimes go unnoticed at surgery and only become apparent when the patient returns postoperatively with cerebrospinal fluid (CSF) drainage from the incision or complaining of postural headaches and is discovered to have a pseudomeningocele.

Once the ligamentum flavum has been removed, the epidural space is explored with the purpose of identifying the nerve root (**Fig. 93.1**). The root is usually seen as a white tubular structure with minute vasculature visible on the surface. The nerve root may be displaced either laterally or medially by disk herniations,

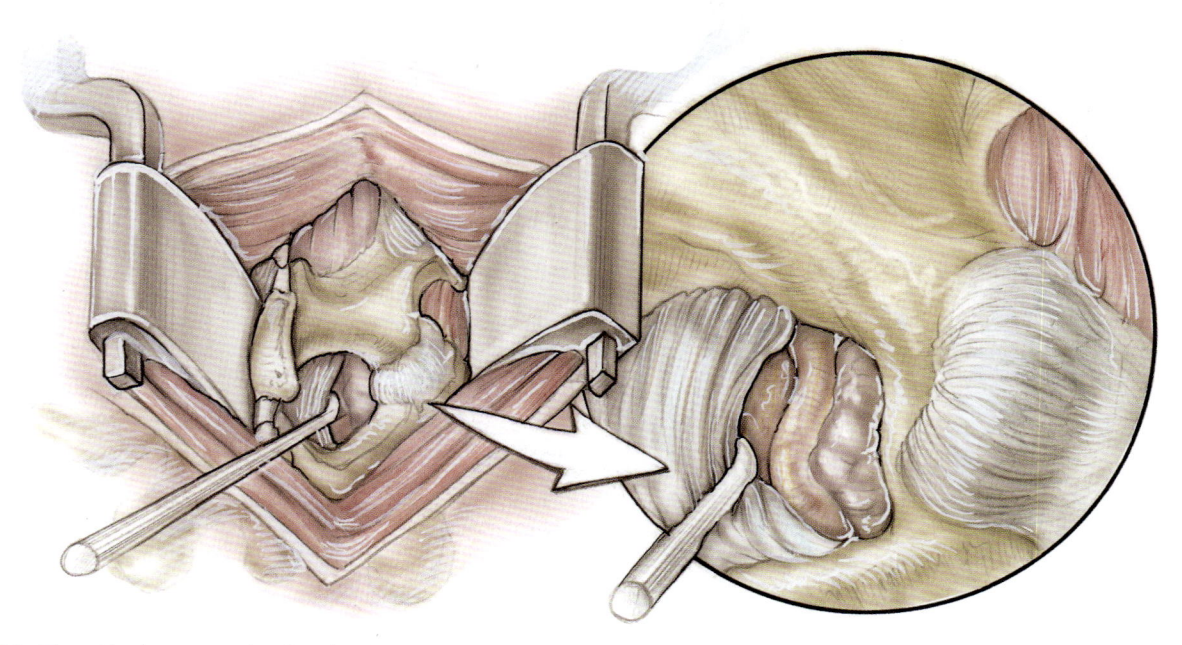

Fig. 93.1 The epidural space is explored to identify the nerve root.

and it is crucial that it be unequivocally identified prior to attempting removal of any disk material. The epidural fat overlying the thecal sac and nerve root can be gently separated and teased out of the way using a Penfield dissector. Epidural veins should be individually coagulated with bipolar cautery on a low setting and sharply divided with microscissors. However, excessive use of the cautery in the epidural space is discouraged. Using a blunt dissector, the lateral gutter of the spinal canal is palpated as far cephalad as possible. By beginning cephalad, one can avoid inadvertent entry into the axilla of a laterally displaced and stretched nerve root. The nerve root is then gently retracted medially and is maintained in this position using a nerve root retractor. This maneuver exposes the underlying disk herniation. If a free fragment of disk material is identified it is removed. If no free fragments are seen, the posterior longitudinal ligament and annulus are then incised in a cruciate fashion and the interspace is entered. Disk material often extrudes spontaneously and this is removed (**Figs. 93.2 and 93.3**). Any disk material that is free in the interspace is also removed. Additional disk material may be freed up by scraping the vertebral end plates with a variety of curettes. We are not convinced that this adds any protection against recurrent disk herniation, and we do not perform this as a routine practice. Moreover, we believe that patients in whom the end plates have been aggressively and excessive scraped suffer significantly more postoperative back pain than patients in whom this step is not performed.

At this point, the spinal canal is explored, looking for any additional free fragments of disk material. Exploration is also performed in the neural foramen above and below the nerve root. This must be done with extreme vigilance in order not to push an occult fragment of disk material further out into the foramen. Then a Valsalva maneuver is performed, and the thecal sac and nerve root are carefully inspected for evidence of a CSF leak. The use of epidural narcotics or steroids at this point has been reported, and should be tailored to the clinical needs of the patient. Placement of a pledget of Gelfoam or fat graft over the nerve root may help prevent epidural fibrosis to the musculature posteriorly. However, the utility of this and whether this truly prevents epidural fibrosis and subsequent recurrent pain is of some question. The wound is then closed in a fashion identical to that described in the previous chapters.

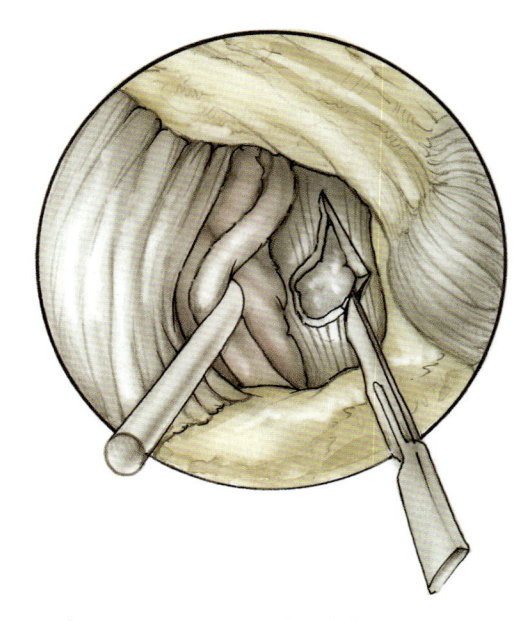

Fig. 93.2 The nerve root is retracted medially to expose the herniated disk. The posterior longitudinal ligament and annulus are incised and the disk interspace is exposed.

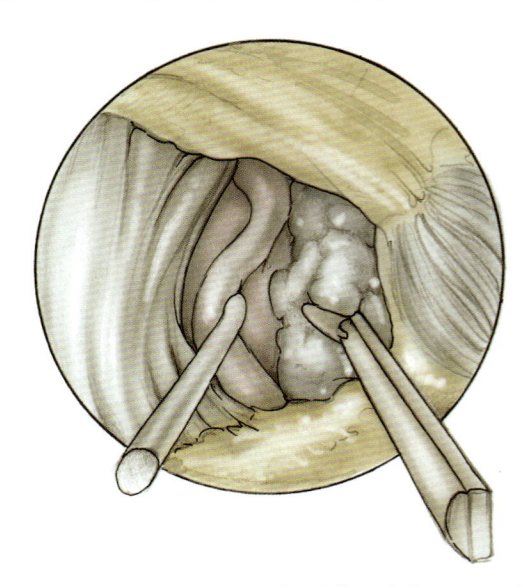

Fig. 93.3 The disk material is removed to sufficiently decompress the neural elements.

Complications

When using a small incision and working in a deep hole, complications can occur. The surgeon can be fooled by the ease of a diskectomy, compared with other more complex, multilevel fusions or deformity corrections. There is nothing worse than underestimating an operation and dealing with an avoidable complication.

During the bony removal, too much of the facet or pars interarticularis can be removed, leading to destabilization of the region. One should avoid removing more than 50% of the facet or pars to preclude needing a subsequent fusion in the future. As is the case with any spine decompression, a durotomy can occur. If repairable, it is best practice to close it primarily with a nonabsorbable suture such as Nurolon. Castro Viejo needle holders may be needed if the operative site is small and deep. Durotomies can be unrepairable if lateral in the foramen. In this case, we prefer to use a mechanical hemostat such as Gelfoam, being mindful of the expansion that will occur, and we close the deep muscle with silk sutures to create a contained pseudomeningocele. Dural sealants can also be used such as DuraSeal (Covidien, Waltham, MA) or Tisseel (Baxter Healthcare Corp., Mountain Home, AR), but does not replace the need for a good closure of the tissue layers.

Nerve root injury can be a serious complication, and it occurs when the nerve root is mistaken for a disk herniation, especially if it is displaced posteriorly. A conjoined nerve root should also be looked for on MRI scan, as the traversing root may lie across the disk space. Cases of spondylolisthesis can push the nerve root toward the operative field, higher than expected, and the surgeon should be wary of this scenario as well. Before the disk is incised, feeling with a Penfield No. 4 or Woodson dental tool is recommended to identify the relevant anatomy and avoid this complication. A life-threatening complication can be vascular damage through the disk space. Damage to the iliac arteries and veins can be encountered during the diskectomy portion of the case. Often when scraping the disk space, the surgeon loses sight of the depth, and these major vessels can be lacerated.[1,11] The damage is often not realized until the patient is flipped supine, and the vessels are no longer tamponaded by the prone positioning and hip rolls. Immediate hypotension is seen, and an emergent call to general surgery for open or endovascular repair must be done expediently.

References

1. Canaud L, Hireche K, Joyeux F, et al. Endovascular repair of aorto-iliac artery injuries after lumbar-spine surgery. Eur J Vasc Endovasc Surg 2011;42:167–171
2. Ducati LG, Silva MV, Brandão MM, Romero FR, Zanini MA. Intradural lumbar disc herniation: report of five cases with literature review. Eur Spine J 2013;22(Suppl 3):S404–S408
3. Williams RW. Microlumbar discectomy: a conservative surgical approach to the virgin herniated lumbar disc. Spine 1978;3(2):175–182
4. Grunhagen T, Wilde G, Soukane DM, Shirazi-Adl SA, Urban JP. Nutrient supply and intervertebral disc metabolism. J Bone Joint Surg Am 2006; 88(Suppl 2):30–35
5. Thompson JP, Pearce RH, Schechter MT, Adams ME, Tsang IK, Bishop PB. Preliminary evaluation of a scheme for grading the gross morphology of the human intervertebral disc. Spine 1990;15:411–415
6. Pfirrmann CW, Metzdorf A, Zanetti M, Hodler J, Boos N. Magnetic resonance classification of lumbar intervertebral disc degeneration. Spine 2001;26:1873–1878
7. Modic MT, Steinberg PM, Ross JS, Masaryk TJ, Carter JR. Degenerative disk disease: assessment of changes in vertebral body marrow with MR imaging. Radiology 1988;166(1 Pt 1):193–199
8. Nickels TJ, Manlapaz MR, Farag E. Perioperative visual loss after spine surgery. World J Orthop 2014;5:100–106
9. Stambough JL, Dolan D, Werner R, Godfrey E. Ophthalmologic complications associated with prone positioning in spine surgery. J Am Acad Orthop Surg 2007;15:156–165
10. Zimmerer S, Koehler M, Turtschi S, Palmowski-Wolfe A, Girard T. Amaurosis after spine surgery: survey of the literature and discussion of one case. Eur Spine J 2011;20:171–176
11. van Zitteren M, Fan B, Lohle PN, et al. A shift toward endovascular repair for vascular complications in lumbar disc surgery during the last decade. Ann Vasc Surg 2013;27:810–819

94 Open Posterior Lumbar Laminectomy

Joseph S. Cheng and Michael D. Dewan

Indications

An open posterior lumbar laminectomy is commonly performed not only for access to the spinal canal, such as for the treatment of tumors, fractures, abscesses, and interbody fusions, but also for decompression of the cauda equina and nerve roots in a patient with lumbar stenosis. The specific type of lumbar stenosis determines the decompression needed, and hence the surgical technique and structures resected. In central canal stenosis, which typically is associated with neurogenic claudication, the laminectomy may span across bilateral medial facet lines with minimal risk of instability as the facet joints are not affected. For lateral recess stenosis, a medial facetectomy is needed to decompress this region from the medial facet line to the medial pedicle border. For foraminal stenosis, which frequently presents with radiculopathy, the surgical technique may require a complete facetectomy to decompress the affected nerve root with a concomitant need for a fusion procedure for the iatrogenic instability caused. This is also seen if the lumbar laminectomy is associated with a more radical exposure, such as a transpedicular or lateral extracavitary approach, or if the lumbar compression is multifactorial (**Box 94.1**). Overall, the extent of the decompression should be tailored to the individual patient. This chapter focuses on the treatment of degenerative spinal stenosis.[1–6]

Box 94.1 Anatomic Factors Contributing to Lumbar Spinal Stenosis

- Congenitally short pedicles
- Facet joint hypertrophy (usually the superior facet)
- Disk space narrowing with upward migration of the superior articular process into the neural foramen
- Acute herniated disk superimposed on an already narrowed canal
- Chronic calcified disk
- Disk margin osteophyte
- Thickening of ligamentum flavum
- Synovial cyst formation
- Degenerative spondylolisthesis

Advantages

- Familiar approach
- Direct access to posterior pathology
- Wide exposure relative to other decompressive techniques

Disadvantages

- Laminectomy is often coupled with partial or complete facetectomy to achieve adequate decompression of the thecal sac and nerve roots.
- May result in spinal instability if the facet joints are disrupted
- Relative to less invasive techniques, involves more extensive dissection and disruption of posterior muscular and ligamentous complexes

Operative Technique

Positioning, the incision, and the initial exposure technique are discussed in Chapter 90. Placement of the lumbar spine into kyphosis, such as with the use of a Wilson frame or sling to flex the hips, may facilitate the exposure of the interlaminar space at the expense of giving the surgeon a false sense of decompression. If there is a concern about adequate decompression, such as for lateral recess decompression, then keeping the patient in lordosis may provide a smaller operating corridor but reflect the natural position of the spine.

After completing the exposure (**Fig. 94.1**), the spinous processes are first removed at the levels to be decompressed. As lumbar stenosis is centered at the motion segment of the spine, the decompression is typically performed at the interspace so that the inferior portion of the spinous process of the level above and the superior portion of the spinous process of the level below are resected to access the ligamentum flavum. This is easily accomplished using a large rongeur or a Horsley bone cutter (**Fig. 94.2**). With either tool, one must avoid biting too deep to avoid entering the posterior spinal canal with the potential for dural injury with cerebrospinal fluid (CSF) leakage or injury to the cauda equina.

The ligamentum flavum is then detached from the inferior aspect of the lamina with a sharp curette where it inserts into

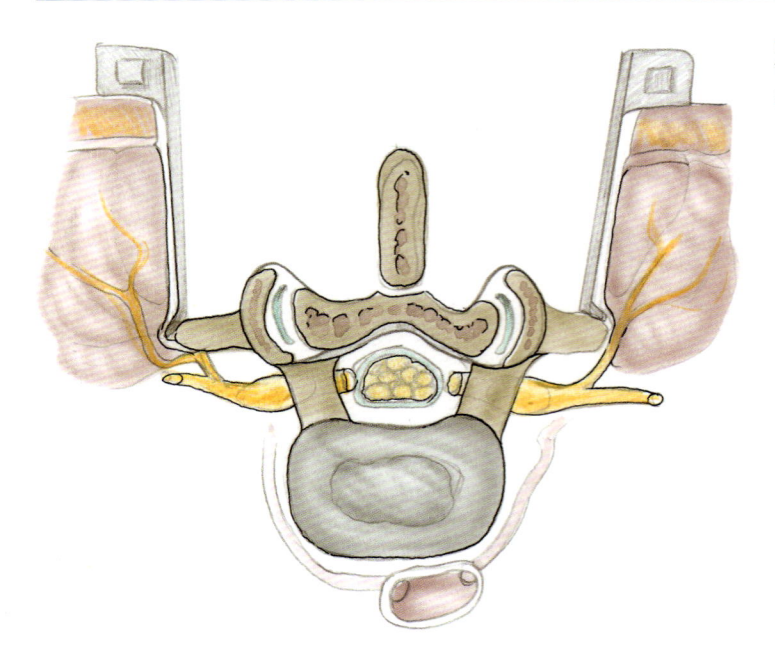

Fig. 94.1 The exposed anatomy of the intertransverse space. The dissection should not go beyond the tip of the transverse process to avoid injury.

the bone (**Fig. 94.3**). A large Leksell rongeur can be used for the initial portion of the laminectomy, with the lower blade placed just beneath the leading inferior edge of the lamina 30 degrees from the vertical or 60 degrees to the long axis of the spine (**Fig. 94.4**). Maintaining the instrument at this angle helps prevent insertion of the lower blade too deep into the spinal canal. Removal of each side is performed in turn, and additional ligamentum flavum is removed as necessary. As the pedicle is approached, the lamina tends to become thicker, and substitution of a narrower instrument facilitates bone removal. Creating a trough with a central laminectomy facilitates removal of the more lateral portions of the lamina and medial facets on each side using a series of Kerrison rongeurs. In many patients, the ligamentum flavum can be removed along with the bone by first separating the ligamentum from the dura. Note that in patients with significant stenosis, the ligamentum (or, in the case of a redo decompression, scar tissue) is not uncommonly adherent to the underlying dura and associated with a CSF leak if the ligamentum has not been completely separated from the dura. This technique can be accomplished by sharp dissection using a scalpel while protecting the underlying dura with a dural elevator (**Fig. 94.5**).

The preceding bone removal produces a central decompression between the medial facet lines. In patients with severe spinal stenosis, this often may not be adequate, and further lateral decompression with undercutting of the facet is required for a medial facetectomy. This is most easily accomplished using 45-degree Kerrison punches (2, 3, and 4 mm). The plane between the ligamentum flavum and the dura should be clearly identified before inserting the footplate of the instrument to avoid dural tears and injury to the nerve roots (**Fig. 94.6**). If possible, the epidural fat should be preserved, although there is often a paucity of fat in patients with very severe stenosis. If epidural bleeding occurs, it should be controlled with warm irrigation, hemostatic agents (Gelfoam, thrombin, Surgicel, etc.) and gentle tamponade, but care should be taken not to create iatrogenic stenosis. Bipolar cautery may be used to address discrete bleeding vessels, although it should be done only after ensuring separation from nearby thecal sac and nerve roots.

Laminectomy performed with high-speed drills has become a popular technique. Indeed, careful use of a drill in experienced hands can greatly facilitate the operation. Conversely, improper use of such an instrument can result in significant morbidity such as dural tears and injury to the cauda equina. There are two basic methods of removing bone using a high-speed drill. The first is to progressively thin the lamina to the thickness of an eggshell using a large cutting bit and then removing the remaining bone in the standard fashion already described (**Fig. 94.7**). The other, and perhaps riskier, technique involves en-bloc removal of the lamina using a footplate inserted beneath the edge of the lamina (**Fig. 94.8**). This technique is not only more dangerous but is probably ill advised in patients with significant canal stenosis.

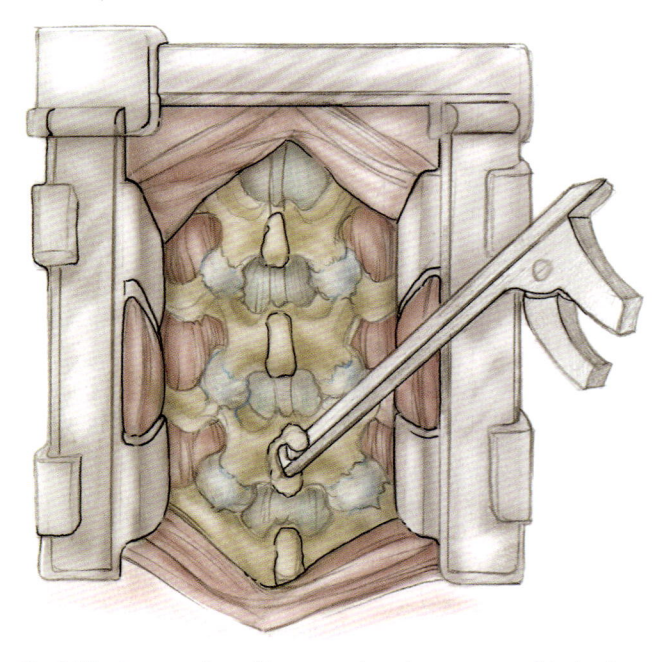

Fig. 94.2 A rongeur is used to remove the spinous process of the levels to be decompressed.

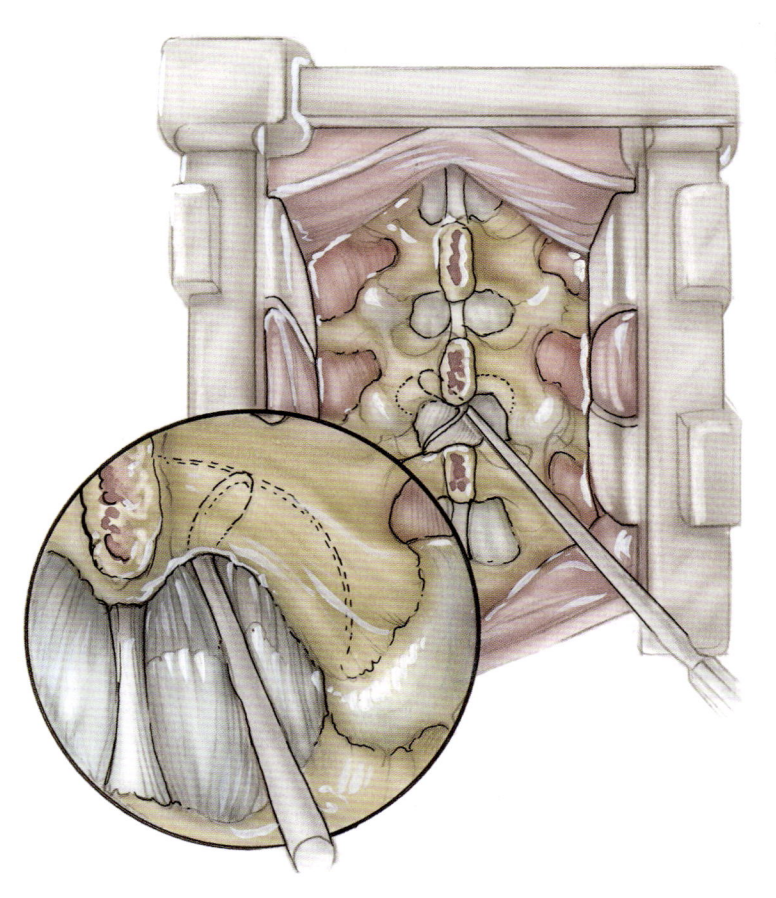

Fig. 94.3 A small curette is used to detach the ligamentum flavum from the inferior aspect of the lamina.

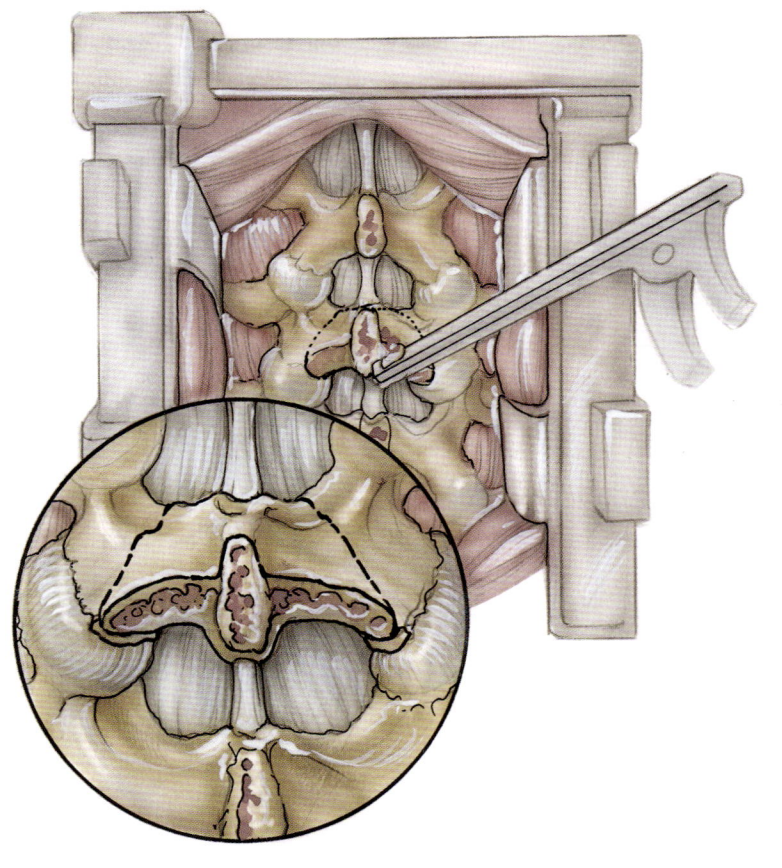

Fig. 94.4 To prevent insertion of the lower blade too deep into the spinal canal, the lower blade of the Kerrison rongeur should be inserted just beneath the leading inferior edge of the lamina at 30 degrees from vertical or 60 degrees from the spine.

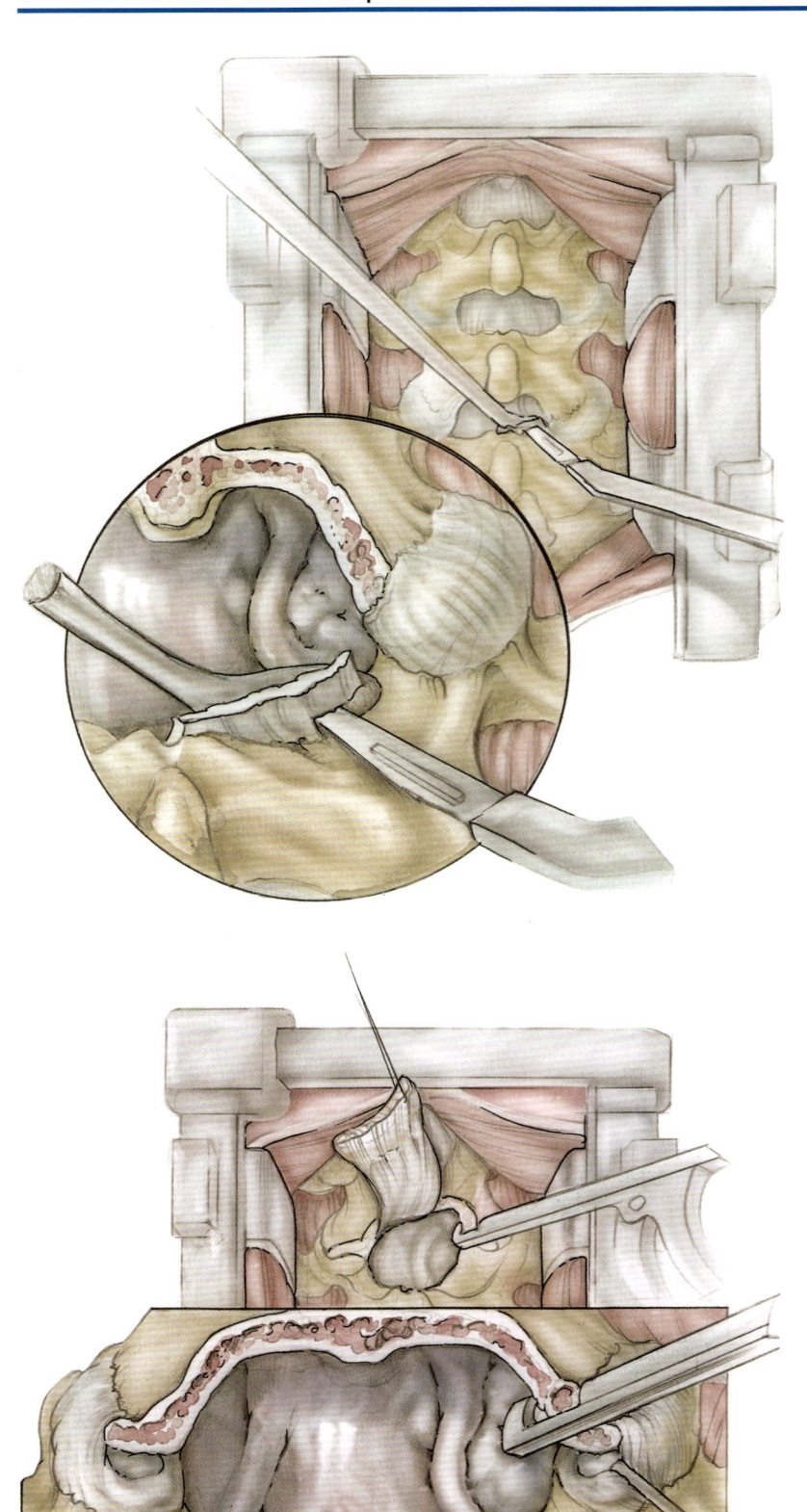

Fig. 94.5 A scalpel is used to remove the ligamentum flavum from the bone while the underlying dura is protected with a dural elevator.

Fig. 94.6 The footplate of the Kerrison punch is inserted between the ligamentum flavum and the dura to avoid dural tears and injury to the nerve roots.

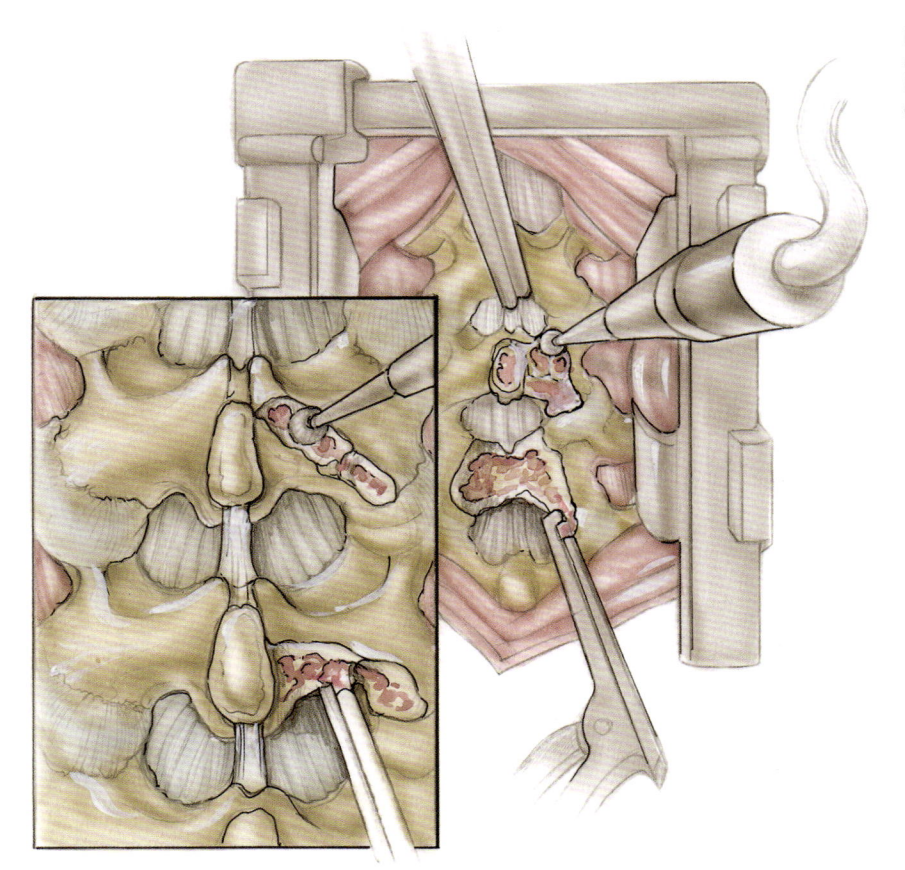

Fig. 94.7 The lamina is thinned to the thickness of an eggshell using a large cutting bit. The bone is then carefully removed using the standard fashion.

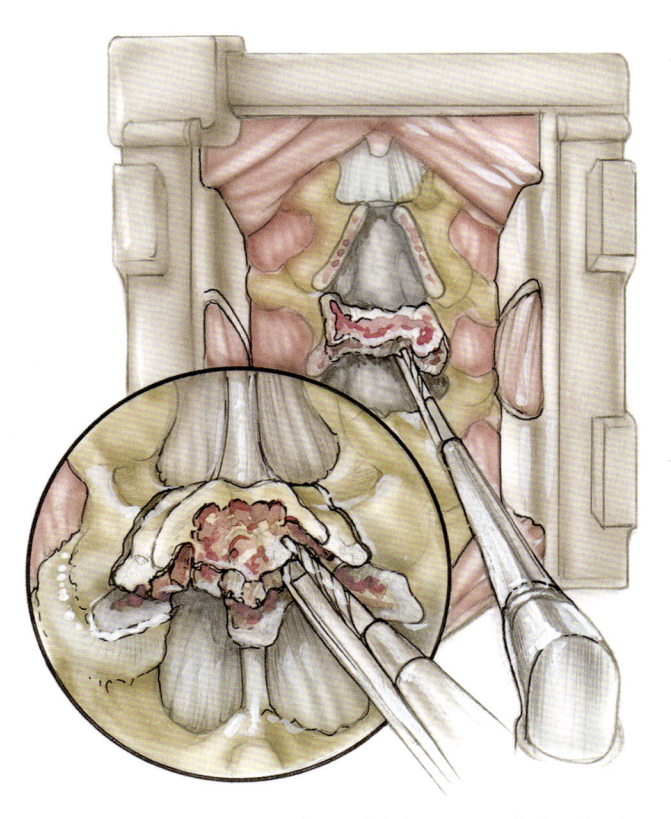

Fig. 94.8 The lamina is removed as a whole by inserting the footplate beneath the edge of the lamina.

Complications

Complications typically include infection, CSF leak, postlaminectomy spondylolisthesis, and postlaminectomy syndrome with inadequate decompression. Neural injury is rare and can almost universally be avoided by attention to proper surgical technique. The incidence of wound infection in a clean, uncomplicated, noninstrumented laminectomy should not exceed 2 to 3%. The risk of wound infection can be reduced by the use of a single dose of a prophylactic antibiotic directed against skin flora. This antibiotic should be chosen based on the infections encountered and drug sensitivities for an individual institution. More recently, topical antibiotic powder administered throughout the wound prior to closure has been shown to reduce the incidence of postoperative wound complications.[7] Other measures that can reduce infectious complications include achievement of meticulous hemostasis and gentle tissue handling.

Dural injury with CSF leakage has been reported to occur in as many as 15% of cases of lumbar laminectomy. Dural tears are better avoided than repaired, and measures to avoid dural tears have been outlined above. If a clean tear occurs in the dorsolateral dura, every attempt should be made at a primary repair. If the tear is irregular and wide, a graft can be utilized. If the tear is ventral, repair is extremely difficult, if not impossible, and attempts at primary repair may only serve to enlarge the defect. In such cases, the dural opening should be covered with a layer of Gelfoam. Alternatively, a piece of fascia can be used and secured in place using fibrin glue. In the latter cases, a lumbar subarachnoid drain provides CSF diversion while the defect heals, and lessens the risk of CSF cutaneous fistula. The incidence of iatrogenic postlaminectomy spondylolisthesis is reported to be 4 to 15%.[8] The risk of listhesis depends on several factors, including the number of levels operated, the extent of the decompression, whether partial or complete facetectomies have been performed, the presence of increased or decreased joint mobility preoperatively, patient age, and the degree of spondylosis. Theoretically, a complete unilateral facetectomy can be safely performed as long as the contralateral joint is intact. The presence of preoperative hypermobility is generally taken as an indication for fusion. Older individuals with markedly degenerated motion segments are less likely to develop a subsequent slip as compared with younger patients.

References

1. Katz JN, Harris MB. Clinical practice. Lumbar spinal stenosis. N Engl J Med 2008;358:818–825
2. Kramer DL, Booth RE, Albert TJ, et al. Posterior lumbar approach. In: Albert TJ, Balderston RA, Northrup BE, eds. Surgical Approaches to the Spine. Philadelphia: WB Saunders; 1997:173–192
3. Long D, McAfee PC, eds. Atlas of Spinal Surgery. Baltimore: Williams & Wilkins; 1992:2–22
4. Watkins RG. Posterior surgical approaches to the lumbar spine. In: Andersson G, McNeill TW, eds. Lumbar Spinal Stenosis. St. Louis: Mosby; 1992:31–45
5. McLain R. Surgical approaches to the lumbar spine. In: Frymoyer JW, ed. The Adult Spine: Principles and Practice, 2nd ed. Philadelphia: Lippincott-Raven; 1997:1723–1744
6. Torrens MJ. Lumbar laminectomy. In: Torrens MJ, Dickson RA, eds. Operative Spinal Surgery. Edinburgh: Churchill Livingstone; 1991:119–124
7. Molinari RW, Khera OA, Molinari WJ III. Prophylactic intraoperative powdered vancomycin and postoperative deep spinal wound infection: 1,512 consecutive surgical cases over a 6-year period. Eur Spine J 2012;21(Suppl 4):S476–S482
8. Shenkin HA, Hash CJ. Spondylolisthesis after multiple bilateral laminectomies and facetectomies for lumbar spondylosis. Follow-up review. J Neurosurg 1979;50:45–47

95 MIS Posterior Lumbar Approach

Russell G. Strom and Anthony K. Frempong-Boadu

Compared with open exposure of the posterior lumbar spine, minimally invasive surgery (MIS) utilizes a smaller incision with less soft tissue injury.[1,2] A series of progressively larger dilators is advanced onto the lamina using a muscle-splitting technique. A tubular retractor is placed over the largest dilator and secured to a table-mounted holder. The tubular retractor serves as a working channel for the operation. Spinal stenosis and disk herniation are treated similarly to open decompression.[2,3] Longer, bayoneted instruments are used for improved visualization through the narrow field. The decompression may be performed with an endoscope or loupes and a headlight, but the operating microscope is typically chosen because of its superior illumination, magnification, and three-dimensional visualization. This chapter describes the MIS posterior lumbar approach for decompression, together with perioperative considerations that apply to all MIS decompressions. The chapters that follow describe specific MIS lumbar decompressive procedures: foraminotomy (Chapter 96), hemilaminectomy (Chapter 97), diskectomy (Chapter 98), and bilateral decompression for stenosis (Chapter 99).

Patient Selection

The ideal surgical candidate has a clinical presentation consistent with lumbar radiculopathy or neurogenic claudication, together with neural compression on imaging corresponding to the level and side of presenting symptoms. Furthermore, because many spinal conditions are self-limited or improve with nonoperative modalities, surgery is generally considered only if symptoms persist despite 6 weeks of conservative management including oral pain medication, physical therapy, and epidural steroid injections. However, expeditious decompression is required for patients with significant motor deficit or cauda equina syndrome. The patient with low back pain should be evaluated for mechanical instability or deformity, which would require a more extensive operation. Patients must be counseled that spinal decompression addresses leg symptoms but not back pain, and the patient with predominantly back pain is a poor candidate for MIS decompression. In appropriately selected patients, lumbar decompression has an 80 to 90% likelihood of improving leg symptoms.

Indications, Goals, and Choice of Operative Approach

Although an MIS posterior approach can be performed for a variety of pathologies, its principal use is to free compressed nerve roots from degenerative disease.[2,3] Degenerative disk disease begins as desiccation of the nucleus pulposus and weakening of the annulus fibrosis. This leads to disk bulge and herniation, and later overgrowth of the ligamentum flavum and facet joints. Neural compression may arise from one or a combination of these processes. The worst compression is typically not in the central spinal canal, but rather in the lateral recess (bordered by the ascending facet, pedicle, and disk). Facet hypertrophy may also compress the nerve root from the level above as it passes through the foramen. Two nerve roots may thus be compressed at one interspace. The root in the lateral recess is called the traversing root, whereas the root in the foramen is called the exiting root.

Most MIS decompressions begin with docking of the tubular retractor onto the lamina, followed by creation of a laminar window (laminotomy) and resection of ligamentum flavum to expose the lateral thecal sac and traversing root.[4] From here, the operation is tailored to the pathology at hand. Often, a patient has multiple types and locations of pathology that can be addressed in the same operation. The most common indications for MIS decompression and the corresponding procedures are as follows:

- Foraminal stenosis secondary to facet hypertrophy: MIS posterior lumbar foraminotomy (Chapter 96)
- Unilateral lateral recess stenosis secondary to facet/ligament hypertrophy: MIS posterior lumbar hemilaminectomy (Chapter 97)
- Primary or recurrent paracentral/foraminal disk herniation: MIS posterior lumbar diskectomy (Chapter 98)
- Bilateral lateral recess stenosis secondary to facet/ligament hypertrophy: MIS posterior lumbar decompression of stenosis (Chapter 99)
- Far lateral disk herniation: far lateral MIS diskectomy (Chapter 101)

Other uses of the tubular retractor approach include transforaminal lumbar interbody fusion, synovial cyst resection, evacuation of epidural abscess, resection of intradural tumors, and tethered cord release.[5–8]

Contraindications

Stand-alone lumbar decompression MIS is contraindicated in the setting of greater than grade I spondylolisthesis, instability on flexion-extension X-rays, significant lateral listhesis, or scoliosis > 30 degrees. Congenital spinal stenosis and profound facet hypertrophy are relative contraindications owing to the narrow laminar space available for docking. Here, the limited working angle with an MIS approach would necessitate greater facet resection to decompress the lateral recess. In contrast, an open approach provides more flexible working angles, enabling facets to be undercut rather than drilled through to free the lateral recess. A predominance of back pain rather than leg pain and severe obesity are also relative contraindications. A previous extensive decompression makes an MIS decompression reoperation more challenging because of the distorted anatomy, and an open procedure should be considered in this case.

Advantages

Lumbar MIS has several advantages over open decompression, including a smaller incision, less muscle injury, lower blood loss, and less postoperative pain.[9,10] These factors lead to faster mobilization and earlier discharge.[11] The dilated paraspinal muscle tends to collapse after MIS, in contrast with an open approach in which the muscle is stripped from its bony attachments. The small dead spine with MIS leads to a low infection risk and a low rate of cutaneous cerebrospinal fluid (CSF) leakage when dural tears occur.[12,13] The learning curve is trivial compared with other MIS techniques.[14] Although the tubular retractor approach differs from open exposure, the operation is similar once the retractor is docked. Spinal decompression is performed using longer and bayoneted versions of the typical instruments (drills, suctions, curettes, nerve hooks, and rongeurs). In experienced hands, MIS exposure of the spine and wound closure are faster than open surgery. The technique is versatile and can address a variety of pathologies. By shifting the tubular retractor cranially and caudally, two adjacent levels can be decompressed through a single small incision. Furthermore, medial angulation of the tubular retractor enables bilateral decompression to be achieved through a unilateral approach.[3] The contralateral facet joints, contralateral paraspinal muscles, and supraspinous and interspinous ligaments are preserved, thereby decreasing the likelihood of postoperative instability.[15,16]

Disadvantages

An MIS decompression involves more fluoroscopy scans than an open approach, with associated radiation risks to the patient and staff. Although MIS has short-term advantages over open decompression, there is little evidence to support superior long-term outcomes.[17] MIS, particularly contralateral decompression, does have a learning curve, and there may be a greater risk of incomplete decompression or dural tear in inexperienced hands. In patients with congenital spinal stenosis or significant facet hypertrophy, limited laminar space is available for docking of the tubular retractor. This issue, combined with the narrow working angle through the tube, can lead to overaggressive facet resection during the lateral recess decompression, with the associated risk of postoperative instability. With profound nerve compression caused by severe spinal stenosis or a massive central disk herniation, the distorted anatomy and narrow portal may raise the risk of a dural tear. Finally, in patients with a coronal plane deformity, the posterior spinal anatomy is rotated, distorted, and more difficult to localize on lateral fluoroscopy. In each of these circumstances, an open approach should be considered.

Preoperative Imaging

Anteroposterior (AP) and lateral lumbar spine X-rays are performed to rule out deformities that would contraindicate stand-alone decompression. For patients with significant back pain or spondylolisthesis, flexion and extension views should be obtained to rule out mechanical instability. Lumbar spine magnetic resonance imaging (MRI) diagnoses the neural compression and details its severity, level, location (central, lateral recess, foramen), and cause (disk, facet, ligament). In patients with prior diskectomy, MRI, with and without contrast, distinguishes between granulation tissue and residual/recurrent disk hernia-tion. Granulation tissue is typically homogeneously enhancing, whereas a disk herniation is nonenhancing, with enhancement only around the periphery. Lumbar spine computed tomography (CT) is not obtained routinely but can demonstrate whether the pathology is calcified or soft. In patients unable to undergo MRI, a CT myelogram delineates the neural compression.

Surgical Procedure

Following endotracheal intubation and application of pneumatic compression stockings, the patient is placed prone onto a Wilson frame or in the knee-chest position on an Andrews table. These positions achieve two goals: First, the lumbar spine is flexed, thereby widening the interlaminar space and facilitating decompression. Second, the abdomen is decompressed partially (Wilson frame) or completely (Andrew table). Minimizing abdominal pressure is critical because it can lead to excessive epidural bleeding. The head is typically supported on a foam headrest. However, in elderly patients and others with cervical spondylosis, use of a Mayfield headholder facilitates positioning in neutral cervical alignment. The shoulders are abducted no more than 90 degrees to avoid brachial plexus injury. The knees are gently flexed to relax the sciatic nerves. Care is taken to ensure that the eyes, axillae, ulnar grooves, breasts, genitals, and bony prominences are free from compression, with foam padding placed as needed. The clamp used to secure the retractor arm is attached to the operating table opposite the side of approach. A dose of intravenous antibiotics is administered, and the lumbar region is widely prepped and draped.

The initial approach is performed under lateral fluoroscopy using one of many possible techniques. We prefer to localize the skin entry point with an 18-gauge needle on a syringe containing 0.25% bupivacaine with 1:100,000 epinephrine (**Fig. 95.1**). The entry point is located where an imaginary line paralleling the disk space meets the skin surface, ~ 1.5 cm off midline on the side of pathology. In obese patients, the entry point is slightly more lateral (2 cm from midline), so that the medial trajectory toward the lamina remains ~ 15 degrees. The skin is infiltrated with local anesthetic, followed by the paraspinal muscles. The skin entry point is adjusted cranially or caudally to be precisely in line with the disk space. A stab incision is then made at the chosen entry point (**Fig. 95.2**). The smallest dilator is inserted through the skin, lumbodorsal fascia, and paraspinal muscle down to the inferior laminar edge (**Fig. 95.3**). Some authors open the fascia sharply or with monopolar electrocautery, but in most circumstances the retractors adequately split the tissue. The lamina is palpated as it drops off inferiorly, connects to the spinous process medially, and merges into the facet laterally. In addition to confirming the anatomy, this step ("wanding") dissects muscle off the lamina. The correct spinal level is assessed on lateral fluoroscopy with the dilator placed on the inferior laminar edge (overlying the disk space). The vertical incision is then widened superiorly or inferiorly as necessary to accommodate a tubular retractor in line with the disk space (**Fig. 95.4**). To prevent skin injury from overstretching, the incision is typically 2 mm larger than the diameter of the planned tubular retractor (typically 14 to 18 mm). For a two-level decompression, the incision can be centered halfway between the two spinal levels; wanding of the dilators provides access to both levels through a single incision.

A series of concentric tubular dilators is advanced onto the inferior laminar edge to achieve a muscle-splitting approach. With one hand used to anchor the preceding dilators on the lamina, each subsequent dilator is advanced using a twisting motion

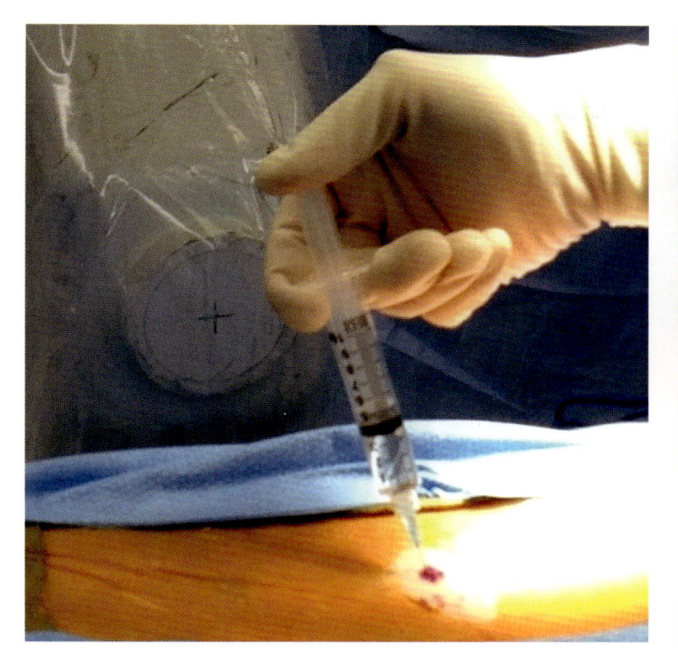

Fig. 95.1 The skin entry point is localized on lateral fluoroscopy using an 18-gauge needle. The skin and muscle are infiltrated with local anesthetic.

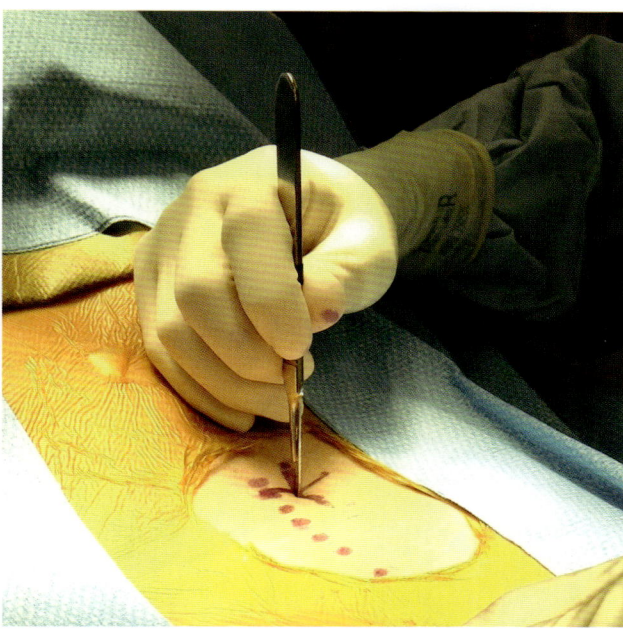

Fig. 95.2 A stab incision is made with a No. 15 blade at the entry point, ~ 1.5 cm off the midline.

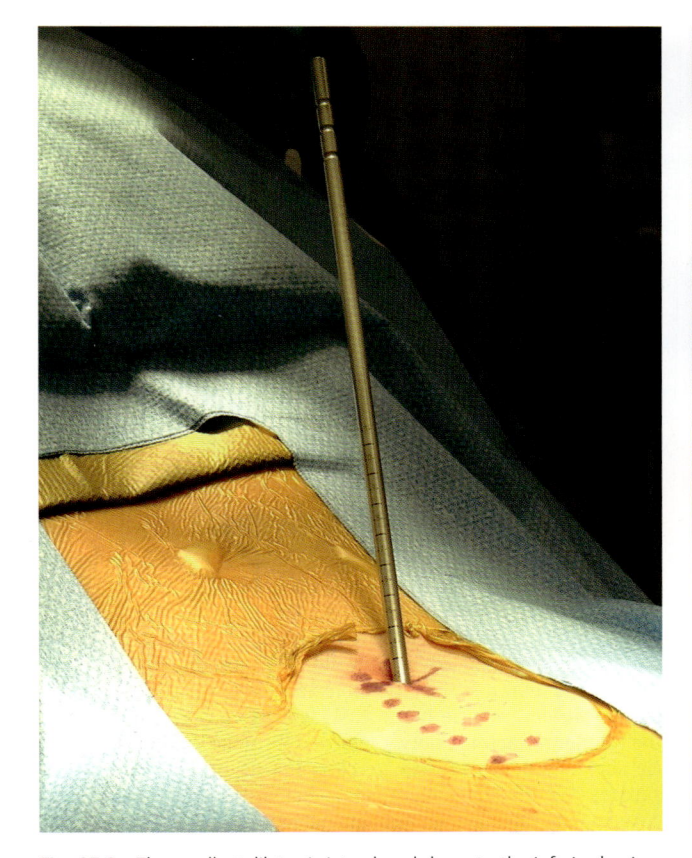

Fig. 95.3 The smallest dilator is introduced down to the inferior laminar edge.

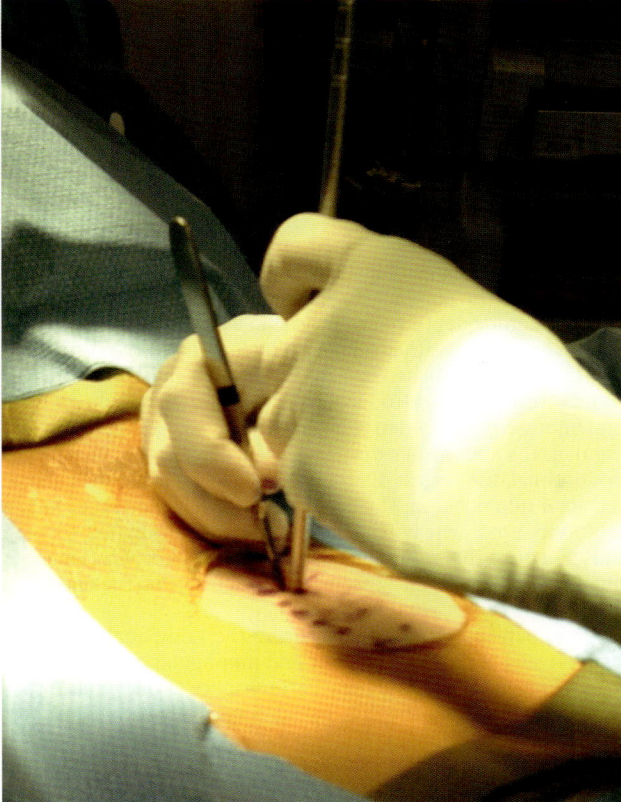

Fig. 95.4 The stab incision is enlarged cranially or caudally to accommodate the tubular retractor without skin tension.

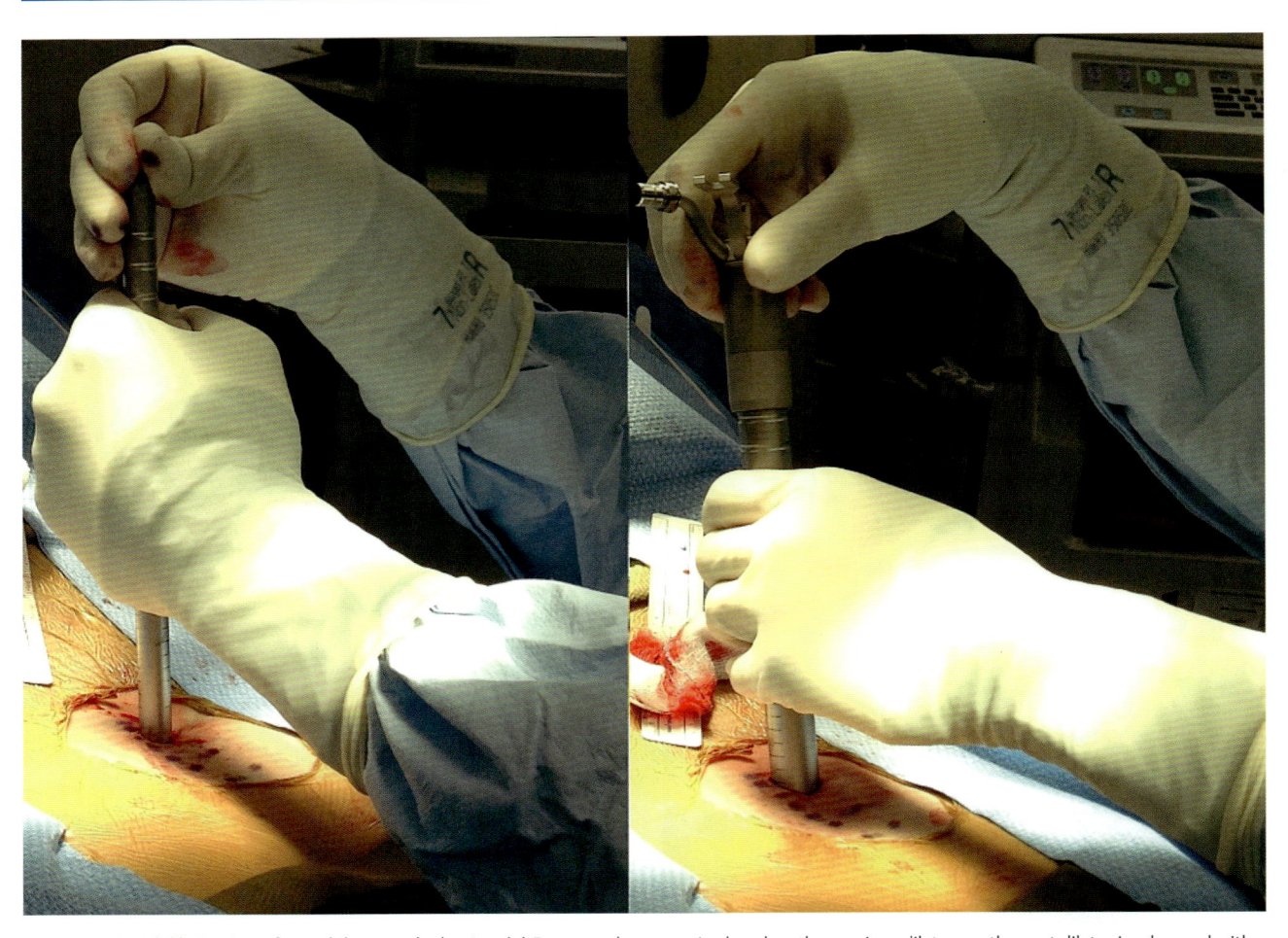

Fig. 95.5 Serial dilation is performed down to the lamina. **(a)** Downward pressure is placed on the previous dilators as the next dilator is advanced with a twisting motion. **(b)** The tubular retractor is placed over the largest dilator.

(**Fig. 95.5**). Applying downward pressure during serial dilation minimizes the degree of muscle creep into the field. The tract is dilated up to the planned diameter of the tubular retractor. The largest dilator's depth ruler at the skin surface indicates the appropriate length for the tubular retractor. The shortest possible length should be chosen to ease instrument manipulation. The tubular retractor is introduced over the largest dilator, and lateral fluoroscopy is used to confirm that it is both centered on and parallels the appropriate disk space (**Fig. 95.6**). If the trajectory is not optimal, the largest dilator can be used to wand the tubular retractor into position. The tubular retractor is then secured to a table-mounted arm with downward pressure applied to keep muscle out of the field (**Fig. 95.7**). A final fluoroscopic image is obtained to confirm an appropriate trajectory, and the operating microscope is brought into position.

Any paraspinal muscle obscuring the bony anatomy is resected using a pituitary rongeur and monopolar cautery with a long, bent tip (**Fig. 95.8**). The inferior aspect of the superior hemilamina (overlying the disk space) is typically near the center of the field. The following anatomic landmarks are defined with a curette or electrocautery: superior aspect of the inferior hemilamina (inferiorly), base of the spinous process (medially), mesial facet joint (laterally), and lateral aspect of pars interarticularis (superolaterally). The tubular retractor can be adjusted as necessary. A more rostral portal is required to treat a superiorly migrated disk or foraminal stenosis at the present interspace, whereas a more caudal portal is required to treat an inferiorly migrated disk or foraminal stenosis at the next interspace.

The degenerative pathology is treated as described in the chapters that follow. A minimally-invasive lumbar discectomy is illustrated in Video 95.1. Regardless of the type of decompression, care must be taken to preserve the pars interarticularis. Resection or excessive thinning of this structure may lead to postoperative instability. A partial facetectomy is generally required to access the lateral recess and foramen, but no more than the medial third should be removed to avoid destabilization. Following the decompression, palpation with a Woodson tool is used to rule out residual stenosis. The wound is copiously irrigated. Bleeding from bone edges is stopped with bone wax. Epidural hemostasis is achieved with bipolar electrocautery and hemostatic agents (FloSeal, Surgiflo, Gelfoam, etc.). The tubular retractor is released from the table-mounted arm. Using bipolar electrocautery, muscle hemostasis is achieved layer by layer as the tubular retractor is slowly removed from the wound. The muscle and lumbodorsal fascia are closed with interrupted 0 Vicryl sutures (**Fig. 95.9**). The dermis is closed with inverted 3-0 Vicryl sutures. The epidermis is approximated with a 3-0 Monocryl suture run in subcuticular fashion. The incision is covered with skin adhesive or Steri-Strips followed by a sterile dressing. The patient is turned supine and extubated.

95 MIS Posterior Lumbar Approach

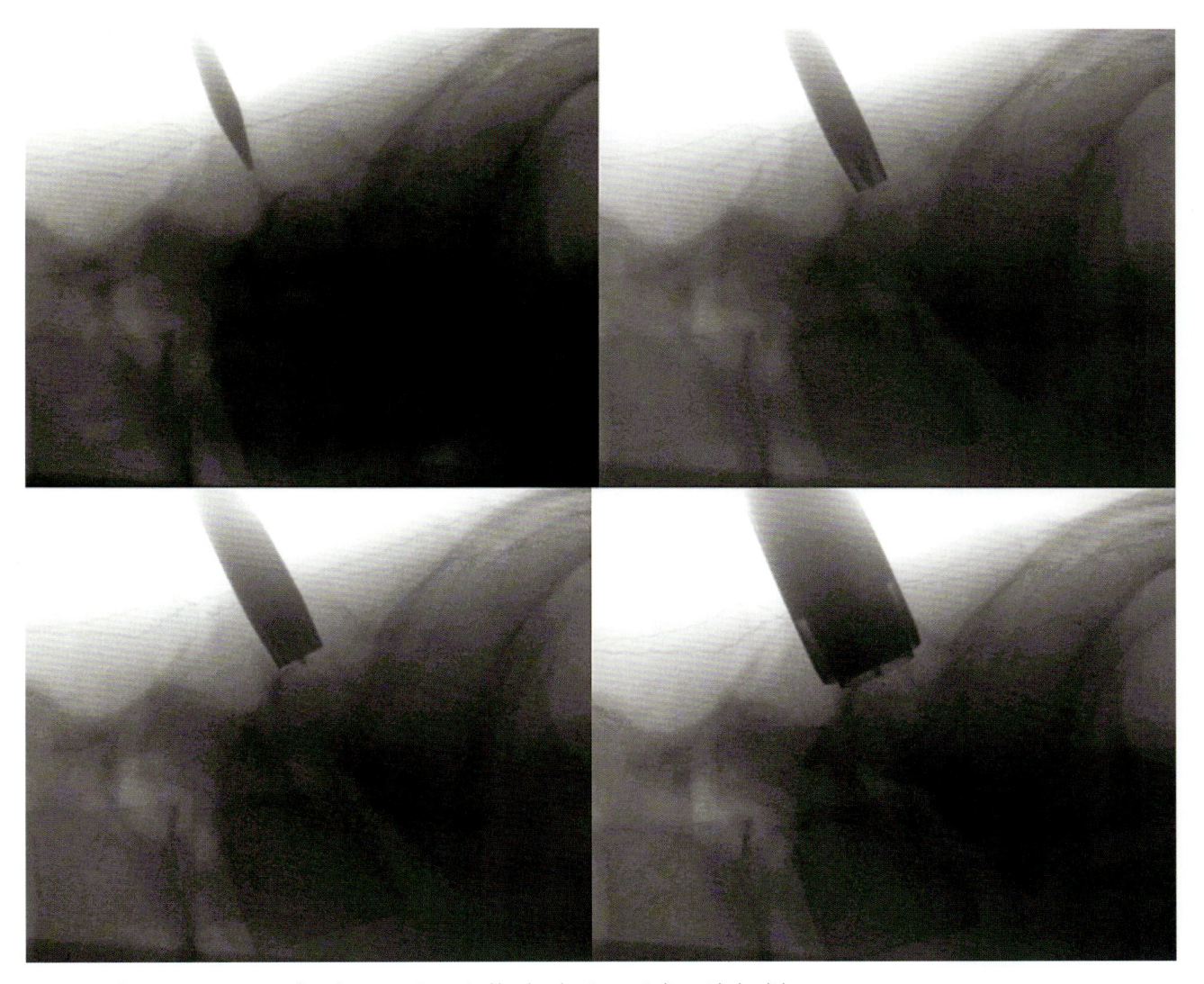

Fig. 95.6 Fluoroscopic images confirm the appropriate spinal level and trajectory in line with the disk space.

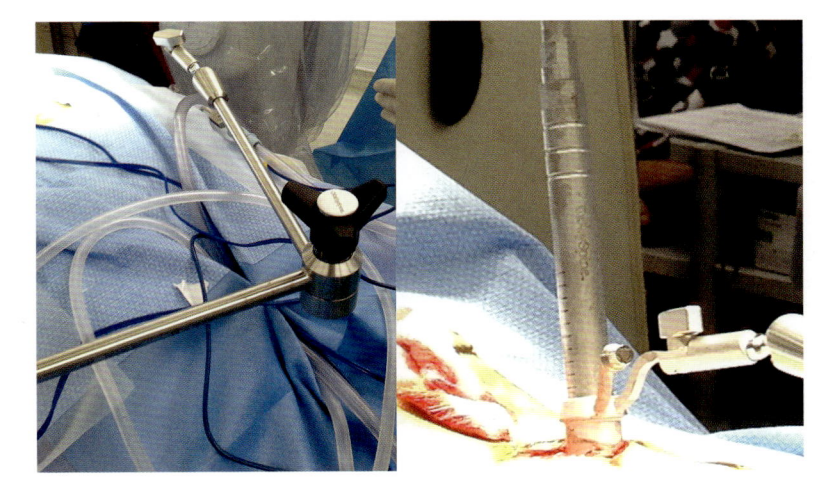

Fig. 95.7 The tubular retractor is secured to a table-mounted arm.

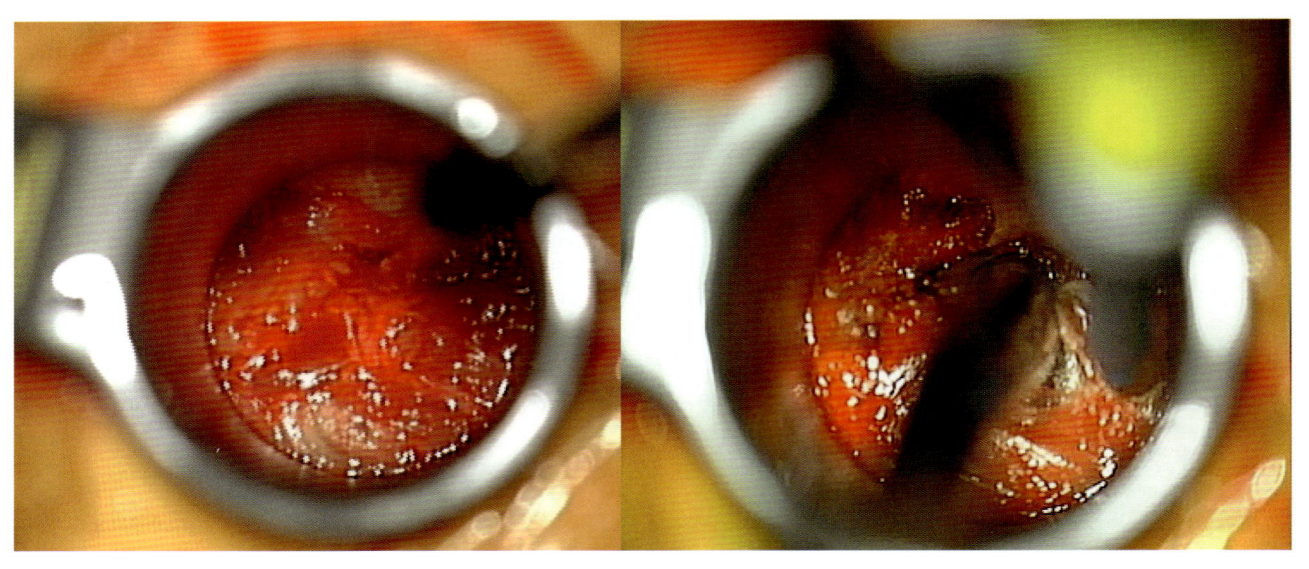

Fig. 95.8 **(a)** Even with careful dilation, some paraspinal muscle may cover the bony anatomy. **(b)** This is cut with electrocautery and removed with a pituitary rongeur.

Postoperative Care

Because less soft tissue disruption occurs with MIS decompression than with open surgery, patients generally have less postoperative pain and earlier mobilization.[9,10] Discharge is generally possible within 4 to 6 hours of surgery if there is adequate pain control, oral intake, voiding, and ambulation. The patient is kept in the hospital overnight if any of these conditions is not met. Furthermore, in the setting of a dural tear, the patient is generally kept flat overnight to minimize the risk of a cutaneous CSF leak. We also elect overnight observation for elderly patients and those with cardiovascular disease.

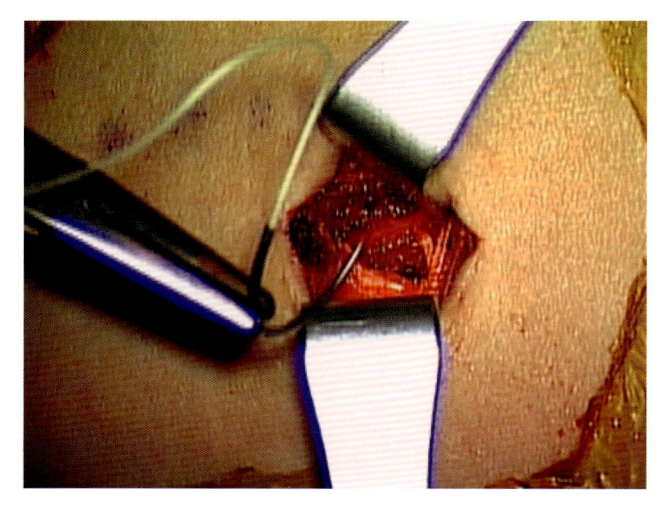

Fig. 95.9 The lumbodorsal fascia and muscle are closed with large absorbable sutures.

Potential Complications and Precautions

If a dural tear occurs, the defect is covered with a cottonoid, and the decompression is continued. In general, the goals of the operation should not be compromised in the setting of a dural tear. Primary repair with 4-0 Nurolon, 6-0 Prolene, or small dural clips can be attempted but is often difficult through a tubular retractor. Despite this issue, the risk of cutaneous CSF fistula is low with MIS decompression because there is little dead space. If primary repair cannot be achieved, a piece of muscle or synthetic collagen matrix is placed over the durotomy at the end of the operation, followed by fibrin glue or polyethylene glycol sealant. Meticulous fascial closure is mandatory after a dural tear, as it provides a strong, watertight barrier to the skin (which often lacks the strength to contain CSF). Although some authors advocate running nylon skin closure in the setting of a dural tear, we have not found this necessary as long as the fascia and dermis are closed well. We approximate the skin as in any other case (running absorbable subcuticular suture and skin adhesive).

Other complications include residual or recurrent nerve compression.[18] This can be prevented by careful inspection and palpation for offending pathology once the decompression is felt to be complete. Occasionally, multiple pathologies may contribute to the compression (e.g., facet overgrowth and disk herniation), and symptoms may persist unless all sources of stenosis are addressed. Postoperative numbness is not uncommon and may result from nerve retraction and manipulation. Often, the numbness was present before surgery but masked by radicular pain; once the nerve root is decompressed, the pain often resolves quickly but the numbness may persist for weeks to months. A new motor deficit from root injury is extremely rare, and immediate imaging should be performed to rule out compressive pathology. A postoperative hematoma can develop in the epidural space, leading to recurrent leg pain or neurologic deficit. Alternatively, a hematoma can occur in the soft tissue and present as a painful mass. Hematoma formation is prevented by meticulous hemostasis with electrocautery and hemostatic agents. It is important to obtain muscle hemostasis as the retractor is slowly withdrawn; once the retractor is removed, bleeding tissue can be difficult to localize. Wound infections are infrequent with MIS decompression,[12] and can be further prevented with the use of copious irrigation prior to closure. Postoperative mechanical instability is more common in the setting of preexisting spondylolisthesis or deformity. With MIS, preservation of the midline tension band and contralateral facet and musculature lowers the risk of instability.[15,19] Iatrogenic instability can be caused by over-resection of the pars and facet. Rarely, bowel or vascular injury may arise from anterior longitudinal ligament violation during diskectomy; these life-threatening injuries mandate expeditious laparotomy.[20]

Conclusion

The MIS posterior lumbar approach is straightforward and versatile. Once the tubular retractor is docked, decompression is performed in similar fashion to open surgery. Reduced soft tissue trauma leads to lower postoperative pain and earlier mobilization. **Box 95.1** lists the key operative steps and the problems that can arise.

Box 95.1 Key Operative Steps and Potential Problems

Step	Problems
Prone positioning	Pressure injury
Skin entry	Wrong spinal level or trajectory
Serial dilation	Muscle creep
Retractor deployment	Poor working angle
Decompression	Pars/facet compromise, dural tear, residual pathology
Closure	Inadequate hemostasis

References

1. Podichetty VK, Spears J, Isaacs RE, Booher J, Biscup RS. Complications associated with minimally invasive decompression for lumbar spinal stenosis. J Spinal Disord Tech 2006;19:161–166
2. Righesso O, Falavigna A, Avanzi O. Comparison of open discectomy with microendoscopic discectomy in lumbar disc herniations: results of a randomized controlled trial. Neurosurgery 2007;61:545–549, discussion 549
3. Palmer S, Turner R, Palmer R. Bilateral decompression of lumbar spinal stenosis involving a unilateral approach with microscope and tubular retractor system. J Neurosurg 2002;97(2, Suppl):213–217
4. Guiot BH, Khoo LT, Fessler RG. A minimally invasive technique for decompression of the lumbar spine. Spine 2002;27:432–438
5. Gandhi RH, German JW. Minimally invasive approach for the treatment of intradural spinal pathology. Neurosurg Focus 2013;35:E5
6. Safavi-Abbasi S, Maurer AJ, Rabb CH. Minimally invasive treatment of multilevel spinal epidural abscess. J Neurosurg Spine 2013;18:32–35
7. Sandhu FA, Santiago P, Fessler RG, Palmer S. Minimally invasive surgical treatment of lumbar synovial cysts. Neurosurgery 2004;54:107–111, discussion 111–112
8. Tredway TL, Santiago P, Hrubes MR, Song JK, Christie SD, Fessler RG. Minimally invasive resection of intradural-extramedullary spinal neoplasms. Neurosurgery 2006;58(1, Suppl):ONS52–ONS58, discussion ONS52–ONS58
9. Brock M, Kunkel P, Papavero L. Lumbar microdiscectomy: subperiosteal versus transmuscular approach and influence on the early postoperative analgesic consumption. Eur Spine J 2008;17:518–522
10. Rahman M, Summers LE, Richter B, Mimran RI, Jacob RP. Comparison of techniques for decompressive lumbar laminectomy: the minimally invasive versus the "classic" open approach. Minim Invasive Neurosurg 2008;51:100–105
11. Mobbs RJ, Li J, Sivabalan P, Raley D, Rao PJ. Outcomes after decompressive laminectomy for lumbar spinal stenosis: comparison between minimally invasive unilateral laminectomy for bilateral decompression and open laminectomy: clinical article. J Neurosurg Spine 2014;21:179–186
12. O'Toole JE, Eichholz KM, Fessler RG. Surgical site infection rates after minimally invasive spinal surgery. J Neurosurg Spine 2009;11:471–476
13. Palmer S. Use of a tubular retractor system in microscopic lumbar discectomy: 1 year prospective results in 135 patients. Neurosurg Focus 2002;13:E5
14. McLoughlin GS, Fourney DR. The learning curve of minimally-invasive lumbar microdiscectomy. Can J Neurol Sci 2008;35:75–78
15. Pao JL, Chen WC, Chen PQ. Clinical outcomes of microendoscopic decompressive laminotomy for degenerative lumbar spinal stenosis. Eur Spine J 2009;18:672–678
16. Tai CL, Hsieh PH, Chen WP, Chen LH, Chen WJ, Lai PL. Biomechanical comparison of lumbar spine instability between laminectomy and bilateral laminotomy for spinal stenosis syndrome—an experimental study in porcine model. BMC Musculoskelet Disord 2008;9:84
17. Ang CL, Phak-Boon Tow B, Fook S, et al. Minimally invasive compared with open lumbar laminotomy: no functional benefits at 6 or 24 months after surgery. Spine J 2015;15:1705–1712
18. Moliterno JA, Knopman J, Parikh K, et al. Results and risk factors for recurrence following single-level tubular lumbar microdiscectomy. J Neurosurg Spine 2010;12:680–686
19. Lee MJ, Bransford RJ, Bellabarba C, et al. The effect of bilateral laminotomy versus laminectomy on the motion and stiffness of the human lumbar spine: a biomechanical comparison. Spine 2010;35:1789–1793
20. Kraemer R, Wild A, Haak H, Herdmann J, Krauspe R, Kraemer J. Classification and management of early complications in open lumbar microdiscectomy. Eur Spine J 2003;12:239–246

96 MIS Posterior Lumbar Foraminotomy

Russell G. Strom and Anthony K. Frempong-Boadu

The intervertebral foramen is bordered superiorly and inferiorly by two adjacent pedicles, anteriorly by the vertebral body and disk, and posteriorly by the pars interarticularis and superior articular process of the facet joint. Foraminal stenosis is most frequently caused by overgrowth of the superior articular process. Lumbar foraminotomy can be a stand-alone procedure, but it is more commonly performed in conjunction with lateral recess decompression. In addition to the medial-to-lateral technique described here, lateral-to-medial foraminal decompression can be performed using an approach similar to far lateral diskectomy (see Chapter 101). Alternatively, a radical foraminotomy involving transaction of the pars and removal of the inferior and superior articulating processes can be performed as part of a transforaminal lumbar interbody fusion (see Chapter 104).

Surgical Procedure

For a stand-alone lumbar foraminotomy, the tubular retractor approach is similar to that described in Chapter 95, but the midportion of the lamina is targeted rather than the inferior laminar edge (**Fig. 96.1**). On lateral fluoroscopy, the tubular retractor should be centered over the compressed foramen, just cephalad to the disk space (**Fig. 96.2**). The mesial facet, lateral border of the pars, and inferior laminar edge are exposed with curettes and electrocautery. The lamina is thinned with a high-speed bur from the inferior laminar edge up to the midportion of the lamina, just medial to the pars interarticularis (**Fig. 96.3**). Drilling continues laterally into the mesial one-third facet, but the pars is preserved (**Fig. 96.4**). Safe drilling requires appreciation of the fact that the ligamentum flavum underlies only the caudal one third to one half of the lamina. We drill the bone full-thickness down to the ligament in the lower one third of the lamina, but more cephalad to that we leave a cortical shell. An upgoing curette is then inserted along the ventral surface of the thinned lamina to free the ligamentum flavum from its laminar attachment (**Fig. 96.5a**). The thinned lamina is removed from caudal to cranial with Kerrison rongeurs. The appearance of fat just cephalad to the ligament attachment signifies entry into the epidural space. Alternatively, the epidural space can be accessed more inferiorly by separating the fibers of the ligamentum flavum with a Penfield No. 4 dissector or nerve hook (**Fig. 96.5b**). Adhesions between the dura and the ligament are freed with an upgoing curette. These adhesions are common and their separation is vital to avoiding a dural tear. The remainder of the thinned lamina, mesial facet, and ligament are removed piecemeal with Kerrison punches until the outer border of the thecal sac is exposed (**Fig. 96.6**). A safe and effective method of ligament and bone removal is to insert a small cottonoid into the epidural dissection plane that was made with the curette. Gentle pressure on the cottonoid with a suction tip in one hand will protect the dura as ligament and bone are removed with a Kerrison in the other hand.

Once the lateral thecal sac is exposed, a Woodson tool is used to palpate the pedicles bordering the foramen superiorly and inferiorly, along with the overgrown superior articular process arising from the inferior pedicle. If desired, the exiting root can be exposed by extending the laminotomy toward the superior laminar edge, where the root is seen exiting the thecal sac, hugging the pedicle, and then turning laterally into the foramen. The overgrown superior articular process is dissected with an upgoing curette and undercut in piecemeal with Kerrison rongeurs. We prefer to use a Kerrison punch with a curved tip; when inserted into the foramen it targets the superior facet while preserving the pars interarticularis (**Fig. 96.7**). The foramen is then palpated with a Woodson tool to search for residual stenosis. Ligament, synovium, disk material, or granulation tissue may need to be removed to complete the decompression.

Foraminotomy is often performed in conjunction with lateral recess decompression (**Fig. 96.8**). If the same root experiences lateral recess and foraminal compression (from two adjacent overgrown facets), the foraminotomy is performed as a *caudal* extension of the initial hemilaminotomy/mesial facetectomy. At the level of lateral recess, the nerve root shoulder is freed from the hypertrophied facet and ligament out to the pedicle. The root is followed under the pedicle, and the overgrown superior articular process from the facet below is undercut with Kerrison rongeurs. More caudal exposure can be achieved by "wanding" the tubular retractor downward and removing more of the inferior lamina. But if one overgrown facet causes both lateral recess and foraminal stenosis (compressing two roots), a foraminotomy is performed as a *cephalad* extension of the lateral recess decompression. After the traversing root is freed via hemilaminotomy and mesial facetectomy, the overgrown superior articular process is identified as it arises from the cephalad aspect of the pedicle. The superior articular process is undercut with Kerrison rongeurs to free the exiting root. More cephalad exposure can be achieved by wanding the tubular retractor upward and removing more of the superior lamina. **Box 96.1** lists the key operative steps and the problems that can arise.

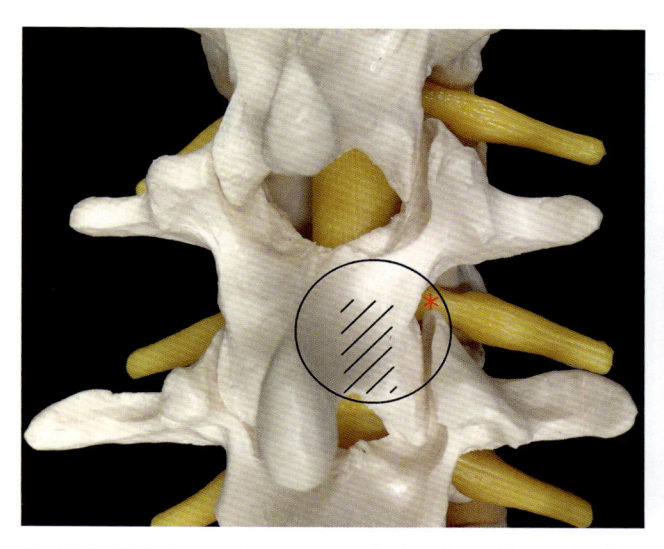

Fig. 96.1 With the tubular retractor docked on the mid-lamina *(circle)*, a hemilaminotomy/mesial facetectomy *(parallel lines)* provides access for foraminal decompression of the exiting root *(asterisk)*.

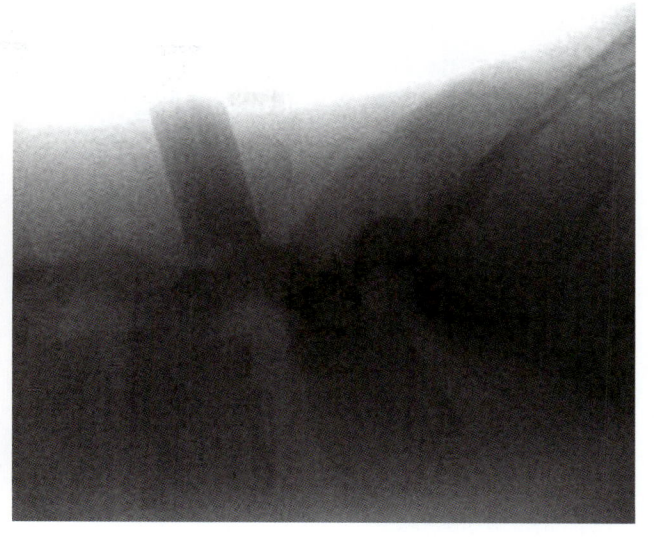

Fig. 96.2 The tubular retractor is centered over the compressed foramen, just cephalad to the disk space.

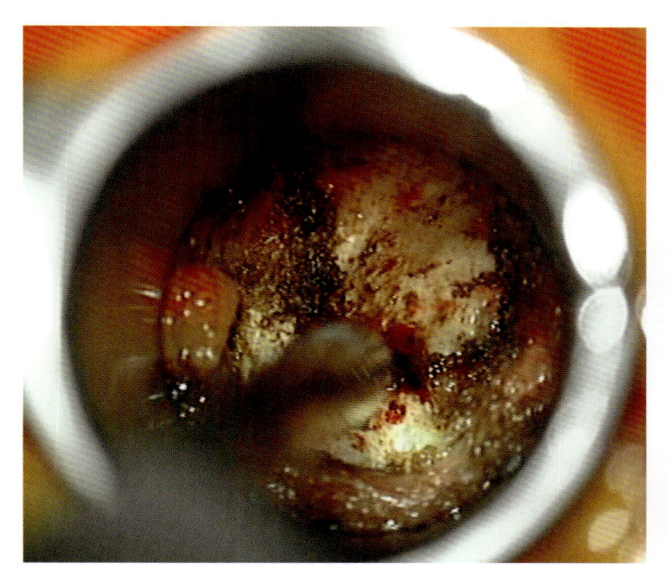

Fig. 96.3 Laminar drilling is performed from the inferior laminar edge *(left of field)* to the midportion of the lamina.

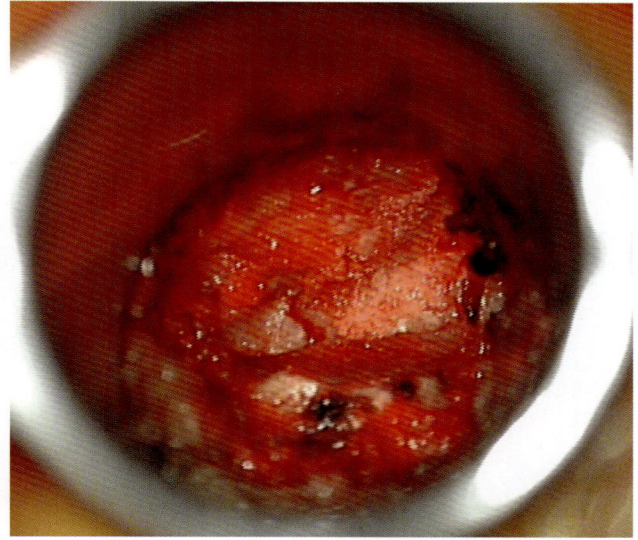

Fig. 96.4 Drilling is performed to the mesial one-third facet *(bottom of field)* to access the lateral recess.

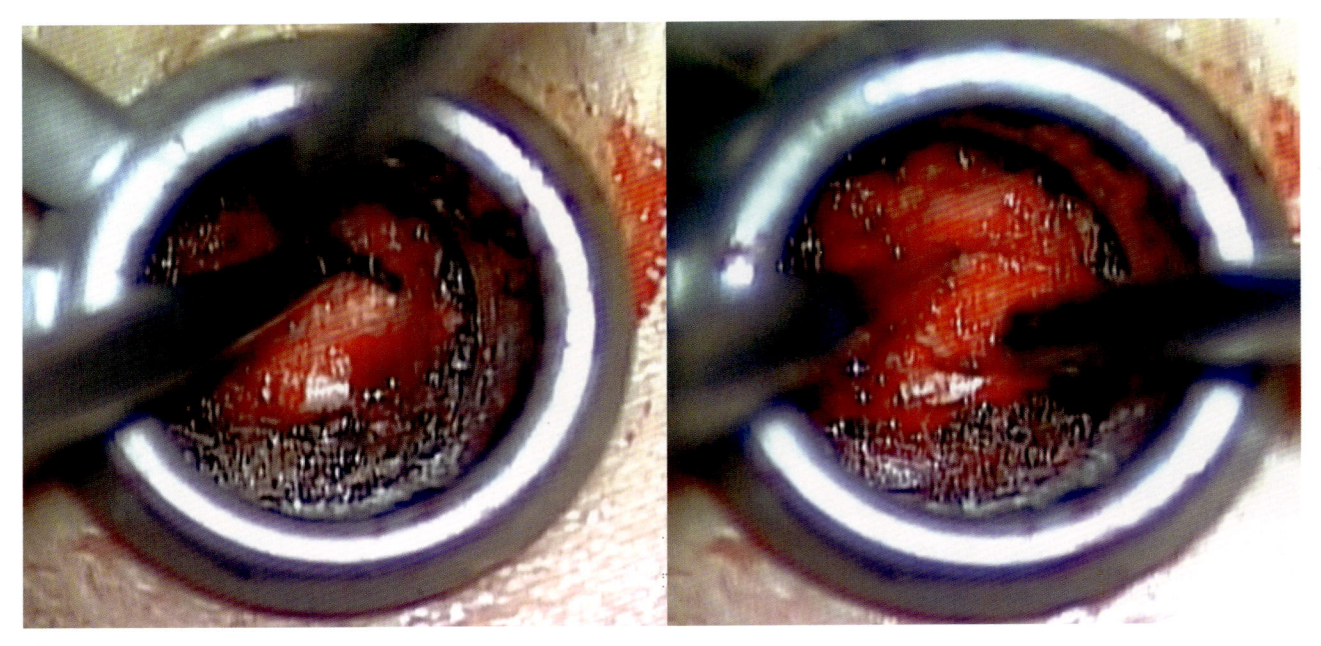

Fig. 96.5 To reach the epidural space, the ligamentum flavum is detached from the ventral lamina using an upgoing curette **(a)** or pierced with a nerve hook **(b)**.

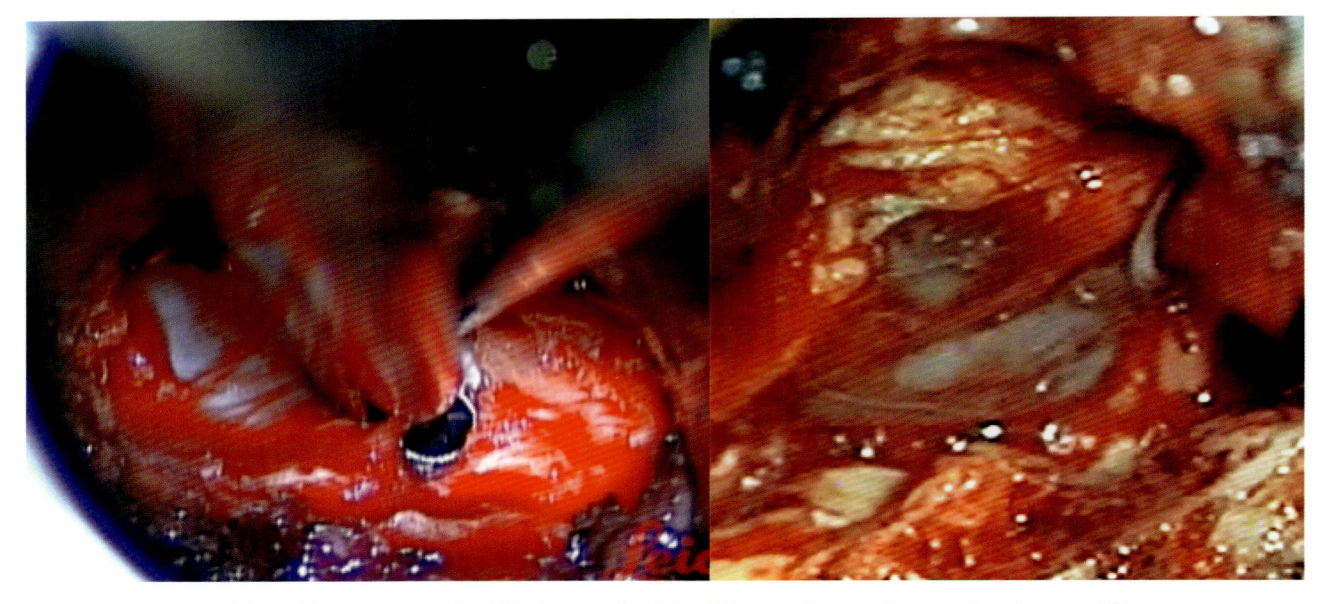

Fig. 96.6 Ligament and thinned bone are removed with Kerrison punches **(a)** until the lateral border of the thecal sac is exposed **(b)**.

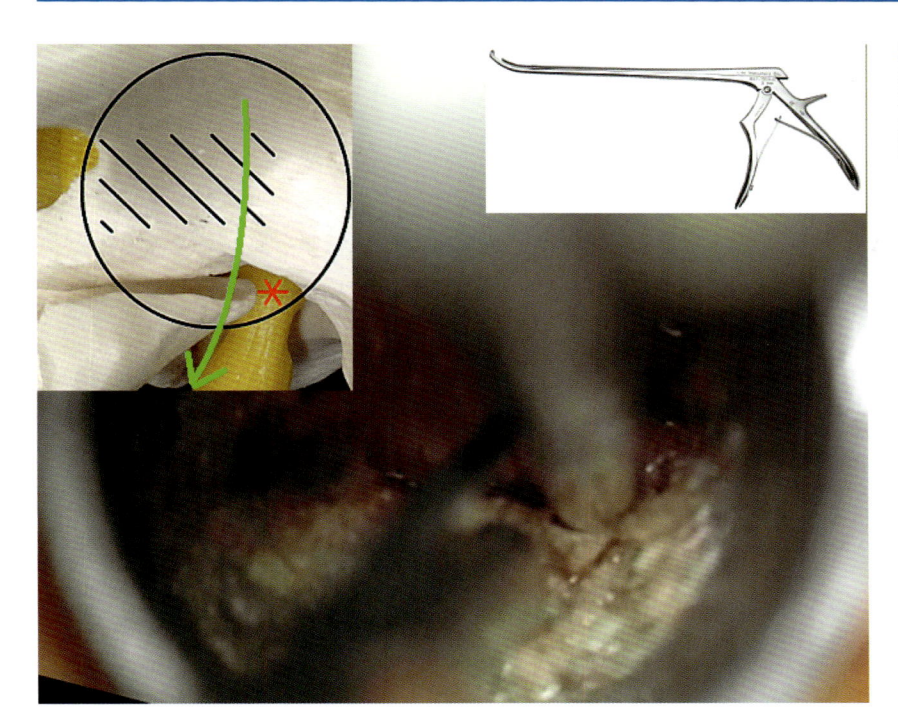

Fig. 96.7 A curved Kerrison rongeur *(upper right inset)* is placed through the lateral recess *(upper left inset)* into the foramen. The hypertrophied superior articular process is undercut, with the pars kept intact.

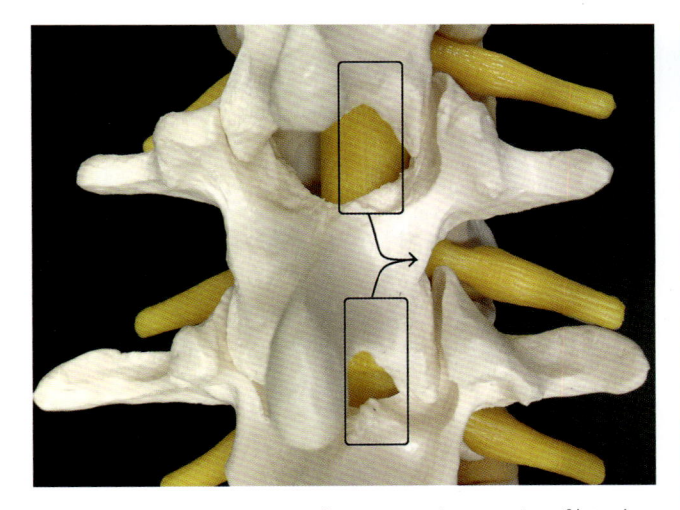

Fig. 96.8 Foraminotomy as an inferior or superior extension of lateral recess decompression.

Box 96.1 Key Operative Steps and Potential Problems

Step	Problems
Localizing the foraminal stenosis	Wrong-level decompression
Tubular retractor placement	Poor working angle
Laminotomy/mesial facetectomy	Over-resection of pars or facet
Ligamentum flavum removal	Dural adhesions and tears
Superior facet undercutting	Incomplete decompression, pars violation

97 MIS Posterior Lumbar Hemilaminectomy

Russell G. Strom and Anthony K. Frempong-Boadu

A minimally invasive surgery (MIS) posterior lumbar hemilaminectomy and mesial facetectomy are used to treat unilateral central/lateral recess stenosis resulting from facet and ligamentum flavum hypertrophy. The procedure is often combined with foraminotomy (Chapter 96), diskectomy (Chapter 98), or contralateral decompression (Chapter 99).

Surgical Procedure

The tubular retractor approach is performed as described in Chapter 95, with the inferior laminar edge in the center of the field (**Fig. 97.1**). The inferior half of the superior hemilamina, mesial facet, and superiormost aspect of the inferior hemilamina are thinned with a high-speed bur (**Fig. 97.2**). Safe drilling requires appreciation of the fact that the ligamentum flavum underlies only the caudal one third to one half of the lamina. We drill the bone full-thickness down to the ligament in the lower one third of the lamina (**Fig. 97.3**), but more cephalad to that we leave a cortical shell. An upgoing curette is inserted along the ventral surface of the thinned lamina to free the ligamentum flavum from its laminar attachment (**Fig. 97.4**). Kerrison punches are then used to remove the thinned lamina from caudal to cranial. The appearance of fat signifies entry into the epidural space just superior to the ligament attachment. Alternatively, the epidural space can be accessed more inferiorly by separating the fibers of the ligamentum flavum with a Penfield No. 4 dissector or nerve hook (**Fig. 97.5**). The fenestration is widened with a Kerrison rongeur to expose epidural fat (**Fig. 97.6**). Adhesions between the dura and the ligamentum flavum are freed with an upgoing curette. These adhesions are common and their separation is vital to avoiding a dural tear. Using Kerrison punches, the ligamentum flavum is resected circumferentially together with its bony attachments that were thinned with the drill (superior and inferior hemilaminae, base of spinous process, mesial one-third facet) (**Fig. 97.7**). A safe and effective method of ligament and bone removal is to insert a small cottonoid into the epidural dissection plane that was made with the curette. Gentle pressure on the cottonoid with a suction tip in one hand protects the dura as ligament and bone are removed with a Kerrison in the other hand.

The outer border of the thecal sac and traversing nerve root are identified in the lateral recess. The dura is dissected from overgrown facet, synovium, and ligament using sharp curettes. The degenerative pathology is undercut laterally with Kerrison punches (**Fig. 97.8**). Decompression continues out to the medial pedicle wall, which can be identified by palpation with a Woodson tool. Once decompressed laterally, the traversing root and thecal sac are mobilized medially, and the disk space is palpated. Rarely, a soft disk herniation contributes to the stenosis, and a diskectomy is performed as described in Chapter 98. A hard disk–osteophyte complex is more common and generally left in place. However, if it causes significant neural compression, the disk–osteophyte complex can be thinned with a high-speed bur. Adequate ventral, lateral, and dorsal decompression of the traversing root is confirmed by inspection and palpation with a Woodson tool (**Fig. 97.9**). The neural foramina above and below the pedicle are palpated, and foraminal decompression (Chapter 96) is performed as necessary. **Box 97.1** lists the key operative steps and the problems that can arise.

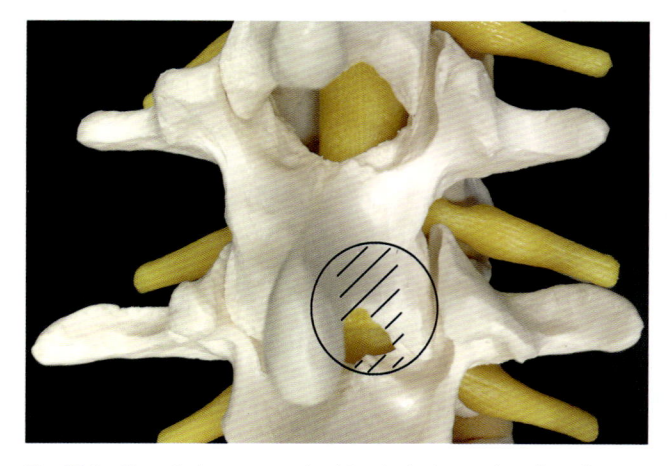

Fig. 97.1 The tubular retractor *(circle)* is docked onto the inferior laminar edge. The *parallel lines* illustrate the bone removal needed for lateral recess decompression: the inferior half of the superior hemilamina, the superiormost portion of the inferior hemilamina, and the mesial one third of the facet.

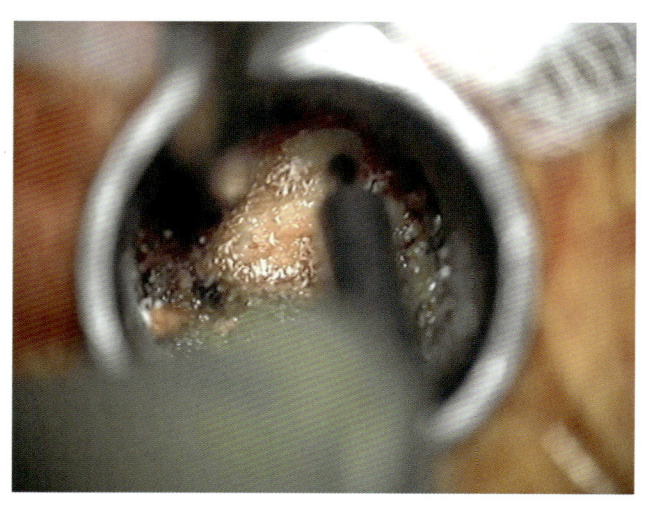

Fig. 97.2 The hemilaminotomy is performed using a high-speed drill with an angled shaft.

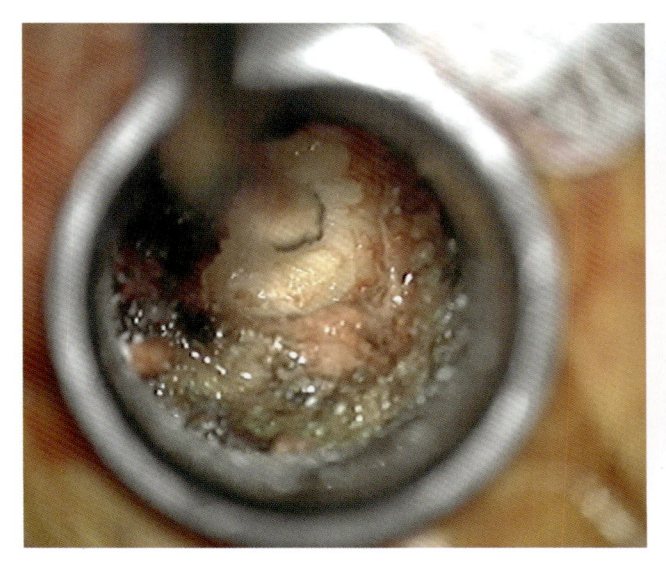

Fig. 97.3 At the inferior one third of the lamina, the ligamentum flavum is safely exposed with the drill alone.

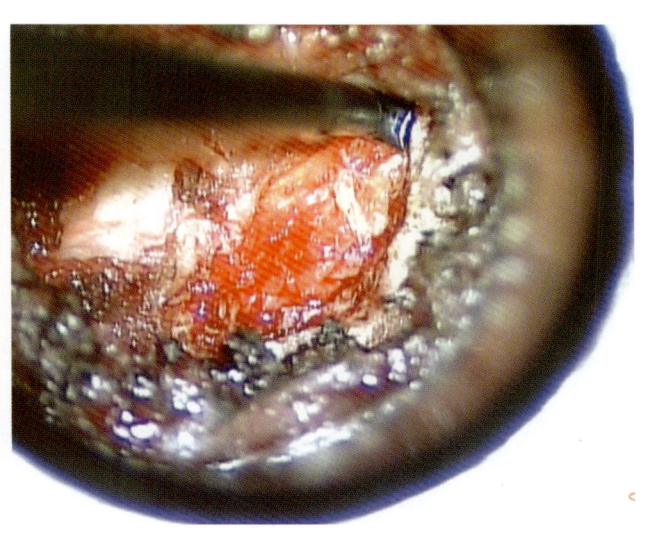

Fig. 97.4 To access the epidural space, the ligamentum flavum's superior attachment on the ventral surface of the lamina can be released with an upgoing curette.

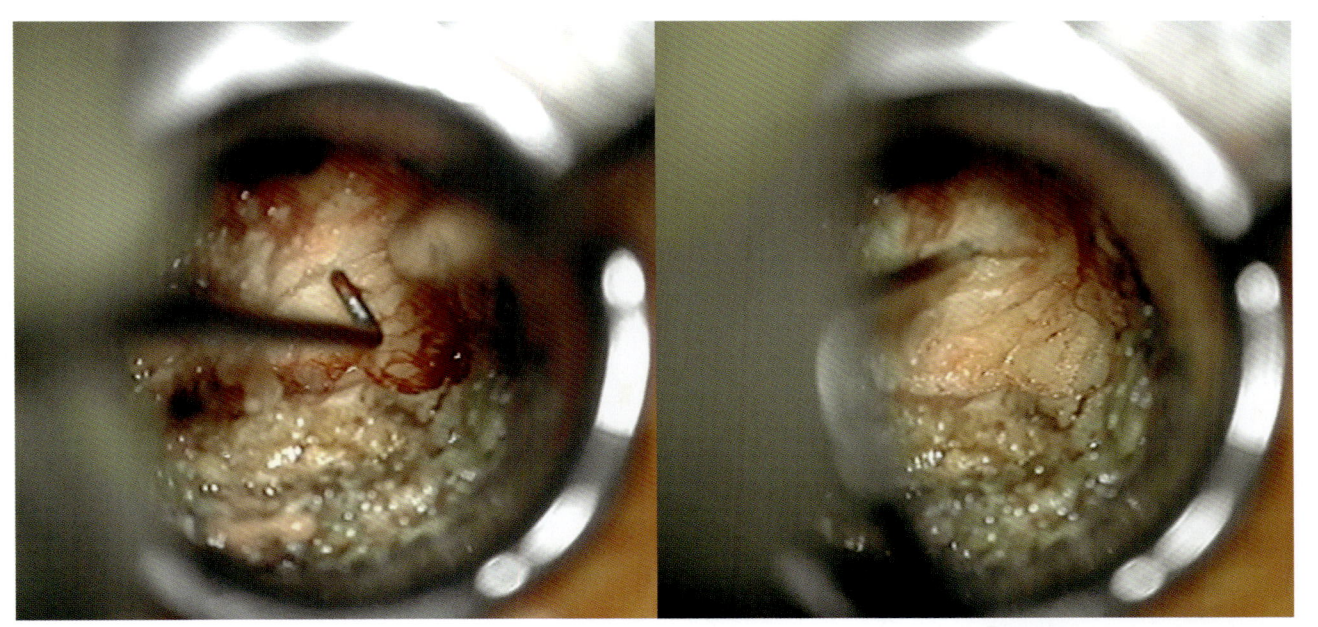

Fig. 97.5 Alternatively, the ligament can be pierced with a nerve hook **(a)**, which is swept side to side to create an opening **(b)**.

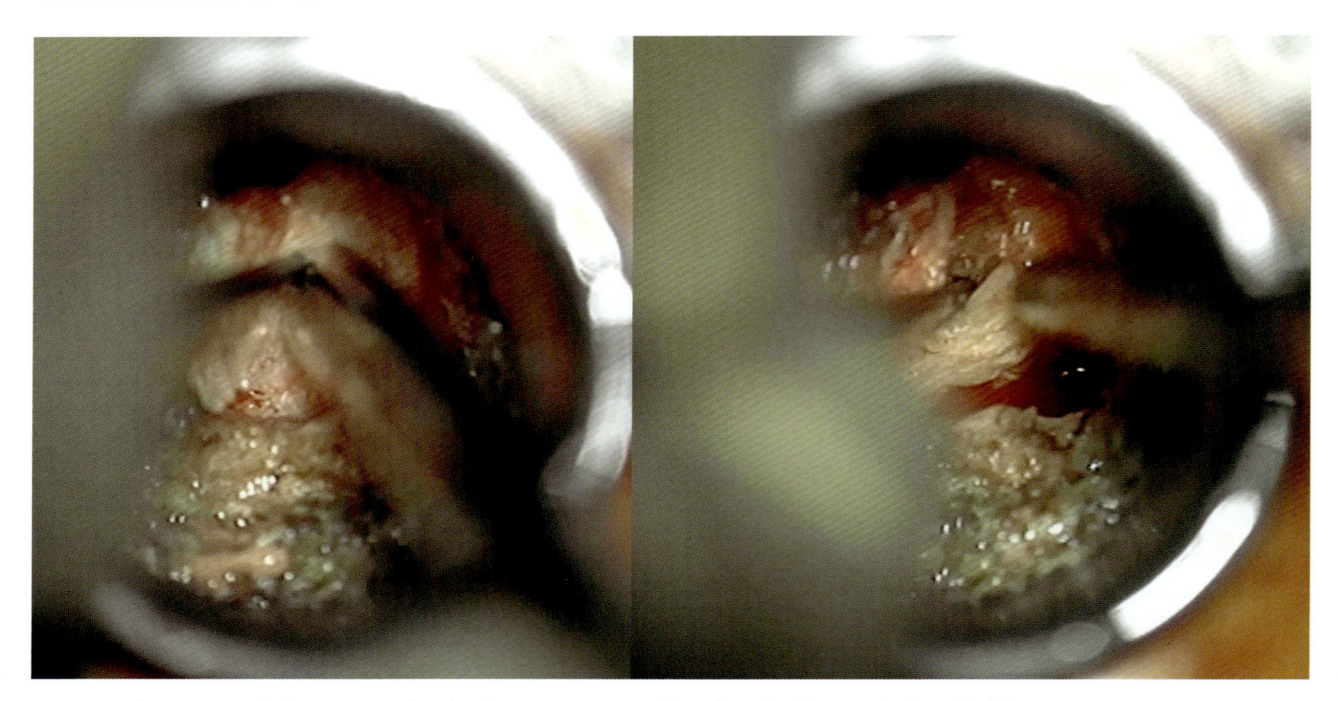

Fig. 97.6 The opening in the ligament is widened with a Kerrison rongeur **(a)**, with epidural fat now clearly visible **(b)**.

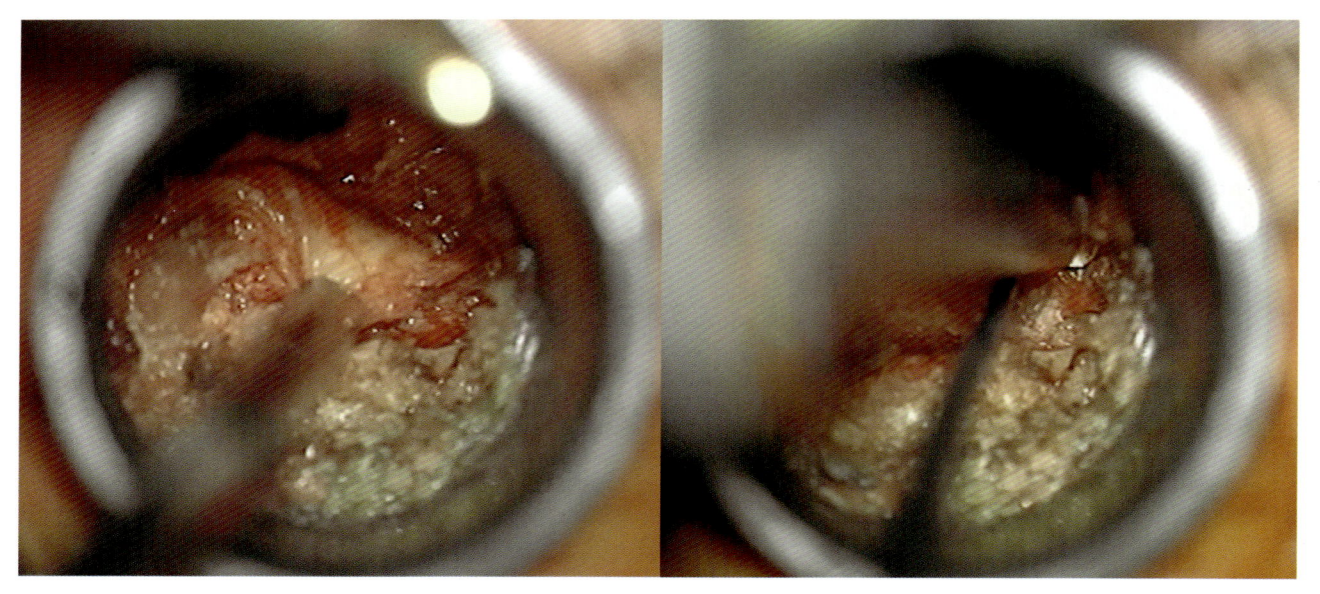

Fig. 97.7 With the freed portion of the ligament retracted with a nerve hook or suction tip **(a)**, the remainder of the ligament is removed together with its thinned bony attachments **(b)**.

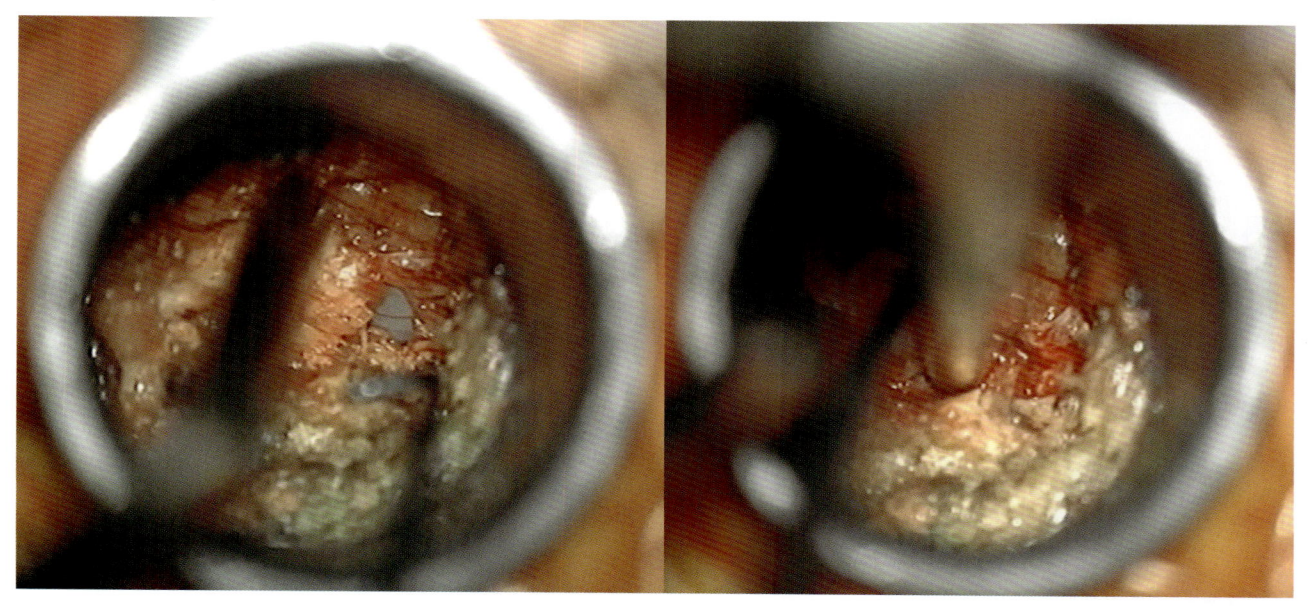

Fig. 97.8 The traversing root is compressed by overgrown ligament and facet **(a)**. The degenerative pathology is undercut with Kerrison rongeurs out to the pedicle **(b)**.

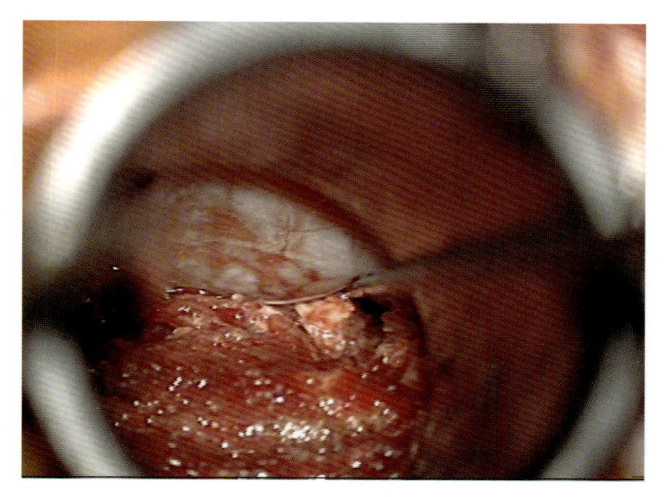

Fig. 97.9 Decompression continues until the traversing root is free on visual and tactile inspection.

Box 97.1 Key Operative Steps and Potential Problems

Step	Problems
Tubular retractor placement	Improper docking over disk space
Laminotomy	Over-resection of pars or facet
Ligamentum flavum removal	Dural adhesions and tears
Lateral recess decompression	Residual stenosis

98 MIS Posterior Lumbar Diskectomy

Russell G. Strom and Anthony K. Frempong-Boadu

A variety of disk herniations can be treated with a tubular retractor approach (primary or recurrent, small or large, paracentral or foraminal). Once the tubular retractor is docked onto the lamina, the operation is nearly identical to an open microdiskectomy. Longer, bayoneted instruments are used for improved visualization through the narrow field.

Surgical Procedure

A tubular retractor approach (Chapter 95) and hemilaminotomy (Chapter 97) are performed over the pathological disk space. Typically only the inferior one third of the superior lamina and superiormost aspect of the inferior lamina need to be drilled, but additional laminar removal may be required for disks migrating cranially or caudally. In the setting of a very large central disk herniation, the laminotomy can be extended medially to include the base of the spinous process and contralateral lamina. This additional bone removal reduces pressure on the thecal sac, enabling it to be more easily mobilized for the diskectomy. The thecal sac and traversing nerve root are identified, and decompression continues into the mesial facet to expose the lateral border of the thecal sac. Insufficient exposure leads to increased tension on the dura during retraction, with the potential for neurologic injury or dural tear.

Once exposed, the traversing root and thecal sac are mobilized medially and protected with a nerve root retractor (**Fig. 98.1**). Epidural fat and vessels are coagulated to reveal the posterior longitudinal ligament overlying the disk space (**Fig. 98.2**). If a large or adherent herniation is visualized, this can be gently dissected away from the dura using a Penfield No. 4 dissector, nerve hook, or down-going curette. Complete mobilization of the traversing root is critical. If the thecal sac is accidentally retracted without the root, the root (often draped over the herniated disk) can be mistaken for disk and cut during the intended annulotomy. **Fig. 98.3** demonstrates a broad, thinned nerve root that resembles a disk herniation. However, no other structure is identified to be the nerve root, and gentle medialization confirms that it is a root flattened by a large disk herniation. If no clear nerve root is seen, further lateral exposure is performed out to the pedicle, and then blunt dissection of the lateral spinal canal is performed from superior to inferior, thereby medializing a thinned or laterally displaced root.

For herniations contained beneath the posterior longitudinal ligament (subligamentous), an annulotomy is made with a bayoneted knife (**Fig. 98.4**). A series of progressively larger downgoing curettes is used to mobilize the disk herniation toward the annulotomy site (**Fig. 98.5**). Disk material is removed with straight and up-biting pituitary rongeurs (**Fig. 98.6**). Medial disk

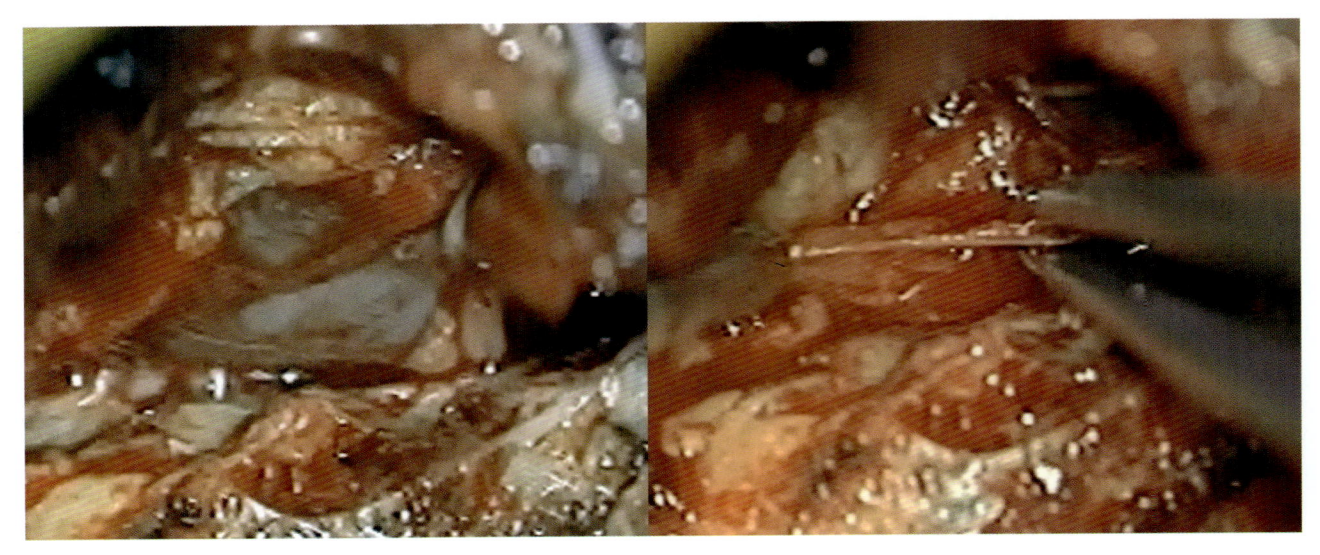

Fig. 98.1 (a) The thecal sac and traversing root are exposed. (b) The root is mobilized medially, and epidural vessels and fat are coagulated with the bipolar.

removal is important for large central disk herniations, whereas lateral disk removal is critical if the disk extends into the foramen.

On the other hand, a disk herniation piercing through the posterior longitudinal ligament (transligamentous) often requires no annulotomy. It can be mobilized free with a nerve hook (**Fig. 98.7**) and then pulled from the annular tear with a pituitary rongeur (**Fig. 98.8**). Gentle outward pressure, with intermittent release to re-grasp the base of the herniation as it is delivered, will sometimes enable the disk herniation to be delivered in one piece (**Fig. 98.9**). Once the herniated fragment is removed and palpation reveals no further compression, the diskectomy is complete. To avoid destabilizing the disk, the annular tear is not widened, and the disk space is not explored unless there is persistent mass effect.

Rarely, the disk pathology is found to be a calcified disk–osteophyte complex that cannot be entered with a knife. In these cases, hemilaminotomy alone is generally adequate to relieve nerve compression. Occasionally, if the disk–osteophyte complex causes significant mass effect, the calcified surface is thinned with a high-speed bur down to soft disk material, which can then be mobilized and resected with the usual instruments.

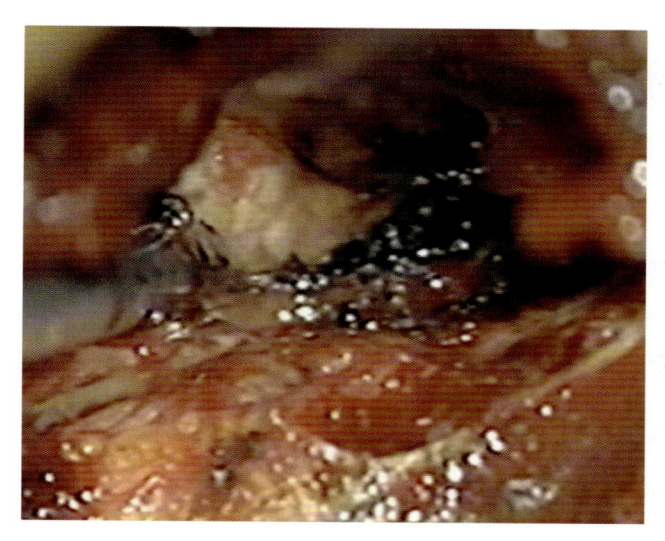

Fig. 98.2 The disk herniation is noted beneath the posterior longitudinal ligament (subligamentous).

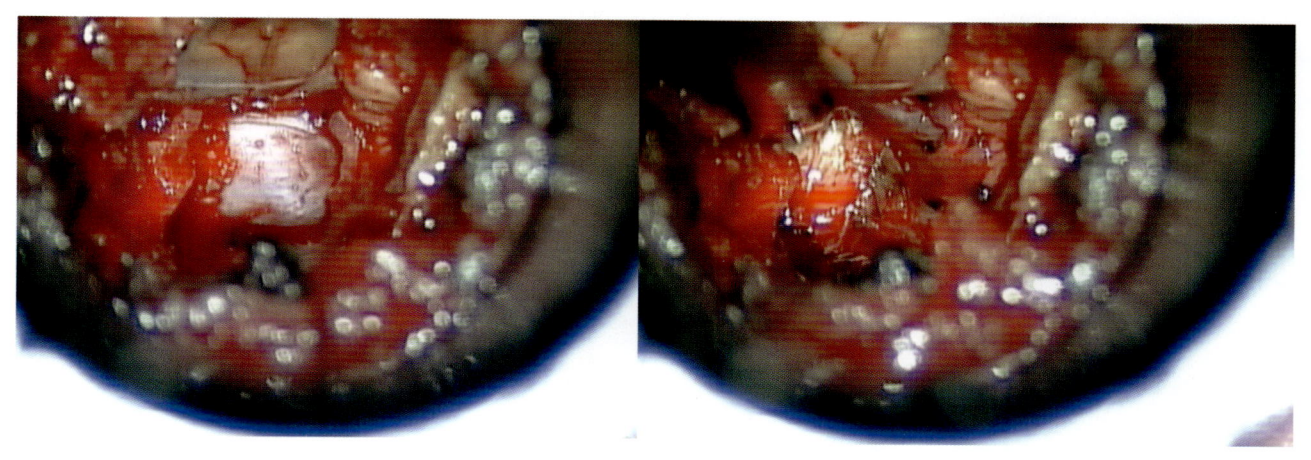

Fig. 98.3 (a) In another patient, the nerve root is flattened and could be mistaken for disk material. (b) Careful medialization of this structure reveals a large underlying disk herniation.

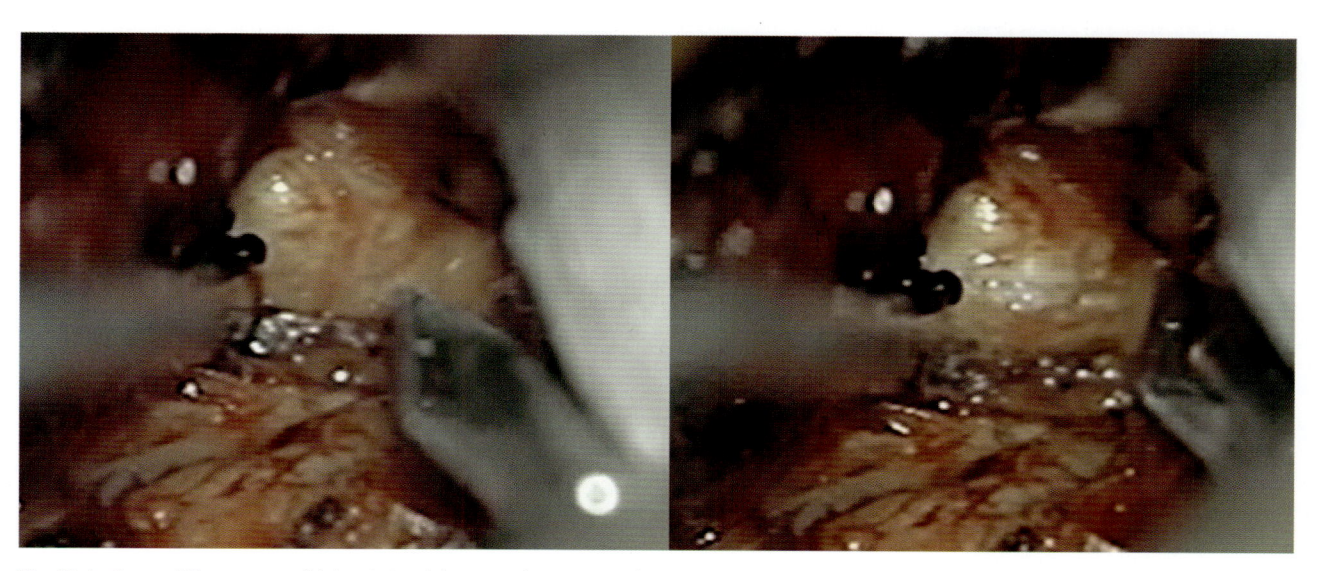

Fig. 98.4 For a subligamentous disk herniation (a), an annulotomy is made with a bayonetted knife (b).

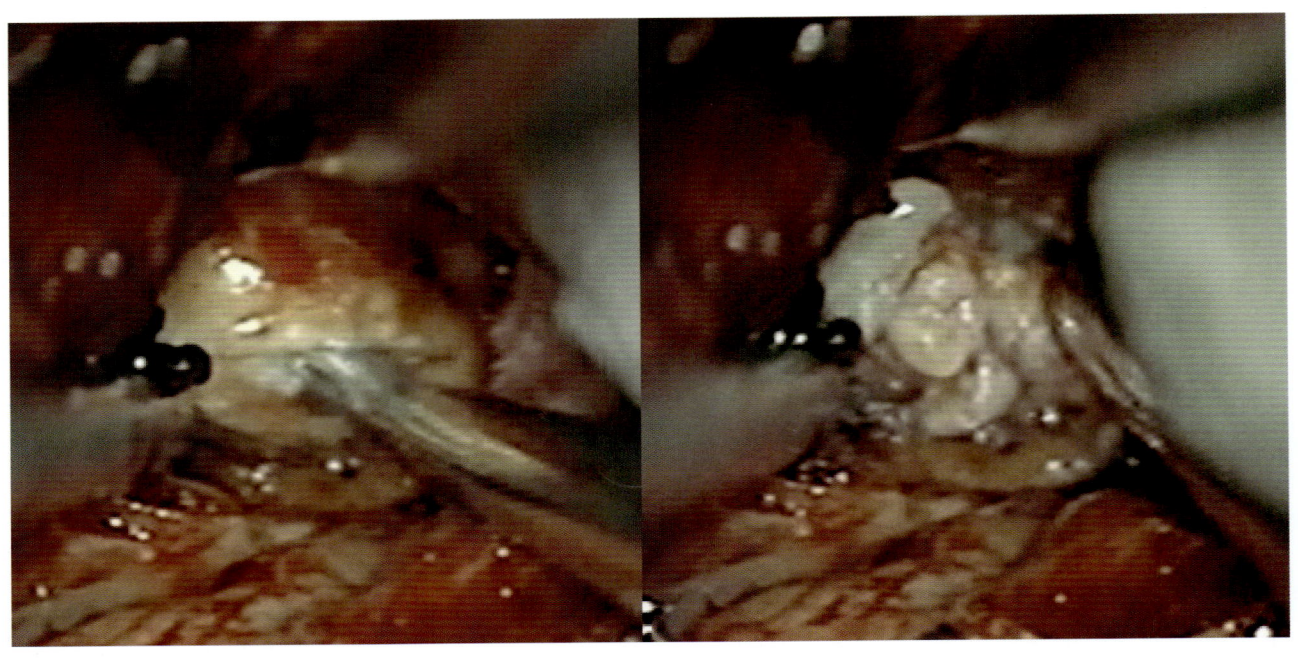

Fig. 98.5 A downgoing curette is inserted **(a)** and delivers disk material toward the annulotomy **(b)**.

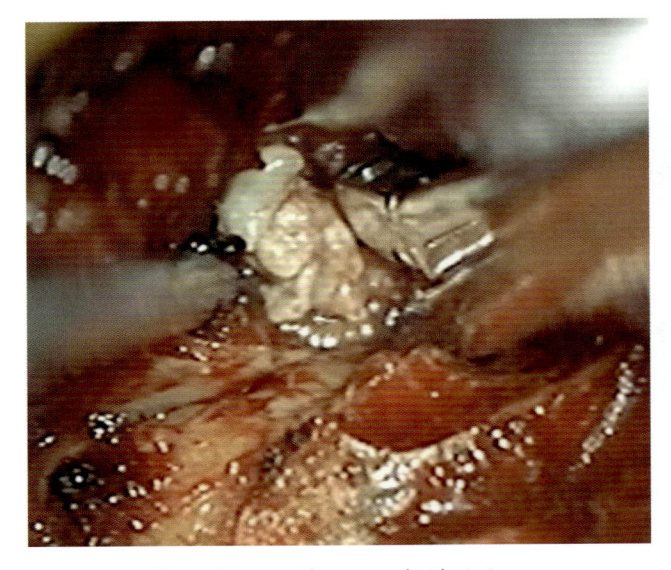

Fig. 98.6 Mobilized disk material is removed with pituitary rongeurs.

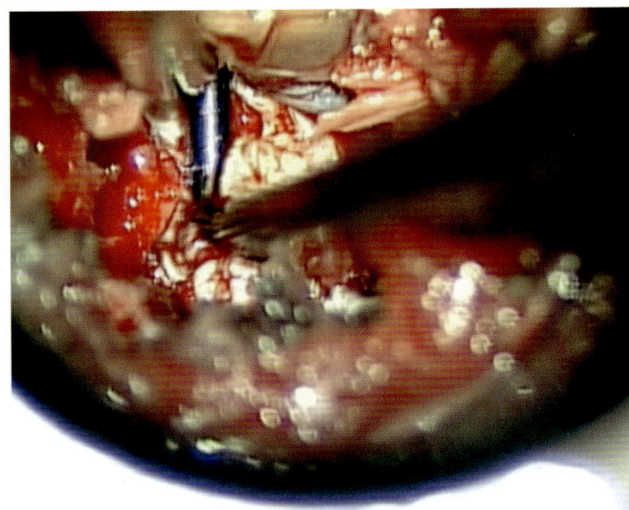

Fig. 98.7 A transligamentous disk herniation is mobilized using a nerve hook. No annulotomy is required.

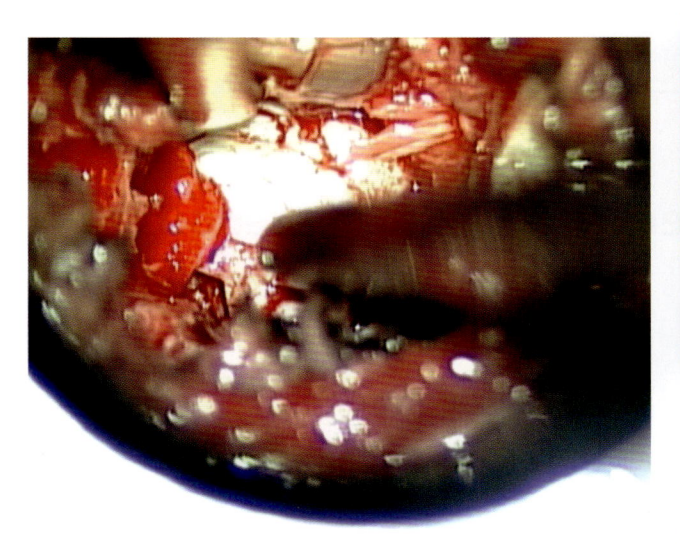

Fig. 98.8 The disk herniation is carefully pulled into the field with pituitary rongeurs.

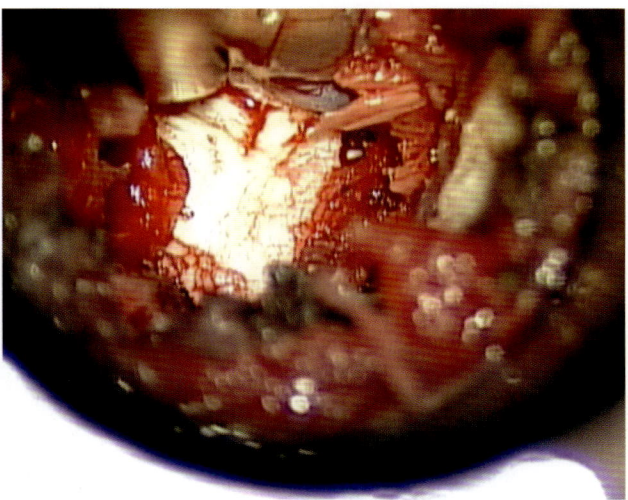

Fig. 98.9 Gentle outward pressure, together with intermittent re-grasping at the base of the herniation, sometimes enables a disk herniation to be delivered in one large piece.

The ventral thecal sac and nerve root are inspected and palpated with a Woodson tool to rule out residual compression. Not uncommonly, further disk material can be found medial, lateral, cranial, or caudal to the working site. To evacuate any remaining free fragments, saline is injected into the disk space using a syringe attached to an angiocatheter. The neural foramina above and below the pedicle are palpated and decompressed as needed. **Box 98.1** lists the key operative steps and the problems that can arise.

Box 98.1 Key Operative Steps and Potential Problems

Step	Problems
Tubular retractor placement	Improper docking over disk space
Laminotomy	Over-resection of pars or facet
Ligamentum flavum removal	Dural adhesions and tears
Nerve root medialization	Neural injury
Diskectomy	Incomplete decompression, destabilization

99 MIS Posterior Lumbar Decompression of Stenosis

Russell G. Strom and Anthony K. Frempong-Boadu

Both sides of the spinal canal can be decompressed through a single paramedian minimally invasive surgery (MIS) approach. Following ipsilateral hemilaminotomy, the tubular retractor is pivoted medially to expose the base of the spinous process and contralateral spinal canal (**Fig. 99.1**). This approach can be used to treat bilateral lateral recess/foraminal stenosis that would otherwise be treated with an open laminectomy or bilateral hemilaminotomies. Compared with these operations, MIS decompression from a unilateral approach preserves the contralateral musculature and facet joint, with less postoperative pain and a lower risk of instability.

Surgical Procedure

The first steps of an MIS bilateral decompression are the tubular retractor approach (Chapter 95) and unilateral hemilaminotomy/mesial facetectomy (Chapter 97). The side with the worse lateral recess stenosis is typically approached and decompressed first. Many surgeons temporarily leave the detached ligamentum flavum over the ipsilateral dura, as this can provide protection during the contralateral decompression. Once the ipsilateral hemilaminotomy is finished, the operating table is rotated away from the surgeon ~ 20 degrees, and the tubular retractor is pivoted medially toward the contralateral side. The base of the spinous process and interspinous ligament are now in view. A high-speed bur is used to remove the base of the spinous process and subsequently the undersurface of the contralateral hemilamina (**Fig. 99.2**).

Once the bony canal is expanded, the contralateral ligamentum flavum is separated from the dura with a curette or nerve hook (**Fig. 99.3**). The ligament and remaining contralateral lamina are undercut with Kerrison punches (**Fig. 99.4**). The stenotic lateral recess is palpated with a nerve hook or Woodson tool (**Fig. 99.5**). The overgrown mesial facet is undercut laterally out to the pedicle to free the traversing root (**Fig. 99.6**). Once clearly seen, the root is decompressed from cranial to caudal as it passes through the lateral recess (**Fig. 99.7**). The root can be protected with a dissector or suction during the decompression (**Fig. 99.8**). Foraminal stenosis is treated by undercutting with a Kerrison rongeur. The lateral recess and foramina are inspected and palpated to rule out residual stenosis (**Fig. 99.9**). Finally, if the ipsilateral ligamentum flavum was left in place for protection, it is now removed and the ipsilateral decompression is completed. **Box 99.1** lists the key operative steps and the problems that can arise.

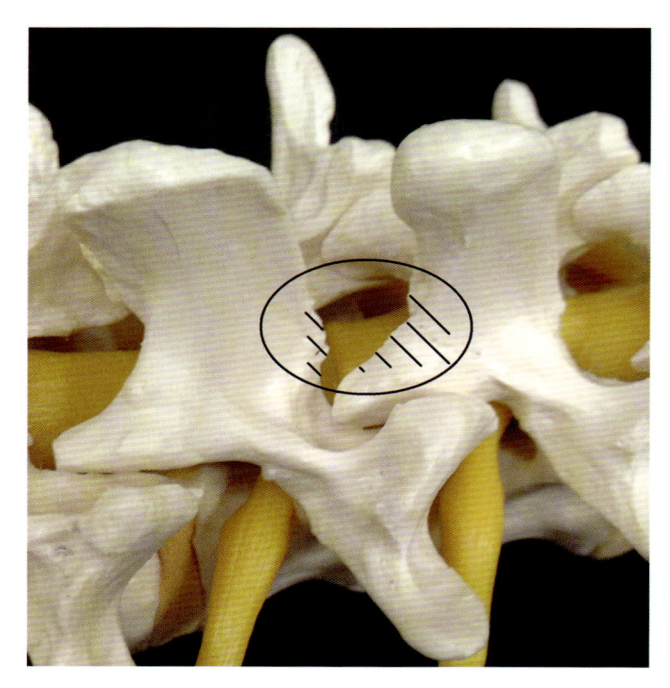

Fig. 99.1 Access to the contralateral spinal canal via ipsilateral hemilaminotomy *(parallel lines)* and angulation of the tubular retractor *(oval)*.

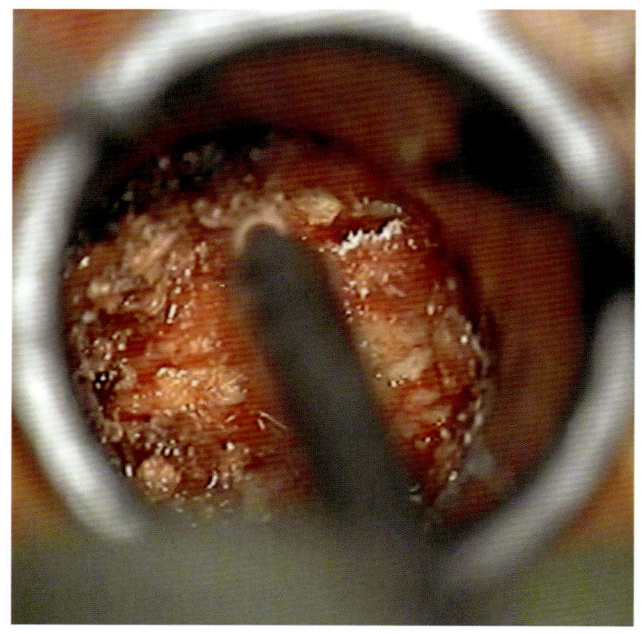

Fig. 99.2 With the ipsilateral ligamentum flavum left over the dura for protection, the base of the spinous process and undersurface of the contralateral lamina are drilled with a high-speed bur.

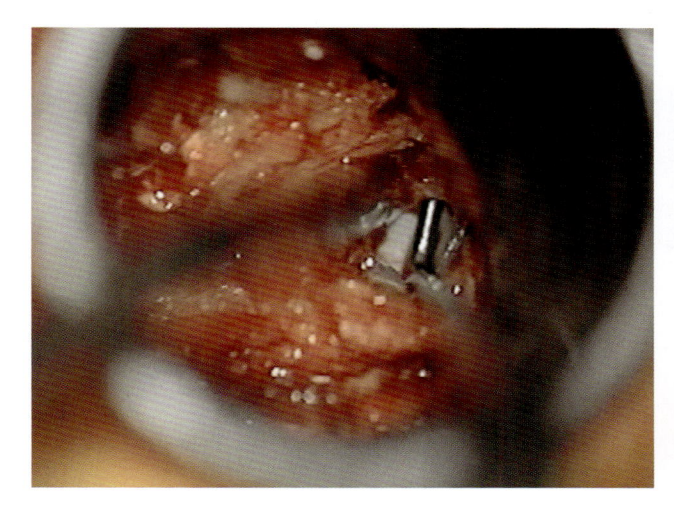

99 MIS Posterior Lumbar Decompression of Stenosis

Fig. 99.3 The contralateral ligamentum flavum is separated from the dura with a nerve hook.

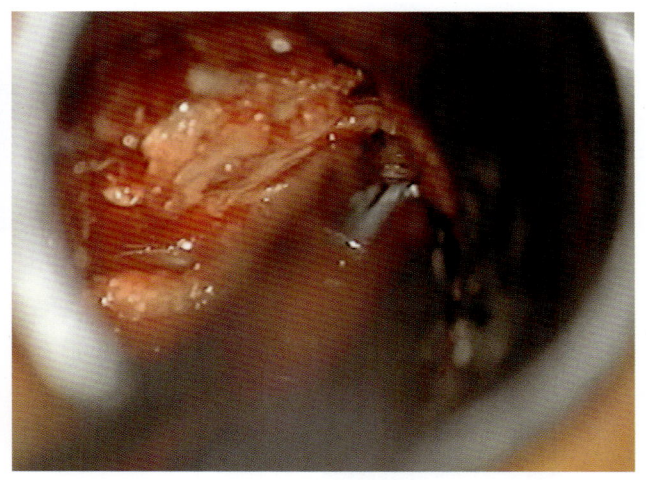

Fig. 99.4 The ligament and remaining contralateral lamina are undercut with Kerrison punches.

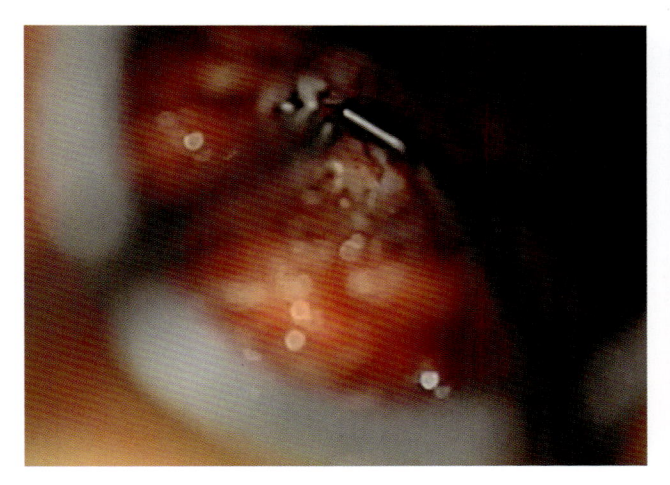

Fig. 99.5 A nerve hook is used to palpate the stenotic contralateral lateral recess out to the pedicle.

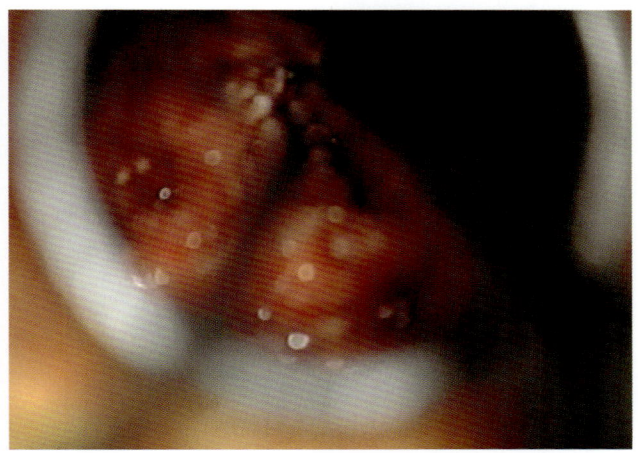

Fig. 99.6 The overgrown contralateral mesial facet is undercut with a Kerrison rongeurs.

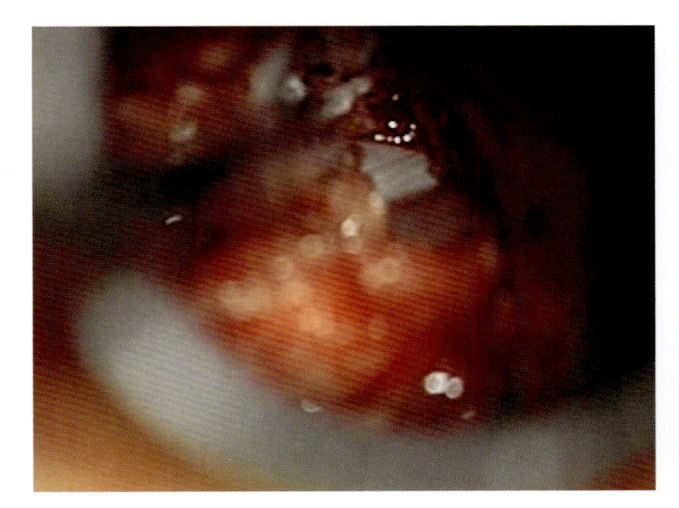

Fig. 99.7 Once clearly identified, the traversing root is freed from ligament and facet from cranial to caudal.

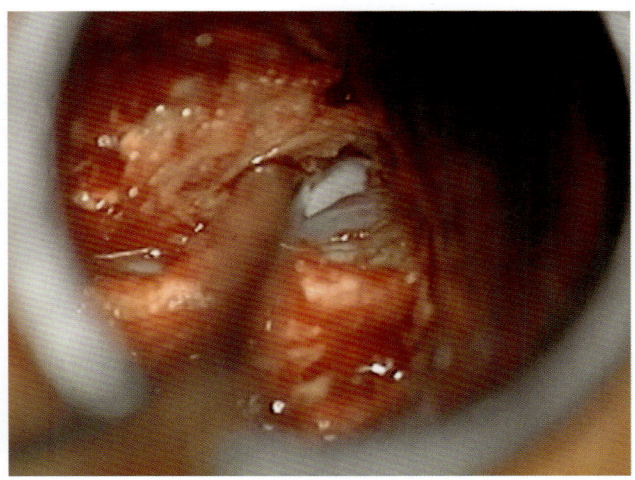

Fig. 99.8 The root can be retracted with a suction tip during the decompression.

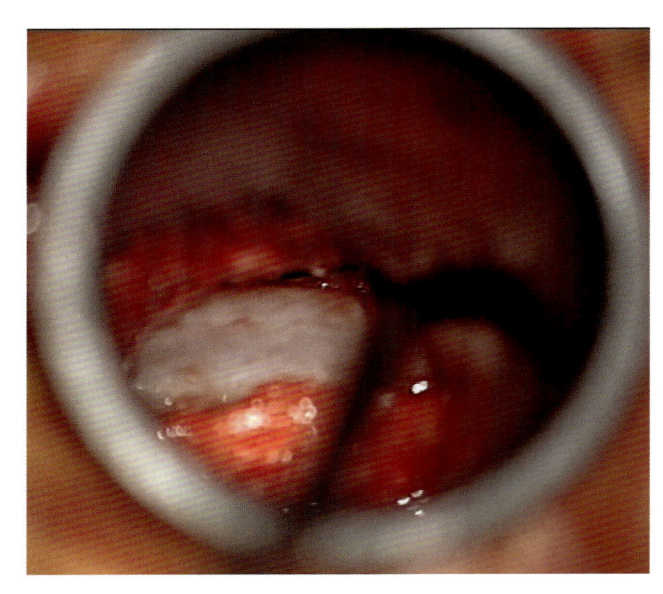

Fig. 99.9 Visual and tactile inspection of the contralateral traversing root ensures no residual compression.

Box 99.1 Key Operative Steps and Potential Problems

Step	Problems
Tubular retractor placement	Improper docking over interspace
Ipsilateral hemilaminotomy	Over-resection of pars or facet
Ligamentum flavum release	Dural adhesions and tears
Lateral recess decompression	Residual stenosis
Contralateral decompression	Unfamiliar working angle leading to durotomy, subtotal decompression

100 Microdiskectomy for Foraminal or Far Lateral Disk Herniations

Olatilewa O. Awe, Andrew James Grossbach, and Patrick W. Hitchon

Indications

- Minimally invasive surgery (MIS) pars approach for foraminal disk herniation (FDH), located lateral to the pedicle

Contraindications

- None

Advantages

- MIS for FDH can be achieved without sacrifice of the inferior or superior facets.
- MIS approach through a tube requires minimal soft tissue dissection, and is associated with less postoperative pain than with an open larger exposure.

Disadvantages

- In cases of reoperation, or where the facets are markedly hypertrophied, and particularly at L5-S1, the pars approach may require patience and can be tedious.
- Repair of a dural tear is difficult through a tube, and when large, the tear may require conversion to an open procedure.

Anatomy and Available Procedures

Far lateral disk herniations (FLDH) or foraminal disk herniations (FDH) account for up to 12% of lumbar disk herniations.[1–4] The disks are found lateral to the pedicle causing foraminal stenosis with exiting nerve root compression. Different surgical techniques can be utilized for excision of the herniated disk and decompression of the affected nerve root with careful consideration of anatomy, patient's body habitus, and feasibility of surgical success.[3,5–12] Despite the numerous options for decompression, the method of choice is increasingly shifting toward MIS, which offers several advantages, including shorter operative time, less blood loss, smaller surgical incisions, reduced postoperative pain, and quicker return to routine activities.[13–15] However, MIS requires extra training that is becoming integral to all residency programs.

Symptoms and Diagnosis

Symptoms of FLDH are often acute and consist of back and leg pain. The back pain usually subsides, and the patient is left with leg pain and numbness. As the involved levels are generally L3-L4 and L4-L5, patients complain of difficulty climbing stairs, and on exam display a depressed knee jerk. The ideal diagnostic test for FDH is magnetic resonance imaging (MRI). Sagittal and axial images reveal the canal stenosis and the displacement of the nerve root and ganglion rostrally and posteriorly. Once the diagnosis is made, and if the deficits are not disabling, a trial of physical therapy, analgesics, and epidural steroid injections is an option. If conservative management fails, surgery can then be undertaken.

Case Examples: Technique

A 33-year-old man who hurt his back while lifting an air conditioner 4 months earlier presented with pain radiating down the left thigh and complained of difficulty climbing stairs. On exam, he had numbness of the anterior thigh, 4/5 motor strength of the quadriceps, and a depressed knee jerk. Sagittal MRI T1- and T2-weighted sagittal and axial images revealed a compromised L4-L5 neural foramen (**Figs. 100.1**). The herniation is better appreciated on the T1 images. Having failed improvement with time and epidural steroids, surgery was recommended.

For lumbar disk surgery, we prefer to use the Mizuho OSI table (Union City, CA) in all cases, particularly with overweight patients (body mass index > 30), and for improved visualization using C-arm fluoroscopy. This open table reduces intra-abdominal pressure and contributes to reduction of vascular distention and possibly of blood loss. Once the level is confirmed with fluoroscopy, a paramedian incision is selected 1 inch from midline. The incision can be farther lateral in large patients; however, lateral incisions make it difficult for the assistant to lean over the patient to assist. The dorsolumbar fascia is incised with Mayo scissors, and a series of dilators culminating with an 18- or 22-mm tube are advanced toward the spinous process and lamina at the appropriate level. Subperiosteal dissection of the paraspinal lumbar musculature (multifidus and longissimus) is carried laterally to the pars interarticularis (**Fig. 100.2**). The shortest working channel is now affixed to the operating table. The procedure requires frequent fluoroscopic confirmation.

For an L3-L4 FLDH, a partial pars resection of L3 is performed under microscopic view with a high-speed drill or narrow rongeurs. Partial resection of the lateral aspects of the L3 inferior

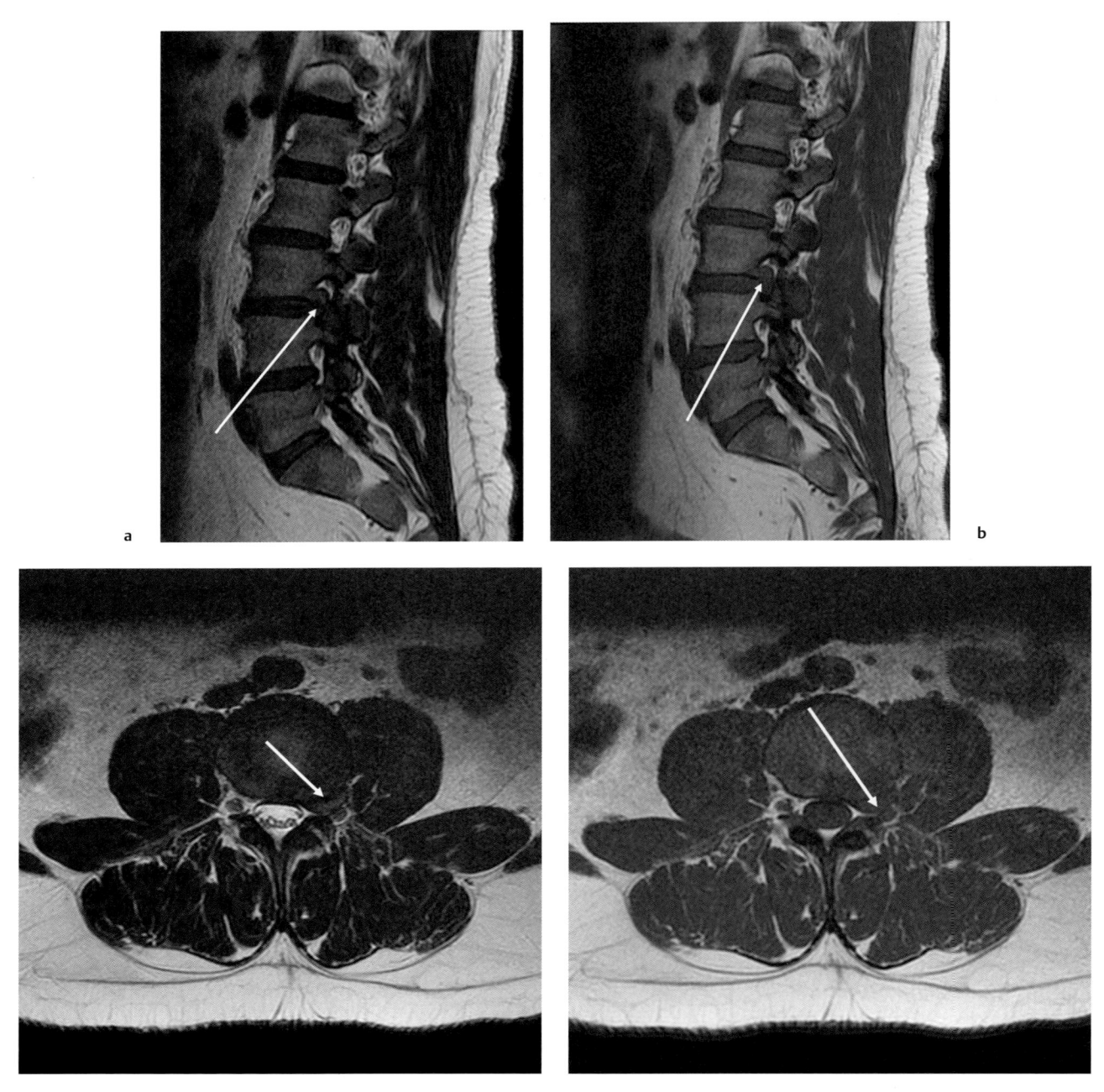

Fig. 100.1 Magnetic resonance imaging (MRI) of a left foraminal L3-L4 herniated disk *(arrow)*: **(a)** sagittal T2-weighted image; **(b)** T1-weighted image; **(c)** axial T2; and **(d)** axial T1. MRI scans are the ideal diagnostic tool for foraminal disks herniation, and in particular the T1 images.

facet and the L4 superior facet also is performed as needed to unroof the foramen and visualize the nerve and ganglion (**Fig. 100.3**). Access to the foramen entails resection of not more than one fourth or one third of the lateral pars. Such limited pars resections have been shown to safeguard spinal stability.[16,17] At more caudal levels of the lumbar spine, the superior facet may have to be partially resected. Because the pars interarticularis is only partially trimmed laterally, the superior and inferior facets of L3 remain attached. With partial resection of the pars, the neural foramen is unroofed, and the swollen, superiorly displaced nerve is visualized. The nerve root is protected and gently retracted superiorly (**Fig. 100.4**), and the disk herniation or loose fragment is identified in the axilla of the nerve (**Fig. 100.5**). In the case of a bulging disk, the annulus is incised in layers from medial to lateral to avoid violating the dura (**Fig. 100.6**). The herniated disk fragment is removed with a pituitary rongeur (**Fig. 100.7**), and the neural foramen explored with a small nerve hook. All loose disk fragments from the L3-4 interspace are excised without an attempt at exenterating the entire disk (**Fig. 100.8**). If there is excessive manipulation of the nerve root, one may instill 30 mg of methylprednisolone acetate onto the nerve root. The fascia is approximated with 2-0 Vicryl (Ethicon, Johnson & Johnson, Somerville, NJ), the dermis with subcutaneous 3-0 suture, and the skin approximated with 4-0 absorbable suture.

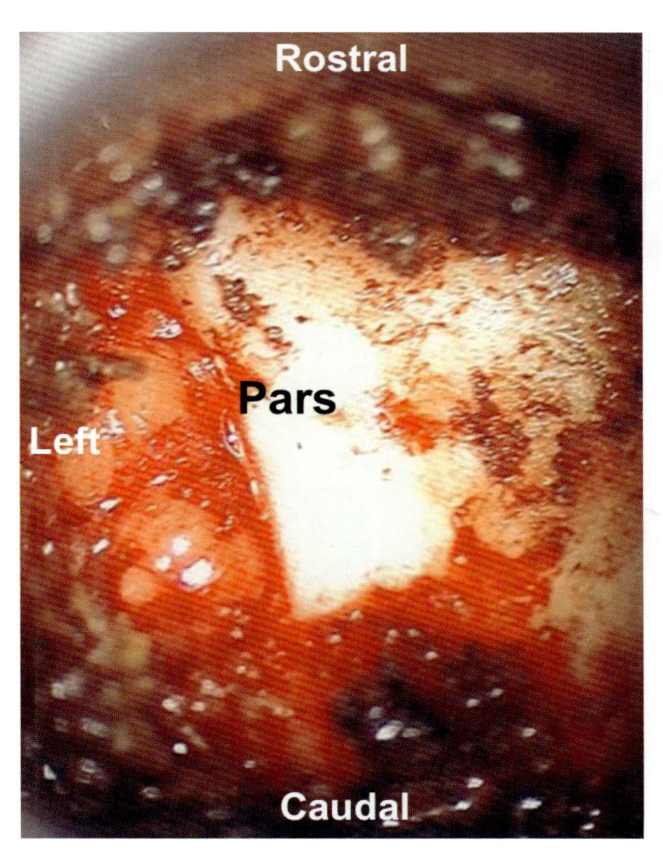

Fig. 100.2 The left L3 pars as seen through the 22-mm tube.

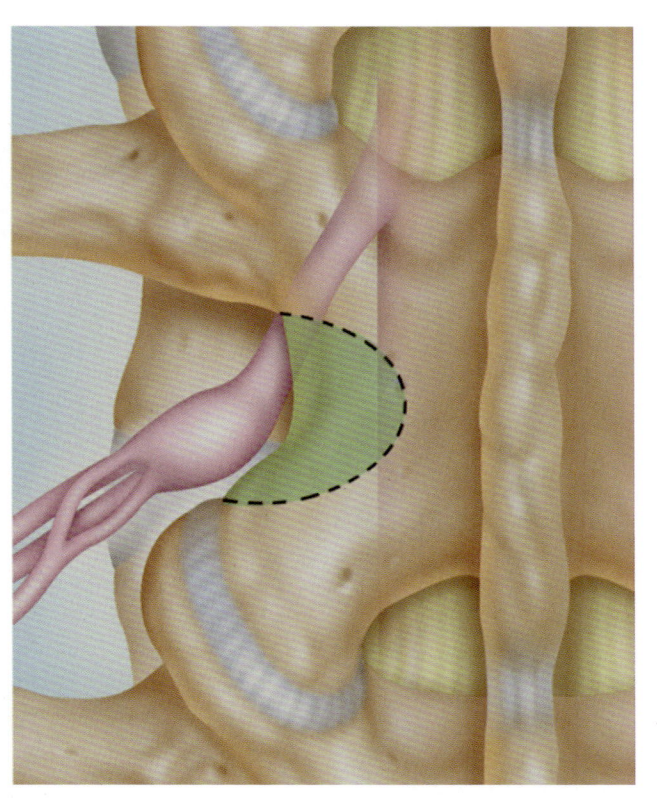

Fig. 100.3 The *green shaded area* is excised using a power drill or punch. A larger tube is not necessarily better, as it catches on the facets and transverse processes and thus prevents the surgeon from docking on the pars.

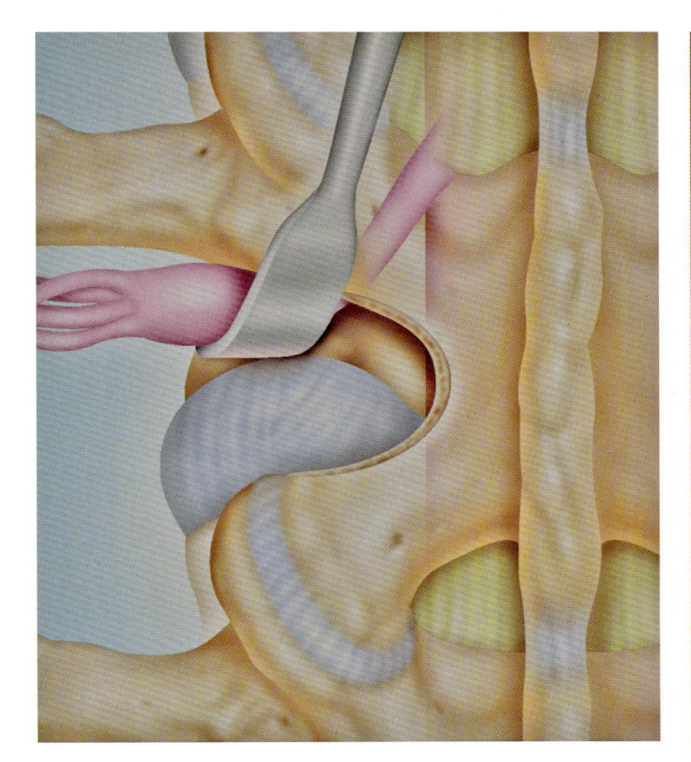

Fig. 100.4 Following excision of the lateral one third of the pars, the neural foramen is unroofed and the nerve root visualized. Elevating the root brings the herniation into view.

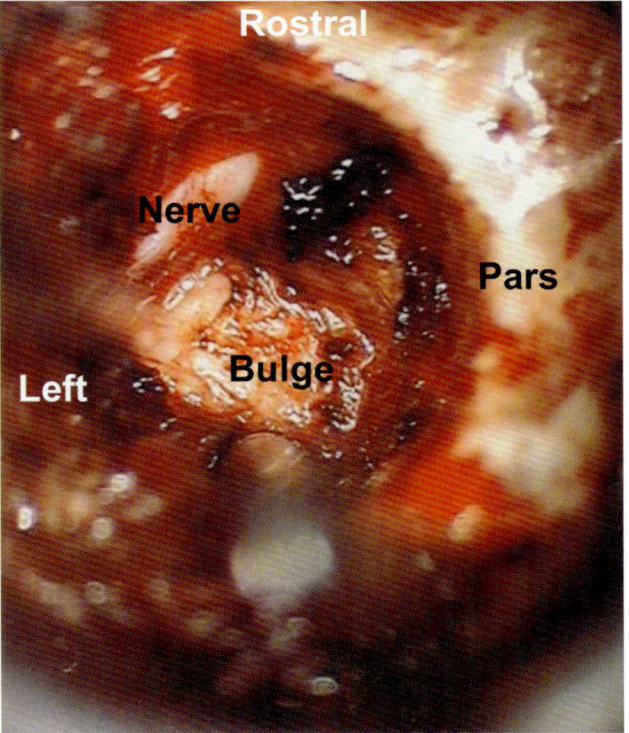

Fig. 100.5 The bulging foraminal disk is visualized displacing the root rostrally.

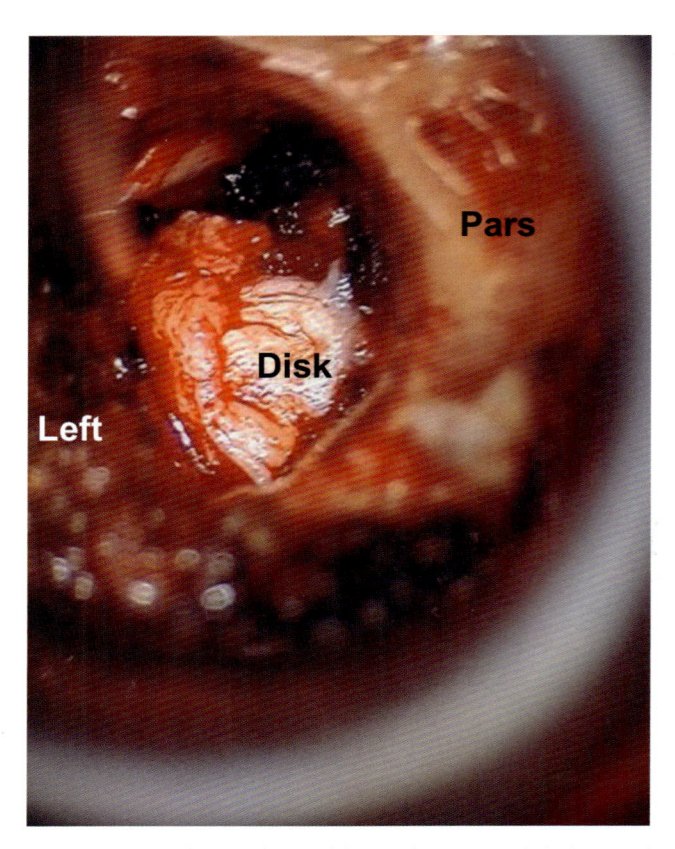

Fig. 100.6 Once the outer layers of the annulus are incised, the herniated disk presents itself.

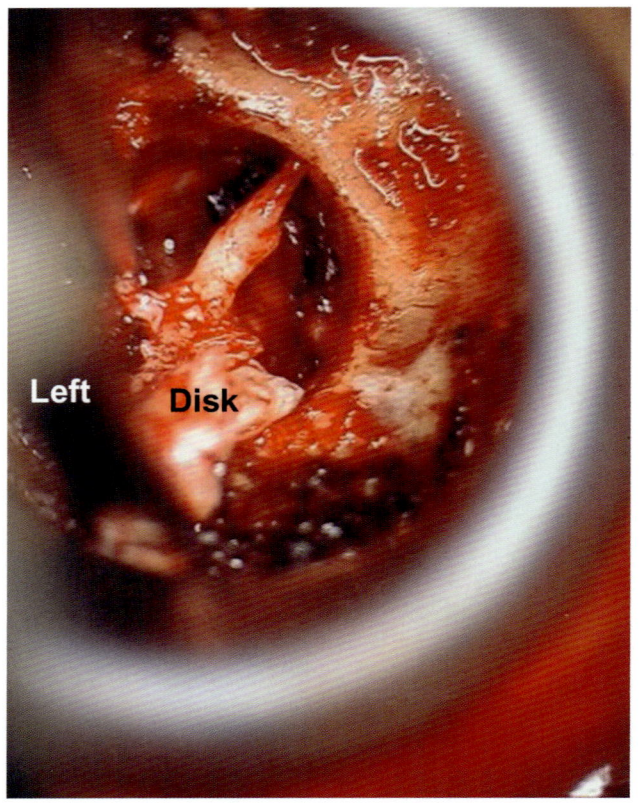

Fig. 100.7 Herniated disk fragments are retrieved easily with a pituitary rongeur.

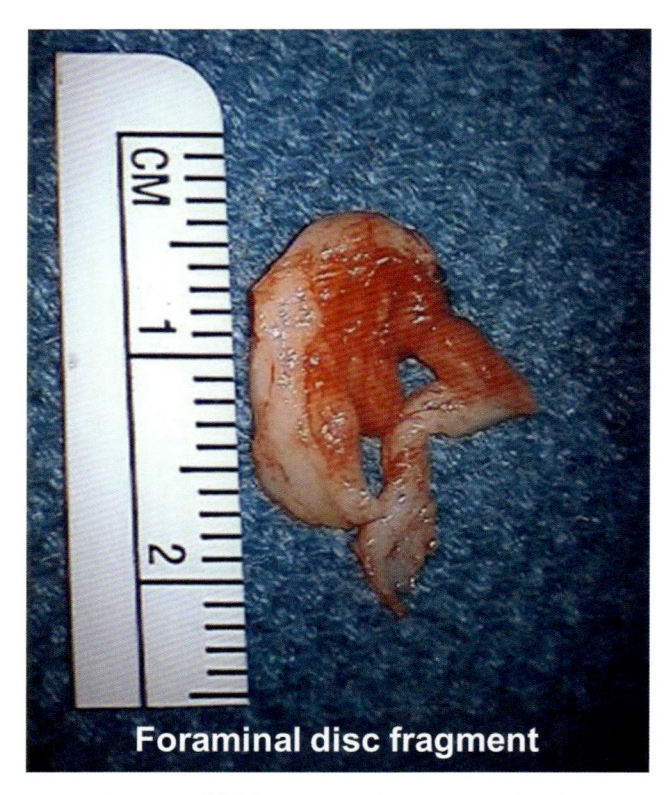

Fig. 100.8 Retrieved disk fragments can be up to 2 cm in length.

Another case example of a foraminal disk herniation is presented in **Fig. 100.9**.

After surgical intervention, patients usually have immediate relief from their preoperative symptoms. Patients should be aggressively mobilized. With minimal comorbidities, the patient is usually discharged the following day, with physical therapy as a useful adjunct.

Results

Since 2004, a total of 38 patients (23 men and 15 women) with FDH have been evaluated. Ages ranged from 33 to 90 years with a mean ± standard deviation of 58 ± 14 years. Duration of symptoms ranged from 2 weeks to 11 months. Fifteen patients had FDH at L4-L5, 11 patients at L3-L4, seven at L2-L3, four at L5-S1, and one at L1-L2. Thirty-four patients underwent MIS, with an average length of hospital stay of 1.0 ± 3 days. There was one *Candida* wound infection. Follow-up periods averaged 1 ± 2 years. With the exception of three workers' compensation cases, the results with MIS have been very gratifying.

Limitations

A potential limitation of MIS is the inability to repair dural tears and structural limitations at the L5-S1 level.[15] Generally, dural tears with MIS under the microscope are sufficiently small that packing with thrombin-soaked Gelfoam and Tisseel (Baxter Healthcare Corp., Mountain Home, AR) is sufficient. If large or persistent, more extensive exploration can be accomplished by extending the same skin incision. In our experience,

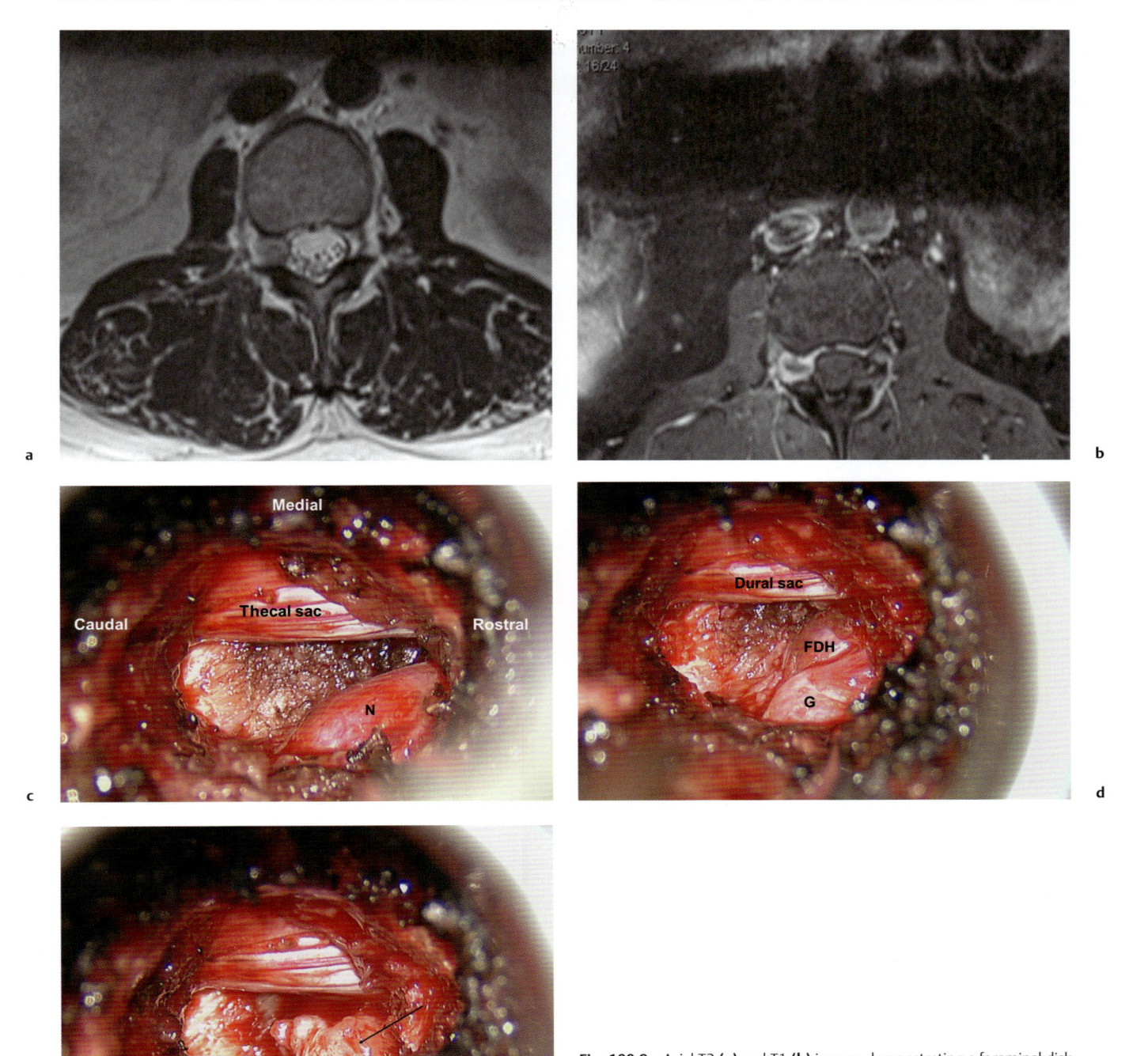

Fig. 100.9 Axial T2 **(a)** and T1 **(b)** images demonstrating a foraminal disk herniation at L2-L3 on the right. **(c)** Following partial resection of the pars of L2, the dural sac and the L2 root (N) are visualized. **(d)** Slight retraction of the nerve and ganglion (G) exposes the foraminal disk herniation (FDH). **(e)** Incising the outer layer of the annulus delivers the disk herniation *(arrow)* in the axilla of the nerve with minimal retraction.

unilateral pars resection and facetectomy at more caudal levels of the lumbar spine has not resulted in instability. MIS is technically challenging but, with encouraging outcomes, is becoming mainstream.

References

1. Sasani M, Ozer AF, Oktenoglu T, Canbulat N, Sarioglu AC. Percutaneous endoscopic discectomy for far lateral lumbar disc herniations: prospective study and outcome of 66 patients. Minim Invasive Neurosurg 2007;50:91–97
2. Siebner HR, Faulhauer K. Frequency and specific surgical management of far lateral lumbar disc herniations. Acta Neurochir (Wien) 1990;105:124–131
3. Epstein NE. Evaluation of varied surgical approaches used in the management of 170 far-lateral lumbar disc herniations: indications and results. J Neurosurg 1995;83:648–656
4. Abdullah AF, Wolber PG, Warfield JR, Gunadi IK. Surgical management of extreme lateral lumbar disc herniations: review of 138 cases. Neurosurgery 1988;22:648–653
5. Epstein NE. Different surgical approaches to far lateral lumbar disc herniations. J Spinal Disord 1995;8:383–394
6. Garrido E, Connaughton PN. Unilateral facetectomy approach for lateral lumbar disc herniation. J Neurosurg 1991;74:754–756
7. Jane JA, Haworth CS, Broaddus WC, Lee JH, Malik J. A neurosurgical approach to far-lateral disc herniation. Technical note. J Neurosurg 1990;72:143–144
8. Kunogi J, Hasue M. Diagnosis and operative treatment of intraforaminal and extraforaminal nerve root compression. Spine 1991;16:1312–1320
9. Maroon JC, Kopitnik TA, Schulhof LA, Abla A, Wilberger JE. Diagnosis and microsurgical approach to far-lateral disc herniation in the lumbar spine. J Neurosurg 1990;72:378–382
10. Wiltse LL, Spencer CW. New uses and refinements of the paraspinal approach to the lumbar spine. Spine 1988;13:696–706
11. Madhok R, Kanter AS. Extreme-lateral, minimally invasive, transpsoas approach for the treatment of far-lateral lumbar disc herniation. J Neurosurg Spine 2010;12:347–350
12. Greiner-Perth R, Böhm H, Allam Y. A new technique for the treatment of lumbar far lateral disc herniation: technical note and preliminary results. Eur Spine J 2003;12:320–324
13. Foley KT, Smith MM, Rampersaud YR. Microendoscopic approach to far-lateral lumbar disc herniation. Neurosurg Focus 1999;7:e5
14. Faust SE, Ducker TB, VanHassent JA. Lateral lumbar disc herniations. J Spinal Disord 1992;5:97–103
15. Salame K, Lidar Z. Minimally invasive approach to far lateral lumbar disc herniation: technique and clinical results. Acta Neurochir (Wien) 2010;152:663–668
16. Ivanov AA, Faizan A, Ebrahim NA, Yeasting R, Goel VK. The effect of removing the lateral part of the pars interarticularis on stress distribution at the neural arch in lumbar foraminal microdecompression at L3-L4 and L4-L5: anatomic and finite element investigations. Spine 2007;32:2462–2466
17. Tender GC, Kutz S, Baratta R, Voorhies RM. Unilateral progressive alterations in the lumbar spine: a biomechanical study. J Neurosurg Spine 2005;2:298–302

101 Far Lateral MIS Diskectomy

Hani R. Malone and Alfred T. Ogden

Lumbar disk herniations are considered "far lateral" when the extruded disk fragment impinges upon the exiting nerve root lateral to the pedicles (**Fig. 101.1**). Although less common than medial disk herniations, which compress nerve roots within the lateral recess, far lateral herniations often cause a more exquisitely painful radiculopathy and are often associated with motor or sensory deficits. The far lateral distinction also has important implications for surgical planning and correct targeting of the offending pathology and affected nerve root. This chapter discusses the evaluation and treatment of far lateral disk herniation and specifically describes the minimally invasive surgery (MIS) approach to far lateral microdiskectomy.

The typical lumbar disk herniation compresses the nerve root that exits the spinal canal a level below the site of herniation. For example, a medial herniation at the L4-L5 level compresses the L5 nerve root at a point called the *axilla* of the root in the lateral recess. This is just when the root diverges from the thecal sac in its own separate root sleeve before continuing inferiorly, around the L5 pedicle, and exiting the spinal canal through the L5-S1 intervertebral foramen. This is not the case for far lateral disk herniations, which extend laterally to compress the rostral lumbar nerve root at the affected level. A far lateral L3-L4 lumbar disk herniation, for example, may compress the L3 nerve root either within the foramen or more distally as the root passes over the extraforaminal disk space.

Far lateral disk herniations account for ~ 10% of all lumbar disk herniations, affect higher lumbar levels, and are more likely to cause objective neurologic deficits.[1–4] A far lateral disk herniation should be suspected with the acute onset of an isolated upper lumbar radiculopathy that affects L3 or L4, causing pain in the thigh or quadriceps weakness. Ganglion irritation is common, causing exquisitely painful symptoms with herniation of even a small disk fragment. Recognition of the far lateral syndrome is important because routine microdiskectomy must be modified to decompress the exiting, rather than traversing, lumbar nerve root.

A midline incision is used in standard surgical approaches to lumbar disk herniation. Exposure of far lateral herniations through a midline incision necessitates a longer skin incision, a wide dissection of the paraspinal muscles, and potentially a greater tendency to perform a more extensive facetectomy. A paramedian, muscle-splitting approach creates a direct posterolateral corridor to the herniated disk with minimal facetectomy (**Figs. 101.1 and 101.2**). Operative morbidity can be further reduced with the use of minimally invasive retractor systems that minimize tissue dissection and blood loss and accelerate postoperative recovery.

Indications and Contraindications

Pain from lumbar disk disease often improves in days or weeks with conservative measures and only a minority of patients require surgery. In the absence of neurologic deficit or intractable pain, conservative treatment should be pursued for at least 6 weeks, as long as the patient continues to improve. Some clinical series suggest that conservative management is less successful for far lateral herniations and surgery is more frequently required.[5] Magnetic resonance imaging (MRI) should be obtained in patients with acute or progressive neurologic deficit, intractable pain, or failure of 6 weeks of conservative therapy. Lumbar diskectomy is indicated in patients with evidence of nerve root compression on neuroimaging and corresponding refractory radicular pain or acute/progressive weakness. A paramedian posterolateral surgical approach is indicated when the offending disk fragment is confined to the far lateral compartment beyond the pedicles. This approach is contraindicated when nerve root compression is medial to the pedicles.

Advantages and Disadvantages

This chapter focuses on the paramedian transmuscular approach to far lateral microdiskectomy using a minimally invasive tubular retractor system, which we believe has significant advantages over traditional midline approaches to far lateral disks.

The primary advantage of the paramedian approach is a surgical trajectory that directly exposes the offending disk and compressed nerve. By comparison, midline approaches require a longer skin incision and extensive muscle retraction to expose the far lateral space, leading to increased blood loss, muscle atrophy and postoperative pain.

The paramedian approach provides excellent exposure of far lateral disks with minimal bony decompression and preservation of the facet joint (**Fig. 101.2**).

The tubular working channel used with minimally invasive systems serves as an efficient retractor. It is placed between muscle fibers, avoiding the need to strip the muscles off their innervation and blood supply, which mitigates postoperative pain and atrophy. Bone resection is minimal or avoided entirely. Smaller incisions contribute to reduced blood loss, rapid healing, and a lower infection rate.

The main disadvantage to the MIS approach to far lateral disk herniation is the learning curve required to master the technique. This is encompassed mostly by the overall reduction in osseous landmarks exposed to the surgeon from the smaller surgical aperture.

622 V Lumbar and Lumbosacral Spine

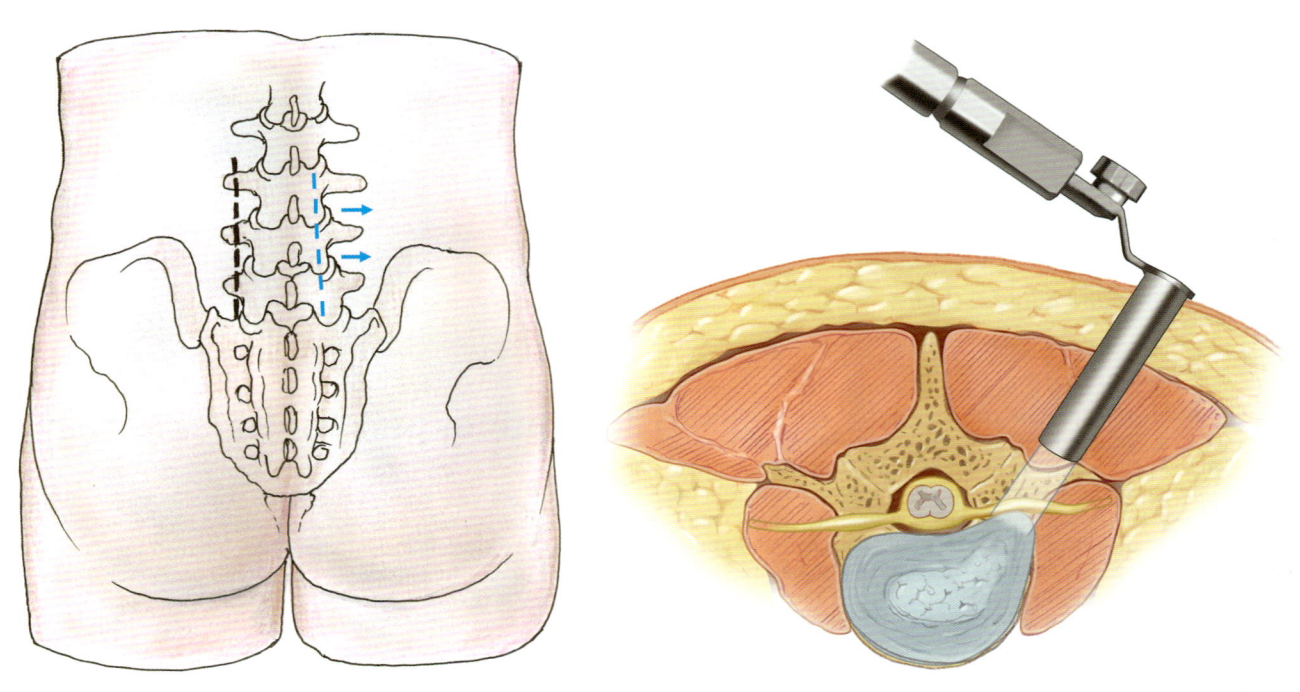

Fig. 101.1 Anatomic localization: **(a)** The "far lateral" distinction refers to disk herniations that occur lateral to the pedicles *(blue dashed line/arrows)*. In the MIS approach to far lateral diskectomy, placement of the tubular retractor system is paramedian, ~ 4 to 6 cm lateral to midline *(black dashed line)*. **(b)** This localization facilitates a direct posterolateral trajectory to the offending disk fragment and exiting nerve root.

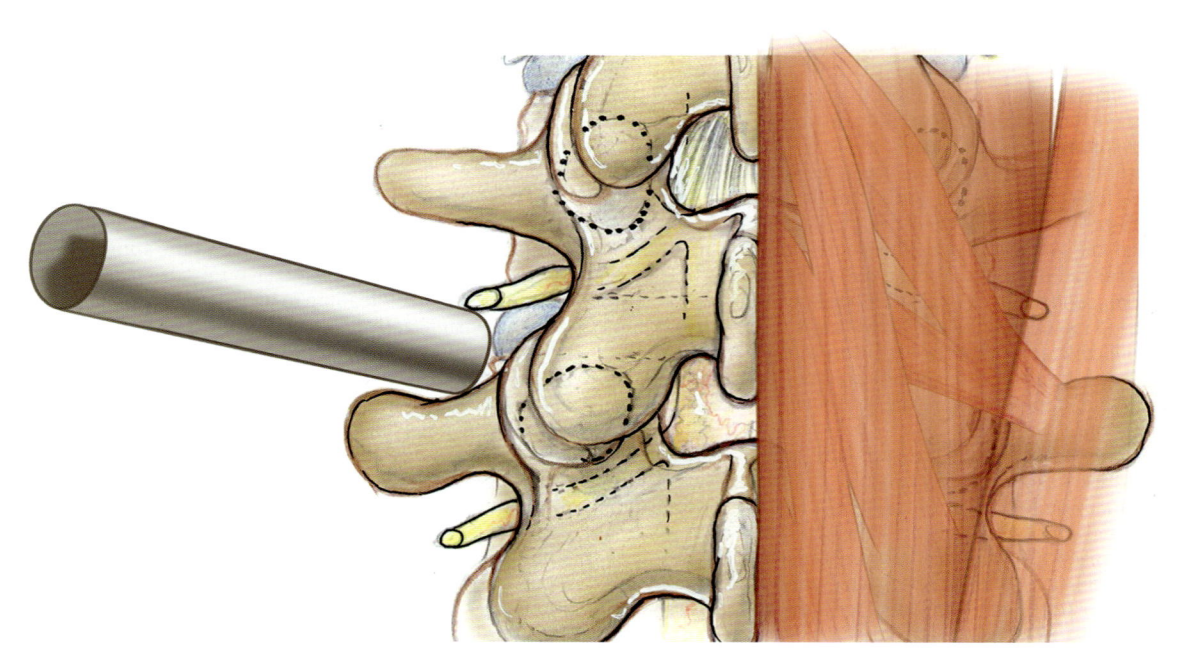

Fig. 101.2 Minimally invasive posterolateral approach. A paramedian posterolateral approach using minimally invasive tubular retractors provides direct access to the far lateral herniated disk fragment and compressed nerve root. This exposure can be achieved with little or no disruption to the facet joint, preserving the biomechanical stability of the segment.

Preoperative Imaging

Magnetic resonance imaging identifies spinal cord/nerve root compression and shows the degree of degenerative change within disks, making it the imaging modality of choice for disk disorders. It is the most effective screening tool for a differential diagnosis that includes structural disorders affecting the nerve roots (**Box 101.1**), as it clearly delineates both intra- and extradural structures. Far lateral disk herniations appear as isointense to hypointense lesions lateral to the pedicles on T2-weighted images (**Fig. 101.3**). Hypointense fat normally surrounds the dorsal root ganglion, and a loss of fat may signal a disk herniation. Parasagittal MRI studies yield the most direct view of the neural foramen and far lateral compartment. Sometimes contrast-enhanced MRI is useful to distinguish between a foraminal or extraforaminal disk and a nerve sheath tumor.

Myelography effectively visualizes spinal nerve roots and their trajectory through the neural foramina, particularly the anatomy of the nerve root sleeve. However, myelography is unrevealing in the evaluation of far lateral disk herniations, as they occur lateral to the spinal canal and root sleeve. In some instances computed tomography (CT), particularly when enhanced with diskography,[6,7] can effectively confirm far lateral disk herniation. Electrodiagnostic studies such as electromyogram (EMG) and a nerve conduction study (NCS) and selective nerve root blocks are seldom essential but useful when radiographic findings do not correlate with clinical presentation.

Box 101.1 Differential Diagnosis of Far Lateral Herniated Nucleus Pulposus

Conjoined roots
Perineural cyst
Neurofibroma
Osteophyte
Prominent venous plexus

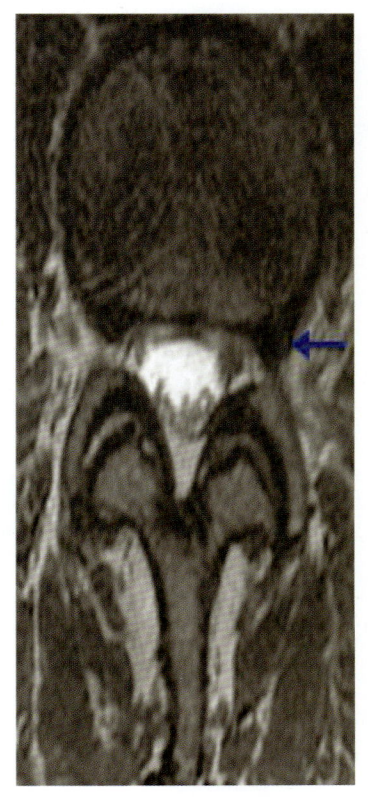

Fig. 101.3 T2-weighted magnetic resonance imaging (MRI) demonstrates a left far lateral disk herniation at the L3-L4 level *(blue arrow)*.

Surgical Procedure: Far Lateral MIS Microdiskectomy

Surgery is performed under general endotracheal anesthesia with the patient in the prone position. Use of the radiolucent Jackson table is preferable but not essential. The Wilson frame may be used for flexion to promote slight distraction of the lumbar disk spaces. In the operating room, the surgical microscope should be positioned ipsilateral to the side of the herniated disk, whereas fluoroscopy and the bed adaptor for the tubular retractor system are contralateral. Perioperative antibiotics should be administered within an hour prior to skin incision; we use cefazolin dosed by weight at our institution. A single intravenous dose of dexamethasone 10 mg preoperatively helps to mitigate potential irritation of the nerve root caused by surgical manipulation. The surgical site is sterilized in standard fashion and should be draped widely. Fluoroscopic localization is used to confirm the level of pathology.

A paramedian incision is planned on the side of the disk herniation (**Fig. 101.1**). The laterality of the incision is dictated entirely by the specifics of the patient's body habitus and the specific facet anatomy of the operated level. In our practice, the simplest way to calculate the optimal distance is to measure about a 30-degree angle from the disk herniation to the skin on axial MRI, and then the distance from that point to the midline. This will typically be 4 to 6 cm. The incision is marked and injected with local anesthetic. A stab incision is made with a No. 11 blade at the center of this mark, enabling a Kirschner wire (K-wire) to be advanced under careful fluoroscopic guidance. After localization with the K-wire, the stab incision is lengthened to 2 cm in whichever direction optimizes the incision. In far lateral disk herniations, the protruding disk fragment generally originates caudal to the affected nerve root and displaces it superiorly against the pedicle of the rostral vertebrae. Thus, our preference is to approach inferiorly, encountering the disk herniation first. With this in mind, the K-wire is advanced first onto the ipsilateral facet and then onto the base of the transverse process (TP) of the caudal vertebrae. This facilitates tubular retractor placement in a caudal-to-rostral trajectory that maximizes exposure of the pathological disk and compressed nerve root.

A "popping" sensation should be felt as the K-wire penetrates the lumbodorsal fascia en route to the facet (**Fig. 101.4a**). Fluoroscopic guidance is used to confirm that the K-wire is securely placed on the caudal TP at the correct level prior to dilation (**Fig. 101.4b**). The first dilator can then be advanced onto the TP in a controlled twisting motion with moderate downward force. With the initial dilator in place, the K-wire can be removed. A series of dilators of incrementally greater caliber are then passed onto the caudal transverse process (**Fig. 101.4c**). Once the final dilator is docked and the appropriate depth established, the tubular retractor system (16- to 18-mm diameter) can be advanced and the dilators removed. The retractor is angled rostrally in the desired trajectory and secured to a flexible articulating arm that is attached to the contralateral side of the bed. Fluoroscopy is repeated to confirm positioning and level (**Fig. 101.4d**).

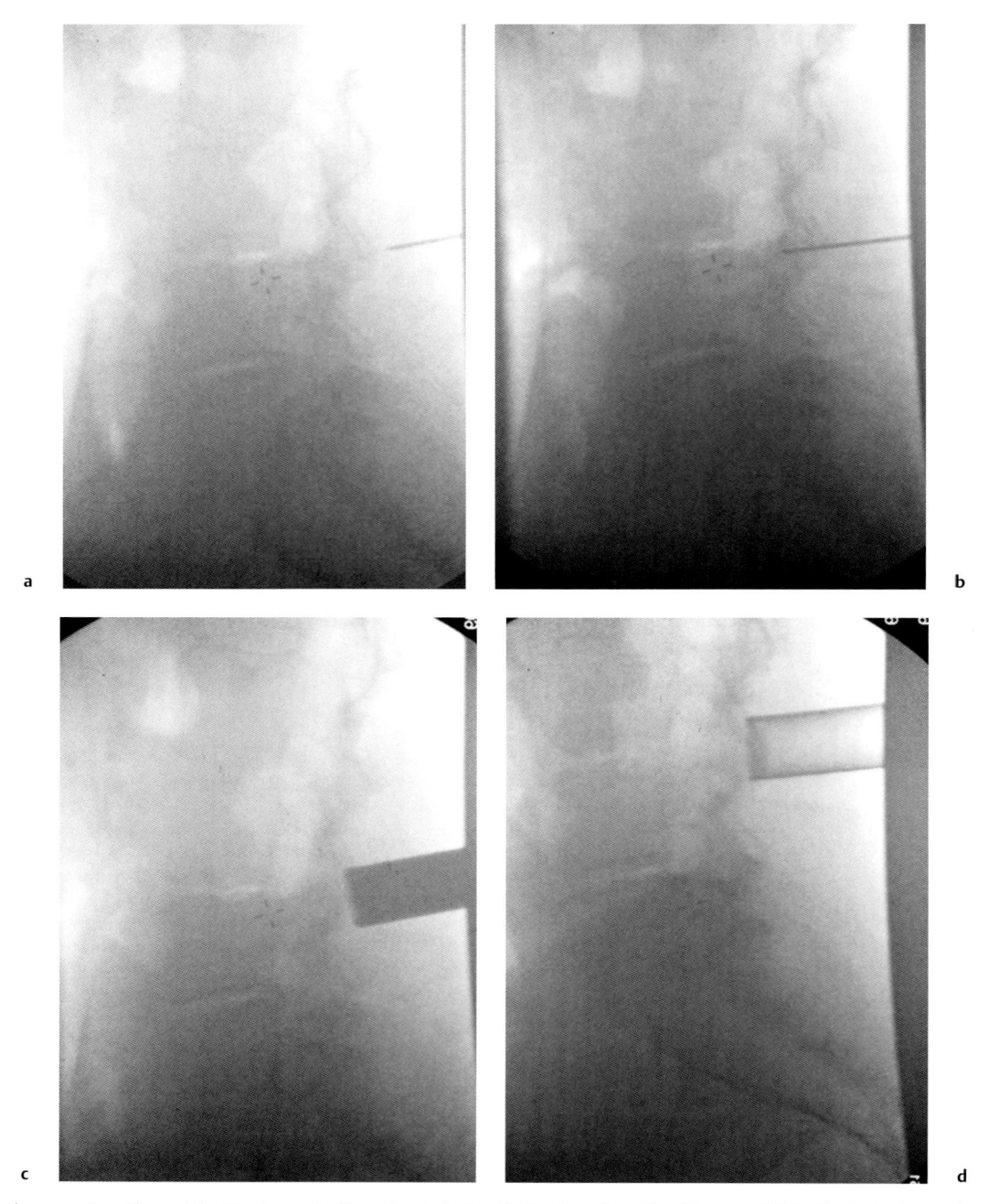

Fig. 101.4 Fluoroscopic guidance. **(a)** A Kirschner wire (K-wire) is docked on the facet overlying the disk space. **(b)** The K-wire is advanced onto the transverse process (TP). **(c)** Dilation over the TP. **(d)** Tubular retractor placement with rostral angulation.

At this point the operative microscope is introduced and focused to the depth of the tubular retractor. A combination of monopolar cautery and pituitary forceps are used to dissect overlying soft tissue and visualize the intertransverse ligament and lateral edge of the facet (**Figs. 101.5 and 101.6**). A portion of the intertransverse ligament is freed from the superior medial edge of the TP and resected over the operative window. A small amount of lateral facet can be removed and undercut with a drill and/or Kerrison rongeur if needed (**Figs. 101.5 and 101.6**).

Once the intertransverse ligaments are divided, the herniated disk may be readily identified; however, usually several minutes of careful microdissection through fat and the foraminal venous plexus are required to safely identify the disk herniation and nerve root. This may require the careful identification and sacrifice of numerous small veins. A microdissector and blunt probe can be used to approach the nerve root working from caudal to cephalad, where the nerve is typically displaced against the rostral pedicle, whereas the caudal pedicle can be used as inferior border to find the disk herniation. Once the disk herniation is identified, the dissection is taken rostrally until the nerve root is identified. The nerve root is then very gently retracted in a rostral and lateral direction to provide greater access to the herniated disk (**Fig. 101.5a**). Care should be taken to limit manipulation of the root and ganglion, which can lead to dysesthetic

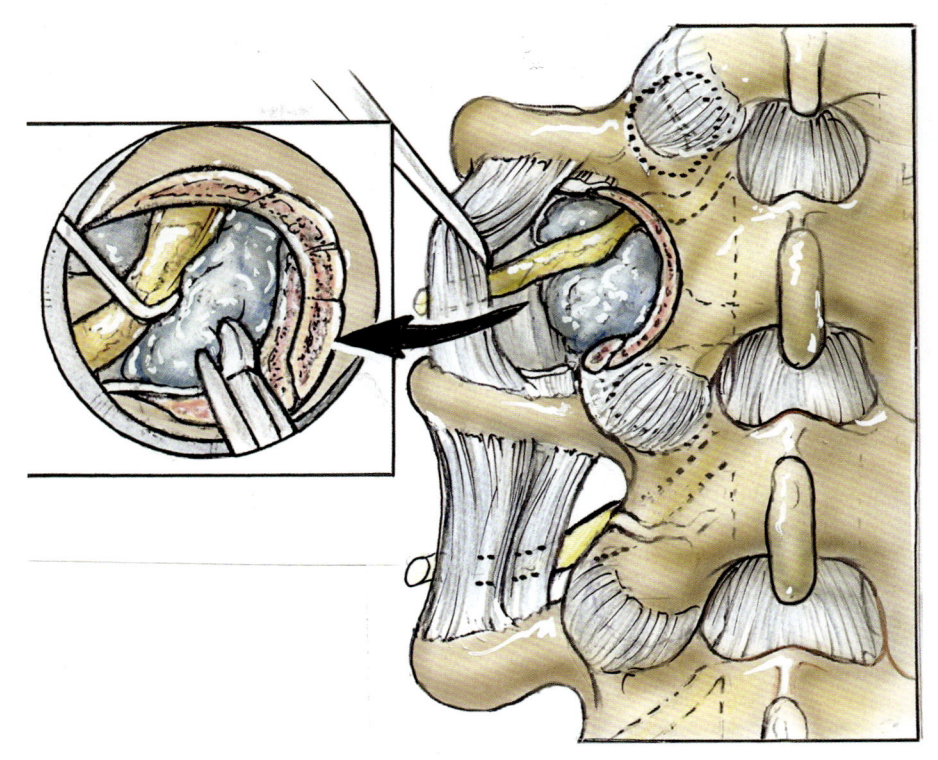

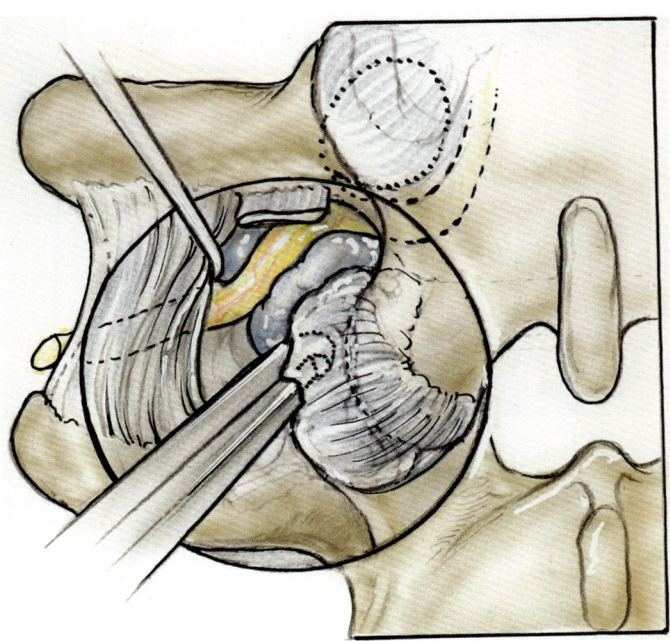

Fig. 101.5 Far lateral diskectomy. **(a)** Anatomy of the posterolateral approach to a far lateral microdiskectomy. A portion of the intertransverse ligament is freed from the superior medial edge of the TP and resected over the operative window. The *inset* depicts a diskectomy with a pituitary rongeur while the nerve root is gently retracted with a nerve hook. **(b)** In some instances, removal of the lateral margin of a hypertrophied superior facet joint is necessary to expose the border of the disk.

pain. The offending disk fragment is often found medial and inferior to the nerve ganglion. Diskectomy is performed with a combination of nerve hooks pituitary forceps, long ball probes, and angled curettes (**Figs. 101.5a and 101.6c,d**).

Following diskectomy, a long nerve hook is used to ensure that the nerve root is decompressed along its length into the neural foramen. Meticulous hemostasis is achieved and followed by copious irrigation. The tubular retractor is removed in a slow twisting motion while any additional bleeding from the dilated paraspinal musculature is cauterized. No fascial sutures are placed given proximity to the nerve root. Skin closure is a matter of surgeon preference. We use subcutaneous 2-0 Vicryl sutures followed by dermal adhesive.

Postoperative Care

Recovery time is most influenced by the duration and severity of preoperative symptoms and the patient's age and medical comorbidities. However, minimally invasive techniques entail smaller incisions and reduced soft tissue trauma, as muscles are split

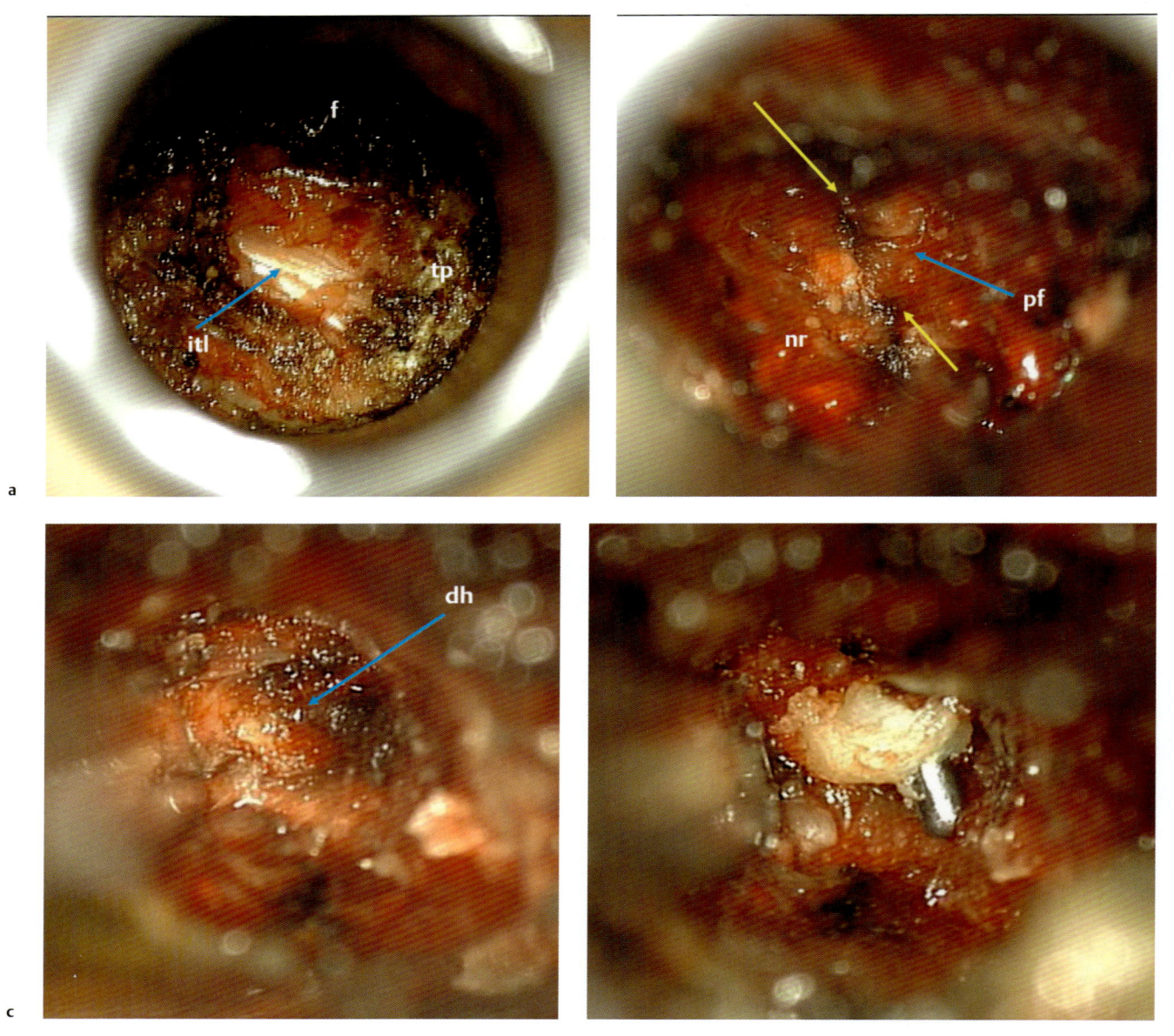

Fig. 101.6 Microscopic view through a minimally invasive retractor. **(a)** Soft tissue is removed with monopolar cautery to reveal the facet (f), transverse process (tp), and intertransverse ligament (itl, *blue arrow*). **(b)** Magnified view with the intertransverse ligament and a small portion of the lateral facet resected, exposing the medial aspect of the exiting nerve root (nr), the perineural fat (pf), and veins. The *yellow arrows* point to the vein that has been coagulated and divided). **(c)** The nerve root is protected with a small retracting suction and the disk herniation (dh) is exposed. **(d)** The disk herniation is incised and removed with a nerve hook.

and not cut by advancing tubular retractors. In our experience, the MIS approach reduces postoperative pain and promotes early mobilization. Postoperative imaging or bracing is not necessary. Surgery can almost always be performed on a same-day outpatient basis, although patients with medical comorbidities may be admitted overnight for observation following general anesthesia.

Potential Complications and Precautions

The posterolateral trajectory inherent to MIS far lateral diskectomy can be disorienting, even among those who are experienced in standard midline lumbar microdiskectomy. Minimally invasive tubular retractor systems also limit the visualization of anatomic landmarks that help with orientation. As a general principle, fluoroscopic guidance should be used liberally as familiarity is gained with MIS approaches. In addition, dilators should be advanced in a controlled-twisting motion. Difficulty may be encountered upon passing dilators through the fascia. Care must be taken to avoid exerting an amount of downward force that could cause a dilator to plunge below the level of the TP where the exiting nerve root is vulnerable to injury.

Far lateral diskectomy is particularly challenging at the level of L5–S1, as the posterolateral trajectory of the tubular retractor system may be obstructed by the sacral ala and iliac crest. The successful use of minimally invasive systems at this level requires a combination of drilling the lateral third of the facet joint, partial resection of the sacral ala, and more medial retractor placement.[8]

Although visceral injury is conceivable with this approach, complications are almost entirely limited to injury or irritation to the nerve root affected by the disk herniation. It is worth emphasizing that lateral disk herniations affect the portion of the nerve root that contains the cell bodies of sensory nerves within the dorsal root ganglion (DRG). The DRG is extremely sensitive to mechanical insult and is not likely to tolerate the same degree of manipulation as the axilla of the nerve root within the lateral recess. Dural tears are exceeding unusual, as this surgery involves the extradural portion of the nerve root. Infection rates are exceedingly low. The risk of indirect medical complications is comparable to that in conventional microdiskectomy.

Conclusion

Minimally invasive far lateral diskectomy is a proven procedure with excellent results and low operative morbidity. Evidence from randomized controlled trials has shown that the long-term substantial improvements in the leg and back achieved with minimally invasive muscle-splitting techniques are comparable to those achieved with standard microdiskectomy.[9] An initial learning curve may be encountered as familiarity is gained using minimally invasive tubular retractor systems to approach far lateral disk herniations. However, once practiced, this approach represents an effective and direct approach to the offending pathology that minimizes perioperative morbidity.

References

1. Abdullah AF, Wolber PG, Warfield JR, Gunadi IK. Surgical management of extreme lateral lumbar disc herniations: review of 138 cases. Neurosurgery 1988;22:648–653
2. Maroon JC, Kopitnik TA, Schulhof LA, Abla A, Wilberger JE. Diagnosis and microsurgical approach to far-lateral disc herniation in the lumbar spine. J Neurosurg 1990;72:378–382
3. Epstein NE. Evaluation of varied surgical approaches used in the management of 170 far-lateral lumbar disc herniations: indications and results. J Neurosurg 1995;83:648–656
4. An HS, Vaccaro A, Simeone FA, Balderston RA, O'Neill D. Herniated lumbar disc in patients over the age of fifty. J Spinal Disord 1990;3:143–146
5. Epstein NE. Foraminal and far lateral lumbar disc herniations: surgical alternatives and outcome measures. Spinal Cord 2002;40:491–500
6. Angtuaco EJ, Holder JC, Boop WC, Binet EF. Computed tomographic discography in the evaluation of extreme lateral disc herniation. Neurosurgery 1984;14:350–351
7. Segnarbieux F, Van de Kelft E, Candon E, Bitoun J, Frèrebeau P. Disco-computed tomography in extraforaminal and foraminal lumbar disc herniation: influence on surgical approaches. Neurosurgery 1994;34:643–647, discussion 648
8. O'Toole JE, Eichholz KM, Fessler RG. Minimally invasive far lateral microendoscopic discectomy for extraforaminal disc herniation at the lumbosacral junction: cadaveric dissection and technical case report. Spine J 2007;7:414–421
9. Dasenbrock HH, Juraschek SP, Schultz LR, et al. The efficacy of minimally invasive discectomy compared with open discectomy: a meta-analysis of prospective randomized controlled trials. J Neurosurg Spine 2012;16:452–462

102 Transverse Process Fusion

Byron C. Branch and Charles L. Branch, Jr.

Intertransverse arthrodesis has been successfully applied to a variety of indications in the thoracolumbar spine, and, prior to the development of interbody fusion techniques, was the primary means of achieving fusion of the lumbar spine. Applicable over a broad range of congenital, degenerative, traumatic, and pathological processes of the lumbosacral spine, the technique can be used in conjunction with internal fixation as a means of immobilizing one or more spinal segments or may be used as an adjunct to interbody fusion. Fusion rates with intertransverse grafting depend on, among other factors, the selection of the graft material, the use of rigid internal fixation, the patient's smoking history, the level(s) fused, and the general health of the patient. Successful clinical outcomes do not always correlate with obtaining a solid arthrodesis and vice versa. Results are more favorable for primary operations than for repeat salvage surgery.

Indications

- Degenerative disk disease
- Traumatic or iatrogenic instability
- Augmentation of anterior fusion
- Fusion following deformity correction

Contraindications

- Inadequate autogenous bone source
- Multiple previous failed posterior fusions
- Anterior column instability

Advantages

- Approach is direct and familiar
- Fusion and instrumentation via a single approach
- Applicable to a broad range of disorders
- May be used in conjunction with instrumentation

Disadvantages

- Extensive muscle dissection
- Significant pain and morbidity
- Possible need for blood transfusion
- Poor resolution of anterior instability
- Unable to place grafts under compression
- Potential for "fusion disease"
- Potential for adjacent-level degeneration

History

Mathieu and Demirleau[1] pioneered intertransverse fusion in 1936, using it as an alternative to dorsal (interlaminar) fusion. Adkins[2] later applied the technique to patients with degenerative spondylolisthesis and pointed out the utility of intertransverse fusion in patients whose laminar arches had been removed, thereby precluding dorsal (interlaminar) fusion. Watkins[3] performed intertransverse fusion via a paramedian incision and approach lateral to the paraspinous muscles, preserving the spinous processes and interspinous ligament. His 1953 report detailed the technique of affixing strips of autologous iliac crest to the transverse processes using screws, resulting in a 68% incidence of solid fusion. Modern techniques of rigid spinal immobilization have improved the fusion rates and clinical outcomes with transverse process fusion, and the technique continues to be a viable means of establishing arthrodesis in the lumbosacral spine.[4-6]

Surgical Technique

Positioning

Paramount to any procedure on the lumbar spine is proper patient positioning. Optimal positioning eliminates external pressure to the abdomen, thereby reducing intra-abdominal and consequently venous pressure. This results in less intraoperative blood loss and is particularly important when working around or lateral to the facet complexes around which exists a network of large anastomotic segmental vessels[7] (**Figs. 102.1 and 102.2**).

The intubated patient is placed prone on chest rolls or any of a variety of commercially available spinal surgery frames, with all pressure points adequately padded and special care given to the spiral groove (ulnar nerve) and eyes. Abduction of the arm should be limited to 80 degrees at most, to avoid stretch injury to the brachial plexus. Pneumatic compression devices are applied to the lower extremities to prevent the development of a deep venous thrombosis in the anesthetized patient. Bladder catheterization is used routinely in most lumbar spinal fusion operations and should be considered for lengthy procedures or in cases where anticipated blood loss is significant. Prophylactic broad-spectrum antibiotics are administered prior to skin incision and with extensive exposure or instrumented fusion are continued for 24 hours postoperatively.

Incision and Dissection (Open and Minimally Invasive)

For the traditional dorsal midline technique, the skin incision is made following the injection of epinephrine-containing local

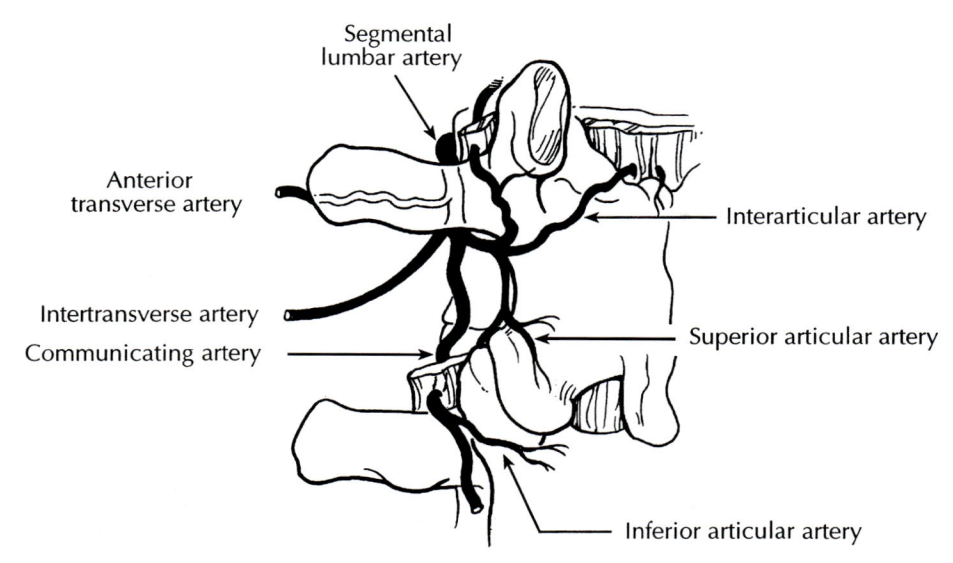

Fig. 102.1 Anteroposterior view demonstrating the vascular anatomy around the facet complexes and transverse processes.

anesthetic. The subcutaneous tissue is dissected sharply or with monopolar electrocautery until the deep dorsal fascia is encountered. The fascia is incised bilaterally immediately adjacent to the spinous process, preserving the supraspinous ligament, which provides a midline anchor for the fascia during wound closure. The fascial incision may be extended beyond the skin incision to facilitate better retraction and improve exposure. The paraspinal muscles are dissected off of the spinous processes and lamina in a subperiosteal fashion using monopolar electrocautery or a second periosteal elevator. Once the muscle dissection is completed bilaterally to the facets, self-retaining retractors are placed to maintain the exposure. With the paramedian, or Wiltse, approach, two separate incisions are made 3 to 4 cm off of the midline and a transmuscular exposure of the transverse processes is achieved.

Intraoperative lateral radiographs should be obtained to verify the correct spinal segment because anatomic landmarks may be unreliable in determining the fusion level in posterolateral lumbar fusion.[8] Once the levels to be fused have been identified, the subperiosteal dissection is performed lateral and ventral to the facet joints, exposing the dorsal surface of the transverse process. The terminal branches of the segmental vessels constitute a rich anastomotic network located above, below, and lateral to the facet joints[7] (**Figs. 102.1 and 102.2**). These vessels should be identified early and coagulated to prevent excessive blood loss. Coagulation should be performed using bipolar electrocautery

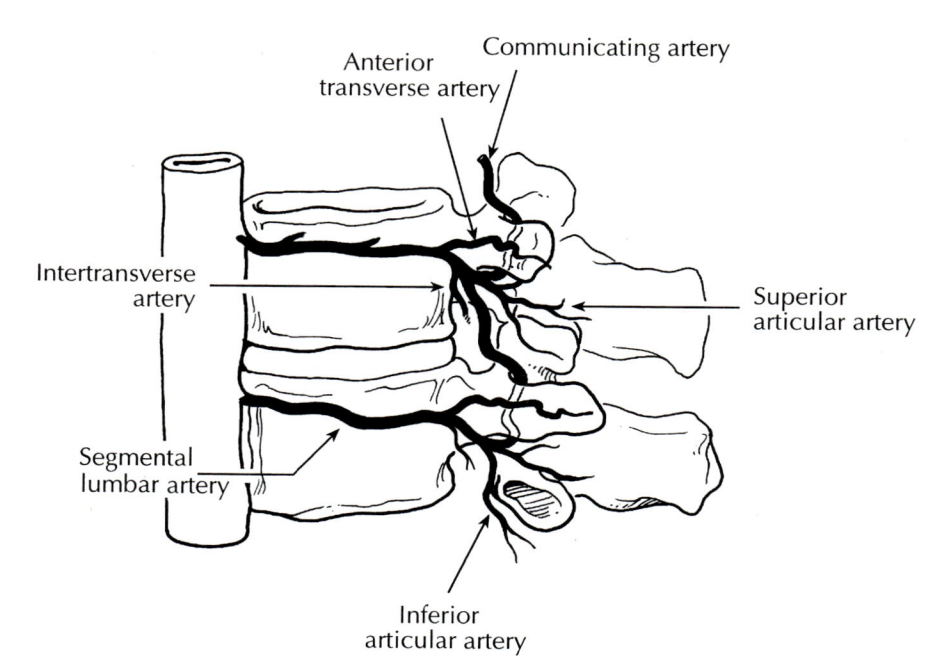

Fig. 102.2 Lateral view demonstrating the vascular anatomy around the facet complexes and transverse processes.

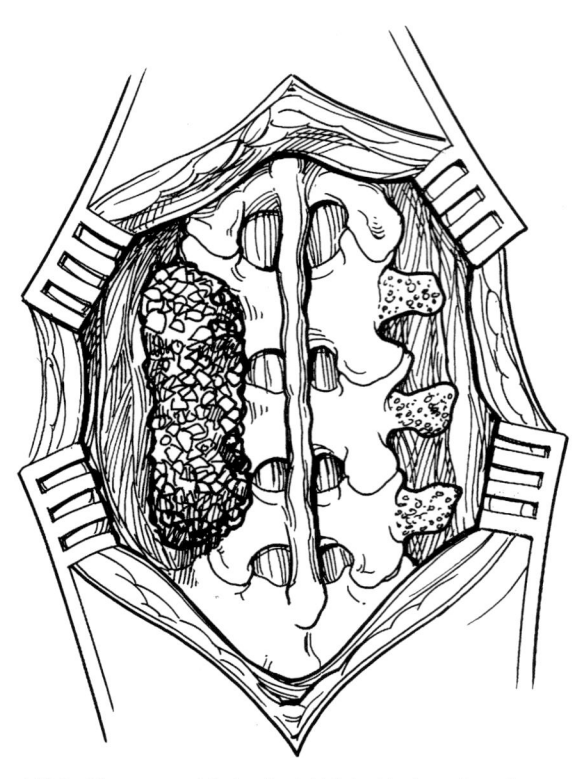

Fig. 102.3 The prepared fusion bed *(right)* with decorticated transverse processes. A morcellized bone graft is seen in place *(left)*.

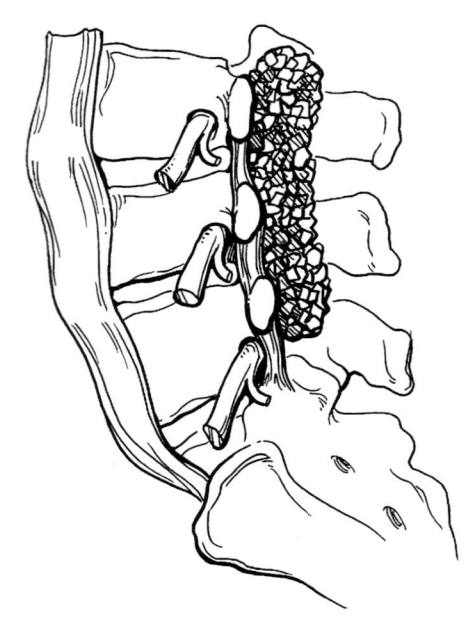

Fig. 102.4 Lateral view of fusion mass consisting of a morcellized graft.

to prevent the transmission of thermal energy to the exiting neural elements in the intervertebral foramen. The pedicle is identified ventral to the junction of the transverse process and superior articular process of the facet complex, and demarcates the rostral extent of the intervertebral foramen below.

Meticulous removal of soft tissue and coagulation debris over the extent of the transverse process should be performed as well as decortication of the dorsal aspect of the transverse process. This provides an optimal grafting surface and can be performed using a combination of periosteal dissectors, osteotomes, and rongeurs. Removal of the facet capsular ligaments and intrafacet synovium with decortication of the dorsal facet surface provides additional graft–host interface. Care should be taken not to fracture the transverse process during dissection and decortication. Dissection should not extend deep to the dorsal aspect of the transverse process, to avoid injury to the anterior transverse artery and exiting nerve root. The intertransverse ligaments and muscles serve as the ventral extent of safe dissection, to avoid injury to the spinal nerve root. Once the fusion surface has been prepared, liberal amounts of corticocancellous bone graft are placed over the decorticated transverse processes and bridging the intertransverse space (**Fig. 102.3**). Graft material can consist of either corticocancellous bone strips or morcellized bone carefully packed onto the facets and transverse processes beneath the overlying muscle (**Fig. 102.4**). A target volume of bone graft for each side of a single intertransverse space should be 40 to 60 mL. Hemostasis should be achieved prior to graft placement to prevent graft migration. The use of bone wax is discouraged because it impairs fusion. Internal fixation can then be performed over the fused segments using transpedicular screws and plates/rods or another fixation device.

In the "open-book" technique, a supraperiosteal exposure of the transverse processes is performed.[9,10] A transverse scoring through the cortical layer of the dorsal transverse process from medial to lateral is accomplished with a dissecting tool. A similar vertical score is made through the cortical layer of the proximal transverse process near the facet interface. The rostral and caudal divisions of the dorsal facet are then reflected open into the intertransverse space using a small curette with the intact periosteum serving as a hinge. Care should be taken not to fracture the transverse process and to maintain continuity of these reflected flaps with the ventral transverse process. Standard decortication of the remaining pars, facet, and laminar edges is then performed. Onlay bone graft material can then be placed directly on this vascularized cancellous bed, in addition to the other decorticated areas. This technique adaptation is most applicable to open fusion procedures, and is not readily performed in minimally invasive surgery (MIS) fusion techniques as they do not require or include an extensive lateral exposure.

The MIS fusion techniques and percutaneous instrumentation provide many advantages over the open techniques. Such techniques are quickly becoming the preferred method of treatment of many thoracolumbar disorders previously treated with open surgery. Most MIS fusion techniques do not require or employ a lateral exposure of the transverse processes. Yet it is still important to achieve bony fusion across the intertransverse space in these techniques. In this regard, we describe an adjunct technique for use with MIS that may augment instrumentation and promote bony fusion across the intertransverse space. Prior to screw placement (direct or percutaneous) a 16- or 18-mm tubular retractor is positioned on the intervening facet joint, using the tubular dilator system and lateral fluoroscopy. (The entry point for the tubular retractor is often through the preexisting MIS incisions.) Bovie electrocautery is then used to expose the facet and delineate the joint capsule. Keep in mind the vertical transition of the lumbar facets with caudal progression. The facet synovium and articular cartilage is quickly shaved using a high-speed drill to create a trough through the synovial space of the facet joint. The trough through the facet joint should follow the natural course of the joint and enable end-plate preparation. Care should be taken not to drill into the facet, completely abolishing the end plate, or to drill too deep and contuse the underlying nerve root. Once an adequate trough has been made, a cancellous bone graft, typically a cancellous block cut to size (which may be soaked in spun marrow aspirate) is packed into the joint space with bayonetted forceps. After placement of the bone graft, the tubular retractor is removed. This process is repeated at all facet joints spanning segments intended for immobilization. Once this graft augmentation for fusion across the intertransverse space has been completed, the patient can then be instrumented.

Closure

The wound is copiously irrigated with antibiotic solution, and meticulous closure is performed in layers. Care should be taken to restore the anatomic relationships and eliminate dead space. A subcutaneous tunneled suction drain is left in place to prevent the accumulation of blood products that could cause migration of the graft material. The drain is left in place for 24 to 48 hours or until output is minimal.

Postoperative Care

Prophylactic antibiotics and bladder catheterization are discontinued on the first postoperative day, and early ambulation in an external orthosis such as a corset or custom-fitted rigid thoracolumbosacral orthosis is encouraged by the second postoperative day.

Postoperative radiographs obtained in the recovery room verify the integrity of the construct and serve as a baseline for evaluating evolving spinal deformity. Plain film evaluation is repeated with the patient upright in an orthosis to again verify the integrity of the construct and ensure that no kyphosis has occurred. Radiographs are repeated at 3 and 9 months postoperatively and at regular intervals thereafter until fusion has been established.

Graft Selection

In addition to meticulous preparation of the fusion surface, careful consideration should be given to the selection of graft material, as the biological properties of the graft affect the eventual development of a solid fusion. An ideal graft should provide four elements: (1) osteoconductive matrix, (2) osteoinductive factors, (3) osteogenic cells, and (4) structural integrity.[11,12] Additional factors to consider include donor-site morbidity and graft immunogenicity. The intended recipient location for the graft will necessitate certain elements and should be taken into account. In the case of intertransverse fusion where grafts are not subjected to stress, the structural integrity element may become less of an issue. Autologous corticocancellous bone from the iliac crest can supply biologically active graft, but procurement may result in donor-site pain, blood loss, infection, or other complications.[13–15] Allograft banked bone may retain some osteoinductive and osteoconductive properties but has the added disadvantage of being subject to immunologic responses from the host. The proliferation of graft extenders or substitutes with a variety of biological and structural components has given the surgeon alternatives to iliac crest autograft, but there is no clearly superior alternative. Compounds that include recombinant human bone morphogenetic protein appear to be effective but remain controversial and do not currently have on-label Food and Drug Administration (FDA) approval.

The volume of bone graft is believed to decrease over time as it forms into a solid bone mass.[16] In particular, in the case of intertransverse fusion grafts in which the construct is not under a stress or load, this volumetric decrease may become even more pronounced. A study by Kim et al[16] in 1999 found that 55% of the initial autograft volume was lost according to volumetric computed tomography (CT) imaging performed at 18 months' follow-up. They also observed a positive correlation between initial autograft volume and residual volume at 18 months, implying a larger fusion mass may occur with larger graft volumes. However, a negative correlation was seen between increasing amounts of initial autograft volume and the fraction that incorporates into the fusion mass, implying a poor efficiency of fusion with increased graft volumes (i.e., more graft does not equate with a better fusion mass). This effect was seen with initial graft volumes exceeding 4,000 mm³ per single-level intertransverse fusion.

Similarly, in the months following surgery, as the graft incorporates into a solid fusion, up to 30% of the original mineral content of the graft may be lost during the first 6 months of bone healing.[17] As remodeling continues up to 1 year, mineral content is restored to within 80 to 90% of baseline levels.[17] Furthermore, vertebral body bone mineral density (BMD) does not necessarily correlate with the BMD of the intertransverse fusion mass.[18] This may be due to the fact alluded to earlier, that intertransverse fusion grafts are not subjected to the same biomechanical forces as the vertebral bodies and their interbody spaces.

Some reports have demonstrated a significantly higher pseudarthrosis rate in patients receiving noninstrumented allograft fusion versus those receiving autograft.[19,20] Jorgenson et al[19] conducted a prospective analysis comparing autograft and allograft in the same patient. Allograft was placed over the intertransverse space on one side and autograft on the other. After 1 year, significantly lower rates of arthrodesis were achieved in the allograft side when compared with the autograft ($p < 0.05$). The potential for an increased rate of pseudarthrosis using allograft must be carefully weighed against the potential for increased morbidity related to autograft procurement. The use of locally harvested bone from the lamina and medial facets provides autograft without the morbidity of harvest at a distant site, but may be inferior to uniform cancellous marrow from the iliac crest.

To Instrument or Not

The lumbar spine, because of its relative high degree of mobility, presents an inherently unfavorable environment for the development of a solid fusion. Despite this, intertransverse grafting without instrumentation results in successful fusion rates ranging from 46 to 100%.[4–6,20,21] Rigid internal fixation using a pedicle screw–rod or screw–plate system has been shown in biomechanical studies to significantly limit motion over the instrumented segments, but there are conflicting data in the literature, summarized in **Table 102.1**, as to whether this results in a higher fusion rate.[4,6,21–23]

Schwab and colleagues[21] reported a 91% fusion rate among patients stabilized with an Edwards instrumentation construct

Table 102.1 Fusion Rates with and Without Internal Fixation

Series	Noninstrumented Fusion Rate (%)	Instrumented Fusion Rate (%)
Zdeblick 1993[4]	65	77–95*
Schwab et al 1995[21]	65	91
Bernhardt et al 1992[6]	78	74

*A 71% fusion rate using a semirigid pedicle screw–plate system, and 95% fusion rate using a rigid pedicle screw–rod construct.

versus a 65% fusion rate in noninstrumented patients. Zdeblick[4] presented prospective randomized patient data also demonstrating significantly higher fusion rates and better clinical outcomes in patients treated with rigid or semirigid fixation compared with noninstrumented fusion. Conversely, Bernhardt et al[6] found no significant difference in the fusion rates among 47 patients undergoing posterolateral fusion with or without the use of a variable spinal plating system. France et al[22] reported prospective randomized data showing no statistical difference in patient-reported outcome in patients undergoing posterolateral fusion with and without pedicle screw instrumentation, despite a statistically nonsignificant trend toward higher fusion rates in instrumented patients.

A higher rate of leg dysesthesias has been reported in patients receiving internal fixation, and up to 15% of instrumentation systems have been removed secondary to so-called hardware-related pain.[6] Although debate exists as to the use of internal fixation in a primary operation, most authors advocate the use of internal fixation in patients with severe degenerative disease, patients who require correction of an existing deformity, or repeat operations for failed fusion.[4]

Intertransverse fusion differs from anterior cervical and lumbar interbody fusion in that axial compressive forces are not exerted upon the graft. Graft compression is thought to promote fusion. Although there is no way to apply axial compression to intertransverse grafts, the addition of internal fixation may enhance fusion by providing rigid immobilization.

Complications and Precautions

Intraoperative

Intraoperative blood loss can be greatly reduced if proper patient positioning is employed. Familiarity with segmental vascular anatomy and early identification and coagulation of anastomotic vessels are essential. Autologous repletion of blood products using a cell saver can reduce transfusion requirements and spare the patient the potential infectious or transfusion-reaction complications associated with banked donor blood.

Compression and traction injuries are avoided by paying careful attention to padding all pressure points, including the knees, anterior superior iliac spines, elbows, feet, and face. Particular attention should be paid to the spiral groove of the humerus wherein lies the ulnar nerve. The eyes should be carefully examined once the patient is in the prone position to ensure that there is no compression. Limiting abduction of the arms to 80 degrees at most can reduce brachial plexus stretch injury.

Postoperative

A troubling syndrome of postoperative pain is thought to result from excessive retraction or devascularization of the paraspinal muscles during lengthy fusion operations. This has been referred to as "fusion disease." The periodic release of self-retaining retractors should be performed to avoid soft tissue compression injury and ischemia.

The incidence of postoperative wound infections increases with the complexity of the procedure and ranges from 1% for simple diskectomy, to 1 to 5% and 3.8 to 9.7% for noninstrumented and instrumented fusions, respectively.[24–27] Preoperative factors associated with an increased incidence of infection include advanced age, prolonged hospital bed rest, diabetes mellitus, obesity, immunosuppressed state, infection at a distant site, cerebral palsy, and myelodysplasia.[26,27] Operative factors increasing the likelihood of infection include procedure length exceeding 5 hours, high volume of personnel traffic through the operating room, the use of internal fixation, wound hematoma, and extension of fusion to the sacrum.[26,27]

Prophylactic broad-spectrum antibiotic therapy should be universally employed in spinal fusion operations.[24–26] Superficial wound infections are most often caused by Staphylococcus aureus and, in some cases, can be managed with parenteral antibiotics alone. Deep wound infections should be treated early with a minimum of 6 weeks of parenteral antibiotic therapy followed by a course of oral antimicrobial therapy tailored to culture results when available. Surgical irrigation and debridement may be necessary, as may the use of a suction-irrigation system. In most cases of deep spinal wound infection, the hardware can be left in place, although it may harbor indolent infection for years. Consideration should be given to removing the hardware following the establishment of a solid arthrodesis.

The prevention of a deep venous thrombosis begins preoperatively and continues until the patient is discharged from the hospital. Patients who have been nonambulatory because of low back pain before surgery should undergo preoperative Doppler evaluation of the lower extremities to rule out a venous thrombosis. Segmental pneumatic compression devices are placed on the patient prior to induction of anesthesia and are maintained until the patient becomes ambulatory. In the event of a deep venous thrombosis during the perioperative period, consideration should be given to a vena cava filter to prevent thromboembolic phenomena while avoiding the bleeding complication of anticoagulation therapy in the postoperative period.

A pseudarthrosis should be suspected clinically in a patient with pain persisting beyond the early postoperative period. It is identified radiographically by the absence of fusion mass on static views or CT as well as the presence of motion on dynamic views. A pseudarthrosis, once identified, may require subsequent surgery with internal fixation. A stable arthrodesis is demonstrated radiographically by the presence of bridging trabecular bone over the intertransverse space and by the absence of motion on dynamic views of the spine. It should be noted that radiographic evaluation of fusion does not always correlate with intraoperative findings in a subsequent "second look" surgery.[28–30]

With a solid arthrodesis comes the potential for accelerated adjacent-segment degenerative change and increased motion secondary to the added biomechanical stress placed on the joints above and below the fusion.[31] The incidence of adjacent-level degenerative problems following fusion with instrumentation is particularly prevalent in postmenopausal women.[32]

Outcomes

Although fusion rates for intertransverse fusion range from 46 to 100%,[4–6,20,21] this does not always correlate with a patient's clinical outcome. Dawson et al[5] reported a 92% fusion rate using autogenous iliac crest intertransverse lumbar arthrodesis, but only a 70 to 80% functional success rate and a limited socioeconomic advantage over internal fixation.[5] When internal fixation is used, the clinical outcome more closely correlates with the development of solid fusion.[21] This may relate to the fact that pedicle screw internal fixation provides biomechanical stability to the anterior and middle columns even after posterolateral fusion is achieved.[23]

Preoperative diagnosis affects outcome in patients treated with intertransverse fusion. Patients with severe degenerative spondylolisthesis or degenerative disk disease fare more poorly than those operated upon for isthmic spondylolisthesis.[4] A history of previous back surgery lowers the clinical success rates independent of whether or not a solid arthrodesis is achieved.[4,5] Successful lumbosacral arthrodesis is more reliably achieved at the L5-S1 level than fusions extending to or above L4.[5] This also holds true for the clinical success rates.[5]

The presence of systemic nicotine has been shown in animal models to adversely affect fusion rates and, when fusion does occur, it consists of biomechanically inferior bone.[9] This evidence is substantiated clinically by a lower fusion rate among smokers.[4]

Although beyond the scope of this technical chapter, certain secondary gain, compensation, or psychological issues may affect patient outcomes after spinal fusion.

Conclusion

Transverse process fusion remains a viable means of achieving arthrodesis in the thoracic and lumbosacral spine. The use of rigid instrumentation systems has improved fusion rates and expanded the indications for transverse process fusion to include spinal deformity correction and severe degenerative pathology. Thorough knowledge of regional anatomy and taking precautions to avoid complications can minimize patient morbidity with the procedure.

References

1. Mathieu P, Demirleau P. Trautement chirugical du spondylolisthesis douloureaux. Rev Orthop 1936;23:352
2. Adkins EWD. Lumbo-sacral arthrodesis after laminectomy. J Bone Joint Surg Br 1955;37-B:208–223
3. Watkins MB. Posterolateral fusion of the lumbar and lumbosacral spine. J Bone Joint Surg Am 1953;35-A:1014–1018
4. Zdeblick TA. A prospective, randomized study of lumbar fusion. Preliminary results. Spine 1993;18:983–991
5. Dawson EG, Lotysch M III, Urist MR. Intertransverse process lumbar arthrodesis with autogenous bone graft. Clin Orthop Relat Res 1981;154:90–96
6. Bernhardt M, Swartz DE, Clothiaux PL, Crowell RR, White AA III. Posterolateral lumbar and lumbosacral fusion with and without pedicle screw internal fixation. Clin Orthop Relat Res 1992;284:109–115
7. Macnab I, Dall D. The blood supply of the lumbar spine and its application to the technique of intertransverse lumbar fusion. J Bone Joint Surg Br 1971;53:628–638
8. Ebraheim NA, Inzerillo C, Xu R. Are anatomic landmarks reliable in determination of fusion level in posterolateral lumbar fusion? Spine 1999;24:973–974
9. Leatherman KD, Dickson RA. The Management of Spinal Deformities. London: Wright; 1988:458
10. Gordon Deen H. The "open book" technique for preparation of the lumbar transverse process for posterolateral fusion. J Neurosurg 2000;93(2, Suppl):332–334
11. Gazdag AR, Lane JM, Glaser D, Forster RA. Alternatives to autogenous bone graft: efficacy and indications. J Am Acad Orthop Surg 1995;3:1–8
12. Zipfel GJ, Guiot BH, Fessler RG. Bone grafting. Neurosurg Focus 2003;14:e8
13. Kurz LT, Garfin SR, Booth RE Jr. Harvesting autogenous iliac bone grafts. A review of complications and techniques. Spine 1989;14:1324–1331
14. Summers BN, Eisenstein SM. Donor site pain from the ilium. A complication of lumbar spine fusion. J Bone Joint Surg Br 1989;71:677–680
15. Younger EM, Chapman MW. Morbidity at bone graft donor sites. J Orthop Trauma 1989;3:192–195
16. Kim KW, Ha KY, Moon MS, Kim YS, Kwon SY, Woo YK. Volumetric change of the graft bone after intertransverse fusion. Spine 1999;24:428–433
17. Hagenmaier F, Kok D, Hol A, Rijnders T, Oner FC, van Susante JLC. Changes in bone mineral density in the intertransverse fusion mass after instrumented single-level lumbar fusion: a prospective 1-year follow-up. Spine 2013;38:696–702
18. Lee JS, Kim KW. Bone mineral densities of the vertebral body and intertransverse fusion mass after instrumented intertransverse process fusion. Spine 2010;35:E1106–E1110
19. Jorgenson SS, Lowe TG, France J, Sabin J. A prospective analysis of autograft versus allograft in posterolateral lumbar fusion in the same patient. A minimum of 1-year follow-up in 144 patients. Spine 1994;19:2048–2053
20. Nugent PJ, Dawson EG. Intertransverse process lumbar arthrodesis with allogeneic fresh-frozen bone graft. Clin Orthop Relat Res 1993;287:107–111
21. Schwab FJ, Nazarian DG, Mahmud F, Michelsen CB. Effects of spinal instrumentation on fusion of the lumbosacral spine. Spine 1995;20:2023–2028
22. France JC, Yaszemski MJ, Lauerman WC, et al. A randomized prospective study of posterolateral lumbar fusion. Outcomes with and without pedicle screw instrumentation. Spine 1999;24:553–560
23. Kotani Y, Cunningham BW, Cappuccino A, Kaneda K, McAfee PC. The role of spinal instrumentation in augmenting lumbar posterolateral fusion. Spine 1996;21:278–287
24. Horwitz NH, Curtin JA. Prophylactic antibiotics and wound infections following laminectomy for lumber disc herniation. J Neurosurg 1975;43:727–731
25. Levi AD, Dickman CA, Sonntag VKH. Management of postoperative infections after spinal instrumentation. J Neurosurg 1997;86:975–980
26. Massie JB, Heller JG, Abitbol JJ, McPherson D, Garfin SR. Postoperative posterior spinal wound infections. Clin Orthop Relat Res 1992;284:99–108
27. Perry JW, Montgomerie JZ, Swank S, Gilmore DS, Maeder K. Wound infections following spinal fusion with posterior segmental spinal instrumentation. Clin Infect Dis 1997;24:558–561
28. Blumenthal SL, Gill K. Can lumbar spine radiographs accurately determine fusion in postoperative patients? Correlation of routine radiographs with a second surgical look at lumbar fusions. Spine 1993;18:1186–1189
29. Brodsky AE, Kovalsky ES, Khalil MA. Correlation of radiologic assessment of lumbar spine fusions with surgical exploration. Spine 1986;11:1942–1943
30. Kant AP, Daum WJ, Dean SM, Uchida T. Evaluation of lumbar spine fusion. Plain radiographs versus direct surgical exploration and observation. Spine 1995;20:2313–2317
31. Eck JC, Humphreys SC, Hodges SD. Adjacent-segment degeneration after lumbar fusion: a review of clinical, biomechanical, and radiologic studies. Am J Orthop 1999;28:336–340
32. Etebar S, Cahill DW. Risk factors for adjacent-segment failure following lumbar fixation with rigid instrumentation for degenerative instability. J Neurosurg 1999;90(2, Suppl):163–169

103 Open Placement of Pedicle Screws: Lumbar, Sacral, and Iliac Screws

Eli M. Baron, Neel Anand, and Doniel Drazin

Pedicle screws are widely used in spinal surgery as a standard method for achieving internal fixation, especially for the treatment of an unstable spine. They were initially described by Harrington and Tullos,[1] and then later popularized by Dick et al,[2] Steffee et al,[3] Roy-Camille et al,[4] and Louis.[5] In most cases, placement of pedicle screws provides a safe and effective method for providing rigid internal fixation and spinal alignment. The screws resist loading in all directions.[6–8] Although the complication rate is low, there have been reports of inaccurate screw placement, dural tear, and screw failure. A screw-related neural injury to the nerve root or spinal cord can result in neurologic or radicular pain after surgery, sometimes requiring revision surgery.[9] It is therefore important to minimize these postoperative complications by verifying the accurate placement of pedicle screws during surgery. Intraoperative imaging and newer navigation technologies are designed to help surgeons improve the accuracy of pedicle screw placement.

Patient Selection

The success of pedicle screws has been linked to the quality of the bone into which they are inserted. Therefore, patient selection is an important consideration. Patients with osteopenia or osteoporosis may not be candidates for pedicle screws, as their bone structure may not support this fixation method. Patients with deformity or abnormal spinal anatomy must also be carefully evaluated, as their anatomic landmarks may not enable the proper placement of pedicle screws. Finally, the pedicle size should also be assessed.

Indications, Contraindications, and Objectives of Surgery

Pedicle screws are indicated for achieving segmental fixation of the lumbar and thoracic spinal column. Using this technique can achieve three-column fixation, appropriate sagittal alignment, and instrumentation of short and long segments for spinal surgery for degeneration, deformity, tumor, and trauma. Additionally, this technique enables short-segment fixation with preservation of lumbar lordosis and adjacent normal motion segments.[10] Osteoporosis may be a relative contraindication (discussed below). Additionally, preoperative imaging should be used to determine pedicle diameter.

The decision to instrument to the pelvis is made typically in situations where a long fusion to the sacrum is being performed. Iliac fixation assists in off-loading sacral pedicle screws. Additionally, they may be used where sacral fixation is poor or impossible and in treatment of L5–S1 pseudarthrosis and high-grade lumbosacral spondylolisthesis.[11]

Advantages and Disadvantages

When pedicle screws are well positioned, they can provide excellent spinal fixation. They also provide segmental instrumentation, enabling the preservation of lordosis. They also can be used for treatment of spinal deformity, listhesis, and abnormal alignment in the setting of trauma. Malpositioned screws, however, can result in neural injuries that affect the patient's quality of life due to radiculopathy, that require costly revision surgeries and rehabilitation, and that put the patient at increased risk secondary to the additional procedures needed to relieve pain and other symptoms.[9] Additionally, screw failure and pseudarthrosis may occur.[12,13]

Choice of Operative Approach

Pedicle screws are inserted posteriorly using a midline or a paramedian approach. The percutaneous technique is another option.

Preoperative Imaging

Typical preoperative imaging includes plain X-ray, magnetic resonance imaging (MRI), and possibly computed tomography (CT). X-rays may include dynamic studies and 36-inch standing films to assess instability and sagittal/coronal balance. MRI provides excellent visualization of soft tissue contrast for simultaneous evaluation of the thecal sac and spinal canal contents,[14] and has supplanted the routine use of CT myelography for this purpose. CT may enable the accurate assessment of complex bony spinal anatomy and the most accurate planning for screw placement.[15] Dual-energy X-ray (DEXA) absorptiometry scanning may demonstrate osteoporosis,[16] enabling the surgeon to appropriately prepare for cement augmentation or other techniques in the operating room.

Lumbar Pedicle Screw Placement

Lumbar pedicle screws have traditionally been placed using a free-hand technique or fluoroscopic assistance. The free-hand technique relies on the proper identification of anatomic landmarks and on surgeon experience. Key anatomic landmarks include the pars interarticularis, the transverse process, the base of the mamillary process, and the accessory process (**Fig. 103.1**). Time should be taken to identify anatomic landmarks and place screws appropriately; revision of inappropriately placed screws results in decreased pullout strength, which can significantly alter the biomechanics of a construct.[17] A hole is made using an awl or high-speed drill at the junction of the pars interarticularis, the

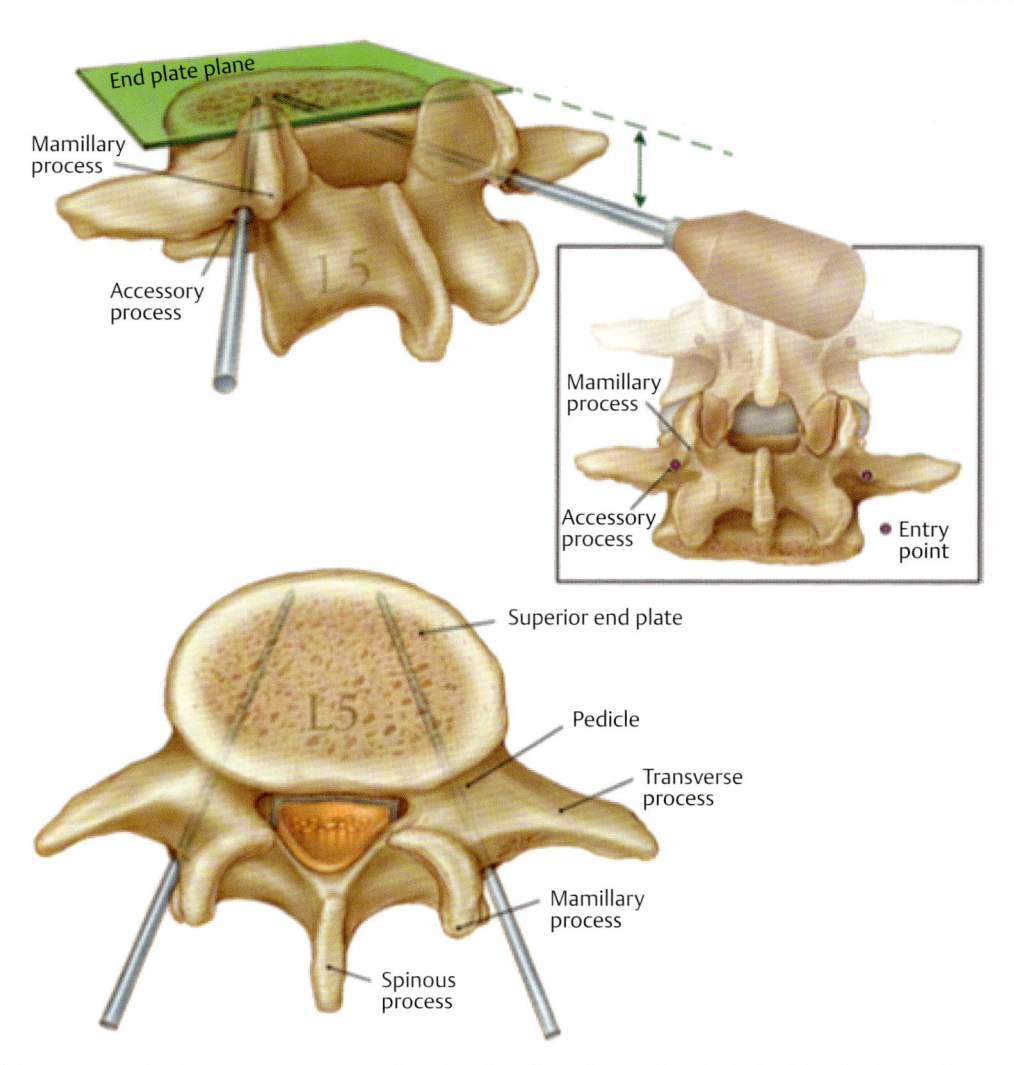

Fig. 103.1 Pedicle entry point for a lumbar segment. Artist's depiction of free-hand pedicle screw placement technique in the lumbar spine with the entry point occurring at the site of the accessory process. The screw trajectory is directed from lateral to medial and parallel with the superior end plate. (From Parker SL, McGirt MJ, Farber SH, et al. Accuracy of free-hand pedicle screws in the thoracic and lumbar spine: analysis of 6816 consecutive screws. Neurosurgery 2011;68(1):170–178, discussion 178. Reprinted with permission.)

mamillary ridge, and transverse process (**Fig. 103.2**). This often corresponds to the accessory process.[18] In a degenerated spine, the actual entry point may be further medial along the inferior border of the mamillary process; using a rongeur to bite off bone and identify cancellous bone may assist entry. An effort should be made to medialize the pedicle screws as much as appropriately possible. as triangulated screws have been shown to have increased pullout strength.[19,20]

A pedicle probe (gear shift) is then used to sound the pedicle. In general, in terms of medial to lateral trajectory, the pedicle inclination angle or transverse angle (angle from the sagittal plane to an axis down the pedicle) has been described as increasingly progressive from L1 to L5. At L1 this has been described, depending on the population studied, as having a mean value of 8.3 to 18.16 degrees, and at L5 this has been described as having a mean value of 21.87 to 28.47 degrees.[21–24] These are general estimates, and individual pedicle anatomy should be assessed on preoperative imaging studies and anatomic findings in the operating room.

The hole is then probed for a breach using a pedicle feeler. At this point, pedicle markers may be placed. Many surgeons use periodic spot fluoroscopy films that may confirm the appropriate rostrocaudal trajectory. If there is a breech, a probe may be used to revise trajectory.[18] Fluoroscopy can be quite useful here too. Anteroposterior (AP) imaging, with the C-arm parallel to the superior end plate enables an appropriate mediolateral trajectory (**Fig. 103.3**).[25] In general, if a probe is advanced 20 to 25 mm into the pedicle without crossing the medial border of the pedicle, it has passed beyond the spinal canal. Its exact depth can be confirmed on lateral fluoroscopy.

The hole is then tapped with an undersized tap relative to the screw, and a screw is placed. Typical lumbar pedicle screws range from 6 to 7.5 mm in diameter and are 50 to 55 mm in length. The screw is placed with its head flush against the mamillary ridge.

Newer technologies may be useful in assisting pedicle screw placement. Chaput et al[26] described the use of a novel local electrical conductivity measurement device, to reduce radiation

Fig. 103.2 (a) Staring point for a lumbar pedicle screw (arrow). This image is after a Wiltse-type paramedian exposure. The point represents the accessory process, which is the junction of the pars interarticularis, the mamillary ridge, and the transverse process. (b) A bur is then used to furnish an entry hole here.

exposure while making a pilot hole for lumbar pedicle screw placement. They demonstrated a 30% reduction of fluoroscopy scans when compared with using fluoroscopy in conjunction with a standard pedicle probe. Additionally, neuronavigation systems may facilitate increased accuracy over free-hand and fluoroscopy-assisted screw placement, with reduced surgeon exposure to radiation.[27–29]

A more recently described pedicle screw trajectory is also known as a cortical trajectory. These cortical screws engage cortical bone rather than the trabecular bone of the vertebral body.[30] This technique's starting point is considerably more medial than a traditional pedicle screw starting point, and thus avoids lateral dissection. These screws are inserted at the lateral part of the pars interarticularis and follow a caudocephalad and a laterally directed path.[31] These screws are typically shorter and of smaller diameter than standard pedicle screws. However, biomechanical testing has demonstrated them to be of equivalent pullout strength to traditional pedicle screws[30,32]

Sacral Pedicle Screws

Fusion to the sacrum has been historically fraught with difficulty. Various interbody techniques have been proposed to increase fusion rates.[33] Additionally, when S1 pedicle screws are used, tricortical fixation has been shown to have significant biomechanical and clinical advantages over unicortical and tricortical screws.[34–36] When tricortical screws are placed, a trajectory directly into the medial sacral promontory is used to gain purchase in the dorsal, anterior, and superior cortices. The medialization also avoids injury to the L5 nerve that travels anteriorly bilaterally over the lateral sacrum.

The sacral ala and L5 second-facet complex should be exposed. The starting point for the S1 screw is just lateral to the base of the superior articular process of S1. As with lumbar screws, a bur or an awl is used to make a starting hole. A slightly curved gearshift is directed anteromedially to the tip of the sacral promontory. This can be confirmed fluoroscopically. The gearshift may be malleted to break through the anterior cortex of the promontory. The appropriate depth of gearshift insertion may be confirmed fluoroscopically with a pelvic inlet view (**Fig. 103.4**). Typically, the sacrum accepts 7.5- to 8.5-mm diameter screws measuring 40 to 55 mm in length.

S1 Alar Screws

This is another type of screw for sacral screw placement. However, these screws may have reduced pullout strength compared with S1 pedicle screws, especially bicortical and tricortical S1 pedicle screws[37] Additionally, sacral alar screws, which are bicortical, risk vascular injury or L4 and L5 root injury in addition to breaching the sacroiliac joint.

The starting point for these screws is halfway between the superior articular process of S1 and the S1 dorsal neuroforamen (in the transverse plane) and in the vertical plane—the lateral crest that is lateral to the S1 superior articular process.

Fig. 103.3 Anteroposterior (AP) fluoroscopic image with the C-arm beam parallel to the L4 end plate. This accommodates fluoroscopic assistance in the placement of the L4 pedicle screw. Note that the gearshift has not passed the medial border of the pedicle as seen on fluoroscopy (arrow).

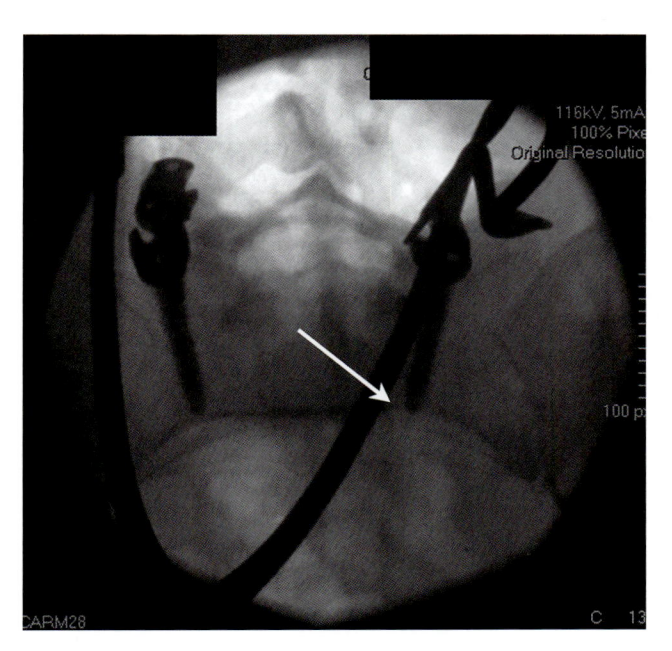

Fig. 103.4 Pelvic inlet view demonstrating tricortical purchase of S1 screw into the sacral premonitory.

A hole is drilled or made with an awl, and a gearshift is angled 20 to 40 degrees laterally and 20 to 25 degrees caudally. The hole is palpated to confirm the lack of breach prior to screw placement.[37,38] Fluoroscopy is very useful here.

S2 Pedicle Screws

These screws may be useful as supplemental sacral fixation and are not usually used alone. Nevertheless, especially in thin patients, their prominence may be bothersome. Additionally, if they are placed bicortically, especially on the left side, there may be a risk of colonic injury.[39] If the screw is angled laterally, the S1 root may be at risk. Also, the sympathetic trunk and iliac vessels may be at risk.[40]

The starting point for these screws is at a point one third of the way to halfway (in the transverse plane) between the S1 and S1 dorsal foramina and halfway between the intermediate and lateral crest in the vertical plane. The screws are typically 25 to 30 mm in length and angled 20 to 30 degrees medially or 30 degrees laterally toward the ala in the vertical plane. The screw is angled ~ 20 degrees caudally or parallel to the S1 end plate.[37,38] Fluoroscopy is very useful here.

Iliac Screws

Iliac fixation provides a fixation moment arm anterior to the spinal axis that enables increased resistance to pullout when compared with sacral instrumentation. It also provides anterior column support[41,42] (**Fig. 103.5**). Although a variety of pelvic fixation techniques have been used with spinal deformity and tumor-related pelvic fixation, the more popular current techniques for iliac screw placement for spine surgery are reviewed here.

The traditional starting point for iliac screws is a point just lateral to the S2 pedicle on the posterior superior prominence of the posterior superior iliac crest.[41] An entry point is furnished with a bur, a rongeur, or an osteotome. If using an osteotome or rongeur, bone can be saved for autogenous bone graft. A gearshift

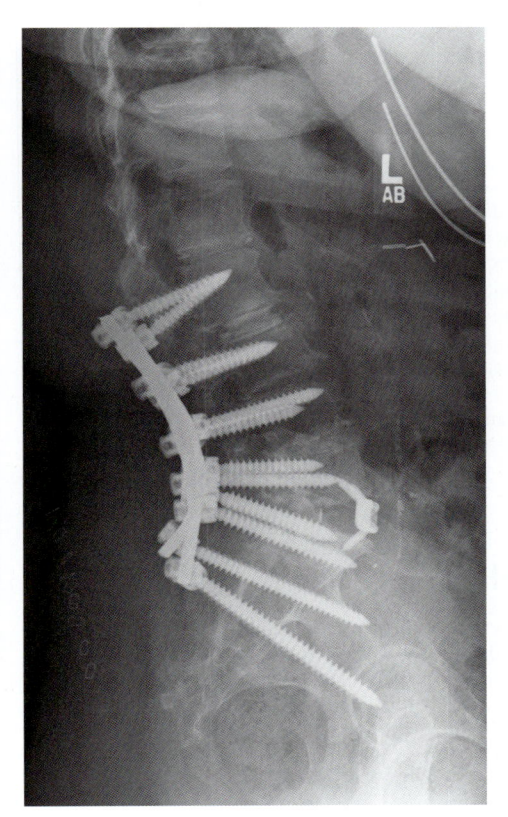

Fig. 103.5 (a) AP and (b) lateral films in a patient with iliac screws. Note that the screws project anterior to the spinal axis and run close to the thicker bone superior to the iliac notch. The technique of Harrop et al[41] was used to enable the screw heads to be in line with lumbosacral rod placement.

is then introduced with a trajectory ~ 20 degrees lateral to the midsagittal plane and 30 to 35 degrees caudal to the transverse plane toward the anterior superior iliac spine (ASIS).[41] Two trajectories for the screws have been postulated, one toward the ASIS and one toward the superior rim of the acetabulum.[43] Aiming for the ASIS may reduce the risk of acetabular violation and enable using longer screws.[44] The gearshift direction is assisted by palpation of the lateral border of the iliac bone with the surgeon's gloved finger. Palpation of the sciatic notch enables placement of the screw 1.5 to 2 cm above the notch. Most commonly, aberrant screw placement involves lateral perforation of the iliac bone.[38] Violation of the sciatic notch is much less common secondary to its thick cortical bone. The downside to this technique is that it often requires a lateral connector. Additionally, instrumentation may be prominent, although a notch could be created in the posterior superior iliac crest starting point, enabling more recessed instrumentation placement.

Harrop et al[41] described a modification of this technique to address this issue, in which an entry point is chosen along the medial border of the posterior iliac crest. With this technique, the tulip head of the iliac screw is in line with lumbosacral rod placement. Thus the need for connectors is avoided, and the screw head is less prominent.

To avoid lateral dissection, and the potential soft tissue disruption and theoretical risks of superior gluteal artery injury, various proposals have been suggested as alternative methods to assist screw placement. Fluoroscopy or image guidance can be used for iliac screw placement.[45–47] The obturator oblique outlet fluoroscopic view is particularly useful. With this technique, the fluoroscopic beam is angled in the sagittal and coronal planes so that the beam is approximately parallel to both the inner and outer tables of the ilium. A teardrop is then visualized that represents a safe passage corridor for screw placement.[45] The C-arm should be positioned with an approximately compound 45-degree anterior and 45-degree cephalad angulation of the beam so that a teardrop is seen with superimposed shadows of the posterior superior iliac spine and anterior inferior iliac spine, and the iliac rim above the sciatic notch.[48] This view should also show the acetabulum so that the surgeon avoids violating it (**Fig. 103.6**). Additionally views, such as pelvic inlet and outlet, help confirm the trajectory, facilitating accurate screw placement.

Fridley et al[44] described the free-hand placement of iliac screws without fluoroscopy, image guidance, or lateral dissection. In their technique, two gearshifts are angled so that their shafts are parallel to the L5 lamina, superior to inferior, with the tip of the probe pointing into a notch created in the ilium. The shafts of the two probes intersect each other over the L5 spinous process. The surgeon makes sure that the probes are still parallel to the lamina. The trajectory that each probe takes after these steps are performed is the path that each iliac screw should take during placement. In their series, a CT scan after surgery verified the accuracy of this method in 10 patients in whom 20 screws were placed.

S2 Alar Iliac Screws

S2 alar iliac screws are a recent form of pelvic fixation that enable lower profile insertion of screws than traditional iliac bolts and that are in line with cephalad instrumentation (**Fig. 103.7**). The starting point is 1 mm inferior and 1 mm lateral to the S1 dorsal foramen. Angulation is directed toward the greater trochanter and ~ 30 degrees anterior to the floor. AP fluoroscopy confirms a probe or a drill cephalad to the sciatic notch. A pelvic inlet view can confirm the probe/drill outside of the pelvis. Additionally, the obturator oblique outlet fluoroscopic view can be used as described above. Typically these screws course 35 to

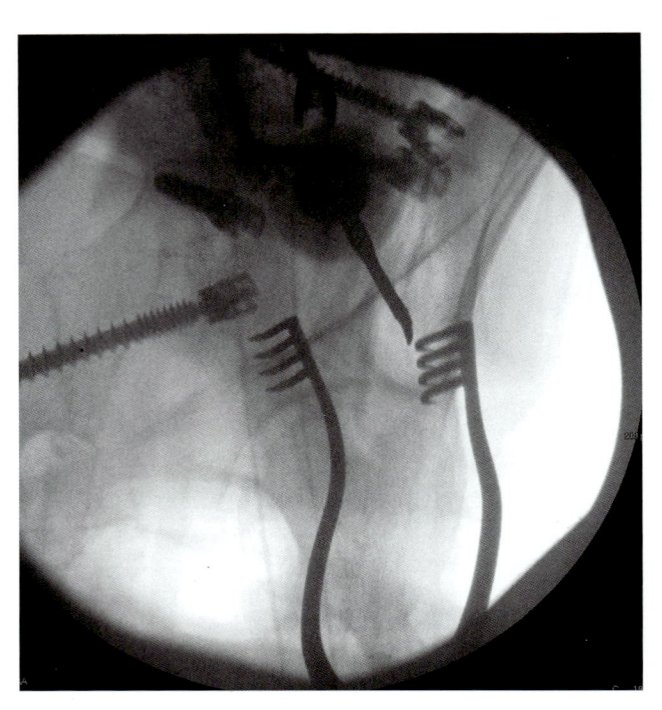

Fig. 103.6 Obturator oblique outlet fluoroscopic view (teardrop) showing the gearshift contained within the iliac bone. Note that this view also shows the acetabulum, so that the surgeon avoids violating it.

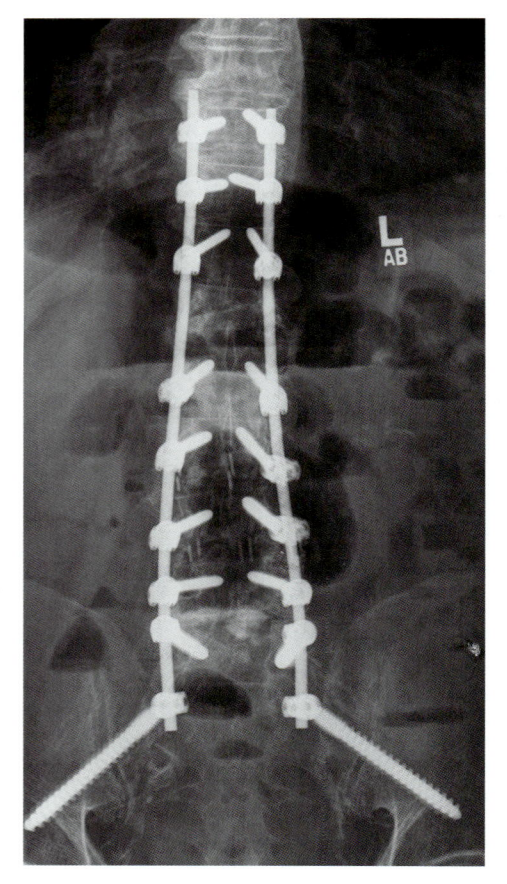

Fig. 103.7 AP X-ray showing well-placed S2 alar iliac screws. Note the in-line starting point relative to the other pedicle screws.

40 mm through the sacrum before the ilium is reached. After advancing the gear shift/drill into the ilium, a ball probe is used to palpate the hole, ensuring no breach, and then to palpate until a cortex is reached. A measurement of the screw length can be made. The screw is then placed with radiographic confirmation.[48-50] S2 alar iliac screws may have a 60% sacroiliac articular cartilage violation.[50] This is in contrast to iliac screws that cross the sacroiliac joint but do not violate the joint. The consequences of this are unknown.[49,50]

Postoperative Care

Postoperatively, we mobilize our patients as soon as possible. Given the rigidity of current instrumentation systems, bracing is not routinely used for degenerative spinal fusions. For deformity and trauma, we are more inclined to brace.

Daily dressing changes are performed until postoperative day 3 or 4.

Follow-up routine radiographs are taken at 10 days, 1 month, 3 to 6 months, and 1 year. They may include 36-inch standing films in cases of deformity correction. We typically obtain a CT scan at 1 year to assess the fusion.

Potential Complications and Precautions

Complications related to lumbosacral screws and pelvic screws can be categorized as acute or chronic, and many complications can be avoided.

Paying close attention to anatomic landmarks gearshift placement and careful palpation of the pedicle tract are critical to avoid screw misplacement. Paying detailed attention to preoperative and intraoperative imaging minimizes the risk of too long a screw being placed. If a screw is acceptably placed but its trajectory is not ideal, for example it could be medialized more, it is often better to leave the original screw, as a redirected screw may have reduced biomechanical strength.[51]

Pedicle screw stimulation (stimulus-evoked electromyography) may have a role in the detection of medial violation of the pedicle wall. This technology has high sensitivity and specificity for detecting a medial breach by the screw.[52-56] Proper technique requires coordination among the surgeon, anesthesiologist, and neuromonitoring technician/clinicians to ensure the patient's appropriate neuromuscular recovery from paralytics and to obtain reliable data with which to make appropriate clinical decisions regarding the possibility of medial wall violation.

Jutte and Castelein[13] reported a 6.5% misplacement rate of pedicle screws in 105 patients. They noted eight cases of durotomy with placement, but only one case of neurologic radicular injury with screw placement.

Lonstein et al[12] reported on complications associated with 4,790 pedicle screws inserted during 915 surgeries on 875 patients, with 76.3 patients undergoing lumbosacral fusion. They noted 2.4% of screws penetrating the anterior cortex, and 11 screws (0.2%) causing neuralgic irritation, most commonly by medially placed screws. Despite removal of the offending screws, three patients remained with neurologic weakness.

Rarely, in the acute setting, life-threatening complications can occur that are directly related to screw placement. Most commonly this is a vascular injury. If brisk bleeding is encountered from an attempt at pedicle screw placement, and it does not readily stop with tamponade and Gelfoam (e.g., in the case of a lateral breech), it may require an emergency laparotomy. Use of a hemostatic matrix down a heavily bleeding pedicle tract should be avoided, as it has been associated with fatal embolism.[57] If arterial bleeding is observed, even if it tamponades, the patient must be observed very closely; any hypotension or hemoglobin drop should prompt an emergency abdominal CT scan. The presence of a retroperitoneal hematoma warrants vascular surgical consultation (or interventional radiology) for a potential arteriogram and embolization or an emergency laparotomy.[58,59] Placement of bicortical sacral screws carries the risk of neurovascular or viscus injury.[60] Great care should be taken to employ an appropriate trajectory when placing bicortical or tricortical sacral screws.

Placement of iliac screws may result in pain or instrumentation prominence. In one series, this was reported to have occurred in 20.8% of 395 adult spinal deformity patients.[61] Removal after a solid fusion may result in significant improvement of these symptoms. When placing iliac screws, the most common complication is lateral perforation of the iliac wing, which is often asymptomatic.[38] A feared common complication is violation of the sciatic notch. Careful attention to either palpation of the notch or fluoroscopy with AP, pelvic inlet, and teardrop views is helpful here. Vascular injury, although very rare, can occur with instrumentation that violates the iliac cortex, as can abdominal injury with instrumentation violating the inner iliac table. As discussed above, iliac screws, especially S2 alar iliac screws, may violate the sacroiliac joint. The long-term consequences of this complication are uncertain.

Osteoporosis represents a challenging environment for the spine surgeon because of several factors: reduced bone stock, resulting in poor fixation with standard instrumentation; potential fracture of instrumented levels; higher incidence of kyphosis in this population; and high pseudarthrosis rate.[62] Various techniques to augment pedicle screws have been proposed, including vertebroplasty (with polymethylmethacrylate or other bone cements), double screws in a single pedicle, bicortical screws, coating screws with hydroxyapatite, expandable screws, and augmentation of spinal fusions with other technologies such as sublaminar hooks, wires, and anterior fixation.[62,63] Additionally, cortical screws, which maintain biomechanical efficacy in poorly trabeculated osteoporotic bone, and screws with double lead and dural thread near the pedicle area may be useful in these patients.[64] All these methods, coupled with advances in pharmacological treatment, are useful in the surgical treatment of the osteoporotic spine.

Screw breakage, loss of fixation, and pseudarthrosis are all delayed complications of pedicle screw placement. Screw fracture may be related to screw design, the presence of pseudarthrosis, and, in the trauma setting, the treatment of burst fractures.[12] Reduction of a spondylolisthesis, especially in cases without anterior load sharing with an interbody graft, may also be a risk factor for screw fracture.[13] A screw trajectory parallel or caudal to the superior end plate can minimize the risk of breakage due to axial loading.[64] Loss of fixation may occur early, as in the failure of a construct that is biomechanically suboptimal, such as a short segment construct, or due to patient risk factors, such as osteoporosis or later in the setting of pseudarthrosis. Occasionally, a screw may loosen or break in a delayed manner without a pseudarthrosis.[12] Risk factors for pseudarthrosis have been described, and include multilevel fusion, fusion material choice, medical comorbidities, poor bone quality, and inadequate surgical planning. Appropriate sagittal balance is an important consideration in avoiding pseudarthrosis, as is the proper use of interbody grafting techniques and consideration of pelvic fixation when fusing to the sacrum.[65]

Conclusion

Lumbosacral pedicle screws and iliac screws have become a mainstay of modern spinal fixation technique. Careful attention to patient selection and to fixation techniques lead to better outcomes and minimization of surgical complications. Preoperative planning with appropriate imaging and anticipation of anatomic anomalies and poor bone stock may reduce the possibility of treatment failure.

References

1. Harrington PR, Tullos HS. Reduction of severe spondylolisthesis in children. South Med J 1969;62:1–7
2. Dick W, Kluger P, Magerl F, Woersdörfer O, Zäch G. A new device for internal fixation of thoracolumbar and lumbar spine fractures: the "fixateur interne." Paraplegia 1985;23:225–232
3. Steffee AD, Biscup RS, Sitkowski DJ. Segmental spine plates with pedicle screw fixation. A new internal fixation device for disorders of the lumbar and thoracolumbar spine. Clin Orthop Relat Res 1986;203:45–53
4. Roy-Camille R, Saillant G, Mazel C. Internal fixation of the lumbar spine with pedicle screw plating. Clin Orthop Relat Res 1986;203:7–17
5. Louis R. Fusion of the lumbar and sacral spine by internal fixation with screw plates. Clin Orthop Relat Res 1986;203:18–33
6. Kim HJ, Kim SG, Lee HM, et al. Risk factors associated with the halo phenomenon after lumbar fusion surgery and its clinical significance. Asian Spine J 2008;2:22–26
7. Marchesi DG, Thalgott JS, Aebi M. Application and results of the AO internal fixation system in nontraumatic indications. Spine 1991;16(3, Suppl):S162–S169
8. Steffee AD, Sitkowski DJ. Posterior lumbar interbody fusion and plates. Clin Orthop Relat Res 1988;227:99–102
9. Mac-Thiong JM, Parent S, Poitras B, Joncas J, Hubert L. Neurological outcome and management of pedicle screws misplaced totally within the spinal canal. Spine 2013;38:229–237
10. Dickman CA, Fessler RG, MacMillan M, Haid RW. Transpedicular screw-rod fixation of the lumbar spine: operative technique and outcome in 104 cases. J Neurosurg 1992;77:860–870
11. Tumialán LM, Mummaneni PV. Long-segment spinal fixation using pelvic screws. Neurosurgery 2008;63(3, Suppl):183–190
12. Lonstein JE, Denis F, Perra JH, Pinto MR, Smith MD, Winter RB. Complications associated with pedicle screws. J Bone Joint Surg Am 1999;81:1519–1528
13. Jutte PC, Castelein RM. Complications of pedicle screws in lumbar and lumbosacral fusions in 105 consecutive primary operations. Eur Spine J 2002;11:594–598
14. Vanderburgh DF, Kelly WM. Radiographic assessment of discogenic disease of the spine. Neurosurg Clin N Am 1993;4:13–33
15. Watura R, Cobby M, Taylor J. Multislice CT in imaging of trauma of the spine, pelvis and complex foot injuries. Br J Radiol 2004;77(Spec. No. 1):S46–S63
16. Placide J, Martens MG. Comparing screening methods for osteoporosis. Curr Womens Health Rep 2003;3:207–210
17. Wadhwa RK, Thakur JD, Khan IS, et al. Adjustment of suboptimally placed lumbar pedicle screws decreases pullout strength and alters biomechanics of the construct: a pilot cadaveric study. World Neurosurg 2015;83:368–375
18. Parker SL, McGirt MJ, Farber SH, et al. Accuracy of free-hand pedicle screws in the thoracic and lumbar spine: analysis of 6816 consecutive screws. Neurosurgery 2011;68:170–178, discussion 178
19. Hadjipavlou AG, Nicodemus CL, al-Hamdan FA, Simmons JW, Pope MH. Correlation of bone equivalent mineral density to pull-out resistance of triangulated pedicle screw construct. J Spinal Disord 1997;10:12–19
20. Ruland CM, McAfee PC, Warden KE, Cunningham BW. Triangulation of pedicular instrumentation. A biomechanical analysis. Spine 1991;16(6, Suppl):S270–S276
21. Mitra SR, Datir SP, Jadhav SO. Morphometric study of the lumbar pedicle in the Indian population as related to pedicular screw fixation. Spine 2002;27:453–459
22. Lien SB, Liou NH, Wu SS. Analysis of anatomic morphometry of the pedicles and the safe zone for through-pedicle procedures in the thoracic and lumbar spine. Eur Spine J 2007;16:1215–1222
23. Karabekir HS, Gocmen-Mas N, Edizer M, Ertekin T, Yazici C, Atamturk D. Lumbar vertebra morphometry and stereological assesment of intervertebral space volumetry: a methodological study. Ann Anat 2011;193:231–236
24. Cheung KM, Ruan D, Chan FL, Fang D. Computed tomographic osteometry of Asian lumbar pedicles. Spine 1994;19:1495–1498
25. Puvanesarajah V, Liauw JA, Lo SF, Lina IA, Witham TF. Techniques and accuracy of thoracolumbar pedicle screw placement. World J Orthop 2014;5:112–123
26. Chaput CD, George K, Samdani AF, Williams JI, Gaughan J, Betz RR. Reduction in radiation (fluoroscopy) while maintaining safe placement of pedicle screws during lumbar spine fusion. Spine 2012;37:E1305–E1309
27. Hodges SD, Eck JC, Newton D. Analysis of CT-based navigation system for pedicle screw placement. Orthopedics 2012;35:e1221–e1224
28. Shin MH, Ryu KS, Park CK. Accuracy and safety in pedicle screw placement in the thoracic and lumbar spines: comparison study between conventional C-arm fluoroscopy and navigation coupled with O-arm® guided methods. J Korean Neurosurg Soc 2012;52:204–209
29. Silbermann J, Riese F, Allam Y, Reichert T, Koeppert H, Gutberlet M. Computer tomography assessment of pedicle screw placement in lumbar and sacral spine: comparison between free-hand and O-arm based navigation techniques. Eur Spine J 2011;20:875–881
30. Santoni BG, Hynes RA, McGilvray KC, et al. Cortical bone trajectory for lumbar pedicle screws. Spine J 2009;9:366–373
31. Rodriguez A, Neal MT, Liu A, Somasundaram A, Hsu W, Branch CL Jr. Novel placement of cortical bone trajectory screws in previously instrumented pedicles for adjacent-segment lumbar disease using CT image-guided navigation. Neurosurg Focus 2014;36:E9
32. Perez-Orribo L, Kalb S, Reyes PM, Chang SW, Crawford NR. Biomechanics of lumbar cortical screw-rod fixation versus pedicle screw-rod fixation with and without interbody support. Spine 2013;38:635–641
33. Bridwell KH. Selection of instrumentation and fusion levels for scoliosis: where to start and where to stop. Invited submission from the Joint Section Meeting on Disorders of the Spine and Peripheral Nerves, March 2004. J Neurosurg Spine 2004;1:1–8
34. Kato M, Taneichi H, Suda K. Advantage of pedicle screw placement into the sacral promontory (tricortical purchase) on lumbosacral fixation. J Spinal Disord Tech 2013;Nov:5
35. Lehman RA Jr, Kuklo TR, Belmont PJ Jr, Andersen RC, Polly DW Jr. Advantage of pedicle screw fixation directed into the apex of the sacral promontory over bicortical fixation: a biomechanical analysis. Spine 2002;27:806–811
36. Orita S, Ohtori S, Eguchi Y, et al. Radiographic evaluation of monocortical versus tricortical purchase approaches in lumbosacral fixation with sacral pedicle screws: a prospective study of ninety consecutive patients. Spine 2010;35:E1230–E1237
37. von Strempel A, Trenkmann S, Krönauer I, Kirsch L, Sukopp C. The stability of bone screws in the os sacrum. Eur Spine J 1998;7:313–320
38. Daftari T, Vaccaro AR, Fishgrund J. Sacropelvic fixation. In: Vaccaro AR, Baron EM, eds. Operative Techniques: Spine Surgery. Philadelphia: Saunders Elsevier; 2008:307–324
39. Mirkovic S, Abitbol JJ, Steinman J, et al. Anatomic consideration for sacral screw placement. Spine 1991;16(6, Suppl):S289–S294
40. Ebraheim NA, Lu J, Yang H, Heck BE, Yeasting RA. Anatomic considerations of the second sacral vertebra and dorsal screw placement. Surg Radiol Anat 1997;19:353–357
41. Harrop JS, Jeyamohan SB, Sharan A, Ratliff J, Vaccaro AR. Iliac bolt fixation: an anatomic approach. J Spinal Disord Tech 2009;22:541–544
42. McCord DH, Cunningham BW, Shono Y, Myers JJ, McAfee PC. Biomechanical analysis of lumbosacral fixation. Spine 1992;17(8, Suppl):S235–S243
43. Berry JL, Stahurski T, Asher MA. Morphometry of the supra sciatic notch intrailiac implant anchor passage. Spine 2001;26:E143–E148
44. Fridley J, Fahim D, Navarro J, Wolinsky JP, Omeis I. Free-hand placement of iliac screws for spinopelvic fixation based on anatomical landmarks: technical note. Int J Spine Surg 2014;8:10.14444/1003
45. Wang MY. Percutaneous iliac screws for minimally invasive spinal deformity surgery. Minim Invasive Surg 2012;2012:173685
46. Schildhauer TA, McCulloch P, Chapman JR, Mann FA. Anatomic and radiographic considerations for placement of transiliac screws in lumbopelvic fixations. J Spinal Disord Tech 2002;15:199–205, discussion 205
47. Hsieh JC, Drazin D, Firempong AO, Pashman R, Johnson JP, Kim TT. Accuracy of intraoperative computed tomography image-guided surgery in

placing pedicle and pelvic screws for primary versus revision spine surgery. Neurosurg Focus 2014;36:E2
48. Kebaish KM, Dafrawy MH. Sacropelvic fixation. In: Vaccaro AR, Baron EM, eds. Operative Techniques: Spine Surgery, Second Edition, 2nd ed. Philadelphia: Elsevier Saunders; 2012:240–255
49. Matteini LE, Kebaish KM, Volk WR, Bergin PF, Yu WD, O'Brien JR. An S-2 alar iliac pelvic fixation. Technical note. Neurosurg Focus 2010;28:E13
50. O'Brien JR, Matteini L, Yu WD, Kebaish KM. Feasibility of minimally invasive sacropelvic fixation: percutaneous S2 alar iliac fixation. Spine 2010; 35:460–464
51. Stauff MP, Freedman BA, Kim JH, Hamasaki T, Yoon ST, Hutton WC. The effect of pedicle screw redirection after lateral wall breach—a biomechanical study using human lumbar vertebrae. Spine J 2014;14:98–103
52. Raynor BL, Lenke LG, Bridwell KH, Taylor BA, Padberg AM. Correlation between low triggered electromyographic thresholds and lumbar pedicle screw malposition: analysis of 4857 screws. Spine 2007;32:2673–2678
53. Toleikis JR, Skelly JP, Carlvin AO, et al. The usefulness of electrical stimulation for assessing pedicle screw placements. J Spinal Disord 2000;13: 283–289
54. Welch WC, Rose RD, Balzer JR, Jacobs GB. Evaluation with evoked and spontaneous electromyography during lumbar instrumentation: a prospective study. J Neurosurg 1997;87:397–402
55. Clements DH, Morledge DE, Martin WH, Betz RR. Evoked and spontaneous electromyography to evaluate lumbosacral pedicle screw placement. Spine 1996;21:600–604
56. Glassman SD, Dimar JR, Puno RM, Johnson JR, Shields CB, Linden RD. A prospective analysis of intraoperative electromyographic monitoring of pedicle screw placement with computed tomographic scan confirmation. Spine 1995;20:1375–1379
57. Skovrlj B, Motivala S, Panov F, et al. Fatal intraoperative cardiac arrest after application of Surgifoam into a bleeding iliac screw defect. Spine 2014;39:E1239–E1242
58. Sandri A, Regis D, Marino MA, Puppini G, Bartolozzi P. Lumbar artery injury following posterior spinal instrumentation for scoliosis. Orthopedics 2011;34
59. Sugimoto Y, Tanaka M, Gobara H, Misawa H, Kunisada T, Ozaki T. Management of lumbar artery injury related to pedicle screw insertion. Acta Med Okayama 2013;67:113–116
60. Ergur I, Akcali O, Kiray A, Kosay C, Tayefi H. Neurovascular risks of sacral screws with bicortical purchase: an anatomical study. Eur Spine J 2007; 16:1519–1523
61. O'Shaughnessy BA, Lenke LG, Bridwell KH, et al. Should symptomatic iliac screws be electively removed in adult spinal deformity patients fused to the sacrum? Spine 2012;37:1175–1181
62. Ponnusamy KE, Iyer S, Gupta G, Khanna AJ. Instrumentation of the osteoporotic spine: biomechanical and clinical considerations. Spine J 2011; 11:54–63
63. Jang SH, Lee JH, Cho JY, Lee HY, Lee SH. The efficacy of hydroxyapatite for screw augmentation in osteoporotic patients. Neurol Med Chir (Tokyo) 2013;53:875–881
64. Cho W, Cho SK, Wu C. The biomechanics of pedicle screw-based instrumentation. J Bone Joint Surg Br 2010;92:1061–1065
65. Ondra SL, Marzouk S. Revision strategies for lumbar pseudarthrosis. Neurosurg Focus 2003;15:E9

104 Minimally Invasive Transforaminal Lumbar Interbody Fusion

Kurt M. Eichholz

Interbody fusion has become a standard surgical treatment for several types of pathology in the lumbar spine. First described by Cloward[1] in 1953 as a treatment for lumbar instability, indications for interbody fusion have been expanded to treat degenerative disk disease and disk collapse, spondylolisthesis, recurrent disk herniation, and spondylosis. This technique enables the removal of a large portion of the intervertebral disk and replacement of the disk space with an intervertebral graft that provides anterior column support. Interbody fusion can be achieved through an anterior approach (either transperitoneal or retroperitoneal), a lateral approach, or a posterior approach, either transforaminal lumbar interbody fusion (TLIF) or posterior lumbar interbody fusion (PLIF). Each of these approaches has advantages and disadvantages. In recent years, TLIF has been performed routinely through a paramedian muscle-splitting approach that has enabled a decreased approach with lower related morbidity, including lower blood loss, lower infection rate, shorter hospitalizations, and faster return to normal activity.[2-4] This chapter describes the minimally invasive, paramedian, muscle-splitting unilateral approach to performing a TLIF, as well as percutaneous pedicle screw fixation.

Patient Selection

Patients who are appropriate surgical candidates for a minimally invasive TLIF include those who present with a grade I or grade II spondylolisthesis, with or without spondylolysis; patients with gross instability in the lumbar spine; patients suffering multiple repeated lumbar disk herniations; and patients with loss of disk height and disk collapse causing significant neural foraminal stenosis that can only be alleviated with a complete facetectomy.

Indications and Contraindications

The primary indications for minimally invasive lumbar fusion include deformity (spondylolisthesis), instability, and central canal or neural foraminal compression. Therefore, the objective of surgery includes adequate decompression of all neural elements, safe removal of the intervertebral disk and its replacement with an interbody graft, and appropriate placement of pedicle screw fixation without violation of the central canal or neural foramen. These objectives can be achieved with careful preoperative planning, meticulous surgical technique, and attention to detail.

Relative contraindications to this approach include high-grade spondylolisthesis (greater than grade II), previously placed instrumentation at the involved level or an adjacent level, and significant coronal plane deformity.

In patients with high-grade spondylolisthesis where the goal of surgery is reduction of the deformity, it may be necessary to utilize an open technique with reduction screws or a "jig" reduction system. I perform TLIF through a minimally invasive approach in patients with up to a fixed, nonmobile, grade II spondylolisthesis. In patients who have previously placed pedicle screw instrumentation, exposure of the previous instrumentation to enable removal of the set screws and rods and interrogation of the pedicle screws is often done more expeditiously through an open approach. In patients who have a concurrent sagittal and coronal plane deformity, the coronal plane deformity may make adequate fluoroscopic visualization of the pedicles for placement of percutaneous instrumentation exceedingly difficult. In addition, bilateral complete facetectomies or osteotomies may be required to appropriately reduce such a deformity, and, therefore, surgeons should consider their experience and comfort level when performing these high difficulty cases through a minimally invasive approach.

Advantages and Disadvantages

There are several advantages of a minimally invasive paramedian approach to the lumbar spine, especially in cases such as TLIF, which enables the placement of an interbody graft with minimal retraction of the thecal sac or traversing nerve roots. This technique reduces the incidence of retraction-induced neurapraxia when compared with a traditional midline PLIF. The posterior or transforaminal approach avoids the potential for vascular or enteric complications, which can occur with anterior approaches. In addition, anterior approaches that are performed above the L4–L5 level may require mobilization of the great vessels to place an interbody graft, which is not necessary with a TLIF approach. Although anterior lumbar interbody grafts typically have larger footprints, a TLIF approach can be combined with a posterolateral fusion to enable anterior and posterior arthrodesis. Pedicle screw instrumentation can be placed at the same setting, whereas with an anterior approach, the patient must be repositioned to place pedicle screw fixation.

The relative disadvantages of a minimally invasive TLIF approach include limited visualization of the targeted anatomy, as well as a relatively steep learning curve. A surgeon who is familiar with open approaches may need to perform many minimally invasive procedures before becoming comfortable with performing a decompression and interbody fusion while visualizing only a limited amount of the patient's anatomy. In addition, percutaneous pedicle screw fixation with fluoroscopy has several more steps than open placement of instrumentation, and new techniques and potential pitfalls must be learned with experience.

Preoperative Planning

Once the decision to surgically intervene is made, appropriate preoperative planning is done. Typically, prior to the scheduling of surgery, the patient has already had an imaging study of the lumbar spine, either magnetic resonance imaging (MRI) or a computed tomography (CT) myelogram. In addition, dynamic radiographs of the lumbar spine should be taken to search for instability; the radiographs can be compared with the supine MRI or myelogram images. In patients with a mobile spondylolisthesis, this imaging enables the surgeon to evaluate how much reduction potentially can be obtained from positioning the patient in the operating room, and can also aid in deciding whether reduction screws should be utilized.

The surgeon should also decide on whether to utilize intraoperative electrophysiological monitoring. Some surgeons routinely use intraoperative somatosensory evoked potential (SSEP) monitoring of the appropriate dermatomes, both above and below the level of interest, as well as electromyograph (EMG) recordings and less often motor evoked potentials (MEPs). This monitoring can help identify a pedicle breach during the placement of instrumentation. The use of electrophysiological monitoring requires the absence of paralytic anesthetic during the operation. The use of intraoperative electrophysiological monitoring is controversial, and is not required for successful TLIF or for the placement of instrumentation.

Surgical Procedure

Radiographic Visualization

Percutaneous pedicle screw instrumentation requires utilization of two- or three-dimensional radiographic visualization. Options include C-arm fluoroscopy or intraoperative CT imaging with navigation. There are advantages and disadvantages to both. C-arm visualization requires the surgeon to be present during fluoroscopy, thereby increasing his or her exposure to X-rays during the procedure. This can be mitigated by proper utilization of lead shielding. Intraoperative CT imaging with navigation (i.e., O-arm with Stealth, Medtronic, Minneapolis, MN) requires both the CT image acquisition device as well as the image guidance system. Although this system enables real-time tracking of instruments during the operation, it increases the patient's exposure to X-rays, and can increase the anesthesia time, because once the images are acquired, they are transferred to the navigation system, and then the operation is planned. Further, there is the cost of acquiring the equipment. Surgeon should decide which visualization options they will use based on the availability of the equipment at their hospital, the skill level of the technicians who operate the devices, and their comfort level with each device. For the purposes of this chapter, percutaneous pedicle screw fixation with fluoroscopy is used.

Positioning

Once the patient is intubated and appropriate intravenous lines are secured, a Foley catheter is placed. The patient is positioned prone onto either a radiolucent Wilson frame or onto gel laminectomy rolls. I prefer to use a radiolucent Wilson frame on a flat Jackson table, to facilitate access of the fluoroscopy equipment. In obese patients, an open Jackson table enables the abdomen to hang between the chest and iliac crest pads, which decreases intra-abdominal pressure, and reduces venous pressure at the operative site. Gentle manual traction between the hips and the shoulders can be applied to reduce mild positional coronal plane deformity prior to draping.

The side of approach should be ipsilateral to the side that has the worse symptoms or pathology. A complete facetectomy is performed on the ipsilateral side, whereas a foraminotomy is performed on the contralateral side. If the patient's symptoms are equal bilaterally, then the left side is typically chosen for a right-handed surgeon, to facilitate the passing of instruments from the scrub nurse. A table mounted arm that holds the tubular retractor in place is attached to the side opposite the surgeon, as is the base of the fluoroscope, which places the equipment opposite the surgeon.

Incision and Localization

Once the patient is prepped and draped, the level is localized. The first dilator is placed lateral to the patient's body parallel to the disk space over the level of interest. A marking pen is then used to draw a line parallel to the disk space of interest. Various retractors are available to enable tubular, muscle-splitting approaches to the lumbar spine. I typically use a 22-mm tube for performing a TLIF. Surgeons who have less experience with this technique may choose to use a larger diameter tubular dilator, or a tube that opens to a larger diameter, until they become more comfortable with this technique. After infiltration of the incision with a Marcaine–epinephrine mixture, a 2.5-cm incision is made 3 to 3.5 cm off the midline. This may need to be further lateral in more obese patients. Once the incision is made, the blade is used to make a linear incision in the lumbosacral fascia, large enough to accommodate the tubular retractor.

After the fascia is incised, the first dilator is used to palpate the patient's posterior spinal elements. Using the dilator, the surgeon is able feel the base of the spinous process, the lamina, and the facet. The first dilator is then placed at the lamino-facet junction. Intraoperative fluoroscopy is used to confirm the level of interest. The rest of the dilators are placed up to the final tube, which is attached to a table mounted arm that holds the retractor in place.

Visualization

Options for visualization through the tubular retractor include operating loupes and microscope. Again, there are advantages and disadvantages of each option. Loupes typically provide up to 3.5× magnification, which is adequate for visualization of the anatomy through the retractor, and do not get in the way of the longer surgical instruments that are used for end-plate preparation. The operating microscope enables the surgeon's assistant to visualize the operating field simultaneously. However, depending on the focal length of the microscope, the head of the microscope may limit the surgeon's ability to place the interbody instruments. The choice of visualization should be made based on the surgeon's level of comfort and experience with each option. I prefer to use loupes for interbody grafting and a microscope for cases that do not require interbody work.

Decompression and Interbody Grafting

Once the retractor is in place, there is a small amount of paraspinal muscle and soft tissue at the base of the tube that is removed with monopolar electrocautery. The trailing edge of the lamina is then delineated with straight and then with angled curettes. An angled curette is placed under the lamina and the level is confirmed with fluoroscopy (**Fig. 104.1**). At this point, an ipsilateral

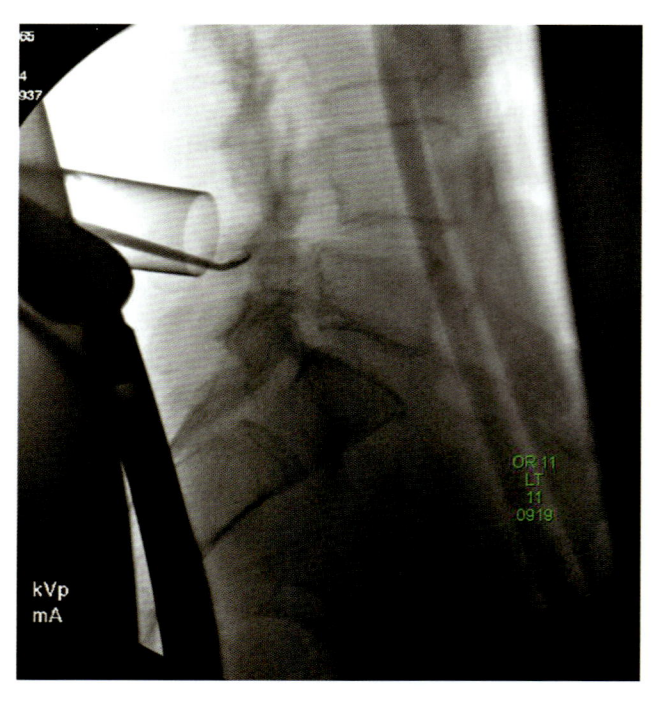

Fig. 104.1 Lateral fluoroscopic view with 22-mm tubular retractor in place over the L4-5 interspace, with an angled curette under the L4 lamina.

hemilaminotomy is performed. This can be done by using Kerrison rongeurs or an osteotome. The laminotomy is then cut laterally across the pars interarticularis, which enables the removal of the inferior articular process of the rostral vertebrae. The remaining ledge of the superior articular process of the caudal level is undercut with Kerrison rongeurs. This is typically done prior to removal of the ligamentum flavum. It is preferable not to use a drill, but rather to use rongeurs to harvest the bone from the decompression for subsequent autografting.

After adequate bony decompression is performed on the ipsilateral side, the tube is tilted toward the contralateral side. In doing so, the medial portion of tube is moved posteriorly, up the base of the spinous process. This exposes the remaining base of the spinous process. The base of the spinous process and contralateral lamina are then undercut with a small high-speed drill. Because of the angle of approach to the lamina, a drill is required for this step to remove this portion of the lamina. This exposes the lateral recess, and some patients may have significant lateral recess stenosis. The footplate of the Kerrison can be placed under the lateral recess to enable good decompression. Typically, the ligamentum flavum is left in place as a barrier to prevent dural violations. Once adequate bony decompression is achieved on both sides, the ligamentum flavum is removed. The ligamentum flavum thins out superiorly, and in patients with lumbar stenosis, the central canal is largest at the midline. Therefore, it is best to use an angled curette to dissect the superior aspect of the ligamentum flavum from the dura in the midline. Once the plane between the dura and ligamentum flavum is delineated, the curette can be used to scrape the ligament along the remaining bony edge. This enables the ligamentum flavum to be disarticulated in one or two pieces, and minimizes the need to use a Kerrison to remove the ligament, thereby reducing the risk of a dural rent.

Once the ligamentum flavum is removed, the thecal sac and traversing nerve root are exposed. The exiting nerve root can be visualized superiorly in the operative field (**Fig. 104.2**). A nerve root retractor is place against the thecal sac for protection during the interbody work. This can be done with a self-retaining arm or with the help of an assistant.

Placing the nerve root retractor exposes the annulus. The annulus should be incised in a rectangular fashion, as large as possible against the end plates superiorly and inferiorly. In patients with a higher grade spondylolisthesis or significant disk collapse, it may be difficult to access the disk space. An osteotome can be used first in this situation to initially open the disk space. Extraneous disk material is removed with pituitary rongeurs. The disk space and cartilaginous end plates are removed using a combination of paddle shavers, box cutters, end-plate

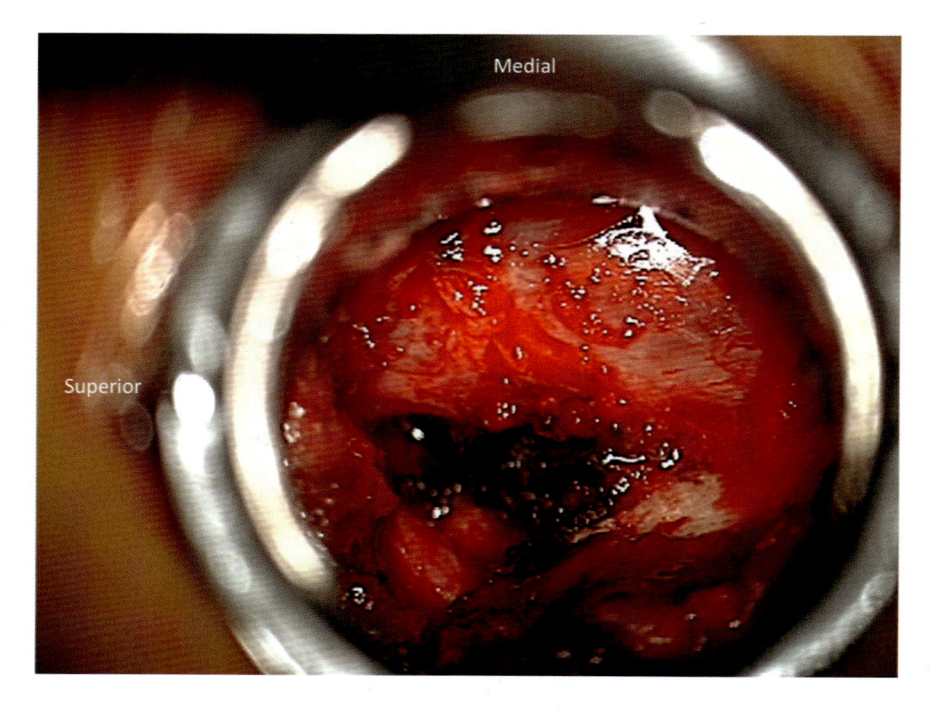

Fig. 104.2 Microscope view through a 22-mm tubular retractor after left-sided decompression at L4-L5. Note the thecal sac with the nerve root exiting from the 9 o'clock position to the 6 o'clock position.

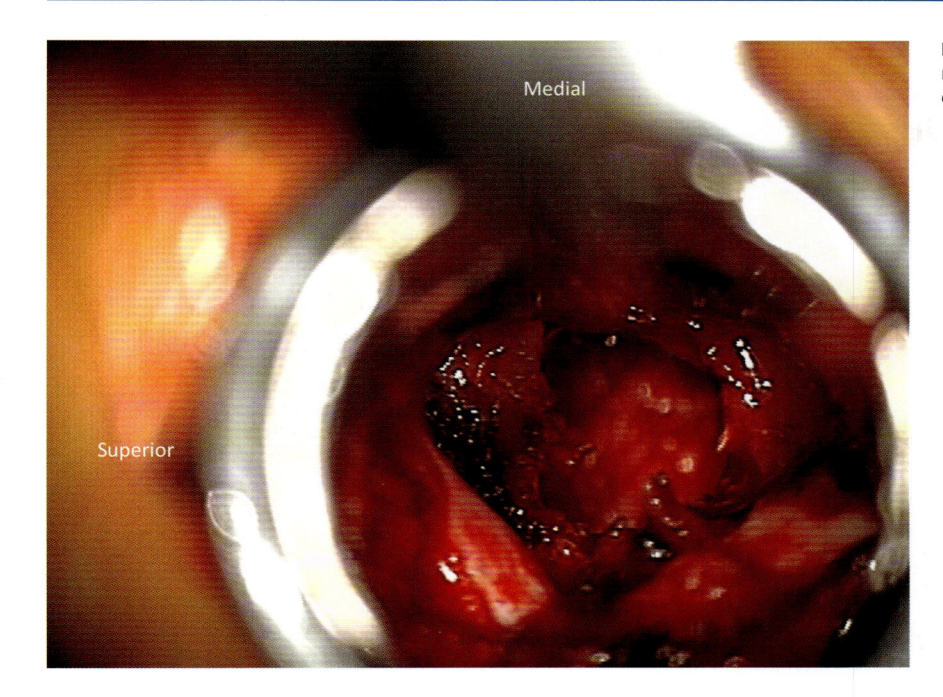

Fig. 104.3 Microscope view with nerve root retractor in place, after interbody space and end-plate preparation.

scrapers, and ring curettes (**Fig. 104.3**). Meticulous end-plate preparation is essential for good arthrodesis, and special care should be taken to remove all of the cartilaginous end plate without violating the bony end plate, which can cause the graft to subside into the vertebral body.

Once the end plates are adequately prepared, the interbody graft is placed. Trials are first placed to assess the appropriate graft size in terms of height and anterior-posterior length (**Figs. 104.4 and 104.5**). The largest graft possible that can be placed without rupturing the anterior longitudinal ligament should be

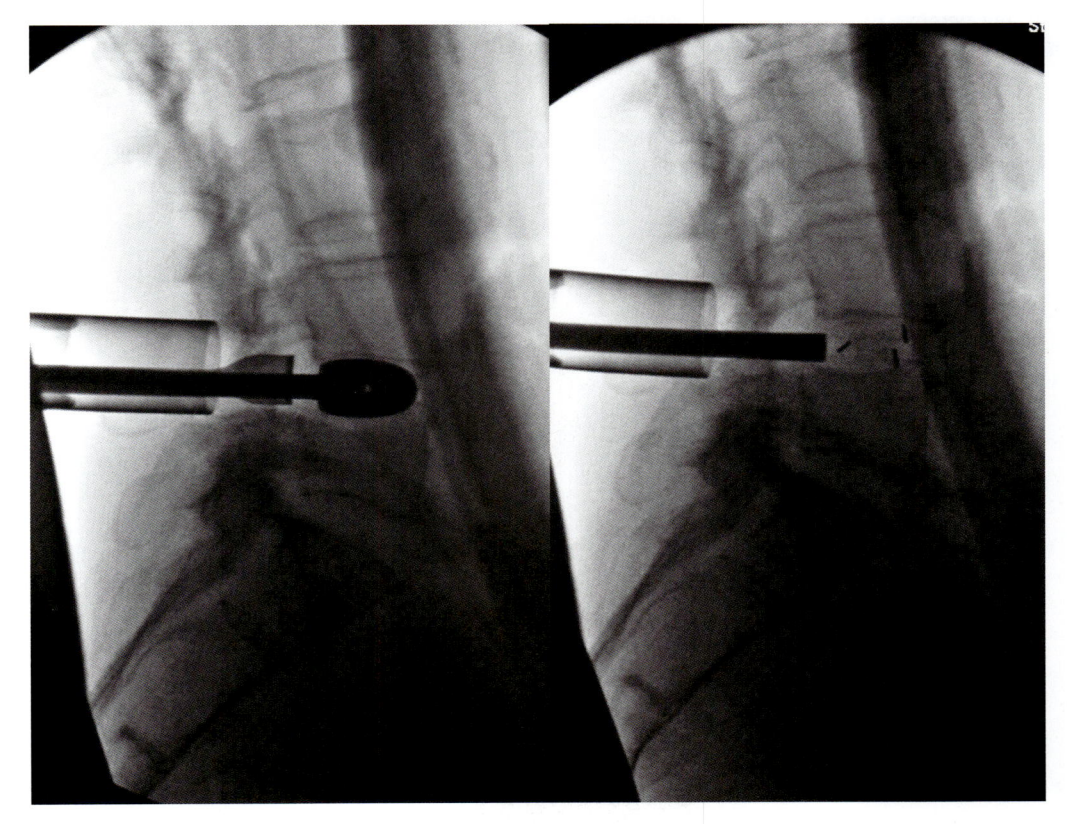

Fig. 104.4 Lateral fluoroscopic images of the L4-L5 trial, and placement of the L4-L5 PEEK interbody graft.

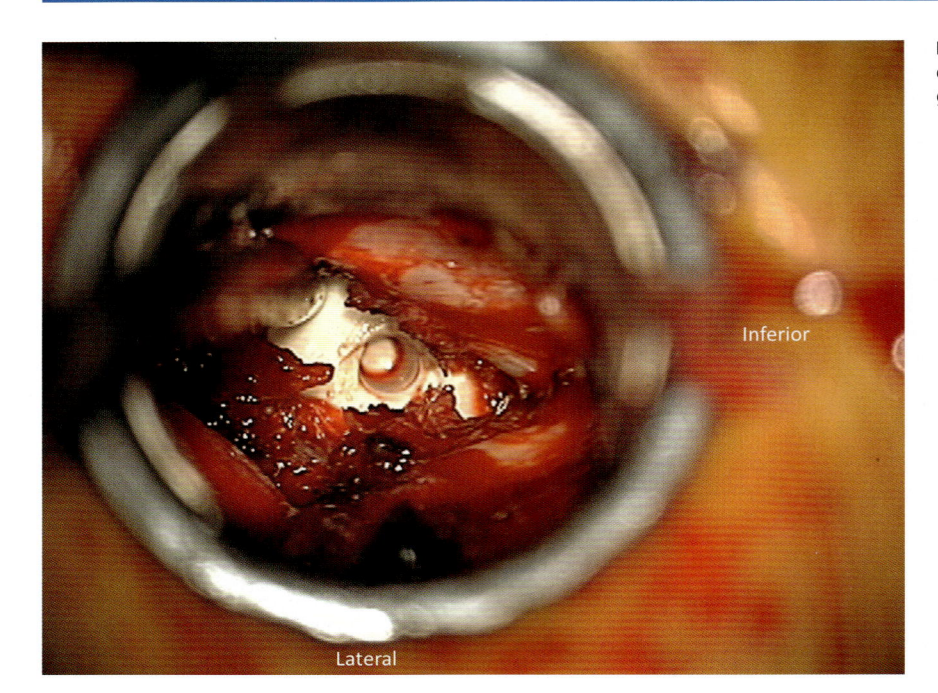

Fig. 104.5 Microscope view after placement of a polyetheretherketone (PEEK) interbody graft.

used. Care should be taken to adequately remove all extraneous disk material so that the graft is able to be adequately countersunk with relation to the end plates. Morcellized autograft from the decompression is placed into the interspace, with bone extender of the surgeon's choice. A variety of interbody grafts are available, including polyetheretherketone (PEEK), carbon fiber, and machined allograft. I prefer PEEK cages filled with morcellized autograft and demineralized bone matrix, although any number of options are acceptable. Once the graft is in appropriate position, hemostasis is obtained, and the tubular retractor is removed for placement of the percutaneous pedicle screws.

Percutaneous Pedicle Screw Placement

After the tube is removed, anteroposterior (AP) fluoroscopy is used. The fluoroscope may need to be tilted to facilitate visualization of the pedicles. Care should be taken to make sure that the end plates are visualized squarely on fluoroscopy, which in

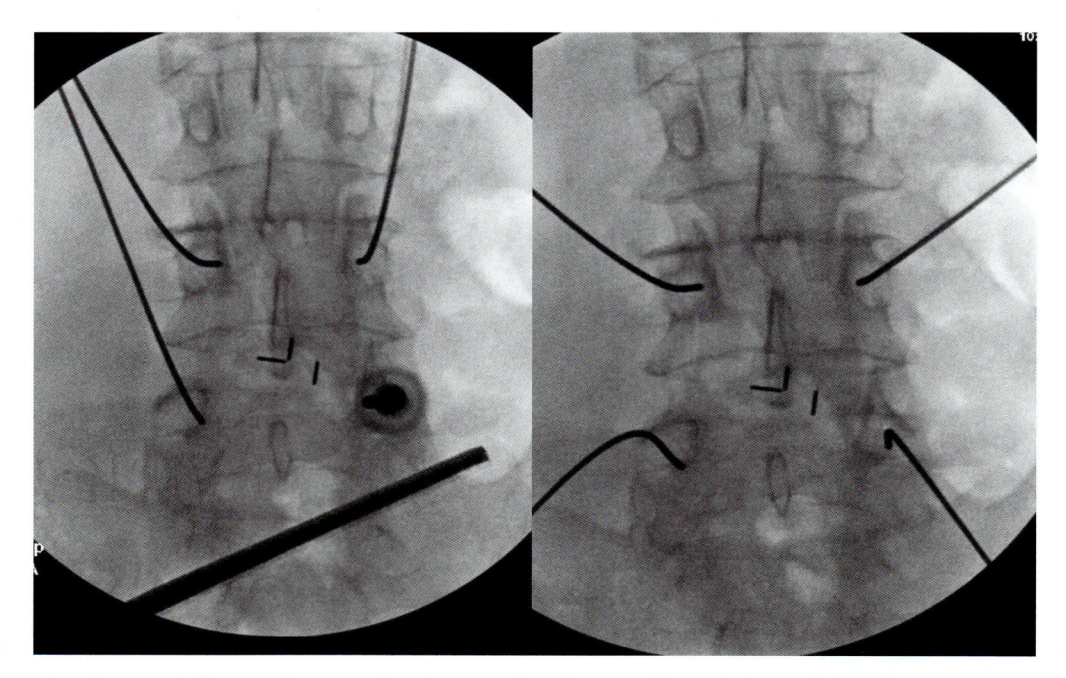

Fig. 104.6 (a,b) Anterior-posterior fluoroscopic images after placement of Kirschner wires (K-wires). The Jamshidi needle is in place (a) prior to placement of the K-wire.

most cases yields the best visualization of the pedicles. In patients with smaller pedicles, the fluoroscope may need to be rotated to see "down the barrel" of the pedicle in an en-face view. When performing an L5-S1 TLIF, the fluoroscope may need to be tilted fairly steeply to be parallel to the L5-S1 end plates, in a Ferguson view. For S1 screws, in many cases, only the medial and inferior walls of the pedicle may be visualized.

Jamshidi needles are placed over the center of the pedicle, with a slight 5- to 10-degree tilt in a lateral to medial direction. The stylet of the Jamshidi needle is removed, and a Kirschner wire (K-wire) is placed with a battery-powered wire driver. The K-wires are advanced 1 to 2 cm through the Jamshidi needle, and then the remaining K-wires are placed (**Fig. 104.6**). The incision from the decompression is used on the ipsilateral side, whereas new stab incisions are made on the contralateral side. Once the K-wires are in appropriate position on AP fluoroscopy, lateral fluoroscopy is used, and the K-wires are advanced with the driver to the junction of the anterior and middle third of the vertebral body.

I prefer long, non-threaded, sharp K-wires. Sharp K-wires have stronger purchase and advance more evenly in the vertebrae than blunt K-wires; non-threaded K-wires are preferred to prevent inadvertently advancing the K-wire when using the drill-tap. If the drill-tap is not completely coaxial to the K-wire, the tip of the drill tap can catch the most proximal threads and cause the K-wire to advance. This is less likely to happen with non-threaded K-wires.

There are several minimally invasive cannulated pedicle screw systems available. The choice of brand and system used should be based on the surgeon's comfort level and training. However, each system has most of the same basic components. Once the K-wire is in position, a set of dilators and then a working channel is placed to prevent soft tissue from advancing with the subsequent instruments. A cannulated combination drill-tap or tap is then placed over the K-wire, through the working channel, down the pedicle. The drill-tap should not be advanced further than 1 cm from the tip of the K-wire. This prevents the K-wire from becoming loose, and potentially being inadvertently removed with the drill-tap. The drill tap must be placed directly coaxial to the path of the K-wire to prevent the K-wire from being advanced or sheared off. If there is a discrepancy between the trajectory of the K-wire and the drill-tap, then the K-wire can be removed and replaced, as long as the tip of the drill-tap is past the pedicle and in the vertebral body. The drill-tap is then used to determine the length of the screw to be used. The drill tap should be undersized compared with the size of the screw to provide good bony purchase of the screw. Once the tip of the screw is in the vertebral body, the K-wire is removed, and the screw is advanced until the base of the polyaxial head abuts the facet joint. The screw should not be overtightened to prevent the polyaxial head from moving, which prevents the rod from being passed. The screw is attached to a screw extender that enables the surgeon to manipulate the polyaxial head for passing the rod. If there is any concern about the placement of the screws, AP fluoroscopy can be used to confirm that there is not a medial breach.

Depending on which system is used, the rod is sized, and then passed either through a separate stab incision, or by passing the rod down one of the screw extenders, and then turning the rod to pass through the extender of the other screw (**Fig. 104.7**). Once the rod is confirmed to be between the screw extenders, fluoroscopy confirms that there is a small amount of rod beyond the polyaxial screw head on both sides. The set screws are placed and counter-torqued to the appropriate tightness. The rod-passing device and screw extenders are then removed, and a final set of AP and lateral fluoroscopy images are obtained.

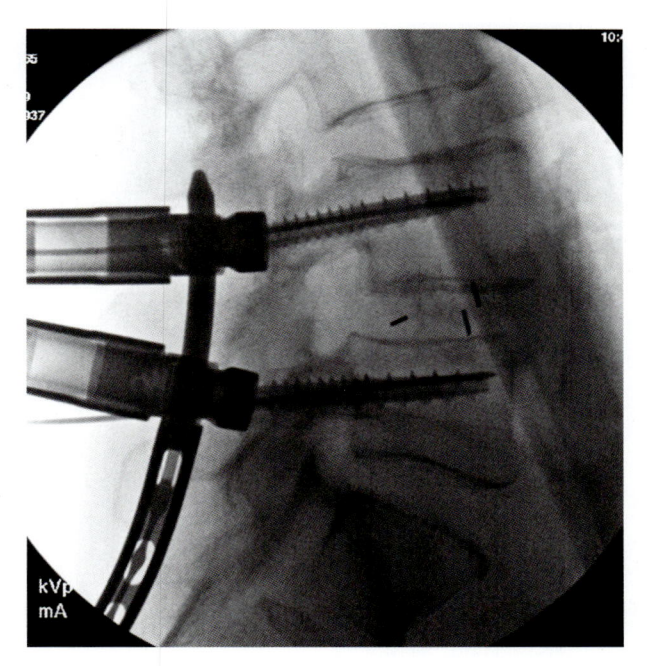

Fig. 104.7 Lateral fluoroscopic image after placement of unilateral pedicle screw instrumentation and rod. K-wires are in place on contralateral side prior to placement of instrumentation.

Standard closure with fascial, subfascial, and subdermal Vicryl sutures is then performed.

Postoperative Care

Postoperative standing radiographs should be obtained within the first day of surgery (**Fig. 104.8**). If there is any concern, CT scan can be performed, which will show the placement of the instrumentation and interbody graft in great detail (**Fig. 104.9**). In the initial learning phase, the surgeon should consider obtaining a CT scan as a learning tool to assess the instrumentation.

Postoperative pain control is performed with intravenous morphine or less often Dilaudid patient-controlled anesthesia for the first 18 to 24 hours. The patient is then switched to oral analgesia, such as hydrocodone or oxycodone. The patient is mobilized with physical therapy, and typically is discharged 2 to 3 days after the procedure. The hospital stay may be longer or shorter depending on the patient's age and medical comorbidities. For patients who require anticoagulation, this can be restarted 24 to 48 hours after surgery. Patients are seen in clinic at regular intervals with standard radiographs for 2 to 3 years postoperatively to assess the fusion. If there is suspicion of pseudarthrosis, a CT scan can be used to assess the interbody fusion or to determine if the instrumentation has been loosened.

Potential Complications and Precautions

Potential complications can be related to the decompression, the placement of the interbody graft, or the placement of the pedicle screw instrumentation. The most common complication related to the decompression is dural violation. Although exposure is limited using a tubular retractor, primary repair is possible using a 4-0 or smaller suture with a micropituitary rongeur. The knot

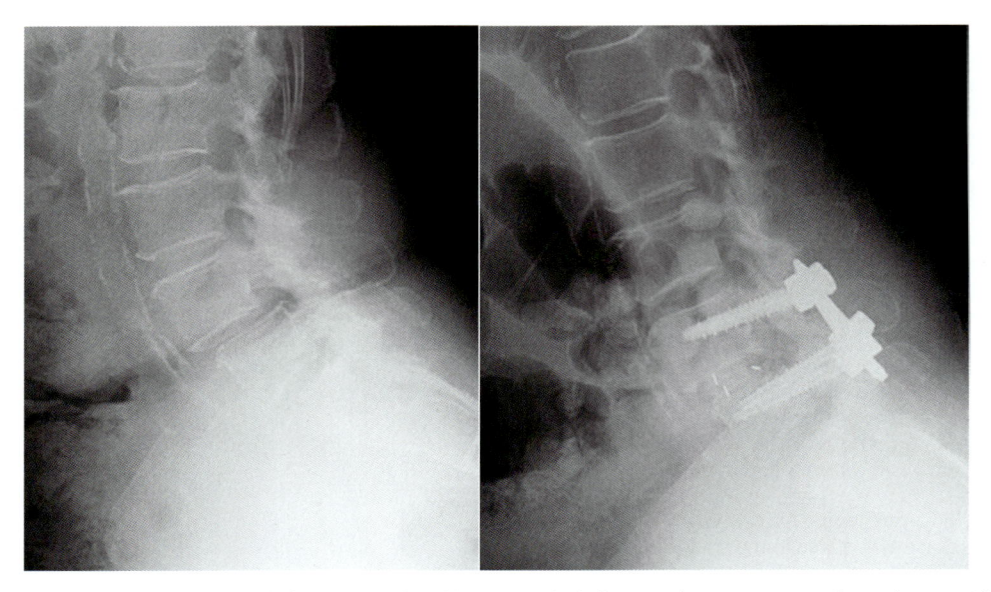

Fig. 104.8 Standing lateral fluoroscopic images before (a) and after (b) L4–5 interbody fusion with instrumentation for grade I spondylolisthesis.

can be pushed with a right-angled ball-tip probe. Smaller violations can be repaired with dural sealant alone.

When placing the interbody graft, potential complications include violation of the bony end plate, which can cause graft subsidence. This can be avoided with careful end-plate preparation, especially in older patients with suboptimal bone quality. In placing the graft itself, careful visualization and maintenance of the trajectory minimizes retraction on the nerve root, and reduces the possibility of retraction-related neurapraxia. The risk of graft displacement or retropulsion is reduced by placing the largest graft possible without violating the end plate, as well as by maintaining compression across the pedicle screws while tightening the set screws.

When using the above technique for placement of percutaneous instrumentation, screw position is entirely dependent on good placement of the K-wires. Ensuring that the K-wires are in the center of the pedicle prevents the risk of a pedicle breach. Maintaining the coaxial trajectory of the cannulated instruments over the K-wire reduces the risk of inadvertently advancing or removing the wire.

Conclusion

Minimally invasive transforaminal lumbar interbody fusion with instrumentation using a paramedian muscle-splitting approach is a safe and effective surgical approach for patients with appropriate pathology. This approach can be used successfully to treat patients with spondylolisthesis, gross instability, spondylolysis, or disk collapse. This approach has been shown to reduce blood loss, postoperative narcotic requirement, and hospital stay, and once the surgeon becomes familiar with this approach, operative time can be reduced significantly compared with that for an open technique. **Box 104.1** lists the key operative steps and the precautions to take to avert problems that can arise.

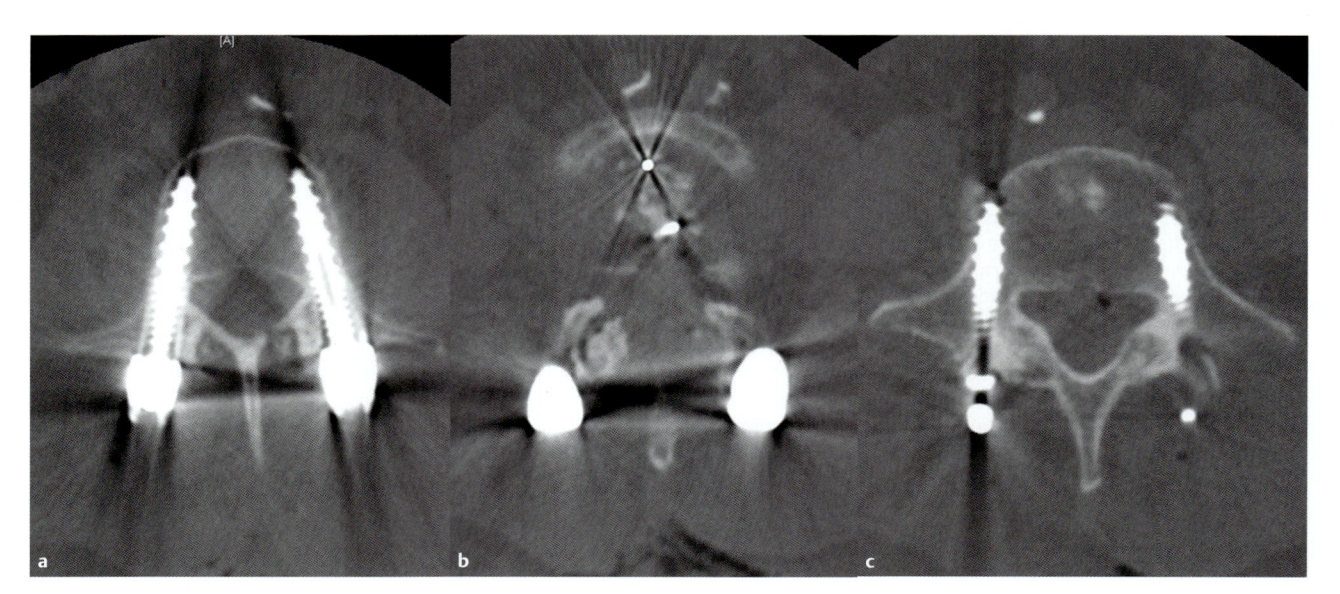

Fig. 104.9 Axial computed tomography (CT) images after percutaneous pedicle screw fixation at L4 (a) and L5 (c), as well as a PEEK interbody graft (b).

Box 104.1 Key Operative Steps and Precautions to Avert Potential Problems

Step	Precautions
Tube placement	3–3.5 cm off midline, based at lamino-facet junction
Decompression	Carefully remove ligament, starting superiorly and toward the midline, where the ligamentum flavum is thinnest
Interbody grafting	Place nerve root retractor medially to protect the dura
	Visualize exiting nerve root to avoid injuring it with interbody preparation instruments
	Avoid violating end plates with graft preparation
	Use largest size graft possible without violating end plates
Percutaneous instrumentation	Use sharp, non-threaded K-wires
	Do not advance the drill or tap past the last 1 cm of K-wire
	Keep drill-tap and screw coaxial to K-wire
	Spend extra time on K-wire placement, as screws placement is dependent on K-wire placement
	Do not overtighten screws, which will lose polyaxial movement of head

References

1. Cloward RB. The treatment of ruptured lumbar intervertebral discs by vertebral body fusion. I. Indications, operative technique, after care. J Neurosurg 1953;10:154–168
2. Park P, Foley KT. Minimally invasive transforaminal lumbar interbody fusion with reduction of spondylolisthesis: technique and outcomes after a minimum of 2 years' follow-up. Neurosurg Focus 2008;25:E16
3. Parker SL, Adogwa O, Witham TF, Aaronson OS, Cheng J, McGirt MJ. Postoperative infection after minimally invasive versus open transforaminal lumbar interbody fusion (TLIF): literature review and cost analysis. Minim Invasive Neurosurg 2011;54:33–37
4. O'Toole JE, Eichholz KM, Fessler RG. Surgical site infection rates after minimally invasive spinal surgery. J Neurosurg Spine 2009;11:471–476

105 MIS Placement of Pedicle Screws: Lumbar, Sacral, and Iliac Wing Screws

Michael Y. Wang

Numerous techniques are available for fluoroscopic-guided pedicle and iliac screw insertion. The use of percutaneous fixation obviated the need for extensive soft tissue exposure to obtain access to the entry sites and trajectories for spinal instrumentation. As such, these techniques represent a significant advance in the practice of spinal surgery.

Patient Selection, Indications, and Contraindications

Percutaneous methods are applicable to patients with a variety of pathologies. These methods may be even more beneficial in the problematic patient, such as those with severe obesity, because the soft tissue exposure is minimized.[1] The only major contraindications would be those related to anatomic localization. For example, fluoroscopy of image guidance are essential for safe screw placement. Because such situations are extremely rare there are few contraindications for percutaneous fixation. The indications would be the same as for any fixation to manage instability due to decompression, deformity, infection, trauma, degeneration, congenital abnormalities, or neoplasia.

Choice of Operative Approach

Several techniques are available for both pedicle screw and iliac screw placement. For pedicle screws, the commonly used methods are discussed in the following subsections.

Anteroposterior View Technique

This technique is described below in greater detail. It has these attributes: (1) it requires only minimal specialized equipment; (2) it can be performed robustly in settings of abnormal anatomy, including axial rotation and deformity[2]; and (3) it entails reduced radiation exposure as compared with other fluoroscopic methods.

Owl's-Eye En-Face Approach

One of the earliest techniques used for pedicle cannulation was described as the "owl's eye," "dead reckoning," or Magerl[3] technique. This method employs the use of fluoroscopic imaging directed along the long axis of the pedicle in all planes. This method became accepted not only for the placement of percutaneous screws (in Europe), but also for cement augmentation (vertebroplasty) techniques. Due to its intuitive nature and the need for only a single fluoroscope, this technique was rapidly adopted during the early years of percutaneous surgery. The disadvantages include the need for fluoroscope repositioning for each pedicle (right and left), and the potentially higher rates of facet joint violation.

Biplanar Fluoroscopy Technique

Use of two fluoroscopic C-arms may be the most approachable technique for the uninitiated. The ability to have a simultaneous anteroposterior (AP) and lateral view is reassuring to many surgeons and requires less mental processing and three-dimensional conceptualization by the surgeon. The disadvantages include increased radiation exposure, obscuration of the operative field by the C-arms, and the need for two fluoroscope machines.

Image-Guided Technique

Image guidance likely has the greatest future potential. The advantages are obvious, as the ability to use previously acquired three-dimensional images gives the surgeon the greatest amount of intraoperative information. Multiple systems are commercially available, and they have great appeal to surgeons unwilling to accept radiation exposure. The disadvantages are also obvious: (1) capital equipment expenses; (2) technological obsolescence; (3) software and image compatibility issues; (4) the need for stereotactic registration; (5) spatial error; and (6) the lack of real-time imaging.

For iliac screws, the commonly used methods are discussed in the following subsections:

Obturator Outlet Approach

This technique was first developed by Ziran et al,[4] and is described in detail below. Similar to the AP pedicle screw technique, the surgeon must acquire high-quality images in the proper alignment in all planes. However, the accuracy of screw placement has also been confirmed in clinical studies.[5]

Mini-Open Approach with Bony Palpation

This is similar to an open approach in that internal palpation of the lateral cortical walls of the ilium is accomplished with a curved pedicle probe to guide the surgeon within the confines of cancellous bone. Placement of a screw with percutaneous extensions then enables a rod–screw hook-up without as much soft tissue exposure. Thus, the placement is similar to the open method but the percutaneous subfascial rod can be connected without a large opening.

Image-Guided Technique

As with pedicle screws, image guidance can be used to assist with iliac screw placement.

Preoperative Imaging

Prior to surgery appropriate imaging studies should be obtained. For relatively normal anatomy, magnetic resonance imaging (MRI) may suffice. However, computed tomography (CT) with three-dimensional (3D) reconstructions gives superior anatomic detail that may affect surgical planning and execution. Details such as the morphology of the facet joints may not be obvious when the spine is not fully exposed (as in percutaneous surgery). This can impact the entry point for pedicle screws. Pedicle and vertebral body size and shape are also important in implant selection and placement. Finally, detail on bone quality and density may affect the surgeon's ability to place screws. Sclerosis of the pedicle or vertebral body may make instrumentation challenging.

Surgical Procedure

Anteroposterior Technique for Thoracolumbar Pedicle Screw Placement

As with other percutaneous techniques, the surgeon should ensure that the operating room table and patient positioning will accommodate high-quality fluoroscopic imaging. Not only do the appropriate levels have to be imaged, but angulation of the C-arm must be accounted for. This occurs in both axial rotation and sagittal angulation, and the image intensifier may thus be obstructed by the table's platform, base, side rails, or radiopaque bolster cushions. This is particularly problematic for C-arm devices with a small diameter. I thus prefer to use a machine with at least a 32.5-inch span between the image intensifier and radiation source. As an alternative, frame-based or frameless navigation devices can be used to guide hardware placement.

For bilateral pedicle screw placement, it is possible to work from only one side of the patient. This is typically the side opposite the fluoroscope. Cannulation of the opposite (C-arm) side is performed first. The fluoroscope is brought into view in line with the disk space and the spinous process centered (**Fig. 105.1**). This "true" AP view enables safe pedicle cannulation on both sides. In the thoracic spine, multiple levels can be captured in one view, allowing for cannulation of multiple levels without C-arm adjustment. This is because there is little change in the vertebral body orientation between levels. However, in the lumbar spine the significant lordosis results in a need to readjust the sagittal plane of the C-arm between levels.

Once the proper images have been obtained, the incision should be made somewhat lateral to the pedicle projection. Jamshidi needle placement onto the bony surface at the transverse process-facet junction is achieved as the starting point. The needle is then inserted 2 cm without passing the medial wall of the pedicle (**Fig. 105.2**). This is followed by Kirschner wire (K-wire) exchange and pedicle preparation/screw placement (**Fig. 105.3**).

At the S1 level the pedicle is not cylindrical. Thus, its projection will appear with only the medial wall visible. Alignment for S1 thus requires the surgeon to first align in the sagittal plane so that the upper sacral end plate is superimposed. Axial rotation is then directed to achieve the highest resolution of the medial pedicle wall. As with the lumbar spine, this angulation can be assisted with measurements on preoperative axial MRI or CT scan images.

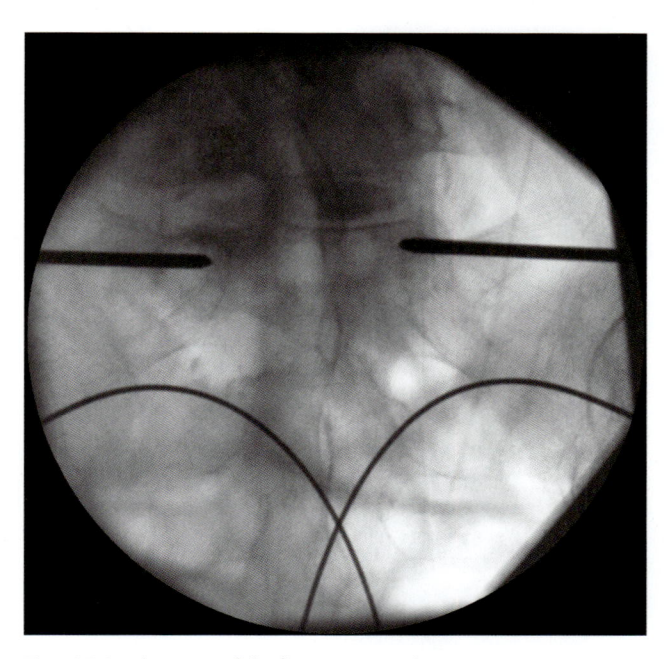

Fig. 105.1 Alignment of the fluoroscope to obtain a true anteroposterior (AP) view with the spinous process in the middle of the X-ray and the upper end plate viewed as a single line (in the plane of the disk space). The Jamshidi needle has been inserted 2 cm without passing the medial walls of the pedicles.

For cases with difficulty in establishing a starting point, a drill can be used to create a bony depression. This is only safe on AP views (**Fig. 105.4**) and should not be done with lateral imaging alone. Adjustment of the trajectory when the bone is too dense can be accomplished using a cannulated pedicle probe (**Figs. 105.5 and 105.6**), which does not deform or bend. Because the screw position can be defined entirely by its starting point

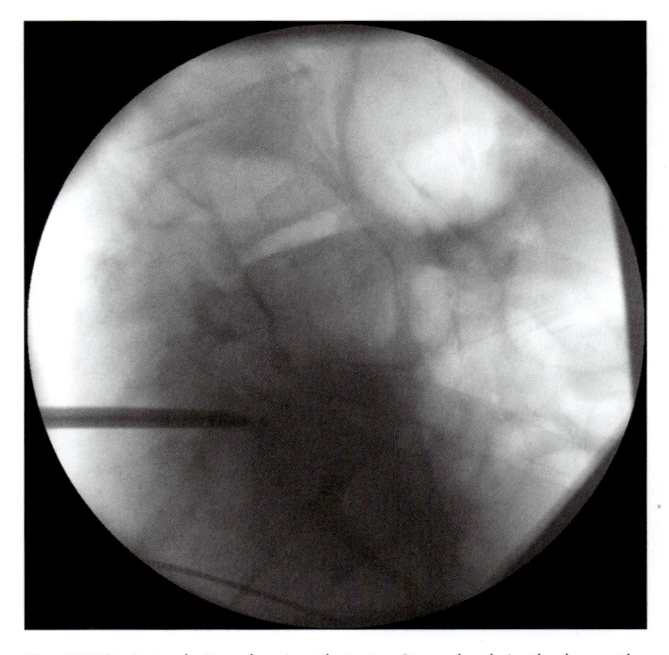

Fig. 105.2 Lateral view showing that at a 2-cm depth in the bone, the Jamshidi needle is passing the pedicle into the vertebral body, confirming safe placement.

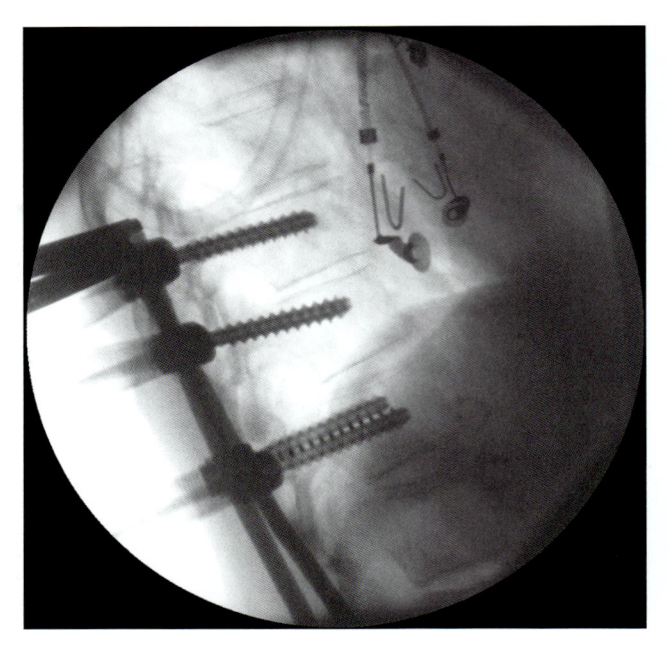

Fig. 105.3 Lateral image showing multiple thoracic pedicle screws with a connecting rod.

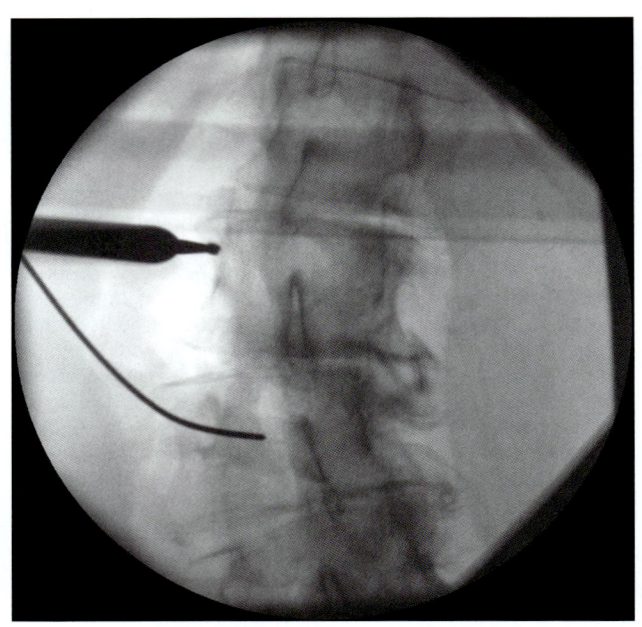

Fig. 105.4 Difficulty with the entry site due to sclerotic bone or challenging anatomy can be overcome by starting the entry point with a drill. This is only safe with AP views and should never be done with lateral imaging alone.

and trajectory, these two tricks can enable successful cannulation in the most challenging cases.

Obturator Outlet View for Iliac Screw Placement

The obturator outlet view is obtained by moving the fluoroscope in both the axial and sagittal planes so as to maximize the size of the "teardrop" view of the ilium. This view is a convergence of the inner and outer tables of the ilium at the proximal and distal sites. It is thus defined by four cortical walls making up the teardrop (**Fig. 105.7**).

A small diagonally placed incision is then made overlying the posterior superior iliac spine (PSIS) of the pelvis. A Jamshidi needle is then docked onto the most superficial aspect of the PSIS and "walked" ventromedially, with care taken not to enter into the sacroiliac joint. The exact starting point along the supero-

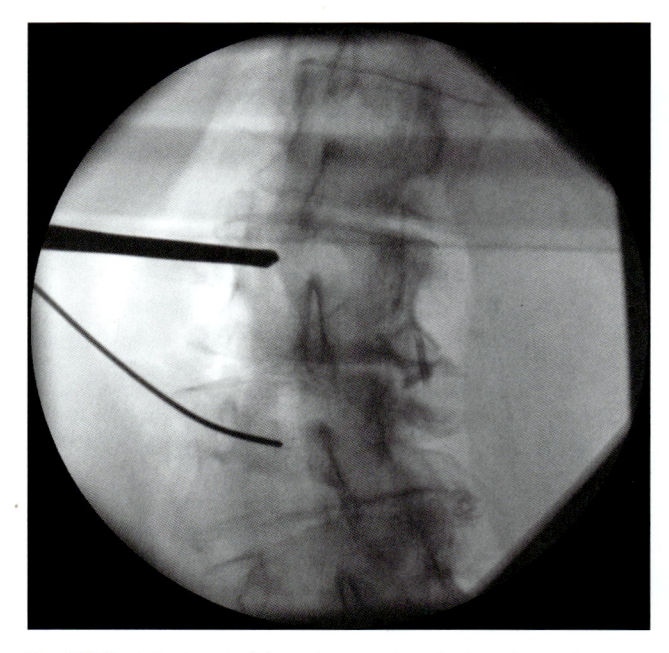

Fig. 105.5 Adjustment of the trajectory when the bone is too dense can be accomplished using a cannulated pedicle probe, which does not deform or bend.

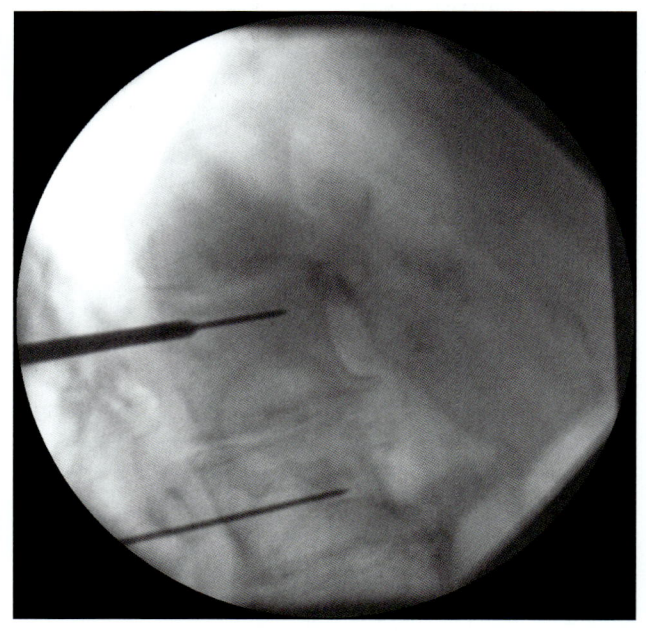

Fig. 105.6 Lateral view of the cannulated pedicle probe.

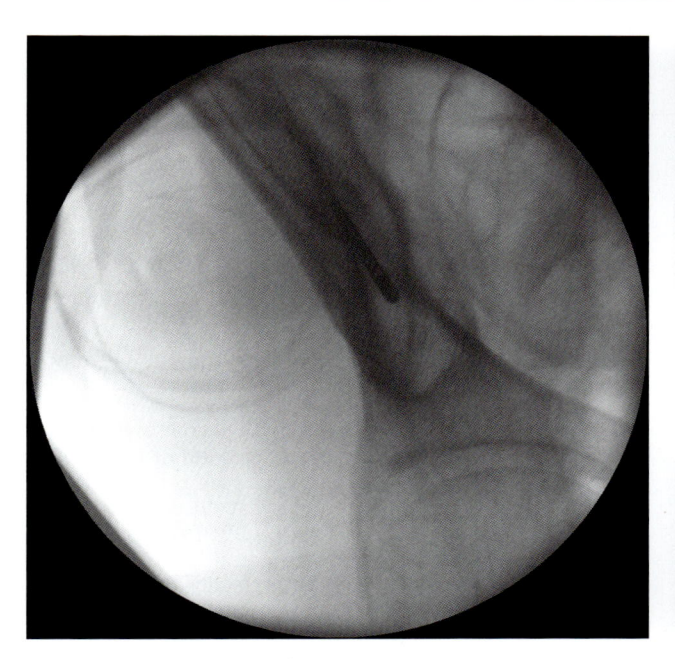

Fig. 105.7 Obturator outlet or "teardrop" view for iliac cannulation.

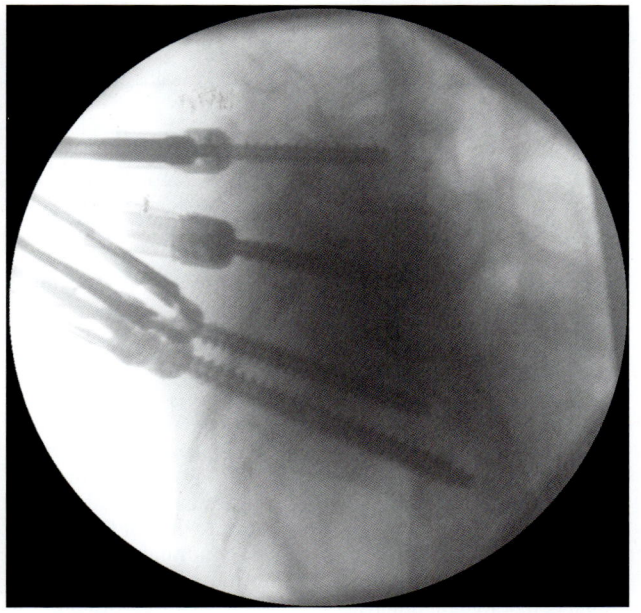

Fig. 105.8 Rod connection to the iliac screws is assisted with the use of extensions on the screws. Note the significant projection effect of two identical iliac screws (right versus left) given their distance on the coronal plane.

inferior plane of the PSIS can vary according to the specific screw trajectory desired, as multiple acceptable paths are acceptable. In this case, the entry point was just beneath the shelf of the ilium underlying the PSIS. A drill or osteotome can be used to create a bony depression to better seat the screw or bolt head to minimize hardware prominence.

The Jamshidi needle is then carefully directed under fluoroscopic guidance with tactile feedback to prevent penetration through the cortical walls. Bony violations are more likely in osteoporotic patients, and a beveled needle tip may be preferable to a diamond tip for this purpose. The Jamshidi needle is then replaced internally with a K-wire and then removed. Cannulated and serially enlarging cancellous screw taps are then placed over the K-wire to the appropriate length (**Fig. 105.8**). Because of the large diameter of iliac screws (7 to 9 mm), after withdrawal of the tap a ball-tipped probe can be used to palpate the internal aspect of the hole thus created with the K-wire still in place.

Screws can then be unilaterally placed using cannulated large-diameter iliac screws or bolts over the K-wire or by using standard iliac screws passed down the now dilated screw path. The contralateral screw is then placed. Screw extension posts can be used to assist with rod passage and screw connection in a manner similar to that used for percutaneous or minimally invasive pedicle screw placement. The extension posts enable pushing the rod onto the polyaxial screw head, acting as a guide. This would have been more difficult to accomplish if the next rod connection point was in closer proximity to the iliac screw (i.e., an S1 pedicle screw).

Postoperative Care

Postoperative care is the same as for standard spinal fusion surgeries.

Potential Complications and Precautions

As with any percutaneous procedure, inadvertent violation of critical neural, vascular, and hollow viscus structures can occur. This risk may be increased due to the lack of direct visualization at the target site. Thus, careful targeting with proper guidance techniques is essential.

Conclusion

Percutaneous techniques are constantly evolving and improving. The goals of a minimally invasive approach are laudable, with reduced pain, disability, blood loss, and infection.

References

1. Fessler RG. Minimally invasive percutaneous posterior lumbar interbody fusion. Neurosurgery 2003;52:1512
2. Ahmad FU, Wang MY. Use of anteroposterior view fluoroscopy for targeting percutaneous pedicle screws in cases of spinal deformity with axial rotation. J Neurosurg Spine 2014;21:826–832
3. Magerl F. Verletzungen der Brust- und Lendenwirbelsaule. Langenbecks Arch Chir 1980;352:428–433
4. Ziran BH, Wasan AD, Marks DM, Olson SA, Chapman MW. Fluoroscopic imaging guides of the posterior pelvis pertaining to iliosacral screw placement. J Trauma 2007;62:347–356, discussion 356
5. Wang MY, Williams S, Mummaneni PV, Sherman JD. Minimally invasive percutaneous iliac screws: Initial 24 case experience with CT confirmation. J Spinal Disord Tech 2012 Sep 25. [Epub ahead of print]

106 Lumbar Osteotomies

Manish K. Kasliwal, Lee A. Tan, and Richard G. Fessler

The ability to maintain an upright posture is fundamental to normal human function. However, the normal sagittal balance can be impaired in patients with spinal deformities.[1] The typical "pitched forward" posture secondary to sagittal imbalance can lead to several debilitating problems including difficulties with forward gaze, compensatory flexion contractures of the hip and the knee, as well as loss of physiological endurance as a result of increased energy expenditure. Studies have demonstrated that global spinal malalignment is a strong predictor of disability in patients with adult spinal deformity.[2]

Fixed sagittal imbalance is a condition that occurs as a result of the loss of the normal lumbar lordosis or the increase in thoracic kyphosis, resulting in the forward displacement of the head relative to the sacrum and pelvis. Research on spinopelvic balance revealed that a normal, harmonious relationship exists between the pelvis and the spine. Various realignment objectives following adult spinal deformity surgery have been developed and include sagittal vertical axis (SVA) < 5 cm, pelvic tilt (PT) < 25 degrees, and lumbar lordosis (LL) proportional to the pelvic incidence (PI) (PI − LL < 9 degrees)[1,3–6] (**Fig. 106.1**).

Spinopelvic balance should be differentiated from sagittal balance; the former describes the global overall sagittal plane relationship between the spine and the pelvis, whereas the latter describes how the individual components of the sagittal plane and the regional curves affect and relate to one another. Restoring this relationship during adult spinal deformity correction may play an important role in determining the surgical outcomes of these patients independent of sagittal balance, and it has been shown to correlate with health-related quality of life (HRQOL).[7]

Although flexible deformity can often be corrected with positioning and instrumentation, treatment of symptomatic rigid sagittal imbalance is potentially complex and often requires one or more osteotomies along with spinal instrumentation and arthrodesis. Conventional correction methods including posterior instrumentation and fusion or combinations of anterior release, posterior instrumentation, and fusion are usually unsatisfactory in rigid deformities, especially if they are severe. The goals of performing an osteotomy in these conditions are to restore sagittal and spinopelvic balance, such that the patient can stand erect without the need to flex the hips or knees, and to reduce the pain and functional disability associated with spinal deformity.[8] Therefore, a solid understanding and mastery of various osteotomy techniques are essential for spine surgeons treating adult spinal deformity.

Historically, the Smith-Petersen osteotomy was first described in 1945 to treat postrheumatoid flexion deformity. This is a posterior column wedge osteotomy that hinges on the posterior longitudinal ligament and causes an opening of the anterior column, and is a true extension osteotomy with shortening of the posterior column and lengthening of the anterior column. Smith-Petersen et al recommended a single-stage posterior wedge resection of the midlumbar spine in a chevron arrangement with controlled fracturing of the ossified anterior longitudinal ligament. Modifications of this technique such as the Ponte procedure and polysegmental osteotomy have been described.[9,10] The posterior closing wedge osteotomy or Ponte osteotomy was first described in 1984 by Alberto Ponte et al[11] for the treatment of flexible Scheuermann's kyphosis in skeletally mature patients. Although the techniques have some differences, often the terms Smith-Petersen osteotomy (SPO), Ponte, and polysegmental osteotomy are used interchangeably, and all these osteotomies will be termed SPO for the remainder of the text. The SPO is generally reserved for smaller sagittal deformities that are long, smooth, and rounded (**Fig. 106.2**). Thomasen[12] first described in 1985 the three-column posterior osteotomy for the management of fixed sagittal plane deformities in patients with ankylosing spondylitis. In contrast to an SPO, the three-column posterior osteotomy maintains the height of the anterior column and hinges on the anterior longitudinal ligament. The posterior pedicle subtraction osteotomy (PSO) is the "workhorse" procedure for correcting fixed sagittal imbalance, enabling a three-column correction of the spine through an entirely posterior approach[13] (**Fig. 106.3**). Vertebrectomy was first described by MacLennan for the treatment of severe scoliotic deformities through a posterior-only approach followed by postoperative casting.[14] A vertebral column resection (VCR) remains the most powerful tool for the correction of spinal deformity and is generally reserved for cases of severe rigid scoliosis where a translation of spinal column is necessary to restore trunk balance and correct deformity (**Fig. 106.4**). Although a VCR can be performed either through a combined anterior and posterior approach or through a posterior approach only, a posterior VCR, as popularized by Suk et al,[15] has various advantages and is the most commonly used technique for VCR.

Patient Selection

Not all patients with sagittal imbalance require surgery. Patients with mild symptoms can often be managed nonoperatively with physical therapy, anti-inflammatory medications, and lifestyle modifications. For those patients with debilitating symptoms due to significant sagittal imbalance, surgical management generally involves spinal instrumentation and fusion in combination with an osteotomy or multiple osteotomies to achieve desired correction in the spinal alignment. The decision of which osteotomy to use depends on the magnitude and character of the deformity, as well as the training and experience of the surgeon.

The key factor for determining the necessity of an osteotomy is the presence of a partially or completely fixed deformity based on the physical examination and radiographic evaluation. In patients with substantial deformities, the initial workup always includes the flexion/extension/lateral bending radiographs of the spine to determine if the deformity is flexible or rigid. They

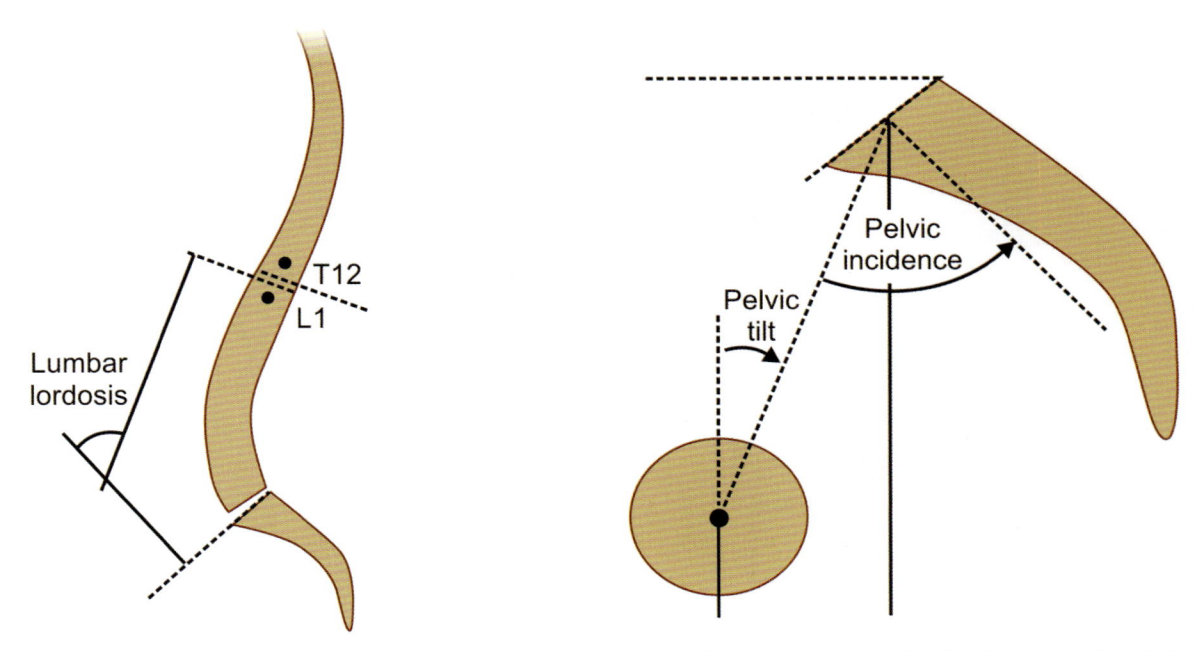

Fig. 106.1 Illustration demonstrating the measurement of lumbar lordosis and spinopelvic parameters. (Reproduced with permission from Kasliwal MK, et al. Posterior only correction of adult thoracolumbar scoliosis. In: In Eck JC, Vaccaro AR, eds. Surgical Atlas of Spinal Operations. New Delhi: Jaypee Brothers Medical Publishers; 2013.)

generally fall into three categories: (1) totally flexible, in which the spinal malalignment corrects entirely with a supine or prone unweighted position; (2) a deformity that only partially corrects through mobile segments; and (3) a totally rigid deformity with no correction in the recumbent position, in which the spine is fused throughout the thoracic and lumbar spine. For patients with partially or completely rigid deformity, osteotomies may be necessary for spinal realignment.

Indications

- Fixed sagittal imbalance
- Smooth and angular kyphosis
- Combined coronal and sagittal imbalance
- Spine pelvic imbalance (LL–PI mismatch or abnormally elevated PT)

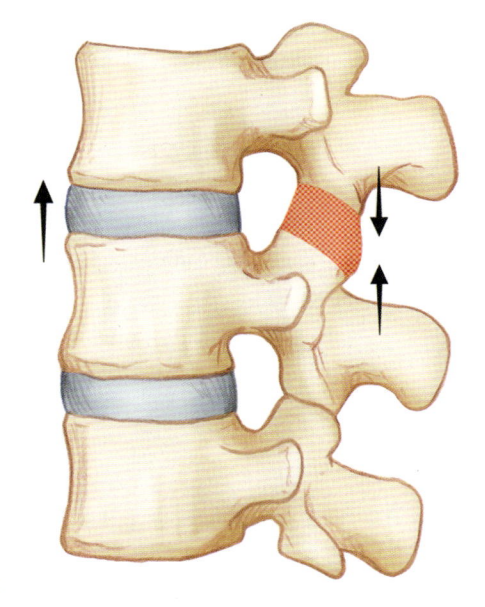

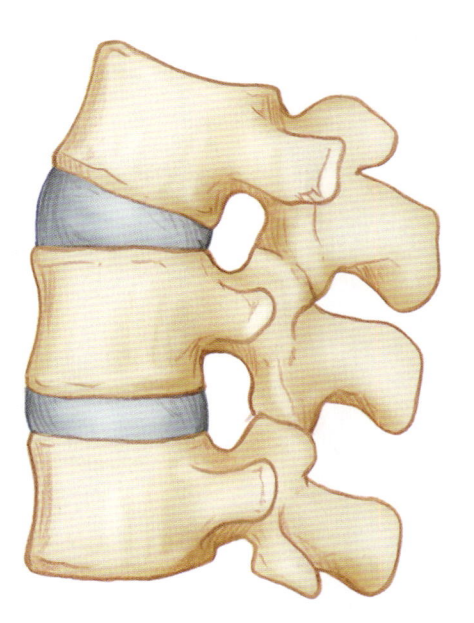

Fig. 106.2 Lateral schematic illustration demonstrating (a) the extent of bone removal for a Smith-Petersen osteotomy (SPO) and (b) closure of the osteotomy.

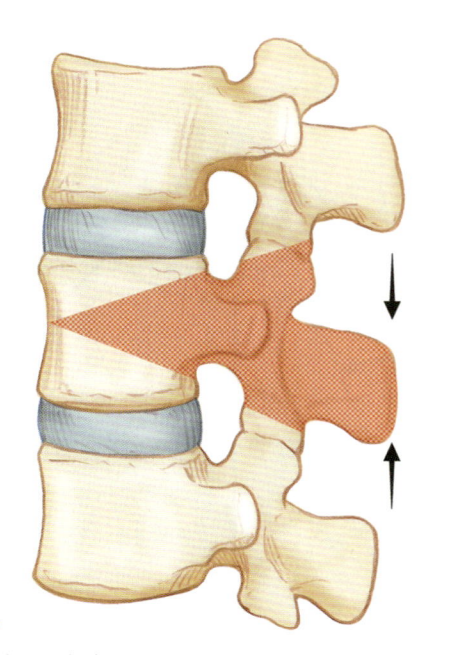

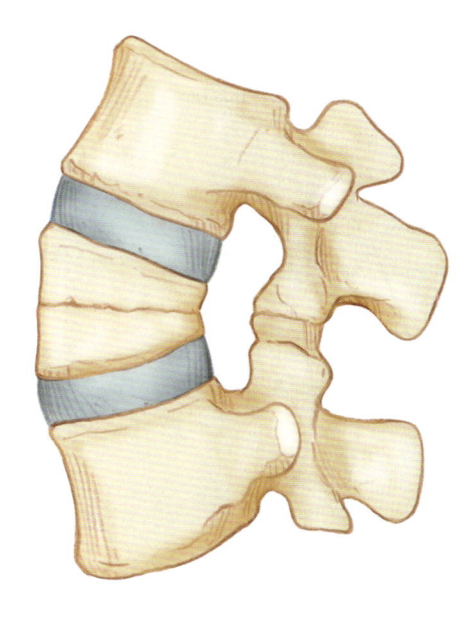

Fig. 106.3 (a) Lateral schematic diagram demonstrating the area of bone resection for a pedicle subtraction osteotomy (PSO). (b) The lordotic segment after the osteotomy is closed. Note how the front of the vertebra is twice the height of the back, causing lordosis.

Contraindications

- Flexible deformity
- Medically unstable patients

Advantages

- An SPO can be performed relatively rapidly, with relatively little blood loss compared with a PSO. Because it does not require neural element manipulation, it can be performed safely at the cord, conus, or caudad levels.
- The PSO is advantageous in that it can produce much more sagittal correction at a single level and has a higher rate of successful bone union due to the three columns of bone contact. It enables a three-column correction of the spine through an entirely posterior approach; more importantly, it does so without lengthening the spinal column and avoids stretching the neural elements.
- A VCR enables correction of more severe coronal and sagittal deformity as compared with SPO and PSO. VCR, by providing translation of spinal column, is the only procedure to restore trunk balance and correct deformity in patients with severe rigid and angular kyphosis.

Disadvantages

- Increased blood loss with different osteotomy techniques (SPO < PSO < VCR)
- Prolonged operating time (VCR > PSO > SPO)

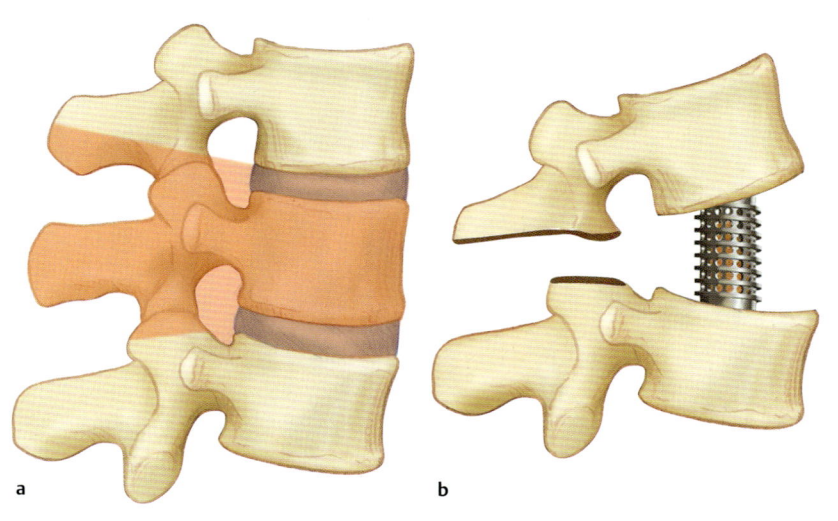

Fig. 106.4 Schematic illustration showing (a) the extent of bone removal and (b) closure following a vertebral column resection.

- Risk of lengthening the spinal cord with SPO
- An open disk space is a prerequisite for closure of the SPO site. Henceforth, an SPO cannot be done at a level at which a spinal arthrodesis has been previously performed, because the disk is no longer mobile. An SPO may exacerbate the concavity of a coronal curve if one is present.

Choice of Operative Approaches

Sagittal imbalance can be classified into type I and type II.[16] In type I imbalance, the patient has a segmental problem with a normal global balance. A portion of the spine is substantially hyperkyphotic, but the patient is able to maintain balance by hyperextending segments above and below. Both a young adult with a prior fusion with Harrington rod instrumentation from T4 to L4 but healthy disks at L4-L5 and L5-S1 and a patient with a posttraumatic kyphosis in which there is a regional kyphosis belong to this category, as these patients are able to maintain global sagittal balance by hyperextending the mobile segments above or below so that the overall sagittal balance is maintained, and on a standing sagittal radiograph the C7 plumb does fall over the sacrum. On the other hand, in patients with a type II imbalance, there is an inability to compensate for the regional hyperkyphosis by hyperextending segments above and below as can be seen in patients with ankylosing spondylitis and the middle-aged or older patient with a Harrington fusion from T4 to L4, with severe disk degeneration at L4-L5 and L5-S1. Other than the presence or type of sagittal imbalance, several factors need to be evaluated for patients with fixed deformity to select the optimal osteotomy technique. These include the number of osteotomies needed, the proposed fusion levels, the number of fixation points needed/available above and below the osteotomy site, and the location of the osteotomy (e.g., thoracic versus lumbar spine, with the risk of surgery around the spinal cord versus the cauda equina). In addition, the presence of prior surgeries may have a huge impact on what osteotomy can be performed. For PSO in particular, it is most useful to perform the osteotomy through a prior fusion mass. The amount of correction needed can be estimated from the preoperative radiographic measurements indicating the degree of curvature in the sagittal plane.

Either multiple SPOs or a single PSO can be used for correction of fixed sagittal imbalance. Although multiple SPOs are preferable in patients with smooth kyphosis and mild sagittal imbalance (5 to 10 cm of positive sagittal balance), a single lumbar PSO may be adequate in patients with angular kyphosis or substantial sagittal imbalance (> 10 cm). In general, the degree of kyphotic correction with a single SPO is 5 to 10 degrees/level or 1 degree/mm of bone resected. On average, 15 to 30 degrees of sagittal plane correction can be achieved with a PSO.[8]

Surgical options for patients with fixed sagittal deformity associated with a coronal deformity includes multiple asymmetric SPOs, one asymmetric pedicle subtraction procedure, or a VCR. The SPO is used in cases where a relatively small amount of correction is required, as well as for patients with mobile anterior columns who need 10 to 20 degrees of correction for each level. A sagittal deformity that is combined with coronal imbalance is better treated with an asymmetric PSO or even a vertebral column resection so that the coronal deformity is corrected rather than exacerbated. A PSO is indicated in sharp, angular deformities and for a more marked sagittal imbalance (> 10 cm positive). They are best performed at L2 or L3, where an adequate number of fixation points can be located above and below the osteotomy. A PSO can be performed in the thoracic spine, but a costotransversectomy approach is then needed, because the thecal sac should not be retracted in cord territory. The ideal candidates for PSO are those patients with a substantial sagittal imbalance of > 10 to 12 cm, those patients with a sharp, angular kyphosis, and those patients who have circumferential fusion between multiple segments.

A VCR is the most aggressive option to correct severe deformities involving both the sagittal and coronal planes, with large amounts of deformity correction achievable with this technique. The indications for VCR are fixed trunk translation, severe scoliosis (congenital scoliosis or neuromuscular scoliosis), spinal tumor, spondyloptosis, rigid spinal deformities > 80 degrees in the coronal plane, and asymmetry between the length of the convex column and concave column of the deformity, which preclude the achievement of balance by a simple osteotomy alone. This procedure is commonly used for cases in which the correction should be performed at an angle of ~ 30 degrees, which is performed mainly at the lumbar level.

Bridwell[17] proposed an algorithm that can serve as a general framework for the selection of the appropriate osteotomy in patients with type I or II sagittal imbalance (**Fig. 106.5**). Essentially, patients with a type I sagittal imbalance with smooth kyphosis can be treated with SPOs, whereas those with sharp angular kyphosis would need a VCR or a PSO depending on the location of the kyphosis in the thoracic or lumbar spine. Similarly, in patients with type II sagittal imbalance, smooth kyphosis with minor imbalance can be treated with SPOs, whereas those with major imbalance need either a PSO or a VCR.

Preoperative Imaging

Assessment of the patient's overall coronal and sagittal balance, both clinically and radiographically, is important. The involvement of the hip joints in a considerable flexion deformity accentuates the sagittal imbalance of the spine. Mobilization of the hips and correction of the fixed deformity by hip arthroplasty should be performed before considering spinal osteotomy in patients with hip contractures.

The following imaging should be considered in patients with adult spinal deformity:

- Standing anteroposterior (AP) and lateral 36-inch radiographs with the hips and knees fully extended
- Supine neutral and supine benders when deemed necessary to assess deformity flexibility in patients with sagittal deformity. Side bending films should be done in patients with significant coronal deformity.
- For patients with prior spinal fusions, oblique AP and lateral radiographs and preferably computed tomography (CT) myelogram should be obtained to evaluate the results and status of prior spinal surgical interventions including the extent of prior decompression, the location and status of prior instrumentation, an assessment of fusion status, and, in revision cases, evidence of prior complications such as pseudomeningocele.
- Magnetic resonance imaging (MRI) and CT myelogram are obtained to investigate areas of spinal stenosis.

Surgical Procedure

Smith-Petersen Osteotomy

The patient is positioned prone on an open Jackson table with the abdomen hanging free to decrease intra-abdominal pressure and epidural bleeding. Use of the Gardner-Wells traction is preferable to keep the face and eyes free of pressure during these lengthy procedures. The arms are maintained on well-padded arm boards in a 90-degree to 90-degree position, with attention

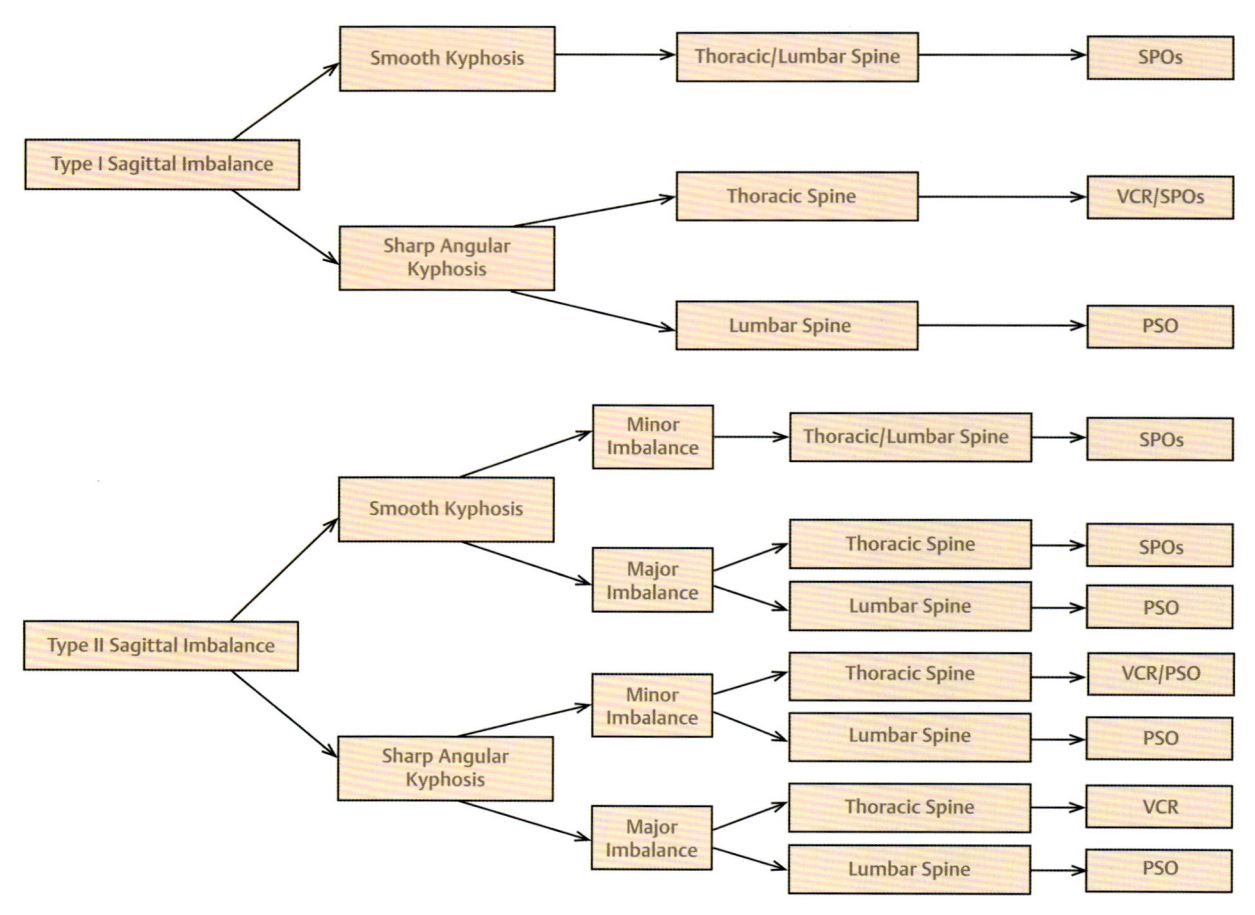

Fig. 106.5 Algorithm for osteotomy type based on the character of the sagittal deformity. PSO, pedicle subtraction osteotomy; SPO, Smith-Petersen osteotomy; VCR, vertebral column resection. (Adapted from Bridwell KH. Decision making regarding Smith-Petersen vs. pedicle subtraction osteotomy vs. vertebral column resection for spinal deformity. Spine 2006;31(19, Suppl):S171–S178)

paid to avoiding shoulder hyperextension. We prefer and recommend intraoperative neuromonitoring, including somatosensory evoked potentials (SSEPs) and motor evoked potentials (MEPs) monitoring for any adult deformity surgery. For major spinal reconstructive procedures the intraoperative administration of antifibrinolytics (aprotinin, tranexamic acid, e-aminocaproic acid) has been gaining increasing popularity. Tranexamic acid (TXA) is a synthetic antifibrinolytic amino acid derivative that inhibits fibrinolysis at the surgical site. We consider the use of TXA with intravenous loading dose of 10 mg/kg followed by a maintenance dose of 1 mg/kg/h administered until skin closure for major deformity cases, especially those involving performance of osteotomies.

Once the patient is positioned, prepped, and draped, standard midline exposure is performed, exposing all the levels to be incorporated in the fusion construct. Dissection is carried down to the level of the thoracodorsal fascia, and self-retaining retractors are placed. The spine is exposed to the tips of the transverse process bilaterally, staying subperiosteally to reduce bleeding and devascularization of the paraspinal muscles. The importance of subperiosteal dissection to keep the blood loss to a minimum cannot be overemphasized. Care should be taken to avoid disruption of the supra-adjacent facet and the interspinous and supraspinous ligaments. Once completely exposed, pedicle screws are inserted from the upper instrumented vertebra to the lower instrumented vertebra except at the level of planned osteotomies.

The osteotomy requires removal of the interspinous ligaments, the ligamentum flavum, and the superior and inferior articular processes bilaterally (**Fig. 106.6**). The interspinous ligaments are removed down to the level of the ligamentum flavum, and the median raphe is identified. The spinous process at the level of osteotomy is resected using a Horsley bone cutter or rongeur. Portions of the spinous processes above and below should also be removed. The lamina and facet joints are then removed. Although this can be performed in several ways, we prefer creating a trough across the lamina and pars on each side and then removing the bilateral inferior facets and part of the lamina as a single piece using a Capener gouge. An osteotome can also be used for this step, depending on the surgeon's preference. The ligament is then removed along with the bilateral superior articular facets until they are flush with the pedicle. In particular, on the lateral end, the structure between the upper and lower pedicles should be removed completely to prevent nerve root impingement during osteotomy closure. Also, both the superior and inferior lamina should be undercut to provide adequate room for neural elements when the osteotomy is closed. The osteotomy is closed by a combination of compression and cantilevering. Compression of the remaining posterior elements can be achieved through gravity from the appropriate intraoperative positioning, the hinging of the operating table, or gentle compression against pedicle screw fixation, although the latter is not advisable in osteoporotic patients. Appropriately contoured rods are then placed, and the final construct is tightened while applying compression during final tightening of the set screws.

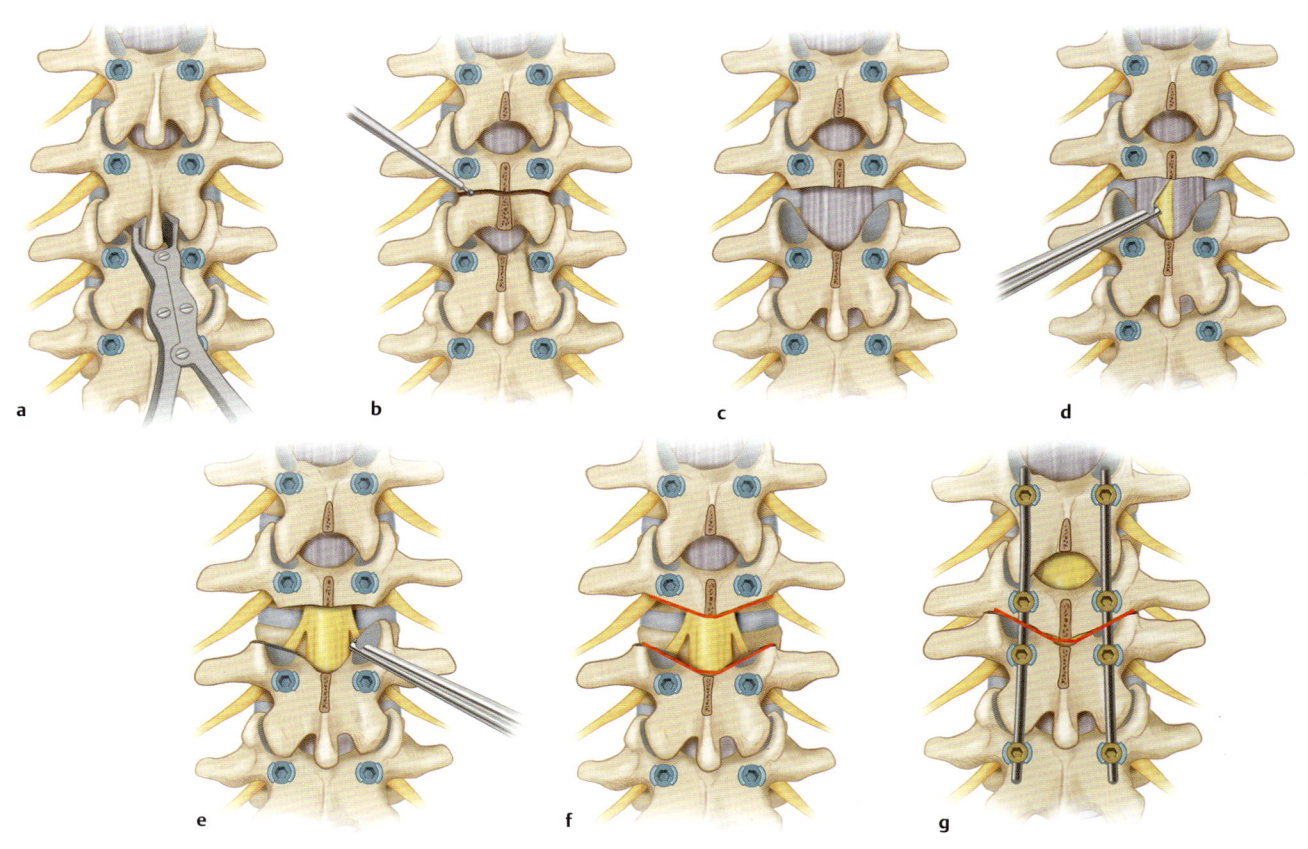

Fig. 106.6 Illustration demonstrating the technique of SPO. **(a)** The spinous process at the level of osteotomy is resected using a Horsley bone cutter or rongeur. Portions of the spinous processes above and below should also be removed. **(b,c)** Removal of the lamina and facet joints by creating a trough across the lamina and pars on each side. **(d–f)** The ligament is then removed along with bilateral superior articular facets until they are flush with the pedicle. Also, both the superior and inferior lamina should be undercut to provide adequate room for the neural elements when the osteotomy is closed. **(g)** The osteotomy is closed by a combination of compression and cantilevering. See text for details.

Pedicle Subtraction Osteotomy

The patient positioning and other details are the same as described for the SPO, above. Once posterior exposure of the spine is done through careful meticulous subperiosteal dissection, attention is directed toward placement of instrumentation and subsequent performance of osteotomy. Before the osteotomy is begun, pedicle screws should be placed cephalad and caudad to the intended osteotomy site, as they will be used to help secure and stabilize the spine after the osteotomy.

The osteotomy requires that all of the posterior elements (spinous process and lamina) at the level of the osteotomy be removed (**Fig. 106.7**). Generally all the posterior elements from 1 cm below the pedicle screws of the vertebra above the osteotomy site to 1 cm above the pedicle screws of the vertebra below the osteotomy site have to be resected. A wide central decompression is completed, followed by exposure of the exiting roots bilaterally. Bone is removed surrounding the pedicles bilaterally. The transverse processes are excised at their bases which can be performed with an osteotome or a Kerrison rongeur. Then, careful dissection of the lateral wall of the vertebral body is performed in a posterior to anterior direction with a small Cobb retractor, taking great care to avoid damage to the segmental vessels. A malleable retractor is placed lateral to the vertebral body in the subperiosteal plane to maintain the exposure. The pedicles are identified bilaterally and are resected with Leksell rongeurs, carefully avoiding the exiting nerve roots.

At this point, the vertebral body osteotomy can be performed. Through the working window of the pedicle, the posterior vertebral body is decancellated. Alternatively, L-shaped or regular osteotomes can also be used to perform the osteotomy, and that is our preferred technique. After this, curettes are used to osteotomize the vertebral body medially, laterally, cranially, and caudally. Care is taken to create a posterior-based triangular wedge. The cortical shell of the vertebral body is left intact to protect neural elements and epidural vessels. The posterior body is then thinned with curved curettes. Temporary fixation should be achieved with a temporary rod before a substantial portion of the body is removed, to prevent neurologic injury due to sudden translation of the spine.

After decancellation has been completed in the posterior aspect of the vertebra extending from lateral wall to lateral wall, the posterior vertebral body wall is then "green-sticked" with a reverse-angle curette, pushing the bone anteriorly into the body. The lateral wall is resected in a wedge shape using a Leksell rongeur working toward the anterior aspect of the spine. Careful attention is paid to ensuring that the removal of bone is uniform throughout the vertebral body unless an asymmetric PSO is intended. This will produce a symmetric closure of the osteotomy site, correcting the sagittal deformity. The anterior cortex must be maintained to prevent subluxation of the spine during closure. The osteotomy can then be closed in a variety of ways, either by hyperextending the patient's hips and knees or using temporary rods and compressors to slowly close the site. Appropriately

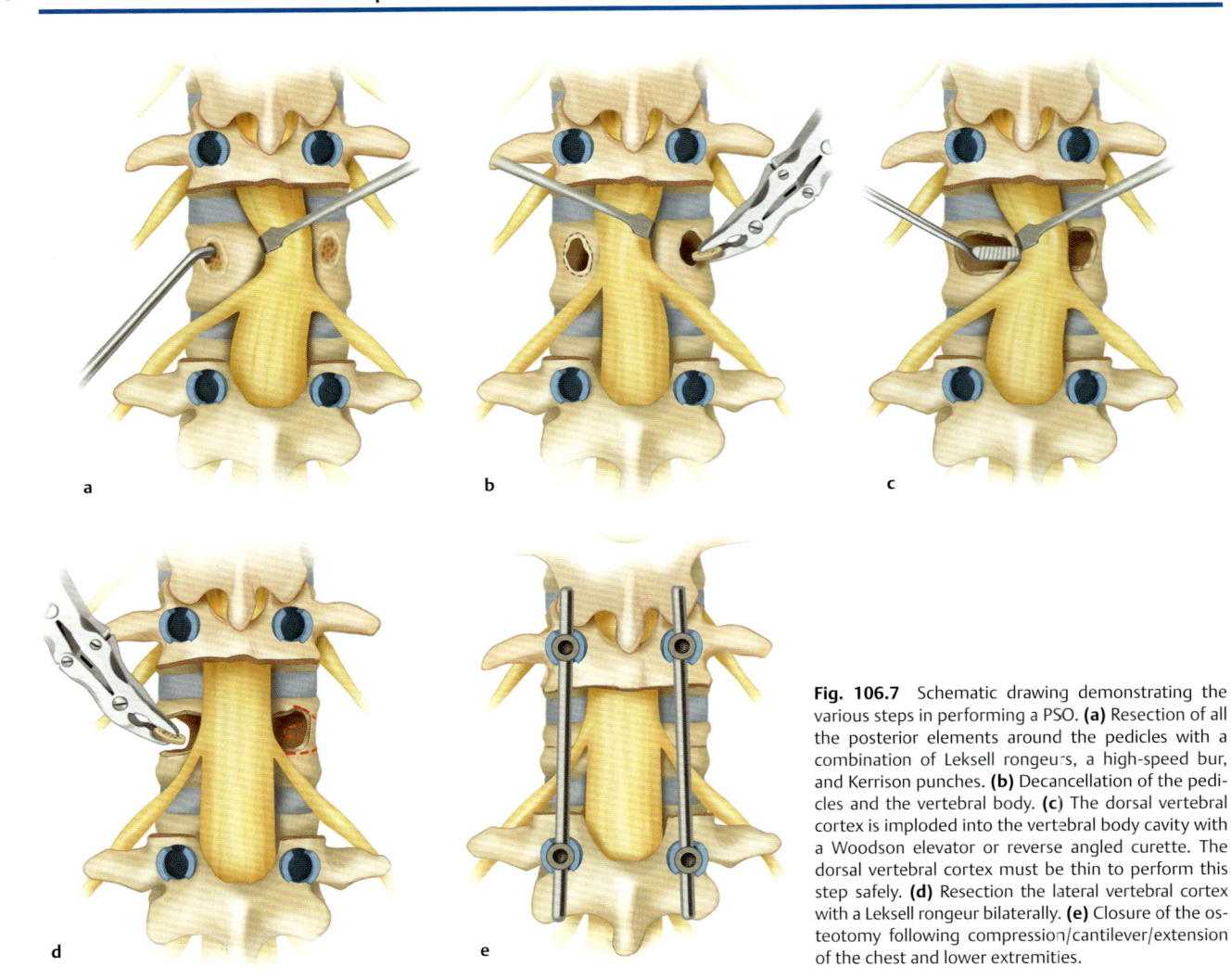

Fig. 106.7 Schematic drawing demonstrating the various steps in performing a PSO. **(a)** Resection of all the posterior elements around the pedicles with a combination of Leksell rongeurs, a high-speed bur, and Kerrison punches. **(b)** Decancellation of the pedicles and the vertebral body. **(c)** The dorsal vertebral cortex is imploded into the vertebral body cavity with a Woodson elevator or reverse angled curette. The dorsal vertebral cortex must be thin to perform this step safely. **(d)** Resection the lateral vertebral cortex with a Leksell rongeur bilaterally. **(e)** Closure of the osteotomy following compression/cantilever/extension of the chest and lower extremities.

contoured rods are then placed, and the final construct is tightened while applying compression during final tightening of the set screws. Separate rods secured to the fixation points proximal and distal to the osteotomy may be connected through dominoes. In this manner, "construct-to-construct" compression may be performed and this may reduce the likelihood of fixation failure.

It is recommended to widely open the canal centrally at the osteotomy site to be able to inspect the dura for buckling and to probe the neural foramina with a Woodson elevator to ensure the absence of any neural compression. We prefer to use iliac screws to protect against S1 pedicle screw pullout or failure in long constructs extending above L2. A variation of the PSO that approaches the next osteotomy to be discussed is the asymmetric PSO. This can be performed to address sagittal imbalance with a coexistent coronal deformity. More bone along the lateral wall of the vertebral body is resected on the side of the convexity compared with the amount of bone resected along the concavity. This not only enables the restoration of sagittal alignment but also helps to restore coronal alignment.

Vertebral Column Resection

The VCR is a powerful technique in deformity correction. Curves with a sharp angle might be best corrected by a resection of a single vertebral body, whereas curves that are broad and sweeping may require a resection of multiple vertebral bodies at the apex to minimize stretching of the neural elements. Once completed, the spinal column can be shortened and the combined sagittal and coronal deformity corrected via a combination of translation and compression. It is recommended that no more than 3.5 cm of spinal shortening should generally be performed to reduce the risk of compromise of the spinal cord. As bone-on-bone contact is not achieved following VCR as the body is completely removed, reconstruction of the spinal column is needed after the deformity is corrected. A metal cage, structural autograft, or allograft may be used to reconstruct the vertebral column after correction of the deformity to bridge the defect left by resection of the vertebral body. Because this procedure circumferentially disconnects the spinal column, obtaining a fusion at this level is paramount.

Following positioning of the patient as described above appropriate posterior exposure of the spine is obtained (**Fig. 106.8**). Complete exposure should be done to both transverse processes to facilitate the removal of the vertebral bodies. Complete removal of the posterior components (spinous processes, lamina, and facet joints) should be performed to the level of the segments that need to be removed, which is often the apex of the deformity. The laminae and facets proximal and distal to the level of the VCR also need to be resected. In the thoracic spine, the rib head is resected from the transverse process. Sacrifice of

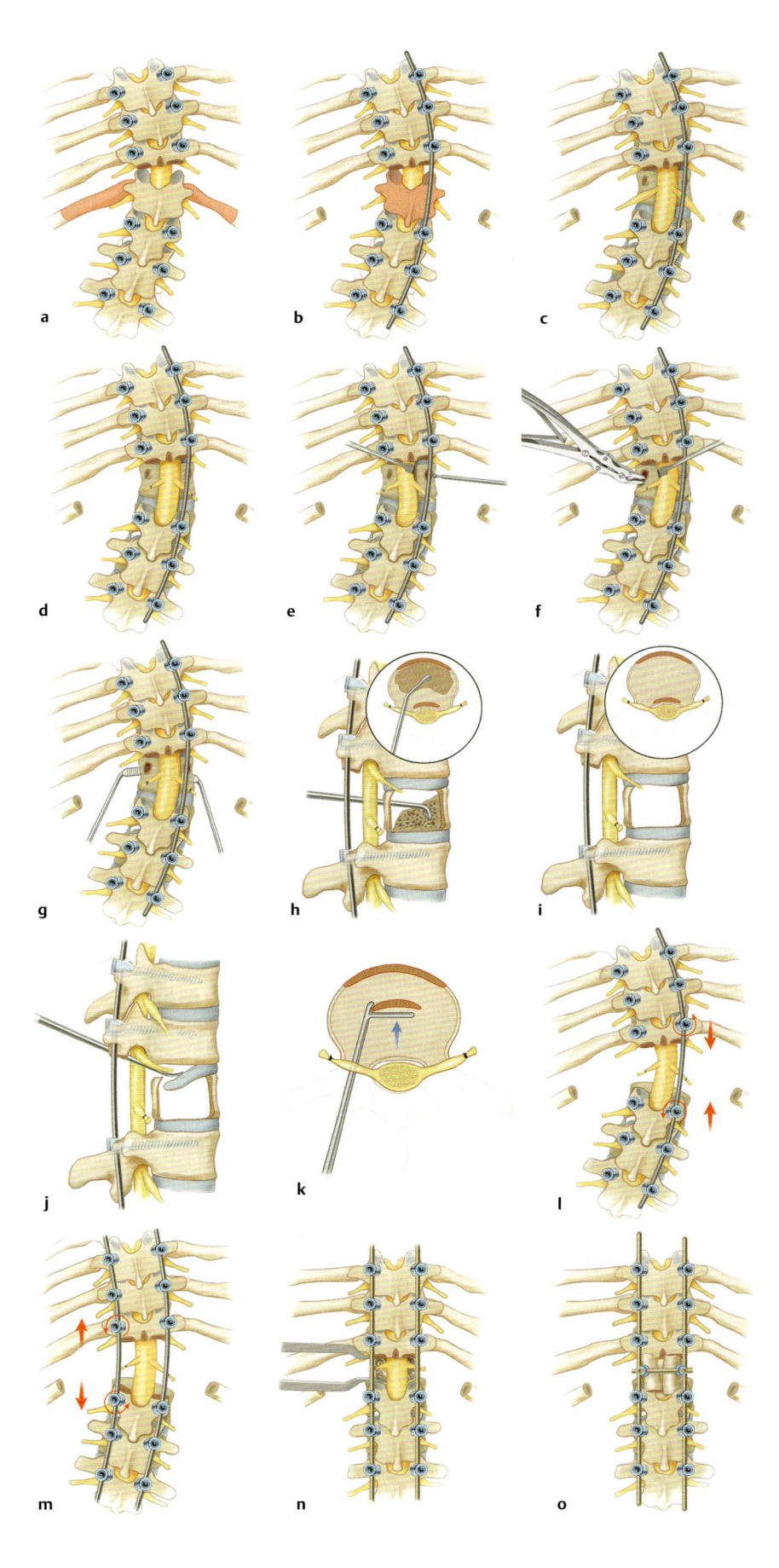

Fig. 106.8 Illustration demonstrating the VCR technique. **(a)** Following exposure of the spine and placement of screws, the inferior facet of the level above the VCR and the superior facets of the caudal vertebrae are removed. **(b)** Bilateral costotransversectomies are performed removing 4 to 5 cm of the adjacent ribs at the apex with placement of a temporary rod on one side of the spine, capturing three levels above and below the planned resection site. **(c,d)** A laminectomy is performed of the entire lamina of the vertebra to be resected extending cephalad to the pars level of the supra-adjacent vertebra. In the thoracic spine, one may elect to sacrifice one or both exiting nerve roots to provide increased exposure for the removal of the vertebral body. **(e,f)** Both pedicles are surrounded and removed down to the base of the vertebral body, carefully protecting the exiting nerve roots that lie against the medial and inferior aspect of the pedicle. The vertebral body is then decancellated. **(g)** The lateral vertebral body walls are then subperiosteally exposed. **(h,i)** The lateral vertebral body walls are then removed, providing an entrance into the remainder of the vertebral body. The remainder of the cancellous portion of the vertebra is completely removed to the end plates of the adjacent disks above and below. **(j)** The disks cephalad and caudad to the resected vertebra are then removed. **(k)** The posterior vertebral body wall is then carefully impaled into the vertebral body using an impactor. **(l,m)** The deformity is then ready for correction by the temporary instrumentation, always beginning with spinal shortening by convex rod compression to avoid excessive stretch on spinal cord. **(n)** An appropriate-sized metallic cage is placed into the anterior defect, filled with bone graft, supplying structural support to the anterior column of the spine. **(o)** Final posterior rod correction is performed with the permanent rods locking in this anterior cage.

exiting nerve roots in the thoracic spine should then be performed; it is well tolerated and makes exposure much easier for working entirely via the posterior approach. In the lumbar region, the nerve roots cannot be sacrificed and thus a VCR may require separate anterior and posterior approaches. Once the rib is removed, a temporary rod is placed opposite the working side to stabilize the spine and protect the neural elements. This can be done later but should be performed before removing a substantial part of the vertebral body. We prefer placing a temporary rod after completing the osteotomy on the first side and before working from the contralateral side. A careful subperiosteal dissection of the soft tissue is performed along the lateral wall of the vertebral body using a small Cobb elevator, as mentioned earlier. The importance of remaining in the subperiosteal plane cannot be overemphasized, because if the segmentals vessels are injured, the bleeding can be massive. It can be controlled by electric cauterization or hemostatic agents such as Surgicel, Gelfoam, and cottonoid.

A malleable retractor is placed lateral to the vertebral body in the subperiosteal plane to maintain the exposure. The pedicles are identified bilaterally and are resected with a Leksell rongeur following by piecemeal resection of the vertebral body and the disks above and below without interfering with the posterior vertebral wall, which is kept intact until the end to protect the thecal sac. This can be performed using the decancellation technique or osteotomies, as mentioned earlier. Osteotomy of the vertebral body is performed on either side of the thecal sac. Bone resection should be wedged in the sagittal plane and may be asymmetric or symmetric in the coronal plane to correct kyphosis and also the scoliosis component. The bone should be removed completely to ensure that anterior cortical breakage occurs. Osteotomy closure is accomplished slowly and steadily using two temporary rods. It is usually necessary to place an anterior structural cage within the defect before complete closure to avoid shortening the spine excessively. The temporary rods are replaced with definitive rods, and the correction is gradually achieved with a combination of cantilevering and compression to correct the deformity.

Closure

Following all the above-mentioned osteotomies, thorough decortication of all exposed bony surfaces and facet joints is performed to maximize the potential for achieving a successful fusion. We prefer placing a morcellized autologous bone graft obtained from the bone harvested during the osteotomy and may extend that with corticocancellous allograft or recombinant human bone morphogenetic protein-2 (rhBMP-2), as establishing fusion is paramount. The use of BMP for posterior lumbar fusion surgery is currently an "off-label" indication, but it is needed to maximize the potential of achieving a successful fusion. We prefer using vancomycin powder during open posterior spinal instrumentation to reduce the risk of wound infection, as has been shown recently in several studies. Muscle and fascia are closed tightly in separate layers, followed by the subcutaneous layer and stapling of the skin.

Postoperative Care

Patients can be extubated right after the surgery or the next day, depending on the intraoperative course, the hemodynamic status, and anesthesia concerns. Thorough immediate neurologic evaluation should be performed as soon as possible, and evidence of any new neurologic deficit should be appropriately investigated. New neurologic deficits can vary from nerve root palsy to dense spinal cord level paralysis. If an anatomic cause of neural impingement is detected, such as screw misplacement, bony encroachment, or compressive hematoma, then an urgent return to the operating room to correct the problem should be considered. Sometimes in a patient with an unexplained deficit with a large deformity correction, the correction may have to be reversed in the absence of any obvious cause. The use of thromboembolic stockings and sequential compression devices should be continued throughout the recovery period. We routinely start pharmacological deep venous thrombosis (DVT) prophylaxis with subcutaneous heparin on postoperative day 1. Physical therapy, including ambulation training and mobilization, should be started as soon as possible.

Suction drains should be removed as the output reduces to less than 30 mL but may have to be kept a bit longer if rhBMP-2 is used. The use of nonsteroidal anti-inflammatory drugs is avoided early in the postoperative period. The patient is seen for follow-up at 2, 6, and 12 weeks, and at 1 year, with periodic radiographs and CT when appropriate. We do not typically recommend the use of a cane or braces following surgery.

Potential Complications and Precautions

Lumbar osteotomies are technically challenging procedures that require extensive training and experience and can be associated with significant complications.[5,18] Potential complications may include neurologic deficit, unintended durotomy, pseudarthrosis, deformity progression, proximal junctional kyphosis, deep wound infection, myocardial infarction, pulmonary embolism, and pneumonia. A thorough and multidisciplinary preoperative evaluation, careful surgical planning, sound judgment, meticulous operative techniques, and early postoperative mobilization can reduce the potential complications associated with lumbar osteotomies.

Considering the high blood loss associated with various osteotomies such as PSO and VCR, use of antifibrinolytics agents such as Tranexamic acid (TXA) and consideration of staging the procedure in cases with excessive blood loss or surgery lasting > 10–12 hours should be considered. Application and development of minimally invasive osteotomy techniques may reduce the risk of the complications associated with open deformity surgery.[19,20] Apart from various general and medical complications following major corrective surgery, certain surgical complications such as proximal junctional kyphosis, rod fracture, and pseudarthrosis warrant special attention. Rod fracture is not uncommon following three-column osteotomies and can be seen in up to 22.0% of patients undergoing a PSO for adult deformity surgery at a minimum of 1-year follow-up.[21] The use of a multi-rod construct should be strongly considered following three-column osteotomy and has been shown to significantly prevent implant failure and symptomatic pseudarthrosis.[22]

Proximal junctional kyphosis (PJK) or failure refers to the development of kyphosis at the segments immediately cephalad to a spinal fusion construct, with an incidence ranging from 9 to 46% in various studies.[23,24] Although development of PJK following various osteotomies remains a challenging and poorly understood complication, several surgical steps have been suggested to reduce its occurrence. These include preserving the superjacent facets and supraspinous ligament; selecting the uppermost instrumented vertebrae (UIV) to be at a level without posterior column deficiency (e.g., laminectomy), listhesis, rotation, or junctional kyphosis; and avoiding a UIV location at the apex of the deformity in either the coronal or sagittal planes. Because of the high risk of pseudarthrosis after a PSO procedure, several strategies, in addition to meticulous surgical technique, may be potentially helpful, such as using bone fusion–enhancing products in addition to excellent bony apposition at the osteotomy site, stabilizing the PSO site with three or four rods, and considering interbody fusion for all large disks adjacent to the PSO site when it is not performed through a prior fusion mass.[25]

Conclusion

Osteotomies are powerful tools that enable spine surgeons to correct rigid spinal deformities. A solid understanding of the principles of spinopelvic alignment and sagittal balance, as well mastery of osteotomy techniques, will enable spine surgeons to restore normal spinal alignment and to improve the quality of life for many patients. Complications associated with this techniques are significant and must be discussed with the patient preoperatively. **Box 106.1** lists the key operative steps.

Box 106.1 Key Operative Steps

- Careful preoperative evaluation and planning are vital to a successful surgery for deformity correction.
- All pressure points must be well padded during positioning.
- Gardner-Wells tongs can be used for traction to avoid pressure on the eyes for a patient in the prone position for prolonged deformity surgeries.
- Intraoperative neuromonitoring changes must be investigated immediately and addressed promptly.
- It is essential to minimize the blood loss during exposure by meticulous subperiosteal dissection.
- Disruption of superjacent facets and supraspinous ligament should be avoided.
- Neural elements must be well decompressed prior to deformity correction to minimize neurologic deficit.
- Disruption of the ventral cortex of the vertebral body during PSO will destabilize the spinal column and should be avoided.
- The importance of creating a central enlargement in the lamina cephalad and caudad to the osteotomy cannot be overemphasized to avoid impingement of the thecal sac and spinal cord during osteotomy closure.
- The lateral wall of the vertebral body during PSO/VCR should be dissected carefully to avoid injuring the segmental vessels and associated blood loss.
- The use of a multi-rod construct should be strongly considered following three-column osteotomy to decrease the risk of implant failure and symptomatic pseudarthrosis.
- Tight fascial and skin closure along with intra-wound vancomycin powder can reduce the risk of wound infection.

References

1. Schwab F, Lafage V, Patel A, Farcy J-P. Sagittal plane considerations and the pelvis in the adult patient. Spine 2009;34:1828–1833
2. Glassman SD, Bridwell K, Dimar JR, Horton W, Berven S, Schwab F. The impact of positive sagittal balance in adult spinal deformity. Spine 2005;30:2024–2029
3. Bess S, Schwab F, Lafage V, Shaffrey CI, Ames CP. Classifications for adult spinal deformity and use of the Scoliosis Research Society-Schwab Adult Spinal Deformity Classification. Neurosurg Clin N Am 2013;24:185–193
4. Klineberg E, Schwab F, Smith JS, Gupta MC, Lafage V, Bess S. Sagittal spinal pelvic alignment. Neurosurg Clin N Am 2013;24:157–162
5. Lowe T, Berven SH, Schwab FJ, Bridwell KH. The SRS classification for adult spinal deformity: building on the King/Moe and Lenke classification systems. Spine 2006;31(19, Suppl):S119–S125
6. Terran J, Schwab F, Shaffrey CI, et al; International Spine Study Group. The SRS-Schwab adult spinal deformity classification: assessment and clinical correlations based on a prospective operative and nonoperative cohort. Neurosurgery 2013;73:559–568
7. Smith JS, Singh M, Klineberg E, et al; International Spine Study Group. Surgical treatment of pathological loss of lumbar lordosis (flatback) in patients with normal sagittal vertical axis achieves similar clinical improvement as surgical treatment of elevated sagittal vertical axis: clinical article. J Neurosurg Spine 2014;21:160–170
8. Yang BP, Ondra SL, Chen LA, Jung HS, Koski TR, Salehi SA. Clinical and radiographic outcomes of thoracic and lumbar pedicle subtraction osteotomy for fixed sagittal imbalance. J Neurosurg Spine 2006;5:9–17
9. Hehne HJ, Zielke K, Böhm H. Polysegmental lumbar osteotomies and transpedicled fixation for correction of long-curved kyphotic deformities in ankylosing spondylitis. Report on 177 cases. Clin Orthop Relat Res 1990;258:49–55
10. Smith-Petersen MN, Larson CB, Aufranc OE. Osteotomy of the spine for correction of flexion deformity in rheumatoid arthritis. Clin Orthop Relat Res 1969;66:6–9
11. Ponte A, Vero B, Siccardi G. Surgical treatment of Scheuermann's hyperkyphosis. In: Winter R, ed. Progress in Spinal Pathology: Kyphosis. Bologna, Italy: Aulo Gaggi; 1984:75–81
12. Thomasen E. Vertebral osteotomy for correction of kyphosis in ankylosing spondylitis. Clin Orthop Relat Res 1985;194:142–152
13. Hyun S-J, Kim YJ, Rhim S-C. Spinal pedicle subtraction osteotomy for fixed sagittal imbalance patients. World J Clin Cases 2013;1:242–248
14. Lenke LG, Sides BA, Koester LA, Hensley M, Blanke KM. Vertebral column resection for the treatment of severe spinal deformity. Clin Orthop Relat Res 2010;468:687–699
15. Suk S-I, Chung E-R, Kim J-H, Kim S-S, Lee J-S, Choi W-K. Posterior vertebral column resection for severe rigid scoliosis. Spine 2005;30:1682–1687
16. Booth KC, Bridwell KH, Lenke LG, Baldus CR, Blanke KM. Complications and predictive factors for the successful treatment of flatback deformity (fixed sagittal imbalance). Spine 1999;24:1712–1720
17. Bridwell KH. Decision making regarding Smith-Petersen vs. pedicle subtraction osteotomy vs. vertebral column resection for spinal deformity. Spine 2006;31(19, Suppl):S171–S178
18. Bianco K, Norton R, Schwab F, et al; International Spine Study Group. Complications and intercenter variability of three-column osteotomies for spinal deformity surgery: a retrospective review of 423 patients. Neurosurg Focus 2014;36:E18
19. Uribe JS, Deukmedjian AR, Mummaneni PV, et al; International Spine Study Group. Complications in adult spinal deformity surgery: an analysis of minimally invasive, hybrid, and open surgical techniques. Neurosurg Focus 2014;36:E15
20. Wang MY. Miniopen pedicle subtraction osteotomy: surgical technique and initial results. Neurosurg Clin N Am 2014;25:347–351
21. Smith JS, Shaffrey E, Klineberg E, et al; International Spine Study Group. Prospective multicenter assessment of risk factors for rod fracture following surgery for adult spinal deformity. J Neurosurg Spine 2014;21:994–1003
22. Hyun S-J, Lenke LG, Kim Y-C, Koester LA, Blanke KM. Comparison of standard 2-rod constructs to multiple-rod constructs for fixation across 3-column spinal osteotomies. Spine 2014;39:1899–1904
23. Buchowski JM, Bridwell KH, Lenke LG, et al. Neurologic complications of lumbar pedicle subtraction osteotomy: a 10-year assessment. Spine 2007;32:2245–2252
24. Reames DL, Kasliwal MK, Smith JS, Hamilton DK, Arlet V, Shaffrey CI. Time to development, clinical and radiographic characteristics, and management of proximal junctional kyphosis following adult thoracolumbar instrumented fusion for spinal deformity. J Spinal Disord Tech 2014
25. Kim Y-C, Lenke LG, Hyun S-J, Lee J-H, Koester LA, Blanke KM. Results of revision surgery after pedicle subtraction osteotomy for fixed sagittal imbalance with pseudarthrosis at the prior osteotomy site or elsewhere: minimum 5 years post-revision. Spine 2014;39:1817–1828

107 Cortical Trajectory Screws

Byron C. Branch and Charles L. Branch, Jr.

Cortical bone screws are a relatively novel screw trajectory introduced in 2009 by Santoni et al.[1] The cortical screw trajectory attempts to orient the load-bearing screw through a denser bone trajectory, anchoring the screw within the pars interarticularis rather than the traditional cancellous tract of the vertebral pedicle and body. This trajectory follows a lateral and cephalad path, obtaining cortical bone purchase at the dorsal cortex at the site of insertion, the medial posterior pedicle wall, the lateral anterior pedicle wall, and the curvature of the vertebral body wall at the dorsolateral superior end plate. These multiple sites of cortical purchase seem to have a critical role in cortical bone screws' stability independent of trabecular bone mineral density.[1,2]

The rationale behind cortical bone screws lies in their potential to avoid the screw loosening and pullout that is seen with traditional pedicle screws, especially in osteopenic bone. Although traditional pedicle screws are the most popular method of instrumentation for the treatment of many spinal disorders, failure due to screw loosening and pullout with resultant pseudarthrosis are well-known complications, particularly prevalent among patients with poor bone quality, such as those with osteoporosis.[3] This is made apparent in studies that analyze the anatomic and biomechanical relationships of traditional pedicle screw coaxial trajectories in an attempt to address the issue of pedicle screw loosening. Several of these studies even propose novel pedicle screw trajectories in an effort to resolve the issue of pedicle screw loosening.[4,5] Another difficulty with traditional pedicle screws lies in the degree of cortical purchase achieved with a pedicle screw. In the clinical setting, it may be presumed that good cortical purchase is achieved if the screw insertion "feels good," but anatomic studies argue that the bulk of pedicle bone is composed of the cancellous type surrounded only by a thin cortical shell. An anatomic study by Misenhimer et al[6] found that, in a majority of cases, cortical bone purchase is not achieved; rather, a cancellous anchored screw with concomitant pedicle expansion is observed.

Biomechanical studies performed on cortical screws placed in the lateral cephalad trajectory have demonstrated statistical equivalence in the pullout load and toggle stress required for failure when cortical trajectory was compared with traditional pedicular trajectory in osteoporotic bone.[1] Although statistical significance was not achieved, there was a substantial trend toward a (~ 30%) higher pullout load required in the cortical trajectory screws.[1] In studies comparing screw–rod fixation constructs with an intact disk, an equivalent construct stability was observed after pedicle screw–rod and cortical screw–rod fixation, except that pedicle screw–rod fixation was stiffer during axial rotation. With direct lateral interbody fusion (DLIF) support, there was no significant difference in stability between pedicle screw–rod and cortical screw–rod fixation. With transforaminal lumbar interbody fusion (TLIF) support, pedicle screw–rod fixation was stiffer than cortical screw–rod fixation during lateral bending only.[7] In vivo studies comparing cortical and pedicle screws have demonstrated a statistically significant higher insertional torque of cortical screws compared with traditional pedicle screws; insertional torque of cortical screws is ~ 1.7 times higher than the traditional technique.[8] This becomes important as insertional torque has been correlated with pullout strength.[9–11]

The cortical screw trajectory is a novel technique that represents an alternative to traditional pedicle screw fixation (**Fig. 107.1**). Biomechanical studies have observed equivalence with pedicle screws with regard to toggle stress, pullout load, and screw–rod construct stability. These studies also suggest the superiority of cortical screws over pedicle screws in regard to pullout load in osteoporotic bone and insertional torque (a correlation with pullout strength). This technique has several uses, including serving as a rescue and revision option and the ability to place cortical screws at the same level as existing pedicle screws, thus permitting adjacent-level fusion without the need for extensive reexposure or removal of preexisting hardware (**Fig. 107.2**).[12]

Indications

- Traumatic or iatrogenic instability
- Augmentation of anterior or interbody fusion
- Fusion following deformity correction
- Treatment of adjacent level disease in patients with existing instrumentation

Contraindications

- Mid- to upper thoracic pedicle fixation

Advantages

- Low profile (thin patients, lower thoracic instrumentation, more room for lateral intertransverse fusion)
- Medial entry point and superolateral trajectory do not require lateral exposure, affording minimal muscle disconnection and smaller incisions. The technique is amendable for minimally invasive surgery (MIS).
- Potentially has better cortical bone purchase and may be more favorable instrumentation for osteoporotic bone
- Trajectory directed away from neural elements
- Can be placed at the same level as the existing pedicle screw, enabling adjacent-level fusion without the need to dissect or remove preexisting hardware

107 Cortical Trajectory Screws

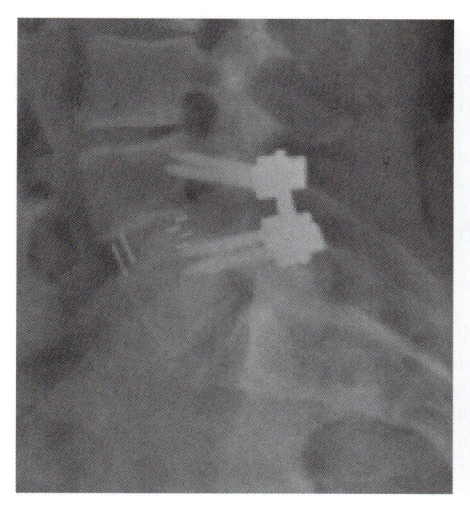

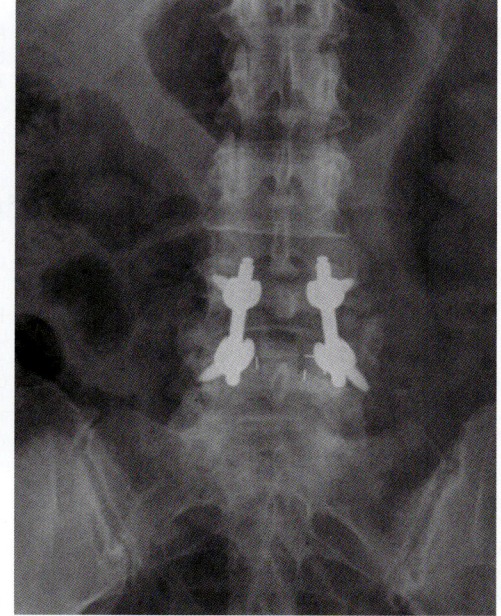

Fig. 107.1 Lateral **(a)** and anteroposterior **(b)** X-ray views of the cortical bone fixation technique with posterior lumbar fusion.

Disadvantages

- Limited research on long-term outcomes with this technique
- Unfamiliar procedure compared with current pedicle insertion
- Currently no method for percutaneous insertion
- Potential risk of entrance point and pedicle fractures during screw insertion due to trajectory through denser bone
- Slightly different entry point and trajectory for L5
- Not applicable at S1
- Increased metal mass over midline may distort magnetic resonance imaging (MRI)

Objective

- Facilitates spinal fusion by immobilizing vertebral segments
- In contrast to traditional open methods, the cortical bone trajectory affords the above objective with less invasive exposures and lower profile constructs.

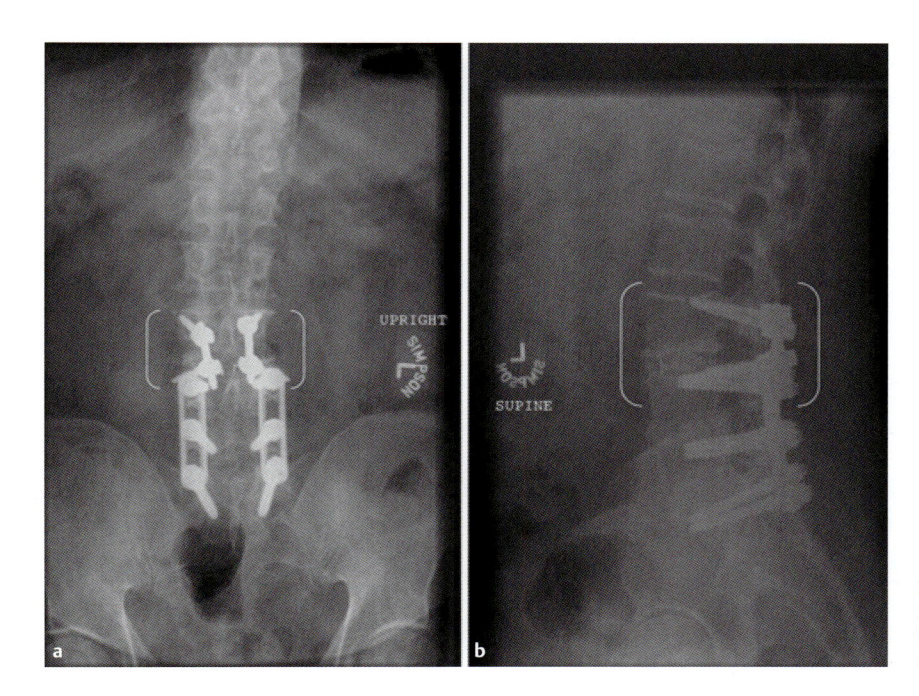

Fig. 107.2 Lateral **(a)** and anteroposterior **(b)** X-ray views of cortical bone fixation technique in adjacent-level fixation with existing instrumentation.

- Facilitates adjacent level spinal fusion without the need for extensive reexposure or removal of existing instrumentation

Patient Selection

- Can be considered for most patients with indications for pedicle screw instrumentation
  - Adjunct to interbody, anterior, intertransverse fusions
- May be advantageous in patients with low bone mineral density (BMD), large patients with potential wound healing issues, thin patients in whom there is a concern about hardware erosion, and patients requiring salvage or adjacent level interventions.

Surgical Technique (Video 107.1)

Positioning

The intubated patient is placed prone on chest rolls or any of a variety of commercially available spinal surgery frames, with all pressure points adequately padded and special care given to the spiral groove (ulnar nerve) and eyes. Abduction of the arm should be limited to 80 degrees at most, to avoid stretch injury to the brachial plexus. Pneumatic compression devices are applied to the lower extremities to prevent the development of a deep venous thrombosis in the anesthetized patient. Bladder catheterization is used routinely in most lumbar spinal fusion operations and should be considered for lengthy procedures or in cases where anticipated blood loss is significant. Prophylactic broad-spectrum antibiotics are administered prior to skin incision, and with extensive exposure or instrumented fusion are continued for 24 hours postoperatively.

Incision

A midline incision with limited separation of the muscles is created comparable to a bilateral microdiscectomy approach. The incision should be 4 to 5 cm to avoid tension at the limits of the incision with adequate retraction.

Technique

After exposure of the dorsal spinal elements, the entry point for the cortical bone trajectory (CBT) is achieved after muscle retraction to the lateral pars. The insertion point is 3 to 4 mm medial to the lateral border of the pars interarticularis at the junction of the caudal border of the transverse process (**Fig. 107.3**). This point may be palpated or visualized on the surface of the lamina with limited muscle dissection or retraction. A pilot hole is initiated with a 2-mm drill, and then the medial to lateral and caudal to cephalad trajectory is established using anteroposterior (AP) and lateral fluoroscopic imaging (**Fig. 107.4**). The sagittal trajectory extends from the insertion point across the pedicle to the apophyseal bone of the vertebra just below the end plate. This is generally 25 to 30 mm. The coronal trajectory extends from the insertion point just caudal and medial to the pedicle, across the pedicle to the apophyseal bone just lateral and superior to the pedicle. This trajectory can be visualized with the pedicle as a clock face that is traversed from the 5 o'clock position to the 11 o'clock position or from the 7 o'clock position to the 1 o'clock position, depending on the side of the fixation (**Fig. 107.5**). Because it is cortical bone over the majority of this track, the drill should be of sufficient length to traverse the entire length of the proposed track (25–35 mm), and the subsequent tap should also be a cortical bone thread that traverses the entire length of the proposed track (**Fig. 107.6**). In general, a screw that is 5.0 mm in diameter is sufficient for fixation. Care is taken to insert the screw to the proper depth and to loosen the screw insertion tool attachment as the final insert occurs to avoid over-insertion and fracture of the bone.

Closure

After fixation, the dorsal fascia is reapproximated to the interspinous ligament if intact, and then routine skin closure is performed.

Revision Technique

Revision of this fixation instrumentation is facilitated by its medial location, so that hardware is accessible with very limited muscular dissection. Because this is a transpedicular approach, this trajectory may be utilized to rescue fixation with a pedicle fracture using a conventional pedicle screw approach.

Another potential application is the avoidance of exposure and removal of existing hardware when performing a fusion at a level adjacent to a fusion with existing fixation hardware. In this case, if there is sufficient room in the instrumented pedicle, a 4.5- or 5.0-mm screw can be inserted using the cortical trajectory with image-guided navigation or conventional fluoroscopy.

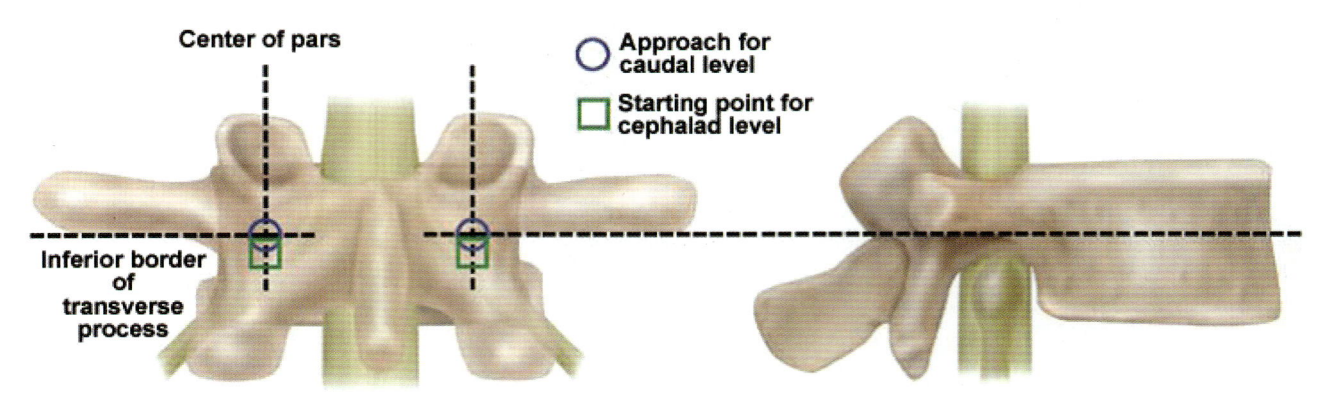

Fig. 107.3 Anatomic landmarks for cortical bone trajectory insertion.

107 Cortical Trajectory Screws 667

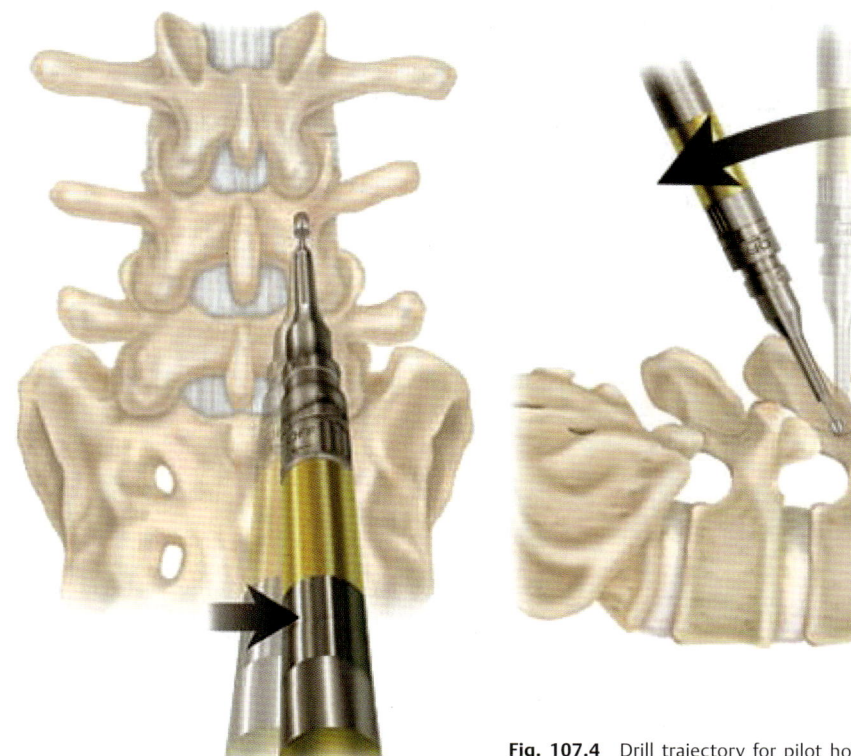

Fig. 107.4 Drill trajectory for pilot hole and tapping **(a)** coronal view and **(b)** sagittal view.

Other Technical Considerations

This technique may be effectively used in conjunction with unilateral or bilateral decompression and the screw trajectory and pilot holes may be drilled and tapped either prior to or after the bony decompression.

This may be effectively used in patients with a pars defect, as the pars defect is generally inferior to the cortical screw starting point.

Paramount to the successful performance of this technique is obtaining the correct entry point and not under-tapping.

Postoperative Care

Prophylactic antibiotics and bladder catheterization are discontinued on the first postoperative day, and early ambulation is encouraged. Some patients may require an external orthosis such as a corset or custom-fitted rigid thoracolumbosacral orthosis for use during weight-bearing activity. Plain film radiographic evaluation is performed during the initial postoperative period with the patient in the upright position to verify the integrity of the construct and to ensure that no deformity has occurred. Radiographs are repeated at 3 and 9 months

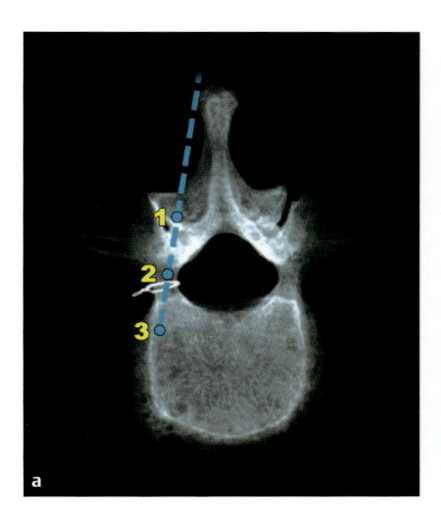

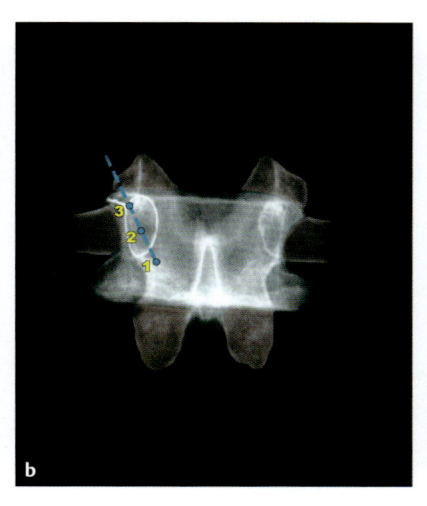

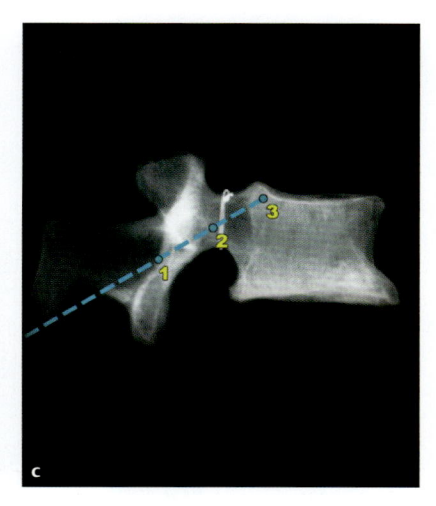

Fig. 107.5 Axial **(a)**, coronal **(b)**, and sagittal **(c)** anatomic trajectory views for the cortical bone technique.

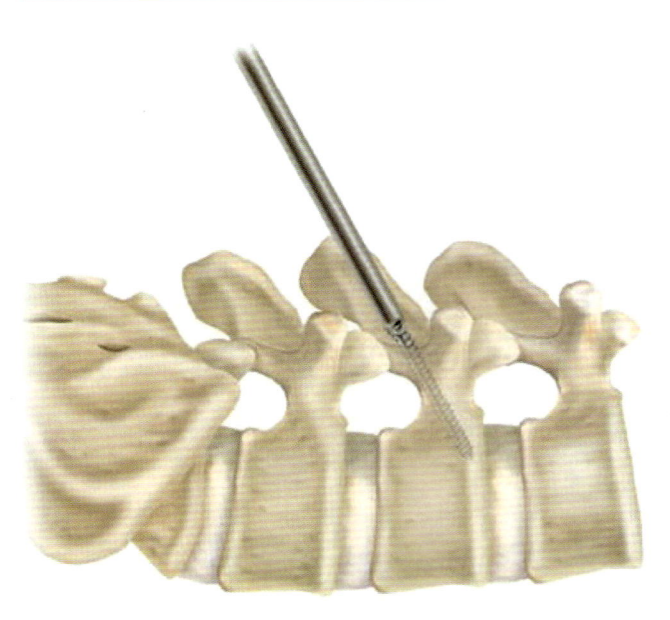

Fig. 107.6 Tap and screw trajectory illustrating the caudal to cephalad approach over the entire proposed screw length.

postoperatively and at regular intervals thereafter until fusion has been established. As this technique affords a minimally invasive approach, a surgical drain is usually not required. If the surgeon elected to place a drain, the drain is removed when output falls below 50 cc within a 24-hour period and should not be left in the surgical bed for more than 3 days postoperatively.

Complications

Excessive screw diameter in relation to the tapped trajectory or under-tapping the entire screw trajectory can result in excessive insertional torques that may cause fractures in the dense cortical bone of the entry point, pars interarticularis, and pedicle. There is the potential for upper nerve root injury by incorrect depth of screw penetration or screw direction, and for lower nerve root injury by insufficient cephalad trajectory because the nerve root is just under the starting point.[2]

References

1. Santoni BG, Hynes RA, McGilvray KC, et al. Cortical bone trajectory for lumbar pedicle screws. Spine J 2009;9:366–373
2. Matsukawa K, Yato Y, Nemoto O, Imabayashi H, Asazuma T, Nemoto K. Morphometric measurement of cortical bone trajectory for lumbar pedicle screw insertion using computed tomography. J Spinal Disord Tech 2013;26:E248–E253
3. Wittenberg RH, Shea M, Swartz DE, Lee KS, White AA III, Hayes WC. Importance of bone mineral density in instrumented spine fusions. Spine 1991;16:647–652
4. Inceoğlu S, Montgomery WH Jr, St Clair S, McLain RF. Pedicle screw insertion angle and pullout strength: comparison of 2 proposed strategies. J Neurosurg Spine 2011;14:670–676
5. Su BW, Kim PD, Cha TD, et al. An anatomical study of the mid-lateral pars relative to the pedicle footprint in the lower lumbar spine. Spine 2009;34:1355–1362
6. Misenhimer GR, Peek RD, Wiltse LL, Rothman SLG, Widell EH Jr. Anatomic analysis of pedicle cortical and cancellous diameter as related to screw size. Spine 1989;14:367–372
7. Perez-Orribo L, Kalb S, Reyes PM, Chang SW, Crawford NR. Biomechanics of lumbar cortical screw-rod fixation versus pedicle screw-rod fixation with and without interbody support. Spine 2013;38:635–641
8. Matsukawa K, Yato Y, Kato T, Imabayashi H, Asazuma T, Nemoto K. In vivo analysis of insertional torque during pedicle screwing using cortical bone trajectory technique. Spine 2014;39:E240–E245
9. Halvorson TL, Kelley LA, Thomas KA, Whitecloud TS III, Cook SD. Effects of bone mineral density on pedicle screw fixation. Spine 1994;19:2415–2420
10. Myers BS, Belmont PJ Jr, Richardson WJ, Yu JR, Harper KD, Nightingale RW. The role of imaging and in situ biomechanical testing in assessing pedicle screw pull-out strength. Spine 1996;21:1962–1968
11. Zdeblick TA, Kunz DN, Cooke ME, McCabe R. Pedicle screw pullout strength. Correlation with insertional torque. Spine 1993;18:1673–1676
12. Rodriguez A, Neal MT, Liu A, Somasundaram A, Hsu W, Branch CL Jr. Novel placement of cortical bone trajectory screws in previously instrumented pedicles for adjacent-segment lumbar disease using CT image-guided navigation. Neurosurg Focus 2014;36:E9

108 MIS Facet Screw

Carter S. Gerard and Richard G. Fessler

The use of facet screws for stabilization of the lumbosacral spine is a well-recognized technique first described by King[1] in 1948. The placement of ipsilateral transfacet screws was later refined by Buocher[2] in 1959 and followed by a depiction of the translaminar transfacet technique by Magerl[3] in 1984. Despite data demonstrating equivalent biomechanical properties to pedicle screws[4] and favorable outcomes for facet screw placement,[5,6] the use of pedicle screws has remained the principal form of posterior fixation of the lumbar spine. However, now with the increasing application of anterior lumbar interbody fusion (ALIF) and direct lateral interbody fusion (DLIF), percutaneous facet screws have become increasingly popular. Multiple studies have shown that ALIF alone does not enable the complete immobilization of the lumbosacral spine, and that posterior fixation is required to limit extension and rotation.[7,8] Grob and Humke[9] first described supplementation of an ALIF with a minimally invasive technique for facet screw placement. Since that time, several studies have refined the method and demonstrated equivalent clinical outcomes when compared with percutaneous pedicle screw fixation.[10–14] In contrast to percutaneous pedicle screws, minimally invasive surgery (MIS) facet screws span adjacent levels, obviating the need for rods or additional screws, and ultimately decreasing the cost and operative time. Minimally invasive facet screws avoid the morbidity of an extensive exposure while offering an attractive adjunct to interbody fusion techniques of the lumbosacral spine.[11,13–15]

Indications
- Supplemental posterior fixation after ALIF or DLIF

Contraindications
- Spondylolysis, kyphotic deformity, high-grade (> grade I) spondylolisthesis
- Absence or fracture of the posterior elements
- Significant osteoporosis (relative contraindication)
- Medical illness precluding surgery
- Life expectancy less than 3 to 6 months

Advantages
- Increased rates of fusion
- MIS form of posterior fixation
- Limited hardware required

Disadvantages
- Requires intact posterior elements
- Does not enable the surgeon to distract or correct alignment prior to fixation
- Does not enable bony preparation for fusion
- Only engages two columns

Objective
- Obtain stabilization of the lumbosacral spine to maintain alignment and promote bony fusion

Preoperative Imaging
- Lateral and anteroposterior (AP) X-rays
- Computer tomography without contrast

Patient Selection
Anesthesia and Positioning

Prior to undergoing any surgical procedure the patient should be evaluated to assess the potential risk and complications associated with anesthesia. The vast majority of patients who are suitable for minimally invasive facet screw placement can undergo general anesthesia, as is required for an ALIF or DLIF. However, those who are opposed to or do not qualify for general anesthesia may have conscious sedation with a controlled dose of fentanyl and midazolam during the procedure.[11] A Foley catheter is typically not required due to the limited operative time and negligible blood loss. A single intraoperative dose of either cefazolin or clindamycin is given 1 hour before incision. Once anesthesia has been induced, the patient is placed in the prone position on a padded radiolucent table. The placement of percutaneous ipsilateral transfacet screws for the patient in the lateral decubitus position has been described for patients undergoing DLIF,[12] but this technique is more challenging and may not be a suitable option for novice practitioners.

Surgical Technique
Percutaneous Ipsilateral Facet Screw

The use of fluoroscopic imaging or computed tomography (CT) with intraoperative guidance now accomplishes the goals of the original facet screw procedure via a minimally invasive technique (**Table 108.1**). The bony imaging must be reviewed preoperatively to plan the screw trajectory and verify the feasibility of fixation across the center of the zygapophyseal joint via a percutaneous approach. Su et al[16] demonstrated that this approach should be limited to L3–S1 because levels cranial to L3–L4 require a trajectory that passes through the spinous process.

Table 108.1 The Major Steps for Percutaneous Placement of an Ipsilateral Transfacet Screw

Step	Description
1	1.5-midline incision two levels above targeted facet
2	Open fascia bilaterally
3	Define starting point • Cranial-caudal dimension: inferior end plate • Medial-lateral dimension: medial pedicle
4	Define trajectory • Through the facet and end in the inferolateral border of the pedicle
5	Introduce Jamshidi needle to starting point
6	Pass Kirschner wire (K-wire) through the facet to the inferior pedicle
7	Introduce tap and drill
8	Introduce screw along the K-wire
9	Remove the K-wire
10	Closure

Once the patient is positioned, the area is prepped and draped in the standard fashion. Fluoroscopy is then used to identify the level of interest. A 1.5-cm midline incision is marked over the spinous process two levels above the targeted facet. The AP fluoroscopy is then adjusted so that the inferior and superior end plates are parallel. The entry point in the AP view is based on the superior level of fixation.

The starting point should be centered over the inferior end plate in the cranial-caudal dimension, and over the medial border of the pedicle in the medial-lateral direction. The lateral view is used to ensure that the trajectory passes through the facet joint and into the pedicle of the inferior lever. The ideal termination of the screw is at the inferolateral border of the pedicle in the AP view and the junction of the pedicle and vertebral body in the lateral view. The usual trajectory results in about 15 degrees of lateral angulation relative to the spinous process in the axial plane and about 30 degrees of angulation relative to the intervertebral disk in the sagittal plane.[12,16] After injection of local anesthetic, the incision is made using a No. 10 bade scalpel and the fascia is opened on both sides of the spinous process with a Bovie cautery. A Jamshidi needle is then advanced to engage the superior level of fixation at the defined entry points cited above (**Fig. 108.1**). A mallet is then used to advance a Kirschner wire (K-wire) across the facet and into the inferolateral aspect of the pedicle of the inferior level of fixation. Once the trajectory is confirmed on lateral and AP imaging, dilators are placed over the K-wire. A cannulated tap is used followed by placement of a cannulated screw. A 35-degree oblique view can then be used to confirm transfacet screw placement. The screw should end in the center of the pedicle or eye of the "Scottie dog"–like shape.[16] Once the screw placement is confirmed, the K-wire is removed and the contralateral side may be completed through the same incision (**Fig. 108.2**).[12] The dorsal lumbar fascia is closed, the subcutaneous tissues approximated, and the skin closed with interrupted subcuticular stitches. The wound is dressed with Dermabond (Ethicon, Johnson & Johnson, Somerville, NJ). The patient is then turned over to the anesthesia team.

Percutaneous Translaminar Facet Screw

The translaminar transfacet technique by was first described Magerl[3] and has been modified to accommodate minimally invasive placement. Grob and Humke[9] initially described percutaneous

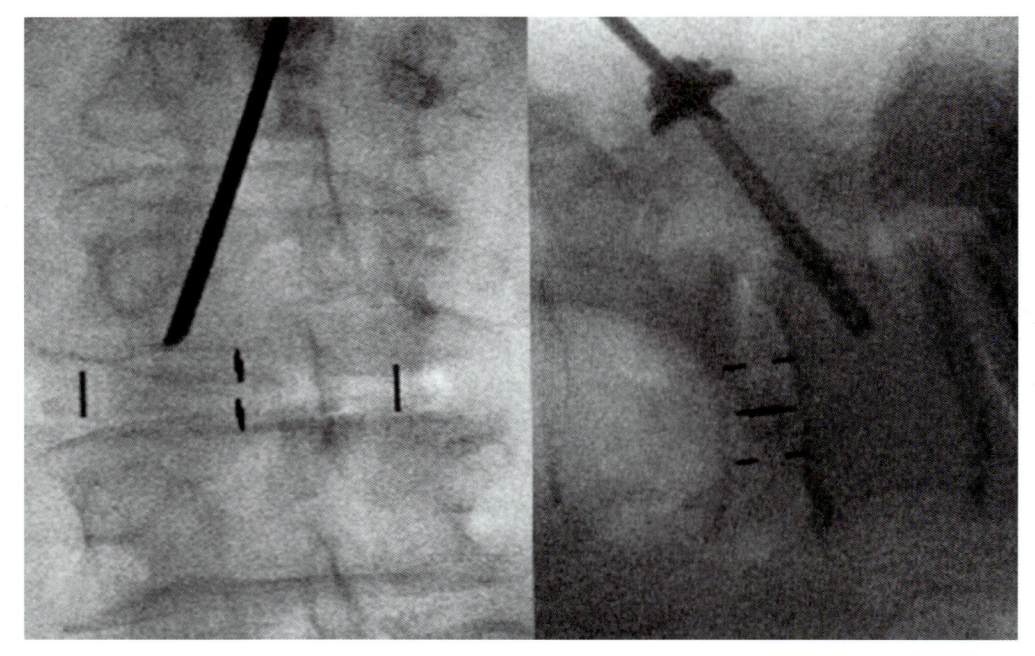

Fig. 108.1 Docking of the needle at the inferior end plate of the superior level and the medial aspect of the pedicle (**a**). The ipsilateral facet screw with the tip in the junction of the pedicle and vertebral body (**b**).

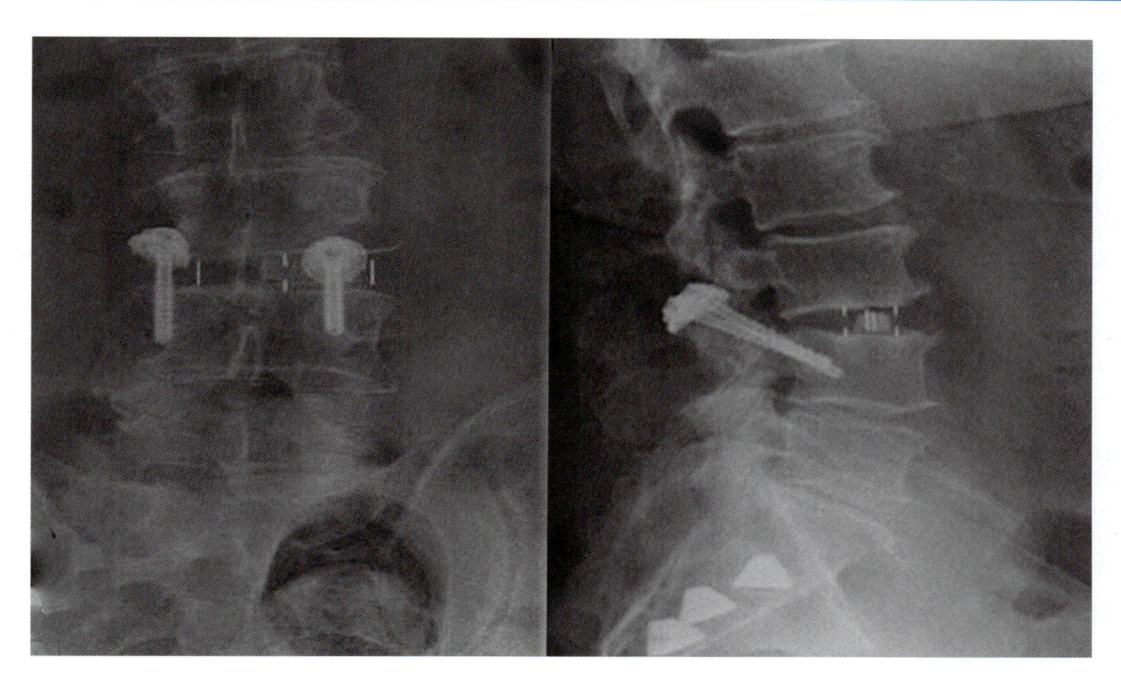

Fig. 108.2 Anteroposterior (AP) **(a)** and lateral **(b)** views of the final placement of bilateral ipsilateral screws after a L3-L4 direct lateral interbody fusion (DLIF) is performed.

translaminar facet screw placement as a supplement to an ALIF. The initial technique required special equipment that was not readily available, and therefore the technique was not universally adopted. Minimally invasive placement of translaminar screws using intraoperative imaging and readily available equipment has since been described by several authors (**Table 108.2**).[13,14]

Although biomechanical studies have shown ipsilateral facet screws and translaminar facet screws to be equally effective,[4] there are advantages and disadvantages to each technique. A defining characteristic of translaminar facet screws is the ability to be placed at more rostral levels, higher than L3-L4, where an ipsilateral facet screw trajectory is obstructed by the spinous process. Translaminar facet screws (**Fig. 108.3**) also enable longer bony fixation when compared with the ipsilateral approach. However, there is also greater risk of breaching the canal and subsequent neural injury. As with any procedure, the imaging must be critically studied preoperatively to ensure that placement of percutaneous tranlaminar facet screws is possible.

Once the patient is positioned, the area is prepped and draped in the standard fashion. Fluoroscopy is then used to identify the level of interest.

The trajectory in the axial plane is determined from preoperative CT beginning at the spinolaminar junction, passing throughout the laminar, facet joint, and the posterior one third of the pedicle (**Fig. 108.4**). This line is continued to the skin, and the distance from the midline is then measured and marked in the operating room. The caudal angle of the screw is determined using fluoroscopy. Using an AP view, a line is drawn from the pedicle of the upper level, traversing the cranial one third of the spinous process, and then to the superolateral quadrant of the contralateral pedicle of the inferior level. The point where this line intersects the previously marked line denoting the axial plane is the site of the skin incision. The skin is infiltrated with local anesthetic and a 1.5-cm incision is made in the skin. A small opening is made in the fascia with Bovie cautery, and the Jamshidi needle is introduced. The needle is then docked on the cranial one third of the spinous process. A K-wire is then introduced and advanced under fluoroscopy through the lamina, facet joint, and finally to the superolateral quadrant of the opposite pedicle. Once the placement is confirmed, the tap and drill are passed over the K-wire. A lag screw is introduced and passed over the K-wire to its final position. The K-wire is removed, and the same procedure can then be repeated for the opposite side. The dorsal lumbar fascia is closed, the subcutaneous tissues

Table 108.2 The Major Steps for Percutaneous Placement of a Translaminar Facet Screw

Step	Description
1	Mark a paramedian line lateral to the midline where the axial trajectory intersects with skin
2	Fluoroscopy is used to define caudal trajectory
3	Incision at the intersection of the paramedian line and caudal trajectory
4	Fascia is opened
5	Introduce Jamshidi needle to the cranial one third of the spinous process
6	Pass K-wire through the lamina, the facet, and into the inferior pedicle
7	Introduce tap and drill
8	Introduce screw along the K-wire
9	Remove the K-wire
10	Closure

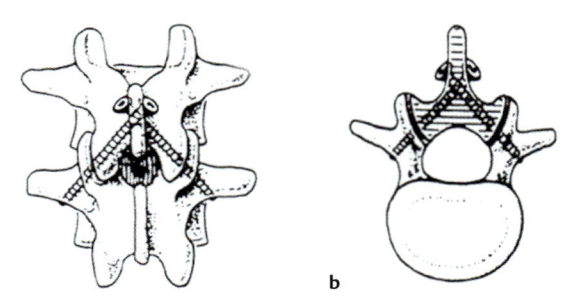

Fig. 108.3 The ideal placement of a translaminar facet screw in the coronal (**a**) and axial (**b**) dimensions.

approximated, and the skin closed with interrupted subcuticular stitches. The wound is dressed with Dermabond. The patient is then turned over to the anesthesia team.

Potential Complications and Precautions

As with all minimally invasive techniques, a limited exposure reduces the potential for related problems such as infection and wound breakdown. However, the technique requires that the surgeon thoroughly understands the relevant anatomy and is able to interpret and adjust to the information provided from intraoperative fluoroscopy or CT. Injury to neural structures typically occurs while passing the K-wire, with inadvertent violation of the spinal canal or foramina. Also, the surgeon must ensure that the wire does not pass anterior to the spine, thereby preventing injury to vascular or visceral structures. This can be avoided by advancing slowly and repeatedly verifying the K-wire position. Another option is to use CT guidance for improved visualization.[11] Attempts to change a trajectory or repeated introduction of the K-wire or screw may result in fracture. If the posterior elements are compromised, a percutaneous pedicle screw may be placed or the surgeon may prefer to convert to an open procedure if there is concern about neural compression.

Conclusion

Facet fixation is a well-described technique with over 50 years of use. Now with minimally invasive techniques, percutaneous facet screws can be placed fluoroscopically with minimal exposure and relative ease. Multiple biomechanical and clinical studies have demonstrated that percutaneous facet screws are a suitable alternative to pedicle fixation as an adjunct to interbody fusion. By understanding the indications, goals, relative anatomy, and potential complications, the surgeon can ensure that this is a safe and effective intervention for patients.

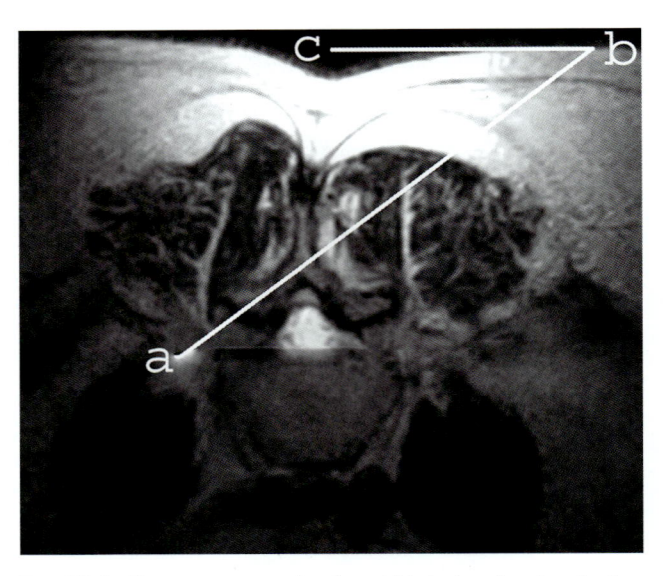

Fig. 108.4 The surgeon must plan the axial trajectory for a translaminar facet screw preoperatively. A line is drawn passing through the facets, through the lamina, and then extended to the skin (line a–b). The distance is then measures from the point on the skin (b) to the midline (c). This distance is then used in the operating room to draw a paramedian line that will intersect with the line of the caudal trajectory and therein mark the site of incision.

References

1. King D. Internal fixation for lumbosacral fusion. J Bone Joint Surg Am 1948;30A:560–565
2. Boucher HH. A method of spinal fusion. J Bone Joint Surg Br 1959;41-B:248–259
3. Magerl FP. Stabilization of the lower thoracic and lumbar spine with external skeletal fixation. Clin Orthop Relat Res 1984;189:125–141
4. Ferrara LA, Secor JL, Jin B-H, Wakefield A, Inceoglu S, Benzel EC. A biomechanical comparison of facet screw fixation and pedicle screw fixation: effects of short-term and long-term repetitive cycling. Spine 2003;28:1226–1234
5. El Masry MA, McAllen CJ, Weatherley CR. Lumbosacral fusion using the Boucher technique in combination with a posterolateral bone graft. Eur Spine J 2003;12:408–412
6. Margulies JY, Seimon LP. Clinical efficacy of lumbar and lumbosacral fusion using the Boucher facet screw fixation technique. Bull Hosp Jt Dis 2000;59:33–39
7. Volkman T, Horton WC, Hutton WC. Transfacet screws with lumbar interbody reconstruction: biomechanical study of motion segment stiffness. J Spinal Disord 1996;9:425–432
8. Tencer AF, Hampton D, Eddy S. Biomechanical properties of threaded inserts for lumbar interbody spinal fusion. Spine 1995;20:2408–2414
9. Grob D, Humke T. Translaminar screw fixation in the lumbar spine: technique, indications, results. Eur Spine J 1998;7:178–186
10. Chin KR, Seale J, Cumming V. Mini-open or percutaneous bilateral lumbar transfacet pedicle screw fixation: a technical note. J Spinal Disord Tech 2015;28:61–65
11. Kang HY, Lee S-H, Jeon SH, Shin S-W. Computed tomography-guided percutaneous facet screw fixation in the lumbar spine. Technical note. J Neurosurg Spine 2007;7:95–98
12. Voyadzis J-M, Anaizi AN. Minimally invasive lumbar transfacet screw fixation in the lateral decubitus position after extreme lateral interbody fusion: a technique and feasibility study. J Spinal Disord Tech 2013;26:98–106
13. Jang J-S, Lee S-H. Clinical analysis of percutaneous facet screw fixation after anterior lumbar interbody fusion. J Neurosurg Spine 2005;3:40–46
14. Shim CS, Lee S-H, Jung B, Sivasabaapathi P, Park S-H, Shin S-W. Fluoroscopically assisted percutaneous translaminar facet screw fixation following anterior lumbar interbody fusion: technical report. Spine 2005;30:838–843
15. Best NM, Sasso RC. Efficacy of translaminar facet screw fixation in circumferential interbody fusions as compared to pedicle screw fixation. J Spinal Disord Tech 2006;19:98–103
16. Su BW, Cha TD, Kim PD, et al. An anatomic and radiographic study of lumbar facets relevant to percutaneous transfacet fixation. Spine 2009;34:E384–E390

109 Transsacral Approach

William D. Tobler

The transsacral (or presacral) approach is a minimally invasive surgical technique to achieve lumbar interbody fusion at L5-S1, or both L4-L5 and L5-S1. Access to the L5-S1 disk is achieved by crossing through the space anterior to the sacrum. The transsacral approach is distinct from any other interbody surgical fusions in its approach, instrumentation, and biomechanics of fixation (**Fig. 109.1**). Benefits offered by the transsacral approach are most notable for minimizing injury to muscular, neural, ligamentous, and vascular structures.[1–5] This chapter discusses the approach, the surgical risks and benefits, and the outcomes reported for the 10-year period since its inception.[1,2] Reengineering of the device, introduction of other refinements,[3] and controversial issues, perhaps affecting the adoption of this approach,[6–13] are also discussed.

Advantages

Compared with other lumbar fusions at L5-S1, the presacral technique is unique in its approach, mechanism of discectomy, biomechanics, and suitability in cases of obesity. First, the anatomic corridor provides access to the spine previously not used for other interbody fusions.[3–8] Its anterior approach to the L5-S1 interbody provides access to the disk space anterior to the sacrum, which is achievable with the patient positioned prone. This is advantageous when compared with the anterior lumbar interbody fusion (ALIF) that requires a transabdominal approach to L5-S1 and two-stage positioning (i.e., supine for the initial part of the procedure and repositioning prone for the posterior stabilization). The presacral approach requires neither patient repositioning nor the assistance of an access surgeon.

Second, interspace preparation uses looped/flat cutters to remove the disk, without direct visualization of the interbody space by the surgeon. Unlike the ALIF opening and retraction of the abdominal wall musculature, the presacral approach divides no muscles or supporting ligaments. Unlike traditional posterior transforaminal lumbar interbody fusion (TLIF) or posterior lumbar interbody fusion (PLIF) approaches, the presacral approach does not disturb, manipulate, or retract the dural sac or the exiting and traversing nerve roots when preparing the disk space and inserting the interbody fixation device.[14]

Third, the biomechanics of the presacral device offer the advantage of an initial superior stabilization. Specifically, patients with a spondylolisthesis and high pelvic incidence face a high risk of construct failure because of the strong shear-force vector acting against the fixation of spinal fusion. Most interbody devices are wedged into the disc space and do not provide resistance against such forces.[15–17] The axial lumbar interbody fusion (AxiaLIF) large threaded rod crosses through the disk space oriented vertically and aligned with the axis of the spine, starting at the sacral interface and extending across L5-S1 into L5, or across the L4-5 interspace, extending up to the L4 vertebra in a two-level fusion (**Fig. 109.1**).

Finally, the presacral fusion technique is suitable for obese patients. Anterior or posterior approaches entail more technical challenges in trying to expose the spine through deeper layers of soft tissues in obesity. The increasing difficulty in performing the ALIF or TLIF thus poses higher risks for patients; in contrast, the presacral approach does not. Rather, it can sometimes be easier to perform in overweight patients. Specifically, access is safe; the distance from the tip of the coccyx/entry point to the L5-S1 disk space does not adversely increase and the typically large presacral fat pad displaces the rectum away from the sacrum.

Disadvantages

Two main disadvantages of the presacral procedure include the risk of bowel injury and failure to maintain distraction and lordosis. However, careful technique and evaluation of the anatomy of the rectum before and after the approach have reduced the risk of unrecognized bowel perforation to very low rates.[6,8,18] The original device, engineered with the capability to distract the interspace when inserted, utilized a reverse Herbert method. The distracting force of the threaded device (L5 and S1 segments of the rod) required a strong bone–device interface that could lead to failure, especially in patients with osteopenia. In some cases, this resulted in subsidence and failure to maintain distraction. Introducing additional lordosis, although possible with the presacral device, was unpredictable. Therefore, the presacral approach should not be used in patients with significant positive sagittal balance that requires interbody fusion and significant restoration of lordosis at L5-S1.

Evolution of the Technique

Since its introduction, the one- and two-level AxiaLIF devices have been reengineered to address subsidence and radiolucencies observed around them. With the second-generation presacral device, design improvements have resolved the stresses that were placed on the vertebral end plates imposed by the original design's reverse Herbert technique. Its modular design, now consisting of L5 and S1 segments and an inner threaded collar, are assembled before insertion (**Fig. 109.1**). Distraction of the interspace occurs after the device is advanced and positioned across the disk space. A torque rod is inserted into the second-generation device, and the inner collar is maximally extended to distract the space. An additional refinement includes

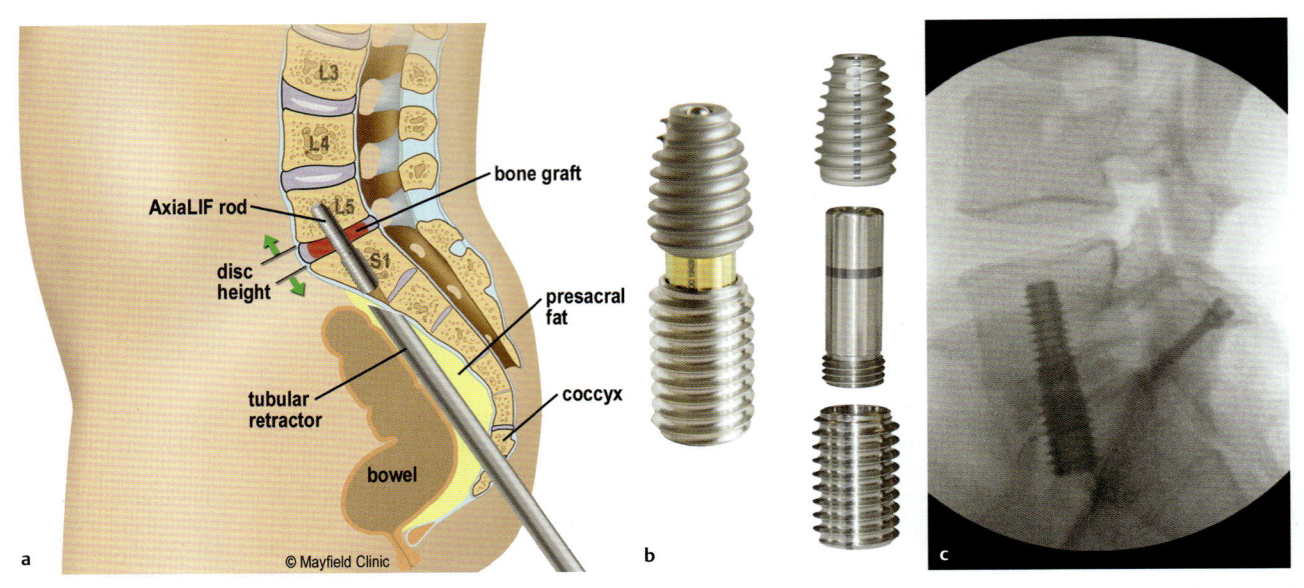

Fig. 109.1 Axial lumbar interbody fusion (AxiaLIF) corridor of approach. **(a)** The approach begins adjacent to the coccyx, moves midline along the avascular sacrum through the presacral fat to access the sacral promontory, and continues transsacral through bone to the L5-S1 disk space. **(b)** Titanium rod is composed of three parts: the S1 segment, inner distraction collar, and tapered L5 segment. When inserted, the distraction rod is adjusted to restore the height of the disk space and indirectly decompresses the neural foramen. **(c)** Facet screws inserted percutaneously achieve a 360-degree stabilization of the motion segment. (Courtesy of the Mayfield Clinic, Cincinnati, OH.)

tapering of the upper end of the device. Application of a porous bead coating can improve fixation and promote arthrodesis. Introducing these changes subsequently eliminated the radiographic halo effect seen around the upper end of the L5 rod, which was often mistaken for loosening of the device or pseudarthrosis on X-ray and computed tomography (CT) imaging.

A presacral access kit to protect the bowel was introduced. This inflatable, soft plastic form inserted into the presacral space and inflated with saline can create a barrier between the instrumentation and retroperitoneal contents during the procedure (**Fig. 109.2**).

A soft rubber gasket has been added to the tip of the exchange cannula, part of the final step of placing the device into the spine. The rubber gasket now forms a soft seal at the distal sacrum. Fixed with two small Steinmann pins, it stabilizes the exchange cannula during device insertion but excludes any soft tissue (e.g., rectum) from becoming entrapped inside it.

Evaluation of the bowel integrity is encouraged. Before the procedure, injecting air into the bowel ensures the surgical position of the rectum. After the procedure, saline injected and aspirated from the rectum can detect any blood that is indicative of bowel perforation. Contrast injected into the rectum at the close of the procedure can demonstrate a fistula. Lastly, a rigid scope can be inserted in the rectum to directly inspect the rectal wall. In conjunction with meticulous surgical technique, these options have reduced the incidence of bowel perforation to < 1%.[18] Intraoperative identification and immediate repair of a perforation can prevent infection and eliminate the need for colostomy.

Indications and Contraindications

The presacral device can be considered for any patient who will undergo interbody fusion with posterior fixation at L5-S1 or L4-L5 and L5-S1. This lumbar fusion is typically indicated for skeletally mature patients who have degenerative disk disease, multiple recurrent disk herniations, or spondylolisthesis. Most patients who have undergone hysterectomies, or bladder or other abdominal surgeries that did not violate the presacral space, can also undergo the presacral approach.

Contraindications include significant scarring in the presacral space that makes mobilization of the rectum and soft tissues impossible. Other contraindications are postsurgical intervention or radiotherapy in the presacral space, and significant inflammatory bowel disease.[6,19]

A large presacral fat pad seen in obese patients provides an already larger space but lack of any fat pad does not create an impediment because the space opens up with blunt finger dissection. T2-weighted sagittal magnetic resonance imaging (MRI) demonstrates the presence and thickness of the presacral fat.

A two-level approach requires very careful evaluation of the potential trajectory before scheduling the procedure. In almost all cases with a two-level device, the cephalad portion of the device comes into close contact with the anterior cortex of the L4 vertebral segment as it passes anteriorly in the L4-5 disk space. Therefore, special care must be exercised in preparing the L4-5 disk space. Specifically, because of the risk of violating the anterior annulus of the L4-L5 disk when using the nitinol cutters, injury to the aortic and iliac vessels is possible.

Patient Selection

Potential candidates for interbody fusion at L5-S1 or L4-L5 and L5-S1 can be evaluated for the presacral approach when the usual conservative measures have failed. The classic course is typically 6 to 12 months of symptoms that fail to respond to anti-inflammatory agents, injection therapy, and lifestyle modification. MRI of the lumbar spine and pelvis as well as standing lateral/flexion extension X-rays are routinely obtained. Bone density studies are important for patients at risk for osteoporosis. However, dual-energy X-ray absorptiometry (DEXA) scan results do not always correlate with the hardness of the shell of the bone, which is necessary for fixation of the implant. As in any surgical planning, medical evaluation identifies any other medical contraindications to a surgical procedure.

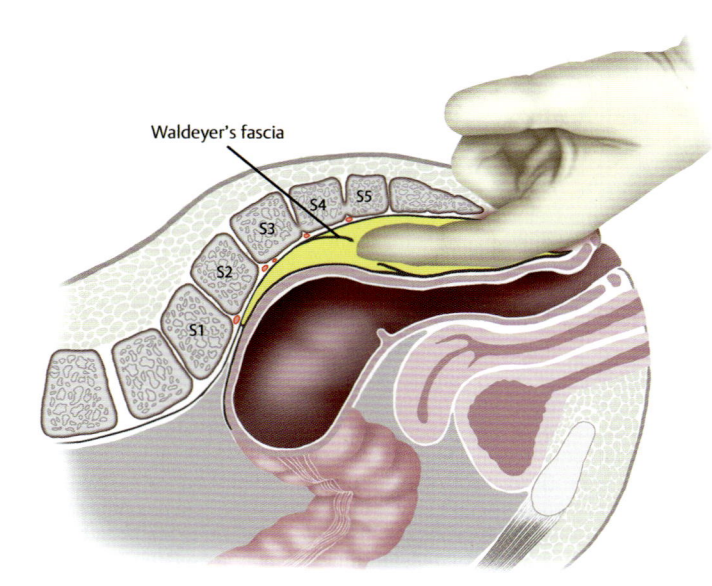

Fig. 109.2 Presacral access. **(a)** Access begins with blunt dissection to penetrate Waldeyer's fascia. **(b)** The presacral access kit is inserted against the sacral surface. Inflation with saline forms a mattress-like device that deflects soft tissues away from the sacrum, making a protective barrier between the bowel and instruments. Fluoroscopic image shows the deployed protective access kit. (Courtesy of Baxano Surgical, Raleigh, NC.)

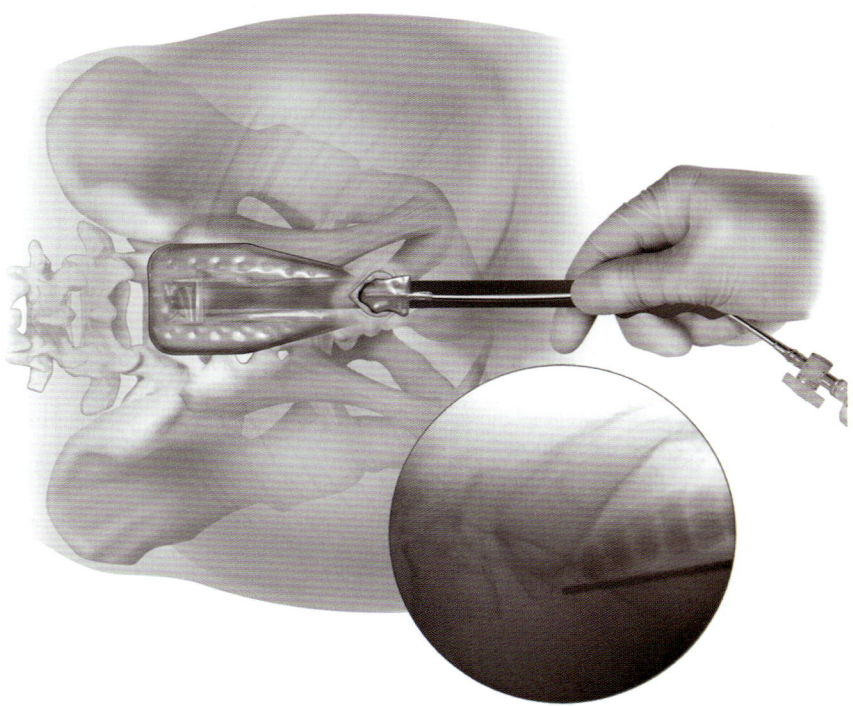

Patient Profile

Ideal candidates for a presacral fusion have a moderate body mass index (BMI) and a classic-shaped sacrum (**Fig. 109.3**). In candidates with degenerative disk disease, Modic end-plate changes without spondylolisthesis represent the best case for good outcomes and minimal technical challenges. Although grade I or II spondylolisthesis is a more difficult scenario, these patients can usually achieve excellent technical results. However, a grade III or higher spondylolisthesis is far more difficult to treat; the procedure is only recommended if the slip can be reduced intraoperatively to obtain the required alignment and trajectory before final placement of the presacral device. This can be accomplished in most cases with posterior osteotomies and the powerful reduction capabilities of most pedicle screw systems. With the patient positioned prone, the surgeon can simultaneously perform portions of the presacral procedure and the posterior portion to achieve reduction of the spine.

The presacral approach may be contraindicated for spondylolisthesis that does not spontaneously reduce or cannot be surgically reduced; in these cases, the rod would advance too posteriorly at L5 and could be misdirected into the spinal canal.

Preoperative Planning

Physical Examination

Complete musculoskeletal and neurologic examinations are required. Gait observation is extremely important to evaluate sagittal balance. Of note, 10 to 14 days before the procedure, patients should discontinue all nonsteroidal anti-inflammatory drug (NSAIDs), antiplatelet agents, minerals, and vitamin supplements.

Radiographic Workup and Preoperative Imaging

Once the decision has been made to perform a spinal fusion, the presacral approach requires evaluation of the presacral space (**Fig. 109.3**). Standing lumbar films with exposure to the tip of the sacrum establish the extent of the patient's lordosis and define the sacral morphology. Evaluation of the lumbosacral anatomy is required for trajectory planning, especially when considering a two-level presacral fusion. Sacral morphology is best evaluated by standing lateral lumbar films with a full view of the sacrum (i.e., lordosis of sacrum and weight-bearing lumbar spine). Vascular anatomy is assessed by MRI of the presacral space/pelvis or computed tomography angiography (CTA) of the pelvis; this confirms the lack of vascularity of the presacral space and the absence of any vascular anomaly (e.g., aberrant iliac vein crossing the S1-S2 entry point).

Sagittal and parasagittal T2-weighted MRI and axial T2 images should be obtained from the L5-S1 disk down to at least the midportion of the sacrum. The presence and thickness of the presacral fat pad can be identified on the T2-weighted sagittal image. However, its absence in a thin person does not contraindicate the surgery; this space devoid of fat will be dissected open early in the procedure.

The trajectory can be defined by overlaying a template onto the X-ray or MRI. Placing a straight rod or pin, the surgeon can examine the path from the tip of the coccyx to the midportion of the L5-S1 disk to determine the feasibility of the procedure. Templating for a two-level procedure is even more critical because of the longer device used (**Fig. 109.3d**). Additionally, if a patient appears to have a sagittal imbalance issue, complete scoliosis films are indicated.

Transsacral Approach: Step-by-Step Procedure

The patient is positioned prone on the operating table, aiming toward maximizing lordosis at L5-S1. With the patient's legs spread, placing 3-inch strips of silk tape onto each buttock provides lateral retraction. A plastic adherent barrier is draped just above the anus (**Fig. 109.4a**). A rectal catheter is inserted into the rectum and remains in place during the procedure.[20]

Surgical Technique

Fluoroscopy Setup

Two fluoroscopy units are preferred: one placed across from the operating surgeon for lateral views and the other set up at a 45-degree angle on the surgeon's same side for the anteroposterior images (**Fig. 109.4b**). Air can be injected to outline the position of the rectum before sterile prep.

Making the Incision

After routine prep of the entire operative field, including the lumbar region, a 20-mm incision is made in the paracoccygeal area, preferably on the right side. The incision, off the midline to the left or right at the coccyx tip, can be based on the surgeon's preference. The trajectory is just inferior to the sacrococcygeal ligament.

Plunging too deeply with a knife or Bovie can lacerate the rectum, which is superficial at this level. Waldeyer's fascia, deep to the subcutaneous layer, can usually be bluntly opened by finger dissection on entering the presacral space (**Fig. 109.2a**). With its oily texture, the periosteum on the sacrum is easily identified. Once the space is opened, the presacral access kit can be placed and inflated with saline.

Accessing and Preparing the Disk Space

Under fluoroscopy, the surgeon advances the guide probe to the entry point usually at the S1-S2 interspace. A series of dilators are advanced into the sacrum, ending with a 12-mm dilator. With the last one placed and its sheath left on, a channel is drilled into the L5-S1 space. The disk is morcellized with various looped nitinol and firm flat cutters, the end plates are scraped and rasped for fusion (**Fig. 109.5**), and wire brushes ensure the complete evacuation of any disk material. The space then can be irrigated with antibiotic solution. Next, bone grafting material is packed radially into the disk space using a beveled cannula. Choice of materials for grafting varies and is determined by surgeon and patient preferences.

Measuring and Placing the Interbody Device

After packing the disk, the surgeon advances a small drill to the L5 end plate and drills open the cortex. A trilator (blunt measuring rod), advanced partially into the L5 vertebra, compacts the bone around the L5 channel rather than drilling it out (**Fig. 109.5d**). Trilator measurements taken from this rod determine the lengths of the L5 and the S1 segments of the device; the device is assembled before insertion. After the 12-mm cannula is removed, the larger two-piece inner and outer exchange cannula is advanced to the sacrum and secured with two fixation pins, thus securing the exchange cannula to the sacrum. The inner cannula of the exchange cannula is removed; the larger Steinmann pin is left in place. The preassembled device is advanced along the Steinmann pin into the sacrum, across the L5-S1 disk, and into the L5 vertebra.

The ideal position of the distal tip is three fourths of the distance from the L5 end plate at L5-S1 toward the end plate at the top of L5 at the L4–5 disk space. A small portion of the proximal rod should protrude from the sacrum. After device placement, the anti-torque and torque rods are inserted into it. Distraction of the disk space can be completed by rotating the torque wrench and visualizing distraction on the fluoroscope. After the torque rods are removed, insertion of a locking pin then completes the procedure.

Closure

The wound is irrigated, and a multilayered closure is performed. Dermabond is usually placed over the incision.

Surgical Technique for a Two-Level Presacral Approach

The two-level procedure is performed similarly to the one-level up to the packing of the L5-S1 disk space. Next, a 9.5-mm channel is drilled across the L5 vertebra into the L4-5 space and the L4-5 disc is evacuated with the cutters as was done for L5-S1.

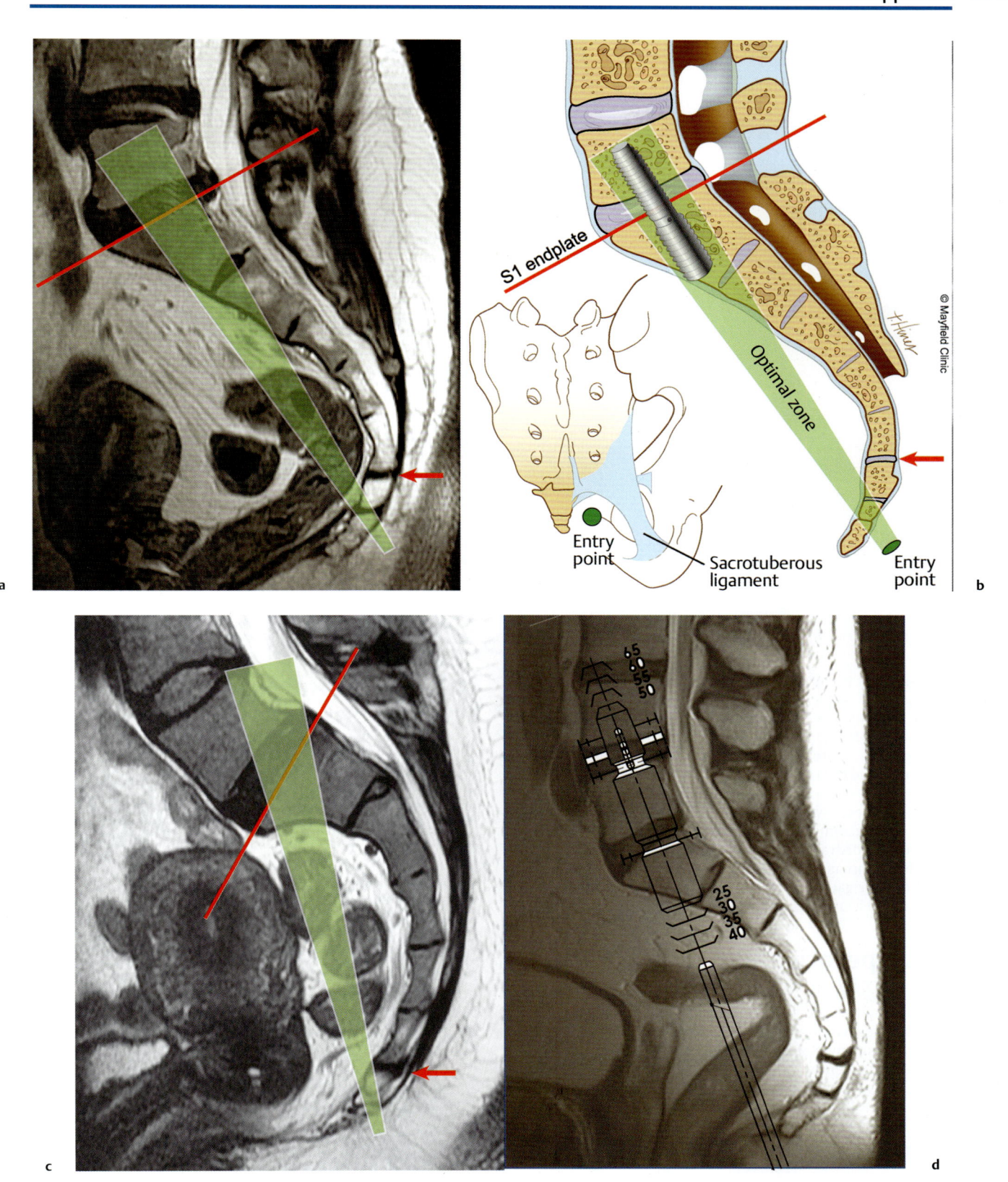

Fig. 109.3 Sacral anatomy and trajectory evaluation. **(a)** Typical sacrum and the trajectory for the approach perpendicular to the angle of the S1 end plate *(red line)*. **(b)** Illustration of the optimal zone *(green)* for placement of the axial rod and the entry point relative to the sacrococcygeal ligament and coccyx. **(c)** A hooked or hyperlordotic sacral curve has an unsatisfactory trajectory that would result in axial rod placement in the spinal canal; this is unsuitable for presacral fusion. **(d)** Template used to plan for a two-level trajectory through S1-L5-L4. (Courtesy of the Mayfield Clinic, Cincinnati, OH.)

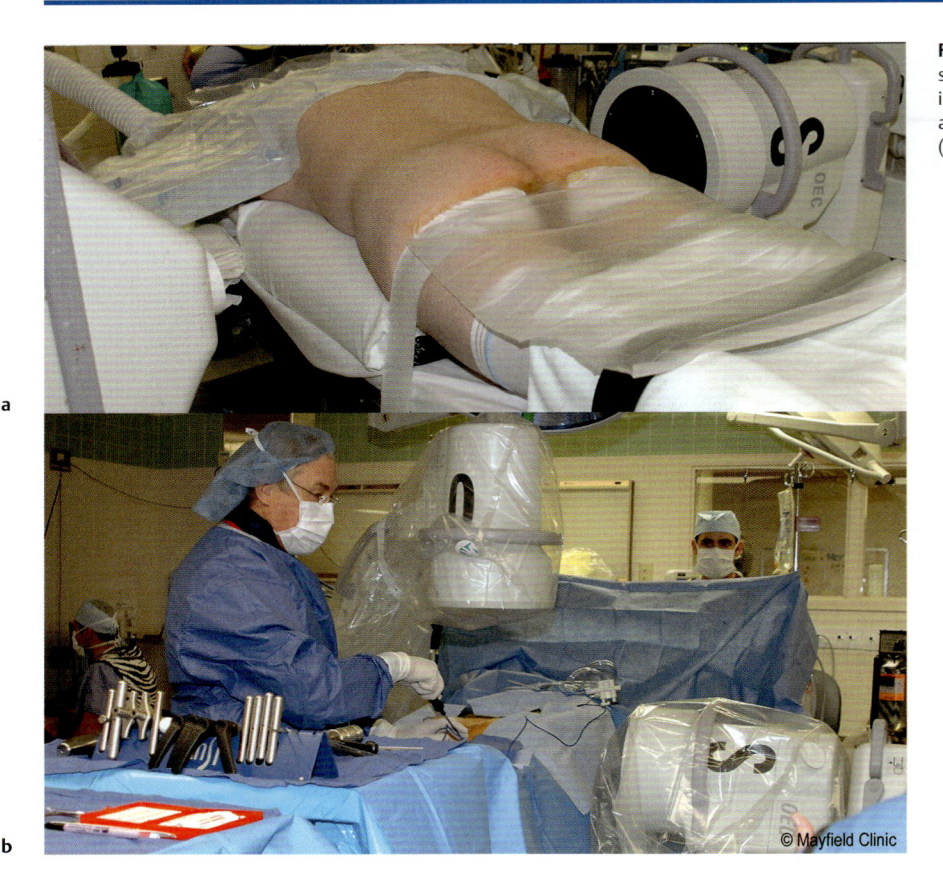

Fig. 109.4 Operating room setup for a presacral fusion. **(a)** Patient positioning and draping. **(b)** Two fluoroscopy units positioned in the anteroposterior (AP) and lateral projections. (Courtesy of the Mayfield Clinic, Cincinnati, OH.)

However, it is important to exercise caution with the cutting instruments at L4 because access in the space is often far anterior at the annulus; the instrument could sweep anteriorly into the space where the aorta and vena cava lie. The L4-5 disk is packed with grafting material. The end plate of L4 is opened with a small drill and the trilator is passed into L4. The two-level device is composed of an L4-L5 segment and S1 segment. Measurements for these two components are similar to the L5-S1 technique. After assembly, the two-level rod is inserted in the same manner, but distraction can only be applied at L5-S1.

The Steinmann pins and exchange cannula are removed. The wound is irrigated, a multilayered closure is performed, and Dermabond is usually placed over the incision.

Postoperative Care

Pain management is routine and with the intent of rapid mobilization. Attention is paid to bowel and bladder management. The paracoccygeal wound and rectum are inspected; in the rare circumstance of any bloody discharge from the rectum, immediate evaluation is required.

Potential Complications and Precautions

The refinements discussed above regarding patient selection, operative technique, the device itself, and radiographic assessments can help in avoiding complications.[19–22] At times, an alternative technique may be needed to achieve interbody lumbar fusion in the event of pseudarthrosis after AxiaLIF.[23]

The complications operatively or immediately after surgery that are of most concern are bowel and vascular injury. Profuse bleeding is rare, especially when preoperative evaluation of the vasculature shows no vascular anomalies. Despite this, brisk venous bleeding can occur while drilling out the sacral channel during the diskectomy. Placement of the device tamponades the bleeding from the sacrum. Making certain that a small portion of the device protrudes from the sacrum adds another point of cortical fixation and seals off any further sacral bleeding. Compression by Flo-Seal or Gelfoam against the sacral entry point can effectively stop bleeding. In the rare event of continued bleeding or development of cardiovascular instability, an emergent vascular consultation is indicated.

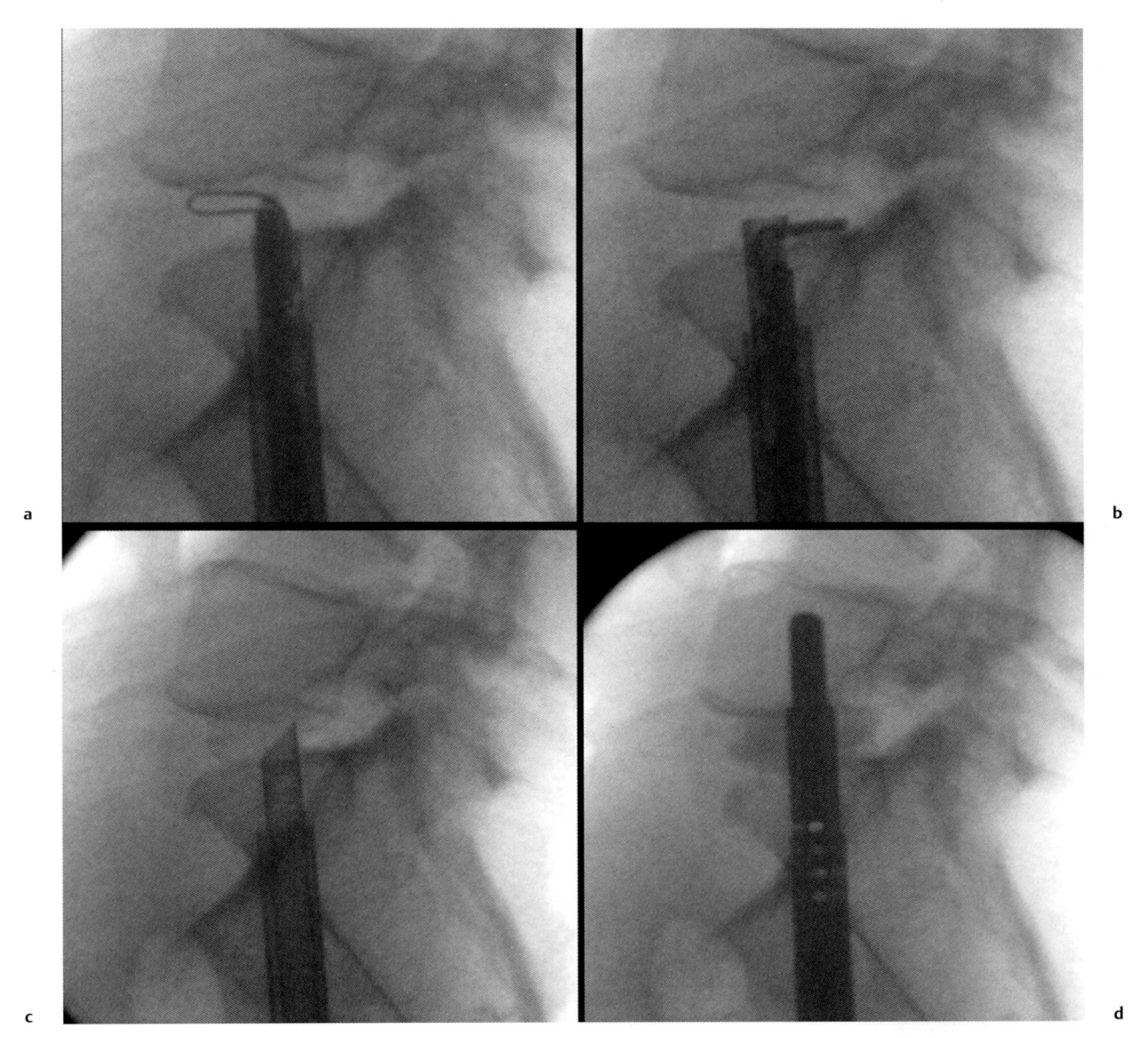

Fig. 109.5 Sequential intraoperative images that show the loop cutter **(a)**, flat cutter **(b)**, beveled bone graft inserter **(c)**, and trilator **(d)** in place. The notches enable direct measurement of the implant to be placed. (Courtesy of the Mayfield Clinic, Cincinnati, OH.)

If bowel perforation occurs, it can present as rectal bleeding, blood in the rectal aspirate, or demonstration of a fistula after contrast injection, and should prompt a consultation with a colorectal surgeon in the operating room. A rectal tear can be primarily repaired under direct visualization with a rigid scope. A small perforation may be treated medically if advised by the colorectal consultant. Immediate recognition and treatment of a bowel perforation can avoid the serious consequences of developing a presacral abscess or peritonitis and the need for a diverting colostomy. Prompt recognition of a bowel perforation can avoid these delayed complications, and importantly, the possible infection that would require removal of the hardware. Such safeguards have reduced the risk of bowel perforation to < 1%.[18]

Clinical Cases

Clinical case examples illustrate the considerations of the transsacral procedure as follows: spondylolisthesis at L5-S1 (**Fig. 109.6**); degenerative disk disease at L5-S1 with long-term follow up (**Fig. 109.7**); and painful pseudarthrosis after ALIF (**Fig. 109.8**).

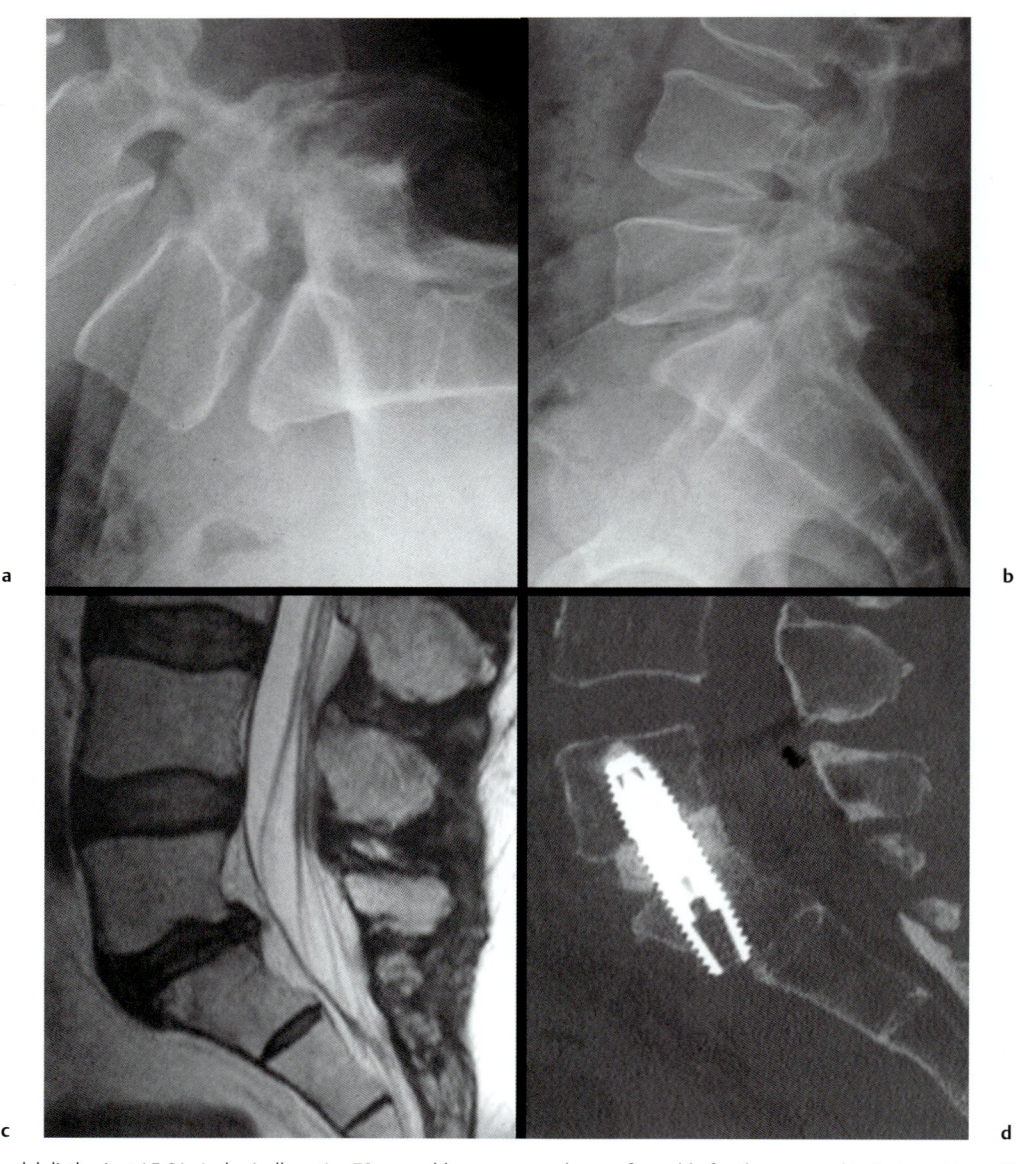

Fig. 109.6 Spondylolisthesis at L5-S1. A physically active 73-year-old man presented with a 1-year history of progressive back and lower extremity pain. The pain radiated into his left calf and heel, and worsened with standing and walking. Physical therapy and two epidural steroid injections brought no lasting relief. Mobility of the spine was normal; neurologic examination demonstrated no deficits. *Imaging findings:* flexion **(a)** and extension **(b)** views demonstrated a mobile spondylolisthesis at L5-S1 and a normal sacral curve favorable for the presacral trajectory. Magnetic resonance imaging (MRI) findings were nearly normal **(c)**. A presacral fusion was performed at L5-S1 with placement of bilateral pedicle screws at L5-S1 and posterior facetectomy at L5-S1 on the right side. *Outcome:* postoperative computed tomography (CT) **(d)** shows ideal device placement, realignment, good lordosis, and full packing of the disk space. (Courtesy of the Mayfield Clinic, Cincinnati, OH.)

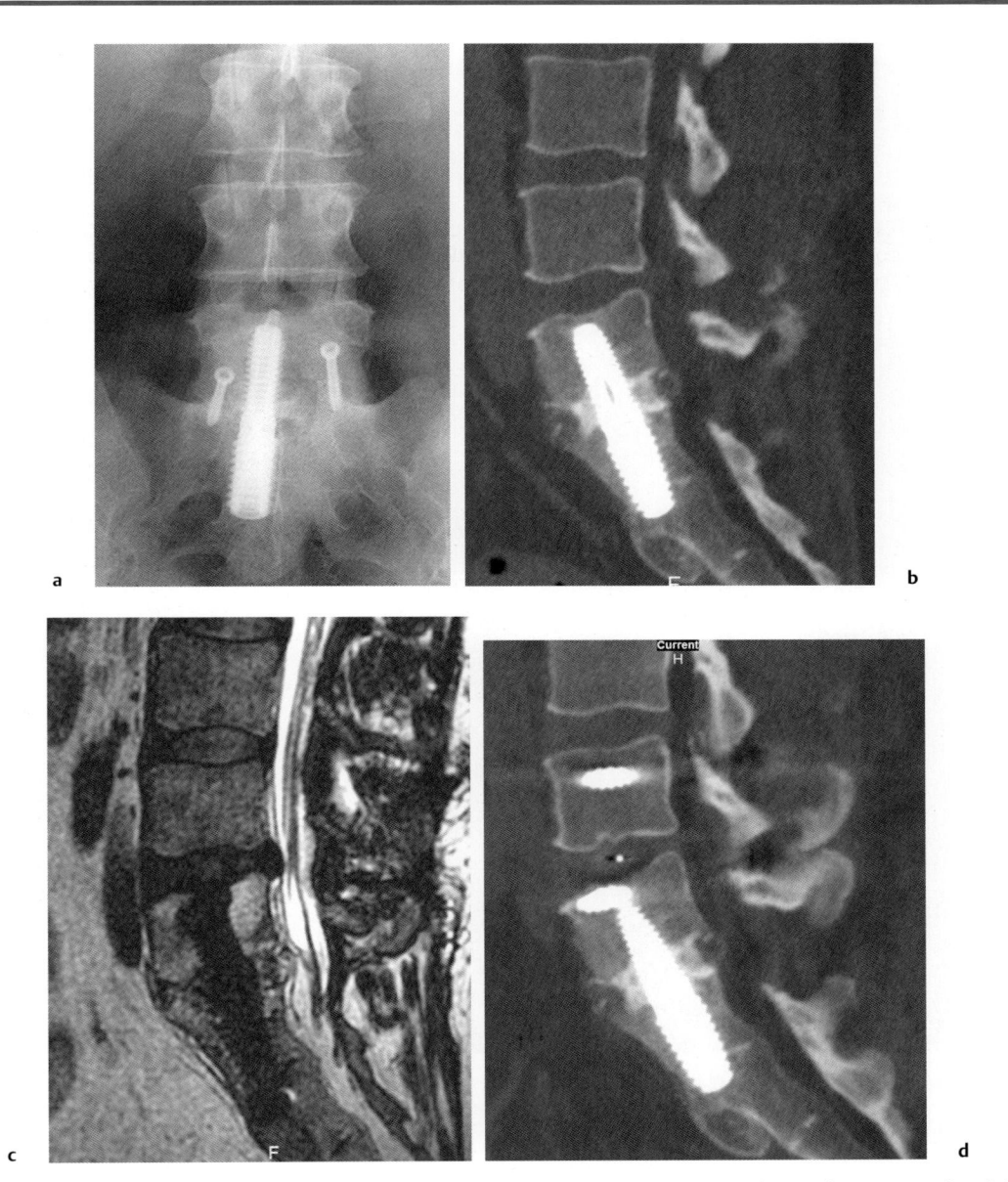

Fig. 109.7 Long-term follow-up after a presacral fusion for degenerative disk disease at L5-S1. A 29-year-old woman presented in 2008 with a third-time noncompressive recurrent disk herniation at L5-S1, located centrally and left sided. Marked degenerative changes were seen at L5-S1. She was too disabled to work or perform physical activities because of mechanical back pain that failed conservative care. No mechanical restriction was found on straight leg raise; she had absent ankle reflex but no motor or sensory deficits. Presacral fusion included posterior stabilization with percutaneously placed facet screws. **(a)** AP image showing the presacral device and facet screws for treatment of an L5-S1 degenerative disk. Surgery was uncomplicated; recovery was excellent, with return to work and all of her activities, including bowling. *Imaging at 6-year follow-up:* with new-onset back and left lower extremity pain, MRI showed a broad disk herniation at L4–5 above the level of the presacral fusion **(c)**. CT images showed solid fusion of the L5-S1 segment with the presacral device and facet screws, specifically a solid arthrodesis with ectopic bone formation in the presacral space, which was asymptomatic **(b)**. Adjacent L4-L5 segment was successfully treated with a transforaminal lumbar interbody fusion (TLIF) and pedicle screw fixation; hardware from the presacral fusion was not removed **(d)**. (Courtesy of the Mayfield Clinic, Cincinnati, OH.)

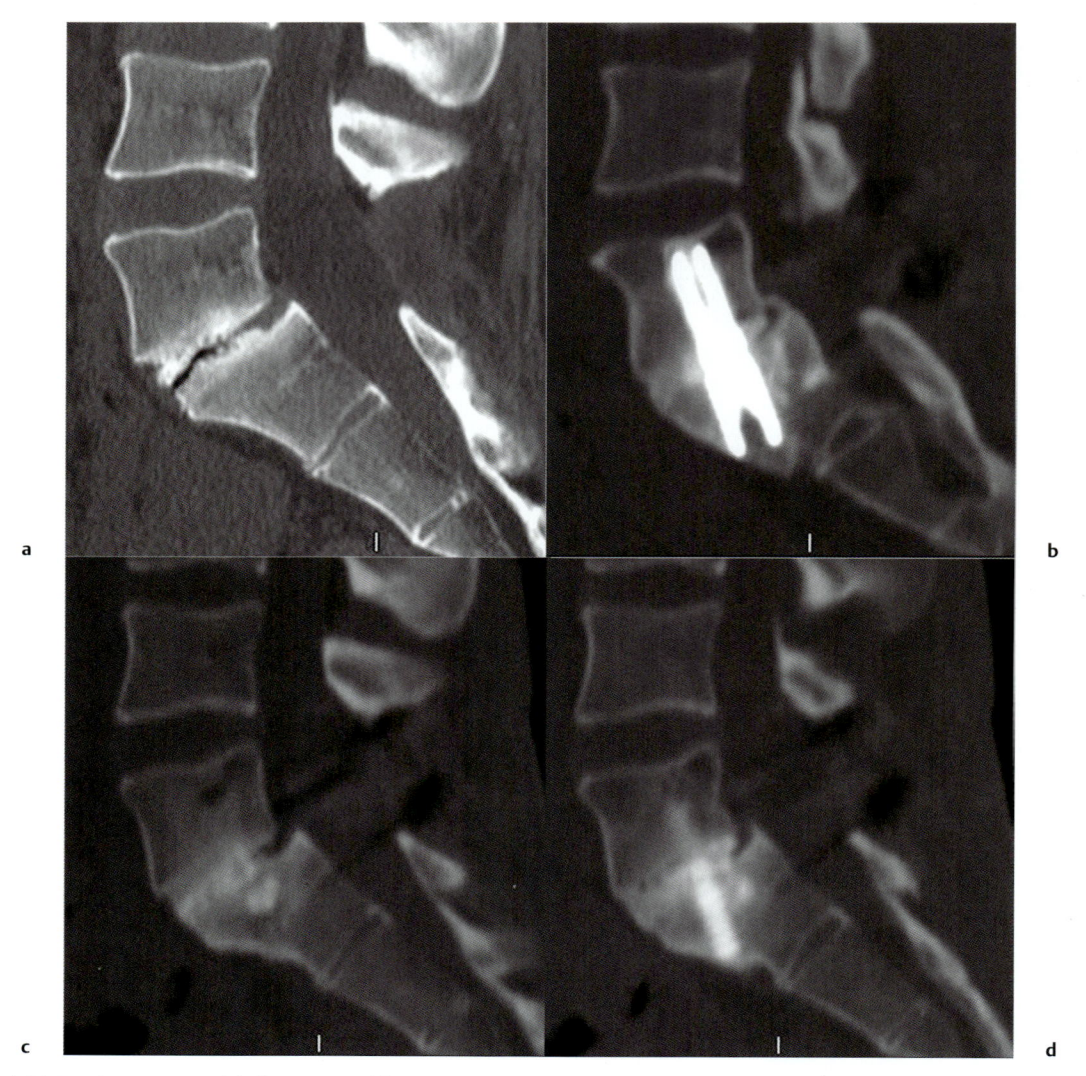

Fig. 109.8 AxiaLIF revision surgery. **(a)** This 42-year-old man presented with painful pseudarthrosis after undergoing anterior lumbar interbody fusion (ALIF) with structural allograft. AxiaLIF revision surgery was performed. **(b–d)** Postoperative CT images at 1-year follow-up demonstrate solid arthrodesis. (Courtesy of the Mayfield Clinic, Cincinnati, OH.)

Conclusion

In the 10 years and nearly 14,000 procedures since its introduction, the transsacral approach is now well understood in terms of risk and outcome profile, especially for one-level fusions. More comprehensive understanding of the two-level fusion is under further investigation. The transsacral operation is technically demanding and requires strict adherence to proper technique to minimize adverse events. Improved technique, careful patient selection, and introduction of other safeguards have decreased the risks; the risk of the most concerning complication—bowel perforation—has been reduced to < 1%. This procedure is particularly well suited for patients with spondylolisthesis and obesity. This minimally invasive procedure can be performed in the ambulatory setting and offers distinct benefits, notably minimizing damage to muscular, neural, ligamentous, and vascular structures.

References

1. Cragg A, Carl A, Casteneda F, Dickman C, Guterman L, Oliveira C. New percutaneous access method for minimally invasive anterior lumbosacral surgery. J Spinal Disord Tech 2004;17:21–28
2. Marotta N, Cosar M, Pimenta L, Khoo LT. A novel minimally invasive presacral approach and instrumentation technique for anterior L5-S1 intervertebral discectomy and fusion: technical description and case presentations. Neurosurg Focus 2006;20:E9
3. Tobler WD, Ferrara LA. The presacral retroperitoneal approach for axial lumbar interbody fusion: a prospective study of clinical outcomes, complications and fusion rates at a follow-up of two years in 26 patients. J Bone Joint Surg Br 2011;93:955–960
4. Ledet EH, Tymeson MP, Salerno S, Carl AL, Cragg A. Biomechanical evaluation of a novel lumbosacral axial fixation device. J Biomech Eng 2005;127:929–933
5. Ledet EH, Carl AL, Cragg A. Novel lumbosacral axial fixation techniques. Expert Rev Med Devices 2006;3:327–334

6. Lindley EM, McCullough MA, Burger EL, Brown CW, Patel VV. Complications of axial lumbar interbody fusion. J Neurosurg Spine 2011;15:273–279
7. Gebauer G, Anderson DG. Complications of minimally invasive lumbar spine surgery. Semin Spine Surg 2011;23:114–122
8. Botolin S, Agudelo J, Dwyer A, Patel V, Burger E. High rectal injury during trans-1 axial lumbar interbody fusion L5-S1 fixation: a case report. Spine 2010;35:E144–E148
9. Hofstetter CP, Shin B, Tsiouris AJ, Elowitz E, Härtl R. Radiographic and clinical outcome after 1- and 2-level transsacral axial interbody fusion: clinical article. J Neurosurg Spine 2013;19:454–463
10. Marchi L, Oliveira L, Coutinho E, Pimenta L. Results and complications after 2-level axial lumbar interbody fusion with a minimum 2-year follow-up. J Neurosurg Spine 2012;17:187–192
11. Tobler WD, Gerszten PC, Bradley WD, Raley TJ, Nasca RJ, Block JE. Minimally invasive axial presacral L5-S1 interbody fusion: two-year clinical and radiographic outcomes. Spine 2011;36:E1296–E1301
12. Bohinski RJ, Jain VV, Tobler WD. Presacral retroperitoneal approach to axial lumbar interbody fusion: a new, minimally invasive technique at L5-S1: Clinical outcomes, complications, and fusion rates in 50 patients at 1-year follow-up. SAS J 2010;4:54–62
13. Mazur MD, Duhon BS, Schmidt MH, Dailey AT. Rectal perforation after AxiaLIF instrumentation: case report and review of the literature. Spine J 2013;13:e29–e34
14. Whang PG, Sasso RC, Patel VV, Ali RM, Fischgrund JS. Comparison of axial and anterior interbody fusions of the L5-S1 segment: a retrospective cohort analysis. J Spinal Disord Tech 2013;26:437–443
15. Hussain NS, Perez-Cruet MJ. Complication management with minimally invasive spine procedures. Neurosurg Focus 2011;31:E2
16. Tender GC, Miller LE, Block JE. Percutaneous pedicle screw reduction and axial presacral lumbar interbody fusion for treatment of lumbosacral spondylolisthesis: A case series. J Med Case Reports 2011;5:454
17. Bartolozzi P, Sandri A, Cassini M, Ricci M. One-stage posterior decompression-stabilization and trans-sacral interbody fusion after partial reduction for severe L5-S1 spondylolisthesis. Spine 2003;28:1135–1141
18. Gundanna MI, Miller LE, Block JE. Complications with axial presacral lumbar interbody fusion: A 5-year postmarketing surveillance experience. SAS J 2011;5:90–94
19. Issack PS, Kotwal SY, Boachie-Adjei O. The axial transsacral approach to interbody fusion at L5-S1. Neurosurg Focus 2014;36:E8
20. Whang PG, Sasso RC, Patel VV, Ali RM, Fischgrund JS. Comparison of axial and anterior interbody fusions of the L5-S1 segment: a retrospective cohort analysis. J Spinal Disord Tech 2013;26:437–443
21. Tobler WD, Melgar MA, Raley TJ, Anand N, Miller LE, Nasca RJ. Clinical and radiographic outcomes with L4-S1 axial lumbar interbody fusion (AxiaLIF) and posterior instrumentation: a multicenter study. Med Devices (Auckl) 2013;6:155–161
22. Zeilstra DJ, Miller LE, Block JE. Axial lumbar interbody fusion: a 6-year single-center experience. Clin Interv Aging 2013;8:1063–1069
23. Louwerens JK, Groot D, van Duijvenbode DC, Spruit M. Alternative surgical strategy for AxiaLIF pseudarthrosis: A series of three case reports. Evid Based Spine Care J 2013;4:143–148

110 Repair of Cerebrospinal Fluid Leaks

Reid Hoshide, Erica Feldman, and William R. Taylor

Lumbar cerebrospinal fluid (CSF) leaks are usually a result of spontaneous dural rupture, iatrogenic durotomy, or dural injuries from traumatic fractures of the spine.[1,2] The potential consequences of durotomies can be very serious, and include durocutaneous fistula formation, arachnoiditis, and infection.[3-6] When a durotomy is encountered intraoperatively, it is important to achieve a meticulous dural closure. However, many durotomies often go unnoticed intraoperatively, and can present in the immediate postoperative period with the appearance of CSF seeping from the wound, high quantities of drain output with the consistency of CSF, or symptoms of low-pressure headaches from a pseudomeningocele formation.[7] There are nonoperative and operative options for the management of posterior lumbar CSF leaks; this chapter discusses the operative options.

Patient Selection

- Patients who have demonstrated symptomatic or clinical evidence of CSF leaks, and who have failed, or are contraindicated for, conservative management

Indications

- Symptomatic CSF leak (unremitting low-pressure postural headaches, CSF seeping through the surgical wound, abscess formation or infection)

Contraindications

- Surgical instability due to comorbid medical problems that require medical optimization first

Objectives of Surgery

- Closure of the dural defect
- Meticulous closure of the soft tissues layers (especially the fascial layer) superficial to the dural defect

Advantages

- Surgical, immediate correction of CSF leak
- Prevention of durocutaneous fistula formation
- Prevention of infection secondary to external CSF communication

Disadvantages

- Surgical morbidity compared with nonoperative management
- May require extension of the previous site of surgical access

Choice of Operative Approach

Approach to a posterior lumbar CSF leak should be centered around the area of known violation (from a fracture, operative site, etc.). A midline incision is used to dissect down to the bony structures in a relatively bloodless plane, and judicious removal of the bony and ligamentous elements reveals the CSF leak without compromising structural stability.

Preoperative Testing and Imaging

- The usual preoperative laboratories and tests to evaluate surgical and anesthetic morbidity
- If a CSF leak is suspected, a β-transferrin test on the expressible fluid can be used to determine the presence of CSF.
- Computed tomography (CT), myelography, or magnetic resonance imaging (MRI) may be useful in determining the proposed site of dural violation if related to trauma or spontaneous rupture.

Surgical Procedure

Preoperative planning entails determining the size and magnitude of the dural defect. A wide surgical exposure of the dural defect needs to be obtained in order to completely identify the defect and to achieve its closure, as an optimal dural closure would be hindered by ligament or bony elements. Therefore, we advocate a wide exposure the provides an adequate view and enables the repair of the dural defect while being mindful of structural stability. Because many of these dural repairs are likely to be revision surgeries, it is also important to begin the approach dissection with the normal cranial-caudal anatomy to safely build a plane of identifiable structures and then to approach the site of previous surgery where such structure might no longer exist. This technique is useful in preventing the propagation of further dural or neural injuries.

There are several suturing techniques for primary dural closure. Several studies have shown no statistical difference in primary repair of leaks when comparing a continuous locking suture versus interrupted sutures placed 1.0 to 1.4 mm apart.[8] The choice of suture, however, was found to have a statistically significant difference on primary repair leaks; 6-0 Prolene sutures were superior to 5-0 Surgilon sutures owing to differences in the needle's bore diameter. The 6-0 Prolene suture needle is only 0.12 mm larger in bore than the thread diameter, whereas the 5-0 Surgilon's needle is 0.20 mm larger in bore than its thread diameter.[8] Some institutions favor the use of 6-0 Gore-Tex for certain properties: monofilamentous suture reducing bacterial wicking, very little structural memory, and the availability of a suture with the ratio of the needle diameter to thread diameter of 1:1.

The use of titanium clips is the latest technique for primary dural closure. The ease and rapidity of clip application makes it an appealing alternative to suturing, especially in a surgical field where suture placement can be difficult and cumbersome. The cost of the titanium clips and the presence of metal artifact on postoperative imaging are a few of the drawbacks associated with clipping a durotomy. No powerful studies to date have compared its clinical benefit with that of other dural closure techniques.

Using a fat or fascial graft for a dural repair has many advantages, as it utilizes the body's native tissue for repair, ensuring that there is no adverse reaction to foreign substances in the body. Also, fat or fascial grafts are useful in situations where dural substitutes are not available or economically feasible. Fascial grafts can sometimes be harvested from the tensor fascia lata or the surgical wound itself. However, caution must be taken with surgical-site fascia harvesting, as this may compromise approximation of the fascia during wound closure, which is important in maintaining a leak-free closure. Harvesting fascia from the tensor fascia lata risks causing weakness in leg abduction. Another disadvantage of fat and fascial grafts is that a second surgical wound may be needed for harvesting.

Fibrin glues in the market have been Food and Drug Administration (FDA) approved as hemostatic agents, but their coagulative properties have been used off-label as a means of sealing dura. Animal models have demonstrated the safety and efficacy of fibrin glues, but there have been no human studies to date.

Polymerizing sealants can also be used as adjuncts to primary closures of dural repairs. The most common sealant is a mixture of polyethylene glycol and trilysine amine, which polymerizes when the two compounds are mixed. These sealants occupy spaces in which primary closure was insufficient, and eventually dissolve in 4 to 8 weeks. Contraindications for its use include the presence of a CSF diversion system (ventriculoperitoneal shunt, lumboperitoneal shunt, or lumbar drain), and extra caution must be exercised when this sealant is placed in a confined area, owing to its expansible properties. There have been case reports in the literature of compression on the spinal cord, causing quadriparesis and cauda equina syndrome following its use in cervical and lumbar surgeries, respectively.[9,10]

When primary closure of a durotomy cannot be achieved due to retraction of the dura, shrinkage of the dura from desiccation or cautery, or large dural defects, dural substitutes can be used as a patch-graft for these defects. Collagenous dura substitutes induce very little inflammatory response, produce little or no adhesions to the spinal structures below, prevent CSF leakage, and are no more susceptible to infection than other forms of patch grafting.[11] Collagen dural matrices seal CSF leaks within 4 to 8 hours after surgery, promote fibroblast proliferation within 3 to 4 days, and becomes fully incorporated into the dura within 14 days after surgery. Theoretically, the use of postoperative steroids arrests the process of fibroblast proliferation and incorporation; therefore, avoidance of postoperative steroids is recommended. Although some manufacturers claim that their dural substitutes do not need to be sutured down, we recommend as close to a watertight suture with the dural substitutes as possible.

Following any repair, the dural closure can be tested by requesting a Valsalva maneuver of 40 mm H_2O pressure from the anesthesia team. Any evidence of leaks should prompt the surgeon to bolster the current closure.

Postoperative Care

Diverting CSF away from the durotomy via lumbar drainage is a useful, though not mandatory, technique for facilitating spontaneous dural and wound healing. Following 3 to 5 days of lumbar drainage at 10 cc per hour, a weaning process should be made over several days with careful attention to the surgical wound, monitoring for any leakage of CSF. Any evidence of a seeping wound would be an indication for reopening the lumbar drain for a prolonged drainage period, or even considering permanent lumbar-peritoneal shunting.

A subfascial wound drain for diversion of CSF is controversial and widely debated in the literature.[12–14] The mechanism of a subfascial drain diverts CSF away from the healing muscle and soft tissue layers. Thus, the muscle and soft tissue layers heal into a watertight seal that would otherwise be patent by the constant egress of CSF. Subfascial drains can also eliminate dead space, preventing the accommodation of CSF collection. Negative suction of a subfascial drain is discouraged because facilitating CSF flow through the durotomy prevents dural healing. Similar to the use of lumbar drains, some institutions favor a weaning process by which the subfascial drain is clamped and the surgical wound is monitored for leaking before committing to discontinuing the drain. The risk of durocutaneous fistula formation from subfascial drains, which had been hypothesized by some authors, has been disproven.[15]

It is important to reduce other factors that can violate the integrity of the dural closure or increase intrathecal pressure. Immediately following surgery, the dural repair should be discussed with the anesthesia team, to ensure that the team is aware of the importance of a careful extubation to prevent intrathecal pressure elevation with violent coughs and vomiting. In the recovery period, vomiting can be controlled by steroids or antiemetics, and the surgeon should have a low threshold to prescribe antiemetics to stay ahead of vomiting episodes postoperatively. Cough suppressants and antitussives should also be utilized. Pain control is also important. Pain may lead to writhing, which can increase intrathecal pressure; therefore, adequate pain control should be provided in the form of opioids and antispasmodics. Caffeine or theophylline may be used if the patient has what appear to be postural headaches secondary to intracranial venodilation from CSF hypovolemia. The common adverse effect of constipation from use of opioid medications can raise intrathecal pressures if the patient is straining to have a bowel movement. Aggressive bowel regimens to include laxatives, stool softeners, and even more aggressive measures like enemas should be considered in the postoperative period. Flat-in-bed positioning to reduce the hydrostatic tension on the dural repair may be contraindicated in patients with positional orthopnea, and can be cumbersome for meals and rehabilitation.

The utilization of prophylactic antibiotics has not been well substantiated in the context of spinal CSF leaks. However, the prophylactic use of antibiotics (cefazolin or vancomycin) while a lumbar or a subfascial drain is present is essential.

When all nonoperative maneuvers and CSF diversionary techniques have failed or have been deemed contraindicated, a reoperation to explore and to repair the dural violation should be performed.

Potential Complications and Precautions

As mentioned above, a surgical approach to a CSF leak following a previous lumbar surgery should be taken with extreme caution so as not to cause further dural and neural injuries from the postsurgical sites where normal anatomic features may no longer exist. We recommend starting the approach from normal anatomy in the cranial-caudal dimension, and working toward the previous surgical site to build planes from normal anatomy to abnormal, postsurgical anatomy.

In the case of the traumatic dural violation from a spine fracture, the surgeon should anticipate the materials and procedures required to address the fracture if instability is a concern. This may include surgical instrumentation and operating room staffing.

In the setting of a suspected infection, wound cultures should be sent to the lab for analysis, and antibiotics should be held preoperatively, if tolerated, to increase diagnostic yield. Once culture specimens are obtained, empiric antibiotics should be started without delay.

Conclusion

Durotomies are encountered many times in lumbar spine surgery. Early identification and anticipation of CSF leaks can prevent the long-term, and often morbid, sequelae of chronic CSF leaks. When conservative management fails or is deemed contraindicated, surgical correction is essential in rectifying this common problem.

References

1. Schievink WI, Meyer FB, Atkinson JL, Mokri B. Spontaneous spinal cerebrospinal fluid leaks and intracranial hypotension. J Neurosurg 1996;84:598–605
2. Bosacco SJ, Gardner MJ, Guille JT. Evaluation and treatment of dural tears in lumbar spine surgery: a review. Clin Orthop Relat Res 2001;389:238–247
3. Verner EF, Musher DM. Spinal epidural abscess. Med Clin North Am 1985;69:375–384
4. Tosun B, Ilbay K, Kim MS, Selek O. Management of persistent cerebrospinal fluid leakage following thoraco-lumbar surgery. Asian Spine J 2012;6:157–162
5. Koo J, Adamson R, Wagner FC Jr, Hrdy DB. A new cause of chronic meningitis: infected lumbar pseudomeningocele. Am J Med 1989;86:103–104
6. Ruban D, O'Toole JE. Management of incidental durotomy in minimally invasive spine surgery. Neurosurg Focus 2011;31:E15
7. Mokri B, Hunter SF, Atkinson JL, Piepgras DG. Orthostatic headaches caused by CSF leak but with normal CSF pressures. Neurology 1998;51:786–790
8. Dafford EE, Anderson PA. Comparison of dural repair techniques. Spine J 2015;15:1099–1105
9. Lee SH, Park CW, Lee SG, Kim WK. Postoperative cervical cord compression induced by hydrogel dural sealant (DuraSeal®). Korean J Spine 2013;10:44–46
10. Thavarajah D, De Lacy P, Hussain R, Redfern RM. Postoperative cervical cord compression induced by hydrogel (DuraSeal): a possible complication. Spine 2010;35:E25–E26
11. Costa BS, Cavalcanti-Mendes GdeA, Abreu MS, Sousa AA. Clinical experience with a novel bovine collagen dura mater substitute. Arq Neuropsiquiatr 2011;69:217–220
12. Hughes SA, Ozgur BM, German M, Taylor WR. Prolonged Jackson-Pratt drainage in the management of lumbar cerebrospinal fluid leaks. Surg Neurol 2006;65:410–414, discussion 414–415
13. Ösün A, Samancıoğlu A, Aydın T, Mutlucan UO, Korkmaz M, Özkan U. Managing The Cerebrospinal Fluid Leaks After Spinal Surgery By Prolonged Subfascial Drainage. J Neurol Sci Turish 2013;30:748–755
14. Patel VV, Patel A, Harrop JS, Burger E. Spine Surgery Basics. New York: Springer; 2013
15. Wang JC, Bohlman HH, Riew KD. Dural tears secondary to operations on the lumbar spine. Management and results after a two-year-minimum follow-up of eighty-eight patients. J Bone Joint Surg Am 1998;80:1728–1732

111 Lumboperitoneal Shunt

Sergei Terterov, Dustin M. Harris, and Marvin Bergsneider

Background

The lumboperitoneal shunt (LPS) provides diversion of cerebrospinal fluid (CSF) from the lumbar intrathecal space to the peritoneal cavity. In general, the LPS is considered in conditions in which there is a free communication between the intracranial ventricular and cisternal CSF compartments and the spinal subarachnoid space. Drainage from the spinal subarachnoid space, in principle, entails drainage of CSF from both those compartments. Worldwide, the LPS operation constitutes less than 5% of CSF shunting procedures, with most neurosurgeons favoring ventricular-based CSF shunts. Although the LPS has its proponents and specific indications, there appears to be a general consensus that it has a higher obstruction rate compared with ventricular shunts, is technically more difficult to place, is less versatile, and poses challenges in regard to the use of adjustable valves. For the appropriately selected patient, however, an LPS can offer advantages over the ventricular counterpart.

Patient Selection

The LPS can be considered for any condition in which CSF diversion is required, with the exception of disorders in which there is the potential for craniocaudal brain herniation. The most common conditions for LPS are as follows:

- *Communicating hydrocephalus.* Conceptually, drainage from the spinal intrathecal compartment in so-called communicating hydrocephalus states could have some advantages. Most reported series of the LPS involve the setting of normal pressure hydrocephalus (NPH). In a small retrospective series of 33 NPH patients treated with an LPS incorporating a horizontal-vertical valve, Bloch and McDermott[1] reported clinical improvement in gait, relief of incontinence, and improvement in memory as 100%, 46%, and 55%, respectively. With a mean follow-up of 19 months, however, the revision rate was 27% with an average time to failure of 11 months. In our practice, we consider using an LPS for communicating hydrocephalus in patients in whom ventricular cannulation carries additional risk, such as patients with poorly controlled seizures, scalp wound issues, or intracranial lesions that limit optimal ventricular catheter placement.
- *Idiopathic intracranial hypertension (IIH), or pseudotumor cerebri.* CSF diversion can be challenging in IIH patients secondary to small or slit-like ventricle size. Even if a well-placed ventricular catheter can be technically achieved, ventricular CSF drainage can lead to further ventricular collapse with resultant intermittent or permanent underdrainage/obstruction. The LPS carries its own technical challenges generally secondary to morbid obesity with most IIH patients. This can result in difficulty cannulating the intrathecal space, accessing the peritoneal space in the lateral body position, and assessing the patency of the shunt. In our experience, shunt patency becomes an automatic concern for patients with any return or continuance of headache symptoms, leading to frequent office or emergency room visits. Nuclear medicine shunt studies and lumbar puncture opening pressures can provide unreliable indicators of shunt failure. In one study by Eggenberger et al[2] of IIH patients undergoing the placement of an LPS, the authors reported that all of the patients had resolution of their symptoms while the shunt was functioning. However, 56% of the cohort required at least one shunt revision, with the number of revisions ranging from 1 to 13. El-Saadany et al[3] reported an LPS revision rate of ~ 30% at 1 year for IIH.
- *Slit-ventricle syndrome (SVS).* The SVS shares some similarities with IIH with regard to technical challenges with shunt placement. In general, the underlying problem with SVS is craniocerebral disproportion, leading to chronic ventricular-shunt overdrainage. An LPS should be considered with caution, as many SVS patients have underlying aqueductal stenosis. Several series demonstrated the efficacy of LPS in the treatment of SVS, albeit with similarly poor mechanical obstruction profiles.[4,5] Some series describe a combined ventriculolumboperitoneal shunting approach for treating SVS because LPS preferentially drains the intracranial subarachnoid space.[6]
- *CSF leak and miscellaneous conditions.* Other indications for LPS include postoperative or traumatic pseudomeningoceles and refractory CSF leaks.[7] Bret et al[8] demonstrated resolution of CSF rhinorrhea in 80% of cases after LPS insertion. Appropriate caution should be taken with anterior cranial fossa CSF leaks treated with spinal CSF drainage with regard to the creation of tension pneumocephalus. In our view, the relatively high obstruction rate of the LPS is in some respects ideal for pseudomeningocele and CSF leak repairs, because the condition usually resolves prior to the time that the LPS fails, and therefore the patient is not left with the potential long-term complications of a working shunt. Lastly, LPS has been used in the setting of refractory syringomyelia, when the subarachnoid obstruction cannot be corrected.[9]

Advantages and Disadvantages

Although an LPS is a management option for the aforementioned conditions, it has some challenging and potentially unfavorable characteristics to consider. First is over-drainage of CSF. This can manifest as postural ("spinal") headaches, which can be quite problematic with LPS due to the long fluid column of the spinal canal in the upright position. To counteract this effect, we routinely use the Horizontal-Vertical (H-V) lumbar valve system (Integra Life Sciences, Plainsboro, NJ). In selected cases, adjustable valves are used, but with the knowledge that it will likely be difficult to change the settings once the system is implanted. Valves with traditional "anti-siphon" or "siphon control" devices will not function as designed because negative catheter intraluminal pressures are not generated with an LPS. The challenge arises from positioning an adjustable valve in a suitable area.[10] If placed over the thoracolumbar fascia, the valve may cause discomfort when the patient is sitting. Over the flank or abdomen, the valve may not be palpable due to the degree of overlying subcutaneous fat. If the valve is placed too superficially, skin breakdown is a risk. Lastly, the valve can easily flip upside down if not secured in place.

It has been theorized that "equal drainage" for the ventricular and cranial subarachnoid spaces would lessen the risk of subdural hematoma, but this has not been demonstrated by any clinical study. Patients with an LPS, particularly elderly ones, are at greater risk of subdural hematoma, and the risk is highest if a lower pressure valve is used. If the valve is carefully selected, subdural hematoma risk can be mitigated. Kamiryo et al,[11] in a retrospective study of 206 patients undergoing LPS for NPH, reported a 2% subdural hematoma rate.

As in all procedures involving implantable hardware, there is a risk of infection of the implanted system. That holds true for both VPS and LPS, and there does not seem to be evidence favoring one over another in this regard.

As noted previously, the LPS appears to carry a generally higher risk of obstruction than its ventricular counterpart. Various studies report a 30% failure rate of LPS at as early as 1 year. Overall, up to 90% of the implanted systems require revision for mechanical failure with long-term follow-up.[1,3,12] It is not clear why the LPS systems are more prone to mechanical failure than their ventricular counterparts.

The development of a secondary Chiari is a complication unique to the LPS.[13] It is seen more commonly in the pediatric population, with as much as 70% of the patients acquiring a radiographic Chiari, but only 5% requiring any treatment for it.[14] In the adult population, only 15% develop a radiographic Chiari, and only 30% of those require treatment.[15] If the Chiari is symptomatic, several options exist for its treatment, but the first step should be to convert the shunt to a ventriculoperitoneal shunt.

Preoperative Planning

There are several factors to consider prior to proceeding with operation. LPS is contraindicated in the following situations:

- Active infectious process involving the low back skin or peritoneum
- Obstructive hydrocephalus in which there is a cranial-caudal pressure gradient
- Existing Chiari malformation

It is technically difficult and relatively contraindicated in patients with history of lumbar fusions or extensive abdominal operations. In those cases, fluoroscopic guidance may be required for accessing the thecal sac, and general surgery assistance may be required for accessing the peritoneum.

Technique

The patient is placed in the lateral decubitus position, with as much flexion as possible without obstructing access to the abdomen (Video 111.1). All pressure points are adequately padded. Three separate incisions are made: (1) for thecal sac access, (2) for peritoneal access, and (3) for placement of the valve in the flank area. A good general principle of shunt operations is that the valve and distal catheters should be situated in place prior to accessing the CSF compartment. If the CSF compartment is cannulated prematurely, then this catheter runs the risk of being damaged, dislodged, or even removed while the surgeon is tunneling and dissecting for the other shunt components. A second general principle is that the distal shunt component should be inserted as the last step, after the proximal catheter and valve have been secured and situated, so as to ensure that there is good spontaneous flow of CSF. Lack of flow typically indicates a kinked catheter or other problem (such as a broken catheter, reversed valve, etc.).

The lumbar incision is vertical (parallel to the spinous processes) and either in the midline or slightly paramedian at the level of the L3-4 or L4-5 interspace, which roughly corresponds to the level of the iliac crest. A paramedian location decreases frictional wear of the catheter with the spinous processes. The incision is taken down to the level of the lumbosacral fascia.

The peritoneal cavity is accessed via a mini-laparotomy using a standard approach. In obese patients, care must be taken not to stray obliquely downward in the subcutaneous fat, missing the rectus fascia completely. At our center, laparoscopic bariatric surgeons have successfully accessed the peritoneum, although using caution because laparoscopic surgery is typically performed with the patient in the supine position.

We prefer to make the flank incision two fingerbreadths above the iliac crest. This incision has to be long enough to be able to anchor catheters on both sides of the H-V valve and accommodate the H-V valve so that it is in the vertical position when the patient is upright. A tunneler is used to pass the peritoneal catheter from the flank to the abdominal incision. The valve is secured to the subcutaneous fat with 2-0 silk sutures to ensure that the long axis of the valve is in line with the long axis of the patient. The peritoneal catheter is connected to the valve and secured with a 2-0 silk tie.

If the surgeon wishes to leave a tapping reservoir, this device is typically situated near the lumbar incision in a pocket.

A 14-gauge Tuohy needle is used to access the lumbar cistern, aiming medially toward midline and 30 to 45 degrees cephalad. Approximately 10 cm of catheter is advanced into the lumbar cistern, and then the needle is withdrawn, taking care not to lacerate the catheter with the sharp tip. The catheter is sutured to the lumbosacral fascia using a silicone butterfly suture clamp. Prior to placing the peritoneal catheter into the peritoneal cavity, the flow of CSF through the valve system is confirmed. All incisions are irrigated copiously with antibiotic irrigation and closed in layers in the standard fashion.

References

1. Bloch O, McDermott MW. Lumboperitoneal shunts for the treatment of normal pressure hydrocephalus. J Clin Neurosci 2012;19:1107–1111
2. Eggenberger ER, Miller NR, Vitale S. Lumboperitoneal shunt for the treatment of pseudotumor cerebri. Neurology 1996;46:1524–1530
3. El-Saadany WF, Farhoud A, Zidan I. Lumboperitoneal shunt for idiopathic intracranial hypertension: patients' selection and outcome. Neurosurg Rev 2012;35:239–243, discussion 243–244
4. Ide T, Aoki N, Miki Y. Slit ventricle syndrome successfully treated by a lumboperitoneal shunt. Neurol Res 1995;17:440–442

5. Le H, Yamini B, Frim DM. Lumboperitoneal shunting as a treatment for slit ventricle syndrome. Pediatr Neurosurg 2002;36:178–182
6. Khorasani L, Sikorski CW, Frim DM. Lumbar CSF shunting preferentially drains the cerebral subarachnoid over the ventricular spaces: implications for the treatment of slit ventricle syndrome. Pediatr Neurosurg 2004;40:270–276
7. Kitchen N, Bradford R, Platts A. Occult spinal pseudomeningocele following a trivial injury successfully treated with a lumboperitoneal shunt: a case report. Surg Neurol 1992;38:46–49
8. Bret P, Hor F, Huppert J, Lapras C, Fischer G. Treatment of cerebrospinal fluid rhinorrhea by percutaneous lumboperitoneal shunting: review of 15 cases. Neurosurgery 1985;16:44–47
9. Oluigbo CO, Thacker K, Flint G. The role of lumboperitoneal shunts in the treatment of syringomyelia. J Neurosurg Spine 2010;13:133–138
10. Kanazawa R, Ishihara S, Sato S, Teramoto A, Kuniyoshi N. Familiarization with lumboperitoneal shunt using some technical resources. World Neurosurg 2011;76:347–351
11. Kamiryo T, Hamada J, Fuwa I, Ushio Y. Acute subdural hematoma after lumboperitoneal shunt placement in patients with normal pressure hydrocephalus. Neurol Med Chir (Tokyo) 2003;43:197–200.
12. Karabatsou K, Quigley G, Buxton N, Foy P, Mallucci C. Lumboperitoneal shunts: are the complications acceptable? Acta Neurochir (Wien) 2004;146:1193–1197
13. Welch K, Shillito J, Strand R, Fischer EG, Winston KR. Chiari I "malformations"—an acquired disorder? J Neurosurg 1981;55:604–609
14. Chumas PD, Armstrong DC, Drake JM, et al. Tonsillar herniation: the rule rather than the exception after lumboperitoneal shunting in the pediatric population. J Neurosurg 1993;78:568–573
15. Johnston I, Jacobson E, Besser M. The acquired Chiari malformation and syringomyelia following spinal CSF drainage: a study of incidence and management. Acta Neurochir (Wien) 1998;140:417–427, discussion 427–428

112 Dorsal Rhizotomy of the Lumbosacral Nerve Roots for the Treatment of Spastic Diplegia in Cerebral Palsy Patients

Marc Sindou, George Georgoulis, and Andrei Brinzeu

Spasticity in diplegic (or quadriplegic) children affected with cerebral palsy (CP) is to a certain extent useful by compensating for the decrease in motor strength. But the spasticity may become excessive and consequently harmful. By limiting passive and active motion and in the extreme by leading to irreducible contractures and deformities, an excess of muscular tone contributes to further incapacity. When hyperspasticity becomes refractory to medical treatment and physical therapy, the recourse to functional neurosurgery may be justified. Besides intrathecal baclofen therapy or peripheral neurotomies when botulinum toxin injections prove insufficient, dorsal rhizotomy (DR) can be a valuable treatment.

The history of DR started in 1898, when Sherrington[1] demonstrated that division of the posterior roots reduced tone in decerebrate cats. On this basis, Foerster[2] applied the technique and in 1913 published his series of posterior root resections in 159 children with CP. The technique consisted of dividing the entire dorsal roots from L2 to S2, excluding the "antigravity root" L4. He used intraoperative electrical stimulation to identify segmental levels and to distinguish between ventral and dorsal roots. In the 1960s, Gros and coworkers[3] in Montpellier, France, separated the dorsal roots into rootlets and performed partial dorsal rhizotomies with nonselective sectioning of 80% of the rootlets of each root to limit postoperative sensory deficits.[3] Later, in the quest for rendering DR more selective in its topographic effects, the Montpellier school developed the "sectorial posterior rhizotomy."[4] After identifying the roots by their topographic muscular responses, sectioning was limited to the roots that corresponded to what the authors categorized as "handicapping" spasticity, as opposed to "useful" spasticity, which is the aspect of spasticity that maintains lower limbs in extension for antigravity.

In 1976, Fasano et al[5] in Turin, Italy, introduced a different concept of dorsal rhizotomy—the functional posterior rhizotomy—based on identification of abnormal muscular responses to electrical stimulation of roots and rootlets. Responses were categorized as abnormal when repetitive dorsal root and rootlets stimulation with a train at a frequency of 50 Hz and a duration of 1 second provoked sustained responses in the corresponding segmental muscles or the spread of response to other territories either ipsilaterally or contralaterally. In Fasano's original technique, the approach consisted of a limited laminotomy.

At the beginning of the 1980s, to achieve more precise identification of the whole lumbar and sacral rootlets, Peacock and Arens[6] and Abbott et al[7] extended the exposure to the entire cauda equina through an L1–S2 laminotomy. Exposure of the entire cauda equina became the most popular modality.[8,9] Extensive laminectomies or laminotomies (from L1-L2 to S1-S2) have the advantage of enabling the complete identification of the roots and rootlets of the entire cauda equina, but they also have the disadvantages of a long and painful postoperative period, and the risk of secondary spine kyphosis and instability. Therefore, it may be preferable to limit exposure to reduce invasiveness.

Limited Approaches

In the 1980s and 1990s we commonly used osteoplastic laminotomy limited to the T11, T12, and L1 vertebrae. Through this approach, the ventral and corresponding dorsal L2 and L3 roots can be reached just before they exit at their respective dural sheaths. The other (dorsal) lumbar and sacral roots/rootlets can be identified at their entry into the dorsolateral sulcus at the conus medullaris.[10] Root functions, in other words their topographical levels, are identified by their muscular responses to electrical stimulation.[11] Stimulation of the L2 ventral root elicits muscular response predominantly in the psoas-iliacus and the adductors, and stimulation of the L3 ventral root elicits muscular response predominantly in adductors and quadriceps. At the conus medullaris, the landmark between the S1 and the S2 medullary segments is located ~ 30 mm from the exit of the (tiny) coccygeal root from the conus.[11] The medullary segments S1, L5, and L4 can be identified according to their evoked motor responses after stimulation (in the triceps surae, extensors of the toes, dorsal flexor of the ankle and quadriceps, respectively). The roots for the bladder (S2-S3) or the anal sphincter (S3-S4) can be identified by cystometry or rectomanometry, or—for the latter—more simply by introducing a glove-protected finger into the anal canal or better by electromyography (EMG) recordings of anal sphincter activity. Usually, on average 60% of the total number of dorsal rootlets are cut. The quantity per root differs with respect to the root level and function and to its involvement in the (harmful) components of the spasticity. It is noteworthy, according to a study from our group, that after an overall 60% sectioning of the dorsal rootlets from L2 to S1(S2), the somatosensory evoked potentials (SSEPs) to tibial nerve stimulation are not altered at long-term postoperative control after DR.[12]

Park and coworkers[13,14] advocated a limited approach at the thoracolumbar junction. By their technique, which they called the "single-level immediately caudal to conus medullaris approach," at the T12-L1-L2 level, the dural sac is exposed. Localization of the conus and adjacent cauda equina are confirmed by an ultrasound probe through the exposed space. The conus appears hypoechogenic and cylindrical, and the cauda equina hyperechogenic and inhomogeneous. Once identification is completed, a single-level laminectomy, or more levels if necessary, is performed. After dural and arachnoid opening, the L1 and L2 roots are identified at the exit of their corresponding foramina. The dorsal root of L2 is separated from the ventral root and followed up to the conus. From the L2 dorsal root at the dorsolateral sulcus, the subjacent dorsal rootlets, from L3 to supposedly S2, are then progressively retracted medially, while being separated from their corresponding ventral roots. The latter are kept apart with a cottonoid placed over them. Then the S3 to S5 roots are identified at their exit from the most caudal part of the conus so that they are spared. The EMG examination is then undertaken at the individual levels of the rootlets, from L2 to S2.

We recently developed a modality that we have termed *keyhole interlaminar dorsal rhizotomy*. This approach has two main objectives:

1. To access the roots to be targeted individually at their exit from the intradural space to the corresponding dural sheath. That is where the dorsal root and ventral root are clearly distinguishable. Under direct vision, identification of the anatomic/topographic level can be precisely verified by electrical stimulation of the (ventral) root. Stimulation of the dorsal root can test its physiological implication in the harmful components of the spasticity and help quantify sectioning.
2. To respect the posterior structures of the spine as much as possible by performing interlaminar (IL) fenestrations in an attempt to reduce invasiveness. The IL fenestrations enable operative vision and maneuvers through the "keyhole" approach. The levels and the number of IL approaches are determined according to patients' clinical presentation and preoperative chart, thus achieving individually tailored surgery.

A detailed description of the procedure follows.

Indications

Before determining if a patient is appropriate for the procedure, the surgeon must discuss with the patient's family the objectives and limitations of the treatment. For diplegic children who are able to ambulate, generally with the so-called scheme of Little,[15] the goals are to improve functional status and autonomy, and prevent or stop the evolution of the deformities. For nonambulatory diplegic or quadriplegic children, the only realistic goal is to facilitate care, provide comfort, and ease pain.

The children most likely to benefit from DR are those with prominent spasticity rather than dystonia, dyskinesia or ataxia, and in whom spasticity limits function. DR is the procedure of choice for children with diplegia, with mild upper limb involvement, and age younger than 10 years **(Fig. 112.1)**. In diplegic patients the main muscles involved are the psoas-iliacus and adductors of thigh (whose corresponding roots are L2 and L3), hamstrings (L5, S1, and S2), triceps surae and tibialis posterioris (S1).

Determination of the appropriate time for surgery is often difficult in children with CP. Too early would be imprudent, as younger children still have the potential for developmental maturation of their central nervous system and the capacity for further locomotion skills. Too late would be unwise, due to the appearance of potentially irreducible contractures and deformities. We advise that the decision be based not on age itself but rather on the deterioration of the child's developmental status, which can be objectively quantified and followed on scoring systems, especially the Gross Motor Function Classification Measure (GMFM) **(Fig. 112.2)**.

For diplegic children who are able to ambulate, the goal of surgery is to improve the quality of locomotion, depending on the preoperative degree of incapacity. For characterization of these degrees, we are currently using the New York University classification:[16]

- Group I: children able to walk independently without assistive devices; the goal is to improve appearance, velocity, and ease of gait
- Group II: children who walk with assistive devices; the goal is to improve ambulation and decrease the dependence on assistive devices
- Group III: quadruped crawlers; the goal is to enable them to reciprocally move the legs in the standing position, using complementary assistive devices
- Groups IV and V: children unable to ambulate even with assistive equipment and a person helping; the goal of enabling them to gain significant improvement in motor function is generally not realistic

In the very disabled groups, a decrease in spasticity may be useful to ease nursing, decrease pain, improve comfort, and prevent worsening of deformities.

Importantly, for children with CP and quadriplegia, dorsal rhizotomies may alleviate spasticity in the upper limbs through

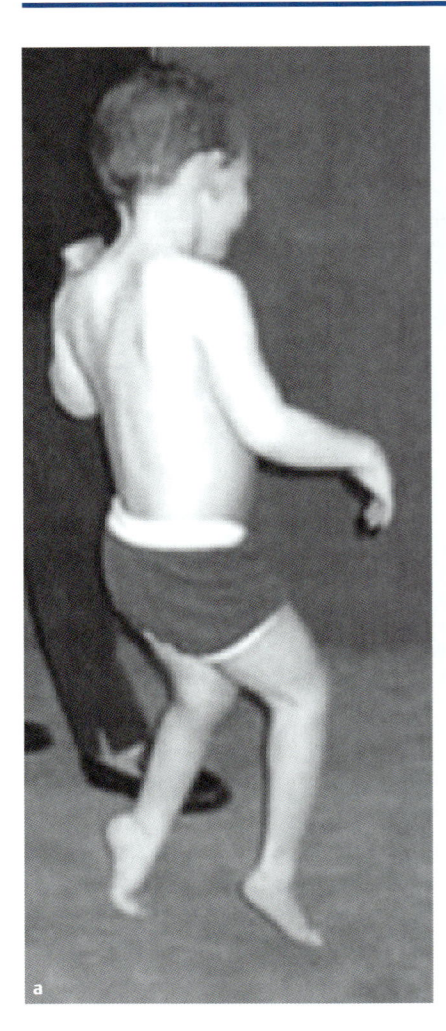

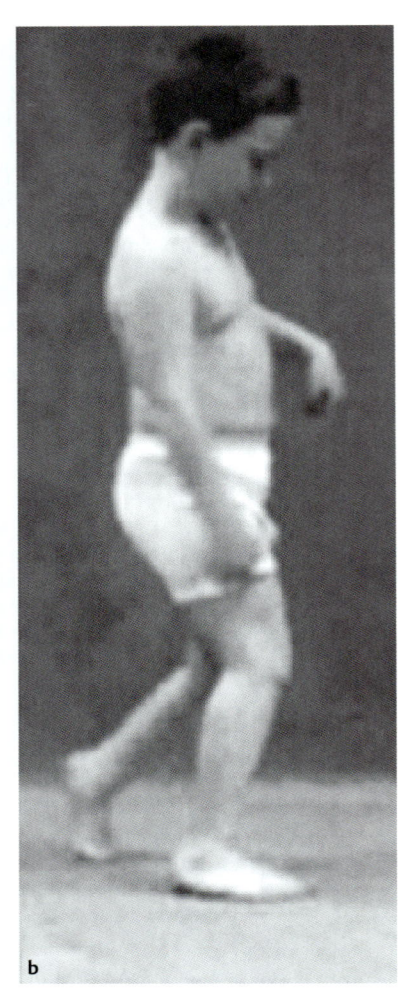

Fig. 112.1 Typical diplegic child with an indication of dorsal rhizotomy. **(a)** Before surgery the child had a jumping gait with true equinus, and he could not ambulate without assistance. **(b)** After surgery the child was able to walk autonomously, with alternate stance and swing phases.

the so-called distant-effect phenomenon, that is, a suprasegmental effect. Those distant effects can be explained by reduction of the inputs originating from the spastic lower limbs onto the brainstem reticular formation, as well as through the propriospinal interneuron system. Through similar mechanisms, DR can also exert favorable influence on swallowing, abnormal postures and movement in neck and trunk, respiratory disturbances, and the emotional overreactivity that is frequently observed in children with CP.

For severely affected children, complementary neuro-orthopedic surgery, especially tendon lengthening, can be useful.

Preoperative Planning

The roots to be targeted are those conveying abnormal hyperactivity in the circuits corresponding to the muscles that harbor "harmful" spasticity. Abnormal clinical patterns in diplegic (or quadriplegic) CP patients with spasticity of the lower limbs, together with the corresponding main muscle groups, nerves, and roots involved, are described in **Fig. 112.3**.

Quantification of rootlet sectioning is established after discussion between the surgeon and the rehabilitation team, and is documented in the patient's preoperative chart (**Table 112.1**).

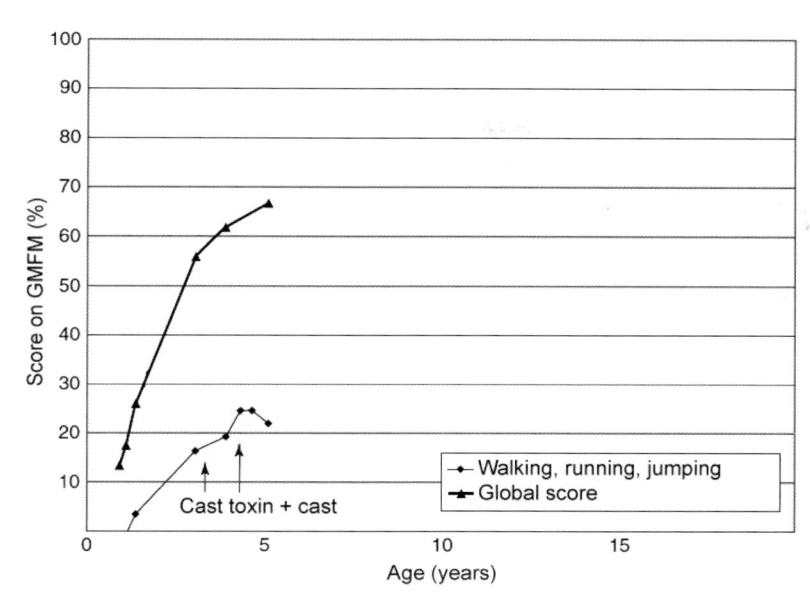

Fig. 112.2 Gross Motor Function Classification System (GMFCM) for the child in **Fig. 112.1** with spastic diplegia from cerebral palsy, showing the time course of the global score and the walking score. **(a)** The timing of the dorsal rhizotomy corresponded to a slow decrease in the GMFM score after a slight and temporary amelioration under a combination of casting and botulinum toxin. **(b)** After the dorsal rhizotomy, note the dramatic improvement in the global score and the walking score.

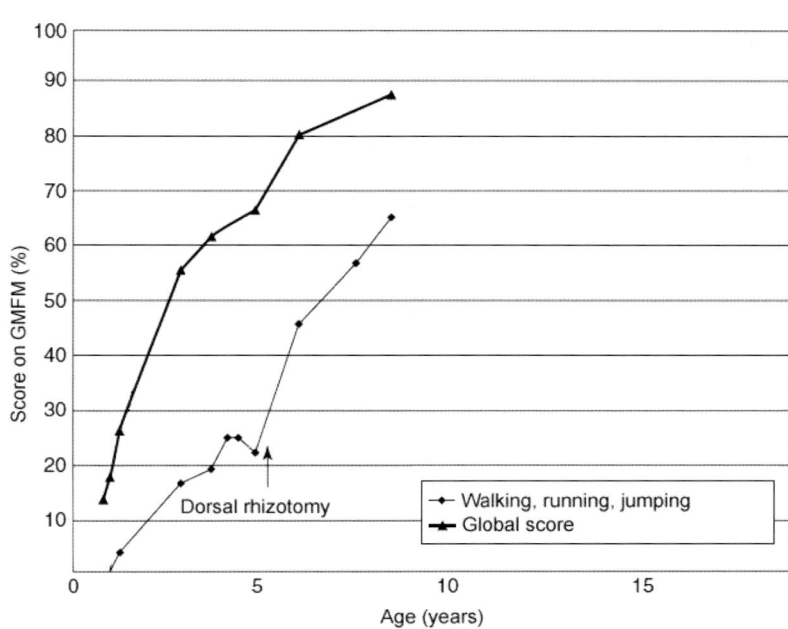

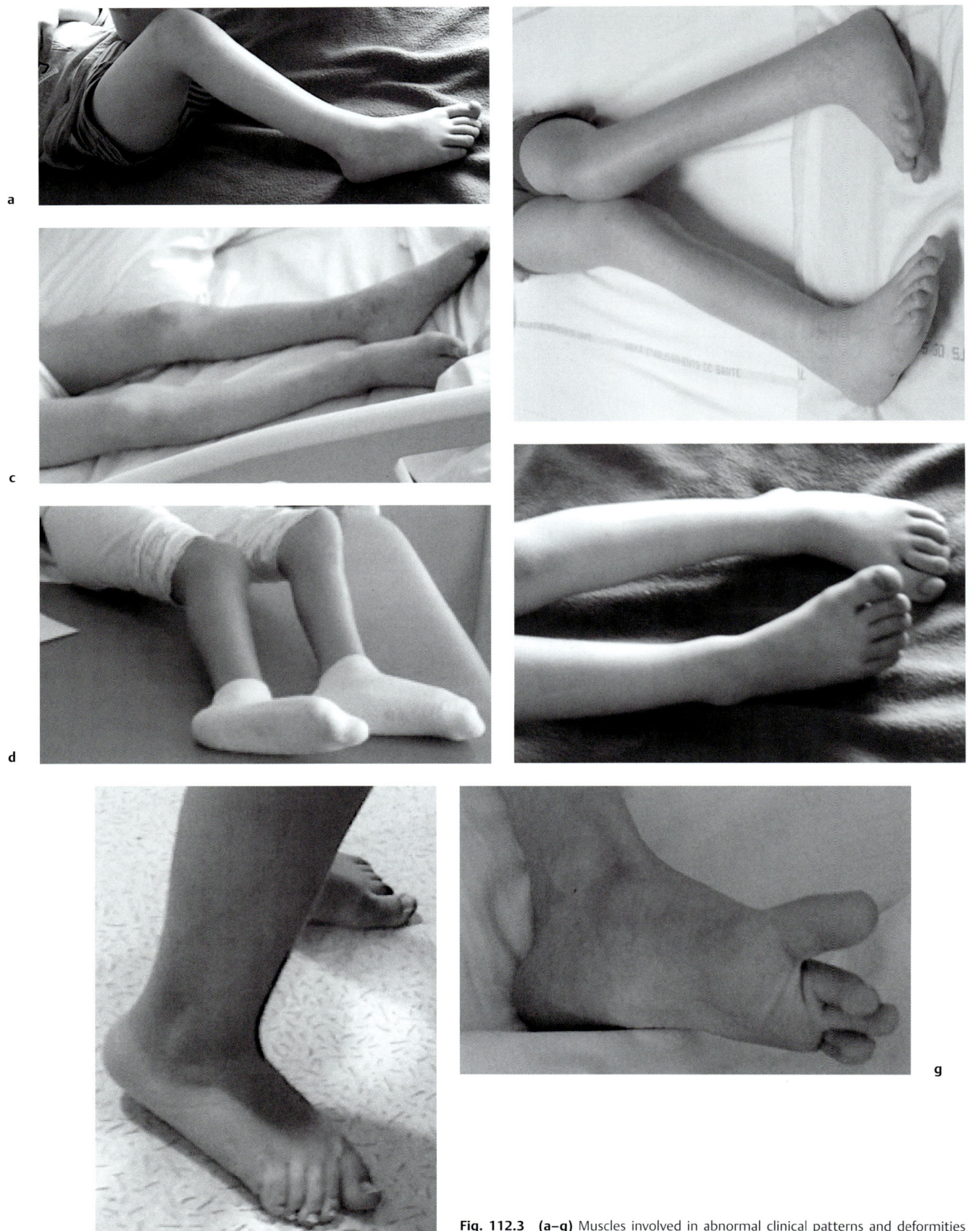

Fig. 112.3 (a–g) Muscles involved in abnormal clinical patterns and deformities observed in severely affected diplegic (tetraplegic) patients.

Table 112.1 Correspondence of Muscles and Nerve/Root Innervation.

Muscles Involved in Spasticity	Nerve(s)	Roots/Segments of Origin	Sectioning Quantification (%)
• Psoas/iliacus • Rectus femoris	Lumbar plexus Femoral	L2-L3 L3-L4	
• Adductor group (longus, brevis, magnus) • Gracilis • Obturator externus • Pectineus	Obturator	L2-L3	
• Quadriceps group (rectus femoris, vastus intermedius, vastus medialis and lateralis)	Femoral	L3-L4	

• Hamstrings
  ○ Biceps femoris
  ○ Semitendinosus
  ○ Semimembranosus
	Sciatic	L5-S2	

• Equinus
  ○ Gastrocnemius
  ○ Soleus
  ○ Popliteal
	Tibial	S1	

• Varus
  ○ Tibialis posterior
  ○ Flexor digitorum longus/brevis
  ○ Flexion of toes
  ○ Flexor hallucis longus
	Tibial
	
	Tibial
		S1
		
		S2	

• Extensor hallucis longus	Peroneal	L4-L5	

Note: The selection and quantification of root sectioning are established by the surgical team, based on the evaluation of the severity of the harmful components of the spasticity. The evaluation is included in the preoperative chart.

The surgical approach is then defined based on the roots to be targeted and their anatomic spine levels as demonstrated in **Fig. 112.4** and illustrated in the case example in **Fig. 112.5**.

The chart should specify the muscular groups to be weakened in tone and to what degree, and those whose tone must be preserved at least partially. Most patients with CP, especially diplegic ones, harbor a posture pattern called the scheme of Little.[15] For patients who are able to ambulate, the muscles contributing to the antigravity function, especially the gluteus and quadriceps, should have their tone and power spared. For wheelchair-dependent or bedridden patients, mostly with severe contractures and deformities, the correspondence between the involved muscles and the root innervation is demonstrated in **Fig. 112.3**.

The surgical program should be specifically tailored to each patient.

The preoperative chart includes (1) the description of the disabling components of spasticity; (2) an enumeration of the muscular groups harboring excess of tone; (3) the designation of the corresponding roots supposed to convey the harmful afferents on the basis of classic anatomic knowledge; and (4) the number of rootlets to be cut for each radicular target, whose estimation is proportional to the excess of tone affecting the corresponding muscle(s). The muscles whose tone needs to be maintained and consequently the corresponding roots that must be preserved should also be carefully noted.

Whatever the modality used, DR must be performed under intraoperative neurophysiological guidance, not only to confirm

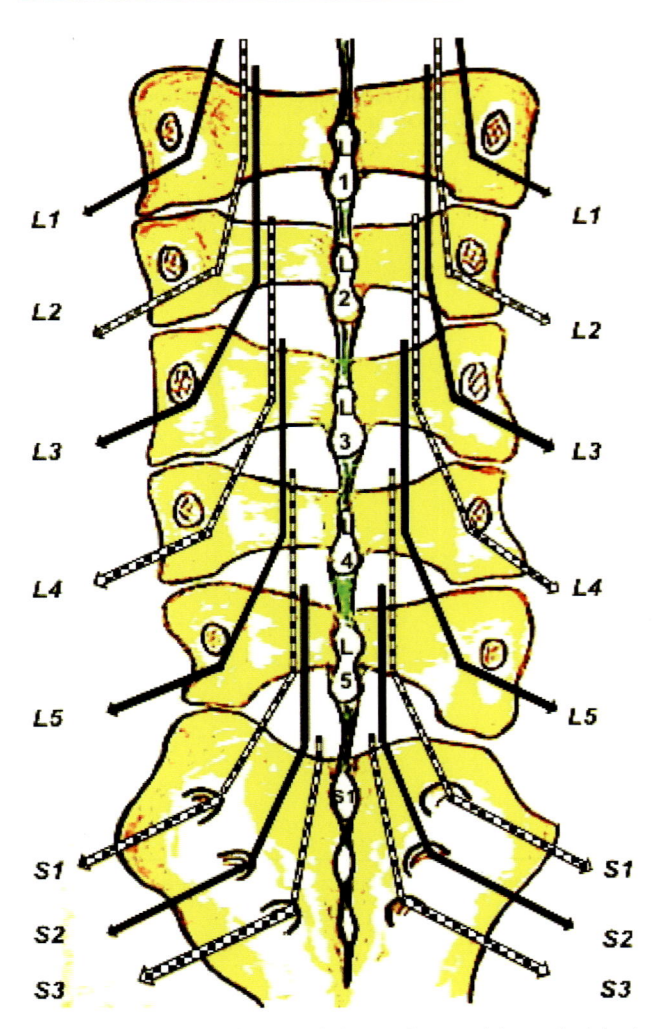

Fig. 112.4 Schematic drawing of the interlaminar (IL) vertebral levels where selected roots can be targeted for dorsal rhizotomy (DR): *L2, L3* at L1-L2; *L3, L4* at L2-L3; *L4, L5* at L3-L4; *L5, S1* at L4-L5; *S1, S2* at L5-S1. The IL spaces to be opened are determined based on the preoperative program for root sectioning (tailored operation).

the topographical level of the roots but also to estimate the degree of excitability of the spinal circuitry of the dorsal roots/rootlets to be targeted. Following Fasano's concept, the criteria for considering dorsal roots/rootlets to be involved in dysfunctional spinal circuits include a low threshold to a single stimulus, a sustained response to a 50-Hz train stimulation at threshold, and a spread of the response outside the myotome corresponding to the stimulated root. The present consensus for grading is to adopt the five-grade classification of abnormal responses modified from Fasano's classification[5] by Phillips and Park[17] (**Table 112.2**). Protocol is as follows: First, the stimulation threshold is determined with current pulses with a duration of 1 ms, beginning with an intensity of 0.1 mA, which is increased until muscular contraction appears. Once the threshold is determined, a stimulus consisting of a train at 50 Hz is delivered with an intensity two to three times that of threshold to recruit a maximum of motor units. Then motor responses are quantified with the five-grade system. Which grade of response would be the most reliable for determining which roots and rootlets should be cut remains a matter of discussion.[18] The first trial is at the dorsal root globally, and a second is at individual dorsal rootlet levels after rootlet dissection, if found useful.

Surgery

Anesthesia and Positioning

Surgery is performed under general anesthesia with endotracheal intubation. It is preferable to place a urinary catheter that will stay in place for a few days after the operation. The patient is placed in the prone position on bolsters to minimize pulmonary and abdominal compression. All pressure points are well padded. Curare is administered at the induction of anesthesia and should be short-lasting to extend only from tracheal intubation and positioning to commencement of the approach. Long-lasting curarization, as well as narcotics or analgesics that could influence neural activities, should be avoided so as not to affect muscular contraction responses to stimulation. The anesthesia protocol uses a combination of inhaled sevoflurane (or 50 to 70% nitrous oxide) and intravenously administered sufentanil (or remifentanil). For elderly patients, the protocol may combine propofol with sevoflurane, although propofol may decrease activities recorded by electromyography (EMG).

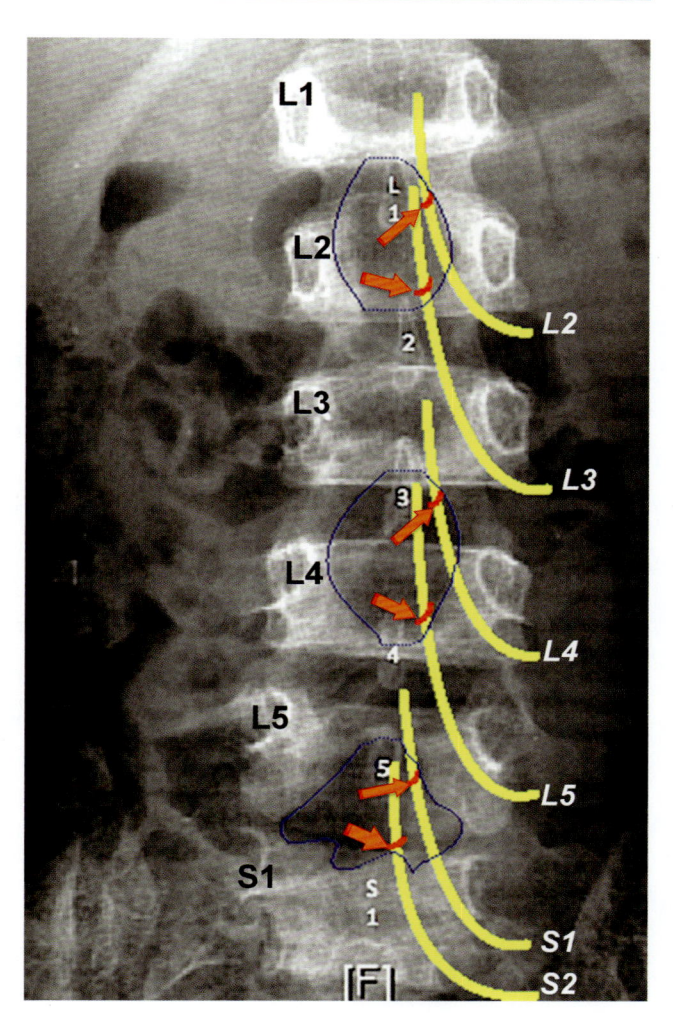

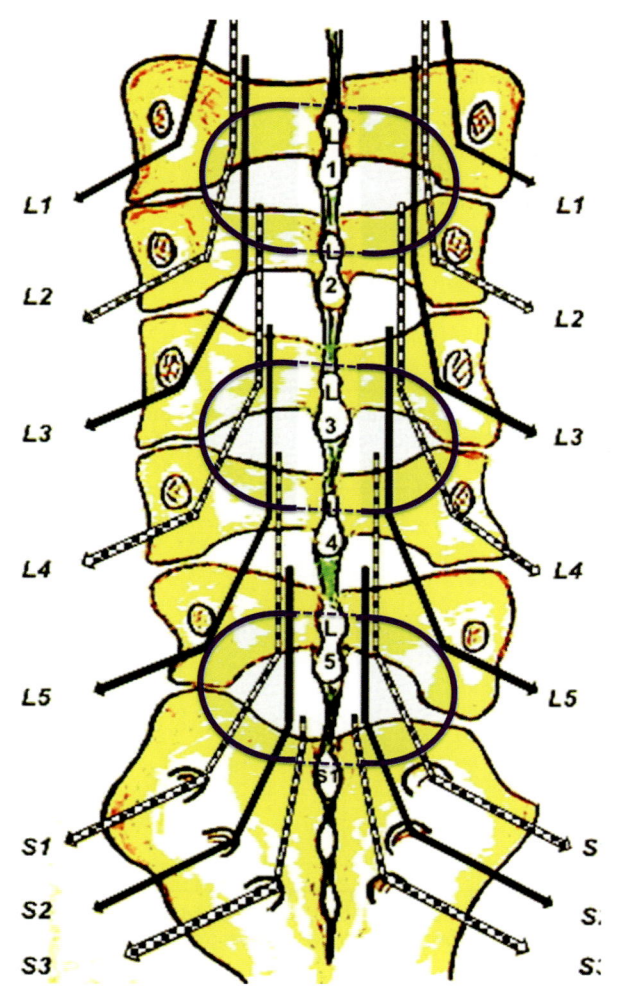

Fig. 112.5 (a) Drawing of the IL vertebral levels where roots were targeted based on the preoperative surgical planning. (b) Postoperative X-ray of the lumbar spine (anteroposterior view) showing enlarged IL fenestrations (delineated by blue-colored ellipses) based on the preoperative surgical planning (tailored operation). Roots L2 and L3 were targeted at the L1-L2 IL space, for treatment of spastic hip and thigh in flexion–adduction. Roots L4 and L5 were targeted at the L3-L4 IL space, for treatment of spastic quadriceps with patella ascension. Roots S1 and S2 were targeted at the L5-S1 IL space, for treatment of spastic foot in equinism and spastic hamstrings. The *red hemicircular arc line* represents the intradural exit of the ventral root/intradural entry of the dorsal root to or from the corresponding dural sheath.

Table 112.2 Intraoperative Neurophysiological Assessment

	Criterion	Grade	
	Unsustained motor response in muscles innervated by segmental level of stimulated dorsal root or rootlet	0	
	Sustained motor response in myotome of stimulated root	1	
	Contraction of muscles in myotomes of adjacent segmental level(s)	2	
	Contraction of muscles in myotomes distant from that of stimulated root	3	
Stimulated Root	**Predominately Responding Muscle(s) (Myotome)**	**Grade of Muscular Response to Dorsal Root Stimulation (as 50 Hz)**	**Amount (%) of Root to Be Sectioned**
L2	Iliopsoas, adductors of hips		
L3	Adductors of hips, quadriceps		
L4	Quadriceps, dorsal flexor of ankle (tibialis anterior)		
L5	Extensors of toes, hamstrings		
S1	Achilles ankle deep tendon reflex, gastrocnemius-soleus group, hamstrings, tibialis posterior		
S2	Flexor digitorum/hallucis		
S3	Anal sphincter		
S4	Anal sphincter		

Note: This form is to be filled out as an operative chart for dorsal rhizotomy sectioning established from intraoperative electrical stimulation of the dorsal roots (using a 50-Hz for 1 second each train). *Upper part (criterion):* grades of excitability as described by Fasano et al[5] and modified by Phillips and Park.[17] *Lower part:* form to be filled out for root/rootlets sectioning.

The operating room setup is schematically illustrated in **Fig. 112.6**. Patient positioning is illustrated in **Fig. 112.7a**. The patient's head should be ~ 10 cm lower than the thorax to minimize cerebrospinal fluid (CSF) loss. The setup of the intramuscular needle electrodes for EMG recordings is illustrated in **Fig. 112.7b**.

Surgical Approach for Keyhole Interlaminar Dorsal Rhizotomy (Fig. 112.6), (Video 112.1)

The lumbar midline incision and muscle separation are extended based on the number and topography of the IL spaces to be reached, which may be one, two, or three, depending on the patient's clinical presentation and preoperative chart. At selected level(s), both the spinous processes and the interspinous ligament are respected. After resection of the flavum ligament of the selected IL space, the IL space is enlarged by resecting the lower two thirds of the upper lamina and the upper two thirds of the lower lamina.

The principles of exposure of lumbar laminae, for example in cases with three IL levels to be approached, are shown in **Fig. 112.7c**. After opening the dura on the midline at the selected IL space, the microscope is installed. The trajectory is oblique at ~ 45 degrees, so that the surgeon's view passes underneath the (respected) interspinous ligament (**Fig. 112.7d**). The goal is to access intradurally the contralateral root, with its ventral and dorsal components, at exit to the corresponding dural sheath (**Fig. 112.7e**). Note that ordinarily two neighboring roots (on a side) can be accessed per interlaminar space, the upper one by going obliquely upward (i.e., rostrally), and the lower one by going obliquely downward (i.e., caudally). The ventral root is first stimulated, with a (bipolar) electrode, to check the anatomic-topographic level. Then the dorsal rootlets, as a whole, are individualized from the ventral root over approximately 1 cm, and stimulated to evaluate the degree of involvement in the "excitability" of the corresponding spinal cord circuitry (which constitutes physiological testing).

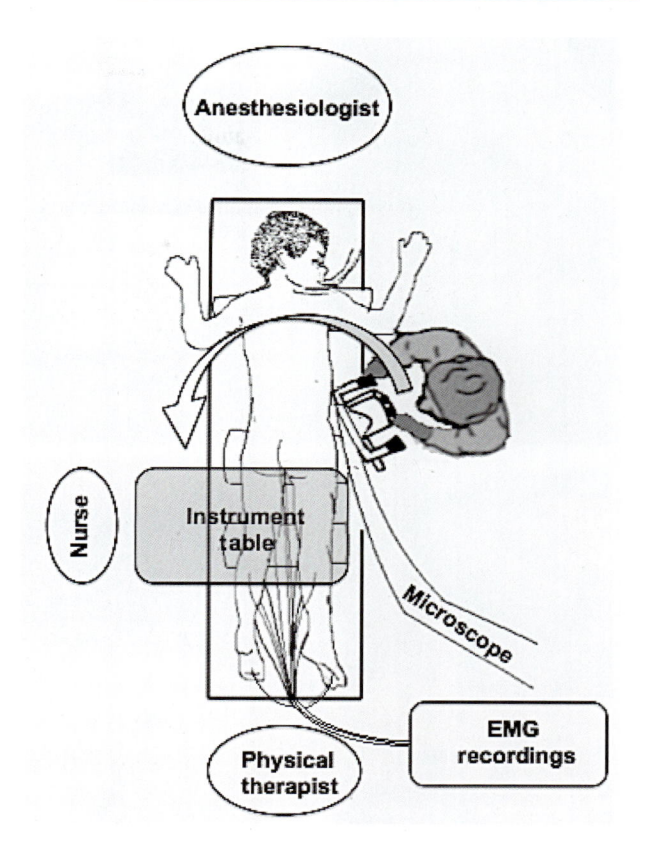

Fig. 112.6 The operating room setup. The *curved arrow* indicates that the surgeon will change side. The microscope is placed in such a way as to enable it to be rotated from one side to the other. The targeted roots should be approached from the contralateral side. The physical therapist must be in a position that provides optimal access to the patient's legs for appropriate clinical examination of muscles during the intraoperative electrical stimulation. EMG, electromyograph.

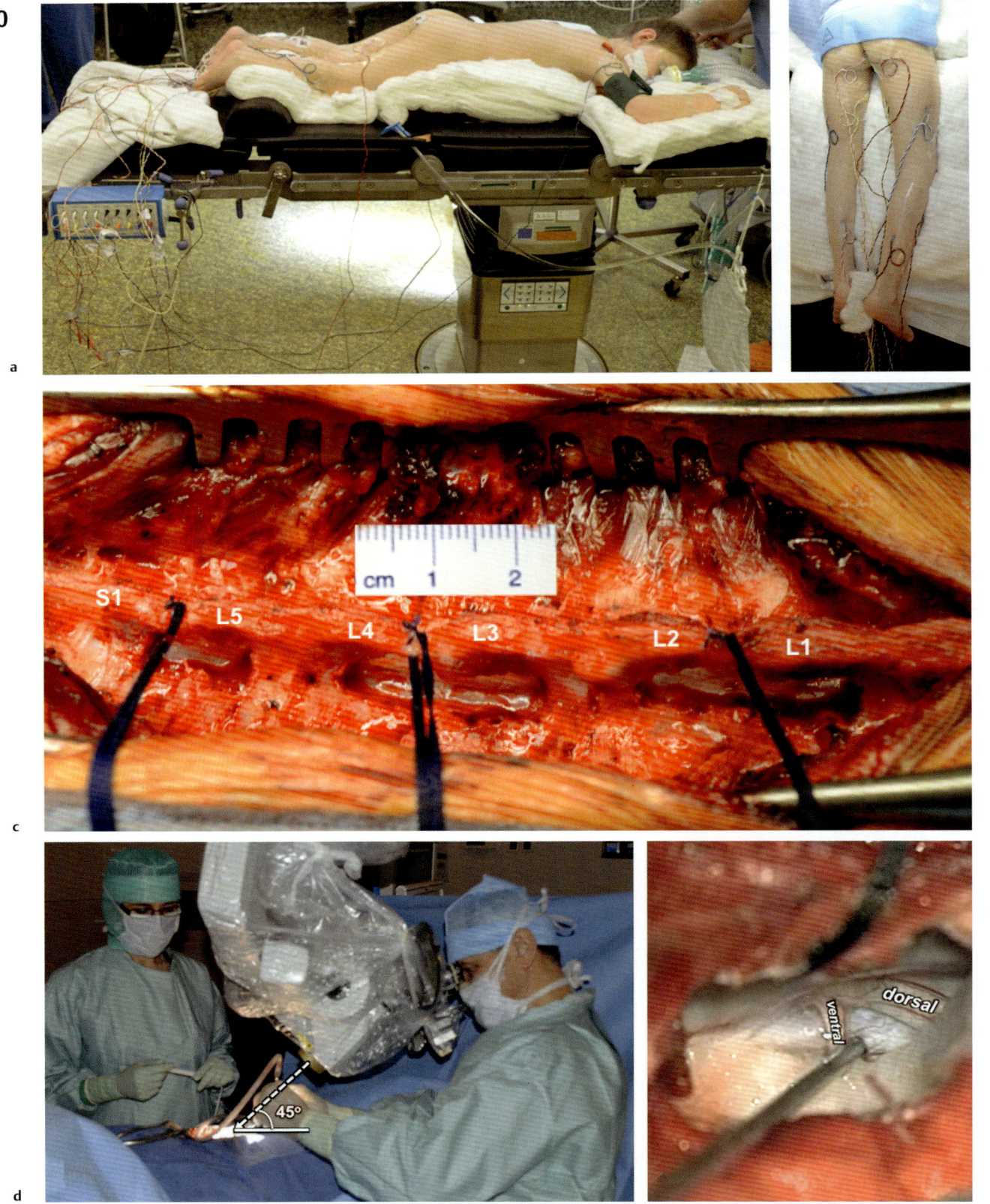

Fig. 112.7 Interlaminar microsurgical dorsal rhizotomy: installation and approach. **(a)** Positioning on table. **(b)** Intramuscular needle electrodes for EMG recordings in the adductors, quadriceps, tibialis anterioris, soleus, biceps femoris, flexor digitorum, anal sphincter (see **Table 112.1** for correspondence between muscles and radicular levels). **(c)** Exposure of L1-S1 laminae, with L1-L2, L3-L4, and L5-S1 IL fenestrations as selected during surgical planning. At each fenestrated level, the inferior two thirds of the upper lamina and the superior two thirds of the lower lamina are rongeured, and the flavum ligamentum is removed to expose the dura, so that the dura and arachnoid are opened on the midline. Note at the fenestrated level(s) the preservation of the spinous processes and the interspinous ligament *(blue tapes)*. **(d)** The surgeon operates from an oblique trajectory, at a 45-degree angle to the target, intradurally, through the IL space, the contralateral root, at the exit to the corresponding dural sheath. **(e)** The trajectory passes underneath the interspinous ligament ("keyhole" surgery) to access the root, with its ventral and dorsal components (well recognizable).

Combined Anatomic Mapping and Physiological Testing

Our own protocol for neurophysiological guidance is as follows.[19]

First, each exposed root is electrically stimulated to identify its innervation territory and thereby confirm its topographic level. This phase is anatomic mapping (**Figs. 112.8a,b** and **112.9**). Stimulation (2 Hz, ~ 200 µA) is first performed on the ventral root component, which is easy when the root is accessible at its exit to its dural sheath. To be noted, a motor response by dorsal root stimulation would require a three to five times higher intensity. Thus the roots corresponding topographically to the muscles harboring "harmful" spasticity are identified prior to sectioning decision.

Then, at the same level, the corresponding dorsal rootlets undergo physiological testing. Stimulation is with a 50-Hz train of 1-second duration for each train. Excitability is considered excessive when stimulation elicits an "exaggerated" (sustained or spreading) response (**Table 112.2; Figs. 112.8c,d** and **112.10**). This testing is to confirm or modify the percentage of the dorsal root to be cut, which was previously indicated in the preoperative chart, in proportion to the severity of the spasticity in the

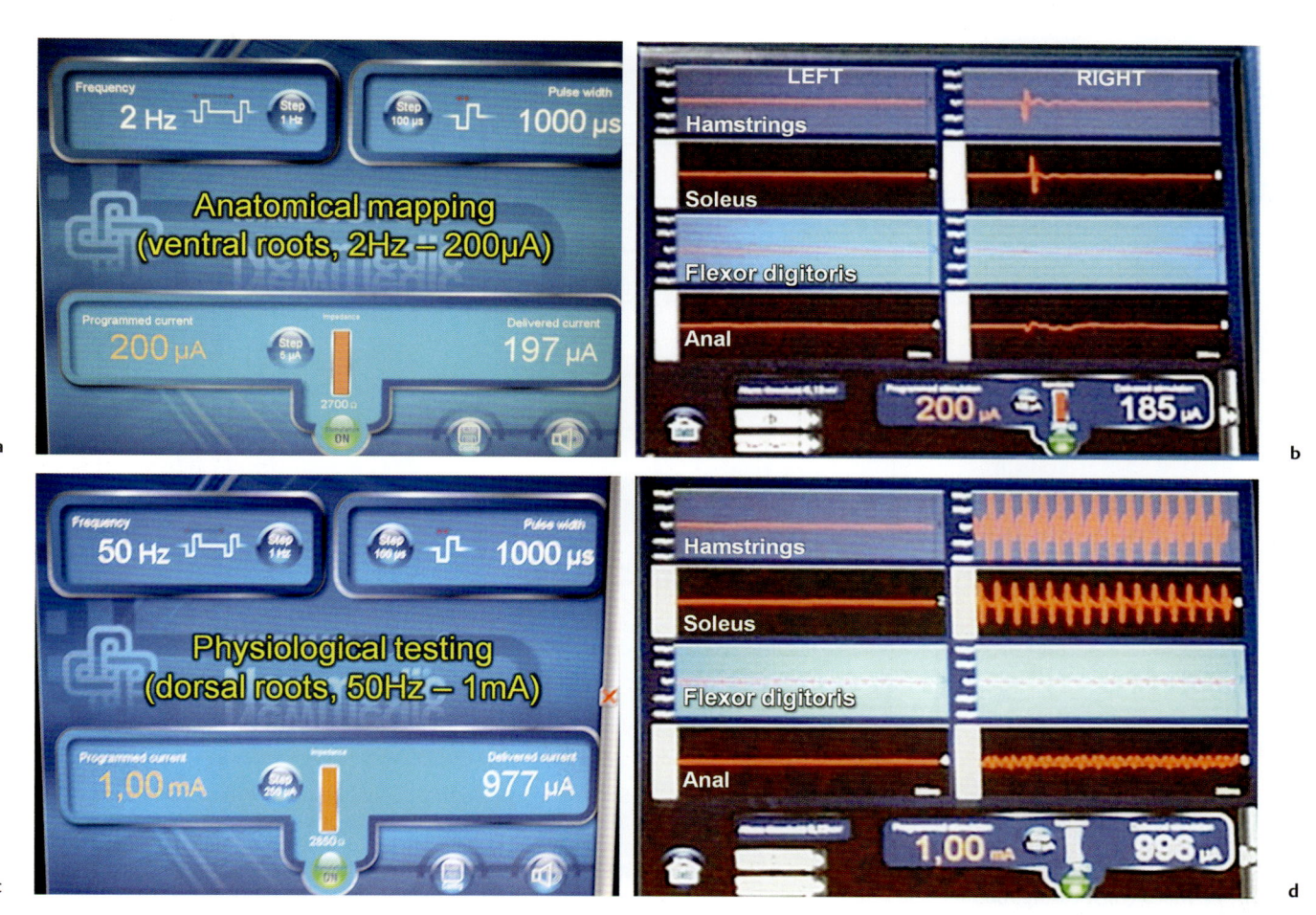

Fig. 112.8 Intraoperative neurophysiological guidance. **(a,b)** Anatomic mapping. Topographic identification of the radicular levels is achieved by electrical stimulation, preferably bipolar, with an intensity of 0.1 to 1 mA, currently at 200 µA for the ventral (motor) root, and at a frequency of 2 Hz. For the dorsal (sensory) root, the required intensity to reach threshold for muscular responses is approximately three to five times higher than that for the ventral root. Muscular responses can be observed by clinical examination or recorded with EMG. Stimulation of a selected root produces predominant, if not specific, motor responses in the corresponding myotomes.[20] In the presented example, which corresponds to stimulation of a (right) S1 ventral root, note the direct muscular response in the soleus and the hamstrings on the right-side recordings. **(c,d)** Physiological testing aims to estimate the level of excitability of the radicular-spinal circuitry, by stimulating the corresponding dorsal roots/rootlets. Following Fasano et al's[5] concept, the criteria for an excess of excitability are a sustained response to a 50-Hz train stimulation (of 1 second each train) at a threshold of ~ 1 mA or a spread of the response outside the myotome corresponding to the stimulated root. In the illustrative example, which corresponds to the stimulation of a S1 (right) dorsal root (in the same patient as in the ventral root stimulation), note the spreading response outside the myotome corresponding to S1, namely to the flexor digitorum and the anal sphincter, the latter two being the tributary to S2-S3.

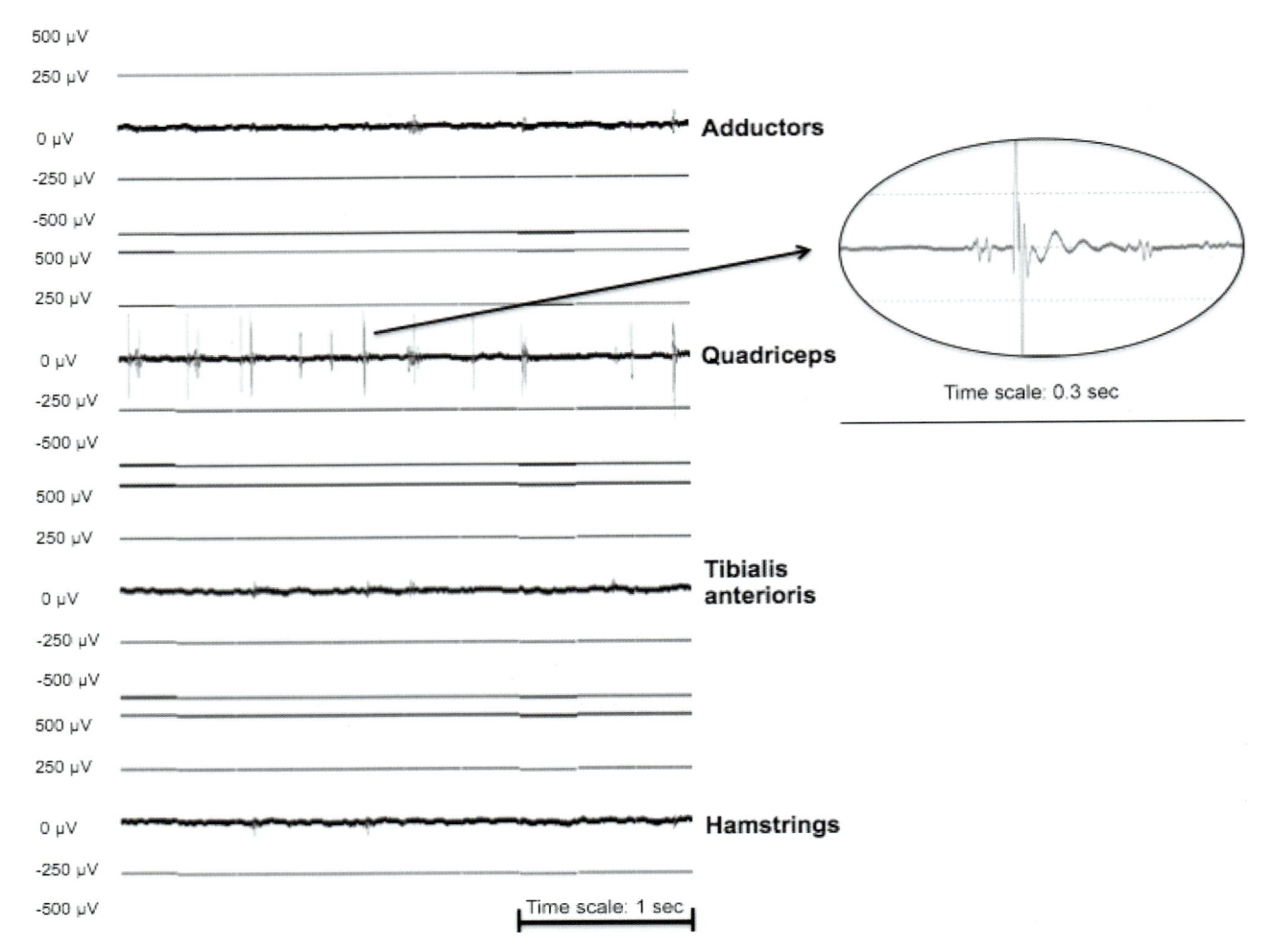

Fig. 112.9 Anatomic mapping for topographic identification of the radicular levels. In this illustrative case, stimulation (at 2 Hz and 200 μA) of the L4 ventral root elicits an EMG response predominantly in the quadriceps muscular group. *Inset:* The graphical element corresponds to magnification of a direct EMG response (time scale: 0.3 s).

corresponding muscular group(s). The number of selected dorsal rootlets to be cut, whose number was also specified in the preoperative chart, is adjusted accordingly. The amount of dorsal rootlets cut generally ranges between one third and four fifths of the root's constituting rootlets. The same protocol is applied at each of the preselected roots to be targeted.

Microsurgical Steps of the "Keyhole" Procedure (Fig. 112.11)

After the dura and the arachnoid are opened on midline for ~ 2 cm at the selected interlaminar space(s), the microscope is installed, contralaterally to the root(s) to be targeted. The trajectory is oblique, on the order of 45 degrees, to reach the root(s) contralaterally at the exit/entry into the corresponding dural sheath. Then microsurgical steps are conducted following the principles of so-called keyhole surgery. At the exit from the dural sheath, the ventral (motor) root is easily identified on its ventral position. The dorsal (sensory) rootlets (on average five per root) are also easily identified; they are grouped posteriorly to the ventral root, often separated from the latter by an arachnoid fold. Then the electrical stimulation protocol is undertaken.

Stimulation preferably should be done with a bipolar electrode to avoid spreading of current and consequently yielding false responses. The ventral root is stimulated first for topographic identification, and then the dorsal root. After confirmation for lesioning of that dorsal root, between one third and four fifths of the constituting dorsal rootlets are cut, based on the preoperative chart and the physiological testing. At the end, the dural incision is sutured in a watertight fashion, and the dural suture line is covered with fat harvested subcutaneously.

Postoperative Management

Currently, the patient stays in the intensive care unit for the following night, then returns to the ward for 5 to 10 days before discharge. The sitting position is resumed next day(s) only progressively to avoid headaches secondary to intraoperative CSF loss. The urinary catheter is removed as soon as the patient is able to use the toilet. Bladder ultrasonography to rule out residue is a wise precaution. Postoperative pain is managed with intravenous infusion of morphine combined with oral acetaminophen and diazepam/clonazepam until discharge. Clonazepam administration may be prolonged for (rare) cases of neuropathic

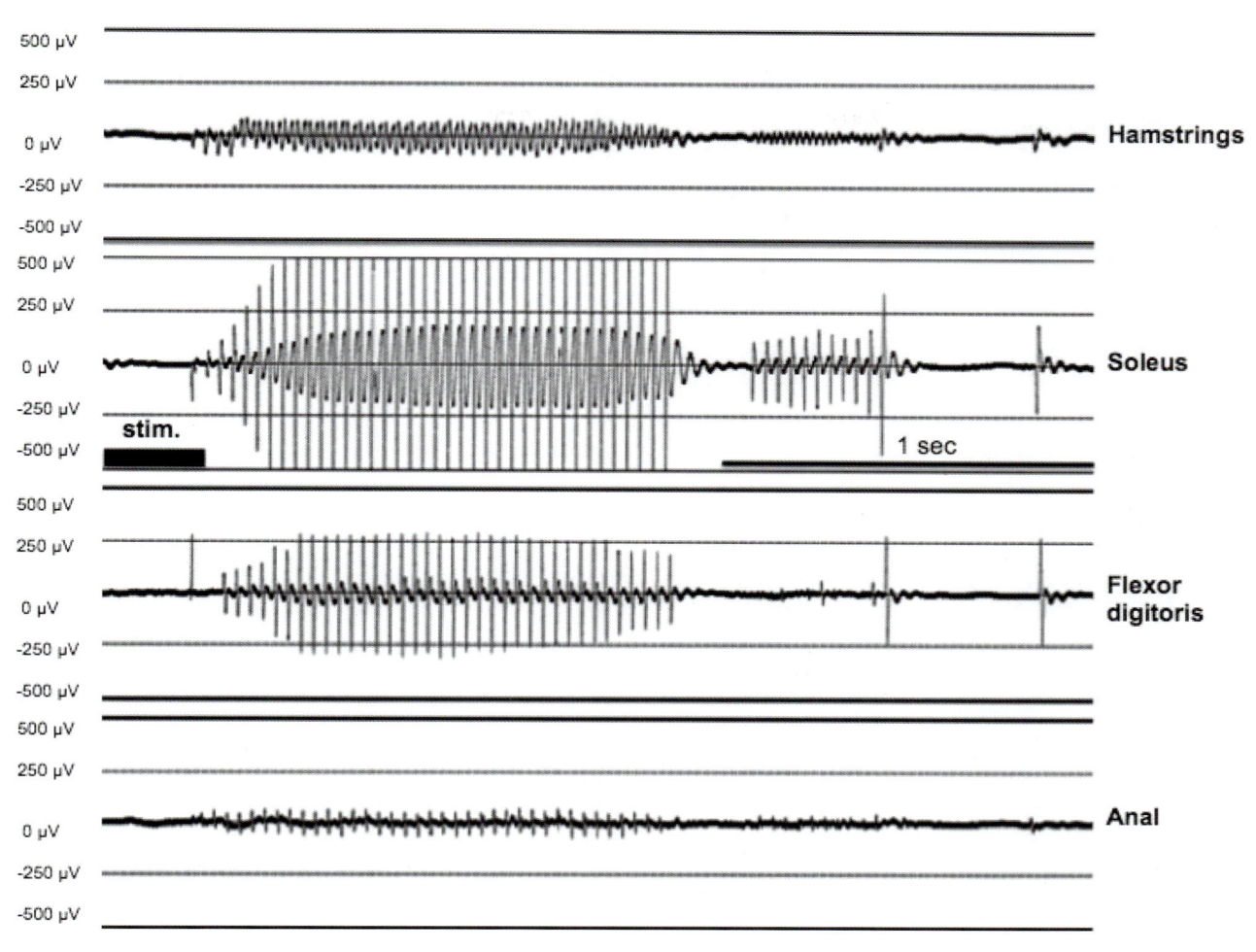

Fig. 112.10 Physiological testing for estimating the excitability of the root–spinal cord circuitry. In this illustrative case, stimulation (at 50 Hz and 1 mA) of the S1 dorsal root elicits an abnormal EMG response: (1) sustained, that is, lasting after the cessation of the stimulation; and (2) spreading, that is, not only at the level of the soleus muscle, but also outside the corresponding S1 myotome. Note the spreading of response to the hamstrings, flexor digitoris, and anal sphincter muscles.

pain, dysesthesias, or disabling paresthesias. It is noteworthy that immediately after surgery, patients may have some flexion spasms until operative pain disappears. The necessity of lumbar immobilization with a corset depends on the type of surgical approach. The interlaminar approach as performed in our most recently operated patients does not necessitate immobilization beyond 10 days, and allows resumption of physical therapy in the early period after surgery. After hospitalization, the patient is transferred to a rehabilitation facility for an average of 1 month of physical therapy program and then is discharged to a community institution or back home under an intensive physical therapy program. Importantly, patients and caregivers must be warned that the procedure generally produces transient excessive hypotonia, which may be responsible for loss of strength that makes doing transfers difficult. The "desirable" satisfactory level is generally reached after 3 to 6 months.

Advantages

Keyhole Interlaminar Dorsal rhizotomy (KIDr) is a patient-tailored procedure that is tailored to the patient's preoperative clinical presentation and the identified harmful components of the excess spasticity.

- KIDr provides maximal accuracy for intraoperative neurophysiological guidance, as the mode of approach offers direct individual access to each one of the roots planned to be targeted, and at the site where ventral and dorsal roots can be anatomically differentiated.
  - Stimulation of ventral roots permits precise anatomic identification of the roots' topographical level and function, by means of clinical observation of the muscular responses by the physical therapist or by EMG recordings.
  - Stimulation of the corresponding dorsal roots helps to evaluate their degree of implication in the triggering of the hyperactive segmental circuits of the spinal cord, and thus to quantify the percentage of dorsal rootlets to be cut in each of the selected roots.
- KIDr reduces the invasiveness of opening the spine by respecting the interspinous ligament(s) as well as part of the laminae. This helps reduce the postoperative

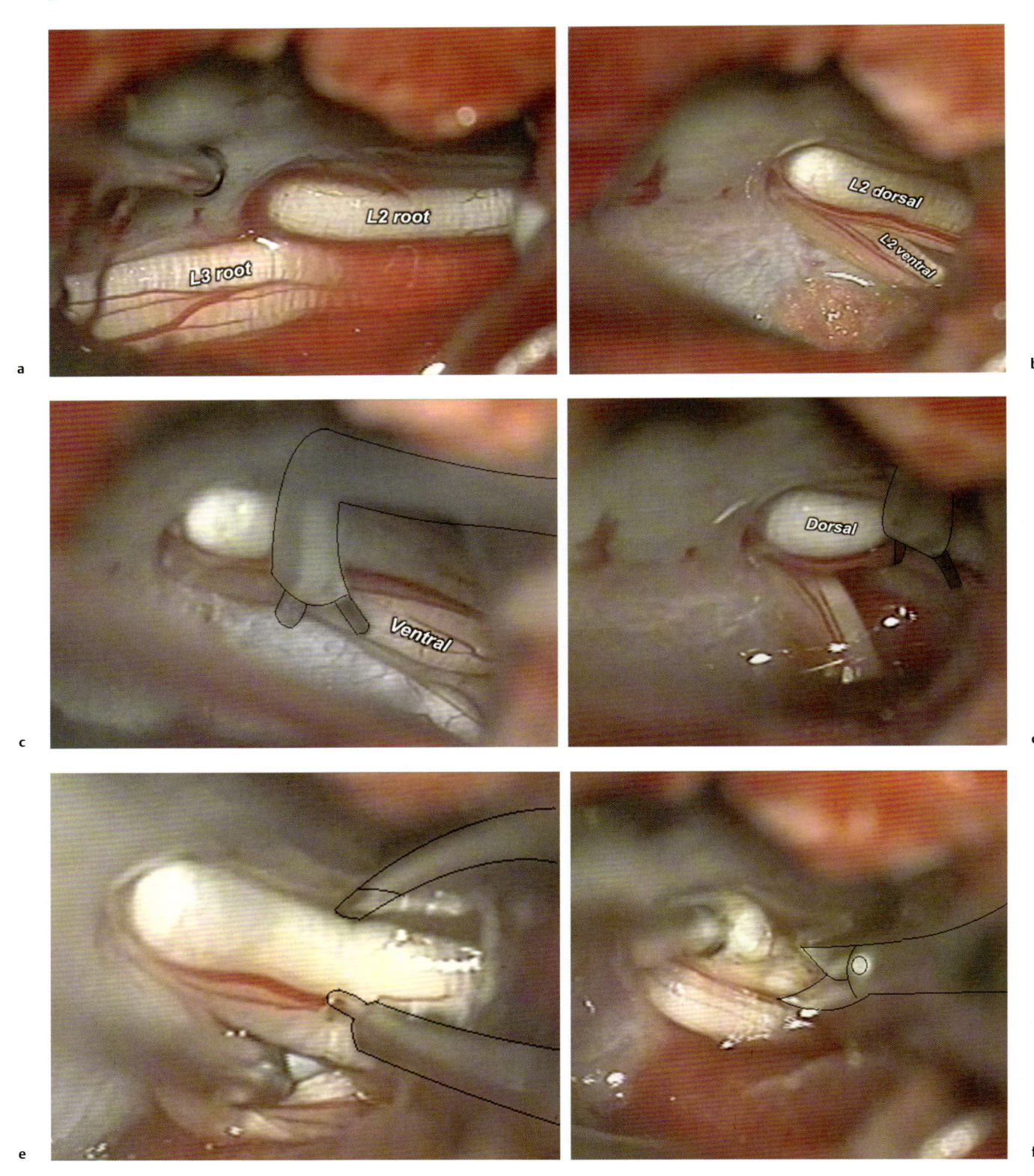

Fig. 112.11 Keyhole interlaminar dorsal rhizotomy: microsurgical steps. This illustrative case is of a patient undergoing surgery at the left L2 root through L1-L2 IL fenestration. **(a)** Exposure of the left L2 dorsal and ventral roots at the entry/exit to/from the dural sheath, obliquely seen under the microscope from the contralateral side. Note the neighboring L3 root going down to the next caudal level; this L3 root will be targeted in the next step through the same IL space (not shown in this figure). **(b)** Individualization of the L2 dorsal root from the L2 ventral root. **(c)** Anatomic mapping: identification of the topographic level of the root by electrical stimulation of the ventral root at 2 Hz and 0.2 mA, using a bipolar electrode. Use of a bipolar electrode is preferable to avoid diffusion of current and consequently false-positive or false-negative responses. **(d)** Physiological testing of the excitability of the dorsal root at 50 Hz and 1 mA, using the same bipolar electrode. **(e,f)** Coagulation with the bipolar forceps **(e)** and sectioning with microscissors **(f)** of the selected dorsal rootlets. In this case, three of the four rootlets, which constitute the dorsal root, were divided.

period of immobilization and decreases the risk of secondary instability.

Disadvantages

- Often the approach involves more than one of interlaminar level, which necessitates an extended skin incision and retraction of paraspinal muscular structures.
- The procedure, which follows the keyhole surgery principles, is demanding and sometimes difficult. When a large number of roots need to be targeted and all of them should be physiologically tested, surgery is time-consuming for the surgical team.

Potential Complications and Precautions

Patients with CP, especially those affected with severe quadriplegia, frequently have disturbances in swallowing and ventilatory command, which are sometimes latent. Preventive respiratory physical therapy is most helpful in this regard.

To avoid postsurgical urinary retention, incontinence, or infections, the urinary catheter should be left in place until the patient is released from bed rest. Absence of residue after withdrawal of the catheter should be checked by suprapubic echography.

A supple lumbar corset may be applied to exert compression on the posterior muscles for about 2 weeks, to decrease the risk of CSF leakage or pseudomeningocele.

Although trophic ulcers in (eventual) hypoesthetic cutaneous areas are rarely observed, prevention should be systematic, especially for patients depending on splints.

In the postoperative long-term, instability may occur, leading to spinal deformity, such as kyphosis, hyperlordosis, or even spondylolisthesis, and generating severe back pain.[21] The risk of instability has been significantly diminished by limiting the extent of the approaches. In spastic hips with subluxation, DR enables stabilization of the situation in most cases; however, decompensation of the subluxation may occur, particularly if the musculature is weak or the patient is overweight.

Prevention of complications is better achieved when the rehabilitation team, physical therapists, and caregivers are well aware of these potential risks.

Spasticity may recur, with varying intensity. However longterm studies show that in the majority of cases the favorable effects of DR are maintained.[8–10,22–27]

Conclusion

When spasticity becomes harmful and threatens to induce irreversible contractures and deformities in spite of intensive physical therapy, an effective neurosurgical armamentarium is available. Peripheral neurotomies for focal spastic (and also to a certain extent dystonic) muscles can be considered if botulinum toxin is not sufficient. When spasticity affects the lower limbs and is rather diffuse, intrathecal baclofen therapy is classically the first option in adults and older children, especially those with strong associated dystonia. For decades, DR has proved to be useful, especially for spastic diplegic children who are able to ambulate. Because of its distant effects, DR may also be indicated in quadriplegic patients; spasticity overreactivity with "parasite" movements in the upper limb and disturbances in swallowing function can be notably improved. Complementary orthopedic surgery is paramount, either as the primary treatment when contractures or deformities predominate, or as an adjuvant to neurosurgical treatment after spasticity had decreased so that orthopedic correction can be more stable. Decision making may be difficult as children are continually developing and the spasticity is evolving. Also, the dystonia that is frequently associated with spasticity has dynamic characteristics. Therefore, working with a multidisciplinary term is of a considerable importance.

References

1. Sherrington CS. Decerebrate rigidity, and reflex coordination of movements. J Physiol 1898;22:319–332
2. Foerster O. On the indications and results of the excision of posterior spinal nerve roots in men. Surg Gynecol Obstet 1913;16:463–474
3. Gros C, Ouaknine G, Vlahovitch B, Frèrebeau P. La radicotomie sélective postérieure dans le traitement neuro-chirurgical de l'hypertonie pyramidale. Neurochirurgie 1967;13:505–518
4. Privat JM, Benezech J, Frerebeau P, Gros C. Sectorial posterior rhizotomy, a new technique of surgical treatment for spasticity. Acta Neurochir (Wien) 1976;35:181–195
5. Fasano VA, Barolat-Romana G, Ivaldi A, Sguazzi A. La radicotomie postérieure fonctionnelle dans le traitement de la spasticité cérébrale Premieres observations sur la stimulation électrique peroperatoire des racines postérieures, et leur utilisation dans le choix des racines à sectionner. Neurochirurgie 1976;22:23–34
6. Peacock WJ, Arens LJ. Selective posterior rhizotomy for the relief of spasticity in cerebral palsy. S Afr Med J 1982;62:119–124
7. Abbott R, Johann-Murphy M, Shiminski-Maher T, et al. Selective dorsal rhizotomy: outcome and complications in treating spastic cerebral palsy. Neurosurgery 1993;33:851–857, discussion 857
8. Farmer JP, McNeely PD. Surgery in the dorsal roots for children with cerebral palsy. Oper Tech Neurosurg. 2004;7:153–156
9. Steinbok P. Selective dorsal rhizotomy for spastic cerebral palsy: a review. Childs Nerv Syst 2007;23:981–990
10. Sindou M. Radicotomies dorsales (postérieures) chez l'enfant. Neurochirurgie 2003;49(2-3 Pt 2):312–323
11. Sindou M, Goutelle A. Surgical posterior rhizotomies for the treatment of pain. In: Krayenbühl H, Brihaye J, Loew F, et al, eds. Advances and Technical Standards in Neurosurgery, vol 10. New York: Springer; 1983: 147–185
12. Parise M, Sindou M, Mertens P, Mauguière F. Somatosensory evoked potentials following functional posterior rhizotomy in spastic children. Stereotact Funct Neurosurg 1997;69(1-4 Pt 2):268–273
13. Park TS, Gaffney PE, Kaufman BA, Molleston MC. Selective lumbosacral dorsal rhizotomy immediately caudal to the conus medullaris for cerebral palsy spasticity. Neurosurgery 1993;33:929–933, discussion 933–934
14. Park TS, Johnston JM. Selective dorsal rhizotomy for spastic cerebral palsy. In: Goodrich JT, ed. Pediatric Neurosurgery, 2nd ed. New York: Thieme; 2008:177–183
15. Little WJ. On the influence of abnormal parturition, difficult labours, premature birth, and asphyxia neonatorum, on the mental and physical condition of the child, especially in relation to deformities. Clin Orthop Relat Res 1966;46:7–22
16. Abbott R. Indications for surgery to treat children with spasticity due to cerebral palsy. In: Sindou M, Abbott R, Keravel Y, eds. Neurosurgery for Spasticity: A Multidisciplinary Approach. New York: Springer; 1991: 215–217
17. Phillips LH, Park TS. Electrophysiologic studies of selective posterior rhizotomy patients. In: Park TS, Phillips LH, Peacock WJ, eds. Management of Spasticity in Cerebral Palsy and Spinal Cord Injury. Neurosurgery: State of the Art Reviews, vol 4. Philadelphia: Hanley & Belfus; 1989:459–470
18. Mittal S, Farmer JP, Poulin C, Silver K. Reliability of intraoperative electrophysiological monitoring in selective posterior rhizotomy. J Neurosurg 2001;95:67–75
19. Sindou M, Georgoulis G, Mertens P. Dorsal rhizotomies for children with cerebral palsy. In: Sindou M, Georgoulis G, Mertens P, eds. Neurosurgery for Spasticity: A Practical Guide for Treating Children and Adults. New York: Springer, 2014:191–212
20. Schirmer CM, Shils JL, Arle JE, et al. Heuristic map of myotomal innervation in humans using direct intraoperative nerve root stimulation. J Neurosurg Spine 2011;15:64–70
21. Yasuoka S, Peterson HA, MacCarty CS. Incidence of spinal column deformity after multilevel laminectomy in children and adults. J Neurosurg 1982;57:441–445

22. Fasano VA, Broggi G, Zeme S, Lo Russo G, Sguazzi A. Long-term results of posterior functional rhizotomy. Acta Neurochir Suppl (Wien) 1980;30:435–439
23. Arens LJ, Peacock WJ, Peter J. Selective posterior rhizotomy: a long-term follow-up study. Childs Nerv Syst 1989;5:148–152
24. Nishida T, Thatcher SW, Marty GR. Selective posterior rhizotomy for children with cerebral palsy: a 7-year experience. Childs Nerv Syst 1995;11:374–380
25. Abbott R. Sensory rhizotomy for the treatment of childhood spasticity. J Child Neurol 1996;11(Suppl 1):S36–S42
26. Hodgkinson I, Bérard C, Jindrich ML, Sindou M, Mertens P, Bérard J. Selective dorsal rhizotomy in children with cerebral palsy. Results in 18 cases at one year postoperatively. Stereotact Funct Neurosurg 1997;69(1-4 Pt 2):259–267
27. Taira T, Hori T. [Selective peripheral neurotomy and selective dorsal rhizotomy]. Brain Nerve 2008;60:1427–1436

113 Resection of Cauda Equina Ependymomas

R. Shane Tubbs and W. Jerry Oakes

Ependymomas are the most common intramedullary spinal cord tumors seen in adults. One variant, myxopapillary ependymoma, is generally seen only in the cauda equina and filum terminale, but rarely can be found in other regions.[1] Myxopapillary ependymomas account for 40 to 50% of spinal ependymomas in adults and 8 to 14% of spinal ependymomas in children younger than 16 years of age.[2,3] Myxopapillary ependymomas are thought to originate from ependymal cell masses in the ventriculus terminalis and filum terminale.[4-8]

Grossly, these tumors are well circumscribed and can compress or envelop the roots of the cauda equina. They are usually cylindrical and have been described as sausage shaped.[4-6] Myxopapillary ependymomas are also highly vascular. Microscopically, these tumors have areas with both rosettes and pseudorosettes intermingled with papillae embedded in a myxoid background. Ultrastructural examination demonstrates adherens junctions and intracytoplasmic lumina with microvilli. These tumors characteristically have a vascular core with a mucoid matrix; necrosis and mitotic figures are variable in their occurrence.[4,7-10] Immunostaining reveals epidermal growth factor receptor (EGFR) expression in some patients. In one study, no correlation between tumor recurrence and EGFR overexpression was found.[10] Myxopapillary ependymomas have unique gene and protein expression patterns compared with other ependymomas. Aberrant expression of HOXB13 suggests the possible recapitulation of developmental pathways in myxopapillary ependymoma tumorigenesis.[11]

Patient Selection

Myxopapillary ependymomas are slow-growing tumors in most patients, presenting in the third to fourth decades of life.[3] Back pain is the commonest presenting symptom.[11] Approximately half of patients report back pain that is made worse by being recumbent.[1] Although not as common, patients may present with leg weakness, subarachnoid hemorrhage, papilledema, and urinary dysfunction.[5] Urinary incontinence at presentation is a poor prognostic sign.[5]

With complete excision, these tumors generally carry a favorable prognosis in the adult population. However, there is a tendency for local recurrence and metastasis. Myxopapillary ependymomas tend to be more aggressive in children; therefore, their prognosis is somewhat worse even with total gross excision.[5]

Indications and Contraindications

The indication for surgery is the presence of tumor in the thecal sac, with imaging indicative of myxopapillary ependymoma. There are no significant contraindications to surgery in a patient with stable cardiopulmonary status.

Advantages and Disadvantages

Surgical excision of the tumor is the primary treatment of choice, although surgery is less curative in tumors that are large, multifocal, or extend outside the thecal sac. Cerebrospinal fluid (CSF) dissemination can occur once the tumor capsule is violated, before or during surgery.[11] If chemotherapy or radiation is used alone, then the common issues seen with these treatments may occur.

Choice of Operative Approach

The operative approach for these lesions is via laminectomy or laminotomy, although with an intraspinal mass, we generally do not replace the laminae to compensate for postoperative swelling or tumor growth.

Preoperative Testing and Imaging

Urodynamics should be obtained to provide the surgeon with a baseline for urinary bladder function. Magnetic resonance imaging (MRI) with and without contrast is obtained to view the anatomy of the tumor. On MRI, myxopapillary ependymomas enhance intensely and are most often intradural, extramedullary lesions. T1-weighted MRI demonstrate these tumors as homogeneous and isointense (**Fig. 113.1**) and T2-weighted images are homogeneous but hyperintense (**Fig. 113.2**).[12] Hemosiderin deposition in the pia and arachnoid is a common finding.[5] Plain radiographs may demonstrate widening of the interpedicular distance, erosion of the posterior elements, and an increase in the size of the intervertebral foramina.[13] MRI is very sensitive (100%) and moderately specific (67%) in detecting direct anatomic contact between the conus and myxopapillary tumors.[6]

Surgical Procedure

The skin is opened in the midline to encompass the length of the tumor. A laminectomy is performed over the lesion using radiographic confirmation of the level, if necessary. The use of a laminotomy can be considered in an attempt to increase the integrity of the spine postoperatively. With the bone removed, the lesion usually can be appreciated through the intact dura mater (**Fig. 113.3**). The dural opening is begun above the lesion and extended over its entire length. The neoplasm itself is usually hemorrhagic, soft, and bluish gray, causing the nerve roots to be displaced laterally (**Fig. 113.4**).

With the dura completely open, the filum is located and cut above the lesion. Using cotton pledgets, the cauda equina is separated from the tumor. Great care is taken to keep the thin capsule of the tumor intact (**Fig. 113.5**). Adhesions from the capsule

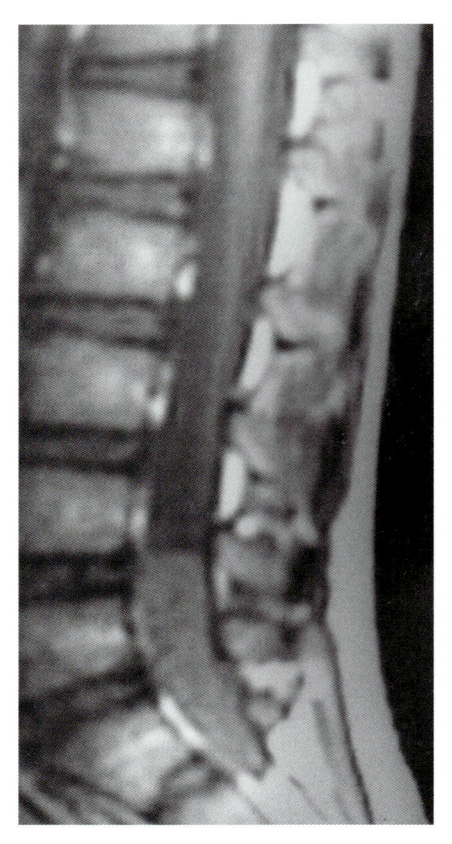

Fig. 113.1 Case example (**Figs. 113.1 to 113.4**). A patient presented with a mass filling the lower lumbar and sacral spine, which is apparent on this midsagittal T1-weighted magnetic resonance imaging scan of the lumbar spine. The lesion is isointense compared with other neural tissue.

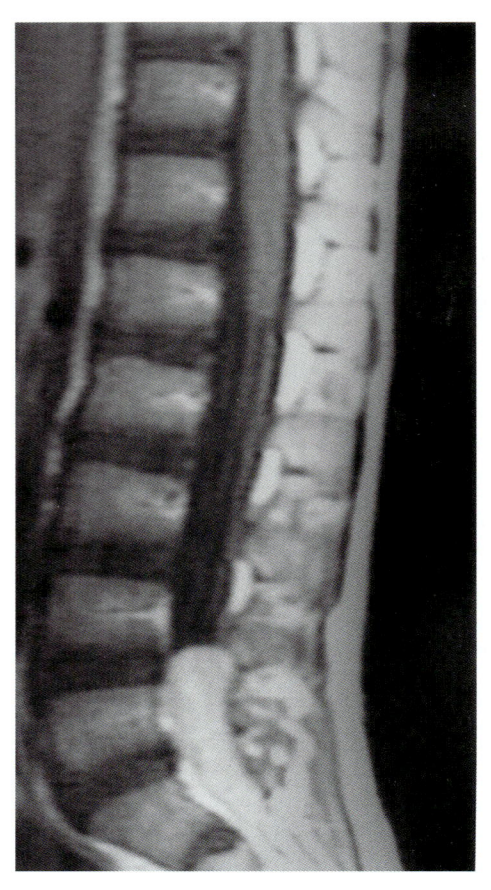

Fig. 113.2 Following intravenous contrast, the tumor enhances homogeneously.

to the surrounding roots are common, and their separation usually can be accomplished. In addition to maintaining the physical integrity of the roots, the vascular supply to these small structures must be maintained. Slowly working around the circumference of the lesion, dealing with points of adhesion, is the best option available. The further caudally the surgeon progresses, the fewer the nerve roots and the easier the dissection. Eventually, the lesion will be freed and delivered. The closure is in the standard manner with or without duraplasty.

Postoperative Care

The standard postoperative care for spinal surgery is given, including monitoring urinary output, providing pain control, and starting physical therapy. Most patients are maintained in a relatively flat position for a few days to enable the best healing of the dura mater.

Radiation therapy (RT) is a controversial treatment option following surgical intervention.[3] Gross total resection of the tumor or subtotal resection followed by radiotherapy is more likely to avoid tumor recurrence than subtotal resection alone.[14] One study found that the 5-year progression-free survival (PFS) was 50.4% and 74.8% for surgery only and surgery with postoperative low-dose (< 50.4 Gy) or high-dose (≥ 50.4 Gy) RT, respectively.[9] Treatment failure was observed in 24 (28%) patients. Fifteen patients presented with treatment failure at the primary site only, whereas two patients presented with treatment failure in the brain and one with distant spinal failure. Age old than 36 years ($p = 0.01$), absence of neurologic symptoms at diagnosis ($p = 0.01$), tumor size ≥ 25 mm ($p = 0.04$), and postoperative high-dose RT ($p = 0.05$) were the factors predictive of improved PFS on univariate analysis. In multivariate analysis, only postoperative high-dose RT was an independent predictors of PFS ($p = 0.04$).

Potential Complications and Precautions

Complications include significant blood loss, neurologic compromise, infection, tumor capsule violation with CSF spread, CSF leak, and postoperative spinal deformation from laminectomy. Such complications can be minimized with strict surgical technique including a watertight dural closure with or without duraplasty and attention to bony removal or replacement.

Conclusion

Myxopapillary ependymomas are slow growing tumors that are often more aggressive in children. Surgery is indicated, with care taken not to allow tumor spread outside of the capsule. Adjunct therapy may improve outcomes. **Box 113.1** summarizes the key operative steps.

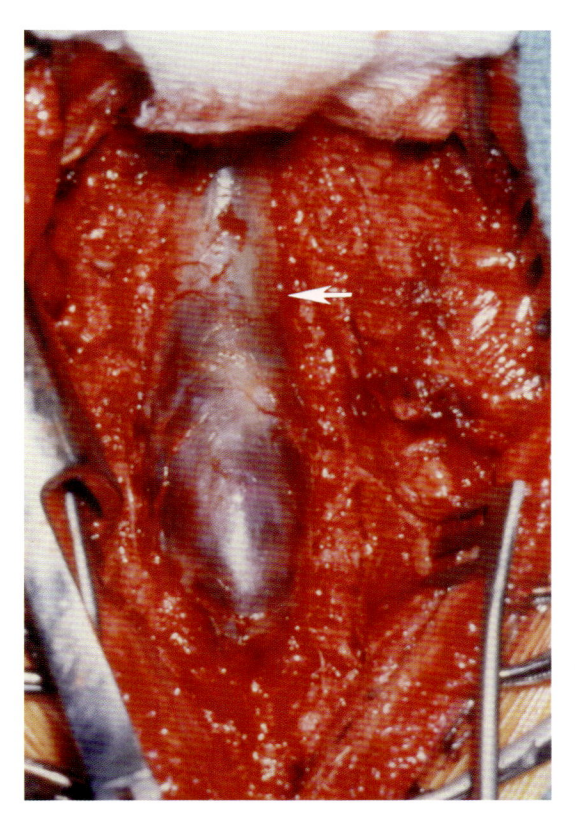

Fig. 113.3 A laminectomy has been performed but the dura is left intact: intraoperative view. The superior pole of the tumor can be appreciated through the dura *(arrow)*.

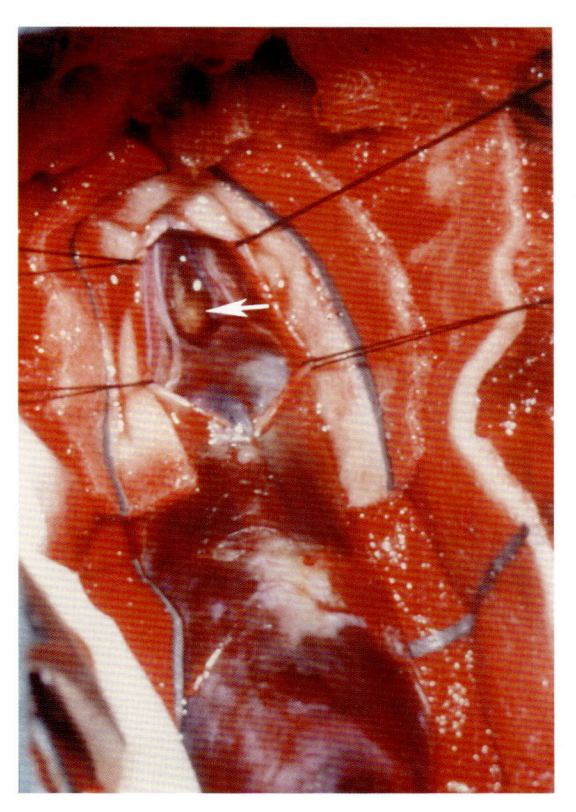

Fig. 113.4 With the dura opened superiorly, the cauda equina can be seen displaced laterally, and the filum terminale is appreciated in the midline *(arrow)* as it enters the superior pole of the tumor.

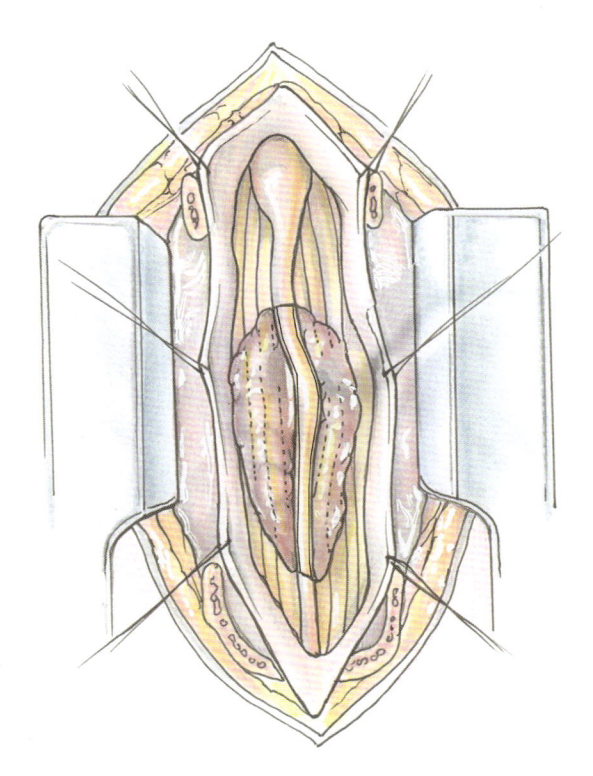

Fig. 113.5 Illustration of the junction of the tumor with the cauda equina.

Box 113.1   Key Operative Steps

- Skin incision
- Laminectomy/otomy over the length of the lesion
- Dural opening
- Dissection of adhesions to tumor capsule/rootlets
- Avoidance of capsule rupture
- Maintain vascular supply to roots
- Removal of lesion/capsule
- Hemostasis
- Dural closure with/without duraplasty
- If laminotomy, secure bone back in place
- Standard fascial/skin closure

References

1. Wiss DA. An unusual cause of sciatica and back pain: ependymoma of the cauda equina. Case report. J Bone Joint Surg Am 1982;64:772–773
2. Gagliardi FM, Cervoni L, Domenicucci M, Celli P, Salvati M. Ependymomas of the filum terminale in childhood: report of four cases and review of the literature. Childs Nerv Syst 1993;9:3–6
3. Nagib MG, O'Fallon MT. Myxopapillary ependymoma of the conus medullaris and filum terminale in the pediatric age group. Pediatr Neurosurg 1997;26:2–7

4. Rubinstein LJ. Myxopapillary ependymomas. In: Russell DS, Rubinstein LJ, eds. Pathology of Tumors of the Nervous System, vol 5. Baltimore: Williams and Wilkins; 1989:203–206
5. Schweitzer JS, Batzdorf U. Ependymoma of the cauda equina region: diagnosis, treatment, and outcome in 15 patients. Neurosurgery 1992;30:202–207
6. Al-Habib A, Al-Radi OO, Shannon P, Al-Ahmadi H, Petrenko Y, Fehlings MG. Myxopapillary ependymoma: correlation of clinical and imaging features with surgical resectability in a series with long-term follow-up. Spinal Cord 2011;49:1073–1078
7. Sonneland PRL, Scheithauer BW, Onofrio BM. Myxopapillary ependymoma. A clinicopathologic and immunocytochemical study of 77 cases. Cancer 1985;56:883–893
8. Specht CS, Smith TW, DeGirolami U, Price JM. Myxopapillary ependymoma of the filum terminale. A light and electron microscopic study. Cancer 1986;58:310–317
9. Pica A, Miller R, Villà S, et al. The results of surgery, with or without radiotherapy, for primary spinal myxopapillary ependymoma: a retrospective study from the rare cancer network. Int J Radiat Oncol Biol Phys 2009;74:1114–1120
10. Wang H, Zhang S, Rehman SK, et al. Clinicopathological features of myxopapillary ependymoma. J Clin Neurosci 2014;21:569–573
11. Barton VN, Donson AM, Kleinschmidt-DeMasters BK, Birks DK, Handler MH, Foreman NK. Unique molecular characteristics of pediatric myxopapillary ependymoma. Brain Pathol 2010;20:560–570
12. Yamada CY, Whitman GJ, Chew FS. Myxopapillary ependymoma of the filum terminale. AJR Am J Roentgenol 1997;168:366
13. Friedman A. Intramedullary tumors and tumors of the cauda equina. In: Rengachary SS, Wilkins R, eds. Principles of Neurosurgery. London: Mosby; 1994:39.2–39.3 and 39.9–39.10
14. Agbahiwe HC, Wharam M, Batra S, Cohen K, Terezakis SA. Management of pediatric myxopapillary ependymoma: the role of adjuvant radiation. Int J Radiat Oncol Biol Phys 2013;85:421–427

114 Release of the Tethered Spinal Cord

R. Shane Tubbs and W. Jerry Oakes

The tethered cord syndrome (TCS) is an increasingly recognized cause of pediatric and adult lower spinal cord dysfunction and disability. Since its original description in the 1950s, this disorder has become more frequently diagnosed because of the increased ease of diagnosis and an expanded definition of the pathology. The recognition of the association of a thickened and taut filum terminale with other forms of occult spinal dysraphism (such as lipomyelomeningocele and split cord malformation) has improved the surgical outcome of numerous patients. Sectioning of the filum terminale is a simple and safe procedure that should be employed at the time the diagnosis is made.

For the purposes of this discussion, the TCS is considered one of the seven pathological entities that make up the family of diseases referred to as occult spinal dysraphism (OSD). It is characterized by excessive tension on the distal spinal cord by a thickened or inelastic filum terminale (**Fig. 114.1**). The pathological filum is almost always infiltrated with fat to the extent that magnetic resonance imaging (MRI) can detect it. The conus usually assumes a low position within the spinal canal reflective of its anticipated position. However, in an extremely small subset of patients, the conus may be located at a normal position. Regardless of position, excessive tension is applied to the spinal cord causing neurologic dysfunction and possibly pain. Traction on the caudal cord results in decreased blood flow causing metabolic derangements that culminate in motor, sensory, and urinary neurologic deficits.

Patient Selection

Patients with the TCS present for clinical attention in a similar manner as patients with other forms of occult spinal dysraphism (such as lipomyelomeningocele). Infants are unlikely to be symptomatic but are brought to clinical attention because of a cutaneous signature of OSD, most commonly capillary hemangioma. However, this is also the least reliable cutaneous sign, with surgically significant pathology occurring in the minority of patients. Associated anomalies that raise the likelihood of a TCS include anorectal atresia and cloacal exstrophy.

After cutaneous signatures, the next most common presenting problems, in order of their occurrence, are neurogenic bladder, orthopedic presentations with foot and leg length discrepancies, scoliosis, and asymmetry of the plantar arches.

The diagnosis and evaluation of patients with TCS is relatively simple. It begins with a history and physical examination. Special attention is paid to the neurologic function of the lower extremities. Imaging usually demonstrates a low-lying conus medullaris or a fatty infiltrated filum terminale.

Indications and Contraindications

The goal of the surgical strategy is to release the tethering structure (fatty filum terminale) and thus the chronic tension on the cord. Early operative intervention is frequently associated with improved outcomes. There are no contraindications to surgery, assuming adequate cardiopulmonary function.

Advantages and Disadvantages

The untethering operation restores blood flow and reverses the clinical picture in most symptomatic cases. Physicians with knowledge in this area understand that neurologic worsening from spinal cord fixation is a constant and ongoing threat, surgical risk is exceedingly low, and recovery from a preoperative neurologic deficit is marginal but dependent on the nature and extent of the deficit. De-tethering may halt or reverse mild scoliotic curvatures. The least likely presentation is with a neurologic deficit, either motor or sensory. Pain as the primary complaint occurs in less than 5% of children but in more than 50% of adults. There are no disadvantages to surgery, as the natural history of continued caudal traction on the spinal cord demonstrates neurologic compromise.

Choice of Operative Approach

A midline incision is used for approaching the midline spine to perform a laminectomy. The surgeon may expose the filum anywhere along its course from the conus to the end of the cul-de-sac. However, we believe that an S1 laminectomy is less likely to result in postoperative pain/instability issues.

Preoperative Testing and Imaging

Evidence of bladder dysfunction can be implied from the history, but much more information can be obtained from urodynamics testing. The position of the conus, the size and character of the filum, and the presence and extent of a potential syrinx can be determined by ultrasound within the first 3 to 4 months of life.

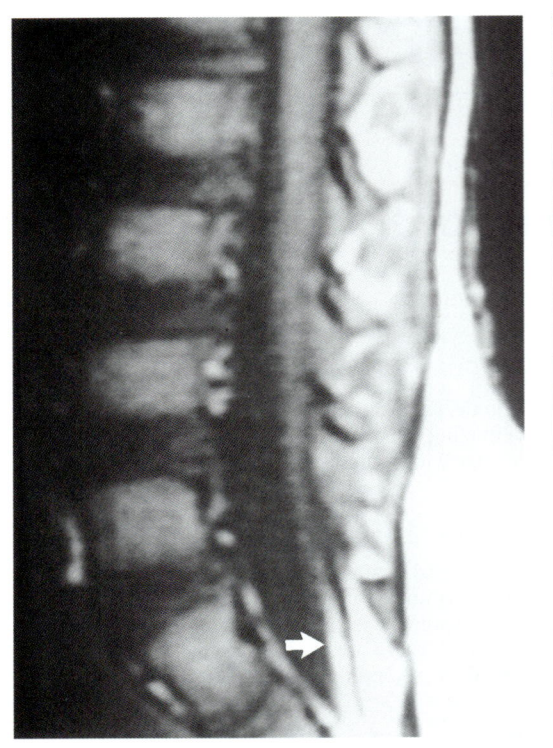

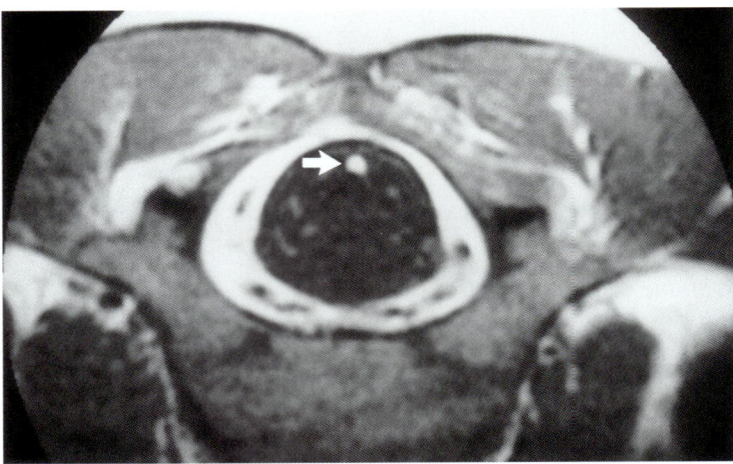

Fig. 114.1 (a) Midsagittal T1-weighted magnetic resonance imaging (MRI) of a typical patient with the tethered cord syndrome. Note the caudal displacement of the conus, its elongated appearance, and the obvious fat in the filum *(arrow)*. (b) Axial MRI of another patient through the sacral region. The enlarged fatty infiltrated filum hugs the dorsal dura *(arrow)*.

After the loss of this acoustical window in the dorsal lumbar spine, MRI is used to assess these variables (**Fig. 114.1**). Routine radiographs of the lumbar spine add information concerning the extent and degree of potential segmentation errors of the spine or bony spina bifida. The normal position of the conus by 3 months of age is at or above the L1-2 disk space. This is true in the vast majority of the population, although in some people it is lower. TCS patients usually have their conus below L3. However, patients may develop symptoms with the conus above L3 with bony spina bifida, fat in an enlarged thickened filum, and an elongated appearance of the conus. The position of the conus is an important criterion for TCS; rarely, patients may be symptomatic and respond to filum sectioning with the conus in a normal position.

Surgical Procedure

The patient is positioned prone with bolsters under the iliac crests and chest to enable free abdominal excursion. A limited midline linear incision is made over S1 and S2 (**Fig. 114.2**) (Video 114.1). Although the dura can be opened between the laminae, we prefer to perform a standard S1 laminectomy and open the dura in the midline. Frequently, the enlarged filum can be appreciated through the intact dura. With the dura open, the roots are seen exiting ventrally and laterally, whereas the fatty infiltrated filum is usually in the midline and exits dorsally. The filum frequently has a bluish hue to help distinguish it from the adherent roots, and on the ventral surface is a characteristic vessel running the length of the structure. If roots are continuing to be significant in number and the cul-de-sac of the subarachnoid space is well below S1, the posterior elements of S2 may be removed to increase visualization.

Once the filum is identified, all neural elements are separated and this structure isolated (**Fig. 114.3**), and with very low settings, the bipolar forceps are used to coagulate and then cut the filum in two places. This enables submitting a specimen for pathological examination and creates a gap between the cut ends of the structure. Care should be taken to avoid contamination of the subarachnoid space with blood to minimize the subsequent risk of arachnoiditis.

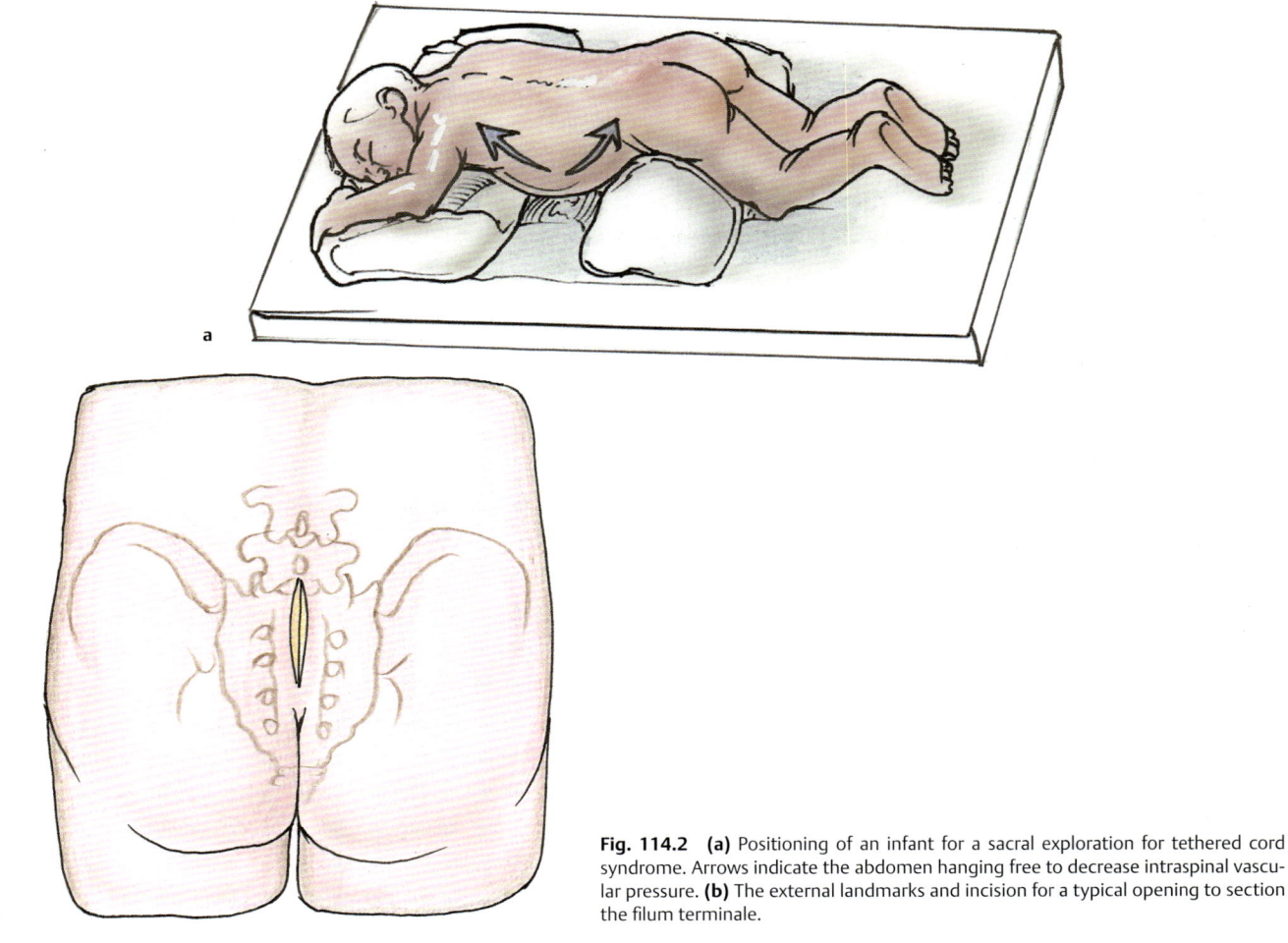

Fig. 114.2 (a) Positioning of an infant for a sacral exploration for tethered cord syndrome. Arrows indicate the abdomen hanging free to decrease intraspinal vascular pressure. (b) The external landmarks and incision for a typical opening to section the filum terminale.

Throughout the operation, no monitoring is performed. With experience, the filum is appreciated as a distinct structure that would be difficult to confuse with any of the surrounding neural elements. All nerve roots have a pathognomonic finding of alternating light and dark banding occurring approximately every millimeter. This banding, easily seen with magnification, is not present in the filum. With the filum cut, the dura and soft tissues are approximated. No drain is necessary.

Postoperative Care

Patients are maintained in a flat position for a few days to enable dural healing without the added effects of orthostatic pressure from an upright posture. This is easily tolerated in small infants but a bit more difficult in children. Pain relief is usually easily accomplished with oral analgesics. Occasionally, bladder catheterization is necessary until the patient is able to assume an upright position.

Potential Complications and Precautions

Very few complications occur with this procedure other then pseudomeningoceles. Care must be taken to open the dura in the area of the cul-de-sac where all neural elements have left the cord and are lateral. Including sacral nerve roots with the section of the filum may result in urinary bladder incontinence and sexual dysfunction. The risk is lower if all the sacral points of exit are in view before selecting the filum for sectioning.

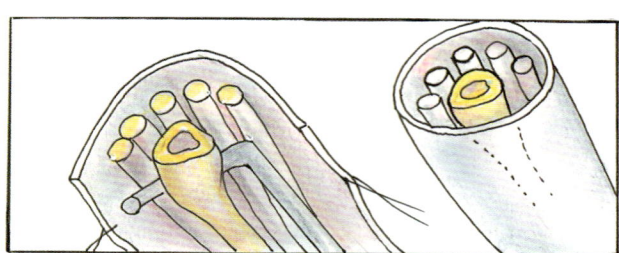

Fig. 114.3 (a) Axial representation of the separation of the fatty infiltrated filum from the surrounding roots. (b) Intraoperative view of the intradural contents. In this case, the filum is quite large and obscures the visualization of the sacral roots. It must be separated from all of these neural elements before (c) the filum is sectioned. (d) Intraoperative view of the sacral intradural contents with a suture around the easily separated and thickened filum terminale. (e) Intraoperative view of a sectioned filum terminale.

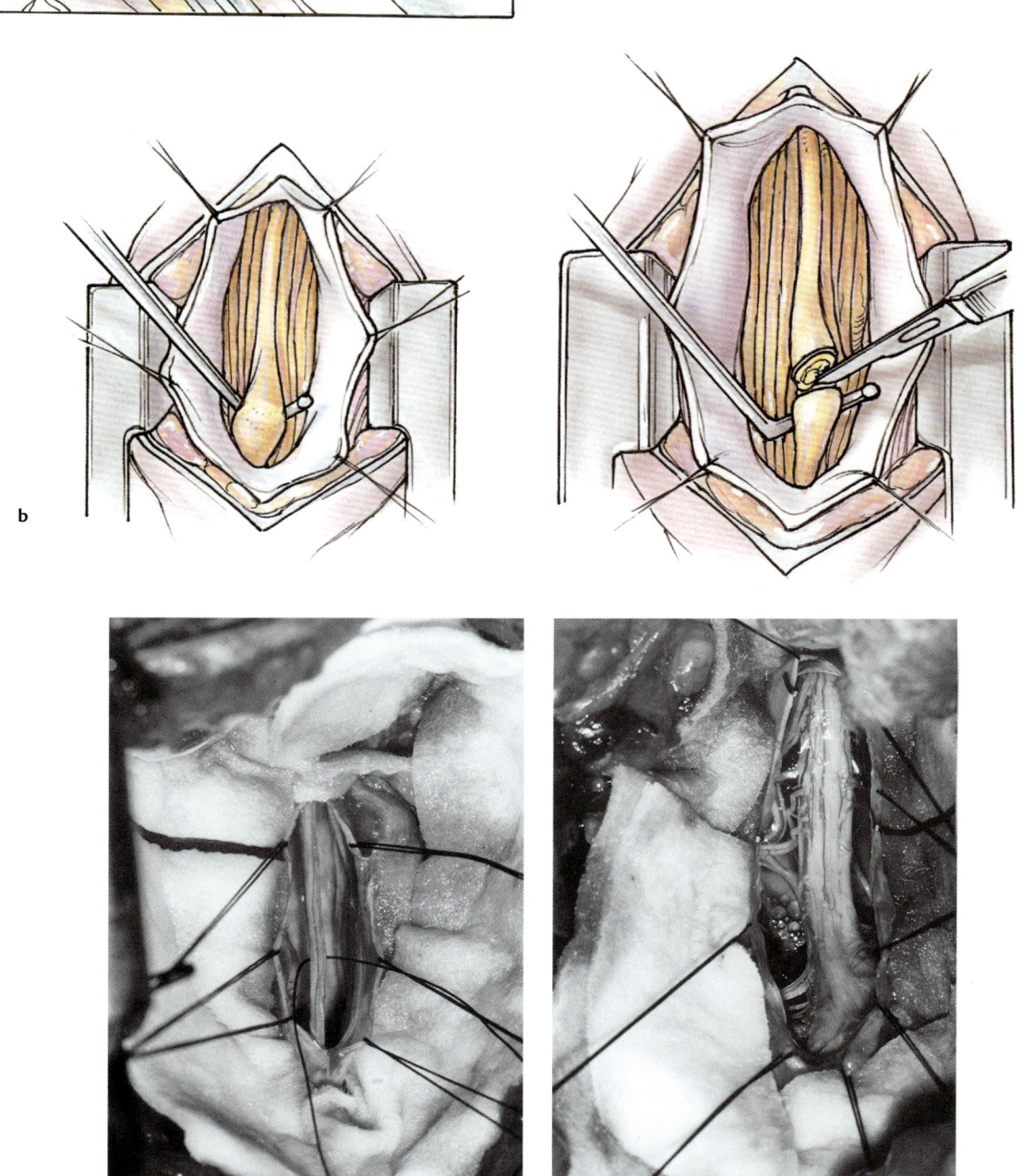

Conclusion

Sectioning of the filum terminale for the TCS is one of the simplest intradural procedures performed by neurosurgeons. The challenge lies in selecting patients for investigation and surgery at the earliest possible time before irreversible symptoms occur. Complications and postoperative problems are minimal. **Box 114.1** summarizes the key operative steps.

Box 114.1 Key Operative Steps

- Midline skin incision over S1 and S2
- S1 laminectomy
- Dural opening
- Identification of filum terminale
- Care in separating attached neural elements
- Careful coagulation of filum at two points
- Transection of coagulated filum
- Specimen for pathology
- Avoid contamination of the subarachnoid space with blood
- Dural closure
- Reapproximate soft tissues in standard manner

Suggested Readings

Chern JJ, Dauser RC, Whitehead WE, Curry DJ, Luerssen TG, Jea A. The effect of tethered cord release on coronal spinal balance in tight filum terminale. Spine 2011;36:E944–E949

Filippidis AS, Kalani MY, Theodore N, Rekate HL. Spinal cord traction, vascular compromise, hypoxia, and metabolic derangements in the pathophysiology of tethered cord syndrome. Neurosurg Focus 2010;29:E9

Lew SM, Kothbauer KF. Tethered cord syndrome: an updated review. Pediatr Neurosurg 2007;43:236–248

McLendon RE, Oakes WJ, Heinz ER, Yeates AE, Burger PC. Adipose tissue in the filum terminale: a computed tomographic finding that may indicate tethering of the spinal cord. Neurosurgery 1988;22:873–876

Sato S, Shirane R, Yoshimoto T. Evaluation of tethered cord syndrome associated with anorectal malformations. Neurosurgery 1993;32:1025–1027, discussion 1027–1028

Sharif S, Allcutt D, Marks C, Brennan P. "Tethered cord syndrome"—recent clinical experience. Br J Neurosurg 1997;11:49–51

Tubbs RS, Wellons JC III, Iskandar BJ, Oakes WJ. Isolated flat capillary midline lumbosacral hemangiomas as indicators of occult spinal dysraphism. J Neurosurg 2004;100(2, Suppl Pediatrics):86–89

Warder DE, Oakes WJ. Tethered cord syndrome and the conus in a normal position. Neurosurgery 1993;33:374–378

Yamada S, Zinke DE, Sanders D. Pathophysiology of "tethered cord syndrome". J Neurosurg 1981;54:494–503

115 MIS Release of the Tethered Spinal Cord

Mena G. Kerolus, Bledi Brahimaj, and Richard G. Fessler

The release of the tethered spinal cord through minimally invasive surgery (MIS) has the following advantages and disadvantages:

Advantages

- Minimizes tissue trauma
- Decreases wound complications
- Minimizes bleeding into the thecal sac, which may lead to retethering
- Minimizes scar tissue, which may lead to retethering
- Decreases the incidence of pseudomeningoceles
- Reduces blood loss
- Results in less postoperative pain
- Leads to a faster recovery
- Entails a shorter hospital stay

Disadvantages

- Entails a significant learning curve
- May limit the length of the durotomy repair

Objective

The ultimate goal of spinal cord detethering is to release the conus from the abnormal filum terminale, providing optimum longitudinal growth and neurologic recovery. The natural history of spinal cord tethering entails neurologic deterioration.[1] Surgery is preferably done before the onset of irreversible neurologic deficits.

In children, early cord detethering prevents deterioration during growth and has been proven to result in significant improvement in neurologic function.[2–5] Children generally have a better outcome if they are younger than 3 years of age at the time of intervention.[6] Timing for treatment in adults is still highly debated. Prognosis is generally better with early intervention, but the degree and duration of neurologic dysfunction ultimately dictates recovery.[2,4,7,8] When compared with the morbidity of the natural progression of the disease, surgical intervention of spinal cord detethering entails low risk and is well tolerated.[8]

Minimally invasive techniques for the tethered cord were designed to provide a safe and efficient method of spinal cord detethering. The added benefits include a reduction in blood loss, shorter hospital stay, fewer activity restrictions postoperatively, and a decreased incidence of retethering. In 2007, Tredway et al[1] described the first minimally invasive approach of spinal cord detethering in three patients of different ages, all of whom experienced neurologic improvement postoperatively.

Clinical Presentation

Tethered spinal cord is a pathological entity involving a developmental abnormality of the spinal cord that is commonly associated with spinal dysraphism, neurologic dysfunction, and orthopedic deformity. Cutaneous physical exam findings typically consist of sacral dimples, hypertrichosis, pigment nevi, nodules, lumbar or sacral hair patches, lipomas, asymmetric gluteal clefts, and midline lumbar hemangiomas. These physical findings tend to be present in childhood, which should prompt further medical workup. In the adult population, cutaneous findings are typically present in only 35% of cases.[2]

Patients with a tethered spinal cord may experience diverse neurologic symptoms. Common symptoms include lower extremity weakness, lower back pain, leg pain, sensory deficits, bladder or bowel symptoms, and sexual dysfunction. Various orthopedic deformities, including neuromuscular scoliosis and asymmetric leg or foot deformities, may be present and are much more common in childhood. Children may experience ataxia, difficulty running, leg cramps, and delayed toilet training with abnormal urodynamics.[4] In the adult population, over 81% of patients experience pain as the primary symptom, followed closely by sensory changes and weakness. Adults either experience initial symptoms as an adult or experience mild symptoms in childhood that become exacerbated with repetitive trauma or degenerative disease. Symptoms are insidious, as many neurologic deficits are nonspecific and do not always correspond to a specific myotome or dermatomal pattern.[2,9]

Preoperative Evaluation

Initial workup should include electrophysiological and urodynamic studies. Plain radiographs may reveal bifid spinous process.[1] In the adult population, plain radiographs demonstrate abnormality in 100% of patients.[1,2] A magnetic resonance imaging (MRI) scan of the thoracic and lumbar spine is still the study of choice for evaluation of tethered cord. MRI findings may include a thoracic syrinx or other abnormalities such as a pathological thickened filum terminale that is greater than 2 mm. A fatty infiltrate is commonly found with a thickened filum or split cord malformation. Additionally, the conus can be identified below the L2 vertebral body.[10] However, not all patients have a low-lying conus. There are several reports of symptomatic patients with a normal-lying conus who improve after tethered cord release.[11]

Description of Procedure

After induction of general anesthesia, the patient is placed in the prone position. With the use of fluoroscopic guidance, the desired level below the level of the conus is localized and marked.

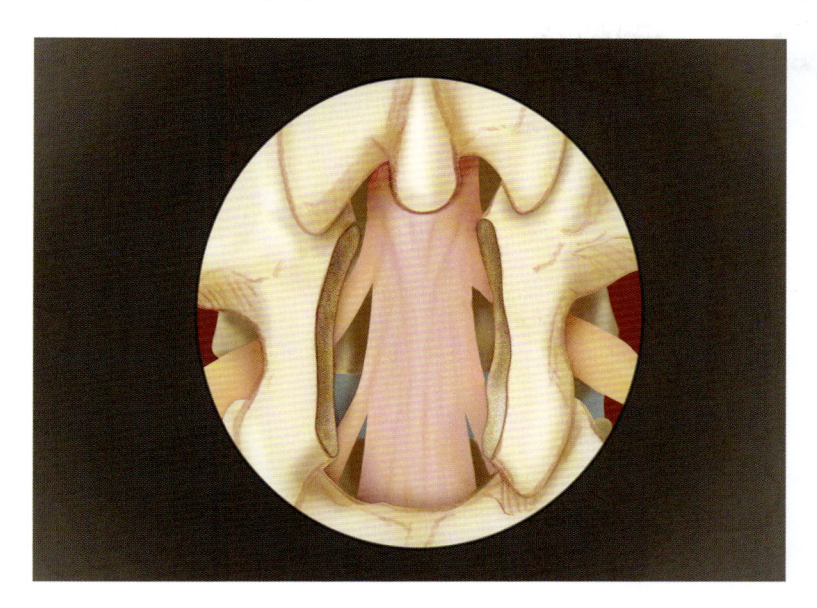

Fig. 115.1 View through the retraction tube showing bilateral laminectomy.

Clear sterile drapes are placed over the lower extremities to visualize stimulation during intraoperative testing. A unilateral minimally invasive approach is used. Using a 15-mm scalpel, a 2-cm incision parallel to the spinous process is made approximately 1 cm lateral to the midline. The fascia is then separated using monopolar electrocautery. Dilators are used to perform a muscle-splitting exposure of the correct interspace. We suggest using an 18- to 22-mm dilator (METRx; Medtronic Inc., Minneapolis, MN). Other tubes, including the X-tube (Medtronic) and Quadrant tube (Medtronic), have been used with similar efficacy in cases with intradural pathology. An important consideration when planning the surgical evaluation of any intradural pathology is that the tube size should be about 0.5 to 1 cm longer than the planned durotomy.[12]

The operative microscope is brought into the surgical field. Using standard minimally invasive techniques as described in previous chapters, a MIS laminectomy is performed. Using a high-speed drill (Midas Rex, Medtronic), a hemilaminectomy is performed on the same side as the dilation, followed by undercutting of the spinous process, and a hemilaminectomy on the other side. The ligamentum flavum is dissected and removed. At this point, the MIS laminectomy provides adequate exposure of the canal and dorsal dural surface of the thecal sac at one particular level (**Fig. 115.1**).

A longitudinal durotomy is opened sharply using an 11-mm scalpel. The dural edges are tacked up with 4–0 Nurolon suture. The suture is pulled through the tube and secured with a hemostat. The sacral nerve roots are dissected from the thickened filum. The filum is easily differentiated from the sacral and lumbar nerve roots. The arachnoid is then dissected using a right angle dissector (**Fig. 115.2**). A nerve root stimulator is used to monitor the bilateral distal lower extremities, and anal sphincter

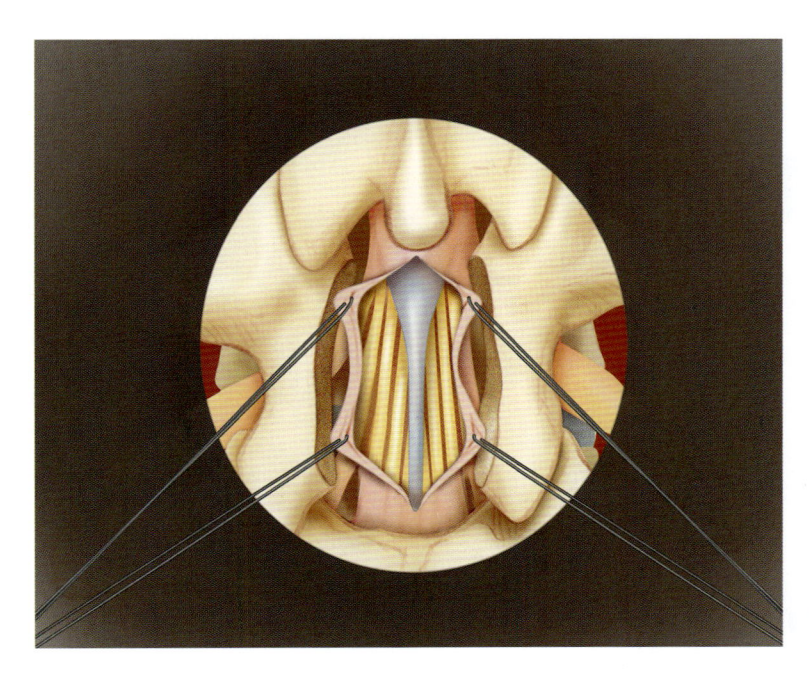

Fig. 115.2 Microscopic MIS view of a 1-cm durotomy revealing the filum terminale.

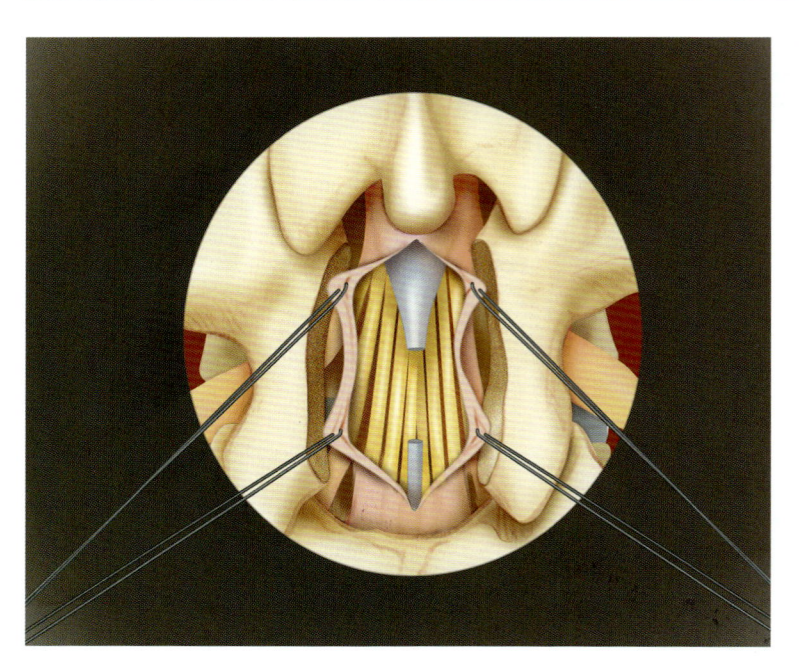

Fig. 115.3 Microscopic view of resected filum terminale.

electromyograms are performed. A control stimulation is done at L5–S1 to assess the expected motor changes. After a successful control stimulation is completed, the filum is stimulated and should fail to produce a response. If the anal sphincter electromyogram is positive, further sacral nerve root dissection is required. After confirmatory identification, the filum is coagulated using bipolar cautery, and a segment is removed. A portion of the filum is sent to the pathology lab for review **(Fig. 115.3)**.

The dura is closed using 5–0 Prolene or 6–0 Gore-Tex sutures (Ethicon, Somerville, NJ) for a watertight closure **(Fig. 115.4)**. Closure and knots are secured using the Scanlan Cardiovasive Chitwood knot pusher (Scanlan International, St. Paul, MN). An intraoperative Valsalva is used to check for a cerebrospinal leak. If a leak is present, the surgeon may use a small piece of harvested muscle for repair of this area.[11] Fibrin glue may be used over the dural repair. The tubular retractor is slowly removed, and hemostasis is achieved using bipolar electrocautery. Interrupted absorbable fascial and subcutaneous sutures are placed and the skin is closed with Dermabond (Video 115.1).

Postoperative Care

Postoperatively, the patient should lie flat for a period of 24 hours prior to sitting up in bed or ambulating. Following open release, patients are required to lie flat for a period of 3 to 5 days (see Chapter 114). However, with MIS the small amount of dead space and the dilating technique of the musculature allow for less activity restriction immediately postoperatively. Tan et al[12] have reported the largest single series of minimally invasive intended durotomy and management. In their series of 23 patients undergoing an MIS approach, none experienced a cerebrospinal fluid (CSF), and all patients were able to ambulate within 24 hours of surgery. Pain is well controlled postoperatively given that a large percentage of patients experience lower back or leg

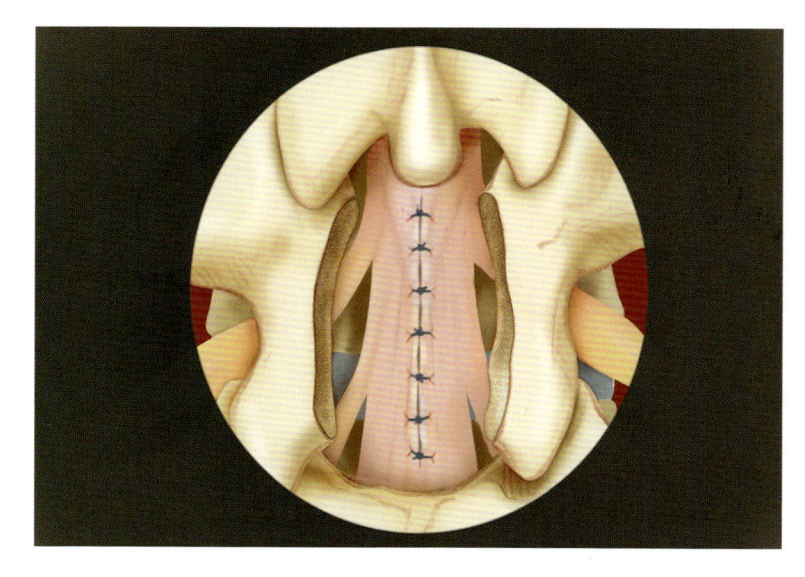

Fig. 115.4 Microscope view of dorsal dura watertight closure.

pain secondary to the tethered cord. When the cord is released, the pain is reduced. Foley placement may be advisable for the first 24 hours after surgery; it can be removed once the patient is upright. Intermittent catheterization may be necessary until urodynamic studies are completed.

Complications

The minimally invasive approach for spinal cord detethering reduces the risk of complications. However, any surgical spine procedure involving intradural pathology may result in a CSF leak that may lead to wound breakdown, meningitis, and the need for reoperation. However, it has been established that MIS durotomy repairs are safe and effective. After an appropriate learning curve, the rate of CSF leak has been reported as low as 0%.[12] Subsequently, the rate of pseudomeningocele formation becomes negligible given minimal tissue disruption.

Conclusion

The consequence of neurologic dysfunction in the setting of a tethered cord may be devastating. Repeated microtrauma during flexion and extension of a mechanically tethered cord can result in permanent injury and neurologic deterioration.[13] Failure of the filum terminale to elongate during growth creates tension along the longitudinal access of the spinal cord.[2,13] Physiological changes due to stretching of the spinal cord and nerve roots result in decreased blood flow. Poor perfusion of the cord leads to ischemic changes due to failure of oxidative metabolism, which may be reversible after detethering.[2,13] Upon detethering of the cord, an increase in blood flow and improvement in nerve conduction studies are noted, especially with early surgical intervention.[14,15]

Open untethering of the spinal cord has yielded excellent results, leading to improvement in lower extremity strength and urologic dysfunction. A minimally invasive approach for treatment of a tethered spinal cord may minimize tissue trauma and bleeding into the thecal sac, and result in a lower incidence of pseudomeningocele because of less dead space, a smaller durotomy, shorter surgical time, shorter hospitalization, earlier ambulation, decreased blood loss, and less postoperative pain.

References

1. Tredway TL, Musleh W, Christie SD, Khavkin Y, Fessler RG, Curry DJ. A novel minimally invasive technique for spinal cord untethering. Neurosurgery 2007;60(2, Suppl 1):ONS70–ONS74, discussion ONS74
2. Aufschnaiter K, Fellner F, Wurm G. Surgery in adult onset tethered cord syndrome (ATCS): review of literature on occasion of an exceptional case. Neurosurg Rev 2008;31:371–383, discussion 384
3. Iskandar BJ, Fulmer BB, Hadley MN, Oakes WJ. Congenital tethered spinal cord syndrome in adults. J Neurosurg 1998;88:958–961
4. Kang J-K, Lee K-S, Jeun S-S, Lee I-W, Kim M-C. Role of surgery for maintaining urological function and prevention of retethering in the treatment of lipomeningomyelocele: experience recorded in 75 lipomeningomyelocele patients. Childs Nerv Syst 2003;19:23–29
5. Pang D, Wilberger JE Jr. Tethered cord syndrome in adults. J Neurosurg 1982;57:32–47
6. Wehby MC, O'Hollaren PS, Abtin K, Hume JL, Richards BJ. Occult tight filum terminale syndrome: results of surgical untethering. Pediatr Neurosurg 2004;40:51–57, discussion 58
7. Cochrane DD, Finley C, Kestle J, Steinbok P. The patterns of late deterioration in patients with transitional lipomyelomeningocele. Eur J Pediatr Surg 2000;10(Suppl 1):13–17
8. Gupta G, Heary RF, Michaels J. Reversal of longstanding neurological deficits after a late release of tethered spinal cord. Neurosurg Focus 2010;29:E11
9. Klekamp J, Raimondi AJ, Samii M. Occult dysraphism in adulthood: clinical course and management. Childs Nerv Syst 1994;10:312–320
10. Bulsara KR, Zomorodi AR, Enterline DS, George TM. The value of magnetic resonance imaging in the evaluation of fatty filum terminale. Neurosurgery 2004;54:375–379, discussion 379–380
11. Warder DE, Oakes WJ. Tethered cord syndrome: the low-lying and normally positioned conus. Neurosurgery 1994;34:597–600, discussion 600
12. Tan LA, Takagi I, Straus D, O'Toole JE. Management of intended durotomy in minimally invasive intradural spine surgery: clinical article. J Neurosurg Spine 2014;21:279–285
13. Yamada S, Won DJ, Pezeshkpour G, et al. Pathophysiology of tethered cord syndrome and similar complex disorders. Neurosurg Focus 2007;23:E6
14. Husain AM, Shah D. Prognostic value of neurophysiologic intraoperative monitoring in tethered cord syndrome surgery. J Clin Neurophysiol 2009;26:244–247
15. Schneider SJ, Rosenthal AD, Greenberg BM, Danto J. A preliminary report on the use of laser-Doppler flowmetry during tethered spinal cord release. Neurosurgery 1993;32:214–217, discussion 217–218

116 Implantation of Spinal Cord Stimulators

Erika A. Petersen and Konstantin V. Slavin

Patients with chronic refractory neuropathic pain often present to neurosurgeons after they have exhausted the medical options for effective pain control. In these situations, neuromodulatory approaches such as spinal cord stimulation (SCS) may be considered. The technique, in which electric current is delivered to the dorsal columns through an implanted epidural electrode array, has been shown to be cost-effective in the treatment of chronic pain in comparison with optimal medical management and with repeat surgery.[1–4] The main benefits of this modality include the possibility of decreased medication side effects and improved pain control and functional status using an alternative and complementary means of pain suppression. Stimulation is thought to affect the neuropathic component of pain at several points along the pain messaging pathway, including its processing at spinal and supraspinal levels, facilitating neurotransmitter release, and modulating internal pain inhibition systems.[5]

Patient Selection

Careful patient selection is essential for identifying candidates most likely to benefit from SCS. Patients with severe chronic neuropathic pain of over 6 months in duration may be candidates for this approach. SCS appears to be a particularly safe and effective tool for the management of multiple specific chronic pain syndromes, most notably failed back surgery syndrome, chronic regional pain syndromes, and vascular and diabetic neuropathy (**Table 116.1**). In general, neuropathic pain responds more favorably than nociceptive pain.

Patients should have first been treated with optimized medical management. If that treatment failed, then they can be considered for an advanced pain therapy such as SCS, and they should have conditions that are not amenable to direct surgical treatment. A randomized clinical study demonstrated the superiority of SCS to reoperation in those patients with persistent or recurrent radiculopathy who were candidates for reoperation.[6] Patients should undergo psychological screening to assess any somatization components of the pain, to ensure that psychological conditions are stable and well treated, and to evaluate their reasonable expectations for pain control with the therapy.[7]

Chronic Neuropathic Pain

Patients with chronic moderate-to-severe neuropathic pain that is refractory to optimized medical and surgical management may benefit from SCS. Pain may be radicular, ischemic, related to injury of the peripheral nerves, or a part of a complex regional pain syndrome. Although most epidural SCS electrodes are placed in the thoracic spine to address back and lower extremity pain, evidence also supports the use of cervical SCS for neuropathic pain in the upper extremities.[8] To qualify for SCS, the patient should demonstrate a clear ability to adhere to treatment regimens. For each patient, the risks of infection, device-related complications, and management complexity should be considered.

Emerging Indications

Recent work has sought to expand the utility of SCS beyond pain modulation to include motor functional improvement,[9,10] congestive heart failure management,[11] and management of cerebral vasospasm.[12] Further developments include the introduction of new electrode designs that are able to focus on specific epidural targets such as the dorsal root ganglion or are able to provide alternative methods of current delivery in patients where perception of paresthesias to accomplish effective pain relief may no longer be necessary.[13]

Indications and Contraindications, and the Objectives of Surgery

Inclusion Criteria

Patients are candidates for SCS if they have pain that is refractory to other treatment measures. Patients should have a favorable psychological profile and a track record of compliance with chronic medical therapy that suggests they are able to comply with the maintenance of an advanced neuromodulation device.

Trial Response

Candidates for SCS placement undergo a trial of stimulation to assess response. Generally, an improvement of over 50% is considered a positive trial. Standardized subjective evaluation tools such as the Visual Analogue Scale (VAS) and the Pain Disability Index (PDI) quantify improvement in pain and function during the course of the trial period and complement pain diary narratives. There are several common trialing techniques. A percutaneous epidural trial consists of placing one or several cylindrical leads, whereas a paddle electrode trial requires a laminotomy or laminectomy. The duration of the trial period varies among practitioners. For a trial to be considered successful, a significant clinical improvement, such as > 50% decrease in the pain VAS score, should be demonstrated.

Exclusion Criteria

Increased Surgical Risk Profile

Patients with active ongoing infection or compromised immune system are at higher risk of infectious complications. SCS surgery is considered contraindicated in patients taking anticoagulants that cannot be suspended in the perioperative period or

Table 116.1 Indications for Spinal Cord Stimulation (SCS) Based on the Strength of the Evidence

Prospective Trials

- Axial back pain
- Chronic ischemic extremity pain
- Complex regional pain syndrome types I and II
- Failed back surgery syndrome
- Refractory angina pectoris

Retrospective Evidence

- Diabetic neuropathy
- Postthoracotomy pain syndrome
- Postherpetic neuralgia
- Raynaud's phenomenon
- Spinal cord injury
- Upper extremity pain
- Visceral pain

Case Reports

- Cluneal neuralgia
- Coccydynia
- Demyelination-related pain
- HIV neuropathy
- Postamputation pain

have other medical comorbidities that would increase anesthesia or perioperative risks. In general, the use of SCS is reserved for patients with a life expectancy exceeding 12 months.

Systemic Concerns

Patients with allergic reactions to certain metals may not be SCS candidates. Furthermore, patients with a body habitus that will not accommodate the device's implantation should not be considered for SCS. Most SCS systems are incompatible with magnetic resonance imaging (MRI). Therefore, thoughtful consideration should be given to device selection for any patient with a clinical condition that necessitates MRI surveillance.

Inability to Comply with the Therapy and the Maintenance Schedule

Patients being considered for the SCS system should be comfortable with the technology and be able to perform device maintenance, including recharging an implanted pulse generator (IPG) on a routine basis. Implantation of a stimulator is discouraged in patients who are unable to comply with the management of the device due to logistical, financial, or cognitive issues.

Advantages and Disadvantages

Unfortunately, any implanted device has certain risks, including the possibility of mechanical failure or infection, and it is estimated that up to 38% of patients with implanted SCS systems will require surgery to address a complication.[7,14,15] Infection rates of between 1% and 15% have been reported. Erosion of the system's components, migration of the electrodes, IPG failure, or lead breakage may occur.[16] The risk of neurologic complications related to SCS paddle electrode placement, including epidural hematoma, sensory deficit, autonomic dysfunction, motor dysfunction, and spinal fluid leak, is less than 0.6%.[17] Patients may also express dissatisfaction with SCS related to their inability to achieve or maintain effective pain relief over time or may express irritation related to unwanted paresthesias outside the anatomic target area.

Choice of Operative Approach

Device Options

Current SCS systems are composed of electrode leads and an IPG. Two categories of leads are available: cylindrical and paddle. A cylindrical lead is inserted in the epidural space through a Tuohy-type needle using a percutaneous, fluoroscopy-guided approach, whereas a paddle lead's larger dimension necessitates a small laminotomy for its placement. A percutaneously introduced slim paddle lead is also available, and prototypes for deployable paddle electrodes that can be placed without a laminotomy are being developed. Each lead type has advantages and disadvantages (**Table 116.2**), but the effectiveness of the two types appears similar.[18] There are numerous electrode designs that carry anywhere between four and 32 separate contacts (**Fig. 116.1**). IPGs can be primary cell (non-rechargeable) or rechargeable, and their dimensions vary (**Fig. 116.2**). Newer IPG technology

Table 116.2 Features of Cylindrical and Paddle Electrodes

Feature	Cylindrical	Paddle
Implantation procedure	Percutaneous, less invasive	Laminotomy (percutaneous for slim paddle)
Migration risk	Moderate	Lower
Lead size	1.3- to 1.4-mm diameter	0.5- to 2.0-cc volume
Complications/risks	Migration, fracture, infection	Infection, fracture, migration
Complexity of programming	Depends on electrode arrangements	May be more efficient due to unidirectional configuration

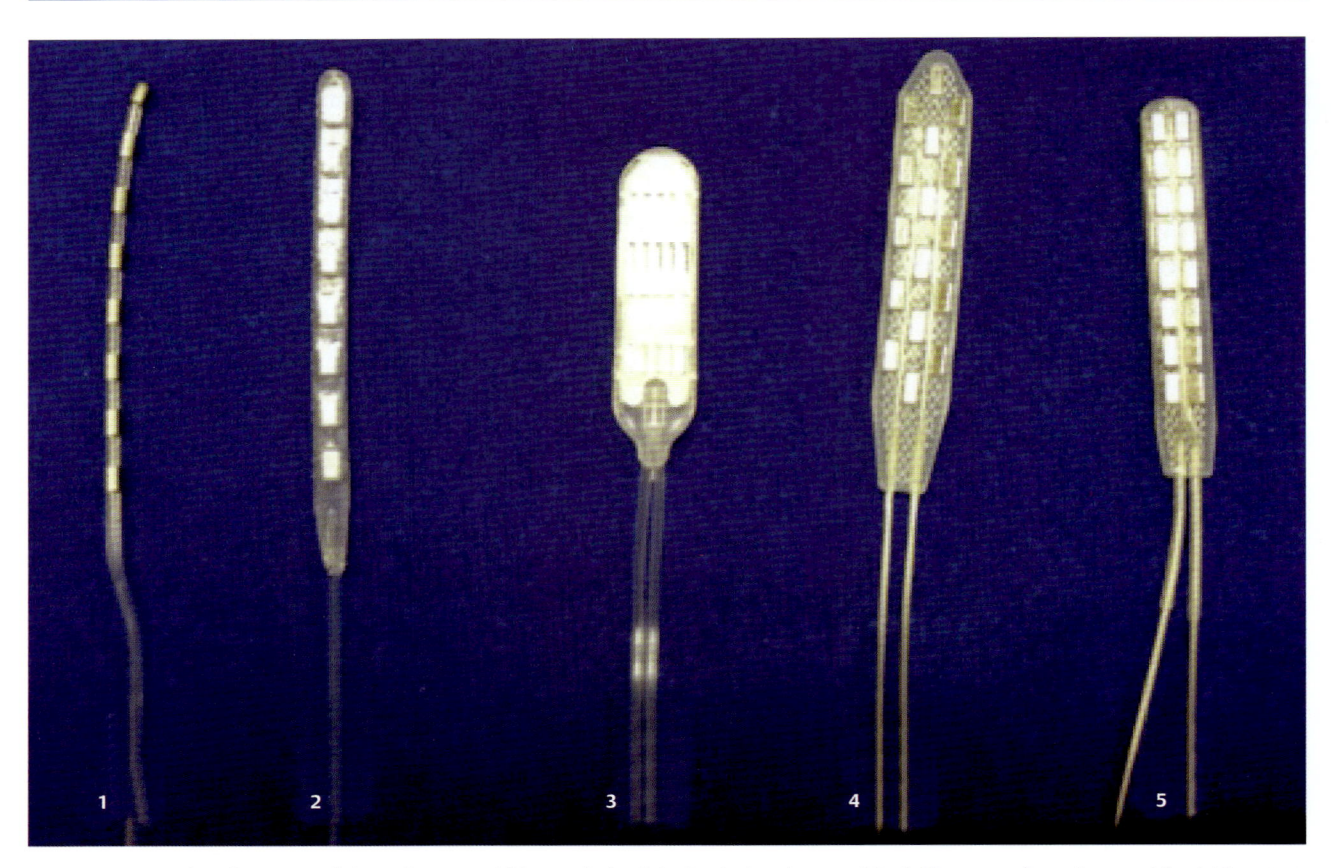

Fig. 116.1 Several configurations of electrodes are available: *1*, cylindrical; *2*, slim single-column paddle; *3*, 20-contact, five-column paddle; *4*, 16-contact, three-column (tripole) paddle; *5*, 16-contact, double-column paddle.

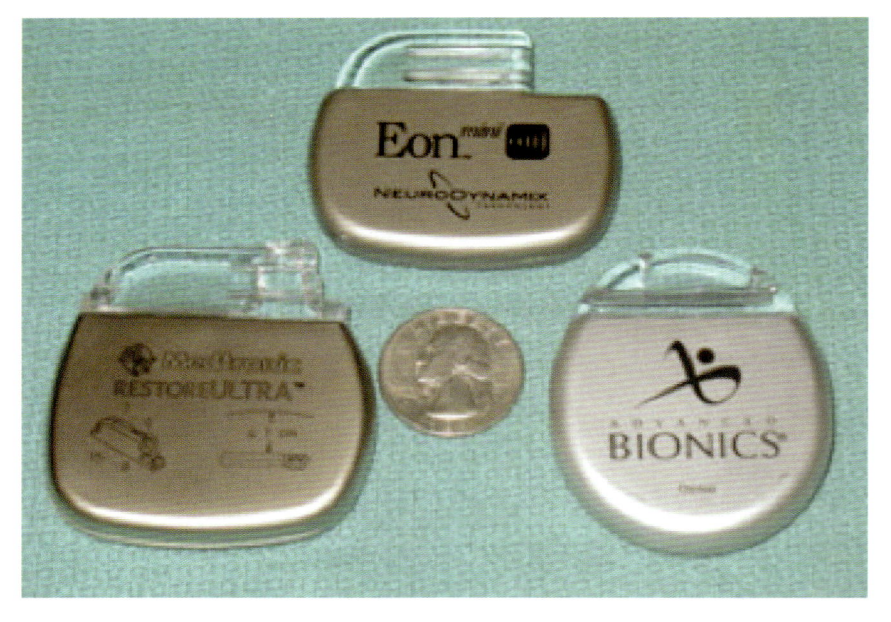

Fig. 116.2 Implanted pulse generators vary in capacity and dimensions.

incorporates more programmable variables for delivery of stimulation current using configurable waveforms across combinations of anodes and cathodes. The lifetime of the primary cell IPG depends on the power demand of the stimulation delivered and the patient's usage pattern. Rechargeable units have an expected lifetime of about 9 years, but the frequency with which they must be recharged varies with usage.

Lead Placement

Percutaneous placement is performed in which the cylindrical lead is introduced through a Tuohy needle into the epidural space and then advanced to the target level using anteroposterior (AP) and lateral fluoroscopy to confirm the location over the dorsal columns. For paddle electrode placement, a small laminotomy is performed to enable access to introduce the electrode. The final electrode position is governed by the patient's pain symptoms and the results of trial electrode placement. The lead is securely anchored to the fascia to minimize the risk of migration.

IPG Placement

The IPG requires placement in a subcutaneous pocket where wireless communication for programming and recharging, if applicable, can be accomplished. The most common locations are in the buttocks or in the abdominal wall, although any subcutaneous location is possible. Care should be taken to ensure that the IPG site does not cause discomfort due to implantation over bony structures or in areas where there is excessive tissue mobility.

Preoperative Testing

Trial Evaluation

All patients undergo a trial period in which a temporary electrode is externalized to enable for several days of test stimulation. Most often these trials are performed using a percutaneous approach to introduce one or several cylindrical leads. In cases where a percutaneous trial is not possible (for example, in patients with significant epidural scarring or a tight stenosis such that leads cannot be safely introduced), a laminotomy trial may be performed. Electrodes are positioned over the dorsal columns to correlate with the location of the afferent fibers for the anatomic region experiencing pain (**Table 116.3**). In each case, the leads are externalized to enable connection to a temporary generator. This may be accomplished by either having temporary electrodes that connect directly to an external pulse generator (EPG) or with a so-called tunneled trial technique in which the electrodes are anchored inside and temporary extension cables are tunneled to a distant exit site for connection to the EPG. The actual technique for trial lead implantation does not differ from permanent lead placement (described below).

The device trial should result in a decrease of over 50% in pain levels, and the patient should experience improvement in daily activities such as mobility and the quality of sleep. At the conclusion of the trial, temporary percutaneous leads can be removed during an office visit. Patients with a successful trial can then proceed to the implantation of a permanent system. In successful laminotomy trials and in tunneled percutaneous trials,

Table 116.3 Spinal Target for Electrode Placement

Anatomic Region of Pain	Spinal Location of Electrode
Angina	T1–T4
Pancreatitis	Midthoracic
Visceral pain	Mid- to high thoracic
Low back	T7-T8
Leg	T8-T9
Pelvic or sacral pain	T12-L1
Foot pain	L1
Sacrum	L1

the patient returns to the operating room for removal of the externalized lead extensions, and the system is converted to a permanent system with the implantation of the IPG. Should a tunneled trial fail, surgical removal of the electrode concludes the trial period.

Imaging

Most patients with chronic pain syndromes have already undergone numerous imaging studies. Prior to implantation of an electrode, particularly the paddle type, appropriate imaging should be obtained to reduce implantation-related risks. Most often an MRI of the spine will aid in assessing neurologic risks related to lead placement. Fluoroscopy is used during the placement of both trial and permanent electrodes.

Permanent SCS Placement Surgical Procedure

The surgical technique for SCS system placement is designed to minimize complications including neurologic deficits, lead migration, and infection. There is no agreement on what is the best anesthesia to use for the procedure. Percutaneous electrode leads are routinely implanted in awake patients with or without sedation, but either general anesthesia or monitored sedation with the use of local anesthetic can be suitable for paddle electrode placement. In placements in awake patients, intraoperative testing of the stimulator is performed to map the patient's perceived paresthesias. The use of neurophysiological monitoring to map stimulation effects can facilitate effective electrode placement in patients receiving general anesthesia.[19] The location of the electrode contacts that provided the most effective pain relief during the trial may be used as a guide for optimal placement of the permanent electrode.

Surgical Preparation

The patient is placed in the prone position using appropriate bolstering and padding (**Fig. 116.3a**). The patient's back and buttocks

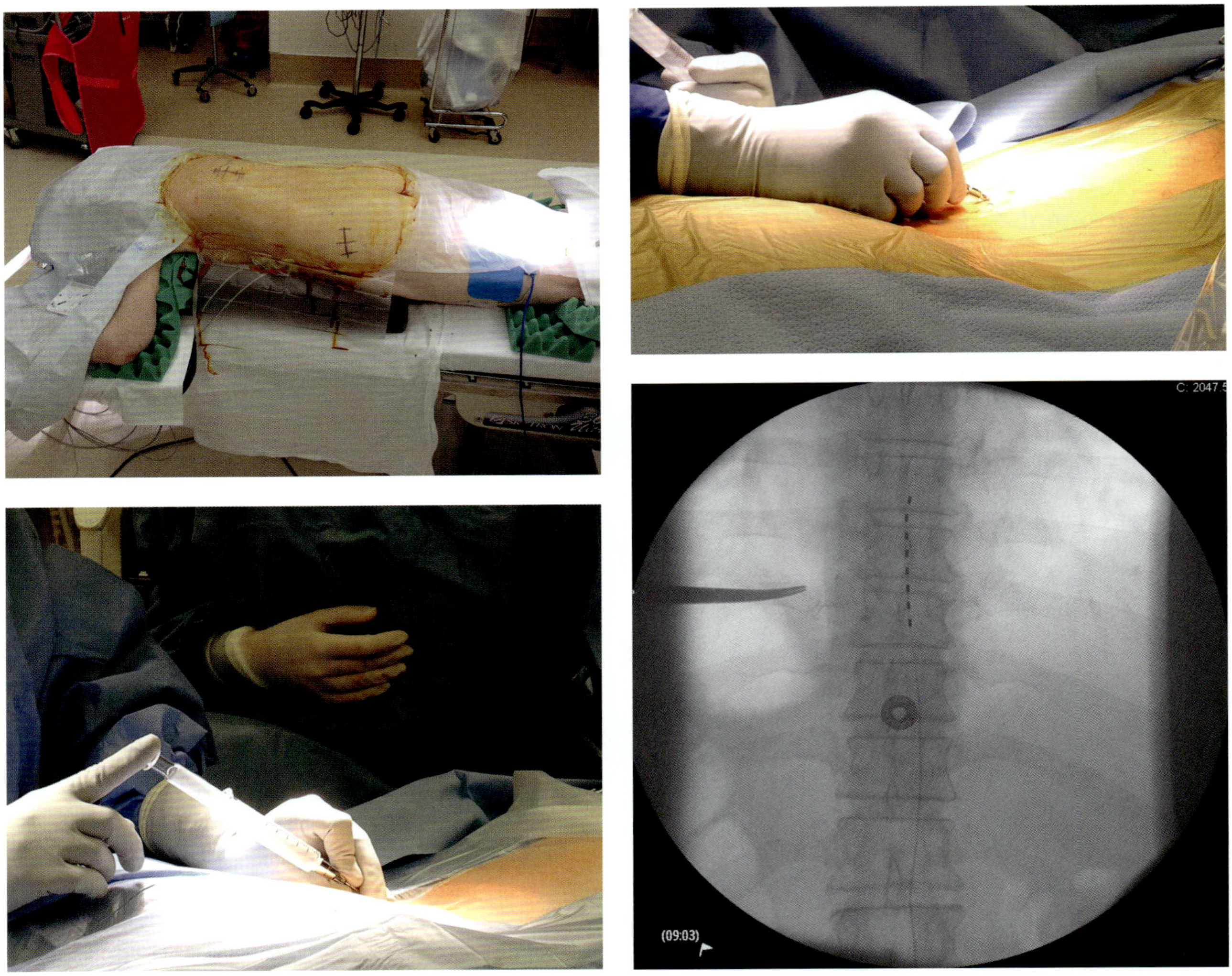

Fig. 116.3 Percutaneous placement of cylindrical electrode. **(a)** Positioning for spinal cord stimulation (SCS) placement. **(b)** The Tuohy needle is advanced at a flat angle (< 45 degrees) to enter the epidural space. **(c)** Loss of resistance technique for needle advancement using a glass syringe. **(d)** Anteroposterior (AP) fluoroscopic image shows the eight-contact cylindrical electrode steered into a midline position overlying T8 and T9. (Courtesy of Dr. Heather Pickard-Dover.)

are prepped and draped. Routine intravenous perioperative antibiotic protocol and antibiotic irrigation should be used.

Placing the Percutaneous Epidural Lead

Using an entry point at L3-L4 just lateral to midline, the Tuohy needle is introduced at a 30-degree angle through a small stab incision (**Fig. 116.3b**) into the spinal canal. The stylet of the Tuohy needle is withdrawn to verify the epidural location of the needle tip by the absence of cerebrospinal fluid (CSF) flow. A loss-of-resistance technique using a glass syringe may be used to confirm the needle entry into the epidural space (**Fig. 116.3c**). The cylindrical lead is advanced through the Tuohy needle, and AP and lateral fluoroscopy is used to navigate the electrode's position within the epidural space, ensuring a dorsal placement overlying the midline (**Fig. 116.3d**). A second electrode may be placed in a similar fashion at the surgeon's discretion. Test stimulation is performed to verify that the perceived paresthesias align with the appropriate anatomic location of the patient's pain targets. The Tuohy needle is withdrawn, taking care to preserve the electrode position. For a trial, the electrode is sewn at the skin exit site to prevent migration, and then a watertight dressing is placed. For a permanent cylindrical lead placement, a small incision is opened down to the fascia surrounding the Tuohy needle to enable placement of an anchor. The lead is secured to the fascia using an anchor and a nonresorbable suture such as Ethibond.

Placing the Laminotomy Epidural Lead

A small midline laminotomy is made at the spinal level just caudal to the intended location of the paddle electrode to facilitate the introduction of the paddle electrode into the epidural space (**Fig. 116.4a**). AP fluoroscopy is obtained to verify the cranial-caudal and medial-lateral position of the electrode (**Fig. 116.4b**). Neurophysiological testing using electromyogram (EMG) and somatosensory evoked potential (SSEP) monitoring while the stimulator is activated can be used to confirm the desired electrode location. The electrode's tails are then anchored to the fascia or supraspinous ligament using an anchor and nonresorbable

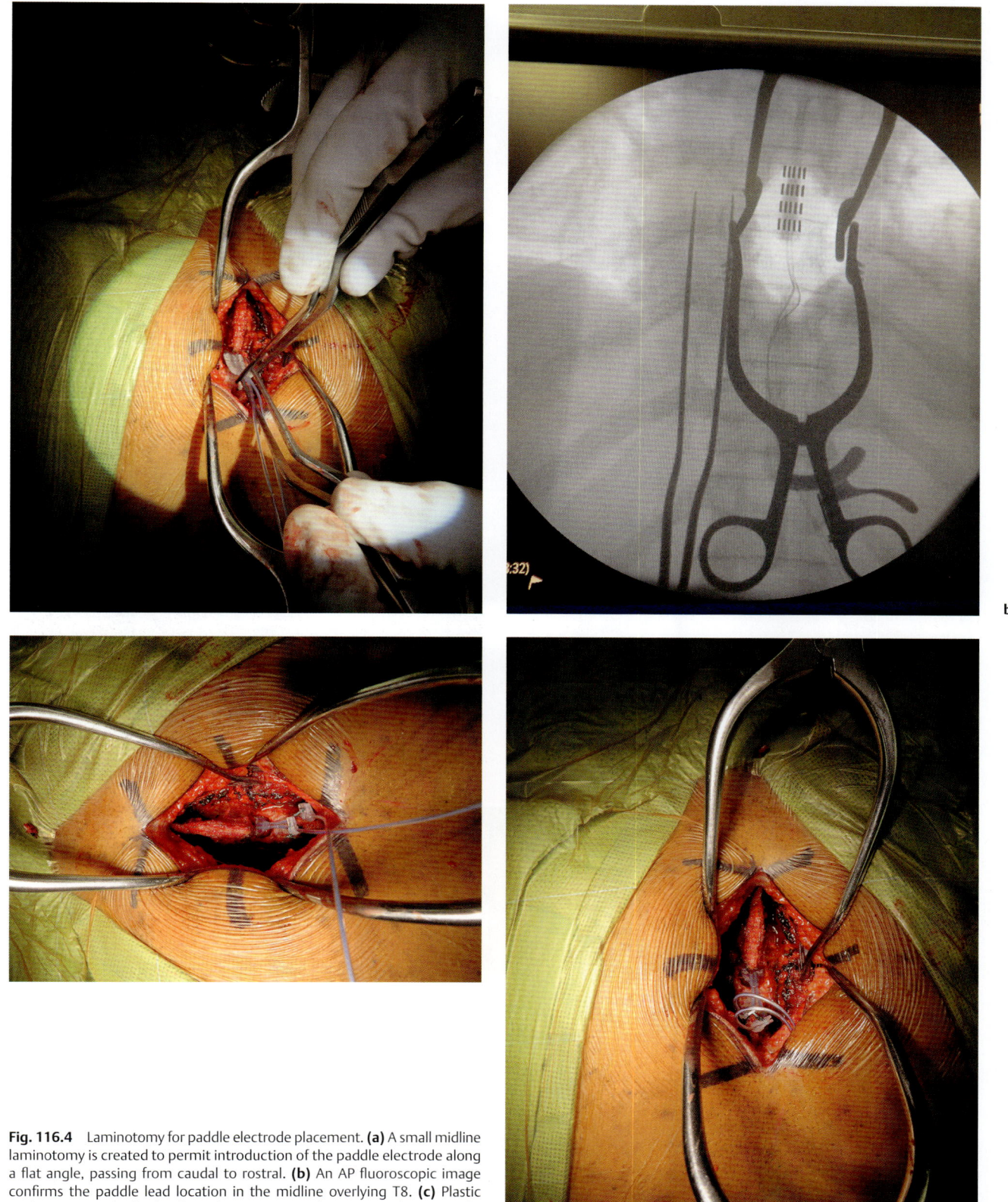

Fig. 116.4 Laminotomy for paddle electrode placement. **(a)** A small midline laminotomy is created to permit introduction of the paddle electrode along a flat angle, passing from caudal to rostral. **(b)** An AP fluoroscopic image confirms the paddle lead location in the midline overlying T8. **(c)** Plastic anchors secure the lead tails to the interspinous ligament with nonresorbable Ethibond sutures (optional step). **(d)** The lead tails are coiled deep to the fascia to form a strain relief loop.

V Lumbar and Lumbosacral Spine

sutures such as Ethibond (**Fig. 116.4c**). A small strain-relief loop is created prior to closure of the fascia (**Fig. 116.4d**).

Creating the IPG Pocket

The IPG should be placed in a location that the patient can reach easily and that does not have excessive soft tissue movement or a high risk of pressing against bone. The lateral buttock, ~ 4 cm inferior to the iliac crest, is a common location. A subcutaneous pocket no more than 1.5 cm deep to the skin surface is created (**Fig. 116.5**).

Connecting the IPG and the Electrode

A subcutaneous tunnel is created with a tunneling rod, and the electrode's leads are threaded from the thoracic incision to the IPG pocket (**Fig. 116.6a,b**). The leads are then coupled to the IPG using a torquing wrench (**Fig. 116.6c**). Prior to final connection, additional fluoroscopic imaging may be obtained to ensure no change in lead position (**Fig. 116.6d**). The system is interrogated

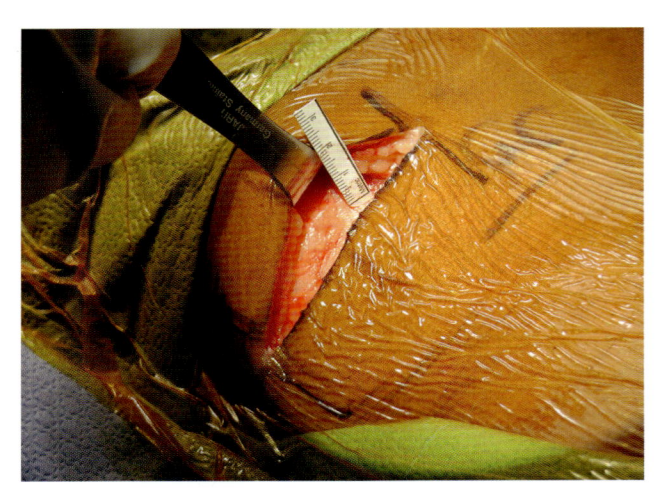

Fig. 116.5 A subcutaneous pocket no deeper than 1.5 cm to the skin surface should be snug around the implanted pulse generator (IPG).

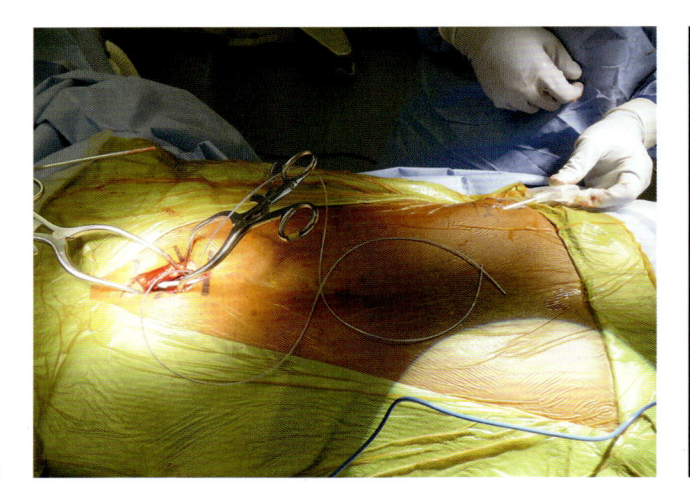

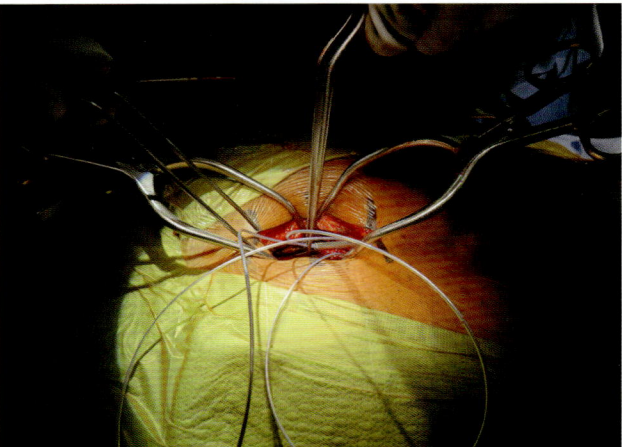

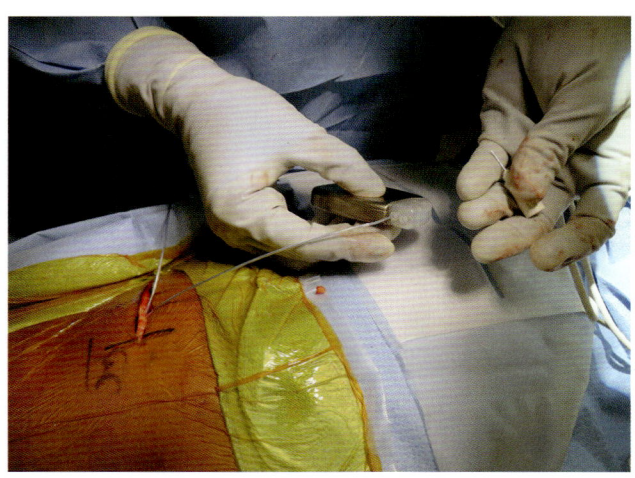

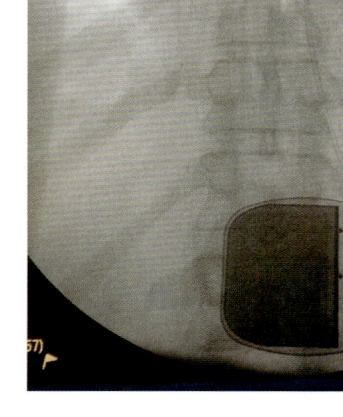

Fig. 116.6 Tunneling and connection of the system. (**a**) A tunneling rod creates a subcutaneous tunnel. (**b**) The leads are threaded from the thoracic incision to the IPG pocket through the hollow core of the tunneling tool. (**c**) The leads are connected within the header of the IPG. (**d**) A final AP fluoroscopic image confirms lead placement and IPG coupling. (Courtesy of Dr. Justin Dowdy.)

to verify that all circuits are satisfactorily connected. The IPG is secured within the pocket using nonresorbable sutures at several anchor points, and a two-layer skin closure is completed.

Starting Therapy

The SCS device can be activated immediately after implantation, but the efficacy of settings may change in the postoperative period. Patients usually undergo several programming sessions over the course of 1 to 2 months to optimize pain relief.

Postoperative Care

Most SCS systems are implanted in an outpatient setting, although some patients may be observed postoperatively due to neurologic or medical concerns. Routine postoperative wound care and perioperative antibiotic protocol should be observed. Patients should be instructed to avoid strenuous activities for 6 to 8 weeks to minimize lead migration risk and enable epidural scar formation around the implanted leads.

SCS Maintenance

The lifetime of an SCS IPG varies by device and by usage pattern. The patient controller unit reports battery status, and clinician programmers can also determine the remaining IPG lifetime. As a patient nears the anticipated IPG end-of-life, an elective replacement of the unit can be scheduled. The surgical procedure to exchange the expiring IPG unit requires opening the IPG site incision, removing the previous IPG from the subcutaneous capsule, disconnecting the leads from the expiring IPG, and inserting the electrode leads into a new unit. Programs can be transferred over from the expiring IPG to the new unit, or new programs can be created after the exchange.

Potential Complications and Precautions

Infection

With an implanted device, infection is the most common complication (**Fig. 116.7**). Infection rates for SCS systems range from 1 to 15%. Steps to reduce the risk of infection can be implemented across the preoperative, intraoperative, and postoperative phases.[20] Patients' comorbidities and nutritional status should be optimized prior to surgery, fastidious infection-reduction precautions and efficient operative technique should be exercised, and healing incisions should be closely monitored. Superficial wound infections and stitch abscesses generally resolve with a course of oral antibiotics but occasionally require surgical intervention. Purulent drainage from incisions should cause immediate concern, and the SCS system should be removed and intravenous antibiotic therapy initiated.

In very thin patients or those with poor nutritional status, device components may erode through the skin. The surgical sites should be inspected at each office visit, but if erosion is detected, removal of the system must be considered.

Mechanical Device Complications

Migration of the electrode, lead fracture or disconnection, and loss of recharging capabilities can occur. Interrogating the system enables one to identify impedance problems that suggest short circuits or lead fractures. Migration or fracture complications should be suspected in a patient who experiences loss of SCS benefit or paresthesias in unwanted regions. Troubleshooting and reprogramming of the SCS system should be attempted, but if effective pain relief and paresthesias cannot be recaptured with further device programming, plain X-ray evaluation may be done to determine the presence of breakage, disconnects, or migration (**Figs. 116.8 and 116.9**). In these circumstances, operative revision of the affected component of the system is necessary. In rare cases the IPG may "flip" within the pocket, creating communication problems for device programming or charging. This inversion is more common in patients with generous subcutaneous tissue. If the IPG's movement provokes untenable device-related pain, relocation of the IPG may be considered.

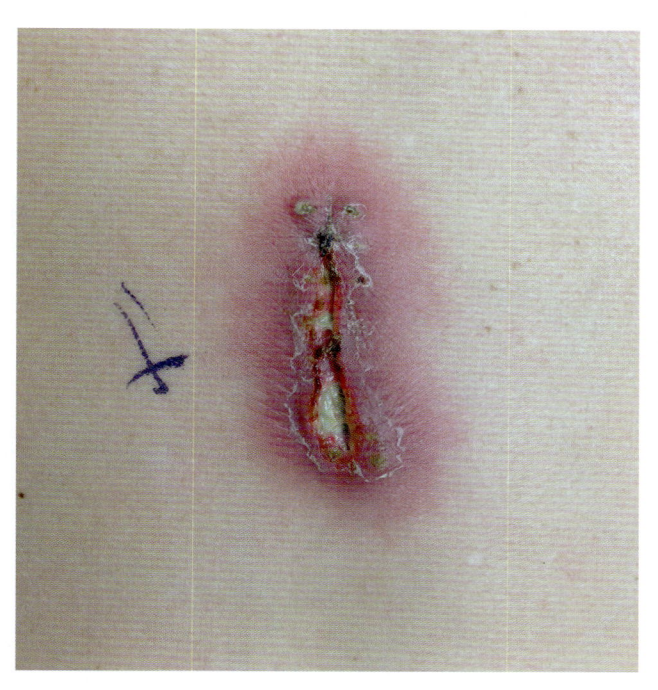

Fig. 116.7 Postoperative infection characterized by erythema and fibrinous exudate at a thoracic incision site.

Subcutaneous Fluid Collection and Seroma

Fluid may sometimes accumulate within the IPG pocket or around the anchors. Fluid noted after surgery may be either a resolving hematoma or, more often, a seroma or CSF collection. These collections can develop within weeks of surgery, especially if dural entry occurred during the electrode placement. Treatment with bed rest, pressure dressings, and fluid aspiration may facilitate the collection's resolution. An epidural blood patch may be performed for persistent CSF leaks.

Conclusion

Spinal cord stimulation is an effective strategy for management of chronic neuropathic pain that is refractory to other medical treatment. Proper patient selection and fastidious technique are essential to good outcomes.

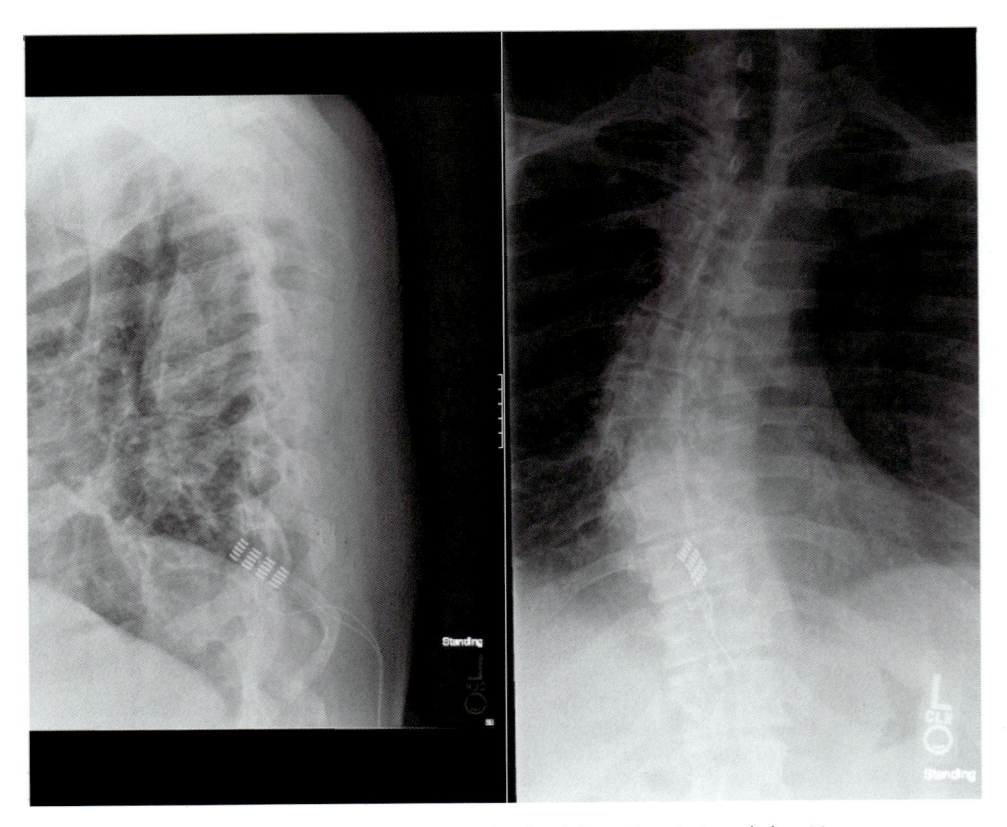

Fig. 116.8 (a) AP and (b) lateral radiographs demonstrating a lead rotated and withdrawn from its intended position.

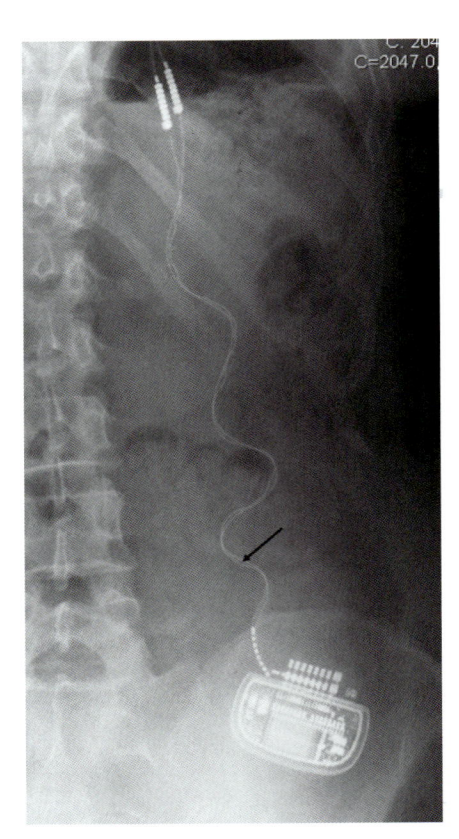

Fig. 116.9 AP radiograph showing electrode lead uncoupled from the IPG header.

References

1. Kumar K, Rizvi S. Cost-effectiveness of spinal cord stimulation therapy in management of chronic pain. Pain Med 2013;14:1631–1649
2. North RB, Kidd D, Shipley J, Taylor RS. Spinal cord stimulation versus reoperation for failed back surgery syndrome: a cost effectiveness and cost utility analysis based on a randomized, controlled trial. Neurosurgery 2007;61:361–368, discussion 368–369
3. Taylor RS, Ryan J, O'Donnell R, Eldabe S, Kumar K, North RB. The cost-effectiveness of spinal cord stimulation in the treatment of failed back surgery syndrome. Clin J Pain 2010;26:463–469
4. Kemler MA, Raphael JH, Bentley A, Taylor RS. The cost-effectiveness of spinal cord stimulation for complex regional pain syndrome. Value Health 2010;13:735–742
5. Oakley JC, Prager JP. Spinal cord stimulation: mechanisms of action. Spine 2002;27:2574–2583
6. North RB, Kidd DH, Farrokhi F, Piantadosi SA. Spinal cord stimulation versus repeated lumbosacral spine surgery for chronic pain: a randomized, controlled trial. Neurosurgery 2005;56:98–106, discussion 106–107
7. Deer TR, Mekhail N, Provenzano D, et al; Neuromodulation Appropriateness Consensus Committee. The appropriate use of neurostimulation: avoidance and treatment of complications of neurostimulation therapies for the treatment of chronic pain. Neuromodulation 2014;17:571–597, discussion 597–598
8. Deer TR, Skaribas IM, Haider N, et al. Effectiveness of cervical spinal cord stimulation for the management of chronic pain. Neuromodulation 2014;17:265–271, discussion 271
9. Sayenko DG, Angeli C, Harkema SJ, Edgerton VR, Gerasimenko YP. Neuromodulation of evoked muscle potentials induced by epidural spinal-cord stimulation in paralyzed individuals. J Neurophysiol 2014;111:1088–1099
10. DiMarco AF, Kowalski KE, Hromyak DR, Geertman RT. Long-term follow-up of spinal cord stimulation to restore cough in subjects with spinal cord injury. J Spinal Cord Med 2014;37:380–388

11. Tse HF, Turner S, Sanders P, et al. Thoracic Spinal Cord Stimulation for Heart Failure as a Restorative Treatment (SCS HEART study): first-in-man experience. Heart Rhythm 2015;12:588–595
12. Slavin KV, Vannemreddy PS, Goellner E, et al. Use of cervical spinal cord stimulation in treatment and prevention of arterial vasospasm after aneurysmal subarachnoid hemorrhage. Technical details. Neuroradiol J 2011;24:131–135
13. Deer TR, Krames E, Mekhail N, et al; Neuromodulation Appropriateness Consensus Committee. The appropriate use of neurostimulation: new and evolving neurostimulation therapies and applicable treatment for chronic pain and selected disease states. Neuromodulation 2014;17:599–615, discussion 615
14. Bendersky D, Yampolsky C. Is spinal cord stimulation safe? A review of its complications. World Neurosurg 2014;82:1359–1368
15. Kumar K, Wilson JR, Taylor RS, Gupta S. Complications of spinal cord stimulation, suggestions to improve outcome, and financial impact. J Neurosurg Spine 2006;5:191–203
16. Levy RM. Device complication and failure management in neuromodulation. Neuromodulation 2013;16:495–502
17. Levy R, Henderson J, Slavin K, et al. Incidence and avoidance of neurologic complications with paddle type spinal cord stimulation leads. Neuromodulation 2011;14:412–422, discussion 422
18. Kinfe TM, Quack F, Wille C, Schu S, Vesper J. Paddle versus cylindrical leads for percutaneous implantation in spinal cord stimulation for failed back surgery syndrome: a single-center trial. J Neurol Surg A Cent Eur Neurosurg 2014;75:467–473
19. Mammis A, Mogilner AY. The use of intraoperative electrophysiology for the placement of spinal cord stimulator paddle leads under general anesthesia. Neurosurgery 2012;70(2, Suppl Operative):230–236
20. Deer TR, Provenzano DA. Recommendations for reducing infection in the practice of implanting spinal cord stimulation and intrathecal drug delivery devices: a physician's playbook. Pain Physician 2013;16:E125–E128

117 Placement of an Intrathecal Drug Delivery System

Erika A. Petersen and Konstantin V. Slavin

Intrathecal delivery of medications offers several advantages to patients. The use of a targeted intrathecal drug delivery system (IDDS) is effective for the treatment of spasticity and for cancer-related and nonmalignant pain when more conservative options have failed. An IDDS has the advantage of a decreased side-effect profile while delivering higher doses directly to the spinal neurons. Furthermore, continuous infusion eliminates some of the fluctuation that occurs with an oral medication schedule. The IDDS is composed of an intrathecal catheter and an implanted pump, which may either have a fixed rate or be adjustable. Improvements in pump technology that enable patients to self-administer boluses of medication may eliminate the need for patients to take supplemental oral medications.

Patient Selection

Spasticity

Patients with severe chronic spastic hypertonia of over 6 months in duration may be candidates for an IDDS. Numerous conditions manifesting with spasticity of both spinal and cerebral origin (**Table 117.1**) may benefit from intrathecal baclofen treatment.[1] Generally, patients should have first been treated with optimized medical management with multiple antispasmodic agents. If that treatment failed, then they can be considered for a pump.

Pain

Cancer Pain

More than half of the patients with pain due to malignancy may be undertreated.[2] A majority of cancer patients with pain also suffer from breakthrough pain.[3] Inadequate treatment may be related to intolerable nausea and other side effects associated with oral or transdermal medications or to patients having refractory severe pain. In patients whose pain medications have been titrated to the limit, intrathecal administration can provide a decreased side-effect profile and continuous delivery.[4] Often these patients can be weaned off of oral pain medications once intrathecal drug delivery has been appropriately dosed, and life expectancy may be extended in patients using an IDDS.[5,6] For each patient, the risks of infection, device complication, and management complexity should be considered. The benefits for the patient's pain control along with improved awareness and cognitive performance side effects outweigh concerns about life expectancy.[7]

Nonmalignant Pain

Patients with chronic moderate-to-severe pain that is refractory to optimized medical and surgical management may also benefit.[8] The types of pain for which an IDDS may be appropriate include refractory low back pain, leg pain, complex regional pain syndrome, pain related to vertebral fractures, and pain related to other etiologies. Patients should have first been tried on more conservative options, which failed, and should demonstrate a clear ability to adhere to treatment regimens. The choice of drugs to administer through the pump varies based on the patient's condition. Although many options exist, only baclofen, morphine, and ziconotide are Food and Drug Administration (FDA) approved for administration through a pump. In practice, however, a large number of chronic pain patients receive intrathecal drug delivery therapy using a variety of medications, often in compounded mixtures. The most common use involves combining morphine with bupivacaine, although combinations including hydromorphone or fentanyl with the possible addition of clonidine are also possible.[7] Long-term follow-up studies have demonstrated statistically significant improvements in measures including pain relief and intensity, coping, and quality of life.[9]

Indications and Contraindications, and the Objectives of Surgery

Intrathecal delivery of medications offers several advantages to patients.

Inclusion Criteria

Patients are candidates for IDDS if they have pain that is refractory to other treatment measures. Patients should have a favorable psychological profile and a track record of compliance with chronic medical therapy that suggests that they are able to comply with the requirements of IDDS maintenance.

Trial Dosing Response

Candidates for IDDS placement undergo a trial administration of medication to assess their response. Generally an improvement of over 50% is considered a positive trial. In the case of spasticity, Modified Ashworth Scale scores are assessed at baseline and then at several time points after administration of a single 50-μg intrathecal dose of baclofen. For pain, several trialing techniques are possible.[10] The trial may use a single intrathecal bolus dose of narcotic or an infusion over time at an escalating dose through an intrathecal or epidural catheter. In both cases, significant clinical improvement, such as more than a 50% decrease in the Visual Analogue Pain (VAS) score, should be demonstrated. A positive correlation between response to a trial dose and long-term pain relief has been demonstrated in patients with post-laminectomy pain syndrome.[11]

117 Placement of an Intrathecal Drug Delivery System

Table 117.1 Clinical Indications for Intrathecal Baclofen Therapy

Spastic cerebral palsy (monoplegia, diplegia, hemiplegia, tetraplegia)
Spasticity after traumatic brain injury
Spasticity due to multiple sclerosis
Post-stroke spastic paresis/paralysis
Spastic paralysis (paraplegia and quadriplegia) after spinal cord injury
Primary dystonia
Secondary (acquired) dystonia
Tardive dystonia
Stiff person syndrome
Spasticity in amyotrophic lateral sclerosis (ALS)
Tetanus
Opisthotonus

Exclusion Criteria

Increased Surgical Risk Profile

Patients with active infectious issues or compromised immune systems may be at higher risk. Surgery is discouraged in patients taking anticoagulants that cannot be suspended in the perioperative period or who have other medical comorbidities that would increase anesthesia or perioperative risks.

Systemic Concerns

Patients with allergic reactions to certain metals or to the medication that the IDDS will supply are not candidates. Furthermore, patients with a body habitus that will not accommodate the pump's implantation should not be considered for a pump.

Inability to Comply with the Therapy and the Maintenance Schedule

The pump reservoir requires periodic refilling in order to continue appropriate delivery of the medication. Implantation of a pump is discouraged in patients who cannot maintain the schedule of frequent visits for management of the device due to logistical, financial, or cognitive issues.

Advantages and Disadvantages

Intrathecal delivery of a small amount of medication may produce the same effect as a larger oral medication dose; therefore, intrathecal drug administration may help minimize side effects that can result from oral therapy. Patients who cannot tolerate the side effects (such as sedation) of higher-dose oral medications or those with inadequate control of their symptoms are potential candidates for an IDDS. Continuous, direct intrathecal administration may enable a patient to be tapered off of oral medication. IDDS treatment is adjustable and reversible, enabling titration of the dose to match the symptoms and side effects. Decreased spasticity can reduce the development of contractures and joint deformities. Reduction in muscle spasms results in decreased muscle pain and fatigue, more consistent sleep patterns, and improvements in the ease of nursing case.[12,13] Patients' pain, psychosocial status, motor functioning, and overall health-related quality of life significantly improve. A survey of 100 patients with cerebral palsy performed between 1 and 4 years after intrathecal baclofen (ITB) pump implantation indicated that most were satisfied with the results, and that they would be willing to undergo pump implantation again.[14]

Unfortunately, any implanted device has certain risks, including the possibility of mechanical failure and of infection. The reservoir of the pump must be refilled at routine intervals to ensure continued effective therapy. If a pump is not refilled, a patient may be at high risk of medication withdrawal. Furthermore, a dry pump may result in a stalled rotor within the pump, resulting in mechanical malfunction.

Choice of Operative Approach

Device Options

The IDDS is composed of an intrathecal catheter and a pump. Two categories of pumps are available: fixed-flow rate and variable programmable rate. A fixed-flow pump relies on changes in the concentration of medication in the reservoir in order to adjust the patient's medication dose. This is usually accomplished by withdrawing the existing medication from the pump reservoir and refilling it with a more concentrated formulation. Changes in the programmed pump flow rate using a variable programmable rate pump alter the medication dose. Variable programmable pumps also enable complex programming and the option of patient-controlled bolus delivery.

Catheter Placement

In most cases a percutaneous placement is performed where the catheter is introduced through a Tuohy needle into the lumbar cistern. In patients where access to the intrathecal space is challenging (because of ankylosing spondylitis, posterior fusion masses, or spinal deformities, for example), a small laminotomy can be performed to enable access to introduce the catheter. The catheter is then advanced within the intrathecal space to the desired level. Generally the tip of the catheter is placed several segments above the targeted level to ensure adequate medication delivery.

Pump Placement

The pump requires placement in a subcutaneous pocket where access for refilling the reservoir is possible. The most common location is in the right lower quadrant of the abdomen. Left lower quadrant and buttocks locations are also possible. The pump dimensions vary by manufacturer. The most common pump, the SynchroMed II (Medtronic, Minneapolis, MN; **Fig. 117.1**) has a diameter of 87.5 mm and a thickness of 19.5 mm for the 20-mL reservoir and 26.0 mm for the 40-mL reservoir. Care should be taken to ensure that the pump site does not interfere with patient mobility or positioning. This is especially important in paraplegics, where sitting positions and wheelchair seatbelts may cause mechanical irritation of the pump site and where the risk of decubitus ulcer formation is elevated.

Preoperative Testing

Intrathecal Trial Evaluation

In the case of spasticity, the Modified Ashworth Scale scores are assessed at baseline and then at several time points after administration of a single 50-μg intrathecal dose of baclofen. For pain, a trial may be with a single intrathecal bolus dose of narcotic or an infusion over time at an escalating dose through an intrathecal or epidural catheter (**Table 117.2**). The type of trial offered for pain pump candidates depends on the type of pain syndrome being treated and on the patient's ability to undergo a prolonged infusion trial.[10] For both pain and spasticity, significant clinical improvement should be demonstrated.

Imaging

In patients with complex spinal anatomy, appropriate imaging should be obtained to assist in preoperative planning for efficient implantation of the device. The use of fluoroscopy to facilitate access to the intrathecal space for delivery of the medication dose during the trial or for placement of the permanent catheter may be helpful.

Permanent IDDS Placement Surgical Procedure

The surgical technique for optimal IDDS placement is designed to minimize complications including cerebrospinal fluid (CSF) leakage, pump or catheter migration, and infection.[15]

Surgical Preparation

General anesthesia is induced, and the patient is placed in the lateral decubitus position using appropriate bolstering and padding (**Fig. 117.2a**). The patient's abdomen, flank, and back are prepped and draped. Routine intravenous perioperative antibiotic protocol and antibiotic irrigation should be used.

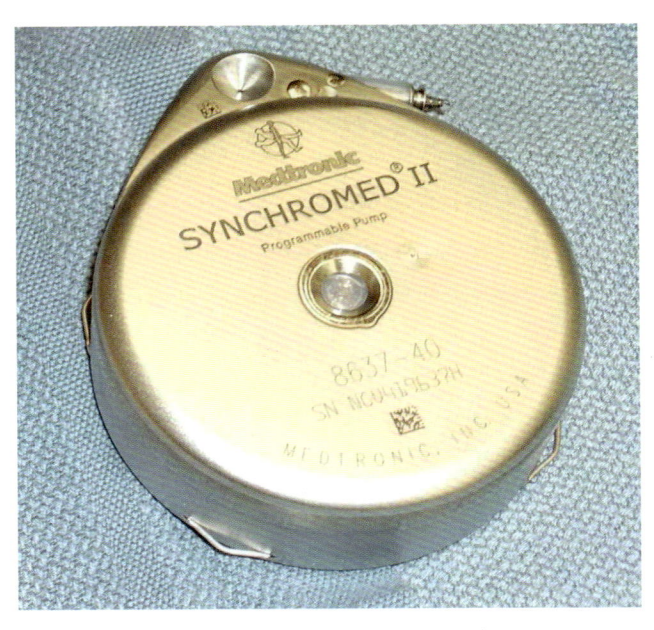

Fig. 117.1 The Medtronic SynchroMed II programmable pump.

Placing of the Intrathecal Catheter

Using a paramedian entry point at L3-L4, the Tuohy needle is introduced at a 30-degree angle through a small stab incision (**Fig. 117.2b**). The stylet of the Tuohy needle is withdrawn in order to verify spontaneous CSF flow. The Silastic intrathecal catheter is advanced through the Tuohy needle, taking careful note of the length of catheter introduced into the intrathecal space (**Fig. 117.2c**). Fluoroscopy can be used to verify the catheter's position (**Fig. 117.2d**). The guidewire is withdrawn from the catheter, and the presence of spontaneous CSF flow at the catheter tip is confirmed. The Tuohy needle entry incision is extended

Table 117.2 Dosing Protocols for Intrathecal Drug Delivery System (IDDS) Trial Evaluations*

Condition	Trial Modality	Dosing	Expected Outcome
Spasticity	Intrathecal baclofen single-dose bolus	50–100 μg	Modified Ashworth Scale score improved 1 to 2 points in lower extremities; subjective improvement in pain and mobility
Nociceptive pain	Intrathecal single-dose bolus	Morphine 1.0 mg or ziconotide 1–5 μg	VAS score improved by 50%
Neuropathic pain	Intrathecal infusion	Morphine 0.025–11 mg/d or ziconotide 2–4 μg/d	VAS score improved by 50%
Neuropathic pain	Epidural infusion	Morphine 4–8 mg with bolus on demand or ziconotide 5–10 μg/h	VAS score improved by 50%

Abbreviation: VAS, Visual Analogue Scale.
*It is recommended to use the lowest possible dose for a trial to avoid possible side effects or drug toxicity.

to a length of 2 cm, and dissection through the subcutaneous tissue is performed until fascia is identified (**Fig. 117.2e,f**). The Tuohy needle is withdrawn, taking care to preserve the catheter's position. The catheter is secured to the fascia using an anchor and a nonresorbable suture such as Ethibond (**Fig. 117.2g**).

Creating the Abdominal Pump Pocket

The pump should be placed lateral to the umbilicus and below the costal margin to decrease the risk of contact with the patient's ribs or iliac crest (**Fig. 117.3**). A subcutaneous pocket approximately 1.5 cm deep to the skin surface is created. Subfascial placement may be considered for patients with low body mass index (BMI) or young age, in whom the pump placement is associated with high erosion risk and cosmetic disfigurement.

Connecting the Pump and the Catheter

A subcutaneous tunnel is created with a tunneling rod, and the intrathecal catheter is threaded around the flank from the lumbar incision to the abdominal pocket (**Fig. 117.2h**). The catheter is then coupled to the pump using the manufacturer's pump segment coupling (**Fig. 117.2i**). Prior to final connection, spontaneous CSF flow should again be confirmed. The pump is secured to the fascia using nonresorbable sutures at several anchor points (**Fig. 117.2j**). After closure of the incisions in two layers and application of sterile dressings, an abdominal binder may be placed in order to increase the resistance to any fluid accumulation under the pump site or spinal incisions.

Starting IDDS Therapy

The pump ships from the manufacturer with a reservoir filled with sterile saline. The pump is brought onto the sterile field where it can be emptied of saline and filled with the treatment drug prior to connection. A low rate is initially selected, and further titration of the dosing can be performed postoperatively during the patient's hospitalization and continuing as an outpatient using the pump programmer.

Postoperative Care

Patients are admitted after IDDS implantation to observe for possible overdose, CSF loss, and other possible complications.

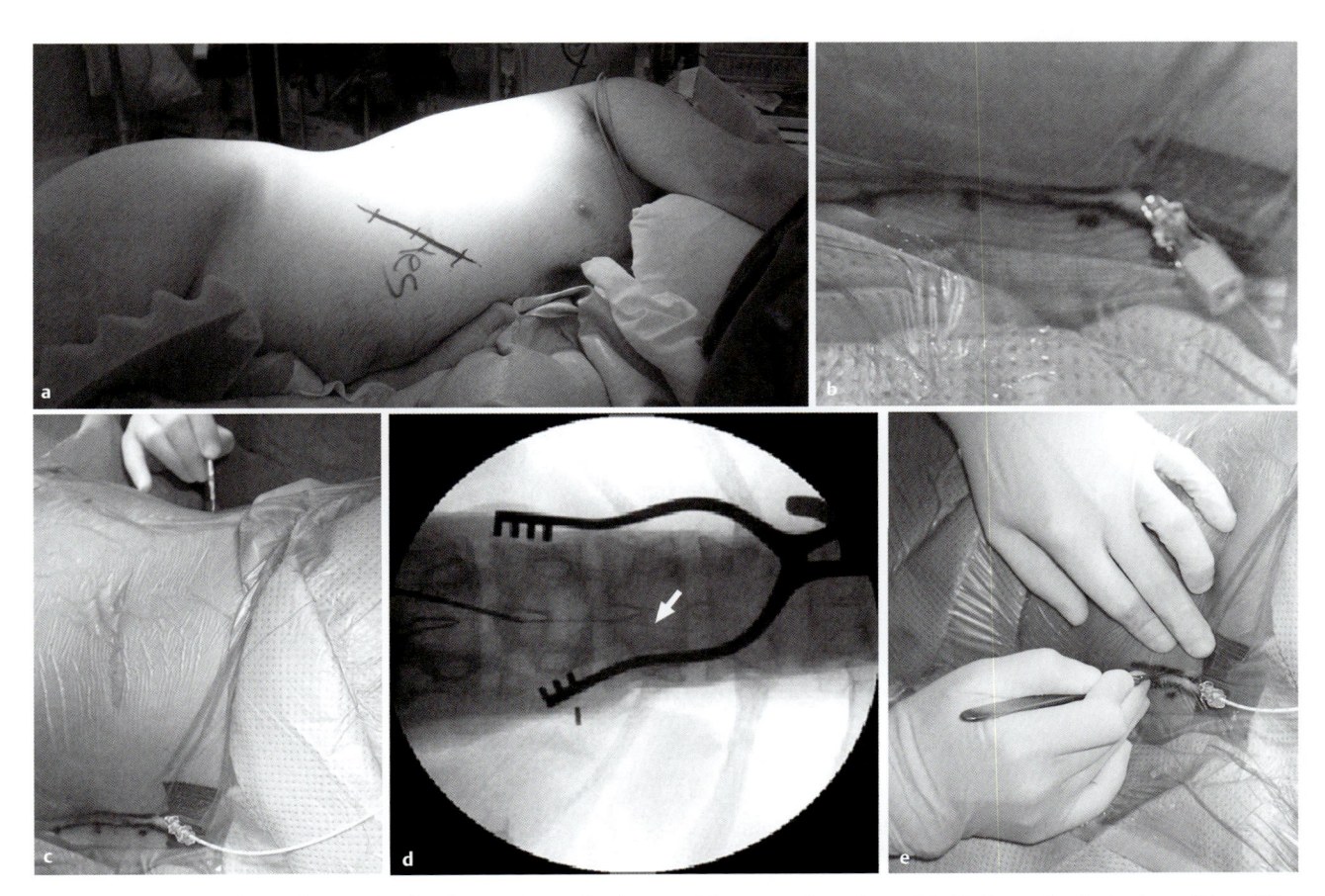

Fig. 117.2 Surgical technique for intrathecal catheter and pump implantation. (**a**) Lateral decubitus positioning with abdominal pocket incision marked. (**b**) Paramedian Tuohy needle insertion with a flat angle of entry. (**c**) Catheter introduction through the Tuohy needle. (**d**) Fluoroscopic image of the paramedian entry point with the angle of entry toward the midline (catheter tip at *arrow*). (**e**) Paramedian lumbar incision about the Tuohy needle entry point. (*continued on page 732*)

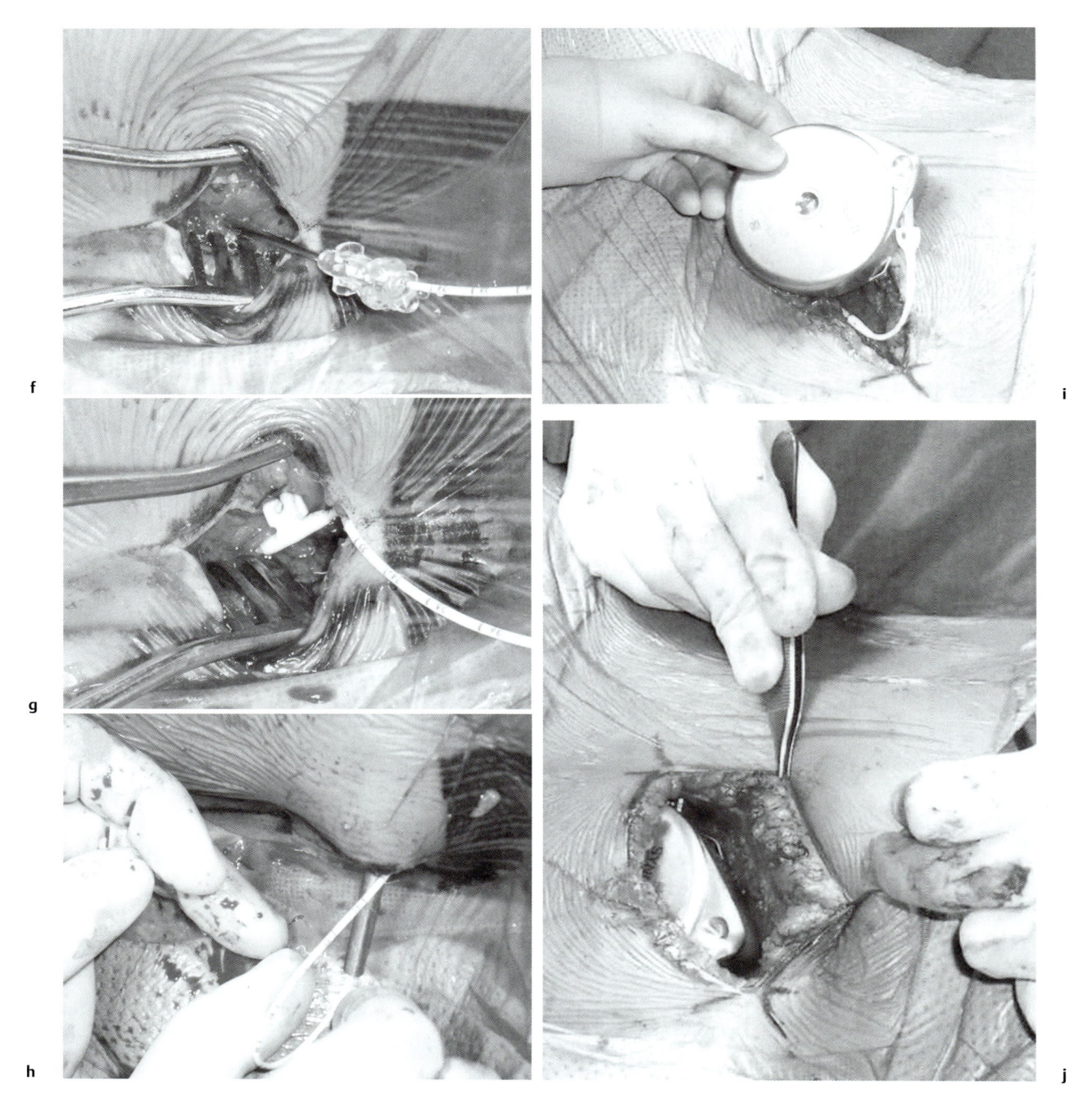

Fig. 117.2 (*continued*) Surgical technique for intrathecal catheter and pump implantation. **(f)** Lumbar incision carried down to the fascia. **(g)** Catheter secured to the fascia with a Silastic anchor. **(h)** Catheter tunneled to the abdominal pocket using a shunt passer. **(i)** Catheter attached to the pump unit. **(j)** Pump positioned within the abdominal pocket.

Telemetry, continuous pulse oximetry, and close neurologic observation are recommended to identify possible early signs of overdose (**Table 117.3**). Patients should be kept horizontal to minimize pseudomeningocele development. Placement of a Foley catheter can facilitate a patient's comfort while remaining flat. The abdominal binder should remain in place for up to 2 weeks. Titration of the IDDS dose should be governed by the response of the patient's symptoms. The anticipated date for refilling the reservoir should be well communicated to the patient and caregivers.

Intrathecal Drug Delivery Dosing

A programming unit that communicates through the skin with the pump can be used to titrate the rate of drug infusion and also query the pump for volumes delivered and estimated time to refill. The frequency with which the pump requires refilling depends on the rate of drug delivery; generally, it ranges between two to six times per year. The pump records an estimated date for the next drug refill, which can be read during an interrogation. The pump sounds an alarm if the drug level declines below

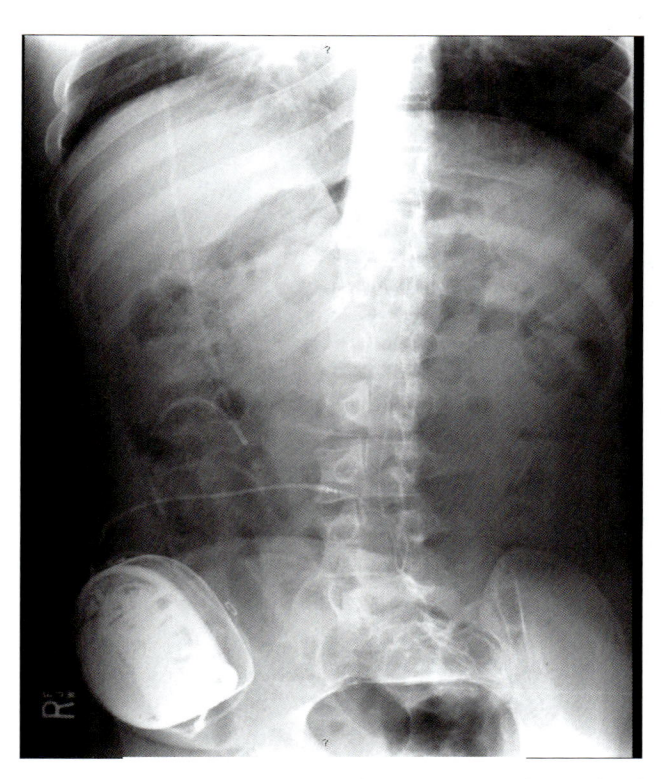

Fig. 117.3 Anteroposterior abdominal film demonstrating the intrathecal pump with the catheter in the correct position.

Table 117.3 Signs and Symptoms of IDDS Drug Overdose

Drug	Signs and Symptoms
Baclofen	Somnolence
	Respiratory depression
	Hypotonia
	Seizures
	Autonomic instability
	Bradycardia
Morphine	Somnolence
	Respiratory depression
	Hypotension
	Nausea and vomiting
	Urinary retention
	Diaphoresis
Ziconotide	Sedation or stupor
	Ataxia
	Nystagmus
	Hypotension
	Myoclonus
	Nausea and vomiting

a set level. Refilling the pump is an in-office procedure that typically takes less than 30 minutes. The central port is accessed using a noncoring (Huber) needle, any excess drug within the pump is drawn off, and the pump is filled with a full volume of medication.

Pump Maintenance

The battery life of the programmable pump is estimated at about 5 years. The pump features a low battery alarm, but as a patient nears the anticipated battery end-of-life, an elective replacement of the unit should be scheduled rather than waiting for the alarm to activate. The surgical procedure to exchange the expiring pump requires opening the pump site's subcutaneous incision, disconnecting the previous pump unit, and inserting a new unit. The new unit must be primed and filled as with the initial pump's insertion. Some surgeons prefer to observe the patient in the hospital overnight for signs of overdose or withdrawal.

Potential Complications and Precautions

Infection

With an implanted device, infection is the most common complication. Infection rates for baclofen pumps range from 0.7 to 1.7%.[16,17] Meningitis rates in patients with implanted pumps range from 0 to 0.7%. The literature reports that infections of the pump, rather than in the reservoir or catheter, appear to be most prevalent, and the most common bacteria cultured are *Staphylococcus aureus* and *Staphylococcus epidermidis*. Superficial wound infections and stitch abscesses generally resolve with a course of oral antibiotics but occasionally require surgical intervention. Purulent drainage from incisions should cause immediate concern, and the pump system should be removed and intravenous antibiotic therapy initiated. In very thin patients or those with poor nutritional status, the pump may erode through the skin (**Fig. 117.4**). The surgical sites should be inspected at each office visit, but if erosion is detected, removal of the system must be considered.

Mechanical Device Complications

Migration of the catheter, catheter fracture or disconnection, and catheter kinking can occur. Catheter-related complications should be suspected in a patient who demonstrates signs of withdrawal or who requires escalating doses of medication in order to obtain the same symptom effect. Plain X-ray evaluation may identify kinking, breakage, disconnects, or migration (**Fig. 117.5**). A pump study using contrast may show extravasation that suggests a crack in the catheter or obstruction. In all these circumstances, operative revision of the catheter is necessary. In rare cases the pump may flip within the abdominal pocket. This inversion is more common in patients with generous subcutaneous tissue. In these instances, implanting the pump within a Dacron pouch may improve anchoring and decrease the likelihood of rotation.

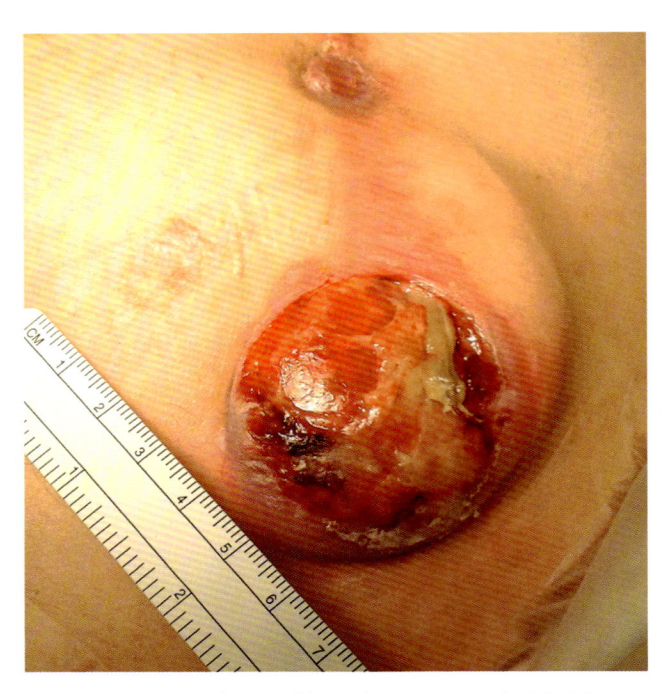

Fig. 117.4 Erosion at the site of the implanted pump in the left abdomen.

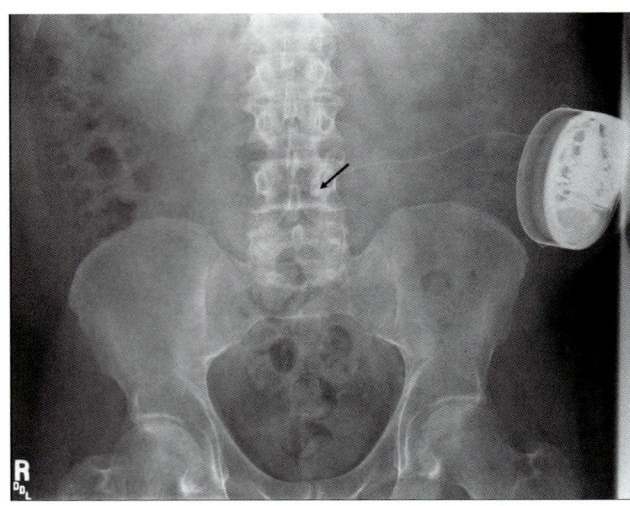

Fig. 117.5 Catheter migration with loops of catheter at the lumbar entry site *(arrow)*.

Subcutaneous Fluid and Seroma

Fluid may collect within the abdominal pocket or under the lumbar incision. These collections can develop within weeks of surgery, or they can arise later, most often in relation to a disruption of an IDDS component. Fluid noted after surgery may be either a resolving hematoma or seroma or CSF that has tracked along the catheter from the point of dural insertion. Treatment with bed rest, pressure dressings, and fluid aspiration may facilitate the collection's resolution. A blood patch may be performed for persistent leaks. In cases in which the effusion persists despite these measures, infection or a problem with the catheter should be suspected. X-rays of the thoracolumbar spine and abdomen may show evidence of catheter disconnection, fracture, or puncture. A contrasted fluoroscopic study in which dye is injected into the pump's side port may also identify a source of fluid leakage.

Drug Overdose

A malfunctioning pump or a transiently kinked catheter may deliver excessive medication, resulting in overdose symptoms (**Table 117.3**). Furthermore, inappropriate programming of bolus dosing may result in overdose. Interrogation of the pump can confirm pump status and screen for any mechanical errors. The programmed dose may be decreased to minimum, and the catheter port of the pump can be accessed to aspirate medication out of the catheter. Although some reversal is possible, supportive care including mechanical ventilation if necessary may be required to treat overdose.

Drug Underdose

The symptoms of withdrawal may develop if inadequate dosing is being delivered into the intrathecal space. A pump stall or failure can usually be identified through interrogation of the device. A kinked or broken catheter can be identified on imaging. Supplemental medication can be delivered intrathecally through a bolus delivered through the pump, through direct access through the catheter port, or through a lumbar puncture. Further supplementation using intravenous or oral medication may be required to prevent worsening withdrawal symptoms.

Catheter Tip Granuloma

The incidence of a granulomatous inflammatory mass developing at the catheter tip is approximately 3%, and occurs most often in patients receiving intrathecal opioid therapy. The granuloma can cause catheter occlusion that can lead to decreased therapeutic effect or even withdrawal symptoms, or the mass may cause cord compression, resulting in neurologic deficits. There is a high risk of permanent neurologic deficits related to such a mass.[18] Computed tomography (CT), myelogram, and magnetic resonance imaging (MRI) can identify an intradural mass, often with compression of the spinal cord, near the distal end of the intrathecal catheter. With discontinuation of the intrathecal infusion, the granuloma may resolve over the next several months.[19] Decompressive laminectomy with removal or repositioning of the catheter should be considered in cases where neurologic deficits are present or there is concern about possible progression.

Conclusion

An IDDS is an effective strategy for management of pain or spasticity that is refractory to other medical treatment. Proper patient selection and fastidious technique are essential to good outcomes.

References

1. Whitworth LA, Petersen EA. Intrathecal baclofen therapy. In: Dewey RB, Chitnis S, eds. Handbook of Movement Disorders. Oxford: Oxford University Press; 2011:159–168
2. Deandrea S, Montanari M, Moja L, Apolone G. Prevalence of undertreatment in cancer pain. A review of published literature. Ann Oncol 2008; 19:1985–1991
3. Deandrea S, Corli O, Consonni D, Villani W, Greco MT, Apolone G. Prevalence of breakthrough cancer pain: a systematic review and a pooled analysis of published literature. J Pain Symptom Manage 2014;47:57–76

4. Hayek SM, Deer TR, Pope JE, Panchal SJ, Patel VB. Intrathecal therapy for cancer and non-cancer pain. Pain Physician 2011;14:219–248
5. Deer TR, Smith HS, Burton AW, et al; Center For Pain Relief, Inc. Comprehensive consensus based guidelines on intrathecal drug delivery systems in the treatment of pain caused by cancer pain. Pain Physician 2011;14: E283–E312
6. Upadhyay SP, Mallick PN. Intrathecal drug delivery system (IDDS) for cancer pain management: a review and updates. Am J Hosp Palliat Care 2012;29:388–398
7. Deer TR, Prager J, Levy R, et al. Polyanalgesic Consensus Conference 2012: recommendations for the management of pain by intrathecal (intraspinal) drug delivery: report of an interdisciplinary expert panel. Neuromodulation 2012;15:436–464, discussion 464–466
8. Hamza M, Doleys D, Wells M, et al. Prospective study of 3-year follow-up of low-dose intrathecal opioids in the management of chronic nonmalignant pain. Pain Med 2012;13:1304–1313
9. Duarte RV, Raphael JH, Sparkes E, Southall JL, LeMarchand K, Ashford RL. Long-term intrathecal drug administration for chronic nonmalignant pain. J Neurosurg Anesthesiol 2012;24:63–70
10. Deer TR, Prager J, Levy R, et al. Polyanalgesic Consensus Conference—2012: recommendations on trialing for intrathecal (intraspinal) drug delivery: report of an interdisciplinary expert panel. Neuromodulation 2012;15:420–435, discussion 435
11. Kim D, Saidov A, Mandhare V, Shuster A. Role of pretrial systemic opioid requirements, intrathecal trial dose, and non-psychological factors as predictors of outcome for intrathecal pump therapy: one clinician's experience with lumbar postlaminectomy pain. Neuromodulation 2011;14: 165–175, discussion 175
12. Kravitz HM, Corcos DM, Hansen G, Penn RD, Cartwright RD, Gianino J. Intrathecal baclofen. Effects on nocturnal leg muscle spasticity. Am J Phys Med Rehabil 1992;71:48–52
13. Hoving MA, Evers SMAA, Ament AJHA, van Raak EPM, Vles JSH; Dutch Study Group on Child Spasticity. Intrathecal baclofen therapy in children with intractable spastic cerebral palsy: a cost-effectiveness analysis. Dev Med Child Neurol 2008;50:450–455
14. Krach LE, Nettleton A, Klempka B. Satisfaction of individuals treated long-term with continuous infusion of intrathecal baclofen by implanted programmable pump. Pediatr Rehabil 2006;9:210–218
15. Albright AL, Turner M, Pattisapu JV. Best-practice surgical techniques for intrathecal baclofen therapy. J Neurosurg 2006;104(4, Suppl):233–239
16. Hsieh JC, Penn RD. Intrathecal baclofen in the treatment of adult spasticity. Neurosurg Focus 2006;21:e5
17. Dickey MP, Rice M, Kinnett DG, et al. Infectious complications of intrathecal baclofen pump devices in a pediatric population. Pediatr Infect Dis J 2013;32:715–722
18. Deer TR, Prager J, Levy R, et al. Polyanalgesic Consensus Conference—2012: consensus on diagnosis, detection, and treatment of catheter-tip granulomas (inflammatory masses). Neuromodulation 2012;15:483–495, discussion 496
19. Deer T, Krames ES, Hassenbusch S, et al. Management of intrathecal catheter-tip inflammatory masses: an updated 2007 consensus statement from an expert panel. Neuromodulation 2008;11:77–91

118 Vertebroplasty and Kyphoplasty

Ricardo B.V. Fontes and Richard G. Fessler

Vertebral body augmentation for osteoporotic vertebral compression fractures (VCFs) is a topic that has been much discussed in the general medical literature in recent years. Since the previous edition of this book was released in 2006, the literature has reported eight randomized controlled trials (RCTs) that compared different forms of vertebral body augmentation and control treatments, producing conflicting results and, consequently, great controversy in both the medical community and the lay public.[1-7] Hospital administrators, third-party payers, policy makers, and general medical practitioners have noted this controversy, and referral and practice patterns have been modified as a result.[8] This chapter reviews the rationale and recent evidence behind two forms of percutaneous vertebral augmentation (vertebroplasty and kyphoplasty), and discusses the controversy, our experience with these techniques, and the relevant technical points.

Natural History, Nonoperative Management and Patient Selection

Percutaneous cement augmentation was originally described for the treatment of symptomatic vertebral body hemangioma; this indication accounts for a minority of cases treated today.[9] Considering the prevalence of osteoporosis in the aging population of developed countries, it is natural that osteoporotic VCFs constitute the majority of cases. Approximately 25% of women in their fifties suffer from osteoporotic VCFs, increasing to 40 to 50% for women in their eighties.[10-12] Olszynski et al[13] demonstrated that VCFs, which were once thought to be a disease affecting mostly females, occur in 40% of male octogenarians. As a direct consequence of this elevated prevalence in an aging population, operative and nonoperative care of osteoporotic VCFs results in an increasing societal burden; in the 1990s, direct medical costs of treating VCFs amounted to $746 million dollars in the United States alone.[12] Ross et al[14] analyzed how the degree of osteoporosis affects a patient's risk of developing VCF, and found that patients with bone mass that is less than two standard deviations from the mean had a fivefold increased risk of developing VCFs. In the presence of two or more VCFs, however, this risk increases to 12-fold.[14] Other predisposing factors for developing osteoporotic VCFs include menopause, prolonged immobility, chronic steroid therapy, diabetes mellitus, rheumatoid arthritis, cirrhosis, renal insufficiency, and malnutrition.[15] Only a third of osteoporotic VCFs become clinically apparent, but they may lead to significant pain and immobility. Patients who become symptomatic are at an elevated risk of experiencing a self-perpetuating process, because immobility and kyphotic deformities are important independent risk factors for new VCFs. Black et al[16] determined that the presence of kyphosis from previous fractures is independently associated with a fivefold increase in the risk of developing new fractures.

Neoplastic disease that is metastatic to the spine is the other important cause of VCF that is pertinent to our discussion. Osseous metastases are a common complication associated with many types of solid tumors, occurring in 30 to 95% of patients with breast, prostate, lung, bladder, and thyroid cancers.[17] Most multiple myeloma patients also present with osteolytic lesions or generalized osteoporosis during the course of their disease. Different forms of radiation therapy may also contribute to cause osteonecrosis, further weakening the bone matrix. The incidence of neoplastic VCFs has been estimated to be 24% in patients with multiple myeloma, and 14%, 8%, and 6%, respectively, in patients with cancers of the breast, lung, and prostate.[17,18]

A majority of patients with osteoporotic VCFs improve within 4 to 6 weeks regardless of the treatment prescribed. Traditional conservative treatment includes analgesia and bed rest; however, these measures accelerate bone loss and increase the risk of developing deep venous thrombosis and pulmonary complications, with important negative impact on the patient.[19] Pharmacological treatment of osteoporotic VCFs includes a 4-week course of calcitonin for patients with acutely diagnosed (within the first 5 days) VCFs, for which moderate-quality evidence exists.[20] Ibandronate and strontium ranelate are considered options to prevent additional VCFs (secondary prevention) in patients presenting with a symptomatic VCF; strontium ranelate, however, is not approved for use in the United States and has severe restrictions in Europe due to its association with cardiovascular disease.[20]

Bracing is often cited as one of the mainstays of nonoperative management of VCFs, but there is little evidence to determine the best type of bracing or how long it should be worn. In theory, bracing is used in VCFs to decrease postural flexion that causes increased load on the painful fractured vertebra and to relieve paraspinal muscle spasm. The brace should be chosen based on the fracture type and level. It should be sufficiently lightweight to ensure patient compliance, should be easy to wear and remove, and should prevent respiratory impairment. For example, although a lumbosacral orthosis (LSO) reduces intervertebral motion in the upper lumbar levels (L1–L3), it actually increases motion in the caudal levels (L4–S1).[21] Several braces are mentioned in the literature as being appropriate to treat VCFs, such as the Cheneau, Taylor, Knight-Taylor, cruciform anterior spinal hyperextension (CASH), Jewett, and custom-made thoracolumbar spinal orthoses (TLSOs), but, to date, only one randomized prospective trial analyzed a TLSO to manage VCFs in postmenopausal women, and it documented an improved quality of life (QOL) and reduced pain levels with brace use.[22] Other supporting evidence stems from studies on nonosteoporotic vertebral burst fractures, which do not exactly mimic the pathophysiology of osteoporotic VCFs.[23] The resulting evidence is so thin that a recent set of guidelines for symptomatic osteoporotic

Table 118.1 Randomized Prospective Trials of Vertebral Augmentation for Osteoporotic Vertebral Compression Fracture (VCFs)

Study	Intervention	Control	No. of Patients at Time of Follow-Up	Results
FREE[7,44]	KP	Nonspecified nonsurgical care, may include bracing	232 at 2 years	KP: improved QOL metrics at 6 months; pain improved at all time points
VERTOS II[4]	VP	Optimal pain management, specified	163 at 1 year	Better VAS pain score with VP, maintained at 1 year; no difference in QOL metrics
INVEST[3,26]	VP	Sham surgery	119 at 1 year	No improvement in first analysis; less pain at 1 year with VP; no difference in functional disability
Blasco et al[45]	VP	Nonoperative treatment, including calcitonin and intrathecal analgesia	95 at 1 year	VAS pain score improvement greater with VP at 2 months; QOL metrics better with VP, but no direct comparisons reported; 14–20% patients at baseline requiring no analgesics
Farrokhi et al[2]	VP	Optimal pain management, specified	76 at 36 months	Better VAS pain score and Oswestry score with VP, maintained over 24 months
Buchbinder et al[1]	VP	Sham surgery	71 at 6 months	No improvement with VP at 6 months
Rousing et al[5]	VP	Optimal pain management, specified, included bracing	55 at 1 year	No difference at most time points; lower VAS pain score at 1 month with VP
VERTOS[6]	VP	Optimal pain management, specified	34 at 2 weeks	Better VAS pain score at 2 weeks with VP; 14 of 16 patients on pain management crossed over to VP

Abbreviations: FREE, Fracture Reduction Evaluation; INVEST, Investigational Vertebroplasty Safety and Efficacy Trial; KP, kyphoplasty; QOL, quality of life; VAS, Visual Analog Scale; VP, vertebroplasty; QOL, quality of life; VERTOS, Vertebroplasty Versus Conservative Treatment in Acute Osteoporotic Vertebral Compression Fractures.

VCFs released by the American Academy of Orthopedic Surgeons was unable to recommend for or against treatment with braces.[20]

In contrast to the lack of evidence supporting nonoperative interventions, eight prospective RCTs have compared vertebral augmentation, either percutaneous vertebroplasty (VP) or kyphoplasty (KP), and different nonoperative management; their characteristics and results are summarized in **Table 118.1**. Except for the study of Rousing et al,[5] they are all thought to be well-controlled for confusion variables.[24] Significant controversy was generated by two large studies that failed to show any benefit of VP over nonoperative management and were published in the same issue of *The New England Journal of Medicine*, a high-impact general medical journal.[1,3] (The controversy is further discussed elsewhere.[25]) One of these two studies (Investigational Vertebroplasty Safety and Efficacy Trial [INVEST]) later demonstrated better pain control at 1 year following VP.[26] The results of these two controversial RCTs were combined to investigate whether a subgroup of patients with acute or more severe pain would have benefited, but it still failed to demonstrate a benefit of VP.[27]

Several problems permeate all of these RCTs: poor definition and heterogeneity of "conservative" (or nonoperative) treatment, utilization of a "sham" procedure as control (which enables a better experimental design and masking of treatment but is not directly applicable to a clinical setting), excessive crossover of patients assigned to control groups (up to 60%), low baseline pain levels (raising issues of external validity), conflict of interests (including industry funding and personal agendas), utilization of questionable metrics (namely, a Visual Analogue Scale [VAS] as an outcome measure), inability to recruit patients, and duration of VCF at the time of the procedure.[28–31] We share the impression of Anderson et al,[24] that the results of INVEST and the Australian trials did not correspond to our clinical experience; great care should be directed to understanding which exact subset of patients with VCFs are being studied in each RCT. Anderson et al combined the results of six of these RCTs to produce a meta-analysis that found that cement augmentation produces a clinically relevant improvement in pain and QOL scores at both early (< 12 weeks) and delayed (1 year) time points. The only routinely observed complication was occurrence of a new fracture, but that was divided evenly among treatment and nontreatment groups, with three studies favoring each. Catastrophic complications of cement augmentation were not seen, and only one neurological adverse event was observed among the more than 500 patients who received intervention in these trials—severe radiculopathy due to a cement leak that required a laminectomy.[2]

Therefore, it is evident from the literature review that cement augmentation is not to be considered for every patient with osteoporotic VCF, and an initial treatment consisting of bed rest for a short period of time and pain control should be tried, which should suffice for most patients. However, for those patients with continued pain, particularly if it results in continued hospital admissions for pain control, cement augmentation is a safe and effective option that produces durable results. The issue of time since the fracture event has not been properly addressed in studies, but it seems that patients with subacute fractures, particularly if demonstrated by an increased short tau inversion recovery (STIR) signal on magnetic resonance imaging (MRI), exhibit greater improvement.[24]

The evidence supporting cement augmentation for neoplastic VCFs is not as robust, even though this treatment has been utilized for neoplastic disease from its inception. Most studies were case series, but then the pivotal Cancer Patient Fracture Evaluation trial was published in 2011 by Berenson et al.[18] This was a multicenter RCT of kyphoplasty versus nonsurgical management for one to three VCFs of neoplastic origin. It demonstrated significant improvement in all QOL metrics analyzed at 1 month post-kyphoplasty, when compared with nonsurgical management. As with most studies of cement augmentation, crossover to the intervention group was significant; at 1 year of follow-up, 80% of the patients still being followed who had been assigned to nonoperative treatment had crossed over.

Indications

- Symptomatic, subacute thoracolumbar vertebral compression fractures of osteoporotic nature refractory to initial medical treatment
- Symptomatic thoracolumbar vertebral compression fracture of proven or suspected neoplastic nature; biopsy may be performed in the same setting, if necessary
- Symptomatic vertebral body hemangiomas

Contraindications

- Coagulopathy
- Underlying vertebral osteomyelitis/spondylodiscitis
- Vertebral collapse of > 90% of the original vertebral height (vertebra plana)
- Myelopathy localizing to the level of fracture
- Inability to lie prone
- Allergy to contrast or cement
- Epidural tumor extension
- Loss of integrity of posterior vertebral body wall with > 20% reduction of spinal canal area (relative contraindication)

Choice of Technique: Vertebroplasty Versus Kyphoplasty

The fundamental principle of cement augmentation for thoracolumbar fractures is the same for both techniques. Even though both VP and KP have been described in the cervical spine, the literature includes only case reports and small series.[32–35] VP accomplishes cement augmentation through direct injection of cement, whereas kyphoplasty involves the creation of a cavity initially and then gradual injection. It has thus been said that although VP is a high-pressure, low-volume injection, KP is low-pressure, higher-volume, although this may not be exactly the case in every situation.[36] The theoretical advantages of KP include restoration of anterior column height and decreased extravasation/embolization of cement. Restoration of height has been demonstrated on the order of 2 to 4 mm initially, losing 1 mm in the first year.[37] The clinical significance of height restoration remains unclear.[38] Reported rates of radiological evidence of extravasation vary widely in retrospective series, ranging from 9.2 to 139% (multiple areas of extravasation per level) for VP and from 0 to 26.3% for kyphoplasty.[37] Symptomatic extravasation is a far less common occurrence; in a 2009 review, 27 reported cases were found.[37] Cardiovascular embolization is a very rare but catastrophic event that is encountered at the case report level. For an accurate assessment of risks, the combined data of the randomized trials is an excellent reference, showing one symptomatic extravasation in over 500 patients.[24] Given the very similar clinical results and risks, it is our preference to perform VP due to a more favorable cost profile.

Preoperative Imaging

Ideally, patients should have MRI of the symptomatic segment including a STIR sequence. Particular attention is directed to the integrity of the posterior wall of the vertebral body; although not an absolute contraindication, a more careful and slow cement injection may be required if the posterior wall is not intact. The STIR sequence can be useful in the context of multiple fractures or uncertain age; the presence of bone marrow edema should indicate the acute/subacute fracture.

Because a large fraction of patients with either osteoporotic or neoplastic VCFs are in very frail condition, obtaining an MRI can be a challenge. For these patients, we have decided at times to forgo the MRI in favor of simply using computed tomography (CT), particularly when the fracture age is not a concern, such as in the event of a clear onset of pain. Finally, standing radiographs may be useful to assess alignment but these are frequently not feasible.

Surgical Procedure

Cement augmentation is a procedure normally performed in patients with many comorbidities; it is therefore our preference to perform VP with the patient under mild sedation and local anesthesia, although the patient can also be under general anesthesia or even just local anesthesia. The ability to interact with the patient and perform a neurologic exam also provides an invaluable form of "neuromonitoring" while avoiding issues related to positive-pressure ventilation. Image guidance is performed with biplanar fluoroscopy. In the interest of minimizing radiation exposure to the surgeon and staff, utilization of navigation during the insertion phase of the procedure has been described. Fluoroscopy is still required, however, for the cement injection phase, when most radiation exposure is utilized.[39,40] Several authors describe performing this procedure in interventional radiology suites; we prefer a full operating room due to the possible need to immediately perform a laminectomy for cement extravasation. Even though this has never been required in our experience, all patients provide informed consent for it prior to undergoing the VP procedure; note that performing the laminectomy by itself would not require conversion from local to general anesthesia[41] **(Figs. 118.1 and 118.2)**.

Once the patient is comfortably placed in the prone position, the fracture site is identified with fluoroscopy. Usual measures to ensure correct localization are taken, particularly in the thoracic spine. The pedicle of interest is marked on the skin, and local anesthetic is infiltrated along the planned track all the way to the periosteum. A wide selection of needles and cement is available for VP, but there is currently only one system available for kyphoplasty (Medtronic Inc., Minneapolis, MN). A trans- or parapedicular approach can be utilized for cement augmentation. We have preferred the latter, aiming for a starting point slightly inferior and lateral to the pedicle, so as to enable a more centered position of the needle tip within the vertebral body **(Fig. 118.3)**. Perfect positioning of the cement is thus achieved with a unilateral injection; other surgeons, particularly if utilizing a transpedicular approach, may opt for a bilateral approach. The inferomedial quadrant of the pedicle should be avoided at all costs as it jeopardizes the exiting nerve root.

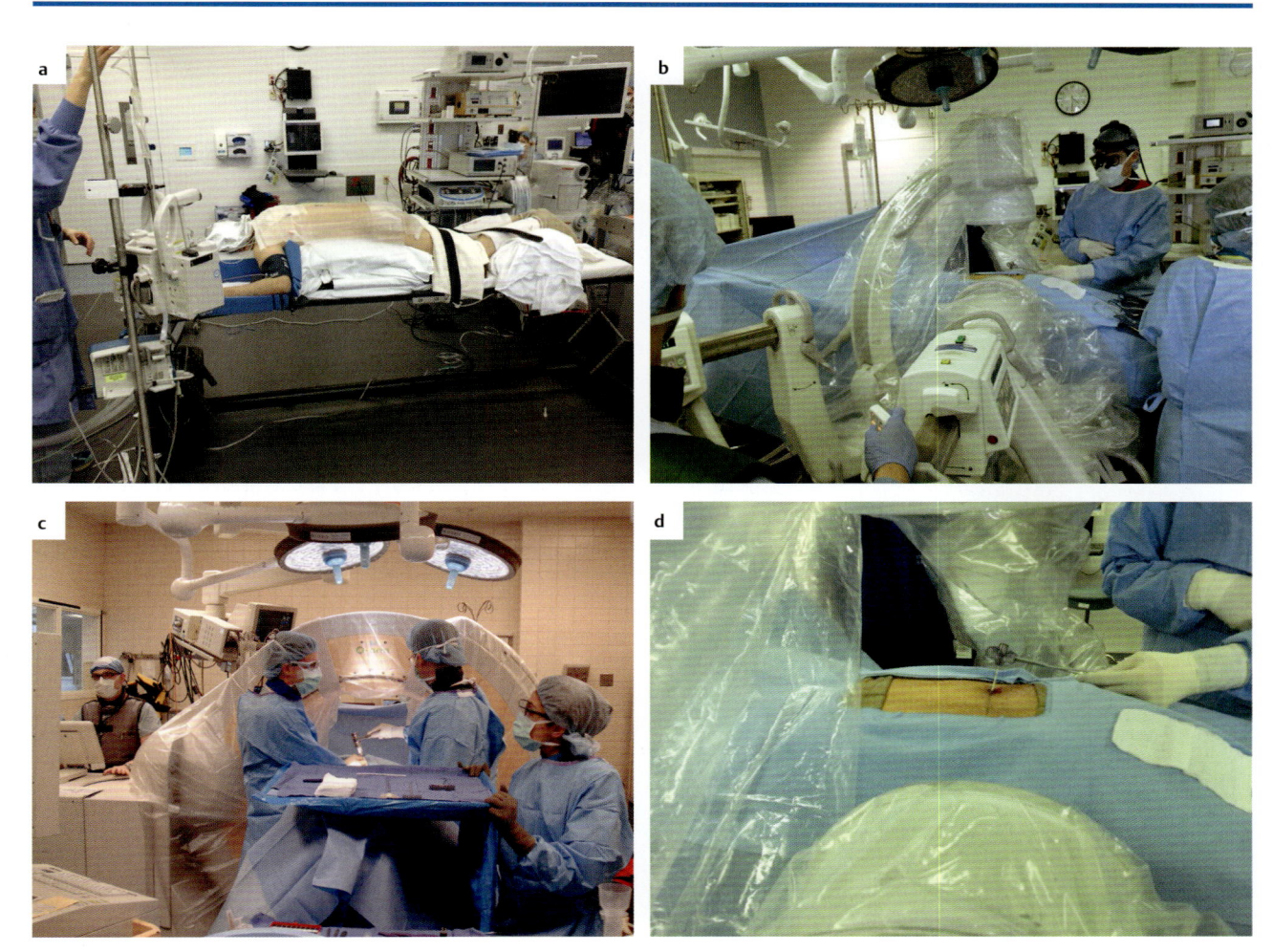

Fig. 118.1 Operating room setup. **(a)** Patient lying prone on a Jackson bed with a Wilson frame, enabling fluoroscopy positioning. Either a biplanar fluoroscopy **(b)** or navigation with O-arm **(c)** setup may be utilized. **(d)** Needle placement, in either setup, is ~ 5 cm off the midline for thoracic cases and 7 cm for lumbar cases. (**c**: Courtesy of Dr. John O'Toole, MD, MS.)

Following a 2-mm skin incision, a Jamshidi-type needle (10- to 15-gauge) is inserted, and contact is made on the vertebra at the above-mentioned target. At this stage, additional local anesthetic can be injected through the needle if desired. Typically, immediately upon insertion, the needle tip touches the transverse process; it is then slowly moved caudally until it reaches the ideal insertion point (**Fig. 118.3**). The needle is advanced into the vertebra, and biplanar fluoroscopy is utilized to ensure that the tip is advanced medial to the pedicle only after it is anterior to the posterior wall of the vertebral body. A midsagittal

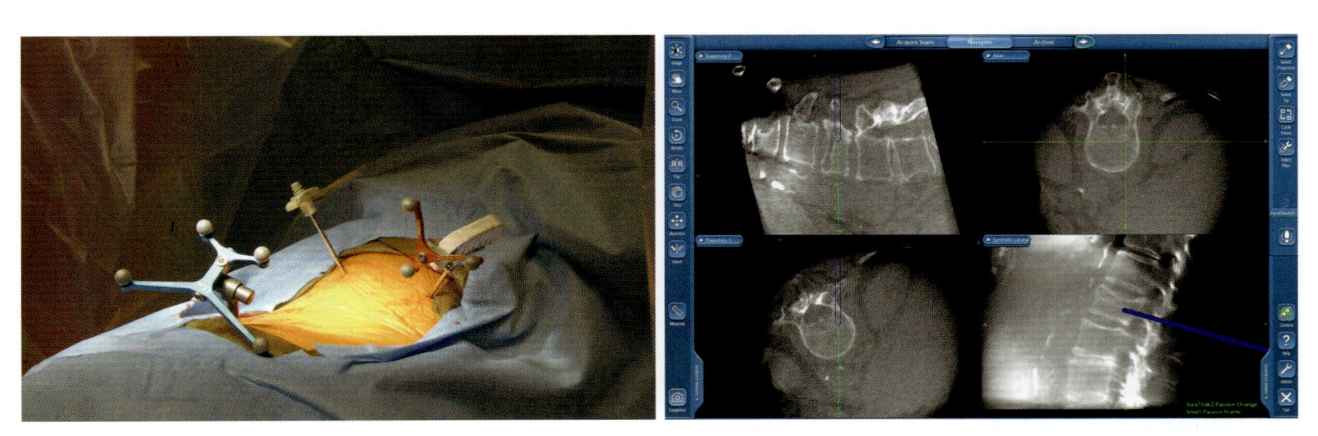

Fig. 118.2 **(a)** Navigation setup for a kyphoplasty case, demonstrating the iliac reference pin and a Jamshidi needle with the navigation tracking attachment. **(b)** The needle trajectory can be followed in three planes during the insertion phase. (Courtesy of Dr. John O'Toole, MD, MS.)

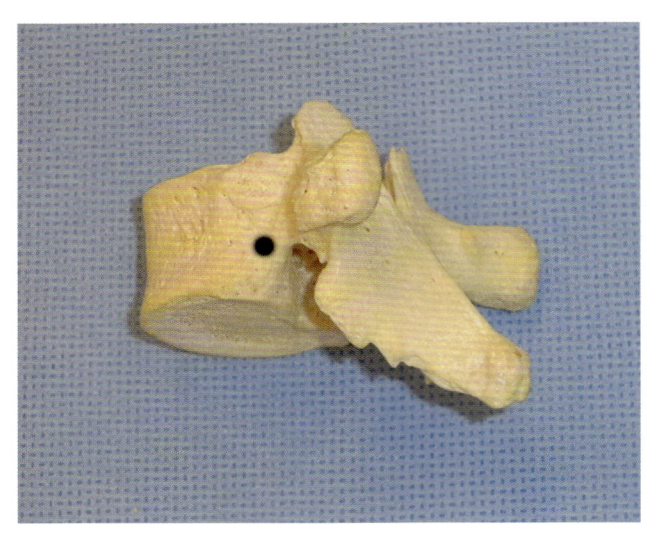

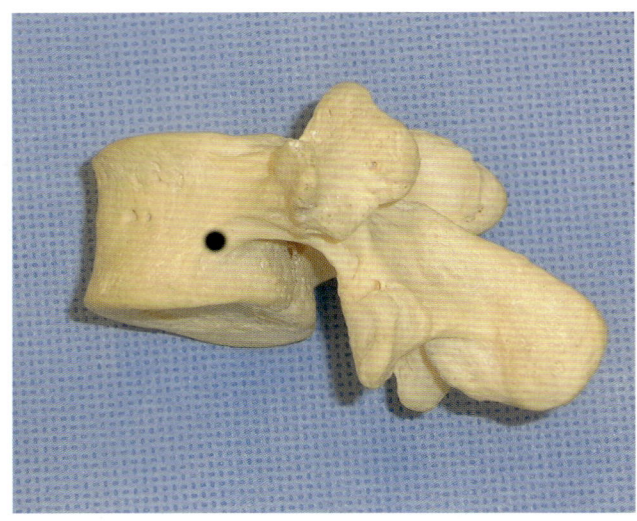

Fig. 118.3 Optimal entry point into the vertebral body for a thoracic (a) and lumbar (b) vertebra. A parapedicular trajectory immediately lateral and inferior to the pedicle avoids the nerve root and enables the central positioning of cement.

position within the anterior half of the vertebral body is desired for the tip of the needle to start cement injection. The Jamshidi trocar is removed, and a biopsy may be performed if neoplastic disease is suspected. We utilize a highly viscous polymethylmethacrylate cement preparation to minimize the risk of embolization or extravasation. This necessitates, on the other hand, the assistance of a hydraulic hand-operated pump to enable cement delivery (Confidence System, DePuy, Raynham, MA). Less complex setups may be utilized with syringes, but injection has to proceed at a slower pace to allow some settling of cement. Typically, cement volumes of 2 to 8 mL are utilized in VP; injection is performed carefully, with fluoroscopy images being obtained every 0.3 to 0.5 mL of cement being injected (**Fig. 118.4**). Injection should be interrupted at any sign of extravasation. The needle may be retracted a centimeter around the midpoint of cement injection, to enable a slightly posterior filling of the vertebral body. Once the needles are removed, a single suture is utilized on the skin.

Kyphoplasty differs in that is has one additional step: Once the needles are positioned inside the vertebral body, the balloons are inserted and inflated gradually. The balloons are filled with contrast medium, so this process may be followed radiographically. A pressure gauge is attached to the system, and pressure during inflation should never exceed 220 psi. Sudden drops

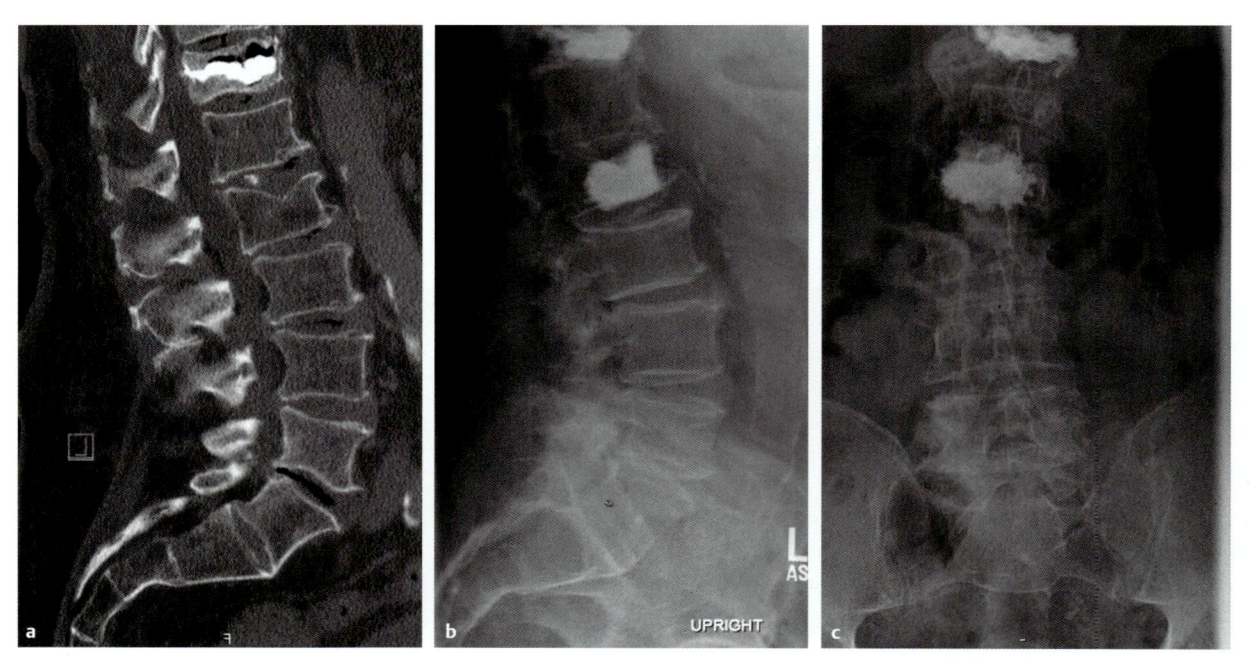

Fig. 118.4 (a) Typical case of an L1 vertebral compression fracture (VCF) of an osteoporotic nature. There is a transitional L5 level, and the patient had already undergone a T11 vertebroplasty (VP) 4 months earlier. Lateral (b) and anteroposterior (AP) (c) radiographs demonstrate a good surgical result with an 8-cc injection of cement.

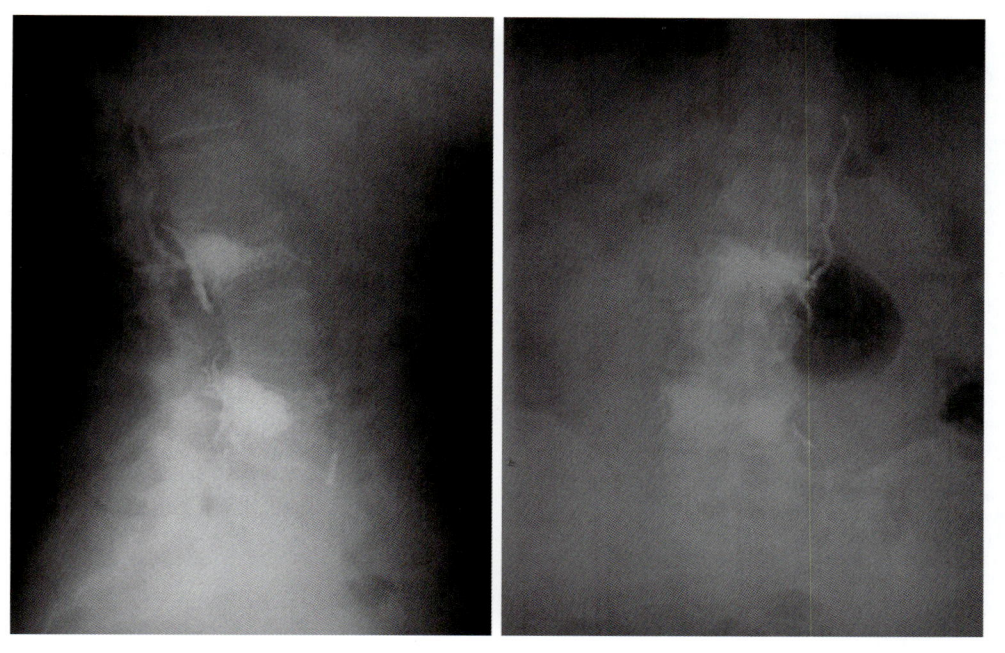

Fig. 118.5 Lateral **(a)** and AP **(b)** radiographs of a two-level VP case, demonstrating asymptomatic embolization of epidural and paravertebral veins. This was caused by injection of excessively liquid cement. The injection was interrupted, and the patient did not have any clinical consequences.

in pressure during inflation may suggest a vertebral body fracture. Inflation in this case should be interrupted. After the cavity is created, balloons are deflated and removed. Cement in injected into the cavity via a cement-filled cannula and its plunger; each cannula contains ~ 1.5 mL of cement. The procedure is interrupted once there is a sign of cement extravasation or a mantle of cement reaches posteriorly about two thirds of vertebral body anteroposterior (AP) length.[42]

Postoperative Care

Two hours after the procedure, patients are encouraged to stand, and standing lateral and AP radiographs of the segment in question are obtained to evaluate the alignment. If it is satisfactory, and if pain is under control, patients are discharged. No further imaging is necessary unless patients become symptomatic. Asymptomatic cement leaks do not require any intervention.

Potential Complications and Precautions

Complications with VP or KP are rare but may be catastrophic. Cement extravasation and embolization are the two most often cited complications. Both can be prevented by assessing cement viscosity prior to injection. While the cement is being mixed, we ensure that it is at least of honey-thick consistency before being prepared for injection into the hydraulic pump (VP) or the cannula (KP). Frequent radiographic assessment is performed every 0.3 to 0.5 mL of cement injection, and the procedure is immediately interrupted if there is evidence of extravasation or embolization (**Fig. 118.5**). The patient is then examined to assess the symptomatology; an emergency laminectomy is performed with the patient under local anesthesia if there is any sign of neurologic compromise. We have not encountered either problem in our practice, but we include the phrase "possible emergency laminectomy" in the consent form. These complications have been reported slightly more frequently in neoplastic VCFs.[43]

Conclusion

It is our experience that patients receiving percutaneous cement augmentation consistently experience rapid and significant pain relief through a safe, minimally invasive approach that is compatible with their often frail state. The literature evidence overwhelmingly supports this surgical option for the treatment of neoplastic and refractory osteoporotic vertebral compression fractures. **Box 118.1** lists the key operative points.

Box 118.1 Key Operative Points

- Prone positioning under sedation and local anesthesia
- Biplanar fluoroscopy guidance
- Map entry point on skin, aim for inferolateral margin of pedicle
- Only advance medial to pedicle when anterior to the spinal canal
- Ideal needle position: midline anterior half of vertebral body
- Cement at least honey-thick consistency
- Inject cement (VP), or inflate balloons, deflate, and inject cement (KP)
- Control for cement extravasation or embolization every 0.5 mL injected
- Check neurologic exam
- Patient may ambulate 2 hours after procedure

References

1. Buchbinder R, Osborne RH, Ebeling PR, et al. A randomized trial of vertebroplasty for painful osteoporotic vertebral fractures. N Engl J Med 2009;361:557–568
2. Farrokhi MR, Alibai E, Maghami Z. Randomized controlled trial of percutaneous vertebroplasty versus optimal medical management for the relief of pain and disability in acute osteoporotic vertebral compression fractures. J Neurosurg Spine 2011;14:561–569
3. Kallmes DF, Comstock BA, Heagerty PJ, et al. A randomized trial of vertebroplasty for osteoporotic spinal fractures. N Engl J Med 2009;361:569–579
4. Klazen CAH, Lohle PNM, de Vries J, et al. Vertebroplasty versus conservative treatment in acute osteoporotic vertebral compression fractures (Vertos II): an open-label randomised trial. Lancet 2010;376:1085–1092
5. Rousing R, Hansen KL, Andersen MO, Jespersen SM, Thomsen K, Lauritsen JM. Twelve-months follow-up in forty-nine patients with acute/semiacute osteoporotic vertebral fractures treated conservatively or with percutaneous vertebroplasty: a clinical randomized study. Spine 2010;35:478–482
6. Voormolen MHJ, Mali WPTM, Lohle PNM, et al. Percutaneous vertebroplasty compared with optimal pain medication treatment: short-term clinical outcome of patients with subacute or chronic painful osteoporotic vertebral compression fractures. The VERTOS study. AJNR Am J Neuroradiol 2007;28:555–560
7. Wardlaw D, Cummings SR, Van Meirhaeghe J, et al. Efficacy and safety of balloon kyphoplasty compared with non-surgical care for vertebral compression fracture (FREE): a randomised controlled trial. Lancet 2009;373:1016–1024
8. Lindsey SS, Kallmes DF, Opatowsky MJ, Broyles EA, Layton KF. Impact of sham-controlled vertebroplasty trials on referral patterns at two academic medical centers. Proc (Bayl Univ Med Cent) 2013;26:103–105
9. Galibert P, Deramond H, Rosat P, Le Gars D. [Preliminary note on the treatment of vertebral angioma by percutaneous acrylic vertebroplasty]. Neurochirurgie 1987;33:166–168
10. Cooper C, Atkinson EJ, Jacobsen SJ, O'Fallon WM, Melton LJ III. Population-based study of survival after osteoporotic fractures. Am J Epidemiol 1993;137:1001–1005
11. Lyles KW. Management of patients with vertebral compression fractures. Pharmacotherapy 1999;19(1 Pt 2):21S–24S
12. Prather H, Hunt D, Watson JO, Gilula LA. Conservative care for patients with osteoporotic vertebral compression fractures. Phys Med Rehabil Clin N Am 2007;18:577–591, xi
13. Olszynski WP, Shawn Davison K, Adachi JD, et al. Osteoporosis in men: epidemiology, diagnosis, prevention, and treatment. Clin Ther 2004;26:15–28
14. Ross PD, Davis JW, Epstein RS, Wasnich RD. Pre-existing fractures and bone mass predict vertebral fracture incidence in women. Ann Intern Med 1991;114:919–923
15. Rao RD, Singrakhia MD. Painful osteoporotic vertebral fracture. Pathogenesis, evaluation, and roles of vertebroplasty and kyphoplasty in its management. J Bone Joint Surg Am 2003;85-A:2010–2022
16. Black DM, Arden NK, Palermo L, Pearson J, Cummings SR; Study of Osteoporotic Fractures Research Group. Prevalent vertebral deformities predict hip fractures and new vertebral deformities but not wrist fractures. J Bone Miner Res 1999;14:821–828
17. Coleman RE. Skeletal complications of malignancy. Cancer 1997;80(8, Suppl):1588–1594
18. Berenson J, Pflugmacher R, Jarzem P, et al; Cancer Patient Fracture Evaluation (CAFE) Investigators. Balloon kyphoplasty versus non-surgical fracture management for treatment of painful vertebral body compression fractures in patients with cancer: a multicentre, randomised controlled trial. Lancet Oncol 2011;12:225–235
19. Lemke DM. Vertebroplasty and kyphoplasty for treatment of painful osteoporotic compression fractures. J Am Acad Nurse Pract 2005;17:268–276
20. Esses SI, McGuire R, Jenkins J, et al. The treatment of symptomatic osteoporotic spinal compression fractures. J Am Acad Orthop Surg 2011;19:176–182
21. Tuong NH, Dansereau J, Maurais G, Herrera R. Three-dimensional evaluation of lumbar orthosis effects on spinal behavior. J Rehabil Res Dev 1998;35:34–42
22. Pfeifer M, Begerow B, Minne HW. Effects of a new spinal orthosis on posture, trunk strength, and quality of life in women with postmenopausal osteoporosis: a randomized trial. Am J Phys Med Rehabil 2004;83:177–186
23. Longo UG, Loppini M, Denaro L, Maffulli N, Denaro V. Conservative management of patients with an osteoporotic vertebral fracture: a review of the literature. J Bone Joint Surg Br 2012;94:152–157
24. Anderson PA, Froyshteter AB, Tontz WL Jr. Meta-analysis of vertebral augmentation compared with conservative treatment for osteoporotic spinal fractures. J Bone Miner Res 2013;28:372–382
25. Georgy B. Can meta-analysis save vertebroplasty? AJNR Am J Neuroradiol 2011;32:614–616
26. Comstock BA, Sitlani CM, Jarvik JG, Heagerty PJ, Turner JA, Kallmes DF. Investigational Vertebroplasty Safety and Efficacy Trial (INVEST): patient-reported outcomes through 1 year. Radiology 2013;259:224–231
27. Staples MP, Kallmes DF, Comstock BA, et al. Effectiveness of vertebroplasty using individual patient data from two randomised placebo controlled trials: meta-analysis. BMJ 2011;343:d3952
28. Aebi M. Vertebroplasty: about sense and nonsense of uncontrolled "controlled randomized prospective trials". Eur Spine J 2009;18:1247–1248
29. Carragee EJ. The vertebroplasty affair: the mysterious case of the disappearing effect size. Spine J 2010;10:191–192
30. O'Toole JE, Traynelis VC. Vertebral compression fractures. J Neurosurg Spine 2011;14:555–559, discussion 559–560
31. Weinstein JN. Balancing science and informed choice in decisions about vertebroplasty. N Engl J Med 2009;361:619–621
32. Blondel B, Litré F, Graillon T, Adetchessi T, Dufour H, Fuentes S. Metastatic odontoid fracture management by anterior screw fixation and kyphoplasty. Neurochirurgie 2013;59:191–194
33. Fransen P, Collignon FP. Direct anterolateral balloon kyphoplasty for a painful C-2 osteolytic malignant lesion. Case illustration. J Neurosurg Spine 2007;6:374
34. Lykomitros V, Anagnostidis KS, Alzeer Z, Kapetanos GA. Percutaneous anterolateral balloon kyphoplasty for metastatic lytic lesions of the cervical spine. Eur Spine J 2010;19:1948–1952
35. Zapalowicz K, Skora P, Myslinski R, Karnicki F, Radek A. Balloon kyphoplasty for painful C-7 vertebral hemangioma. J Neurosurg Spine 2008;8:458–461
36. Eichholz KM, O'Toole JE, Christie SD, Fessler RG. Vertebroplasty and kyphoplasty. Neurosurg Clin N Am 2006;17:507–518
37. Mendel E, Bourekas E, Gerszten P, Golan JD. Percutaneous techniques in the treatment of spine tumors: what are the diagnostic and therapeutic indications and outcomes? Spine 2009;34(22, Suppl):S93–S100
38. Bastian L, Schils F, Tillman JB, Fueredi G; SCORE Investigators. A randomized trial comparing 2 techniques of balloon kyphoplasty and curette use for obtaining vertebral body height restoration and angular-deformity correction in vertebral compression fractures due to osteoporosis. AJNR Am J Neuroradiol 2013;34:666–675
39. Kang JD, An H, Boden S, Phillips F, Foley K, Abdu W. Cement augmentation of osteoporotic compression fractures and intraoperative navigation: summary statement. Spine 2003;28(15, Suppl):S62–S63
40. Villavicencio AT, Burneikiene S, Bulsara KR, Thramann JJ. Intraoperative three-dimensional fluoroscopy-based computerized tomography guidance for percutaneous kyphoplasty. Neurosurg Focus 2005;18:e3
41. Ames WA, Songhurst L, Gullan RW. Local anaesthesia for laminectomy surgery. Br J Neurosurg 1999;13:598–600
42. Garfin SR, Yuan HA, Reiley MA. New technologies in spine: kyphoplasty and vertebroplasty for the treatment of painful osteoporotic compression fractures. Spine 2001;26:1511–1515
43. Barr JD, Jensen ME, Hirsch JA, et al; Society of Interventional Radiology; American Association of Neurological Surgeons; Congress of Neurological Surgeons; American College of Radiology; American Society of Neuroradiology; American Society of Spine Radiology; Canadian Interventional Radiology Association; Society of Neurointerventional Surgery. Position

statement on percutaneous vertebral augmentation: a consensus statement developed by the Society of Interventional Radiology (SIR), American Association of Neurological Surgeons (AANS) and the Congress of Neurological Surgeons (CNS), American College of Radiology (ACR), American Society of Neuroradiology (ASNR), American Society of Spine Radiology (ASSR), Canadian Interventional Radiology Association (CIRA), and the Society of NeuroInterventional Surgery (SNIS). J Vasc Interv Radiol 2014;25:171–181

44. Boonen S, Van Meirhaeghe J, Bastian L, et al. Balloon kyphoplasty for the treatment of acute vertebral compression fractures: 2-year results from a randomized trial. J Bone Miner Res 2011;26:1627–1637

45. Blasco J, Martinez-Ferrer A, Macho J, et al. Effect of vertebroplasty on pain relief, quality of life, and the incidence of new vertebral fractures: a 12-month randomized follow-up, controlled trial. J Bone Miner Res 2012;27:1159–1166

119 Resection of Lumbosacral Lipomas

Carter S. Gerard, Lee A. Tan, Robert G. Kellogg, and Lorenzo F. Muñoz

Congenital lipomas that arise in the lumbosacral area are one of the most common forms of spinal dysraphism, with an incidence estimated at 1 in 4,000 births.[1] Lumbosacral lipomas are a heterogeneous group of lesions that may be organized in three main anatomic groups: lipomas of the filum, subpial lipomas, and lipomas arising from the conus. This chapter discusses the classification, presentation, and management of lipomas arising from the conus. Lipomas of the conus medullaris have received the greatest amount of attention as they are the most common, making up as high as 86% of spinal lipomas,[2] and are the most challenging to treat. Children with lumbosacral lipomas typically have normal neurologic function at birth and then gradually develop deficits over time. There remains considerable controversy as to the natural history of lumbosacral lipomas, which has resulted in disagreement on the management of asymptomatic patients.[2–4] However, multiple series have shown that symptomatic patients stabilize or improve after surgical intervention, but are unlikely to regain normal function.[2,5–7] The damage to neural elements is likely due to ischemic changes caused by hypoperfusion of the tethered spinal cord.[8,9] Therefore, the goal of surgical intervention is to protect neurologic function by removal of the fatty mass and untethering of the spinal cord while preserving neurologic tissue.

Indications

- Symptomatic lumbosacral lipomas
- Asymptomatic lesions in patients of ages < 3 months with radiographic evidence of tethering

Advantages

- Stabilization/reversal of neurologic deficits associated with tethering
- Possible prevention of neurologic deficits in asymptomatic patients

Disadvantages

- Potential for new neurologic deficits
- Re-tethering after lipoma resection and untethering

Definition

Multiple classification systems and terms have been devised in an attempt to accurately describe the full range of lumbosacral lipomas.[1,5,10,11] Chapman[12] outlined the three-tier classification that is the most commonly used and widely recognized system for describing conus medullaris lipomas. The system includes dorsal, caudal, and transitional subtypes. The caudal subtype, also known as the terminal lipoma, is joined to the caudal aspect of the conus and may enter into the central canal. These lipomas may replace the filum entirely or may be separated from the conus by a short thickened filum terminale. The dural sac and dorsal fascia are not violated.

The dorsal type arises from the dorsal aspect of the lumbar spine, always sparing the distal conus. The junction between the lipoma and spinal cord can be defined along the dorsal root entry zone (DREZ) with the dorsal roots laterally. The dorsal lipoma is void of nerve roots. The lipoma extends from the neural placode through a dural defect to join extradural fat. Although the distal conus is not involved, it is often associated with a thickened or fatty filum terminale.[1,13] Transitional lipomas are similar to the dorsal type as there is an identifiable border at the lateral margin between the lipoma and the DREZ. However, unlike the dorsal variant, the transitional lipomas continue caudally to involve the conus. The asymmetric nature often results in a blurred lipoma–cord interface and may result in rotation of the neural placode. Despite the irregular orientation, the nerve roots are always lateral or ventral to the lipoma–cord interface. The irregular nature and large size of these lipomas can make it extremely difficult to define the anatomy, which inhibits safe resection.[13]

Pang et al[5] described the "chaotic" lipoma, which has a caudal portion that extends ventral to the neural placode, with involvement of the neural roots and the neural placode. The name is derived from the variable nature of the anatomy and the indistinct relationship among the neural placode, roots, and lipoma. It is an uncommon lesion that is characteristically seen with sacral agenesis.[5]

Dorsal and transitional lipomas occur as a result of premature dysjunction, that is, separation from the neural tube from the surrounding ectoderm. The neural tube is then open posteriorly and mesenchymal cells are able to enter the abnormal cleft.[14,15] These mesodermal elements are then induced to become adipocytes and occupy the space between these embryological tissues, impeding the development of dura and closure of the laminae and lumbosacral fascia. The mesodermal elements mature into fat that often connects the subcutaneous space to the distal spinal cord.

Caudal lipomas, also referred to as terminal lipomas, are a result of an error in secondary rather than primary neurulation. Therefore, the lumbar and upper sacral nerve roots in addition to the dura and dorsal structures that are formed during primary neurulation are never affected. Often these lesions are found to have disorganized neural elements that suggest that they are due to incomplete or failed apoptosis.[16,17]

Presentation

The majority of infants are brought to medical attention due to a visible lumbosacral mass (**Fig. 119.1**) or other cutaneous finding, such as focal hirsutism, a rudimentary tail, or a dermal sinus

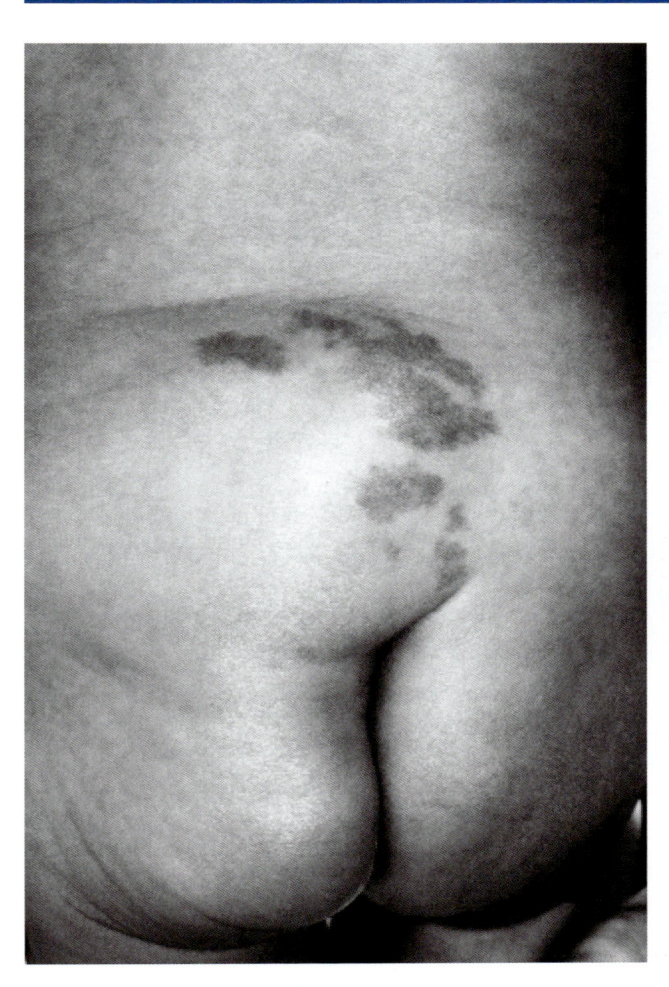

Fig. 119.1 A visible lumbosacral mass.

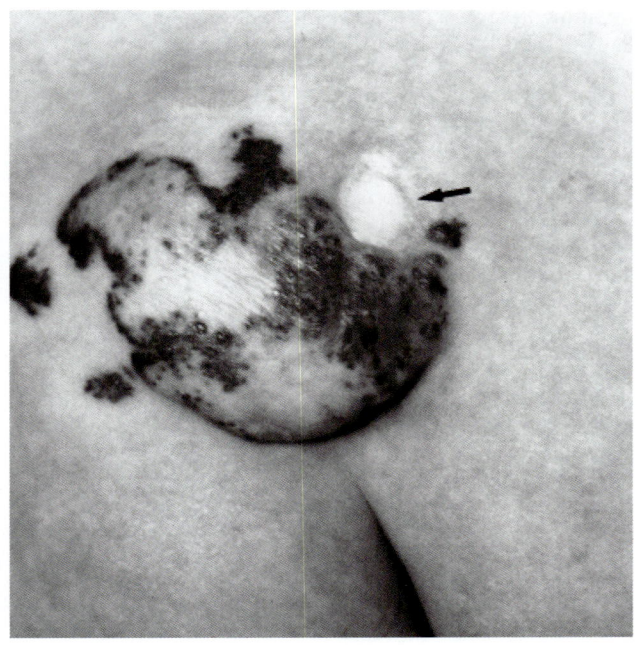

Fig. 119.2 A typical mass with an overlying hemangioma. The lipoma may result in deviation or asymmetry of the upper portion of the gluteal crease; if the mass is subtle, an asymmetric crease may be the only external finding.

tract. A subcutaneous mass is the most common clinical finding. The mass is covered with intact skin and may have an overlying hemangioma (**Fig. 119.2**). The lipoma may result in deviation or asymmetry of the upper portion of the gluteal crease; if the mass is subtle, an asymmetric crease may be the only external finding.[2]

Symptomatic patients present with a wide array of syndromes including urologic dysfunction, neurologic impairment, pain, and orthopedic malformations.[2] Urologic dysfunction in patients with lumbosacral lipomas is closely correlated with older age and with the sensitivity of the test used to assess dysfunction; urodynamic testing is more sensitive than clinical assessment.[18] Foster et al[19] used urodynamic studies in patients with lumbosacral lipomas to demonstrate abnormal bladder function, and found that 79% of patients older than 18 months but only 42% of patients younger than 18 months were abnormal. Clinically, urinary dysfunction may be difficult to diagnose in an infant. However, as impairment progresses, the child may develop repeated urinary tract infections, incomplete voiding, or complete incontinence.[20] If the urinary dysfunction is severe, rectal incontinence may follow, but this is uncommon.[21]

Although multiple series have demonstrated the progressive neurologic decline in patients with lumbosacral lipomas, early deficits are subtle and are rarely the primary complaint at presentation.[2] This is especially true in infants because normal function is difficult if not impossible to confirm. Although the majority of patients with a midline lipoma are intact at birth, those patients with an asymmetric mass have a greater risk of neurologic impairment in the lower extremity ipsilateral to the lesion. Patients who have clinical findings typically show progressive asymmetric weakness with patchy sensory loss in the lower extremities. The exam may show upper and lower motor neuron deficits in the same extremity.[21] Electromyographic abnormalities are present in half the asymptomatic patients and in all the symptomatic patients.[2]

Orthopedic deformity is a well-recognized sequela of lumbosacral lipomas and is often the primary complaint upon presentation in early childhood.[21] In a series of 291 patients with lumbosacral lipomas and lipomas of the filum, Pierre-Kahn et al[2] reported that 31% of patient had an orthopedic deformity at presentation, mostly affecting the lower limb and to a lesser degree the spine. Clubfoot, with equinovarus and clawing of the toes, was the most common deformity.[2] Other findings of the extremity may include asymmetric foot and leg length, muscle mass discrepancies, and joint deformity.[21] Scoliosis is present in 10% of children and may progress as a result of spinal cord tethering. Multiple authors have reported arrested progression and even reversal of scoliosis after untethering.[6,22]

Although uncommon in infants and young children, pain is the most common presenting symptom in adolescence and adults. The patient may complain of low back pain and asymmetric pain in the legs that changes with time; occasionally, a Lhermitte sign is seen.[1,23,24] The pain is often exacerbated by activity, including bending, walking, and running, or by trauma.

Natural History and Surgical Outcome

The decision to operate is clear in patients with symptomatic lumbosacral lipomas. Large series have shown that loss of neurologic function is unlikely to be regained completely in the majority of cases.[2,6,22] Symptomatic patients who undergo untethering have a 67 to 90% likelihood of symptom stabilization and occasional reversal.[2,6,11,25] Pain, if short lived, is likely to resolve, whereas orthopedic deformity and bladder dysfunction are unlikely to improve once present.

However, due to the imperfect understanding of the natural history of this disease, there is still some controversy as to the best course for asymptomatic patients. Some authors have advocated a conservative approach after weighing the real risk of perioperative insult versus the possible risk of decline. Studies have shown that 33 to 40% of asymptomatic infants are likely to deteriorate over the course of 10 years.[4,25] Wykes et al[4] followed 56 asymptomatic patients for 10 years and found a median age of 1.9 years at the time of deterioration, and identified female sex, the presence of an associated syrinx, and the presence of transitional lipomas as being the factors that entailed the highest risk of deterioration. Due to the progressive nature of this disease and the irreversible nature of the deficits, prophylactic surgery was previously performed on the majority of asymptomatic patients. However, in a large series Pierre-Kahn et al[2] reported that more than half of asymptomatic patients who underwent prophylactic surgery went on to have neurologic decline within 120 months of surgery. The lack of efficacy coupled with a 4% rate of immediate postoperative decline led the senior author to warn against prophylactic surgeries and to endorse careful surveillance, including serial electromyography (EMG), urodynamics, and magnetic resonance imaging (MRI), coupled with timely intervention, for asymptomatic patients.

In 2010, Pang et al[26] reported the long-term neurologic status of a group of 86 asymptomatic patients who had undergone total resection and a group of 116 patients who had undergone partial resection. The results for the group of patients with a partial resection were in keeping with the Pierre-Kahn study and with later natural history studies, with a progression-free survival of 43% at 12 years. However, the cohort of asymptomatic patients with total resections produces an impressive progression-free survival of 98.4% at 16 years. The results of this study would suggest that prophylactic surgery is able to change the natural history of the disease only if a total resection is accomplished.

Preoperative Evaluation

All patients with a confirmed or suspected lumbosacral lipoma should undergo a full physical and neurologic evaluation. This includes special evaluation of the lumbar region, and neurologic exam of the extremities, perineum, and sphincter. The extremities are inspected to assess muscle mass and bony anatomy. Prior to surgery patients should undergo urodynamics and EMG. This is important in establishing a baseline, and it also may aid in communicating the risk and expected outcomes of the surgery to the patient and family.

Imaging for patients with lumbosacral lipomas is designed to assist in both diagnosis and surgical planning. Spinal ultrasound is a valuable tool to screen for lumbosacral lipomas in the neonate. However, the ability to evaluate the anatomy of the malformation is limited, and all patients who have a positive ultrasound will require an MRI. Routine X-rays demonstrate the presence and the level of a bony defect or other malformation such as diastematomyelia, in addition to the presence or absence of scoliosis. Lack of ossification in newborn patients makes the interpretation of X-rays difficult and therefore of questionable value. The primary form of imaging for lumbosacral lipomas is MRI (**Fig. 119.3**). MRI in axial and sagittal views with T1- and T2-weighted sequences are obtained. This is essential to understand the relationship between the lipoma and the spinal cord. Although the sagittal view confirms the level of the lesion in relationship to the spinal cord and vertebra, the axial sequence demonstrates any rotation and the relationship of the lipoma to

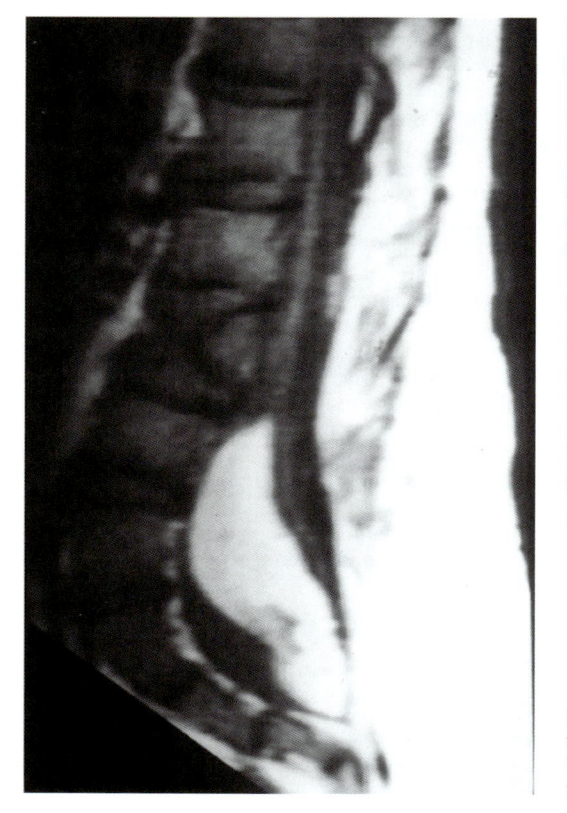

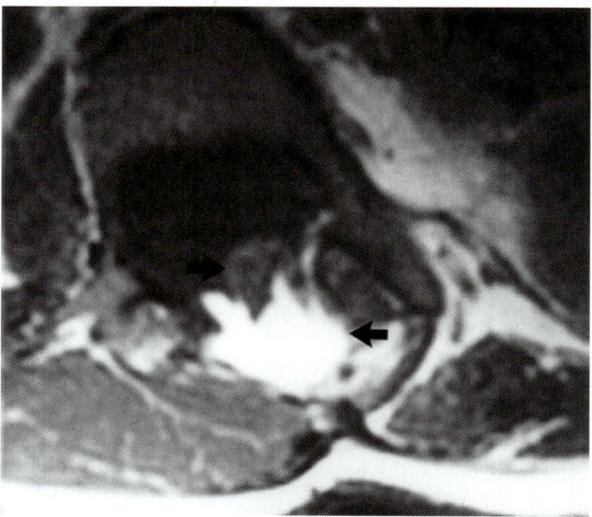

Fig. 119.3 (a) Sagittal T1-weighted magnetic resonance imaging (MRI) shows ventral extension of the lumbosacral lipoma into the enlarged lumbar cistern. (b) Axial T1-weighted MRI shows the interdigitated relationship *(arrow)* between the lipoma and placode with minimal rotation of the neural elements.

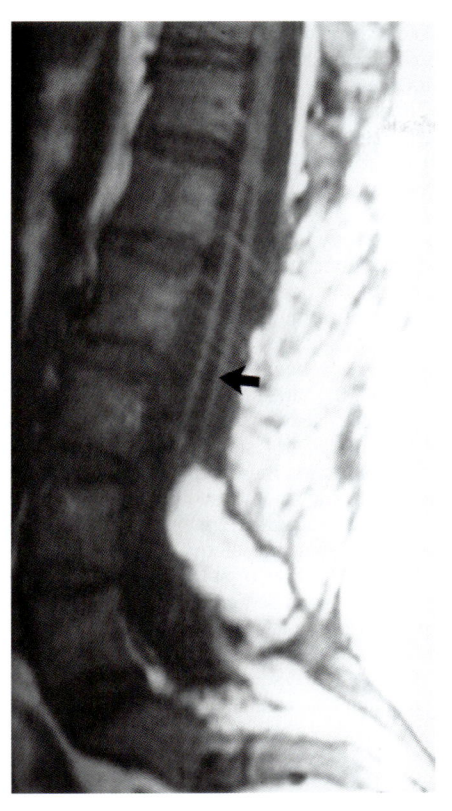

Fig. 119.4 Sagittal T1-weighted MRI demonstrates a dorsal lipoma with an associated syrinx *(arrow)*.

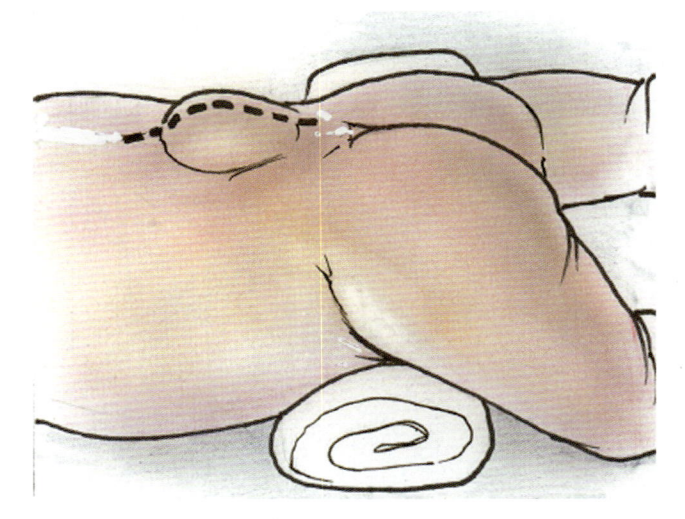

Fig. 119.5 The patient is positioned prone and bolsters are placed under the iliac crest and chest to minimize intra-abdominal pressure. The incision is made beyond the lipoma both rostrally and caudally.

the nerve roots. MRI also enables preoperative evaluation of an associated syrinx (**Fig. 119.4**).

Surgical Technique

Goals

The goals of surgical intervention are to untether and decompress the spinal cord, avoid damage to functional neural tissue, and prevent the re-tethering of the cord. These goals can be accomplished by separating adhesions, removing as much of the lipoma as possible, with the goal of complete lipoma resection. Finally, re-tethering may be avoided by enlarging the dural sac prior to closure.

Positioning

After induction of general anesthesia, appropriate intravenous access is placed. A Foley catheter is inserted and secured. A single intraoperative dose of either cefazolin or clindamycin is given 1 hour before incision and redosed every 6 hours. After the initial induction of anesthesia, neuromuscular paralytics are avoided to enable improved feedback from the nerve root during the operation. After the patient is positioned prone, bolsters are placed under the iliac crest and chest to minimize intra-abdominal pressure (**Fig. 119.5**). At this time, monitoring of somatosensory evoked potentials (SSEPs) and evoked EMG can be established. Although we routinely use monitoring, this is in no way mandatory. Surgeons who do not use monitoring argue that a change in signals should not preclude the surgeon from completing the operation.

Incision and Dissection

Once the patient is in position, a midline incision is made over the lipoma that provides access to the entire length of the pathology. This incision may be curved at the caudal aspect to gain access to low-lying asymmetric lipomas. A curved incision has the added benefit of avoiding the intergluteal cleft and avoiding the risk of fecal contamination. Once the skin is open, the subcutaneous fat is identified and removed from the skin flaps, with care taken not to devascularize the skin. Often, a fatty stalk connects the subcutaneous potion to the intraspinal lipoma through a defect in the lumbosacral fascia. When the fascial defect is identified, the fat lateral and dorsal can be removed with scissors and bipolar cautery. If the neural placode lies dorsal to the spinal canal, ultrasonic aspiration should be used to prevent potential damage to the underlying neural structures. During removal, the surgeon should be careful not to apply excessive tension to the fatty stalk, as it is firmly attached to the spinal cord (**Fig. 119.6**). Once the subcutaneous portion is debulked and the neck of the lipoma is freed from the surrounding fascial defect, the fascia is opened in the midline to expose the adjacent lamina and spinous process. Care must be taken to identify the bifid spinous process or laminar defects. A subperiosteal dissection can then be performed to remove musculature from the lamina and medial facet. The lower extent of the bony exposure should extend 1 cm past the neural placode rather than the lipoma. Caudal fat may extend down into the thecal sac, which becomes irrelevant once the conus has been detached.[5] A generous laminectomy is then performed to enable visualization of the dura caudal to the lipoma.

The dura rostral to the lipoma is then opened in the midline and retracted to expose the spinal cord (**Fig. 119.7**). The dural edge is then followed caudally to identify the dural attachment to the neck of the lipoma. Working in the subdural space, sharp dissection is then used to cut the dural attachments from the lipoma. The dural cuts may be joined caudal to the lipoma, thereby completing the dorsal release. The dura lateral to the lipoma can then be retracted to expose the full extent of the intradural involvement. Then, the intersection of the lipoma, pia, and spinal cord, also referred to as the fusion line, can be identified. The fusion line is always medial to the DREZ and the nerve roots.

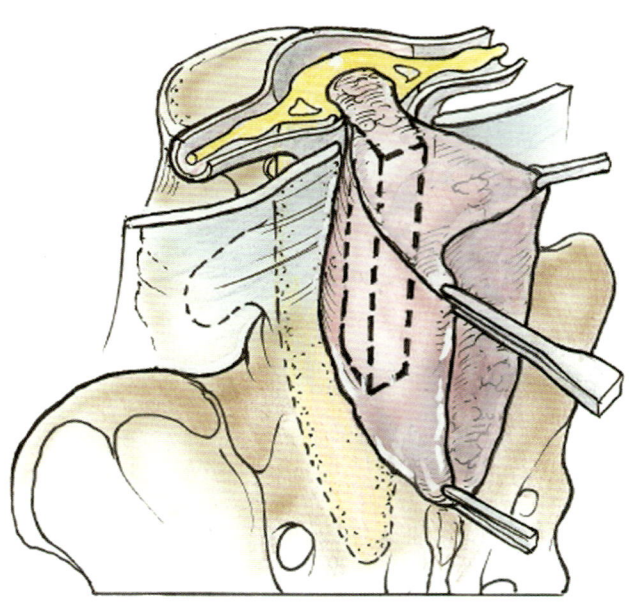

Fig. 119.6 Oblique drawing of a subcutaneous lipoma. The planned removal of the subcutaneous lipoma is marked with *dashed lines*.

Once the fusion line is recognized, the course and location of the nerve roots can be safely identified.

Using low settings on the ultrasonic aspirator, the central mass of fat is debulked (**Fig. 119.8**). Alternatively, a CO_2 laser may be used, although some authors discourage it, stating that the charred surface makes final removal of the lipoma more difficult.[5] During dural opening and debulking, the sensory nerve roots are at greatest risk of injury. It is vital to review the preoperative MRI to fully understand the symmetry of the lipoma and the degree of rotation of the neural elements. The debulking is continued until the neural placode can be identified, leaving only a thin layer of remaining fat. Another technique is to use sharp dissection to separate the lipoma from the placode (**Fig. 119.9**). The dissection begins rostrally where the anatomic relationships among the fat, spinal cord, and nerves are clear. Microscissors are then used to identify a white plane between the lipoma and placode. The incision is continued caudally, with attention paid to remaining medial to the fusion line. If neural tissue is found within the lipoma, evoked EMG is used to evaluate the functionality. If there is extension of the mass into the central canal, causing thinning of the spinal cord, a myelotomy may be made in the midline or at the site that has been thinned. Limit debulking can then be performed with the ultrasonic aspirator. Once the lipoma is removed, the neural placode can be reapproximated.

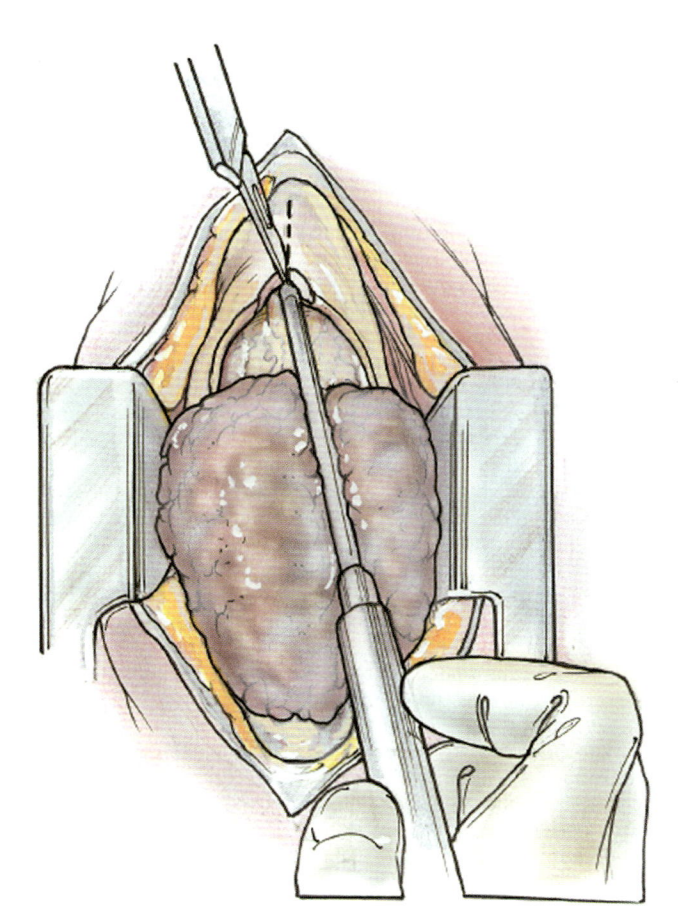

Fig. 119.7 The surgeon opening the dural band that surround the neck of the lipoma. The rostral dura is opened in the midline and retracted to expose the spinal cord.

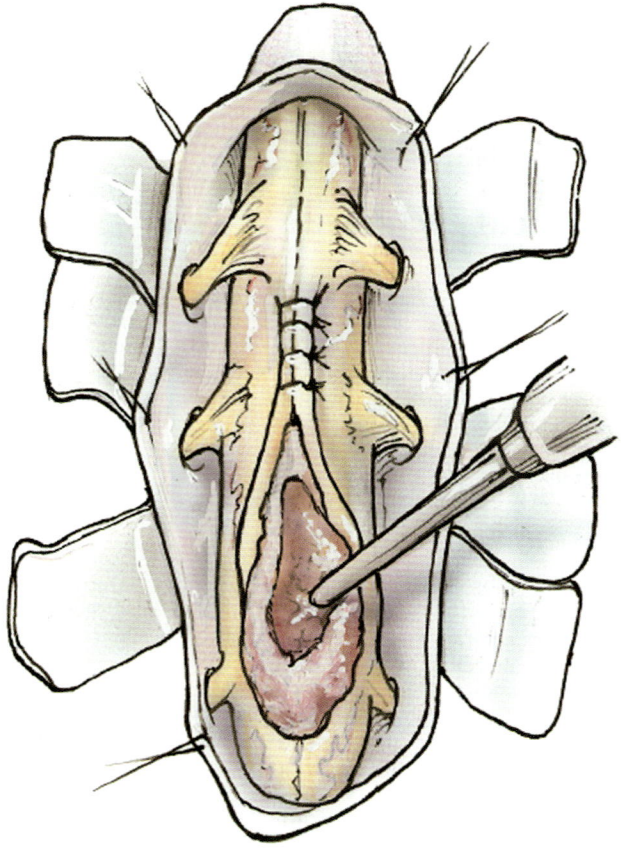

Fig. 119.8 The surgeon using an ultrasonic aspirator to debulk a dorsal lipoma.

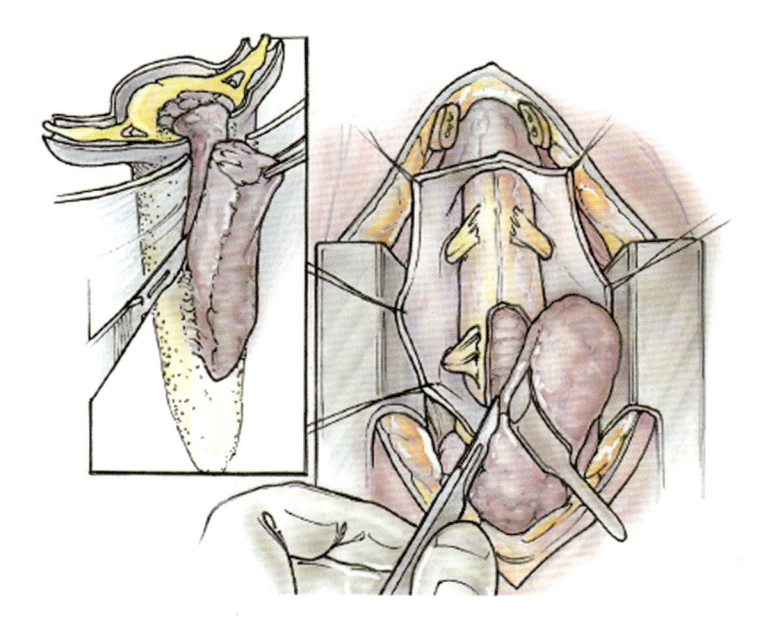

Fig. 119.9 Sharp dissection separates the lipoma from the placode (see Chapter 123, Fig. 123.9). The dissection begins rostrally where the anatomic relationship among the fat, spinal cord, and nerves is clear. Microscissors or a scalpel is then used to identify and separate the plane between the lipoma and placode.

A series of inverted interrupted 8-0 nylon sutures is then used to reapproximate the pial edges of each side of the placode (**Fig. 119.10**). Special care should be taken to limit the amount of tension placed on the placode. Once the neural tube is reconstructed, the filum terminale is identified. Once again, evoked EMG is used to exclude the possibility of injury a nerve root. The filum is then coagulated and cut. The reconstituted neural tube is placed in the spinal canal and should be in contact with the ventral dura to ensure a degree of movement within the canal. If there is sufficient dura remaining, a primary closure may be performed. However, if there is a considerable defect or a concern about re-tethering, a soft graft such as bovine pericardium may be used to enlarge the intradural space. The graft is placed with a running Prolene suture, and a Valsalva maneuver is performed to ensure a watertight closure. Once the dura is closed, the lumbosacral fascia is approximated. If there is a large defect that cannot be closed, a fascia lata graft may be used. The remainder of the soft tissue is closed in the standard fashion.

Postoperative Care

The patient receives antibiotics for 24 hours after the procedure. Perioperative pain can be considerable and requires aggressive management. Development of a pseudomeningocele is always a concern after resection of a lumbosacral lipoma. The risk of pseudomeningocele is increased if there is a history of prior surgery or if there is a poor dural closure. The patient is kept flat for 3 to 5 days to enable the dural close to mature prior to challenging it with normal cerebrospinal fluid (CSF) pressure. Some surgeons place a lumbar drain intraoperatively to allow for controlled CSF drainage to promote dural healing.

After the postoperative period, the patient is seen for regular follow-up with a multidisciplinary team for careful surveillance and monitoring of the existing deficit and to establish a new functional baseline. Clinical exams, urodynamics, EMG, and repeat imaging are done on these visits. Patients with an associated syrinx need especially close monitoring. The surgeon may decide to

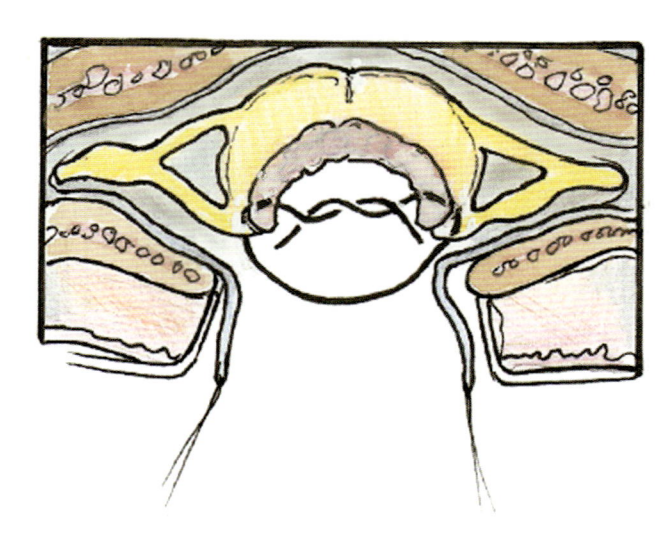

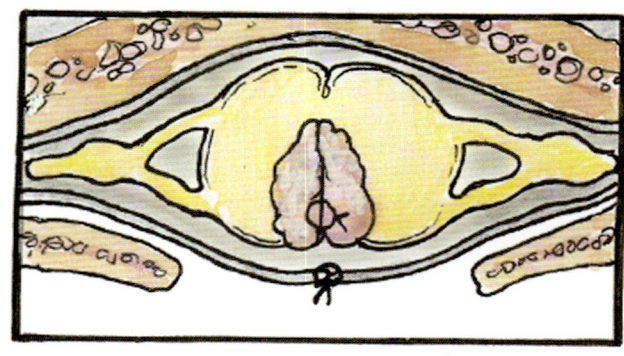

Fig. 119.10 (a,b) The inverted interrupted 8-0 nylon sutures used to reapproximate the pial edges on each side of the placode. Special efforts are made to limit the amount of tension placed on the reconstructed neural tube.

treat the syrinx with an syringosubarachnoid shunt during the lipoma resection. Another option is to perform the lipoma resection and then follow the syrinx with serial imaging. If the patient does not improve after successful de-tethering or if there is syrinx enlargement, a shunting procedure may be required.

Potential Complications and Precautions

Complications that may occur during the acute postoperative period include new neurologic deficits, neuropathic pain, wound infection, CSF leak, and re-tethering. The cited rates of new neurologic or urologic deficits range from 4 to 10%.[2,26,27] The potential for neurologic injury is increased when there is challenging or obscure anatomy. This is especially true if there is a history of prior surgery where normal planes of dissection are blurred. The risk of injury is also increased in cases of transitional lipomas where there is considerable rotation of the neural elements. When rotation is present, special attention must be given to the dural opening to prevent injury to the underlying dorsal roots or placode. Neuropathic pain may result after the use of bipolar cautery to the DREZ. When bleeding occurs lateral to the fusion line, thrombin-soaked Gelfoam can be used to avoid this rare complication.

A CSF leak is the most common complication, occurring in 2 to 47% of patients.[26] Some of the postoperative techniques for pseudomeningocele prevention have been discussed above, but the most effective form of prevention is with a watertight dural close. If a reliable closure is not possible, organic or synthetic tissue glues may be used to supplement the dural construct. Other authors have recommended removal of the subcutaneous lipoma at a later date to prevent the creation of a large amount of dead space and thereby discourage pseudomeningocele formation.[13]

After the initial surgical intervention, there is a 10 to 50% chance of re-tethering.[1] The rates of re-tethering increase with time and have been found to be around 40% in two large studies.[2,28] It has also been shown that patients with transitional lipomas are also at greater risk for re-tethering that is thought to be due to the larger raw surface area of these lesions.[28] Regardless of the initial success of the surgery, a patient with a history of lumbosacral lipomas requires close follow-up for many years.

Conclusion

Lumbosacral lipomas are complex congenital anomalies that are associated with progressive loss of neurologic function. The outcomes for a symptomatic patient can be stabilized or even improved with removal of the lipoma and de-tethering of the neural structures. Because the natural history is not completely understood, there remains controversy regarding management of asymptomatic patients. However, if the goals of surgery can be accomplished with a relatively low rate of complications, there is likely to be significant benefit to the patient and maintenance of the preoperative neurologic status.

References

1. Finn MA, Walker ML. Spinal lipomas: clinical spectrum, embryology, and treatment. Neurosurg Focus 2007;23:E10
2. Pierre-Kahn A, Zerah M, Renier D, et al. Congenital lumbosacral lipomas. Childs Nerv Syst 1997;13:298–334, discussion 335
3. Oi S, Nomura S, Nagasaka M, et al. Embryopathogenetic surgicoanatomical classification of dysraphism and surgical outcome of spinal lipoma: a nationwide multicenter cooperative study in Japan. J Neurosurg Pediatr 2009;3:412–419
4. Wykes V, Desai D, Thompson DNP. Asymptomatic lumbosacral lipomas—a natural history study. Childs Nerv Syst 2012;28:1731–1739
5. Pang D, Zovickian J, Oviedo A. Long-term outcome of total and near-total resection of spinal cord lipomas and radical reconstruction of the neural placode: part I-surgical technique. Neurosurgery 2009;65:511–528, discussion 528–529
6. Byrne RW, Hayes EA, George TM, McLone DG. Operative resection of 100 spinal lipomas in infants less than 1 year of age. Pediatr Neurosurg 1995;23:182–186, discussion 186–187
7. Hoffman HJ, Taecholarn C, Hendrick EB, Humphreys RP. Management of lipomyelomeningoceles. Experience at the Hospital for Sick Children, Toronto. J Neurosurg 1985;62:1–8
8. Kang JK, Kim MC, Kim DS, Song JU. Effects of tethering on regional spinal cord blood flow and sensory-evoked potentials in growing cats. Childs Nerv Syst 1987;3:35–39
9. Schneider SJ, Rosenthal AD, Greenberg BM, Danto J. A preliminary report on the use of laser-Doppler flowmetry during tethered spinal cord release. Neurosurgery 1993;32:214–217, discussion 217–218
10. Chapman PH, Frim DM. Symptomatic syringomyelia following surgery to treat retethering of lipomyelomeningoceles. J Neurosurg 1995;82:752–755
11. Muthukumar N. Congenital spinal lipomatous malformations: part II—clinical presentation, operative findings, and outcome. Acta Neurochir (Wien) 2009;151:189–197, discussion 197
12. Chapman PH. Congenital intraspinal lipomas: anatomic considerations and surgical treatment. Childs Brain 1982;9:37–47
13. Pang D, Zovickian J, Wong S-T, Hou YJ, Moes GS. Surgical treatment of complex spinal cord lipomas. Childs Nerv Syst 2013;29:1485–1513
14. McLone DG, Naidich TP. Terminal myelocystocele. Neurosurgery 1985;16:36–43
15. Naidich TP, McLone DG, Mutluer S. A new understanding of dorsal dysraphism with lipoma (lipomyeloschisis): radiologic evaluation and surgical correction. AJR Am J Roentgenol 1983;140:1065–1078
16. Pang D, Zovickian J, Moes GS. Retained medullary cord in humans: late arrest of secondary neurulation. Neurosurgery 2011;68:1500–1519, discussion 1519
17. Talwalker VC, Dastur DK. "Meningoceles" and "meningomyeloceles" (ectopic spinal cord). Clinicopathological basis of a new classification. J Neurol Neurosurg Psychiatry 1970;33:251–262
18. Caruso R, Cervoni L, Fiorenza F, Vitale AM, Salvati M. Occult dysraphism in adulthood. A series of 24 cases. J Neurosurg Sci 1996;40:221–225
19. Foster LS, Kogan BA, Cogen PH, Edwards MS. Bladder function in patients with lipomyelomeningocele. J Urol 1990;143:984–986
20. Satar N, Bauer SB, Shefner J, Kelly MD, Darbey MM. The effects of delayed diagnosis and treatment in patients with an occult spinal dysraphism. J Urol 1995;154(2 Pt 2):754–758
21. Blount JP, Elton S. Spinal lipomas. Neurosurg Focus 2001;10:e3
22. Herman JM, McLone DG, Storrs BB, Dauser RC. Analysis of 153 patients with myelomeningocele or spinal lipoma reoperated upon for a tethered cord. Presentation, management and outcome. Pediatr Neurosurg 1993;19:243–249
23. Pang D, Wilberger JE Jr. Tethered cord syndrome in adults. J Neurosurg 1982;57:32–47
24. McGillicuddy GT, Shucart W, Kwan ES. Intradural spinal lipomas. Neurosurgery 1987;21:343–346
25. Kulkarni AV, Pierre-Kahn A, Zerah M. Conservative management of asymptomatic spinal lipomas of the conus. Neurosurgery 2004;54:868–873, discussion 873–875
26. Pang D, Zovickian J, Oviedo A. Long-term outcome of total and near-total resection of spinal cord lipomas and radical reconstruction of the neural placode, part II: outcome analysis and preoperative profiling. Neurosurgery 2010;66:253–272, discussion 272–273
27. La Marca F, Grant JA, Tomita T, McLone DG. Spinal lipomas in children: outcome of 270 procedures. Pediatr Neurosurg 1997;26:8–16
28. Colak A, Pollack IF, Albright AL. Recurrent tethering: a common long-term problem after lipomyelomeningocele repair. Pediatr Neurosurg 1998;29:184–190

120 Repair of Myelomeningoceles

Lorenzo F. Muñoz

Myelomeningocele is a neural tube defect that can affect the entire nervous system. It occurs after a failure of primary neurulation in the fourth week of embryogenesis. The caudal neuropore fails to fuse dorsally, leaving a flat plate of neural tissue known as the neural placode. The central groove is the remnant of the central canal of the spinal cord. Surrounding the defect lies dysplastic skin edges.

These defects occur mostly in the thoracolumbar spine (85%), followed by the thoracic spine (10%) and the cervical spine (5%). They frequently occur in concert with other abnormalities, such as absence of spinous processes and lamina, increased interpedicular distances, decreased pedicle height, and small vertebral bodies.[1] These structural changes may result in kyphotic deformities at birth. Delayed neurologic deficits and adult back pain may occur later in life.

Myelomeningocele is often cited as having a 100% association with Chiari II malformation. The morbidity and mortality associated with this entity are attributed to cranial disease and hindbrain herniation.[2] The effects of hindbrain herniation include apnea, cyanosis, bradycardia, dysphagia, nystagmus, stridor, vocal cord paralysis, hypotonia, spasticity, and opisthotonos. A theory that has gained favor in the literature, the "two-hit" hypothesis, posits that the neurologic deficits are a secondary insult as a result of the continued exposure of the neural placode to the amniotic environment,[3] and so a limited number of specialized centers now perform prenatal myelomeningocele repair. This effort is collectively known as the Management of Myelomeningocele Study (MOMS). Initial results have shown promise in reducing the number of shunt-dependent patients, and perhaps improving long-term functional outcomes.[4,5] Of course, prenatal surgery requires a multidisciplinary team of highly specialized professionals.[6] Expectantly, after prenatal surgery, there is an elevated peripartum risk of low birth weight, neonatal respiratory distress syndrome, and higher rates of maternal/obstetric complications, including pulmonary edema, placental abruption, spontaneous preterm labor, transfusion at delivery, and hysterotomy-site complications.

Ventriculoperitoneal shunting trends have varied significantly. One review of the literature cited a published post-repair shunt rate of 85%.[7] That same group in the United Kingdom employed more stringent shunting criteria to produce a shunt rate of only 52% in patients after myelomeningocele repair. Interestingly, in the MOMS trial, the postnatal surgery group had a shunt rate of 82% compared with the prenatal surgery group rate of 40%. A review of Medicaid claims data found that rate of shunting during the same hospitalization for repair was only 57%.[8]

Fortunately, the overall prevalence of myelomeningocele has declined,[8] which may be due to increased folate supplementation and earlier in-utero recognition. In a review of the Nationwide Inpatient Sample database from 1988 to 2010, repairs peaked at 1,260 in 1988, and the numbers have plateaued at around 860 for the last four observed years.

Indications

- Presence of a myelomeningocele in an infant who is not chronically ill or comatose

Contraindications

The Child Abuse Prevention Act[9] mandates that all patients with myelomeningoceles be repaired except in cases of the following contraindications:

- The infant is chronically and irreversibly comatose.
- The treatment would merely prolong dying.
- The treatment would be virtually futile in terms of the survival of the infant and inhumane under such circumstances.

When considering prenatal surgery, several additional contraindications are of important consideration:

- Maternal systemic factors such as obesity, diabetes, uncontrolled hypertension, and positivity of blood-borne viruses
- Maternal gynecologic and obstetric history including short cervix, uterine abnormality, history of premature delivery or incompetent cervix, and maternal-fetal Rh isoimmunization
- Pregnancy factors including multigravida, placenta previa, or placental abruption
- Fetal factors such as concomitant anomaly or kyphosis > 30 degrees.

Advantages

The repair can eliminate cerebrospinal fluid leakage and decrease the risk of infection. Additionally, a prenatal myelomeningocele repair can prevent the theoretical "second hit" that may cause secondary neurologic deficits including hydrocephalus.

Disadvantages

The treatment could potentially prolong death if the child is terminally ill. Additionally, in the case of prenatal myelomeningocele repair, the patient risks include low birth weight and neonatal respiratory distress syndrome. Maternal risks include pulmonary edema, placental abruption, spontaneous preterm

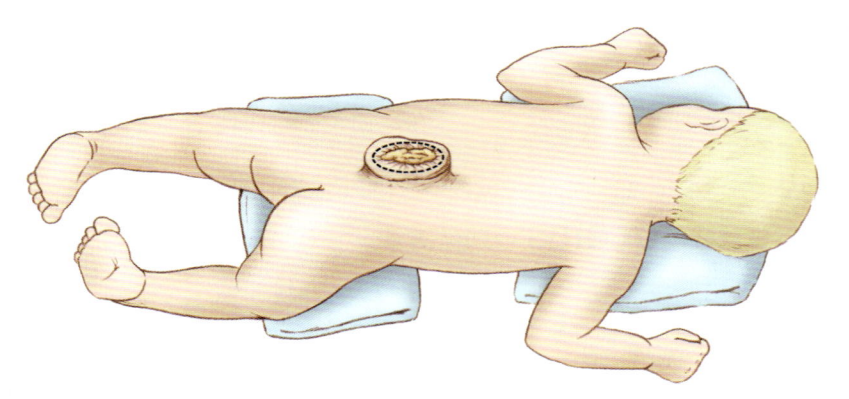

Fig. 120.1 Positioning for repair of a myelomeningocele. Note the chest and hip rolls.

labor, necessity of transfusion at delivery, and hysterotomy-site complications.

Preoperative Planning

In the neonate, a myelomeningocele should be covered with a sterile, saline-moistened Telfa pad. The patient is maintained in the prone position. Prophylactic broad-spectrum intravenous antibiotics should be started and continued through the perioperative period. The patient should be medically optimized so that the surgical repair can be performed within 48 hours of birth.[10] Latex products should be avoided because of the risk of allergen exposure.

A comprehensive initial assessment should be performed. A neurologic exam with special attention to function in the lower extremities as well as clinical signs of hydrocephalus should be noted. Some infants with myelomeningoceles require immediate shunt placement.

Prenatal repair requires several additional studies. Evaluation by an experienced maternal–fetal medicine obstetrician and anesthesiologist with experience in prenatal surgery is necessary. A comprehensive obstetrical ultrasound examination, a fetal magnetic resonance imaging (MRI), and an echocardiogram will elucidate maternal and fetal surgical anatomy and identify other potential fetal surgical risk factors.

Surgical Technique

Anesthesia and Positioning

The patient is induced with general anesthesia. Intravenous broad-spectrum antibiotics are continued. The patient is placed supine on a foam doughnut for endotracheal intubation. The patient is then positioned prone with transverse rolls placed under the hips and chest (**Fig. 120.1**). The surgical area should be prepared widely to allow for a potentially long incision should a flap or advancement be utilized for closure. Contact of the neural placode with povidone-iodine solution should be avoided.

Again, in prenatal surgery, several additional considerations must be incorporated. In addition to antibiotics, indomethacin is administered to maintain the patency of the ductus arteriosus. General and epidural anesthesia is induced for the mother. After dissection and exposure, intramuscular fentanyl and vecuronium are administered to the fetus. Continuous fetal echocardiography is performed throughout the procedure.

Repair of the Defect

Maternal exposure begins with a low transverse laparotomy. The uterus is exteriorized. Ultrasound is utilized to locate the fetus and placenta and to plan the hysterotomy. The fetus is manually positioned within the uterus such that the myelomeningocele sac is centered in the hysterotomy. After entry with sharp dissection, a uterine stapling device is used to apply absorbable polyglycolic acid staples while ensuring that the incision is free of fetal tissue. About a 7-cm incision is made, large enough to expose the myelomeningocele.

Closure of the meningomyelocele defect is essentially identical when done prenatally or postnatally. Magnification should be utilized. A nerve stimulator may be helpful in identifying neural tissue.

The initial incision is made circumferentially at the junction of the arachnoid and the skin to isolate the neural placode (**Fig. 120.2**). The rostral aspect of the incision is extended to the level of the next intact caudal lamina. The lumbosacral fascia is identified, incised bilaterally, and dissected from the sacrospinalis muscle. The viable skin is dissected free from the placode membrane. Next, a blunt dissection is carried circumferentially through the subcutaneous fat to define a plane between the fascia and dura at the junctional zone.[11]

Next, the lateral edges of the neural placode are approximated, and the pial surfaces of the placode are sutured together with a 7-0 absorbable suture (**Fig. 120.3**). Occasionally, the placode is too wide, and repairing the neural tube defect compromises the perfusion of the tissue. Without closure of the pial layer, there may be an increased risk of tethered cord syndrome later in life.[12] The intact dura is then identified and reapproximated at midline with a 5-0 nonabsorbable suture to reconstruct the

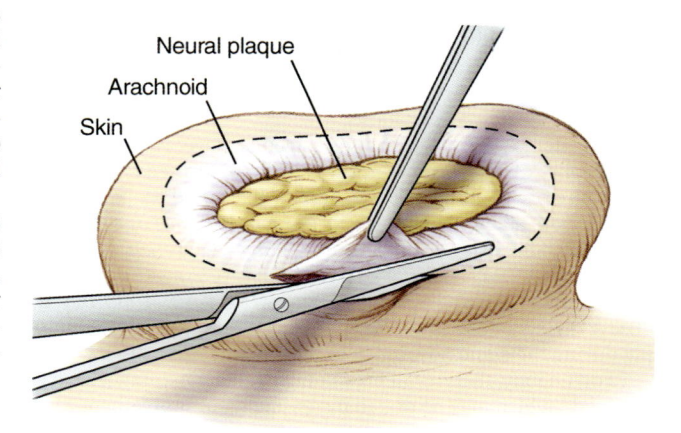

Fig. 120.2 Isolation of the neural placode. The initial incision is made along the circumferential line formed by the junction of the arachnoid and the skin.

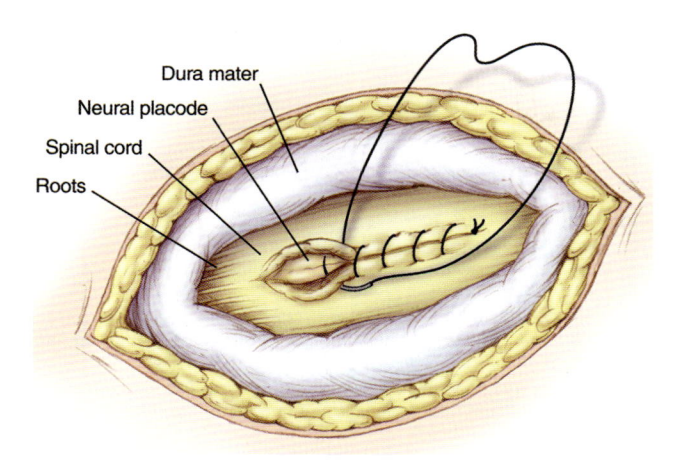

Fig. 120.3 Approximation of the lateral edges of the neural placode with a 7-0 absorbable suture.

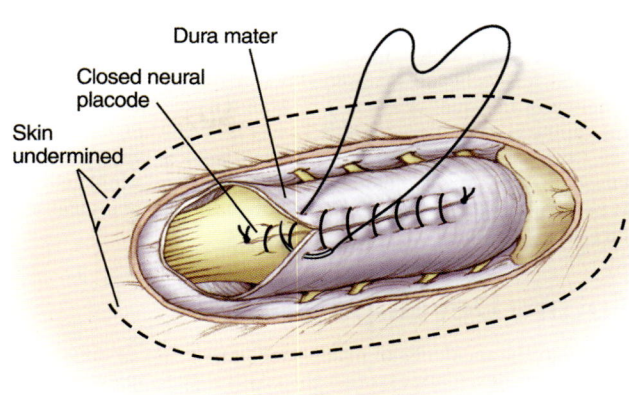

Fig. 120.4 The dura is reapproximated in the midline with a 5-0 nonabsorbable suture.

thecal sac (**Fig. 120.4**). Occasionally, large defects may require a synthetic dural patch. If possible, the lumbosacral fascial edges are then reapproximated with a 5-0 absorbable suture (**Fig. 120.5**). A tension layer is then created with the previously defined junctional zone. The final step in the closure of the defect is reapproximation of the subcutaneous tissue and skin. If possible, the subcutaneous tissue is reapproximated and closed with a 5-0 interrupted absorbable suture. The skin is undermined bilaterally and then reapproximated at midline with a 5-0 running nylon suture (**Fig. 120.6**). Again, if the size of the defect does not permit primary closure, a synthetic dermal substitute may be used.

In prenatal surgery the additional step of uterine repair is performed. The first layer should incorporate the absorbable staples and uterine membranes. A secondary imbricating layer should incorporate the initial suture line. Prior to final sutures, amniotic fluid is replaced with lactated Ringer's mixed with nafcillin or vancomycin to restore a normal amniotic fluid index. The abdominal fascia and dermis are closed in the standard fashion.

Postoperative Care

Antibiotics should be continued for 24 hours. The postnatal patient should be positioned prone. Special attention is paid to minimizing pressure to the repair and to maintain cleanliness. A sterile drape or "mud flap" should be utilized to maintain a barrier between the incision and anus. The wound should be closely monitored for leakage, dehiscence, and infection. The patient should be monitored closely for signs of hydrocephalus. Increasing head circumference, bulging fontanelle, splaying of the sutures, or the "sun-setting" sign (downward deviated gaze) should warrant further investigation. Weekly serial head ultrasonography is typically employed for this purpose. Additionally, symptomatic Chiari signs (respiratory and swallowing difficulty, bradycardia), cerebrospinal fluid leak, or pseudomeningocele at the repair site are also criteria for shunting. Most shunts are placed in the first 6 months of life.

Prenatal repair has additional peripartum management challenges. In addition to antibiotics, magnesium sulfate and indomethacin are continued for up to 48 hours postoperatively.

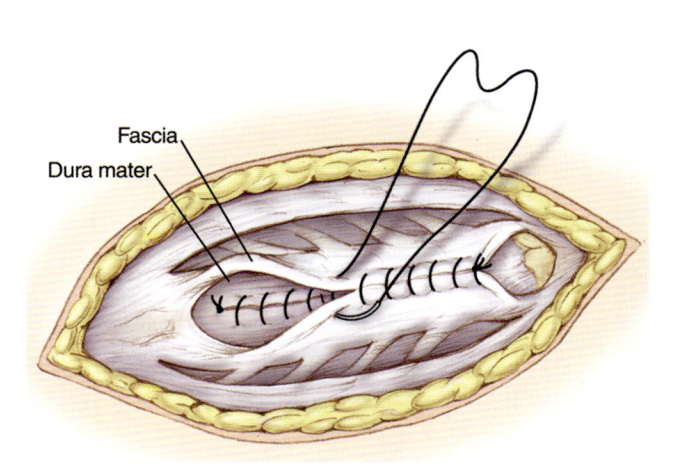

Fig. 120.5 The fascial edges are approximated with a 5-0 absorbable suture.

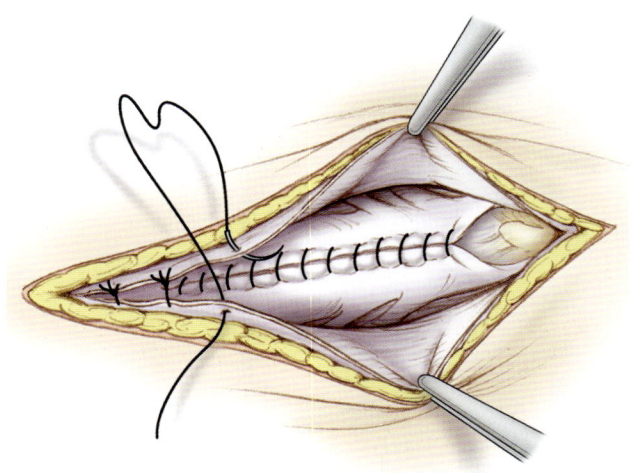

Fig. 120.6 The skin is undermined and reapproximated in the midline with a 5-0 nylon suture.

Magnesium is prescribed as needed for preterm contractions occurring longer that 1 hour apart. While the patient is in the hospital, fetal echocardiography is performed daily to ensure the patency of the ductus arteriosus. Maintenance therapy of oral nifedipine is continued up until 37 weeks' gestation.

Outpatient follow-up is scheduled weekly with brief, focused ultrasound examinations. At 37 weeks' gestation, delivery is performed by cesarean section through the prior surgical skin incision.

Future Developments

Although the incidence of myelomeningocele has declined over several decades, it appears that the post-folate supplementation era has led to a stable rate of new myelomeningocele cases. Longitudinal data from the MOMS group will have further implications in how myelomeningocele is treated. Although this surgery is performed in three highly specialized centers, further data may lead to expansion of such programs to selected geographic areas to best distribute care. Additionally, new intrauterine techniques such as endoscopic and robot-assisted surgery need further study to determine if they may lower the risks involved with prenatal surgery.[13]

References

1. Cohen A, Robinson S. Early management of myelomeningocele. In: McClone D, ed. Pediatric Neurosurgery. Philadelphia: WB Saunders: 2001:241–259
2. McLone D, Dias L, Kaplan W. Continuing concepts in the management of spina bifida. In: Marlin A, ed. Concepts in Pediatric Neurosurgery. New York: Karger; 1985:97–106
3. Heffez DS, Aryanpur J, Hutchins GM, Freeman JM. The paralysis associated with myelomeningocele: clinical and experimental data implicating a preventable spinal cord injury. Neurosurgery 1990;26:987–992
4. Adzick NS, Thom EA, Spong CY, et al; MOMS Investigators. A randomized trial of prenatal versus postnatal repair of myelomeningocele. N Engl J Med 2011;364:993–1004
5. Bruner JP, Tulipan N, Paschall RL, et al. Fetal surgery for myelomeningocele and the incidence of shunt-dependent hydrocephalus. JAMA 1999; 282:1819–1825
6. Cohen AR, Couto J, Cummings JJ, et al; MMC Maternal-Fetal Management Task Force. Position statement on fetal myelomeningocele repair. Am J Obstet Gynecol 2014;210:107–111
7. Chakraborty A, Crimmins D, Hayward R, Thompson D. Toward reducing shunt placement rates in patients with myelomeningocele. J Neurosurg Pediatr 2008;1:361–365
8. Kshettry VR, Kelly ML, Rosenbaum BP, Seicean A, Hwang L, Weil RJ. Myelomeningocele: surgical trends and predictors of outcome in the United States, 1988-2010. J Neurosurg Pediatr 2014;13:666–678
9. Department of Health and Human Services. Federal Registry part VI. 1985
10. Heimburger RF. Early repair of myelomeningocele (spina bifida cystica). J Neurosurg 1972;37:594–600
11. Cheek WR, Laurent JP, Cech DA. Operative repair of lumbosacral myelomeningocele. Technical note. J Neurosurg 1983;59:718–722
12. Park T. Myelomeningocele. In: Albright L, Pollack I, Adelson P, eds. Principles and Practice of Pediatric Neurosurgery New York: Thieme; 1999: 291–320
13. Aaronson OS, Tulipan NB, Cywes R, et al. Robot-assisted endoscopic intrauterine myelomeningocele repair: a feasibility study. Pediatr Neurosurg 2002;36:85–89

121 Excision of a Spinal Congenital Dermal Sinus Tract/Dermoid

Robert G. Kellogg, Carter S. Gerard, Lee A. Tan, and Lorenzo F. Muñoz

Dermal sinus tracts (DSTs) are a form of spinal dysraphism that results from an aberration in dysjunction during fetal development, with an estimated incidence of ~ 1 in 2,500 live births.[1–3] The pathology is hypothesized to occur when there is failure of separation of the neural ectoderm from the cutaneous ectoderm between the third and eighth weeks of gestation.[4,5] The tract, lined by stratified squamous epithelium, can terminate anywhere between the subcutaneous tissue and the spinal cord itself, depending on the severity of separation failure.[3,6] DSTs are most commonly located in the lumbar (40%) or lumbosacral (45%) region and are much less common in the cervical (< 1%) or thoracic (10%) region.[3,6,7]

Typical clinical manifestations may include skin stigmata, central nervous system (CNS) infections, and neurologic deficits.[2–5] In one recent case series, 43.7% of patient presented with skin abnormalities, 12.5% with motor weakness, 6.2% with an epidural abscess, and 6.2% with an intradural abscess.[2] The clinical manifestations are largely dependent on the depth to which the tract penetrates. In the absence of a frank infection, the contents of a dermoid cyst spilling into the subarachnoid space can produce chemical meningitis and arachnoiditis. Recurrent meningitis can impair cerebrospinal fluid (CSF) absorption and over time result in hydrocephalus.

A DST may be solitary or found in combination with other forms of spinal dysraphism. One case series found that 26% of patients with DSTs harbored an intradural dermoid cyst and 39% of these patients had another form of dysraphism such as lipomyelomeningocele, diastematomyelia, and tethered spinal cord.[5]

Indications

- Presence of a DST on physical examination or imaging study

Advantages

- Repair prevents CNS infection.
- Resection of associated intradural masses or repair of dysraphism can prevent neurologic deficit.
- Reduces the risk of chronic meningitis and hydrocephalus

Disadvantages

- Cerebrospinal fluid (CSF) leak postoperatively
- Recurrence of inclusion tumors in the setting of subtotal resection
- Risk of surgical morbidity in the form of a new neurologic deficit

Preoperative Tests

- Magnetic resonance imaging (MRI) with contrast of the affected region

Preoperative Planning

Patients with a DST are typically referred to the neurosurgeon by the child's pediatrician after discovery of cutaneous stigmata, orthopedic deformity, urologic problems, or a neurologic deficit. Cutaneous findings are common and can include a sinus ostia dorsal to the spine, skin tags, hypertrichosis, abnormal skin pigmentation, angioma, and symptoms of a superficial infection such as erythema or induration (**Fig. 121.1**). The opening of the sinus tract may be difficult to identify except with close inspection, and should be looked for in a child having recurrent bouts of meningitis of an unknown etiology.

A detailed history should be taken and a physical examination should be performed for all patients. However, exploring the tract in an office setting with a probe or by injecting contrast material followed by imaging is contraindicated, as it may introduce infection or damage neural tissue if there is a communication between the tract and the spinal canal. The tract is typically palpated as well; if the coccyx is felt, then this is typically another indication of a benign entity. It is important to distinguish a DST from a sacrococcygeal pit or dimple, as the latter typically does not require further workup or intervention (**Fig. 121.2**). Sacrococcygeal dimples are thought to occur in 2 to 4% of all infants and are classified as intergluteal dorsal dermal sinuses.[8] An intergluteal position of the dimple has historically been used to determine that a sacrococcygeal dimple has no intraspinal communication, whereas dimples that occur above the gluteal fold are thought to require further workup.[8,9] More recent studies have found that even if a patient with an intergluteal dimple

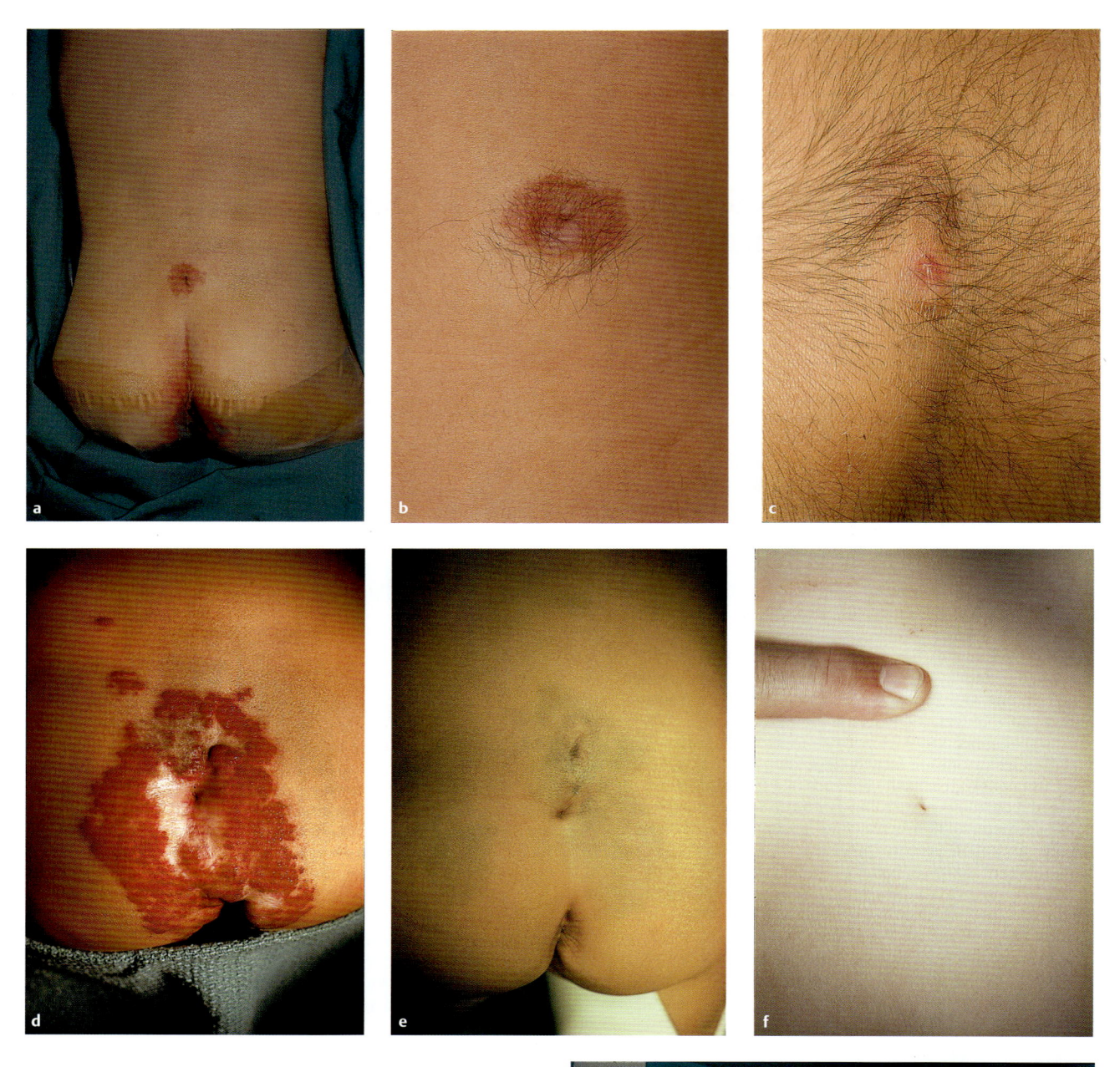

Fig. 121.1 (a) Typical midline lumbosacral location of a congenital dermal sinus. (b) A dermal sinus surrounded by an area of capillary telangiectasia and a mild hypertrichosis. (c) The opening of a tract that has just a very small area of capillary telangiectasia. There is an altered pattern to the hair in the region. (d) A sinus opening is surrounded by an area of hyperpigmentation and an extensive capillary hemangioma. (e) Two separate tracts that are surrounded by areas of hyperpigmentation. Only one tract extended intradurally. (f) A sinus opening with no cutaneous stigmata. (g) A tract associated with a subcutaneous lipoma that extended through a defect in the fascia and posterior neural arches. The lipomatous malformation involved the conus that was low lying and tethered. A capillary telangiectasia of the skin is also present.

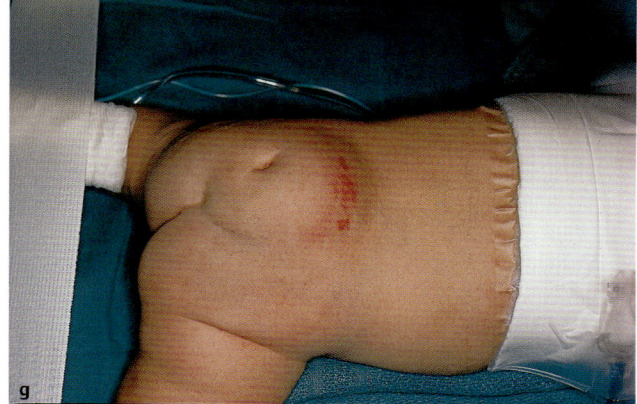

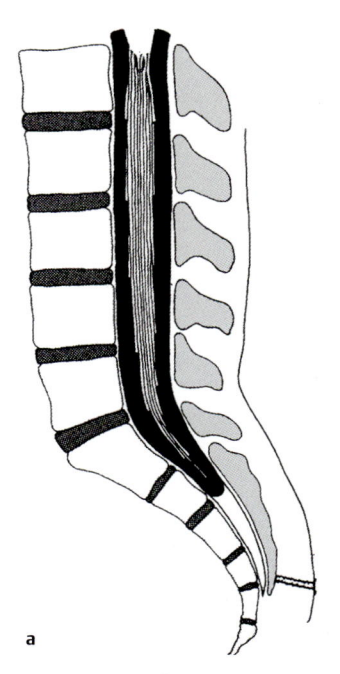

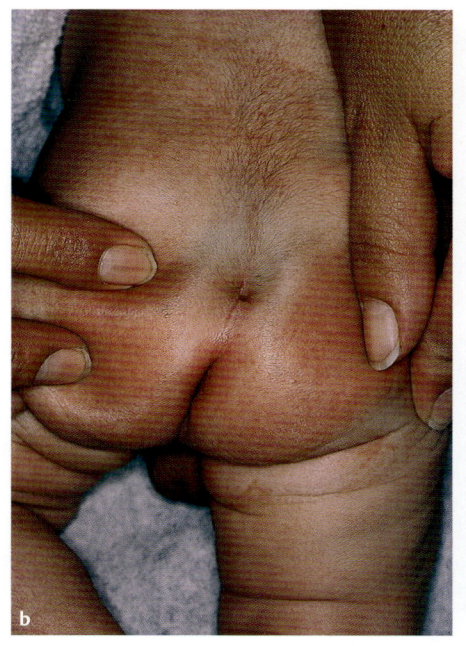

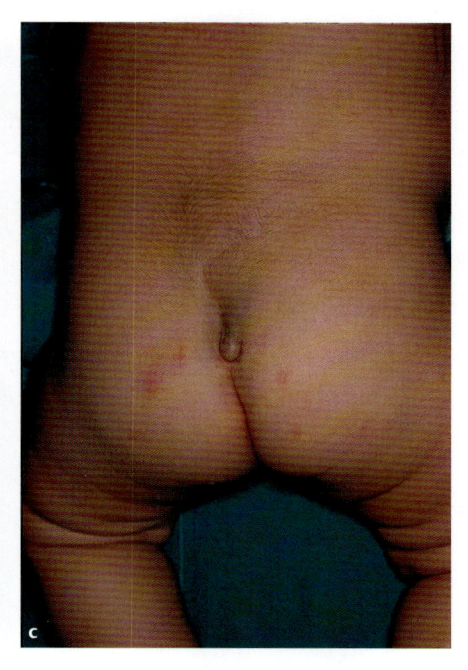

Fig. 121.2 **(a)** A tract located in the coccygeal region. A tract in this location will end in the fascia and has no chance of extending into the subarachnoid space. Dimples in this location are fairly common and need not be excised. **(b)** A typical dimple in the coccygeal region. No neurocutaneous stigmata present. **(c)** Another example of a dimple in the coccygeal region that is also associated with a small skin tag.

is found to have a thickened filum terminale or filum lipoma on imaging, surgery is not likely to be indicated.[9]

Plain X-ray films and spinal ultrasound have been used in the past to characterize DSTs, but the contrast-enhanced MRI scan has become the diagnostic modality of choice. MRI can often identify the extent of the tract through the subcutaneous tissue but fails to show exactly how far the tract penetrates. However, MRI can identify epidural/intradural abscesses and associated intradural tumors, such as a dermoid that is important for operative planning (**Fig. 121.3**). A negative imaging study, however, does not necessarily preclude the need for operative exploration, as the diagnosis of a DST is based on clinical findings with imaging results playing a supportive role only.

The clinical status of the patient and the presence or absence of acute meningitis must be taken into account when considering operative exploration of a DST. Patients who present with meningitis but are neurologically stable should be treated with appropriate antibiotic therapy prior to surgery. Patients with a deteriorating condition should be taken to surgery urgently, with the goal of preserving neurologic function.

Surgical Technique

The patient is placed prone on the operating table after induction of general anesthesia and placement of an endotracheal tube. All pressure points including the axillae, iliac crests, knees, and abdomen are well padded. Careful attention should be paid to minimizing or eliminating pressure on the eyes during the procedure. A paralytic agent may be used with induction of anesthesia but then should be allowed to wear off so that nerve monitoring and stimulation can be utilized. A dose of preoperative antibiotic should be given prior to incision if the patient is not already receiving antibiotics.

A No. 15 blade scalpel is used to make an elliptical incision about the ostia of the sinus. Subcutaneous dissection is then performed with Metzenbaum scissors to avoid entering the DST. Steady traction is applied to the tract while dissecting on alternate sides until the deep fascia is reached, taking care to minimize manipulation of the tract, as this may inadvertently put traction on the spinal cord[10] (**Fig. 121.4**). The fascia should be inspected for penetration of the tract and, if the deep fascia is intact, the operation can be terminated at this point. In most cases, however, there is a defect in the fascia through which the tract passes, and it often involves the interspinous ligament. The deep fascia is incised in the midline just caudal to the tract with cranial extension of the incision as needed for visualization. Kerrison rongeurs are then used to remove the spinous process and lamina rostral to the tract. Dissection is followed down to the dura mater and is carefully inspected. In most cases there will be violation of the dura mater by the tract. The dura mater is opened and explored, and the tract removed (**Fig. 121.5**).

Dermoid cysts can be identified on preoperative MRI scan and must be removed in total if encountered during the exploration to prevent recurrence and potential chemical meningitis or arachnoiditis (**Fig. 121.6**). If the dermoid is found to be embedded in the conus medullaris or adherent to the cauda equina, it must be meticulously dissected using microsurgical techniques and the operating microscope. Nerve stimulation is always used to identify neural structures during dissection.[11,12] Frequently, there is extensive scarring from inflammation that can make this dissection challenging. Upon completion of the resection, the thecal sac is extensively irrigated with saline solution to remove any debris that could cause postoperative chemical meningitis. The dura mater is then closed in a watertight fashion using a 6-0 running Prolene suture. The anesthesia team is asked to perform a Valsalva maneuver to document a watertight closure. Provided there is an adequate dural closure, no collagen matrix repair material or surgical glue need be utilized to augment the closure. The deep fascia and subcutaneous tissues are closed with interrupted absorbable sutures. The skin is closed with a 4-0 running

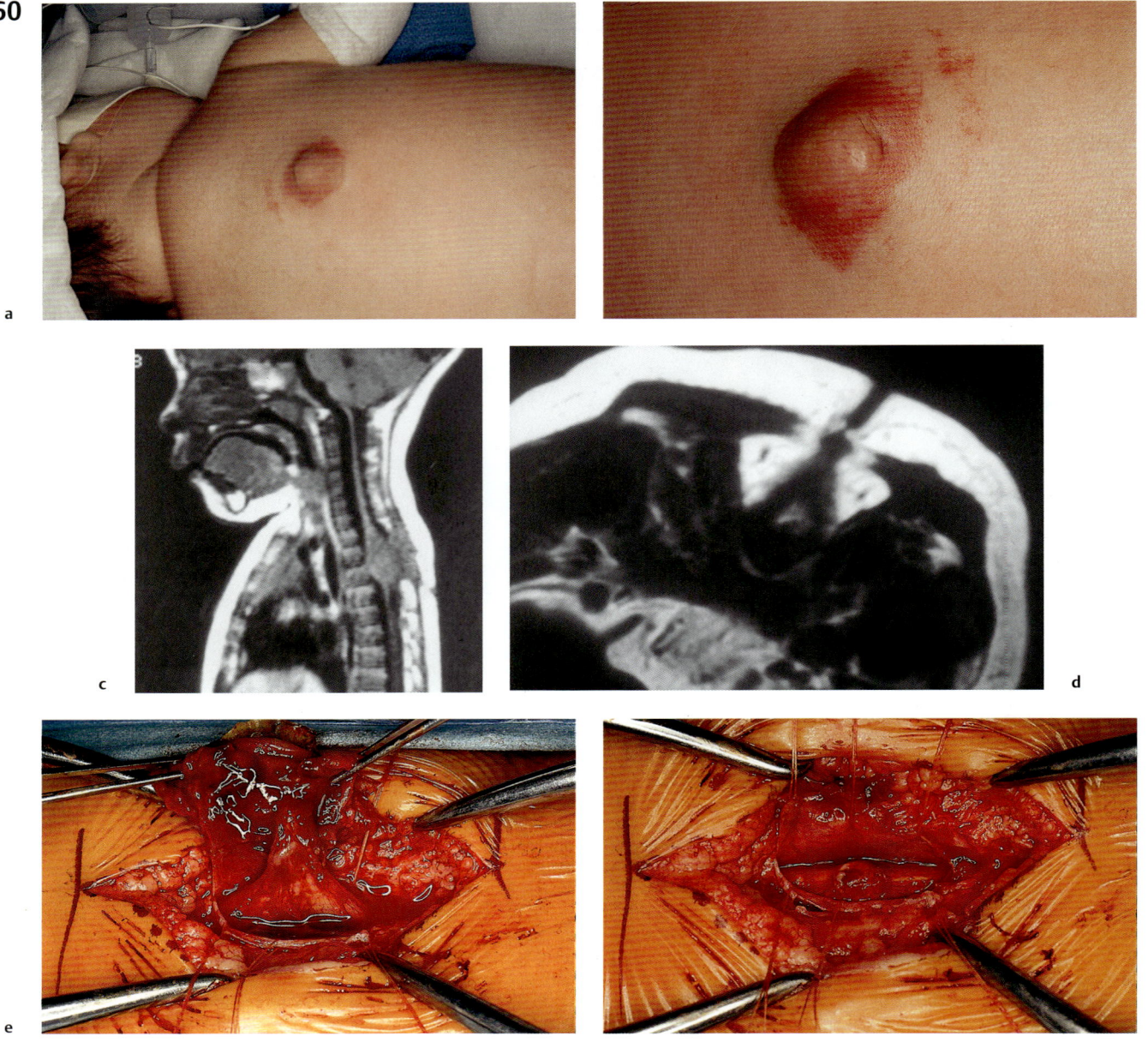

Fig. 121.3 (a) A 14-month-old with a thoracic congenital dermal sinus. This lesion went unnoticed until it became infected. (b) The opening of the tract. The skin is red primarily because of abscess formation. (c) T1-weighted sagittal magnetic resonance imaging (MRI) study showing the tract and abscess extending into the thoracic spinal cord. (d) T1-weighted axial MRI study showing the tract going into the spinal canal. (e) Intraoperative photograph showing the extent of the tract, which was quite large. (f) The spinal cord following the excision of the tract.

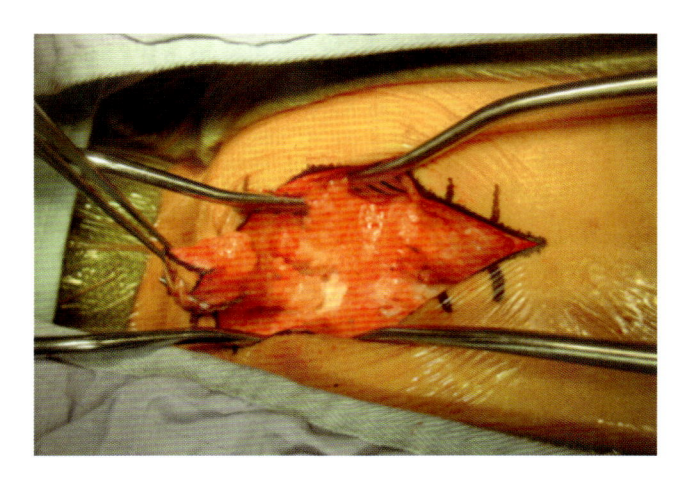

Fig. 121.4 An intraoperative photograph showing dissection of the soft tissues, enabling the formation of an excision pedicle.

Fig. 121.5 (a) A congenital dermal sinus (CDS) with subcutaneous abscess. Purulent drainage is present on the buttocks from the sinus located at the inferior aspect of the subcutaneous area of redness and swelling. (b) Intraoperative photograph showing epidural abscess associated with an infected CDS. (c) Intraoperative photograph showing extensive scarring of the cauda equina and conus medullaris associated with a previous infection. Also present is a dermoid cyst embedded in the conus. The presence of the extensive inflammatory reaction and scarring can make removal quite difficult.

Fig. 121.6 A patient presented with acute paraplegia and sepsis. (a) Magnetic resonance imaging shows the abscess and the enhancement of inflammatory process with gadolinium. Due to anatomic distortions, the intradural dermoid and thick filum observed intraoperatively are not obvious. (b) Tethered cord due to the stalk extending from the sinus to the intradural space and attached to the distal part of cord. (c) Intradural dermoid tumor attached to the thin stalk extending from the sinus to the intradural space producing a tumor far from the sinus location, which is apparent on (d) T2-weighted image. (e) Tethered cord is an associated anomaly without any relation to dermal sinus and tract. The cord is tethered with a thick filum.

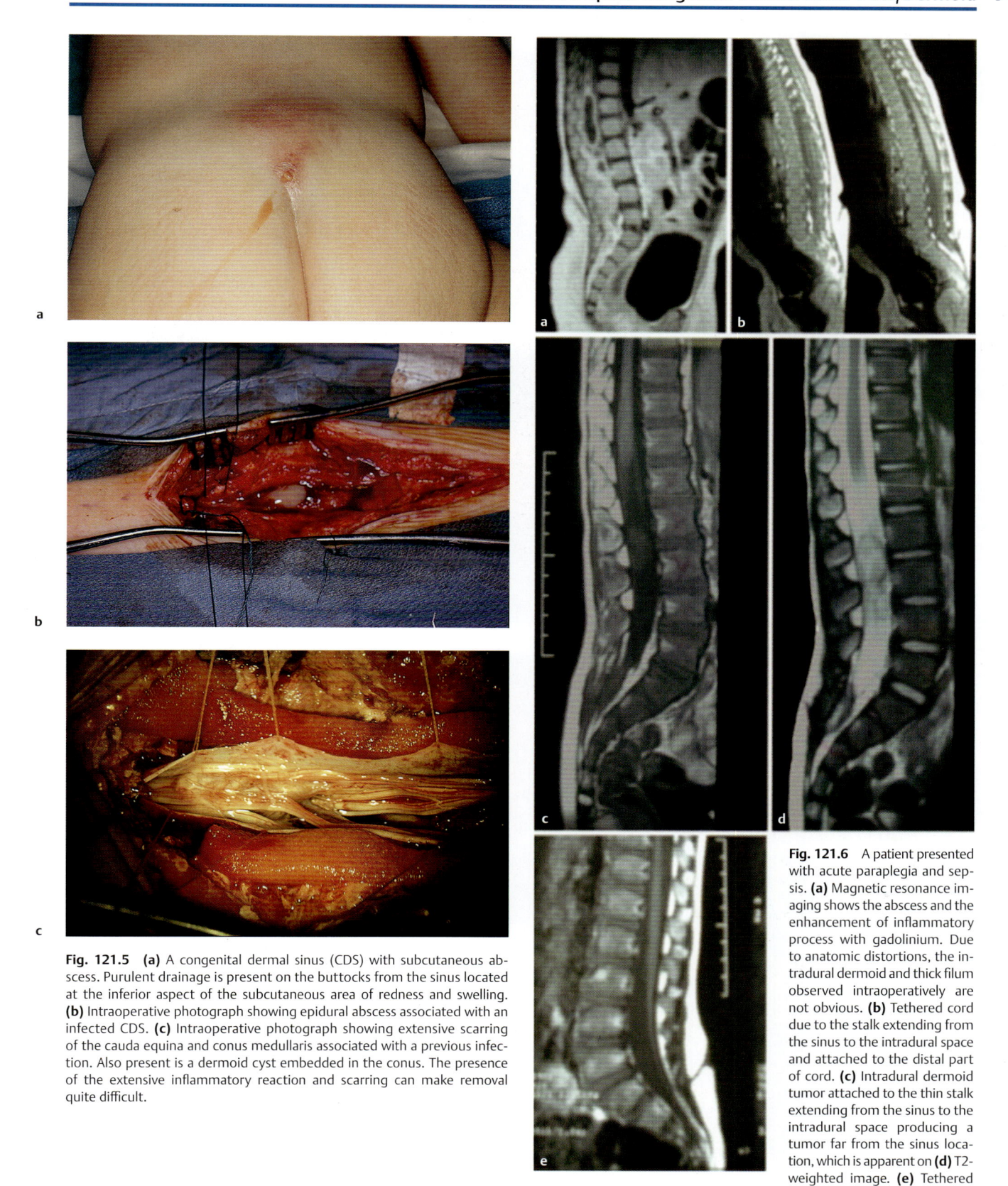

monocryl or nylon suture depending on surgeon preference. A sterile dressing is applied to the incision prior to turning the patient supine for extubation.

Postoperative Care

The patient is encourage to remain flat as much as possible for the first few days after the procedure to minimize the risk of CSF leakage. Antibiotics may be terminated or tapered depending on the preoperative presence of infection and in accordance with intraoperative cultures if they were obtained.

Potential Complications and Precautions

Postoperative complications following surgery for resection of a DST or a dermoid cyst may include CSF leak, wound infection, neurologic injury, chemical meningitis, and recurrence of infection or dermoid. Many of these complications can be avoided by adhering to a meticulous microsurgical technique. Nerve monitoring should be utilized during resection of dermoid cysts and during dissection of adhesions from the cauda equina and conus medullaris. Careful inspection and irrigation of the thecal sac prior to closure can minimize the risk of chemical meningitis and subtotal resection.

Conclusion

Dermal sinus tracts and dermoid cysts of the pediatric spine are relatively rare entities that must be approached in a systematic fashion for each patient. Performing a thorough physical examination and obtaining proper and adequate preoperative imaging studies are of the utmost importance. The surgical procedure, when indicated, is guided by these findings and must be performed with precision and care. Adherence to these guidelines will ensure that the patient has the highest chance for cure and will minimize postoperative complications.

References

1. De Vloo P, Lagae L, Sciot R, Demaerel P, van Loon J, Van Calenbergh F. Spinal dermal sinuses and dermal sinus-like stalks analysis of 14 cases with suggestions for embryologic mechanisms resulting in dermal sinus-like stalks. Eur J Paediatr Neurol 2013;17:575–584
2. Mete M, Umur, AS, Duransoy YK, Barutçuoğlu M, Umur N, Gurgen SG, et al. Congenital dermal sinus tract of the spine: experience of 16 patients. J Child Neurol 2014;29:1277–1282
3. Radmanesh F, Nejat F, El Khashab M. Dermal sinus tract of the spine. Childs Nerv Syst 2010;26:349–357
4. Ackerman LL, Menezes, AH. Spinal congenital dermal sinuses: a 30-year experience. Pediatrics 2003;112(3 Pt 1):641–647
5. Elton S, Oakes, WJ. Dermal sinus tracts of the spine. Neurosurg Focus 2001;10:e4
6. Martínez-Lage JF, Almagro MJ, Ferri-Ñiguez B, Izura Azanza V, Serrano C, Domenech E. Spinal dermal sinus and pseudo-dermal sinus tracts: two different entities. Childs Nerv Syst 2011;27:609–616
7. Jindal A, Mahapatra AK. Spinal congenital dermal sinus: an experience of 23 cases over 7 years. Neurol India 2001;49:243–246
8. Weprin BE, Oakes WJ. Coccygeal pits. Pediatrics 2000;105:E69
9. Gomi A, Oguma H, Furukawa R. Sacrococcygeal dimple: new classification and relationship with spinal lesions. Childs Nerv Syst 2013;29:1641–1645
10. Coumans JV, Walcott BP, Redjal N, Kahle KT, Nahed, BV. En bloc excision of a dermal sinus tract. J Clin Neurosci 2011;18:554–558
11. Hoving EW, Haitsma E, Oude Ophuis CMC, Journée HL. The value of intraoperative neurophysiological monitoring in tethered cord surgery. Childs Nerv Syst 2011;27:1445–1452
12. Beyazova M, Zinnuroglu M, Emmez H, Kaya K, Ozkose HZ, Baykaner MK, et al. Intraoperative neurophysiological monitoring during surgery for tethered cord syndrome. Turk Neurosurg 2010;20:480–484

122 Resection of Sacrococcygeal Teratoma

David Jimenez and Byron C. Branch

Sacrococcygeal teratoma (SCT) is the most common germ cell tumor and the most common newborn and fetal neoplasm, occurring at a reported incidence of 1 in 20,000 to 1 in 40,000 live births.[1,2] These tumors appear to occur more frequently in females, with an observed 2–4:1 female predominance.[1-3] Sacrococcygeal teratomas are thought to arise from perturbed or displaced nests of pluripotent cells originating from the primitive knot in the caudal end of the embryo. These cells become displaced during their migration along the midline dorsal mesentery of the hindgut around the fifth week of gestation.[1,2] As the tumor grows it protrudes through the space between the anus and coccyx, typically presenting in the newborn as a palpable sacral mass. More occult SCT tumors can be located entirely within the pelvis.

The Altman classification of SCTs categorizes these tumors based on the degree of intra- and extrapelvic extension (**Fig. 122.1**).[3] The majority of SCTs are benign lesions that can be cured with complete surgical resection. The incidence of malignancy is reported to be around 20%, and has been correlated with the anatomic Altman classification and the age at presentation. However, it has not correlated with the size of the tumor. Older age at presentation and higher Altman class (III and IV) are associated with an increased likelihood of malignancy.[1,3,4] The majority of SCTs present with a palpable sacral mass in the neonatal period, with over 50% presenting on the first day of life. Early presenting masses tend to be benign tumors, whereas those with occult masses (Altman class IV) may present later (around 2 to 4 years of age) with urinary/renal dysfunction, constipation, or fecal frequency, and they have a higher incidence of malignancy.[1-3] Coexisting anomalies are present in 10 to 20% of patients presenting with SCTs.[1,3] The most common approach for the removal of SCTs is the posterior approach, as the majority of these tumors are extrapelvic or have a relatively smaller intrapelvic component.[3]

Indication
- Palpable sacral mass with imaging characteristics that are suspicious for SCT (benign or malignant) with primarily extrapelvic extension (Altman class I and II)

Contraindications
- The presence of associated anomalies that preclude survival (e.g., severe fetal hydrops, congenital syndromes with severe phenotype, hydrencephaly, certain cardiac malformations)
- Evidence of distant metastases (malignant SCT) in the setting of an invasive pelvic tumor that carries high surgical morbidity

Advantages
- Can be curative when complete resection and total coccygectomy is performed
- Direct approach providing immediate access to the tumor, coccyx, and surrounding musculature
- Can be combined with anterior approaches for resection of intrapelvic SCT

Disadvantages
- Adequate cosmetic result may be difficult
- Higher risk of wound infection at this location due to proximity to anus
- Low threshold for blood loss in neonates in a well-vascularized tumor and increased risk of blood transfusion
- Relatively high incidence of urogenital and anorectal dysfunction
- Tumor vascular supply exists ventral to the mass, necessitating extensive tumor dissection to access
- Requires combination with anterior approach for intrapelvic SCTs (Altman class III and IV)

Objective
- Complete surgical resection of SCT
- Complete surgical resection of coccyx
- Preservation of urinary and fecal continence and neurologic function
- Obtain adequate skin and subcutaneous closure

Preoperative Planning

Preoperative evaluation and surgical planning should account for the possible involvement of the gastrointestinal, neural, and vascular elements. Additional consideration should be given to planning for hemorrhage control and evaluation of a need for urinary diversion or colostomy. The latter usually is required in an SCT with a high Altman class, with a large intrapelvic component and symptoms of colonic obstruction. Adherent bowel should be resected en bloc along with the tumor. In these situations an anterior approach is typically performed. When suspecting SCT, an initial serum α-fetoprotein (AFP) should be obtained, which aids in diagnosis and serves as a baseline value for follow-up.

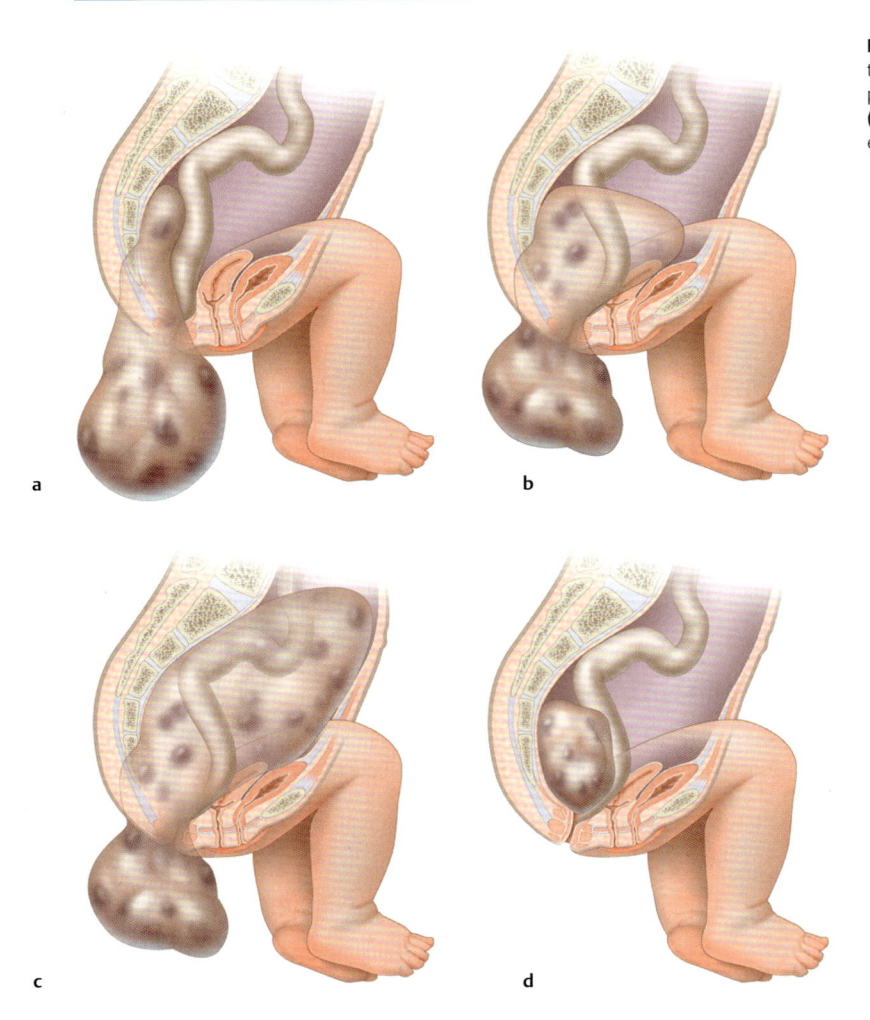

Fig. 122.1 Altman classification of sacrococcygeal teratoma. **(a)** Class I: primarily extrapelvic mass. **(b)** Class II: predominate extrapelvic mass with intrapelvic extension. **(c)** Class III: predominant intrapelvic mass with extrapelvic extension. **(d)** Class IV: primarily intrapelvic mass.

Timing of Surgery

Early resection on an elective basis within the first 2 months of life is recommended for most SCTs, as there appears to be a lower incidence of malignancy and better long-term outcomes among those with early diagnosis and resection.[2] Additionally, with surgical delay, the risk for coagulopathy, pressure necrosis, infection, and hemorrhage within the tumor may increase.

Preoperative Hemorrhage Control

Surgical procedures in newborns present a particularly difficult challenge to the surgical team. Extremely low blood volume (80 cc/kg), low hemodynamic reserve, and large vascular lesions may lead to significant intraoperative challenges. Sacral coccygeal teratomas can be very difficult lesions to treat, given their vascularity and extension into surrounding structures. One large series on the surgical treatment of SCTs reported a mean estimated blood loss of 207 cc for posteriorly approached SCT resections.[2] Gaining sufficient central and intravenous (IV) access and having blood available for transfusion are important preparations for this surgery. Other reported noninvasive techniques to manage blood loss include hemodilution, controlled hypotension, and hypothermia.[5] When preoperative evaluation identifies a highly vascular tumor, or in cases with an exceptionally high risk of high blood loss, some reports have described the use of extracorporeal membrane oxygenation, preoperative suturing of Teflon pledgets across the exophytic neck of the sacral mass, or anterior placement of a controllable vascular loop around the abdominal aorta prior to the start of surgery.[1,5–7] Staged resections have also been described, but surgical delay or prolongation may carry a theoretical risk of malignant transformation.

Preoperative Imaging

The differential diagnosis of SCT includes myelomeningocele, neuroblastoma, hemangioma, leiomyoma, and lipoma. Preoperative imaging is selected to aid in diagnosis, in the detection of metastasis, in the characterization of the mass and related anatomy, and in the detection of coexisting anomalies. Multimodal imaging evaluation is recommended for evaluation of a newly discovered sacral mass in the newborn with select imaging studies performed based on exam findings. Most patients should undergo an abdominopelvic computed tomography (CT) or magnetic resonance imaging (MRI) and ultrasound with color-flow Doppler.

Postnatal ultrasound with color-flow Doppler is typically performed in all patients and is useful for identifying spinal, abdominal, or pelvic extension; the nature of tumor (solid, cystic); the degree of vascularity; spinal dysraphism; and differentiation of SCT (cystic) from other pathologies such as myelomeningocele. Plain radiographs should be taken in most patients as a useful screening tool for identifying sacral defects, pulmonary metastasis, and congenital abnormalities. CT with IV and rectal contrast is useful for delineating intrapelvic extension, identifying urinary tract displacement or obstruction, and identifying bony invasion and metastatic disease. An MRI can be useful if spinal involvement is suspected or if the diagnosis is in doubt. A barium enema is helpful when there is suspicion for pelvic or colonic invasion. Intravenous urography can be useful when there is suspicion for extension to bladder or urethra.

Preoperative Exam

In addition to a neurologic exam, patients should undergo (1) a cardiac exam to rule out congenital disease, arteriovenous shunts, or heart failure; and (2) a rectal exam to evaluate anal tone and anal patency, and to detect intrapelvic extension. Patients harboring a sacral mass may have other regional anomalies that need to be accounted for as they may impact surgical planning. One such constellation is the Currarino triad of sacral defect, anorectal malformation, and presacral mass. The presence of hydrops, polyhydramnios, or premature birth (before 32 weeks) correlates with increased mortality.[1]

Surgical Technique

Anesthesia

All patients are placed under general endotracheal anesthesia in a temperature-controlled environment. Preoperative urinary catheter insertion and preoperative bowel prep are recommended. Gaining sufficient central and IV access and having blood available for transfusion are important preparations for this surgery. Preoperative antibiotic should be administered and a surgical "time-out" should be conducted prior to the skin incision.

Positioning

Positioning is dependent on the approach. Surgical approaches are planned based primarily on the location and type of SCT (Altman classification) corresponding with the degree of presacral extension. Anterior or combined approaches necessitating supine positioning are often utilized for giant SCTs, high Altman classification (III or IV), and in patients with high-output heart failure. For combined approaches, the anterior approach should be performed first to address the intrapelvic components and free them from their attachments, when possible avoiding partial resection, and the subsequent posterior approach should then address the posterior and extrapelvic elements and complete an en-bloc tumor resection.[8]

For the posterior approach, the patient should be placed in the prone jackknife position with the hips abducted and flexed at 90 degrees (**Fig. 122.2**). A gel roll or rolled blanket may be placed ventrally to elevate and support the pelvis, permitting relaxed hip abduction, such that the abdomen is relaxed and not in contact with the operating table. This is the position of choice to be used in the more frequent low Altman classification (I and II) SCTs and in patients with normal cardiac function. Placement of adhesive bands over either gluteal cheek provides additional exposure to the sacrococcygeal area and gluteal cleft. The rectum can be irrigated with a prep solution and should be packed (e.g., with a Hegar dilator or Vaseline pack) to aid in its identification and to prevent injury during dissection. The dilator may be soaked in antiseptic and should be positioned such that it can be manipulated during surgery to provide the surgeon with constant awareness of rectal location.

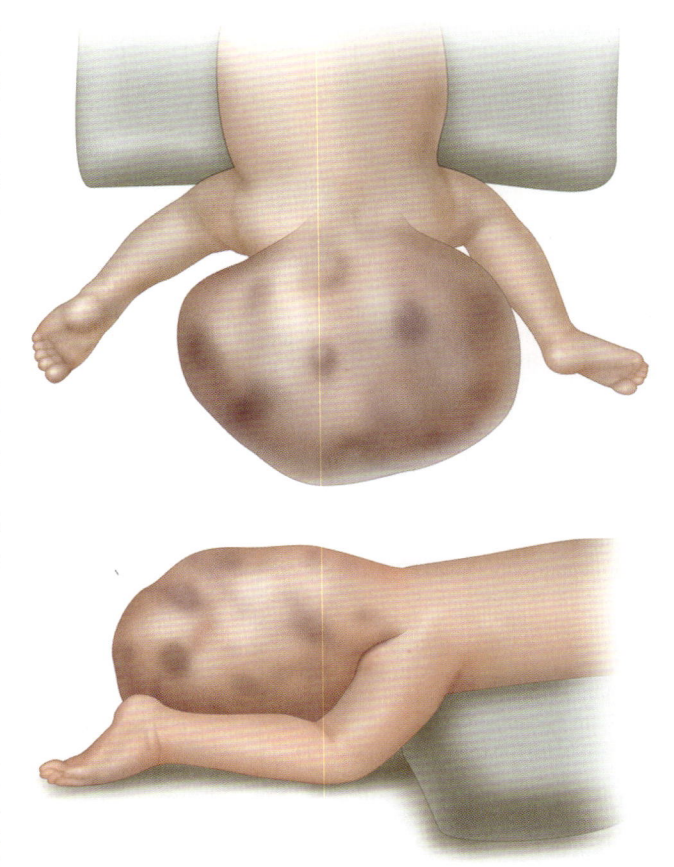

Fig. 122.2 Prone jack-knife positioning for posterior approach.

Incision

The traditional incision described for the posterior approach is an inverted U- or V-shaped incision made transversely across the lower sacrum and gluteal cheeks, superior to the mass (**Fig. 122.3**).[1,4,9,10] The coccyx can be palpated beneath the mass, facilitating appropriate incisional planning at or near the level of the

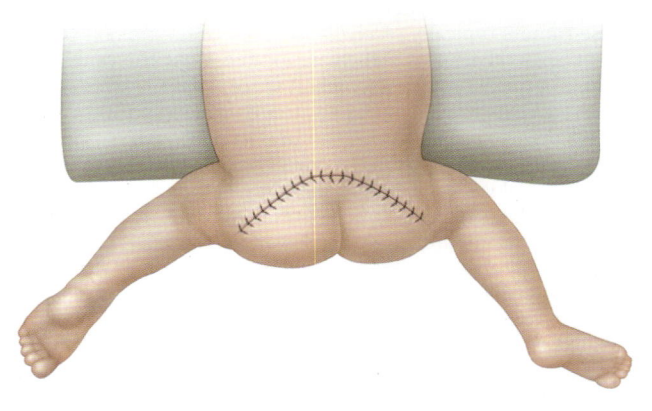

Fig. 122.3 Traditional incision for posterior approach.

sacrococcygeal junction. This incision helps keep wound closure at a distance from the anus. The incision can be made with a Bovie unit set at 15 W, in the blend mode with the needle tip attachment, which is used to bloodlessly dissect the skin and subcutaneous tissues. After creating this incision, dissection should proceed caudally in the subcutaneous tissue layers circumferentially dissecting the margins of the tumor, so as to create a caudally reflected flap. Self-retaining retractors can be positioned at the skin edges on either side of the tumor to maintain exposure. Other incisions described for this approach include a Chenon-shaped transverse incision between the coccyx and anus,[2] and a midline sagittal incision between the sacrum and prox anus.[2,11] Although these latter incisions produce a more favorable cosmetic result, they are placed in close proximity to the anus and may carry an increased risk for wound infection or sphincter damage.

Tumor Resection

Paramount to obtaining the best outcome and least amount of morbidities and complications is a thorough knowledge of the regions anatomy (**Fig. 122.4**). Engaging the assistance of a pediatric general surgeon is extremely important for achieving a successful outcome. After creation of the skin incision, dissection proceeds circumferentially around the tumor capsule, separating it from the gluteal muscles laterally. This can often be performed bluntly with coagulation of small perforating vessels as they are encountered entering the tumor. Care should be taken to excise the mass without spill or rupture of tumor. In the case of a cystic SCT, needle aspiration and decompression of the cyst can aid in visualization for tumor resection. During ventral and inferior dissection it is important to maintain awareness of the location of the anus and attempt to preserve perianal musculature (retrorectal and anal levator ani muscles), which is critical for fecal continence. Blunt dissection is often adequate to delineate and separate the plane between the tumor, perianal musculature, and rectum during inferior and ventral dissection.

After freeing the tumor from the ventral rectum and adjacent perianal musculature, it can be elevated cephalad, such that the only remaining attachments are those to the coccyx. Superiorly a subperiosteal exposure of sacral margins and coccyx from rostral to caudal helps prevent inadvertent rectal injury. The sacrococcygeal junction is identified at the interbody space between S5 and the coccyx. Coccygectomy at this level is recommended in all cases, as it has been reported to prevent recurrence. The coccyx is resected so that it is maintained in continuity with the tumor, and the entire complex is elevated free of the rectum (ventrally) and removed together as one unit.[2,4,9,10,12] Failure to remove the coccyx has been reported to result in a 30 to 40% recurrence rate with a higher probability of malignancy.[2,12] These tumors typically receive a majority of their blood supply from the sacral arteries, which are located along the ventral sacrum and coccyx in the retrorectal space. These vessels can be observed in the retrorectal space after coccygectomy.

Following coccygectomy, the presacral components of the tumor can be bluntly dissected. Identification and control of the feeding sacral vessels is important, but whether they are ligated before or after dissection of the presacral tumor mass remains debatable. Be mindful that sacral tumors can have significant collateral circulation. After coccygectomy, ligation of the blood supply and circumferential dissection of the pre- and postsacral tumor mass are performed, and the tumor and coccyx are then elevated en bloc. It is important to attempt the removal of all gross evidence of the tumor.[9] If needed, due to tumor invasion, a more rostral resection of the sacrum may be performed up to and including S2 without the need for sacral reconstruction. However, if S1 is compromised sacral reconstruction is required.[13]

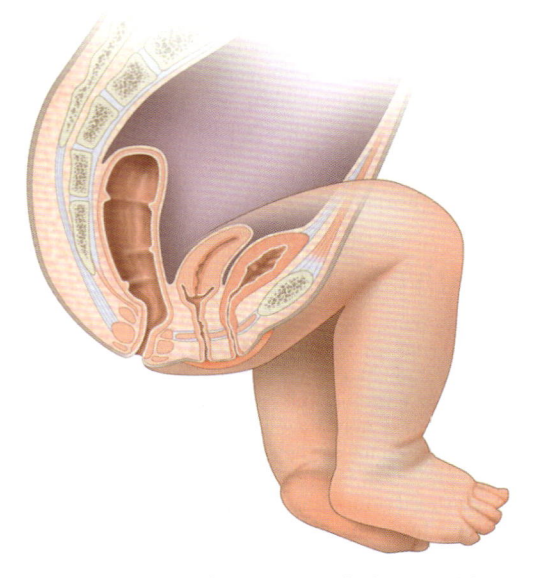

Fig. 122.4 Anatomic considerations. Note the location of the coccyx and the attaching pelvic floor musculature. The retrorectal space exists ventral to the sacrum and coccyx, wherein lies the sacral arteries.

Reconstruction and Closure

Upon the conclusion of tumor resection and the achievement of hemostasis, wound closure must attempt to reconstruct a normal pelvic floor, anal location, and symmetric gluteal cheeks. Elevating and repositioning the rectum and anus to a normal location typically requires reattachment of the supportive rectal musculature to the caudal sacrum. The levator ani musculature and anococcygeal ligament, which attach to the coccyx, are located and removed from their coccygeal attachment and reinserted onto the caudal sacrum. Absorbable sutures may be placed approximating the presacral fascia (superiorly) to the cuff of the levator ani (inferiorly) to elevate the anus to a normal position.[4] In older children or in those in whom it is not possible to locate adequate presacral fascia, the levator ani cuff may be tacked to the sacrum using a cranial bone plating system.

Incision closure and gluteal reconstruction begins by excising excess thin cutaneous layers that stretched over the dome of the tumor in the sacral region, while trying to preserve the more robust cutaneous margins for incorporation into a Chevron shaped or π-shaped closure (**Fig. 122.5**).[14] The type of closure should be determined based on the amount of available skin robust enough for closure relative to the size of defect. Care should be taken when excising the skin flap caudally near the anus so as to prevent damage or perforation while also retaining enough tissue to perform a closure that maintains the anus at a distance from the wound closure. Subcutaneous/suprafascial dissection over the gluteal cheeks and superiorly over the dorsal lumbar fascia can facilitate additional mobilization of robust and healthy skin for use in wound closure. The wound is then irrigated with sterile antibiotic solution and closed in layers with absorbable suture. A drain may be placed below the skin flap, and the skin is closed with running monofilament suture. A vascularized gluteal or latissimus muscle flap can be harvested and rotated into or over the defect and secured in place. These flaps are not always necessary, but they are useful for closing dead space, positioning a healthy vascularized tissue barrier between the underlying structures and the skin incision, and cosmetic reconstruction.

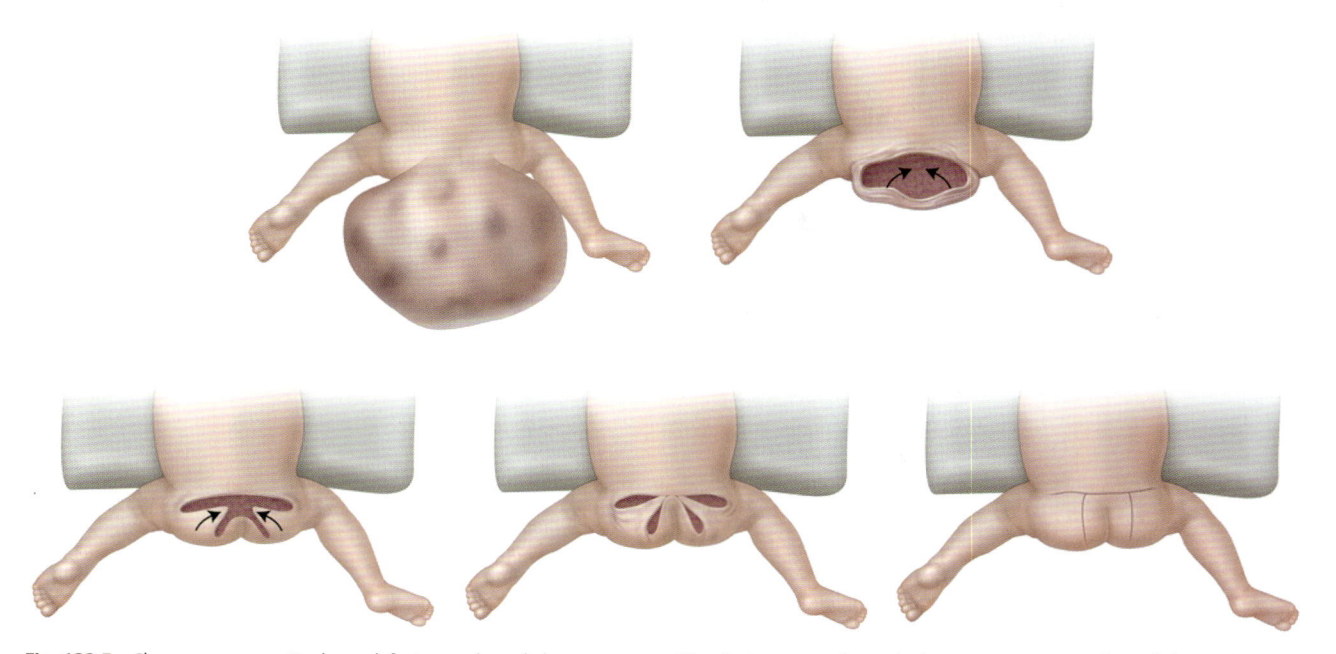

Fig. 122.5 Closure sequence. For large defects a p-shaped closure may provide a better cosmetic result than attempting a traditional closure (see **Fig. 122.3**).

Complications

- Intraoperative hemorrhage and excessive blood loss is the most worrisome complication.
  - Intraoperative hemorrhage leading to death reported at 0.8%[3]
- Wound infection reported to occur in 18%[2,9]
- Rectal injury reported at 1.4%[15]
  - Once identified can be managed with colostomy and antibiotics
- Necrosis of the flap reported at 1.4%[15]
- Perioperative/postoperative mortality reported to occur in 4.1 to 4.5%[2,15]
- Overall mortality among SCT patients is related to malignancy, Altman class, size of tumor, and age at presentation, and is reported at 7 to 60%[3]
- Urinary dysfunction reported to occur in 9.1 to 33%[2,12,16]
  - Neurogenic bladder (most common)
- Anorectal dysfunction reported to occur in 9.2 to 29%[12,16]
  - Chronic constipation (most common)
- Poor cosmesis reported to occur in as high as 40.3%[12]

Postoperative Course

Newborn patients may begin feeding within a few hours of surgery. The Foley catheter is continued, and patients are kept prone for several days to help maintain wound cleanliness. A postoperative MRI can be obtained to evaluate the extent of resection and serve as a baseline for comparison. Following discharge, patients are followed with serial MRI and serial AFP measurements at 6 months, and then annually. Recurrence rates of benign and malignant SCTs are reported at 0 to 10% and 7.5 to 30%, respectively.[2,13] In the case of tumor recurrence, reoperation is recommended.[9,10] Chemotherapy regimens used for malignant SCTs have included cisplatin, etoposide, and bleomycin.[1,2]

References

1. Azizkhan R. Teratomas and other germ cell tumors. In: O'Neill JA, Coran AG, Fonkalsrud E, Grosfeld JL, eds. Pediatric Surgery, 6th ed. New York: Elsevier Health Sciences; 2006:554–563
2. Barakat MI, Abdelaal SM, Saleh AM. Sacrococcygeal teratoma in infants and children. Acta Neurochir (Wien) 2011;153:1781–1786
3. Altman RP, Randolph JG, Lilly JR. Sacrococcygeal teratoma: American academy of pediatrics surgical section survey—1973. J Pediatr Surg 1974;9:389–398
4. Hendren WH, Henderson BM. The surgical management of sacrococcygeal teratomas with intrapelvic extension. Ann Surg 1970;171:77–84
5. Hase T, Kodama M, Kishida A, et al. Techniques available for the management of massive sacrococcygeal teratomas. Pediatr Surg Int 2001;17:232–234
6. Lindahl H. Giant sacrococcygeal teratoma: a method of simple intraoperative control of hemorrhage. J Pediatr Surg 1988;23:1068–1069
7. Smithers CJ, Javid PJ, Turner CG, Klein JD, Jennings RW. Damage control operation for massive sacrococcygeal teratoma. J Pediatr Surg 2011;46:566–569
8. Gokaslan ZL, Romsdahl MM, Kroll SS, et al. Total sacrectomy and Galveston L-rod reconstruction for malignant neoplasms. Technical note. J Neurosurg 1997;87:781–787
9. Ein SH, Mancer K, Adeyemi SD. Malignant sacrococcygeal teratoma—endodermal sinus, yolk sac tumor—in infants and children: a 32-year review. J Pediatr Surg 1985;20:473–477
10. Gross RW, Clatworthy HW Jr, Meeker IA Jr. Sacrococcygeal teratomas in infants and children; a report of 40 cases. Surg Gynecol Obstet 1951;92:341–354
11. Jan IA, Khan EA, Yasmeen N, Orakzai H, Saeed J. Posterior sagittal approach for resection of sacrococcygeal teratomas. Pediatr Surg Int 2011;27:545–548
12. Derikx JPM, De Backer A, van de Schoot L, et al. Long-term functional sequelae of sacrococcygeal teratoma: a national study in The Netherlands. J Pediatr Surg 2007;42:1122–1126
13. Deutsch H, Mummaneni PV, Haid RW, Rodts GE, Ondra SL. Benign sacral tumors. Neurosurg Focus 2003;15:E14

14. Fishman SJ, Jennings RW, Johnson SM, Kim HB. Contouring buttock reconstruction after sacrococcygeal teratoma resection. J Pediatr Surg 2004;39:439–441, discussion 439–441
15. Wakhlu A, Misra S, Tandon RK, Wakhlu AK. Sacrococcygeal teratoma. Pediatr Surg Int 2002;18:384–387
16. Partridge EA, Canning D, Long C, et al. Urologic and anorectal complications of sacrococcygeal teratomas: prenatal and postnatal predictors. J Pediatr Surg 2014;49:139–142, discussion 142–143

123 Surgical Management of Spinal Dysraphism

Mena Kerolus, Ravi Nunna, and Lorenzo F. Muñoz

Open Spinal Dysraphism (Myelomeningoceles)

Open spinal dysraphism, or open myelomeningocele, is considered the most complex and serious congenital defect of the central nervous system that is compatible with survival. Due to advances in prenatal care, screening, and folate supplementation, the incidence has decreased tremendously.[1] Outcome studies have shown that patients are living into early adulthood with adequate supportive care.[2] Myelomeningoceles are caused by a midline defect in the embryological stage of neurulation that results in exposure of intradural neural elements to the outside world. It is also important to recognize that there are multiple conditions associated with this neurologic anomaly, including hydrocephalus, shunt dependence, late brainstem dysfunction, Chiari malformation type II, hydrosyringomyelic cysts, and tethered cord syndrome.[3]

Normal Embryogenesis

Embryogenic formation of the spinal cord occurs in three stages: gastrulation, neurulation, and caudal regression. The gastrulation stage completes on postovulatory days 16 to 18 with the release of mesenchymal factors that promote the differentiation of the neuroectoderm and formation of the neural plate (**Fig. 123.1**). The neuroectoderm is composed of pseudostratified columnar epithelium that is continuous with the cutaneous ectoderm. The neuroectoderm appears on day 16, followed by the formation of the neural groove on days 18 to 19. During weeks 3 to 4, the neuroectoderm undergoes thickening, narrowing, and elongation with the aid of microtubules regulated by the mesoderm. The neural groove folds deepen and begin forming a cleft (**Fig. 123.2**). Development of the neural tube occurs in four stages: formation, shaping, bending, and fusion (**Fig. 123.3**). The formation and shaping of the neural tube involves multiple intrinsic forces of actin-like filaments. Fusion involves many molecular cell–cell interactions at the dorsal portion of the neural folds with the formation of intercellular junctions and surface glycoproteins. As the neural tube closes, it enters a phase of disjunction that involves separation of the cutaneous ectoderm from the once continuous neuroectoderm. Neural crest cells initially located at the neural folds migrate to form the dorsal root ganglion (**Fig. 123.4**). Paraxial mesoderm differentiates into its respective tissue depending on the adjacent neuroectoderm.

The first portion of the neural tube to close is the cranial spinal cord at the sixth cervical somite. The neural tube closes in separate segments over the next 6 days. It was once thought that closure occurs in a zipper-like fashion, but that is no longer thought to be true.[4] The rostral portion of the neural tube closes by day 24, and the caudal portion, the sacral vertebral level adjacent to somite 30, closes by days 26 to 28 to form the primary neural tube. The paraxial mesoderm ventral to the neuroectoderm differentiates into the meningeal layers and travels circumferentially to cover the neural tube.

Secondary neurulation begins with the condensation of a cluster of pluripotent primitive stem cells called the "caudal cells" or "tail-bud cells," which form the medullary cord through a process of canalization. The medullary cord is a continuous extension of the primary neural tube,[5] and it is thought that a secondary neural tube occurs independent of primary neurulation.[6] The final formation of the neural tube occurs during a process of retrogressive differentiation. The caudal portion of the neural tube becomes smaller and thinner in diameter, forming the conus and filum terminale. The final position of the conus medullaris occurs in the first postnatal month.

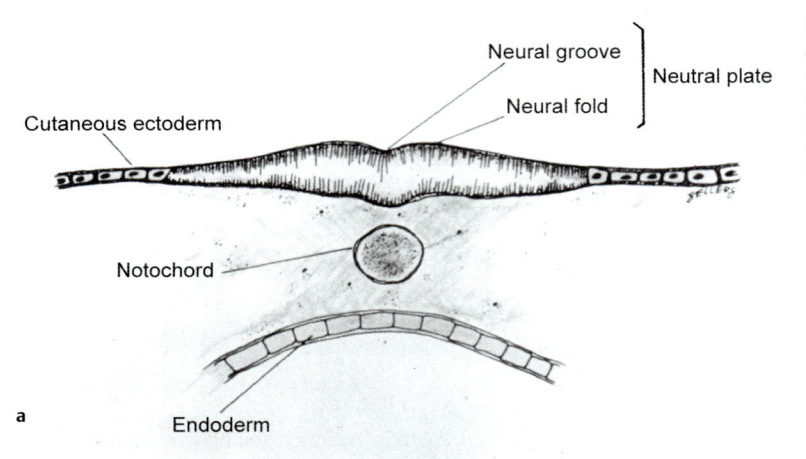

Fig. 123.1 Primary neurulation. **(a)** Normal neurulation. A neural groove is noted on the dorsal surface of the neural plate. **(b)** Elevation of the neural folds, which occurs as the paraxial mesoderm enlarges. As elongation of the neural plate occurs, stretching of the overlying cutaneous ectoderm aids in bringing the neural folds together. Note the emergence of the neural crest cells.

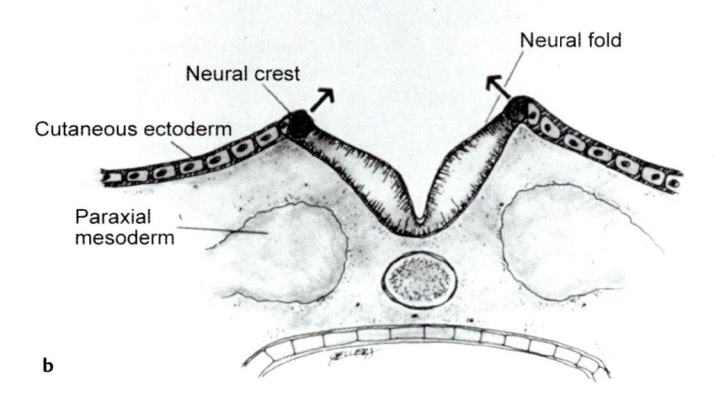

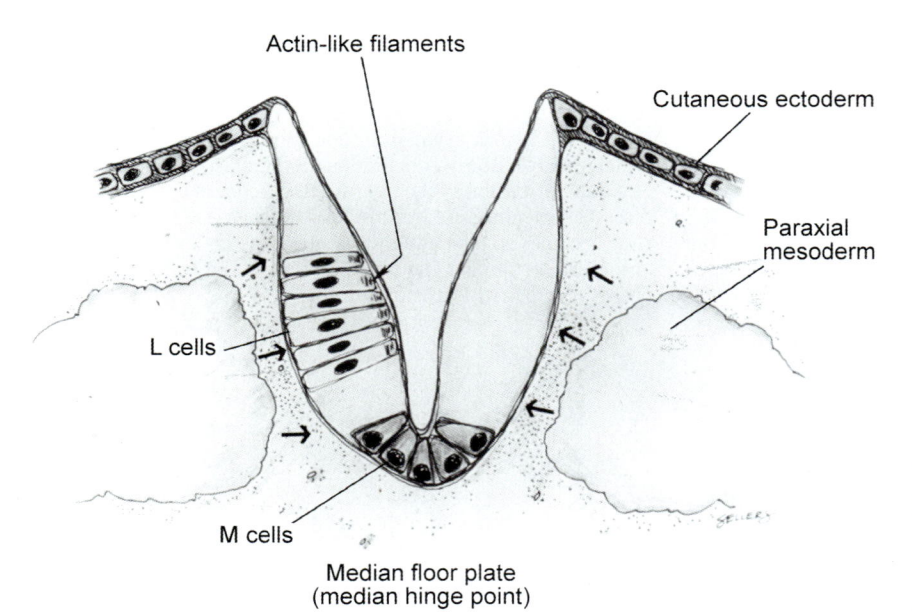

Fig. 123.2 Primary neurulation. The neural groove folds deepen and begin formation of a cleft aided by actin-like contractile filaments within L cells located in the lateral portions of the neural folds. The wedge-shaped M cells at the median hinge point specify the dorsal direction of cleft formation.

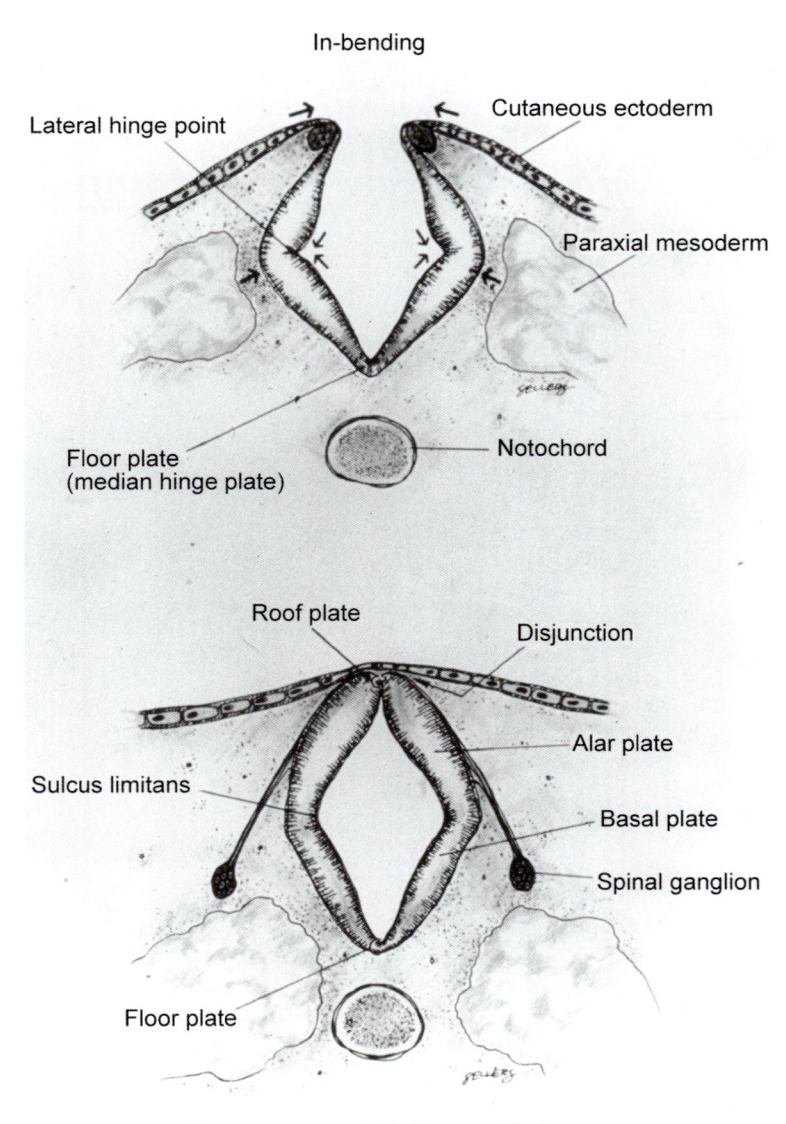

Fig. 123.3 Primary neurulation. Bending and fusion of the neural folds lead to dorsal midline fusion. Fusion involves many molecular cell–cell interactions at the dorsal portion of the neural folds. Glycosaminoglycan molecules appear to be active in the recognition process between the approaching lips of the neural folds. Segregation of neurons within the primitive neural tube into the dorsal alar plate and the ventral basal plate are separated by the sulcus limitans.

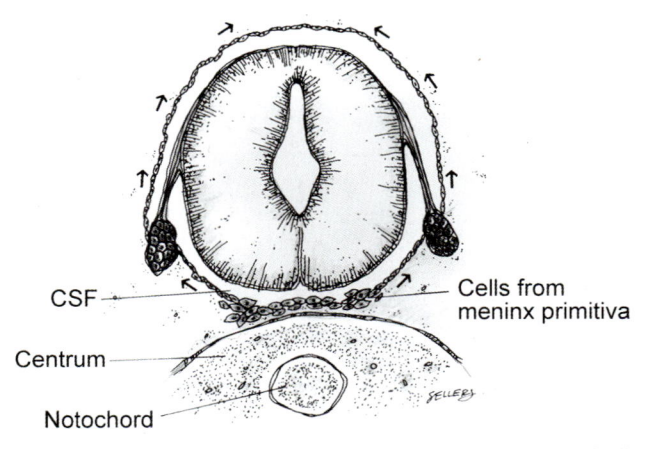

Fig. 123.4 Primary neurulation. Dura is formed from dorsally located cells from the meninx primitiva, which travels circumferentially. The neural crest cells migrate ventrally to form the dorsal root ganglia and the dorsal nerve root. CSF, cerebrospinal fluid.

Embryogenesis of Open Myelomeningoceles

Open myelomeningoceles contain a flat neural placode that remains continuous with the cutaneous ectoderm (**Fig. 123.5**). The flat dorsal placode is considered the inner lining of the cord if the neural tube has completely formed. The ventral placode contains the medial ventral nerve roots and the lateral sensory dorsal nerve roots. The junctional zone is the region between the arachnoid membrane of the neural placode and the cutaneous ectoderm. The meninges form in the basal aspect of the neuroepithelium, and therefore the dorsal surface does not have meningeal covering. The ventral aspect of the neural placode is displaced dorsally by cerebrospinal fluid (CSF) accumulation forming a distended cyst (**Fig. 123.6**). The arachnoid membranes still connect the cutaneous ectoderm to the neural placode. Dura is also present in the ventral portion of the neural sac but fuses with the underlying fascia, muscle, and failed lamina of the periosteum.[7] The presence of a ventral CSF collection differentiates a myelomeningocele from a myelocele.

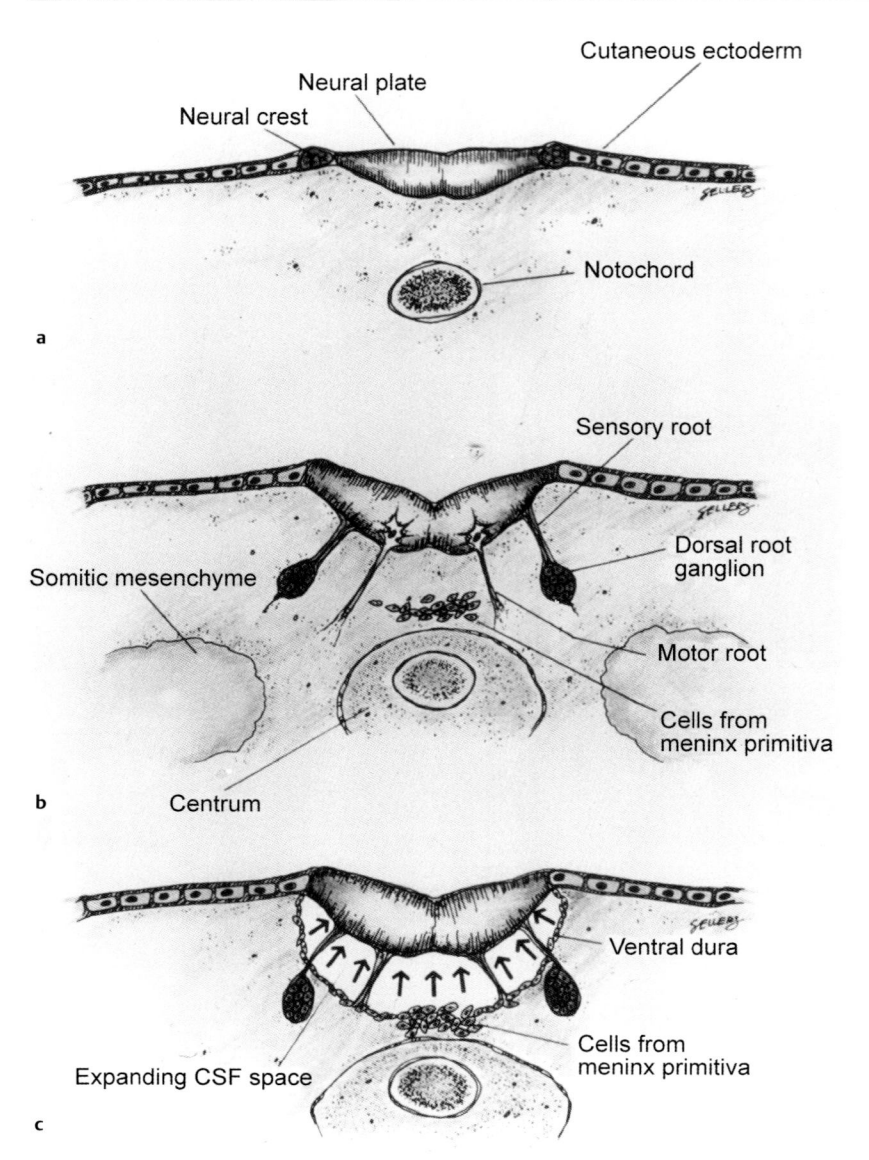

Fig. 123.5 Formation of open myelomeningocele. **(a)** Elevation of the neural folds does not take place. **(b)** The ventral surface of the neural placode contains the medial ventral nerve roots and the lateral sensory dorsal nerve roots. **(c)** Failure of the meninx primitive cells to travel circumferentially around the forming neural tube inhibits formation of the dural covering of the dorsal surface of the neural placode.

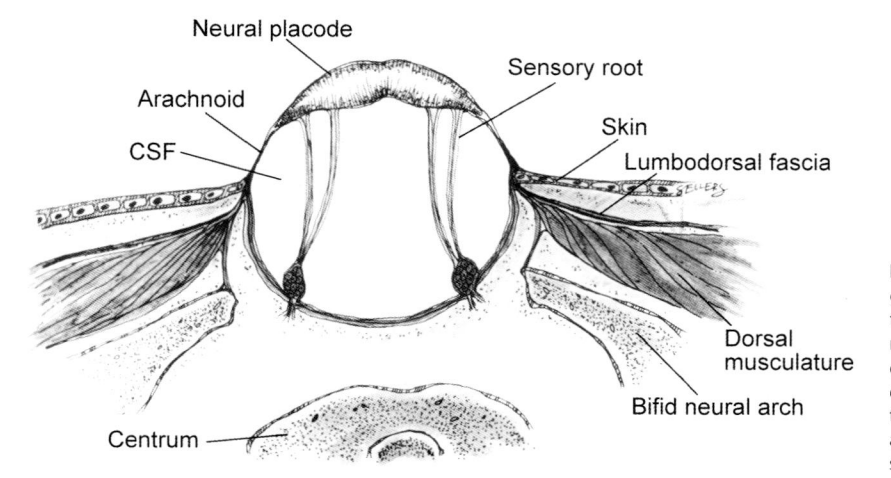

Fig. 123.6 Formation of an open myelomeningocele. Cerebrospinal fluid (CSF) accumulates on the ventral side of the neural placode and ultimately pushes the placode, forming an enlarging cyst. The leptomeninges stretch between the lateral margins of the neural placode to the edges of the abnormal skin. The lateral edges of the dura attaches to skin, lumbodorsal fascia, dorsal paraspinous muscles, and periosteum.

Goals of Surgery

When repairing an open myelomeningocele defect, the goal of surgery is to restore the neural tube's intended anatomy and doing so in a timely manner, preventing CSF leakage, and preserving as much neurologic function as possible while promoting wound healing.

Preparation for Surgery

A comprehensive history should be taken and a full physical examination should be performed prior to surgical intervention, with special attention given to the level of the lesion, lower extremity function, and urologic function. We prefer head ultrasound as a diagnostic tool for evaluation of the ventricles and subsequent shunt placement. Computed tomography (CT) and magnetic resonance imaging (MRI) are also options; the latter provides a more detailed evaluation of congenital anomalies that may aid in the discussion of the prognosis with the family.[8] Head circumference and assessment of the anterior fontanelle should be measured daily. Due to an increase in prenatal planning and the use of routine ultrasound in the prenatal period, diagnosis of an open myelomeningocele defect and the subsequent discussion with the family enable prompt treatment upon birth. Although it is beyond the scope of this chapter, intrauterine surgery for repair of open myelomeningocele defects is proving to result in a decreased incidence of ventricular peritoneal (VP) shunts and improved neurologic function.[9-11] Cesarean section is likely to be pursued in the event that prenatal ultrasound reveals enlarged ventricles; however, the use of cesarean section over vaginal delivery has not been shown to have a significant benefit in terms of outcome after delivery.[12,13]

Once delivery occurs, the infant should be placed in the prone position and the defect covered with moist sterile nonadhesive dressings such as Telfa to prevent contamination and dehydration of the thin covering membrane. We recommend starting preoperative cefazolin and gentamicin to prevent infection. A multidisciplinary approach to treatment should include the urology, nephrology, neurology, and orthopedic teams. Other congenital malformations, although uncommon, may require cardiology or gastroenterology evaluation. In these cases, genetic testing should be performed to rule out an underlying chromosomal abnormality. Comprehensive care is essential to successful rehabilitation for these infants. Therapies are lifelong and demanding, but with adequate care the prognosis is good.[3] The intervention entails minimal risk of infection if it is done within the first 48 to 72 hours after birth.[8] Randomized trials of "immediate" surgical intervention prior to initial admission to the neonatal intensive care unit (NICU) did not show lower rates of postoperative infections.[14]

Positioning

In a latex-free operating room, the neonate should undergo induction of general anesthesia. A soft roll or surgical jelly donut may be placed distal to the defect at the level of the pelvis during intubation. Alternatively, intubation may be performed in the lateral position. It is not uncommon, however, that children born with open myelomeningocele defects are intubated and placed on positive pressure ventilation from birth. Once the airway is secured, the infant is placed in the prone position for surgery. The use of a soft rolled towel is placed at the level of the pelvis perpendicular to the long axis of the torso. Meticulous sterile preparation is done using povidone iodine solution with avoidance of the neural placode. During sterilization, Telfa may be used to prevent iodine-induced toxicity. The neural placode is cleaned with sterile normal saline. In cases of a large defect or suspected difficulty in skin closure, a large myocutaneous flap may be needed. There may be multiple folds in the dorsal membrane that need to be sterilized, as careful preparation will minimize recontamination with dissection. A bare hugger or warm blankets should be placed under the infant to maintain normal body temperature.

Skin Incision and Opening

Once the patient is appropriately positioned and prepped, the neural placode is identified in the midline of the dorsal defect as a thin, pink membrane (**Fig. 123.7**). An incision with a No. 11 scalpel is made at the junction of the skin and the edge of the arachnoid membrane that surrounds the neural placode (**Fig. 123.8**). Careful dissection in a circumferential manner is done until the entire arachnoid membrane is free. During this step, careful attention is paid to underlying the bridging veins, which are treated with 1- to 2-mm fine-tipped bipolar cautery or the use of cottonoids and pressure (**Fig. 123.9**). Minimal use of the bipolar is suggested so that the skin margins may heal appropriately. The dorsal root entry zone is displaced laterally, so care must be taken in identifying the border of the neural placode. Upon completion of full circumferential dissection, the neural placode will be free from the surrounding arachnoid. During dissection, one may encounter epidermal or dermal ectopic tissue that will need to be removed to prevent dermoid/epidermoid cyst formation. Multiple feeding arteries will be identified and mobilized under the arachnoid membrane. Careful dissection is crucial because thrombosis of these vessels may interfere with tissue vascularization, and increased tension may impede wound healing. At the caudal aspect of the defect the filum is identified with meticulous microsurgical dissection. At the rostral end, dissection to one or two vertebral levels above the defect is advised to visualize the normal cord and to aid in continuous closure of the neural placode (**Fig. 123.10**).

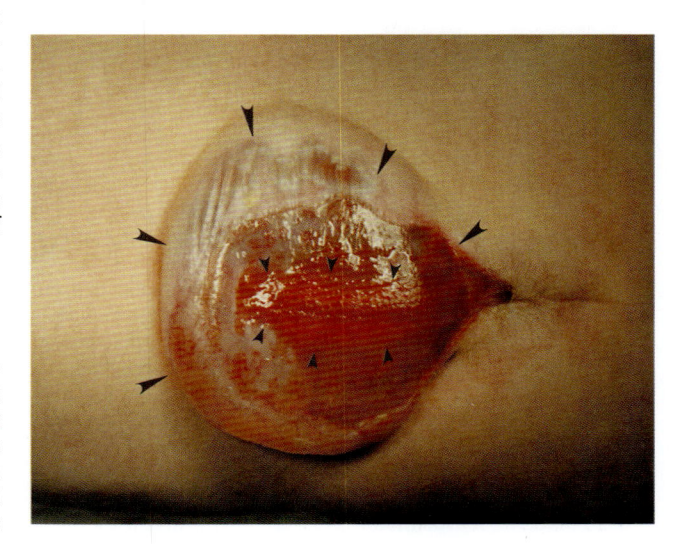

Fig. 123.7 Open myelomeningocele with a terminal neural placode. *Small arrowheads* outline the margin of the neural placode. The pink leptomeningeal membrane stretches between the placode and the skin. *Large arrowheads* outline the skin edge. The right end of the figure points toward the anus.

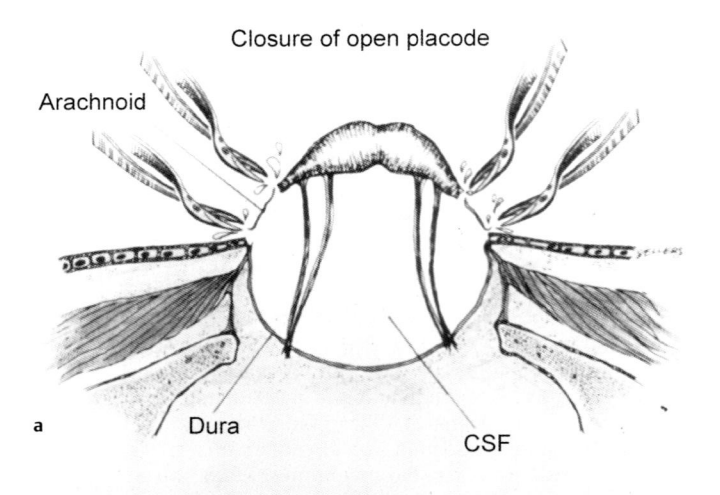

Fig. 123.8 Steps of surgical repair of an open myelomeningocele. **(a)** Initial incision occurs at the junction between the membrane and the healthy skin. **(b)** After excision of the arachnoid membrane, the neural placode is attached together using microsutures. The dura is closed at the dorsal midline surface after careful dissection of the lateral dural margins from its lateral attachments. **(c)** Final closure includes muscle, fascia, and skin over the dural tube (triple-layer closure).

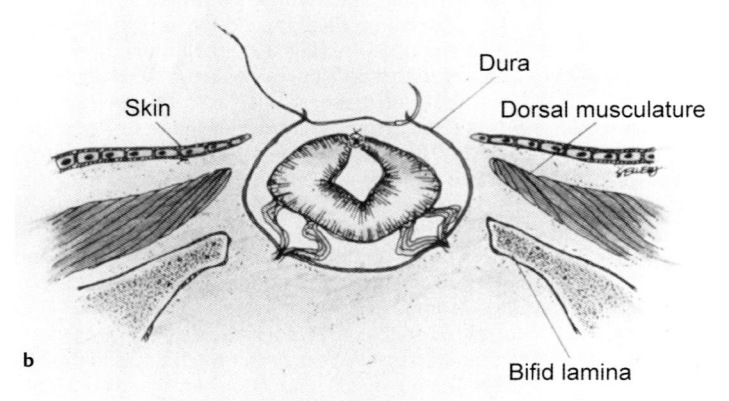

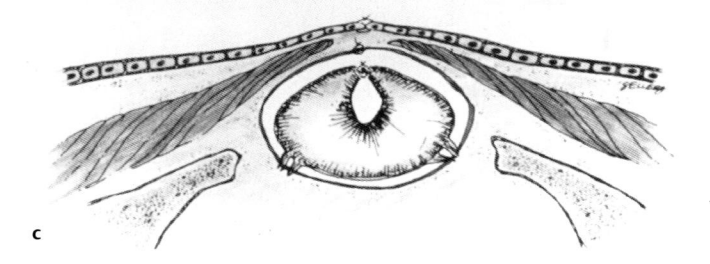

Handling of the Neural Placode

Careful dissection of the neural placode is essential to prevent bleeding and tearing of the pia-arachnoid. Often after freeing of the neural tissue from the healthy epithelium, the placode inherently rolls into its natural tube-like structure, especially at the rostral end of the defect (**Fig. 123.11**). Attention to the stiffness and manipulation of the neural placode should remain minimal as mechanical or vascular compromise may risk neurologic function. On the ventral aspect of the pia ventral or dorsal nerve roots may be encountered. These nerve roots should be kept in place, as sensorimotor function may return. If the placode is thin, it may roll into its natural tubular shape and the pia-arachnoid membranes are closed at midline. We favor using a 6-0 blue Prolene stitch for closure of the neural placode. This facilitates identification when returning to the operating room for untethering of the cord. The final step involves forming a "normal" neural tube similar to the one that would have formed if secondary neurulation had occurred properly. The presence of normal-appearing neurulated cord in a segment of the open defect may be a segmental placode. Careful handling of this tissue is crucial to maintain a normal neural placode. Although debated, formation of a tubular neural placode may aid in the reduction of late tethering.

Dural Closure

Dural dissection is best started close to the midline at the rostral end of the incision (**Fig. 123.12**). Epidural fat may be appreciated and may aid in initial dissection. Sharp dissection is used in a circumferential manner until both dural sheets are mobilized. The ultimate goal of dural closure is to prevent CSF leakage and promote a "normal" environment for the neural placode. We generally use a 5-0 monofilament running suture, as it produces better closure. Dural substitutes may need to be used if the tubular neural placode is too large or if the mobilized dural sheets

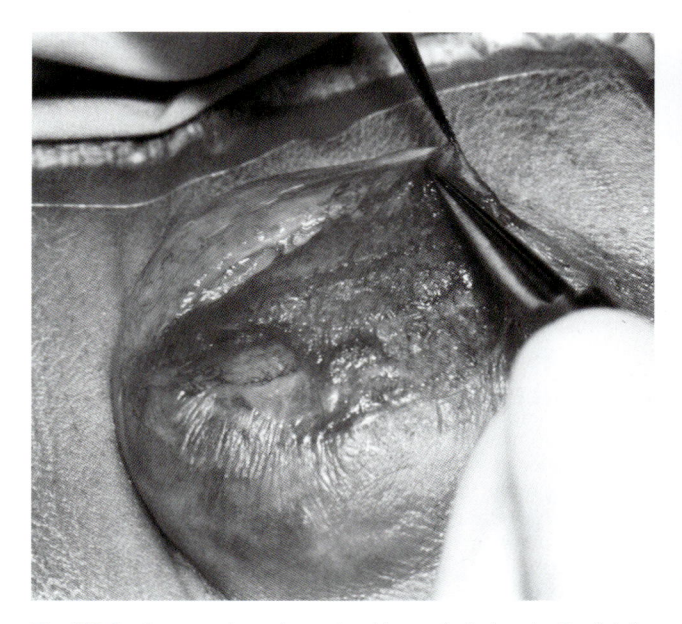

Fig. 123.9 Open myelomeningocele with terminal placode. Careful dissection of the leptomeningeal membrane just outside the margin of the placode.

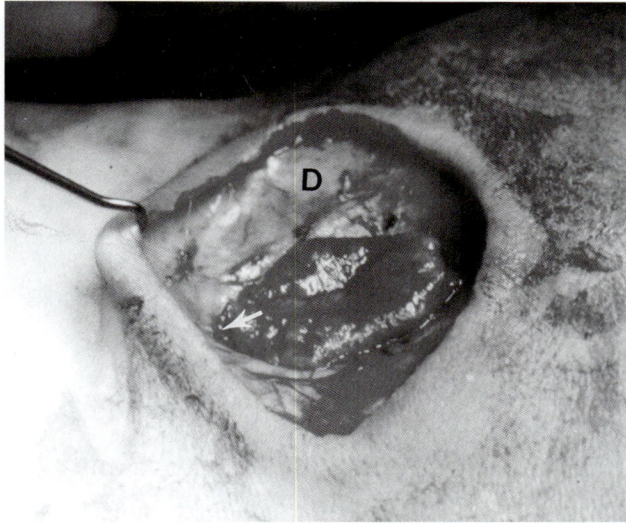

Fig. 123.10 Open myelomeningocele after leptomeningeal membrane has been removed. The dissected neural placode lies in the bottom of the original sac. Ventral dura *(D)* lines the bottom of the sac and fuses with the skin margin *(hook)*. Rostral margin of the placode *(white arrow)* is continuous with the normal spinal cord.

are insufficient to cover the neural placode. Valsalva maneuver should be performed upon closure of the dura to ensure no CSF leak. If leaking is observed, another attempt at closure should be made, or dural glue may be required. Even slow egress of CSF is problematic, as it can cause tension upon the myocutaneous closure and disrupt wound healing (**Fig. 123.8**).

Skin and Myofascial Closure

The most important and dreaded complications can occur during the final stage, which involves skin and myofascial closure. The true defect of a myelomeningocele is not fully appreciated until the dura is finally closed and the surrounding dermis is evaluated. Simple undermining of the skin is sufficient for small defects with minimal tension. However, in large defects, stay sutures are used in the underlying fascial plane to help approximate the skin. Regardless of the extent of the closure, coagulation or sacrifice of perforating vessels should be minimized so as not to compromise the essential blood supply needed for wound healing. The subcutaneous layer is approximated using interrupted 4-0 Vicryl, and the skin is closed with a running 4-0 nylon. In severe cases of large defects, a bipedicle flap, multiple rotational flaps, or a myocutaneous flap may be needed for closure (**Fig. 123.13**). Myocutaneous flaps offer an advantage because of the vasculature supplying the muscles; the multiple layers of closure, preventing the tension on the final skin layer;

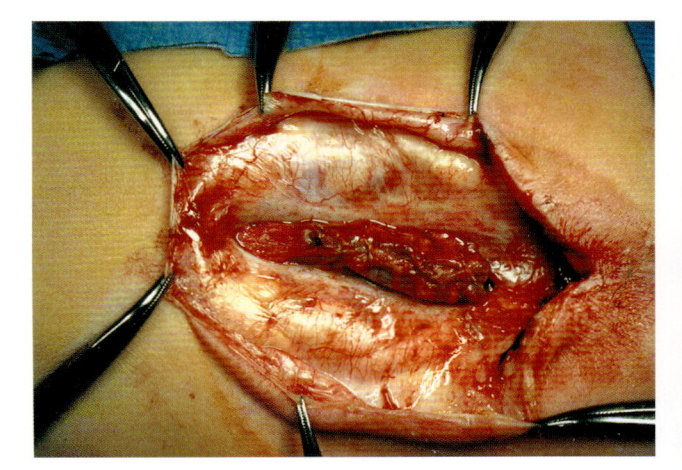

Fig. 123.11 Open myelomeningocele. Attempt at formation of a neural tube with 8-0 microsutures stitching pia to pia. The sensory (dorsal) nerve roots lie on each side of the placode margin. To the right of the image lies the terminal placode. To the left side of the image lies the spinal cord–neural placode transition.

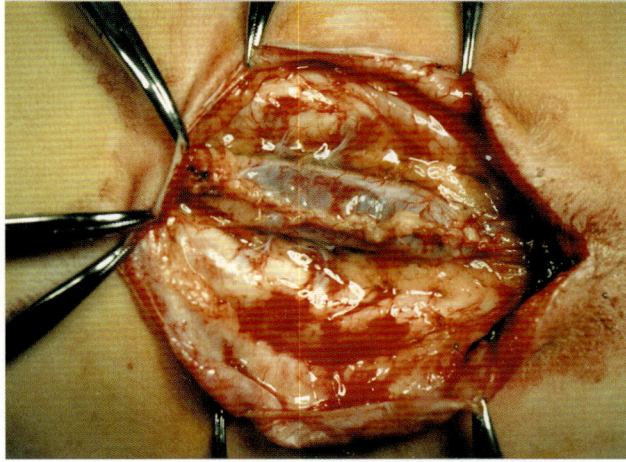

Fig. 123.12 Open myelomeningocele. Closure of the overlying dural tube. The paraspinous muscles and periosteum of the bifid neural arch are exposed on each side of the closed dural tube. The anus is to the right of the figure.

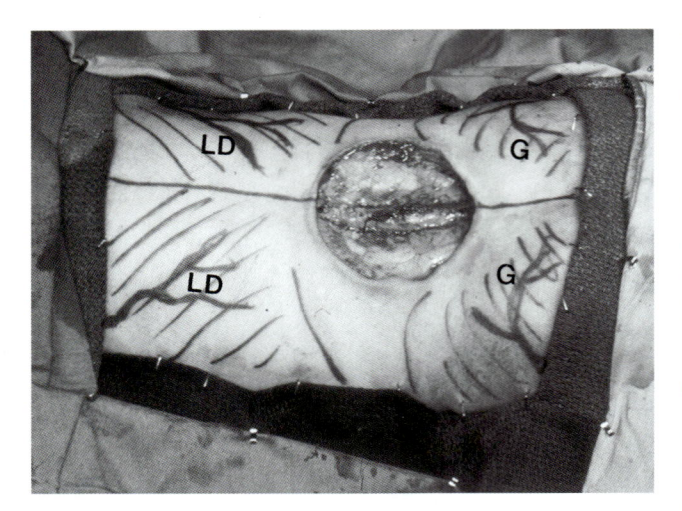

Fig. 123.13 Myocutaneous flaps closure of a large skin defect. The thoracodorsal and gluteal arteries are noted and their respective flaps.

and a blockade preventing CSF leak and formation of a fistula. Closure may be delayed, resulting in a longer duration of general anesthesia; however, the results are favorable. Meticulous hemostasis is essential to prevent seroma or hematoma formation. A drain is rarely used. Plastic surgery assistance is generally not needed; one study reported it was used in only two of 600 patients.[15] Topical nitroglycerin may be used to promote vasodilation in cases of skin tension and blanching. Its use must be carefully monitored in the NICU and removed immediately if hemodynamic instability occurs.

Postoperative Care

Wound care is the most important aspect of postoperative care after surgery. Placement of Xeroform with underlying bacitracin is suggested. Telfa is applied followed by a sterile occlusive dressing using Tegaderm. A mud flap on the caudal aspect of the incision is encouraged to prevent fecal contamination of the wound. The infant is monitored in the NICU for development of hydrocephalus, and is kept prone for the first week and then placed in the lateral position until sutures are removed 14 days after surgery. Postoperative antibiotics are suggested for 24 hours after surgery and prolonged in cases of higher risk of infection. Urologic care is essential, as increased bladder pressure also places increased pressure on the wound. Straight cauterization or Foley placement is suggested.

Developing hydrocephalus commonly needs to be addressed in the postoperative period. VP shunt placement remains a comorbid condition associated with repair of myelomeningocele defects. Ventricular shunt placement is reported in 75 to 92% of patients with postnatal myelomeningocele repair.[9,16] Attempts of determining predictors of the need for VP shunt include fontanelle assessment and an increased rate of 3 mm/day head growth.[16] In studies of long-term management of hydrocephalus, over 64% of infants with open myelomeningocele repair and shunt placement experience initial shunt failure, with a median time of 300 days postoperatively, and up to a quarter of these failures are due to shunt infection.[17] Placement of a VP shunt prior to, during, or after the myelomeningocele defect repair is open to much debate. Radmanesh et al[18] reported a series of 127 infants with open myelomeningocele defects; 65 patients had shunt placement after repair of the open tube defect, 46 patients underwent shunt placement concurrently with repair of the defect, nine patients had only shunt placement, and seven underwent shunt placement first. There was no statistical difference in infection rate between patients who underwent shunt placement concurrently with the repair of the open myelomeningocele defect and patients who underwent shunt placement after the repair. However, infants who underwent only shunt placement or infants whose initial procedure was placement of shunt rather than repair of the myelomeningocele defect had a higher rate of infection and mortality. A general consensus supports the timely placement of a ventricular shunt system in patients with evident hydrocephalus, as it is generally a precursor to increased tension along the wound.

Complications

Operative mortality is low in infants undergoing open myelomeningocele repair.[7] Wound dehiscence is the most common complication, and it occurs during the first week postoperatively. There have been some reports in the literature that defects greater than 44 cm^2 have higher wound tension and increased in CSF morbidity.[19] It is not uncommon to see dark red along the suture line, which may be due to venous stasis that resolves after several days. Sloughing of the epidermis and dermal layers heals by secondary intention. However, if full-thickness necrosis occurs, reconstruction with a flap may be needed. A demarcation between healthy and necrotic tissue forms. Eventually the skin sloughs away from the midline suture associated with fat necrosis and exudate along the incision. If full-thickness necrosis occurs and the dura is exposed, operative measures must be taken to prevent meningitis and desiccation. It is important that the infant is obtaining adequate nutrition in the immediate postoperative period to promote wound healing.[7]

Wound Infection

An open defect with an exposed neural placode at birth would suggest that wound infection would be a common complication in spinal dysraphism repair. If repair occurs within 48 hours of birth, the rate of infection is much lower. Intradural infections occur more often than extradural infections. A contributing factor in intradural infections is a large neural sac with multiple membranes. Upon closure of the neural tube, the redundant membranes are discarded, but recontamination occurs due to the additional neural folds. In the setting of meningitis, there are early signs of poor feeding and lethargy occurring 1 to 3 days after closure. Formation of an intradural abscess is not as common but may occur. If infection or intradural abscess is suspected, prompt diagnosis with a CSF sample from a ventricular shunt or external drain is crucial. If an infection is expected in the intradural space, the wound will often be elevated, become fluctuant, and express purulence. The skin may also become erythematous and edematous. It is very important to note that the infant may not have signs of systemic infection. Prompt identification is necessary to aspirate the material, irrigate with antibiotic solution, and close with suction drains if an infection is found. A new flap may be needed to bring a new vascular supply to the healing wound. Dura may or may not be needed depending on whether there is suspicion of an intradural abscess. If a ventricular system was already placed, it will need to be removed. Broad-spectrum antibiotics are started.

Cerebrospinal Fluid Leakage

The dura in a neonate is thin, and careful closure is of the utmost importance. Common areas of dural defect occur at the lateral aspect of the dural attachment to the periosteal defects of the vertebrae. A small amount of transdural CSF may leak through the suture holes and is self-limited. It is common to have slight fullness of the skin flap during the first 1 to 3 postoperative days. This is attributed to venous stasis but may also be due to an accumulation of CSF. If CSF is suspected and fluid leaks through the skin barrier, immediate treatment and antibiotics must be initiated. An external ventricular drain should be considered to divert CSF flow to an external source, allowing time for the wound to heal. The skin edges can be re-sutured and the incision monitored. Most leaks are managed without reoperation. If leaking continues despite placement of an external ventricular drain, reoperation and exploration of the dural sac is done for primary repair.

Open Myelomeningocele with Segmental Placode

The presence of a normal spinal cord within a segment of the neural placode is termed segmental placode (**Fig. 123.14**). The mechanism is unknown, but this is recognized to occur in 10 to 15% of all open neural tube defects during primary neurulation.[7] The importance of this finding is crucial to the surgeon preoperatively so that during dissection, normal neural tissue is handled with care. This finding is often associated with other congenital malformations such as split cord malformation and spinal cord lipomas. MRI may be needed prior to surgical intervention. A segmental placode is most likely to be identified in the midthoracic or thoracolumbar region. A careful neurologic examination is essential for discovery of these segments of normal neural tissue; distal lower extremity motor function should be a clue that there may be normal neural tissue distal to the open defect. The surgical planning and approach for a segmental placode is similar to an open myelomeningocele. The continuous closure of the remaining "tubular" neural placode with the segmental placode should be attempted. The initial goal of repair of an open myelomeningocele at birth is to prevent infection and to attempt to preserve as much neural tissue as possible; a tethered cord or lipoma may need to be repaired at a later time.

Open Myelomeningocele and Kyphectomy

Along with failure of neural tube formation, varying degrees of the support system of the spinal column may be defective as well. Failure of vertebral arch formation and defective paraspinal musculature can lead to kyphosis of the thoracolumbar spine, which is reported in 21% of patients with myelomeningocele defects.[20,21] Treatment of these patients is essential due to the associated comorbid medical conditions, such as decreased lung capacity; respiratory distress leading to fatal pneumonia; decreased abdominal volume; urogenital and skin complications, including infections, pressure ulcers, and sores; and underlying osteomyelitis.[21] Rehabilitation after repair of an open myelomeningocele is essential to providing an adequate quality of life. Severe kyphosis must be addressed and corrected to facilitate these needs. Nonoperative management including bracing for these infants is generally not successful.[22]

Upon assessment of an infant with an open myelomeningocele defect, overlying kyphosis should be suspected in those with obvious abnormal spinal curvature and those with a worse neurologic exam than one would expect. Lateral radiographs are used for appropriate assessment prior to surgical intervention in the neonate (**Fig. 123.15**). Carstens et al[20] analyzed a series of 719 patients with open myelomeningoceles and found that 151 had lumbar kyphosis. The kyphosis was categorized into three groups: paralytic, sharp-angled, and congenital. The mechanisms involved included normal spine curvature with failure of adequate paraspinal muscle formation leading to spinal instability, curvature > 90 degrees with unopposed pathological muscles (e.g., psoas muscle), and vertebral anomalies that fail to form a normal spinal column. The degree of kyphosis may worsen with age.[20] If extensive spinal correction is needed due to underlying scoliosis or kyphosis, which is commonly the case, major corrective surgery is postponed until the infant enters childhood.

The primary goal of the initial repair of an open myelomeningocele defect is closure of the neural tube to prevent CSF leak and subsequently to decrease infection. Ensuring an adequate skin closure is crucial to a successful surgery. However, if the underlying kyphosis prevents adequate closure, resection will need to be pursued during the initial surgery. Postoperative complications after correction of kyphosis in the setting of myelomeningocele repair has been reported as high as 90%.[23–26] Complications include high blood loss, longer anesthesia times, hardware failure requiring removal, delayed wound healing, and disruption of CSF flow requiring the use of a shunt or reevaluation of a shunt system. Some patients died.

After the initial surgical dissection of a neural placode, as described earlier in this chapter, the rostral dural sac of the normal spinal cord is identified (**Fig. 123.16**). This portion of

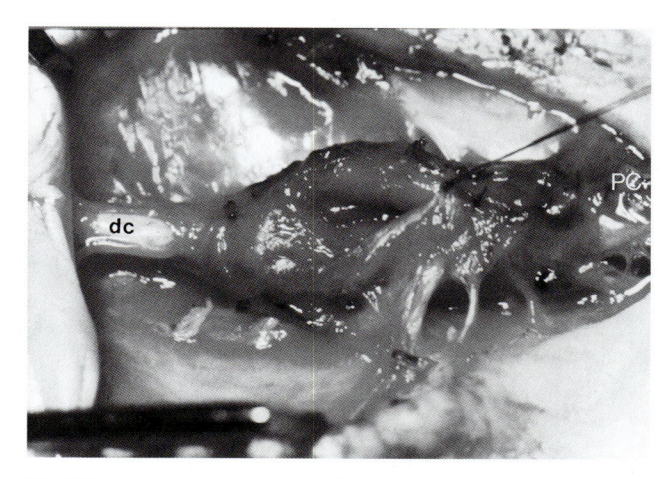

Fig. 123.14 Open myelomeningocele with segmental neural placode. The neural placode has been rolled up and sutured. The placode lies between the fully neurulated proximal cord *(PC)* and equally well-neurulated distal cord *(dc)*.

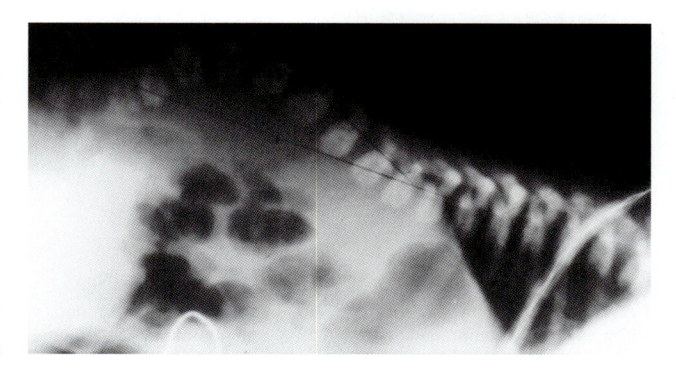

Fig. 123.15 Thoracolumbar kyphosis. Lateral radiograph demonstrating multiple vertebral bodies involved in the kyphotic deformity.

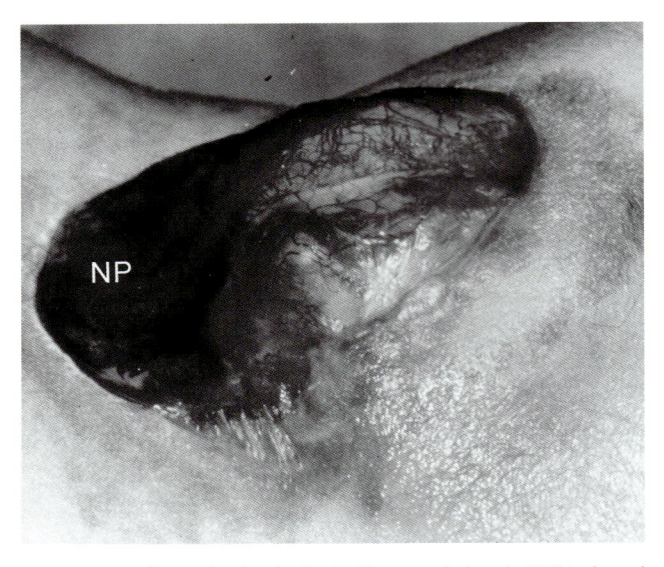

Fig. 123.16 Thoracolumbar kyphosis. The neural placode (NP) is draped over the kyphotic deformity. This neural placode lacks a true cyst or sac.

the spinal cord proximal to the kyphectomy is ligated. There has been discussion in the literature that ligation of the distal sac prevents CSF leak and helps with wound healing, whereas preservation may decrease the rate of excess CSF accumulation, leading to shunt failure and hydrocephalus.[25,27] The vertebral body segments and posterior elements undergo periosteal dissection, removing all musculocutaneous tissue, ligament, veins, and dura (**Fig. 123.17**). All intervertebral disks in the involved area are removed. The anterior great vessels and organs should be appreciated. Once all the tissue has been removed and the end plates cleared, wire loops are used to facilitate fusion (**Figs. 123.18 and 123.19**). During the initial reconstruction, the wire loops are placed under a tremendous amount of tension. Adequate purchase of hard bone is needed rather than cartilaginous or soft bone, as the multiple stressors of the newborn place distracting tension on the wire loops, resulting in shortening of the wires and failure of repair. Placement in a surgical brace postoperatively for 6 months to 2 years may be necessary. The use of anterior or posterior fusion, anterior or posterior plates, Harrington rods, the Galveston technique, Dunn-McCarthy fixation, cables, hooks, wires, pins, transcorporeal screws, and more recently pedicle screws has been described but generally is reserved for large corrections in childhood.[21,28] Although these children undergo

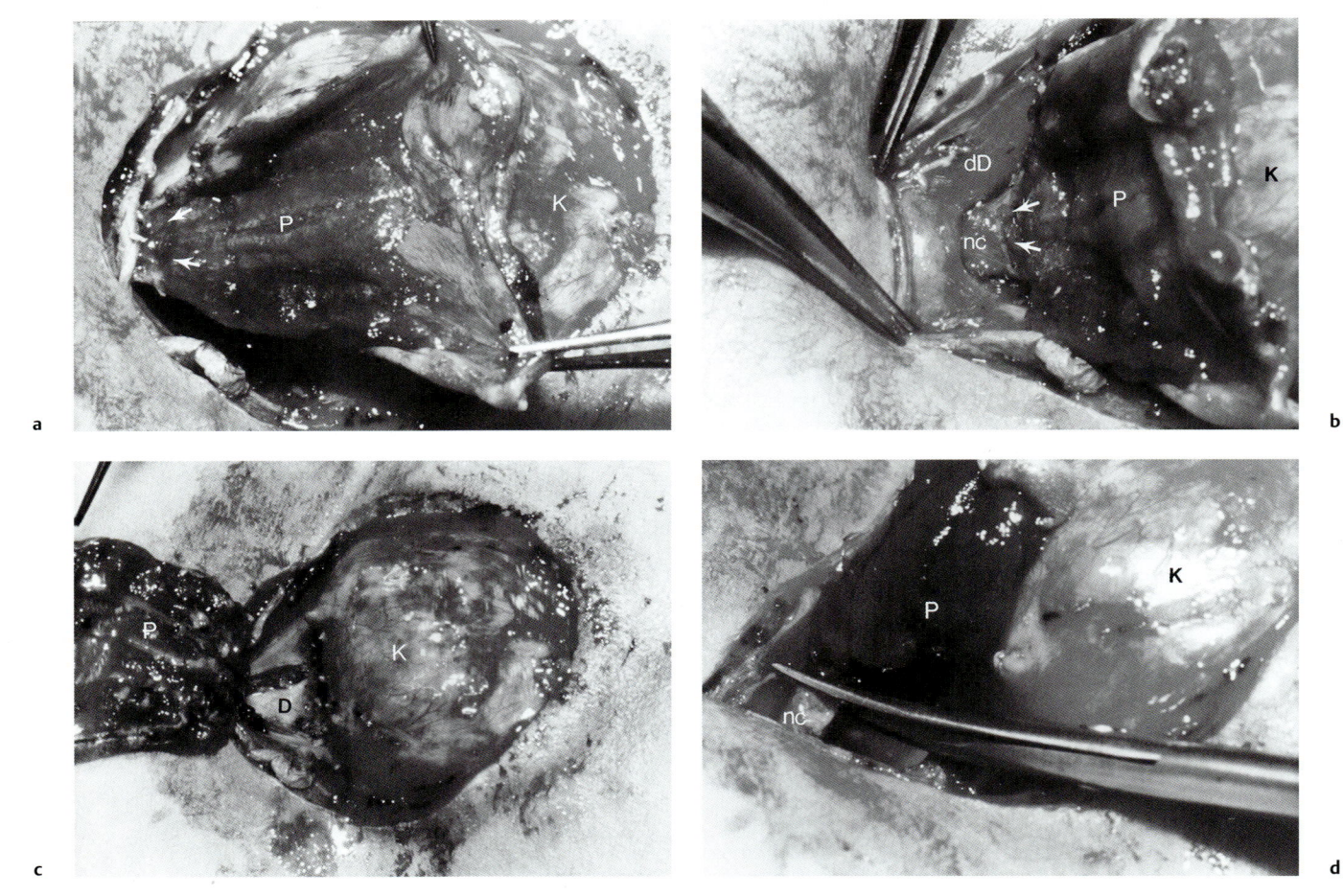

Fig. 123.17 Open myelomeningocele with a kyphos. **(a)** The surrounding leptomeningeal membrane is removed and a thin neural placode is dissected and held with forceps. **(b)** Rostral view reveals a normal cord and the cord–neural placode transition. **(c)** The neural placode is flipped up to reveal the ventral dura extending over the kyphotic deformity. **(d)** The thin neural placode is resected from normal cord. K, kyphos; P, placode; nc, normal cord; D, ventral dura; dD, dorsal dura; *white arrows* point to cord-placode transition.

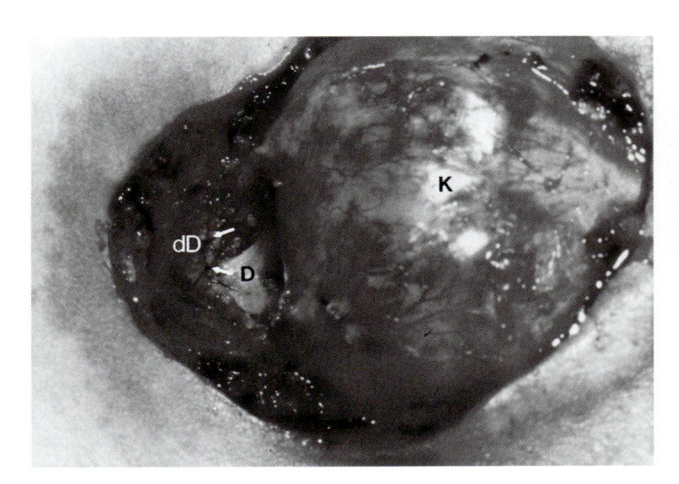

Fig. 123.18 Open myelomeningocele with kyphos (K). The neural placode has been resected. Dorsal dura (dD) and ventral dura (D) have been closed with sutures (arrows) to form a blind stump.

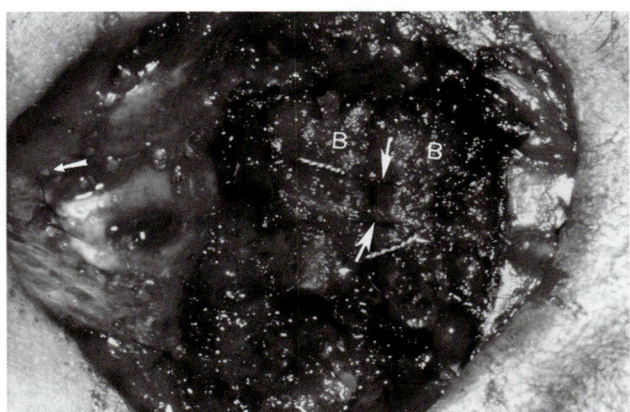

Fig. 123.19 Open myelomeningocele with a kyphos. After removal of the kyphotic deformity, the remaining vertebral bodies (B) are stabilized using sutured wire loops (large arrows) forced through the bodies by sharp needles. Small arrow points to a blind dural stump.

extensive surgical resection and a long and complicated postoperative course, it has been reported that long-term clinical outcomes, both radiographically and clinically, are excellent and provide a better quality of life.[18,21]

Spinal Cord Lipomas

Spinal cord lipomas most often occur in the lumbosacral region due to a defect in early disjunction during primary neurulation or a defect in secondary neurulation, either in formation of the medullary cord or during retrogressive differentiation. Patients present with an obvious lumbosacral mass or with cutaneous findings such as a rudimentary tail, dermal sinus tract, or focal hirsutism (**Fig. 123.20**). Symptomatic patients may present with neurologic impairment, back and leg pain, urologic dysfunction with either spastic or atonic bladders, or orthopedic malformations. By removing the abnormal fatty tissue and untethering of the spinal cord, neurologic function can be maintained.[29]

Anatomy and Classification

Chapman[30] categorized spinal cord lipomas into three anatomic classifications: dorsal, transitional, and terminal. The common encompassing pathology involves a defect in the dorsal portion of the spinal column and its overlying tissue in the presence of pathological fatty tissue that blends with the spinal cord. The fibro-adipose stalk connects the intramedullary and extradural component of the fatty tissue. The dorsal nerve roots are never encompassed by the fatty tissue; however, the dorsal nerve roots may lie on the ventral or lateral surface of the fatty tissue as the roots travel caudally.[31]

The dorsal lipoma arises from the dorsal aspect of the spinal column and never involves the caudal portion of the cord. Although not directly involved, it may have a thickened filum. The transitional lipoma also involves a portion of the cord similar to that of the dorsal lipoma but also involves the conus. The amount of fatty tissue varies and may result in a rotation of the spinal cord, making dissection difficult. A terminal or caudal lipoma affects the filum and the caudal portion of the conus. It also never involves the spinal cord or dorsal roots. It may attach directly to the spinal cord or be separated by a short thickened filum. In this type, the overlying dura and fascia are intact.[31,32]

Embryogenesis of Spinal Cord Lipomas

Dorsal and transitional lipomas are both thought to be due to a defect in primary neurulation, especially the phase involving disjunction (**Fig. 123.21**). In addition, a defect in secondary neurulation is thought to contribute to formation of a transitional lipoma, given its involvement of the conus. Terminal lipomas are

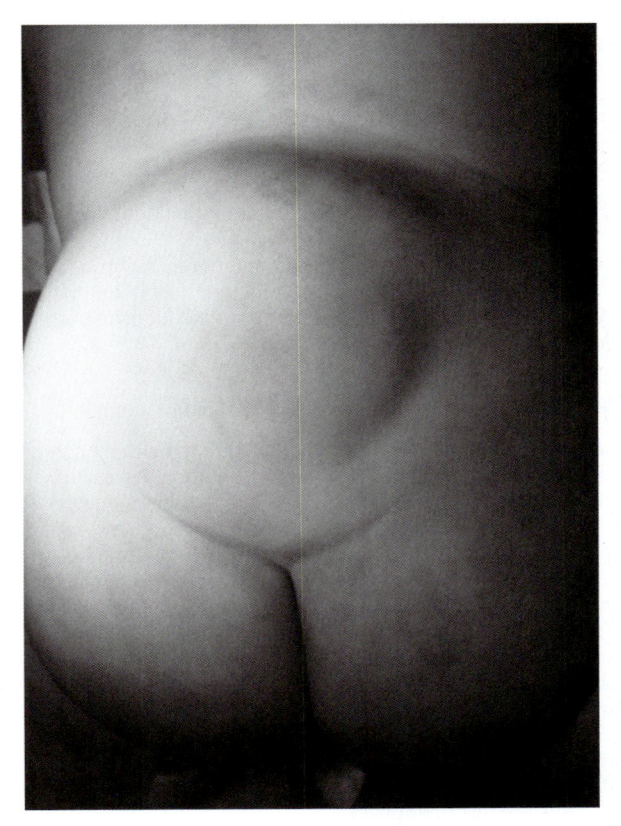

Fig. 123.20 Subcutaneous lipoma overlying dorsal lipoma.

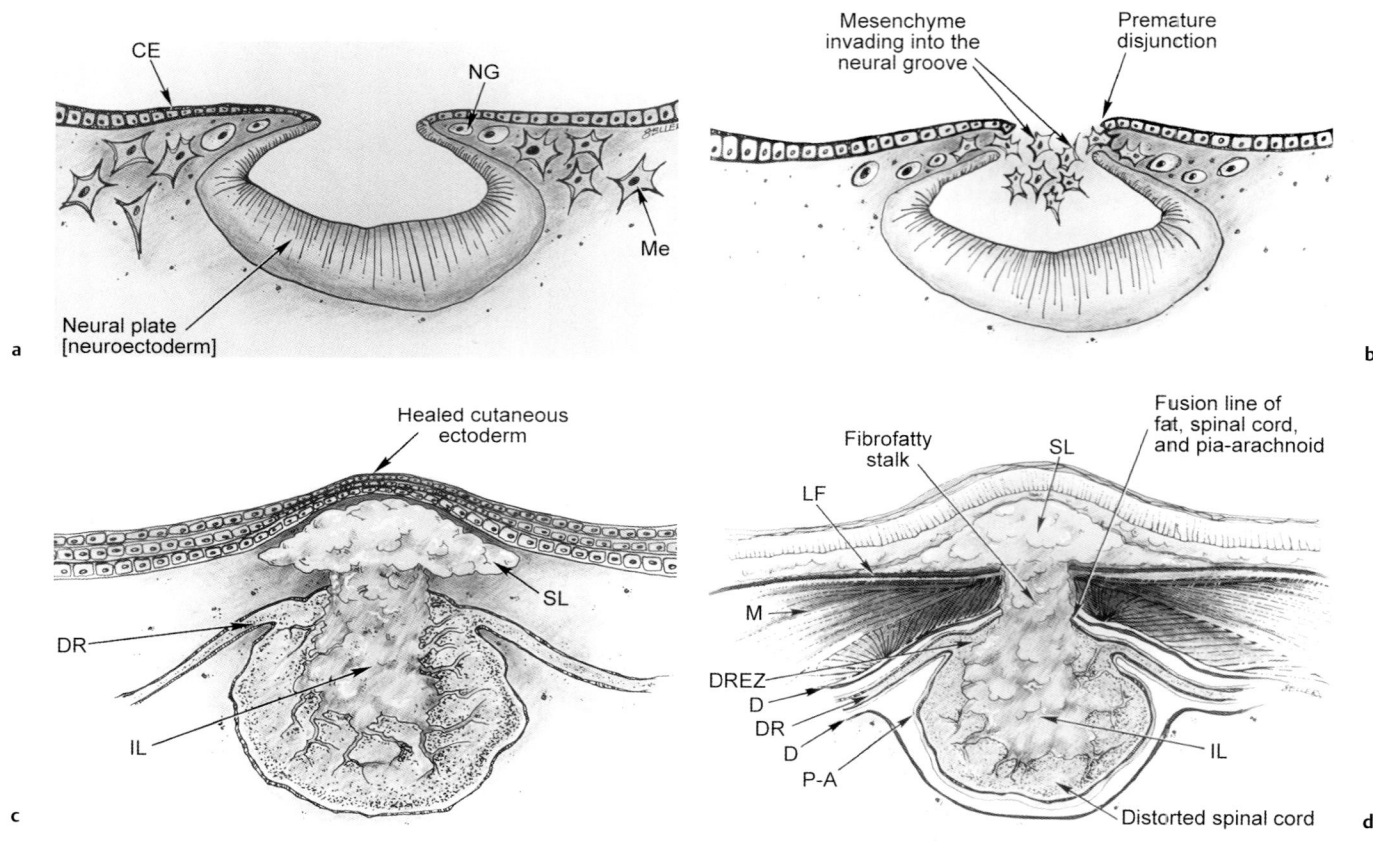

Fig. 123.21 Embryogenesis of dorsal and transitional lipomas. **(a)** The end of the neural tubes migrates toward the midline. At this stage, due to the continuous ectodermal *(CE)* layer, mesenchymal *(Me)* cells are excluded from the neural groove *(NG)*. **(b)** Premature disjunction of cutaneous and neural ectoderms occurs. Mesenchymal cells invade the closing neural folds and enter the central canal of the neural tube. **(c)** Mesenchyme within the central canal form adipose tissue which is continuous with the subcutaneous adipose layer through a fibrofatty stalk. Cutaneous ectoderm heals over the subcutaneous lipoma (SL) to form overlying skin. DR, dorsal root. **(d)** Mesenchymal tissue is induced to form meninges that surround the cord except at the fusion line. Dorsal nerve roots exit from the spinal cord just lateral to the fusion line joining cord, lipoma, and leptomeninges. D, dura; DREZ, dorsal root entry zone; IL, intradural lipoma; LF, lumbar fascia; P-A, pia-arachnoid; SL, subcutaneous lipoma; M, muscle.

thought to be an error in retrogressive differentiation, a specific phase in secondary neurulation. Adequate formation of overlying dura and fascia are evidence of a successful primary phase and the initial secondary phase of neurulation.

Dorsal and Transitional Lipomas

Dorsal and transitional lipomas are thought to be caused by premature disjunction during primary neurulation. As described at the beginning of this chapter (see Normal Embryogenesis), disjunction of the cutaneous and neuroectoderm occurs during the first phase of primary neurulation. Premature disjunction results in incomplete fusion of the neural plate and a dorsal defect that allows mesenchymal cells to enter this abnormal cleft.[32,33] Mesenchymal cells differentiate based on the adjacent neuroectoderm. In this case, the neuroectoderm promotes differentiation of the mesenchymal cells in the abnormal cleft into pathological adipose tissue. Mesenchymal cells ventral to the neuroectoderm differentiate into meninges that still form but fail to fuse at the dorsal midline, along with the overlying muscle and fascia. The dural defect allows a fibrofatty stalk to form that connects the intramedullary and extramedullary adipose tissue that is tethered to the subcutaneous tissue.

Another key finding in dorsal and transitional lipomas involves the location of the dorsal root ganglion. The space between the lipoma and dorsal root ganglion is referred to as the fusion line. Due to incomplete fusion of the neural folds, the dorsal root ganglion remains open in a ventrolateral position from its intended position. The dorsal root entry zone is the location of the dorsal root ganglion lateral to the fusion line.

Dorsal lipomas are similar in characteristics to that of a segmental placode: normal neural tissue rostral and caudal to the defect. Unlike dorsal lipomas, transitional lipomas extend caudally to involve the conus due to an error in secondary neurulation. Secondary neurulation is much less understood and disorganized in comparison to primary neurulation. What is called a "chaotic" lipoma arises from fat that is present on both the dorsal and ventral aspect of the neural placode, as described by Pang et al.[34]

Terminal Lipoma

Formation of a terminal lipoma is thought to be due to failure of retrogressive differentiation in the last stage of secondary neurulation. Because primary neurulation is not responsible for this defect, terminal lipomas never involve the lumbar or upper

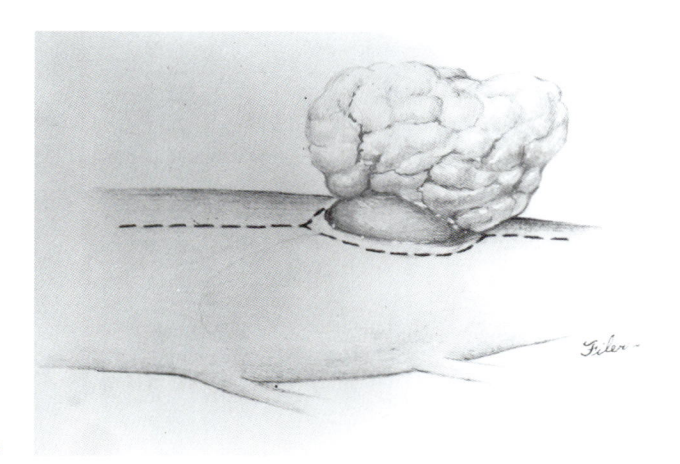

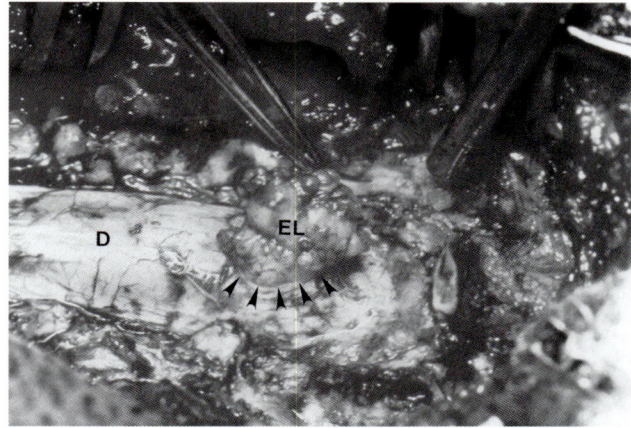

Fig. 123.22 Dorsal lipoma. **(a)** A discrete circumferential midline defect reveals the extradural component of the lipoma. **(b)** Intraoperative view of dural defect *(D)* with an extradural lipoma *(EL)* outlined by *arrowheads*.

sacral portions of the cord. Terminal lipomas either replace or form a portion of the thickened filum. Due to the disorganized and not well understood nature of secondary neurulation, it is not completely unexpected that multiple tissues of mesodermal origin may be identified as the result of the failed apoptosis of these tissues.

Operative Treatment

General anesthesia is induced and the patient is placed prone with the standard pressure points protected. A midline incision is made in both the rostral and caudal orientation above the lesion. A scalpel is used to incise the skin, and the subcutaneous adipose tissue is debulked with scissors and electrocautery. The key to a successful lipoma repair is the identification of the fusion line. The fusion line is the exact location where the fat, spinal cord, and meningeal layers meet. Working medial to the fusion line prevents the involvement of the dorsal root entry zone and potential neurologic morbidity. Although their benefit remains unclear, the use of intraoperative monitoring with rectal electromyography (EMG), urethral EMG, somatosensory evoked potentials (SSEPs), and rectal and bladder pressures continues to be debated.[29]

Dorsal Lipoma

When planning surgical resection of a dorsal lipoma, the normal cord is easily identified in both the rostral and caudal orientation (**Fig. 123.22**). The dorsal root entry zone is identified lateral to the fusion line. The fibrofatty stalk and the circular dural defect surrounding the stalk are identified. In some circumstances, the rostral intradural portion of the fibrofatty stalk has migrated upward with the spinal cord in relationship to the dural opening. Careful attention should be paid to elevating the dura, as it may be adherent at the fusion line (**Figs. 123.23 and 123.24**).

After removal of the subcutaneous fat, the fascial defects are widened, and periosteal dissection of the paraspinal muscles is performed along the lamina in both the rostral and caudal direction. The lamina one level above and one level below the lipoma is removed. The dura is then cut open with enough room to expose the fusion line and dorsal root entry zone. The lipoma is removed with a cut along the fusion line. Then attention

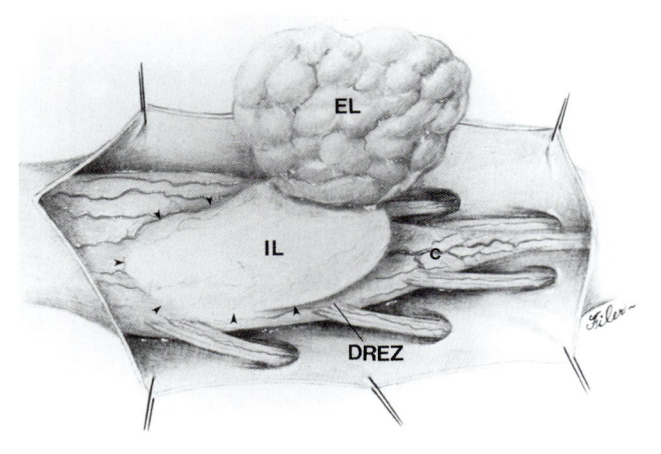

Fig. 123.23 Dorsal lipoma. **(a)** Drawing of the extradural and intradural component of the lipoma. **(b)** A circumferential fusion line (outlined by *arrowheads*) between fat, pia-arachnoid, and the spinal cord. The dorsal root entry zone (DREZ) and dorsal rootlets are lateral to the fusion line. C, conus; EL, extradural lipoma; IL, intradural lipoma.

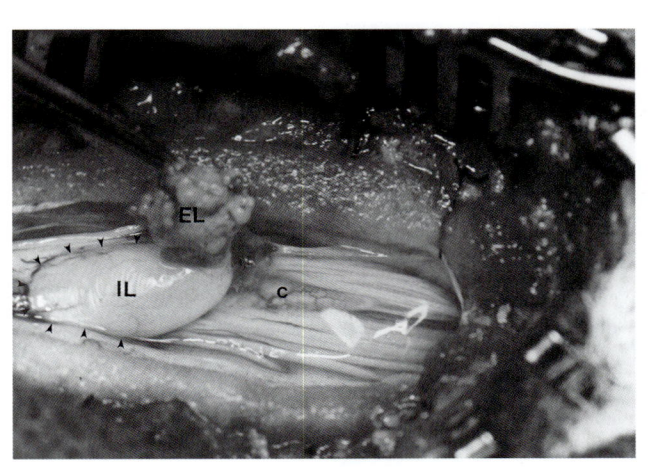

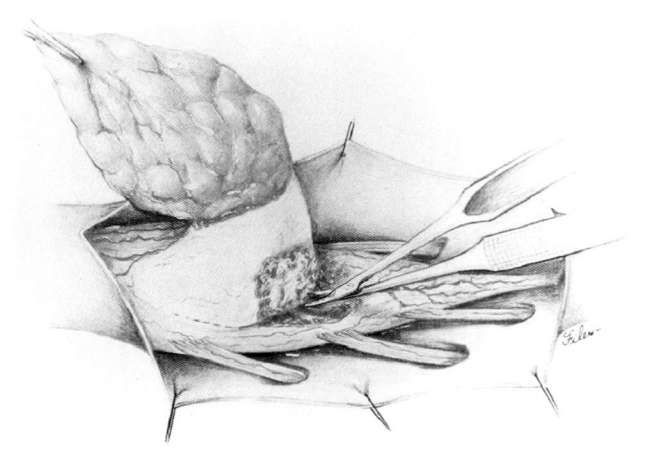

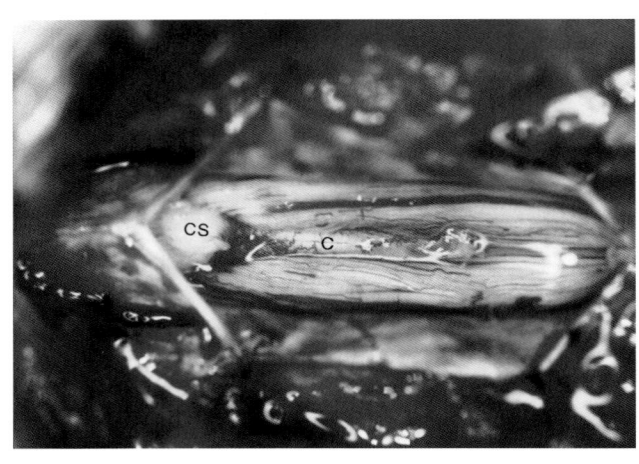

Fig. 123.24 Dorsal lipoma. **(a)** Resection of the lipomatous stalk. Note that the stalk is medial to the fusion line. **(b)** Intraoperative postresection of the cut surface *(CS)* of lipoma stump and normal conus *(C)* distally.

is turned toward identifying the filum; if it is thickened, it is divided.

Transitional Lipoma

The dissection and removal of the rostral portion of a transitional lipoma is the same as for a dorsal lipoma (**Figs. 123.25 and 123.26**). Continued appreciation of the fusion line and lateral dorsal root entry zone is important. However, at the caudal portion of the transitional lipoma, the fusion line is displaced ventrally and in an oblique fashion as the lipoma invades the terminal conus (**Fig. 123.27**). Although the transitional lipoma may be rotated and although it may be difficult to identify the fusion line, the dorsal nerve roots are never involved within the fatty tissue. It is common to find asymmetry of the lipoma not only in the rostral and caudal orientation but on either side of the spinal cord. Physical examination findings of worsening deficits in one lower extremity may correspond to a more aggressive lipoma infiltration or a more ventrally oriented lipoma on that particular side. It is generally easier to advance from a rostral to caudal dissection and then to the side of less invasion of the lipoma. Freeing the easier side facilitates rotating the cord as the

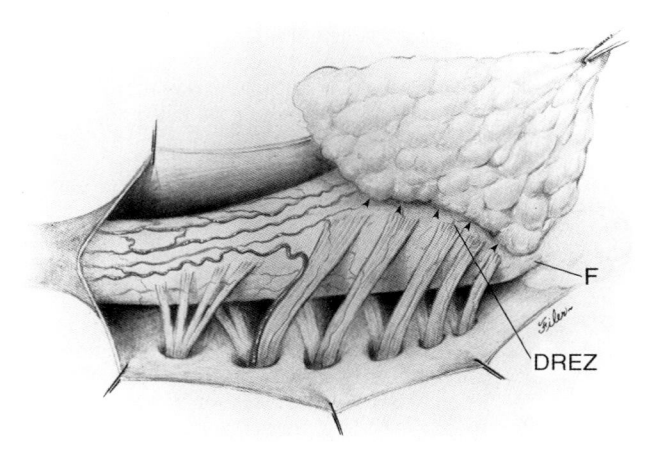

Fig. 123.25 Transitional lipoma. Caudally the lipoma merges with general extradural fat. The oblique fusion line stretches from a rostral-dorsal point to a caudal-ventral point at the tip of the conus. The fat involves most of the distal conus, but a discrete filum (F) is still identified. DREZ, dorsal root entry zone.

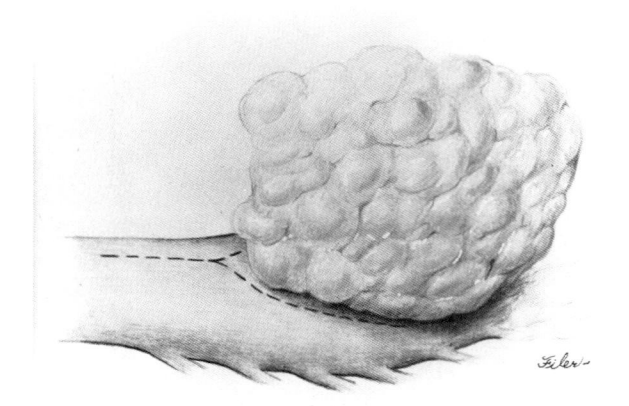

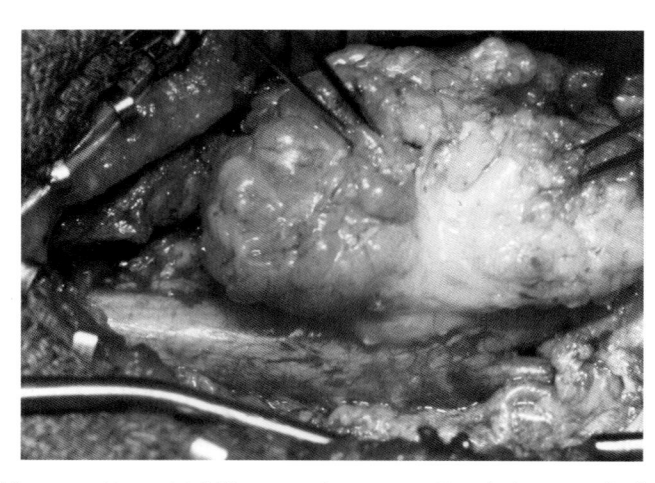

Fig. 123.26 Transitional lipoma. **(a)** The planned dural opening *(dashed line)* from rostral to caudal. **(b)** Intraoperative exposure. Note the large extradural fat. The dural and lipoma planes blend together, making dissection challenging.

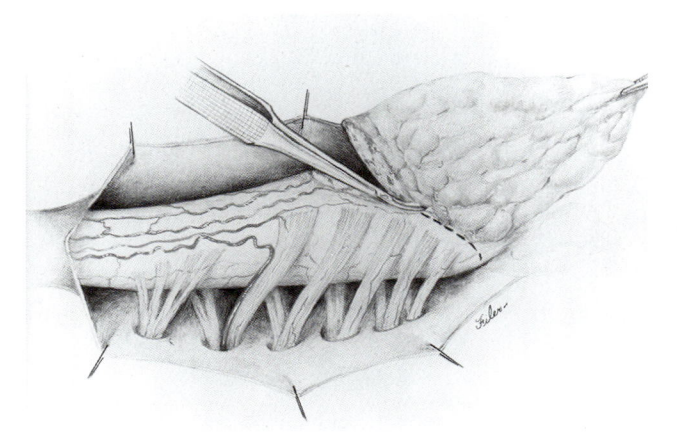

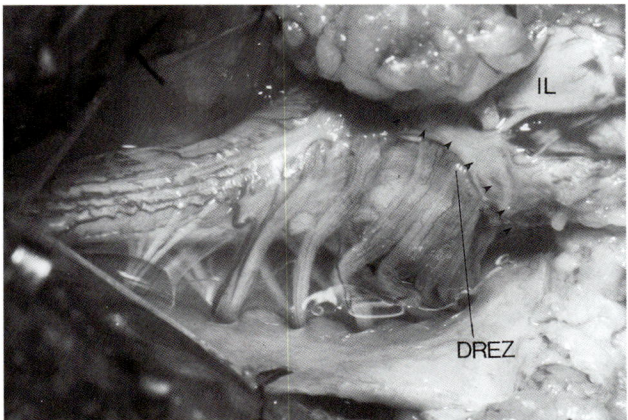

Fig. 123.27 Transitional lipoma. **(a)** The fusion line *(dashed line)*. There is always a distinct plane between fat and the spinal cord. **(b)** Intraoperative view of the fusion line *(arrowheads)* and DREZ just outside of the fusion line.

side with more fatty infiltration is dissected. It is important to note that ventral to the fusion line is the dorsal root entry zone and ventral CSF. When removing the fibrofatty stalk, a sharp cut is made in the dorsoventral oblique plane in the rostral to caudal direction **(Fig. 123.28)**. The thickened filum at the ventral portion of the neural placode is cut. The neural placode is rolled into its natural "tubular" orientation and closed with 8-0 nylon sutures. Suture tension should not be constricting to reduce the risk of re-tethering. A dural graft is used to create a large dural sac.[7,31,34]

Terminal Lipoma

The dura and posterior superficial layers involved with a terminal lipoma remain intact and there is no adherence between the lipoma and dura **(Fig. 123.29)**. The terminal lipoma is either a direct extension of the conus or separated by a short segment of thickened filum **(Figs. 123.30 and 123.31)**. In the direct extension variation of terminal lipoma, the lipoma is easily identified as adipose tissue due to its inherent yellow color versus the pink, velvety appearance of the spinal cord. When a filum separates the conus from the terminal lipoma, it may be difficult to identify the beginning of the lipoma. However, as with the dorsal and transitional lipoma, the terminal lipoma is never involved at the dorsal root entry zone. Noting the location of the sacral nerve roots helps in identifying the conus. Care must be taken during dissection of the nerve roots as they may come in contact with the ventral or lateral surface of the lipoma.

After initial dissection at the rostral portion of the lipoma, the next incision is made at the conus–lipoma junction. The filum is identified and pulled in the rostral direction. The ventral veins and filum are then coagulated. The shortening of these structures causes an instantaneous tension between the conus and lipoma that can be detrimental. The cord should be rendered without tension to prevent this from occurring.[31,34] Once the vein and filum are coagulated and cut, the tension resolves, and the filum and the conus are free **(Fig. 123.32)**. The distal lipoma is cut and removed. The dura is closed primarily.

Outcome

Lipoma resection can be accomplished with minimal morbidity. Patients who are symptomatic are candidates for surgery. However, improvement of already lost neurologic function is unlikely to occur.[29,35] The sharp, radicular, perineal pain diminishes within the first 3 months but many patients will be left with back pain. Improvement in sensorimotor function is mixed, but the progression of symptoms is often halted. New neurologic and urologic

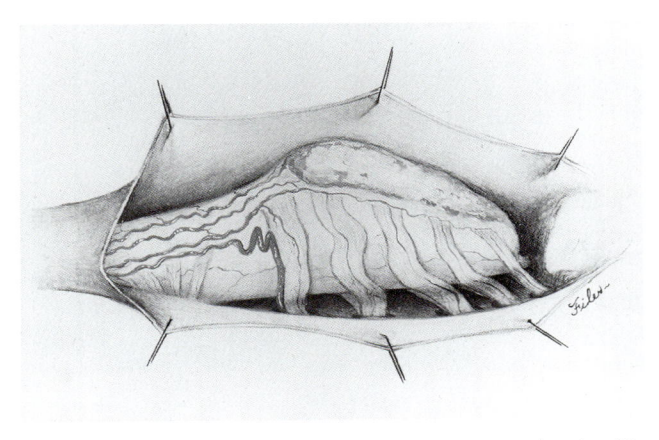

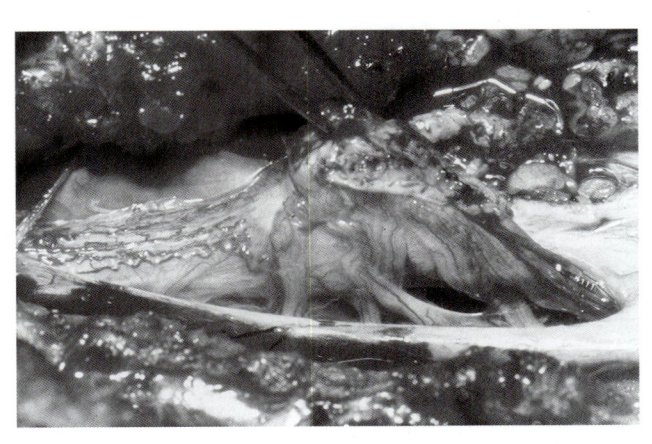

Fig. 123.28 Transitional lipoma. **(a)** Removal of lipoma revealing the oblique surface of the neural placode. **(b)** Intraoperative view.

784 V Lumbar and Lumbosacral Spine

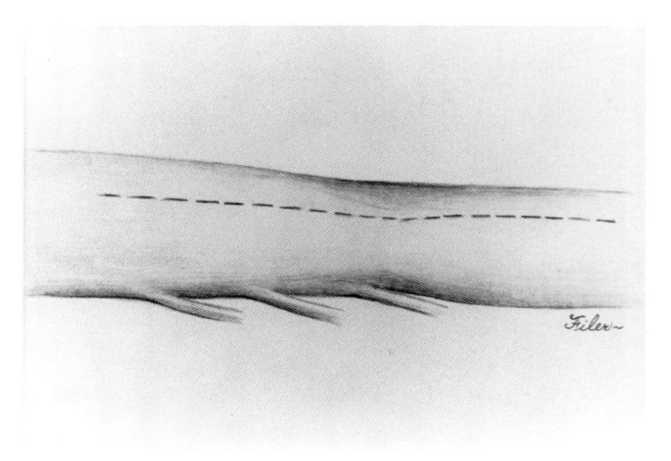

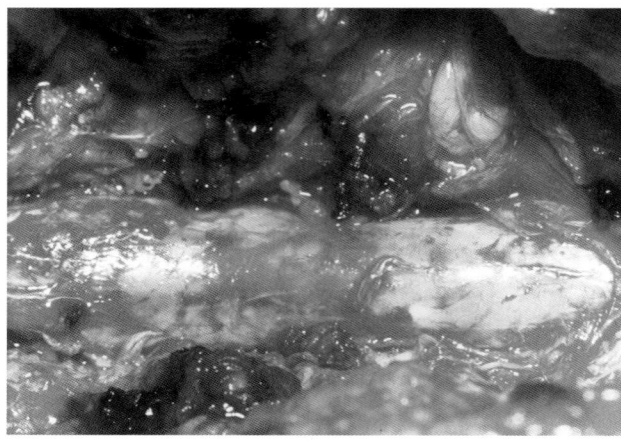

Fig. 123.29 Terminal lipoma. **(a)** Dural opening *(dashed line)*. **(b)** Intraoperative view of dural opening

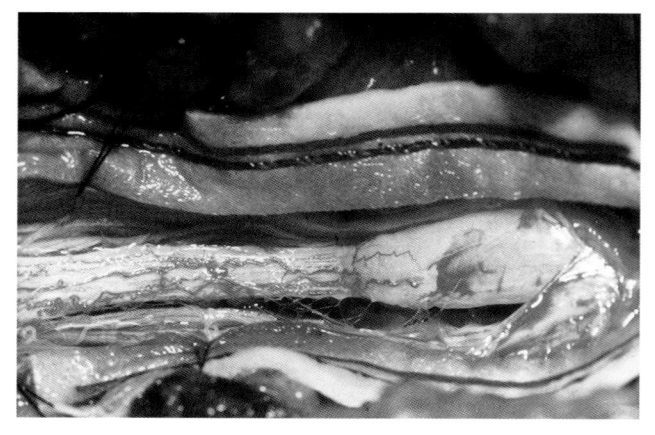

Fig. 123.30 Terminal lipoma (direct insertion type) revealing a distinct junction between the conus and lipoma. All nerve roots exit rostral to this junction.

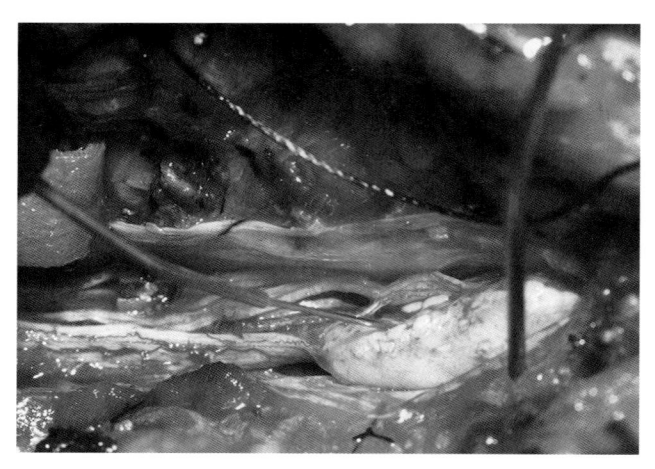

Fig. 123.31 Terminal lipoma (direct insertion type) revealing adjacent and caudal nerve roots that will need to be detached prior to lipoma resection.

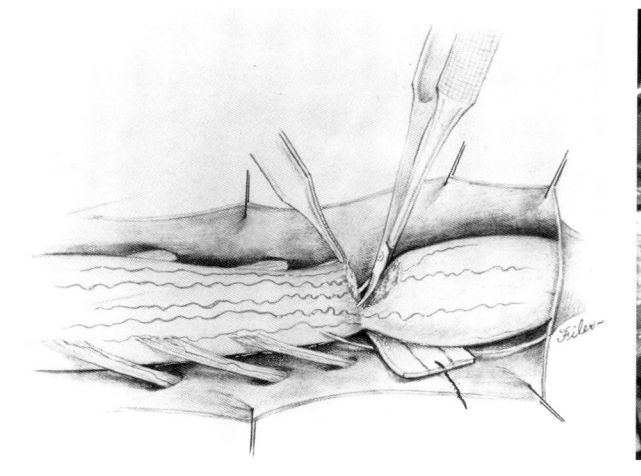

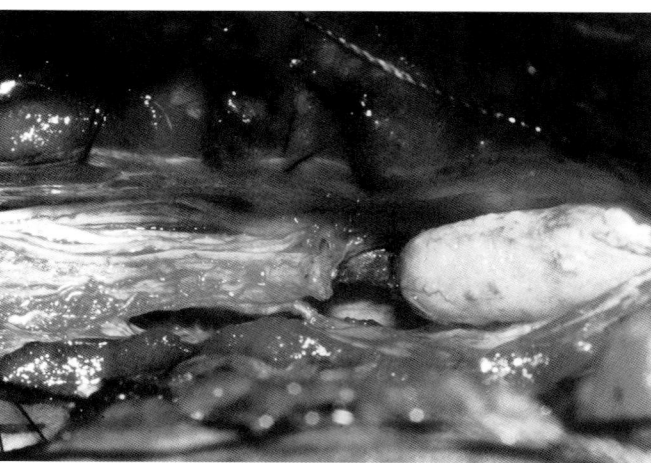

Fig. 123.32 Terminal lipoma. **(a)** Transition line demarcates the separation of the lipoma from the conus. **(b)** The relaxation of the conus vessels after removal of the lipoma.

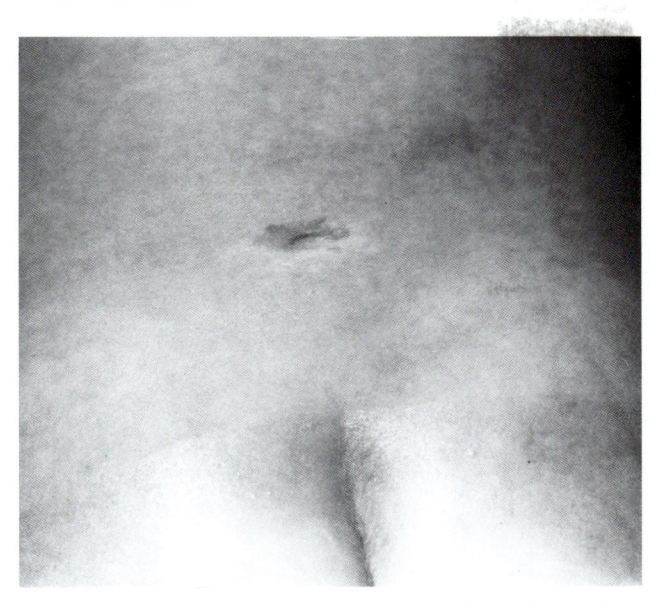

Fig. 123.33 Skin dimple overlying a lumbar limited dorsal myeloschisis with a surrounding capillary hemangioma.

Limited Dorsal Myeloschisis

Limited Dorsal Myeloschisis (LDM) is a form of spinal dysraphism characterized by two primary features: a pseudo-closed small midline skin defect and a fibroneural stalk that links this lesion to the dorsal aspect of the spinal cord via a small dorsal dural opening. LDMs can be thought to occupy a middle ground in the spectrum of spinal dysraphism between the rather extreme open neural tube defect and the more subtle closed anatomic variants that lack apparent signs on skin examination.

A LDM is generally easily identifiable by its cutaneous findings: a flat and thickened skin, a small midline indentation or pit, or a CSF-filled sac with either thick or thin skin on the surface (**Figs. 123.33 and 123.34**).[36,37] The underlying defect extends to the cutaneous ectoderm, preventing full closure of the underlying tissue. As CSF develops around the normal neural tube, it is pushed out of the small dorsal dural defect and frequently distends this fragile skin and forms the CSF-filled sac with overlying skin.[36] Internally, CSF may also distend the most dorsal segments of the fibroneural stalk, resulting in the formation of a myelocystocele (**Fig. 123.35**). In all cases, the dorsal spinal cord is tethered to the dorsal musculature and fascia of the back by the fibroneural stalk and the overlying meninges. Neurologic deficits associated with LDMs primarily develop due to this tethering effect. LDMs are most frequently found in the thoracolumbar and lumbar spine. Cervical LDMs, although rare, also cause hydrocephalus and Chiari II malformations in about half of all cases.[36]

Embryogenesis of Limited Dorsal Myeloschisis

The embryogenesis involving LDM is due to failure in primary neurulation, specifically during the stage disjunction (**Fig. 123.36**). The neural placode undergoes formation, which entails shaping and bending it. However, the dorsal tube is unable to completely fuse at the midline, and consequently it remains attached to the overlying cutaneous ectoderm. A fibroneural stalk forms between

deficits have been reported to occur in as high as 10% of patients, and even higher in patients with complex anatomy and in patients who require reoperations because the normal dissection planes are obscured.[29,34] The transitional type of lipoma has the worst outcome given its rotational position and its difficult anatomy. CSF leak is the most common complication, occurring in 2 to 47% of lipoma resections.[34] Surgeons are encouraged to obtain a watertight closure and to use dural glues if necessary. Long-term monitoring of bladder function helps determine if further urologic intervention is necessary.

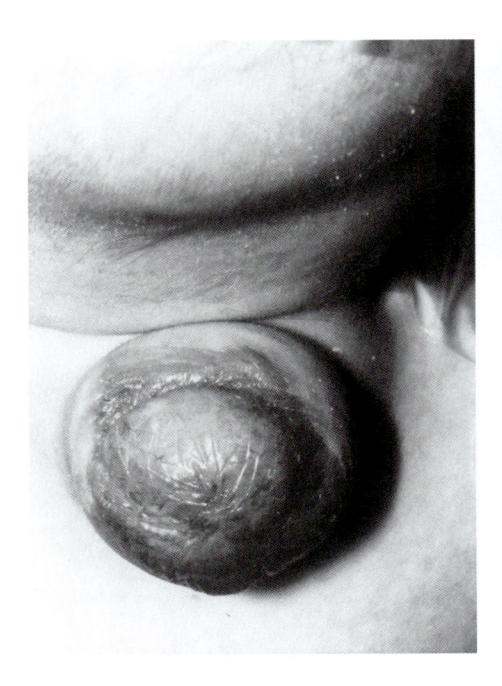

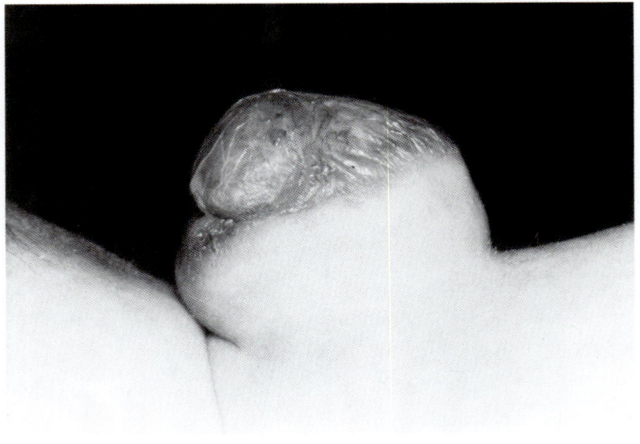

Fig. 123.34 Cervical limited dorsal myeloschisis. Fluctuant fluid-filled prominence that is covered with skin at the base with a thick, purplish squamous epithelial membrane. **(a)** Dorsal view. **(b)** Lateral view.

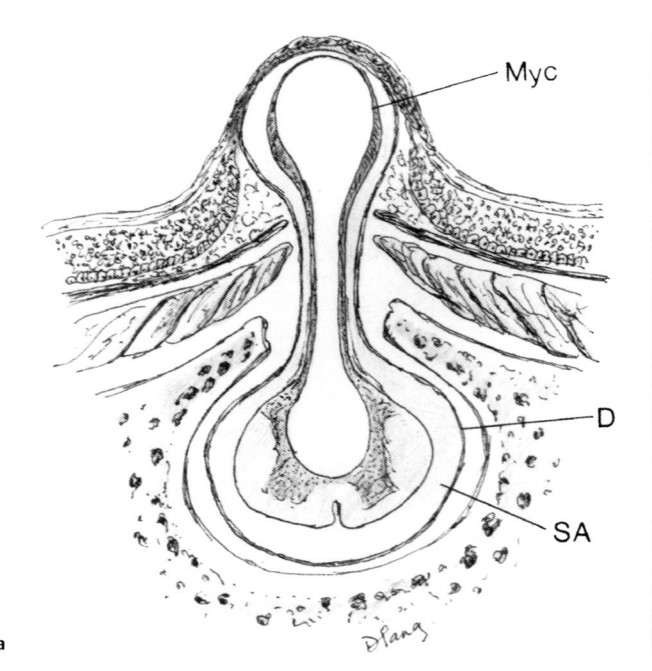

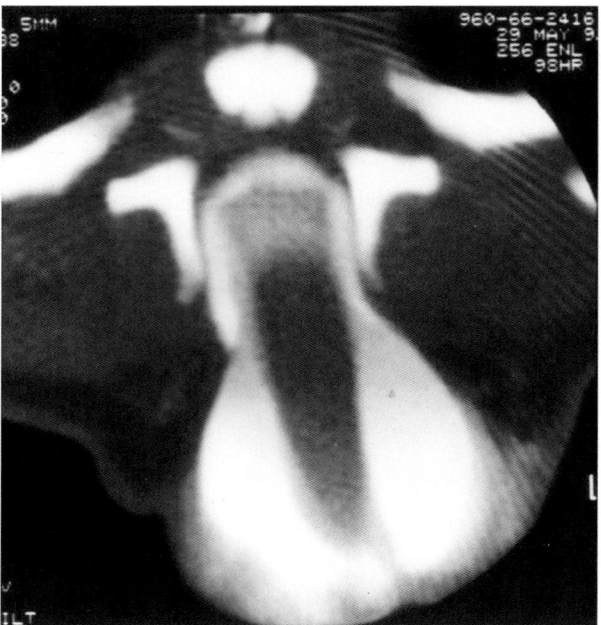

Fig. 123.35 Limited dorsal myeloschisis with myelocystocele. **(a)** A limited dorsal myeloschisis sac that consists of two chambers. The outer chamber is a meningocele continuous with the subarachnoid space of the dural stalk and spinal cord. The inner chamber is the myelocystocele sac continuous with a small hydromyelic distention of the underlying cord. It is lined by an atrophic, ependymal-lined neural membrane. D, dura; Myc, myelocystocele; SA, subarachnoid space. **(b)** Computed tomography (CT) myelogram demonstrating an outer chamber meningocele sac filled with contrast, continuous with spinal subarachnoid space. The inner myelocystocele sac is not contrast filled.

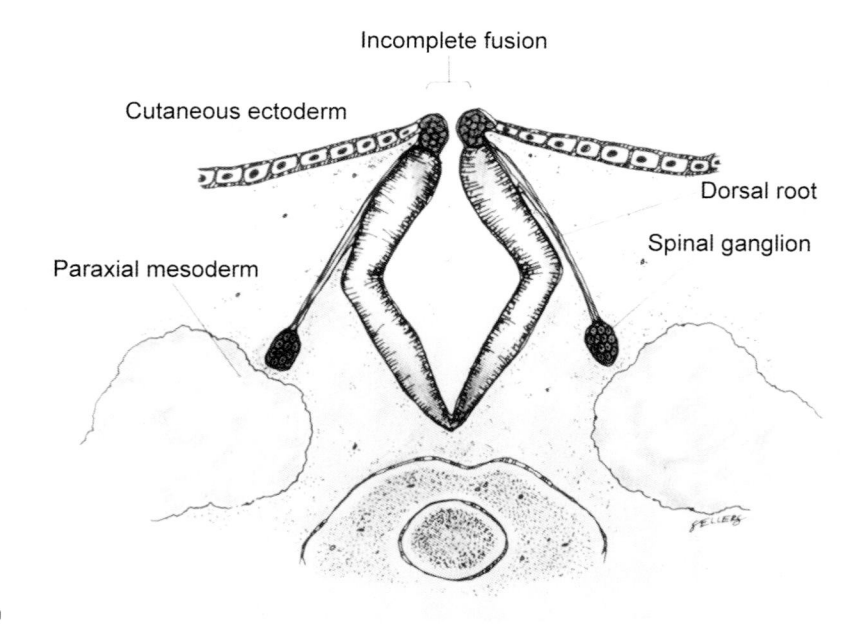

Fig. 123.36 Formation of limited dorsal myeloschisis. **(a)** The dorsal open neural tube remains attached to the overlying skin due to an incomplete dorsal midline fusion and junction between cutaneous and neural ectoderms. Neural crest cells remain and form the dorsal nerve roots and ganglia in the future fibroneural stalk.

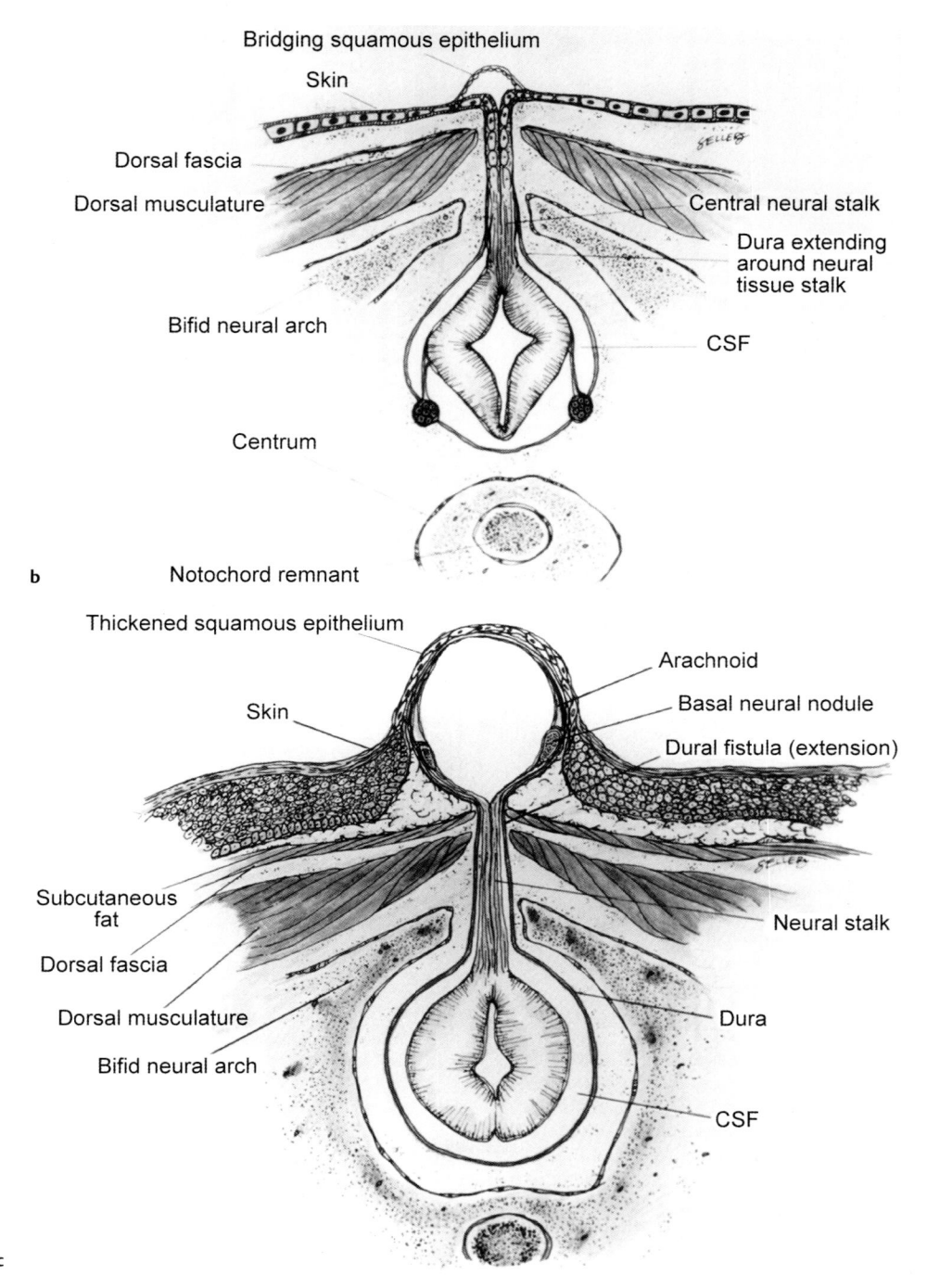

Fig. 123.36 (*continued*) **(b)** Growth of dorsal myofascial tissues progressively displaces the neural tube ventrally away from the skin. The cutaneous-neural attachment remains in position as the lengthening neural stalk containing central and peripheral neural tissues. Squamous epithelium covers the failed overlying gap. **(c)** A skin-covered cerebrospinal fluid (CSF) dome forms that courses around the distal fistula and out the epithelium. The dorsal neural stalk ends in basal neural nodules that mark the original cutaneous-neural attachment. The cord is tethered by this fibroneural stalk.

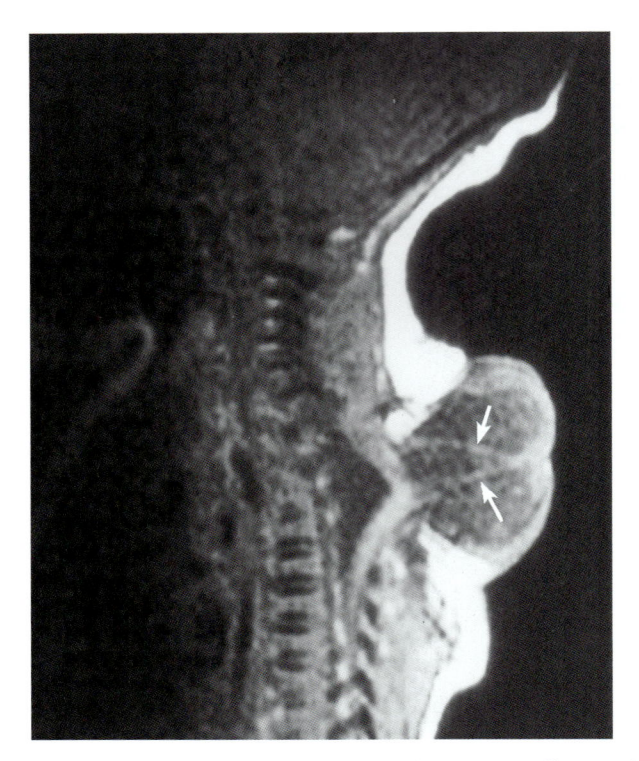

Fig. 123.37 Limited dorsal myeloschisis revealing a narrow fibroneural stalk (arrows) that is visible within the dome of the sac. The underlying cord is tethered up toward the base of the sac.

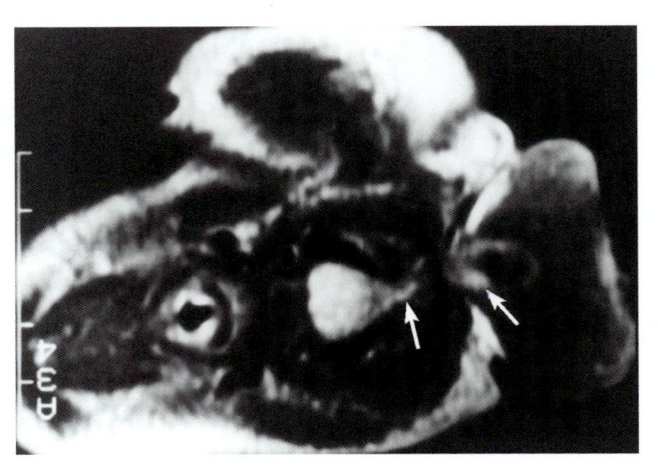

Fig. 123.38 Limited dorsal myeloschisis with basal neural nodule (arrow) on magnetic resonance imaging (MRI). The placode lacks a true cyst or sac.

the dorsal neural tube and the overlying cutaneous ectoderm. The superficial dorsal layers continue to form but are unable to fuse at midline. Normal meninges develop around the neural tube and the fibroneural stalk. CSF may track along this fibroneural stalk, and a saccular balloon of CSF forms on the cutaneous surface. As the CSF builds, the neural tube becomes tethered.

Surgical Indications and Treatment

The primary indication for surgical management of LDMs is elimination of the cord tethering secondary to the tension placed by the fibroneural stalk (**Figs. 123.37 and 123.38**). This tethering effect causes neurologic deficits based on the level where the fibroneural stalk meets the dorsal spinal cord. Given that LDMs are nonleaking in nature, emergent surgery is rarely a necessity. However, early surgery is certainly a prudent option, especially in cases where a large membranous sac makes the safe handling of an infant difficult or if the membranous sac has ruptured.

The surgical technique for the various cutaneous manifestations of LDMs differs only in the size of the initial incision. An elliptical incision is made surrounding the margin of the cutaneous lesion. Careful dissection renders the fibroneural stalk, which may be distended. This stalk is traced through the dorsal musculature and fascia as it enters in between the bifid laminae. Care is taken at this point to perform a laminectomy one level caudal and one level rostral to the fibroneural stalk to enable the junction between the stalk and cord to be completely exposed. This junction is always a small distance rostral to the initial dissection.

The dorsal dura is then incised to expose the stalk, which is typically attached to a linear spot or cleft in the midline. The stalk is then cut flush with the surface of the cord. Careful examination of the surrounding tissue may reveal small nerves, blood vessels, or connective tissue that surrounds the stalk, which are cut. Complete detachment of the fibroneural stalk is then followed by en-bloc resection of the extradural stalk and cutaneous lesion. Special care is taken in cases of lumbar LDMs to explore in the rostral direction as the filum terminale may be thickened and, if identified, should be cut during initial resection. Finally, inspection of the spinal cord, in both cervical and thoracolumbar LDMs, is frequently associated with type II split cord malformations. (Type I malformations are composed of two dural sacs and a bony or fibrocartilaginous spur; Type II malformations are composed of a single dural sac and intradural fibrous septum.) The fibroneural stalk is typically nearly contiguous with the fibrous septum that separates the cord in these cases.

References

1. Mathews TJ, Honein MA, Erickson JD. Spina bifida and anencephaly prevalence—United States, 1991-2001. MMWR Recomm Rep 2002;51(RR-13):9–11
2. Bowman RM, Boshnjaku V, McLone DG. The changing incidence of myelomeningocele and its impact on pediatric neurosurgery: a review from the Children's Memorial Hospital. Childs Nerv Syst 2009;25:801–806
3. Talamonti G, D'Aliberti G, Collice M. Myelomeningocele: long-term neurosurgical treatment and follow-up in 202 patients. J Neurosurg 2007;107(5, Suppl):368–386
4. Dias MS, Partington M. Embryology of myelomeningocele and anencephaly. Neurosurg Focus 2004;16:E1
5. Müller F, O'Rahilly R. The development of the human brain, the closure of the caudal neuropore, and the beginning of secondary neurulation at stage 12. Anat Embryol (Berl) 1987;176:413–430
6. Costanzo R, Watterson RL, Schoenwolf GC. Evidence that secondary neurulation occurs autonomously in the chick embryo. J Exp Zool 1982;219:233–240
7. Pang D. Surgical complications of open spinal dysraphism. Neurosurg Clin N Am 1995;6:243–257
8. Perry VL, Albright AL, Adelson PD. Operative nuances of myelomeningocele closure. Neurosurgery 2002;51:719–723, discussion 723–724
9. Adzick NS, Thom EA, Spong CY, et al; MOMS Investigators. A randomized trial of prenatal versus postnatal repair of myelomeningocele. N Engl J Med 2011;364:993–1004
10. Bruner JP, Tulipan N, Paschall RL, et al. Fetal surgery for myelomeningocele and the incidence of shunt-dependent hydrocephalus. JAMA 1999;282:1819–1825
11. Tulipan N, Sutton LN, Bruner JP, Cohen BM, Johnson M, Adzick NS. The effect of intrauterine myelomeningocele repair on the incidence of shunt-dependent hydrocephalus. Pediatr Neurosurg 2003;38:27–33

12. Luthy DA, Wardinsky T, Shurtleff DB, et al. Cesarean section before the onset of labor and subsequent motor function in infants with meningomyelocele diagnosed antenatally. N Engl J Med 1991;324:662–666
13. Merrill DC, Goodwin P, Burson JM, Sato Y, Williamson R, Weiner CP. The optimal route of delivery for fetal meningomyelocele. Am J Obstet Gynecol 1998;179:235–240
14. Pinto FCG, Matushita H, Furlan ALB, et al. Surgical treatment of myelomeningocele carried out at "time zero" immediately after birth. Pediatr Neurosurg 2009;45:114–118
15. Caldarelli M, Di Rocco C, La Marca F. Shunt complications in the first postoperative year in children with meningomyelocele. Childs Nerv Syst 1996;12:748–754
16. Phillips BC, Gelsomino M, Pownall AL, et al. Predictors of the need for cerebrospinal fluid diversion in patients with myelomeningocele. J Neurosurg Pediatr 2014;14:167–172
17. Tuli S, Drake J, Lamberti-Pasculli M. Long-term outcome of hydrocephalus management in myelomeningoceles. Childs Nerv Syst 2003;19:286–291
18. Radmanesh F, Nejat F, El Khashab M, Ghodsi SM, Ardebili HE. Shunt complications in children with myelomeningocele: effect of timing of shunt placement. Clinical article. J Neurosurg Pediatr 2009;3:516–520
19. Lee B-J, Sohn M-J, Han S-R, Choi C-Y, Lee D-J, Kang JH. Analysis of risk factors and management of cerebrospinal fluid morbidity in the treatment of spinal dysraphism. J Korean Neurosurg Soc 2013;54:225–231
20. Carstens C, Koch H, Brocai DRC, Niethard FU. Development of pathological lumbar kyphosis in myelomeningocele. J Bone Joint Surg Br 1996;78:945–950
21. Garg S, Oetgen M, Rathjen K, Richards BS. Kyphectomy improves sitting and skin problems in patients with myelomeningocele. Clin Orthop Relat Res 2011;469:1279–1285
22. de Amoreira Gepp R, Quiroga MRS, Gomes CR, de Araújo HJ. Kyphectomy in meningomyelocele children: surgical technique, risk analysis, and improvement of kyphosis. Childs Nerv Syst 2013;29:1137–1141
23. Hall JE, Poitras B. The management of kyphosis in patients with myelomeningocele. Clin Orthop Relat Res 1977;128:33–40
24. Ko AL, Song K, Ellenbogen RG, Avellino AM. Retrospective review of multilevel spinal fusion combined with spinal cord transection for treatment of kyphoscoliosis in pediatric myelomeningocele patients. Spine 2007;32:2493–2501
25. McMaster MJ. The long-term results of kyphectomy and spinal stabilization in children with myelomeningocele. Spine 1988;13:417–424
26. Kaplan SÇ, Ekşi MŞ, Bayri Y, Toktaş ZO, Konya D. Kyphectomy and pedicular screw fixation with posterior-only approach in pediatric patients with myelomeningocele. Pediatr Neurosurg 2015;50:133–144
27. Hwang SW, Thomas JG, Blumberg TJ, et al. Kyphectomy in patients with myelomeningocele treated with pedicle screw-only constructs: case reports and review. J Neurosurg Pediatr 2011;8:63–70
28. Niall DM, Dowling FE, Fogarty EE, Moore DP, Goldberg C. Kyphectomy in children with myelomeningocele: a long-term outcome study. J Pediatr Orthop 2004;24:37–44
29. Byrne RW, Hayes EA, George TM, McLone DG. Operative resection of 100 spinal lipomas in infants less than 1 year of age. Pediatr Neurosurg 1995;23:182–186, discussion 186–187
30. Chapman PH. Congenital intraspinal lipomas: anatomic considerations and surgical treatment. Childs Brain 1982;9:37–47
31. Pang D, Zovickian J, Wong S-T, Hou YJ, Moes GS. Surgical treatment of complex spinal cord lipomas. Childs Nerv Syst 2013;29:1485–1513
32. Finn MA, Walker ML. Spinal lipomas: clinical spectrum, embryology, and treatment. Neurosurg Focus 2007;23:E10
33. McLone DG, Naidich TP. Terminal myelocystocele. Neurosurgery 1985;16:36–43
34. Pang D, Zovickian J, Oviedo A. Long-term outcome of total and near-total resection of spinal cord lipomas and radical reconstruction of the neural placode: part I-surgical technique. Neurosurgery 2009;65:511–528, discussion 528–529
35. Kulkarni AV, Pierre-Kahn A, Zerah M. Conservative management of asymptomatic spinal lipomas of the conus. Neurosurgery 2004;54:868–873, discussion 873–875
36. Pang D, Zovickian J, Oviedo A, Moes GS. Limited dorsal myeloschisis: a distinctive clinicopathological entity. Neurosurgery 2010;67:1555–1579, discussion 1579–1580
37. Pang D, Zovickian J, Wong S-T, Hou YJ, Moes GS. Limited dorsal myeloschisis: a not-so-rare form of primary neurulation defect. Childs Nerv Syst 2013;29:1459–1484

124 Repair of Diastematomyelia

Sandi K. Lam and Andrew Jea

Diastematomyelia is an uncommon congenital malformation of the spinal cord and spinal column. It is characterized by a focal (single segment) longitudinal (sagittal) division of either the spinal cord or the cauda equina with an interposed septum. This osseous, cartilaginous, or fibrous septum usually in the midline of the spinal canal may invaginate the dura and divide the spinal cord.[1]

Based on the state of the thecal sac and the nature of the median septum, two types of split cord malformation have been proposed by Pang et al[2]: type I, diastematomyelia, in which each hemicord has its own dural tube; and type II, diplomyelia, in which two hemicords are contained in a single dural tube. The term *diastematomyelia*, however, refers to both types of split cord malformation.[1]

The septum adhering to the medial aspect of the hemicords may represent a tethering lesion, which could result in progressive neurologic deterioration due to both stretching and compression of the spinal cord.[3] The severity of symptomatology varies from asymptomatic to tethered cord syndrome, including pain syndrome, lower extremity weakness, gait disturbance, and bladder and bowel dysfunction.

One management approach is to address these lesions prophylactically, to prevent the possibility of irreversible and progressive neurologic damage.[1] However, the natural history of diastematomyelia is not clearly delineated; therefore, much like other forms of spinal dysraphism, the timing of treatment is controversial: prophylactic versus that based on the development of symptoms.[4]

Indications and Contraindications

Clinical indications for surgery include tethered cord syndrome, scoliosis, foot deformity, intractable back and leg pain, leg weakness, spasticity, changes in gait, and bowel and bladder dysfunction or detrusor-sphincter dyssynergy on formal urodynamic studies. Syringomyelia is a radiographic indication for surgical treatment.

Surgical treatment is not necessary for asymptomatic type I diastematomyelia, as patients who were treated conservatively showed no worsening of their neurologic status over an average follow-up of 4.5 years.[1] Moreover, there is no significant difference in outcome between surgical treatment and nonsurgical treatment for patients with type II diastematomyelia.[1]

Objectives of Surgery

Type I diastematomyelia may be accompanied by secondary tethering at the filum terminale.[1,5] Consideration should be given not only to resecting the problematic septum but also to sectioning the filum terminale in the same surgical setting to fully mobilize the spinal cord. Note that sectioning the filum terminale should be performed after the removal of the septum.[1,5]

Syringomyelia is presumed to be a local disturbance of hydrodynamics of cerebrospinal fluid (CSF) in the subarachnoid compartment, Virchow-Robin spaces, and central canal. The ideal treatment of syringomyelia has not been determined. However, with the restoration of normal CSF dynamics by elimination of tethering lesions of the spinal cord, the syringomyelia may slowly resolve, and it may be more prudent to manage this condition conservatively with regular monitoring rather than directly intervene on the syrinx itself.

Preoperative Imaging

The diagnosis of diastematomyelia should be established by myelography, computed tomography (CT), magnetic resonance imaging (MRI), or a combination of these modalities. Myelography shows a typical "island-like" filling defect formed by contrast medium around the septum (**Fig. 124.1**). CT may help to differentiate a bony or cartilaginous septum (**Fig. 124.2**). MRI may demonstrate asymmetric splitting of the spinal cord and, associated with syringomyelia, a thickened or fatty filum, dermoid cyst, or spinal lipoma. Most patients have a widened interpedicular distance without erosion of the pedicles at the level of the septum. Rarely a patient will have multiple septa at different vertebral levels (1.3%).[1] The lumbar region (46%) is the most common site for diastematomyelia, followed by the thoracolumbar area (40%), the thoracic region (13%), and the cervical spine (1%).[1] Most spinal cords are split over an average of six vertebral segments.[1]

Surgical Procedure

Positioning

As with any spine surgery, the patient is placed in the prone position with appropriately padded bolsters that extend from the shoulder/clavicular area to the iliac crest. To minimize venous bleeding at the operative site, the abdominal cavity should be allowed to hang free between the bolsters. This position prevents retrograde venous flow into the epidural and spinal venous systems, thus decreasing bleeding at the surgical site.[6] General endotracheal anesthesia is used with a combination of narcotics and inhalation agents. A single dose of the antibiotic of choice (nafcillin, cefazolin, or vancomycin) is given prior to skin incision and repeated if the procedure lasts for more than 4 hours. Care must be taken to prevent skin pressure sores, nerve compression/stretching, or ocular injury when the head is placed on a cerebellar or doughnut-shaped headrest. Intraoperative neurophysiological monitoring (IONM) including somatosensory

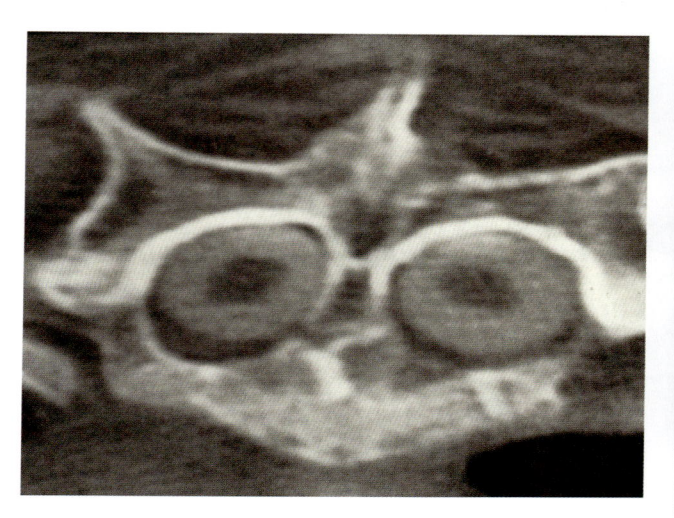

Fig. 124.1 Myelographic image of diastematomyelia with two hemicords and a midline filling defect.

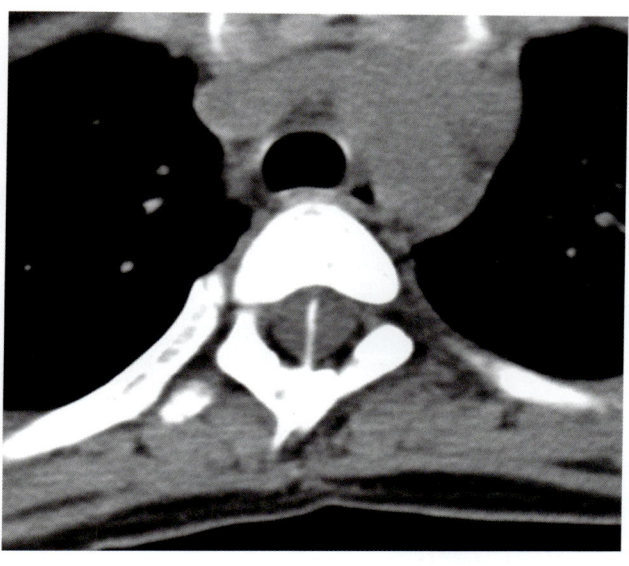

Fig. 124.2 Computed tomography (CT) scan showing midline bony septum, helping to distinguish between a bony or cartilaginous septum.

evoked potentials (SSEPs), motor evoked potentials (MEPs), and spontaneous electromyography (EMG) actively, should be performed, and the electrodes properly placed and tested prior to draping. This surgical adjunct has been applied to the youngest of patients and those with baseline neurodevelopmental abnormalities.[7,8]

Incision

The surgeon must thoroughly identify the exact location of the median septum and its vertebral level prior to making a skin incision. Localization of the appropriate level may be done with fluoroscopy or plain X-ray films. A posterior midline approach is used. The affected laminae are removed. In type I malformations, not uncommonly, the spinous processes and lamina overlying the septum may be abnormal.[6] They may present with bifid or eccentric spinous processes or dysmorphic and hypertrophic laminar arches. The spinous processes and lamina may be removed with Leksell and Kerrison rongeurs in a piecemeal fashion. Extreme care must be taken when removing the lamina over the septum in this type of malformation because the traversing midline septum is often fused with the undersurface of the lamina and the base of the spinous process (**Fig. 124.3**).

Dural Opening and Septum Resection of the Split Cord Malformation Type I (Diastematomyelia, Bony Spur)

The midline bony septum, which is always located extradurally, should be left in situ after circumferential removal of the overlying lamina is performed (**Fig. 124.4**). A helpful anatomic factor for intraoperative localization is that the septum can be consistently located where the spinal canal is widest. A blunt dissecting tool can be used to carefully separate the surrounding dural sleeve from the bony spur (**Fig. 124.5**). Not uncommonly, the widest area of the bony septum is located at its junction with the overlying lamina. Occasionally, but not uncommonly, the septum may be manipulated so as to fracture its narrow ventral

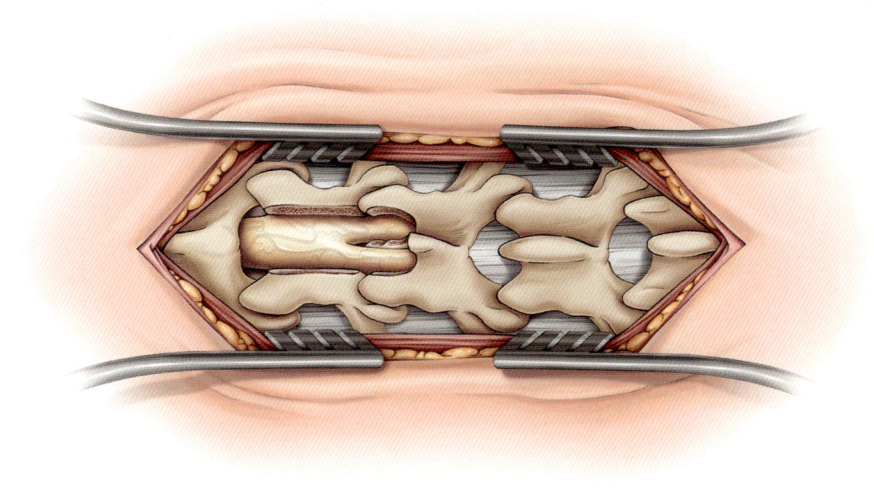

Fig. 124.3 Laminectomy exposure demonstrates a bony spur splitting the spinal cord and its dural sleeves. The bony spur extends to the ventral surface of the canal.

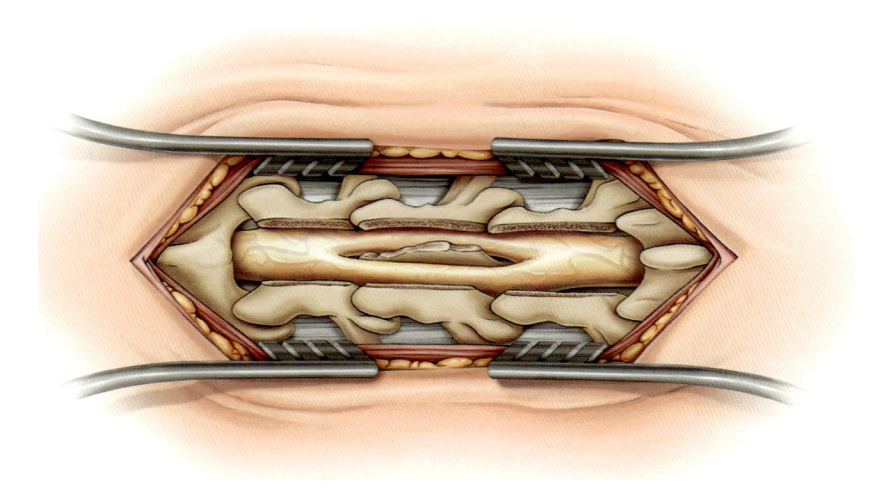

Fig. 124.4 Following laminectomies, the bony spur is left in place after its attachment to the posterior elements. Fibrous dural attachments to the bony spur are freed in a circumferential fashion.

base for complete removal (**Fig. 124.6a**). However, most commonly it has to be removed in a piecemeal fashion using small rongeurs or a micro-drill with a diamond bur (**Fig. 124.6b**).

The septum often contains relatively large blood vessels at its ventral attachment, which frequently cause brisk bleeding. Such bleeding can be easily controlled by applying a piece of bone wax, placed at the tip of a Kittner dissector, and gently applying pressure to the base. When using a micro-drill, the assistant should use thin retractors such as brain ribbon metal bands to protect the dura and the spinal cord from injury. Following complete resection of the bony septum, the dura is opened in the midline above the level of the diastematomyelia, and the incision is carried medially along both dural sleeves and continued caudally in the midline as well (**Fig. 124.7**). Care must be taken when exploring the medial dural sleeves because fibrous adhesions and nonfunctional paramedian nerve roots may tightly adhere to the dural sleeve. These adhesions should be sharply dissected and cut (**Fig. 124.8**). Due to the mechanics of bone and spinal cord growth, the septum is closely pressed against the caudal end of the split dural sacs. Consequently, the two hemicords are similarly tightly adhered to the caudal end of the split dural sac. Freeing of the hemicord and dural dissection of this area carries the possibility of injury to the spinal cord. Following resection of the dura of the ventral surface, a dural defect may be created. If it is possible and easily done, the dural edges may be approximated primarily. However, often it is not possible to primarily close the dural defect, which may be left alone. CSF leaks are uncommon due to the abundant adhesions present ventrally to the posterior longitudinal ligament.[6]

Closure

The intradural space is irrigated with saline solution, and adequate hemostasis is obtained. The dorsal aspect of the dura is closed with 5-0 Prolene in a running, simple, watertight fashion. This maneuver in split cord malformation type I leads to the reconstitution of the two dural sacs into a single dural tube. The epidural space is also irrigated, and careful hemostasis of the

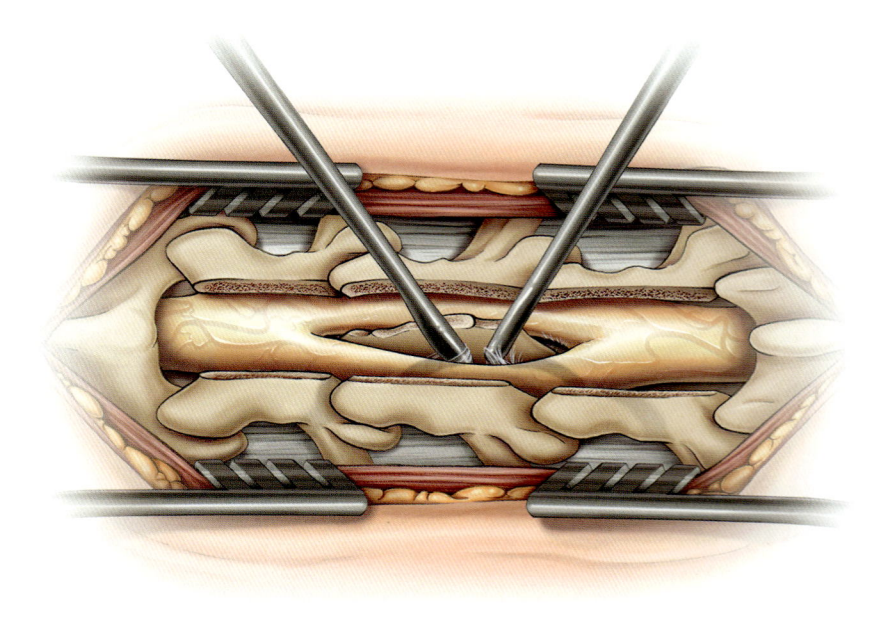

Fig. 124.5 A bony spur splits the dural sac in two. Blunt dissectors are used to carefully free the surrounding dural sac from the bony spur prior to its removal.

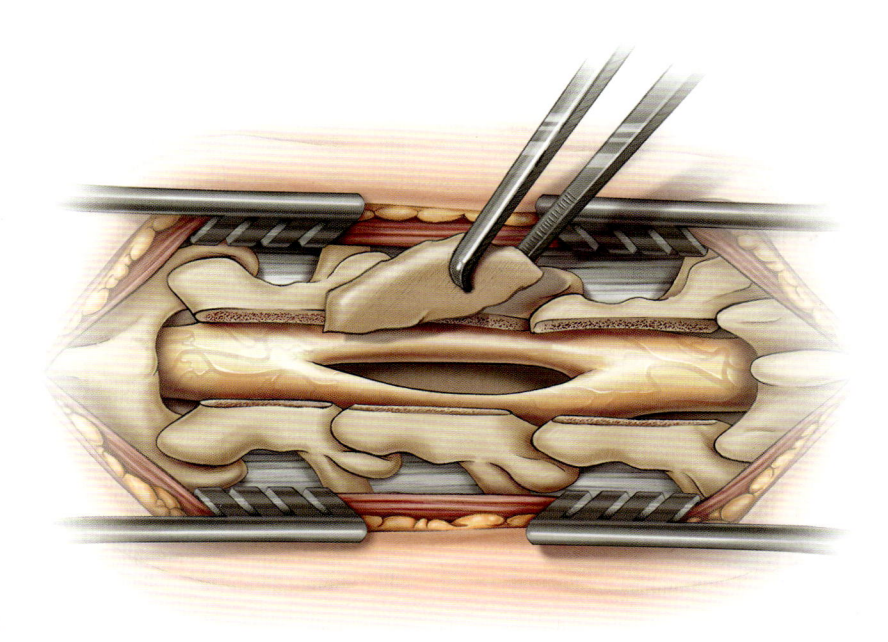

Fig. 124.6 (a) The bony spur may be removed by fracturing its base and removing it as a single unit. (b) When the attachment is too wide and unable to be removed in a single piece, the bony spur may be removed using micro-drills and pituitary rongeurs to reach its ventral surface.

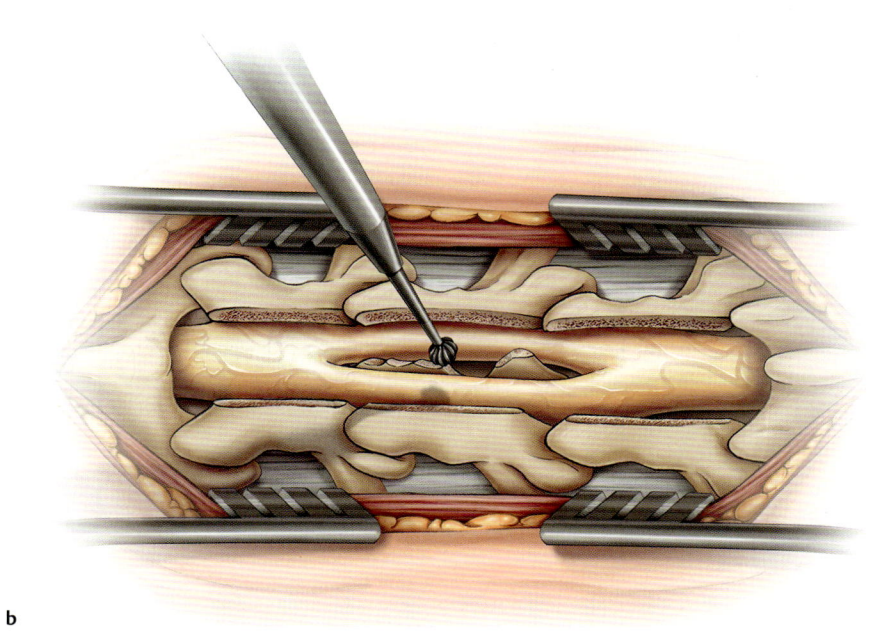

epidural veins is obtained with bipolar electrocautery and other hemostatic agents as needed. A Valsalva maneuver is performed to ensure a watertight dural closure. The paraspinous muscles are closely approximated with 2-0 absorbable sutures (Vicryl) along with the dorsal lumbar fascia. Marcaine 0.25% may be injected into the muscle and subcutaneous tissue. Subcutaneous tissue closure can be done with 3-0 absorbable suture, and the skin is closed with a running vertical mattress suture using 4-0 Monocryl or other suture of choice.

Postoperative Care

The patient is mobilized early after surgery. A longer hospital stay for maintaining patients flat may not prevent a CSF leakage.[9]

A Foley catheter is left in place to improve patient comfort until fully mobilized; it is not uncommon for the patient to experience temporary urinary retention in the immediate postoperative period necessitating straight catheterization. In patients over 12 years of age, sequential compression pneumatic stocking and prophylactic doses of low molecular weight heparin should be used to minimize venous thrombosis development until they are moving and ambulating well. If significant muscular spasms are present, antispasmodics may be given to control pain and increase comfort. The patient may be discharged from the hospital when ambulating and voiding without difficulties.

Temporary neurologic worsening (2.5%) and CSF leak (1.3%) are the two most common complications of surgical treatment.[1] Meticulous planning, knowledge of anatomy, and attention to detail are imperative.

794 V Lumbar and Lumbosacral Spine

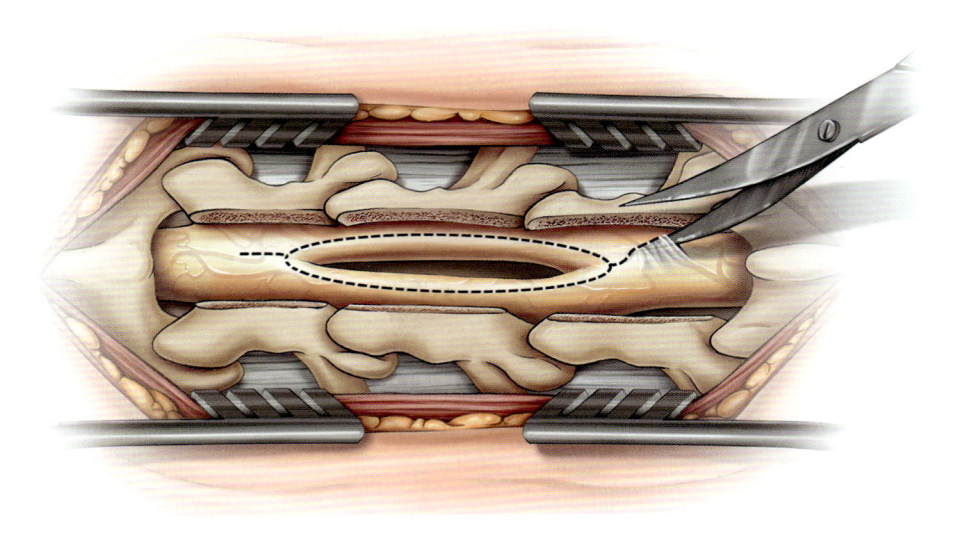

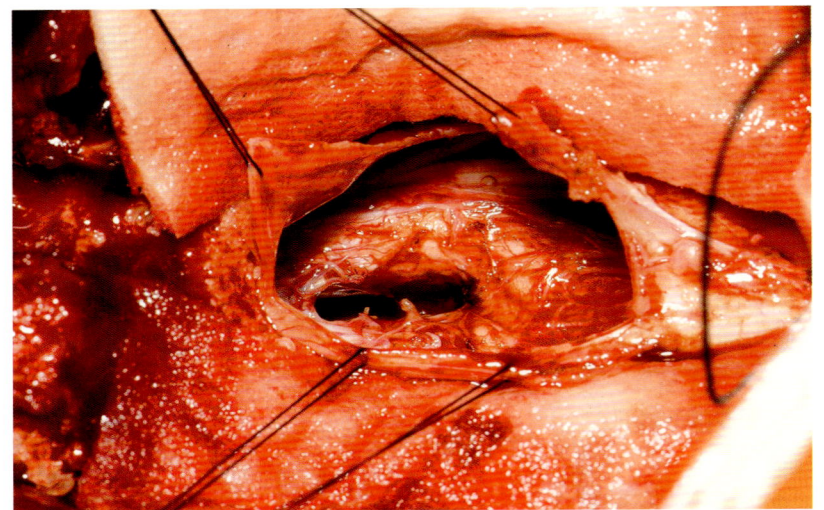

Fig. 124.7 (a) Following resection of the bony spur, the dural opening is performed. (b) Intraoperative view.

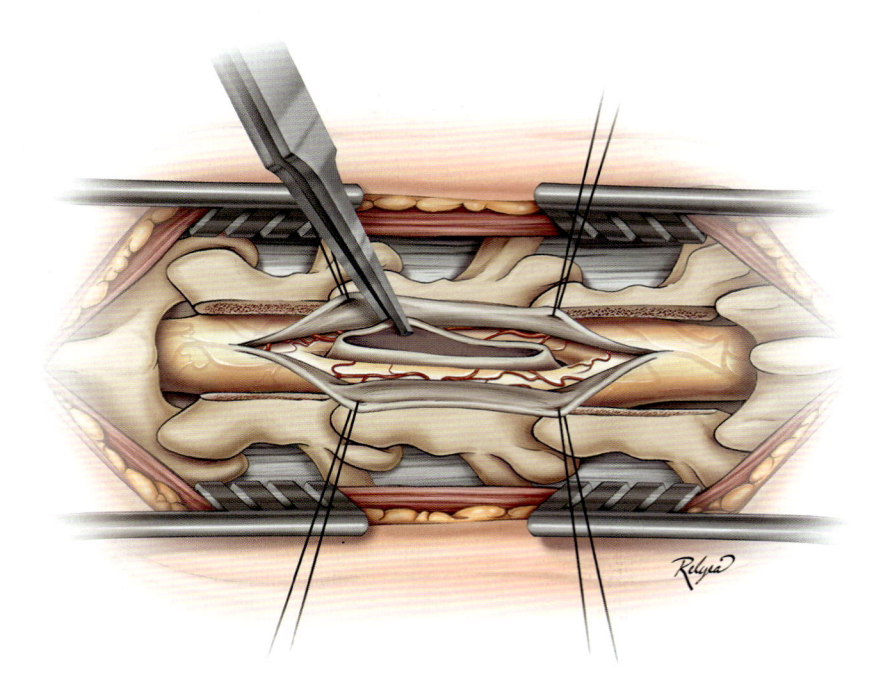

Fig. 124.8 After the dural sac has been completely opened, the medial dural sleeves need to be resected flush with the ventral surface with the spinal canal. Often it is not necessary to repair the dural defect of the ventral surface because abundant adhesions to the bony elements preclude cerebrospinal fluid leaks.

Conclusion

Surgical treatment is not necessary for asymptomatic Pang type I diastematomyelia. Similarly, there is no significant difference in outcome between operative and nonoperative treatment for Pang type II diplomyelia. Laminectomy and resection of the septum form the basic tenets of surgical treatment for diastematomyelia. The split head of the dura and abnormal fiber bundles should be resected as well to reconstitute and reconstruct a single thecal sac. Diastematomyelia may be associated with additional symptomatic tethering at the filum terminale. Associated syringomyelia should be managed expectantly as there is opportunity for resolution of the syringomyelia with restoration of normal CSF dynamics.

References

1. Huang S-L, He XJ, Wang KZ, Lan BS. Diastematomyelia: a 35-year experience. Spine 2013;38:E344–E349
2. Pang D, Dias MS, Ahab-Barmada M. Split cord malformation: Part I: A unified theory of embryogenesis for double spinal cord malformations. Neurosurgery 1992;31:451–480
3. Huang S-L, Shi W, Zhang LG. Characteristics and surgery of cervical myelomeningocele. Childs Nerv Syst 2010;26:87–91
4. Kulkarni AV, Pierre-Kahn A, Zerah M. Conservative management of asymptomatic spinal lipomas of the conus. Neurosurgery 2004;54:868–873, discussion 873–875
5. Cheng B, Li FT, Lin L. Diastematomyelia: a retrospective review of 138 patients. J Bone Joint Surg Br 2012;94:365–372
6. Jimenez DF, Nottmeier E. Repair of diastematomyelia. In: Fessler R, Sekhar L, eds. Atlas of Neurosurgical Techniques: Spine and Peripheral Nerves, 1st ed. New York: Thieme; 2006:759–764
7. DiCindio S, Theroux M, Shah S, et al. Multimodality monitoring of transcranial electric motor and somatosensory-evoked potentials during surgical correction of spinal deformity in patients with cerebral palsy and other neuromuscular disorders. Spine 2003;28:1851–1855, discussion 1855–1856
8. Fulkerson DH, Satyan KB, Wilder LM, et al. Intraoperative monitoring of motor evoked potentials in very young children. J Neurosurg Pediatr 2011;7:331–337
9. Chern JJ, Tubbs RS, Patel AJ, et al. Preventing cerebrospinal fluid leak following transection of a tight filum terminale. J Neurosurg Pediatr 2011;8:35–38

125 Sacral Agenesis

David Jimenez and Asif Maknojia

Sacral agenesis is part of a spectrum disorder known as caudal regression syndrome. This syndrome involves agenesis or the absence of the caudal segments of the spine, which could include the lower thoracic, lumbar, sacral, or coccygeal spine. Williams and Nixon initially described the term in 1957. Renshaw[1] further classified the disorder into five types based on radiological findings: type I, with total or partial unilateral sacral agenesis; type II, with variable lumbar and total sacral agenesis and the ilia articulating with sides of the lowest vertebrae; type III, with variable lumbar and a total sacral agenesis, the caudal end plate of the lowest vertebra resting above either a fused ilia or an iliac amphiarthrosis; type IV, with fusion of soft tissues of both the lower limbs; and type V, with sirenomelia with only a single femur and tibia.[1] Anatomically, patients can be divided into simple groups that have differing clinical presentations. In a select group of patients, the conus lies at the level of L1. This group of patients often presents with severe sacral malformations and a club-shaped cord with a decreased number of anterior horn cells and dilation of the central canal. A second group of patients presents with low-lying conus, a tethered cord, spinal dysraphisms, and lipoma. The sacral agenesis is milder in this second group.[2]

Incidence and Prevalence

Caudal regression syndrome is a nonfamilial, mostly sporadic, disease with an incidence estimated as 1:25,000 to 1:60,000 births.[3] However, the incidence increases to 1:350 in diabetic mothers. The cause of this is unclear. The incidence of sacral agenesis is estimated to be 0.01 to 0.05 per 1,000 live births.[4]

Pathophysiology

Sacral agenesis is associated with other syndromes including VACTERL (*v*ertebral, *a*norectal, *c*ardiac, *t*racheo-*e*sophageal fistula, *r*enal, and *l*imb anomalies), the OEIS complex (*o*mphalocele, cloacal *e*xstrophy, *i*mperforate anus, and *s*pinal malformation), and the Currarino syndrome, which is a autosomal dominant congenital disorder caused by mutation in the *HLXB9* homeobox gene. It is hypothesized that sacral agenesis results from failure of secondary neurulation where the medullary cord fails either to form or to cavitate and merge with the neural canal of the more cranial neural tube.[5] Genetic association studies have suggested that mutations in the *HLXB9, HOXD13*, or *CYP26A1* are involved in sacral agenesis.[6] Another theory of the development of caudal regression syndrome includes abnormal shunting from the vitelline artery during fetus development, but this theory remains controversial.

Embryologically, the caudal eminence, a mass of pluripotent cells that is continuous with the primitive streak, gives rise to the caudal spine, hindgut, and genitourinary system. On day 26 of embryogenesis, when the caudal neuropore closes, the primitive streak regresses and the caudal eminence takes its place spanning between Henson's node and the cloacal membrane analage.[7] Through the process of secondary neurulation, the caudal eminence lays down a solid neural cord in comparison to the spinal cord formed by primary neurulation up to the lumbosacral junction. The process by which the caudal neural cord joins with the primary neural tube is still not well understood. Caudal eminence is also responsible for the formation of somite 31 and below, whereas the primitive streak gives rise to somite 30 and above. This corresponds to the S1-S2 junction, with S1 being developed from end-stage primary neurulation and S2–S5 arising from caudal eminence. It is hypothesized that errors in the formation of caudal eminence, which would give rise to the severe defects seen in caudal regression syndrome, or more local defects in the caudal neural cord and axial mesoderm result in subtotal sacral defects.

Clinical Presentation

In sacral agenesis it is estimated that one fifth of the patients are not diagnosed before the age of 3. The average age of diagnosis is 2.2 years, with a range as broad as from birth to 9 years of age.[4] Patients usually present to orthopedic, urologic, gastrointestinal, or neurosurgical services. Causes include myelomeningocele, tethered cord with progressive neurologic deficits, dermal sinus tract, diastematomyelia, urinary incontinence, repeated urinary tract infection (UTI), urinary ascites, rectovaginal fistula, imperforate anus, and congenital dislocation of the hip or a foot deformity. The most common causes of referral to the neurosurgical service were myelomeningocele, followed by progressive neurologic deficits due to a tethered cord.[4]

Patients with sacral agenesis can be difficult to diagnose, and thus the physician must maintain a high level of suspicion. Pediatric patients with urinary incontinence, difficulty voiding, constipation, or recurrent UTIs should raise suspicion for sacral agenesis. Delayed diagnosis is associated with worsening renal and neurologic outcomes. Physical exam can reveal flattening of the buttocks, a palpable sacral defect, absence of the gluteal cleft, widely space buttock dimples, pes cavus, or a flatfoot widebase gait.[8]

Neurologic presentation of patients was varied, with 46% of patients presenting with lower limb weakness, mostly distal. Most weakness was usually bilateral, but in patients with myelomeningocele or diastematomyelia, unilateral limb weakness was often seen as the dominant feature. Sensory dysfunction was less common in sacral agenesis and could involve autonomic dysfunction.[9] Less commonly patients presented with low back pain or scoliosis. In a case series of 50 patients, 42% presented with associated myelomeningocele or lipomyelomeningocele, 20% with diastematomyelia, and 20% with syrinx or hydromelia. Progressive neurologic symptoms were associated with the presence of tethered cord, which was seen in 58% of the patients.[4,10,11] Patients are also reported to have cervical abnormalities, including odontoid abnormalities, occipito-atlantal joint instability, and congenital fusions of the cervical spine. Spinopelvic instability and scoliosis of the spine are also often seen in these patients.

Other nonneurosurgical presentations, which were more common, included urinary incontinence in 85% of patients and UTI in 74% of patient. Imperforate anus and fecal incontinence were seen in 22% patients.

Management

Neurosurgical management of patients with sacral agenesis is often delayed until other nonneurologic symptoms, which are more life threatening, are treated, with the exception of open myelomeningocele. Of primary concern are urinary symptoms, because early treatment is important in improving outcomes. The main goals of urologic intervention are preserving renal function, preventing infection, and establishing continence.[12]

Most neurosurgical intervention is due to the presence of either myelomeningocele or progressive neurologic deficits secondary to tethered cord. In Pang's[12] series, patients were classified into three groups: (1) patients with open myelomeningocele, lipomyelomeningocele, or a dorsal dural effect, all of which require early surgical treatment; (2) patients with a tethered cord presenting with progressive neurologic deficits, for which surgical treatment can be delayed; and (3) patients with spinal cord compression presenting with progressive neurologic deficits, for which surgical treatment can be delayed. In Pang's results, no group 1 patients had worsening of their neurologic deficits. In group 2, 60% of the patients had improvement in their neurological status after surgery and 40% remained stable, and all patients had no progressive symptoms and stable neurologic deficits after surgery. Also, group 2 patients with no progressive symptoms for whom conservative management was selected had no worsening in their deficits.

Preoperative Planning and Considerations

Indications

- Dorsal spinal lesions with open myelomeningocele, lipomyelomeningocele, or dorsal dural effect
- Spinal lipomas
- Progressive neurologic defects resulting from dural sac stenosis or tethered cord
- Spinopelvic instability in patients with potential for ambulation

Contraindications

- Associated anomalies present that preclude survival
- No absolute contraindications

Objectives

- Prevention of worsening of progressive neurologic deficits
- Closure of open lesions that risk infections of the nervous system
- Decompression of neural elements
- Stabilization of the spine in patients with potential for ambulation

Timing of Surgery

Surgical consideration in patients should account for other associated anomalies and should determine the urgency of the underlying problem requiring surgical intervention. Open myelomeningocele and lipomyelomeningocele require immediate intervention. Patients with tethered cord and progressive neurologic deficits can have surgery on a nonurgent basis. Similar to patients with lumbar stenosis, dural sac stenosis in patients with sacral agenesis should be surgically managed with progressive symptoms. Spinopelvic instability should be managed as soon as possible to provide the maximal opportunity for early rehabilitation in patients with the potential for ambulation.

Preoperative Imaging

Patient should have plain films obtained of the lumbosacral spine in the anteroposterior and lateral views to evaluate the bony anatomy and curvature of the spine. Plain films of the cervical spine should also be obtained to rule out any osteochondral (O-C) abnormalities that would affect the positioning of the patient r risk cervical injury. Computed tomography (CT) can evaluate the bony anatomy. Finally, magnetic resonance imaging (MRI) of the spine should be obtained in all patients to identify any stenosis or the presence of abnormalities, including spinal lipoma, diastematomyelia, tethered cord, and a thickened filum. Furthermore, MRI would also reveal where the conus lies in regard to the bony anatomy. MRI of the head and craniocervical junction should also be obtained to rule out hydrocephalus or scoliotic neck.

Surgical Technique

Anesthesia

Given the variety of anomalies in patients with sacral agenesis, anesthesia can be challenging. Although the literature is sparse regarding anesthesia in patients with sacral agenesis, anesthesia should be based on a complete understanding of the patient's other anomalies. In one published case report of induction with ketamine in a pediatric patient, fentanyl and vecuronium were used along with ketamine, with or without benzodiazepine for maintenance.[13] Patients requiring intraoperative electrophysiological monitoring should not be given long-acting muscle relaxants.

Patient Positioning

The patient is intubated in the supine position, with a head ring placed around the lesion to prevent compression. Intubation can also be performed with the patient in the lateral position. The patient is then placed in the prone position, with small gel rolls on the chest and hip. The abdomen should be allowed to hang freely to enable adequate venous drainage to prevent bleeding during surgery. The hips and knees should be flexed and the upper extremities flexed at the elbows. Pressure points are padded with towels or foam. The skin is sterilized with povidone iodine, with care taken to prevent contact of the povidone iodine with neural tissue.

Myelomeningocele

Operative Procedure

The area between the dysplastic epidermis and the neural placode is identified and marked circumferentially. The epidermis can be infiltrated with lidocaine and epinephrine to minimize bleeding. The incision is made between the arachnoid of the neural placode and the epidermis (junctional zone) using sharp dissection. The use of electrocautery is minimized to prevent damage to the neural tissue. The incision should be carried down until the dura is observed. The base of the sac should be mobilized from the surrounding tissue until it is seen entering the fascial defect. With the neural placode mobilized, a moist Telfa should be placed on it while performing the next step. The dysplastic skin that previously surrounded the placode is incised using either sharp dissection or monopolar electrocautery. Care should be taken to remove all of the skin to prevent the development of an epidermoid cyst. The placode then should be reconstructed using 4-0 or 5-0 absorbable sutures bringing in approximation the pial layer. This ensures that the neural tissue fits well into the dural sac and also decreases the incidence of tethering. Next, the dura is released from the fascia and closed using nonabsorbable sutures. The dura should be located at the last intact lamina and mobilized from there down to facilitate identification and plane formation. In certain circumstances, duraplasty using synthetic materials or fascia is required to prevent cerebrospinal fluid (CSF) leak. Care should be taken to ensure that the closure of the dura does not compress the neural elements. Next the fascia is closed over the dura after undermining to allow for a stress-free closure. With the fascia closed, the subcutaneous tissue and finally the skin are closed over. In cases with a large defect, fasciocutaneous flaps or intraoperative acute tissue expansion can be used for closure.

Complications

The most common complication is superficial wound dehiscence. Some surgeons keep the patient in the prone position to prevent any pressure on the wound. Others opt for early shunting or CSF diversion to prevent leakage leading to wound healing failure. Other complications include superficial wound infections, for which dressing changes and intravenous antibiotics are recommended. Venous congestion secondary to a tight wound closure might require placement of leeches or revision of the wound.

References

1. Renshaw TS. Sacral agenesis. In: Weinstein SL, ed. The Pediatric Spine: Principles and Practice, vol 1. New York: Raven Press; 1994:2214
2. Jadav V, Gandhi J, Soni H, Desai S. Caudal regression syndrome. Gujarat Medical Journal. 2012;67:129–131
3. Singh SK, Singh RD, Sharma A. Caudal regression syndrome—case report and review of literature. Pediatr Surg Int 2005;21:578–581
4. Emami-Naeini P, Rahbar Z, Nejat F, Kajbafzadeh A, El Khashab M. Neurological presentations, imaging, and associated anomalies in 50 patients with sacral agenesis. Neurosurgery 2010;67:894–900, discussion 900
5. Schoenwolf GC, Bleyl SB, Brauer PR, Francis-West PH. Larsen's Human Embryology, 4th ed. New York: Elsevier; 2008
6. Semba K, Yamamura K. Etiology of caudal regression syndrome. Hum Genet Embryol 2013:3
7. Müller F, O'Rahilly R. The first appearance of the major divisions of the human brain at stage 9. Anat Embryol (Berl) 1983;168:419–432
8. Wilmshurst JM, Kelly R, Borzyskowski M. Presentation and outcome of sacral agenesis: 20 years' experience. Dev Med Child Neurol 1999;41:806–812
9. Sarnat HB, Case ME, Graviss R. Sacral agenesis. Neurologic and neuropathologic features. Neurology 1976;26:1124–1129
10. Muthukumar N. Surgical treatment of nonprogressive neurological deficits in children with sacral agenesis. Neurosurgery 1996;38:1133–1137, discussion 1137–1138
11. Harlow CL, Partington MD, Thieme GA. Lumbosacral agenesis: clinical characteristics, imaging, and embryogenesis. Pediatr Neurosurg 1995;23:140–147
12. Pang D. Sacral agenesis and caudal spinal cord malformations. Neurosurgery 1993;32:755–778, discussion 778–779
13. Yegin A, Sanli S, Hadimioglu N, Sahin N. Anesthesia in caudal regression syndrome. Paediatr Anaesth 2005;15:174–175

126 Iliac Crest Bone Grafting

Lee A. Tan and Richard G. Fessler

The autologous iliac crest bone graft (ICBG) is an ideal graft material for spinal fusion procedures given its osteoconductive, osteoinductive, and osteogenic properties. However, with the recent advances in spinal fusion technology, and considering the postoperative complications associated with ICBG harvesting, such as pain, hematoma formation, and infection at the donor site, many surgeons have switched to using allografts and synthetic cages, occasionally with recombinant human bone morphogenetic protein (rhBMP) supplementation, to achieve satisfactory fusion rates.[1] However, ICBG is still considered the "gold standard" for fusion, and it is an essential tool that all spine surgeons should have in their armamentarium. This chapter discusses the anterior and posterior approaches for ICBG harvesting. The operative nuances are emphasized to minimize potential complications associated with ICBG harvesting.

Patient Selection

Most patients undergoing anterior or posterior spinal fusion procedures are candidates for ICBG harvesting. Either the anterior or posterior iliac crest can be used for bone graft harvesting, depending on patient positioning for the indexed procedure.

Indications

- Anterior cervical diskectomy and fusion
- Spinal deformity
- Spondylolisthesis
- Spinal instability
- Vertebral fractures

Contraindications

- Infection involving the donor site
- Tumor involving the donor site
- Prior graft harvesting from the same site (relative contraindication)
- Radiation or compromised vasculature of the donor site (relative contraindication)

Advantages

- Ideal graft material with osteogenic, osteoinductive, and osteoconductive properties
- The iliac crest can be easily accessed with the patient in the prone, supine, or lateral position.
- Minimal risk of injury to critical neurovascular structures
- Relatively large reserve of both cortical and cancellous bones
- No risk of transmissible disease
- Lower cost compared with its alternatives

Disadvantages

- Postoperative pain at the donor site
- Hematoma formation at the donor site
- Infection at the donor site
- Abdominal hernia through the iliac crest defect
- Pelvic instability/fractures
- Cosmetic deformity
- Injury to the contents of the greater sciatic notch including the sciatic nerve and superior gluteal artery
- Injury to the traversing nerves
  - Anterior approach: injury to the lateral femoral cutaneous nerve, resulting in postoperative lateral thigh pain or numbness
  - Posterior approach: injury to the cluneal nerves, resulting in postoperative buttock pain or numbness

Choice of Operative Approach

The choice of operative approach for ICBG harvesting largely depends on the surgical approach selected for the indexed spinal fusion procedure. Anterior iliac crest is easily accessible for anterior spinal procedures with the patient placed in the supine position; the posterior iliac crest is readily accessible for posterior spinal procedures with the patient in the prone position.

Preoperative Testing

Routine preoperative testing for the indexed spinal procedure is often sufficient; no additional testing specific to ICBG harvest is usually necessary.

Surgical Procedure

Anesthesia and Positioning

The patient is brought into the operating room and placed under general endotracheal intubation anesthesia. Either the anterior or posterior iliac crest graft can be used for bone graft harvesting depending on whether the patient is positioned supine or prone for the indexed procedure. For anterior iliac crest graft harvesting in the supine position, it is often helpful to place a folded towel under the patient to elevate the pelvis and rotate the ipsilateral ilium medially and more superficially. The anterior superior iliac spine (ASIS) is usually clearly visible and easily accessible during the procedure. In the prone position, the posterior superior iliac spine (PSIS) is readily palpable in most cases. All pressure points should be well padded in the standard fashion. The iliac harvest sites can be prepped and draped separately from the indexed procedure or contiguously if the primary procedure is in the lower lumbar region.

Approach to the Anterior Iliac Crest

An important anatomic relationship to keep in mind during the approach to the anterior iliac crest is the location of the lateral femoral cutaneous nerve (LFCN) relative to the ASIS. The LFCN usually exits from the pelvis ~ 2 to 3 cm medial to the ASIS, although occasionally it can exit 2 cm lateral to the ASIS.[2,3] To minimize the risk of LFCN injury, the surgical incision should begin at least 2 to 3 cm posterior and lateral to the ASIS[3] and parallel and distal to the iliac crest margin (**Fig. 126.1**). The anterior iliac tubercle (AIT), which is the thickest portion of the iliac crest (up to 15 mm), is typically located ~ 3 to 5 cm posterior to ASIS; it is an optimal site for bone graft harvesting.[4] Furthermore, the risk of ASIS avulsion by the action of the tensor fascia lata or the sartorius muscle is much less if the graft is harvested from at least 3 cm posterior to the ASIS.[5] This is an important point to keep in mind because the ASIS plays an important role in cosmesis as well as in comfort when wearing pants with belts.

The gluteus minimus, medius, and tensor fascia latae are all supplied by the superior gluteal nerve, and they originate along the iliac crest and the external aspect of ilium. The iliacus muscle fills the iliac fossa medially, and is innervated by the femoral nerve. The length of the bone graft is usually limited to 35 mm to avoid potential complications associated with extensive soft tissue dissection, detachment of abductor muscles (tensor fascia lata and gluteus muscles), and to avoid injuring the LFCN as it traverses the medial aspect of the iliac crest during exposure of the inner table of the ilium. It is also important not to extend the exposure over the anterior tip of the ASIS because separation of the inguinal ligament from its attachment can occur, leading to hernia.

Keeping these important anatomic considerations in mind, the anterior iliac crest can be safely exposed by making an incision 2 to 3 cm posterior to the ASIS and along the iliac crest margin. The incision should center over the anterior iliac tubercle where the quantity of corticocancellous bone is greatest, as discussed above. Because there are no intervening vital structures, exposure of the anterior iliac crest can be readily achieved by using a monopolar cautery in a subperiosteal fashion. Given that the anterior crest has far less overlying soft tissue and musculature, a medium-sized self-retaining retractor is typically sufficient to maintain the exposure.

Approach to the Posterior Iliac Crest

The posterior superior iliac spine (PSIS) and the superior and middle cluneal nerves are important anatomic structures to keep in mind during the approach to posterior iliac crest. The PSIS is usually palpable under the buttock dimple in the medial and superior portion of the buttock region. The posterior iliac crest has a natural contour that curves upward and laterally from the PSIS. Several anatomic studies have shown that the most medial branch of the superior cluneal nerves generally cross the posterior iliac crest ~ 7 cm anterolateral to the PSIS.[6,7] Consequently, if the incision is kept within 7 cm anterolateral to the PSIS, the superior cluneal nerves are typically safe from iatrogenic injury during dissection.

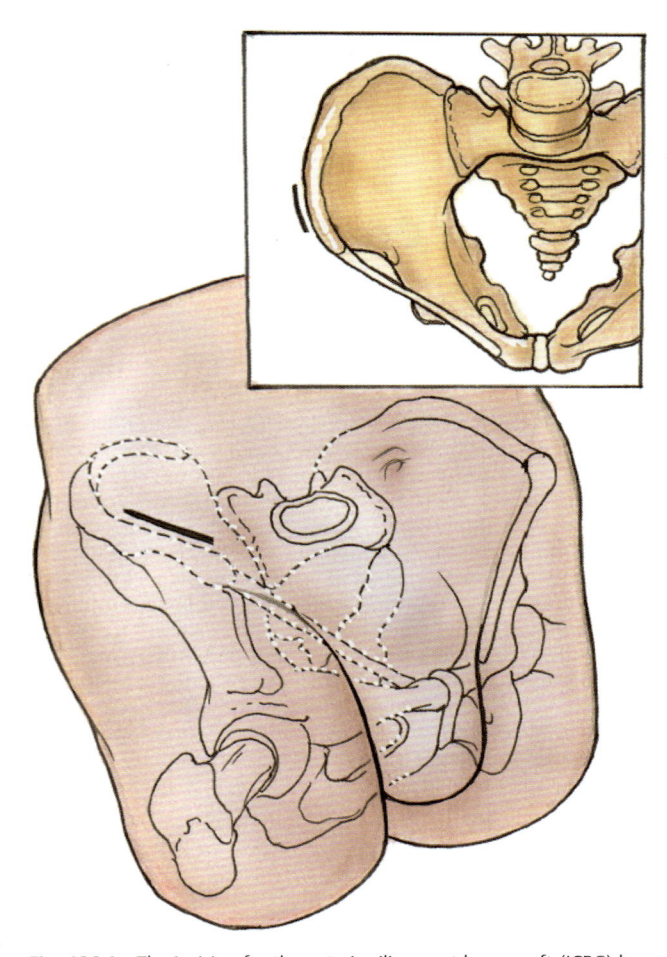

Fig. 126.1 The incision for the anterior iliac crest bone graft (ICBG) harvest should begin at least 2 to 3 cm posterior-lateral to the anterior superior iliac spine (ASIS) and parallel to the iliac crest margin (see inset) to minimize the risk of injury to the lateral femoral cutaneous nerve (LFCN), detachment of the inguinal ligament, and ASIS avulsion.

The middle cluneal nerves usually traverse just inferior to the PSIS, and injuries to these nerves typically can be avoided by keeping the incision above the PSIS. Therefore, an oblique, curved, or vertical incision can be used according to the surgeon's preference, with the incision centered over or just slightly anterior to the PSIS (**Fig. 126.2**). However, one study demonstrated that the most medial branch of the superior cluneal nerves can sometimes cross as close as 5 cm anterolateral to the PSIS, and the middle cluneal nerves can cross 2 cm superior to PSIS.[8] These findings have led the authors to advocate using an incision perpendicular to the iliac crest margin and centered at 2.5 cm from the PSIS; they believe that this incision minimizes the risk of injuries to the superior and middle cluneal nerves and reduces the incidence of painful neuromas and pain/numbness in the buttock region postoperatively (**Fig. 126.3**). If a midline posterior lumbar incision has already been made for the indexed procedure, the incision can be simply extended to the sacrum, and the subcutaneous tissue and fat elevated off the lumbodorsal fascia laterally to the iliac crest. This plane should be identified at the level of the midline incision and then opened and mobilized. As this plane is avascular, this medial to lateral exposure of the PSIS can usually be accomplished bluntly under mild tension of the musculocutaneous flap.

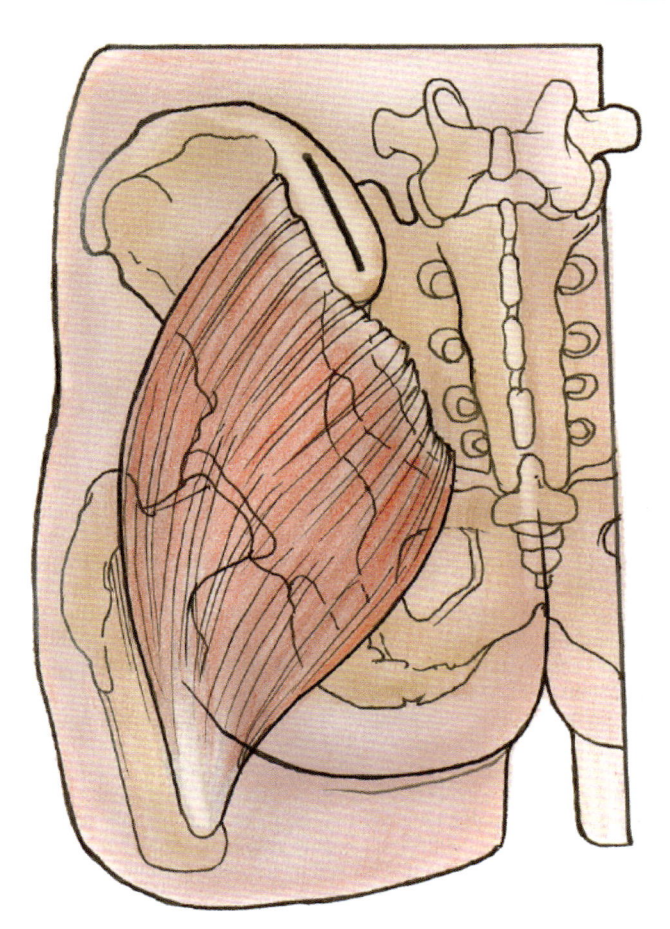

Fig. 126.2 The incision for the posterior ICBG harvest (solid black line) can be oblique, curved, or vertical, based on the surgeon's preference, with the incision centered over or just slightly anterior to the posterior superior iliac spine (PSIS) and kept within 7 cm of the PSIS anterolaterally to avoid injury to the superior cluneal nerves.

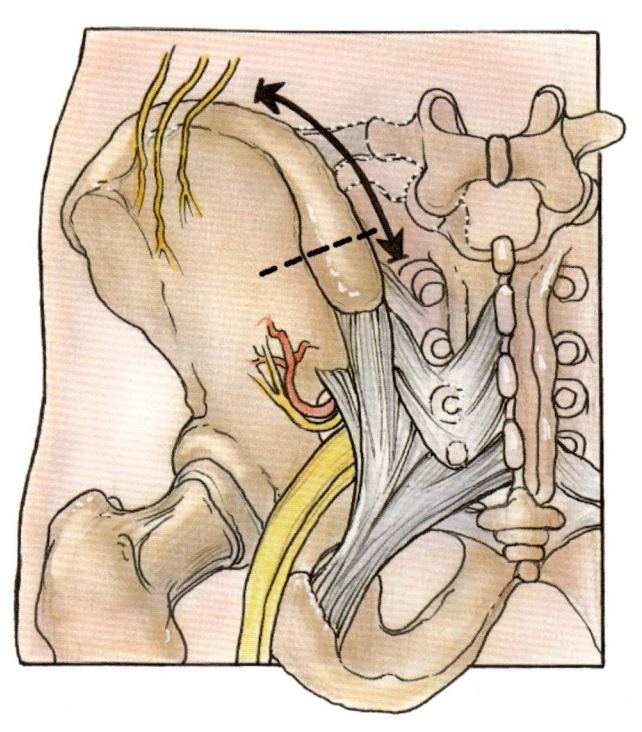

Fig. 126.3 Some surgeons advocate using an incision perpendicular to the iliac crest margin and centered at 2.5 cm from the PSIS (dashed line) as opposed to the traditional incision parallel (solid line), to minimize the risk of injuries to the superior and middle cluneal nerves and reduce the incidence of painful neuromas and pain/numbness in the buttock region.

The fascia overlying the PSIS and posterior iliac crest can then be incised. The thickest portion of the posterior iliac crest is directly anterolateral to the PSIS along the posterior gluteal line and the tubercle. This area is ideal for harvesting cancellous bone graft. The gluteus maximus, medius, and minimus originate from the lateral surface of the ilium. The superior gluteal nerve innervates the medius and minimus, whereas the inferior gluteal nerve supplies the maximus. The posterior gluteal line, which separates the gluteus maximus and medius attachments to the ilium, is then identified. An incision is made sharply along this line, and the muscles are then dissected off both surfaces of the crest. Subperiosteal dissection is performed in the outer cortex caudally. Hemostasis can be maintained using monopolar cautery, Surgicel, Gelfoam, and bone wax as needed.

Dissection should not extend to the greater sciatic notch. The sciatic nerve and superior gluteal artery are at risk if the dissection is taken close to or beyond the sciatic notch (**Fig. 126.4**). An imaginary horizontal line can be created from the PSIS out laterally and perpendicular to the vertical spinal axis (**Fig. 126.5**). Keeping the dissection cephalad to this level protects the sciatic notch and its contents. After appropriate mobilization of the muscles and periosteum has been completed to expose the ilium, retractors can be placed to maintain the exposure. Because the primary angle of retraction is caudal and lateral, a Taylor

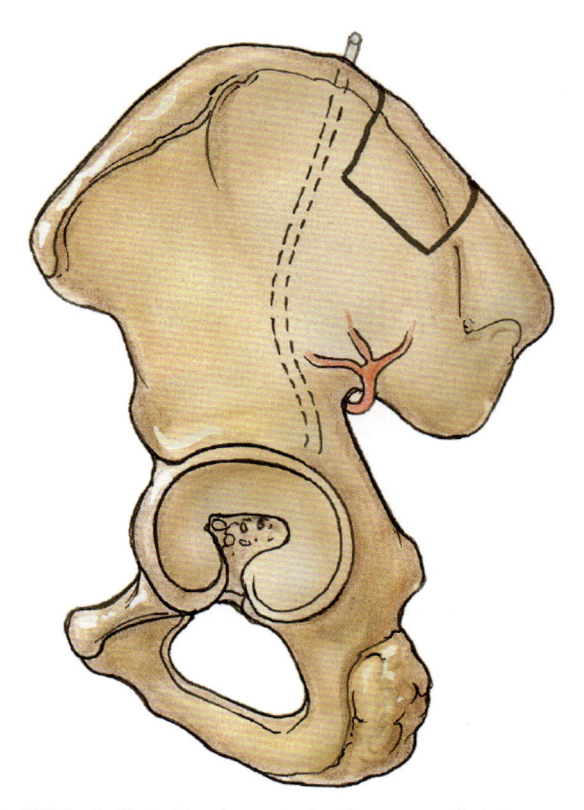

Fig. 126.4 An illustration demonstrating the courses of sciatic nerve and superior gluteal artery. Both structures are at risk if the dissection is take too close to or beyond the sciatic notch.

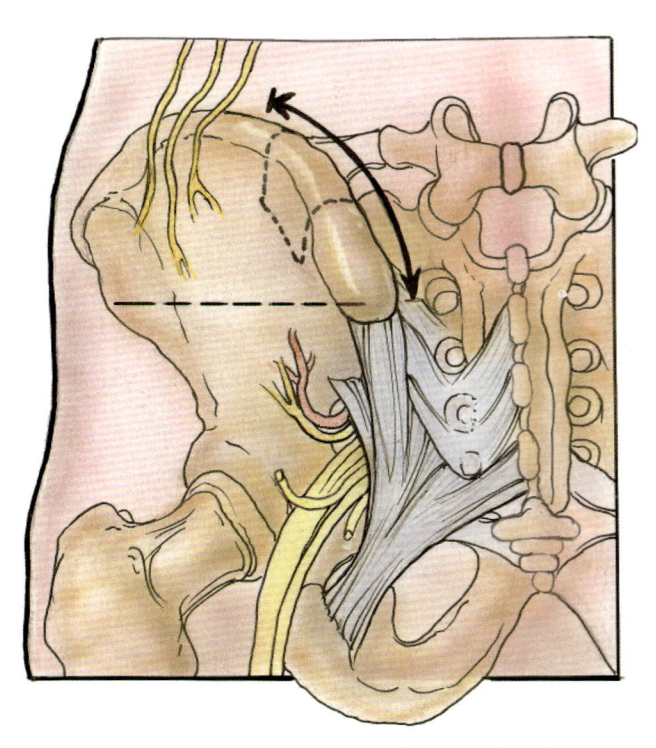

Fig. 126.5 An imaginary horizontal line can be created from the PSIS out laterally and perpendicular to the vertical spinal axis (dashed line); dissection should never be carried below this line to avoid injury to the contents of the sciatic notch. In addition, the incision should be kept within 7 cm of PSIS (solid line with arrows) to avoid injury to the superior cluneal nerves.

retractor can be placed with its point along the inferolateral face of the posterior iliac wing. Using a lap sponge anchored to the bed, gentle yet firm retraction of the gluteal musculocutaneous flap can be obtained. Caution should be exercised to avoid placing the Taylor too deep within the sciatic notch.

The key to safety in this approach is keeping the dissection subperiosteal. If the dissection strays into the gluteal musculature, excessive bleeding and injury to the neurovascular structures are more likely to occur. Also the large vascular structures leave the pelvis via the sciatic notch. Laceration of the superior gluteal artery typically occurs near this region and can cause vessel retraction into the pelvis. If the sacroiliac joint is visualized, the dissection has been brought in too medial a direction.

Graft Harvesting Techniques

Depending on the nature and type of bone graft desired, the exact technique of crest harvesting varies. For cases where primarily cancellous bone graft is desired, a small window can be made along the iliac tubercle in the region of the PSIS or ASIS. Only a small exposure of the crest line is made with minimal muscular stripping, to enable the creation of the window. Gouges and curettes are then used to remove the cancellous bone from between the cortical walls, thus sparing their muscular and soft tissue attachments (**Fig. 126.6**). This approach helps to minimize postoperative graft-site pain by decreasing scarring and maintaining the anatomic musculotendinous insertions around the ilium.

For cases where corticocancellous chips are desired, an osteotome can be used to create a cortical window below the actual crest line. Preservation of the outer crest margin is beneficial for both cosmetic and functional reasons. If corticocancellous bone strips are needed, longitudinal parallel cuts can be made using the osteotome (**Fig. 126.7**). The osteotome should be visualized carefully during this maneuver to avoid making fractures through the sciatic notch and sacroiliac joint. Additionally, care should be taken not to violate the inner table to decrease the risk of postoperative hernia. Generally, bone harvesting from the inner table is associated with a higher risk of peritoneal violation, perforation, and retroperitoneal hematoma.

When large wedge-shaped grafts or plugs are needed, careful exposure of the medial wall of the ilium should be completed prior to bone harvesting. Direct visualization and the avoidance of blind cuts are essential to prevent deep pelvic and retroperitoneal injury and bleeding. Use of an oscillating saw in such cases may also be helpful in creating smooth parallel cuts and to help prevent microfractures, thereby increasing the integrity of the graft. Whenever possible, bone graft should be harvested near the time when the operative site is ready. As the harvesting process disconnects the graft from its blood supply, prolonged intervals between harvesting and actual grafting can cause desiccation and ischemia of the bone. Maintenance of the health and moisture of the graft are thus essential in improving the chance of a successful fusion. As such, wrapping of the graft(s) in wet normal saline gauze and decreasing the out-of-body time are important surgical goals.

Closure

In cases where the crestal margin has been violated, it may be desirable to reconstruct the cosmetic edge with titanium plates

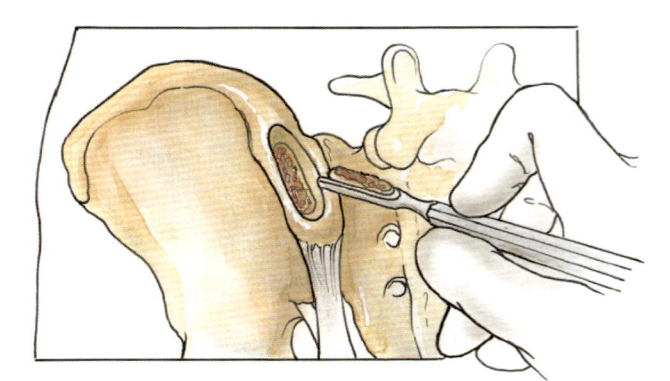

Fig. 126.6 Gouges and curettes can be used to remove the cancellous bone from between the cortical walls, thus sparing their muscular and soft tissue attachments.

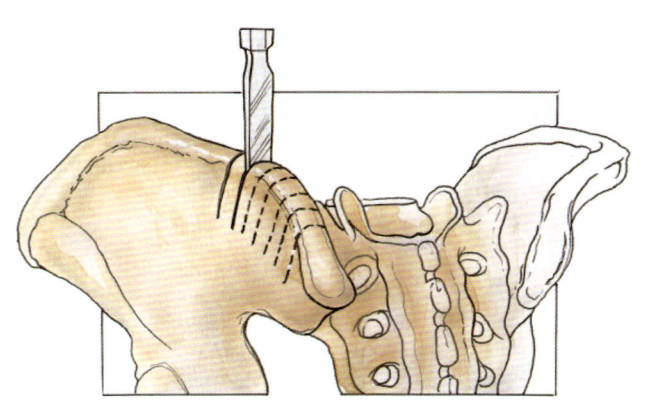

Fig. 126.7 The osteotome can be used to make longitudinal parallel cuts to obtain corticocancellous bone strips.

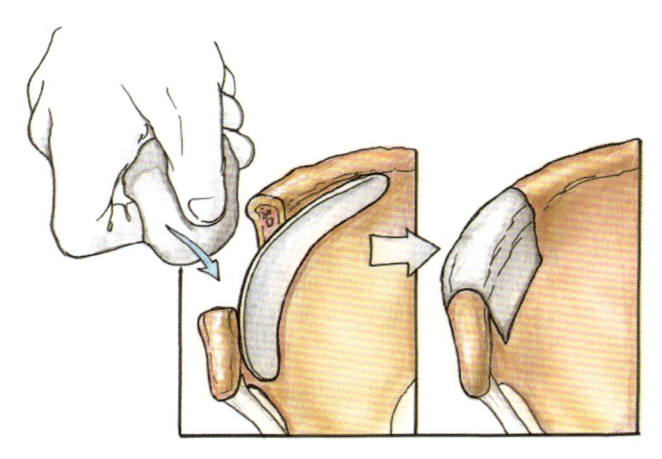

Fig. 126.8 The iliac wing defect can be reconstructed with bone cement, and malleable blades can be used to repair the iliac wall as shown.

or mesh. Similarly, when large defects of the medial iliac wall have been created, repair with mesh, plates, or bioabsorbable materials can help to significantly reduce the risk of an abdominal hernia (**Fig. 126.8**). Reconstruction of large crestal defects has also been reported to decrease the incidence of chronic pain due to musculotendinous incompetency. Meticulous hemostasis is essential in the graft site. Excessive use of bone wax to control bleeding in the cancellous edges should be avoided because this will retard bone healing and has been associated with a higher incidence of seroma formation. Typically, the use of thrombin-impregnated Gelfoam, Avitene, or similar substances is effective to stop bleeding. For large defects, a closed suction drainage system is often used to minimize the risk of postoperative hematoma. The muscle and fascia are then sutured to their original anatomic positions to minimize the risk of hernia. Restoration of the musculotendinous gluteal and abdominal attachments over some type of solid support (e.g., bone or metal plates) is important to decrease pain and prevent cosmetic dimpling. The wound is then dressed in the usual fashion. Drains should be left in place until their output is minimal, but generally should not remain for longer than 2 to 3 days.

Postoperative Care

- Pain management
- Monitor for hematoma at the donor site

Potential Complications and Precautions

Potential complications associated with ICBG harvesting include injury to the LFCN or the superior and middle cluneal nerves, hematoma formation, infection, injury to the contents of the sciatic notch, abdominal hernia, and ASIS avulsion. A thorough understanding of local anatomy and meticulous surgical techniques as detailed in this chapter will help surgeons to minimize the potential complications associated with ICBG.

Conclusion

Iliac crest bone graft harvesting is an essential tool that all spine surgeons should keep in their armamentarium. A solid understanding of the anatomic relationships between the ASIS and the LFCN, and between the PSIS and the superior cuneal nerves, as well as meticulous surgical techniques, can minimize complications associated with this procedure and optimize patient outcome. **Box 126.1** lists the key operative steps.

Box 126.1   Key Operative Steps

- Properly position the patient and pad all pressure points.
- Locate the ASIS or PSIS for anterior or posterior ICBG harvesting, respectively.
- Mark the incision at the appropriate locations to minimize the risk of injuries to the LFCN or cluneal nerves, as detailed in this chapter.
- Use subperiosteal dissections to minimize bleeding and the risk of neurovascular injury.
- Be aware of the location of the sciatic notch and its contents.
- Perform meticulous closure of the fascia to minimize the risk of hernia.
- Consider iliac crest reconstruction if the defect is large.

References

1. Cabraja M, Kroppenstedt S. Bone grafting and substitutes in spine surgery. J Neurosurg Sci 2012;56:87–95
2. Aszmann OC, Dellon ES, Dellon AL. Anatomical course of the lateral femoral cutaneous nerve and its susceptibility to compression and injury. Plast Reconstr Surg 1997;100:600–604
3. Ropars M, Zadem A, Morandi X, Kaila R, Guillin R, Huten D. How can we optimize anterior iliac crest bone harvesting? An anatomical and radiological study. Eur Spine J 2013
4. Ebraheim NA, Yang H, Lu J, Biyani A, Yeasting RA. Anterior iliac crest bone graft. Anatomic considerations. Spine 1997;22:847–849
5. Hu R, Hearn T, Yang J. Bone graft harvest site as a determinant of iliac crest strength. Clin Orthop Relat Res 1995;310:252–256
6. Colterjohn NR, Bednar DA. Procurement of bone graft from the iliac crest. An operative approach with decreased morbidity. J Bone Joint Surg Am 1997;79:756–759
7. Lu J, Ebraheim NA, Huntoon M, Heck BE, Yeasting RA. Anatomic considerations of superior cluneal nerve at posterior iliac crest region. Clin Orthop Relat Res 1998;347:224–228
8. Xu R, Ebraheim NA, Yeasting RA, Jackson WT. Anatomic considerations for posterior iliac bone harvesting. Spine 1996;21:1017–1020

Section VI   Peripheral Nerves

A. Pathology of the Brachial Plexus

127 Neoplasms of Peripheral Nerves

Carlos E. Restrepo Rubio and Robert J. Spinner

Peripheral nerve tumors are relatively rare, making their diagnosis and management challenging for inexperienced radiologists and surgeons. Still, surgical resection of these tumors is and needs to be part of a neurosurgeon's armamentarium. In the general population, these peripheral nerve tumors are estimated to account for 10 to 12% of the benign soft tissue neoplasms.[1,2]

The most common tumors affecting the peripheral nerves are benign nerve sheath tumors, that is, schwannomas (neurilemomas or even "neuromas") and neurofibromas. These tumors may arise from any peripheral nerve with a Schwann cell, including distal portions of cranial nerves.[3] They may occur sporadically or in association with syndromes. In our experience, patients with a solitary nerve sheath tumor more commonly have a schwannoma than a neurofibroma. The finding of several nerve sheath tumors (schwannomas or neurofibromas) can be associated with syndromes: (1) multiple schwannomas can be associated with neurofibromatosis type 2 (NF2), which is a syndrome characterized by bilateral acoustic neuromas or (2) a newer form of NF, called schwannomatosis distinguished by multiple schwannomas more commonly located in the periphery than intracranially, and not not usually associated with acoustic neuromas; and (3) multiple neurofibromas in subcutaneous or deep tissues can be associated with neurofibromatosis type 1 (NF1).[4] The tumors involving small cutaneous nerves may appear as numerous subcutaneous nodules. If surgical intervention is required, they are easily resected from surrounding tissues. There are few or no sequelae associated with sacrificing the sensory nerve containing the neurofibroma. When tumors involve large nerves, elephantiasis neuromatosa or local gigantism can occur.

A benign peripheral nerve sheath tumor often presents as a slow-growing mass that can be found incidentally during self-examination; it can also be accompanied by a mild to moderate degree of pain or radiating dysesthesias in the nerve distribution. Physical examination reveals a soft, mobile mass. The presence of motor impairment is not a common feature in benign nerve sheath tumors as the tumor tends to displace fascicles. Both schwannomas and neurofibromas have the potential to develop into large tumors with an intra- and extraspinal component connected through the intervertebral foramen by a narrowed segment of tumor; hence the descriptive term *dumbbell tumor*. Neurologic symptoms occur in more than 60% of these patients.[5] The slow growth of the tumor can result in extensive bony erosion.

Other rarer benign nerve lesions exist, including perineuriomas, intraneural ganglion cysts, and adipose lesions. These tend to present with neurologic deficit. Their magnetic resonance imaging (MRI) features can generally be readily distinguished from a conventional benign nerve sheath tumor (schwannoma, neurofibroma) or malignant peripheral nerve sheath tumor (MPNST). In many cases, experienced radiologists can diagnose these lesions based on their radiological appearance, thus making biopsy unnecessary.

Primary or secondary malignant nerve lesions, though rare, also occur. Malignant nerve sheath tumors may occur in patients sporadically, in those who have been radiated, and are well known in those with NF1; transformation of plexiform neurofibromas to MPNSTs has been estimated to occur in 8 to 13% of patients with NF1.[6] Schwannomas, whether solitary or syndromic, entail essentially no risk of malignant transformation. Secondary forms of malignancy can affect peripheral nerve by direct, hematogenous, or perineural spread.

In contrast, malignant lesions must be suspected especially when patients develop new-onset severe pain that is poorly controlled with medications, a rapidly enlarging mass that is not mobile, and a progressive neurologic deficit. Imaging studies can provide information concerning the size, extent, anatomic location, and the relationship of the tumor to the surrounding structures. High-resolution MRI can provide some useful information about the nature of the tumor type, but cannot reliably differentiate schwannomas from neurofibromas, or benign from malignant nerve sheath tumors. Positron emission tomography (PET) scanning can be a helpful adjunct in patients with malignant lesions.[7]

This chapter discusses the surgical treatment of benign nerve sheath tumors—schwannomas and neurofibromas—and how to distinguish them from MPNSTs. The operative management of MPNSTs is beyond the scope of this review. Recent advances in the surgery of benign nerve sheath tumors have shown that, with the appropriate use of microsurgical techniques, the majority of these lesions can be safely resected with few or no neurologic sequelae.

Indications

The main indications for tumor surgery are the presence of pain, any type of neurologic symptoms (e.g., paresthesias, dysesthesias, and weakness), or compressive symptoms from adjacent tissues. Cosmetic reasons can also can be considered. Asymptomatic or mildly symptomatic lesions may be resected after careful consideration of the risks and benefits, knowing that larger tumors are associated with more presenting symptoms and a higher surgical complication rate of temporary or permanent neurologic sequelae.

Occasionally, tumors are operated on for a definitive diagnosis or suspicion of malignancy, including progressive neurologic deficit or tumors that show significant growth during the imaging follow-up.

Advantages

The primary advantages of surgery are that it removes the tumor, reduces the pain, and improves the sensory symptoms. In rare cases where a benign lesion is causing compression over the neighboring fascicles or adjacent structures resection, the resection can help improve the motor weakness and restore function. Definitive tissue diagnosis is obtained. If appropriate total resection is done, uninvolved fascicles are preserved and long-term imaging follow-up is generally not necessary, because recurrence from benign lesions is negligible. Resection of tumors avoids further tumor growth. In neurofibromas, it prevents the risk of malignant transformation.

Disadvantages

The major disadvantage of surgical resection is that it creates unintended neurologic complication by injuring uninvolved fascicles, potentially resulting in neuropathic pain, sensory impairment, and motor weakness.

Management

The natural history of benign nerve sheath tumors is that they are slow growing. The treatment of symptomatic lesions is operative excision (**Figs. 127.1, 127.2, 127.3**). Generally, asymptomatic lesions that are not growing do not need to be resected. Unless the tumor is massive, or prior surgery has been performed, operative excision can be accomplished with little or no injury to the parent nerve. Recurrences after removal are infrequent.

Patients suffering from NF-related syndromes can have hundreds of tumors; thus, the management of a particular lesion must take into consideration the severity of the symptoms associated with it, the size of the lesion, and the suspected pathology. Conventional globular schwannomas or neurofibromas are most

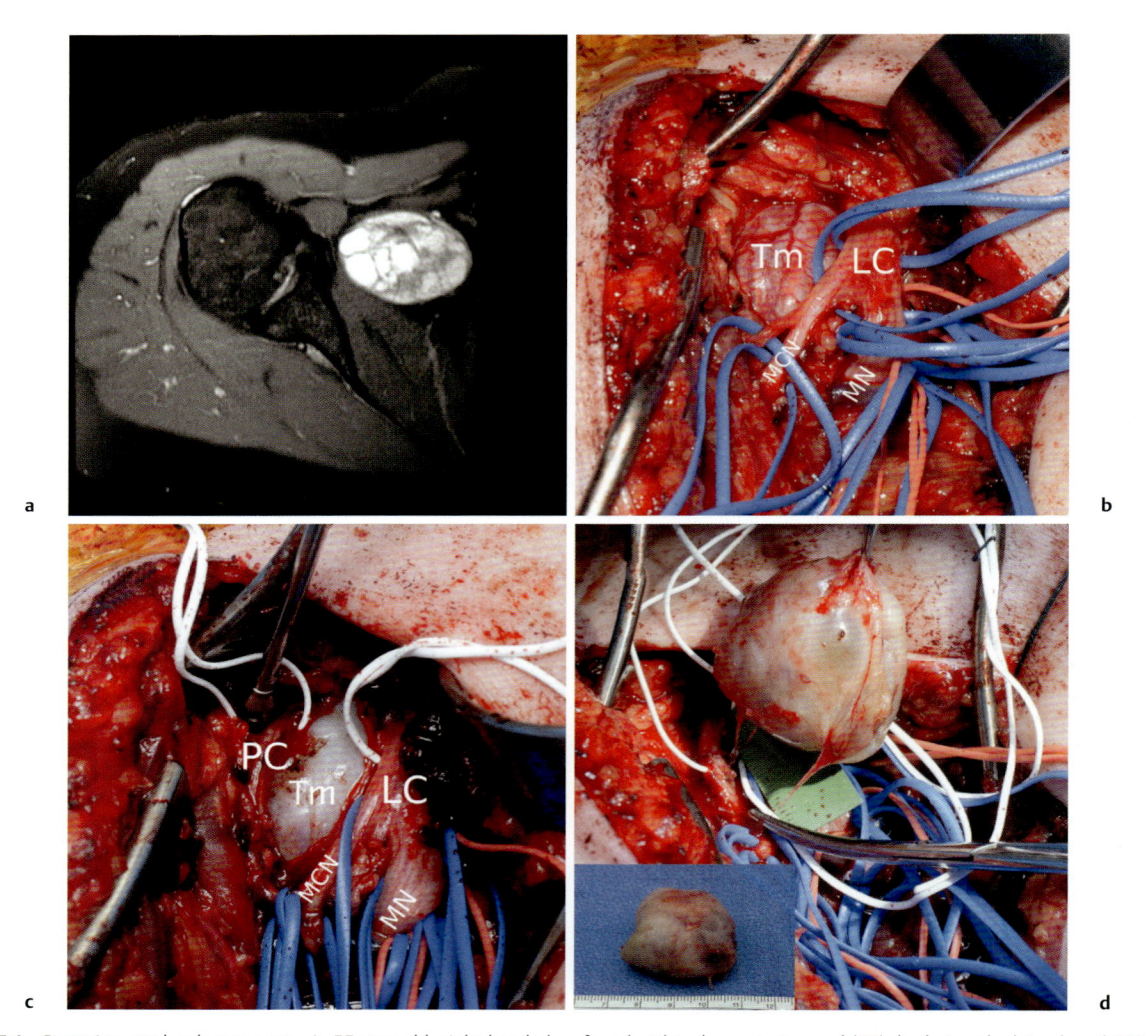

Fig. 127.1 Posterior cord schwannoma. A 55-year-old right-handed woman presented with severe progressive pain radiating into her dorsal wrist. **(a)** T2-weighted axial magnetic resonance imaging (MRI) demonstrated a heterogeneous cystic mass in her axilla intimately related to the infraclavicular brachial plexus. A biopsy of the lesion done at an outside institution had revealed a schwannoma. **(b,c)** A deltopectoral incision was made to approach the infraclavicular brachial plexus. The tumor (Tm) was found within the posterior cord (PC) displacing the lateral cord (LC) anteriorly. MCN, musculocutaneous nerve; MN, median nerve. **(c)** After a longitudinal opening in the epineurium was made, circumferential dissection was done to free up the mass. **(d)** The entering and exiting fascicle was isolated and then cut. A complete resection of the lesion was achieved, sparing the rest of the fascicles of the posterior cord. Neurologic function was preserved and pain was resolved.

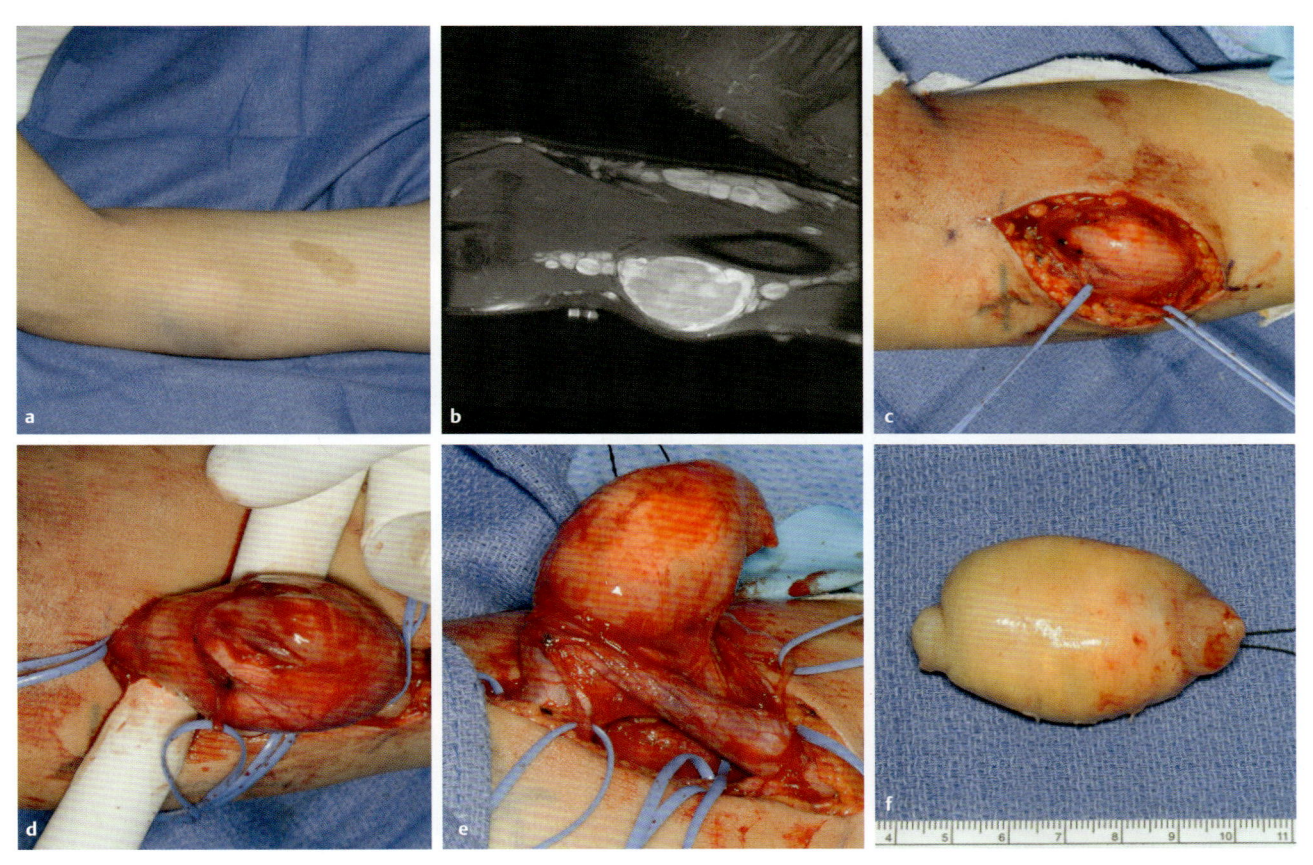

Fig. 127.2 Radial nerve plexiform neurofibroma. **(a)** A 17-year-old left-handed boy with a history of neurofibromatosis type 1 (NF1) presented with a slowly but steadily enlarging mass involving the radial nerve in the distal left arm near a café-au-lait spot. Neurologic examination was normal. There was moderate pain with percussion of the tumor. **(b)** T2-weighted sagittal MRI of the arm revealed plexiform lesions involving several nerves, including the radial nerve in which there was a large nodule admixed with multiple smaller ones. **(c)** A 7-cm skin incision was made centered over the palpable tumor using an anterolateral approach to the distal arm between the brachioradialis/brachialis and triceps. **(d)** Proximal and distal control of the radial nerve was obtained. The radial nerve was enlarged. Stimulation of the plexiform lesions produced forearm extensor muscle contraction. **(e)** The large nodule was then mobilized circumferentially. It had two or three smaller fascicles that were worm-like but were part of this large tumor. **(f)** The tumor was then resected in toto. It measured over 6 cm in size. The other nodular plexiform lesions were left behind. Pathology revealed a neurofibroma. The patient remained neurologically intact postoperatively.

often slowly enlarging, painless masses. Typically, conventional globular lesions involve small sensory fascicles and can be excised without creating a meaningful neurologic deficit. Even when globular tumors involve a major nerve, often only one or two fascicles are involved. In these situations, sacrifice of the involved fascicle(s) is not associated with further loss of neurologic function. Nerve graft repair should be considered in rare situations when the nerve sheath tumor involves a larger percentage of the nerve.

The situation for plexiform lesions is quite different. Plexiform neurofibromas are well known in patients with NF1, but plexiform schwannomas also occur in patients with NF2 or schwannomatosis. These lesions are typically asymptomatic, but, on occasion, pain is prominent. This occurs particularly when the lesion is trapped in a compartment. These lesions extend over considerable lengths of the nerve, coursing into multiple branches. Separate tumors of different sizes tend to develop on multiple fascicles; occasionally, a predominant mass may occur in the setting of innumerable smaller tumors. Either the same or different fascicles can be involved, with tumor at multiple points along the course of the nerve, creating a string-of-pearls appearance. If only one or several fascicles are involved with the tumor, excision is possible of this particular lesion (**Fig.** 127.2); however, complete removal of all of the tumors from a major mixed nerve will result in a neurologic deficit. Debulking the sizable tumor may ameliorate symptoms while preserving function. In rare situations, it may be possible to improve the symptoms by performing an external neurolysis of the nerve combined with enlarging the surrounding (e.g., foraminotomy).

Prior to planning removal of an intraspinal nerve sheath tumor, it is essential to evaluate the lesion for the possible presence of a dumbbell tumor. MRI is especially important for distinguishing a nerve root sheath tumor from an intra/extraforaminal intervertebral disk prolapse. Computed tomography (CT)/myelography enables the delineation of the bony anatomy and its relation to the neural elements. If the tumor is located in the lower thoracic region, spinal arteriography can be performed to determine the blood supply of the spinal cord. In addition, very large tumors can be embolized to ease surgical removal. If evidence exists of proximal tumor involvement, then preoperative investigation of the spine is performed to delineate the intraspinal extension of the tumor.[8]

If there is concern about an MPNST based on clinical and radiological features, then we perform percutaneous image-guided biopsy prior to surgical resection. In these specific situations, the advantages of knowing the definitive diagnosis preoperatively

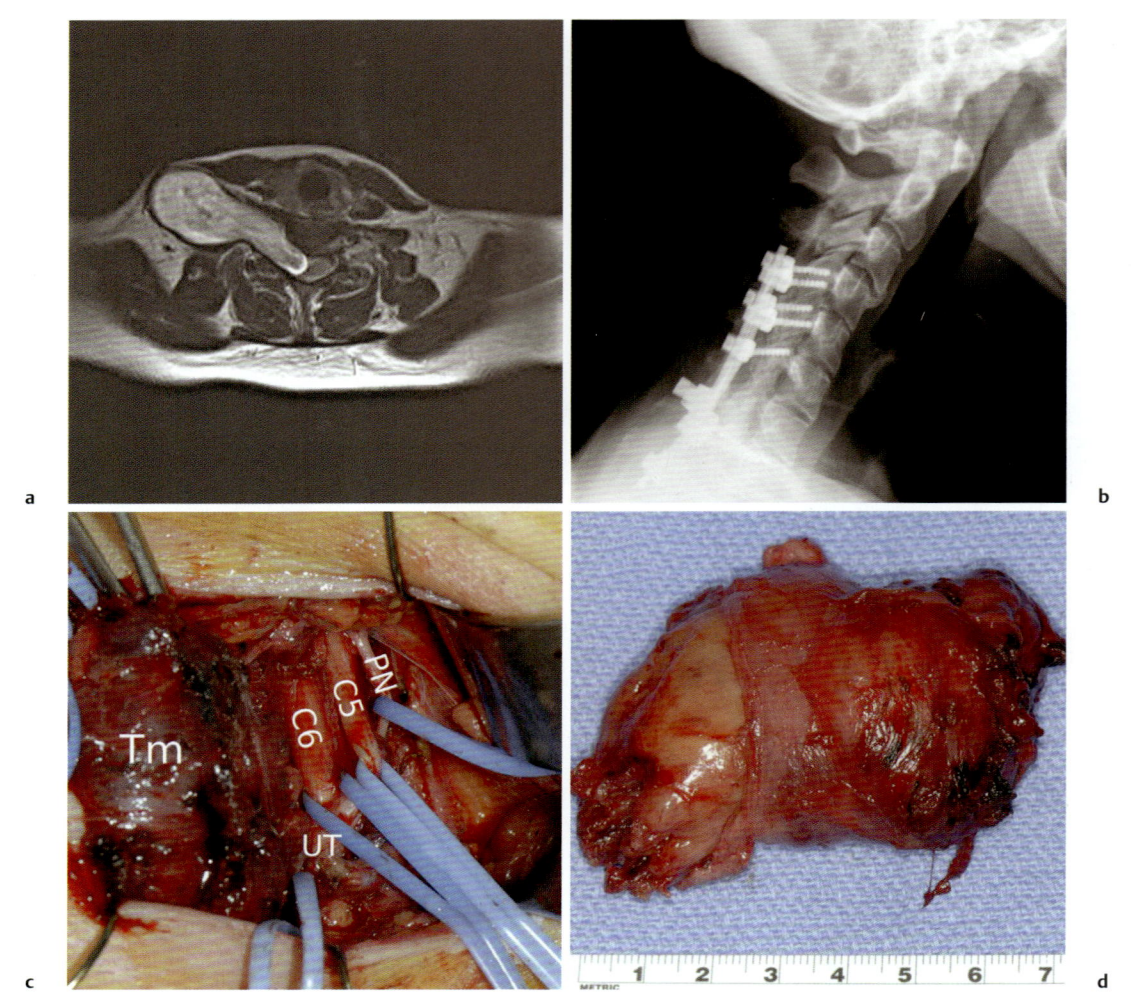

Fig. 127.3 Dumbbell schwannoma of C7 and middle trunk. A 34-year-old right-handed woman presented with a slow-growing mass in the anterior right neck that was previously biopsied and consistent with a schwannoma. She had no neurologic impairment. She had a Tinel's sign radiating from the supraclavicular fossa to the middle finger. **(a)** An axial T2-weighted MRI demonstrated a large dumbbell tumor involving the middle trunk and extending through the right C6-C7 neural foramen into the spinal canal, moderately compressing the spinal cord. **(b)** A two-stage operation was performed starting with a decompression of the spinal cord with a partial removal of the tumor through a C6 and C7 hemilaminectomy, facetectomy and subsequent instrumentation. **(c)** The second stage was done through an anterior supraclavicular approach. The phrenic nerve (PN), C5 and C6 nerves, and upper trunk (UT) were identified and protected. The tumor (Tm) was dissected circumferentially and followed to the upper and lower poles. **(d)** The entering fascicles were identified and the tumor was resected in toto.

and making management decisions far outweighs the small risks associated with the biopsy (pain or deficit from neural injury, tissue sampling errors, or tumor seeding).[9] A patient with a suspected or confirmed MPNST should undergo staging studies with CT of the chest, abdomen, and pelvis or PET scanning as part of the planning before the review of a treatment plan with medical and radiation oncologists and sarcoma surgeons. In patients without metastatic disease, wide surgical resection is generally performed in combination with radiation by itself or with chemotherapy (**Fig. 127.4**).

Surgical Removal of Benign Nerve Sheath Tumors

Anesthesia and Positioning

General, regional, or local anesthesia can be used; however, only general or regional anesthesia enables the use of a tourniquet, which greatly facilitates the dissection by providing a dry field. Muscle relaxant is avoided because it precludes the use of nerve stimulation. The patient is positioned to maximize the exposure of the tumor. In the rare case where nerve grafting is considered, positioning may require attention to the possible need for harvesting of a donor nerve.

Incision and Dissection

A skin incision is made that provides safe exposure of the nerve tumor with identification of normal anatomy. For smaller lesions, this can be done through shorter incisions, enabling a short segment of proximal and distal control of the nerve tumor and the nerve tumor itself. For larger lesions, a more extensile approach would be necessary. Incisions should be planned centered on the lesion, which can be palpated or localized by imaging (MRI or ultrasound).

Dissection continues through the subcutaneous tissues, with close attention paid to hemostasis. As the nerve is approached,

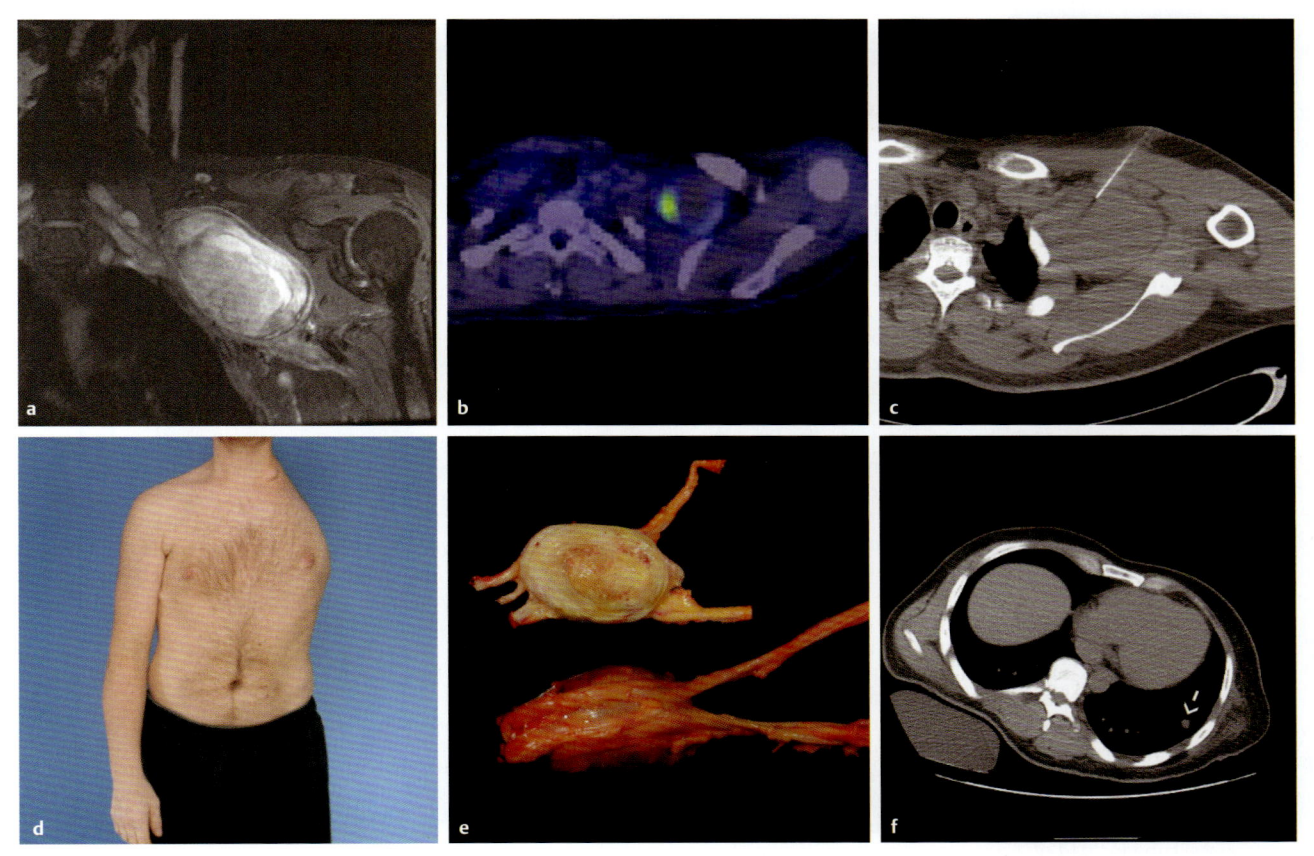

Fig. 127.4 An NF1-related malignant peripheral nerve sheath tumor (MPNST) of the posterior cord of the brachial plexus. A 37-year-old, right-handed man with history of NF1 presented with a progressive severe burning pain in his left shoulder that radiated down the dorsal arm and wrist. There was weakness in the radial innervated muscles as well as numbness in dorsum of his hand. **(a)** Coronal T2-weighted MRI revealed a heterogeneous mass at the level of the divisions and cords of the left brachial plexus that affected primarily the posterior cord. **(b)** A positron emission tomography (PET)–computed tomography (CT) scan showed increased avidity of the left brachial plexus mass. **(c)** A CT-guided biopsy confirmed the presence of an MPNST. Despite chemotherapy, the mass increased in size. **(d)** A forequarter amputation was performed, with transaction of the spinal nerves at the foramina. **(e)** Negative margins were achieved. Immediately following the surgery, pain improved significantly. **(f)** One year postoperatively, the patient developed a left lung metastasis *(white arrow)*.

the exposure begins in a region of normal anatomy and extends into the region of tumor formation. Loupe magnification or an operating microscope is essential for identification of the fascicles coursing over the tumor. Electrical nerve stimulation is also used to differentiate fascicles from tumor. A dissection plane is now established by gently separating and elevating the fascicles from the surface of the tumor. There may be a thin capsule (epineurium) that requires opening to facilitate the dissection of the tumor from the nerve. A second deeper tissue plane may be present that also has to be entered to enable the dissection of the tumor from the nerve. In many circumstances the tumor is enveloped with fascicles, and the appearance on first inspection may suggest that the tumor cannot be resected. An internal neurolysis with careful separation of the fascicles will reveal that the tumor can be separated from the fascicles. If required, to ease the dissection or manipulation, the capsule can be opened and the tumor debulked from within and removed in a piecemeal fashion. Very large tumors may require debulking with the aid of an ultrasonic aspirator.

Most conventional globular tumors can be removed en bloc. Although often splayed and thinned, the uninvolved fascicles are functioning and must be preserved. The surface of the tumor may be mapped to determine the location of functioning fascicles with a nerve stimulator. If ongoing electromyographic (EMG) activity is being monitored from muscles innervated by the nerve, feedback can be gained concerning aggressive manipulation of the fascicles. As the tumor is mobilized, there may be a single fascicle seen entering and exiting the mass. Electrical stimulation will determine if this is a motor fascicle and still functional or if fascicles enlarged by tumor provide motor function (**Fig. 127.1**), typically is not functional.

A plexiform neurofibroma may be encountered, which may limit the ability to fully excise the tumor. Once the region of the nerve containing the dominant nodule is exposed, magnification is employed. If the tumor is not visible on the surface of the nerve, an internal neurolysis is required. As the epineurium is opened, the tumor can be identified. Frequently, there is a pseudocapsule enveloping the tumor that requires opening. Once the correct plane has been entered, the surgeon will usually be able to preserve the vast majority of the fascicles by separating the tumor from the nerve. One or more fascicles will be seen entering and exiting the tumor and will have to be sacrificed. The tumor can then be gently dissected away from the remaining fascicles (**Fig. 127.2**).

For dumbbell tumors, more than one approach may be needed to remove all aspects of the tumor; the approach should be individualized. In many cases, the intradural and intraspinal components should be removed first because spinal cord compression is often the major source of concern. Once the intraspinal component is removed, the paraspinal approach is addressed. In some cases, especially when the intervertebral foramen is expanded from bony erosion over the course of years, a soft tumor may be safely removed from an anterior approach alone. A small intra- or extraspinal component remnant need not always be resected; it can also be monitored for growth. Once the tumor removal is complete, the dura mater is sealed (often requiring a graft). Unilateral loss of a facet joint in the thoracic spine is easily tolerated. In the cervical or lumbar spine, a dumbbell tumor resection often requires stabilization of the spine utilizing bony fusion techniques **(Fig. 127.3)**.

The tumor specimen and the tumor bed are inspected for any evidence of divided fascicles. If a divided fascicle is found, the distal end can be electrically stimulated to determine if it is a motor fascicle and what muscles are innervated by the fascicle. Nerve grafting should be considered anytime a significant fascicle is sacrificed. The decision as to the need for a nerve graft repair is based on the degree of anticipated deficit from the divided fascicle. The need for a nerve graft repair after removal of a schwannoma or neurofibromas by experienced surgeons is rare. Depending on the clinical scenario, the surgeon will determine if sacrifice of the fascicle necessitates a nerve graft repair. Unlike the fascicles entering a schwannoma, those entering a neurofibroma may still be functioning. If there is concern about neurologic sequelae, a nerve graft repair is performed. Individual fascicles can be grafted using a perineurial technique; alternatively, if the entire cross section of nerve has been damaged, an epineurial repair is performed. A 9-0 nonabsorbable filament suture or fibrin glue may be utilized to secure the grafts. The sural nerve frequently serves as the donor nerve, although local cutaneous nerves may also be utilized. Some surgeons have opted to use a nerve tube instead of a nerve graft in these circumstances.

No attempt is made to remove the remaining tumor capsule because the presence of tumor capsule is not associated with tumor recurrence. Frozen section of the tumor is obtained to determine if a malignancy (MPNST) is present. Wound closure is performed in layers, taking care not to entrap the nerve in a tight compartment. If a nerve graft was required, splinting is employed for 3 weeks.

Pathology

Schwannoma

On gross examination the tumor appears shiny, tan-yellow, and encapsulated. It is distinguished from other nerve sheath tumors histologically by the presence of only Schwann cells; perineural cells and fibroblasts are not present.[2] Tumor cells can be arranged in alternating hypercellular palisading regions (Antoni A) and hypocellular loosely meshed (Antoni B) regions, or there can be a predominance of only one pattern. A crucial histological feature is that, unlike neurofibromas, these lesions grow within the nerve sheath, displacing the fascicles, and typically do not envelop the axonal processes.[10] Despite this characterization, one can almost always find a small fascicle entering or exiting the proximal and distal poles of the tumor.[11] Schwannomas become well encapsulated by the epineurium and push aside adjacent fascicles.[2] They are frequently soft to palpation and can be cystic.

Neurofibroma

The globular tumors are well circumscribed, ovoid, pale gray, and translucent. On histological evaluation, neurofibromas are unencapsulated tumors. Based on gross appearance and resectability, it appears that most neurofibromas do indeed have a capsule (likely perineurium), and fascicles are often peripherally enclosed in its layers.[10,11] Neurofibromas are composed of a mixture of proliferating nerve sheath cells likely arising from the perineural fibroblast and are intimately associated with the nerve fibers. Proliferating cells expand the fascicle and envelop the axonal processes. A crucial histological feature is that, unlike schwannomas, the tumor involves the entire cross section of the fascicle, resulting in a lack of surgical cleavage plane between the nerve fibers and the tumor. Thus, by necessity, when neurofibromas are removed, the axons enveloped by the tumor must also be removed. Fortunately, in many instances fascicles that are not expanded by tumors can be spared.

References

1. Kransdorf MJ. Benign soft-tissue tumors in a large referral population: distribution of specific diagnoses by age, sex, and location. AJR Am J Roentgenol 1995;164:395–402
2. Enzinger FM, Weiss SW. Benign tumors of peripheral nerves. In: Enzinger FM, Weiss SW, eds. Soft tissue tumors, 3rd ed. St. Louis: Mosby; 1995: 821–888
3. Asthagiri AR, Parry DM, Butman JA, et al. Neurofibromatosis type 2. Lancet 2009;373:1974–1986
4. Koontz NA, Wiens AL, Agarwal A, Hingtgen CM, Emerson RE, Mosier KM. Schwannomatosis: the overlooked neurofibromatosis? AJR Am J Roentgenol 2013;200:W646-53
5. Grillo HC, Ojemann RG, Scannell JG, Zervas NT. Combined approach to "dumbbell" intrathoracic and intraspinal neurogenic tumors. Ann Thorac Surg 1983;36:402–407
6. Evans DG, Baser ME, McGaughran J, Sharif S, Howard E, Moran A. Malignant peripheral nerve sheath tumours in neurofibromatosis 1. J Med Genet 2002;39:311–314
7. Ahlawat S, Chhabra A, Blakely J. Magnetic resonance neurography of peripheral nerve tumors and tumorlike conditions. Neuroimaging Clin N Am 2014;24:171–192
8. Dorsi MJ, Belzberg AJ. Paraspinal nerve sheath tumors. Neurosurg Clin N Am 2004;15:217–222, vii
9. Resnick JM, Fanning CV, Caraway NP, Varma DG, Johnson M. Percutaneous needle biopsy diagnosis of benign neurogenic neoplasms. Diagn Cytopathol 1997;16:17–25
10. Rodriguez FJ, Folpe AL, Giannini C, Perry A. Pathology of peripheral nerve sheath tumors: diagnostic overview and update on selected diagnostic problems. Acta Neuropathol 2012;123:295–319
11. Donner TR, Voorhies RM, Kline DG. Neural sheath tumors of major nerves. J Neurosurg 1994;81:362–373

128 Traumatic Peripheral Nerve Injuries

Zarina S. Ali, Gregory G. Heuer, and Eric L. Zager

Traumatic peripheral nerve injuries (PNIs) affect 360,000 people each year in the United States, resulting in a significant lifelong disability in most patients.[1] The majority of these injuries are due to automobile and motorcycle accidents, followed by gunshot wounds, stabbings, and birth trauma.[1,2] Up to 73.5% of PNIs occur in the upper extremities, with the ulnar nerve being the most commonly affected.[2] Evaluation and treatment of PNIs require a thorough understanding of the pathophysiology of nerve injury and repair, the classification and grading schemes for PNI, clinical assessment, and nerve repair strategies.

Mechanisms of Peripheral Nerve Injuries

The general mechanisms of traumatic PNI can be classified as penetrating, crush or mechanical compression, stretch or traction, and ischemic injury.[3,4] Less common etiologies include radiation, thermal, electric, and vibration injuries. Of these, stretch injuries are the most common and are a result of supraphysiological levels of nerve elongation, resulting in mechanical trauma to neural integrity, as well as nerve ischemia.[5] Penetrating injuries, such as lacerations, in contrast, result in direct complete or partial axotomy, with variable degrees of nerve degeneration at the proximal stump. Another common mechanism of PNI is mechanical compression. This etiology is implicated in acute, crush injuries as well as chronic entrapment neuropathies. As compression progresses, demyelination of axons ensues, and can result in distal axonal degeneration and compromise of normal nerve function. Ischemic nerve injury can be a result of other mechanisms of PNI or it can be the primary cause of nerve injury.[6,7]

Classification and Grading

An appreciation of axonal anatomy is critical to understanding the classification and grading schemes used for PNIs.[8] Each individual myelinated axon and groups of unmyelinated axons are surrounded by endoneurium, which is a loose, gelatinous collagen matrix.[9] Individual axons join together to form fascicles that are surrounded circumferentially by perineurium, which consists of collagen fibrils dispersed among perineural cells.[10] An internal epineurium then surrounds nerve fascicles; finally, an external epineurium that is formed by primarily collagen and elastic fibers encircles the nerve (**Fig. 128.1**).[11]

The Seddon[12] and Sunderland[13] classification schemes for peripheral nerve injury are the most commonly used systems to grade PNI (**Table 128.1**). In the Seddon classification, neurapraxia refers to a loss of axonal conduction due to focal demyelination, and corresponds to Sunderland type I PNI. Motor fibers tend to be affected more than sensory fibers due to conduction block. The lack of axon disruption or wallerian degeneration favors spontaneous recovery of nerve function once remyelination takes place over days to weeks. It is important to appreciate that since axons may be remyelinated at different rates and to different degrees, function may be regained heterogeneously.[14]

The hallmark of axonotmesis is axonal injury. Varying degrees of surrounding connective tissue may also be compromised, and this heterogeneity distinguishes Seddon grades II to IV (**Fig. 128.2**). Grade II injuries maintain some potential for reasonable recovery, because the endoneurium is still intact. In contrast, grade III injuries exhibit variable reinnervation, with a return of only 60 to 80% of normal function. Grade IV injuries exhibit more serve disruption of the axon and surrounding connective tissue, resulting in extensive scarring and neuroma formation without effective reinnervation.

Neurotmesis is characterized by the most severe PNI, in which the nerve is no longer in continuity. No reinnervation occurs in fourth- and fifth-degree injuries without surgical repair.

Pathophysiology of Nerve Injury and Regeneration

Following axonal injury, wallerian degeneration occurs in the distal portion of the axon.[15] This process is characterized at the ultrastructural level by cell membrane compromise and breakdown of the axonal cytoskeleton. However, because the surrounding endoneurium, perineurium, and epineurium are preserved, a path for regenerating axons exists from the proximal injured nerve to the distal target. Schwann cells are instrumental in the regenerative process and transform into a regenerative phenotype after axonal injury, lining up within the basal lamina to form the bands of Büngner, which provide guidance cues for regenerating axons.[16] A robust inflammatory response, characterized by macrophage infiltration and phagocytosis of axonal and myelin debris, also occurs.[17-20] The process of wallerian degeneration begins within hours of injury and is complete by 6 to 8 weeks.[21,22] Schwann cells become atrophic if axonal regeneration does not occur.[23] However, the presence of regenerating axonal interactions can alter their phenotype back into remyelinating cells.[24]

Reinnervation is a highly variable process and depends, in part, on the degree of internal disorganization, and the distance to the muscle.[14] Regenerative and repair processes must occur at a variety of foci, including the nerve cell body, the proximal nerve stump, the injury site, the distal nerve stump, and the end organ.[25] There are three major mechanisms for PNI repair: remyelination, collateral sprouting distally from preserved axons, and regeneration from the site of injury.[14] Collateral sprouting, in the setting of partial nerve injury, in which only 20 to 30% of axons are injured, is an effective strategy for reinnervation and occurs

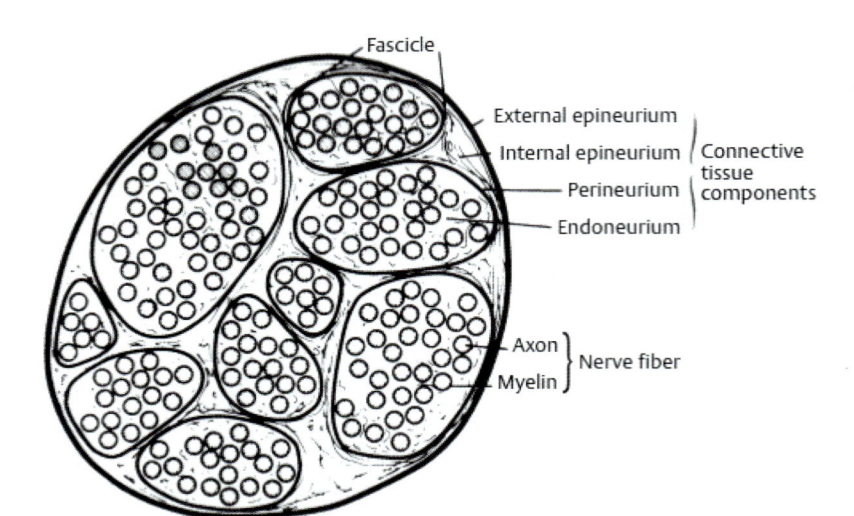

Fig. 128.1 Diagrammatic representation of the cross section of a normal peripheral nerve, demonstrating the connective tissue and nerve tissue components. (Adapted from Mackinnon SE, Dellon AL. Surgery of the Peripheral Nerve. New York: Thieme, 1988:36. Reprinted with permission.)

over 2 to 6 months.[14] In contrast, with more severe injuries affecting a greater majority of axons, regeneration from the site of injury is the primary mechanism of repair. Therefore, the timing of recovery of function is highly dependent on the distance from the site of injury to the target organ.

There are several imposed barriers to successful nerve regeneration. One critical factor is the size of the gap between the proximal and distal nerve stumps. Regenerating axons that are unable to enter the distal nerve stump cannot form functional end-organ connections. In addition, connective tissue scar within the site of regeneration impedes regenerating nerve fiber growth. In these cases, some nerve fibers may be misdirected, resulting in aberrant regeneration. The rate of axonal regeneration, on average, is 1 mm/day, or 1 inch/month. However, recovery of function may be delayed beyond this due to the process of remyelination of regenerating axons, enlargement and maturation of regenerating fibers, and the formation of functional connections with the end organ. Nevertheless, the neuron's ability to sustain regenerative attempts persists for at least 12 months after injury.[14]

Clinical Assessment

The appropriate clinical assessment of the PNI patient begins with a thorough history and physical examination to determine the timing and mechanism of injury, the nerves affected, the extent and severity of injury, and whether the injury is open or closed (**Figs. 128.3 and 128.4**).

The timing and mechanism of injury are extremely relevant to the surgeon's decision as to whether surgical repair is indicated acutely or not. For example, in the case of a sharp penetrating injury, most authors recommend early exploration and acute surgical repair, ideally within 48 to 72 hours. In contrast, a motor vehicle accident, resulting in a stretch injury of the brachial plexus with variable clinical deficits, is typically managed conservatively until the full extent of nerve dysfunction is elucidated over the course of several weeks. Even then, repair is often delayed after several months due to a variety of reasons.

Table 128.1 Seddon and Sunderland classification of Peripheral Nerve Injuries

Seddon Classification	Sunderland Classification	Neuropathology
Neurapraxia	I	Segmental demyelination
Axonotmesis	II	Axon severed, endoneurium intact
Axonotmesis	III	Axon and endoneurium injured, perineurium and fascicular arrangement preserved
Axonotmesis	IV	Axon, endoneurium, and perineurium injured, epineurium intact
Neurotmesis	V	Loss of continuity of entire nerve

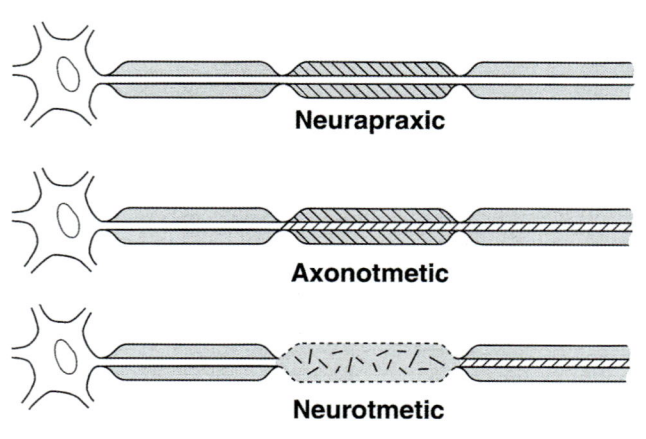

Fig. 128.2 Seddon's three grades of traumatic peripheral nerve injury. A neurapraxic grade of injury is characterized by focal demyelination and conduction block. In an axonotmetic injury, both the myelin sheath and axon are disrupted, resulting in distal wallerian degeneration. However, parts of the surrounding connective tissue are preserved, thereby enabling some regenerating. In a neurotmetic injury, there is complete disruption of the nerve and surrounding connective tissue, with no chance for spontaneous recovery of function.

128 Traumatic Peripheral Nerve Injuries

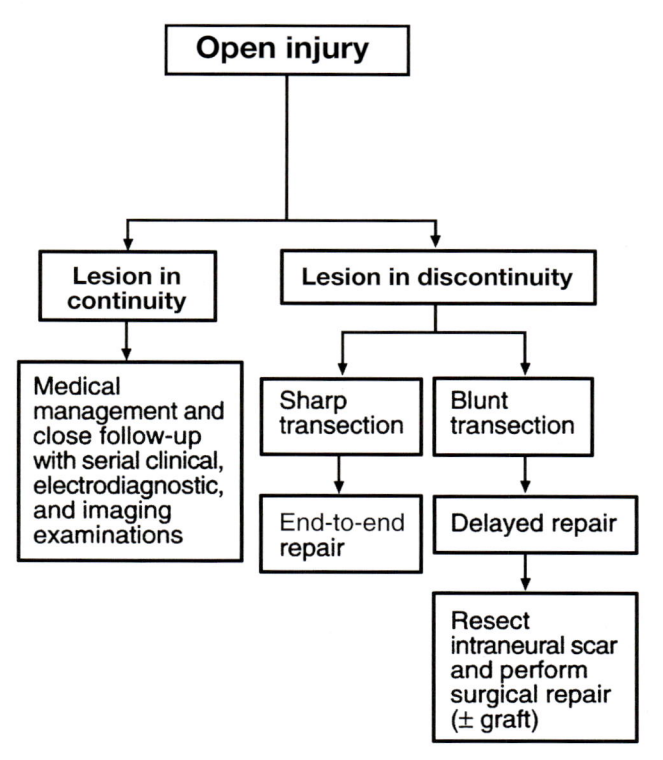

Fig. 128.3 Guidelines for the management of open traumatic peripheral nerve injuries.

A systematic physical examination is paramount in identifying the injured nerves and severity of dysfunction. The neurosurgeon should begin the examination with visual inspection and palpation of the musculoskeletal system, then assess the passive joint range of motion, and then proceed to a neurologic assessment. Serial examinations can be critical in distinguishing complete from incomplete injuries, which may have dramatically different treatment implications. The technique for examination of each muscle group is beyond the scope of this chapter, but is discussed elsewhere.[26] Muscle power is important to grade using a universal system. Most clinicians use the British Medical Research Council (BMRC) system, which grades motor strength on a scale of 0, indicating complete loss of function, to 5, indicating normal muscle power. In pediatric patients with brachial plexus injuries, the Toronto Active Movement Scale (AMS)[27] is often used along with functional scales such as the Mallet test[28] and the Gilbert and Raimondi scales.[29] Sensation is assessed using response to light touch and pinprick. The Tinel sign should be elicited to localize the point of lesion, but it has varying specificity and sensitivity depending on nerve pathology and the specific nerve injured. The pupils should also be carefully examined for evidence of a Horner's sign, which typically indicates nerve discontinuity at the level of the spinal root, also known as a nerve root avulsion, and usually involves T1. Additionally, a physical exam should be performed and imaging should be obtained to determine the functionality of the phrenic nerve.

Electrodiagnostic studies can also be a valuable source of information about the nature of the PNI. Most electrodiagnostic studies are obtained 3 to 4 weeks after the injury, because changes associated with wallerian degeneration may not be apparent before then. Also, the presence of a sensory nerve action

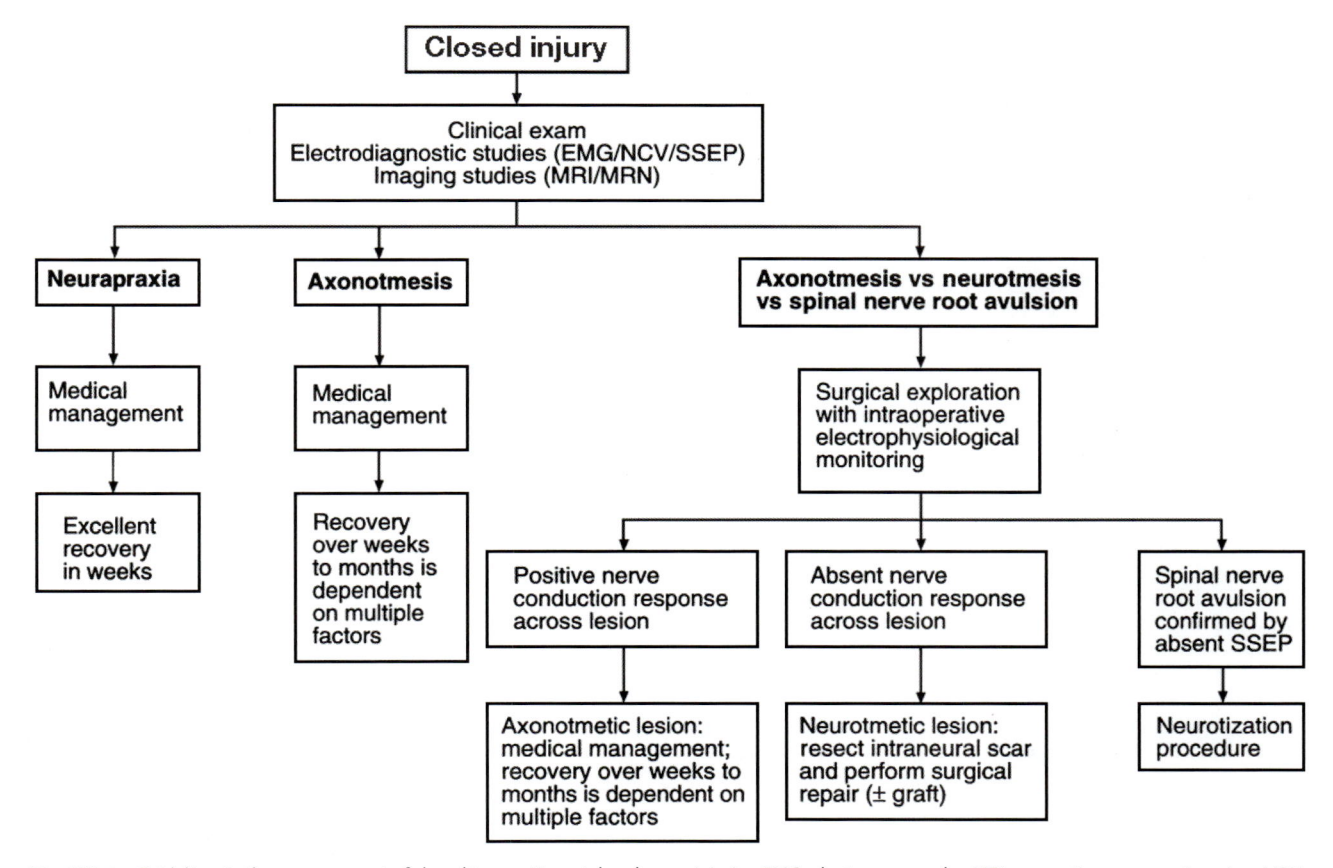

Fig. 128.4 Guidelines in the management of closed traumatic peripheral nerve injuries. EMG, electromyography; MRI, magnetic resonance imaging; MRN, magnetic resonance neurography; NCV, nerve conduction velocity; SSEP, somatosensory evoked potential.

potential (SNAP), in the setting of clinical loss of sensation, can be an important diagnostic clue as to the location of injury. In this case, the injury is proximal to the sensory nerve cell body, housed in the dorsal root ganglion because the SNAP is present. Again, this indicates a nerve root avulsion injury. On electromyography (EMG) studies, denervated muscle exhibits typical positive sharp waves and fibrillations as the motor nerve undergoes wallerian degeneration. More importantly, EMG can also identify signs of early reinnervation. For example, the presence of nascent motor units or polyphasic action potentials, which may precede functional recovery, may be the first evidence of reinnervation. Care should be taken not to overinterpret the electrical studies, particularly in children, as the studies may not correlate with clinically significant recovery.

Diagnostic imaging studies are capable of detecting the presence of nerve root avulsions. For example, a computed tomography (CT) myelogram is able to detect nerve root avulsions with a sensitivity of 85% and a specificity of 95%.[30] Magnetic resonance imaging (MRI) has also been used to identify both evidence of avulsion injury and the precise location of injury.[31]

Nerve Repair Techniques

Depending on the pathology of nerve injury, many surgical nerve repair strategies exist. Nerve grafting was first introduced by Seddon[32] in 1963 and remains the most commonly employed technique in nerve reconstruction surgery. It involves primary exploration of the nerve injury site, which is often disrupted with neuroma formation and dense scar tissue. Neurolysis is employed when the nerve injury is in continuity, implying that some healthy axons are present and capable of undergoing spontaneous recovery. External neurolysis, in which dissection is performed around the epineurium, and internal neurolysis, in which an interfascicular dissection is performed, are options to decompress the injured neural elements. Nerve grafting is employed when direct suture coaptation of ruptured nerve ends cannot be achieved without tension. Most commonly, this is performed using a free nerve graft, such as the autologous sural nerve graft, although recently cadaveric options have become available.[33]

In the case of a nerve in continuity with neuroma formation, intraoperative nerve action potentials (NAPs) are recorded across the lesion to determine the extent of axonal regeneration. Lesions with positive NAPs typically only undergo external neurolysis, because spontaneous functional recovery occurs in ~ 90% of cases. However, if negative NAPs are identified intraoperatively, the neuroma is resected and nerve grafts are used to bridge a normal healthy proximal nerve stump to the distal nerve. Common examples of interpositional nerve grafting include coaptation of the C5 root to the suprascapular nerve or axillary nerve (for shoulder abduction), C6 to the musculocutaneous nerve (for elbow flexion), and C7 to the triceps or radial nerve (for elbow extension and wrist extension).[34] Outcomes following nerve grafting are highly dependent on the length of the graft, the presence of scar tissue at the wound site, the number of grafts used, and the presence of a healthy proximal stump available for grafting.[35] Despite the improved outcomes with autologous nerve grafting, the donor nerve supply is limited. Therefore, vein grafts and manufactured conduits are also used.[36-38]

In severe PNIs, such as root avulsions, the options for recovery of function rely on the use of nerve transfers and other palliative approaches. As with nerve grafting procedures, the goal is to supply the denervated muscle with functioning motor axons. Nerve transfers are founded on the principal that the sacrifice of a physiologically healthy nerve can be used to regenerate within a distal, more functionally important, injured nerve.[39] This process is known as neurotization. Several donor nerves exist. For upper extremity nerve transfers, these donor nerves can originate from within the brachial plexus neural elements, known as intraplexal nerve transfers, or can come from other sources, termed extraplexal nerve transfers (Video 128.1). Some examples of extraplexal donor nerve sources include the phrenic nerve, spinal accessory nerve, deep motor branches of the cervical plexus, hypoglossal nerve, intercostal nerves, and the contralateral C7 spinal nerve.[34,40,41] Free muscle transfers, particularly the gracilis myocutaneous transfer, as well as tendon transfers, can also be important palliative surgical options.

In cases of penetrating injuries, direct nerve repair with suture and/or fibrin glue coaptation can be performed. In some instances, jagged lacerations of the nerve can be tagged for delayed repair, which enables appropriate trimming of the injured nerve stumps and grafting, if necessary.

Postoperative Considerations

Nerve reconstruction strategies are highly individualized to each patient, because the mechanism of injury, the pathophysiology of the nerve damage, and the surgical repair strategy may be unique in each case. Still, some common postoperative sequelae should be avoided, including poor wound healing or infection, especially of sural nerve harvest incision sites. Patients in high-risk populations, such as diabetic and renal failure patients, should be counseled appropriately in the preoperative setting about wound care. Donor-site morbidity from nerve harvesting is also a recognized complication nerve grafting. Management of neuropathic pain due to PNI is an important consideration after trauma and usually requires the involvement of pain management specialists.[42,43] Sometimes procedural interventions, such as stellate ganglion blocks, peripheral nerve stimulator, and dorsal column stimulator placement are required.[43-46]

References

1. Midha R. Epidemiology of brachial plexus injuries in a multitrauma population. Neurosurgery 1997;40:1182–1188, discussion 1188–1189
2. Kouyoumdjian JA. Peripheral nerve injuries: a retrospective survey of 456 cases. Muscle Nerve 2006;34:785–788
3. Robinson LR. Traumatic injury to peripheral nerves. Muscle Nerve 2000;23:863–873
4. Robinson LR. Traumatic injury to peripheral nerves. Suppl Clin Neurophysiol 2004;57:173–186
5. Lundborg G, Rydevik B. Effects of stretching the tibial nerve of the rabbit. A preliminary study of the intraneural circulation and the barrier function of the perineurium. J Bone Joint Surg Br 1973;55:390–401
6. Lewis T, Pickering GW, Rothschild P. Centripetal paralysis arising out of arrested bloodflow to the limb, including notes on a tingling. Heart 1931;16:1–32
7. Rydevik B, Lundborg G. Permeability of intraneural microvessels and perineurium following acute, graded experimental nerve compression. Scand J Plast Reconstr Surg 1977;11:179–187
8. Maggi SP, Lowe JB III, Mackinnon SE. Pathophysiology of nerve injury. Clin Plast Surg 2003;30:109–126
9. Olsson Y, Reese TS. Permeability of vasa nervorum and perineurium in mouse sciatic nerve studied by fluorescence and electron microscopy. J Neuropathol Exp Neurol 1971;30:105–119
10. Reale E, Luciano L, Spitznas M. Freeze-fracture faces of the perineurial sheath of the rabbit sciatic nerve. J Neurocytol 1975;4:261–270
11. Mackinnon SE, Dellon AL. Surgery of the Peripheral Nerve. New York: Thieme; 1988
12. Seddon HJ. Three types of nerve injury. Brain 1943;66:237–288
13. Sunderland S. A classification of peripheral nerve injuries producing loss of function. Brain 1951;74:491–516

14. Campbell WW. Evaluation and management of peripheral nerve injury. Clin Neurophysiol 2008;119:1951–1965
15. Waller A. Experiments on the section of the glossopharyngeal and hypoglossal nerves of the frog and observations of the alterations produced thereby in the structure of their primitive fibers. Philos Trans R Soc Lond, B 1850;140:423–429
16. Stoll G, Müller HW. Nerve injury, axonal degeneration and neural regeneration: basic insights. Brain Pathol 1999;9:313–325
17. Taskinen HS, Röyttä M. The dynamics of macrophage recruitment after nerve transection. Acta Neuropathol 1997;93:252–259
18. Brück W. The role of macrophages in wallerian degeneration. Brain Pathol 1997;7:741–752
19. Liu HM, Yang LH, Yang YJ. Schwann cell properties: 3. C-fos expression, bFGF production, phagocytosis and proliferation during wallerian degeneration. J Neuropathol Exp Neurol 1995;54:487–496
20. Stoll G, Griffin JW, Li CY, Trapp BD. Wallerian degeneration in the peripheral nervous system: participation of both Schwann cells and macrophages in myelin degradation. J Neurocytol 1989;18:671–683
21. Hall SM. Regeneration in the peripheral nervous system. Neuropathol Appl Neurobiol 1989;15:513–529
22. Kang H, Tian L, Thompson W. Terminal Schwann cells guide the reinnervation of muscle after nerve injury. J Neurocytol 2003;32:975–985
23. Hall SM. The biology of chronically denervated Schwann cells. Ann N Y Acad Sci 1999;883:215–233
24. Sulaiman OA, Gordon T. Effects of short- and long-term Schwann cell denervation on peripheral nerve regeneration, myelination, and size. Glia 2000;32:234–246
25. Burnett MG, Zager EL. Pathophysiology of peripheral nerve injury: a brief review. Neurosurg Focus 2004;16:E1
26. M OB. Aids to the Examination of the Peripheral Nervous System, 5 ed. Philadelphia: Saunders; 2000
27. Curtis C, Stephens D, Clarke HM, Andrews D. The active movement scale: an evaluative tool for infants with obstetrical brachial plexus palsy. J Hand Surg Am 2002;27:470–478
28. Mallet J. [Obstetrical paralysis of the brachial plexus. II. Therapeutics. Treatment of sequelae. Priority for the treatment of the shoulder. Method for the expression of results]. Rev Chir Orthop Repar Appar Mot 1972;58(Suppl 1):1, 166–168
29. Haerle M, Gilbert A. Management of complete obstetric brachial plexus lesions. J Pediatr Orthop 2004;24:194–200
30. Carvalho GA, Nikkhah G, Matthies C, Penkert G, Samii M. Diagnosis of root avulsions in traumatic brachial plexus injuries: value of computerized tomography myelography and magnetic resonance imaging. J Neurosurg 1997;86:69–76
31. Yoshikawa T, Hayashi N, Yamamoto S, et al. Brachial plexus injury: clinical manifestations, conventional imaging findings, and the latest imaging techniques. Radiographics 2006;26(Suppl 1):S133–S143
32. Seddon HJ. Nerve grafting. J Bone Joint Surg Br 1963;45:447–461
33. Brooks DN, Weber RV, Chao JD, et al. Processed nerve allografts for peripheral nerve reconstruction: a multicenter study of utilization and outcomes in sensory, mixed, and motor nerve reconstructions. Microsurgery 2012;32:1–14
34. Giuffre JL, Kakar S, Bishop AT, Spinner RJ, Shin AY. Current concepts of the treatment of adult brachial plexus injuries. J Hand Surg Am 2010;35:678–688, quiz 688
35. Chuang DC. Brachial plexus injury: nerve reconstruction and functioning muscle transplantation. Semin Plast Surg 2010;24:57–66
36. Chiu DT. Autogenous venous nerve conduits. A review. Hand Clin 1999;15:667–671, ix
37. Chiu DT, Strauch B. A prospective clinical evaluation of autogenous vein grafts used as a nerve conduit for distal sensory nerve defects of 3 cm or less. Plast Reconstr Surg 1990;86:928–934
38. Whitlock EL, Tuffaha SH, Luciano JP, et al. Processed allografts and type I collagen conduits for repair of peripheral nerve gaps. Muscle Nerve 2009;39:787–799
39. Fox IK, Mackinnon SE. Adult peripheral nerve disorders: nerve entrapment, repair, transfer, and brachial plexus disorders. Plast Reconstr Surg 2011;127:105e–118e
40. Gu Y, Xu J, Chen L, Wang H, Hu S. Long term outcome of contralateral C7 transfer: a report of 32 cases. Chin Med J (Engl) 2002;115:866–868
41. Chuang DC. Neurotization procedures for brachial plexus injuries. Hand Clin 1995;11:633–645
42. Schwartzman RJ, Maleki J. Postinjury neuropathic pain syndromes. Med Clin North Am 1999;83:597–626
43. Merritt WH. The challenge to manage reflex sympathetic dystrophy/complex regional pain syndrome. Clin Plast Surg 2005;32:575–604, vii–viii
44. Bittar RG, Teddy PJ. Peripheral neuromodulation for pain. J Clin Neurosci 2009;16:1259–1261
45. Novak CB, Mackinnon SE. Outcome following implantation of a peripheral nerve stimulator in patients with chronic nerve pain. Plast Reconstr Surg 2000;105:1967–1972
46. North R, Shipley J, Prager J, et al; American Academy of Pain Medicine. Practice parameters for the use of spinal cord stimulation in the treatment of chronic neuropathic pain. Pain Med 2007;8(Suppl 4):S200–S275

129 Compressive Lesions of the Peripheral Nerve

Shane V. Abdunnur and Daniel H. Kim

Compression neuropathies can occur both acutely and chronically due to excessive pressure on a nerve. This typically takes the form of an entrapment that occurs at or near joints, where a fibrous band, either a tendon or ligament, attaches to a nearby osseous structure. There are several causes of and predispositions for entrapment neuropathy, including congenital narrowing of the osseous tunnel, thickening of overlying tissue, and enlarged muscles. Surgical intervention has high success rates with relatively low morbidity, and therefore is a good option.

Pathophysiology

The physiological effect of compression on a nerve results in ischemia and edema and concordant interruption of the normal propagation of action potentials and neural feedback mechanisms. During the early stages of compression, segmental demyelination occurs even in the absence of macroscopic changes. Edema, epineural fibrosis, and further thickening of the nerve occur with chronic compressive lesions. Damage to the nerve eventually becomes permanent as the myelin sheath cannot be repaired and axonal damage occurs. As such, impaired membrane permeability results in conduction block and wallerian degeneration. Not all fibers are equally susceptible, as large-diameter fibers resist compression less than small-diameter fibers. Centrally located fibers are typically spared at the expense of peripherally located ones.

Median Nerve Entrapment

Anatomy

The median nerve originates from branches of the medial and lateral cords. Motor fibers are contributed by the medial cord primarily, whereas the lateral cord contributes mostly sensory fibers. The two branches unite superficial to the brachial artery, and the nerve and artery retain this close relationship throughout their course in the arm. The median nerve courses first lateral and then medial to the brachial artery. This transition occurs at the level of the insertion of the deltoid. The median nerve in the distal arm and the cubital fossa lie medial to the biceps and its tendon and medial to the brachial artery as the nerve courses over the brachialis muscle (**Fig. 129.1**). At the level of the elbow, it lies behind the bicipital aponeurosis or lacertus fibrosis. The two heads of the pronator teres insert into the radius via a common tendon. The median nerve runs between these two heads and can be a source of compression neuropathy. As the median nerve courses through the two heads of the pronator teres, it typically gives off the anterior interosseous nerve from its lateral/posterior surface. Emerging from the distal border of the pronator teres, the median nerve passes under the tendinous origin of the flexor digitorum superficialis muscle, and the nerve courses down the forearm posterior to the undersurface of the flexor digitorum superficialis, on the lateral aspect of the flexor digitorum superficialis tendons. Below this point, the median nerve courses in a straight line to the wrist.

Just proximal to the wrist, the median nerve lies deep in the space between the flexor digitorum superficialis and palmaris longus tendons. The median nerve then courses deep to the flexor retinaculum, accompanying the flexor tendons in the carpal tunnel. In the carpal tunnel, the median nerve lies lateral to the flexor digitorum superficialis to the middle finger and medial to the flexor carpi radialis, which is in its own compartment. After the median nerve emerges from the distal end of the flexor retinaculum, the nerve divides into the recurrent motor and sensory digital nerves.

Entrapment neuropathies of the median nerve can occur at the supracondylar process, in the cubital fossa, or at the flexor retinaculum at the wrist. The supracondylar process is an anomaly that occurs in less than 2% of the population and is rarely symptomatic. It is a small bony prominence that arises 5 to 7 cm proximal to the medial epicondyle. The ligament of Struthers extends from the supracondylar process to the medial epicondyle, enclosing a foramen through which the median nerve and brachial artery and vein run. Compression of the median nerve can occur at the ligament of Struthers (**Fig. 129.2**). In the cubital fossa, the lacertus fibrosis, two heads of the pronator teres, and the flexor digitorum superficialis tendinous origin can all cause median nerve compression neuropathy. More distally, the carpal tunnel is the most common cause of all compression neuropathies in the body and, by far the most common compression neuropathy of the median nerve.

Carpal tunnel syndrome (CTS) is caused by compression of the distal median nerve within the flexor retinaculum or transverse carpal ligament (**Fig. 129.3**). This fibro-osseous tunnel is bounded laterally by the scaphoid and trapezium, medially by the hamate and pisiform, dorsally by the carpal bones and flexor tendons, and ventrally by the transverse carpal ligament. Common predisposing factors to the development of CTS are listed in **Box 129.1**.

Presentation and Diagnosis

Ligament of Struthers compression presents with pain over the elbow with weakness of pronation and hand grip. Dysesthesia occurs in the lateral three fingers. On exam, the surgeon may palpate a fibrous mass just proximal to the medial epicondyle along with weakness of the pronator teres, flexor carpi radialis, flexor pollicis longus, and digital finger flexion. Sensory loss is in the median distribution. Pronator weakness distinguishes ligament of Struthers compression from other syndromes. Nerve conduction studies show slowing of the velocity in the median nerve in the arm. Electromyography (EMG) may show denervation

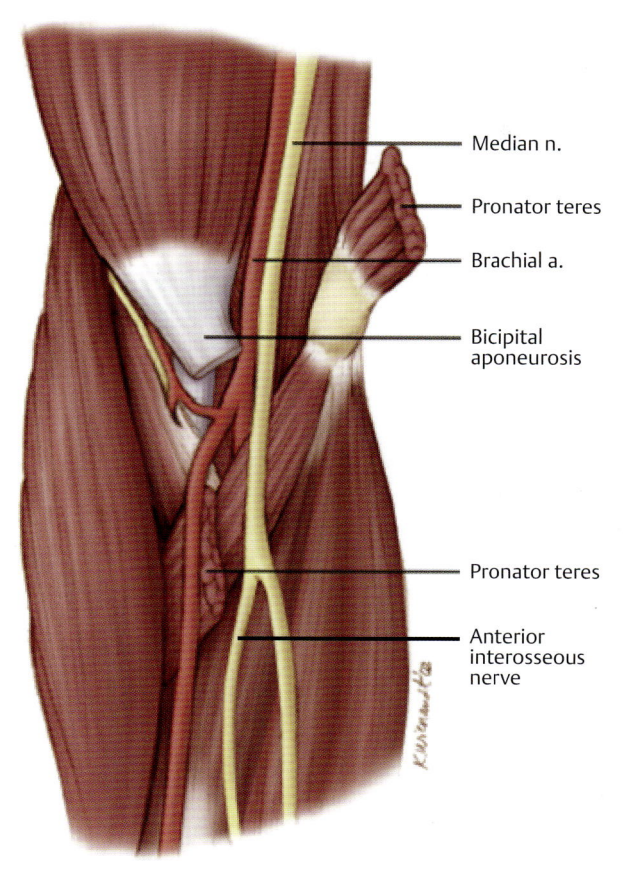

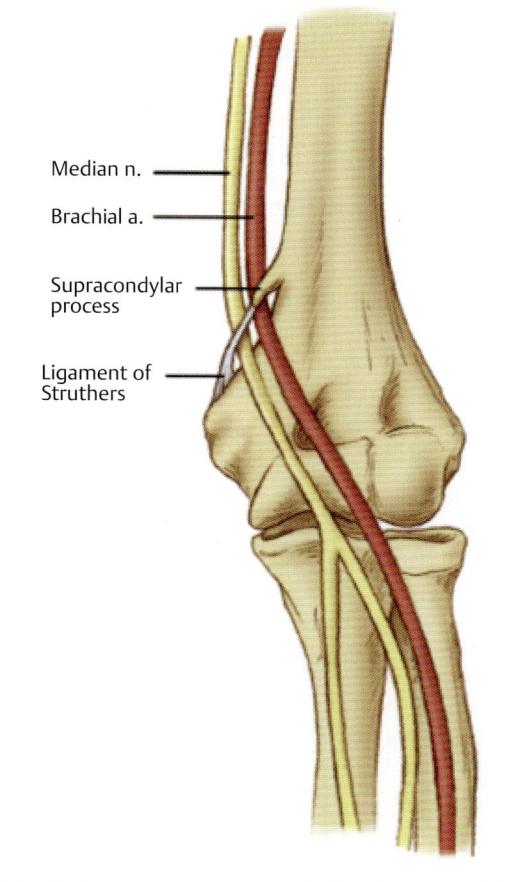

Fig. 129.1 The median nerve in the antecubital fossa. The relationship of the median nerve to the brachial artery is demonstrated as well the origin of the anterior interosseous nerve.

Fig. 129.2 Median nerve entrapment proximal to the supracondylar process at the ligament of Struthers.

potentials in the weak muscles. Diagnosis is often clinical, and relies on pronation weakness as the key feature.

Cubital fossa entrapment occurs due to three structures, and their clinical consequence is identical. It is not typically possible to differentiate the exact cause of entrapment clinically or electrodiagnostically, and therefore the true lesion can only be appreciated intraoperatively. The three structures include the lacertus fibrosis, the two heads of the pronator teres, and the flexor digitorum superficialis tendinous insertion. Exploration should address all three locations. Patients may experience weakness in the forearm muscles and hand grip with dysesthesia in the first two digits. CTS can be distinguished due to increasing symptomatology at night and a history of repetitive supination and wrist motion. Weakness is most notable in the flexor pollicis longus and abductor pollicis brevis. Importantly, nerve conduction velocity should be slowed in the forearm, but the distal

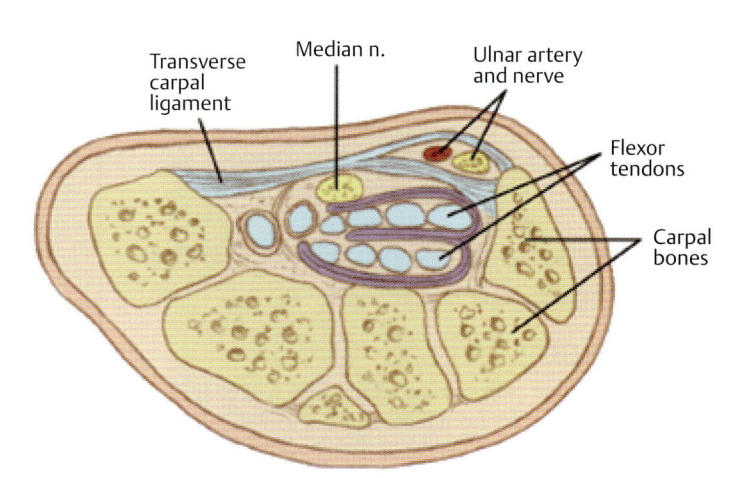

Fig. 129.3 Entrapment neuropathy at the wrist. The median and ulnar nerves are both vulnerable to compressive lesions at the wrist.

Box 129.1 Risk Factors for Carpal Tunnel Syndrome

Local Factors

Reduction in the Capacity of the Carpal Canal

Idiopathic or familial thickening of the transverse carpal ligament

Congenitally small carpal canal

Malunion or callus following Colles' fracture or fracture of the carpal bones

Improper immobilization of the wrist ("cotton loader position")

Unrestricted dislocations of the wrist or intercarpal joints

Compression by cast

Increased Volume of the Contents of the Carpal Canal

Anomalous muscles and tendons

Hypertrophic tenosynovitis

Persistent median artery with or without thrombosis, aneurysm, arteriovenous malformation

Acute palmar space infections

Masses: neurofibroma, hemangioma, lipoma, ganglion cyst, gouty tophus, xanthoma

Systemic Factors

Inflammatory and Autoimmune Disorders

Rheumatoid arthritis

Dermatomyositis

Scleroderma

Polymyalgia rheumatica

Increased Susceptibility of Nerves to Pressure

Amyloidosis

Hereditary neuropathy with liability to pressure palsies

Alcoholic or diabetic polyneuropathy

Proximal lesions of the median nerve ("double crush" syndrome)

Other polyneuropathies

Metabolic Disorders

Mucopolysaccharidoses

Mucolipidoses

Amyloidosis

Gout

Factors Unique to Women

Pregnancy and lactation

Contraceptive pills

Menstrual cycles

Menopause

Toxic shock syndrome

Eclampsia

Other Hormonal Factors

Myxedema

Acromegaly

Other Systemic Factors

Obesity

Raynaud's disease

---

sensory and motor latencies are normal, unless there is an overlying CTS.

Carpal tunnel syndrome affects women more often than men in a ratio of 7:3. Although it varies, patients are typically between the ages of 40 and 60 at the onset of symptoms. Patients most typically complain of burning, aching, and tingling in the fingertips of the first three fingers of the hand. But some patients state that the pain is in all the fingers, and this should not throw the surgeon off the diagnosis. Pain is usually maximal at night or early in the morning or with repetitive movements of the wrist. Patients may shake or massage their hand to relieve their symptoms. Subjective muscle weakness in the hand is a late finding, but it can often be elicited during physical examination. Atrophy of the thenar compartment may also be present. Tinel's sign can be assessed by tapping over the median nerve at the wrist. A positive sign reproduces symptoms. A Phalen's test is positive if flexing the wrist to 90 degrees for 1 minute results in exacerbation of symptoms. Both tests have a high false-positive rate, and diagnosis is always confirmed with EMG and nerve conduction studies. Sensation is decreased in the median nerve distribution as well. The most important electrodiagnostic study is prolonged sensory latency, although this may be normal in 25%. Sensory nerve action potentials are typically very low amplitude or absent. EMG of the abductor pollicis brevis and opponens pollicis may show fibrillation potentials or polyphasic motor potentials indicative of neuropathy as opposed to myopathy.

Anterior Interosseous Nerve Syndrome

Anatomy

The anterior interosseous nerve (AIN) is predominantly a motor nerve that arises from the posterior/lateral aspect of the median nerve just prior to its passage between the two heads of the pronator teres muscle, 5 cm above the medial epicondyle. It traverses the anterior interosseous membrane between the flexor digitorum profundus and the flexor pollicis longus, supplying both muscles. AIN terminates in the pronator quadratus just proximal to the wrist. There are several possible sites of injury, but most are related to a traumatic fracture in the forearm. Natural points of compression include the two heads of the pronator teres, between the flexor digitorum profundus and flexor pollicis longus, and the accessory head of the flexor pollicis longus.

Presentation and Diagnosis

Although the AIN is a motor nerve, some patients complain of aching pain in the elbow and forearm. There is no sensory deficit. Most commonly, patients present with isolated motor findings of weakness in the flexor pollicis longus and flexor digitorum profundus, leading to the most recognized clinical finding of an abnormal pinch posture. This finding is demonstrated when the patient is asked to pinch the thumb and the index finger together. The clinician will note extension/hyperextension of the metacarpophalangeal joint of the thumb and interphalangeal joint of the index finger. Pronator quadratus weakness exists but can be difficult to evaluate clinically. The elbow should be flexed as to isolate the pronator quadratus from the pronator teres. Subtle weakness in wrist pronation can be demonstrated in this way. EMG shows irritation with loss of motor units in the flexor digitorum profundus, flexor pollicis longus, and pronator quadratus.

Radial Nerve Entrapment

Anatomy

The radial nerve takes its origin from the posterior cord of the brachial plexus, which is composed of the posterior divisions of all three trunks. C5, C6, C7, C8, and T1 are all represented in the radial nerve. The motor component primarily supplies extensor muscles of the arm, forearm, and hand. The radial nerve gives off the posterior cutaneous nerve of the arm and then proceeds to give a branch to the long and medial heads of the triceps as it runs between the axilla and spiral groove of the humerus. The nerve to the lateral head of the triceps is given off in the spiral groove. The nerve is often separated from the spiral groove of the humerus by 1 to 5 cm of muscle. After giving off a branch to the triceps, the radial nerve courses from the posterior aspect of the humerus to the anterolateral aspect along the intermuscular septum; 2 cm proximal to the lateral epicondyle, the brachioradialis and extensor carpi radialis branches are given off. Importantly, the radial nerve crosses the posterior aspect of the humerus 20 cm proximal to the medial epicondyle and 15 cm proximal to the lateral epicondyle (**Fig. 129.4**). In the proximal forearm, the radial nerve divides into two major branches. The sensory nerve innervates the skin over the dorsum of the radial side of the hand, thumb, and index and middle fingers. The sensory component is termed the superficial branch of the radial nerve and passes into the forearm deep to the brachioradialis muscle. The motor branch of the radial nerve is known as the posterior interosseous nerve (PIN) due to its relationship with the interosseous membrane in the forearm. This is the deep branch of the radial nerve. The PIN passes backward through the supinator muscle at the arcade of Frohse to supply nine muscles of the forearm extensors. The distal course of the PIN is diminutive and continues to the wrist joint where it supplies the seven finger extensors.

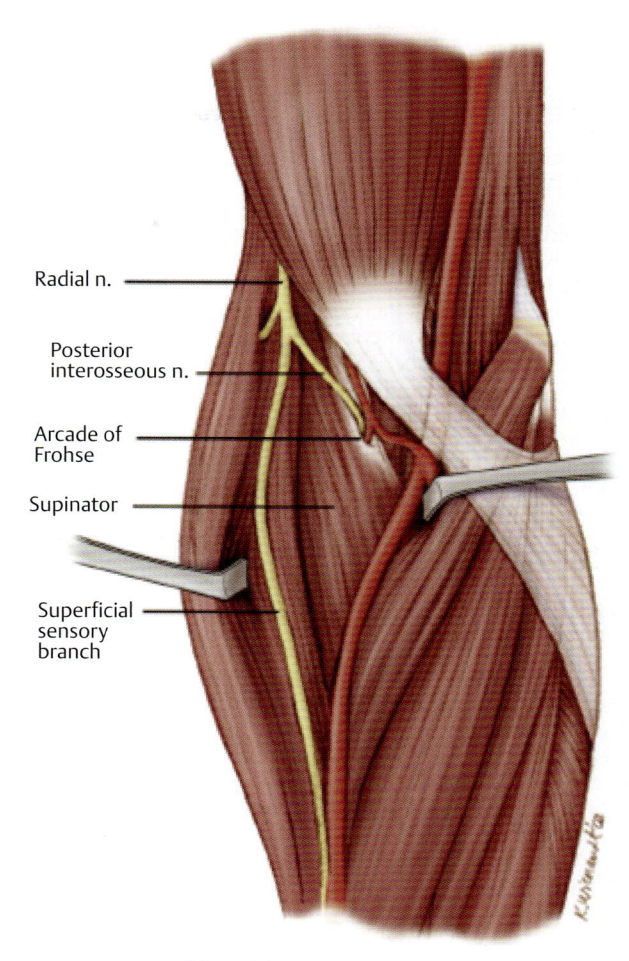

Fig. 129.4 Course of the radial nerve.

Presentation and Diagnosis

The radial nerve is most commonly compressed above the elbow due to the humeral shaft in the spiral groove fractures that require operative intervention. Presentation is that of "Saturday night palsy." Patients commonly present with wrist drop and decreased sensation over the lateral aspect of the dorsum of the hand. Finger extension is affected as well. Brachialis function is compromised; however, patients can still flex the elbow due to the intact function of the biceps. It is important to assess the strength of elbow flexion to distinguish radial nerve palsy from PIN syndrome, in which elbow flexion is unaffected. Nerve conduction studies and EMG may aid in making the correct diagnosis if the history and physical exam are not entirely clear.

Posterior Interosseous Nerve Syndrome

Anatomy

The PIN is the motor branch of the radial nerve below the elbow. Its origin is at the level of the lateral epicondyle between the biceps and triceps muscles. It gives off branches to the extensor carpi radialis brevis and the supinator muscles prior to entering the arcade of Frohse, which is a tough fibrotendinous band at the origin of the supinator muscle.

Presentation and Diagnosis

There are several distinguishing features that enable the diagnosis of PIN syndrome from radial nerve palsy. The sensory branch of the radial nerve does not pass through the arcade of Frohse, and therefore there is no sensory disturbance with PIN syndrome as opposed to radial nerve palsy above the elbow. With PIN syndrome, there is no wrist drop as the radial nerve supplies the extensor carpi radialis longus muscle prior to the PIN. The patient's wrist extension occurs with concordant radial deviation due to weakness of the PIN-innervated extensor carpi ulnaris muscle. The cardinal finding of PIN syndrome is metacarpophalangeal joint weakness of the fingers and thumb with normal strength at the interphalangeal joint. Physical exam and history remain the cornerstone of diagnosis, with EMG and nerve conduction studies supporting the diagnosis.

Ulnar Nerve Entrapment

Anatomy

The ulnar nerve takes its contribution from the C7, C8, and T1 nerve roots that continue through the medial cord of the brachial plexus and finally give rise to the ulnar nerve. At its origin, the ulnar nerve lies between the axially artery and vein, with the medial antebrachial cutaneous nerve ventral to it. Traveling between the coracobrachialis and triceps muscles, the ulnar nerve courses straight down to the medial epicondyle. At the level of insertion of the deltoid, the ulnar nerve leaves the flexor compartment of the arm by running posterior to the medial intermuscular septum. The nerve is accompanied by the superior ulnar collateral artery and a motor branch to the triceps muscles from the radial nerve. The ulnar nerve runs along the medial head of the triceps and occasionally within the muscle. As it courses inferiorly, the ulnar nerve traverses the fascial structure known as the ligament of Struthers 8 cm proximal to the elbow. The postcondylar groove marks the entry of the ulnar nerve into the elbow, at which point the nerve gives off an articular branch. The cubital tunnel is bounded by the olecranon laterally and the medial epicondyle medially. The roof is formed by the arcuate ligament of Osborne, which extends from the tip of the olecranon to the medial epicondyle. The floor is formed by the medial collateral ligament. This is the most common site of compression of the ulnar nerve (**Fig. 129.5**).

Osborne's fascia is the distal continuation of the arcuate ligament of Osborne, where it fuses with the aponeurosis of the flexor carpi ulnaris muscle. This is another potential site of entrapment and compression. The ulnar nerve enters the forearm by passing between the humeral and ulnar heads of the flexor carpi ulnaris. As it descends the ulnar aspect of the arm, the nerve lies on the surface of the flexor digitorum profundus. The nerve supplies the flexor carpi ulnaris and the flexor digitorum profundus to the fourth and fifth digits. The palmer cutaneous branch of the ulnar nerve originates 16 cm proximal to the ulnar styloid and provides sensation to the ulnar aspect of the forearm. The ulnar nerve emerges superficially from the flexor carpi ulnaris muscle just proximal to the wrist, lying medial to the ulnar artery and lateral to the tendon. The dorsal cutaneous branch of the ulnar nerve passes medial to the tendon and emerges on the dorsal ulnar aspect of the hand.

The ulnar nerve enters the hand through Guyon's canal, which is a fibrotendinous passage between the hook of the hamate and the pisiform. The floor of Guyon's canal is formed by the pisohamate ligament. The roof is the superficial volar carpal ligament. Within the canal, the ulnar nerve branches into a deep and superficial branch. The superficial branch carries all sensory fibers of the ulnar nerve. Guyon's canal is another potential site of entrapment (**Fig. 129.3**).

As described above, there are three anatomic sites of possible entrapment of the ulnar nerve. In the arm, Struthers's arcade/medial intermuscular septum can cause entrapment. At the elbow, the nerve can become entrapped at the postcondylar groove. Guyon's canal at the wrist is the final possible location of entrapment.

Presentation and Diagnosis

Patients with ulnar nerve entrapment in the arm and elbow complain of paresthesias in the fourth and fifth digits with elbow pain and hand weakness. Because the ulnar nerve carries a preponderance of motor fibers, motor symptoms can occur early.

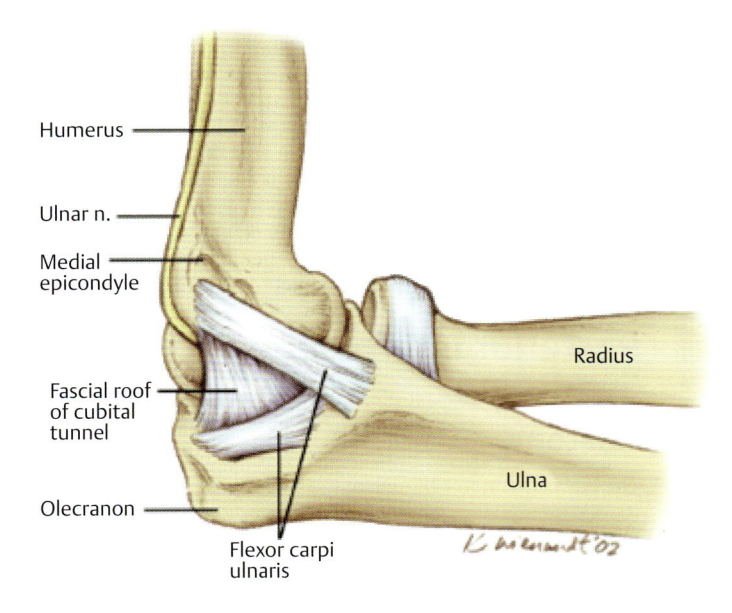

Fig. 129.5 Ligaments of the cubital tunnel. The most common site of ulnar neuropathy is along the medial epicondyle as the ulnar nerve passes through the cubital tunnel.

The history may reveal occupations or hobbies with repetitive elbow flexion. The physical exam shows decreased sensation over the palmer and dorsal aspects of the fourth and fifth fingers with the fifth finger being most clearly defined. When the dorsal cutaneous branch of the ulnar nerve is spared, the clinician should immediately suspect entrapment at Guyon's canal. The fifth lumbrical shows weakness as well as the abductor digiti minimi muscle. Proximal muscle weakness of the flexor carpi ulnaris and flexor digitorum profundus occur later in the course of disease. Muscle wasting is common and can be noted over the first dorsal interosseous and hypothenar compartment. Lumbrical weakness occurs late and results in clawing of the fourth and fifth digits. The Wartenberg sign may occur due to weakness of the third volar interosseous muscle, which allows abduction of the fifth digit at rest. Diagnosis is made by the history and physical exam. The elbow pressure-flexion test is sensitive and specific for cubital tunnel syndrome and consists of placing the patient's elbow in flexion with manual pressure over the cubital tunnel for 30 seconds. When positive, the patient complains of pain in the ulnar distribution and over the elbow. Thoracic outlet syndrome and C8 radiculopathy should be ruled out as well.

Electrodiagnostic evaluation with EMG and nerve conduction studies are reliable for helping localize the site of ulnar entrapment. Cubital tunnel syndrome results in prolonged motor and sensory latency across the elbow but normal latency in the distal forearm. Ulnar innervated muscles may show reduced voluntary motor units and fibrillations. Studies should be conducted with the elbow in flexion, as this puts the greatest compression on the ulnar nerve. False-negative tests occur, and the clinician needs to maintain a high index of suspicion.

Thoracic Outlet Syndrome

Anatomy

The boundaries of the thoracic outlet include the vertebral column medially, the first rib laterally, and the clavicle inferiorly/anteriorly. The anterior scalene muscle originates from the anterior tubercles of C2 through C6 and inserts on the anterior superior surface of the first rib. The posterior tubercles of C2 through C7 give rise to the middle scalene muscle, which inserts on the superior surface of the first rib as well. In addition to the subclavian artery, the brachial plexus travels between the anterior and middle scalene muscles in the thoracic outlet. Any entrapment of the neurovascular structures traversing the thoracic outlet can lead to symptoms, although this is most commonly in the form of neural compression.

Three distinct sites can cause entrapment. The brachial plexus can be compressed in its course between the anterior and middle scalene muscles by the first rib, between the first rib and the clavicle, and lastly beneath the pectoralis minor muscle. The lower trunk (C8 and T1 roots) of the brachial plexus is most commonly affected (**Fig. 129.6**). A detailed anatomic description of the course of the supraclavicular brachial plexus is presented in Chapter 130.

Presentation and Diagnosis

Thoracic outlet syndrome (TOS) is a constellation of disorders that are defined as a neurovascular compression in the anatomic thoracic outlet. The lower trunk (C8 and T1 roots) of the brachial plexus is most commonly affected, and results in medial forearm pain with decreased sensation along the medial forearm down to the fourth and fifth digits. Motor signs and symptoms may include thenar wasting, hypothenar wasting, and intrinsic hand weakness. Chest X-ray may show a cervical rib, a prominent C7 transverse process, or a Pancoast tumor. EMG and nerve conduction studies demonstrate low-amplitude motor responses in the median and ulnar distribution and decreased ulnar sensory responses more than median nerve responses. Taken in context with the history, physical exam, and X-rays, the EMG and nerve conduction studies are essential to differentiate TOS from median and ulnar neuropathy and tandem lesions of the two nerves.

Lateral Femoral Cutaneous Nerve Entrapment

Anatomy

The lateral femoral cutaneous nerve takes its origin from the ventral rami of L2 and L3, and travels inferiorly and laterally to

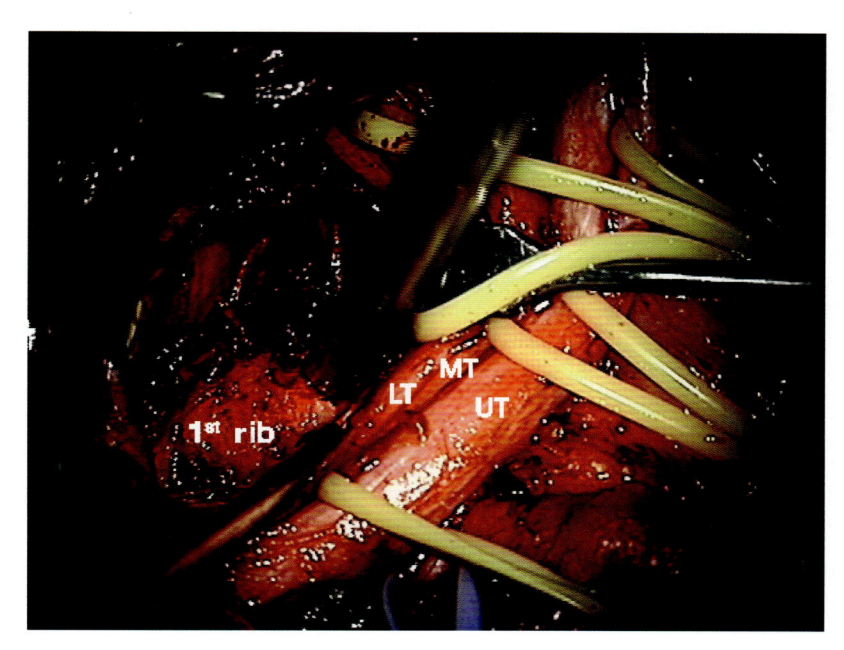

Fig. 129.6 Prominent first rib resection due to compression of the lower trunk (LT). MT, middle trunk; UT, upper trunk.

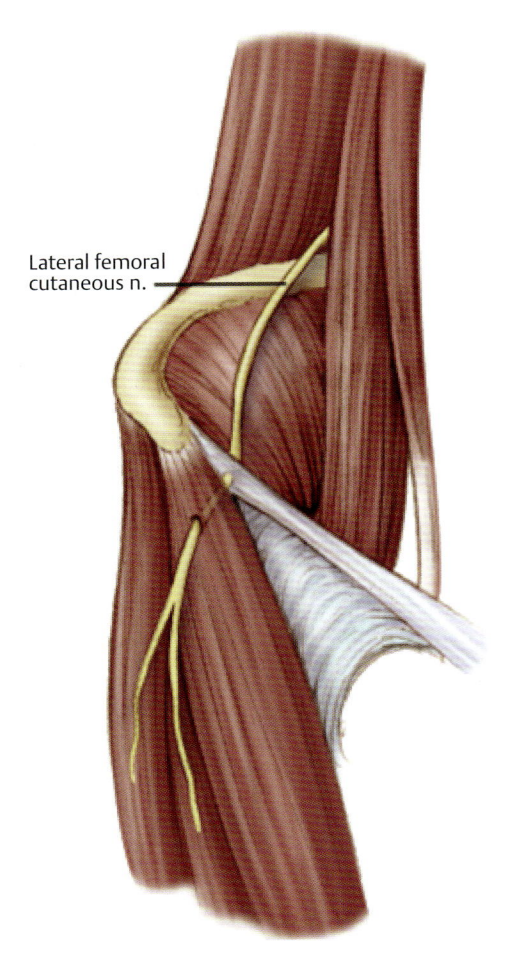

Fig. 129.7 The lateral femoral cutaneous nerve is compressed as it pierces the inguinal ligament.

emerge from the lateral border from the psoas at the level of the iliac crest. It travels on the ventral surface of the iliacus muscle, descending to pass behind and through the inguinal ligament 1 cm medial to the anterior superior iliac spine (ASIS). After piercing the inguinal ligament, the nerve courses deep to the fascia lata for 0.5 cm where it penetrates the fascia lata and becomes subcutaneous. It innervates the lateral aspect of the thigh down to the knee inferiorly.

The lateral femoral cutaneous nerve can be compressed at any of the fascial bands; however, the most common location for symptomatic entrapment occurs at the inguinal ligament (**Fig. 129.7**). Causal factors include stretching or compression of the inguinal ligament such as in obesity, prolonged standing, or iatrogenic injury, and compression after hernia repair. Tight-fitting jeans and pregnancy have also been identified as causal factors.

Presentation and Diagnosis

Meralgia paresthetica is the clinical term for numbness over the lateral femoral cutaneous nerve distribution of the lateral thigh from the hip down to the knee. Patients complain of numbness, tingling, and abnormal sensation. Rarely is pain associated unless there has been direct trauma to the nerve. The sensory fibers lie in the anterior portion of the nerve as it traverses the inguinal ligament, and thus patients' symptoms are typically in the anterolateral thigh.

Because the lateral femoral cutaneous nerve is a purely sensory nerve, there are no object findings on physical exam. Any motor or reflex abnormalities on exam should either clue the physician to another diagnosis or an additional diagnosis. EMG and nerve conduction studies are not warranted for meralgia paresthetica. The best diagnostic test is to administer local anesthetic 1 cm medial to the ASIS where the lateral femoral cutaneous nerve penetrates the inguinal ligament. The diagnosis is confirmed if the symptoms are relieved.

Common Peroneal Nerve Entrapment

Anatomy

The common peroneal nerve is formed at the bifurcation of the sciatic nerve in the lower third of the posterior compartment of the thigh. Fibers from L4, L5, S1, and S2 travel in the common peroneal nerve. In the thigh, the nerve gives off an articular nerve to the knee and a lateral sural cutaneous nerve, which provides sensation to the posterolateral aspect of the leg just below the knee. As the common peroneal nerve courses inferiorly across the lateral portion of the popliteal fossa, it runs downward and laterally toward the neck of the fibula. At the neck, the common peroneal nerve runs under the arching peroneus longus fibers. The edge of this arch may be fibrous, and is the site of potential entrapment of the nerve (1 to 2 cm distal to the fibular head). After crossing the fibula, the common peroneal nerve lies lateral to the lateral head of the gastrocnemius muscle and medial to the biceps tendon.

Division of the common peroneal nerve into its superficial and deep components occurs within the substance of the peroneus longus muscle at the level of the neck of the fibula. Three articular branches to the knee are also noted in this location. The superficial nerve spirals around the neck of the fibula and supplies the muscles of the peroneal compartment. The sensory branches continue down the fibula and are seen and palpated on the dorsal aspect of the ankle. Sensory branches from the superficial peroneal nerve also supply the dorsum of the foot. The deep branch of the peroneal nerve supplies the tibialis anterior, extensor hallucis longus, extensor digitorum longus, and peroneus tertius muscles (all L5-derived axons). From its origin at the neck of the fibula, the deep branch runs deep to the extensor digitorum longus, between the muscle and the tibialis anterior with the anterior tibial vessels. The deep peroneal nerve penetrates the lateral intermuscular septum to enter the anterior compartment of the leg, supplying the muscles of the compartment as well as sensory to the web of the first interspace.

Presentation and Diagnosis

Common peroneal nerve entrapment occurs just as the nerve pierces the fibrous bands of the peroneus longus muscle. The space is bordered medially by the periosteum of the fibula and laterally by the peroneus longus muscle fibers. Patients with entrapment may complain of pain over the fibular neck with radiation down the lateral ankle, the dorsum of the foot, and the web of the first interspace. The deep peroneal nerve is responsible for ankle dorsiflexion, ankle eversion, and toe extension. Weakness in these muscles manifests clinically as footdrop or frequent tripping. It is important to distinguish peroneal neuropathy from L5 pathology and tibial neuropathy. L5 is responsible for foot inversion and great toe flexion, which are readily assessed by manual muscle testing. The biceps femoris is innervated by the tibial nerve, and weakness should prompt the evaluation of the proximal common peroneal nerve and sciatic nerves. The Tinel sign is

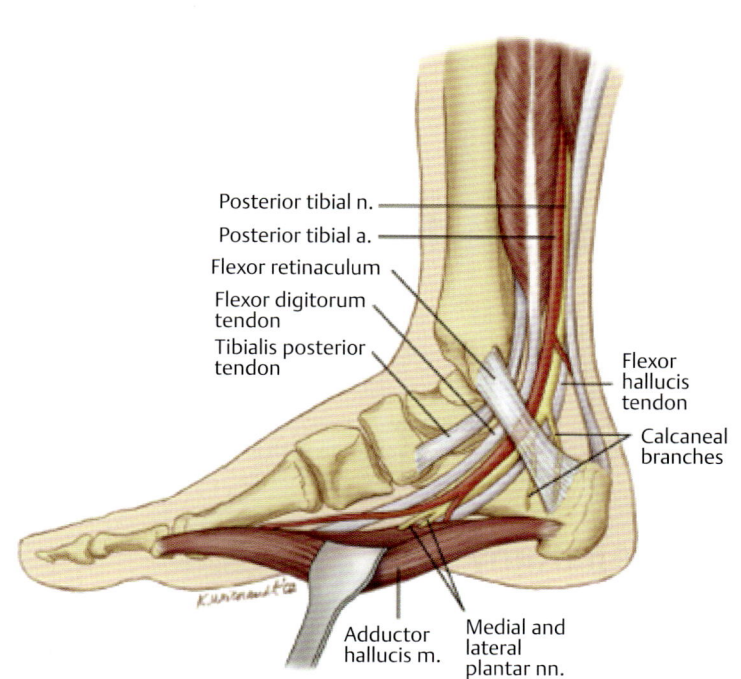

Fig. 129.8 Posterior tibial nerve compression at the tarsal tunnel.

usually present over the fibular neck for a common peroneal nerve entrapment.

Electrodiagnostics are useful in distinguishing L5 pathology from sciatic, peroneal, and tibial neuropathies. Sensory nerve action potentials (SNAPs) of the superficial peroneal nerve may be reduced, in contrast to L5 radiculopathy where they are normal. There is frequently focal slowing and temporal dispersion over the common peroneal nerve. The tibialis posterior and flexor digitorum are L5-innervated muscles and they are normal with common peroneal nerve entrapment. Imaging studies are useful adjuncts if a tumor is suspected. Ultrasound can show compressive lesions of the common peroneal nerve; however, imaging adds little information to the history, physical exam, and electrodiagnostics in typical cases.

Posterior Tibial Nerve Entrapment
Anatomy

The tibial nerve is formed at the bifurcation of the sciatic nerve in the lower third of the posterior compartment of the thigh. Fibers from L4, L5, S1, S2, and S3 travel in the tibial nerve. Because entrapment neuropathy at the tarsal tunnel is the most clinically recognized syndrome to effect the posterior tibial nerve, the anatomic description of the posterior tibial nerve focuses on its distal course.

The posterior tibial nerve descends in the posterior aspect of the leg deep to the soleus muscle and enters the tarsal tunnel just behind the posterior tibial vessels on the medial aspect of the medial malleolus. Just distal to the medial malleolus, the posterior tibial nerve divides into the calcaneal, medial plantar, and lateral plantar nerves. The calcaneal branch has a variable origin and number of branches. The latter two nerves pierce and innervate the abductor hallucis muscle, an intrinsic muscle of the foot, and then continue to provide sensory innervation to the sole of the foot. The calcaneal branch is purely sensory to the medial aspect of the heel.

The tarsal tunnel is located posterior and inferior to the medial malleolus. The roof is formed by the flexor retinaculum, and the floor is formed by the periosteum of the medial malleolus and calcaneus. The contents of the tarsal tunnel, from anterior to posterior, are the tendon of the tibialis posterior muscle, the tendon of the flexor digitorum longus muscle, the posterior tibial artery and vein, the posterior tibial nerve, and the tendon of the flexor hallucis longus muscle. There are also numerous fibrous bands that compartmentalize the tarsal tunnel and that vary from patient to patient and can predispose to a compressive neuropathy (**Fig. 129.8**).

Presentation and Diagnosis

Fifty percent of patients who present with tarsal tunnel syndrome have a history of trauma to their ankle. The most common presenting complaint is burning pain over the planar surface of the foot. The pain may radiate up the posterior compartment of the leg along the course of the posterior tibial nerve. The heel of the foot is variably affected as the calcaneal branches off the posterior tibial nerve may arise prior to the nerve entering the tarsal tunnel. The Tinel test is positive over the nerve as it courses past the medial malleolus. Abduction of the hallucis may be weak if clinically tested.

Diagnosis is primarily by history and physical exam. EMG and nerve conduction shows prolonged distal motor latency and decreased motor amplitudes in the abductor hallucis and abductor digiti quinti muscles.

B. Surgery of the Brachial Plexus

130 Supraclavicular Approach to Brachial Plexus Surgery

Shane V. Abdunnur and Daniel H. Kim

Trauma is the most common etiology of supraclavicular brachial plexus pathology that necessitates surgical intervention. Typically, these traumas are sustained in high-speed motorcycle or automobile accidents, sports injuries, or work-related accidents. Most of these traumas result in stretch injury to the brachial plexus.[1–4] Other known causes of brachial plexus injury requiring the need for surgical intervention are listed below. Parsonage-Turner syndrome, or acute brachial plexitis, is the most common brachial plexus pathology that can masquerade as a surgical lesion and should be ruled out prior to surgery. Obtaining a detailed history is therefore critical.

Indications

- Traction injury
- Laceration injury (sharp knife or glass, blunt transection from propeller or chain saw)
- Penetrating injury from gunshot wound (GSW) or metal fragments)
- Iatrogenic injury
- Injection injury (regional anesthesia)
- Compression injury (thoracic outlet syndrome)
- Obstetric injury (birth palsy)
- Nerve sheath tumor, metastatic tumor
- Radiation injury

Contraindications

- Brachial plexitis
- Transient radiation plexopathy
- Multiple pseudomeningocele on myelogram

Advantages

- Complete access to the entire high cervical plexus; the spinal nerves, trunks, and their branches; the phrenic, dorsal scapular, long thoracic, and suprascapular nerves; as well as the spinal accessory nerve
- Partial access to the anterior and posterior divisions; the lateral, posterior, and medial cords of the brachial plexus and their branches
- Access to the C5 to T1 roots

Disadvantage

- Technically complex exposure of the roots, trunks, or branches of the brachial plexus, which lie beneath the clavicle or distal segment of the brachial plexus. In cases where this disadvantage is present, combining the supraclavicular approach with an infraclavicular approach will resolve this risk.

Anatomy

The brachial plexus is formed by the union of the ventral rami of C5, C6, C7, C8, and T1. The supraclavicular portion of the brachial plexus includes the C5 to T1 spinal nerves and the three trunks of the plexus. The anterior and posterior divisions lie beneath the clavicle and are only partially accessible via the supraclavicular approach. Lateral, posterior, and medial cords are infraclavicular, where they provide the origin of the major nerves of the upper extremity (**Fig. 130.1**).

The spinal nerve, or root of the plexus, begins as multiple sensory rootlets from the dorsal root entry zone, and usually includes one ventral motor rootlet from the spinal cord. The dorsal root ganglion is located at the intraforaminal level, and both roots come together to form the spinal nerve. The primary posterior branches go to the paraspinal muscles and the large anterior branch contributes to the brachial plexus.

The extraforaminal course of C5 is along the lateral edge of the anterior scalene muscle, where it unites with C6, which runs between the anterior and middle scalene muscles, to form the upper trunk of the plexus.

The dorsal scapular nerve arises from the proximal portion of C5, lateral to the contribution of the long thoracic nerve near the foramen, and then pierces through the middle scalene muscle to reach the deep surface of the levator scapulae. The dorsal scapular nerve runs parallel with the dorsal scapular artery along the medial border of the scapula to innervate the rhomboids.

C5 also supplies a branch to the phrenic nerve, running anteriorly to the brachial plexus on the lateral border of the anterior scalene muscle. The subclavian nerve arises from the anterior surface of the upper trunk and passes anteriorly to the lower portion of the plexus, innervating the subclavius muscle.

The long thoracic nerve arises from the dorsal surface of C6 distally, close to the junction of the upper trunk, and also receives contribution from C5 and C7. It runs posterior to the brachial plexus, then descends laterally and distally into the thoracic wall to innervate the serratus anterior muscle.

The suprascapular nerve arises from the posterolateral portion of the upper trunk and runs beneath the posterior belly of the omohyoid, parallel to the suprascapular vessels, running distally through the scapular notch to innervate the supraspinatus and infraspinatus muscles.

The C7 spinal nerve emerges from the posteromedial edge of the anterior scalene muscle to form the middle trunk. The C8 spinal nerve, combined with T1, forms the lower trunk, which lies behind the subclavian artery and on top of the middle and posterior scalene muscles. The middle and lower trunks do not

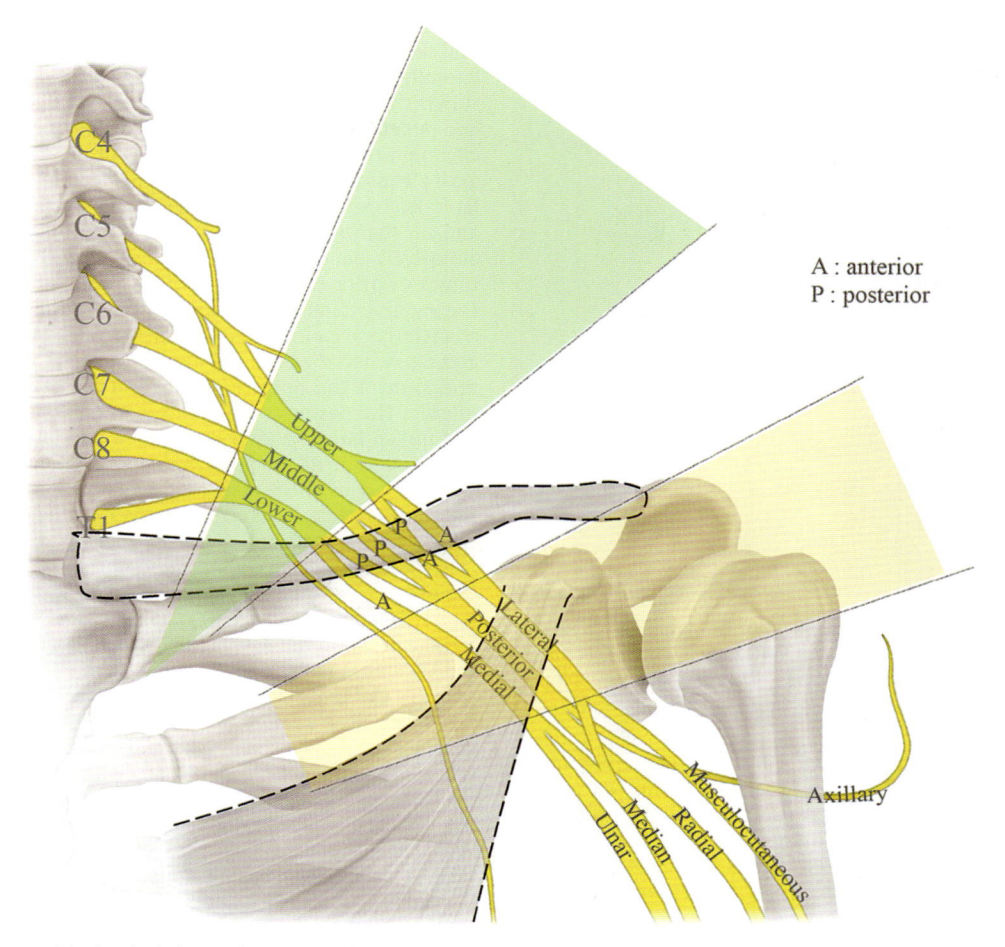

Fig. 130.1 Overview of the brachial plexus. The roots, trunks *(green)*, and proximal divisions are accessible via the supraclavicular approach.

generate branches prior to their terminations. The trunks of the brachial plexus lie in the posterior cervical triangle area, bounded by the posterior border of the sternomastoid muscle, the anterior border of the trapezius, and the superior border of the clavicle. The middle trunk is smaller in caliber than the upper or lower trunks as it takes its origin from the C7 root alone.

The vertebral artery originates from the subclavian artery, ascending anteriorly toward the lower trunk to enter the foramen transversarium of C6. Small branches from the vertebral artery supply the spinal nerves and eventually anastomose with spinal cord vasculature. Suprascapular and transverse cervical arteries from the thyrocervical trunk run laterally across the anterior surface of the lower plexus, and branches of ascending cervical and deep cervical arteries anastomoses with vertebral arteries. Beneath the clavicle, each trunk separates, forming anterior and posterior divisions.

Objective

The goal of the supraclavicular approach is to expose and obtain direct access to the supraclavicular portion of the brachial plexus, including the spinal roots or nerves, and the trunks and their branches for the purpose of neurolysis, direct end-to-end suture or graft repairs, or nerve sheath tumor resection.

Surgical Technique
Anesthesia and Positioning

General anesthesia is recommended. The neuromuscular blockade used for induction must wear off during the early phase of the dissection so that the intraoperative electrical output of the effects of muscle contraction from stimulation can be recorded and tested. Local anesthetic should be utilized judiciously and administered with care, as it has been reported to cause errors in intraoperative nerve recordings if infiltrated improperly or in excess.

The patient is placed in the supine position, with the head resting on a circular roll, away from the side of the lesion. The patient's shoulder and clavicle are brought superiorly by placing a small roll or bolster behind the scapula on the ipsilateral side. The head of the bed should be elevated 20 degrees, creating a semi-seated position, to decrease bleeding into the operative field. Because the brachial plexus is found deep to the lateral aspect of the sternocleidomastoid, the incision is planned over its lateral boarder, which is easily palpable (**Fig. 130.2**). Depending on the details of the case, it is often prudent to prepare for a combined supraclavicular and infraclavicular approach.

The entire upper extremity of the patient's surgical side should be prepped and draped free, and the patient's arm extended onto

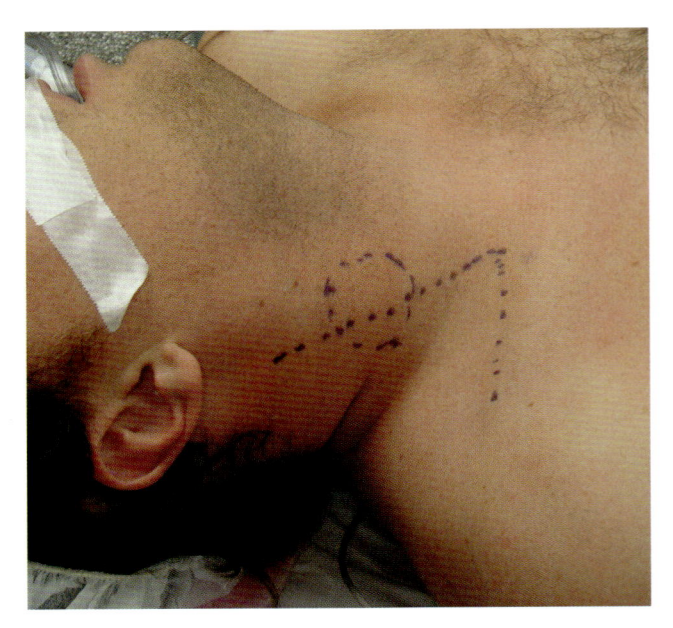

Fig. 130.2 Location of the supraclavicular brachial plexus deep to the sternocleidomastoid muscle. A planned incision over the lateral aspect of the sternocleidomastoid muscle provides access to the supraclavicular plexus.

a board at the side of the operating table. The surgeon should be able to manipulate the position of the arm to improve surgical exposure. Meticulous hemostasis can be achieved through the use of bipolar cautery throughout the dissection. The placement of tourniquets around the extremities is seldom required, and their use can cause ischemia to tissue or further compressive and ischemic damage to an already injured nerve.

Our generally preferred method of nerve grafting is to use the sural nerve due to its length and minimal morbidity from harvesting. In cases where it is known or highly anticipated that a graft will be needed, we prefer to harvest the graft with the patient in the prone position prior to starting the brachial plexus operation. Preoperative physical examination and electrodiagnostic studies are critically important for predicting the intraoperative electrical recordings and thus the need for a graft. In cases where it is difficult to predict the need for nerve grafting, we prefer to make this decision intraoperatively at the time of brachial plexus exploration. The sural nerve graft harvest can then be performed in another step with subsequent interfascicular graft repair. Appropriate preoperative planning greatly alleviates this occurrence.

Incision

After the site is marked with crosshatched lines, a No. 10 blade is used to make an oblique incision along the posterior border of the sternocleidomastoid muscle toward the medial portion of the clavicle. The incision curves parallel to the clavicle toward the proximal part of the deltopectoral groove. A pure supraclavicular approach does not require an incision past the lateral third of the clavicle. That being said, the marked line should also extend below the clavicle, toward the axillary crease, if it becomes necessary to expose the infraclavicular portion of the brachial plexus.

Dissection

After the skin incision is made, a thin layer of platysma muscle is encountered and sharply incised. The posterior cervical triangle is bound by the posterior border of the sternocleidomastoid muscle medially, the anterior border of the trapezius muscle laterally, and the clavicle at the base. After sharply incising the superficial investing fascia layer, supraclavicular fat is dissected and pulled away laterally from the posterior edge of the sternocleidomastoid muscle. The branches of the supraclavicular cervical plexus and external jugular vein are identified and dissected laterally. Larger vessels may need to be ligated with silk suture and cut sharply. The external jugular vein and larger vessels can almost always be mobilized safely unless they are encased in tumor or prior exposure to radiation complicates the situation. During dissection along the upper part of the posterior cervical triangle, great caution must be taken to avoid injury to the spinal accessory nerve where the nerve emerges from just above the midpoint of the posterior border of the sternocleidomastoid muscle. The posterior belly of the omohyoid muscle is divided and pulled laterally after it is tagged with sutures for later reapproximation. As the posterior cervical triangle fat is dissected from the edges of the sternocleidomastoid muscle and clavicle, the transverse cervical artery and vein, which cross the plexus, can be seen, ligated, and divided.

When the sternocleidomastoid muscle is retracted medially, the phrenic nerve can be identified as it runs along the superolateral border on the ventral surface of the anterior scalene muscle. The phrenic nerve is an important landmark for locating the C5 spinal nerve, which unites with C6 to form the upper trunk of the brachial plexus (**Fig. 130.3**). The nerve stimulator, set at 1 mA, can be used to stimulate the phrenic nerve, causing contraction of the ipsilateral hemidiaphragm. The phrenic nerve is dissected and mobilized medially with a vascular loop around the nerve so that the upper trunk can be dissected.

Another helpful anatomic landmark to identify is the transverse cervical rami. It emerges from the posterior border of the sternocleidomastoid muscle, loops around it, and can be traced proximally to identify C4 inferiorly to the C5 spinal nerve.

Proximal dissection of the C5 nerve requires the resection of the transverse process with a high-speed drill or a No. 2 Kerrison punch. Venous plexus around the spinal nerve close to the foramen requires meticulous hemostasis with bipolar, Gelfoam with thrombon, or Surgicel. Special attention is required during dissection of C5 at the foramen to avoid injuring the dorsal scapular nerve, which originates from the posterior aspect of C5, lateral to the small branch given off, forming the long thoracic nerve.

The long thoracic nerve arises from the dorsal surface of the C6 spinal nerve with contributions from C5 and C7. It pierces through the middle scalene muscle and runs posterior to the brachial plexus and continues inferiorly to innervate the serratus anterior muscle in the chest wall.

The nerve to the subclavius muscle arises from the anterior aspect of the upper trunk. This nerve has no clinical significance except that it is the origin of the phrenic nerve. If necessary, it can be sacrificed distal to the origin of the phrenic nerve.

During dissection along the posterolateral aspect of the upper trunk, the suprascapular nerve can be identified and isolated from the upper trunk. It runs toward the scapular notch, level with the clavicle and the suprascapular artery and vein.

The C7 spinal nerve emerges from between the anterior and middle scalene muscles inferior to the C5 and C6 spinal nerves (**Fig. 130.4**). To improve the exposure of the proximal middle trunk and C7 spinal nerve, the anterior scalene muscle can be resected while protecting the phrenic nerve.

The C8 and T1 spinal nerves are located posterior to the subclavian artery. The lateral portion of clavicular insertion of the sternocleidomastoid muscle is detached from the clavicle, and retraction of the subclavian artery inferiorly by using a vein retractor can further expose C8, T1, and the lower trunk (**Fig. 130.5**). At times, the clavicle must be temporarily removed,

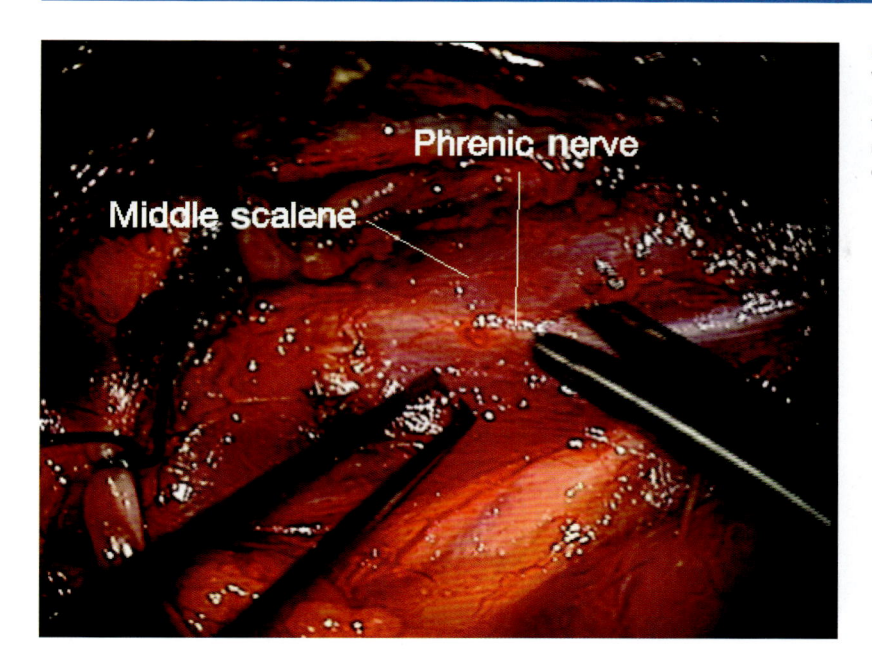

Fig. 130.3 Initial superior exposure of the supraclavicular brachial plexus. After the sternocleidomastoid muscle is retracted medially, the phrenic nerve is found overlying the superficial surface of the scalenus medius. The phrenic nerve can be traced proximally to define C4 and C5 spinal nerves from C6.

which provides excellent access to the most inferior nerve roots. Resection of the anterior scalene muscle facilitates the mobilization of the subclavian artery. Special caution must be taken when dissecting around the T1 spinal nerve to prevent injury to the vertebral artery, cervicothoracic ganglion (stellate ganglion), apex of pleura, and thoracic duct in left-side dissection. If the surgeon inadvertently enters the pleura during dissection of the T1 spinal nerve, the pleura can be repaired with 4-0 silk sutures and controlled ventilation by the anesthesiologist. Plan to obtain an intraoperative chest X-ray in the operating room after closure for chest tube placement if there is significant pneumothorax.

There are no nerve branches originating from the middle or lower trunks in the supraclavicular region. The clavicle is dissected circumferentially by isolating both the subclavius muscle and the vessel beneath the clavicle. The segment of the subclavius muscle and vessel are ligated and resected. A moistened sponge gauze is placed around the clavicle and clamped with a large hemostat, which can be used to pull the clavicle inferiorly, giving a better view of the structures underneath the clavicle. Anterior and posterior divisions from three trunks are located under the clavicle.

Donor Nerve Graft Harvesting

The most common sources of donor nerve grafts are the sural nerves from both lower extremities. A longitudinal incision is made at ankle level between the Achilles tendon and medial malleolus toward the popliteal fossa, and then along the posterior calf where it lies subcutaneously. The entire length of the sural nerve can be harvested as it generally forms from the peroneal

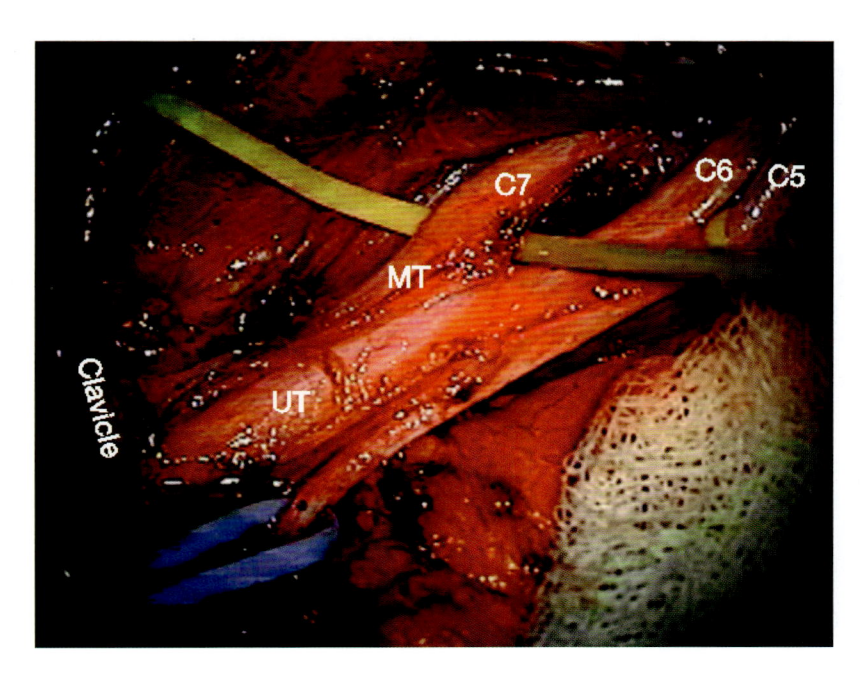

Fig. 130.4 Supraclavicular brachial plexus. Further dissection through the fat pad reveals spinal roots C5 and C6, which join to form the upper trunk (UT). C7 forms the middle trunk (MT). Suprascapular nerve is shown (*blue vessel loop*).

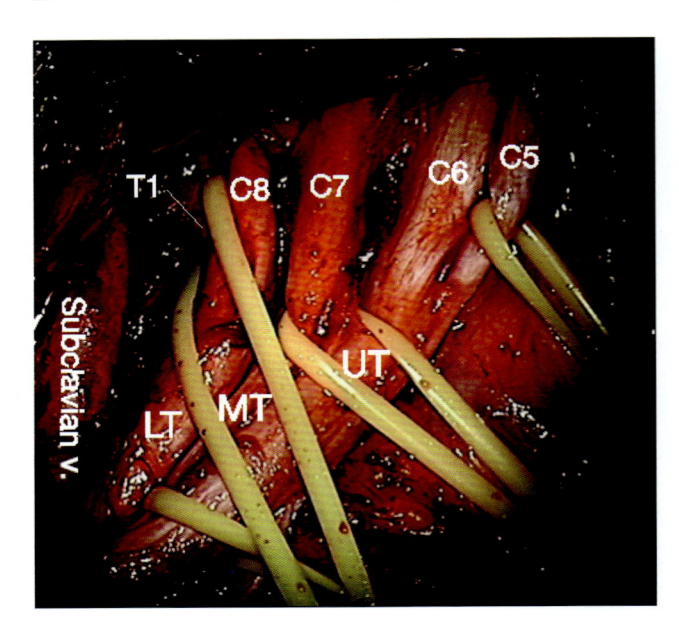

Fig. 130.5 Exposure of the entire supraclavicular brachial plexus.

nerve. An average length of 25 to 35 cm of sural nerve can be harvested from each leg.

Surgical Repair

Laceration

Transection or acute laceration injuries to the plexus are best repaired immediately while inflammation and nerve regeneration has not yet begun. Acute exploration and direct end-to-end suture repair (neurorrhaphy) of supraclavicular brachial plexus injuries that are the result of sharp laceration have very favorable functional surgical outcomes.

If bluntly transected injuries from motor blades or chain saws are observed during acute exploration for vascular repair, each stump needs to be tacked down to the adjacent soft tissue for future repair. This will maintain the length of the lesion and minimize the length of any nerve grafts that are required after resection of both ends of the nerve stumps. Posttraumatic neuromas must be resected until healthy fascicles can be observed in subsequent surgeries.

Penetrating Injury

Most penetrating injuries, such as GSWs, produce complete or incomplete lesions. A small number result in total physical disruption. If no signs of reinnervation are seen after several months, exploration should be performed and intraoperative nerve action potentials (NAPs) should be recorded. External neurolysis is performed only if NAPs are recorded across the lesion. If no NAPs are recorded, a segment of the lesion is resected until healthy fascicles are noted and then repaired with direct end-to-end suture repair; more frequently, nerve graft repair is necessary.

Stretch Injury

Most stretch or traction injuries do not avulse or pull the plexus elements away completely. Most injuries are lesions in continuity, along with severe internal disruption and formation of the neuroma mass. The dissection should be extended proximally and distally to the injured nerve segment, as well as to other neural elements of the brachial plexus, so as to understand the extent of the injury and its relationship to the surrounding anatomy. It is essential that the surgeon record intraoperative NAP across the lesion to determine internal fascicular disruption and to assess the extent of axonal regeneration.

Because spontaneous recovery may be expected, lesions in continuity with positive NAP should not be resected after external neurolysis is performed to free the nerve from the surrounding dense fibrotic scar tissue.

Large neuromas, combined with the absence of NAPs, indicate internal disruption of fascicles. These are resected with a sharp No. 15 blade until healthy-appearing fascicular patterns are observed on the cross sections of both nerve stump ends. Nylon sutures (8-0 or 9-0) are used to perform interfascicular graft repair. It is essential that proper decisions are made as to which proximal lead-out grafts go with what distal segments. Determining the number of nerve grafts to be used and their proper lengths will minimize tension at the repair sites. These are important factors to address, as they have a significant impact on functional recovery. The length of the nerve gap can be shortened by mobilizing the nerve. This is done by extending the dissection of the nerve longitudinally along the nerve, mobilizing the joint, and performing nerve transposition, which provides a more direct route to the nerve.

Most stretch injuries of the supraclavicular brachial plexus cannot be repaired by direct suture repair. Autologous interfascicular nerve grafts are required to repair the gap, after resection of the nonrecordable NAP portion of the nerve.

If avulsed spinal nerves are identified, proximal dissection at the level of the foramen is necessary so that the surgeon may find a potential lead-out stump for nerve graft repair.

If complete spinal root avulsion is encountered, it may not be possible to identify proximal lead-outs for direct nerve grafting, in which case the surgeon must perform neurotization using the descending cervical plexus, distal spinal accessory nerve, or intercostal nerves to the musculocutaneous nerve.

Surgeons must be prepared to extend their exploration into the infraclavicular brachial plexus to obtain adequate access when necessary. Proper preoperative planning including physical examination, electrodiagnostic studies, and magnetic resonance imaging are critical in obtaining good long-term neurologic outcomes.

References

1. Kline DG, Hackett ER, Happel LH. Surgery for lesions of the brachial plexus. Arch Neurol 1986;43:170–181
2. Kline DG. Perspectives concerning brachial plexus injury and repair. Neurosurg Clin N Am 1991;2:151–164
3. Lusk MD, Kline DG, Garcia CA. Tumors of the brachial plexus. Neurosurgery 1987;21:439–453
4. Kline DG, Hudson AR. Nerve Injuries: Operative Results for Major Nerve Injuries, Entrapments, and Tumors. Philadelphia: WB Saunders; 1995

131 Infraclavicular Approach to Brachial Plexus Surgery

Shane V. Abdunnur and Daniel H. Kim

Infraclavicular brachial plexus injury is caused by stretch injuries, contusive injuries to the cords, cords and nerve lesions with associated axillary artery injury, shoulder dislocation or fracture, and humeral fracture. Infraclavicular stretch injuries often spare shoulder function, but damage extends from divisions of the cords to more distal nerves.[1,2] Isolated axillary nerve palsy associated with injuries to cords or nerves is also common. With the infraclavicular approach, the surgeon has complete access to the anterior and posterior divisions; the lateral, posterior, and medial cords of the brachial plexus and their branches; and the musculocutaneous, subscapular, thoracodorsal, axillary, radial, ulnar, median, lateral, and medial pectoral nerves.

Indications

- Traction injury (motorcycle or automobile accident, or sports or work related)[2,3]
- Laceration injury (sharp knife or glass, or blunt transection from propellers or chain saws)[2,3]
- Contusive injury (associated shoulder or humeral fractures)
- Penetrating injury from gunshot wound (GSW) or metal fragments[2,3]
- Iatrogenic injury (head and neck, shoulder orthopedic surgeries)
- Compression injury
- Injection injury (regional anesthesia)
- Nerve sheath tumor, metastatic tumor[4]
- Radiation injury

Contraindications

- Brachial plexitis
- Transient radiation plexopathy

Advantages

- Complete access to the anterior and posterior divisions of the brachial plexus
- Good exposure of the lateral, posterior, and medial cords
- Ability to visualize the cord branches from proximally to distally; the lateral cord's lateral pectoral and musculocutaneous nerves; the posterior cord's thoracodorsal, subscapular, axillary, and radial nerves; the medial cord's ulnar nerve; and the lateral and medial cord's formation of the median nerve

Disadvantage

- Difficult to visualize or obtain full access to the roots, trunks, or branches of the brachial plexus without extending the incision supraclavicularly

Objective

- To expose and obtain direct access to the infraclavicular portion of the brachial plexus, including divisions, cords, and their branches; to perform neurolysis, direct end-to-end suture or graft repairs, or nerve sheath tumor resection

Anatomy

Beneath the clavicle, each trunk separates into anterior and posterior divisions. The anterior division contains fibers to the flexor muscles or anterior surface of the arm and forearm, whereas the posterior division distributes fibers to the extensor muscles and dorsal surface of the upper extremities. The divisions of all three trunks help form the three cords of the brachial plexus.

The anterior divisions of the upper and middle trunks unite to form the lateral cord, distal to the clavicle. The lateral cord is the first neural element to be encountered during infraclavicular dissection. It is situated in the anterolateral aspect of the axillary artery. The anterior division of the lower trunk continues to form the medial cord, which is medial to the axillary artery. All posterior divisions of the three trunks unite to form the posterior cord of the brachial plexus, which is situated behind the axillary artery.[3] Cords are named relative to their proximity to the axillary artery at the level of the pectoralis minor.

The lateral cord runs in a medial to lateral direction over the axillary artery and terminates to form the musculocutaneous nerve after giving off a lateral contribution to the median nerve. The musculocutaneous nerve descends into the biceps and the brachialis after supplying branches to the coracobrachialis muscle. The lateral pectoral nerve arises from the lateral cord and sends a ramus to the medial pectoral nerve, which forms a loop and penetrates through the clavipectoral fascia to innervate the pectoralis major muscle.[1,3]

The posterior cord is situated posterior to the axillary artery and gives off upper subscapular, thoracodorsal, lower subscapular, axillary, and terminal branch radial nerves in that order. The upper subscapular nerve is a small branch that runs posterior to the axillary artery and innervates the upper part of the subscapular muscle. The thoracodorsal nerve emerges between the upper

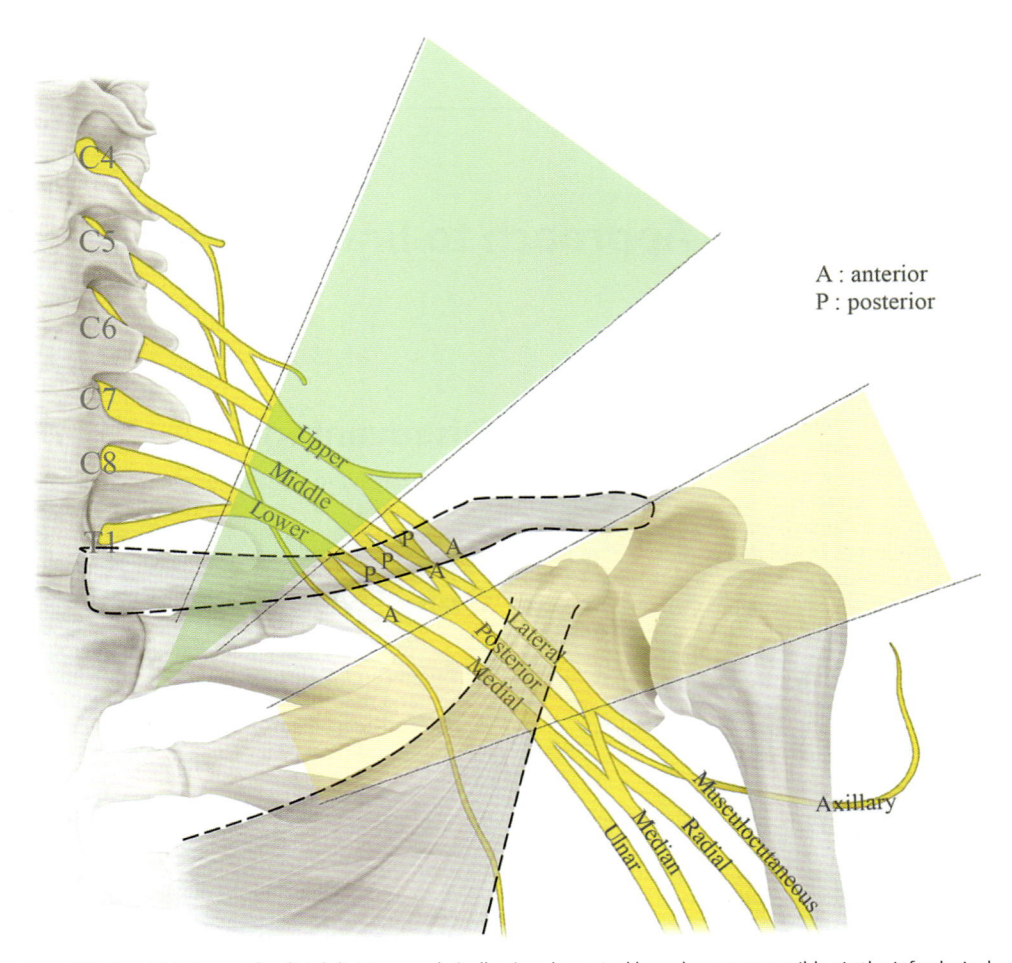

Fig. 131.1 Overview of the brachial plexus. The distal division, cords (yellow) and terminal branches are accessible via the infraclavicular approach.

and lower subscapular nerves and runs in the posterior axillary wall, innervating the latissimus dorsi muscle. The lower subscapular nerve innervates the lower part of the subscapularis and teres major muscles. The axillary nerve generally arises from the posterior cord but can also arise from the posterior divisions of the upper and middle trunks. It runs anterior to the subscapularis muscle and passes through the quadrilateral space, which is bounded above by the subscapularis and teres minor muscles, below by the teres major muscle, medially by the long head of the triceps, and laterally by the surgical neck of the humerus. The axillary nerve innervates the articular shoulder joint, the deltoid and teres minor muscles, and the skin overlying the deltoid. The radial nerve is a large terminal branch of the posterior cord, which runs inferiorly toward the humeral groove and wraps around the humerus.[1]

The medial cord provides the major contribution to the median nerve, the medial brachial cutaneous nerve, the medial antebrachial cutaneous nerve, and the ulnar nerve.[3] The medial pectoral nerve arises from the medial cord and connects with the lateral pectoral nerve through a communicating loop.[3] It divides into several branches and innervates both pectoralis major and minor muscles (**Fig. 131.1**).

Surgical Technique

Anesthesia and Positioning

General anesthesia is recommended. The neuromuscular blockade used for induction must wear off during the early phase of the dissection so that the intraoperative electrical output of the effects of muscle contraction from stimulation can be recorded and tested. Local anesthetic should be utilized judiciously and administered with care, as it has been reported to cause errors in intraoperative nerve recordings if infiltrated improperly or in excess.[1,3,4]

The patient is placed in the supine position with the head resting on a circular roll, away from the side of the lesion. The patient's shoulder and clavicle are brought superiorly by placing a small roll or bolster behind the scapula on the ipsilateral side. The head of the bed should be elevated 20 degrees, creating a semi-seated position, to decrease bleeding into the operative field. The affected upper limb is supported on an extended arm board in a 60-degree abducted position (**Fig. 131.2**). Depending on the details of the case, it is often prudent to prepare for a combined supraclavicular and infraclavicular approach (**Fig. 131.3**).

131 Infraclavicular Approach to Brachial Plexus Surgery

The surgeon should be able to manipulate the position of the arm to improve surgical exposure. Meticulous hemostasis can be achieved through the use of the bipolar cautery throughout the dissection. Placement of tourniquets around the extremities is seldom required, and their use can cause ischemia to tissue or further compressive and ischemic damage to an already injured nerve.

Incision

After the site is marked with crosshatched lines, a No. 10 blade is used to make an incision that follows the deltopectoral groove, beginning proximally at the clavicle and extending distally toward the axillary crease. The lateral border of the pectoralis major muscle is dissected from the clavicle and split along the deltopectoral groove. The cephalic vein is typically ligated as it crosses the axillary vein close to the clavicle.

Dissection

After the subclavicular muscle and vein are dissected and ligated, the clavicle can be mobilized and retracted superiorly by using a moistened sponge, which is placed under and around the clavicle to expose the infraclavicular portion of the brachial plexus.

After self-retaining retractors, such as an Adson, are placed between the deltoid and pectoralis major muscles along the deltopectoral groove, the clavipectoral fascia is identified and then divided to expose the origin of the pectoralis minor muscle at the coracoid process (**Fig. 131.4**). The tendon belonging to the pectoralis minor muscle is divided after being tagged with two sutures on either side for later approximation. Distal exposure is gained by elevating and pulling the pectoralis major muscle inferiorly on a sling with a sponge gauge to expose a broad expanse of the infraclavicular space.

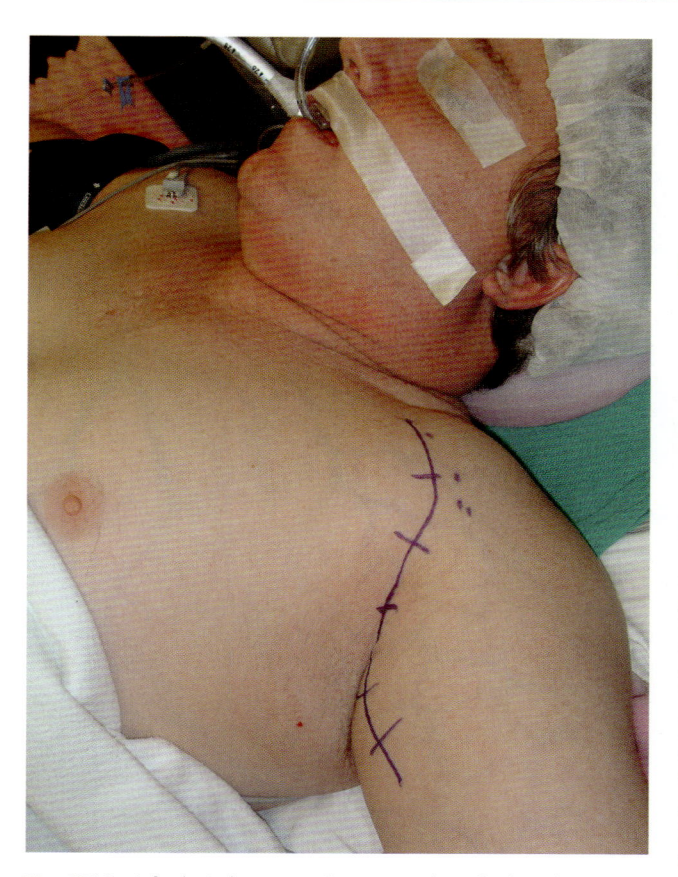

Fig. 131.2 Infraclavicular approach incision. The infraclavicular incision starts at the superior margin of the deltopectoral groove and extends distally to the axillary crease.

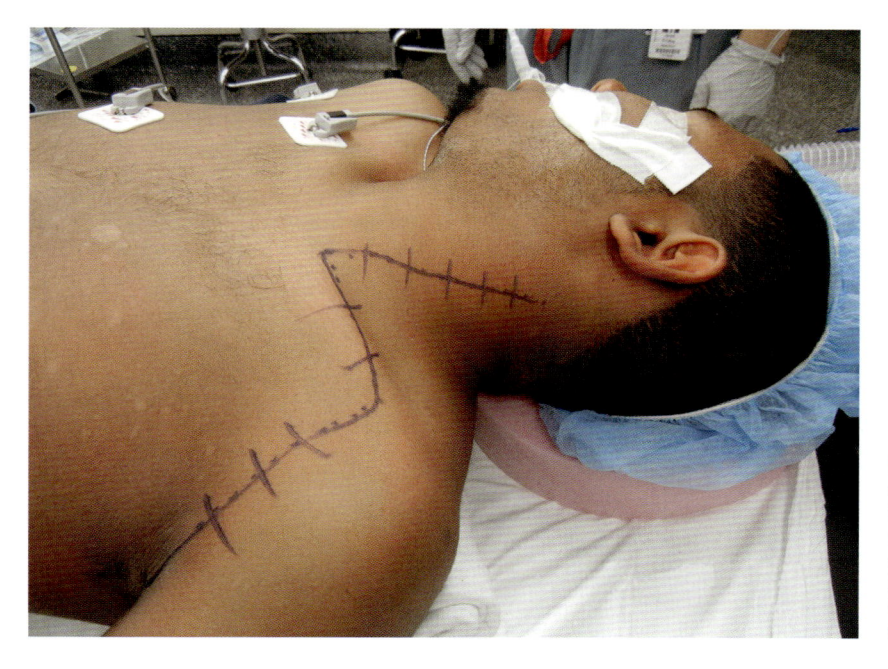

Fig. 131.3 Combined supraclavicular and infraclavicular approach incision. The infraclavicular incision starts at the superior margin of the deltopectoral groove and extends distally to the axillary crease. The supraclavicular portion should always be planned as it courses over the lateral aspect of the sternocleidomastoid muscle down to its attachment at the clavicle.

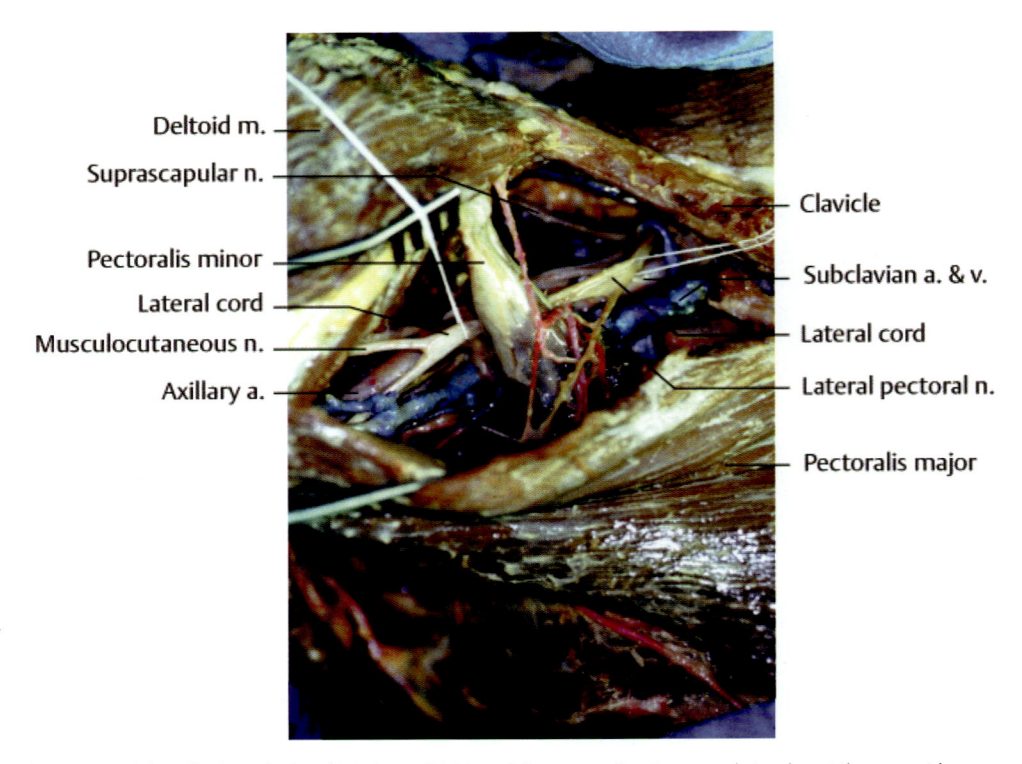

Fig. 131.4 Initial exposure of the infraclavicular brachial plexus. Division of the pectoralis minor muscle tendon at the coracoid process enables complete dissection of the infraclavicular brachial plexus.

The first neural element the physician encounters is the lateral cord, which is created from contributions from the anterior divisions of the upper and middle trunks, which lie superficial and lateral to the axillary artery. The lateral cord gives off the lateral pectoral nerve and branches into the musculocutaneous nerve and lateral cord and contributes to the median nerve. The musculocutaneous nerve, a terminal branch of the lateral cord, dives into the biceps and brachialis after piercing and supplying the coracobrachialis muscle.

The posterior cord is formed by the posterior divisions of all three trunks and lies posterior to the axillary artery. The posterior cord gives off subscapular, thoracodorsal, axillary, and radial nerves. Several subscapular branches arise, usually from the posterior cord or axillary, and run inferiorly and obliquely, innervating the subscapularis and teres major muscles. The thoracodorsal nerve arises from the posterior cord, innervating the latissimus dorsi.

The posterior cord then divides into its two major branches, the axillary and the radial nerves. The axillary nerve dives down into the quadrilateral space, with the posterior humeral circumflex vessel, innervating the deltoid and teres minor muscles. The terminal outflow of the posterior cord is the radial nerve, which runs inferiorly toward the humeral groove and winds around the humerus. A very important anatomic landmark is the medial relation between the radial nerve and the profundus branch of the axillary artery. This can be used to locate the proximal radial and differentiate it from the more lateral axillary nerve.

The medial cord is formed from the lower trunk, which emerges between the axillary artery and vein. It gives off the medial pectoral nerve; the medial brachial cutaneous nerve; the

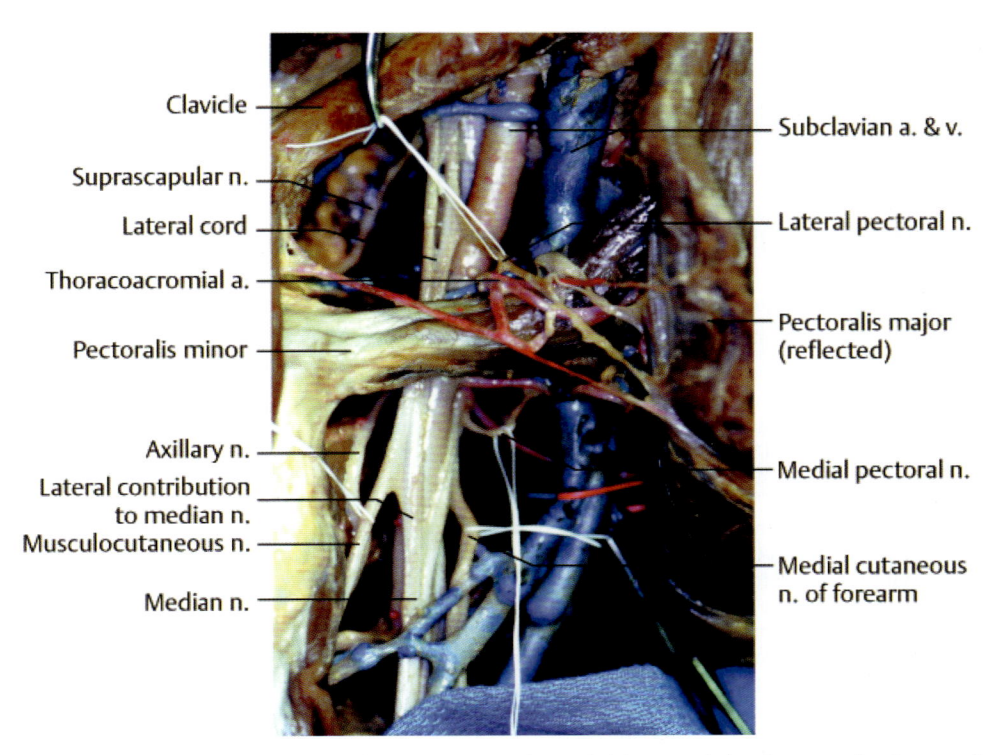

Fig. 131.5 Complete exposure of the infraclavicular brachial plexus. Deeper and extended dissection below the pectoralis minor muscle reveals the terminal branches of the infraclavicular brachial plexus. The pectoralis minor muscle has been left intact for orientation purposes.

medial antebrachial cutaneous nerve (a major contribution to the median nerve, which wraps around the medial and superior side of the axillary artery); and its terminal branch, the ulnar nerve. These neural structures remain medial to the brachial artery as they begin to descend the upper arm (**Fig. 131.5**).

Thus, the infraclavicular brachial plexus is explored lateral to medial unless pathology dictates otherwise. If there is extensive scarring, exploration should begin as distally as possible, locating normal tissue prior to proceeding proximally.[3,4]

Surgical Repair

Methods of recording intraoperative nerve action potentials and of performing neurolysis, and direct end-to-end suture and graft repair were described in Chapter 130.

References

1. Kline DG, Hackett ER, Happel LH. Surgery for lesions of the brachial plexus. Arch Neurol 1986;43:170–181
2. Kline DG. Perspectives concerning brachial plexus injury and repair. Neurosurg Clin N Am 1991;2:151–164
3. Kline DG, Hudson AR. Nerve Injuries: Operative Results for Major Nerve Injuries, Entrapments, and Tumors. Philadelphia: WB Saunders; 1995
4. Lusk MD, Kline DG, Garcia CA. Tumors of the brachial plexus. Neurosurgery 1987;21:439–453

132 Surgical Approach to the Spinal Accessory Nerve

Tene A. Cage, Arnau Benet, Erron W. Titus, and Michel Kliot

The spinal accessory nerve (SAN), cranial nerve XI, provides motor innervation to the sternocleidomastoid (SCM) and trapezius muscles. It is composed of lower motor neurons (LMNs) that arise from rootlets at the C1 to C5 levels of the spinal cord. The SAN ascends through the foramen magnum, runs rostrally through the skull base, turns to exit the skull through the jugular foramen, and then descends into the neck to innervate the ipsilateral SCM and trapezius muscles. Injuries to the SAN anywhere along its course result in a lower motor neuron lesion, but it is most vulnerable to injury in its distal and more superficial segment in the neck. From loss of trapezius function, patients experience ipsilateral shoulder drop, winging of the scapula, and difficulty with shoulder abduction. From loss of SCM function, patients experience weakness when turning the head toward the contralateral side.

Indications for Surgery and Lesions of the Spinal Accessory Nerve

Injury to the SAN can lead to significant functional disability. Shoulder drop presents with downward and lateral rotation of the scapula, inability to raise the shoulder, as well as winging of the scapula with attempted lateral shoulder abduction. The physical asymmetry is apparent, and patients are unable to abduct the arm above the shoulder. Surgical repair of the nerve may restore function and independence to patients. Depending on the mechanism of injury, surgical repair may involve neurolysis, direct end-to-end nerve anastomosis, or interposition nerve grafts with or without the aid of nerve tubes. In addition, the intact SAN is an important donor nerve in distal neurotization procedures to restore function after brachial plexus injury.[1] This chapter discusses the approach to injuries of the cervical portion of the nerve after it exits the skull base through the jugular foramen.

Trauma

The SAN can be damaged by penetrating trauma, a blunt impact, or as the result of stretch or avulsion. One series found that 24% of injuries to the nerve were the result of trauma.[2] Gunshot or knife wounds to the neck have been described as causes of penetrating SAN injury.[3] Blunt injuries such as a blow to the neck during contact sports (e.g., wrestling) can also lead to SAN palsies.[4] Mechanisms of injury involving traction on the nerve include whiplash from a car accident,[5,6] stretch during diving accidents, and brachial plexus birth injuries. In the latter case, it is also common for patients to suffer upper trunk brachial plexus injuries without injury to the SAN. In these patients, the intact SAN can be leveraged as a donor in neurotization for an avulsed or otherwise injured upper trunk. Most commonly, SAN to suprascapular nerve neurotization procedures have proven successful.[7-9] However, SAN to musculocutaneous nerve neurotization has also been reported.[10] When successful, these techniques have restored shoulder rotation function.[11]

Iatrogenic Injury

Perhaps the most common etiology of SAN injury is iatrogenic, noted to be as high as 71% in one series.[2] The SAN runs through the posterior triangle of the neck, which is bounded anteriorly by the posterior border of the SCM, laterally by the anterior border of the trapezius, and at the base by the middle third of the clavicle (**Fig. 132.1**). Therefore, any surgical procedure in this area carries the risk of injuring the SAN. Procedures with reported SAN injury complications include neck dissection for carotid endarterectomy, lymph node biopsy, and parotidectomy. Scarring resulting from radiation therapy to the posterior triangle can also injure the SAN.

Tumor

Tumors affecting the SAN itself can also be the cause of SAN palsy. Although rare, schwannomas, malignant peripheral nerve sheath tumors, inflammatory myofibroblastic tumors, meningiomas, and even cavernous malformations of the SAN have been reported.[12-17] As well, tumors arising at or near the jugular foramen, such as a glomus jugulare, have been associated with SAN neuropathy.[18]

Contraindications to Surgical Repair

Not all injuries of the SAN require direct surgical repair of the nerve. Injury to the supranuclear or nuclear portion of the SAN in the brain or spinal cord, respectively, is not an indication for surgical repair. For example, amyotrophic lateral sclerosis (ALS), syringomyelia, polio, or high cervical cord intrinsic tumors may cause nuclear injury to the nerve that cannot be repaired surgically. In addition, more proximal lesions along the course of the nerve, such as jugular foramen tumors, parotid gland tumors, carotid body tumors, high cervical lymphadenopathy, and skull base fractures through the jugular foramen, may compress the nerve and thereby compromise its function. Such lesions must be treated by debulking or removing the primary lesion to enable nerve decompression along its course.

Advantages of Surgical Repair

In addition to paralysis or weakness of the trapezius and SCM, injury to the SAN can also cause significant stiffness and pain. Pain is thought to be secondary to shoulder drop in the setting of

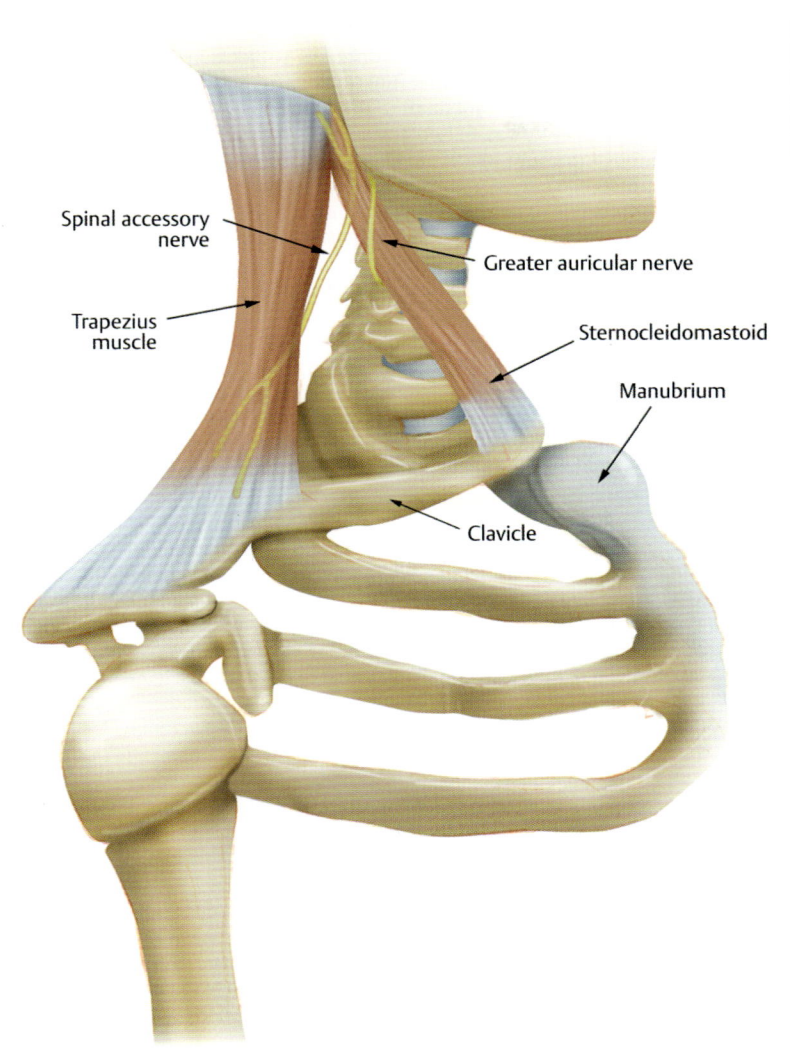

Fig. 132.1 Relationship of the spinal accessory nerve (SAN) to the greater auricular nerve as they emerge from the deep surface of the sternocleidomastoid (SCM) muscle. The posterior triangle is bounded anteriorly by the posterior border of the SCM, posteriorly by the anterior border of the trapezius muscle, and inferiorly by the clavicle.

trapezius weakness. The weight of the shoulder puts excessive stretch on the ipsilateral brachial plexus, resulting in pain that starts in the neck and radiates down the arm.[19] Successful repair of the SAN improves shoulder strength and function and can reduce the pain associated with the subsequent secondary brachial plexopathy. Therefore, advantages to surgical repair of the SAN include not only restoration of motor function but also, in some cases, reduction of pain. The anterior approach to the SAN enables the direct exposure and visualization of the nerve along its course through the posterior triangle of the neck. This is most commonly the choice for proximal nerve tumors or iatrogenic injuries during neck dissection. The posterior approach to the SAN allows for dissection and mobilization of the distal portion of the nerve. Here it is anatomically closest to the suprascapular nerve, which is imperative when performing a SAN to suprascapular nerve transfer operation.

Disadvantages of Surgical Repair

Depending on the degree and mechanism of injury, surgical repair following nerve injury may not be able to restore partial or full function to the trapezius or SCM muscles. Preoperative electromyography (EMG) and nerve conduction studies (NCSs) can be helpful in predicting possible functional benefit from nerve repair. If electrodiagnostic and imaging studies indicate complete wasting of the trapezius muscle in the setting of a complete and chronic (usually present for at least 1 year) nerve injury, the likelihood of a successful return of function is very low. In this case, muscle transfers or scapular fixation may be required to restore shoulder elevation.[20] The anterior approach provides a more difficult exposure to the distal portion of the nerve after it has crossed through the posterior triangle of the neck. The posterior approach to the SAN similarly does not provide access to the proximal portion of the nerve, before it reaches the trapezius muscle.

Choice of Operative Approach and Surgical Objectives

Surgical exploration of the SAN is most commonly performed via an anterior approach and is necessary to localize and expose the cervical segment of the nerve after it exits the skull base through the jugular foramen. With this accomplished, the nerve can be accessed for neurolysis, direct end-to-end repair, grafting, or distal neurotization in which the SAN is a donor nerve.

SAN-to–suprascapular nerve neurotization is commonly utilized for upper trunk avulsion injury repair, and for this, the posterior approach to the SAN may be more favorable.

Anatomy

The SAN is composed of lower motor neurons whose cell bodies arise from the accessory nucleus. This nucleus is located in the lateral portion of the ventral horn of the spinal cord spanning the C1 to C5 levels (**Fig. 132.2a,b**). The SAN receives cortical input from neurons of the motor cortex whose axons travel via the internal capsule, across the decussation of the pyramids, and into the contralateral lateral corticospinal tract to synapse in the accessory nucleus with cranial nerve XI LMN axons. The LMN axons form rootlets that exit the spinal cord laterally, dorsal to the dentate ligament, and join together to form one SAN fiber that ascends through the skull base and through the foramen magnum and into the posterior fossa of the skull. The nerve then then turns lateral and caudal to exit the skull base via the jugular foramen along with cranial nerves IX and X (**Fig. 132.2c**).

Just before the SAN exits the jugular foramen, fibers that arise from the lower nucleus ambiguus of the medulla join the SAN briefly as it courses through the jugular foramen. After exiting the skull, these fibers quickly split off to join up with the vagus nerve. The greater portion of these fibers were historically referred to as the cranial roots of cranial nerve XI, on the assumption that they contributed to the function of the SAN. A study involving a small number of subjects appears to confirm that these fibers belong functionally to the vagus nerve and contribute little or not at all to the function of the SAN.[21]

Once it has exited the jugular foramen, the SAN descends posterior and medial to the styloid process and runs for a short distance between the internal carotid artery and internal jugular vein. From there, it continues through the stylohyoid muscle and the posterior belly of the digastric muscle to reach the deep border of the SCM. The nerve then passes along the deep surface of the SCM in a caudal direction parallel to the muscle fibers. Some SAN fibers branch off early to pierce and innervate this muscle while others continue to travel along the deep surface of the muscle until they reach a point approximately midway between the muscle's origin at the mastoid process and its insertion at the clavicle and manubrium of the sternum. Here, the SAN emerges from the posterior border of the muscle to cross the posterior triangle of the neck, and its remaining fibers continue on to innervate the trapezius.

To locate the region in which the SAN crosses the posterior triangle, the surgeon may use the greater auricular point as a landmark (**Fig. 132.1**). The posterior triangle is bounded anteriorly by the posterior border of the SCM, posteriorly by the anterior border of the trapezius muscle, and inferiorly by the clavicle (**Fig. 132.1**). The greater auricular nerve wraps around the SCM from the deep to superficial surfaces of the muscle near the mid-

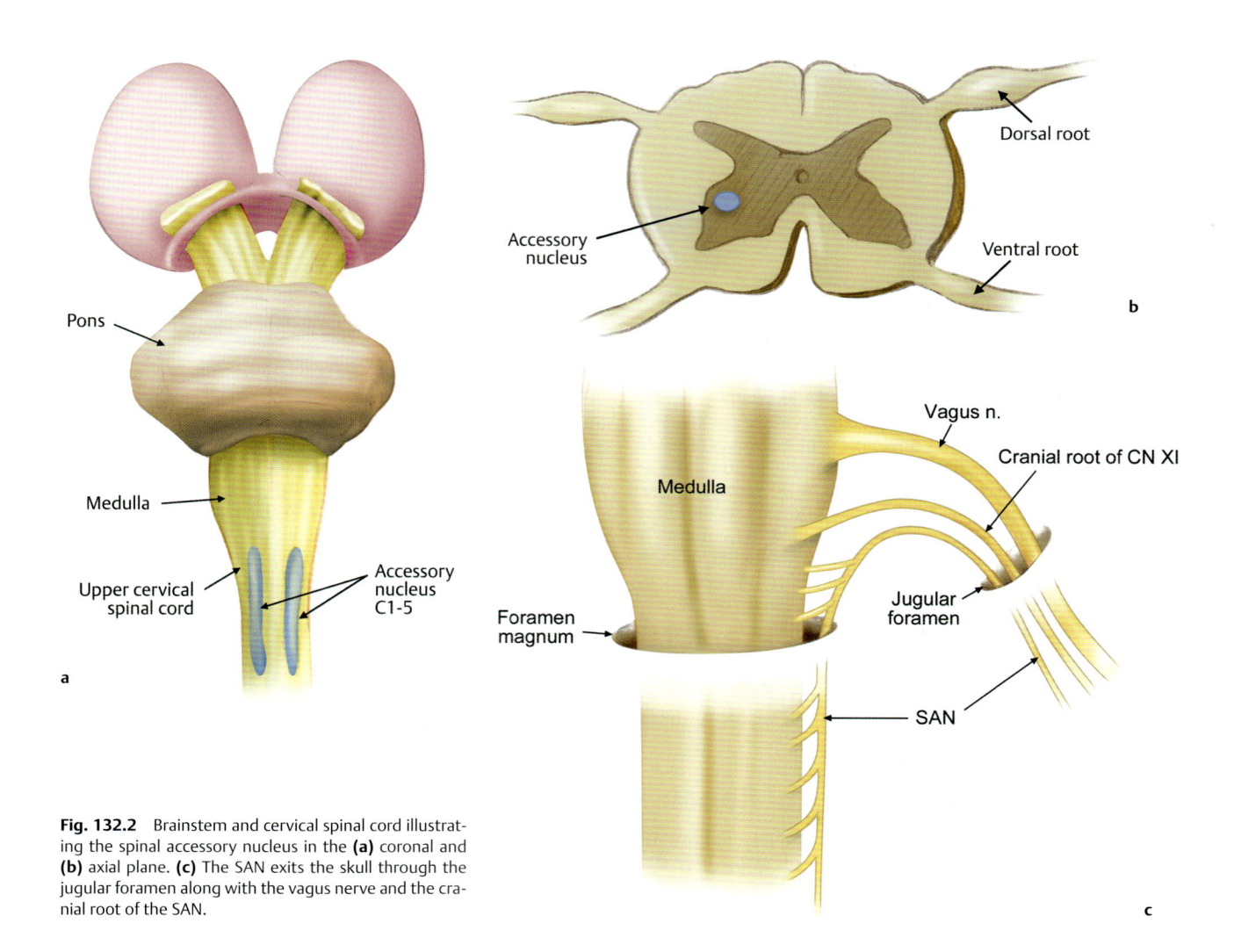

Fig. 132.2 Brainstem and cervical spinal cord illustrating the spinal accessory nucleus in the (**a**) coronal and (**b**) axial plane. (**c**) The SAN exits the skull through the jugular foramen along with the vagus nerve and the cranial root of the SAN.

point of the muscle. Where the greater auricular nerve emerges on the superior surface of the SCM is called the greater auricular point. The SAN emerges from the posterior border of the muscle to cross the posterior triangle approximately 1 to 2 cm cranial to the greater auricular point.[15,22,23] These fibers, which go on to innervate the trapezius, run lateral and inferior through the posterior triangle and superficial to the levator scapulae muscle. The terminal branches from these fibers enter the trapezius muscle deep to its anterior border. This point where the nerve enters the trapezius muscle can be estimated by measuring the distance along the trapezius muscle above the clavicle, which is, on average, 5 cm.[15] It should be noted that this is a less reliable landmark than the relationship of the proximal SAN to the greater auricular point. Along this distal part of its course, the nerve is quite superficial and vulnerable to injury.

Preoperative Tests and Considerations

Imaging and electrodiagnostic studies can provide considerable information about the injured SAN prior to surgical exploration. Neuromas or tumors may be visualized as an enlargement of the nerve. Transection sites may be identified as a discontinuity of the nerve. Magnetic resonance imaging (MRI) and magnetic resonance neurography (MRN) are helpful in visualizing the SAN and any nerve lesions prior to surgical exploration. Ultrasound is also useful in identifying the SAN and potential sites of injury along the course of the nerve.[24] In general, MRN is the preferred modality where available, whereas ultrasound is a useful adjuvant tool for preoperative and intraoperative localization of the lesion. EMG and NCS permit interrogation of SCM and trapezius muscle function as an indirect measure of SAN function. These may also be valuable preoperative tests.

Surgical Procedure and Technique

Anesthesia

It is critical for the surgeon and the anesthesiologist to work together to ensure accurate nerve identification, preservation, and response during the operation. Accessory nerve repair or exploration is done with the patient under general anesthesia and endotracheal intubation. Nerve identification relies on the ability to directly stimulate and monitor intact electrical function and motor responses to both the sternocleidomastoid and trapezius muscles via both antidromic and orthodromic impulses. Thus, it is important to ensure that the effects of paralytic agents are terminated before surgical dissection begins. In addition, if the surgeon chooses to use any local anesthetic, it is recommended that only a minimal amount be used, taking care to limit it to the superficial dermal and subdermal layers. The distal segment of the SAN is very superficial, and inadvertent injection of the nerve with local anesthetic can easily occur. In the event that this happens, intraoperative neuromonitoring and nerve identification will be compromised.

Positioning

Anterior Approach

Patients are positioned supine with the head resting on a donut headholder and turned to the contralateral side of the surgery. This serves to make the area between the angle of the mandible and the clavicle accessible, in particular providing access to the posterior triangle of the neck. The upper portion of the body can then be raised, usually ~ 30 degrees, in relation to the hip and lower portion of the body until the jugular vein collapses to minimize bleeding. A horizontal incision can be marked out on the skin along the course of the SAN. The incision should be long enough to enable adequate skin retraction to access the posterior triangle of the neck.

Posterior Approach

Patients are positioned prone with the arms adducted. A line between the midline and the acromion is marked along the superior border of the scapula on the posterior shoulder. A point 40% of the distance from the midline is marked, as it corresponds to the location of the SAN.[25] Then, a horizontal incision can be marked over this area spanning the SAN site and the suprascapular nerve site (50% of the distance between the SAN and acromion) in the case of a SAN-to–suprascapular nerve transfer.[25]

Neuromonitoring and Electrophysiological Considerations

Intraoperative neurophysiological monitoring includes motor evoked potentials (MEPs) and somatosensory evoked potentials (SSEPs) from the SCM and trapezius muscles as well as direct SAN electrical stimulation intraoperatively. Direct stimulation of the nerve using EMG signals intraoperatively can be especially useful when identifying the proximal or distal stump of the nerve. Identifying the distal stump of the nerve in the setting of a complete transection injury depends on the time since injury. Electrical studies have shown that by 3 to 5 days after transection, MEPs have dropped by 50% in the distal stump as axons undergo wallerian degeneration.[26,27]

Dissection, Nerve Identification, and Neurolysis

The skin is incised sharply from the posterior border of the SCM to the anterior border of the trapezius muscle. Using monopolar cautery, the platysma is divided and the subplatysmal space dissected bluntly using curved Metzenbaum scissors. Self-retaining or handheld retractors can be placed beneath the platysma to expose the SCM (**Fig. 132.3a**). This blunt dissection should be continued laterally to identify the anterior border of the trapezius muscle and medially to identify the posterior border of the SCM, so that the transverse cervical nerves and the greater auricular nerve, as well as the external jugular veins, are protected in the approach to the posterior border of the SCM. When the greater auricular nerve is identified, the proximal SAN end can be found exiting on the deep surface of the SCM approximately 1 to 2 cm cranial to the greater auricular point (**Fig. 132.1**). Once the proximal stump of the nerve is identified, the nerve stimulator should be used to verify its identity. By directly stimulating the nerve, antidromic impulses will activate axons, resulting in contraction of the SCM.

The course of the nerve should then be traced under direct visualization distally to the site of pathology (e.g., neuroma, tumor, or transection). If there is a neuroma or tumor, the lesion should be isolated carefully with a combination of blunt and sharp dissection to identify the lesion. Once isolated, a neuroma should be resected using a sharp No. 15 blade scalpel, exposing viable nerve fascicles on either end of the remaining nerve. For a nerve tumor, the surface or capsule of the lesion should be stimulated with a nerve stimulator probe to identify where the nerve fascicles run so that they can be avoided. Once a window on the tumor capsule, free of nerve fibers, is found, a No. 11 blade scalpel

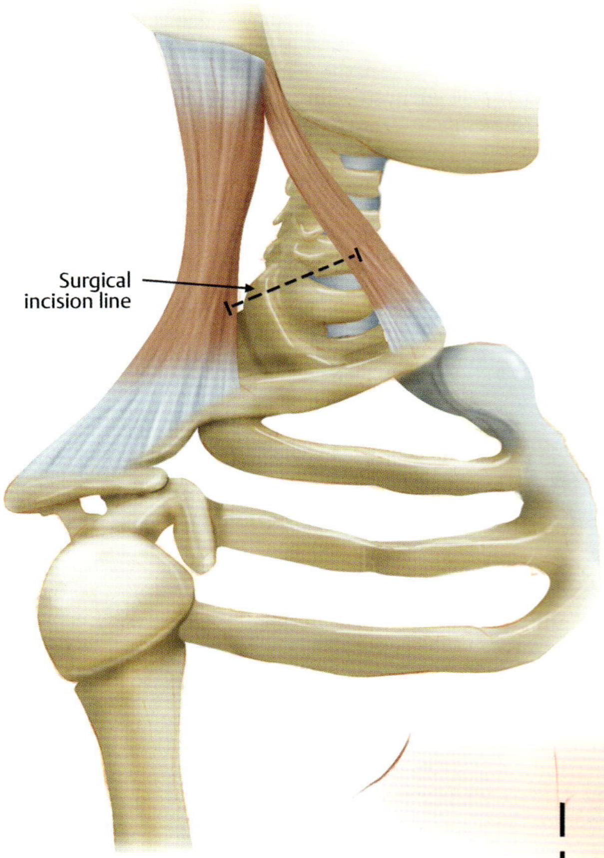

Fig. 132.3 **(a)** The anterior approach to the SAN. **(b)** The posterior approach to the SAN.

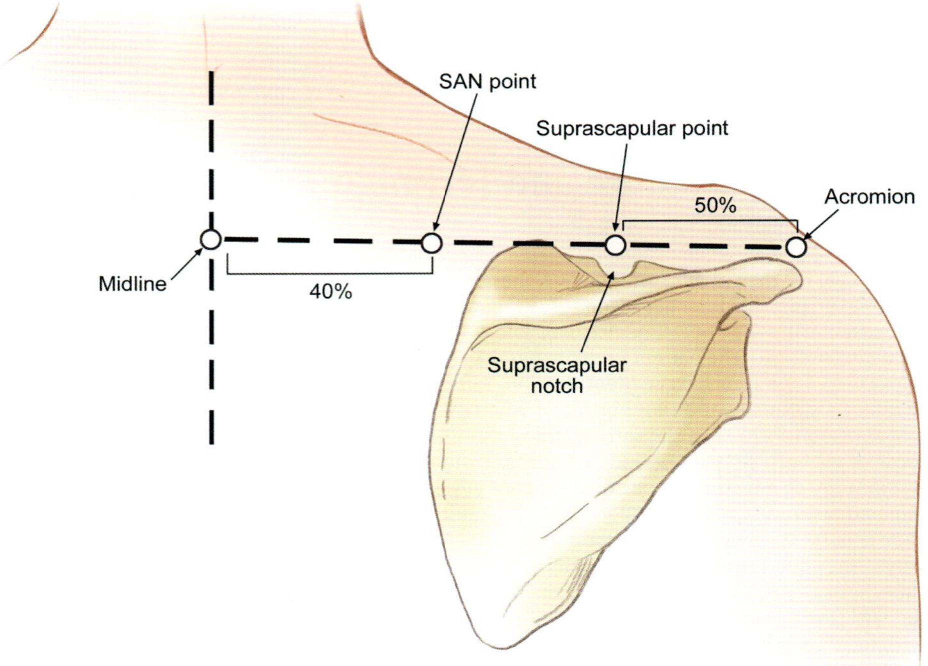

should be used to enter the capsule and a blunt Penfield No. 4 dissector can be used to define a plane between the nerve fibers and the tumor. Then, the tumor can be removed either piecemeal or en bloc, preserving surrounding nerve fascicles.

In the case of nerve transection, the proximal end should be marked with a vessel loop or suture and attention then turned to locating the distal end of the nerve. If the injury occurred less than 3 days prior to the surgery, direct nerve stimulation can aid in searching for the distal end of the SAN, as the nerve should still produce robust contractions of the trapezius muscle.[28] However, if the injury is more remote in time from the repair, the distal end of the nerve must be explored and identified with careful blunt and sharp dissection between the proximal stump and the anterior border of the trapezius muscle. When both ends are identified, the nerve should be carefully inspected and trimmed back sharply using a No. 15 blade scalpel in both directions until viable axon fascicles are identified at each end.

Nerve Repair

Once viable fascicles are visualized at the proximal and distal ends of the nerve, the nerve is then ready to be repaired. It is important that the nerve not be placed under tension when reconnecting the proximal and distal ends. If the injury was from a knife or other sharp cut and the viable nerve ends have not contracted or formed scar, the two ends can be reapproximated and repaired primarily via an end-to-end anastomosis.

However, it is more often the case that there is a gap between the two ends, requiring that an interposition graft be placed between the two ends. The options for grafts include autograft or allograft. Autograft utilizes a piece of a donor nerve from the patient as an interposition graft. Commonly, a segment of the patient's own sural nerve is chosen. An alternative to the sural nerve, however, is to use a piece of a local cervical plexus sensory nerve to bridge the gap between the two cut ends of an injured SAN, which will produce some numbness.[7] The donor sural nerve or local sensory nerve can be cut as long or short as is necessary to bridge the two ends of the SAN. The donor nerve is cut to size and sutured at the proximal and distal ends with one or two 7-0 Prolene sutures at each end to achieve a good approximation followed by wrapping with a layer of Surgicel (**Fig. 132.4a**). Another option if the gap between the proximal distal ends of the SAN is less than 7 cm is to use an allograft that is nerve harvested and treated from human cadavers to produce decellularized nerve grafts such as Avance® Nerve Graft (AxoGen Inc., Alachua, FL). Similar to an autograft, the donor graft is simply cut to size and secured to the proximal and distal ends of the nerve with 7-0 sutures (**Fig. 132.4a**). Alternatively, if the gap between the proximal and distal ends of the SAN is 4 cm or less, then a synthetic bioabsorbable tube may be used instead, for example, the NeuraGen™ (Integra, Plainsboro, NJ) collagen tube or wrap. The two ends of the nerve are prepared and the tube is placed with the ends of the wrap encasing both proximal and distal ends. This is then secured with a single 7-0 suture through the tube and the nerve on each end (**Fig. 132.4b**).

For all interposition grafts the mode of nerve repair is the same. The graft provides a highway along which the axons in the SAN can regrow. After the graft is secured in place and the wound carefully irrigated, a layer of fibrin glue can be applied over the interface of the graft and the nerve.

Closure and Postoperative Considerations

Meticulous hemostasis should be obtained followed by copious irrigation of the surgical bed with antibiotic-containing (e.g., Bacitracin) saline irrigation prior to closure of the wound. Usually, the tissues are closed by suture-reapproximation of three distinct layers: (1) the platysma, (2) the subcutaneous tissues, and (3) the skin. The arm can be suspended in a sling when the patient is out of bed to support the shoulder for 2 to 3 weeks. However, gentle neck and shoulder range of motion exercises are encouraged starting in the immediate postoperative period to prevent scarring and adhesion formation at the surgical site.

Although the surgical repair restores gross anatomic continuity to a transected or otherwise injured SAN, the functional regeneration of the nerve takes place in the postoperative period. As the axons regenerate through the repaired segment of nerve, function returns in a proximal to distal direction. For example, in patients with proximal injuries to the SAN, clinical reinnervation of the nerve will be observed as return of function first in the upper portion of the trapezius muscle, then in the middle portion, and finally in the lower portion. Postoperative

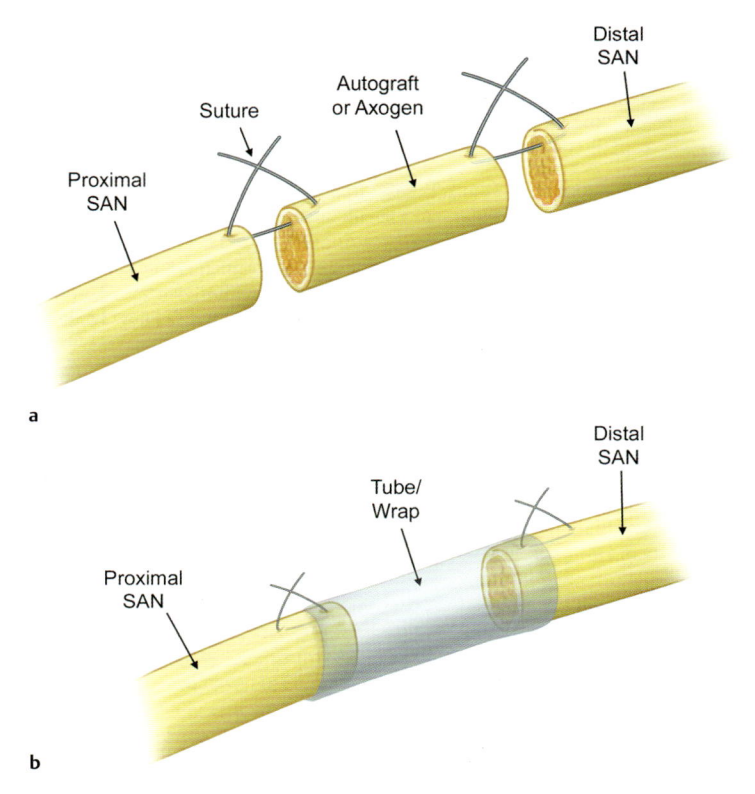

Fig. 132.4 Interposition grafts using **(a)** autograft and **(b)** nerve tube or wrap allograft.

EMG and NCS can be used to monitor nerve regrowth and reinnervation of the affected muscles. Because the nerve is expected to grow approximately 1 inch per month, the more proximal the injury, the longer it will take to see distal return of motor function. These patients can be followed with serial EMG and NCS testing. Patients will also benefit from daily physical therapy on their own to maintain and improve range of motion and muscle strength as successful muscle reinnervation occurs supplemented by intermittent formal physical therapy where deemed beneficial.[29] **Box 132.1** lists the key operative points.

> **Box 132.1 Key Operative Points in the Approach to the SAN**
>
> - Just before reaching the SCM, some fibers of the SAN pierce the SCM to innervate it, whereas others course behind the SCM to innervate the trapezius muscle distally.
> - The SAN emerges from the deep surface of the SCM ~ 1 to 2 cm rostral to the greater auricular point (where the greater auricular nerve runs superficially to the SCM) to enter the posterior triangle of the neck.
> - The SAN traverses the posterior triangle of the neck running inferolaterally from above the greater auricular point to send terminal branches deep to the anterior border of the trapezius muscle, where these fibers then terminate to innervate this muscle.
> - As the SAN runs through the posterior triangle of the neck, it is quite superficial, and care must be taken to preserve and protect the nerve.

References

1. Guan SB, Hou CL, Chen DS, Gu YD. Restoration of shoulder abduction by transfer of the spinal accessory nerve to suprascapular nerve through dorsal approach: a clinical study. Chin Med J (Engl) 2006;119:707–712
2. Donner TR, Kline DG. Extracranial spinal accessory nerve injury. Neurosurgery 1993;32:907–910, discussion 911
3. Kabataş S, Bayrak Y, Civelek E, Imer SM, Hepgül TK. Spinal accessory nerve palsy following gunshot injury: a case report. Ulus Travma Acil Cerrahi Derg (Turkish Trauma Journal) 2008;14:76–78
4. Ozçakar L, Erol O, Kara M, Kaymak B. Accessory nerve injury during amateur wrestling: silent but not overlooked. Br J Sports Med 2003;37:372
5. Bodack MP, Tunkel RS, Marini SG, Nagler W. Spinal accessory nerve palsy as a cause of pain after whiplash injury: case report. J Pain Symptom Manage 1998;15:321–328
6. Omar N, Alvi F, Srinivasan MS. An unusual presentation of whiplash injury: long thoracic and spinal accessory nerve injury. Eur Spine J 2007;16(Suppl 3):275–277
7. Ruchelsman DE, Ramos LE, Alfonso I, Price AE, Grossman A, Grossman JA. Outcome following spinal accessory to suprascapular (spinoscapular) nerve transfer in infants with brachial plexus birth injuries. Hand (NY) 2010;5:190–194
8. Tse R, Marcus JR, Curtis CG, Dupuis A, Clarke HM. Suprascapular nerve reconstruction in obstetrical brachial plexus palsy: spinal accessory nerve transfer versus C5 root grafting. Plast Reconstr Surg 2011;127:2391–2396
9. van Ouwerkerk WJ, Uitdehaag BM, Strijers RL, et al. Accessory nerve to suprascapular nerve transfer to restore shoulder exorotation in otherwise spontaneously recovered obstetric brachial plexus lesions. Neurosurgery 2006;59:858–867, discussion 867–869
10. Bhandari PS, Sadhotra LP, Bhargava P, et al. Surgical outcomes following nerve transfers in upper brachial plexus injuries. Indian J Plast Surg 2009;42:150–160
11. Grossman JA, Ruchelsman DE, Schwarzkopf R. Iatrogenic spinal accessory nerve injury in children. J Pediatr Surg 2008;43:1732–1735
12. Hazzard MA, Patel NB, Hattab EM, Horn EM. Spinal accessory nerve cavernous malformation. J Clin Neurosci 2010;17:248–250
13. Kohli R, Singh S, Gupta SK, Matreja PS. Schwannoma of the spinal accessory nerve: a case report. J Clin Diagn Res 2013;7:1732–1734
14. Liechty P, Tubbs RS, Loukas M, et al. Spinal accessory nerve meningioma in a paediatric patient: case report. Folia Neuropathol 2007;45:23–25
15. Salgarelli AC, Landini B, Bellini P, Multinu A, Consolo U, Collini M. A simple method of identifying the spinal accessory nerve in modified radical neck dissection: anatomic study and clinical implications for resident training. Oral Maxillofac Surg 2009;13:69–72
16. Sheikh OA, Reaves A, Kralick FA, Brooks A, Musial RE, Gasperino J. Malignant nerve sheath tumor of the spinal accessory nerve: a unique presentation of a rare tumor. J Clin Neurol 2012;8:75–78
17. Yasumatsu R, Nakashima T, Miyazaki R, Segawa Y, Komune S. Diagnosis and management of extracranial head and neck schwannomas: a review of 27 cases. Int J Otolaryngol 2013;2013:973045
18. Lee S, Yang S, Lee J, Kim I. Spinal accessory neuropathy associated with the tumor located on the jugular foramen. Ann Rehabil Med 2013;37:133–137
19. Walker H. Cranial nerve VI: the spinal accessory nerve. In: Walker H, Hall WD, Hurst JW, eds. Clinical Methods: The History, Physical, and Laboratory Examinations, 3rd ed. Boston: Butterworths; 1990
20. Wills AJ, Sawle GV. Accessory nerve palsies. Pract Neurol 2010;10:191–194
21. Ryan S, Blyth P, Duggan N, Wild M, Al-Ali S. Is the cranial accessory nerve really a portion of the accessory nerve? Anatomy of the cranial nerves in the jugular foramen. Anat Sci Int 2007;82:1–7
22. Chen DT, Chen PR, Wen IS, et al. Surgical anatomy of the spinal accessory nerve: is the great auricular point reliable? J Otolaryngol Head Neck Surg 2009;38:337–339
23. Hone SW, Ridha H, Rowley H, Timon CI. Surgical landmarks of the spinal accessory nerve in modified radical neck dissection. Clin Otolaryngol Allied Sci 2001;26:16–18
24. Lucchetta M, Pazzaglia C, Cacciavillani M, et al. Nerve ultrasound findings in two cases of spinal accessory nerve palsy. Muscle Nerve 2014;49:293–294
25. Colbert SH, Mackinnon S. Posterior approach for double nerve transfer for restoration of shoulder function in upper brachial plexus palsy. Hand (NY) 2006;1:71–77
26. Chaudhry V, Cornblath DR. Wallerian degeneration in human nerves: serial electrophysiological studies. Muscle Nerve 1992;15:687–693
27. Lee CH, Huang NC, Chen HC, Chen MK. Minimizing shoulder syndrome with intra-operative spinal accessory nerve monitoring for neck dissection. Acta Otorhinolaryngol Ital 2013;33:93–96
28. Harper CM. Intraoperative cranial nerve monitoring. Muscle Nerve 2004;29:339–351
29. Shimada Y, Chida S, Matsunaga T, Sato M, Hatakeyama K, Itoi E. Clinical results of rehabilitation for accessory nerve palsy after radical neck dissection. Acta Otolaryngol 2007;127:491–497

133 Surgical Approach to the Axillary Nerve

Arnau Benet, Tene A. Cage, and Michel Kliot

This chapter discusses the anatomy of the axillary nerve, clinically correlates its lesions, and describes the anterior and posterior approaches for neurolysis, direct suture, or nerve graft repair.

Indications

- Stretch/contusive injury
- Laceration
- Penetrating injury
- Iatrogenic injury (in orthopedic surgery)
- Compression injury
- Injection injury
- Nerve sheath tumor

Contraindications

- Brachial plexitis
- Transient radiation plexopathy

Advantage of the Anterior Approach

- Direct exposure of the axillary nerve at its origin at the posterior cord and of the thoracodorsal and subscapular nerves

Disadvantage of the Anterior Approach

- Difficulty of exposure of the distal portion of the axillary nerve distal to the quadrilateral space

Advantages of the Posterior Approach

- Optimal delineation of the distal axillary nerve as it exits the quadrangular space
- Direct exposure of the surgical neck of the humerus

Disadvantages of the Posterior Approach

- Difficulty in tracing the damaged portion of the nerve to healthy proximal tissue within the posterior cord
- Difficulty reaching the pre-quadrangular segment of the axillary nerve

Surgical Anatomy

The axillary nerve plays a very important role in arm abduction and lateral rotation of the humerus. It innervates the deltoid muscle, which is responsible for arm abduction against resistance and arm swinging while walking, and provides synergistic components to other shoulder movements. The axillary nerve also innervates the teres minor muscle, whose main action is lateral rotation and stabilization of the humerus in the glenoid fossa during shoulder movements. Thorough knowledge of the course and spatial relationships of the axillary nerve is key to determining the anatomic location of a lesion affecting the axillary nerve. The origin, course, and innervation of the axillary nerve are described in this section.

In most cases, the axillary nerve arises from C5-C6, although it can also have a minimal C7 component, especially in a postfixed brachial plexus configuration. Its fibers run in the upper trunk of the brachial plexus until the subclavicular region, where they merge to give rise to posterior division, which forms the posterior cord of the brachial plexus. After taking off from the brachial plexus, the axillary nerve runs posterior to the axillary artery, lateral to the radial nerve, and anterior to the subscapular muscle toward the humeroscapular articular capsule. When the axillary nerve reaches the inferior border of the subscapular muscle, it gives off a branch to the shoulder joint before entering the quadrangular space. The limits of the quadrangular space are the surgical head of the humerus laterally; the long head of the triceps medially; the teres major inferiorly; and the subscapular muscle, capsule of the shoulder, and teres minor superiorly, as the nerve passes through the space. In the quadrangular space, the axillary nerve coexists with the posterior circumflex humeral vessels (**Fig. 133.1**).

At the quadrangular space, the axillary nerve divides into two branches: anterior and posterior. The anterior branch curves around the surgical neck of the humerus together with the posterior circumflex artery and vein. The main function of the anterior branch is innervating the deltoid muscle, although it is also responsible for a small part of the sensory innervation of the skin over the inferior rim of the deltoid.

The posterior branch follows the long head of the triceps and runs intimately related to the shoulder joint capsule (**Fig. 133.2**). At this point, the posterior branch of the axillary nerve innervates the teres minor muscle and branches into the upper lateral cutaneous nerve of the arm (sensory) and gives off a small nerve to the posterior third of the deltoid muscle (motor). The upper lateral cutaneous nerve of the arm pierces the deep fascia at the posterior aspect of the deltoid and supplies the superior

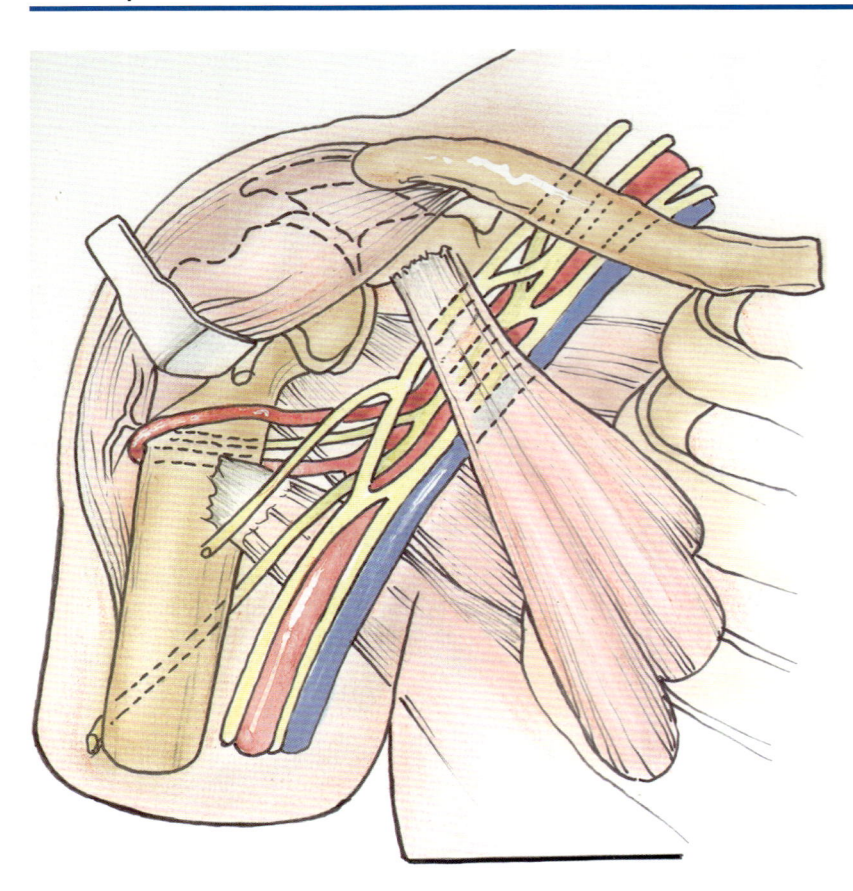

Fig. 133.1 Overview anterior anatomy of the axillary nerve.

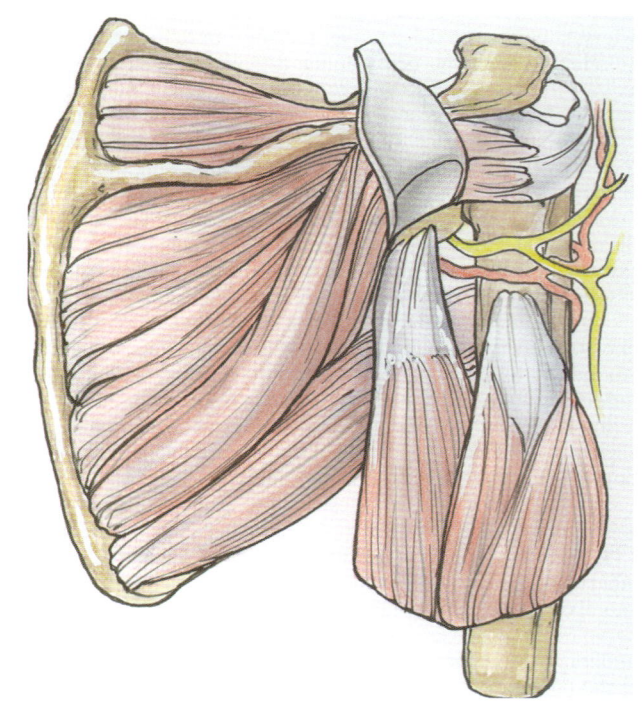

Fig. 133.2 Overview posterior anatomy of the axillary nerve.

lateral brachial cutaneous dermatome (inferior and lateral aspect of the deltoid area).

Surgical Landmarks

- The axillary nerve takes off from the posterior cord of the brachial plexus and runs posterior to the axillary artery.
- At the quadrangular space, the axillary nerve divides into anterior and posterior branches.
- The anterior branch of the axillary nerve runs around the surgical neck of the humerus and is responsible for the main innervation of the deltoid muscle.
- The posterior branch of the axillary nerve is intimately related to the shoulder joint capsule.
- The posterior branch of the axillary nerve innervates the teres minor and the superior lateral brachial cutaneous dermatome.

Anatomic-Clinical Correlation

The most common causes of axillary nerve injury are shoulder dislocation, stretch or contusive injury related to humeral neck fracture, and a sharp upward blow directly under the armpit. Lesions affecting the anterior aspect of the neck of the humerus, such as anterior dislocation of the shoulder or a fracture of the surgical neck of the humerus, could damage the anterior branch of the axillary nerve as it wraps around the humerus in its course toward the deltoid muscle. An isolated lesion of the anterior branch of the axillary nerve could be clinically identified, as the patient would show very limited abduction of the shoulder above 15 degrees, deltoid muscle atrophy, and subluxation of the glenohumeral joint. The posterior branch of the axillary nerve runs very close to the glenoid articular capsule, which places it at risk of entrapment or stretch during capsular plication. Also, a sharp upward blow to the inferior aspect of the armpit or a pseudoganglion involving the branch to the teres minor could damage the posterior branch, which may result in an unstable shoulder, limited lateral rotation, and loss of sensation in the area around the inferior and lateral edge of the deltoid. A posterior dislocation of the shoulder, a complex humeral fracture, a gunshot wound, or the quadrilateral space syndrome could potentially damage the main trunk or both branches of the axillary nerve at the quadrangular space, resulting in complete loss of axillary function. Other injuries at or above the infraclavicular space typically include deficits related to other nerves.

Preoperative Tests and Assessment

Although the clinical assessment and physical exploration may be sufficient for the diagnosis of axillary nerve injury, both radiological studies and electromyography may aid the surgeon in identifying the level of the lesion, the etiology, and the anatomic features. Moreover, a good preoperative evaluation is essential for optimal surgical planning and approach selection. Magnetic resonance imaging (MRI) and magnetic resonance neurography (MRN) are the radiological techniques of choice. In cases of transection of the axillary nerve, total discontinuity of the nerve may be observed in axial series on MRI. Also, tumors or lesions associated with trauma may be identified and anticipated on MRI. Electromyography is performed preoperatively to establish the baseline function of the upper arm and to monitor the surgical procedure and recovery.

Surgical Technique
Anesthesia and Positioning

General anesthesia is recommended because brachial plexus surgery may require extensive operative time and involves electrophysiological stimulation and recording from nerves and muscles. Preoperatively, the surgeon needs to advise the anesthetist that the neuromuscular blockade used in induction must wear off during the early phase of the procedure so that intraoperative electrical recording may be performed, which include direct stimulation of nerve and recording from muscle, nerve-to-nerve stimulation and recording, and the recording of somatosensory evoked potentials (SSEPs) and motor evoked potentials (MEPs). Local anesthetic should be avoided or limited to the superficial subcutaneous layers to avoid producing a nerve conduction block, which may compromise the intraoperative monitoring of motor and sensory responses during the procedure.

Electrophysiological Considerations

To ensure the maximum standards of safety and electrophysiological function preservation, the assessment of the axillary nerve is initiated before the skin incision and continued frequently thereafter. The axillary nerve is a branch of the posterior cord of the brachial plexus with predominant motor function. The electrophysiological surveillance of the axillary nerve involves MEPs, which test all axonal segments from the cerebral cortex to the muscle innervation point. One to three electrodes are placed in the deltoid muscle (posterior, middle, and anterior portions) for continuous recording and surveillance. Additional electrophysiological techniques for a thorough assessment of the nerve conductivity include direct nerve-to-nerve stimulation and direct nerve recording of MEPs while the patient is paralyzed.

The patient is placed in the lateral decubitus position with the affected side up. A semi-sitting position with a bump under the patient's ipsilateral shoulder may also be used with the arm flexed and positioned over the chest. The patient's head is placed on a horseshoe holder or donut, and the entire shoulder and upper extremity of the surgical site should be prepped, draped free, and placed along the patient's side. The surgeon should be able to manipulate the position of the patient's arm to improve surgical exposure. The patient's leg is prepped for possible sural nerve graft harvesting.

Incision and Dissection: Anterior

The optimal patient positioning for an anterior approach to the axillary nerve should provide wide access to the infraclavicular space and brachial plexus in the surgical procedure. To that purpose, the patient is placed supine with the head tilted to the contralateral side and the prepped arm on an armboard (**Fig. 133.3a**). The skin incision is started proximally at the clavicle and extends distally through the deltopectoral groove toward the axillary crease (**Fig. 133.3b**). The lateral border of the pectoralis major muscle is dissected from the clavicle and split along the deltopectoral groove. The cephalic vein (deltopectoral vein) is ligated close to the axillary vein to gain surgical exposure. The subclavicular muscle and vessels are dissected and ligated to expose the clavicle, which is retracted superiorly. At this point, the infraclavicular segment of the brachial plexus is exposed. Care must be taken to avoid damaging the infraclavicular artery when dissecting in this region by using sharp dissection and thorough hemostasis. Also, the clavicle must be elevated gently, and applying progressive increments of force to prevent dislocation of the shoulder.

Next, self-retaining retractors are applied to both the deltoid and pectoralis major muscles to split the deltopectoral groove (**Fig. 133.3c,d**). Then, the claviculopectoral fascia is identified and opened to expose and divide the tendon of the pectoralis minor muscle at the coracoid process. At this point, the infraclavicular space is widened inferiorly by elevating and pulling the pectoralis major muscle inferiorly.

The first neural element encountered in this procedure is the lateral cord, which lies superficially and laterally to the axillary artery. The musculocutaneous nerve is dissected and protected as it arises from the lateral cord. The axillary artery is then dissected and mobilized inferiorly and laterally with the vein retractor, which provides exposure of the posterior cord and axillary and radial nerves at the level of the coracoid process (**Fig. 133.3e**). To prevent complications in this part of the dissection, the axillary artery should not be directly touched by the self-retracting retractors and the musculocutaneous nerve should be kept in a bundle of fascia and its feeding vessels—the vasa nervorum.

Dissection should follow the axillary nerve as it runs along the anterior aspect of the subscapular muscle into the quadrilateral space (**Fig. 133.3e**). The most damaged segment of the axillary nerve should be identified proximally before entering the quadrangular space. Dissection should occur proximally into the infraclavicular portion of the brachial plexus to evaluate the extent of the injury. If the full extent of the injured segment of nerve can be seen through this approach, then either a neurolysis or repair can be performed.

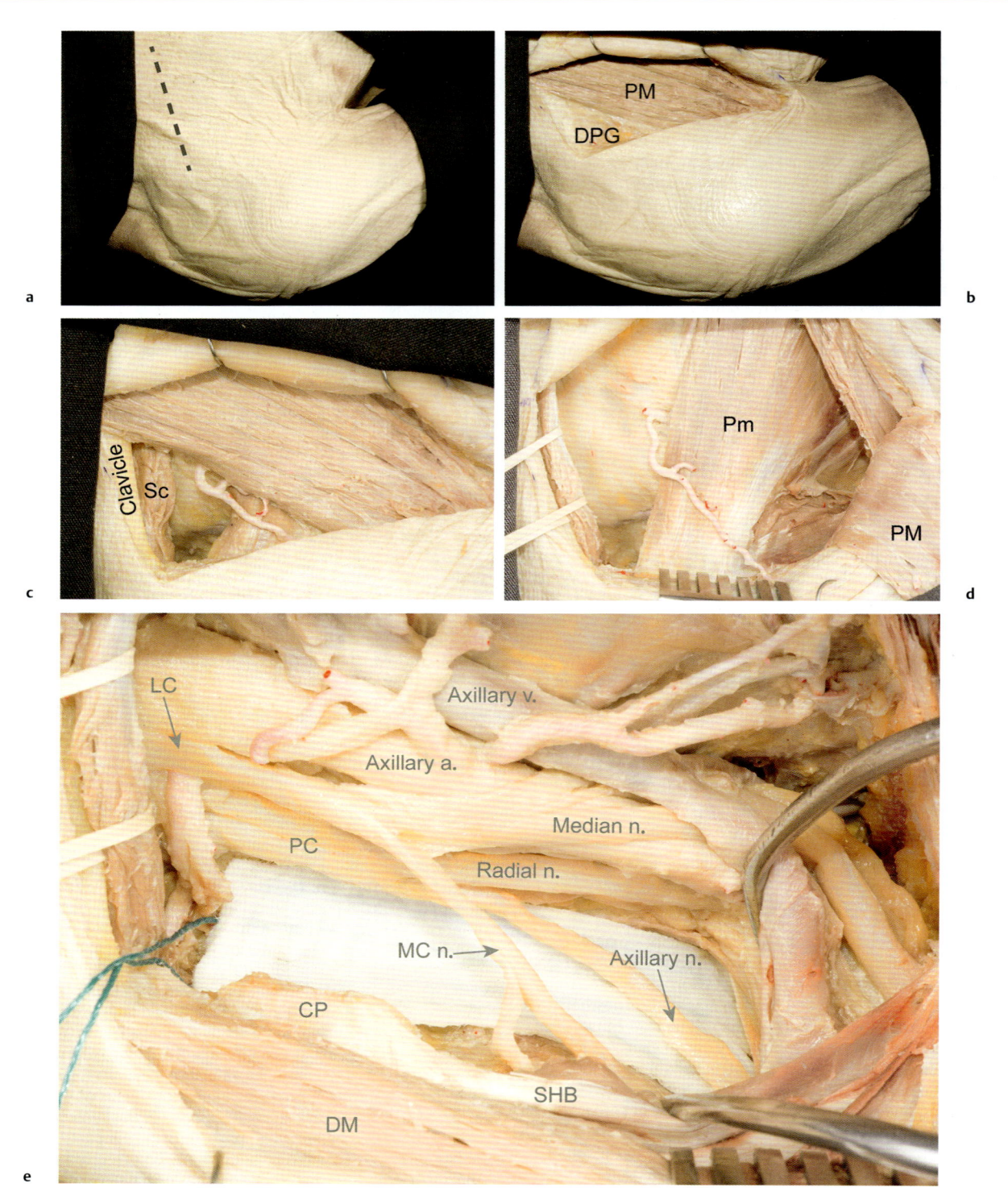

Fig. 133.3 Surgical simulation of the anterior approach to the axillary nerve. **(a)** The right shoulder is prepped and draped, exposing the deltopectoral groove and axillary depression completely and the lateral aspect of the clavicle *(dashed line)*. **(b)** The skin incision was started in the lateral third of the clavicle and continued through the deltopectoral groove, and the initial skin dissection was done to expose the pectoralis major. DPG, deltopectoral groove; PM, pectoralis major muscle. **(c)** Further dissection in the deltopectoral groove exposed the clavicle and subclavicular muscle. Sc, subclavian muscle. **(d)** The pectoralis major was dissected away from the clavicle and reflected inferolaterally, exposing the pectoralis minor and its tendon at the coracoid process. Pm, pectoralis minor muscle. **(e)** The superior and lateral aspects of the brachial plexus were dissected and exposed along with the axillary artery and vein. The deltoid muscle is exposed and retracted laterally together with the short head of the biceps muscle. LC, lateral cord; PC, posterior cord; CP, coracoid process; DM, deltoid muscle; MC, musculocutaneous; SHB, short head of the biceps muscle; a, artery; v, vein; n, nerve. (Courtesy of the University of California–San Francisco Skull Base and Cerebrovascular Laboratory.)

Incision and Dissection: Posterior

The patient positioning for a posterior approach to the axillary nerve should provide optimal exposure of the quadrangular space and the distal branches of the axillary nerve. To that purpose, the patient is tilted anteriorly (modified supine position or semi-sitting position) and the arm is brought forward across the chest, which enables direct, comfortable dissection over the lateral and posterior aspect of the shoulder.

An incision is made along the posterior border of the deltoid muscle from the spine of the scapula and extends toward the posterior axillary fold. At this point, the deltoid muscle interferes with exposing the distal branches of the axillary nerve. However, detaching the lateral half of the posterior deltoid muscle may be deemed unnecessary in those cases with marked deltoid denervation wasting. If the specific features of the patient require splitting the posterior half of the deltoid muscle, the surgeon must identify and protect the distal branches of the axillary nerve to prevent surgical morbidity.

As the surgeon dissects along the teres minor, the quadrangular space can be exposed, and the axillary nerve and the posterior humeral circumflex artery can be identified (**Fig. 133.4**).

Decompression/Neurolysis

If scar tissue is encountered during the exploration of the axillary nerve, external neurolysis and mobilization of the nerve are performed. Stimulating and recording electrodes are then used to measure the nerve action potentials (NAPs) across the lesion. If positive NAPs are recorded, neurolysis is usually sufficient for a favorable recovery.

Suture Repair

If transection of the axillary nerve is recognized during surgery, then direct end-to-end suture repair is possible. However, significant tension at the suture repair site is often encountered as a result of distal retraction at both ends of the nerve stumps and might jeopardize successful repair.

Graft Repair

Discontinuous lesions require nerve graft repairs to reestablish continuity between the proximal and distal nerve stumps. In most cases, a sural nerve is used as the donor nerve. Other options include cadaveric nerve graft for gaps less than 7 cm long and NeuroGen bioabsorbable tubes for gaps less than 4 cm in length; ½ to 1 cm is added to the gap length when harvesting the nerve graft to ensure that no tension is encountered during the suturing process.

If neuroma in continuity is encountered, NAPs across the lesion are recorded. If NAPs (nerve-to-nerve stimulation) are not obtained across the lesion, a sharp No. 15 blade is used to cut the injured segment until grossly healthy fascicles are observed on the cross sections in both the proximal and distal segments. Graft repair is then performed to reestablish continuity. If the lesion extends through the quadrangular space, posterior exposure is necessary to identify the distal extent of the lesion. After

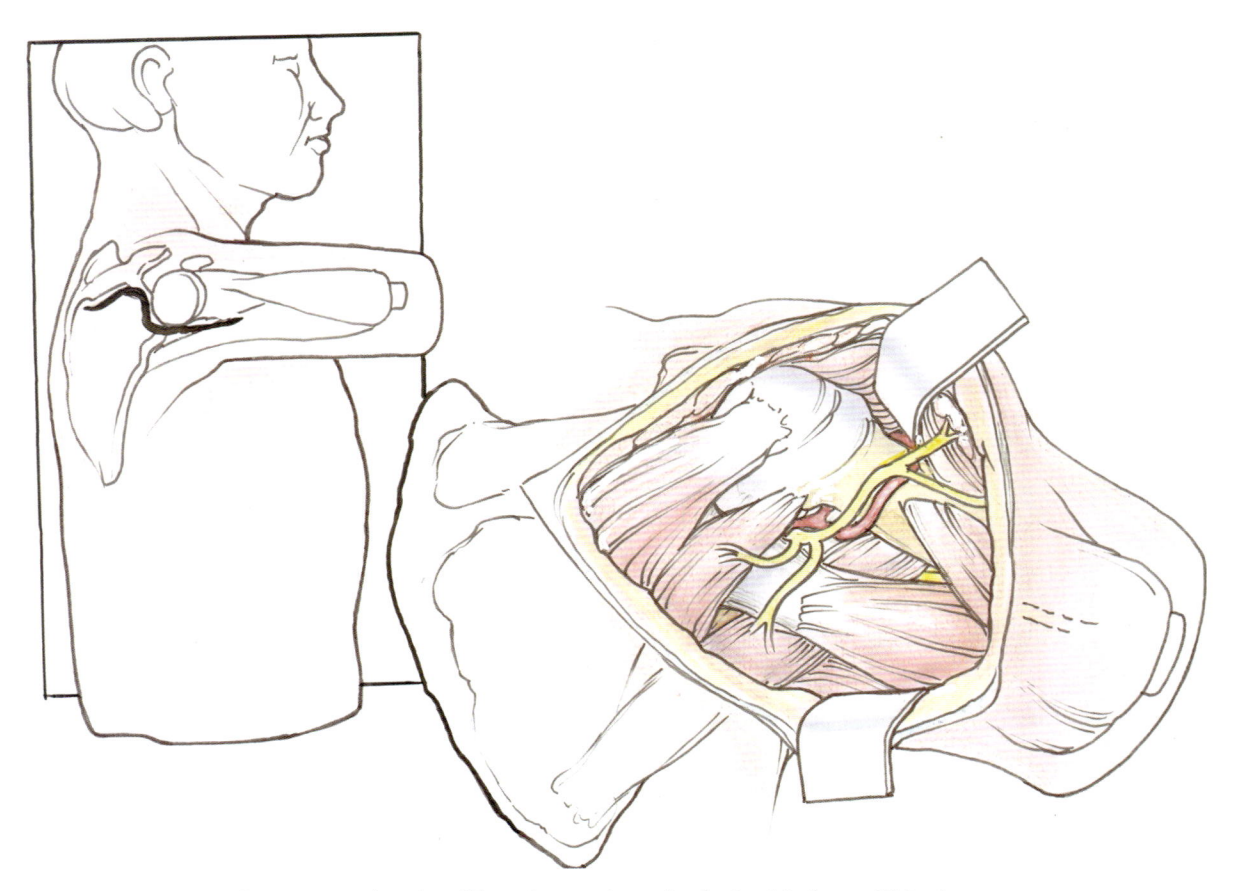

Fig. 133.4 Exposure of the axillary nerve as it branches off from the posterior cord and enters into the quadrilateral space.

preparation of the distal stump, the grafts are sutured to the distal segment and then passed through the quadrangular space from posterior to anterior. The posterior incision is then closed, and the operating table is rotated for better anterior exposure of proximal graft anastomosis.

Neurotization

When there is traumatic injury affecting the upper trunk of the brachial plexus, an avulsion of C5 and C6 roots, or in cases where the damage to the axillary nerve is deemed not repairable by means of nerve anastomosis or grafting, a nerve transfer—neurotization—might be an option.

There is evidence that the medial pectoral nerve to axillary nerve neurotization can provide good results in well-selected patients. The medial pectoral nerve is a branch of the medial cord and its axons belong to C8 and T1 in the majority of cases. It can be harvested during the dissection of the infraclavicular space and connected to the axillary nerve directly or with an interpositional graft from the medial antebrachial cutaneous nerve.

Another surgical strategy to regain deltoid function after axillary nerve damage is a radial nerve transfer. In such cases, the radial nerve branch for the lower triceps medial head and anconeus is transferred to the anterior division of the axillary nerve. Dissection of the radial branch and exposure of the axillary nerve are performed through a larger skin incision than that of the posterior approach to the axillary nerve. The anterior division of the axillary nerve is exposed and prepared first, and the dissection continues inferiorly to harvest the branch of the radial nerve. The nerve to the lower triceps medial head and anconeus is dissected distally, then sectioned and flipped 180 degrees to be sutured to the axillary nerve. Bertelli and Ghizoni[1] recently reported a deltoid recovery rate of 100% with maintained fully functional elbow extension using this nerve transfer technique in nine patients. Other nerves that can be used for axillary nerve neurotization include the long thoracic, intercostals, thoracodorsal, suprascapular, and distal accessory nerve.

Closure and Postoperative Care

The detached pectoralis minor muscle may be reapproximated to the coracoid process, and then the deltopectoral groove is closed in layers for the posterior approach. Exhaustive hemostasis is combined with generous irrigation of saline solution containing antibiotic agents during standard multilayer closure.

Postoperatively, an arm sling is used to immobilize the shoulder for 3 weeks, and then passive to progressive range-of-motion therapy may be started with close monitoring by the physical therapy team.

An early postoperative electromyography analysis followed by a series of delayed combined electromyography and neural conductivity stimulation studies may be used to monitor recovery of function and predict prognosis. Continued progressive physical therapy has been identified as one of the most important factors for successful recovery of function, especially proximal arm abduction, and evidence of recovery is observed in the late electromyography tests.

Conclusion

Lesions of the axillary nerve limit the abduction of the arm and cause loss of sensation in the superior lateral brachial cutaneous dermatome. Depending on the features of the lesion and the anatomic location, an anterior or posterior approach may be selected. MRI, MRN, and electromyography may aid in the identification of the anatomic level of the lesion and surrounding structures and in setting the baseline for surgery and posterior recovery. The surgeon treating a discontinuing lesion of the axillary nerve may be familiar with the different neurotization techniques for reconstruction. Early involvement of the physical therapy team is essential for optimal recovery of function.

Reference

1. Bertelli JA, Ghizoni MF. Nerve transfer from triceps medial head and anconeus to deltoid for axillary nerve palsy. J Hand Surg Am 2014;39:940–947

Suggested Readings

Dahlin LB, Cöster M, Björkman A, Backman C. Axillary nerve injury in young adults—an overlooked diagnosis? Early results of nerve reconstruction and nerve transfers. J Plast Surg Hand Surg 2012;46:257–261

Leechavengvongs S, Teerawutthichaikit T, Witoonchart K, et al. Surgical anatomy of the axillary nerve branches to the deltoid muscle. Clin Anat 2014; Feb:4

Ray WZ, Murphy RK, Santosa K, Johnson PJ, Mackinnon SE. Medial pectoral nerve to axillary nerve neurotization following traumatic brachial plexus injuries: indications and clinical outcomes. Hand (NY) 2012;7:59–65

134 Surgical Treatment of the Musculocutaneous Nerve

Angela M. Bohnen, Joseph Weiner, and Aruna Ganju

The upper limb is innervated by the anterior rami of spinal nerves C5 to T1. Collectively, these rami form a network of nerves referred to as the brachial plexus, which extends from the neck and courses distally through the axilla, providing motor and sensory innervation to the upper limb. As the plexus courses distally, it forms roots, trunks, divisions, cords, and terminal branches (**Fig. 134.1**).[1] The lateral cord, thusly named because of the relationship to the axillary artery, provides two terminal branches deep to the pectoralis muscles: the musculocutaneous nerve (MCN) and a contribution to the median nerve.[2]

The MCN innervates the coracobrachialis muscle, diving into it, and continues laterally between the biceps brachii and brachialis muscle. Branches from the MCN supply these muscles as well.[3] As the MCN approaches the cubital fossa, it pierces the fascia lateral to the biceps tendon and becomes the lateral cutaneous nerve of the forearm[4] (**Fig. 134.2**). In the proximal arm, it receives the majority share of its blood supply from the anterior circumflex humeral artery and from the brachial artery more distally.[3]

As is expected, great variation in the MCN exists in regard to its branching pattern and anatomic course in the upper arm.[5]

The MCN is a mixed nerve, containing both motor and sensory fibers. It provides motor innervation to anterior compartment muscles, including the coracobrachialis, brachialis, and biceps brachii. On the contrary, the sensory innervation of the MCN lies below the cubital fossa and receives input from the superficial portion of the lateral forearm (**Fig. 134.3**).[3] Hence, presenting symptoms of nerve palsy include weak arm flexion, decreased bicep tendon reflex, paresthesias, and decreased sensation to the lateral forearm.[5,6]

Pathology of Injury

Due to its anatomic course and origin in the brachial plexus, the MCN is rarely injured in isolation. It tends to be involved in upper brachial plexus injuries resulting from downward traction on the arm or excessive lateral neck flexion. Though uncommon, isolated lesions of the MCN have been reported with an incidence of 2%.[7] The etiology of injury can be divided into two categories: traumatic and nontraumatic. The mechanism of nontraumatic lesions can be further subdivided into proximal (involving the entire nerve) and distal (only the lateral cutaneous nerve).[8]

Sharp lacerations or stab wounds to the anterior shoulder or upper arm may result in nerve transection. More commonly, the MCN can be damaged through traction injuries such as those caused by excessive lateral flexion of the neck or downward traction of the arm. As a consequence of the anatomy and muscular attachments, hyperextension of related muscles can cause stretching or even tearing of the nerve. Extensive stretching can occur during traumatic hyperextension, improper arm positioning during sleep, or positioning during surgical procedures.[9,10]

Nontraumatic lesions of the MCN tend to occur with a much higher frequency than those of a traumatic nature. These palsies tend to arise as a consequence of the nerve's course through and between large muscles of the anterior compartment of the upper arm. In competitive athletes and weight lifters, the nerve can become entrapped within the coracobrachialis or in between the biceps brachii and brachialis muscle.[11] It is postulated that entrapment of the nerve causes damage primarily via external compression, either due to repetitive contraction of the muscle or secondary to hypertrophy of the muscle.[8,9] Damage is caused by both mechanical and ischemic insult to the nerve with subsequent focal demyelination.

More distally, in the antebrachial region, the lateral cutaneous nerve of the forearm can become entrapped in the superficial antebrachial fascia or compressed by the biceps tendon.[12] Given its primary sensory innervation to the forearm, patients usually present with sensory deficit or dysesthesia.

Iatrogenic MCN injury can occur after orthopedic repair of a distal humerus fracture; both the radial and lateral cutaneous nerve of the forearm are at risk during internal fixation of fracture.[13]

Patient Selection

Patient selection depends on the underlying etiology of injury. For traumatic injuries, patients who have not regained motor or sensory function may benefit from an exploration and repair via reanastomosis or nerve grafting/transfer.

The MCN can become entrapped or compressed by any of the structures in proximity to it, such as the coracobrachialis, the biceps, or the fascia. With such neuropathies, patients usually complain of pain and lateral forearm paresthesias. When conservative management has failed, decompression can be attempted. Davidson et al[14] described a 12-week period of treatment consisting of 6 weeks of nonsteroidal anti-inflammatory drugs (NSAIDs) and rest followed by injection and then splinting, with unsuccessful cases treated with decompression.

Preoperative Testing and Imaging

The most useful diagnostic modality is a thorough neurologic exam, which can help localize the site of injury. Magnetic resonance imaging (MRI) and computed tomography (CT) myelogram can help diagnose nerve root avulsion by the presence of a small pseudomeningocele at the level of injury, whereas magnetic resonance neurography (MRN) helps identify the ends of a transected nerve. Electromyography (EMG) and nerve conduction velocity (NCV) are performed in a delayed manner, typically 2 to 3 weeks postinjury, confirming the diagnosis.[15]

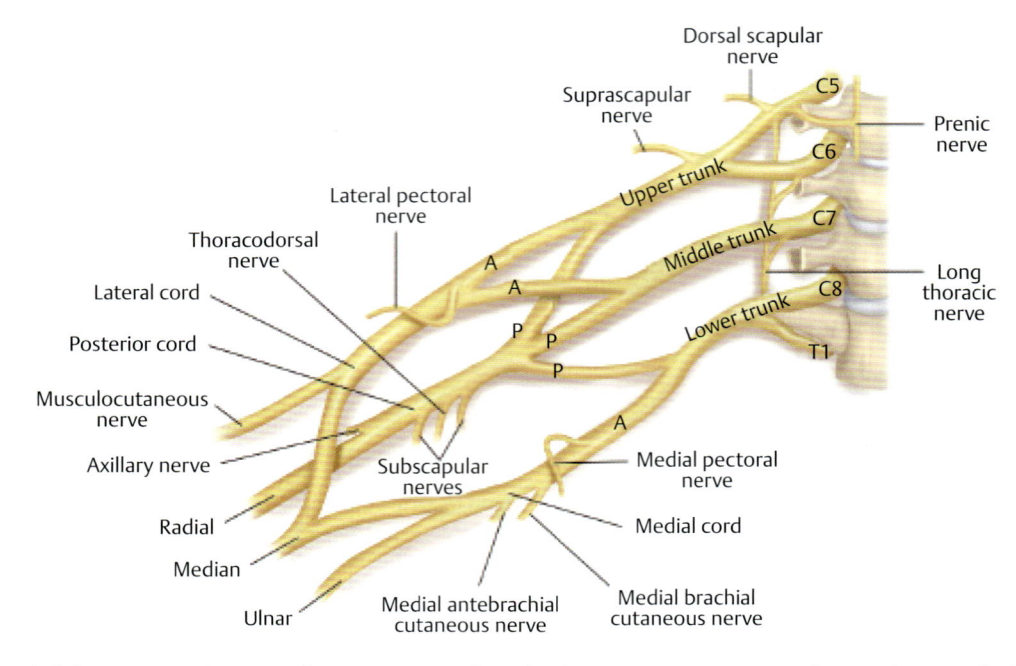

Fig. 134.1 Brachial plexus anatomy. (From Russell SM. Examination of Peripheral Nerve Injuries: An Anatomical Approach. New York: Thieme; 2015.)

Surgical Indications and Timing[7,8,16]

Clinical manifestations of MCN injury depend on the location of the injury and the presence of anatomic variations. This can make localizing the lesion to one peripheral nerve in this region challenging. Furthermore, due to its origin in the brachial plexus, the MCN is rarely injured in isolation. However, there are situations where sole exposure of the nerve is warranted (**Table 134.1**).

Contraindications

- Evidence of recovery on diagnostic physiological testing
- Nerve root avulsion

Advantages[6,8]

- Restores motor function of the involved nerve and distal musculature
- Restores sensory function

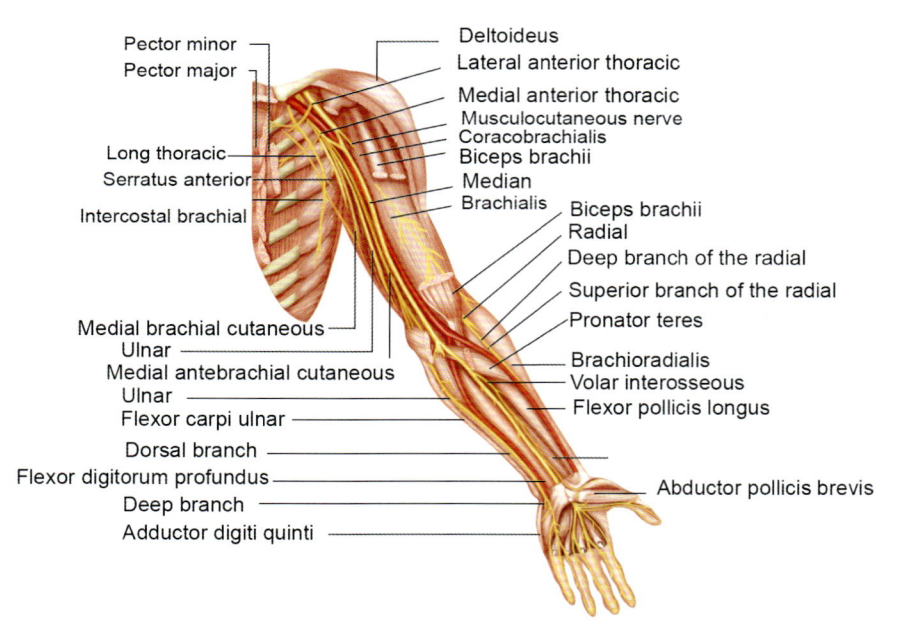

Fig. 134.2 Anatomic course of the musculocutaneous nerve.

- Nerve grafting provides quicker recovery times by eliminating the time for nerve recovery to restore reinnervation.[6]
- Nerve grafting enables shorter and less complicated operations because the surgical bed resides in an uninjured area.

Disadvantages[6,17]

- Nerve grafting requires growth of axons across suture lines.
- Donor nerve may not have good expendability.

Surgical Procedure

Peripheral nerve repair is dependent on many factors and has a limited supply of surgical options. The surgical procedure is dictated by the etiology of the injury. When a known skeletal injury has occurred, this gives the surgeon an idea of the location of nerve damage. However, in a stretch or hyperextension injury, it may be more difficult to localize the area of injury, and an exploratory approach may need to be taken. If compression is suspected, conservative management may be provided prior to surgical intervention.

Patient Positioning

The patient is placed supine on the operating table and placed under general anesthesia. Short-acting paralytic agents are used for induction and intubation but long-acting paralytics should be avoided, so that muscle stimulation can be observed during surgery. The patient's arm is placed on an arm board in an extended and supinated position. It is critical that the arm be placed at the patient's side and not in an abducted position that can lead to tension on the brachial plexus. The shoulder should be elevated by placing a folded sheet underneath the scapula.[2,18]

Exposure for Exploration

The location of the operative field is directed toward the point of injury. To identify the branch point of the MCN from the lateral cord, an infraclavicular approach is used. This incision starts at the lateral third of the clavicle and follows the deltopectoral groove (**Fig. 134.4**). This incision line may be used as an extension of the supraclavicular approach or continued down the medial aspect of the arm for more distal exposure (this step is discussed further in the respective procedures). The dissection toward the cords can be either transpectoral, where the fibers of the pectoralis muscle are split, or directed between the pectoralis and deltoid muscles via blunt dissection. Angled retractors are inserted for visualization. Beneath the pectoralis major lies the pectoralis minor. Its insertion at the coracoid process can be palpated, at which point the muscle should be dissected from the surrounding fatty tissue, revealing the distal plexus structures. Most often, the lateral cord is first exposed and the MCN terminal branch will be seen running medial to lateral.[2]

During dissection, the cephalic vein can be preserved by working inferiorly and medially to the structure. Vascular structures traversing the field are often ligated without consequence. Vessel loops or Penrose drains are used to identify and isolate plexus structures, aiding in dissection of the dorsal surface.[2]

For sufficient exposure, the biceps tendon may need to be dissected. A small portion can be split without subsequent repair; however, sometimes the pectoralis major may need to be dissected and mobilized. Tagging sutures may be used to help in reapproximation. Further mobilization of the MCN can be achieved by dissecting its branches to the coracobrachialis

Anterior   Posterior

▪ Lateral antebrachial cutaneous nerve

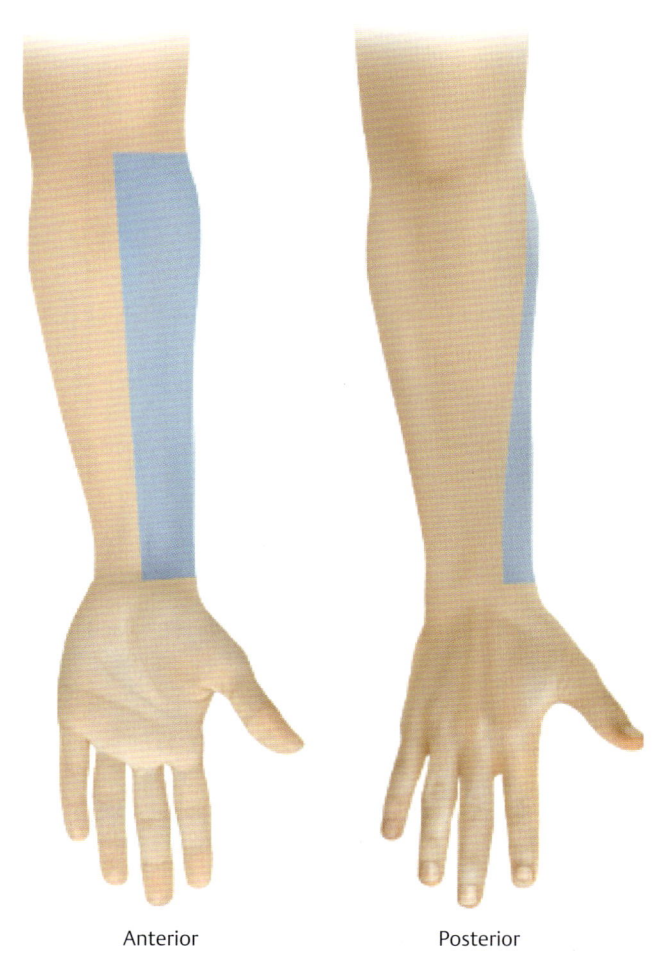

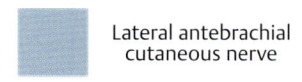

Fig. 134.3 Sensory distribution of the musculocutaneous nerve. (From Russell SM. Examination of Peripheral Nerve Injuries: An Anatomical Approach. New York: Thieme; 2015.)

Table 134.1 Surgical Timing of Exploration of the Musculocutaneous Nerve

Injury	Surgical Timing
Sharp lacerations/stab wounds	Acute
Blunt/open wounds	Delayed, 2–3 weeks
Traction/stretch/gunshot wound	Delayed, 3–4 months
Nerve transfers for root avulsions to restore elbow flexion/nerve sheath tumors	Nonacute

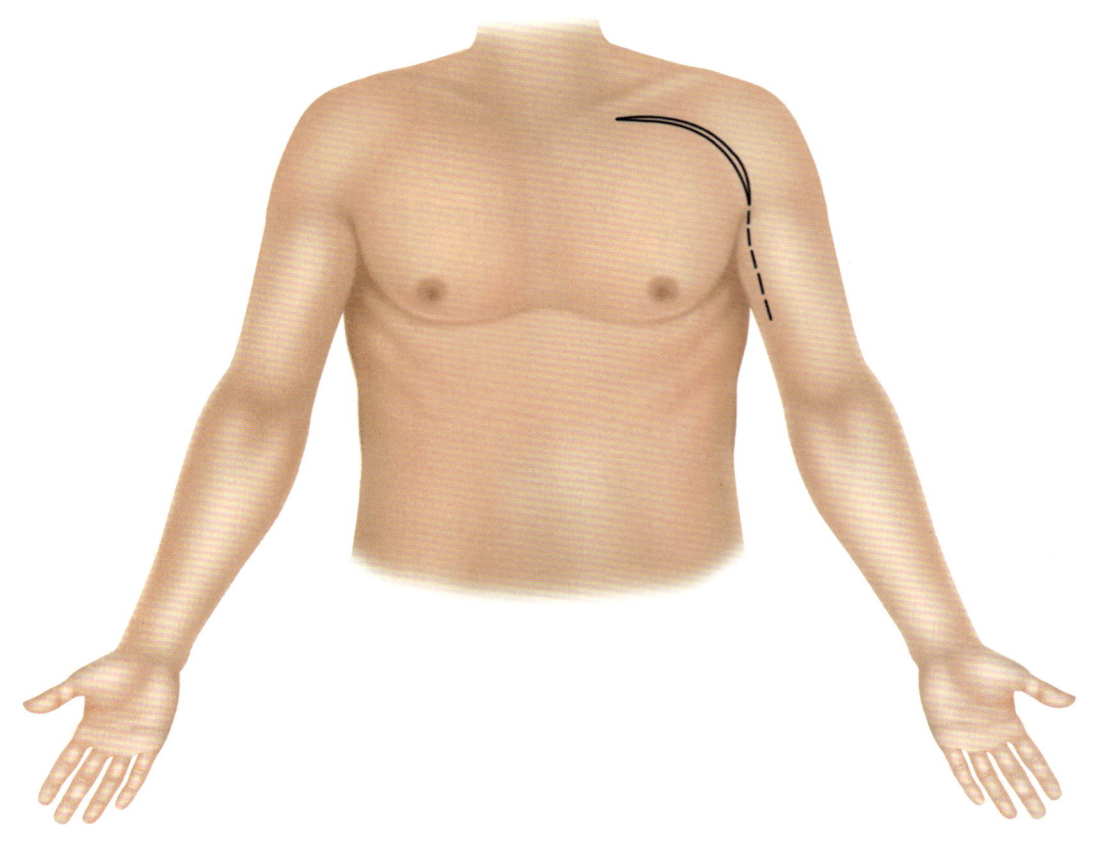

Fig. 134.4 Illustration showing the skin incision for the infraclavicular approach; the skin incision follows the deltopectoral groove and then the medial edge of the biceps muscle.

muscle to prevent traction injury. Furthermore, if the injury has caused retraction of the distal nerve into the coracobrachialis, this muscle will need to be dissected.[8]

Dissection should continue distal between the biceps and brachialis muscles to the antecubital fossa. At this point, the nerve from proximal to distal can be explored for injury. Nerve action potential (NAP) recordings may be used and if appropriate, repair via neuroma resection, anastomosis, or grafting may proceed.[8]

Nerve Repair

If nerve dysfunction is secondary to compression, the site is visualized by a flattened nerve with decreased vascular markings. Resection of the overlying muscle or aponeurosis is performed. Verification of decompression is tested via intraoperative supination and pronation and verbal cues from the awake patient.[14]

For nerve transfer (either grafting or via neurolysis), the ulnar nerve is often harvested. The ulnar nerve should be identified 3 to 4 cm from the area of concern and dissection of the fascicle(s) should extend distal enough to allow for direct transfer.[16] Furthermore, if the biceps and brachialis branches are the main concern, double fascicle transfer is a good option. Here, an incision 4 cm distal to the axilla reaching 4 cm proximally to the medial epicondyle, extending down the bicipital sulcus, is utilized. The ulnar and median nerves can be identified near the biceps and brachialis branches of the MCN. Neurolysis at appropriate locations to enable single transfer from donor to recipient, allowing for accurate length and size match, can be performed.[6] Coaptation is done utilizing 11-0 nylon sutures.[15]

Closure

After the nerve is repaired, retractors and vessel loops/Penrose drains may be removed and hemostasis can be achieved via bipolar cautery. If the pectoralis muscle was dissected and mobilized, it should be reapproximated.[8] The superficial layers should be closed in the normal fashion

Postoperative Management

In the postoperative period, patients should be monitored for hematoma development. The affected arm should be kept in a sling for about 3 weeks to prevent tension on the healing nerves.[15] Physical therapy can commence once movement restrictions are lifted.

Conclusion

The MCN is an important branch of the brachial plexus and is responsible for arm flexion and sensation to the lateral forearm. Although solitary injury to the MCN is uncommon, the reparative techniques described herein can be used universally for nerve injuries. Reparative technique should be decided on a patient-specific basis; however, function can be regained when injury is recognized in a timely fashion and appropriately treated.

References

1. Morton DA, Foreman KB, Albertine KH. Gross anatomy the big picture. In: McGraw-Hill's Access Medicine Lange Educational library: Basic Science. New York: McGraw-Hill; 2011
2. Tender GC, Kline DG. The infraclavicular approach to the brachial plexus. Neurosurgery 2008;62(3, Suppl 1):180–184, discussion 184–185
3. Macchi V, Tiengo C, Porzionato A, et al. Musculocutaneous nerve: histotopographic study and clinical implications. Clin Anat 2007;20:400–406
4. Standring S. Gray's Anatomy: The Anatomical Basis of Clinical Practice, 39th ed. London: Churchill Livingstone; 2004
5. Besleaga D, Castellano V, Lutz C, Feinberg JH. Musculocutaneous neuropathy: case report and discussion. HSS J 2010;6:112–116
6. Mackinnon SE, Novak CB, Myckatyn TM, Tung TH. Results of reinnervation of the biceps and brachialis muscles with a double fascicular transfer for elbow flexion. J Hand Surg Am 2005;30:978–985
7. Osborne AW, Birch RM, Munshi P, Bonney G. The musculocutaneous nerve. J Bone Joint Surg Br 2000;82:1140–1142
8. Fessler RG, Sekhar LN. Atlas of Neurosurgical Techniques: Spine and Peripheral Nerves. New York: Thieme; 2006
9. Inaba A, Yokota T. Isolated musculocutaneous nerve palsy during sleep. Muscle Nerve 2003;28:773–774
10. Dundore DE, DeLisa JA. Musculocutaneous nerve palsy: an isolated complication of surgery. Arch Phys Med Rehabil 1979;60:130–133
11. DeFranco MJ, Schickendantz MS. Isolated musculocutaneous nerve injury in a professional fast-pitch softball player: a case report. Am J Sports Med 2008;36:1821–1823
12. Belzile E, Cloutier D. Entrapment of the lateral antebrachial cutaneous nerve exiting through the forearm fascia. J Hand Surg Am 2001;26:64–67
13. Blyth MJ, Macleod CM, Asante DK, Kinninmonth AW. Iatrogenic nerve injury with the Russell-Taylor humeral nail. Injury 2003;34:227–228
14. Davidson JJ, Bassett FH III, Nunley JA II. Musculocutaneous nerve entrapment revisited. J Shoulder Elbow Surg 1998;7:250–255
15. Midha R, Zager EL, ed. Surgery of Peripheral Nerves. New York: Thieme; 2008
16. Rohde RS, Wolfe SW. Nerve transfers for adult traumatic brachial plexus palsy (brachial plexus nerve transfer). HSS J 2007;3:77–82
17. Chan KM, Olson JL, Morhart M, Lin T, Guilfoyle R. Outcomes of nerve transfer versus nerve graft in ulnar nerve laceration. Can J Neurol Sci 2012;39:242–244
18. Kim DH, Hudson AR, Kline DG. Atlas of Peripheral Nerve Surgery. New York: Elsevier Health Sciences; 2012

135 Open and Endoscopic Decompression of the Median Nerve

Ahmed Alaqeel, Albert M. Isaacs, and Rajiv Midha

Median Nerve Anatomy

Axilla and Arm

The median nerve is derived from medial and lateral cords that are adjacent to the axillary to brachial artery junction in the axilla. The medial cord provides mainly motor fibers, and the lateral cord provides mainly sensory fibers to the hand, but also some motor contribution to pronator and flexor muscles in the forearm and wrist. The main nerve is easily seen during the initial brachial plexus exposure in the axilla, but the motor contribution from the medial cord may be posteromedial to the artery and only obviously seen when dissected away from the vessel. In rare cases, lateral or medial cord input to median nerve may pass posterior to the axillary artery. The median nerve maintains a close relationship with the brachial artery to the midhumerus before running in a groove between the brachialis and biceps, crossing the antecubital fossa anterior to the brachial artery from lateral to medial at the level of insertion of the coracobrachialis, under the bicipital aponeurosis. A supracondylar process is present 5 to 7 cm above the medial epicondyle, and may connect with the medial epicondyle via a fibrous ligament (Struthers's ligament). It is not a constant ligament, present in only 1% of humans, and it may be acquired or congenital.[1,2] The median nerve may be subject to compression there, especially if the coracobrachialis inserts on Struthers's ligament or the pronator teres originates there. Because the median nerve has not yet branched at the level of the supracondylar process, entrapment at this level affects all median innervated muscles.[2]

Forearm and Wrist

In the proximal forearm, the nerve maintains its medial relation to the brachial artery, and runs beneath the aponeurosis, anterior to the brachialis muscle. The median nerve lies between the flexor digitorum superficialis (FDS) and flexor digitorum profundus (FDP) before going between the FDS and the flexor pollicis longus, and giving off the anterior interosseus nerve (AIN) and muscular branches to the FDS, flexor carpi radialis (FCR), and pronator teres (PT).[3,4] The anterior interosseous nerve runs along the anterior surface of the interosseous membrane and gives branches to the FDP (digits two and three) and the flexor pollicis longus, and finally ends in the pronator quadratus near the wrist joint. In the wrist, the median nerve overlies the radius, deep to and between the tendons of the palmaris longus muscle and the flexor carpi radialis muscle. The palmar cutaneous branches typically arises before the carpal tunnel at the distal part of the forearm, ~ 5 to 6 cm proximal to the distal wrist creases, and supplies sensory innervation to the lateral cutaneous aspect of the palm (but not the digits), although some variations have been reported.[5] The carpal tunnel is ~ 4 to 6 cm in length and contains nine tendons, four FDPs, four FDSs, and the flexor pollicis longus tendon, in addition to the median nerve. The carpal canal floor and lateral wall is formed by carpal bones, and its roof is formed by the transverse carpal ligament (TCL). The TCL usually is 4 cm in length and 2.5 to 3.5 mm in thickness; it is attached medially to the hamate and pisiform and laterally to the trapezium and scaphoid tuberosity.[6]

Hand

The median nerve enters the hand through the carpal tunnel under the flexor retinaculum, along with the FDS, FDP, and flexor pollicis longus. The terminal motor branches serve the abductor pollicis brevis (APB), opponens pollicis (OP), flexor pollicis brevis (FPB), and the first and second lumbricals. The terminal sensory digital cutaneous branches serve the lateral three and a half digits on the palmar side, and the index, middle, and ring fingers on the dorsum of the hand.

Important Findings

- The recurrent motor branch to the thenar muscles usually arises off the median nerve extraligamentous position distal to the transverse carpal ligament (46–90%). There can be considerable variation, so that the motor branch may arise subligamentous in up to 31% or transligamentous in up to 23%.[7]
- Martin Gruber anastomosis (10–15%) can occur when motor fibers from the median nerve cross over to the ulnar nerve.
- Riche-Cannieu anastomosis occurs when there is a connection between the deep ulnar and recurrent branch of the median nerve in the hand.
- Pronator syndrome is very uncommon when compared with carpal tunnel syndrome (CTS). It results from the compression of the median nerve as it passes between the two heads of the PT or under the fibrous edge of the FDS arch. Usually the sensation in the palmar cutaneous nerve distribution is affected, so it is very helpful in distinguishing between this syndrome and CTS, as this nerve branch arises proximal to the carpal tunnel.[8,9] Affected patients usually show the benediction attitude due to the inability to flex the lateral three finger while doing a fist.

- Anterior interosseous syndrome (Kiloh-Nevin syndrome) is a rare entrapment of the anterior interosseous nerve (AIN), resulting from the isolated compression of the AIN under the fibrous arch of the FDS or the PT. It presents with a weakness of the FPL and FDP of the index and middle fingers. Patients with complete palsy cannot use the fingers to make a pinch or the "OK" sign.[10,11] They usually do not present with sensory loss, and it is estimated that this syndrome account for 1% of all upper extremity neuropathies.[10,11] It should be noted that the median nerve is almost straight, and not much length can be gained by mobilization.[12]

Entrapment of the Median Nerve in the Arm

Patient Selection and Preoperative Imaging

This rare diagnosis should be considered when the patient presents with a spontaneous median neuropathy involving the complete distribution of the nerve. Because tumors and other mass lesions are much more common than an entrapment by a rare Struthers's ligament, imaging of the arm with magnetic resonance imaging (MRI) or ultrasound is recommended. A plain X-ray may show the supracondylar process. Once the diagnosis is made, excising Struthers's ligament enables nerve decompression for the relief of symptoms.[13,14]

Surgical Procedure

The treatment of median nerve entrapment in the arm is straightforward. The patient is placed in the supine position with the arm straight and supinated. An incision is made in a lazy-S shape in the medial arm along the intermuscular septum between the biceps and triceps muscles. The median nerve and the brachial artery are isolated first, and then followed until they pass under Struthers's ligament. Decompression is achieved by excising the ligament (**Fig. 135.1**).

Entrapment of the Median Nerve in the Elbow and Forearm

Patient Selection and Preoperative Testing and Imaging

Diagnosis rests on taking a careful history, performing a physical exam, and ordering supportive electrodiagnostic studies. The latter may show that other nerve distributions are involved, thus suggesting a more generalized brachial neuritis, and in this case surgical decompression is contraindicated. If a structural mass lesion is suspected, then appropriate MRI or ultrasound imaging is recommended. Surgical treatment for pronator syndrome and AIN syndrome is indicated if nonsurgical management fails to relieve symptoms and reverse the neuropathy.

Surgical Procedure

The patient is placed in the supine position with the arm and forearm supinated. A zigzag or lazy-S incision is made over the antecubital fossa, with the transverse component in line with elbow flexion crease; it continues distally along the lateral side of the nerve to avoid its branches (**Fig. 135.2**) The nerve is identified just proximal to the antecubital crease, which in turn easily identifies the median nerve. The nerve is followed distally until it passes under the bicipital aponeurosis. Then it is dissected free from the overlying lacertus fibrosus, which is incised.[15] The median nerve is then followed into the PT. The superficial head of the PT is incised medially, releasing any fibrous bands, to visualize the median nerve. The interval between the PT and FCR is then opened to gain more distal dissection, which requires division of the FDS fibrous arch, if seen. By the end of this exposure, the median nerve and the AIN will be readily visualized and decompressed over a considerable length. Almost all of the median nerve's branches course off its ulnar (medial) side at this level, with the notable exception being the AIN, which branches off the radial side of the nerve.

Generally, most studies report that 85 to 90% of patients have good to excellent outcomes for operative management of these isolated syndromes.[16,17]

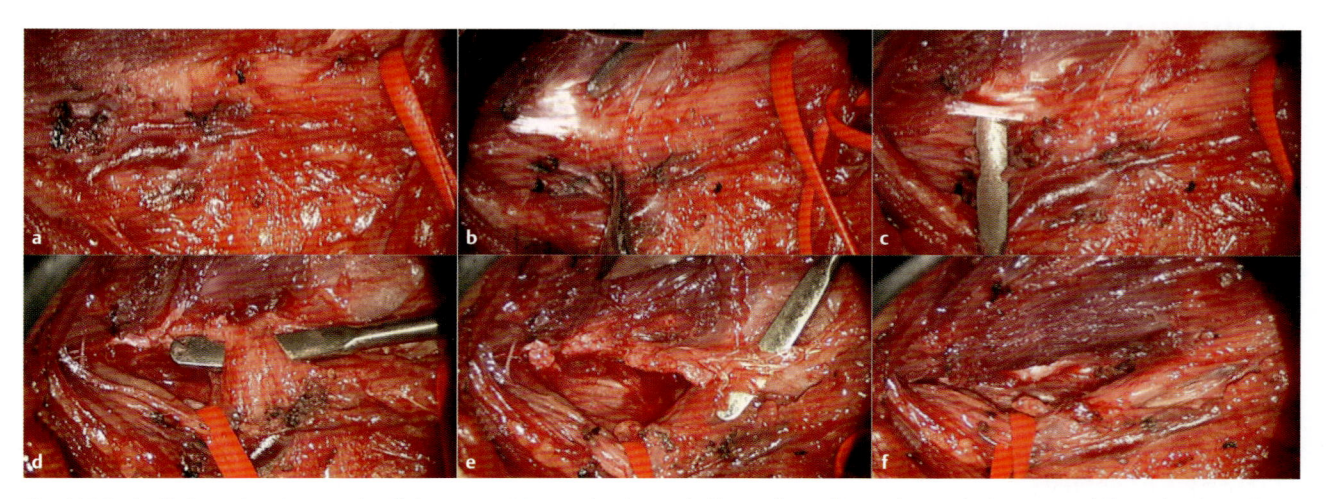

Fig. 135.1 (a–f) Operative photographs of the sequential steps for the surgical decompression of median nerve entrapment by a Struthers's ligament and a band (prominent to the left in **b,c**). The median nerve is encircled by a red vessel loop, whereas the ligament and fibrous bands are shown with a Penfield dissector pointing at or under them. **(f)** Complete decompression of the nerve was achieved by excising the ligament and bands.

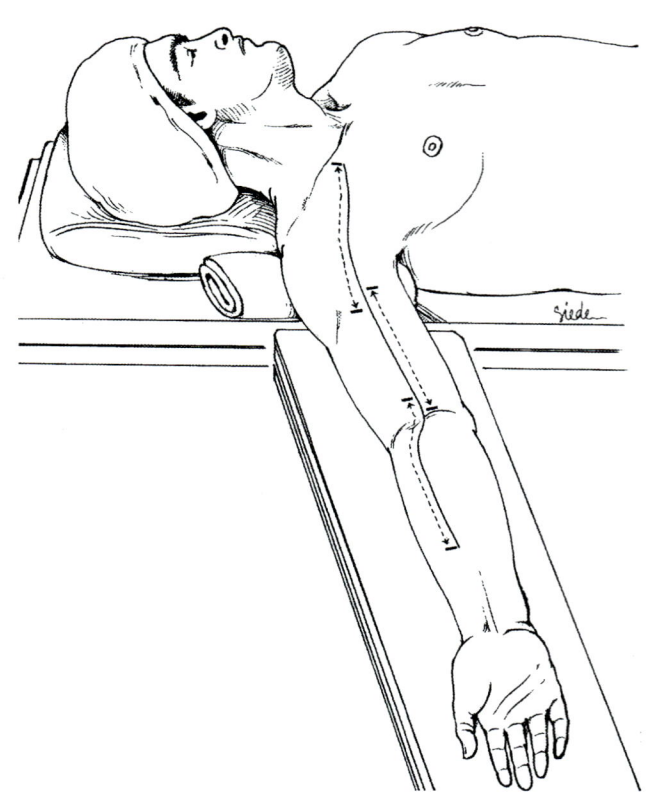

Fig. 135.2 The brachial exposure starts at the distal groove and extends to the midarm level just above the cubital crease. Cubital exposure starts above the cubital crease just medial to the distal biceps, curves medially over the cubital crease, and extends distally down the mid-arm. (From Tiel R. The median nerve. In: Fessler RG, Sekhar L, eds. Atlas of Neurosurgical Techniques, 1st ed. Spine and Peripheral Nerves. New York: Thieme; 2006: 932–936. Reprinted with permission.)

Entrapment of the Median Nerve at the Wrist: Carpal Tunnel Syndrome

Carpal tunnel decompression is the most common operation for peripheral nerves.[18] Studies show that the prevalence of CTS is 1% in the general population.[19] The underlying pathological process is thought to be increased pressure within the canal that exceeds the perfusion pressure of the nerve, causing compromised circulation and nutrition of the nerve fibers.[20] Surgical decompression of the carpal tunnel via transection of the transverse carpal ligament (TCL) was first explained by Sir James Learmonth in 1933, and multiple series since then have reported good to excellent patient satisfaction rates with the procedure.[21] Okutsu et al[22] introduced the use of an endoscope to cut the transverse carpal ligament in patients with CTS. Since then, at least six types of procedures have been reported, and two of the most popular techniques are the single-portal and dual-portal systems.[23–25]

Patient Selection

Surgery is the treatment of choice when nonsurgical treatments have been unsuccessful or when the initial presentation is advanced progressive weakness or sensory denervation.[26] The aim of surgery is to divide the TCL and decompress the median nerve while preserving its recurrent motor and palmar cutaneous branches.

Conventional (Open) Carpal Tunnel Release Technique

Advantages

The open technique operation is typically performed as a day-surgery procedure with optional mild conscious sedation anesthesia; it has been shown to be safe and cost-effective, and it is our preferred method.[27,28]

Surgical Procedure

Video 135.1 describes a step-by-step approach to an open decompression of the median nerve at the carpal tunnel. The patient is placed in the supine position with the arm abducted and the forearm supinated on an arm board. We usually do not use a tourniquet (to avoid unnecessary ischemia), but some surgeons prefer to use it (**Fig. 135.3**). We often place a roll under the wrist to provide some degree of wrist extension.

Following a sterile prep and drape, a 1.5- to 2-cm incision is marked starting a few millimeters distal to the distal wrist crease and extending to the palm but no further than the intercepting point of the imaginary Kaplan's cardinal line drawn from the distal border of the outstretched thumb obliquely toward the pisiform prominence in line with the radial border of the ring finger paralleling and ~ 2 mm ulnar to the midpalmar crease. A local anesthetic with epinephrine is infiltrated in the marked incisional site. Incision is made with a No. 15 knife blade (**Fig. 135.4**). Deep to the skin, the incision is then carried down through the subcutaneous fat and the palmar aponeurosis, exposing the TCL, with care taken to protect the palmar cutaneous branch of the median nerve, which is not consistently visualized (**Fig.**

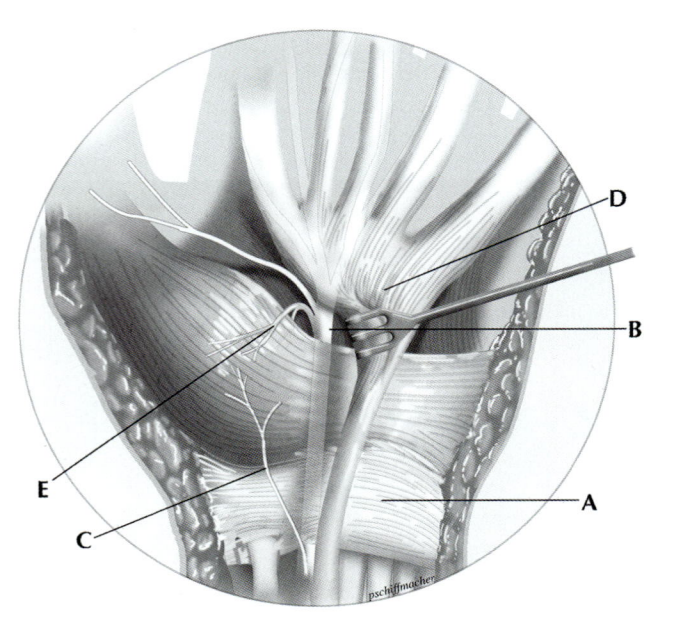

Fig. 135.3 Surgical anatomy of the carpal tunnel (left hand). *A*, transverse carpal ligament; *B*, median nerve; *C*, palmar cutaneous branch; *D*, palmaris longus tendon; *E*, recurrent motor branch. (From Huang JH, Whitmore RG, Zager EL. Carpal tunnel release. In: Wolfa CE, Resnick DK, eds. Neurosurgical Operative Atlas, 2nd ed. Spine and Peripheral Nerves. New York: Thieme; 2007:317–322.)

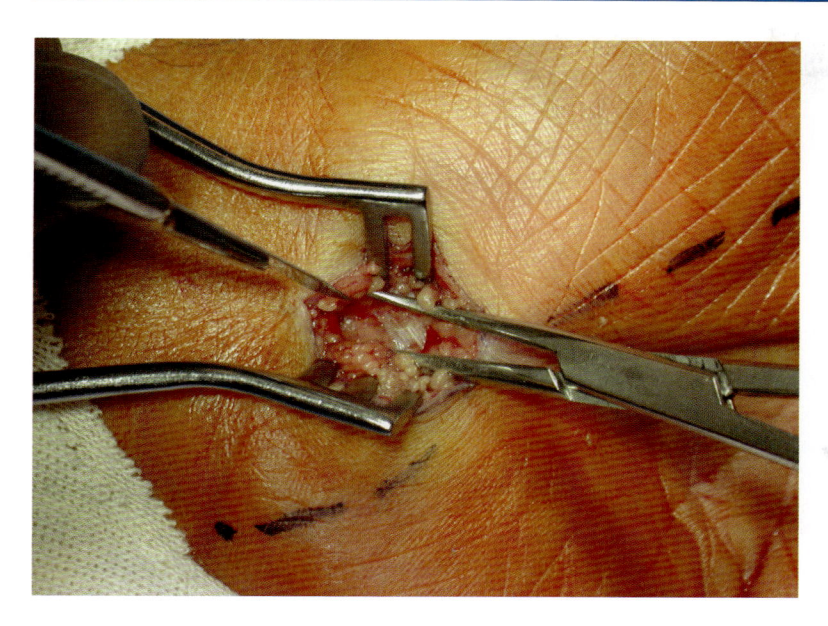

Fig. 135.4 Initial dissection through the palmar fascia using a dissector and No. 15 scalpel. (From Huang JH, Whitmore RG, Zager EL. Carpal tunnel release. In: Wolfa CE, Resnick DK, eds. Neurosurgical Operative Atlas, 2nd ed. Spine and Peripheral Nerves. New York: Thieme; 2007: 317–322.)

135.5). A small retractor is then placed to help for the deeper dissection.

The TCL is divided at its midpoint in layers with a No. 15 scalpel, with the aid of a fine instrument such as a flat or fine pointed dissector to elevate each layer. Once the edge of the transverse carpal ligament is seen and the median nerve is visualized, a dissector is placed above the nerve, and the TCL is incised both proximally and distally using a knife and small sharp tenotomy scissors, with the assistant retracting on the skin edges proximally and distally to gain direct visualization. Being cautious with retraction is important, as the ulnar nerve lies superficial to the TCL just medially, and forceful retraction can accidentally cause compression of the ulnar nerve in Guyon's canal and result in distal ulnar nerve palsy. Proximally, the skin is elevated to permit visualization 2 to 3 cm into the forearm, so that further division of the TCL 1 to 2 cm proximal to the wrist crease into the deep fascia of the forearm confirms complete proximal decompression.

The most common cause of surgical failure is incomplete division of the proximal aspect of the ligament.[29] The distal TCL is incised until the distal edge is visualized and the deep palmar fat pad is encountered. No attempt to dissect or manipulate within the fat space is needed and indeed can be dangerous to branches of the median nerve along with the vascular arcade. Neurolysis of the median nerve is not recommended if this is the initial operation of the carpal tunnel. Before closure, the wound is inspected for hemostasis, and any bleeding points are coagulated with bipolar coagulation set on low current; if used, the tourniquet should be released at this point. The wound is irrigated with sterile saline solution and then approximated with several 3-0 interrupted and inverted Vicryl sutures. The skin is closed with simple interrupted or vertical mattress 4-0 nylon suture (**Fig. 135.6**).

Postoperative Care

We often apply a bulky hand dressing, and the patient is encouraged to do gentle range-of-motion exercises.[30] Postoperative splinting is not usually recommended and has not shown a benefit.[31] The patient is prescribed an oral analgesic.

Studies show that open carpal tunnel release is associated in general with good to excellent relief of symptoms. One study reported reductions in pain (in 87% of patients), in paresthesia (92%), in numbness (56%), and in weakness (42%). Major symptoms persisted in 6% of patients.[32] Studies have shown enhancements in grip and pinch strengths by 12 weeks after surgery and improvement in conduction velocities and distal latencies.[33,34]

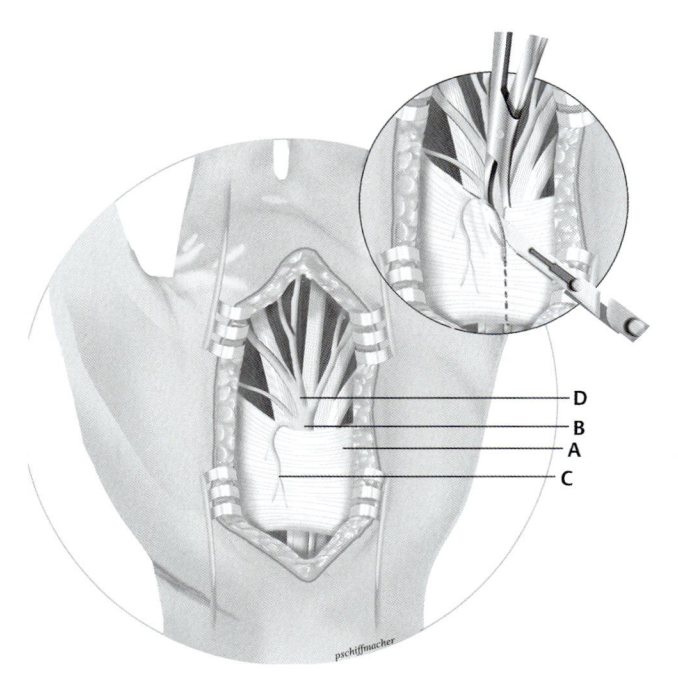

Fig. 135.5 Artist's drawing demonstrating important anatomic landmarks during open carpal tunnel release (left hand). A, transverse carpal ligament; B, median nerve; C, recurrent motor branch; D, cutaneous sensory branch to the radial palm, thumb, index, middle, and radial half of ring fingers. (From Huang JH, Whitmore RG, Zager EL. Carpal tunnel release. In: Wolfa CE, Resnick DK, eds. Neurosurgical Operative Atlas, 2nd ed. Spine and Peripheral Nerves. New York: Thieme; 2007:317–322.)

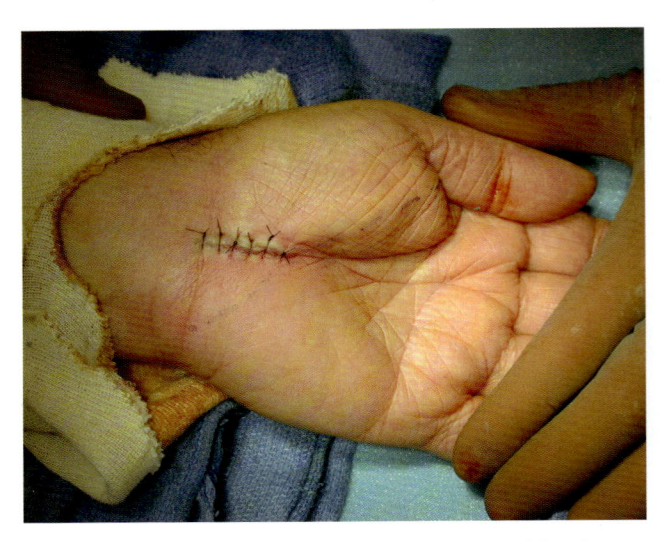

Fig. 135.6 Skin closure with interrupted 4-0 nylon suture, although a running stitch may also be used. (From Huang JH, Whitmore RG, Zager EL. Carpal tunnel release. In: Wolfa CE, Resnick DK, eds. Neurosurgical Operative Atlas, 2nd ed. Spine and Peripheral Nerves. New York: Thieme; 2007: 317–322.)

Potential Complications

Complications after surgery include the development of painful neuroma of the palmar cutaneous nerve, section of the motor branch with resulting weakness, postoperative fibrosis, tender scarring, wound infections, reflex sympathetic dystrophy, and hematoma.[32,33] Patient-related systemic factors that affect the outcome after surgery include diabetes mellitus and advanced muscle weakness at the time of surgery.[33]

Endoscopic (Closed) Carpal Tunnel Release Technique

Advantages and Disadvantages

Potential advantages include a smaller incision that may decrease the patient's postoperative pain as well as avoid cutting the superficial palmar fascia, thus yielding better postoperative grip strength when compared with the open technique.[35] Disadvantages include a steep learning curve, less visibility, increased neurovascular injury, and increased cost associated with endoscopic instruments.

Surgical Procedure

The patient is placed in the supine position and the affected arm is place on an arm board.[36] A tourniquet is placed above the elbow and either local anesthesia or Bier blocks are used. The hand and forearm are carefully prepped and draped. Before starting the procedure, the instrumentation should be checked to be sure it is ready, and it should include a television monitor, camera, recorder, synovial elevator, an obturator, a hook knife, and a set of short endoscopes.

A line perpendicular to the distal palmar crease along the ulnar side of the fourth digit and Kaplan's line are drawn. The intersection between the two lines indicates the location of the hook of hamate or the most medial end of the TCL. The distal wrist crease is marked.[36] The patient is asked to flex the wrist and oppose the thumb and fifth digit to help visualize the palmaris longus tendon. The proximal incision part is between 1 and 2 cm proximal to the distal crease ulnar to the palmaris longus tendon, taking care not to extend more than 1 cm medially.

After induction, the arm is elevated and a rubber Esmarch bandage is applied to exsanguinate the extremity. The tourniquet is inflated to 80 to 100 mm Hg above the present systolic value of the systemic blood pressure, and the Esmarch bandage is removed. This produces a blood-operating field and enhances the visibility with the endoscope.

A small transverse incision 10 to 15 mm in length is made on the ulnar side of the palmaris longus tendon. Usually the median nerve is on the radial side of the palmaris longus tendon outside the incisional site as well as the superficial sensory and recurrent motor branches. Two points are marked, the first is 3 cm distal to the distal crease in a link directed toward the third web space, and the second is 4 cm distal to the distal crease where the distal stab incision can be safely made (**Fig. 135.7**).

The antebrachial fascia is exposed and divided bluntly to gain entrance into the carpal tunnel. One or two superficial veins may be faced and may be bluntly mobilized and moved laterally. An elevator is placed deep to the antebrachial fascia and superficial to the flexor tendons. An obturator and slotted cannula are then inserted into the carpal tunnel while staying superficial to the median nerve and flexor tendons and beneath the TCL, and the hand is maintained in a neutral position. Pressure should be applied to the obturator to ensure that the tip is immediately lateral to the hook of hamate, and once it passes the hook of the hamate the wrist is extended to 30 degrees. In the dual-portal

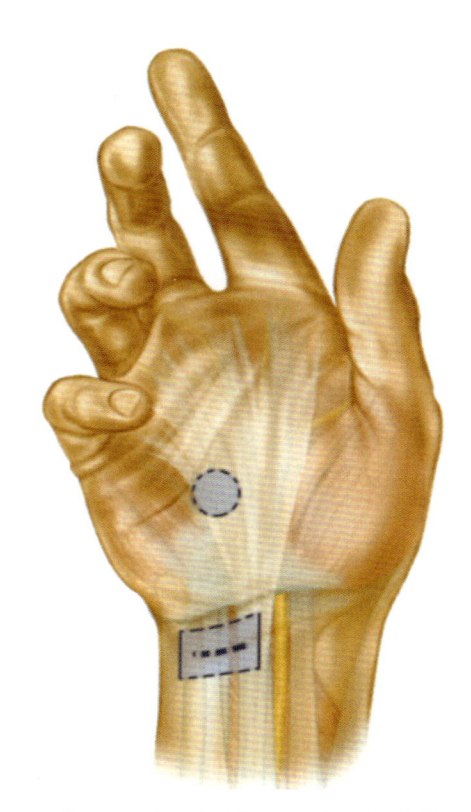

Fig. 135.7 Safe areas where incisions can be placed. Two points are marked; the first is 3 cm distal to the distal crease in a link directed toward the third web space, and the second is 4 cm distal to the distal crease where the distal stab incision can be safely made. (From Jimenez DF. Endoscopic carpal tunnel release via a biportal approach. In: Wolfa CE, Resnick DK, eds. Neurosurgical Operative Atlas, 2nd ed. Spine and Peripheral Nerves. New York: Thieme; 2007:323–330.)

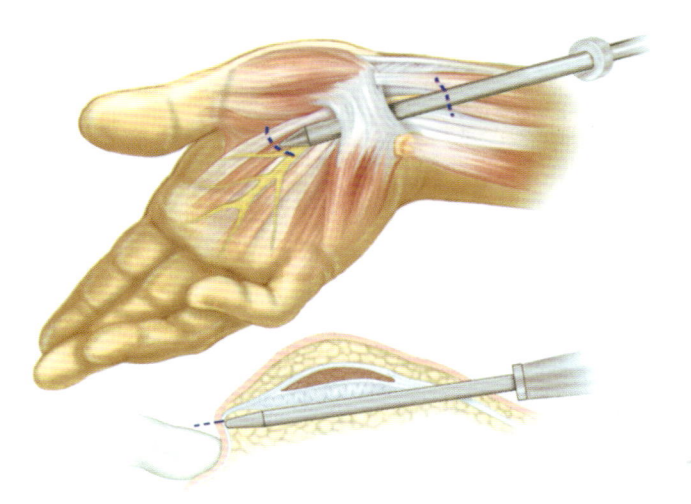

Fig. 135.8 The obturator-cannula assembly is inserted into the carpal tunnel while staying superficial to the median nerve and flexor tendons and beneath the transverse carpal ligament, and the hand is maintained in a neutral position. A stab incision is placed in the distal area over the obturator's tip. The surgeon's nondominant hand is used to apply pressure over this area. (From Jimenez DF. Endoscopic carpal tunnel release via a biportal approach. In: Wolfa CE, Resnick DK, eds. Neurosurgical Operative Atlas, 2nd ed. Spine and Peripheral Nerves. New York: Thieme; 2007:323–330.)

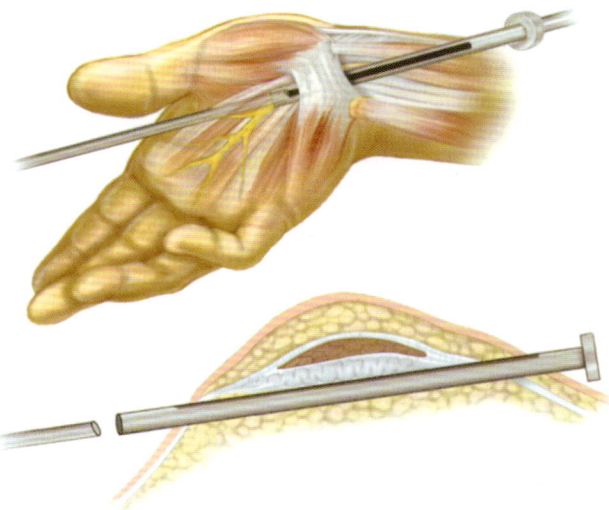

Fig. 135.9 The obturator is removed, and an endoscope is placed through the distal opening. The cannula is slotted to gain passage of a blade. The transverse carpal ligament fibers are split along their natural direction to enter the carpal tunnel. (From Jimenez DF. Endoscopic carpal tunnel release via a biportal approach. In: Wolfa CE, Resnick DK, eds. Neurosurgical Operative Atlas, 2nd ed. Spine and Peripheral Nerves. New York: Thieme; 2007:323–330.)

technique, the obturator and cannula are brought through the skin ~ 4 cm distal to the distal wrist crease, the obturator is removed, and an endoscope is placed through the distal opening **(Figs. 135.8 and 135.9)**.[36] The cannula is slotted to gain passage of a blade. The transverse carpal ligament fibers are split along their natural direction to enter the carpal tunnel **(Fig. 135.10)**.[36] In the uniportal technique, the endoscope camera follows the blade.

Once the TCL has been completely divided, the cannula is removed, the tourniquet is deflated, hemostasis is obtained, the operative field is irrigated with warm saline solution under endoscopic vision, and the skin incisions are closed with two or three simple nylon sutures.

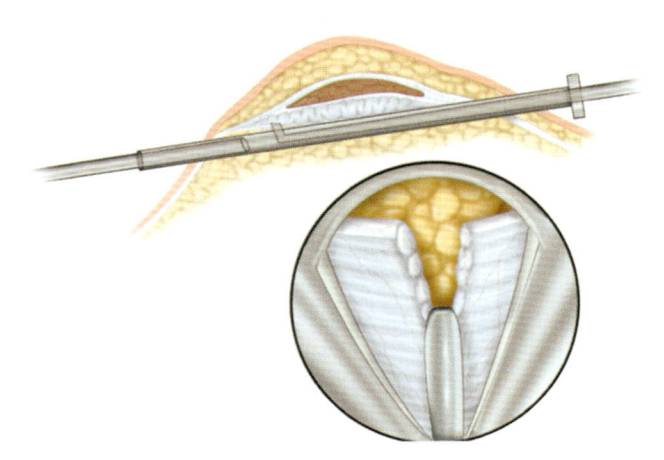

Fig. 135.10 A hooked blade is used to cut the ligament distal to the proximal incision. (From Jimenez DF. Endoscopic carpal tunnel release via a biportal approach. In: Wolfa CE, Resnick DK, eds. Neurosurgical Operative Atlas, 2nd ed. Spine and Peripheral Nerves. New York: Thieme; 2007:323–330.)

Choice of Surgery (Open) Versus (Endoscopic)

A recently published meta-analysis of 28 studies found that at short-term follow-up (≤ 3 months), grip strength was increased after endoscopic open carpal tunnel release (ECTR) when compared with open carpal tunnel release (OCTR). This corresponds to a mean difference of 4 kg when compared with OCTR, which is probably not clinically significant.[37] However, the authors concluded that in the long term (> 3 months postoperatively) there was no significant difference in overall improvement between ECTR and OCTR, and that OCTR and ECTR are about equally effective in relieving symptoms and improving hand function in CTS. Additionally, they found that ECTR probably has lower rates of minor complications (such as scar pain and infections) than OCTR but similar rates of major complications.[37] Also, patients treated with ECTR returned to work and daily activities 8 days earlier than did the patients treated with OCTR. ECTR more frequently resulted in transient nerve problems (e.g., neurapraxia, numbness, and paresthesias), whereas OCTR resulted in more wound problems (e.g., infection, hypertrophic scarring, and scar tenderness).[37]

Conclusion

Reports have shown no difference in long-term outcomes between the open and closed techniques, so the choice of technique should be guided by patient and surgeon preference.[37–41]

References

1. Hommel U, Bellée H, Link M. [The validity of parameters in neonatal diagnosis and fetal monitoring of breech deliveries. 1. Neonatal status after breech delivery]. Zentralbl Gynakol 1989;111:1293–1299
2. Struthers J. On a peculiarity of the humerus and humeral artery. J Hand Surg Eur Vol 2007;32:54–56

3. Hollinshead WH. Anatomy for Surgeons, 2nd ed. New York: Hoeber Medical Division; 1968
4. Sunderland SS, Walshe F. Nerves and Nerve Injuries. Edinburgh and London: E & S Livingstone; 1968
5. Lindley SG, Kleinert JM. Prevalence of anatomic variations encountered in elective carpal tunnel release. J Hand Surg Am 2003;28:849–855
6. Rotman MB, Donovan JP. Practical anatomy of the carpal tunnel. Hand Clin 2002;18:219–230
7. Davlin LB, Aulicino PL, Bergfield TL. Anatomical variations of the median nerve at the wrist. Orthop Rev 1992;21:955–959
8. Seyffarth H. Primary myoses in the M. pronator teres as cause of lesion of the N. medianus (the pronator syndrome). Acta Psychiatr Neurol Scand, Suppl 1951;74:251–254
9. Tetro AM, Pichora DR. High median nerve entrapments. An obscure cause of upper-extremity pain. Hand Clin 1996;12:691–703
10. Kiloh LG, Nevin S. Isolated neuritis of the anterior interosseous nerve. BMJ 1952;1:850–851
11. Spinner M. The anterior interosseous-nerve syndrome, with special attention to its variations. J Bone Joint Surg Am 1970;52:84–94
12. Tarlov IM. How long should an extremity be immobilized after nerve suture? Ann Surg 1947;126:366–376
13. Laha RK, Dujovny M, DeCastro SC. Entrapment of median nerve by supracondylar process of the humerus. Case report. J Neurosurg 1977;46:252–255
14. Varlam H, St Antohe D, Chistol RO. [Supracondylar process and supratrochlear foramen of the humerus: a case report and a review of the literature]. Morphologie 2005;89:121–125
15. Swiggett R, Ruby LK. Median nerve compression neuropathy by the lacertus fibrosus: report of three cases. J Hand Surg Am 1986;11:700–703
16. Werner CO, Rosén I, Thorngren KG. Clinical and neurophysiologic characteristics of the pronator syndrome. Clin Orthop Relat Res 1985;197:231–236
17. Tsai TM, Syed SA. A transverse skin incision approach for decompression of pronator teres syndrome. J Hand Surg [Br] 1994;19:40–42
18. Owings MF, Kozak LJ. Ambulatory and inpatient procedures in the United States, 1996. Vital Health Stat 13 1998;139:1–119
19. Jimenez DF, Gibbs SR, Clapper AT. Endoscopic treatment of carpal tunnel syndrome: a critical review. J Neurosurg 1998;88:817–826
20. Sunderland S. The nerve lesion in the carpal tunnel syndrome. J Neurol Neurosurg Psychiatry 1976;39:615–626
21. Louis DS, Greene TL, Noellert RC. Complications of carpal tunnel surgery. J Neurosurg 1985;62:352–356
22. Okutsu I, Ninomiya S, Takatori Y, Ugawa Y. Endoscopic management of carpal tunnel syndrome. Arthroscopy 1989;5:11–18
23. Piccirilli CB, Shaffrey CI, Young JN, Lovell LR. Two-portal endoscopic carpal tunnel release surgery: report of early experience. Neurosurg Focus 1997;3:e5
24. Agee JM, McCarroll HR Jr, Tortosa RD, Berry DA, Szabo RM, Peimer CA. Endoscopic release of the carpal tunnel: a randomized prospective multicenter study. J Hand Surg Am 1992;17:987–995
25. Chow JC. Endoscopic release of the carpal ligament: a new technique for carpal tunnel syndrome. Arthroscopy 1989;5:19–24
26. Verdugo RJ, Salinas RA, Castillo JL, Cea JG. Surgical versus non-surgical treatment for carpal tunnel syndrome. Cochrane Database Syst Rev 2008;4:CD001552
27. Gebhard RE, Al-Samsam T, Greger J, Khan A, Chelly JE. Distal nerve blocks at the wrist for outpatient carpal tunnel surgery offer intraoperative cardiovascular stability and reduce discharge time. Anesth Analg 2002;95:351–355
28. Lalonde D, Bell M, Benoit P, Sparkes G, Denkler K, Chang P. A multicenter prospective study of 3,110 consecutive cases of elective epinephrine use in the fingers and hand: the Dalhousie Project clinical phase. J Hand Surg Am 2005;30:1061–1067
29. Huang JH, Zager EL. Mini-open carpal tunnel decompression. Neurosurgery 2004;54:397–399, discussion 399–400
30. Midha R, Zager EL. Surgery of Peripheral Nerves: A Case-based Approach. New York: Thieme; 2008
31. Finsen V, Andersen K, Russwurm H. No advantage from splinting the wrist after open carpal tunnel release. A randomized study of 82 wrists. Acta Orthop Scand 1999;70:288–292
32. Kim DH, Cho Y-J, Tiel RL, Kline DG. Outcomes of surgery in 1019 brachial plexus lesions treated at Louisiana State University Health Sciences Center. J Neurosurg 2003;98:1005–1016
33. Aulisa L, Tamburrelli F, Padua R, Romanini E, Lo Monaco M, Padua L. Carpal tunnel syndrome: indication for surgical treatment based on electrophysiologic study. J Hand Surg Am 1998;23:687–691
34. Seror P. Nerve conduction studies after treatment for carpal tunnel syndrome. J Hand Surg [Br] 1992;17:641–645
35. Kohanzadeh S, Herrera FA, Dobke M. Outcomes of open and endoscopic carpal tunnel release: a meta-analysis. Hand (NY) 2012;7:247–251
36. Wolfla CE, Resnick DK. Neurosurgical Operative Atlas: Spine and Peripheral Nerves, 2nd ed. New York and Rolling Meadows, IL: Thieme and the American Association of Neurosurgeons; 2007
37. Vasiliadis HS, Georgoulas P, Shrier I, Salanti G, Scholten RJ. Endoscopic release for carpal tunnel syndrome. Cochrane Database Syst Rev 2014;1:CD008265
38. Katz JN, Keller RB, Simmons BP, et al. Maine Carpal Tunnel Study: outcomes of operative and nonoperative therapy for carpal tunnel syndrome in a community-based cohort. J Hand Surg Am 1998;23:697–710
39. Brown RA, Gelberman RH, Seiler JG III, et al. Carpal tunnel release. A prospective, randomized assessment of open and endoscopic methods. J Bone Joint Surg Am 1993;75:1265–1275
40. Dumontier C, Sokolow C, Leclercq C, Chauvin P. Early results of conventional versus two-portal endoscopic carpal tunnel release. A prospective study. J Hand Surg [Br] 1995;20:658–662
41. Wong KC, Hung LK, Ho PC, Wong JM. Carpal tunnel release. A prospective, randomised study of endoscopic versus limited-open methods. J Bone Joint Surg Br 2003;85:863–868

136 Decompression of the Ulnar and Radial Nerve

Ahmed Alaqeel, Albert M. Isaacs, and Rajiv Midha

Ulnar Nerve

Structural Anatomy

Axilla and Arm

The ulnar nerve arises as a direct continuation from the medial cord of the brachial plexus just distal to the origins of the medial cutaneous nerves of the arm and forearm and the medial head of the median nerve, receiving contribution from C8 and T1 spinal roots (and occasionally C7). At the axillary level, the ulnar nerve lies between the axillary artery and axillary vein, with the medial antebrachial cutaneous nerve anterior to it. The nerve lies deep and posteromedial to the axillary brachial artery segment up to the middle of the arm. At the level of insertion of the deltoid in the middle third of the arm, the ulnar nerve leaves the flexor compartment of the arm by running either posterior or pierces the medial intermuscular septum (MIS) to enter the posterior compartment of the arm, which is a potential, albeit rare, site for nerve compression. The ulnar nerve is accompanied by the superior ulnar collateral artery. Then the nerve runs obliquely across the head of triceps, which if hypertrophied would be another potential site of nerve compression. The nerve then passes through the arcade of Struthers, which is a musculofascial band that is ~ 1.5 to 2 cm wide and ~ 8 cm proximal to the medial epicondyle and occurs in 68 to 70% of limbs; it is another potential, although rare, site of ulnar nerve compression. In the lower arm, there is a close relationship of the ulnar nerve to the olecranon notch.

Elbow and Forearm

The ulnar nerve descends in the groove between the medial epicondyle of the humerus and the ulnar olecranon process accompanied by the superior ulnar collateral artery within the cubital tunnel, the most common site of ulnar nerve entrapment.[1] The nerve enters the cubital tunnel by passing under Osborne's ligament, a 4-mm-wide ligament that extends between the medial epicondyle and the tip of the olecranon.[1] The nerve is surrounded by fat throughout the cubital tunnel except adjacent to the medial epicondyle. The cubital tunnel ends just proximal to the heads of the flexor carpi ulnaris (FCU) muscle. The roof of the cubital tunnel is formed by the cubital tunnel retinaculum and the arcuate ligament of Osborne, which extends from the tip of the olecranon to the medial epicondyle, and the floor is formed by the capsule of the elbow joint and the medial collateral ligament; the walls are formed by the medial epicondyle and olecranon. The distal extent of the retinaculum fuses with the common aponeurosis of the FCU muscle, known as Osborne's fascia, another potential site of entrapment.[2] The ulnar nerve then enters the forearm by passing between the two heads (humeral and ulnar) of the FCU lying under the aponeurosis of the flexor pronator, another potential site of nerve compression.[2,3] The palmar cutaneous branch of the ulnar nerve originates ~ 16 cm proximal to the ulnar styloid and provides sensation to the distal ulnar aspect of the forearm.[4] The nerve lies on the surface of the flexor digitorum profundus (FDP) and descends to supply the ulnar part of the FDP that sends tendons to digits 4 and 5 and traveling deep to the FCU in the upper half of the forearm and lateral to the FCU in the lower half, accompanied by the ulnar artery, giving off the volar and the dorsal cutaneous branches 5 cm above the wrist. The dorsal branch is sensory and goes deep to the FCU tendon, to gain the extensor surface.

Wrist and Hand

In 1861, Jean Casimir Felix Guyon described an anatomic canal now named Guyon's canal in the palmar-ulnar side of the wrist that is a potential cause of nerve compression.[5] Other potential sites of compression include the distal ulnar tunnel and the carpal ulnar neurovascular space. At the wrist level, the ulnar nerve and the ulnar artery and vein pass lateral to the pisiform bone through the Guyon canal, a 4-cm-long triangular tunnel. The roof of the tunnel is formed from the distal extension of the antebrachial fascia and the palmaris brevis, where the floor is composed of the hypothenar muscles and the medial portion of the transverse carpal ligament. The ulnar nerve divides into superficial and deep branches. The distal ulnar tunnel is divided into three zones. Zone 1 is the area where the ulnar nerve is proximal to its divisions into terminal branches; usually the nerve bifurcates or trifurcates at the middle of the canal. Zone 2 is the deep branch, and zone 3 is the superficial branch. The clinical presentation corresponds with the zone in which compression is occurring.[6] The superficial branch gives off cutaneous branches to the volar surfaces of the medial one and a half digits and the palmaris brevis.[7] The deep branch supplies the hypothenar muscles (abductor, opponent, and flexor digiti minimi), the medial two lumbricals, the adductor pollicis, and all the dorsal and palmar interossei, and ends in the thenar area, within the adductor pollicis and the medial (deep) head of the flexor pollicis brevis.[7,8]

Important Findings

- Martin-Gruber anastomosis (10–15%) can occur when motor fibers from the median nerve cross over to the ulnar nerve in the forearm.
- Riche-Cannieu anastomosis occurs when there is a connection between the motor branch of the ulnar nerve and the recurrent motor branch of the median nerve,[9] hence returning the motor fibers to the median nerve before their terminal innervation.
- It is important to distinguish clinically between compression of the nerve at the elbow and compression at the wrist. A sensory deficit over the dorsoulnar aspect of the hand and dorsum of the little finger benefits in

this differentiation. Compression at Guyon's canal spares the dorsal sensation, as this area is innervated by the dorsal sensory branch of the ulnar nerve, which has already branched off ~ 5 to 6 cm proximal to Guyon's canal in the wrist.

Distal Entrapment of the Ulnar Nerve

Patient Selection and Preoperative Imaging

Given its rarity, this condition has good outcomes if diagnosed early and a complete decompression is performed. Usually patients present with pain, hand weakness, or sensory deficit on the ulnar sided digits, with sparing of the dorsal cutaneous distribution. Electrodiagnostic assessment confirming the conduction change at the wrist versus the elbow level is critical. The most common etiologies include idiopathic, degenerative, posttraumatic, various muscles and fibrous bands, and various masses. Because several of the conditions entail mass lesions (variant muscles, ganglion cyst, and nerve tumors), imaging of Guyon's canal with either ultrasound or magnetic resonance imaging (MRI) is recommended. When any of the above conditions is identified, surgical exposure and nerve decompression is indicated when a trial of nonoperative management has failed.[10-12]

An outline of the arm can be used in preoperative evaluation to facilitate a more accurate localization of the site of the radial or ulnar entrapment. If surgical decompression is indicated, different surgical approaches are applicable, with good outcomes.

Surgical Procedure

The procedure is typically performed as a day-surgery operation, under local, regional, or general anesthesia. Video 136.1 demonstrates a step-by-step approach to performing ulnar nerve decompression at the elbow. The patient is positioned supine, with the limb on a hand table. The shoulder is abducted and externally rotated with the arm in full supination, and a small rounded towel is placed under the wrist to keep the fingers in an extended position. We usually do not use a tourniquet, but if it is used, the limb should be elevated and exsanguinated with an Esmarch bandage. Following a sterile prep and drape, a 7-cm curvilinear skin incision is marked to decompress the Guyon's canal in the interval between the palmar cutaneous branches of the median and ulnar nerve, 4 cm into the ulnar aspect of the palm and 3 cm into the distal forearm between the pisiform and the hook of hamate (**Fig. 136.1**). The incision crosses the transverse wrist crease between the pisiform and the hook of the hamate at an oblique angle. Crossing the wrist crease at right angles should be avoided.

It is easiest to identify the nerve first in the junction of the distal forearm and wrist. The FCU tendon is identified in the distal forearm and retracted medially. Then the ulnar nerve and artery are exposed. The artery is typically located volar and radial to the nerve. These neurovascular structures are traced from proximal to distal, where they enter Guyon's canal, and the ulnar nerve is tagged with a rubber dam and the artery with a vessel loop. The volar carpal ligament, palmaris brevis, and hypothenar fat and fibrous tissue are incised, decompressing the nerve along its entire course through the canal. The neurovascular structures should be mobilized before addressing any underlying pathoanatomic problem, and if a Ganglion cyst is identified, its stalk is traced to a neighboring joint and obliterated. Before closure, the wound is inspected for hemostasis, and any bleeding points are treated with bipolar coagulation set on low current; if a tourniquet was used, it should be released at this point. The wound is irrigated with sterile saline solution and then approximated with several 4-0 Prolene simple and horizontal mattress sutures.

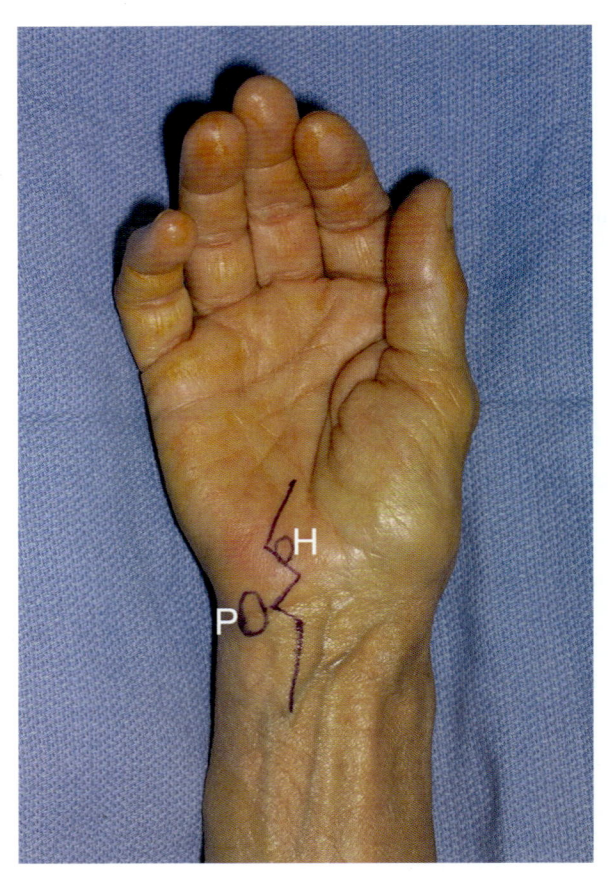

Fig. 136.1 The planned skin incision is shown. The ulnar nerve is located between the pisiform (P) and the hook of the hamate (H). (From Spinner RJ, Bishop AT. Surgical treatment of ulnar nerve entrapment at the wrist. In: Wolfa CE, Resnick DK, eds. Neurosurgical Operative Atlas, 2nd ed. Spine and Peripheral Nerves. New York: Thieme; 2007:344–349.)

Postoperative Care

We often apply a bulky hand dressing, and the patient is encouraged to do gentle range-of-motion exercises.

Entrapment of the Ulnar Nerve at the Cubital Tunnel

Patient Selection and Preoperative Testing and Imaging

The cubital tunnel syndrome was first named by Feindel and Stratford in 1958.[13] Diagnosis rests on taking a careful history, performing a physical exam, and ordering supportive electromyography and nerve conduction studies. Usually the sensory fibers are affected before the motor fibers in the cubital tunnel syndrome, and therefore they may present first with sensory deficit along the ulnar nerve distribution before weakness of grip occurs. On examination, tenderness at the elbow joint and a positive Tinel's sign, Wattenberg's sign, and Froment's paper sign as well as a positive elbow flexion test are demonstrated. We reserve elbow plain X-ray to exclude fracture or osteophyte formation for those with a history of trauma or severe arthritis, accompanied by elbow deformity. The main etiologies of ulnar nerve damage at the elbow joint are due to compression, ischemia, traction, longitudinal strain, and friction.[13-17] Interestingly it was observed that there is six times increased cubital tunnel pressures with elbow flexion, wrist extension, and shoulder abduction.[18] Friction on the nerve may result from subluxation or dislocation of the nerve because of congenital or developmental laxity of the soft tissue surrounding the ulnar nerve in its groove at the cubital tunnel.[17] If nonsurgical management fails to relieve symptoms and reverse the neuropathy, then a surgical release should be considered.[19]

Surgical Options

Several surgical options are available to treat compression of the ulnar neuropathy at the elbow, including simple or in-situ decompression, medial epicondylectomy, subcutaneous transposition, intramuscular transposition, and submuscular transposition.

Simple Ulnar Nerve Decompression

The simple ulnar nerve decompression procedure is typically performed as day surgery under local, regional, or general anesthesia. The patient is placed supine, with the shoulder abducted to 90 degrees and externally rotated, and the arm placed on an arm board with the elbow extended, with a folded towel placed under the elbow; the forearm is supinated and slightly flexed. Although some surgeons prefer the use of a tourniquet during the surgery, we do not use it at our center.

Following a sterile prep and drape, an ~ 8 to 10 cm curvilinear skin incision is marked over the course of the ulnar nerve centered at the elbow on the medial distal arm; it extends along the medial edge of the triceps muscle and goes between the medial epicondyle and the olecranon process of the ulna along the medial volar elbow to the proximal medial forearm between the heads of the FCU (**Fig. 136.2**). Recently, the use of smaller incisions with the aid of an endoscope has been reported in the literature.

Dissection is performed with a No. 15 scalpel blade, after the site is infiltrated with 0.25% Marcaine with epinephrine in a 1:100,000 concentration, to expose the subcutaneous tissues, taking care to preserve the medial antebrachial cutaneous nerve branches because injury may result in neuroma formation that may cause elbow pain, numbness around the elbow, and tender scarring.[20,21] Usually the ulnar nerve is found proximal to the level of the olecranon notch. The deep fascia overlying the nerve is incised with either scissors or a No. 15 scalpel blade. The nerve is then exposed proximal to the postcondylar groove, to inspect for possible potential compression at the arcade of Struthers and the medial intermuscular septum to unroof it and decompress it.

Dissection is then carried distally through the postcondylar groove, and the fibrofascial cubital retinaculum overlying the nerve. The nerve is followed distally by dividing Osborne's fascia. The groove is the site of maximal nerve compression in most cases. Distal to the postcondylar groove, the ulnar nerve is followed as it courses deep to the aponeurosis between the two heads of the flexor carpi ulnaris muscle, where the aponeurosis is divided to explore the ulnar nerve (**Fig. 136.3**). With simple decompression, neurolysis of the nerve is not indicated. Once decompression is completed, the elbow is flexed and extended to look for nerve dislocation across the medial epicondyle. If there is significant dislocation, then a transposition procedure is warranted. In practice, we find this to be the case in only about 5% of cases. We intentionally do not perform an external neurolysis of the nerve so as to prevent iatrogenic dislocation. Before closure, the wound is inspected for hemostasis and any bleeding points are treated with bipolar coagulation set on low current. The wound is irrigated with sterile saline solution and then approximated with absorbable sutures.

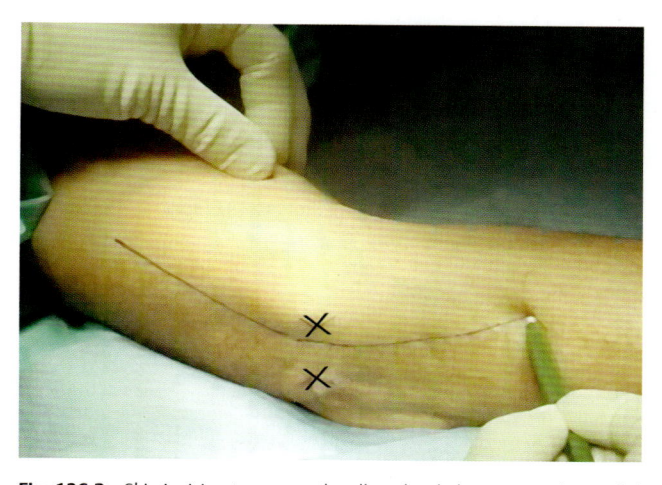

Fig. 136.2 Skin incision to expose the elbow level ulnar nerve. The medial epicondyle is marked with an X on the top and the lower X marks the olecranon process. (From Murovic JA, Kim DH, Kline DG. Ulnar neurolysis for cubital tunnel syndrome. In: Wolfa CE, Resnick DK, eds. Neurosurgical Operative Atlas, 2nd ed. Spine and Peripheral Nerves. New York: Thieme; 2007: 331–335.)

Postoperative Care

We often apply a bulky elbow dressing, and the patient is encouraged to do gentle range-of-motion exercises.[22]

Ulnar Nerve Neurolysis

If a subcutaneous, submuscular, or intramuscular transposition is indicated, complete external neurolysis of the ulnar nerve is performed.[23] The nerve is dissected free on the posterior side; small articular branches and small vessels tethering the ulnar nerve often need to be sectioned, taking care to preserve as much blood supply as possible. Nerve branches to the FCU should be preserved if possible. Following and dissecting the branches back proximally and separating them from the ulnar nerve enable more mobility. Distally, the nerve is followed in the plane deep to the fibrous band of fascia between the heads of the FCU muscle. This band is often a site of nerve entrapment and is dissected.

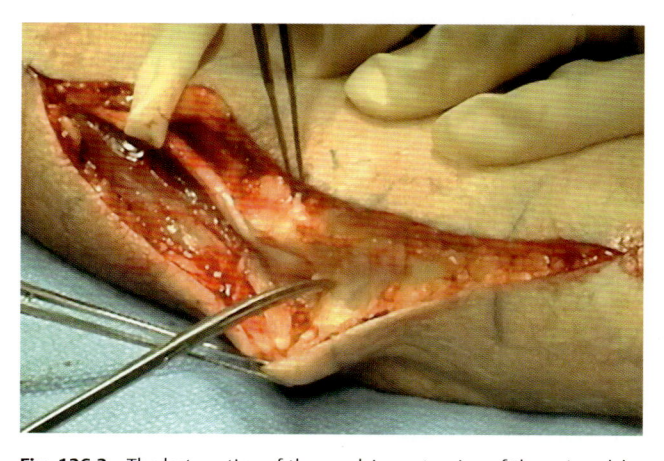

Fig. 136.3 The last portion of the overlying extension of the epicondylar fascia is being sectioned. (From Murovic JA, Kim DH, Kline DG. Ulnar neurolysis for cubital tunnel syndrome. In: Wolfa CE, Resnick DK, eds. Neurosurgical Operative Atlas, 2nd ed. Spine and Peripheral Nerves. New York: Thieme; 2007:331–335.)

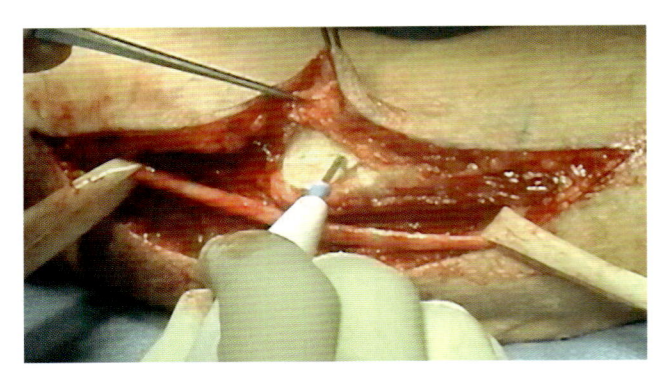

Fig. 136.4 In a subcutaneous transposition, the plane between the flexor carpi ulnaris muscle and the subcutaneous tissue is dissected. (From Murovic JA, Kim DH, Kline DG. Ulnar neurolysis for cubital tunnel syndrome. In: Wolfa CE, Resnick DK, eds. Neurosurgical Operative Atlas, 2nd ed. Spine and Peripheral Nerves. New York: Thieme; 2007:331–335.)

A distal segment of the medial intermuscular septum must be fully resected to prevent tethering or compression of the transposed nerve, with the base sharply incised and devascularized with bipolar coagulation and, if not excised adequately, this would be the most common cause of transposition failure.

Subcutaneous Transposition

Should subcutaneous transposition be chosen, after a complete external neurolysis, the nerve is brought anterior to the medial epicondyle between the subcutaneous tissue and the fascia of the flexor pronator muscles, and a fascial sling is fashioned by raising a layer from the flexor tendons found on top of the medial epicondyle and secured by suturing it to the subcutaneous tissue, and in this way the nerve is prevented from returning to its position in the ulnar groove (**Fig. 136.4**).[24] In this new location, it must be ensured that the nerve is free from any point of adhesion or pressure that may irritate the nerve.

Advantages and Disadvantages

The advantages of this transposition technique compared with submuscular transposition are that the subcutaneous transposition include shorter incision, shorter operative time and less postoperative pain.[25,26] The reported disadvantages of subcutaneous transposition include a relative avascularity and vulnerability to trauma, mainly in patients with little subcutaneous tissue.[27]

Submuscular Transposition

After the nerve has undergone a complete neurolysis, the origin of the flexor-pronator muscles is isolated and divided in a stepcut or Z-plasty configuration using a scalpel, with a proximal cuff of muscle and fascia left intact. Laterally, care must be taken to avoid the brachial artery and median nerve, so identifying these before incising the flexor pronator muscle is mandatory. The proximal attachment of the volar FCU to the ulna needs to be incised to prevent distal kinking of the ulnar nerve.[23] The ulnar nerve is brought anteriorly and placed deep to the flexor-pronator mass in an oblique and slightly curved fashion through the pronator teres and proximal portion of the FCU muscle on a fascial bed over the brachialis (**Fig. 136.5**).[28] The nerve must not be kinked or compressed over its new course. The flexor-pronator mass is then reapproximated by using the step cut to provide lengthening. Then the nerve is pulled gently back and forth to ensure that there is no tension on the nerve. Before closure, the wound is inspected for hemostasis, and any bleeding points are treated with bipolar coagulation set on low current. The wound is irrigated with sterile saline solution and then the subcutaneous tissue is approximated with 2-0 sutures, and a subcuticular running suture is used for skin approximation. We often apply a bulky arm dressing, and the patient is encouraged to do gentle range-of-motion exercise.

Advantage and Disadvantage

The advantage is that this is the only technique that addresses nerve compression at all five potential sites. The disadvantage is that occasionally the procedure can result in perineural scarring.[29]

Subfascial/Intramuscular Transposition

After the nerve has undergone a complete neurolysis, the nerve is placed in a shallow muscular trough shaped in the pronator teres and flexor carpi ulnaris.

Advantage and Disadvantage

The advantage is that this technique entails less muscular dissection. The disadvantage is that recurrent symptoms secondary to postoperative scarring are more commonly reported with this technique.[27,30]

Choice of Surgical Technique

The literature review from 1970 to 1997 that was done by Bartels et al[31] concluded that, irrespective of patients' preoperative status, a simple decompression had the most favorable outcomes and that patients with subcutaneous and submuscular transpositions had the worst outcomes. We prefer simple in-situ decompression, unless transposition is indicated, because it involves a shorter operative time and recovery time, does not require sacrifice of any vessels or nerve branches, and preserves the anatomic course of the nerve.

A meta-analysis of four randomized controlled trials that compared simple decompression and ulnar nerve transposition found no significant difference in clinical outcome or postoperative nerve conduction velocity between these techniques.[32]

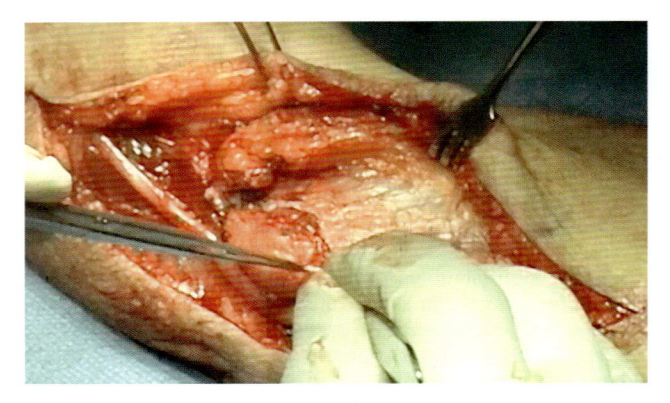

Fig. 136.5 In a submuscular transposition, the common flexor tendon of the flexor carpi ulnaris and pronator teres is incised. (From Murovic JA, Kim DH, Kline DG. Ulnar neurolysis for cubital tunnel syndrome. In: Wolfa CE, Resnick DK, eds. Neurosurgical Operative Atlas, 2nd ed. Spine and Peripheral Nerves. New York: Thieme; 2007:331–335.)

Significantly fewer complications occurred in patients who underwent simple decompression than in those who underwent anterior transposition, with a total median cost 2.5 times that of simple decompression.[33–35]

Endoscopic surgery for simple decompression or neurolysis has been described.[36–39] The procedure focuses on the division of Osborne's arcuate ligament. Several series showed good or excellent results with endoscopic procedures, ranging from 80 to 92%.[36,37,40–42] However, direct comparison to an open procedure is lacking in these reports.

Radial Nerve

Structural Anatomy

Axilla and Arm

The radial nerve is the largest branch of the brachial plexus. It is derived from the posterior cords of the brachial plexus, receiving contribution from C5 to T1 spinal roots because the posterior cord is made from divisions derived from the upper, middle, and lower trunks of the brachial plexus. The radial nerve lies posterior to the third portion of the axillary artery at its origin, behind the upper part of the brachial arteries. The coracoid process is an important landmark at which the radial nerve continues as the main outflow of the posterior cord, posterior to the axillary artery. In its proximal course, the subscapular artery crosses the nerve. The nerve passes dorsally toward the upper end of the spiral groove deep to the long head of the triceps and between the lateral and medial heads and gives off a variable number of branches to the triceps at the axillary level. Then the nerve deviates from the brachial artery and goes around the posterior aspect of the humerus from the medial to the lateral side of the arm. This is the point at which it has the fewest number of fascicles (approximately four or five) in its entire course. The heads of the triceps are supplied by the radial nerve, and the surgeon should be aware that these motor branches leave the dorsal aspect of the radial nerve close to its origin, are variable in number, and run obliquely to supply one or more of the three heads of the triceps muscle. The surgeon should be very careful during dissection in the deep axilla where these branches may be encased within a scar tissue.

The profunda brachial, also called the deep brachial artery, a branch of the axillary artery, travels with the radial nerve as it leaves the axilla. The anconeus is supplied by a long branch of the radial nerve in the spiral groove. Although this small muscle is of little importance during the clinical examination, an electrode can be placed into it on electromyography studies and helps to determine the location of denervation, which is proximal to the outflow of this branch. The radial nerve also gives off a branch to the brachialis from its medial aspect, to the brachioradialis 2 to 3 cm proximal to the elbow and extensors carpi radialis longus (ECRL) muscles and cutaneous branches to supply the skin along the posterior aspect of upper arm.

Elbow and Forearm

In the distal arm, the radial nerve emerges from the spiral groove on the lateral aspect of the humerus lying in the groove between the brachialis medially and the brachioradialis laterally, an excellent location to find the nerve at surgery. The nerve then runs through the lateral intermuscular septum to reenter the anterior compartment, and passes anteriorly to the lateral epicondyle and continues in the forearm. The nerve divides into two major branches, the superficial sensory radial nerve (SSRN), and the posterior interosseous nerve (PIN), an exclusively motor nerve.

The SSRN branch lies under the brachioradialis, lateral to the radial artery, and supplies sensation to the dorsum of the thumb, the first web space (anatomic snuffbox), and the dorsoradial aspect of the carpus, extending up to the index and middle fingers. The PIN is a motor-only nerve that supplies the extensor muscles and abductor pollicis longus distal to the elbow. The PIN travels along the radial tunnel, a 5-cm space defined by the capsule of the radiocapitellar joint dorsally, the ECRL and extensor carpi radialis brevis (ECRB) muscles laterally, the biceps tendon and brachialis muscles medially, and the brachioradialis volarly. The PIN pierces the supinator muscle and the posterior extensor muscles and comes to lie on posterior interosseous membrane just below the extensor pollicis brevis, and ends as a pseudoganglion below the extensor retinaculum on the dorsum of the wrist.

Within the area of the radial tunnel there are five potential sites of compression: (1) fibrous bands to the radiocapitellar joint between the brachialis and brachioradialis; (2) the recurrent radial vessels, or so-called leash of Henry; (3) the leading tendinous edge of the ECRB; (4) the proximal edge of the supinator, known as the arcade of Fröhse; and (5) the distal edge of the supinator.[43–47] The arcade of Fröhse is the most common site of PIN compression. It is a tough fibrous ring where the nerve enters the supinator. Compression of the PIN gives rise to two different compression syndromes—the PIN syndrome and the radial tunnel syndrome. The surgical exposure for these two syndromes is identical.

Wrist and Hand

The SSRN branch curves around the wrist deep to the brachioradialis tendon. The nerve pierces the deep fascia and breaks into four or five branches when it reaches the hand, crossing the anatomic snuffbox. These terminal branches supply the dorsal aspect of the thumb, index finger, and radial side of the middle finger except the nail beds, which are supplied by proper digital branches of the median nerve.

Exposure of the Radial Nerve in the Arm

Patient Selection

Injury to the radial nerve at the arm level owing to humeral fracture is the most common mechanism for radial injury.[48,49] In most cases the nerve is injured at the time of initial trauma and recovers well. In rare cases, the radial nerve can be compressed at the lateral intermuscular septum or the triceps muscle at this region. The origin and course of the radial nerve make exposure of the radial nerve difficult with a single surgical approach.

Surgical Procedure

For the exposure of the infraclavicular plexus, an anterior deltopectoral incision is recommended, which can be extended along the groove between the biceps and triceps. For more distal decompression in the posterior arm, an incision is made between the long and lateral head of the triceps and extended distally, ventral and medial to the lateral epicondyle (**Fig. 136.6**). If any difficulty is encountered in finding the nerve, the surgeon should not hesitate to expose the nerve first in the intermuscular sulcus between the brachioradialis and brachialis (**Fig. 136.6**). The nerve is explored to look for and decompress the nerve at any potential site of compression under the lateral intermuscular septum or by the triceps muscle (**Fig. 136.6**). Care must be taken to avoid an injury to the posterior cutaneous nerve of the arm.

866   VI   Peripheral Nerves

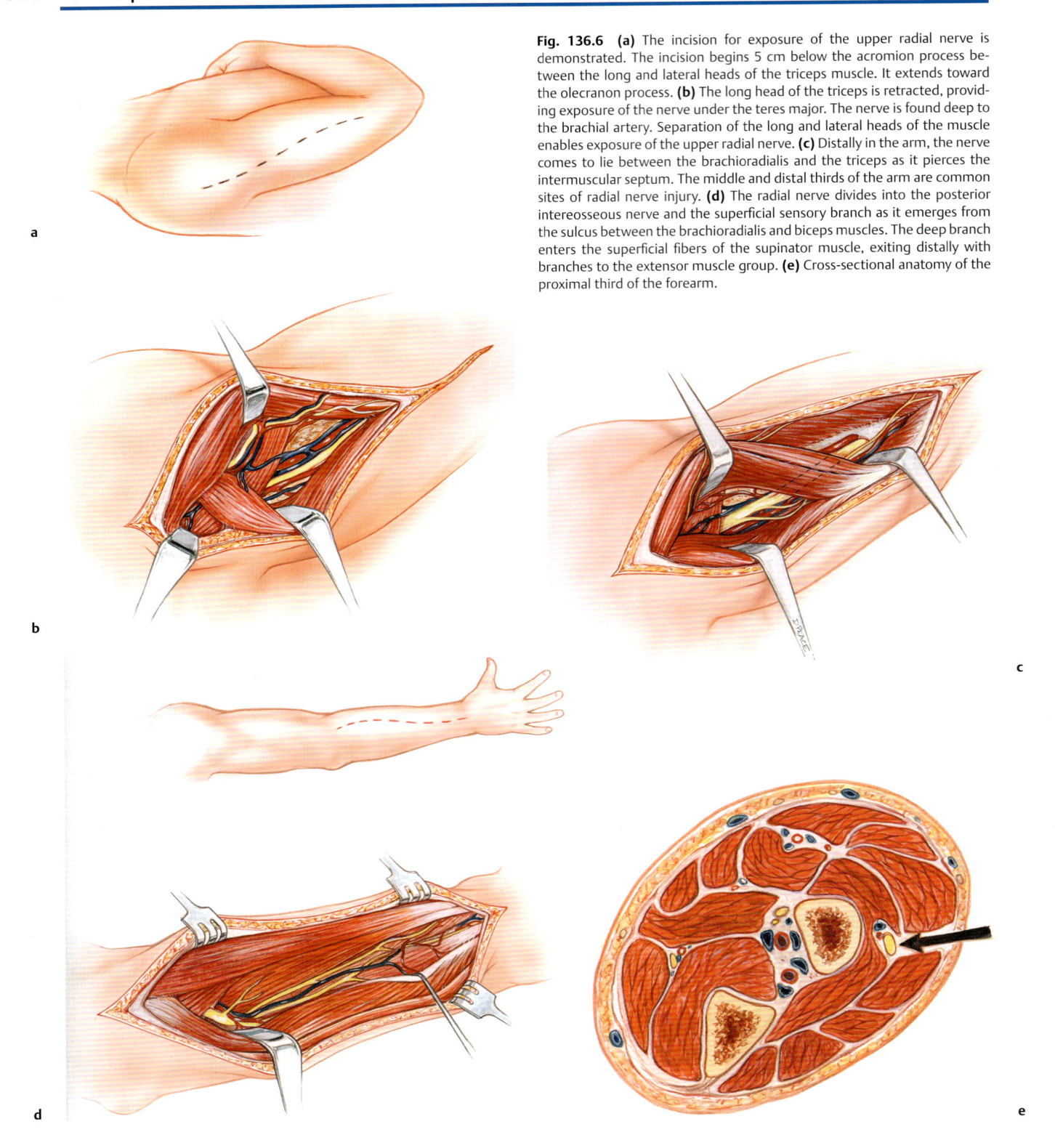

Fig. 136.6 (a) The incision for exposure of the upper radial nerve is demonstrated. The incision begins 5 cm below the acromion process between the long and lateral heads of the triceps muscle. It extends toward the olecranon process. (b) The long head of the triceps is retracted, providing exposure of the nerve under the teres major. The nerve is found deep to the brachial artery. Separation of the long and lateral heads of the muscle enables exposure of the upper radial nerve. (c) Distally in the arm, the nerve comes to lie between the brachioradialis and the triceps as it pierces the intermuscular septum. The middle and distal thirds of the arm are common sites of radial nerve injury. (d) The radial nerve divides into the posterior interosseous nerve and the superficial sensory branch as it emerges from the sulcus between the brachioradialis and biceps muscles. The deep branch enters the superficial fibers of the supinator muscle, exiting distally with branches to the extensor muscle group. (e) Cross-sectional anatomy of the proximal third of the forearm.

Entrapment of the Deep Branch of the Radial Nerve (Posterior Interosseous Nerve)

Patient Selection

Patients with the PIN syndrome present with weakness in all muscles innervated distal to the supinator, causing loss of finger and thumb extension, most frequently due to compression of the PIN at the arcade of Fröhse.[50] Wrist extension is preserved, with radial wrist deviation, as innervation to the extensor carpi ulnaris muscle is affected, whereas that to the radial extensors (ECRL AND ECRB) is spared.[51] Patients usually do not present with pain. Because the nerve contains only motor fibers, sensory symptoms do not occur in this disorder.

Radial tunnel syndrome, like PIN syndrome, results from compression of the PIN, but in contrast to PIN syndrome, patients complain of lateral proximal forearm pain with no noticeable motor weakness. Usually patients complain of pain with resisted supination of the forearm and resisted extension of the middle finger. The syndrome must be distinguished from the much more common lateral epicondylitis. Unfortunately, electrophysiology is often not helpful in radial tunnel syndrome, and one study found that the accuracy of diagnosis can only be improved to 50% even with detailed studies.[52] Differential injections may be useful in distinguishing lateral epicondylitis from radial tunnel syndrome, whereas imaging studies are only helpful if a mass lesion is suspected as the causative factor.[53-55] Weitbrecht and Navickine[56] reported an incidence of 1% in a large series of compression neuropathies of the upper limb. This reflects the difficulty in making an accurate diagnosis, with many cases being wrongly diagnosed as resistant tennis elbow.[57]

Surgery is the treatment of choice for the PIN syndrome when nonsurgical treatments have been unsuccessful for more than 3 months with avoidance of aggravating activities, rest, splinting, and stretching.[53,58] If surgery is delayed for ~ 18 months, fibrosis of muscles innervated by the PIN will occur, making tendon transfers a reasonable option.

Surgical Procedure

Both anterior and posterior approaches have been reported for decompression of the PIN. For the anterior (modified Henry) approach, the patient is placed in the supine position with the arm slightly flexed, rotated medially, and prone on an arm table. A curvilinear or zigzag incision is fashioned beginning proximal to the lateral epicondyle and continuing in the interval between the biceps and brachioradialis muscles, and then curving 2 cm above the elbow flexion crease, back over the mobile (supinator-extensor muscle) wad, and medial to the ulnar border of the brachioradialis muscle. The cutaneous nerves are identified and protected. The fascia along the brachioradialis muscle is divided and retracted while retracting the biceps and pronator teres medially. The radial nerve is identified with a gentle lateral retraction of the brachioradialis muscle (**Figs. 136.7 and 136.8**). The nerve is followed distally until the supinator muscle is pierced (**Fig. 136.7**). The recurrent radial vessels of Henry are ligated, and the arcade of Fröhse is released. Decompression is attained by dividing the fibrous ring and the superficial head of the supinator to expose the nerve to its terminal branches, to exclude any other potential sites of compression.

A posterior (Henry or Thompson) approach is done with the patient's forearm pronated. A 10-cm straight skin incision is made along an imaginary line extending from the lateral epicondyle to Lister's tubercle. The incision can be prolonged proximally onto the lateral ridge of the epicondyle as needed. The posterior cutaneous nerve of the forearm is identified and protected. The brachioradialis and extensor carpi radialis longus interval is identified by a fascial stripe as well as by the darker color of the brachioradialis, where blunt dissection is carried down to the radial nerve. The superficial sensory radial nerve is found on the undersurface of the brachioradialis and protected. The arcade of Fröhse is readily identified and divided. The supinator is identified deep to the extensor muscles in the proximal third of the incision. The posterior interosseous nerve can then be found at the proximal edge of the supinator, and the fibrous leading edge of the extensor carpi radialis brevis and the tendinous leading edge of the supinator are released. The recurrent leash of the vessels of Henry are ligated. The superficial head of the supinator muscle should be released to its distal border. Other points of compression are identified and released.

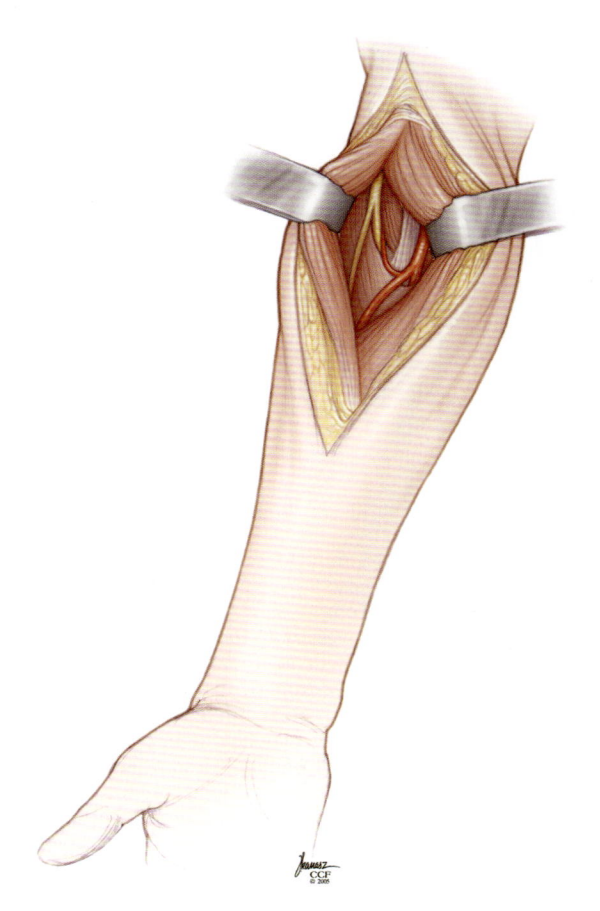

Fig. 136.7 The radial nerve divides into the posterior interosseous nerve (PIN) and the superficial radial nerve proximal to the supinator muscle, and the PIN passes under the supinator. (From Borsellino SR, Lastra-Powers JJ, Boulis NM, Benzel EC. Surgical exposure of peripheral nerves of the upper extremity; radial nerve. In: Wolfa CE, Resnick DK, eds. Neurosurgical Operative Atlas, 2nd ed. Spine and Peripheral Nerves. New York: Thieme; 2007: 363–367.)

Postoperative Care and Outcome

Good to excellent result may be expected in 90% of patients who undergo surgical decompression of the PIN after symptom onset.[59] Vrieling et al[60] noted a good to excellent response in 75% in patients in a smaller study. The differences in outcomes may be due to the fact that in the former study patients underwent

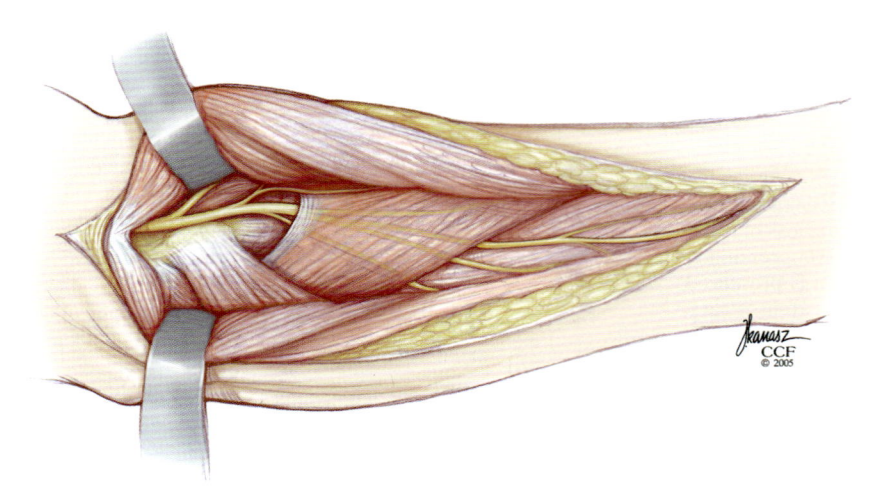

Fig. 136.8 The radial nerve is identified after gentle retraction of the brachioradialis muscle. (From Borsellino SR, Lastra-Powers JJ, Boulis NM, Benzel EC. Surgical exposure of peripheral nerves of the upper extremity; radial nerve. In: Wolfa CE, Resnick DK, eds. Neurosurgical Operative Atlas, 2nd ed. Spine and Peripheral Nerves. New York: Thieme; 2007:363–367.)

surgery at a mean of 2.5 months sooner following symptom onset than in the latter study.

The role of surgical decompression in radial tunnel syndrome remains unclear and controversial. In their systematic review of observational studies, Huisstede et al[61] noted that the success of surgical decompression ranged from 67 to 92%. Good to excellent relief of symptoms has been reported in 51 to 92% of cases.[62,63] This variability in success rates may be due in part to the existence of concomitant lateral epicondylitis in some patients; other studies have shown poorer outcomes among patients with coexistent lateral epicondylitis.[64] Likewise, poorer outcomes following surgical decompression for radial tunnel syndrome have been reported among patients receiving workers' compensation.[65]

Entrapment of the Superficial Sensory Radial Nerve Branch

Patient Selection

This syndrome is also known as Wartenberg's disease. Diagnosis rests on a careful history, physical exam, and supportive electrodiagnostic studies. Patients usually have paresthesias in the dorsal aspect of the thumb, index finger, and the radial side of the middle finger. Surgery is the treatment of choice when nonsurgical treatments have been unsuccessful for more than 6 months with avoidance of repetitive wrist deviation and elimination of tight bands (tight watches, wrist jewelry and handcuffs, as examples). A contraindication is de Quervain's tenosynovitis, which often entails an irritation of the radial sensory nerve and should be treated before considering decompression.

Surgical Procedure

For decompression, the forearm is positioned midway between supination and pronation. An incision is made 2 cm proximal to the radial styloid along the lateral border of the brachioradialis muscle, avoiding injury to the lateral antebrachial nerve and avoiding tethering of the incision scar over the superficial radial nerve. The SSRN is identified as it exits from under the tendon of the brachioradialis (**Fig. 136.8**). The overlying fascia is divided, taking care not to disturb the nerve.

Postoperative Care and Complications

Surgery usually relieves the symptoms, with an overall good outcome.[66,67] The main complication is related to iatrogenic nerve injury at the time of surgery, which may lead to postoperative scarring and neuroma formation of the nerve. Early joint mobilization is highly encouraged after surgery.

References

1. Khoo D, Carmichael SW, Spinner RJ. Ulnar nerve anatomy and compression. Orthop Clin North Am 1996;27:317–338
2. Amadio PC, Beckenbaugh RD. Entrapment of the ulnar nerve by the deep flexor-pronator aponeurosis. J Hand Surg Am 1986;11:83–87
3. Gonzalez MH, Lotfi P, Bendre A, Mandelbroyt Y, Lieska N. The ulnar nerve at the elbow and its local branching: an anatomic study. J Hand Surg [Br] 2001;26:142–144
4. McCabe SJ, Kleinert JM. The nerve of Henlé. J Hand Surg Am 1990;15:784–788
5. Guyon F. Note sur une disposition anatomique propre à la face antérieure de la région du poignet et non encore décrite. Bull Soc Anat Paris 1861; 6:184–186
6. Posner MA. Compressive neuropathies of the ulnar nerve at the elbow and wrist. Instr Course Lect 2000;49:305–317
7. Atkins SE, Logan B, McGrouther DA. The deep (motor) branch of the ulnar nerve: a detailed examination of its course and the clinical significance of its damage. J Hand Surg Eur Vol 2009;34:47–57
8. Polatsch DB, Melone CP Jr, Beldner S, Incorvaia A. Ulnar nerve anatomy. Hand Clin 2007;23:283–289, v
9. Dumitru D, Walsh NE, Weber CF. Electrophysiologic study of the Riche-Cannieu anomaly. Electromyogr Clin Neurophysiol 1988;28:27–31
10. Zoch G, Meissl G, Millesi H. Results of decompression of the ulnar nerve in Guyon's canal. Handchir Mikrochir Plast Chir 1990;22:125–129
11. Kaiser R, Houšťava L, Brzezny R, Haninec P. [The results of ulnar nerve decompression in Guyon's canal syndrome]. Acta Chir Orthop Traumatol Cech 2012;79:243–248
12. Hacke W. Sensory conduction in the syndrome of Guyon's tunnel. J Neurol 1981;226:195–198
13. Feindel W, Stratford J. Cubital tunnel compression in tardy ulnar palsy. Can Med Assoc J 1958;78:351–353
14. Osborne G. Ulnar neuritis. Postgrad Med J 1959;35:392–396
15. Pechan J, Julis I. The pressure measurement in the ulnar nerve. A contribution to the pathophysiology of the cubital tunnel syndrome. J Biomech 1975;8:75–79
16. Vanderpool DW, Chalmers J, Lamb DW, Whiston TB. Peripheral compression lesions of the ulnar nerve. J Bone Joint Surg Br 1968;50:792–803
17. Aoki M, Takasaki H, Muraki T, Uchiyama E, Murakami G, Yamashita T. Strain on the ulnar nerve at the elbow and wrist during throwing motion. J Bone Joint Surg Am 2005;87:2508–2514
18. Apfelberg DB, Larson SJ. Dynamic anatomy of the ulnar nerve at the elbow. Plast Reconstr Surg 1973;51:79–81

19. Nakamichi K, Tachibana S, Ida M, Yamamoto S. Patient education for the treatment of ulnar neuropathy at the elbow. Arch Phys Med Rehabil 2009; 90:1839–1845
20. Sarris I, Göbel F, Gainer M, Vardakas DG, Vogt MT, Sotereanos DG. Medial brachial and antebrachial cutaneous nerve injuries: effect on outcome in revision cubital tunnel surgery. J Reconstr Microsurg 2002;18:665–670
21. Dellon AL, MacKinnon SE. Injury to the medial antebrachial cutaneous nerve during cubital tunnel surgery. J Hand Surg [Br] 1985;10:33–36
22. Huang JH, Samadani U, Zager EL. Ulnar nerve entrapment neuropathy at the elbow: simple decompression. Neurosurgery 2004;55:1150–1153
23. Kim DH, Midha R, Murovic J, Spinner R, Teil R. Kline and Hudson's Nerve Injuries. Philadelphia: Saunders; 2008
24. Eaton RG, Crowe JF, Parkes JC III. Anterior transposition of the ulnar nerve using a non-compressing fasciodermal sling. J Bone Joint Surg Am 1980; 62:820–825
25. Jaddue DA, Saloo SA, Sayed-Noor AS. Subcutaneous vs submuscular ulnar nerve transposition in moderate cubital tunnel syndrome. Open Orthop J 2009;3:78–82
26. Zarezadeh A, Shemshaki H, Nourbakhsh M, Etemadifar MR, Moeini M, Mazoochian F. Comparison of anterior subcutaneous and submuscular transposition of ulnar nerve in treatment of cubital tunnel syndrome: a prospective randomized trial. J Res Med Sci 2012;17:745–749
27. Broudy AS, Leffert RD, Smith RJ. Technical problems with ulnar nerve transposition at the elbow: findings and results of reoperation. J Hand Surg Am 1978;3:85–89
28. Janjua RM, Fernandez J, Tender G, Kline DG. Submuscular transposition of the ulnar nerve for the treatment of cubital tunnel syndrome. Neurosurgery 2008;63(4, Suppl 2):321–324, discussion 324–325
29. Dellon AL, MacKinnon SE, Hudson AR, Hunter DA. Effect of submuscular versus intramuscular placement of ulnar nerve: experimental model in the primate. J Hand Surg [Br] 1986;11:117–119
30. Inserra S, Spinner M. An anatomic factor significant in transposition of the ulnar nerve. J Hand Surg Am 1986;11:80–82
31. Bartels RH, Menovsky T, Van Overbeeke JJ, Verhagen WI. Surgical management of ulnar nerve compression at the elbow: an analysis of the literature. J Neurosurg 1998;89:722–727
32. Zlowodzki M, Chan S, Bhandari M, Kalliainen L, Schubert W. Anterior transposition compared with simple decompression for treatment of cubital tunnel syndrome. A meta-analysis of randomized, controlled trials. J Bone Joint Surg Am 2007;89:2591–2598
33. Bartels RH, Verhagen WI, van der Wilt GJ, Meulstee J, van Rossum LG, Grotenhuis JA. Prospective randomized controlled study comparing simple decompression versus anterior subcutaneous transposition for idiopathic neuropathy of the ulnar nerve at the elbow: Part 1. Neurosurgery 2005;56:522–530, discussion 522–530
34. Bartels RH, Termeer EH, van der Wilt GJ, et al. Simple decompression or anterior subcutaneous transposition for ulnar neuropathy at the elbow: a cost-minimization analysis—Part 2. Neurosurgery 2005;56:531–536, discussion 531–536
35. Gervasio O, Gambardella G, Zaccone C, Branca D. Simple decompression versus anterior submuscular transposition of the ulnar nerve in severe cubital tunnel syndrome: a prospective randomized study. Neurosurgery 2005;56:108–117, discussion 117
36. Krishnan KG, Pinzer T, Schackert G. A novel endoscopic technique in treating single nerve entrapment syndromes with special attention to ulnar nerve transposition and tarsal tunnel release: clinical application. Neurosurgery 2006;59(1, Suppl 1):ONS89–ONS100, discussion ONS89–ONS100
37. Ahčan U, Zorman P. Endoscopic decompression of the ulnar nerve at the elbow. J Hand Surg Am 2007;32:1171–1176
38. Hoffmann R, Siemionow M. The endoscopic management of cubital tunnel syndrome. J Hand Surg [Br] 2006;31:23–29
39. Heinen CP, Richter HP, König RW, Shiban E, Golenhofen N, Antoniadis G. [The endoscopic management of the cubital tunnel syndrome—an anatomical study and first clinical results]. Handchir Mikrochir Plast Chir 2009;41:23–27
40. Tsai TM, Chen IC, Majd ME, Lim BH. Cubital tunnel release with endoscopic assistance: results of a new technique. J Hand Surg Am 1999;24:21–29
41. Kim DH, Han K, Tiel RL, Murovic JA, Kline DG. Surgical outcomes of 654 ulnar nerve lesions. J Neurosurg 2003;98:993–1004
42. Filippi R, Farag S, Reisch R, Grunert P, Böcher-Schwarz H. Cubital tunnel syndrome. Treatment by decompression without transposition of ulnar nerve. Minim Invasive Neurosurg 2002;45:164–168
43. Millender LH, Nalebuff EA, Holdsworth DE. Posterior interosseous-nerve syndrome secondary to rheumatoid synovitis. J Bone Joint Surg Am 1973; 55:753–757
44. Frohse F, von Bardeleben KH, Fick R, Fränkel M. Die muskeln des menschlichen Armes. Fischer; 1908
45. Riordan DC. Radial nerve paralysis. Orthop Clin North Am 1974;5:283–287
46. Comtet J, Chambaud D. "Spontaneous" paralysis of the posterior interosseous nerve by unusual lesions. Rev Chir Orthop Repar Appar Mot 1975; 61:533–541
47. Konjengbam M, Elangbam J. Radial nerve in the radial tunnel: anatomic sites of entrapment neuropathy. Clin Anat 2004;17:21–25
48. Holstein A, Lewis GM. Fractures of the humerus with radial-nerve paralysis. J Bone Joint Surg Am 1963;45:1382–1388
49. Shah JJ, Bhatti NA. Radial nerve paralysis associated with fractures of the humerus. A review of 62 cases. Clin Orthop Relat Res 1983;172:171–176
50. Suematsu N, Hirayama T. Posterior interosseous nerve palsy. J Hand Surg [Br] 1998;23:104–106
51. Lubahn JD, Cermak MB. Uncommon nerve compression syndromes of the upper extremity. J Am Acad Orthop Surg 1998;6:378–386
52. Albrecht S, Cordis R, Kleihues H, Noack W. Pathoanatomic findings in radiohumeral epicondylopathy. A combined anatomic and electromyographic study. Arch Orthop Trauma Surg 1997;116:157–163
53. Tsai P, Steinberg DR. Median and radial nerve compression about the elbow. J Bone Joint Surg Am 2008;90:420–428
54. Roles NC, Maudsley RH. Radial tunnel syndrome: resistant tennis elbow as a nerve entrapment. J Bone Joint Surg Br 1972;54:499–508
55. Sarhadi NS, Korday SN, Bainbridge LC. Radial tunnel syndrome: diagnosis and management. J Hand Surg [Br] 1998;23:617–619
56. Weitbrecht WU, Navickine E. [Combined idiopathic forearm entrapment syndromes]. Z Orthop Ihre Grenzgeb 2004;142:691–696
57. Stanley J. Radial tunnel syndrome: a surgeon's perspective. J Hand Ther 2006;19:180–184
58. Eaton CJ, Lister GD. Radial nerve compression. Hand Clin 1992;8:345–357
59. Hashizume H, Nishida K, Nanba Y, Shigeyama Y, Inoue H, Morito Y. Non-traumatic paralysis of the posterior interosseous nerve. J Bone Joint Surg Br 1996;78:771–776
60. Portilla Molina AE, Bour C, Oberlin C, Nzeusseu A, Vanwijck R. The posterior interosseous nerve and the radial tunnel syndrome: an anatomical study. Int Orthop 1998;22:102–106
61. Huisstede B, Miedema HS, van Opstal T, de Ronde MT, Verhaar JA, Koes BW. Interventions for treating the radial tunnel syndrome: a systematic review of observational studies. J Hand Surg Am 2008;33:72–78
62. Vrieling C, Robinson PH, Geertzen, JHB. Posterior interosseous nerve syndrome: literature review and report of 14 cases. Eur J Plast Surg 1998; 21(4):196–202
63. Ritts GD, Wood MB, Linscheid RL. Radial tunnel syndrome. A ten-year surgical experience. Clin Orthop Relat Res 1987;219:201–205
64. Lee JT, Azari K, Jones NF. Long term results of radial tunnel release—the effect of co-existing tennis elbow, multiple compression syndromes and workers' compensation. J Plast Reconstr Aesthet Surg 2008;61:1095–1099
65. Sotereanos DG, Varitimidis SE, Giannakopoulos PN, Westkaemper JG. Results of surgical treatment for radial tunnel syndrome. J Hand Surg Am 1999;24:566–570
66. Lanzetta M, Foucher G. Entrapment of the superficial branch of the radial nerve (Wartenberg's syndrome). A report of 52 cases. Int Orthop 1993; 17:342–345
67. Dellon AL, Mackinnon SE. Radial sensory nerve entrapment in the forearm. J Hand Surg Am 1986;11:199–205

C. Pathology of the Lumbosacral Plexus

137 Trauma to the Lumbosacral Plexus

Debora Garozzo

Anatomy

The lumbosacral plexus was first identified by Giulio Casserio in 1632.[1] For descriptive purposes, anatomists usually distinguish three plexuses (the lumbar, the sacral, and the pudendal) that provide motor and sensory innervation for the pelvis and the lower limb, but their anatomic adjacency and interconnection as well as their simultaneous involvement in various clinical syndromes justify including them in a single entity.

The lumbosacral plexus (**Fig. 137.1**) is formed by the anterior divisions of the spinal nerves from L1 to S4; near their origins they receive gray rami communicantes from the lumbar ganglia of the sympathetic trunk. In contrast with its brachial counterpart, where these structures form an intricate interlacement, within the lumbosacral plexus they divide into anterior and posterior branches from which several nerves of distribution arise.

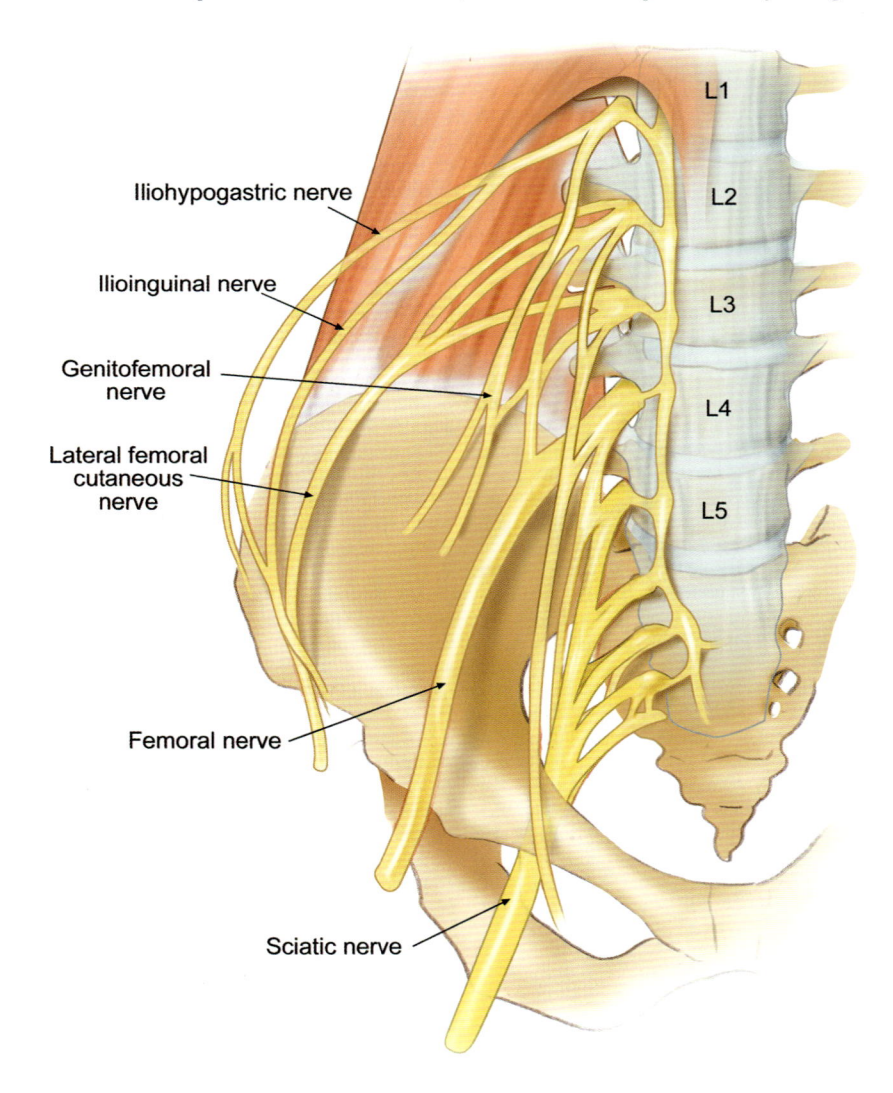

The lumbar plexus (**Fig. 137.2**) originates from the ventral primary rami of the L1–L4 spinal nerves that pass downward and laterally from the lumbar spine and enter the psoas major muscle to form the plexus. The L1 anterior division, usually supplemented by a twig from the last thoracic nerve, splits into two

Fig. 137.1 The lumbosacral plexus.

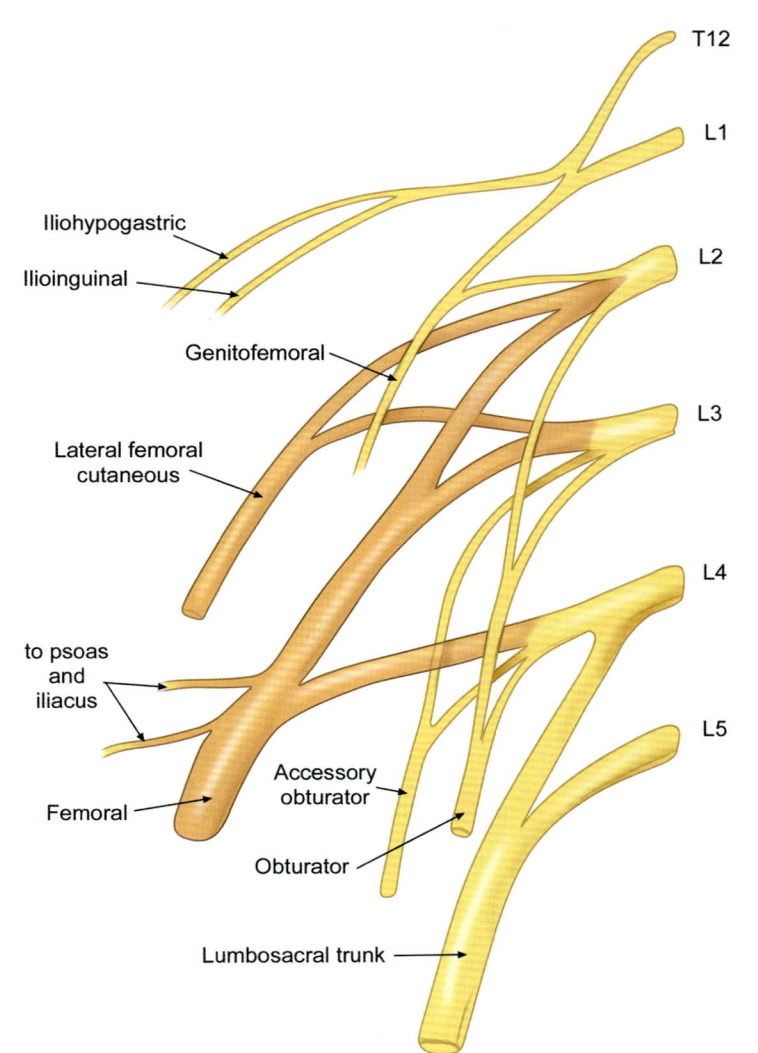

Fig. 137.2 The lumbar plexus.

branches: the upper, and larger, one divides into the iliohypogastric and ilioinguinal nerves; the lower, and smaller, one joins a branch from the second lumbar nerve, giving origin to the genitofemoral nerve.

The remainder of the second lumbar nerve and the third and fourth nerves split into ventral and dorsal branches. The three ventral divisions (the one from the third division is the largest, whereas the branch from the second nerve is generally very thin) of the L2–L4 nerves join together and branch off the obturator nerve, which emerges from the medial border of the psoas muscle near the brim of the pelvis and then runs behind the common iliac vessels, on the lateral side of the hypogastric vessels (that separate the nerve from the ureter), along the wall of the lesser pelvis in proximity with the obturator vessels. Through the upper obturator foramen, it enters the thigh where it divides into two branches. The obturator nerve is responsible for the sensory innervation of the medial aspect of the thigh; it also innervates the adductor muscles of the lower extremity (external obturator, adductor longus, abductor brevis and magnus) and the pectineus (variably) and gives off branches for the hip joint.

Each dorsal division of the second and third lumbar nerves splits into two branches—one small and one large. The two small branches form the lateral femoral cutaneous nerve. The large branches, joining the dorsal division from the fourth ventral nerve, give origin to the femoral nerve, which is the largest nerve of the lumbar plexus. It emerges from the lower part of the lateral border of the psoas muscle, passes between the psoas and iliacus muscles, courses deep to the inguinal ligament lateral to the femoral artery and vein, and reaches the anterior thigh. Within the abdomen, it gives off small branches to the iliacus muscle and a branch distributing to the femoral artery. In the upper thigh it splits into its terminal branches: an anterior division giving off sensory branches for the anterior surface of the thigh and muscular branches for the pectineus and sartorius, and a posterior division that supplies the four parts of the quadriceps femoris and also provides articular branches for the knee joint. It ends in the saphenous nerve that descends in Hunter's canal, emerges through the fascia above the knee, and runs down the medial side of the tibia, providing sensory innervation for the medial surface of the leg, ankle, and arch of the foot.

Table 137.1 details the collateral and terminal branches of the lumbar plexus.

The lumbar plexus communicates with the sacral plexus via the lumbosacral trunk. This structure is formed by some fibers from the fourth and all of those from the fifth lumbar ventral branch of the spinal nerve. It passes over the ala of the sacrum

Table 137.1 Collateral and Terminal Nerves of the Lumbar Plexus: Motor and Sensory Innervation

Nerve	Nerve Roots	Innervated Muscles	Sensory Innervation
Iliohypogastric nerve	T12-L1	Transversus abdominis, abdominal internal oblique	Skin of the lateral hip and above the inguinal ligament
Ilioinguinal nerve	L1	Transversus abdominis, abdominal internal oblique	Skin over the pubic symphysis and the lateral aspect of the labra majora or scrotum
Genitofemoral nerve	L1-L2	Cremaster (in males)	Scrotal skin or labra majora
Lateral femoral cutaneous nerve	L2-L3		Anterolateral skin of the thigh
Obturator nerve	L2–L4	Obturator externus, adductors (magnus, longus, brevis), gracilis, pectineus	Medial thigh
Femoral nerve	L2–L4	Iliopsoas, quadriceps, pectineus, sartorius	Anterior thigh, medial leg
Direct branches from the plexus	T12–L4	Psoas major, quadratus lumborum, lumbar intertransverse	

adjacent to the sacroiliac joint and its union with the ventral rami arising from the S1–S4 nerves and gives origin to the sacral plexus.

The sacral plexus (**Fig. 137.3**) lies on the posterior and posterolateral walls of the pelvis and converges toward the sciatic notch; it has only one terminal branch—the sciatic nerve. This is the largest nerve of the human body, measuring 2 cm in breadth; it supplies nearly all the skin of the leg, the muscles of the back of the thigh, and those of the leg and foot.

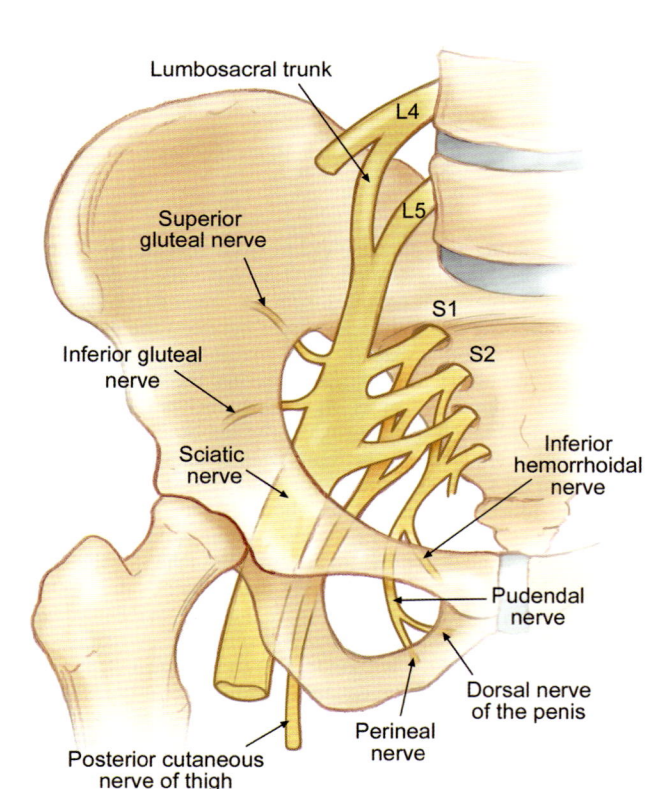

The sciatic nerve is made up of two distinct nerve trunks—medial and lateral. Like their lumbar counterpart, the sacral ventral rami split into ventral and dorsal branches. From the union of the lumbosacral trunk and the dorsal branches of the S1 and S2 spinal nerve ventral rami, the sciatic lateral trunk arises. The ventral branches of the same ventral rami (L4–S2) join and form the medial trunk.

The two trunks generally run together, sharing a common sheath from their origin to the lower third of the back of the thigh: at this level they separate from each other, continuing as the terminal branches of the sciatic nerve. Sometimes they can run in close proximity but separately for all or part of their course.

Once formed, the sciatic nerve leaves the pelvis through the greater sciatic notch. In the buttock, it runs downward between the ischial tuberosity and the greater trochanter, lying close to the capsule of the hip joint; it is covered by the gluteus maximus muscle. It continues distally deep in the thigh branching off for the hamstring muscles and then eventually splitting into the tibial nerve and the common peroneal nerve just proximal to the popliteal fossa; the former is the medial, thicker branch and provides sensory and motor innervation to the anterior compartment of the leg, whereas the latter is the thinner common peroneal nerve that innervates the skin and muscles of its posterior compartment.

The collateral nerves of the sacral plexus are the gluteal nerves, the posterior cutaneous nerve of the thigh, and the pudendal nerve.

Table 137.2 details the sensory and motor innervations provided by the collateral and terminal branches arising from the sacral plexus.

The above description is of the most common presentation of the anatomy of the lumbosacral plexus. However, dissection studies have demonstrated high variability in the findings; the prevalence of anatomic variations in the individual nerves can range from 8.8 to 44.1%, with a mean prevalence of 20.1%. Variations include the absence of the iliohypogastric nerve, the

Fig. 137.3 The sacral plexus.

Table 137.2 Collateral and Terminal Branches of the Sacral Plexus: Motor and Sensory Innervation

Nerve	Nerve Roots	Innervated Muscles	Sensory Innervation
Superior gluteal nerve	L4–S1	Gluteus medius and minimus, tensor fascia latae	
Inferior gluteal nerve	L5–S2	Gluteus maximus	
Posterior cutaneous femoral nerve (also known as small sciatic nerve)	S1–S3		Gluteal skin, perineum, posterior thigh and leg
Direct branches from plexus	S1-S2	Piriformis	
Direct branches from plexus	L5–S2	Obturator internus and superior gemellus	
Direct branches from plexus	L4–S1	Quadratus femoris and inferior gemellus	
Sciatic nerve	L4–S3	Semitendinous, semimembranous, biceps femoris, adductor magnus	
Common peroneal nerve: superficial branch	L4–S2	Peronei longus and brevis	Anterolateral aspect of the lower leg and dorsum of the foot
Common peroneal nerve: deep branch		Tibialis anterior, extensors digitorum longus and brevis, extensor hallucis longus and brevis, peroneus tertius	
Tibial nerve	L4–S3	Triceps surae, plantaris, popliteus, tibialis posterior, flexor digitorum longus, flexor hallucis longus	Sole of the foot
Tibial nerve: medial plantar		Abductor hallucis, flexor digitorum brevis, flexor hallucis brevis (medial head), I-II lumbricals	
Tibial nerve: lateral plantar		Flexor hallucis brevis (lateral head), quadrates plantae, abductor digiti minimi, flexor digiti minimi, III-IV lumbricals, plantar and dorsal interossei, adductor hallucis	
Pudendal nerve	S2–S4	Muscles of the pelvic floor	

presence of the accessory obturator nerve, variations in the origin or splitting of several collateral nerves, as well as the above-mentioned variations in the course of the sciatic nerve.[2]

Causative Mechanisms of Lumbosacral Plexus Injuries

A posttraumatic injury of the lumbosacral plexus was first described in 1960.[3] Since then, these injuries have received less attention in the medical literature in comparison with other nerve lesions, probably due to their presumed rarity; however, their actual incidence is unknown.

Because of its protected position within the pelvis, posttraumatic injuries of the lumbosacral plexus are undoubtedly far less common than their brachial counterparts and generally occur in massive life-threatening traumas. Therefore, when these patients are admitted to the hospital, the physicians' attention is usually drawn to the life-threatening injuries, and a thorough neurologic examination is difficult or impossible to conduct; furthermore, as the patients are often unconscious or uncooperative, they do not demonstrate palsy. Therefore, the neurologic complication associated with the pelvic trauma easily goes unrecognized. If it is noted, the motor impairment is attributed to the bone injuries; less than 50% of lumbosacral plexus injuries (LSPIs) are detected during early diagnostic assessment.[4–7] Thus they may actually be more frequent than thought until now; the literature reports an incidence of LSPIs of between 40% and 52% in pelvic ring traumas,[4,8] and some authors recommend obtaining an early electromyogram (EMG) to determine the presence of neurologic complications in these patients.[9]

The LSPIs occur during automobile accidents in ~ 60% of the cases.[7] This explains why there are no relevant differences in gender incidence and no specific age peak (in contrast to brachial plexus injuries, which mainly occur during motorcycle accidents and therefore generally affect young men in their second or third decade of life). The automobile accidents often are due to driving off the road, or they involve a frontal or lateral impact with another vehicle, the guardrail, or trees lining the road. The patient becomes trapped in the car and sustains a crush injury, such as a pelvic ring fracture or a perforating injury of the internal organs. Although every kind of pelvic bone injury can occur (including comminuted pelvic fractures), iliac iliopubic fractures, sacral fractures, femoral fractures and dislocations (**Fig. 137.4**)

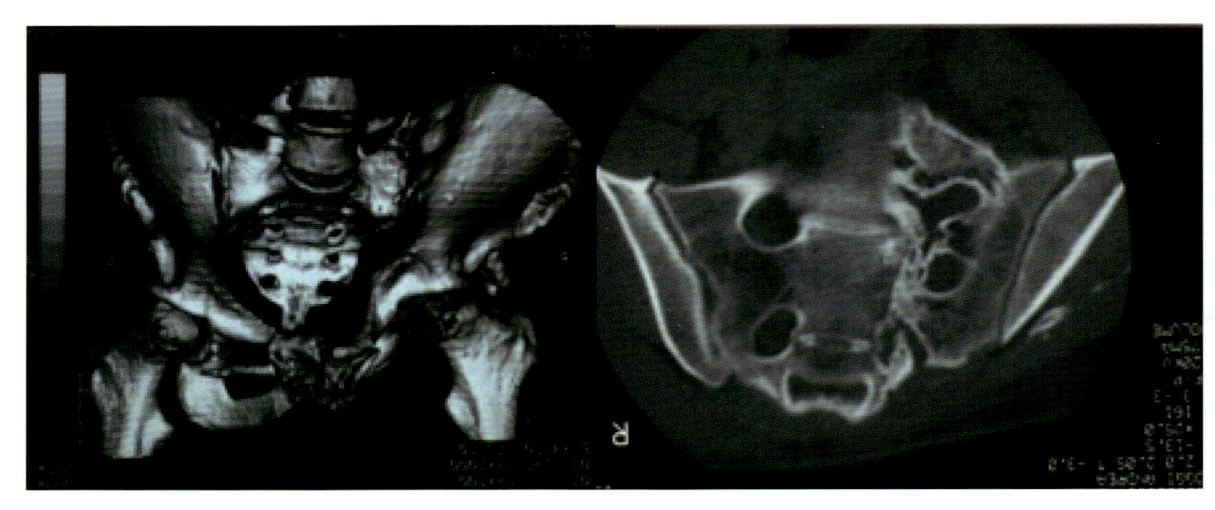

Fig. 137.4 (a) Acetabular fracture. (b) Sacral fracture.

are more frequent; the latter type is generally due to the fact that the driver often stomps forcefully on the brake trying to avoid the impact or instinctively braces the foot against the floor in an attempt to hold oneself back. In these patients, neurologic complications are generally the consequence of compression injuries caused by fractures or dislocated bone fragments, whereas traction injuries and in particular avulsions are less likely to occur.

In the orthopedic literature,[4,10–14] transection of nerve roots and avulsions are seldom associated with sacral fractures, whereas compression injuries of the spinal nerves are well recognized. In Denis's classification,[15] zone 1 fractures (**Fig. 137.5a**), accounting for 50% of sacral fractures, are associated with an L5 (which runs on the top of the sacral wing) injury in 6% of cases; zone 2 fractures (**Fig. 137.5b**) (34% of sacral fractures) present neurologic complications in 28% of cases due to injuries of L5, S1, and S2; zone 3 fractures (**Fig. 137.5c**) (16% of sacral fractures) result in sacral root injuries in up to 58% of cases. Transverse fractures (**Fig. 137.5d**) (considered a subtype of zone 3 fractures) are associated with nerve injuries in up to 97% of cases, one third of which are transections. Upper transverse fractures involving S1–S3 cause urinary dysfunction more frequently than do lower transverse fractures.

Femoral fractures are also associated with compression injuries; a perifracture hematoma may form inside the inextensible space delimited by the iliac fascia anteriorly and the internal surface of the hip bone posteriorly, resulting in compression on the lumbar plexus roots.[4,7]

Compression injuries of the lumbosacral plexus also occur during other types of causative events that are responsible for crushing pelvic traumas: the literature reports LSPIs occurring in pedestrians who are run over by motor vehicles and in manual laborers accidently crushed by silos or asphalt slabs during work accidents.

Motorcycle accidents are less common causative events but they are responsible for more severe injuries to the lumbosacral plexus.[7] These accidents always involve high kinetic energy; during the traumatic impact at high speed, the patient is often hurled off the cycle and thrown to the ground. Forced flexion-abduction of the hip, posterior dislocation of the hip, and hyperextension of the thigh with external rotation of the fractured or dislocated part of the pelvis are associated with severe traction injuries that often result even in root avulsions. In motorcycle accidents, the most common bone injuries are sacroiliac joint dislocations, found in more than 50% of cases; these bone injuries are almost invariably associated with root avulsions.[4,7]

Severe traction injuries also result during traumas from falling from a height, such as in work accidents (e.g., falling from a scaffold) or suicide attempts.

Traction injuries may also occur in breech delivery, although there is a dearth of information on their natural history due to their extreme rarity.

Concerning other causative mechanisms, LSPIs due to gunshots are rarely described in the literature, probably because gunshot injuries are often fatal; in contrast, iatrogenic injuries of the lumbosacral plexus are often reported. Gunshot and iatrogenic injuries entail greater involvement of the upper portion of the lumbosacral plexus,[10] whereas LSPIs that result from motor vehicle accidents generally damage the lower plexus.

Most gunshot injuries are caused by high-velocity bullets. The nerve damage is the result not only of the direct action of the bullet but also of the shock waves and cavitation effects that have impact on the surrounding soft and muscular tissues, bones, and internal organs. Therefore, the initial picture always appears to be more severe during the first evaluation and then there is a progressive, partial recovery during the following weeks of observation.

Iatrogenic injuries of the lumbar plexus have been described after hip arthroplasty or pelvic and abdominal surgery; the neurologic complication is usually the consequence of a nerve ischemia due to excessive traction by self-retaining retractors. However, surgical revisions have occasionally demonstrated accidental nerve transections.

The literature also reports lumbar plexus injuries following surgical fusion of the lumbosacral spine. Extreme lateral interbody fusion (XLIF) is associated with a 3% incidence of lumbar plexus injuries that rises to 3.8% if the L4-L5 level is included in the procedure,[16] despite the use of continuous and evoked EMG monitoring; these lesions are the consequence of a combination of compression (resulting from posterior retraction) and stretch of the lumbar plexus from aggressive table flexion to facilitate access to the disk in anatomically challenging situations. Lumbar plexus injuries are more likely to occur in lateral lumbar interbody fusion when recombinant human bone morphogenetic protein-2 (rhBMP-2) is used, although the mechanism remains to be determined.[17]

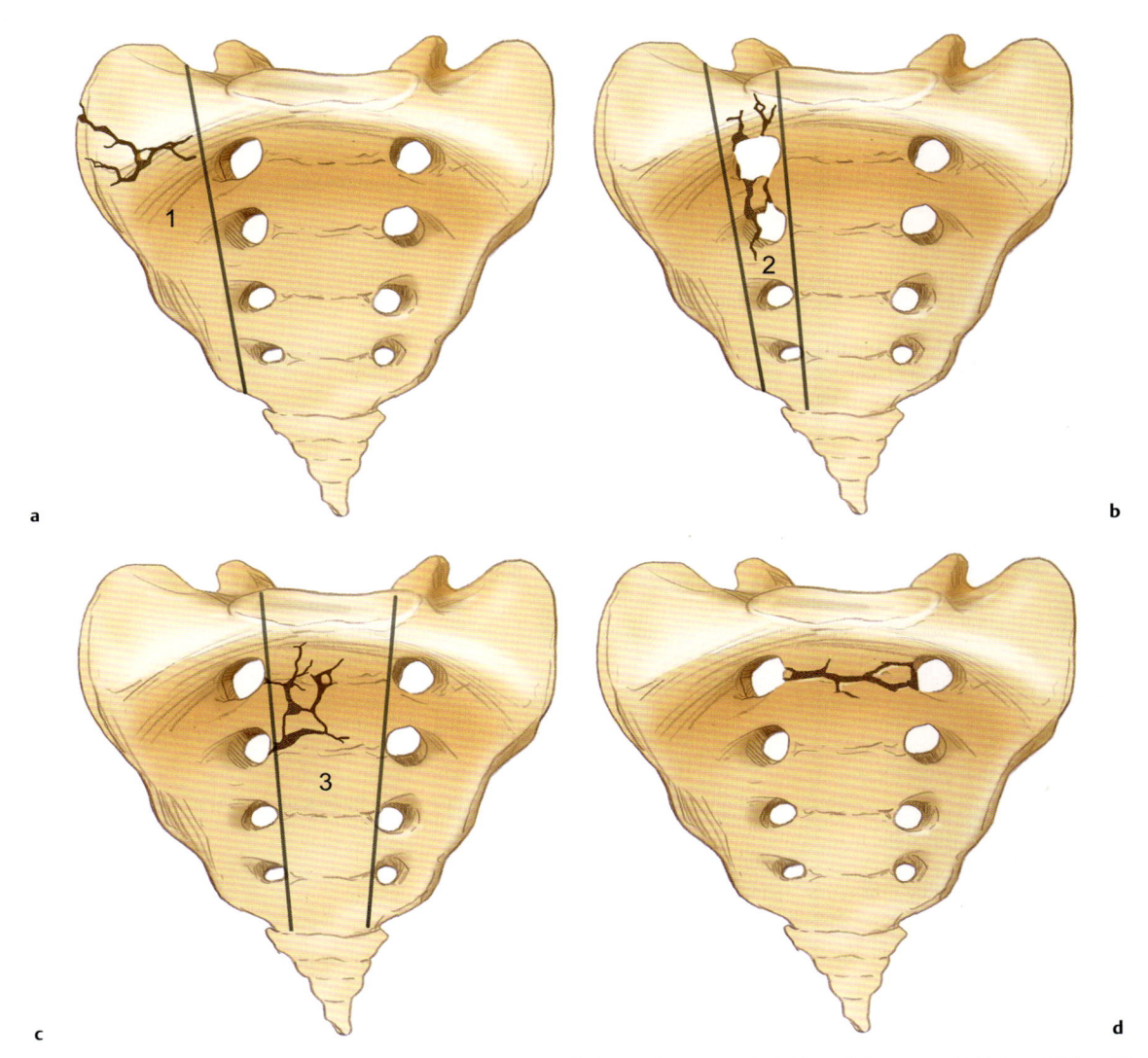

Fig. 137.5 umbosacral plexus injuries associated with sacral fractures classified according to Dennis. **(a)** Zone 1 fracture and L5 injury. **(b)** Zone 2 fractures and L5, S1 and S2 injuries. **(c)** Zone 3 fractures and sacral root injuries. **(d)** Transverse sacral fracture and sacral root transection.

Clinical Presentation

As previously mentioned, LSPIs generally occur during severe, massive life-threatening traumas. Bone fractures and dislocations of the pelvis and the proximal lower limb, vascular lesions, and injuries of the endopelvic organs are directly correlated, and highly so, with damage to the lumbosacral plexus.

Bone injuries have been found in up to 90% of patients.[7] As previously mentioned, although every kind of pelvic bone injury is likely to occur, some fractures are statistically more prevalent, and there is a correlation between the causative mechanism and the bone injury associated with the plexal lesion.

Up to 30% of these patients present with injuries of the endopelvic organs.[7] The most common internal lesion is an extraperitoneal bladder rupture that is clinically revealed by hematuria, abdominal pain, or swelling. It is caused by direct penetration of a bone fragment after ischiopubic or symphysis fractures or rupture or stretch injury of the puboprostatic ligament, and is more likely to happen when the organ is full. Intestinal perforation of the terminal sigmoid colon or rectum frequently occurs as well. Injuries of the endopelvic organs generally require urgent surgery.

In 10% of these cases, a rupture of the gluteal or iliac artery/vein causing a retroperitoneal bleeding that requires urgent embolization has been described.[7]

A thorough neurologic examination is difficult to perform in the acute phase of the injury.[4,7] In contrast to its brachial counterpart, bilateral impairment of the lumbosacral plexus often occurs.[5,7]

A careful examination of the hip girdle and leg muscles usually enables determining whether the injury involves the spinal roots, the plexus, or individual peripheral nerves (**Table 137.3**). Occasionally, when several peripheral nerves have been simultaneously injured by the trauma, it might be almost impossible to distinguish this condition from one that involves the plexus. Evaluating the proximal muscles (iliopsoas, hip adductors, and gluteal muscles) is particularly helpful in making an accurate diagnosis. For example, in lumbar plexus injuries the most striking clinical abnormality is the functional impairment of the quadriceps, with numbness of the skin over the anterior thigh. When

876 VI Peripheral Nerves

Table 137.3 Differential Diagnosis of Neurologic Deficit in the Lower Limb

	Muscle Involvement	Sensory Loss	Reflex Loss
Roots			
L4	Quadriceps, hip adductors, gluteus medius, tibialis anterior	L4 dermatome (medial lower leg and ankle)	Knee
L5	Gluteus medius and maximus, tibialis anterior and posterior, extensors digitorum and hallucis longus, peronei, hamstrings	L5 dermatome (anterolateral lower leg and dorsum of foot)	Ankle
S1	Gluteus medius and maximus, hamstrings, peronei, gastrocnemius, flexor digitorum longus, intrinsic foot muscles	S1 dermatome (sole and lateral surface of foot and ankle)	Ankle
Plexus			
Lumbar plexus	Iliopsoas, quadriceps, hip adductors	Anterior, medial, and lateral surfaces of the thigh and medial aspect of the lower leg	Knee
Lumbosacral trunk	Glutei, peronei, tibialis anterior and posterior, extensors digitorum and hallucis longus	Mainly L5 dermatome	
Sacral plexus	Glutei, hamstrings, peronei, gastrocnemius, tibialis anterior and posterior, extensors digitorum and hallucis longus	Buttock and perineum, posterior surfaces of thigh and calf, anterolateral aspect of the lower leg, sole of foot	Ankle
Nerves			
Femoral nerve	Quadriceps	Anterior surface of the thigh and anteromedial surface of the lower leg	Knee
Obturator nerve	Hip adductors	Upper medial thigh	
Sciatic nerve	Hamstrings, peronei, gastrocnemius, tibialis anterior and posterior, extensors digitorum and hallucis longus, intrinsic foot muscle	Leg and foot	Ankle

testing the proximal muscles, they demonstrate weakness in the iliopsoas and the hip adductors, and the clinical presentation points to a lumbar plexopathy more than just a femoral nerve injury. If the glutei muscles are not carefully evaluated (**Fig. 137.6**), a sacral plexus injury can easily be mistaken for a sciatic nerve injury. Loss of activity in the glutei muscles impairs pelvic stability, resulting in a positive Trendelenburg's sign (**Fig. 137.7**).

Lumbosacral trunk injuries are generally more difficult to diagnose. The most striking clinical sign is a foot drop that easily fools the uninitiated into thinking that the injury involves the common peroneal nerve. Yet in the latter case, weakness of the glutei and the tibialis posterior muscles is not present.

Care should be taken also in analyzing sensation along the lower limb. If sensation on the dorsal aspect of the thigh is preserved (due to intact function of the posterior cutaneous nerve) in association with abolished function of the hamstrings and muscles distal to the knee, then a sacral plexus injury must be ruled out and the diagnosis is a proximal sciatic injury.

To assess the function of the lower nerves of the plexus, it is necessary to rule out sensory deficits in the perianal and perineal areas and to test the anal and bulbocavernosus reflexes too.

Clinical examination identifies four injury patterns: lumbar plexus injury, lumbosacral trunk injury, sacral plexus injury, and complete lumbosacral plexus injury.

As previously mentioned, lumbar plexus injuries have been more frequently described after gunshot or iatrogenic injuries, whereas they have been seldom found after motor vehicle accidents or sports injuries, which are associated with femoral fractures in more than 50% of cases.[4,7] In the literature, in the absence of bone injuries, lumbar plexus lesions have been occasionally described in association with a bulky hematoma in the psoas muscle as demonstrated on a computed tomography (CT) scan.[7]

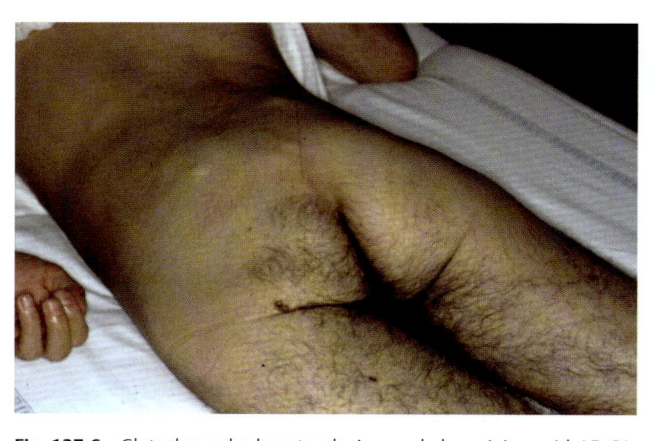

Fig. 137.6 Gluteal muscles hypotrophy in sacral plexus injury with L5, S1, and S2 avulsions

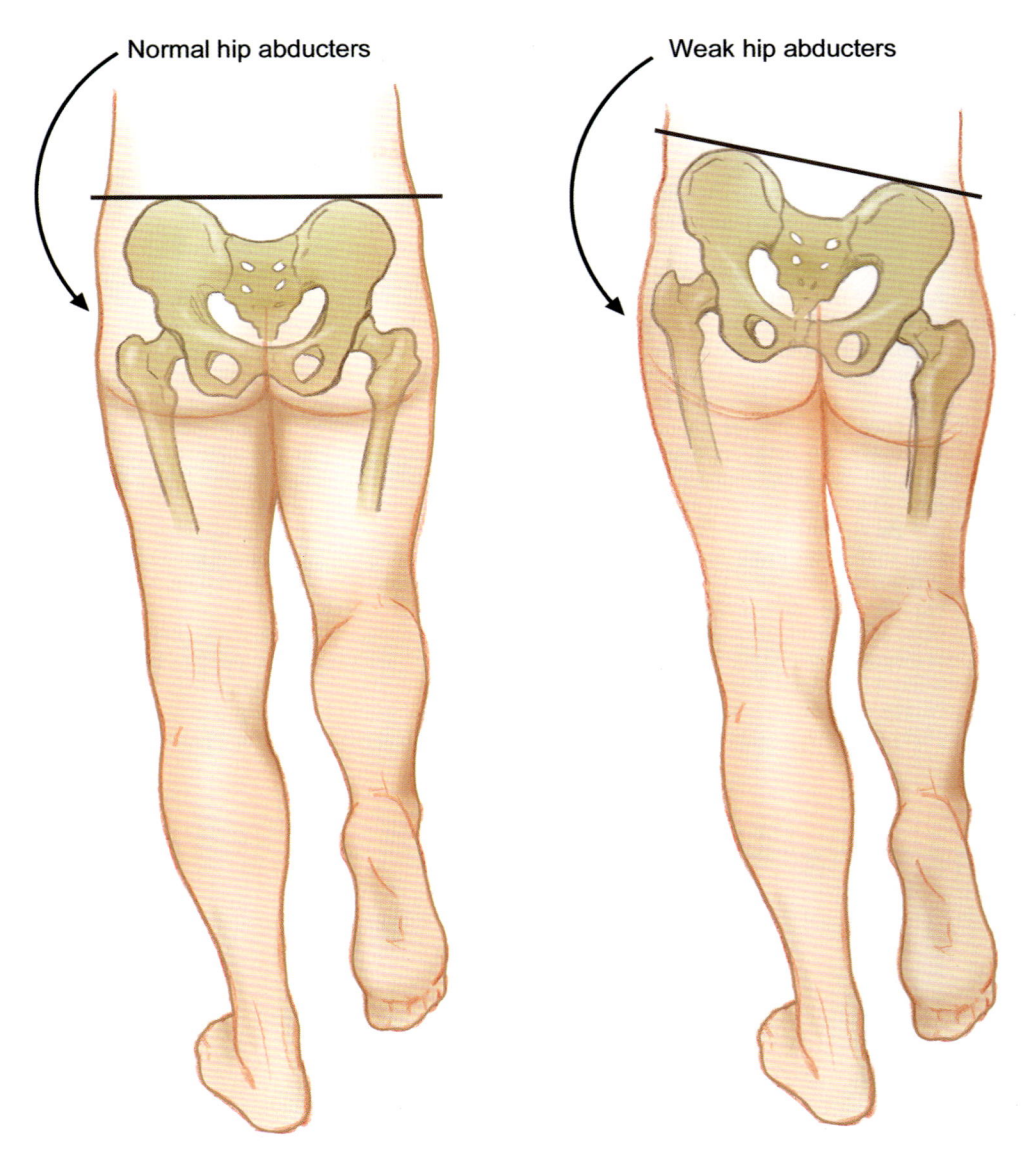

Fig. 137.7 Trendelenburg's sign.

The typical neurologic presentation includes iliopsoas muscle weakness associated with quadriceps palsy. An impairment of the adductors is seldom described. Sensory loss involves anterior, lateral, and medial surfaces of the thigh.

Lumbosacral trunk injuries are the most frequent injury pattern: the patient generally presents an impairment of the lateral sciatic trunk (peroneal muscles, tibialis anteriori, extensor digitorum and extensor hallucis longus) and a partial impairment of the medial trunk (tibialis posterior) associated associated with Trendelenburg's sign due to gluteal muscle weakness. Sensory loss is distributed mainly along the L5 dermatome.

Sacral plexus injuries are the second most statistically common injury pattern. The function of the iliopsoas, hip adductors, and quadriceps is preserved, but all the other muscles of the thigh and leg are paralyzed; sensory loss occurs on the skin covering the buttock, perineum, posterior aspect of the thigh and calf, anterolateral lower leg, and sole of foot. Abolished sphincter control and severe, shooting pain (providing clinical evidence of root avulsions) along the lower limb may complete the clinical presentation.

Total palsies, fortunately, are rare; they are responsible of severe invalidity as they involve loss of function in all the muscles of the hip, thigh, leg, and foot. Loss of sphincter control sometimes is also associated with impairment of sexual function in patients with this injury pattern; moreover, these patients often suffer from excruciating leg pain.

Management of Lumbosacral Plexus Injuries

The LSPIs should always be suspected in pelvic traumas, and a careful neurologic examination should be attempted in spite of its limits during the acute phase.

In sacral fractures allegedly associated with neurologic complications, experience has demonstrated that early traction, limiting the rise of the hip bone and the lateral fragment of the aileron, reduces the compression, which, together with surgical realignment, favors neurologic recovery.[4]

In gunshot injuries, the bullet wound should receive immediate treatment to avoid complications, in particular infections.

If the clinical examination raises the suspicion of a posttraumatic injury of the lumbosacral plexus, the patient should undergo electrodiagnostic and neuroradiological studies to assess the extent and severity of the nerve damage.

The main purpose of these examinations is to determine the presence of root avulsions: preganglionic injuries cannot recover spontaneously.

It is better to perform electrodiagnostic studies 3 to 4 weeks after the traumatic event, as early EMG cannot distinguish between neurapraxia and more severe forms of nerve damage (axonotmesis or neurotmesis). Information given by such techniques is anyway inferred and not directly demonstrated; thus, imaging is actually the core of the diagnostic assessment. But it must be emphasized that the absence of pseudomeningocels does not exclude avulsions and viceversa (intact roots have been visualized inside meningoceles), yet it must be emphasized that these bulky, mushroom-shaped images consequent to the dural tear occurring when the roots are violently pulled out from the spinal cord are still fundamental in the diagnostic assessment of plexal injuries. Therefore, neuroradiological studies also should be performed at least 3 weeks after the trauma, due to the fact that pseudomeningoceles need a few weeks to form.

Three-dimensional magnetic resonance imaging (MRI) (**Fig. 137.8**) should be considered the modality of choice, because of its high diagnostic accuracy and the advantage of not being an invasive investigation like a CT myelogram (**Fig. 137.9**). It can also give information on the muscle denervation in correlation with the signal intensity.[18]

Whereas in brachial plexus injuries neuroradiological examinations reveal root avulsions in more than 70% of cases, they seem to occur in less than 25% of LSPIs[7] and have been found only in sacral plexus and complete lumbosacral plexus injuries (**Figs. 137.8 and 137.9**). L5 and S1 are the most frequently avulsed roots; L3 and L4 avulsions are less common and the upper roots are never found avulsed.

Once the diagnostic assessment is completed, patients should be referred to a peripheral nerve surgeon, who will ultimately determine whether the injury is amenable to spontaneous recovery or requires surgical treatment.

Regardless of the indications for surgery or conservative treatment, patients should start rehabilitation as soon as possible. Intensive physiotherapy is absolutely mandatory to prevent muscle degeneration and joint stiffness with further worsening of the initial clinical picture. A kick-up brace should be prescribed whenever needed.

In severe, devastating LSPIs pain management is of paramount importance. Uncontrolled, excruciating pain is extremely detrimental, as it renders rehabilitation impossible and completely disrupts the patient's life. It must be emphasized that in LSPIs pain is not only the consequence of the orthopedic lesions associated with the nerve injuries but also is due to the deafferentation following root avulsions.

A multidisciplinary approach is necessary to obtain adequate pain control, including medical therapy, physical treatments,

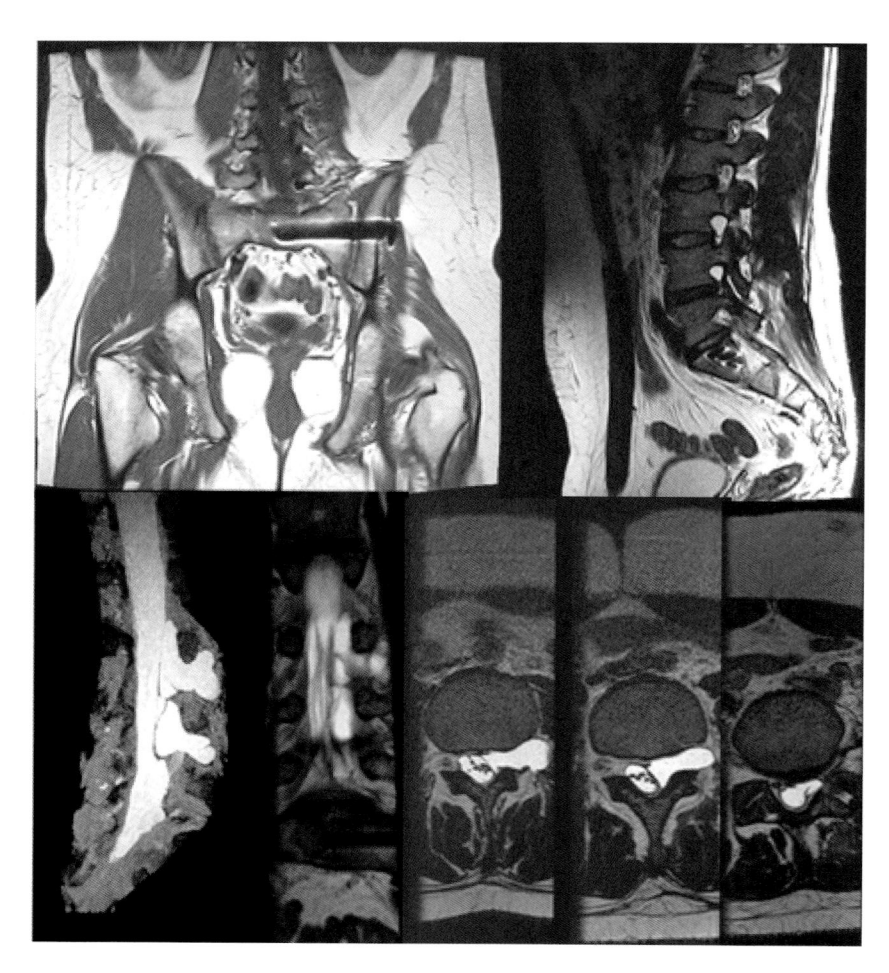

Fig. 137.8 Magnetic resonance imaging (MRI) studies of a complete lumbosacral plexus injury with multiple avulsions. The patient had previously undergone iliosacral screwing

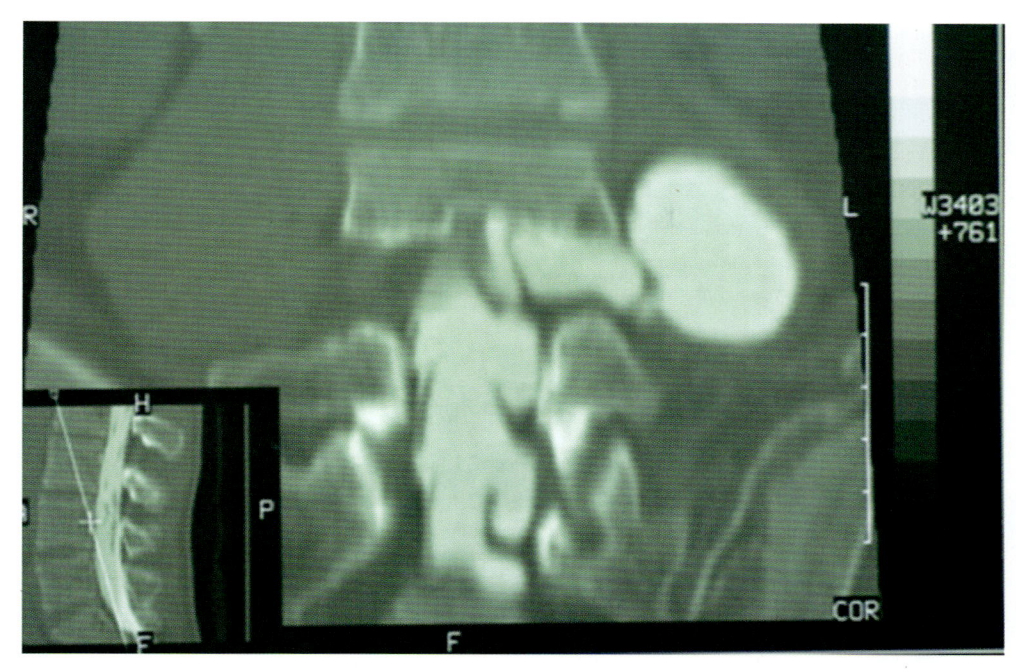

Fig. 137.9 Computed tomography myelogram in a lumbosacral plexus injury with avulsions.

and psychological support. Tricyclic antidepressants, opiates, and more recently pregabalin (which has almost completely replaced gabapentin) and tapentadol are the medications more frequently prescribed (often in combination) for the treatment of neuropathic/deafferentation pain.

It has been largely demonstrated that reintegrating the patient as soon as possible into an active life, both socially and professionally, has a positive effect on pain control. Mirror visual feedback treatment gives favorable results in chronic pain of central origin, and could possibly be applied in these cases, although no such use has been reported. Nevertheless, it must be acknowledged that in severe deafferentation pain only some degree of symptom control is possible, and in some cases treatment is ineffective; in such cases, surgical options (e.g., dorsal root entry zone [DREZ]otomy) should be advocated.

Sildenafil is also offered to patients with impaired sexual functions.[4]

Natural History

Spontaneous recovery of LSPIs occurs in 50 to 70% of cases at between 8 and 36 months (average, 18 months).[4,7,13]

Complete, spontaneous recovery seems to be the rule in lumbar plexus injuries associated with femoral fractures with the reabsorption of the perifracture hematoma. Lumbar plexus injuries associated with detection of an hematoma in the psoas are also invariably susceptible to spontaneous recovery.

Iatrogenic injuries normally present spontaneous recovery when caused by traction of self-retaining retractors. Lumbar plexus injuries complicating XLIF always recover well in 6 to 8 months.[16]

Lumbosacral trunk injuries as well as sacral plexus and complete lumbosacral injuries with no avulsions also recover spontaneously in a high percentage, although complete restitution to the original condition is unlikely, as minor sequelae such as hallux extensor and gluteus medius deficits are extremely frequent.[4,13] In some cases, spontaneous recovery only involves the sciatic medial trunk, and the foot drop remains as permanent deficit.[7]

The low rate of avulsions in comparison with the brachial counterpart is not the only explanation for the high frequency of spontaneous recovery of LSPIs.[5] As previously mentioned, the lumbosacral plexus frequently presents anatomic variations, occurring as extradural or intradural anastomosis as well as extradural nerve root divisions. Some of the recovery is likely to occur as collateral sprouting from healthy or less severely injured neighboring nerves.

References

1. Casserio G. Tabulalae Anatomicae. Bucretius; 1632
2. Anloague PA, Huijbregts P. Anatomical variations of the lumbar plexus: a descriptive anatomy study with proposed clinical implications. J Manual Manip Ther 2009;17:e107–e114
3. Finney LA, Wulfman WA. Traumatic intradural lumbar nerve root avulsion with associated traction injury to the common peroneal nerve. Am J Roentgenol Radium Ther Nucl Med 1960;84:952–957
4. Tonetti J, Cazal C, Eid A, et al. [Neurological damage in pelvic injuries: a continuous prospective series of 50 pelvic injuries treated with an iliosacral lag screw]. Rev Chir Orthop Repar Appar Mot 2004;90:122–131
5. Lang EM, Borges J, Carlstedt T. Surgical treatment of lumbosacral plexus injuries. J Neurosurg Spine 2004;1:64–71
6. Hersche O, Isler B, Aebi M. [Follow-up and prognosis of neurologic sequelae of pelvic ring fractures with involvement of the sacrum and/or the iliosacral joint]. Unfallchirurg 1993;96:311–318
7. Garozzo D, Zollino G, Ferraresi S. In lumbosacral plexus injuries can we identify indicators that predict spontaneous recovery or the need for surgical treatment? Results from a clinical study on 72 patients. J Brachial Plex Peripher Nerve Inj 2014;9:1
8. Lindahl J, Hirvensalo E. Outcome of operatively treated type-C injuries of the pelvic ring. Acta Orthop 2005;76:667–678
9. Weis EB Jr. Subtle neurological injuries in pelvic fractures. J Trauma 1984;24:983–985
10. Chiou-Tan FY, Kemp K Jr, Elfenbaum M, Chan KT, Song J. Lumbosacral plexopathy in gunshot wounds and motor vehicle accidents: comparison

of electrophysiologic findings. Am J Phys Med Rehabil 2001;80:280–285, quiz 286–288
11. Stoehr M. Traumatic and postoperative lesions of the lumbosacral plexus. Arch Neurol 1978;35:757–760
12. Rai SK, Far RF, Ghovanlou B. Neurologic deficits associated with sacral wing fractures. Orthopedics 1990;13:1363–1366
13. Majeed SA. Neurologic deficits in major pelvic injuries. Clin Orthop Relat Res 1992;282:222–228
14. Sabiston CP, Wing PC. Sacral fractures: classification and neurologic implications. J Trauma 1986;26:1113–1115
15. Denis F, Davis S, Comfort T. Sacral fractures: an important problem. Retrospective analysis of 236 cases. Clin Orthop Relat Res 1988;227:67–81
16. Coe J, Meyer S. Lumbar plexus palsy after XLIF. An avoidable complication? Presented at the Society for Minimally Invasive Spine Surgery (SMISS) 2009 Annual Conference, Las Vegas
17. Lykissas MG, Aichmair A, Sama AA, et al. Nerve injury and recovery after lateral lumbar interbody fusion with and without bone morphogenetic protein-2 augmentation: a cohort-controlled study. Spine J 2014;14:217–224
18. Bendszus M, Koltzenburg M, Wessig C, Solymosi L, Sequential MR. Sequential MR imaging of denervated muscle: experimental study. AJNR Am J Neuroradiol 2002;23:1427–1431

138 Tumors of the Lumbosacral Plexus

Carlos E. Restrepo Rubio, Scott P. Zietlow, and Robert J. Spinner

Tumors of the lumbosacral plexus are relatively uncommon. The natural history of these tumors is unpredictable. The indications and techniques for operative intervention of these lesions are not well described.[1–4] Operative management requires consideration of many factors, including the age and health of the patient, the presence of clinical symptoms and findings, the imaging characteristics, the size and histology of the lesion (if available), as well as the accessibility of the tumor and the estimated risks of surgery.

In our experience, the most common benign nerve sheath tumor in patients overall is a schwannoma if you exclude patients with neurofibromatosis type 1 (NF1). Patients with NF1 develop neurofibromas much more commonly than schwannomas. The plexiform neurofibroma is characterized by its producing a diffuse enlargement of the plexus or nerve trunks and branches and is almost pathognomonic of NF1; it entails a 5 to 10% risk of developing malignant peripheral nerve sheath tumors (MPNSTs); however, MPNSTs may also occur sporadically or in those who have had prior radiation. The lumbosacral plexus also may be invaded by the malignant tumors of pelvic organs (so-called neoplastic lumbosacral plexus lesion), including rectal, prostate, cervical, and bladder cancer; involvement may be from direct, contiguous spread, or from perineural spread from the primary organ that was affected.[5]

This chapter discusses distinguishing benign masses from malignant nerve sheath tumors; exposing and obtaining direct access to the lumbosacral plexus, including their major branches; resecting a benign nerve sheath tumor safely; and improving symptoms and preserving normal function. The management of malignant lesions is controversial and beyond the scope of this review.

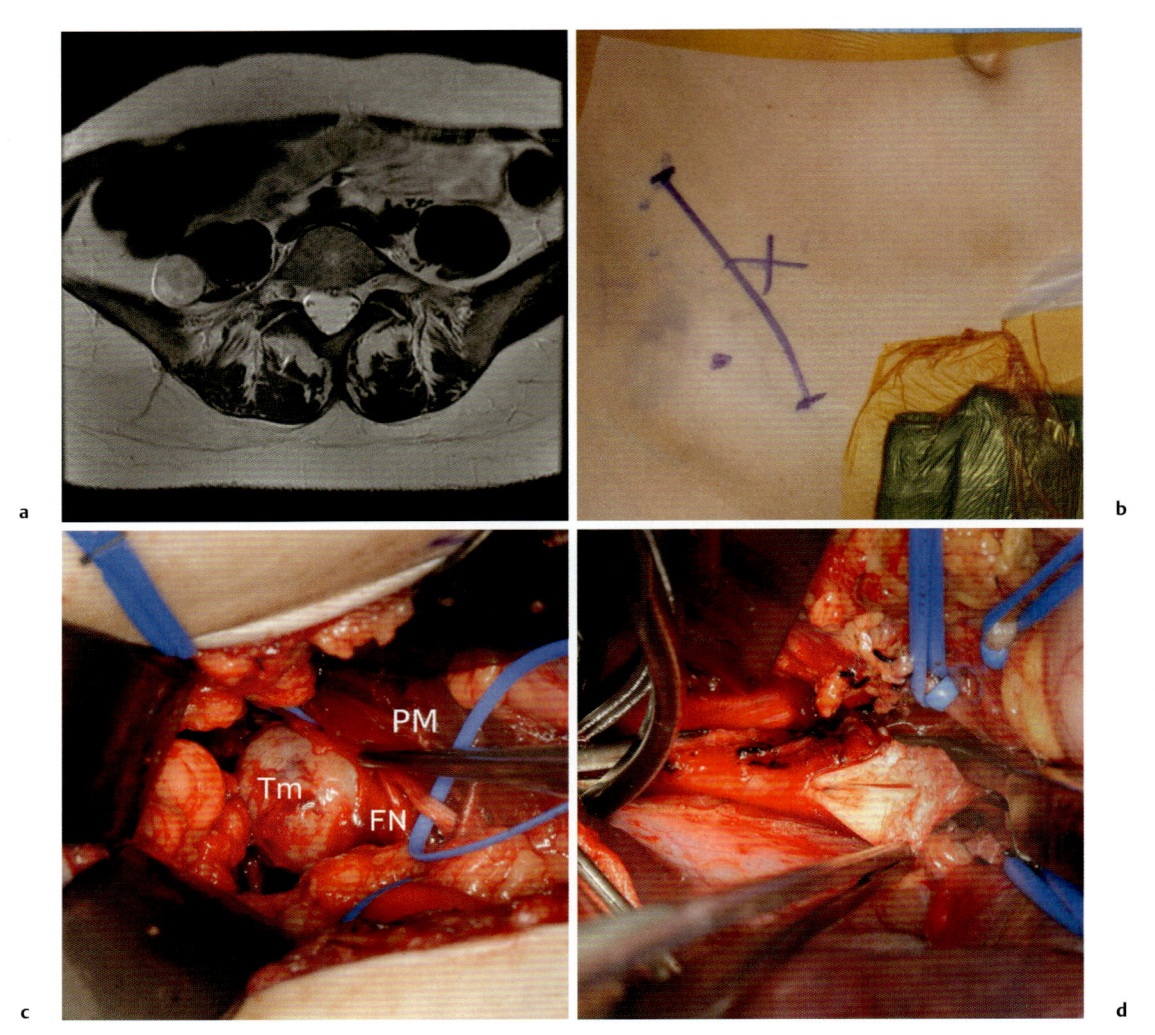

Fig. 138.1 A 39-year-old woman presented with persistent right thigh and medial leg pain. She had subjective sensory loss on the anterior thigh and medial leg. **(a)** An axial T2-weighted magnetic resonance imaging (MRI) of the pelvis demonstrated a 3-cm psoas mass suggestive of a benign peripheral nerve tumor in the femoral nerve (note the "target" sign). **(b)** An ilioinguinal retroperitoneal approach was done. **(c)** The tumor (Tm) was found within the psoas muscle (PM). Proximal and distal control of the femoral nerve (FN) was obtained. Genitofemoral nerve was identified (in a vasoloop). A small longitudinal opening in the bare area (i.e., away from fascicles) enabled a fascicular level resection of this tumor. **(d)** Total resection was achieved, sparing the nerve. Pathology was consistent with a schwannoma. Postoperatively the patient noticed immediate improvement in her pain, and her motor function was intact.

Indications

Benign nerve sheath tumors (e.g., schwannomas, neurofibromas) can be treated surgically if they cause local pain, radiating paresthesias or dysesthesias (**Figs. 138.1 and 138.2**), as well as other compressive symptoms from mass effect on other pelvic organs. Masses that enlarge while being observed or those presenting at a large size also should be surgically resected. There is a relative advantage to resecting asymptomatic or minimally symptomatic tumors that needs to be considered when weighing the risk/benefit ratio of surgery. Larger tumors are more difficult to resect safely and often present with more symptoms. Many benign nerve sheath tumors tend to grow slowly, and young patients may be at some increased risk of having tumors enlarge as they age. Tumors often present at a large size in the pelvic region because they have a wide space in which to grow before becoming symptomatic. Benign nerve sheath tumors generally have characteristic features on magnetic resonance imaging (MRI).

Patients with malignant lesions (either primary or secondary) tend to present differently. They often have severe pain (typically refractory to medications and narcotics) and neurologic deficits (predominantly weakness). Malignancies often demonstrate atypical MRI findings, such as irregular contours (**Fig. 138.3a**) and enhancement as well as necrosis (**Fig. 138.3b**). These patients undergo positron emission tomography (PET) scans, which characteristically show increased avidity (**Fig. 138.3c**). We recommend close collaboration with experienced radiologists who can be of tremendous help in distinguishing benign from malignant nerve sheath tumors and in distinguishing tumors from other lesions that may have tumor-like appearances (including inflammatory or systematic infiltrative lesions). Patients in whom there is a suspicion of malignancy based on clinical or

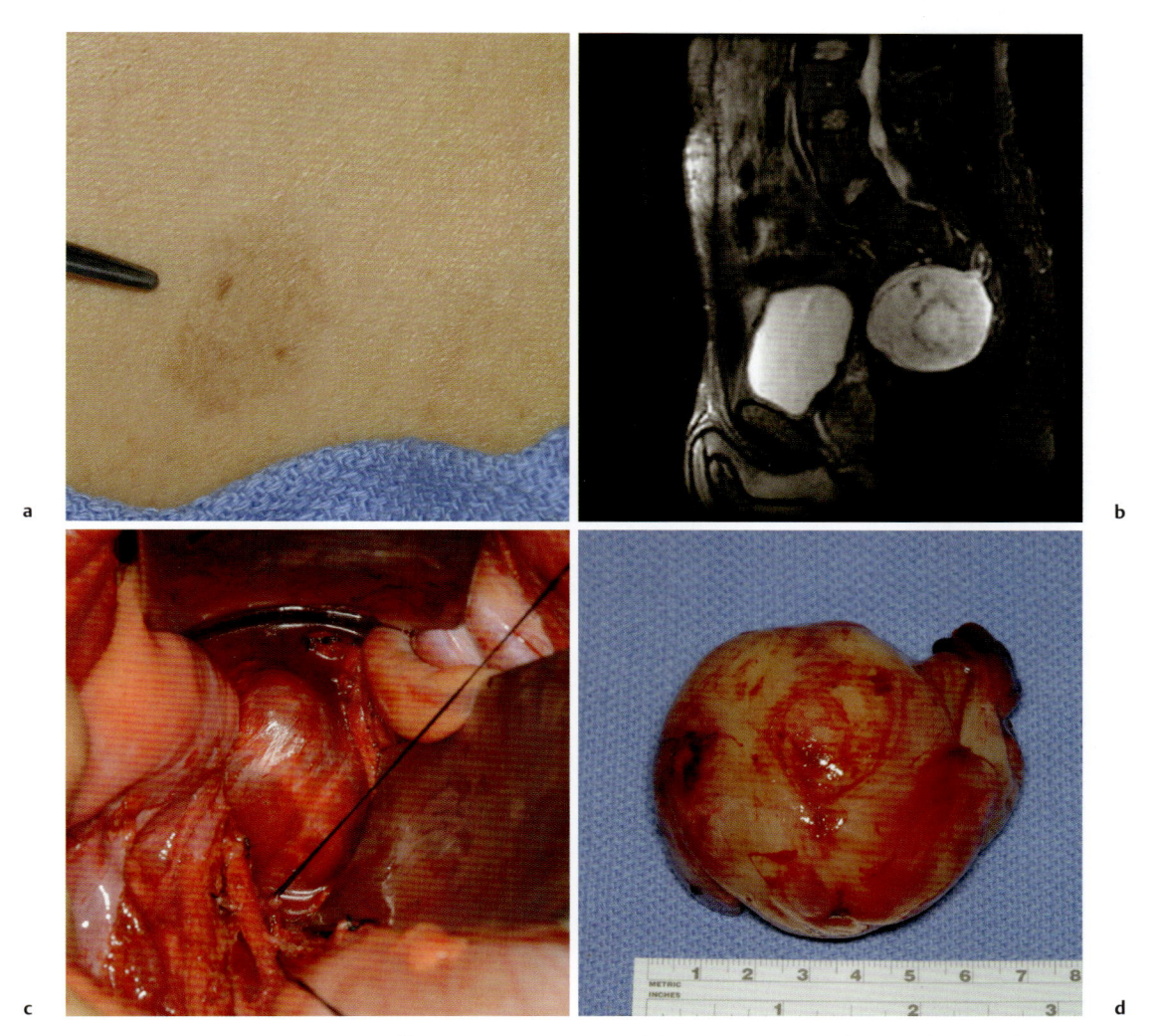

Fig. 138.2 A 40-year-old man with a history of neurofibromatosis type 1 (NF1) presented with transient problematic dysesthesias in the left leg and lower abdominal discomfort. **(a)** On physical examination, he had stigmata of NF1 including a café-au-lait spot and cutaneous neurofibroma near the planned abdominal incision. Motor testing was normal. **(b)** Sagittal T2-weighted MR showed a presacral lesion originating from the left S3 root. A transabdominal transperitoneal approach was made using a midline incision. **(c)** The large mass was visualized displacing the rectum to the right. The sheath of the tumor was opened and peeled off of the tumor with its accompanying nerve fibers. **(d)** Total resection was accomplished. Histology was consistent with a neurofibroma.

radiological features should undergo a preoperative biopsy; for suspected MPNSTs, this is often done percutaneously by image guidance (**Fig. 138.3d**); for suspected secondary lesions, this may be done by an open biopsy.

Contraindications

- Absolute: intrapelvic tumors with extensive invasion
- Relative: elderly age, medical comorbidities, asymptomatic small lesions that have been stable on serial imaging

Advantages

Benign nerve sheath tumors can often be resected completely and safely. Resection of these tumors by experienced surgeons typically leads to clinical improvement without additional neurologic sequelae. Long-term radiological follow-up is unnecessary. The recurrence rate after gross total resection is negligible.

Disadvantages

The lumbosacral plexus exposure is difficult; it requires assistance from surgical colleagues. Neurosurgeons may have limited exposure to this type of lesion due to its rarity.

Surgical Technique

Anesthesia

General anesthesia is utilized. Preoperatively, the surgeon should advise the anesthetist that the neuromuscular blockade used in induction must wear off during the early phase of the dissection so that intraoperative electrical recording can be done and the

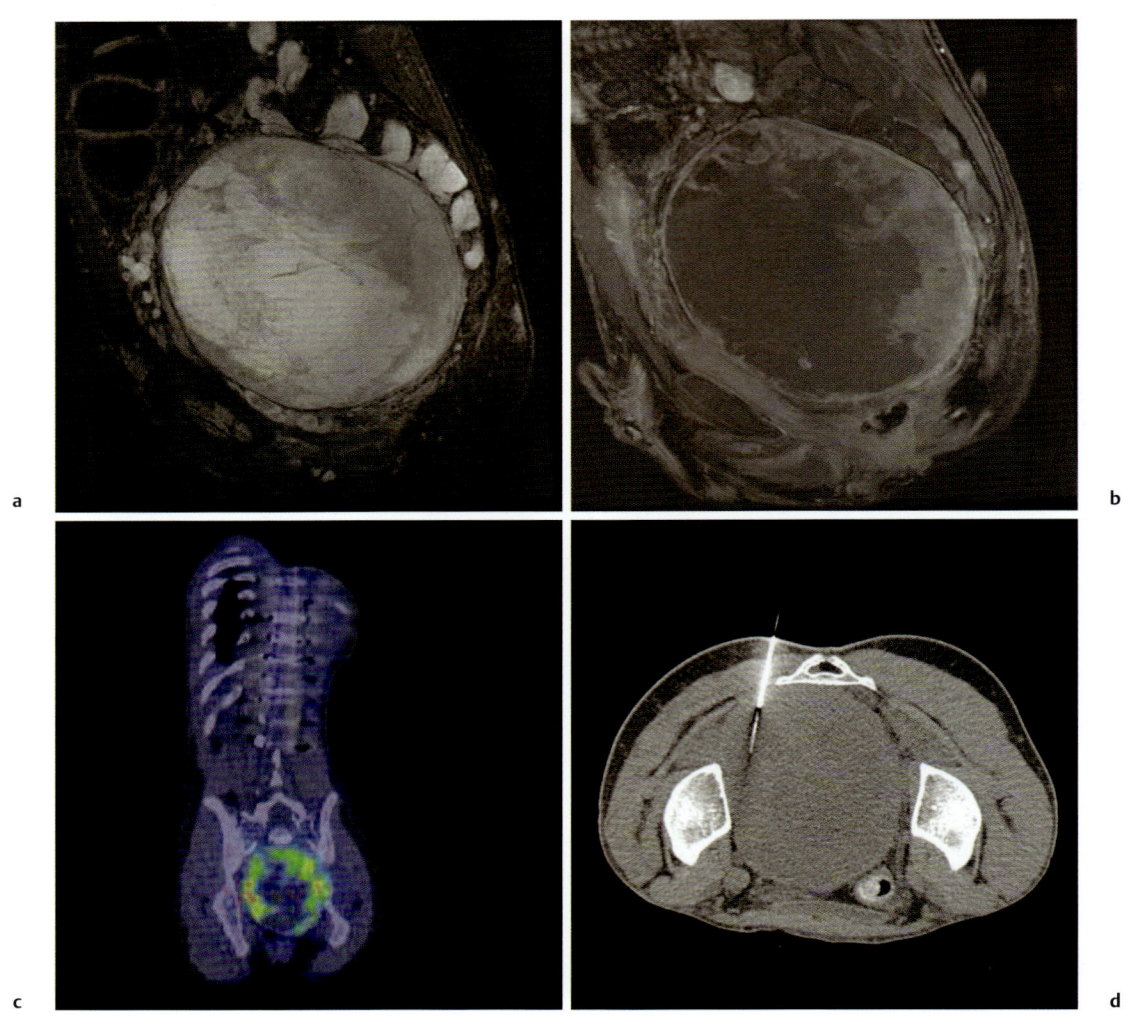

Fig. 138.3 A 22-year-old patient with NF1 presented with left leg pain and progressive weakness that had gradually intensified. The pain was not relieved with narcotic medications. **(a)** T2-weighted sagittal MRI of the pelvis demonstrated a plexiform neurofibroma affecting the lumbosacral plexus along with a large presacral heterogeneous mass. **(b)** The tumor enhanced heterogeneously with gadolinium and showed areas of necrosis. **(c)** A positron emission tomography (PET)/computed tomography (CT) scan showed intense avidity of the tumor, suggesting malignancy. **(d)** A CT-guided needle biopsy was performed confirming an malignant peripheral nerve sheath tumor (MPNST) with rhabdomyoblastic differentiation.

effects of appropriate muscle contraction from the stimulation can be tested. Local anesthetic should be avoided due to the possibility of a nerve conduction block, which may cause errors in recording intraoperative nerve action. For large tumors, especially those in the presacral space, needle electromyography (EMG) monitoring of lumbosacral muscles in the limbs and perineum is performed. Occasionally, stent placement may be helpful in identifying the ureters intraoperatively in cases where the anatomy is distorted.

Positioning and Exposure

Tumors involving the lumbar plexus are treated slightly differently depending on anatomic considerations, such as the nerve of origin or standard bony landmarks including the anterior superior iliac spine, iliac crest, pubic symphysis, and 12th rib. For lower lumbar plexal lesions, the patient is placed in the supine position with a slight bump placed behind the lowerback/lumbar area using a rolled towel. For more proximal lesions, an increasingly lateral position is used.

In our practice, an access general surgeon exposes tumors involving the lumbar plexus through a retroperitoneal approach (as described in Chapter 89). A relatively limited skin incision is made based on the location of the tumor (**Fig. 138.1b**). A modified ilioinguinal approach is used for central or lower lumbar plexal tumors. A muscle-splitting approach is used, staying lateral to the rectus abdominis. A 2-cm width of fascia attached to the iliac crest is maintained to prevent hernia formation and to decrease pain postoperatively. Occasionally, a more posterolateral flank-type incision may be used exclusively or in conjunction with the previous incision over the iliac crest for more proximal tumors or when additional exposure is needed. For proximal exposure, the 12th rib can be resected in an extraperitoneal and extrapleural fashion. Our neurosurgical team assists with the exposure, initially to help identify and preserve cutaneous branches (including the subcostal and lateral femoral cutaneous nerves for the more proximal tumors) and later to safely identify the tumor and its parent nerve. The retroperitoneal space is entered and the peritoneal contents (and the kidney, if necessary) are retracted medially. In general, the tumors are located within the psoas muscle, and blunt dissection is performed directly toward the tumor, sparing more superficially located sensory nerves (including the genitofemoral, ilioinguinal, and iliohypogastric nerves).

Tumors involving the lumbosacral plexus are surgically treated with the patient in the supine position. The approach to these tumors involving the lumbosacral plexus is done by a colorectal surgeon, sometimes with the assistance of a vascular surgeon. A transabdominal transperitoneal approach is used typically through a midline incision for bigger tumors, but a Pfannenstiel incision can be used for smaller ones or in some thinner patients. Abdominal and pelvic contents are mobilized, and the presacral space is entered inbetween the bifurcation of the iliac vessels (**Fig. 138.2c**). As necessary, major vessels are mobilized. The position of the ureters must be appreciated during the exposure and prior to tumor dissection and resection.

On rare occasion, dumbbell tumors need to be treated individually via differing approaches, incorporating exposure of either the spine (laminectomies) or the sciatic notch region.

In general, for benign lesions, nerve grafting is not necessary.

Tumor Resection

Once the surgical approach is done, the tumor is easily recognizable and palpable because of its size. Whenever possible, proximal and distal control of the parent nerve of the tumor is obtained to identify the normal anatomy. The nerve is enveloped in vasoloops and gently suspended. Other neighboring nerves or communicating branches are also identified to avoid their injury. At this time the nerve stimulator can be helpful in distinguishing among the motor and sensory nerves.

Conventional nerve sheath tumors are generally resectable and should be approached with the intent of complete extirpation. An often achievable goal is the resection without neurologic sequelae. The majority of lesions can be removed in toto as a single specimen separating the tumor from the nerve (**Fig. 138.1d**).

A longitudinal opening is made in the tumor capsule in a bare zone (i.e., away from fascicles). The pseudocapsule is identified and maintained. The usual finding is of a tumor growing within the substance of the nerve with uninvolved fascicles splayed around the center of the mass. Schwannomas tend to be more eccentrically located and neurofibromas more centrally located. With a microsurgical technique, fascicles are gently dissected free of the tumor in the extracapsular plane. As the tumor is thus gradually exposed and the proximal and distal poles are approached, care should be taken to isolate any fascicles. Schwannomas are noted to have fascicles that run within the capsule but are unlikely to have intratumoral fascicles of significance, although they occur in the superficial layers of very large tumors. The entering and exiting fascicle(s) at the poles are sought. In deep dissections, they may not always be identified. Schwannomas are thought to have a single fascicle at each pole, whereas neurofibromas may have more fascicles entering and exiting the substance of the tumor at their poles. Resection of any fascicle should not be done until the late stage of the procedure when the tumor itself is about to be definitively removed and the surgeon is confident that any fascicle cannot be maintained. The redundant tumor capsule is not resected.

Occasionally, for larger lesions, intracapsular enucleation and a piecemeal approach may be used. A longitudinal incision is made in the capsule between fascicles, and the tumor is debulked from within. The smaller, remaining tumor can then be mobilized more readily and resected. We favor removing the tumor in one piece as we believe the debulking method entails a higher risk of leaving tumor behind. For plexiform lesions, debulking predominant tumor nodules may be the goal, as complete resection may not be realistic.

Immaculate hemostasis in the tumor bed is achieved. Closure is done in layers. A drain is not utilized. Patients are advised to avoid heavy lifting and strenuous activity for 6 weeks. Follow-up visits are scheduled at 3 months and at 1 year. A single postoperative MRI may be useful in documenting complete resection and serving as a baseline should there be a symptomatic recurrence.

References

1. Benzel EC, Morris DM, Fowler MR. Nerve sheath tumors of the sciatic nerve and sacral plexus. J Surg Oncol 1988;39:8–16
2. Kim DH, Midha R, Murovic JA, Spinner RJ. Kline & Hudson's Nerve Injuries: Operative Results for Major Nerve Injuries, Entrapments, and Tumors, 2nd ed. Philadelphia: Saunders Elsevier; 2008
3. Robertson JH, Gropper GR, Dalrymple S, Acker JD, McClellan GA. Sacral plexus nerve sheath tumor: case report. Neurosurgery 1983;13:78–81
4. Donner TR, Voorhies RM, Kline DG. Neural sheath tumors of major nerves. J Neurosurg 1994;81:362–373
5. Capek S, Howe BM, Tracy JA, García JJ, Amrami KK, Spinner RJ. Prostate cancer with perineural spread and dural extension causing bilateral lumbosacral plexopathy: case report. J Neurosurg 2015;122:778–783

D. Surgery of the Lumbosacral Plexus

139 Approach to the Nerves of the Lower Extremity

Jonathan D. Choi and Allan H. Friedman

The nerves of the lower extremity are the "neglected stepsister" of the nerves of the upper extremity. Nerve entrapment syndromes of the lower extremity are less well appreciated, and nerve injuries in the lower extremity are thought to have a poorer prognosis. Publications by Kline et al[1-3] have demonstrated that repair of the nerves in the lower extremity can be successful. This chapter discusses the anatomy and surgical exposure of the nerves in the lower extremity, including new approaches designed to decrease approach-related morbidity.

Patient Selection

Patients present with compression neuropathies, tumors, and trauma, with injury to the nerve. Selection for surgery is based on multiple factors, including the underlying disease process, the severity of the neurologic symptoms such as severe pain or motor weakness, the focality of the pathology, and the ability of the patient to undergo surgery. The clinical aspects of nerve entrapment syndrome and the techniques of peripheral nerve repair are not discussed in this chapter.

Indications and Contraindications

Indications include injury to a nerve (partial or complete transection), tumor (benign or malignant), and entrapment syndrome. Contraindications include medical causes of neuropathy not amenable to surgical decompression, and patient health not amenable to undergoing surgery.

Advantages and Disadvantages

There are multiple ways to approach the peripheral nerves of the lower extremity. The larger incision approaches provide better visualization of the nerve and associated anatomy at the expense of increased approach-related morbidity from disruption of normal tissue and anatomic planes. More recent approaches have been focused on minimizing the disruption of normal tissue and decreasing the approach-related morbidity. These procedures are technically more challenging due to the decreased visualization of anatomy and the smaller opening in which to work. Both types of approaches are discussed.

Choice of Operative Approach

The anatomy and choice of surgical approach for each major peripheral nerve of the lower extremity are discussed below in separate sections for each peripheral nerve.

Preoperative Testing and Imaging

A complete history is taken and a physical exam is performed, including a detailed neurologic workup. Laboratory tests are ordered to evaluate the metabolic causes of neuropathy. A nerve conduction study, electromyography (EMG) testing, and magnetic resonance imaging (MRI) are ordered when appropriate to determine the presence of a possible tumor and to narrow the differential diagnosis.

Surgical Procedure

In the following subsections, each major peripheral nerve of the lower extremity is discussed, including the pertinent anatomy and the surgical approaches.

Lateral Femoral Cutaneous Nerve

The lateral femoral cutaneous nerve originates most frequently from the ventral rami of the second and third lumbar nerve roots. After emerging from behind the psoas muscle, the nerve lies on the iliacus muscle, passing just under the pelvic brim to exit under the inguinal ligament and over the sartorius muscle approximately one fingerbreadth medial to the anterior superior iliac spine (**Figs. 139.1 and 139.2**).[4] The nerve may run through the inguinal ligament or through the attachment of the sartorius muscle. Rarely, the nerve may run over the top of the anterior superior iliac spine. In the upper thigh the nerve travels in a tunnel within the deep fascia. Approximately 5 cm beyond the iliac crest it divides into an anterior and a posterior branch, both of which pierce the fascia lata, ~ 10 cm distal to the inguinal ligament.

Exposure of the lateral femoral cutaneous nerve in the pelvis is rarely indicated. When lateral femoral cutaneous nerve muscle is found in the pelvis, it is exposed by opening the abdominal wall along the anterior pelvis brim. The lateral femoral cutaneous nerve is found lying on the iliacus muscle lateral to the femoral nerve beneath the iliac fascia. The first author (J.D.C.) and Robert Isaacs have removed a schwannoma from a patient's lumbar plexus using the NuVasive MaXcess extreme lateral interbody fusion (XLIF) retractor system (NuVasive, San Diego, CA) to approach the tumor through a 3-cm incision laterally at the iliac crest. The small incision and the approach through the retroperitoneal fat minimizes blood loss and approach-related morbidity.

Most frequently the surgeon is interested in identifying the nerve as it passes under the inguinal ligament. Because it is often difficult to find the nerve at the level of the inguinal ligament,

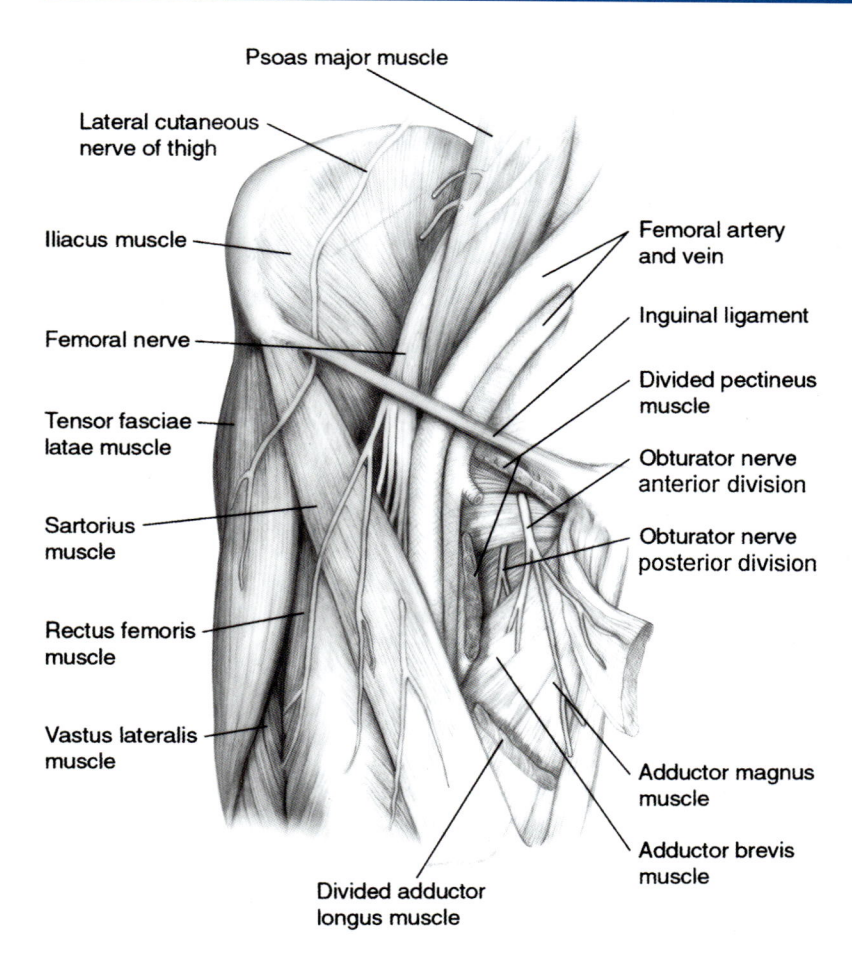

Fig. 139.1 The lateral femoral cutaneous nerve travels under the iliacus fascia just beneath the pelvic brim emerging over the medial border of the sartorius muscle. The obturator nerve travels lateral to the internal iliac vessel. The anterior branch of the obturator nerve travels behind the pectineus and adductor longus muscles and in front of the adductor brevis and longus. The posterior branch of the obturator nerve travels behind the adductor brevis.

the nerve is best identified 2 or 3 inches beyond the ligament by opening the deep fascia over the sartorius muscle. A branch of the lateral femoral cutaneous nerve identified at this level can be followed proximally by the surgeon to the tunnel under the inguinal ligament.

Femoral Nerve

The femoral nerve is formed in the substance of the psoas muscle from the dorsal portion of the ventral rami of the second, third, and fourth lumbar nerve roots. The nerve emerges from the psoas major muscle at the pelvic brim and travels in the groove between that muscle and the iliacus muscle under the cover of the iliac fascia (**Fig. 139.2**). The femoral nerve enters the thigh from under the inguinal ligament lateral to the femoral artery. Prior to reaching the inguinal ligament, the sensory fibers migrate anteriorly and the motor fibers migrate posteriorly within the nerve. At the level of the ligament, a small branch innervates the pectineus muscle; 1 to 2 inches distal to the ligament the nerve divides into anterior and posterior divisions, which quickly subdivide into the terminal branches of the femoral nerve.[5]

The anterior division innervates the sartorius muscle and provides sensation to the anterior thigh as far distally as the knee through the medial cutaneous nerve and the intermediate cutaneous nerve.

The posterior division innervates the quadriceps femoralis muscle through a splay of branches and gives origin to the saphenous nerve. The saphenous nerve is the longest branch of the femoral nerve, providing sensation to the medial leg. The saphenous nerve passes behind the sartorius muscle where it travels with the femoral artery in the adductor canal. The saphenous nerve gives rise to the infrapatellar branch, which pierces the tendon of the sartorius muscle to innervate the skin just below the knee. The saphenous nerve then passes between the tendons of the gracilis and sartorius muscles, entering the subcutaneous tissue and innervating the medial leg to the medial malleolus and the top of the medial foot, extending toward the large toe. In the distal third of the leg, the saphenous nerve bifurcates into two terminal branches, one paralleling the medial tibia to the malleolus and the second passing anterior to the malleolus and continuing over the medial foot. Throughout its subcutaneous course, the saphenous nerve is intimately related to the saphenous vein.

The femoral nerve can be exposed from its appearance at the edge of the psoas muscle to its exit under the inguinal ligament through an anterior lateral extraperitoneal approach (**Fig. 139.3**). A skin incision is made just above and parallel to the iliac crest, and the abdominal wall is opened in layers, exposing the pre- and retroperitoneal fat. It is wise to tack the edges of the cut muscle layers so that they can be reapproximated at the time of

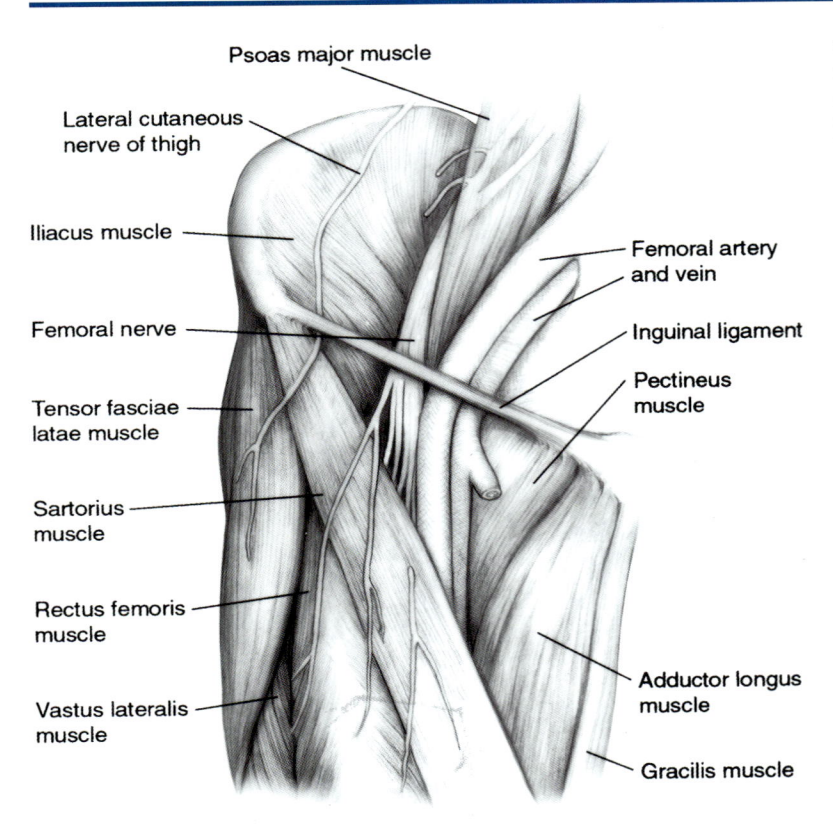

Fig. 139.2 The lateral femoral cutaneous nerve exits under the inguinal ligament and travels over the sartorius muscle in a tunnel in the deep fascia. The femoral nerve emerges from within the psoas muscle and passes under the inguinal ligament lateral to the femoral artery.

closure. Retracting the peritoneal contents anteriorly will readily expose the lateral femoral cutaneous and femoral nerves, which lie under the iliac fascia and the branches of the genitofemoral nerves as they perforate the psoas muscle. This exposure can be extended anteriorly to expose the femoral nerve in the thigh. If the inguinal ligament is severed in the exposure, the ligament's ends should be tacked so that they can be reapproximated at the end of the operation.

Several modifications of this approach have been described that offer a better exposure of the more proximal intrapsoas portion of the femoral nerve; the upper lumbar roots, which form the femoral nerve; or the proximal lower lumbar roots, which contribute to the sciatic nerve. More proximal exposure of the upper lumbar plexus is achieved by an incision that begins just below the lateral rib cage and extends transversely to just below the umbilicus. The external oblique muscle is split and the deeper abdominal wall layers are cut. Again the peritoneal contents are swept forward, allowing the upper lumbar roots to be traced through the psoas muscle to their exit from the spine. Dissection within the psoas muscle is facilitated by flexing the patient's hip, releasing the tension on that muscle. In male patients, care should be taken not to injure the sympathetic chain, which lies in the gutter between the psoas muscle and the vertebral body, because this can result in retrograde ejaculation. The cutaneous nerve is found lying on the iliacus muscle lateral to the femoral nerve beneath the iliac fascia. As mentioned in the lateral femoral cutaneous nerve section, the lumbar plexus and femoral nerve can be approached through a small incision in the lateral flank by using the NuVasive MaXcess XLIF retractor system to approach focal lesions. The small incision and the approach through the retroperitoneal fat minimize blood loss and approach-related morbidity.

The femoral nerve can be exposed in the thigh by a vertical incision made parallel and lateral to the femoral artery. The incision can be carried as far distally as necessary. Proximal exposure of the femoral nerve is obtained by curving the incision laterally along a line connecting the anterior superior iliac spine with the pelvis symphysis. The more proximal femoral nerve is exposed by opening the muscular abdominal wall into the retroperitoneal space. Care should be taken to identify and protect the ilioinguinal nerve.

The saphenous nerve can be exposed at the knee by an incision made parallel and lateral to the tendon of the sartorius muscle. The main trunk of the saphenous nerve may be hidden behind the saphenous vein because these two structures maintain an intimate relationship down the leg. The infrapatellar branch travels from lateral to medial just below the level of the tibial plateau.

Obturator Nerve

The obturator nerve takes its origin from the ventral division of the ventral rami of L2, L3, and L4. The nerve forms in the psoas major muscle, but unlike the femoral nerve it passes behind the common femoral vessels lateral to the internal iliac artery. The nerve travels through the lesser pelvis to the obturator foramen. It exits the obturator foramen, passing over the obturator internus muscle. As it passes through the obturator foramen into the anterior thigh, the nerve divides into an anterior and a posterior branch (**Fig. 139.1**).[6]

The anterior branch travels anterior to the adductor brevis and behind the pectineus and adductor longus muscles. A branch joins the medial cutaneous nerve, providing sensation to the medial upper thigh. In some cases this area of sensory innervation extends down to the knee. Motor branches pass to the adductor longus, adductor brevis, and gracilis muscles. The nerve ends at the femoral artery.

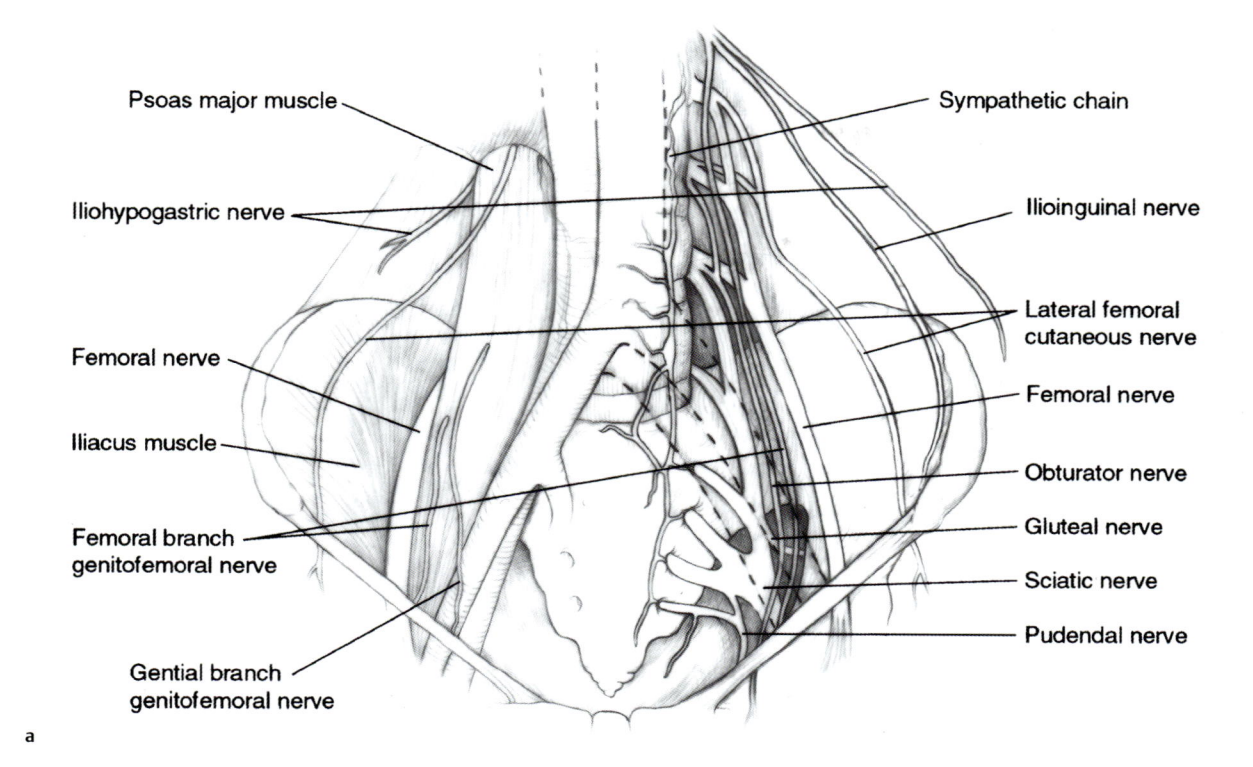

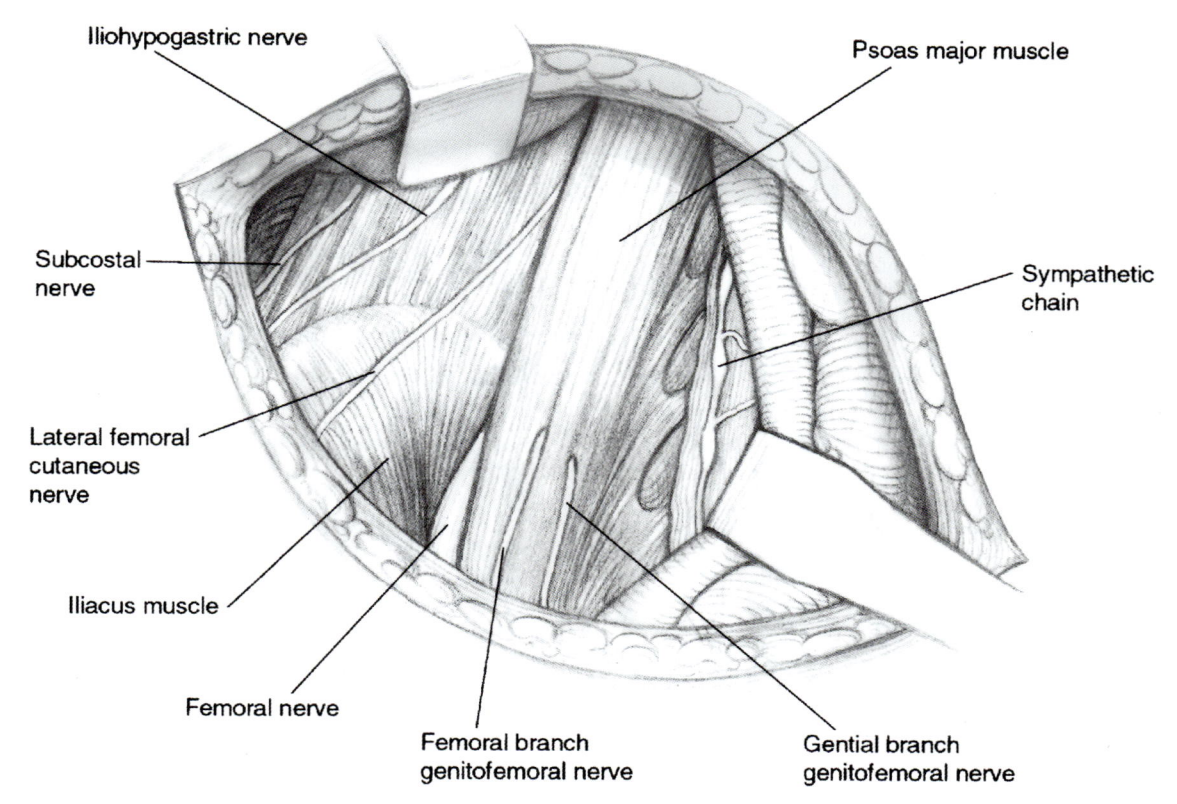

Fig. 139.3 (a) The lumbar and sacral plexus. (b) Retroperitoneal exposure of the upper lumbar plexus.

The posterior branch passes behind the adductor brevis and in front of the adductor magnus. This nerve enters the popliteal fossa along with the femoral artery to innervate the knee joint.

Fortunately, surgeons rarely need to repair the nerve within the pelvis, where its deep location makes repair quite difficult. The obturator mononeuropathy most frequently occurs after urologic, gynecologic, or orthopedic procedures.[7] The proximal portion of the obturator nerve can be exposed by a transabdominal, laparoscopic, or extraperitoneal approach to visualize the nerve from its origin from the psoas muscle to its exit from the pelvis at the obturator foramen.[8]

Extrapelvic exposure of the obturator nerve is accomplished through a linear incision, which begins over the pubic tubercle and extends down the medial leg. The interval between the pectineal and the adductor longus, both of which originate from the pectineal line of the pubis, is developed. If it is difficult to open this plane, the medial interval between the adductor longus and adductor magnus can be opened and the adductor longus can be mobilized. The proximal pectineus may need to be detached to afford a good look at the nerve. The anterior division of the obturator nerve is seen passing over the obturator brevis muscle. Exposure of the posterior division may require partial sectioning of the obturator brevis muscle. The posterior branch is seen behind this muscle.

Sciatic Nerve

The sciatic nerve is composed of contributors from L4–S3. The two lumbar nerves L4 and L5 combine to form the lumbosacral branch, which crosses the ala of the sacrum to join the upper three sacral roots forming the sciatic nerve. From its inception, the sciatic nerve contains the tibial division, which is formed by the ventral division of L4–S3, and the peroneal division, which is formed by the dorsal division of L4–S3. The sciatic nerve exits through the greater sciatic notch below the piriformis muscle and above the superior gemellus under the cover of the gluteus maximus muscle. The fibers destined to form the peroneal nerve segregate lateral to the fibers destined to form the tibial nerve.

The sciatic nerve travels down the thigh posterior to the exterior rotators of the hip (the obturator internus, the gemellus, and the quadratus femoris) and the adductor magnus. The nerve is flanked medially by the semitendinosus muscle and laterally by the short head of the biceps femoralis, and is crossed posteriorly by the long head of the biceps femoralis muscle because that muscle makes its way from the ischial tuberosity to the head of the fibula. Soon after exiting the sciatic notch, the sciatic nerve provides innervation to the hamstring muscles with branches to the semimembranous, semitendinous, long head of the biceps, and adductor magnus originating from the tibial division, and branches to the short head of the biceps originating from the peroneal division.

Most commonly the sciatic nerve divides into a medial tibial division and a smaller lateral peroneal division in the lower third of the thigh proximal to the popliteal fossa.[9] The tibial nerve passes behind the knee joint covered only by adipose tissue, fascia, and skin. As the nerve enters the popliteal fossa, it lies lateral to the artery, but in the midfossa it passes behind the artery to continue distally on the artery's medial side. The nerve leaves the popliteal fossa, passing between the heads of the gastrocnemius muscle, and continues distally, sandwiched anterior to the soleus muscle and behind the posterior tibialis muscle, emerging 4 cm above the ankle from the medial side of the tendon calcaneus.

Muscular branches to the gastrocnemius and soleus muscles originate at approximately the level of the medial epicondyle of the femur, and 3 to 5 cm proximal to the knee joint the tibial nerve contributes to the sural nerve. This cutaneous branch passes between the head of the gastrocnemius muscle before perforating the deep fascia and communicating with the sural communicating branch of the peroneal nerve. The combined sural nerve then travels along the lateral border of the Achilles tendon, passing between that tendon and its lateral malleolus. Motor branches from the tibial nerve are given to the posterior tibialis, flexor hallucis longus, and flexor digitorum longus muscles, and the nerve travels behind the soleus muscle.

The tibial nerve emerges from the medial side of the tendon calcaneus to pass between that tendon and the lateral malleolus under the flexor reticulum.[10] In most cases the nerve divides into the medial and lateral plantar nerves within 1 cm of the medial malleolus. The calcaneal branch to the heel can originate from the posterior tibial nerve, the lateral plantar nerve, and, rarely, from the medial plantar nerve.[11] The calcaneal branch can be duplicated. Beneath the flexor retinaculum the tibial nerve lies posterior to the posterior tibial artery. Two veins accompany the artery and nerve through the tarsal tunnel.

The medial and lateral plantar nerves enter the foot within adjacent but separate canals. The roof of the canal for the lateral plantar nerve is the aponeurosis of the foot, and the roof for the canal of the medial plantar nerve provides the origin of the abductor hallucis brevis.

Exploration of the Intrapelvic Sciatic Nerve

Because of the slope of the sacrum away from the surgeon, exploration of the sacral plexus is difficult through the retroperitoneal approach. A transperitoneal approach affords a good exposure of the proximal sciatic nerve and control of the adjacent vasculature. The peritoneal cavity is opened through a midline or transverse approach, and the peritoneal contents are displaced superiorly with moist sponges exposing the posterior peritoneum. The posterior peritoneum is opened, exposing the lower lumbar and sacral plexus. The descending portion of L4 joins the L5 root anterior to the promontory of the sacrum. The three upper sacral roots join this trunk, separated from the sacrum by the origin of the piriformis muscle. Branches of the internal iliac artery and the superior gluteal, inferior gluteal, and internal pudendal arteries pass through the proximal sacral plexus.

Exposure of the Proximal Extrapelvic Sciatic Nerve

An extensive approach described by Henry[12] lifts the gluteus maximus muscle to expose the entire proximal portion of the sciatic nerve. A question mark–shaped incision is made in the skin passing 3 cm inferior and parallel to the iliac crest, down to the greater trochanter parallel with the femur to the inferior edge of the gluteus maximus muscle, medial and just inferior to the gluteal fold to the midline of the thigh, and then inferiorly along the midline of the thigh. The posterior femoral cutaneous nerve, which travels down the posterior midthigh, must be avoided. The gluteus muscle is detached from its insertion into the femur and the iliotibial track, the interval between the gluteus medius and gluteus maximus is developed, and the gluteus maximus muscle is lifted, hinged on its medial origin, into the posterior gluteal line of the ileum and the dorsal sacrum. The sciatic, superior gluteal, inferior gluteal, posterior femoral cutaneous, and pudendal nerves can be seen. The sciatic and posterior femoral cutaneous nerves are seen exiting the pelvis under the piriformis muscle and then traveling caudally over the short external rotators of the hip.

For lesions localized to the gluteal region, a transgluteal approach can be accomplished by a muscle-splitting approach through the gluteus maximus muscle (**Fig. 139.4**).[13] This approach

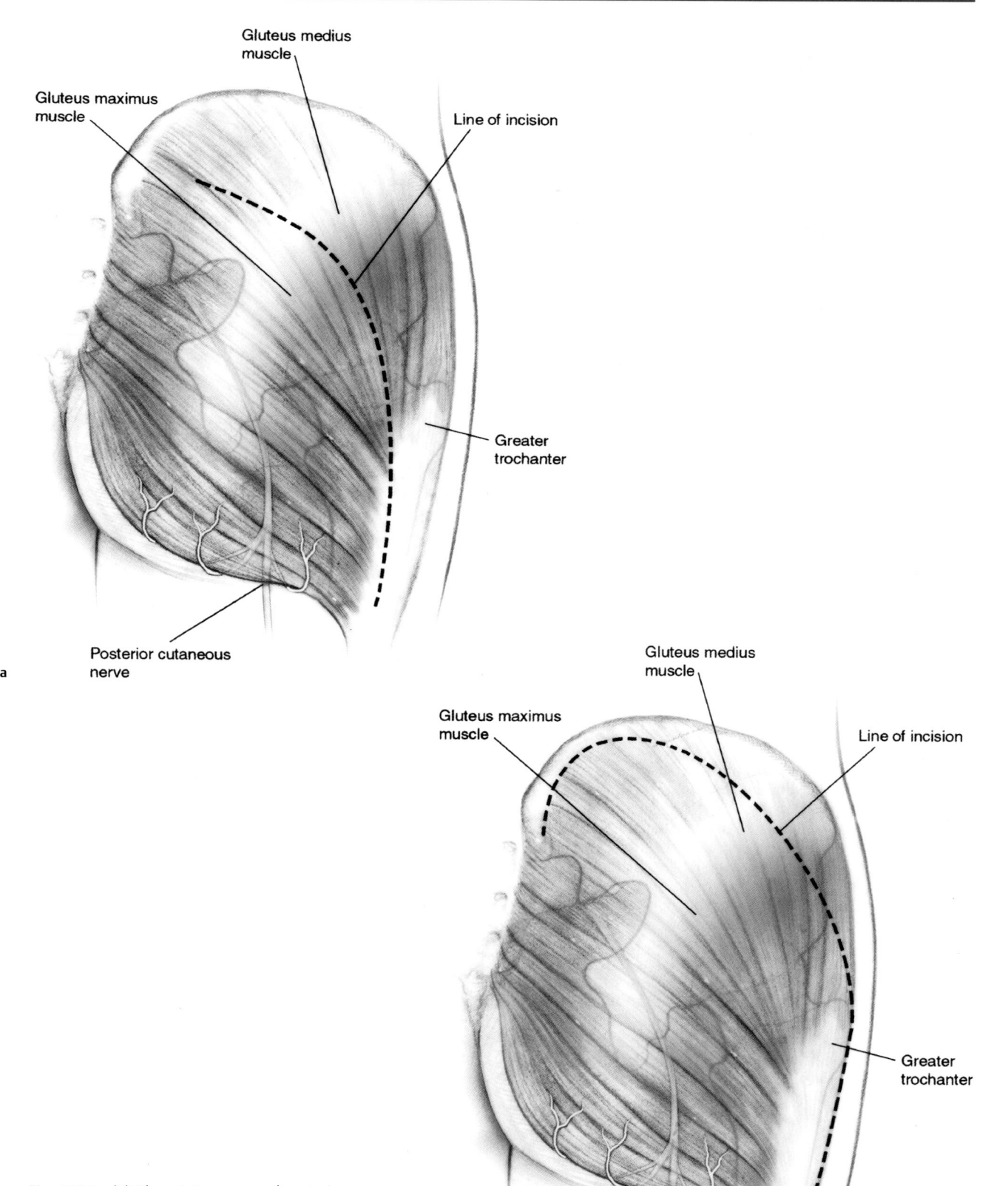

Fig. 139.4 (a) The sciatic nerve and posterior cutaneous nerve of the thigh are covered by the gluteus maximus. A limited view of the sciatic nerve can be obtained by splitting the fibers of the gluteus maximus. (b) A more extensive exposure requires detaching the gluteus maximus from the iliac crest and cutting the insertion of the muscle into the femur and the iliotibial track. (*continued on page 892*)

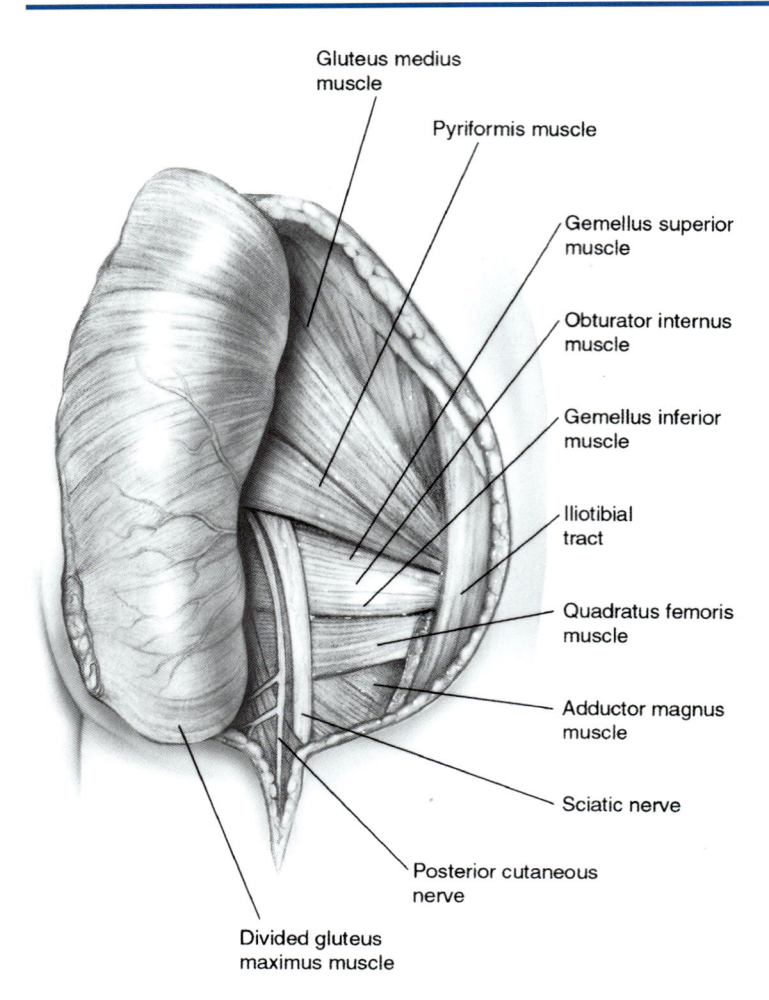

Fig. 139.4 (*continued*) **(c)** The sciatic nerve emerges under the piriformis muscle and over the short external rotators of the hip.

is similar to the posterior approach in the hip. The patient is placed in the three-quarter prone position with the affected side up. An 8- to 10-cm incision begins at the greater trochanter and extends medially in line with the fibers of the gluteus maximus. The fascia over the gluteus maximus is cut in line with a skin incision, and the muscle fibers of the gluteus maximus are split revealing the short external rotators of the hip. Further exposure can be obtained by extending the fascial incision into the fascia lata. The nerve is found encased in fat lying upon the short external rotators of the hip (the obturate extensor, the two gemelli, and the quadratus femoris). A sufficient length of piriformis muscle is exposed so that that muscle can be cut through this exposure. The transgluteal approach has the advantage of being easier, faster, and less structurally disruptive than the large question mark–shaped incision and approach.[13]

Martin et al[14] describe the use of endoscopy to decompress the sciatic nerve in the gluteal region through two to three small skin portals. Through the anterolateral and posterolateral portals, the peritrochanteric space was explored in 35 patients using 70-degree standard and long arthroscopes. Various sciatic nerve compression pathologies were managed endoscopically, including the resection of fibrovascular scar bands, the release of the piriformis tendon, and the resection of scarred hamstring tendon. The advantage of a much shorter skin incision length and less disruption to the surrounding tissue must be balanced with decreased visualization of the nerve and the technical difficulty of using the endoscope.

In the thigh, the sciatic nerve runs between the semitendinous muscle medially and the biceps femoris laterally. Exposure can be obtained by a longitudinal incision in the center of the posterior thigh. Care should be taken not to injure the posterior femoral cutaneous nerve that runs over the long head of the biceps femoris beneath the deep fascia. Once the deep fascia is opened, only the long head of the biceps, which crosses the nerve from medial to lateral, stands between the surgeon and the sciatic nerve. In the distal thigh the skin incision curves laterally along the medial border of the tendon of the biceps femoralis. If exposure below the knee joint is needed, the skin incision returns to the midline along the posterior cutaneous crease of the knee joint and then down the midcalf. Care should be taken not to injure the sural communicating nerve or the lateral cutaneous nerve of the calf, both of which branch from the common peroneal nerve as it travels parallel to the biceps femoris tendon or the sural nerve, which exits from the tibial nerve between the heads of the gastrocnemius muscle.

Exposure of the Tibial Nerve in the Leg

The proximal tibial nerve is exposed between the heads of the gastrocnemius muscle (**Fig. 139.5**). The midpoint of the gastrocnemius is marked by the short saphenous vein external to the deep fascia and the sural nerve deep to the deep fascia. Once the deep fascia is opened, the muscle bellies of the gastrocnemius can be separated with finger dissection. The tibial nerve can be followed distally to where it dives behind the soleus arch.

Distally the tibial nerve emerges from the medial edge of the Achilles tendon where the gastrocnemius and soleus merge to form that tendon ~ 4 cm proximal to the medial malleolus. The tibial nerve can be isolated behind the posterior tibial artery after it emerges from under the Achilles tendon through a vertical incision placed halfway between the Achilles tendon and the medial malleolus (**Fig. 139.6**). To expose the nerve behind the soleus muscle, the soleus bridge must be cut from proximal to distal, and the fibers of the soleus muscle divided or, if more

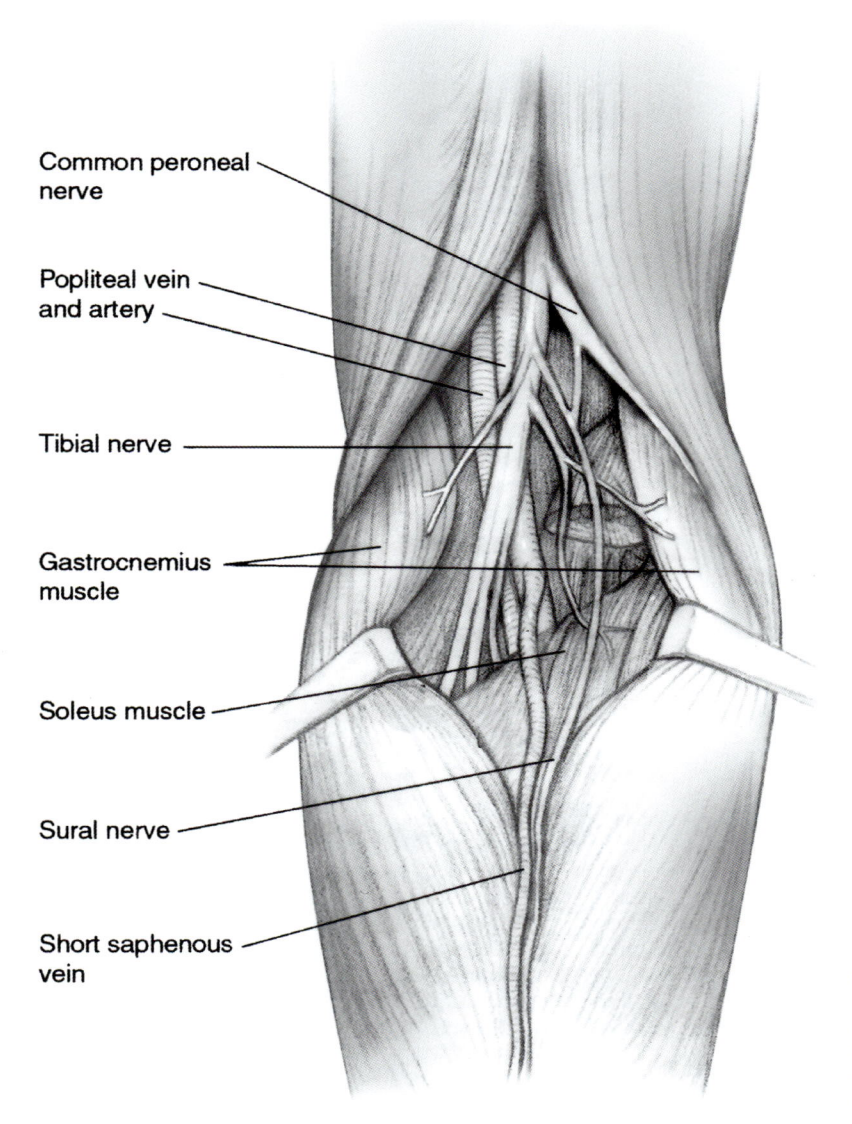

Fig. 139.5 In the upper leg, the posterior tibial nerve can be exposed down to the soleus bridge between the heads of the gastrocnemius muscle. The interval between the heads is marked superficially by the short saphenous vein and below the deep fascia by the contribution from the posterior tibial nerve to the sural nerve.

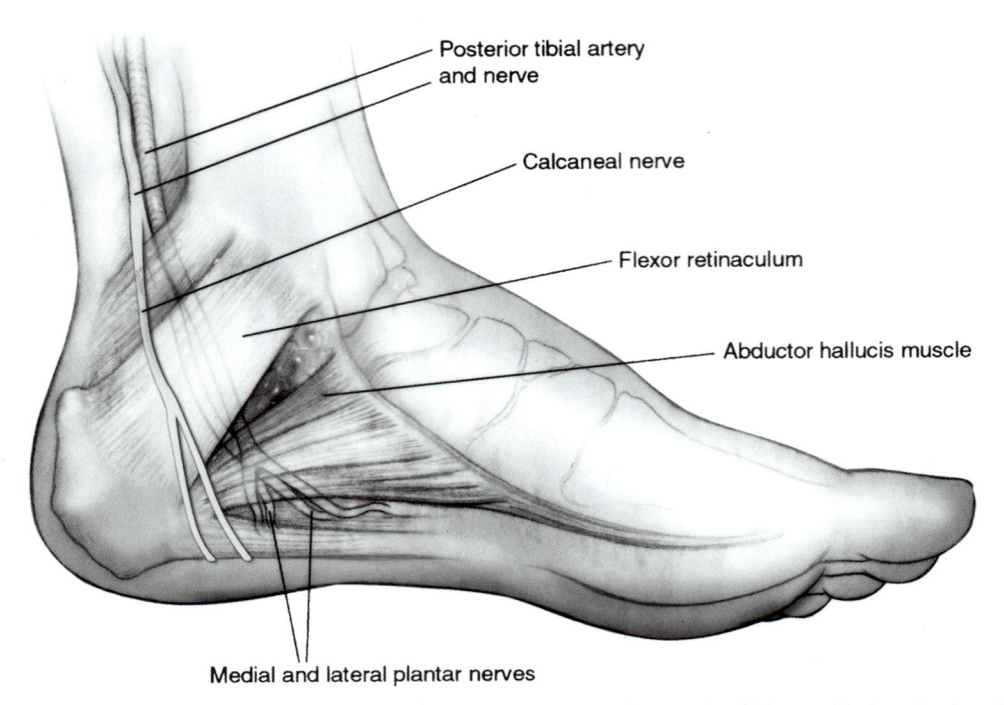

Fig. 139.6 The posterior tibial nerve is freed in the tarsal tunnel where it runs posterior to the posterior tibial artery. The lateral and medial plantar nerves are followed into their respective canals. Care is taken to identify and preserve the calcaneal branch.

extensive exposure is required, the soleus muscle can be detached from the tibia (**Fig. 139.7**).[12] The detachment of the soleus muscle from the middle third of the tibia is performed from distal to proximal. The distal neurovascular bundle is identified and followed behind the Achilles tendon. Using the index finger to protect this bundle, the attachment of the soleus muscle is first detached from the medial edge of the tibia. Two thirds of the way up the tibia, the attachment becomes thicker and more fibrous and passes obliquely to the lateral (inner) edge of the tibia. After freeing the tibia attachment, the soleus muscle can be rotated laterally, exposing the tibial nerve. This is analogous to the exposure of the median nerve behind the flexor digitorum sublimis muscle.

Exposure of the Tibial Nerve in the Ankle

The posterior tibial nerve is best located under an incision that begins 3 to 4 cm proximal to the medial malleolus and travels distally along a course halfway between the medial malleolus and the tendon calcaneus (**Fig. 139.6**). Care must be taken to avoid the terminus of the saphenous nerve.

The incision curves forward to terminate at the edge of the plantar aspect of the foot. The origin of the adductor hallucis muscle may be seen. The deep fascia is opened, and the nerve is identified behind the anterior tibial artery proximal to the flexor retinaculum. The flexor retinaculum is released from proximal to distal. Care is taken to preserve the calcaneus branch of the tibial nerve. The plantar nerves are followed into their respective tunnels, which requires cutting the fascia underlying the adductor hallucis.

Ducic and Felder[15] advocate the use of lighted retractors to minimize the skin incision and aid direct visualization of the nerve subcutaneously approximately 4 cm proximal and distal to the skin incision. With the light retractor, the typical skin incision length is 5 cm for the proximal calf and 4.5 cm for the tarsal tunnel.

Peroneal Nerve

The peroneal nerve travels over the lateral head of the gastrocnemius, under cover of the thick popliteal fascia and the medial edge of the biceps tendon. It passes around the neck of the fibula and, prior to diving between the two heads of the peroneus longus muscle, the common peroneal nerve gives off a lateral cutaneous nerve, which innervates the upper posterior leg and a communicating branch to the sural nerve.[16] Two articular branches to the knee joint originate at the peroneus longus bridge.

The peroneal nerve bifurcates under the cover of the peroneus longus muscle into the superficial and deep peroneal nerves. The superficial peroneal nerve passes between the peroneus longus and the extensor digitorum longus, innervating the peroneus longus and brevis. Two thirds of the way down the leg, the nerve emerges from between those two muscles to pierce the deep fascia and bifurcate into the medial dorsal and intermediate dorsal cutaneous nerves of the leg, which supply skin sensation to the dorsum of the ankle, foot, and toes.[17] In the middle third of the leg, the superficial peroneal nerve has been found to have variability in its course. Ducic et al[18] examined 111 legs, and found that in 69% the nerve coursed in the expected positioned in the lateral compartment, in 16% the nerve split and had branches in both the anterior and lateral compartment, in 6% the nerve was in the intermuscular septum, and in 8% the nerve traveled only in the anterior compartment.[18]

The deep peroneal nerve passes under the tendinous origin of the extensor digitorum longus and travels distally on the anterior interosseous membrane between the extensor digitorum longus muscle and the anterior tibialis muscle. The deep peroneal nerve innervates the extensor digitorum longus and the anterior tibialis through short branches, which tether the nerve

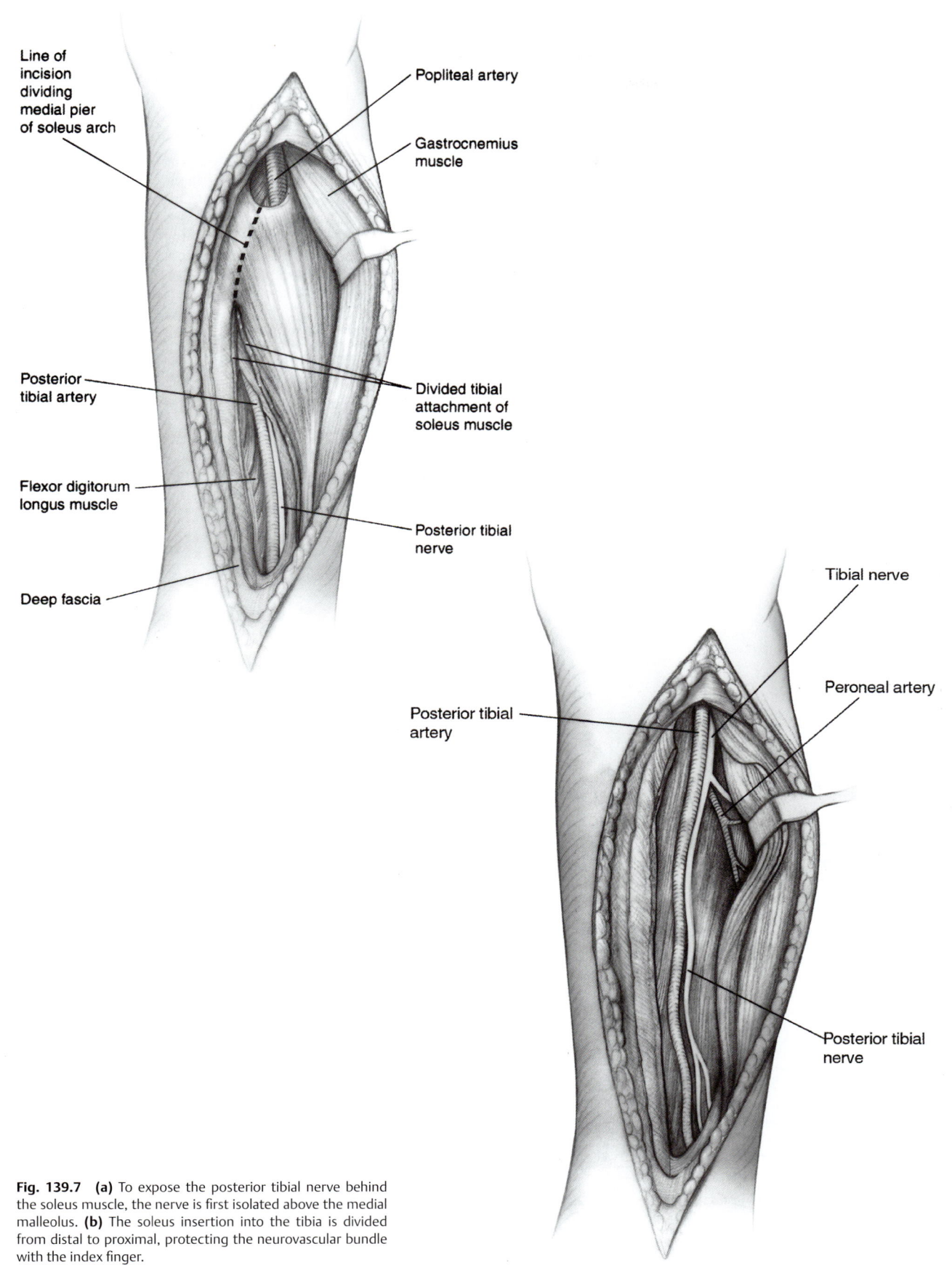

Fig. 139.7 (a) To expose the posterior tibial nerve behind the soleus muscle, the nerve is first isolated above the medial malleolus. (b) The soleus insertion into the tibia is divided from distal to proximal, protecting the neurovascular bundle with the index finger.

proximally. More distally it innervates the extensor hallucis longus and peroneus tertius muscles. The anterior tibial artery accompanies the nerve in the distal two thirds of the leg. The deep peroneal nerve emerges lateral to the tendon of the extensor hallucis longus and medial to the tendon of the extensor digitorum longus, and passes under the extensor retinaculum of the ankle lateral to the anterior tibial artery. The nerve branches, with its lateral branch innervating the extensor digitorum brevis and its medial branch passing under the tendon of the extensor hallucis brevis to innervate the first dorsal web space.

Exposure of the Common Peroneal Nerve at the Knee

The peroneal nerve can be exposed as it passes around the head of the fibula by an extension of the sciatic nerve exposure or by an S-shaped incision that begins medial to the tendon of the biceps femoris muscle, curves over the inferior aspect of the fibular head, and passes over the interval between the peroneus longus and the extensor digitorum longus (**Fig. 139.8**).[19] The common peroneal nerve can be palpated as it passes around the head of the fibula. The deep fascia over the nerve is divided, taking care not to injure the sural communicating and lateral cutaneous nerves as they pierce the fascia. The fibrous edges of the peroneus longus and the extensor digitorum longus are cut, exposing the bifurcation of the nerve. As with decompression of the tibial nerve, Ducic and Felder[20] recommend the use of lighted retractor to limit the skin incision length to 3.5 cm for decompression of the common peroneal nerve.

Exposure of the Superficial Peroneal Nerve

The superficial peroneal nerve passes anterior to the peroneus brevis and pierces the deep fascia of the leg 10 to 12 cm above the ankle. To expose this potential site of entrapment, a linear incision is made lateral to the extensor digitorum longus from 7 to 12 cm proximal to the ankle. One of the two branches of the superficial peroneal nerve, the medial dorsal cutaneous nerve or the intermediate dorsal cutaneous nerve, can be identified superficial to the deep fascia and followed proximally to where the superficial peroneal nerve pierces the fascia and passes behind the peroneal brevis muscle.[16]

Exposure of the Deep Peroneal Nerve at the Ankle

The deep peroneal nerve travels down the leg between the extensor hallucis longus and the anterior tibialis muscles (**Fig. 139.9**). An inch above the ankle, the nerve emerges lateral to the tendon of the extensor hallucis longus and medial to the ten-

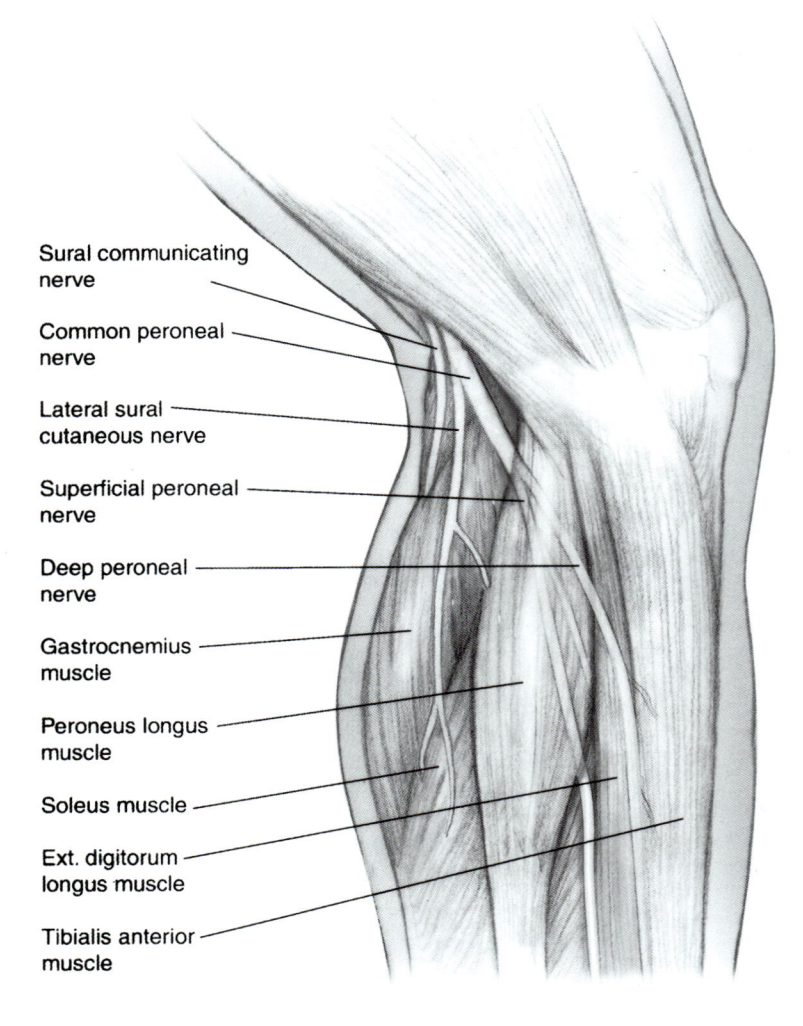

Fig. 139.8 The deep peroneal nerve passes under the extensor retinaculum of the foot between the tendons of the extensor hallucis longus and the extensor digitorum longus. The nerve continues under the tendon of the extensor hallucis brevis to innervate the first dorsal web space.

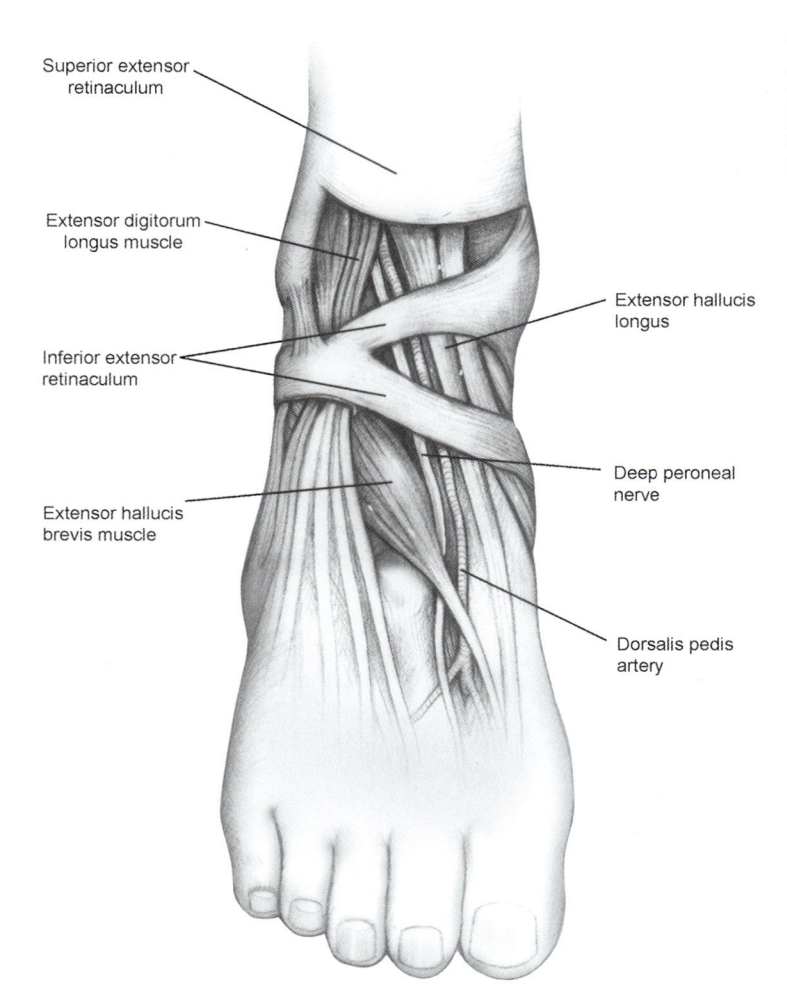

Fig. 139.9 The common peroneal nerve gives rise to the lateral cutaneous nerve of the calf and the sural communicating nerve prior to passing around the fibula. After parting from the superficial peroneal nerve, the deep peroneal nerve passes under the fibrous origins of the peroneus longus and extensor digitorum longus muscles.

dons of the extensor digitorum brevis. The nerve can become entrapped under the extensor retinaculum at the ankle or under the tendon of the extensor hallucis brevis.[10,21] The nerve can be identified by palpating the pulse of the anterior tibial artery or the movement of the extensor hallucis longus tendon. The lateral portion of the nerve, which innervates the extensor digitorum brevis, can be biopsied to provide motor fascicles. The extensor retinaculum can be cut to relieve entrapment of the distal deep peroneal nerve. This can be performed through an open approach or through an endoscopic approach.[22]

Postoperative Care

In addition to general wound care, postoperative care specific to peripheral nerve surgery of the lower extremity includes careful diet advancement when the abdominal contents have to be manipulated and retracted as part of the approach. For more distal extremity surgery, elevation of the extremity helps decrease postoperative swelling.

Potential Complications and Precautions

Complications include nerve injury, vascular injury, injury to intra-abdominal and intrapelvic contents, compartment syndrome, wound infection, deep venous thrombosis, other medical complications of surgery, and complications caused by decreased mobility. A thorough understanding of the anatomy is necessary to minimize potential complications. Also, minimizing disruption of normal tissues and performing a smaller, more focal procedure decreases complications associated with the approach.

Conclusion

There are multiple approaches for surgery of the peripheral nerves of the lower extremity. By understanding the advantages and disadvantages of the various approaches, the surgeon can tailor the approach to best treat the patient's specific pathology.

References

1. Kim DH, Kline DG. Surgical outcome for intra- and extrapelvic femoral nerve lesions. J Neurosurg 1995;83:783–790
2. Kline DG, Kim D, Midha R, Harsh C, Tiel R. Management and results of sciatic nerve injuries: a 24-year experience. J Neurosurg 1998;89: 13–23
3. Kline DG, Hudson AR. Nerve Injuries: Operative Results for Major Nerve Injuries, Entrapments, and Tumors, 1st ed. Philadelphia: WB Saunders; 1995
4. Edelson JG, Nathan H. Meralgia paresthetica. An anatomical interpretation. Clin Orthop Relat Res 1977;122:255–262

5. Sunderland S. Femoral nerve. In: Sunderland S, ed. Nerves and Nerve Injuries, 2nd ed. Edinburgh; New York: Churchill Livingstone; 1978: 999–1006
6. Sunderland S. Obturator nerve. In: Sunderland S, ed. Nerves and nerve injuries, 2nd ed. Edinburgh; New York: Churchill Livingstone; 1978: 992–998
7. Kitagawa R, Kim D, Reid N, Kline D. Surgical management of obturator nerve lesions. Neurosurgery 2009;65(4, Suppl):A24–A28
8. Rigaud J, Labat JJ, Riant T, Bouchot O, Robert R. Obturator nerve entrapment: diagnosis and laparoscopic treatment: technical case report. Neurosurgery 2007;61:E175, discussion E175
9. Sunderland S, Ray LJ. The intraneural topography of the sciatic nerve and its popliteal divisions in man. Brain 1948;71(Pt 3):242–273
10. Marinacci AA. Neurological syndromes of the tarsal tunnels. Bull Los Angeles Neurol Soc 1968;33:90–100
11. Dellon AL, Mackinnon SE. Tibial nerve branching in the tarsal tunnel. Arch Neurol 1984;41:645–646
12. Henry AK. Extensile Exposure, 2nd ed. Edinburgh: Churchill Livingstone; 1973
13. Patil PG, Friedman AH. Surgical exposure of the sciatic nerve in the gluteal region: anatomic and historical comparison of two approaches. Neurosurgery 2005;56(1, Suppl):165–171, discussion 165–171
14. Martin HD, Shears SA, Johnson JC, Smathers AM, Palmer IJ. The endoscopic treatment of sciatic nerve entrapment/deep gluteal syndrome. Arthroscopy 2011;27:172–181
15. Ducic I, Felder JM III. Tibial nerve decompression: reliable exposure using shorter incisions. Microsurgery 2012;32:533–538
16. Mackinnon SE, Dellon AL. Surgery of the Peripheral Nerve. New York; Stuttgart: Thieme; 1988
17. Kopell HP, Thompson WAL. Peripheral entrapment neuropathies. Baltimore, Williams and Wilkins; 1963
18. Ducic I, Dellon AL, Graw KS. The clinical importance of variations in the surgical anatomy of the superficial peroneal nerve in the mid-third of the lateral leg. Ann Plast Surg 2006;56:635–638
19. Mont MA, Dellon AL, Chen F, Hungerford MW, Krackow KA, Hungerford DS. The operative treatment of peroneal nerve palsy. J Bone Joint Surg Am 1996;78:863–869
20. Ducic I, Felder JM III. Minimally invasive peripheral nerve surgery: peroneal nerve neurolysis. Microsurgery 2012;32:26–30
21. Dellon AL. Deep peroneal nerve entrapment on the dorsum of the foot. Foot Ankle 1990;11:73–80
22. Lui TH. Endoscopic anterior tarsal tunnel release: a case report. J Foot Ankle Surg 2014;53:186–188

140 Exposure and Biopsy of the Sural Nerve

Ahmed Alaqeel and Rajiv Midha

Structural Anatomy

The sural nerve in humans is a purely sensory nerve that supplies the skin of the posterior and lateral side of the distal third of the leg, as well as the lateral malleolus and lateral side of the foot up to the fifth toe. The sural nerve carries mainly S1 sensory fibers and is formed primarily from two components originating from the posterior tibial (medial sural cutaneous nerve) and peroneal (lateral sural cutaneous nerve or the communicating fibular branch) in the popliteal fossa.[1–3] Some authors describe the sural nerve as a direct branch of the tibial nerve and occasionally from the peroneal alone.[4,5] Before the tibial nerve goes beneath the gastrocnemius, the tibial nerve gives off a small cutaneous branch, the medial sural cutaneous nerve, which lies between the two heads of the gastrocnemius, deep to the fascia.[3] The peroneal nerve courses laterally after dividing from the sciatic nerve and courses parallel to the distal portion of the biceps femoris muscle toward the fibular head, where it gives off the lateral sural cutaneous nerve and is superficial to the gastrocnemius fascia. The medial sural nerve descends deep to the gastrocnemius fascia in the proximal lower leg, running in the posterior midline, and emerges from the fascia into the subcutaneous plane about halfway down the leg, an average of 16 cm proximal to the lateral malleolus.[6]

Shortly after the medial sural nerve emerges from the fascia, there is an anastomosis with the lateral sural nerve that is found in 75 to 84% of cadaveric dissections at the distal third of the gastrocnemius, as the lateral and medial sural nerves run superficial to it to form the main sural nerve.[3,6] The point of junction of the two component nerves varies from immediately proximal to the lateral malleolus to the popliteal fossa. The nerve then continues in a slightly oblique course from the initial midline position down the leg on the posterior lateral side, then anterior to the Achilles tendon and posterior to the lateral malleolus, where it lies in a close relation to the small saphenous vein (**Fig. 140.1**). The standard zone of sensory innervation (and sensory loss following injury, biopsy, or nerve harvesting) is to the dorsal lateral foot (**Fig. 140.1**). Distal to the lateral malleolus, the sural nerve runs along the lateral border of the foot and ends at the lateral side of the little toe. The sural nerve terminal branches include the lateral dorsal cutaneous nerve and the lateral calcaneal branches.[2]

Indications

Sural nerve biopsy is indicated only in a small subset of patients with peripheral neuropathy who meets the following three criteria: (1) There is evidence of a disease other than diabetic peripheral neuropathy. (2) The suspected disease is capable of causing diagnostically relevant changes in the nerve. (3) Identification of the neuropathy is likely to influence subsequent treatments.[7]

Patient Selection and Preoperative Testing

A sural nerve biopsy is not required to diagnose most peripheral neuropathies, and conventional methods of detailed clinical investigation and laboratory workup should be performed before embarking on this procedure.[8] Sensory nerve conduction studies are used to electrically evaluate the sensory axonal loss in distal neuropathies, mainly due to the fact that mononeuropathy is rarely encountered in the sural nerve.[9] The sural nerve is the most frequently biopsied peripheral nerve, for several reasons[10]: It has a reliable anatomic course. It is a pure sensory and autonomic nerve, leaving no loss of motor function and is usually well tolerated with low morbidity; for example, its sensory distribution is located on the dorsolateral aspect of the foot, so permanent anesthesia in this area is not likely to dispose a patient to a plantar ulcer. Finally, the sural nerve has an appropriate anatomic makeup, including the presence of vessels and connective tissue, a reasonable caliber and number of fascicles, and lack of intertwining fascicles over a 6- to 10-cm distance, so that individual fascicles can be dissected out for tease mount preparation to facilitate neuropathological interpretation.[5,11]

Sural Nerve Exposure and Biopsy Surgical Procedure

Sural nerve biopsy is performed as an outpatient procedure, using local anesthetic only, in the majority of cases. The sural nerve is most easily biopsied with the patient in a lateral position, with the side being biopsied facing upward. Placing a pillow or padding between the dependent knee and the upper one aids patient

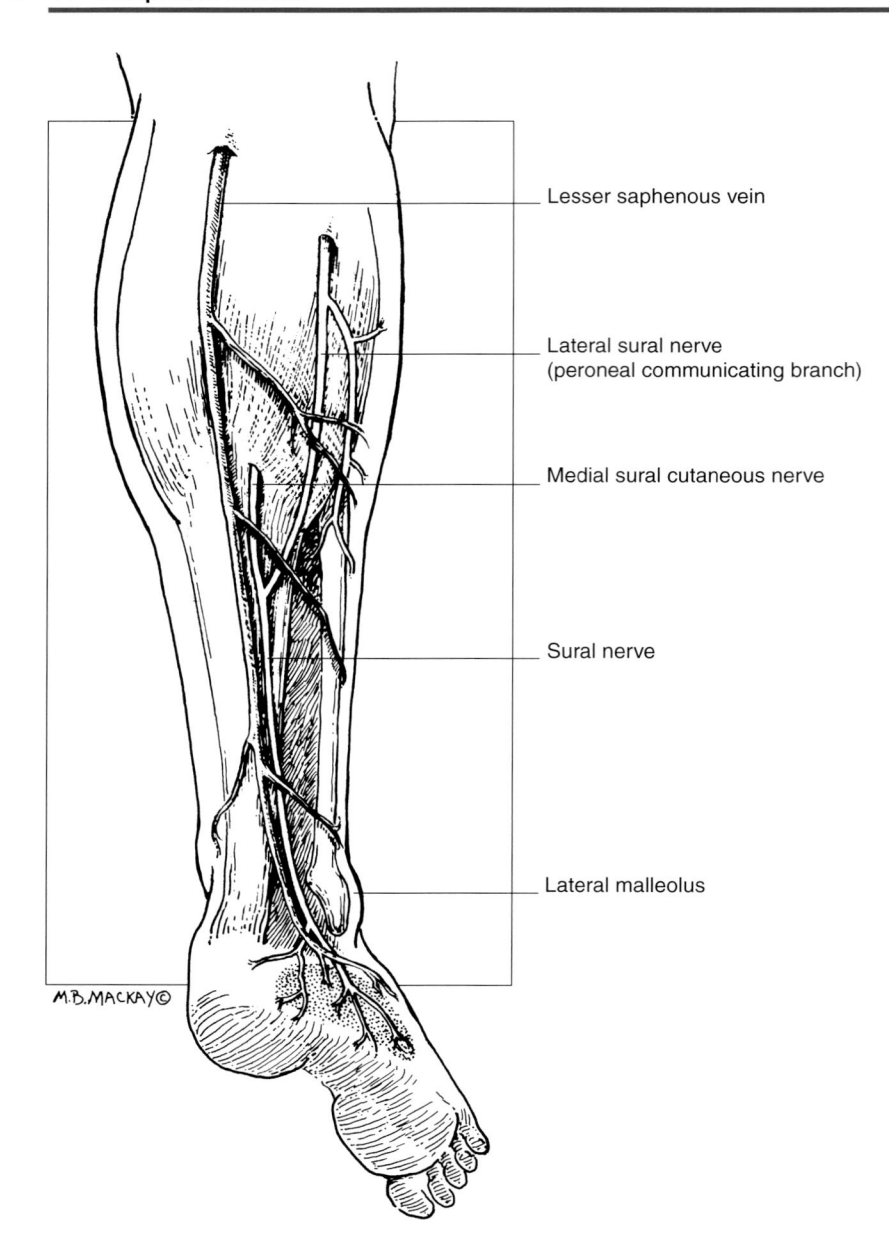

Fig. 140.1 The sural nerve, with the contribution from the tibial (medial sural) and peroneal (lateral sural or communicating branch) nerve, along with the relationship of the nerve to the lesser saphenous vein and lateral malleolus. The typical sensory zone of the sural nerve is illustrated *(stippling)*.

comfort. The lateral lower leg and ankle region is suitably prepped and draped, following which 1% lidocaine with 1:200,000 epinephrine is infiltrated subcutaneously in the region between the lateral malleolus and Achilles tendon. No tourniquet is used, and bipolar cautery is used for hemostasis to avoid damage to adjacent structures.

A 10-cm longitudinal skin incision is made equidistant between the lateral malleolus and the Achilles tendon, extending distally and ending just proximal to the lateral malleolus (**Fig. 140.2**). The incision follows the course of the lesser saphenous vein because it is the most reliable anatomic landmark in the area, lying immediately deep to the semitransparent Scarpa's fascia (**Fig. 140.3a**). The sural nerve lies immediately adjacent or deep to the lesser saphenous vein at this level. The incision is then deepened until the lesser saphenous vein is identified. The vein must be retracted to visualize the sural nerve (**Fig. 140.3b**). A small branch or two from the vein adjacent to the lateral malleolus may need to be coagulated and incised to facilitate nerve exposure and procurement. Approximately 10 cm of the sural nerve is exposed.

The decision to perform a whole or fascicular nerve biopsy is based on whether the underlying neuropathy may have a multifocal basis and on the severity of neuropathy. Thus, if the underlying cause is likely to result in patchy pathology and the neuropathy is severe, then a complete nerve biopsy should be done. If, however, the neuropathy is likely to result from a diffuse cause, which involves all the fascicles, and the neuropathy, and hence sensory deficit before biopsy, is mild, then a fascicular biopsy may be performed carefully under loupe magnification. The patient is then warned that the nerve is to be cut because this step causes severe but transient pain. For this reason, the proximal end of the sural nerve segment being harvested is first cut. Using gentle traction, the nerve is sharply and quickly divided. The stump of the sural nerve remaining in the patient is allowed to retract into deep subcutaneous tissue proximal to the apex of the wound, minimizing the risk of painful neuroma formation. Then the final removal of the nerve proceeds with any further distal dissection and cutting of the nerve. It is important not to coagulate directly into the nerve, and to handle it gently at all times; grasp the nerve with forceps only at its cut end to avoid crush and injury artifact. The fresh nerve specimen is directly handed to the pathology technologist.

Closure and Postoperative Care

The wound is closed in layers using 2-0 or 3-0 absorbable suture on a cutting needle in a running fashion for the subcutaneous tissue, and a 3-0 subcuticular suture for skin closure. A strip dressing is applied to the incision, bolstered by a 4-inch by 4-inch gauze pad and Kling rolled gauze wrapped in a circumferential fashion around the lower leg and ankle to apply gentle pressure. The patient is instructed to ambulate immediately and to elevate the leg at night and when sitting. The dressing is removed after 5 days, and the incision is left exposed to air thereafter.

Other Considerations and Potential Complications

The time the specimen must remain in the fixing solution is based on laboratory protocol and varies from 5 minutes to 3 hours. The most important point is that the surgeon immediately places the specimen in the fixative and does not allow it to sit or coil. On occasion, the neurosurgeon has to do both a nerve and muscle biopsy. Harvesting the sural nerve in midcalf enables doing a simultaneous gastrocnemius muscle biopsy. The drawback is that the sural nerve here is often smaller in diameter, and consists of four to eight fascicles because it is devoid of the contribution of the peroneal. This information should be conveyed to the neuropathologist. On the plus side, there may be little or no sensory loss, and the risk of a painful neuroma is lessened

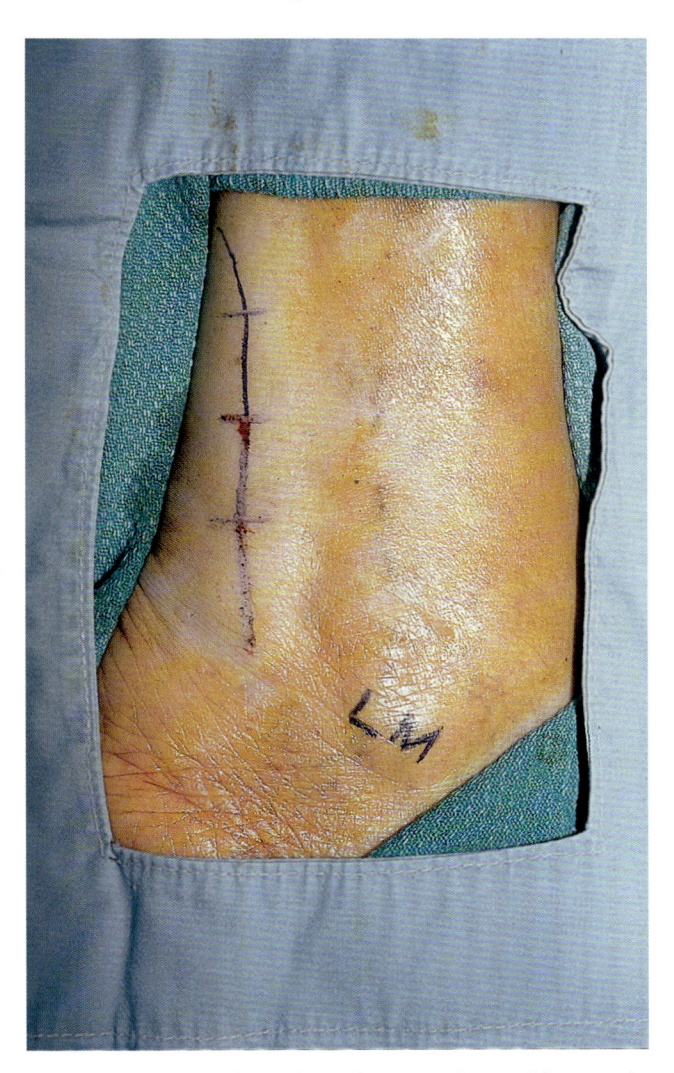

Fig. 140.2 The incision for sural nerve biopsy is in the trough between the lateral malleolus (LM) and Achilles tendon.

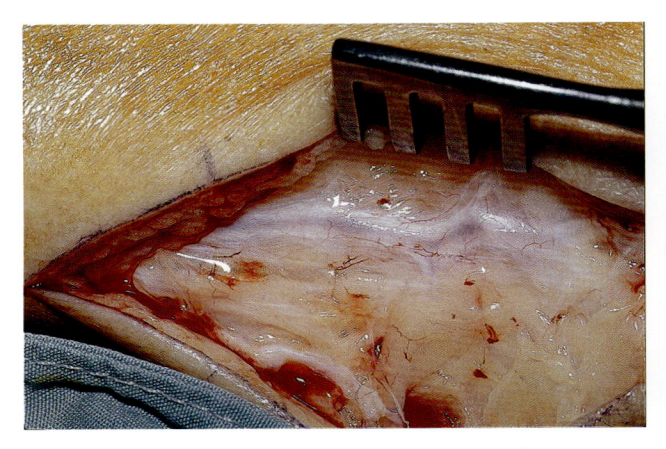

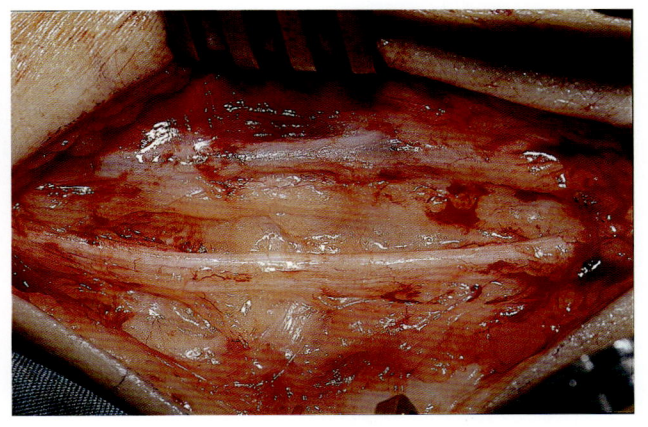

Fig. 140.3 (a) The lesser saphenous vein serves as an excellent anatomic landmark for the sural nerve, which lies just deep to it and slightly posterior. (b) The sural nerve is exposed just deep to the saphenous vein.

because the proximal sural nerve stump is deep to the fascia, within an intermuscular plane. With the patient prone, a 10-cm longitudinal incision is made in the posterior calf midline. The sural nerve is immediately deep to the fascia covering the gastrocnemius muscle here. After incising the fascia, the lesser saphenous vein and nerve should be sought. After harvesting the nerve, a generous sample of the gastrocnemius muscle may be removed for biopsy from the superior part of the exposure, where the muscle is fleshier and less tendinous.

Conclusion

Sural nerve biopsy is indicated only in a small subset of patients with peripheral neuropathy. A detailed clinical investigation and laboratory workup should be performed before embarking on this procedure.

References

1. Kosif R, Arifoglu Y, Diramali M. Bilateral variations in the formation of sural nerve. IJAV 2010;3:118–121
2. Standring S, Ellis H, Healy J, Jhonson D, Williams A, Collins P. Gray's anatomy: the anatomical basis of clinical practice. AJNR Am J Neuroradiol 2005;26:2703
3. Coert JH, Dellon AL. Clinical implications of the surgical anatomy of the sural nerve. Plast Reconstr Surg 1994;94:850–855
4. Uluutku H, Can MA, Kurtoglu Z. Formation and location of the sural nerve in the newborn. Surg Radiol Anat 2000;22:97–100
5. Ortigüela ME, Wood MB, Cahill DR. Anatomy of the sural nerve complex. J Hand Surg Am 1987;12:1119–1123
6. de Moura W, Gilbert A. Surgical anatomy of the sural nerve. J Reconstr Microsurg 1984;1:31–39
7. Dyck PJ, Thomas PK. Diabetic Neuropathy. Philadelphia: WB Saunders; 1999
8. McLeod JG. Sural nerve biopsy. J Neurol Neurosurg Psychiatry 2000;69:431
9. Pimentel ML, Fernandes RMP, Babinski MA. Anomalous course of the medial sural cutaneous nerve and its clinical implications. Braz J Morphol Sci 2005;22:179–182
10. Dyck P, Giannini C, Lais A. Pathologic alterations of nerves. In: Dyck PJ, Thomas PK, Griffin JW, eds. Peripheral Neuropathy, 3rd ed, vol 1. Philadelphia: WB Saunders; 1998:514–595
11. Midroni G, Bilbao J. Normal anatomy of peripheral (sural) nerve. In: Midroni G, Bilbao J, eds. Biopsy Diagnosis of Peripheral Neuropathy. Boston: Butterworth-Heinemann; 1995:13–33

141 Approach to the Lumbosacral Plexus

incision on the dura. The graft may course above the facet joint or inside the neuroforamen, although the latter is technically more difficult. The dural incision must be sealed with blood and fibrin glue to avoid CSF leakage.

In multiple avulsions, motor rootlets from the contralateral healthy side are selected, cut, and sutured to the distally avulsed roots via interposition grafts (**Fig. 141.2**).

Occasionally, the roots are found to be severely scarred or stretched and twisted (**Fig. 141.3**), and neurolysis is performed.

Advantages

The procedure offers the possibility to perform a direct root repair. When interposition grafts are needed, they are short. In cases in which severe scarring is found, neurolysis significantly reduces the pain.

Disadvantages

The procedure entails no specific theoretical disadvantages but it is statistically uncommon that the intraoperative findings allow its feasbility. Retrieving the proximal and distal stumps after their intradural rupture and correctly coapting them for each root is technically unlikely in our experience. Intraoperative electrodiagnostic tests help to exclude the possibility to cause any additional functional deficit when an ipsilateral or contralateral root is selected and harvested but CSF leaks and infections are certainly possible to occur in high percentage due to the wide dural opening and long time of surgery.

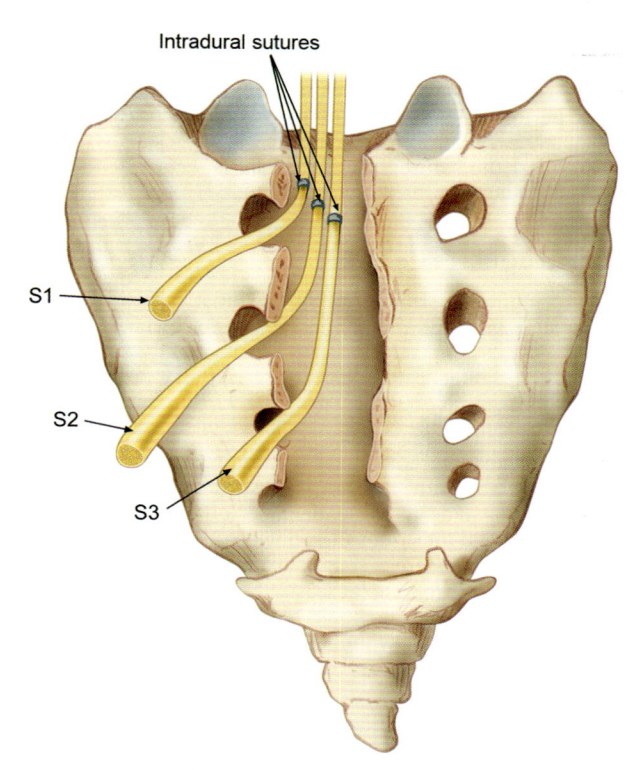

Fig. 141.1 Intradural repair of ruptured ventral roots.

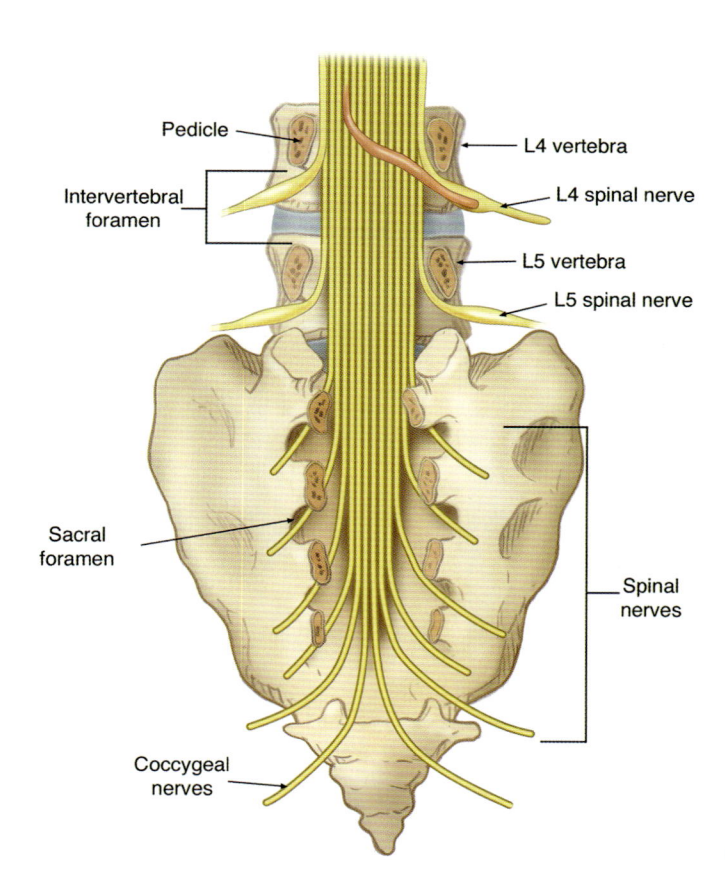

Fig. 141.2 Intradural-extradural repair.

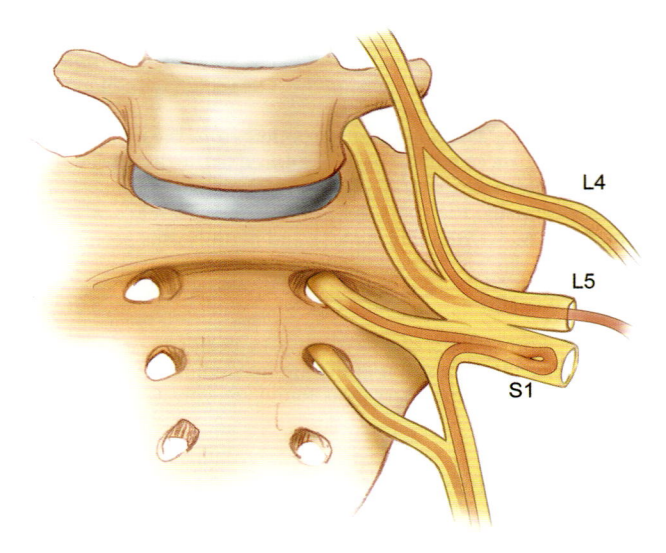

Fig. 141.3 The S1 root twisted and intercepted at L5 level.

Intradural to Extradural Intraplexal Nerve Transfer

When distal stumps are not found at exploration, the surgeon may proceed with a technique to restore hip stability and knee flexion.

From two to four motor fascicles are harvested from the homolateral L3 or L4 rootlets (usually intact in L5-S1 avulsions) or from the contralateral healthy side in cases of multiple avulsions and then sutured to two sural strands passing through the dura. After a waterproof dural closure is achieved, exposure of the recipient gluteal nerves and medial sciatic trunk is performed via Henry's approach **(Fig. 141.4)**.[12]

The sural grafts then must be tunneled subcutaneously and through the displaced gluteus maximus. A dissecting/ligature forceps is first carefully forced through to open the way and then is used to delicately pass the strands from the intradural area so that their distal tips reach the exposed recipients. Neurotization can be performed either to both gluteal nerves or to the superior gluteal nerve and the medial trunk of the sciatic nerve **(Fig. 141.5)**. After the sutures, the gluteal lid is reapproached to its insertion by nonresorbable sutures (0 Vicryl).

Advantage

This procedure is certainly the most statistically feasible one among all those requiring an intradural exploration to retrieve the roots.

Disadvantages

This techinique is extremely time consuming and technically demanding. Intraoperative electrodiagnostic tests allow the procedure to be safe and not cause any additional functional deficit but CSF leaks and infections due to wide dural opening and the long time of surgery are certainly major risks. Moreover the interposition grafts are long (at least 20 cm), highly jeopardizing the outcome. Therefore it should be offered only when surgery is performed within a few months from the injury and in young and very motivated patients.

Intra-Abdominal Exposure and Direct Repair of the Femoral Nerve

The patient is placed in the supine position with the hip and knee slightly flexed or in the lateral decubitus position on the contralateral side to the affected plexus. **Fig. 141.6** illustrates the intra-abdominal exposure of the femoral nerve. If the proximal course of the femoral nerve must be explored, through a dissection over the psoas the lateral aspect of the lumbar column can be exposed, and then the lumbar roots that give origin to the nerve (L2, L3, and L4) are identified. Once the exposure is completed, the nerve injury is assessed to determine whether it is amenable to neurolysis only or if a graft repair (after excision of

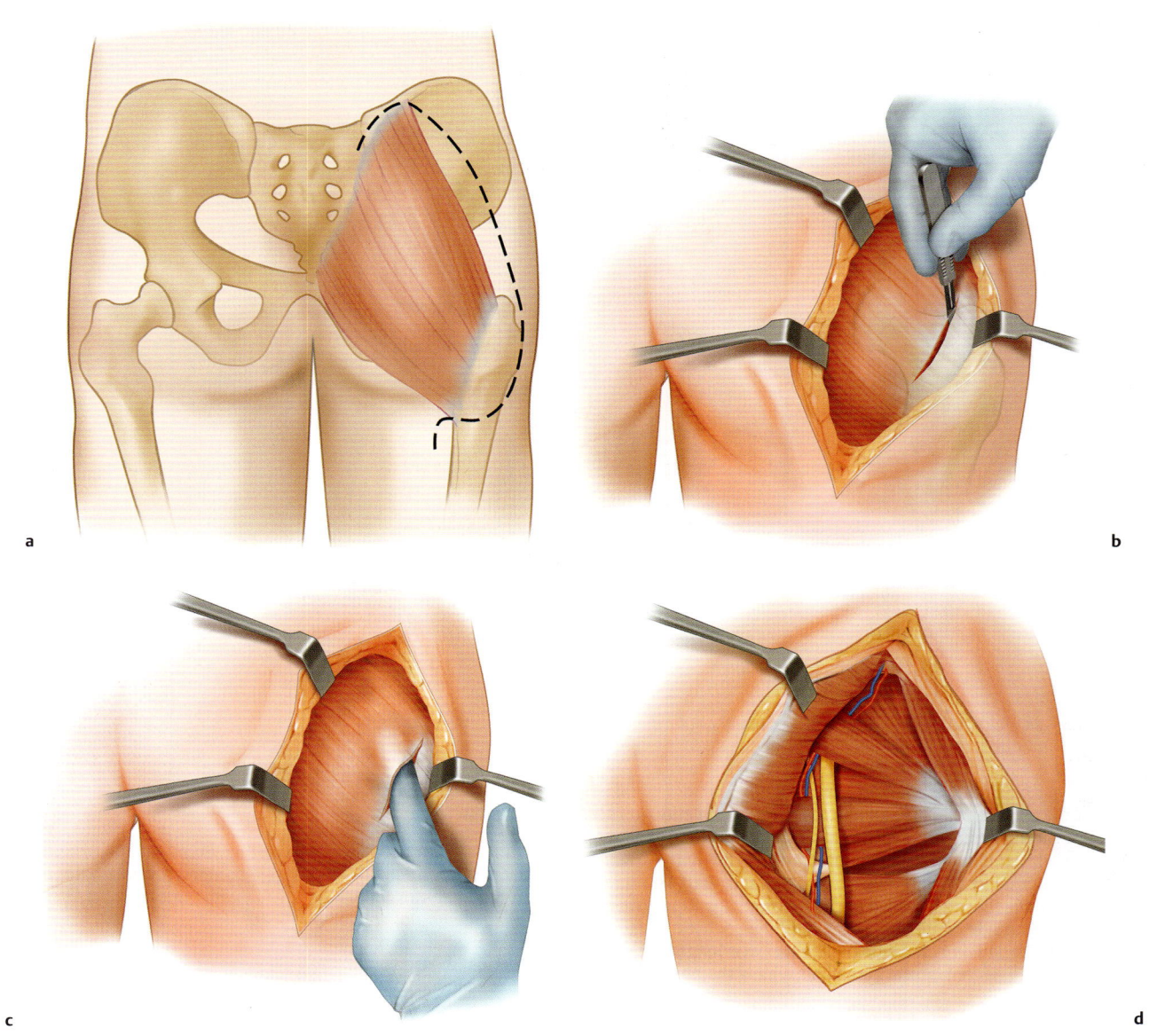

Fig. 141.4 Henry's approach to expose the sciatic nerve course under the buttock. The leg must be externally rotated at the hip joint to relax the gluteal muscles. **(a)** A question mark–shaped skin incision is drawn following the five illustrated anatomic landmarks: it starts from the posterior superior spine, partly follows the iliac crest, reaches the great trocanter, and along the gluteal fold and then it is extended to the posterior midline of the thigh. The skin incision must reach but not trespass the deep fascia to preserve the posterior cutaneous nerve that runs immediately below it and then at the level of the gluteal fold gives off sensitive collaterals for the posterior thigh skin and the perineum. **(b,c)** Detachment of the gluteus maximus. The gluteal fascia is vertically incised on the external surface of the great trochanter. The surgeon slides an index finger into the incision and palpates the posterior surface of the great trochanter that separates the planes. Moving the finger under the fascia, the lateral insertion of the gluteus maximus is progressively detached. The superior external border of the muscle (corresponding to the fusion of its superficial and deep aponeurosis) is delimited by a yellow-white line from the border of the gluteus medius. Following this line, the gluteus maximus must be completely detached from the iliac crest, otherwise the surgeon will be constantly hampered in visualizing the proximal sciatic nerve exiting the notch. Distally, the muscle must be detached from its insertion on the femoral shaft, cutting down to the bone. Every 5 to 6 cm, the fascial edges are marked by 0 Vicryl stitches that are useful for reapproximating the gluteus maximus during closure. **(d)** Exposure of the course of the sciatic nerve. Once its insertion is completely cut, the whole gluteal "lid" can be gently lifted and medially displaced, and the course of the sciatic nerve is clearly exposed. The anatomic landmark to identify the gluteal nerves is the piriformis muscle. Its edges are not always clear, as a deep fold in the gluteus medius occasionally can be mistaken for a replicating piriformis. The superior gluteal vessels and nerve are found above the piriformis muscle. The nerve runs forward off the vessels. Its identification is not straightforward as it is concealed by the gluteus medius. The inferior gluteal vessels are easily identified, being the most superficial structures to emerge at the lower edge of the piriformis. During the dissection the gluteal vessels must be carefully respected. In the event that they are stretched and torn during dissection, once the "gluteal lid" is hinged back they can become a source of bleeding.

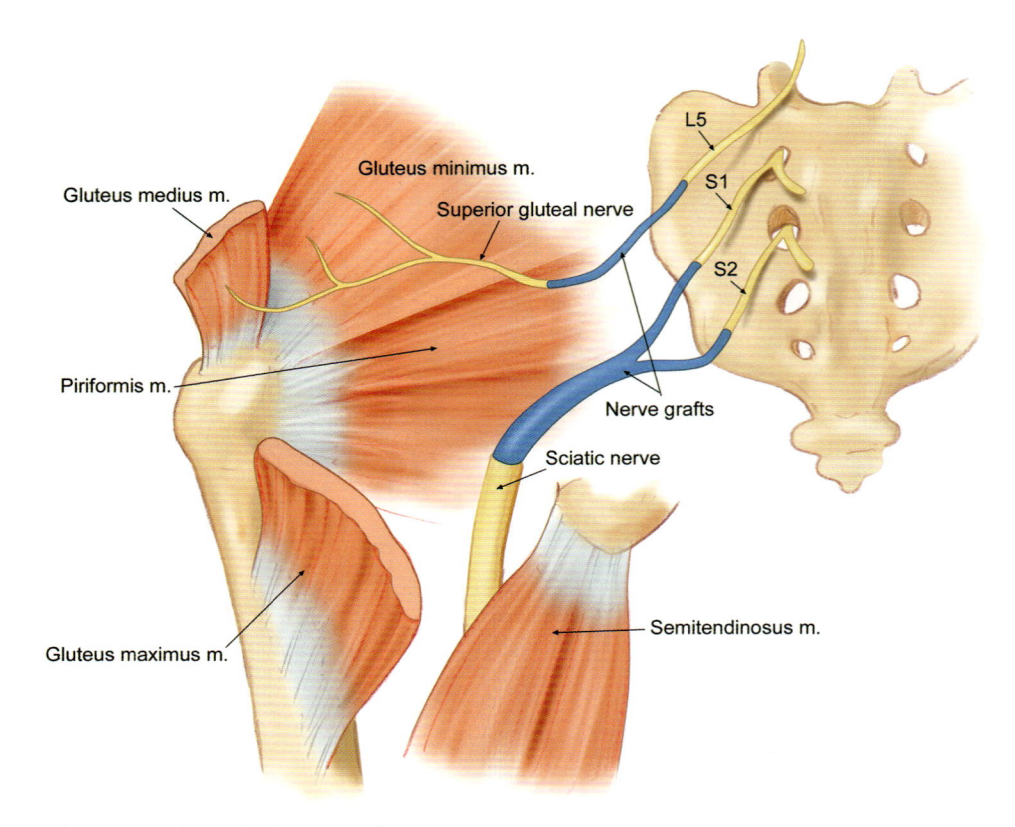

Fig. 141.5 Intraspinal to extraspinal intraplexal nerve transfer.

a neuroma) is needed (**Fig. 141.7**). Depending on the surgical findings, the surgeon may expose the extra-abdominal course of the femoral nerve as well (see below), and perform an intra- to extra-abdominal graft repair. In such cases the graft should be tunneled under the lateral third of the inguinal ligament to avoid injury to the funicle content.

If direct repair is ruled out (e.g., excessive length of interposition graft), nerve transfers (see below) are the best option.

Advantage

Depending on the length of the grafts, intra-abdominal or intra- to extra-abdominal repair of the femoral nerve is generally favorable even if complete recovery is unlikely.

Disadvantage

Proximal, intra-abdominal exposure of the femoral nerve may require a multidisciplinary team, including a general or urologic surgeon.

Obturator to Femoral Nerve Transfer

Intra-Abdominal Procedure

The surgical approach is the same as that described to expose the proximal femoral nerve. The obturator nerve courses in close proximity to the femoral nerve at the level of the middle of the psoas muscle; therefore, it can be identified and coapted with the former (**Fig. 141.8**). One third of the population has an accessory obturator nerve arising from L3-L4 (the main nerve comes from L2, L3, and L4) that can be preferably chosen as the donor.

Advantage

When found, an accessory nerve is an excellent donor as it innervates only the pectineus muscle (otherwise normally innervated by the femoral nerve).

Disadvantages

This exposure requires the help of a gynecologist or a general surgeon. If no accessory obturator nerve is found, the procedure causes loss of adduction.

Extra-Abdominal Procedure

The patient is placed in the supine position with the thighs slightly apart. A vertical skin incision is drawn from the inguinal line on the anterolateral surface of the thigh to the opening of the fascia lata, providing exposure of the femoral vessels. Opening the iliacus fascia lateral to the femoral artery exposes the femoral nerve, which splits into its four terminal branches just 2 to 3 cm distal to the inguinal ligament.

After opening the fascia and following the lateral edge of the longus adductor, the obturator nerve can be identified medial to the femoral vein. Following the lateral edge of the adductor brevis muscle (located deeper than and superior to the adductor longus), the nerve can be traced back to its bifurcation into the anterior and posterior divisions, the latter coursing behind the adductor brevis muscle. Stimulation is used to determine the most suitable donor branch for a direct suture with the femoral recipient. The choice should be made carefully to avoid significant denervation of the adductor muscles.

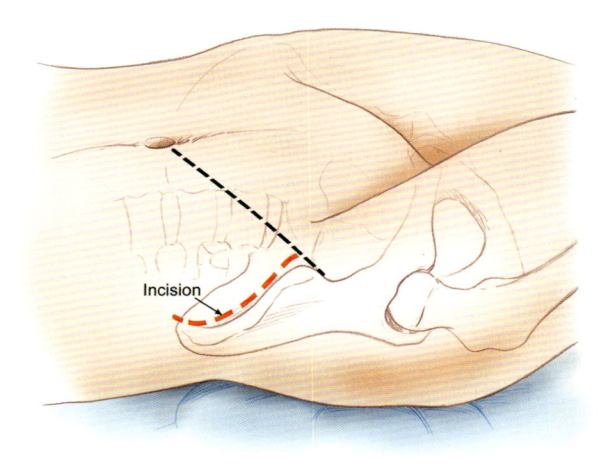

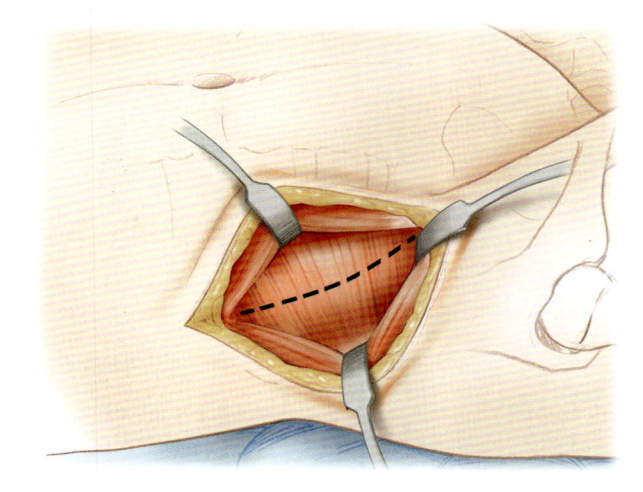

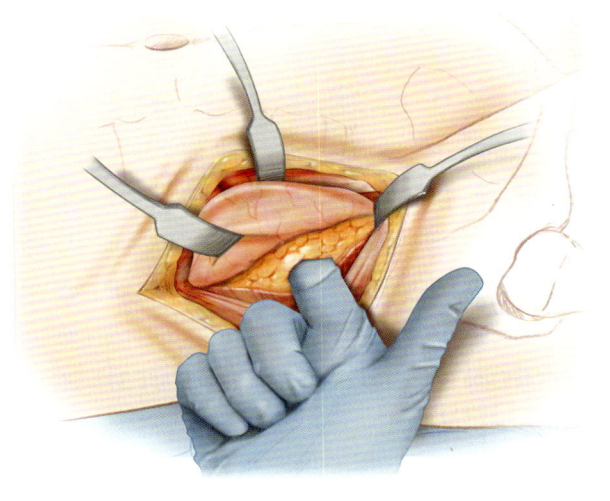

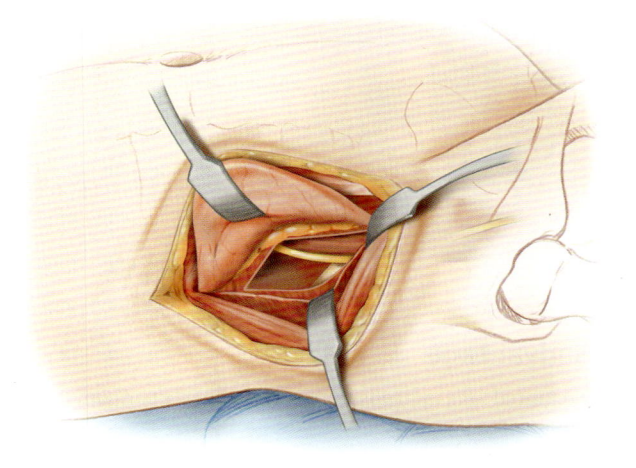

Fig. 141.6 Intra-abdominal exposure of the femoral nerve. **(a)** A flank incision starting at the medial point of the iliac crest and 1 cm above and in line with it is drawn down to the anterior superior iliac spine. **(b)** The muscles of the abdominal wall (external and internal oblique muscles and the transversalis muscle) are dissected following the direction of their fibers as long as possible to access the endoabdominal space. **(c)** A blunt dissection of the retroperitoneal fat and medial retraction of the peritoneum and viscera with large retractors enable entering the retroperitoneal space. **(d)** The psoas muscle can be easily identified, and at its lateral border the femoral nerve looks like a white ribbon that runs toward the inguinal ligament. The urethra must be identified and carefully preserved.

Advantages

This procedure provides easy access to both nerves and offers the possibility of performing direct transfer due to their proximity.

Disadvantages

The denervation of some muscles that are useful for adduction can occur in correlation with the number of donor fascicles. In cases of unsuccessful outcomes, an adjunctive impairment of hip adduction may add to the previous disability.

Femoral Nerve to Gluteal Nerve Transfer

The patient is placed in the lateral decubitus position, lying on the contralateral side to the affected lumbosacral plexus. The femoral nerve and the course of the sciatic nerve (including identification of the gluteal nerves) under the buttock must be exposed, as previously discussed. Once the femoral nerve is isolated, its lateral fascicles (supplying the lateral portions of the quadriceps) must be dissected from its main trunk and then severed to serve as donor fascicles. The distance between the femoral donor fascicles and the gluteal recipients requires an interposition graft whose length can be measured by passing a suture thread with a dissecting/ligature forceps that is carefully tunneled under the tensor fascia lata muscle. Two sural strands matching the measured length are prepared with two tips glued together. They are then tunneled under the tensor fascia lata muscle. On the anterior thigh, the glued tips are sutured to the donor femoral fascicles; at the buttock each strand is coapted with a gluteal nerve. Alternatively, one strand can be coapted to the medial trunk of the sciatic nerve to regain hamstring reinnervation.

Advantages

This procedure is not technically demanding and there is no risk of complications. Exposure of both the sciatic and the femoral nerves can be performed by two surgeons at the same time.

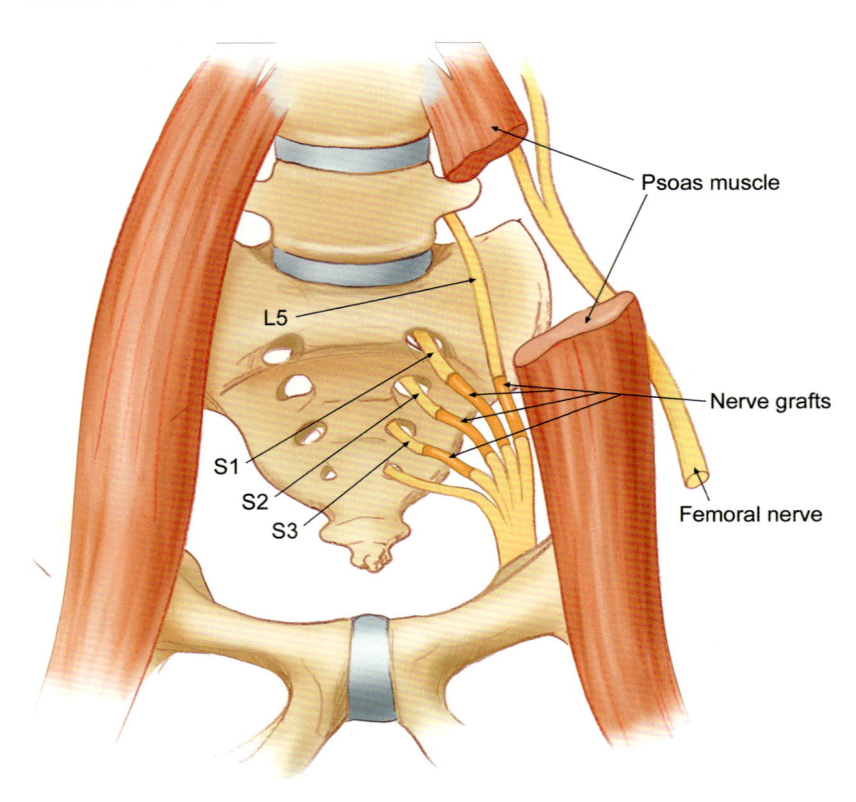

Fig. 141.7 Intrapelvic repair of the femoral nerve.

Disadvantage

The required long interposition grafts are likely to doom the procedure to an unsuccessful outcome.

Postoperative Care After Nerve Transfers

Bed rest is advised for at least 10 days, and anti-thromboembolism prophylaxes must be administered. Physiotherapy is intensely resumed at the end of the immobilization period.

Surgical Technique for Persisting Foot Drop

Anesthesia

Surgery can be performed with the patient under general or spinal anesthesia, and there are no contraindications to the use of muscular blocks.

The patient is placed in the supine position, with the foot placed at the lower edge of the operating table, to enable the

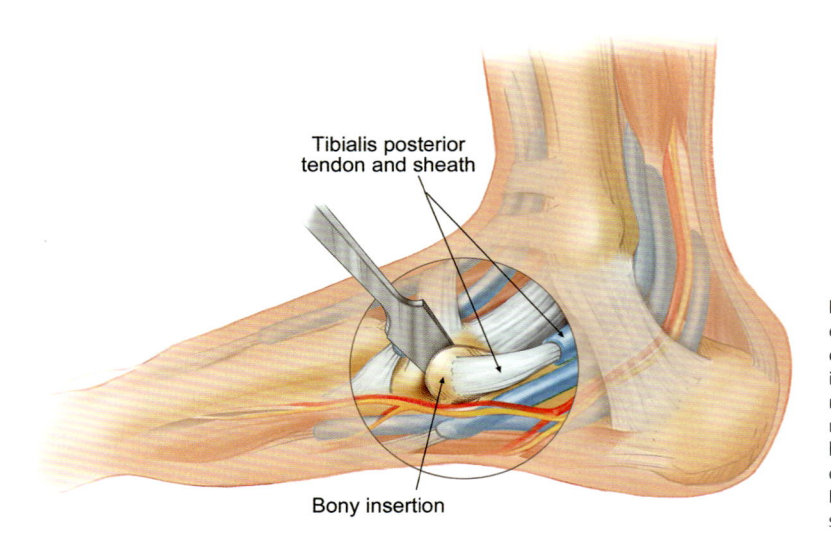

Fig. 141.8 The flexor digitorum longus tendon can be easily mistaken for the posterior tibialis tendon (PTT). To correctly identify the PTT, it can be pulled to demonstrate its action. The flexor digitorum longus tendon is also thinner than the PTT. The PTT fan-like insertion on the scaphoid must be carefully detached. It is preferable to avoid prolongation of the incision on the malleolar skin (due to occasional poor healing of the wound) and to pull out the PTT at the retromalleolar level, and palpate and expose its subcutaneous course toward the plantar arc.

assistant to push the foot up to 90 degrees when required during the procedure.

Surgical Technique

Through a proximally extended retromalleolar incision on the medial aspect of the ankle, after opening of the fascia the posterior tibialis tendon (PTT) is identified (**Fig. 141.8**). After the detachment of its insertion, the flexor retinaculum is subcutaneously opened to enable the proximal pulling out of the tendon. A Kocher forceps is passed through the interosseus membrane, to create an adequate opening, and extending to the lateral malleolus. Through a small skin incision at this level, another Kocher forceps is passed, following the reverse course of the first tool to hook and pull out the PTT. An incision on the dorsum of the foot exposes the third cuneiform; the extensor hallucis longus and extensor digitorum longus tendons are identified, encircled by Penrose drains and displaced. A gouge is used to induce decortication on the bone surface to favor osteosynthesis, which will encompass the new PTT insertion. The tendon is subcutaneously tunneled under the extensor retinaculum and pulled out to reach the third cuneiform with the foot at 90 degrees. Two Mitek anchors are used to insert the tendon on the dorsum of the foot that must be mantained at 90 degrees of flexion. To avoid Claw toes, an Extensor hallucis longus and extensor digitorum longus tenodesis is performed on the newly inserted tendon; alternatively, the flexor digitorum longus tendon is passed together with the PTT, and a Pulvertaft suture with the toe extensors tendons is performed.

In injuries of long duration, severe hypertrophy of the Achilles tendon can render the 90-degree posture of the foot difficult to achieve; this can be overcome with a Z elongation. A talocalcaneal posterior capsulotomy is seldom necessary.

A cast with the foot at 90 degrees and the toes slightly extended is applied at the end of the surgery.

Postoperative Care

The procedure requires immobilization for 4 to 6 weeks (the latter in cases of Achilles tendon elongation). The foot must be kept elevated for 5 days, after which the patient can resume walking with crutches, avoiding weight-bearing on the operated limb. Anti-thromboembolism prophylaxes and a calcium-rich diet are prescribed. Once the cast is removed, a short period of rehabilitation may be needed to train the patient to appropriately use the transfer.

Advantages

Learning to use the transfer is generally almost automatic and the patient regains normal gait.

Disadvantages

The procedure normally reduces the full range of plantar flexion; when the tendon is short (such as in injuries of long duration or due to an anatomic condition of the patient), plantar flexion can be severely impaired.

Some patients occasionally complain of ankle instability after Achilles tendon elongation.

A long-term supinated flatfoot may occasionally ensue.

The flexor digitorum longus transfer to toe extensors normally turns out to work as a passive tenodesis. Although learning to perform inversion to regain foot dorsiflexion is easy, learning to flex the toes to obtain their extension is not that simple. In our experience, only very young patients acquire this ability.

Conclusion

Lumbosacral plexus injuries have a high rate of spontaneous recovery, and the selection of surgical candidates is less straightforward than with other posttraumatic nerve injuries. If surgery is indicated, the surgeon must be well versed in the priorities in functional restoration, and the repair strategy must be carefully tailored to the patient. These lesions are complex and variable due to the multiple factors influencing the nerve injury (such as the causative mechanism and the associated vascular and musculoskeletal lesions). The time at which the injury is evaluated for surgical treatment is crucial in the choice of the repair strategies, which include a wide variety of techniques ranging from direct nerve microreconstruction to tendon transfers. Therefore, the surgeon who is willing to take up the challenge presented by these lesions must be highly experienced in peripheral nerve surgery in order to choose the treatment most likely to offer the best possible outcome.

After the introduction of nerve transfers, postprocedural complications are less frequent than they were in the past, and nowadays this surgery can be considered rather safe. But the functional outcomes are uncertain, and the success rate is lower than with surgery of the counterpart.

References

1. Sedel L. Voies d'abord des nerfes du member inferieur. Med Chir Techn Chirurg Orthop (Paris) 1975;44530:1–8
2. Linarte R, Gilbert A. Trans-sacral approach to the sacral plexus. Periph Nerve Repair Regen 1986;4:17–20
3. Stoehr M. Traumatic and postoperative lesions of the lumbosacral plexus. Arch Neurol 1978;35:757–760
4. Campbell AA, Eckhauser FE, Belzberg A, Campbell JN. Obturator nerve transfer as an option for femoral nerve repair: case report. Neurosurgery 2010;66(6, Suppl Operative):375, discussion 375
5. Tung TH, Chao A, Moore AM. Obturator nerve transfer for femoral nerve reconstruction: anatomic study and clinical application. Plast Reconstr Surg 2012;130:1066–1074
6. Goubier JN, Teboul F, Yeo S. Transfer of two motor branches of the anterior obturator nerve to the motor portion of the femoral nerve: an anatomical feasibility study. Microsurgery 2012;32:463–465
7. Lang EM, Borges J, Carlstedt T. Surgical treatment of lumbosacral plexus injuries. J Neurosurg Spine 2004;1:64–71
8. Zhao S, Beuerman RW, Kline DG. Neurotization of motor nerves innervating the lower extremity by utilizing the lower intercostal nerves. J Reconstr Microsurg 1997;13:39–45
9. Penkert G, Fansa H. Peripheral nerve lesions. In: Penkert G, Fansa H, eds. Nerve Surgery and Secondary Reconstructive Repair. New York: Springer; 2004:164–166
10. Wiltse LL, Bateman JG, Hutchinson RH, Nelson WE. The paraspinal sacrospinalis-splitting approach to the lumbar spine. J Bone Joint Surg Am 1968;50:919–926
11. Warren A, Prasad V, Thomas M. Pre-operative planning when using the Wiltse approach to the lumbar spine. Ann R Coll Surg Engl 2010;92:74–75
12. Henry AK. Extensile Exposure Applied to Limb Surgery. Edinburgh: E & S Livingstone; 1950.

E. Other Nerves

142 The Intercostal Nerves

Allan D. Nanney III, Karina Nieto, and Aruna Ganju

The intercostal nerves are part of the somatic nervous system; together, they innervate the majority of the cutaneous and subcutaneous tissue, thoracic and abdominal musculature, and visceral coverings such as the thoracic pleura and the abdominal peritoneum. They innervate many of the muscles of respiration, with the exception of the diaphragm, which is primarily serviced by the phrenic nerve. They also relay sensory information from both the superficial soft tissues and deeper viscera of the thoracic and abdominal compartments. Appreciation of the intercostal nerves is critical for neurosurgeons as various pathological processes and pain syndromes affect this nerve. Additionally, the intercostals can be utilized as donor nerves during brachial plexus surgery. This chapter discusses the anatomy and clinical implications of the intercostal nerves.

Anatomy and Function[1,2]

The Thoracic Spinal Nerves and the Proximal Intercostal Nerves

As the thoracic spinal nerves exit their intervertebral foramina, they divide into dorsal and ventral rami. The dorsal rami innervate the paraspinous musculature, joints, bones, and cutaneous tissues of the trunk. The intercostal nerves represent the anterior, or ventral ramus, of the first 11 spinal nerves of the thoracic spine.

The first and second intercostal nerves supply fibers to the upper limb via the brachial plexus, but also, with intercostal nerves 3 to 6, supply the thorax. Intercostal nerves 7 to 11 supply the thorax and the abdomen. The 12th thoracic spinal nerve is named the *subcostal nerve* as it runs not between two ribs but rather below the last rib; this nerve innervates the abdominal wall and skin overlying the buttocks.

Following its origination from the anterior ramus, the intercostal nerves give rise to two branches—the gray and white rami communicantes. These branches convey unmyelinated and myelinated fibers, respectively, to and from the sympathetic ganglion related to the corresponding intercostal space. The gray ramus typically joins the intercostal nerves medial to the point at which the white ramus leaves it.

Unlike the peripheral nerves that travel from the spine to the upper and lower extremities, each intercostal nerve pursues an independent course without forming a plexus with neighboring nerves. Anatomically, each intercostal nerve exits laterally from the spine and courses around the thoracic cavity in the inferiorly located costal groove of its respectively numbered rib. Within these grooves, the nerves run in parallel with the intercostal arteries and veins of the corresponding level in the following superior-to-inferior order: vein, artery, and nerve (**Fig. 142.1**). This anatomic arrangement is pertinent when chest tube insertion and thoracentesis are performed; to avoid the neurovascular bundle, the thorax should be entered above a rib. In contrast, in an intercostal nerve block, the neurovascular bundle is the target of the procedure, and injection should be performed infracostally. What is presented here is somewhat simplified; in reality, the true journey of each intercostal nerve as it exits the spinal canal is more complex.

After exiting the neuroforamina, dividing into a dorsal and ventral ramus and receiving autonomic supply via the gray and white communicantes, each intercostal nerve lies within an intercostal space formed by the parietal pleura internally, and the posterior intercostal membrane externally. As the nerve moves laterally and enters its costal groove, its internal boundary transitions from the parietal pleura to the subcostal muscle and then to the innermost intercostal muscle, also known as the intracostal muscle. Likewise, as the nerve moves laterally, its external boundary transitions from the posterior intercostal membrane to the internal intercostal muscle. The nerve travels in the subcostal groove for a long distance, sandwiched between the innermost intercostal and internal intercostal muscles (**Fig. 142.2**). In general, the typical intercostal nerve follows this predictable and reproducible anatomic course as described above, and gives off important named branches. These branches and classic deviations of individual nerves are discussed in the following subsections.

Intercostal Nerve Branches (Fig. 142.2)

Along its course, the main intercostal nerve gives off predictable branches. As this intercostal nerve travels in its costal groove, proximal to the rib angle, it gives off a collateral branch that travels parallel but inferior to the main nerve. A communicating branch on the main intercostal nerve below may connect these branches anywhere between the midaxillary line and the anterior end of the rib; these nerves can also coalesce prior to dividing again. These nerves travel anteriorly to terminate as anterior cutaneous branches that innervate the midline thoracic cutaneous region and may further divide into medial and lateral branches. Hence, each intercostal may provide two anterior cutaneous branches, the collateral nerve being the lower of the two anterior branches.

The lateral cutaneous branch generally branches from the main nerve mid-rib, between the vertebrae and the sternum, but may branch at any point between the angle of the rib and the midaxillary line. It continues to run in the space between the innermost and internal intercostal muscles until it obliquely pierces the internal and external intercostal muscles and serratus anterior to innervate the skin on the lateral thoracic wall. These nerves further divide into anterior and posterior branches.

The anterior branch of the lateral cutaneous nerve courses anteriorly to the side and front of the chest, supplying the cuta-

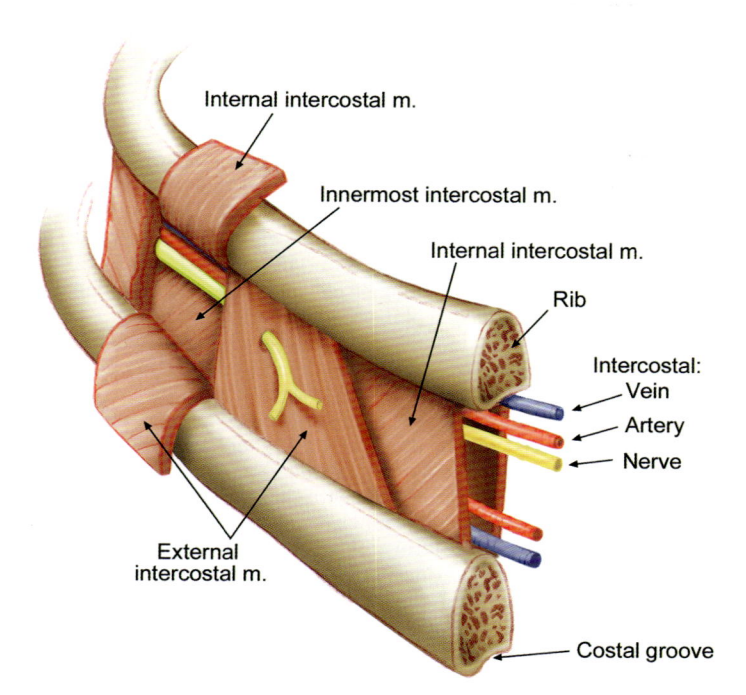

Fig. 142.1 The orientation of the vein-artery-nerve bundle in a superior to inferior order as these structures travel within their respective costal grooves between the innermost and internal intercostal muscles.

neous and mammary tissue in this region. As the name suggests, the posterior branches of the lateral cutaneous nerve course posteriorly after their origin supplying the skin over the scapula and the latissimus dorsi muscle.

The intercostals give rise to many other branches including muscular, pleural, and peritoneal branches. Muscular branches are small branches that supply the muscles of the intercostal spaces. Pleural branches are the afferent sensory branches from the parietal pleura. Peritoneal sensory branches are similar to the pleural branches but arise from the lower intercostal nerves.

Several branches specific to certain levels are worthy of note. The first intercostal nerve is connected to the brachial plexus by its equivalent of the lateral cutaneous nerve. Additionally, the first intercostal nerve has no anterior cutaneous branch owing to its short length. The lateral cutaneous branch of the second intercostal nerve does not branch; it is known as the intercostobrachial nerve. This nerve joins the medial brachial cutaneous nerve to supply the skin of the upper half of the medial and posterior arm.

The First and Second Intercostal Nerves (Fig. 142.2)

The first thoracic nerve divides into a large and a small branch. The large branch, akin to the lateral cutaneous branch, exits the thorax anterior to the first rib and enters the brachial plexus. The smaller branch, the true first intercostal nerve, runs in the first intercostal space and terminates in the anterior cutaneous tissues in front of the thorax. Because of its small size, the first intercostal nerve typically lacks a true anterior cutaneous branch.

The second intercostal nerve supplies the second intercostal space, the skin of the armpit, and the proximal medial arm. The

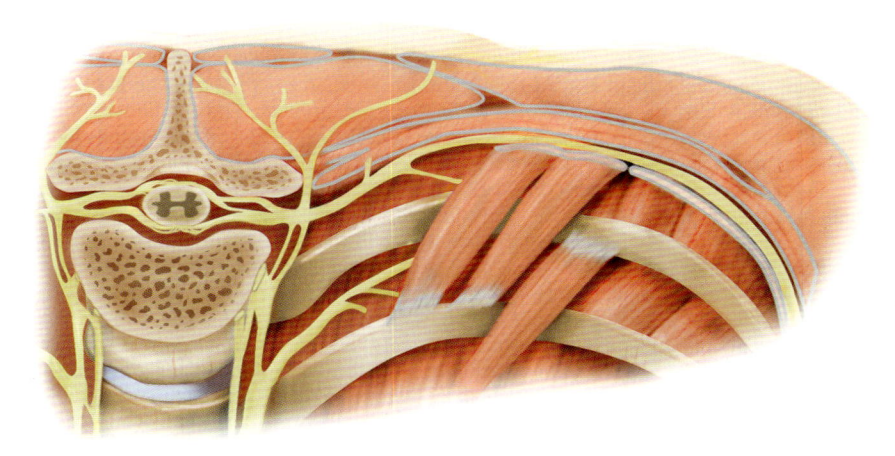

Fig. 142.2 The classic anatomic relationship of the intercostal nerves from the point at which they arise from the ventral ramus of the thoracic spinal nerves and their journey around the thoracic cage or abdominal wall as it travels in the costal groove between known muscular structures and gives off expected branches.

second intercostal nerve may give rise to an intercostobrachial nerve that contributes to the medial cutaneous nerve of the arm.

The Upper Thoracic Nerves (Fig. 142.2)

The second to sixth intercostal nerves are collectively known as the upper thoracic or thoracic intercostal nerves. These nerves course around the thorax, supplying respiratory muscles such as the intercostales, subcostales, levatores costarum, serratus posterior superior, and transversus thoracis. The first six intercostal nerves receive sensory pleural branches and terminate within their respective intercostal spaces.

The Lower Thoracic Nerves (Fig. 142.2)

The seventh to 11th intercostal nerves are collectively known as the lower thoracic, thoracoabdominal, or thoracicoabdominal intercostal nerves. Anteriorly, they travel behind the costal cartilages and between the obliquus internus and transversus abdominis to supply the rectus abdominis muscle. Upon termination, as anterior cutaneous branches, they supply the skin of the anterior abdomen. As each muscle and skin segment may receive innervation from two or three intercostal nerves, there is an unpredictable degree of collateral plexus formation in the abdominal wall. These nerves also carry afferents from the peritoneum.

The seventh, eighth, and ninth intercostal nerves exit the intercostal space ventrally and enter the anterior abdominal wall by traveling between the costal cartilages and the transversus abdominis muscle. In contrast, the 10th and 11th intercostal nerves pass directly into the abdominal wall. The last three lower thoracic nerves send branches to the serratus posterior inferior. Their lateral cutaneous branches give rise to anterior and posterior branches. The former supplies the obliquus externus abdominis to the lateral margin of the rectus abdominis. The posterior branches course dorsally supplying the skin over the latissimus dorsi.

The Twelfth Thoracic Nerve/The Subcostal Nerve (Fig. 142.2)

The anterior ramus of the 12th thoracic nerve is the largest, traveling along the lower border of the 12th rib and ending as the subcostal nerve. It can contribute a branch to the first lumbar nerve as well as the iliohypogastric nerve of the lumbar plexus. In addition, the subcostal nerve gives rise to a large lateral cutaneous branch that supplies sensory innervation to the skin over the hip.

Neurosurgical Considerations

The neurosurgeon typically encounters the intercostal nerves clinically when treating patients with pain syndromes or when considering alternate nerve graft options for neurotization procedures of the brachial plexus and its peripheral branches. The literature is replete with reports of intercostal pain syndromes and the use of the nerve in reinnervation attempts for treatment of brachial plexus injuries (**Table 142.1**).

The intercostal nerves are the culprit in several relatively common pain syndromes including postthoracotomy, postherpetic, posttraumatic, and postneoplastic neuralgias. Despite the segmental distribution of the intercostal nerves, overlap of cutaneous innervation results in complete anesthesia only being achieved when two or three nerves are sectioned.

A variety of therapeutic options are available for intercostal nerve pain syndromes. Although intercostal nerve blocks can provide temporary relief,[3] spinal cord and peripheral nerve stimulation is an option for more definitive treatment of chronic, intractable pain.[4] Lesioning procedures, such as dorsal rhizotomies and dorsal root ganglionectomies, can also be utilized in the treatment of select chronic pain patients.[5]

Brachial plexus injuries and upper extremity peripheral nerve palsies are seen as a result of gunshot and knife wounds, and in infancy as a result of obstetric complications.[6,7] Intercostal nerves have been used for neurotization procedures to reinnervate the brachial plexus, phrenic nerve, and lumbosacral plexus.[8–26] Intercostal nerves have a long history of being used in the neurotization of the brachial plexus and its peripheral nerves used to restore elbow flexion[10–12,16,24,26]; this involves transposition of one or more intercostal nerves to the musculocutaneous nerve, thereby reinnervating the biceps brachialis muscle.

Recent studies suggest that good deltoid and bicep function can be restored with an intercostal graft,[15] although the spinal accessory nerve may be a better option for biceps reinnervation.[24] Outcomes may be comparable with those of ulnar transposition for biceps function.[26] Interestingly, by using the intercostal nerves, one may expect the return of some motor and sensory function.[24] The intercostal nerves have been used in reinnervation procedures for restoration of sensory deficit; variable results have been reported.[23] Restoration of elbow extension with intercostal nerve grafting has been less successful.[15,18] When compared with other grafting techniques, intercostal nerve harvesting does not increase surgical morbidity[16,24] unless several nerves are harvested simultaneously.[17]

The best results are achieved if neurotization is performed within 6 months after initial injury.[21] If it is successful, patients notice a return of biceps brachialis function around 8 months after surgery. Initially, the muscle action is not under voluntary control, with contractions elicited during coughing, but with training and observed motor nerve plasticity, patients can gain voluntary control, full range of motion, and the ability to hold the arm steadily flexed through the respiratory cycle.[13]

Surgical Technique for Intercostal Nerve Transposition to the Musculocutaneous Nerve

The patient is placed in the prone position. Surgical prep extends from the spine to the sternum and from the jaw to the inferior costal margin on the side of the injury. The proximal brachial plexus is explored through a standard supraclavicular approach, checking for any intact nerve roots. If no intact nerve roots are found, then an incision in the deltopectoral groove is made from the clavicle to the pectoralis major muscle. The plane is deepened, and the pectoralis is divided near its insertion into the humerus. Next, the pectoralis minor is divided from the conjoined ligament. At this point, the median nerve should be identified ~ 2 inches below the coracoid process. The median nerve is traced proximally to the lateral cord to identify the musculocutaneous nerve; this should be explored to rule out any preexisting injury (**Fig. 142.3**).

Once the musculocutaneous nerve is isolated, the patient is positioned in the lateral decubitus position. An incision is made from the lateral border of the paraspinous muscles to the midaxillary line just inferior to the inferior border of the scapula. This incision is deepened through the latissimus dorsi and serratus anterior muscles (**Fig. 142.3**). The third through fifth intercostal nerves are then dissected from the costal groove in the inferior margin of their respective ribs as far proximally and distally as possible. The lateral cutaneous branch of the intercostal nerves may be identified at its takeoff just proximal to the poste-

Fig. 142.3 Neurotization of biceps brachialis using intercostal nerves. **(a)** An incision is made in the deltopectoral groove. **(b)** The deltopectoral groove is dissected and the pectoralis major is divided just proximal to its insertion into the humerus. **(c)** The musculocutaneous nerve is identified and **(d)** the transposed intercostal nerves (dissected from a thoracic incision made just below the tip of the scapula) are then anastomosed to it.

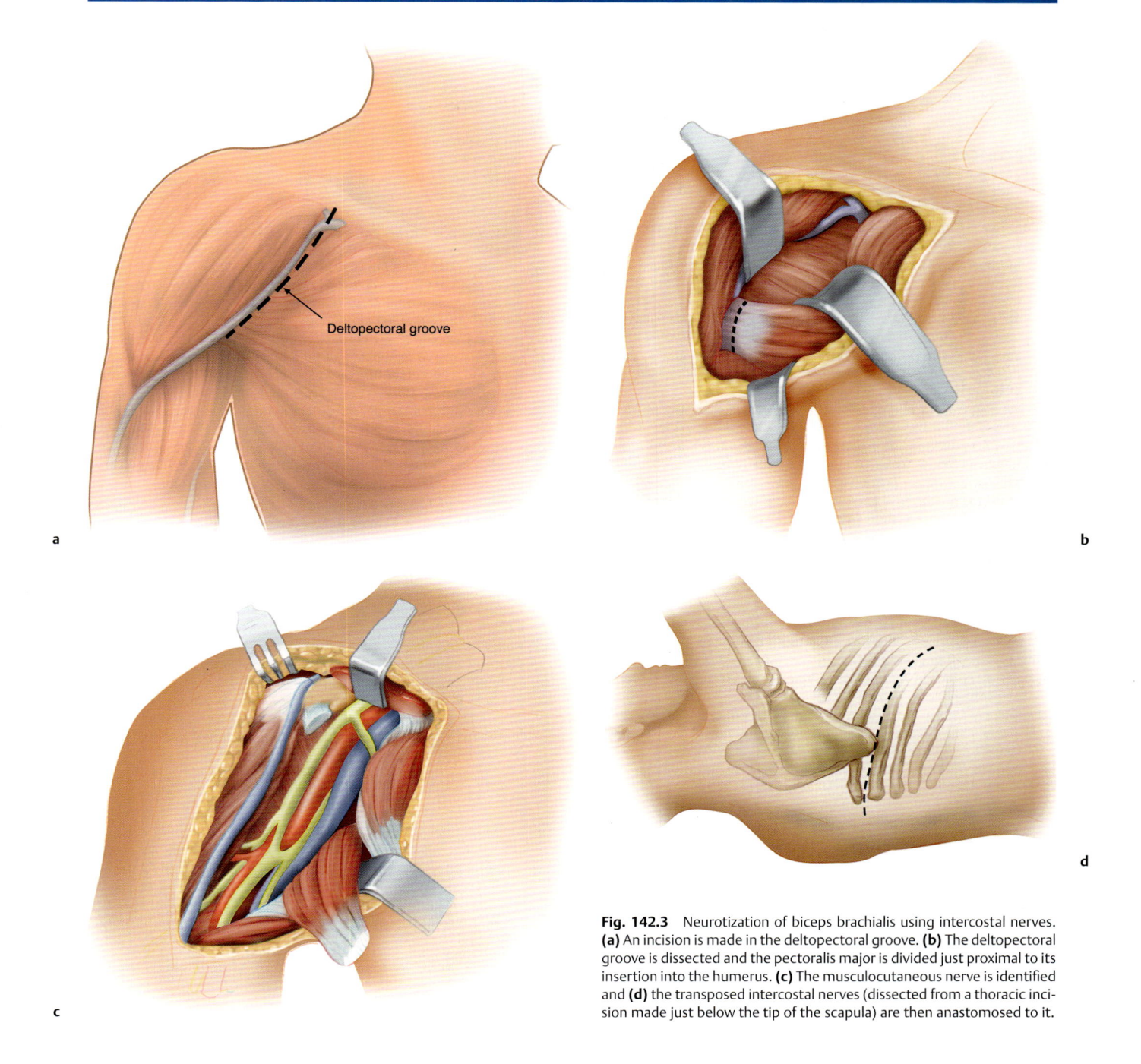

rior axillary line. It should be noted that the lateral cutaneous branch might be larger than the distal intercostal nerve.

Next, a tunnel is created from the lateral incision to the anterior incision. Once the distance to the musculocutaneous nerve is measured and a satisfactory length of intercostal nerve has been mobilized, the intercostal nerves are divided distally and tunneled to the anterior incision. The lateral wound is then irrigated and closed. Chest tubes may be necessary if the pleura has been violated. After closure, the patient is again positioned prone. The musculocutaneous nerve is incised close to the coracobrachialis muscle without putting undue tension on the transposed intercostal nerves. End-to-end anastomosis of the three intercostal nerves to the end of the transected musculocutaneous nerve is performed using a 10-0 nylon. The wound is copiously irrigated and then closed. After 6 weeks of immobilization, passive range-of-motion physical therapy may begin.

Conclusion

The intercostal nerves, with some exceptions, follow a predictable anatomic course as it exits the spine and travels around the thoracic and abdominal walls. It innervates a vast area and is responsible for supplying many of the muscles of respiration in addition to the cutaneous and muscular layers of the thorax and abdomen. The intercostals are also responsible for relaying superficial and visceral sensory information from these compartments.

The peripheral nerve surgeon should be familiar with the intercostal nerves and their surgical anatomy as they can be good donor candidates, in certain cases, for neurotization procedures and brachial plexus re-innervation.

References

1. Snell RS. Clinical Anatomy for Medical Students, 3rd ed. Boston: Little, Brown; 1981:63-71
2. Netter FH. Atlas of Human Anatomy. Summit, NJ: CIBA Geigy Corporation; 1989:237-241
3. Brechner VL. Management of pain by conduction anesthesia techniques. In: Youmans JR, ed. Neurological Surgery, 3rd ed. Philadelphia: WB Saunders; 1990:4007-4025
4. Johnson RD, Green AL, Aziz TZ. Implantation of an intercostal nerve stimulator for chronic abdominal pain. Ann R Coll Surg Engl 2010;92:W1-3
5. Young RF. Dorsal rhizotomy and dorsal root ganglionectomy. In: Youmans JR, ed. Neurological Surgery, 3rd ed. Philadelphia: WB Saunders; 1990: 4026-4035
6. Yeoman PM. Traction Injuries of the Brachial Plexus. Nurs Mirror Midwives J. 1971;132(4):26-27
7. Friedman AH. Surgical management of peripheral nerve injury and entrapment. Neurosurg Clin N Am 1991;2:165-174
8. Krieger AJ, Gropper MR, Adler RJ. Electrophrenic respiration after intercostal to phrenic nerve anastomosis in a patient with anterior spinal artery syndrome: technical case report. Neurosurgery 1994;35:760-763, discussion 763-764
9. Zhao S, Beuerman RW, Kline DG. Neurotization of motor nerves innervating the lower extremity by utilizing the lower intercostal nerves. J Reconstr Microsurg 1997;13:39-45
10. Friedman AH, Nunley JA II, Goldner RD, Oakes WJ, Goldner JL, Urbaniak JR. Nerve transposition for the restoration of elbow flexion following brachial plexus avulsion injuries. J Neurosurg 1990;72:59-64
11. Malessy MJ, Thomeer RT. Evaluation of intercostal to musculocutaneous nerve transfer in reconstructive brachial plexus surgery. J Neurosurg 1998;88:266-271
12. Malessy MJ, van der Kamp W, Thomeer RT, van Dijk JG. Cortical excitability of the biceps muscle after intercostal-to-musculocutaneous nerve transfer. Neurosurgery 1998;42:787-794, discussion 794-795
13. Narakas AO, Hentz VR. Neurotization in brachial plexus injuries. Indication and results. Clin Orthop Relat Res 1988;237:43-56
14. Zheng MX, Qiu YQ, Xu WD, Xu JG. Long-term observation of respiratory function after unilateral phrenic nerve and multiple intercostal nerve transfer for avulsed brachial plexus injury. Neurosurgery 2012;70:796-801, discussion 801
15. Malungpaishrope K, Leechavengvongs S, Witoonchart K, Uerpairojkit C, Boonyalapa A, Janesaksrisakul D. Simultaneous intercostal nerve transfers to deltoid and triceps muscle through the posterior approach. J Hand Surg Am 2012;37:677-682
16. Luo PB, Chen L, Zhou CH, Hu SN, Gu YD. Results of intercostal nerve transfer to the musculocutaneous nerve in brachial plexus birth palsy. J Pediatr Orthop 2011;31:884-888
17. Kovachevich R, Kircher MF, Wood CM, Spinner RJ, Bishop AT, Shin AY. Complications of intercostal nerve transfer for brachial plexus reconstruction. J Hand Surg Am 2010;35:1995-2000
18. Zheng MX, Xu WD, Qiu YQ, Xu JG, Gu YD. Phrenic nerve transfer for elbow flexion and intercostal nerve transfer for elbow extension. J Hand Surg Am 2010;35:1304-1309
19. Durand S, Oberlin C, Fox M, Diverrez JP, Dauge MC. Transfer of the first intercostal nerve to supra- and infraspinatus muscles: an anatomical study and report of the first case. J Hand Surg Eur Vol 2009;34:196-200
20. Wahegaonkar AL, Doi K, Hattori Y, Addosooki AI. Technique of intercostal nerve harvest and transfer for various neurotization procedures in brachial plexus injuries. Tech Hand Up Extrem Surg 2007;11:184-194
21. Moiyadi AV, Devi BI, Nair KP. Brachial plexus injuries: outcome following neurotization with intercostal nerve. J Neurosurg 2007;107:308-313
22. Boulouednine M, Allieu Y. Intercostal nerve transfer classification. Chir Main 2001;20:136-137
23. Schultes G, Gaggl A, Kärcher H. Neuronal anastomosis of the cutaneous ramus of the intercostal nerve to achieve sensibility in the latissimus dorsi transplant. J Oral Maxillofac Surg 2000;58:36-39
24. Waikakul S, Wongtragul S, Vanadurongwan V. Restoration of elbow flexion in brachial plexus avulsion injury: comparing spinal accessory nerve transfer with intercostal nerve transfer. J Hand Surg Am 1999;24:571-577
25. Honey RJ, Ghiculete D, Ray AA, Pace KT. A randomized, double-blinded, placebo-controlled trial of intercostal nerve block after percutaneous nephrolithotomy. J Endourol 2013;27:415-419
26. Kakinoki R, Ikeguchi R, Dunkan SF, et al. Comparison between partial ulnar and intercostal nerve transfers for reconstructing elbow flexion in patients with upper brachial plexus injuries. J Brachial Plex Peripher Nerve Inj 2010;5:4

143 Surgical Treatment of Ilioinguinal Neuralgia

Angela M. Bohnen, Joseph Weiner, Aruna Ganju

Postoperative neuropathy is a recognized consequence of many pelvic surgeries. Although the incidence rates cited in the literature are variable, the rate of inguinodynia, or chronic groin pain, after surgery has been estimated to be as high as 63%.[1,2] The nerves typically involved in this complex syndrome are those of the lumbar plexus: the ilioinguinal nerve, the iliohypogastric nerve, the genital branch of the genitofemoral nerve, and the lateral femoral cutaneous nerve.[1] Specifically, the ilioinguinal nerve (IIN), sometimes in combination with the iliohypogastric nerve, is the second most common neuropathy, representing 22% of all neuropathies in women undergoing pelvic surgery.[3,4]

Inguinal herniorrhaphy is one of the most common elective surgeries performed worldwide,[1,5–7] and is the most common cause of postoperative IIN.[6,8,9] Although IIN typically affects 1 to 2% of herniorrhaphy patients,[5] some studies report an incidence as high as 57%.[7] The pathogenesis is unknown,[10] but the mesh used to provide a tension-free closure[5] can entrap the nerve, resulting in both primary and secondary damage. Additional mechanisms of nerve damage include partial or complete transection, stretching, contusion, crushing, entrapment within a suture, damage by trocar placement, tacking during laparoscopy, and electrocautery-induced thermal injury.[1,4,8,11,12] Secondary injury occurs as a result of inflammation and can include formation of granulomas, neuromas, or fibrosis.[1,4]

Although appendectomy is the second most common cause of postoperative inguinodynia,[8] IIN can be the result of any surgical procedure in the lower abdominal quadrant. IIN has been reported following Pfannenstiel incision (hysterectomy, cesarean), urologic procedures for incontinence (needle suspensions, tension-free vaginal tap), and even iliac bone crest harvesting.[4,13] Nonsurgical and infectious etiologies of IIN include blunt abdominal trauma, Pott's disease, and psoas abscess.[2]

Anatomy

Understanding the course and variation of the IIN may prevent its damage and facilitate successful treatments. The IIN is a mixed nerve sharing both motor and sensory fibers.[8] It classically arises from the ventral ramus of L1 but occasionally receives some contribution from neighboring levels T12 or L2[4,8,13,14] (**Fig. 143.1**). Following its exit from the spinal column, the nerve runs subperitoneally lateral to the psoas muscle and anterior to the quadratus lumborum.[8,15] At the iliac crest, the nerve pierces the transversus abdominis ~ 1 cm superior to the anterior superior iliac spine (ASIS) before crossing the internal oblique in a medial direction. While staying dorsal to the external oblique muscle, the nerve continues with the spermatic cord or round ligament and enters the inguinal ring[4,8,14] (**Fig. 143.2**). After piercing the external oblique, the nerve provides sensory innervation to the proximal medial thigh, base of the penis and scrotum, and skin of the female genitalia.[4,8,14,16] These nerve endings can usually be found near the lateral aspect of the rectus muscle.[15]

Important clinical variations exist and lead to difficulty in both diagnosing and treating IIN. In Ndiaye et al's[16] dissection and study of 100 cadaverous specimens, anatomic variation was observed in 20% of specimens; 7% of cadavers lacked an IIN. In 14% of the specimens, the IIN shared a common trunk with the iliohypogastric nerve[16]; other authors have noted a common trunk rate as high as 46%.[17] Anatomic variation of the nerve in relation to the internal abdominal oblique muscle, inguinal ligament, and termination was also noted.

Diagnosis

Diagnosis is mostly based on clinical findings and the history. Nerve blocks can be utilized to confirm the clinical suspicion via injection at the trigger spot.[18]

Because of its anatomic variation, diagnosis of IIN can be challenging.[1,8,16] The overlapping dermatomes can make precise identification of the affected nerves difficult,[11,19] leading to misdiagnosis and unsuccessful treatment.[1] It is not uncommon for the chronic pain patient to manifest a varied symptomatology including neuropathic, nonneuropathic, visceral, or somatic pain.[1]

Neuropathic pain typically presents in a sensory distribution; a positive Tinel's sign at the ASIS may be seen.[1,11] IIN is usually described as lancinating, sharp, or stabbing pain[1,14,15] that radiates toward the pubic region or upper leg.[11,15] In contrast, nonneuropathic pain, caused by fibrosis formation or mesh entrapment, usually presents as a dull ache and can be exacerbated by walking and sitting.[1,11] Patients may also complain of pain with upper body twisting movements.[15]

Indications[1,18,19]

- Failure of conservative management
- Persistent pain
- Excessive scarring of nerve
- Successful nerve block

Contraindications

- Lymphadenopathy
- Strain of the abdominal muscle or the pectineal muscle
- Periostitis of the pubic tubercle
- Broad ligament neuritis
- Pelvic sympathetic syndrome[14]

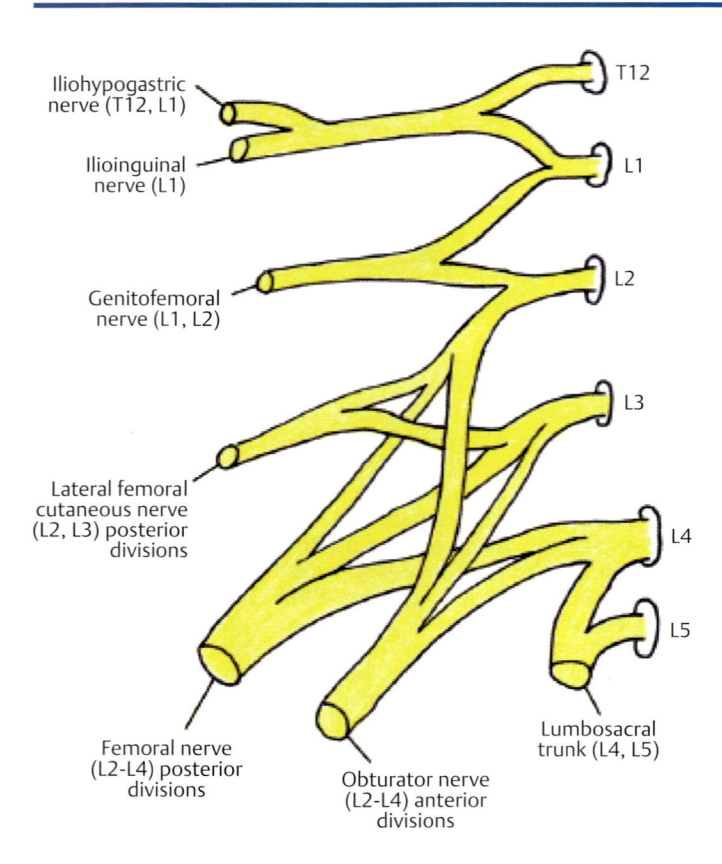

Fig. 143.1 The lumbar plexus. (From Russell SM. Examination of Peripheral Nerve Injuries. New York: Thieme; 2008.)

Advantages[18]

- Decompression of entrapped nerve
- Pain alleviation
- Neurolysis enables preservation of sensory function

Disadvantages[18]

- Neurectomy leads to loss of sensation
- Lack of pain relief

Preoperative Testing and Imaging

Ancillary testing, such as computed tomography (CT), magnetic resonance imaging (MRI), and electromyography (EMG) can be used to further evaluate difficult cases.[1] Imaging may help with diagnosing the etiology of nonneuropathic pain, particularly in the setting of mesh-related pathology, recurrent hernias, and neuroma formation.[1] The use of EMG can help differentiate specific nerve involvement and should specifically test for denervation of the pyramidalis muscle when assessing IIN damage.[7,8]

Treatment

Chronic groin pain can be difficult to treat; success is dependent on determining the correct etiology and making an accurate diagnosis. Initial management should take a conservative approach,[18] including nonsteroidal anti-inflammatory drugs (NSAIDs), muscle relaxants, transcutaneous electrical nerve stimulation (TENS), pulsed radiofrequency, cryoablation, and nerve blocks.[1,7] If this conservative management fails, surgical intervention should be considered, such as neurectomy, nerve stimulation, neurolysis, mesh excision,[1] and dorsal root ganglionectomy.[18]

Nerve Block

Nerve blocks may provide temporary pain relief by interfering with normal neuronal transmission and resetting the pain threshold.[19] Injections of local anesthetic, glycerol, alcohol, and phenol have been described; all are potentially harmful to the nerve and surrounding tissues.[1]

Nerve blocks should be performed proximal to the site of injury.[1] Although the use of ultrasound increases the success rate, a failure rate of 10 to 30% has been reported.[16] Opinion varies as to the optimal injection site; some authors suggest a location 2 inches medial and inferior to the ASIS,[8] whereas others postulate that diffusion under the external oblique aponeurosis will accommodate the varied anatomy.[16] With this in mind, Ndiaye et al[16] suggest an injection point 3.3 cm ventral to the ASIS.[16] Eichenberger et al[20] and Jamieson et al[21] recommend injecting 5 cm superior and posterior to the ASIS[16,20,21]; at this location, the nerve is larger and easier to target.[20]

Exposure

The patient is placed in the supine position. An incision is made parallel to the inguinal ligament extending from the medial and superior aspect of the ASIS down to the pubic tubercle[18] (**Fig. 143.3**). The incision should incorporate the previous surgical scar. The external oblique muscle is divided parallel to its fibers to expose the external inguinal ring. The IIN is identified and dissected along its course.[18]

Decompression and Neurolysis

The nerve is often encased with scarring. The nerve itself is freed surgically; however, the subsequent healing process only produces more scar.[11,14] Hence, the original pathology is ultimately

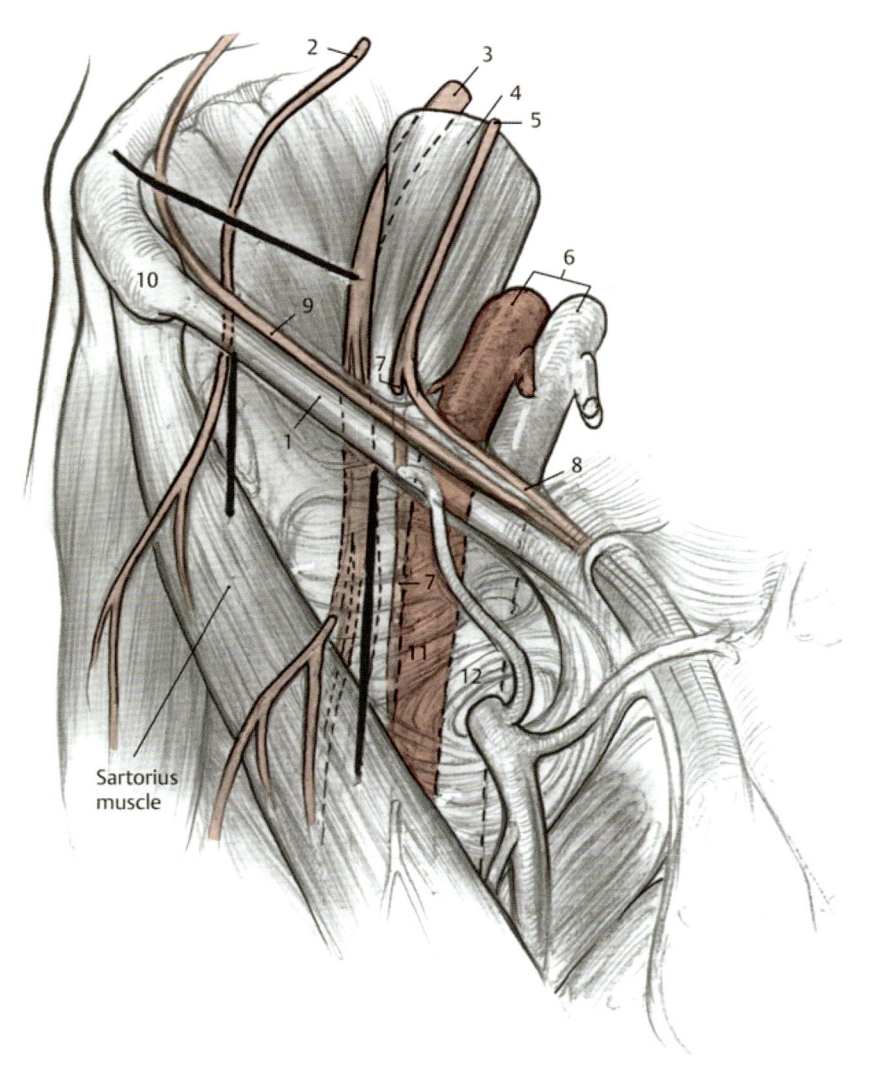

Fig. 143.2 The course of the ilioinguinal nerve. 1, inguinal ligament; 2, lateral femoral cutaneous nerve; 3, femoral nerve; 4, psoas nerve; 5, genitofemoral nerve; 6, external iliac artery and vein; 7, femoral branch of genitofemoral nerve; 8, genital branch of genitofemoral nerve; 9, ilioinguinal nerve; 10, anterior superior iliac spine; 11, femoral artery; 12, femoral vein. (From Nader R, Gragnaniello C, Berta SC, Sabbagh AJ, Levy ML (eds.). Neurosurgery Tricks of the Trade — Spine and Peripheral Nerves. New York: Thieme; 2014.)

not treated. Stulz and Pfeiffer[14] describe this procedure, in which the old scar is lengthened toward the ASIS and the nerve is excised close to where it is entrapped with scar tissue.[14]

Removal of mesh may be unnecessary as well, unless a meshoma or densely fibrotic collection has encased the nerve, leading to compression and damage.[11]

Neurectomy

Since 1982, neurectomies for chronic IIN have been performed with varied success rates of 70 to 100%.[1,10,14,19] There is no consensus in the literature regarding the timing of a neurectomy, the selection of the pelvic nerves to be severed, and whether mesh removal is necessary.[1,6] Details of surgical treatment, pathology found intraoperatively, and decision making are rarely reported, and when it is reported it varies among studies, making the evidence hard to interpret.[1]

The nerve is resected from its trigger point to a proximal portion near the ASIS. The nerve endings should be cauterized and buried in the local musculature to prevent neuroma formation.[7,11,19] All compressive materials should be removed at this time (e.g., mesh, suture, staple).[11] Given the variability in nerve contribution and anatomic course, some surgeons resect multiple adjacent nerves, including the iliohypogastric and genitofemoral nerves.[9,11]

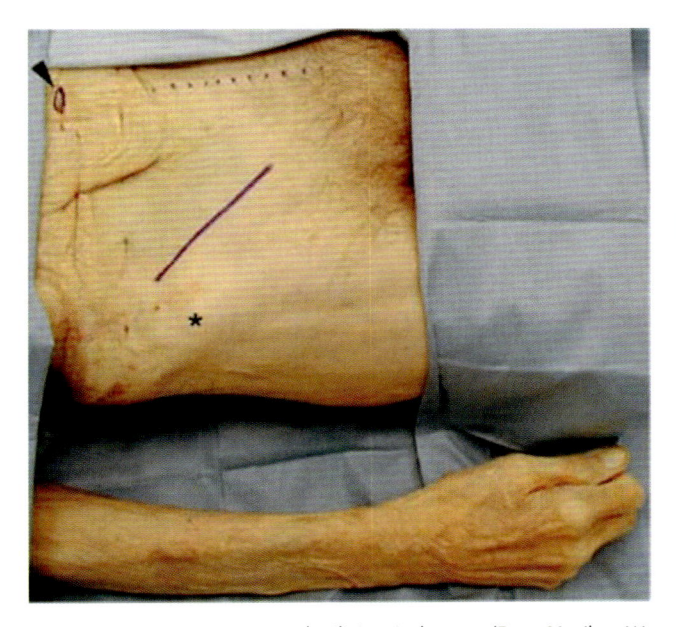

Fig. 143.3 Incision to expose the ilioinguinal nerve. (From Manikar AH. Operative Exposures in Peripheral Nerve Surgery. New York: Thieme; 2005.)

Neuromodulation

Nerve root stimulation (NRS), which relies on electrical and magnetic stimulation to alter nerve conduction, is typically most effective for patients who have pharmacologically and surgically unresponsive chronic pain.[2,22,23] Comparatively, NRS may provide more benefit than spinal cord stimulation (SCS) alone, particularly when there is only one nerve involved and when the pain is in an area difficult to treat with SCS, such as the foot, lower back, buttocks, and pelvic region.[23] Alo et al[23] placed percutaneous leads in the transforamen of the affected nerve roots under light sedation to provide relief from neuralgia.

Peripheral nerve stimulation (PNS) entails dermatomal stimulation and inhibition of nociceptive first-order neurons, providing relief of pain due to central sensitization. With PNS, an electrode is tunneled under the skin, subcutaneously, in the area of greatest pain.[2]

Pulsed Radiofrequency

Radiofrequency (RF) ablation is another noninvasive measure that uses a constant high temperature and electrical energy to destroy nervous tissue.[24] Surgically, the nerve root is cannulated under local anesthesia and direct visualization with fluoroscopy. Sensory and motor stimulus is used to confirm the levels followed by pulsed RF.[24,25] The procedure is well tolerated, and in one study patients experienced 75 to 100% pain relief for 6 to 9 months.[24]

Cryoablation

Cryoablation uses extreme temperature to destroy the peripheral nerve, creating a local conduction block.[12] A small incision is made under local anesthesia, and a cryoprobe is placed using a nerve stimulator for localization. For ilioinguinal neuralgia, it is suggested to use three 2-minute cryo-cycles to deliver subthermal temperature to the involved nerve.[12] When used as an adjunctive treatment during an open procedure, the cryoprobe is maneuvered under direct visualization. Two 1-minute freezes are considered sufficient.[12] One published study supported the use of cryoneurolysis, reporting less postoperative pain,[25] whereas others have found no statistical difference in its use.[26,27]

Postoperative Care

Postoperatively, normal wound care should commence, with observation for possible hematoma development. Movement should be restricted to prevent tension on sutures and possible dehiscence.

Complications

- Wound infection
- Nerve injury
- Vascular injury
- Hematoma

Conclusion

Ilioinguinal neuralgia is a chronic pain syndrome that leads to disability and to poorer quality of life. The syndrome is diagnostically challenging, so surgeons must have a comprehensive understanding of and familiarity with the anatomic variations of the nerve and the levels of contribution. Misdiagnosis of the syndrome can lead to mismanagement and ultimate sensitization, thus precluding successful treatment. Although conservative therapy is usually the starting point, it is often ineffective. Surgically, neurectomy has shown the most promising results for pain relief; however, an understanding of all treatment modalities is necessary, and treatment should be tailored to the needs of each patient.

References

1. Hakeem A, Shanmugam V. Current trends in the diagnosis and management of post-herniorraphy chronic groin pain. World J Gastrointest Surg 2011;3:73–81
2. Rauchwerger JJ, Giordano J, Rozen D, Kent JL, Greenspan J, Closson CW. On the therapeutic viability of peripheral nerve stimulation for ilioinguinal neuralgia: putative mechanisms and possible utility. Pain Pract 2008;8:138–143
3. Cardosi RJ, Cox CS, Hoffman MS. Postoperative neuropathies after major pelvic surgery. Obstet Gynecol 2002;100:240–244
4. Whiteside JL, Barber MD, Walters MD, Falcone T. Anatomy of ilioinguinal and iliohypogastric nerves in relation to trocar placement and low transverse incisions. Am J Obstet Gynecol 2003;189:1574–1578, discussion 1578
5. Miller JP, Acar F, Kaimaktchiev VB, Gultekin SH, Burchiel KJ. Pathology of ilioinguinal neuropathy produced by mesh entrapment: case report and literature review. Hernia 2008;12:213–216
6. Johner A, Faulds J, Wiseman SM. Planned ilioinguinal nerve excision for prevention of chronic pain after inguinal hernia repair: a meta-analysis. Surgery 2011;150:534–541
7. Kim DH, Murovic JA, Tiel RL, Kline DG. Surgical management of 33 ilioinguinal and iliohypogastric neuralgias at Louisiana State University Health Sciences Center. Neurosurgery 2005;56:1013–1020, discussion 1013–1020
8. Viswanathan A, Kim DH, Reid N, Kline DG. Surgical management of the pelvic plexus and lower abdominal nerves. Neurosurgery 2009;65(4, Suppl):A44–A51
9. Wijsmuller AR, van Veen RN, Bosch JL, et al. Nerve management during open hernia repair. Br J Surg 2007;94:17–22
10. Aasvang E, Kehlet H. Surgical management of chronic pain after inguinal hernia repair. Br J Surg 2005;92:795–801
11. Amid PK. Causes, prevention, and surgical treatment of postherniorrhaphy neuropathic inguinodynia: triple neurectomy with proximal end implantation. Hernia 2004;8:343–349
12. Trescot AM. Cryoanalgesia in interventional pain management. Pain Physician 2003;6:345–360
13. Klaassen Z, Marshall E, Tubbs RS, Louis RG Jr, Wartmann CT, Loukas M. Anatomy of the ilioinguinal and iliohypogastric nerves with observations of their spinal nerve contributions. Clin Anat 2011;24:454–461
14. Stulz P, Pfeiffer KM. Peripheral nerve injuries resulting from common surgical procedures in the lower portion of the abdomen. Arch Surg 1982;117:324–327
15. Bischoff JM, Koscielniak-Nielsen ZJ, Kehlet H, Werner MU. Ultrasound-guided ilioinguinal/iliohypogastric nerve blocks for persistent inguinal postherniorrhaphy pain: a randomized, double-blind, placebo-controlled, crossover trial. Anesth Analg 2012;114:1323–1329
16. Ndiaye A, Diop M, Ndoye JM, et al. Emergence and distribution of the ilioinguinal nerve in the inguinal region: applications to the ilioinguinal anaesthetic block (about 100 dissections). Surg Radiol Anat 2010;32:55–62
17. Papadopoulos NJKE, Katritsis ED. Some observations on the course and relations of the iliohypogastric and ilioinguinal nerves (based on 348 specimens). Anat Anz 1981;149:357–364
18. Midha R, Zager EL. Surgery of Peripheral Nerves. New York: Thieme; 2008
19. Loos MJ, Scheltinga MR, Roumen RM. Surgical management of inguinal neuralgia after a low transverse Pfannenstiel incision. Ann Surg 2008;248:880–885
20. Eichenberger U, Greher M, Kirchmair L, Curatolo M, Moriggl B. Ultrasound-guided blocks of the ilioinguinal and iliohypogastric nerve: accuracy of a selective new technique confirmed by anatomical dissection. Br J Anaesth 2006;97:238–243

Surgical Anatomy
Anatomy of the Nerve

Attention to the underlying anatomy of the nerve is paramount in achieving satisfactory clinical outcomes after nerve repair. Motor nerves are primarily myelinated and outnumbered by sensory unmyelinated structures by 4:1.[6] Nerves are further classified as monofascicular, oligofascicular, or polyfascicular, and may exhibit each form in their course. Monofascicular nerves are typically located distally, such as the terminal nerves of the digits and are composed of one fascicle with solely sensory or motor fibers. Oligofascicular nerves are composed of a few fascicles and may be pure or mixed sensorimotor, whereas polyfascicular nerves are composed of many fascicles. As an example of the transition between these categories, the ulnar nerve is classified as polyfascicular in the axilla, oligofascicular in the olecranon, and purely motor monofascicular in the palm.

Fascicles are composed of three distinct layers: outer epineurium, perineurium, and endoneurium. The epineurium is constituted of loose areolar connective tissue and a longitudinal vascular plexus as well as an inner layer extending within. The perineurium encircles each fascicle and is the smallest structure capable of accepting sutures. Lastly, the inner endoneurium circumscribes individual nerve fibers and contains within it endoneurial fluid. This fluid may accumulate with peripheral nerve injury; such pathology may be assessed using MRN.[7,8]

Anatomy of the Nerve Injury

Nerve injury is subdivided into three types as described by Seddon et al[9] in 1943; in order of increasing severity, they are neurapraxia, axonotmesis, and neurotmesis. Neurapraxia involves a disruption of impulse conduction and can be due to ischemia or compression, but no wallerian degeneration occurs. Recovery generally takes hours to weeks. Axonotmesis is mainly seen in crush injury and involves disruption of the axon with maintenance of the surrounding myelin sheath; this is subdivided further by the Sunderland classification to account for endoneurial and perineurial element involvement. In a second-degree Sunderland injury, the endoneurium and perineurium are intact; regeneration and neurologic recovery are expected but take several months. In cases of very proximal injury with distal targets, muscle atrophy or motor end-plate degeneration may occur before regeneration is completed, and prevents functional recovery. In a third-degree Sunderland injury, the endoneurium is disrupted, whereas the perineurium is additionally disrupted in a fourth-degree Sunderland injury. Third- and fourth-degree injuries likely require surgical intervention. Finally, neurotmesis is the most severe lesion, occurring because of laceration, stretch, or severe contusion, involving disruption of the axon, endoneurium, perineurium, and epineurium. Neurotmesis corresponds to a fifth-degree Sunderland injury. Fifth-degree injuries cannot recover spontaneously without surgical intervention.[10,11]

Surgical Procedure
Goals of Surgery

Procedurally, the goal of nerve repair is to function at the connective tissue level to coapt healthy proximal and distal nerve stumps. Grafting is a means of augmenting repair by providing a conduit for proximal and distal endoneurial tubes to grow. The choice of repair method requires careful specification by the surgeon according to both the type of nerve, be it monofascicular, oligofascicular, or polyfascicular, and the tension of the repair site. Tension may in turn be influenced by the size of the nerve gap, longitudinal excursion, and the timing and quality of the injury.[12] Large gaps between proximal and distal nerve stumps are prone to neuroma formation and fibrosis, and generally do not predispose to spontaneous reinnervation; thus, grafting may be necessary in these cases.[13] Longitudinal excursion refers to the degree of nerve extension induced by extremity movement; for example, significant longitudinal excursion may be produced in the upper extremity from wrist and finger extension with concurrent elbow flexion.[14] In cases with a superimposed large nerve gap, the surgeon must carefully consider the degree of longitudinal excursion a nerve may undergo and appropriately choose a corresponding repair modality. Lastly, the caliber of injury is important in determining the treatment method, as blunt injury with resultant scarring may necessitate graft repair, whereas simple transections may be feasibly restored directly.

Generally, in performing a nerve repair, certain principles are followed irrespective of the method chosen. Surgically, dissection must proceed from the normal nerve toward the region of pathology to ensure proper anatomic identification. Scarred and adjacent connective tissue should be sharply dissected to adequately categorize nerve stumps, resecting tissue until fresh fascicles are visualized under trimmed epineurium. It is particularly important to remove this nonviable tissue, whether identifying it microscopically or via frozen-section pathological evaluation, as persistent scarring may induce painful neuroma formation[13] and hinder regeneration. Bleeding from sectioned stump surfaces may be irrigated away with isotonic saline, and, if necessary, controlled with a muscle patch or Gelfoam, or, in certain circumstances of uncontrolled arterial bleeding, coagulated with fine-tipped bipolar forceps under magnification. To ensure adequate coaptation of nerve stumps without tension, mobilization of the affected extremity is imperative in minimizing distractive forces. If such distraction persists in spite of mobilization, grafting may be necessary. Finally, the fewest sutures possible should be used, as excessive suturing may lead to increased scarring and diminished functional recovery.

Keeping these tenets in mind, one may then decide on the method of repair, be it direct repair or via nerve graft harvesting. Nerve grafting should be used in conditions where mild tension cannot be overcome, but in other cases, an easier, faster, direct repair may suffice.

Types of Repair

Nerve repair may be performed at different anatomic levels, each with associated strengths and weaknesses. If the injury site is devoid of tension, an epineurial repair may be considered. This method involves passing suture through the epineurial sheath, thereby theoretically preserving nerve stump continuity without tension and with proper anatomic alignment, the latter of which may be facilitated by utilizing the longitudinal epineurial vasculature as a landmark. Technically, this method involves placing two orienting lateral 8-0 or 9-0 monofilament sutures within the epineurium 180 degrees apart. The tails of these sutures can be held with hemostats to confer rotation after the lateral sutures are tied, thus further aiding coaptation. A small gap should be left in this connection to avoid mismatch, malalignment, or protrusion of fascicles. However, if the nerve gap is too large or the distracting forces are too great, direct epineurial repair may be inferior compared with the use of a graft. Most polyfascicular nerve repair is possible with epineurial repair.[12]

Grouped fascicular repair is a more accurate technique best applied with direct visualization of fascicles within the main nerve. By placing 8-0 to 10-0 sutures in the interfascicular epineurium after dissecting the external epineurium and identifying the adjacent fascicular groups, the fascicle ends may be appropriately coapted. This method, although more technically demanding, decreases physical manipulation, disruption of the nerve's vascular environment, and scar formation, and may have greater potential than epineurial repair for the regenerating fibers to enter the correct endoneurial tube on the distal stump.[12,15,16]

Fascicular repair involves suturing corresponding fascicles. This reconstitution is performed by placing perineurial sutures after stripping the external epineurium for a length double the diameter of the cross-sectional nerve area. Preservation of perineurial connective tissue is ideal to maintain vascular integrity and cover the repair site. After dissection of interfascicular epineurium proximal and distal to the lesion, fascicles may be visualized by recognizing the spiral bands of Fontana in the perineurium. These bands maintain proper fascicular structure and disappear under significant tension; preservation is imperative for good clinical results.[17] Meticulous trimming removes protruding intrafascicular material from the perineurial edge and engenders adequate coaptation. Two to three 10-0 or 11-0 sutures should then be placed 180 degrees from one another in the perineurium, avoiding the endoneurial content, with a knot tied under minimal tension to minimize protrusion of internal elements. This method is easily achieved in oligofascicular and monofascicular repair, but its potential has not been realized due to an increased incidence of intrafascicular scar formation stemming from greater manipulation. Furthermore, the time-consuming nature of this repair limits its practical use.[18]

Grafting

Grafting is a helpful adjunct when tension or a nerve gap may limit postoperative functional recovery; the gold standard in these cases involves harvesting a nerve autograft. As with other means of repair, the surgeon must debride damaged areas of the divided nerves and nonfunctioning neuromas in continuity after a longitudinal epineurial incision, carefully trimming fibrotic fascicular components with fine, sharp dissection. Graft lengths should be 10% longer than the repaired gap to allow for retraction and graft shrinkage.[12] Also, careful attention should be paid to the sensorimotor components of individual fascicles at the proximal and distal repair sites. Although proximal components are largely mixed sensory and motor, function is more explicit distally, and by using topographical cues, fascicular alignment may be optimally achieved. After graft harvesting, the nerve must be kept moist and manipulated delicately, but may be cut into segments of the required length. It is also crucial to place the nerve into a healthy tissue bed to confer proper nourishment and minimize scarring. Interfascicular tissue is first resected back to expose fascicles, and then graft segments may be placed with two lateral sutures to widen the graft edges, akin to a fish-mouth shape (because the cross-sectional area of the nerve graft is generally smaller than the recipients stumps to which it is sewn). Sutures are passed through the graft epineurium to the interfascicular epineurium or perineurium remaining on the surface of the isolated fascicular group. Grafts are usually sutured proximally first and then distally, to complete the repair more easily, and when no tension remains on the suture site, the repair is sufficiently strong. Upon completion of grafting, reexamination of all repair sites is imperative, as some ends may be easily distracted when others are sewn into place.[19]

In cases where the diameter of the required nerve graft exceeds the diameter of the donor (e.g., in proximal brachial plexus reconstruction with sural nerve grafting), multiple cables can be created from one lengthy donor nerve. These can be coapted proximally and distally and collected together using fibrin glue. In certain instances of primary repair or nerve grafting, suture coaptation sites can be further reinforced with fibrin glue and collagen conduits, as per surgeon preference.[11]

Donor Site

When selecting a donor nerve, one must consider the cross-sectional area, the length of the nerve gap, and donor-site morbidity. The larger a nerve's cross-sectional area, the more limited its use as a nerve graft, as poor central revascularization leads to necrosis and axonal nerve growth failure. Conversely, small-diameter nerve grafts obtain their nourishment at the surface. The use of these nerves is preferable, and multiple small-diameter grafts may be used as a standard method of repair for major nerve injuries. It is also important to minimize the loss of sensory function adjacent to the damaged area; for this reason, grafts are usually chosen from a distant site.

The most common nerve chosen for graft repair is the sural nerve. Other possible donors include the median antebrachial cutaneous nerve (MACN), lateral antebrachial cutaneous nerve (LACN), and superficial radial sensory nerve.[12] The sural nerve is by far the most common, due to its appropriate diameter (2.5 to 4.0 mm proximally, 2.0 to 3.0 mm distally), relatively fast revascularization, and potential harvests of 30 to 50 cm in nerve graft material. Histological studies have reported nine to 14 fascicles embedded in the sural nerve with a nutrient artery and vein.[20] The peroneal communicating branch lies superficial to fascia, and in cases where less harvesting is required, may be solely taken to preserve medial sural cutaneous nerve sensation in its distribution, and minimize disturbing anesthesia. The bulk of the nerve may be harvested with the patient in the supine position, the lower extremity flexed 40 degrees at the knee and internally rotated at the hip, and the ankle dorsiflexed. A longitudinal incision is made extending from the lateral ankle to the popliteal fossa; this ensures that all communicating branches are identified, no damage is done to the donor graft, and maximal material is obtained.[21]

Postoperative Care

Dressings are changed on postoperative day 2; when applied, they provide gentle compression on the site.[12] The strength of the construct plateaus at 3 weeks. In cases of tenuous repair, a short course of immobilization may be in order. Movement is resumed gradually, and it is necessary for nerve recovery; thus, the patient must be encouraged to work with a physical therapist to optimize neuromuscular recovery and to prevent contracture and disuse atrophy.

Potential Complications and Precautions

Complications from nerve harvesting include dysesthesia and neuroma formation.[22] Neuroma formation may be minimized with attention to the proximal nerve stump, suture ligating its end, and cauterizing patulous fascicles with the bipolar forceps. Protecting the stump by enveloping it in a muscle flap may further prevent neuromas.[23] Diligent physical therapy is also vital to prevent painful contractures from forming and to optimize the range of motion of the affected area.[24]

Future Directions

Other methods of graft repair are on the horizon. Tissue and molecular engineering have provided several biological and synthetic components that may augment nerve repair. Such methods include scaffolds, support cells, growth factors, and specialized extracellular matrix.[6,25]

Conclusion

Peripheral nerve injury is a complex process, and the use of techniques such as nerve grafting and harvesting may confer significant benefit due to the need for tension-free repair. **Box 146.1** lists the key operative points and steps to take to avoid complications.

Box 146.1 Key Operative Points and Ways to Avoid Complications

- Nerve repair may be performed at different anatomic levels for epineurial, grouped fascicular, or fascicular repair.
- Grafting is useful when tension or the nerve gap may limit postoperative functional recovery.
- The most common nerve chosen for graft repair is the sural nerve.
- Sural nerve harvesting occurs with the patient in the supine position, with the lower extremity flexed 40 degrees at the knee and internally rotated at the hip, and the ankle dorsiflexed.
- Grafts are sutured proximally first and then distally; when no tension remains on the suture site, the repair is sufficiently strong.
- Suture coaptation sites can be reinforced with fibrin glue and collagen conduits.
- Protecting the stump by enveloping it in a muscle flap, suturing the ligating ends, and cauterizing the patulous fascicles may prevent neuroma formation.
- Structural analogues such as nerve tubes or conduits are now available for clinical use and have been used in small gap pathology.

References

1. Sanborn M, Jackson EM, Zager EL. Nerve repair with conduits. In Midha R, Zager EL (eds.). Surgery of Peripheral Nerves. New York: Thieme; 2008:153–156
2. Millesi H, Zöch G, Reihsner R. Mechanical properties of peripheral nerves. Clin Orthop Relat Res 1995;314:76–83
3. Spinner RJ, Kline DG. Surgery for peripheral nerve and brachial plexus injuries or other nerve lesions. Muscle Nerve 2000;23:680–695
4. Zaidman CM, Seelig MJ, Baker JC, Mackinnon SE, Pestronk A. Detection of peripheral nerve pathology: comparison of ultrasound and MRI. Neurology 2013;80:1634–1640
5. Dubuisson A, Kline DG. Indications for peripheral nerve and brachial plexus surgery. Neurol Clin 1992;10:935–951
6. Evans GR. Peripheral nerve injury: a review and approach to tissue engineered constructs. Anat Rec 2001;263:396–404
7. Lundborg G, Myers R, Powell H. Nerve compression injury and increased endoneurial fluid pressure: a "miniature compartment syndrome." J Neurol Neurosurg Psychiatry 1983;46:1119–1124
8. Filler AG, Maravilla KR, Tsuruda JS. MR neurography and muscle MR imaging for image diagnosis of disorders affecting the peripheral nerves and musculature. Neurol Clin 2004;22:643–682, vi–vii
9. Seddon HJ, Medawar PB, Smith H. Rate of regeneration of peripheral nerves in man. J Physiol 1943;102:191–215
10. Sunderland S. A classification of peripheral nerve injuries producing loss of function. Brain 1951;74:491–516
11. Spinner RJ, Shin AY, Herbert-Blouin M, Elhassan BT, Bishop AT. In: Wolfe SW, Hotchkiss RN, Pederson WC, Kozin SH, eds. Green's Operative Hand Surgery, 6th ed. Philadelphia: Elsevier; 2011:1235–1292
12. Matsuyama T, Mackay M, Midha R. Peripheral nerve repair and grafting techniques: a review. Neurol Med Chir (Tokyo) 2000;40:187–199
13. Lewin-Kowalik J, Marcol W, Kotulska K, Mandera M, Klimczak A. Prevention and management of painful neuroma. Neurol Med Chir (Tokyo) 2006;46:62–67, discussion 67–68
14. McLellan DL, Swash M. Longitudinal sliding of the median nerve during movements of the upper limb. J Neurol Neurosurg Psychiatry 1976;39:566–570
15. Orgel MG. Epineurial versus perineurial repair of peripheral nerves. Clin Plast Surg 1984;11:101–104
16. Ogata K, Naito M. Blood flow of peripheral nerve effects of dissection, stretching and compression. J Hand Surg [Br] 1986;11:10–14
17. Zachary LS, Dellon ES, Nicholas EM, Dellon AL. The structural basis of Felice Fontana's spiral bands and their relationship to nerve injury. J Reconstr Microsurg 1993;9:131–138
18. Zhong SZ, Wang GY, He YS, Sun B. The relationship between structural features of peripheral nerves and suture methods for nerve repair. Microsurgery 1988;9:181–187
19. Whitcomb BB. Separation at the suture site as a cause of failure in regeneration of peripheral nerves. J Neurosurg 1946;3:399–406
20. Ortigüela ME, Wood MB, Cahill DR. Anatomy of the sural nerve complex. J Hand Surg Am 1987;12:1119–1123
21. Strauch B, Goldberg N, Herman CK. Sural nerve harvest: anatomy and technique. J Reconstr Microsurg 2005;21:133–136
22. Staniforth P, Fisher TR. The effects of sural nerve excision in autogenous nerve grafting. Hand 1978;10:187–190
23. Chim H, Miller E, Gliniak C, Cohen ML, Guyuron B. The role of different methods of nerve ablation in prevention of neuroma. Plast Reconstr Surg 2013;131:1004–1012
24. Russell SM, Kline DG. Complication avoidance in peripheral nerve surgery: preoperative evaluation of nerve injuries and brachial plexus exploration—part 1. Neurosurgery 2006;59:441–447
25. Anton ES, Weskamp G, Reichardt LF, Matthew WD. Nerve growth factor and its low-affinity receptor promote Schwann cell migration. Proc Natl Acad Sci U S A 1994;91:2795–2799

147 Superficial Peroneal Nerve Biopsy

Brian D. Dalm and Chandan G. Reddy

The sural nerve is the single most commonly biopsied nerve for diagnosis of peripheral neuropathy,[1] but the superficial peroneal nerve (SPN) is also occasionally requested for biopsy. This may especially be the case when a simultaneous nerve and muscle combination are of interest, owing to the close proximity of the SPN with the peroneus brevis muscle. But given the infrequency of biopsy request, and thus less surgeon familiarity, combined with anatomic variation, the SPN biopsy is technically more challenging than the sural nerve biopsy. A thorough understanding of the anatomic variation and the surgical technique facilitates a successful surgical outcome.

Patient Selection

Generally, patients for whom an SPN biopsy has been requested have been thoroughly evaluated by the referring neurologist for an underlying cause of peripheral neuropathy. Although nerve biopsy may be the next logical step in the diagnostic workup, the surgeon must be carefully attuned to potential risk factors that can lead to complications in this relatively higher risk population. Many of these patients have multiple risk factors for poor wound healing, including advanced age, immunosuppression, advanced diabetic or other peripheral neuropathy, and anticoagulation. In consultation with the referring physicians, appropriate precautions should be taken in the perioperative period to optimize the patient's condition, including withholding anticoagulants, optimizing diabetic control, and pausing the use of immunosuppressive medications. In cases of extreme risk for wound complication or patient morbidity, the possibility of empiric treatment without biopsy should be discussed with the referring physician.

Indications

The search for a treatable cause of neuropathy is the main indication for a nerve biopsy, with vasculitis being the major clinical diagnosis for which a nerve biopsy is requested.[2] Other diagnoses of peripheral neuropathy may be reached by alternate means, but the nerve biopsy may be indicated to guide the physician toward the appropriate investigation, for example, the spontaneous presentation of a hereditary neuropathy with no prior family history, leading to further specific workup based on nerve pathology.[3] Finally, a nerve biopsy may be necessary to characterize a previously unknown disease entity.[4]

Advantages and Disadvantages

The ideal nerve for biopsy should be easy to access surgically, have minimal deficits following removal, have a predictable anatomic location and course, and be involved in the neuropathic process. Typically, neuropathic processes involve nerves more distally located in the extremities. For this reason, in addition to its relatively superficial location, low frequency of anatomic variability, purely sensory modality, and abundant normative morphological data, the sural nerve in the leg is most commonly targeted.[1] When a muscle biopsy is also requested, however, various nerve and muscle combinations can be chosen. The SPN represents one such target that also provides easy access to the peroneus brevis muscle through a single small incision.

Compared with sural nerve biopsy alone, the addition of the peroneus brevis muscle biopsy may increase the diagnostic sensitivity in cases of suspected vasculitis to 60% (from less than 50%), and the complication rate may be comparable between the two procedures.[5-9] Correspondingly, the peroneal nerve is the most frequently affected peripheral nerve in vasculitic neuropathy, presenting with potential concurrent motor deficits.[6,10]

Theoretically, there should be fewer wound complications due to a more proximal incision of the SPN biopsy compared with the sural nerve biopsy. However, the SPN is generally a smaller caliber nerve than the sural nerve.[11]

Choice of Approach

The SPN has a relatively consistent anatomic course, but certain anatomic variants should be recognized. The common peroneal nerve typically bifurcates into the superficial and deep peroneal branches within 0.5 to 6 cm after coursing around the fibular neck (**Fig. 147.1**). The SPN then courses through the lateral compartment of the leg between the peroneus longus and extensor digitorum longus muscles. As the nerve courses more distally in the leg, it becomes more superficial and eventually passes between the peroneus longus and peroneus brevis muscles. More distally, the SPN pierces the crural fascia between the middle and distal third of the leg.[12] Measuring proximally from the lateral malleolus, the point where the SPN emerges from the crural fascia is reported with wide variation, between 3 and 18 cm (average, 13 cm).[13,14] From this point, the SPN usually bifurcates into the medial and intermediate dorsal cutaneous nerves of the foot within 2 cm of piercing the fascia.[14] In a study of 85 cadaver legs, 73% of SPNs follow this course. In 14%, however, the SPN exits from the anterior compartment, and in 12%, the SPN bifurcates more proximally and exits from both the lateral and anterior compartments.[14] These variations are important, especially if the initial dissection does not readily reveal the SPN, warranting a more proximal dissection to accurately trace the course of the nerve.

Preoperative Testing and Imaging

It should be noted that any nerve biopsy should only be pursued after a thorough and exhaustive evaluation has failed to yield a diagnosis, and the patient's symptoms continue to cause significant impairment.[2,3] As part of the thorough neurologic workup,

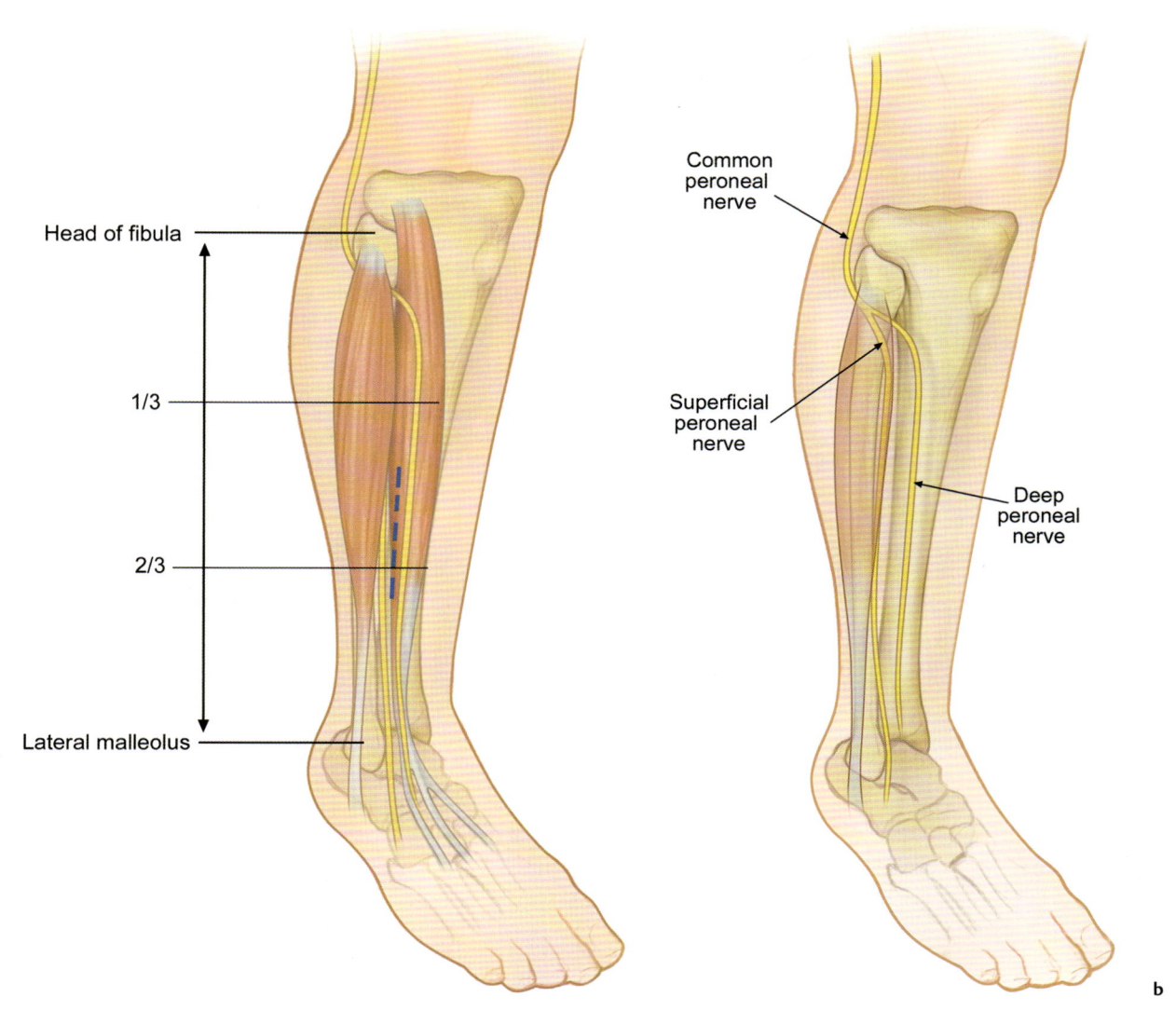

Fig. 147.1 (a,b) Anterolateral view of the right leg showing the superficial peroneal nerve emerging from the fascia between the middle and distal third of the leg. The lateral malleolus and fibular head are marked with the fibula outlined. Proposed incision is marked with the dashed line and care should be taken to avoid the deep peroneal nerve which is more medial and likely deeper. In this location, the nerve is found above the muscle fascia overlying the anterior muscle group between the tibia and fibula.

prior investigations may include electromyography, nerve conduction studies, and screening serum laboratories. Depending on the differential diagnosis, genetic testing, cerebrospinal fluid investigations, or noninvasive imaging may be performed prior to nerve biopsy.[11] With regard to preoperative planning, anticoagulation status should be established and the risk factors mitigated.

On occasion, the lateral portion of the extensor digitorum brevis may be innervated by an anomalous innervation from the SPN, called the accessory deep peroneal nerve. This is the most frequent anomaly of the lower extremity, with a prevalence ranging from 12%[15] up to 20 to 28%.[16] The anomaly, when inherited, shows a dominant trait.[17] Occasionally, the extensor digitorum brevis may receive exclusive supply from this communication.[18] The presence of this anomaly may be elucidated by preoperative electrodiagnostic testing, if stimulation of the deep peroneal nerve at the ankle gives rise to a much smaller compound muscle action potential than electrical stimulation applied at the knee. Stimulation of the accessory deep peroneal nerve behind the lateral malleolus can confirm this diagnosis by activating the anomalously innervated lateral portion of the muscle.[16] Injury to the deep peroneal nerve that ordinarily causes weakness of the entire extensor digitorum brevis would spare its lateral portion in the presence of this anastomosis.[19] Conversely, biopsy of the SPN could potentially lead to motor weakness of the lateral portion of the extensor digitorum brevis, but this has not been reported.

Surgical Procedure

As with other nerve biopsy procedures, SPN biopsy is performed as an outpatient procedure. It is important to perform this operation when a neuropathologist is readily available to ensure proper postoperative handling. Attempts should be made to use local or regional anesthesia, unless the patient's condition would require general anesthesia for safety concerns during the surgical procedure. Given the increased technical challenges of biopsy of the SPN compared with that of the sural nerve, the surgeon, especially in the early stages, should allot more time and should plan for a greater depth of anesthesia than would be required for a standard sural biopsy.

The biopsy of the SPN (**Fig. 147.2a,c**) is most easily performed with the patient in the lateral or semilateral position, with a pillow placed between the patient's legs for support. This orients the surgical field parallel to the floor, and provides a comfortable position for both the patient and the surgeon. Alternatively, the supine position may be used, with the affected leg gently flexed at the hip and knee, and slightly internally rotated at the hip. A pillow may be used for support of the flexed knee, and a strap may be used to help hold the lower extremity in internal rotation. This position holds the biopsied leg over the opposite leg, and exposes the anterolateral surface of the biopsied leg for easy access from either a standing or sitting position.

Given that the SPN may pierce through the crural fascia from 3 to 18 cm proximal to the lateral malleolus with an average distance of 13 cm, we recommend planning an initial incision of 6 cm from 9 to 15 cm proximal to the lateral malleolus, between the midpoint and distal third of the leg (**Fig. 147.2b**). The lateral tibial border and lateral surface of the fibula should be easily palpable. An incision is proposed ~ 1.5 cm anterior to the lateral border of the fibula (**Fig. 147.3**). On occasion, in larger patients, the fibula is difficult to palpate, and the incision should be planned two thirds of the distance from the lateral tibial border to the suspected location of the fibula.

The SPN is often just deep to the crural fascia around this area, and care should be taken to avoid injuring it during opening. For surgeons with limited experience with this biopsy, a wider area should be draped to plan for the possibility of additional exposure, especially in the rostral direction.

The exposed leg is then prepped and draped in the usual sterile fashion. A stocking net cap or Coban™ can be used to cover the foot, based on surgeon preference. Local anesthetic consisting of 1% lidocaine or 0.5% bupivacaine with 1:200,000 epinephrine is infiltrated into the subcutaneous tissue. An incision is made with a No. 10 scalpel. Dissection should be carried down sharply through the skin, until either the SPN is identified superficial to the crural fascia or the crural fascia is encountered (**Fig. 147.4**). If the SPN is identified in the subcutaneous space superficial to

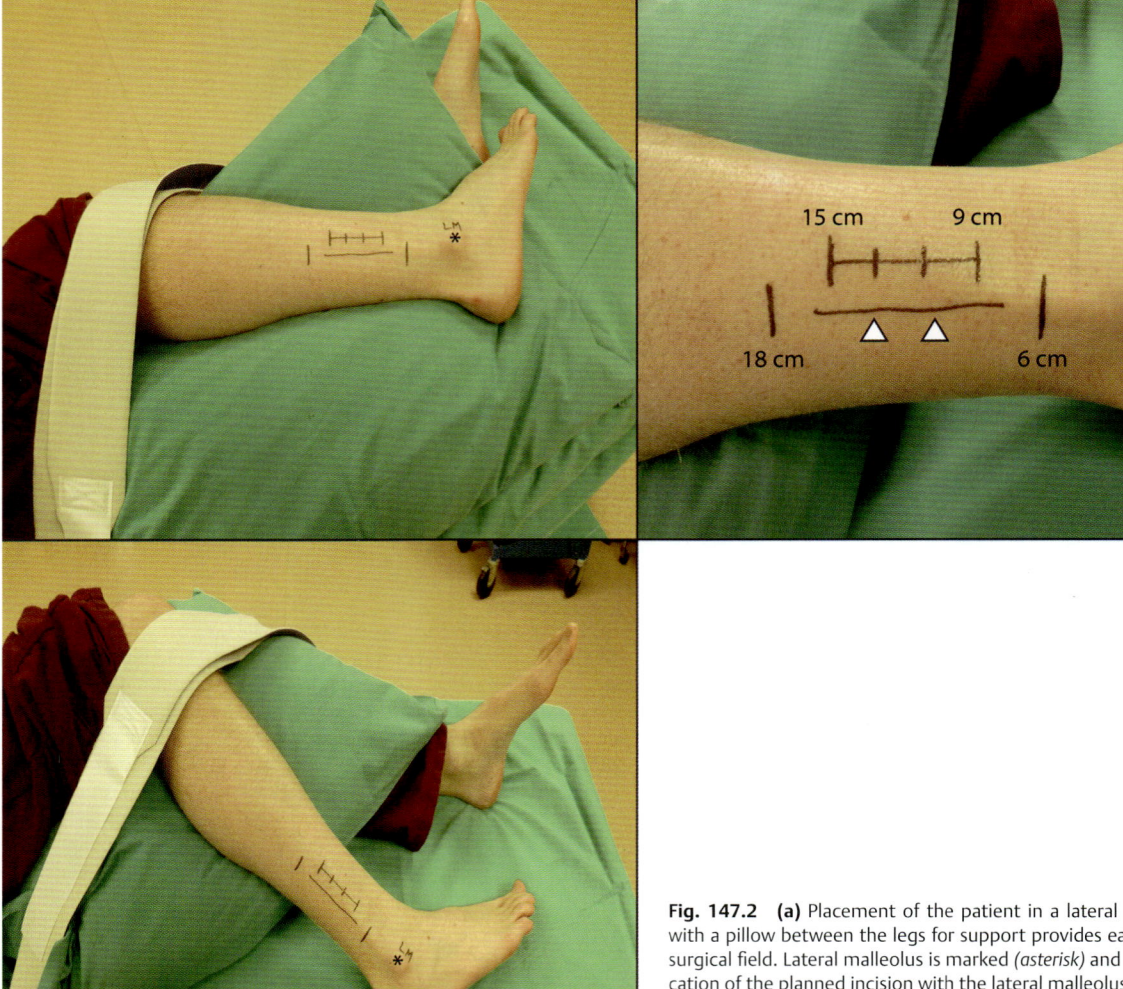

Fig. 147.2 **(a)** Placement of the patient in a lateral decubitus position with a pillow between the legs for support provides easy exposure of the surgical field. Lateral malleolus is marked *(asterisk)* and labeled *LM*. **(b)** Location of the planned incision with the lateral malleolus and fibular border *(white arrowheads)* demarcated. Vertical line marking between 6 and 18 cm proximal to the lateral malleolus are delineated. The incision is then proposed from 9 to 15 cm proximal to the lateral malleolus. **(c)** Placement of the patient in the supine position with a pillow between the legs also provides easy exposure of the surgical field.

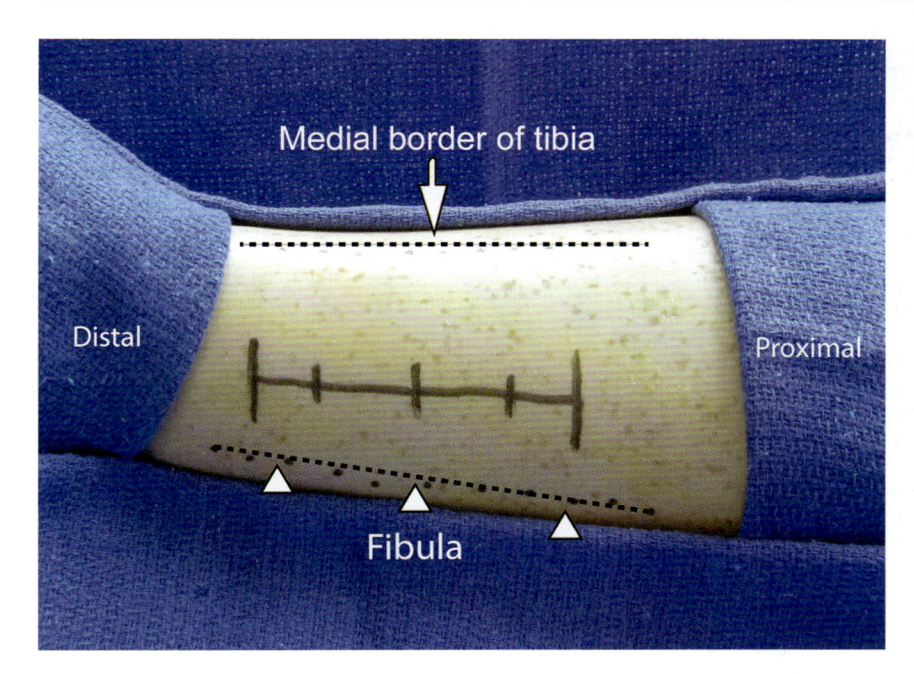

Fig. 147.3 Cadaveric specimen of the left leg. The tibial and fibular borders should be palpable and marked. The planned incision should be ~ 1.5 cm anterior to the fibular margin. The medial border of tibia *(white arrow)* and the anterior margin of the fibula *(white arrowheads)* are shown.

the crural fascia, the nerve should be traced proximally to its exit point from the fascia, and the fascia should be opened sharply to expose the nerve in the lateral compartment of the leg overriding the peroneus brevis muscle (**Fig. 147.5**). If the crural fascia is identified first, this fascia should be opened sharply, and the lateral compartment gently dissected to identify the SPN (**Fig. 147.6**). The SPN and peroneus brevis muscle can then be inspected in the lateral compartment to identify any potential nerve branches from the SPN innervating the peroneus brevis muscle. If no branches are seen, the nerve can be biopsied within the lateral compartment, or it can be traced to its exit point from the crural fascia and biopsied there. Depending on institutional preference, a 4-cm length of full-thickness nerve biopsy should be obtained. If muscle is also required, an associated biopsy of the peroneus brevis muscle can be taken after opening the crural fascia. The patient should be warned prior to cutting the nerve that this is a painful step, but that the pain is transient. It is recommended to make the proximal cut of the nerve first as this subjects the patient to only one painful cut. Little hemostasis is often needed, as large veins such as the greater and lesser saphenous veins typically do not course through the involved surgical site.

Given the variation of the exit site of the SPN from the crural fascia, it is possible to dissect down to the fascia, without first identifying the nerve (**Fig. 147.3**). If the initial incision is kept ~ 1.5 cm anterior to the lateral fibular margin, then opening the fascia at this level should give access to the lateral compartment of the leg (**Fig. 147.5**). However, in patients with a difficult-to-palpate fibular margin, the incision may be more anteriorly located than originally planned, and opening the crural fascia may cause inadvertent entrance into the anterior compartment. This can usually be avoided by palpating the lateral edge of the

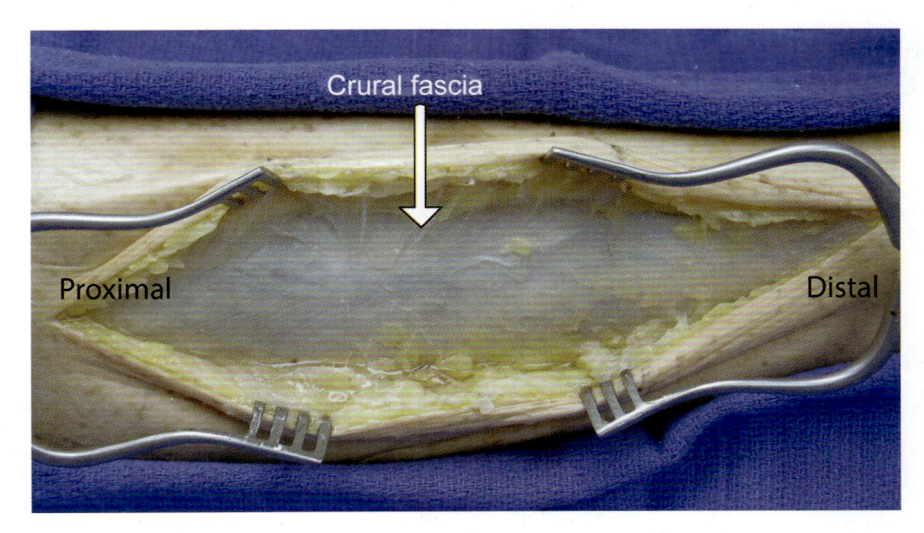

Fig. 147.4 Cadaveric specimen of the right leg. Exposure of the crural fascia *(white arrow)* as seen by a thick layer of white connective tissue. In this particular specimen, the superficial peroneal nerve (SPN) was not seen piercing the crural fascia within the expected area.

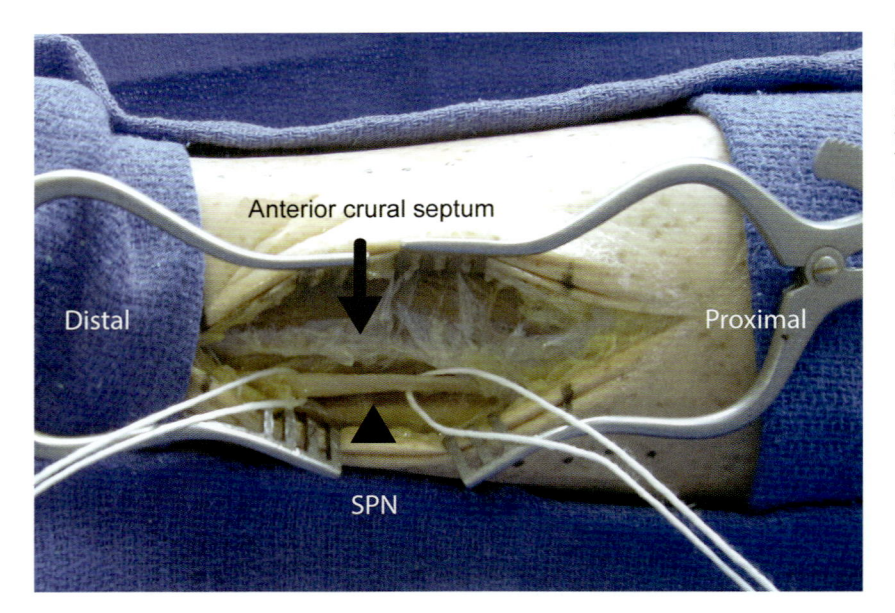

Fig. 147.5 Cadaveric specimen of the left leg (same patient as in **Fig. 147.2**). The crural fascia has now been opened both above and below the anterior crural septum *(arrow)*, which separates the anterior and lateral compartments of the leg. The SPN *(arrowhead)* can be seen in the lateral compartment just over the peroneus brevis muscle.

tibia, which is easily palpable in most patients, and planning the incision approximately two thirds of the distance between the tibia and where the fibula would be expected. If the anterior compartment is inadvertently entered, posterior dissection deep to the crural fascia and superficial to the musculature should lead to the interfascial septum, which verifies the location within the anterior leg compartment. Care should be taken not to biopsy the deep peroneal nerve, which travels more medially in the anterior compartment and provides motor innervation to the extensor digitorum brevis and extensor hallucis brevis, as well as sensation to the first dorsal webspace. Fascia of the anterior compartment, if entered, should then be closed and dissection performed in a more posterior location. If the nerve is not readily visible in the lateral compartment, consideration should be given to the anatomic variation where the nerve emerges from the anterior compartment.

Nerve Handling

It is important to handle the nerve with care both during and after the surgical procedure as nerves are easily damaged with unwanted pinching, twisting, and pulling, lowering the yield of the biopsy. Toothed forceps should be avoided. Fine-tipped De-Bakey forceps are suitable for this type of fine tissue manipulation. During biopsy, the nerve should be transected sharply. The nerve should be placed in saline immediately. If the neuropathologist prefers, prior to biopsy of the nerve, a suture may be placed through the proximal end of the cut nerve. This suture is then used to suspend the nerve in a container of saline, which keeps it moist and prevents unwanted crush injury or bending that may occur during processing and transporting to the neuropathologist. Intraoperative frozen section may used in cases where the nerve may be confused with a sclerotic vein, and is

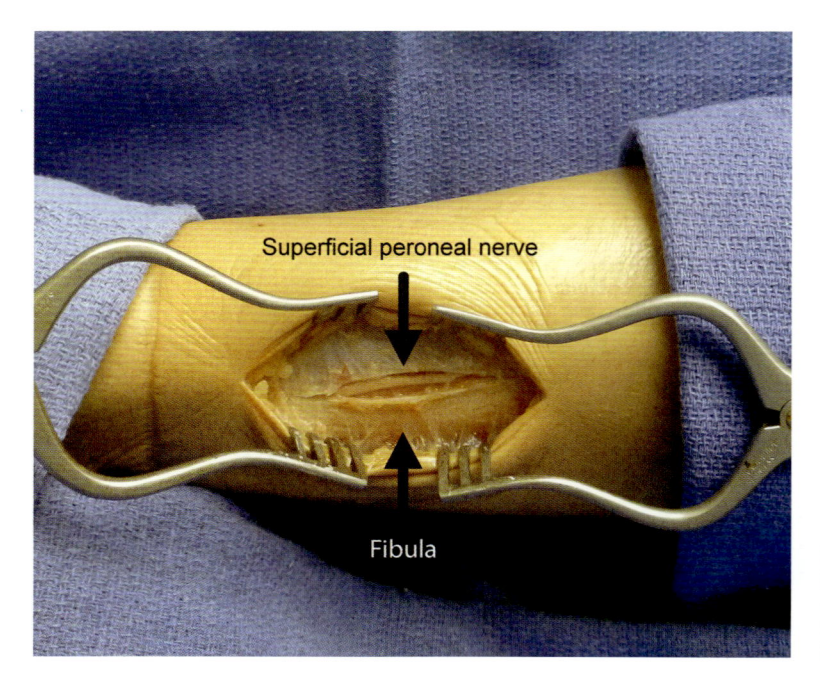

Fig. 147.6 In this cadaveric specimen of the left leg, the SPN runs just deep to the crural fascia in the distal portion of the leg prior to piercing the fascia. Care should be taken to open the fascia carefully to avoid injury to the nerve. The SPN and fibula are marked.

especially helpful in children, whose fibro-adipose tissue may render dissection relatively more difficult, or elderly patients whose disease state may cause the nerve to be embedded in dense aggregates of connective or inflamed tissue.[1] This practice, while not routine, may obviate the need to return to the operating room for failure to locate the nerve. Some surgeons advocate inspection of the cut end of the nerve under magnification to look for axons as opposed to luminal structures.

Closure

Patients with peripheral neuropathy may have difficulty with wound healing for many reasons, including loss of sensation to the area, rendering the wound susceptible to trauma and dehiscence; vascular ischemia; malnutrition; immunodeficiency from systemic disease or medications; and others. For these reasons, care should be taken to close the wound well. The wound should be well irrigated with bacitracin. The wound should be closed in layers. We typically close the crural fascia with a 2-0 or 3-0 polyglycolic acid absorbable suture in an interrupted fashion. The subcutaneous fascia is closed in a similar manner using inverted suture. For skin, we recommend using a 3-0 nylon suture on a cutting needle in a simple running fashion, taking care not to cause ischemia of the approximated skin edges. Following skin closure, the incision should be cleaned and dried. Bacitracin ointment is placed over the incision, and a 4 × 4 gauze is applied. Alternately, skin can be closed with a monofilament undyed subcuticular closure followed by cyanoacrylate adhesive, in which case a dressing may be avoided. A Kling wrap is lightly applied circumferentially for gentle pressure.

Postoperative Care

The patient is encouraged to ambulate but should keep the leg elevated while at rest or in bed for 48 hours. The patient should keep the dressing on for a minimum of 2 days, and let the incision be exposed to air from that point forward. If sutures have been used, these are typically left in for 10 to 14 days, with close inspection planned for wounds at risk.

Potential Complications and Precautions

As mentioned earlier, the inexperienced surgeon should plan for a longer operating time and potentially greater depth of anesthesia than for the standard sural nerve biopsy. Knowledge of anatomic variation facilitates inspecting the anterior compartment, with care taken to avoid the deep peroneal nerve. Anomalous innervation of the lateral portion of the extensor digitorum brevis through the SPN has been reported, with a prevalence of up to 28%, but there are no reports of new weakness following SPN biopsy.

The most common symptom after SPN biopsy is numbness, which is present almost uniformly adjacent to the site of incision, extending to the dorsum of the foot. Due to the overlap in cutaneous innervation, sensation over the dorsum of the foot may be absent or merely diminished to a varying extent. Over time, this usually becomes less noticeable as sprouting from adjacent nerves compensates.[9]

In a review of sural and peroneal nerve biopsies in 50 patients in the United Kingdom,[9] of 26 peroneal nerve biopsies, 15% of patients reported postoperative pain, 12% reported dysesthesias, and 54% reported paresthesias. Respective comparisons from the sural nerve biopsy group were 29% pain, 29% dysesthesias, and 38% paresthesias. Combining both groups, nine patients (18%) had delayed wound healing of greater than 3 weeks. Of these, five patients were treated postoperatively with immunosuppressive medications, and one was diabetic. Four (8%) of these patients were treated for a wound infection. Two patients (4%) suffered from a postoperative hematoma, and in one patient (1%) a postoperative neuroma was identified. These numbers are consistent with other published data.[20-27]

The relatively high rate of complication after nerve biopsy in general underscores the importance of only pursuing a biopsy if all other methods of identifying the cause of the peripheral neuropathy have proven inconclusive. Further complicating this is the observation that the diagnostic yield of a combined SPN and peroneus brevis muscle biopsy has been variably reported as 30 to 58%.[3,6-8,28-30]

Conclusion

Superficial peroneal nerve biopsy is a technically more demanding operation than the sural nerve biopsy, but may have higher yield in cases of vasculitis, especially in combination with biopsy of the peroneus brevis muscle. Thorough knowledge of anatomic variation helps preclude inadvertent entry into the anterior compartment or biopsy of the deep peroneal nerve. Frozen section may be useful in difficult or equivocal cases, due to the smaller caliber of the SPN relative to the sural nerve. Given that patients referred for nerve biopsy in general are a higher risk subpopulation, the surgeon should additionally screen for risk factors that would complicate wound healing, and should optimize the patient's condition for surgery. **Box 147.1** lists the key operative steps and the problems that can arise.

Box 147.1 Key Operative Steps and Potential Problems

- Surgeon should screen referrals and optimize patient's perioperative status.
- SPN biopsy is more technically demanding than sural nerve biopsy.
- Incision should be planned between 9 and 15 cm rostral to lateral malleolus and 1.5 cm anterior to the fibula.
- The SPN arises from the crural fascia on average 13 cm rostral to the lateral malleolus, with wide variation (between 3 and 18 cm), in 73% of cases.
- In 14% of specimens, the SPN arose from the anterior compartment.
- In 12% of specimens, the SPN bifurcates more proximally and exits from both the anterior and lateral compartments.
- The portion of the deep peroneal nerve which innervates the foot musculature, while traveling through the anterior compartment, should not pierce through the fascia at this level.

References

1. Katirji B. Neuromuscular Disorders in Clinical Practice. Boston: Butterworth-Heinemann; 2002
2. Said G. Value of nerve biopsy? Lancet 2001;357:1220–1221
3. King R, Ginsberg L. The nerve biopsy: indications, technical aspects, and contribution. Handb Clin Neurol 2013;115:155–170
4. Staff NP, Engelstad J, Klein CJ, et al. Post-surgical inflammatory neuropathy. Brain 2010;133:2866–2880

5. Agadi JB, Raghav G, Mahadevan A, Shankar SK. Usefulness of superficial peroneal nerve/peroneus brevis muscle biopsy in the diagnosis of vasculitic neuropathy. J Clin Neurosci 2012;19:1392–1396
6. Collins MP, Mendell JR, Periquet MI, et al. Superficial peroneal nerve/peroneus brevis muscle biopsy in vasculitic neuropathy. Neurology 2000; 55:636–643
7. Said G, Lacroix-Ciaudo C, Fujimura H, Blas C, Faux N. The peripheral neuropathy of necrotizing arteritis: a clinicopathological study. Ann Neurol 1988;23:461–465
8. Vital C, Vital A, Canron MH, et al. Combined nerve and muscle biopsy in the diagnosis of vasculitic neuropathy. A 16-year retrospective study of 202 cases. J Peripher Nerv Syst 2006;11:20–29
9. Hilton DA, Jacob J, Househam L, Tengah C. Complications following sural and peroneal nerve biopsies. J Neurol Neurosurg Psychiatry 2007;78: 1271–1272
10. Dyck PJ, Benstead TJ, Conn DL, Stevens JC, Windebank AJ, Low PA. Non-systemic vasculitic neuropathy. Brain 1987;110(Pt 4):843–853
11. Hart MG, Santarius T, Trivedi RA. Muscle and nerve biopsy for the neurosurgical trainee. Br J Neurosurg 2013;27:727–734
12. Sunderland S. Nerves and Nerve Injuries, 2nd ed. Edinburgh; New York: Churchill Livingstone; distributed by Longman; 1978
13. Flanigan RM, DiGiovanni BF. Peripheral nerve entrapments of the lower leg, ankle, and foot. Foot Ankle Clin 2011;16:255–274
14. Adkison DP, Bosse MJ, Gaccione DR, Gabriel KR. Anatomical variations in the course of the superficial peroneal nerve. J Bone Joint Surg Am 1991; 73:112–114
15. Rayegani SM, Daneshtalab E, Bahrami MH, et al. Prevalence of accessory deep peroneal nerve in referred patients to an electrodiagnostic medicine clinic. J Brachial Plex Peripher Nerve Inj 2011;6:3
16. Kimura J. Electrodiagnosis in Diseases of Nerve and Muscle: Principles and Practice. Philadelphia: F.A. Davis; 1983
17. Crutchfield CA, Gutmann L. Hereditary aspects of accessory deep peroneal nerve. J Neurol Neurosurg Psychiatry 1973;36:989–990
18. Neundörfer B, Seiberth R. The accessory deep peroneal nerve. J Neurol 1975;209:125–129
19. Dyck PJ, Thomas PK. Peripheral Neuropathy, 4th ed. Philadelphia: Saunders; 2005
20. Kumar S, Jacob J. Variability in the extent of sensory deficit after sural nerve biopsy. Neurol India 2004;52:436–438
21. Ruth A, Schulmeyer FJ, Roesch M, Woertgen C, Brawanski A. Diagnostic and therapeutic value due to suspected diagnosis, long-term complications, and indication for sural nerve biopsy. Clin Neurol Neurosurg 2005; 107:214–217
22. Perry JR, Bril V. Complications of sural nerve biopsy in diabetic versus non-diabetic patients. Can J Neurol Sci 1994;21:34–37
23. Flachenecker P, Janka M, Goldbrunner R, Toyka KV. Clinical outcome of sural nerve biopsy: a retrospective study. J Neurol 1999;246:93–96
24. Pollock M, Nukada H, Taylor P, Donaldson I, Carroll G. Comparison between fascicular and whole sural nerve biopsy. Ann Neurol 1983;13: 65–68
25. Neundörfer B, Grahmann F, Engelhardt A, Harte U. Postoperative effects and value of sural nerve biopsies: a retrospective study. Eur Neurol 1990;30:350–352
26. Gabriel CM, Howard R, Kinsella N, et al. Prospective study of the usefulness of sural nerve biopsy. J Neurol Neurosurg Psychiatry 2000;69:442–446
27. Dahlin LB, Eriksson KF, Sundkvist G. Persistent postoperative complaints after whole sural nerve biopsies in diabetic and non-diabetic subjects. Diabet Med 1997;14:353–356
28. Said G, Lacroix C. Primary and secondary vasculitic neuropathy. J Neurol 2005;252:633–641
29. Collins MP, Periquet MI, Mendell JR, Sahenk Z, Nagaraja HN, Kissel JT. Non-systemic vasculitic neuropathy: insights from a clinical cohort. Neurology 2003;61:623–630
30. Chia L, Fernandez A, Lacroix C, Adams D, Planté V, Said G. Contribution of nerve biopsy findings to the diagnosis of disabling neuropathy in the elderly. A retrospective review of 100 consecutive patients. Brain 1996; 119(Pt 4):1091–1098

Index

Note: Page references indicated by *b*, *f*, and *t* indicate boxes, figures, and tables, respectively.

A

Abducens nerve, paralysis of, 139
Ablative procedures
    cryoablation, for ilioinguinal neuralgia, 920
    radiofrequency ablation, for ilioinguinal neuralgia, 920
Abscess
    epidural, 333–338, 334*f*–338*f*
        osteomyelitis associated with, 338
    retropharyngeal pyogenic, 70
Accident-related injuries, lumbosacral, 873–874
Adduction relief sign, 148
Adolescents
    atlantoaxial rotatory subluxation in, 32
    fibrous dysplasia in, 547
    scoliosis in, 293*t*, 500, 501*f*, 502*f*, 503, 504
Airway management
    in cervical trauma, 173
    postoperative, 81
Alar ligament, anatomy and function of, 28
Altman classification, of sacrococcygeal teratomas, 763, 764*f*
American/British/French (ABF) classification, of spinal vascular malformations, 344, 344*t*
American Spinal Injury Association (ASIA) Impairment Scale, 554, 555*t*
Amyotrophic lateral sclerosis (ALS), 150, 153, 161
Anastomoses
    Martin-Gruber, 854, 861
    Riche-Cannieu, 854, 861
Anatomic mapping, in dorsal keyhole interlaminar rhizotomy, 701–702, 701*f*–702*f*
Anesthesia
    for anterior cervical diskectomy and fusion (ACDF), 186–187
    for anterolateral retroperitoneal approach, 564
    for benign nerve sheath tumor removal, 810
    for brachial plexus surgery, 827, 832
    for cervical stabilization, 174
    for costotransversectomy, 436
    for decompressive thoracic laminectomy, 493
    for dermal sinus tract excision, 759
    for dorsal rhizotomy, 696
    for endoscopic lateral transthoracic approach, 370
    for endoscopic lateral transthoracic diskectomy, 385, 386*f*
    for endoscopic lateral transthoracic vertebrectomy, 385, 386*f*
    for endoscopic thoracic sympathectomy, 379, 379*f*
    for facet screw fixation, 669
    for far lateral microdiskectomy, 623
    for foot drop correction surgery, 910
    for intradural extramedullary tumor resection, 461
    in Klippel-Feil syndrome, 143
    for lateral mass screw fixation, 244
    for lateral transthoracic approach, 357
    for lumbar/lumbosacral surgery, 570
    for lumbosacral plexus injury repair, 904
    for minimally invasive posterior lumbar approach, 594, 595*f*
    for minimally invasive retroperitoneal lateral interbody fusion, 417
    for minimally invasive retroperitoneal vertebrectomy, 423–424
    for minimally invasive thoracic decompression, 524
    for myelomeningocele repair, 754
    for open lateral transthoracic approach, 361
    for pediatric spondylolisthesis surgery, 534
    for pedicle screw-rod instrumentation, 497
    for posterior cervical foraminotomy, 217
    for posterior surgical techniques, in cervical spine, 206, 209
    for retropharyngeal approach, 72
    in sacral agenesis, 797
    for sacrococcygeal teratoma surgery, 765
    for screw fixation of odontoid fractures, 130
    for spinal accessory nerve surgery, 839
    for spinal cord compression, 283
    for tethered cord release, 716
    for transforminal interbody fusion, 643
    for vertebral cement augmentation, 740
Aneurysms, arteriovenous malformation-associated, 341, 345
Angiography, spinal. *See also* Computed tomography angiography; Magnetic resonance angiography
    of arteriovenous fistulas and malformations, 343–344
    of spinal vascular malformations, 340
    of thoracic/thoracolumbar tumors, 315–316
    of thoracolumbar congenital abnormalities, 291–292
Ankylosing spondylitis
    of craniovertebral junction, 19
    extension injuries associated with, 327
Annulotomy, in lumbar diskectomy, 608–609, 609*f*–610*f*
Annulus fibrosus, 538
    tears of, 584
Anterior approaches
    anterior cervical diskectomy with fusion (ACDF), 186–192
        advantages/disadvantages, 186
        alternative to, 193
        comparison with laminoplasty, 228, 232
        comparison with transcorporeal tunnel approach, 202, 203
        complications of, 191, 191*b*, 228, 232
        corpectomy in, 186, 189–190, 190*f*
        indications/contraindications, 186
        instrumented *versus* noninstrumented, 190
        patient positioning for, 186–187, 187*f*
        patient selection for, 186
        right *versus* left-sided approach in, 187–188, 187*f*
        surgical procedure, 186–190
        without fusion, 190
    to atlantoaxial instability, 118
    to axillary nerve, 843, 845, 846
    to cervical spine
        in cervical arthroplasty, 194–195
        for cervical spondylotic myelopathy, 151
        for cervical stabilization, 173–178, 175*f*–178*f*
        decompression and arthrodesis, 174–177, 175*f*–176*f*, 178*f*
        indications for, 207*t*
        in trauma, 173–178
            anatomic plane in, 174, 175*f*
            cervical plating in, 177–178, 178*f*
            diskectomy, 176, 177*f*
            incisions in, 174, 175*f*
    to cervicothoracic junction
        for corpectomy, 274–275
        supraclavicular approach, 263–267
    to lumbar/lumbosacral junction, 558–562, 559*f*, 560*f*, 561*f*
    to lumbar/lumbosacral spine
        lumbar interbody fusion
            with facet screw placement, 669
            for lumbar lordosis restoration, 560, 561*f*
            pseudarthrosis after, 682*f*
            revision surgery following, 682*f*
        open retroperitoneal approach, 412–415, 413*f*, 414*f*, 415*f*
    occipitocervical anterior fusion and instrumentation, 80
    to spinal accessory nerve, 839, 840*f*
    to thoracic/thoracolumbar spine
        after cervicothoracic corpectomy, 275–276, 275*f*
        anatomic basis for, 389
        in cervicothoracic corpectomy, 275, 275*f*
        lateral transthoracic
            endoscopic, 369–377, 385–390, 386*f*–388*f*
            open approach, 356–368, 357*f*, 358*f*, 359*f*, 362*f*–367*f*
        versus posterior approaches, 389
        for trauma, 555–556

939

Anterior atlantodental interval (ADI), in rheumatoid arthritis, 17
Anterior atlanto-occipital ligament, anatomy, 28
Anterior column reconstruction
 after cervicothoracic corpectomy, 280–282, 281f
 after vertebrectomy or diskectomy, 364–365, 367f
 of burst fractures, 327, 328f
 with cages, 388
 with endoscopic lateral transthoracic diskectomy, 388
 lateral graft and plate technique, 400–403, 401f, 402f, 403b
 with polymethylmethacrylate, 365, 366
Anterior column release, during lateral transpsoas lumbar interbody fusion, 518, 520
Anterior interosseous nerve syndrome (AIN), 820–821, 855, 856f
Anterior longitudinal ligament (ALL)
 anatomy and function of, 146, 147, 552
 in anterolateral retroperitoneal approach, 566–567
Anterior spinal artery, anatomy of, 341
Anterior superior iliac spine (ASIS), in ilioinguinal neuralgia, 917, 918, 919
Anterolateral approach, to lumbar/lumbosacral spine, combined with retroperitoneal approach, 563–568, 564f, 565f, 566f, 567f
Anterolateral transthoracic approach, 356–360
AO (Arbeitsgemeinschaft fur Osteosynthesefragen) classification system, for thoracic/thoracolumbar fractures, 326
AOSpine Spinal Cord Injury and Trauma Knowledge Forum, 552
Apert's syndrome, 139
Arachnoid dissection, with suboccipital craniectomy, 91
Arcuate foramen, 107–108
Arterial system, of spinal cord, 341
Arteriovenous malformations (AVMs), thoracic/thoracolumbar
 clinical presentation, 345
 of conus medullaris, 342, 344, 344f, 345
 dural, 340, 345
  differential diagnosis, 150
 endovascular treatment, 348t–349t, 352
 glomus, microvascular treatment, 348f–349f, 350, 351f
 imaging of, 342–344
 intradural, perimedullary, 340
 intradural/intramedullary, 345
 microvascular treatment, 346, 348t–349t, 350
 treatment outcomes, 354
Artery of Adamkiewicz
 anatomy, 341, 341f, 443, 566
 angiography of, 315–316
 in anterolateral retroperitoneal approach, 566
 in minithoracotomy-transsdiaphragmatic approach, 411
 in thoracic diskectomy, 457
 in thoracolumbar surgery, 291–292

Arthritis. See also Rheumatoid arthritis
 psoriatic, 19
 reactive, 19
Arthrodesis techniques
 atlantoaxial
  Brooks and Jenkins method, 115, 116f
  Gallie's method, 115, 115f
  interspinous C1-C2 method, 115–116, 116f
  posterior, 18, 18f, 109–117
  in rheumatoid arthritis patients, 18
 for cervical trauma, 173
 occipitocervical, 104
 with retropharyngeal approach, 79–83
  advantages/disadvantages, 79
  complete neural decompression in, 80, 80f
  complications, 82–83
  dural closure in, 80
  indications/contraindications, 79
  intraoperative craniovertebral stabilization in, 80, 81f
  postoperative care, 81–82
  retraction in, 80, 80f
Arthroplasty
 cervical, 193–200
  advantages/disadvantages, 193–194
  complications, 198–199
  indications/contraindications, 193
  patient positioning for, 194
  surgical technique, 194–197, 198f
  ProDisc-C prosthesis implantation, 195–197, 196f–198f
 for lumbar degenerative disk disease, 543
Astrocytomas, intramedullary, 153, 155, 156f, 158
 of filum terminale, 162
 surgical resection of, 467, 468–470
Atlantal posterior foramen, 107–108
Atlantoaxial dislocation
 Down syndrome-related, 6f
 transoral approach to, 37
 into ventral cervicomedullary junction, 9f
Atlantoaxial instability, 5b
 anterior approaches to, 118
 atlantodental interval in, 109
 C1-C2 screw fixation of
  C1-C2 transarticular screw fixation, 118–122
  C1 lateral mass-C2 pars screw fixation, 123–128
 causes of, 5b
 as contraindication to C1-C2 posterior approach, 106
 inflammatory bowel disease-related, 19
 occipitocervical fusion for, 100
 posterior C1-C2 junction exposure in, 106
 posterior wiring in, 118
 retropharyngeal approach to, 70
 rheumatoid arthritis-related, 17
Atlantoaxial junction
 irregular segmentation of, 5b
 malformations of, 5b
Atlantoaxial subluxation
 anterior C1-C2, rheumatoid arthritis-related, 16
 lateral, 16
 posterior C1-C2, rheumatoid arthritis-related, 18

 rheumatoid arthritis-related, 13, 16–18
 rotatory (AARS), 29
  in children and adolescents, 32
  radiographic presentation, 32, 32f
  rheumatoid arthritis-related, 18
  treatment algorithm, 35f
  treatment options, 32
Atlantodental interval (ADI)
 in atlantoaxial instability, 109
 in transverse ligament disruption, 31, 34f
Atlanto-occipital dislocation (AOD), 5b, 28
 classification, 28
 as mortality cause, 28, 30
 radiographic presentation, 30–31, 31f
 treatment options, 32
Atlanto-occipital junction
 dislocation of. See Atlanto-occipital dislocation (AOD)
 malformations of, 5b
Atlas-axis fractures, 30
 combined, 30
 radiographic findings in, 34f
 treatment options for, 32
Atlas-axis subluxation, transverse atlantal ligament disruption in, 31
Atlas (C1). See also C1-C2 junction
 anatomy, 110–111, 110f, 146
 arches
  anterior
   in C1-C3 strut arthrodesis, 80–81, 81f
   median tubercle, in retropharyngeal approach, 75–76, 77f
   reduction of, 38
   transoral-transpalatopharyngeal approach to, 45, 45f, 46f
  aplasia of, 5b
  posterior, bony exposure of, 86–89, 86f, 87f
 assimilation (occipitalization) of, 5b, 10
 biomechanics of, 147
 fractures, 29
  combined atlas-axis, 30
  Jefferson, 110
  as posterior atlantoaxial wiring contraindication, 110
  radiographic findings in, 34f
  treatment options for, 32
 malformations, 5b
 rotary subluxation, 10
 variants, 5b
Atlas vertebra, pathologies of, 4t
Atrial septal defects, Klippel-Feil syndrome-related, 141
Axillary hyperhidrosis, endoscopic thoracic sympathectomy for, 382t
Axillary nerve, surgical approach to, 843–848, 846f, 847f
 anatomic considerations in, 843–845, 844f
Axis (C2). See also C1-C2 junction; Dens
 anatomy, 111–113, 111f, 112f, 123, 146
 biomechanics of, 147
 fractures, 29–30
  combined atlas-axis, 30
  hangman's, 19, 30, 32
  treatment options for, 32
 malformations, 5b
 pathologies, 4t
Axonotmesis, 813, 814f

Index

B

Babinski sign, 147
Baclofen, intrathecal drug delivery system for, 730–737
  overdose with, 735*t*
Basilar impression. *See* Basilar invagination
Basilar invagination, 5*b. See also* Cranial settling
  determination of presence of, 15*f*
  natural history of, 70
  pre-operative imaging of, 10
  retropharyngeal approach to, 70
  rheumatoid arthritis-related, 13, 14*f*
  transoral-transpalatopharyngeal approach to, 42
Basilar migraine, 7*f*
Basion, in basilar invagination, 14, 15*f*
Basion-dental interval (BDI), 31*f*
Benediction sign, 148
Biceps brachialis, neurotization of, 914–915, 915*f*
Biopsy
  of peripheral nerve sheath tumors, 809–810, 882–883, 884*f*
  of spinal tumors, 316
  of superficial peroneal nerve, 932–938
    anatomical considerations in, 933*f*
    complications, 937, 937*b*
    with sural nerve biopsy, 932
    surgical procedure, 933–937, 933*f*–937*f*, 937*b*
  of sural nerve, 899–902, 901*f*, 932
Bisphosphonates, as giant cell tumor treatment, 167, 168*f*
Bladder, lumbosacral trauma-related rupture of, 875
Bladder cancer, metastatic, 881
Blue cell tumors, 169*f*
Bone grafts. *See also* Iliac crest bone grafts
  for anterior cervical decompression, 176
  in children, 143
  for occipitocervical arthrodesis, 80, 81, 81*f*
  for posterior C1-C2 fixation, 115, 116
  thoracic/thoracolumbar
    for in-situ fusion, 492, 494, 495*f*
    for pedicle screw-rod instrumentation, 496
    for thoracoabdominal/retroperitoneal graft and lateral plating, 431–434, 432*f*, 433*f*, 434*f*
    for transverse process fusion, 628, 630–631, 630*f*
Bone plates, for cervical spine stabilization, 182, 182*f*
Bone scans, of thoracic/thoracolumbar tumors, 315
Bone screws, cortical, 664–668, 665*f*–668*f*
Bone tumors, of cervical spine, 167–172
  benign tumors, 167, 168*f*
  malignant tumors, 167–171, 169*f*, 170*f*
  metastatic tumors, 170, 171*f*
Brachial plexus
  anatomy, 826–827, 827*f*, 849, 850*f*
  infraclavicular approach, 831–835, 832*f*
    anatomical considerations in, 831–832, 832*f*
    dissection techniques, 833–834, 834*f*
    incision, 833, 833*f*
  injuries to
    neurotization for, 914
    radiographic evaluation of, 928
    root avulsions in, 878
  supraclavicular approach, 826–830
    anatomical considerations in, 826–827, 827*f*
    dissection techniques, 828–829, 829*f*
    donor nerve graft harvesting, 829–830
    incision, 828
    laceration repair, 830
    stretch injury repair, 830
Bracing, as vertebral compression fracture treatment, 738–739
Brainstem, cranial settling-related dysfunction of, 14
Breast cancer, metastatic, 170
Brooks and Jenkins method, of cable fixation, 115, 116*f*

C

C1-C2 junction
  exposure of, 106–108
  fusion at
    effect on neck mobility, 84
    with posterior suboccipital/upper cervical exposure, 84–90
  instability. *See* Atlantoaxial instability
  pannus formation, 5*b*, 13, 14, 16, 70
  posterior approach to, 106–108, 107*f*, 108*f*
  screw fixation at, 123–128
    with C1 lateral mass-C2 pars screws, 123–128, 126*f*, 128*b*
    with pedicle screws, 123, 124*f*, 125, 126*f*, 127*b*
Cable fixation
  Brooks and Jenkins method, 115, 116*f*
  Gallie method, 115, 115*f*
  interspinous C1-C2 method, 115–116, 116*f*
  with multistranded titanium braided cables, 115–116
  types of, 115–116
Café-au-lait spots, 883*f*
Cages
  for anterior cervical diskectomy with fusion, 190
  for anterior column reconstruction after vertebrectomy or diskectomy, 364–365, 367*f*
  with endoscopic lateral transthoracic diskectomy, 388
  for cervicothoracic junction anterior reconstruction, 280–281
  failure of, 260
  for lateral graft and plate reconstruction, 400–403, 401*f*, 402*f*, 403*b*
  polyetheretherketone (PEEK), 190
  for post-spondylectomy reconstruction, 259, 259*f*, 260
  as strut graft alternative, 176
  for thoracoabdominal/retroperitoneal graft and lateral plating, 432–433, 432*f*, 434*f*
Calcium pyrophosphate deposition, 5*b*, 19, 19*f*
Canalis vertebralis, 107–108
Carotid artery, in anterior cervical diskectomy and fusion (ACDF), 187–188
Carotid sheath, in supraclavicular approach, 264, 265*f*
Carpal tunnel release
  endoscopic (closed) technique, 858–859, 858*f*–859*f*
  open technique, 856–858, 856*f*–858*f*
Carpal tunnel syndrome, 818, 820, 820*t*
  differentiated from pronator syndrome, 854
Caspar titanium plate-and-screw fixation, 81, 81*f*
Cauda equina tumors, 161
  ependymomas, 461, 465, 707–710, 708*f*, 709*b*, 709*f*
  extramedullary tumors, 161
  paragangliomas, 162
Caudalis dorsal root zone entry (DREZ) operation, 482–484, 483*f*
Caudal regression syndrome, 796
Cavernomas, imaging of, 342, 343*f*
Cavernous malformations, 341
  clinical presentation, 345–346
  of filum terminale, 162
  microvascular treatment for, 350–351
  treatment outcomes, 354
Cement augmentation, vertebral. *See also* Kyphoplasty; Vertebroplasty
  randomized controlled trials of, 738, 739*t*
Central cord syndrome, 182*f*
Cerebral palsy, spastic diplegia treatment in, 690–706
Cerebrospinal fluid
  diversion of, 82–83
  focal obstruction of, 485*b*
Cerebrospinal fluid leaks, intraoperative/postoperative, 260, 376
  Chiari I malformation treatment-related, 91, 95
  lipoma resectioning-related, 752
  lumbar/lumbosacral surgery-related, 572, 573–574
  myelomeningocele repair-related, 776–777
  repair of, 684–686
  shunt placement-related, 487–488, 489, 490
  transoral approach-related, 40
Cervical cancer, metastatic, 881
Cervical disk replacement (CDR). *See* Arthroplasty, cervical
Cervical spine
  anatomy, 146–147, 206, 208*f*
  anterior surgical approaches
    in cervical arthroplasty, 194–195
    for cervical spondylotic myelopathy, 151
    for cervical stabilization, 173–174, 175*f*–178*f*
    decompression and arthrodesis, 174–177, 175*f*–176*f*, 178*f*
    indications for, 207*t*
    in trauma, 173–178
      anatomic plane in, 174, 175*f*
      cervical plating in, 177–178, 178*f*
      diskectomy, 176, 177*f*
      incisions in, 174, 175*f*
  arthroplasty of, 193–200
    advantages/disadvantages, 193–194
    complications, 198–199
    indications/contraindications, 193
    patient positioning for, 194

Cervical spine (continued)
    surgical technique, 194–197, 198f
        ProDisc-C prosthesis implantation, 195–197, 196f–198f
  biomechanics of, 147
  bone tumors, 167–172
    benign tumors, 167, 168f
    malignant tumors, 167–171, 169f, 170f
    metastatic tumors, 170, 171f
  degenerative disease, 146–152. See also Spondylosis, cervical
  distraction-flexion injuries, 239–242
    closed reduction of, 239–242
      advantages/disadvantages, 239–240
      complications, 241, 242b
      indications/contraindications, 239
      key operative points in, 242b
      surgical procedure, 241
  mid- and lower cervical spine
    congenital osseous anomalies, 137–145. See also Klippel-Feil syndrome
      classification, 137–138
      phenotypic features of, 138
      sagittal plane deformities, 141
      torticollis associated with, 138
    trauma, 173–185
      anterior approach to, 173–185
      initial assessment and stabilization, 173
      posterior approach to, 173–174, 178–185
      surgical techniques for, 173–185
  rheumatoid arthritis of, 13, 14
  stabilization
    anterior approach, 174–178, 175f–178f
    with clamp and hook systems, 183
    combined anterior and posterior approach, 185
    with facet wiring, 183
    with interspinous wiring, 183–184, 184f
    with lateral mass fixation, 243–246
    with occipitocervical arthrodesis, 82
    posterior, 178–185, 179f–182f, 185f
    in retroperitoneal approach to occipitocervical junction, 80, 81f
    with sublaminar wiring, 185
  stenosis of, 146–152
    minimally invasive posterior cervical laminoforamiotomy for, 221–227
  tumors
    bone tumors, 167–172
      benign tumors, 167, 168f
      malignant tumors, 167–171, 169f, 170f
      metastatic tumors, 170, 171f
    intramedullary extramedullary, 153, 161–166
      clinical features, 161
      differential diagnosis, 161
      treatment, 166
      types of, 161–163
  upper cervical spine. See also Atlas (C1); Axis (C2)
    minimally invasive endoscopic approaches to, 56–62
    endoscopic endonasal approach, 57–58
    endoscopic transcervical approach, 58–62, 59f–61f
    endoscopic transoral approach, 56–57
Cervical Spine Injury Severity Score (CISS), 239

Cervicomedullary angle, 15
Cervicomedullary junction
  compression of, 42
  sensory and motor tracts at, 483f
Cervicothoracic curve, 141
Cervicothoracic junction
  anterior supraclavicular approach to, 263–267
  corpectomy of, 274–279, 275f, 277f, 278f
    anterior approach, 274–275
    anterior reconstruction following, 280–282, 281f
    anterior thoracic approach, 275, 275f
    endplate preparation in, 276–277
    following anterior thoracic approach, 275–276, 275f
    indications/contraindications, 274
    posterolateral approach, 277–278, 277f–278f
  definition of, 268
  fixed sagittal malalignment of, 253–256
  posterior instrumentation and fusion for, 283–288, 285f, 286f, 287f
    with C7 pedicle screws, 284–285, 285f, 286
    construct design challenges in, 286–287
    with lateral mass screws, 284, 285f, 287f
    length of construct, 286
    rod placement and fusion surface preparation, 285–286
    with thoracic pedicle screws, 285, 287f
    with translaminar screws, 285, 286f
  transmanubrial-transclavicular approach to, 268–270, 269f, 270f, 271f
  transsternal approach to, 268–269, 270–272
Chamberlain's line, 14, 15f
Chest intubation
  in endoscopic thoracic sympathectomy, 380–381
  in lateral transthoracic diskectomy, 398
  in retropleural approach, 358, 359–360
  in transthoracic approach, 393, 394
Chiari, Hans, 91
Chiari 1 malformations
  suboccipital craniectomy and cervical laminectomy for, 91–95
  syringomyelia associated with, 91, 92, 92f, 306–307
Chiari 2 malformations
  limited dorsal myeloschisis-related, 785
  myelomenigoceles associated with, 753
  prenatal surgery for, 299
  syringomyelia associated with, 207, 306
Chiari malformations
  craniovertebral junction abnormality-related, 5, 8, 8f, 11f
  syringomyelia associated with, 485
Children
  anterior arthrodesis in, 143
  astrocytomas in, 155
  atlantoaxial rotatory subluxation in, 29, 32
  atlanto-occipital dislocation in, 28
  brachial plexus injury grading in, 815
  congenital spinal tumors in, 156
  dermal sinus tracts/dermoids in, 757–762
  dorsal rhizotomy in, for spastic diplegia, 690–706
  ependymomas in, 155
  fibrous dysplasia in, 547

  Grisel's syndrome in, 29
  intramedullary tumors in, 153
  lumbosacral lipomas in, 746–752
  median labiomandibular glossotomy in, 50–51, 50f–51f
  osteoblastoma in, 547
  osteoid osteoma in, 547
  preoperative craniocervical reduction in, 43–44
  preoperative nutritional support in, 42–43
  sacral agenesis in, 796–798
  scoliosis in, 50
  spinal vascular malformation in, 345
  spondylolysis and spondylolisthesis in, 529–536
  tethered cord release in, 716
  transoral approach in, 39, 40
Chondromas
  lumbar/lumbosacral, 545–546
  thoracic/thoracolumbar, 318
Chondrosarcomas
  cervical, 170
  of occipitocervical junction, 25
  thoracic/thoracolumbar, 320
Chordomas
  cervical, 167, 169
  of the clivus, 24
  lumbar/lumbosacral, 548, 549f
  of occipitocervical junction, 24–25, 25f, 70
  thoracic/thoracolumbar, 318, 319f
Circumferential approach, for cervical stabilization, 174
Clamp and hook systems, for cervical spine, 183
Clival/pharyngeal tubercle, in retropharyngeal approach, 76–77
Clivus
  chordomas of, 224
  pathologies of, 4t
  segmentations of, 5b
Closed reduction techniques, in lateral mass fixation, 244
Cluneal nerves, in iliac crest bone graft harvesting, 800, 801f, 802f, 803b
Cobb syndrome, 340, 345
Coccyx, teratomas of, 763–768
Colitis, ulcerative, 19
Collagen, in disk degeneration, 540, 541f
Combined anterior-posterior approach
  to cervical spine, indications for, 207t
  for spondylectomy in midcervical spine, 257–260
  to thoracolumbar trauma, 555–556
Common peroneal nerve entrapment, 824–825
Computed tomography
  of aneurysmal bone cysts, 167, 545
  for anterolateral retroperitoneal approach, 563
  of atlantoaxial rotatory subluxation, 32, 32f
  of atlantoaxial subluxation, 17
  for C1-C2 screw fixation, 125
  for C1-C2 transarticular fixation, 119
  for cervical arthroplasty, 193, 194
  of cervical spondylotic myelopathy, 149
  of cervical trauma, 173
  of craniovertebral junction, 8, 9f, 10, 10f, 42
  for craniovertebral junction reduction, 44
  of disk herniations, 311–312
  of encephaloceles, 96

for endoscopic approach to upper cervical spine, 56
of eosinophilic granulomas, 545–546
of Ewing's sarcoma, 549
for extended maxillotomy approach, 63, 63b
of fibrous dysplasia, 547
of fixed sagittal cervicothoracic malalignment, 254
of giant cell tumors, 167
of hemangiomas, 547
of ilioinguinal neuralgia, 918
of intradural extramedullary tumors, 163
in Klippel-Feil syndrome, 142, 143, 144
for lateral transthoracic vertebrectomy or diskectomy, 396
of locked facet joints, 240, 241
for lumbar/lumbosacral anterior approach, 558
for lumbar/lumbosacral decompression, 595, 623
for lumbar/lumbosacral posterior approach, 570
of lumbar/lumbosacral tumors, 545
of neurofibromas, 23
of odontoid fractures, 130, 133f
of osteoid osteomas, 548
of osteosarcomas, 549
of pediatric spondylolisthesis/spondylolysis, 531
for pedicle screw fixation, 651
of sacrococcygeal teratomas, 764
for spondylectomy, 257
for thoracic laminectomy, 443
for thoracic pedicle screw fixation, 497
of thoracic/thoracolumbar congenital abnormalities, 291
of thoracolumbar trauma, 555
of transverse atlantal ligament disruption, 34f
for vertebral cement augmentation, 740
Computed tomography angiography
of cervical trauma, 173
of craniovertebral junction abnormalities, 10
of locked facet joints, 241
for transsacral approach, 676
of vascular malformations, 343
Computed tomography myelography
of brachial plexus injury-associated injuries, 928
for cervical radiculopathy, 223
of disk herniations, 311–312
of fixed sagittal cervicothoracic malalignment, 254
of lumbosacral plexus injuries, 879f
of musculocutaneous nerve injury, 849
of nerve sheath tumors, 809
for pedicle screw fixation, 634
of thoracic disk herniation, 455, 456
for thoracic laminectomy, 447
of thoracolumbar trauma, 555
for transforminal interbody fusion, 643
Congenital anomalies
of craniovertebral junction, 4t
of mid- and lower cervical spine, osseous anomalies, 137–145. *See also* Klippel-Feil syndrome
classification, 137–138
phenotypic features of, 138

torticollis associated with, 138
spinal tumors, 156–157
of thoracic/thoracolumbar spine, 291–309
dermal sinus tracts, 301–302, 301f
diastematomyelia (split spinal cord malformations), 299–301, 300f, 301f
dysplastic (congenital) spondylolisthesis, 297, 298f
embryology of, 292–293
formation errors, 293, 293f, 294, 294t
intraspinal cysts, 304–305, 304f, 305f
Klippel-Feil syndrome, 297
kyphosis, 295–296, 296f, 297f
lipoma of the terminal filum, 302
lipomyelomeningoceles, 302–303, 303f
lordosis, 296–297
meningoceles, 299, 300f, 304f
myelomeningoceles, 298–299, 299f
neuroendothelial cysts, 305–306
neuroenteric cysts, 303–304, 304f
radiological evaluation of, 291–292
scoliosis, 293–294, 293t, 294f, 295t
segmentation defects, 293–296, 293t, 294t, 296f
spinal dysraphism, 297–298, 302f
syringomyelia, 306–307, 306f
tethered cord syndrome, 302
of vertebral body, 293–304
Conus medullaris
arteriovenous malformations of, 342, 344, 344f, 345
congenital tumors of, 156–157
embryogenesis of, 769
lipomas of, 747
in tethered cord syndrome, 712, 712f, 716
Cordotomy, thoracic/thoracolumbar open anterolateral, 476–477
Corpectomy
anterior approach, 186, 189–190, 190f, 274–275
C2, with/without C1 anterior arch resection, 77, 77f
cervicothoracic, 274–279, 275f, 277f, 278f
anterior approach, 274–275
anterior reconstruction following, 280–282, 281f
anterior thoracic approach, 275, 275f
end-plate preparation in, 276–277
following anterior thoracic approach, 275–276, 275f
indications/contraindications, 274
posterolateral approach, 277–278, 277f–278f
endoscopic, 388
lateral transthoracic approach, 365–366, 367f, 397, 398f, 399b
lateral graft and plate reconstruction following, 400–403
retropleural, lateral graft and plate reconstruction following, 400–403
with thoracoabdominal/retroperitoneal graft and lateral plating, 432, 432f
Cortical bone screws, 664–668, 665f–668f
Costotransversectomy
cervicothoracic, 277
minimally invasive, 440–442, 441f
for thoracic epidural abscess, 336f, 337, 337f
thoracic open, 435–439, 439b

for disk herniations, 435–437, 436f, 437f, 438f
for sympathectomy, 435, 437–439, 438f
Cranial footplates, in thoracic laminoplasty, 451, 452f, 454, 454f
Cranial nerves, occipitocervical junction lesion-related dysfunction of, 30, 71
Cranial settling, rheumatoid arthritis-related, 13, 14–15, 14f, 15f, 70
irreducible, 15, 16f
occipitoatlantoaxial pannus formation in, 16
partially reducible, 17f
Craniectomy, suboccipital, for Chiari I malformation, 91–95
Craniocervical junction. *See* Craniovertebral junction
Craniotomy footplate, in thoracic laminectomy, 447
Craniovertebral junction
abnormalities of, 3–12
acquired, 4t, 5b
anatomy of, 86f, 87f
classification of, 4, 5b
congenital, 4t
developmental, 4t, 5b
diagnosis of, 4–5
irreducible, 12, 38–39
neuroradiological investigations of, 5–10
osteoligamentous, 10, 11f
radiographic criteria for, 30–31
reducibility of, 5, 10
signs and symptoms of, 4–5, 5b
treatment decision making for, 5, 8, 10
treatment strategy for, 10–12, 11f
with ventral cervicomedullary compression, 3
anatomy, 3, 37
endoscopic endonasal approach to, 42
instability, 100
rheumatoid arthritis of, 13–19
atlantoaxial subluxation in, 16–18
cranial settling in, 13, 14–15, 14f, 15f, 70
pannus formation in, 5b, 13, 14, 16, 70
treatment outcomes, 18–19
rheumatologic and degenerative disease of, 13–20
seronegative spondyloarthropathies of, 19
stability, 28
surgical approaches to, 12, 12b
transmandibular-median labiomandibular approach, 39
transoral approaches to, 37–41
complications, 37, 38
development and history of, 37–38
endoscopic approach, 56–62, 59f–61f
extended approaches, 38, 38t, 39, 48–51
for intradural pathology, 40
standard approaches, 38–39, 38t
transmandibular-median labiomandibular approach, 38t, 39
transmaxillary-Le Fort I osteotomy
with down-fracture of maxilla, 38t, 39, 40, 49
with palatal split, 38t, 40, 49–50, 64, 66f, 67f
transoral-transpalatopharyngeal approach, 38–39, 38t
transoral-transpharyngeal approach, 37

Craniovertebral junction (continued)
  trauma, 29
  treatment algorithm, 38, 42
Crohn's disease, 19
Crouzon's syndrome, 139
Crown-halo traction, 43–44
  for cervical closed reduction, 234, 235f, 236–237, 238b
Cruciate ligament, in transoral odontoidectomy, 45
Cryoablation, as ilioinguinal neuralgia treatment, 920
CT. *See* Computed tomography
Cubital tunnel syndrome, 818, 819–820, 823
  surgical treatment, 862–863, 863f
CyberKnife radiosurgery, for spinal vascular malformations, 352
Cysts
  aneurysmal bone, 21, 167
    embolization of, 21, 545, 546f
    lumbosacral, 545, 546f
    thoracic/thoracolumbar, 316, 317f
  dermoid, 156–157, 159f, 757, 759, 761f, 762
  inclusion, 158, 161
  intradural arachnoid, laminoplasty for, 451, 453f
  intramedullary, 153, 161
  intraneural ganglion, 807
  intraspinal, 304–305
    extradural meningeal, 304
    extradural meningeal with spinal nerve root fibers, 305
    intradural spinal meningeal, 305, 305f
    sacral meningoceles, 304–305, 304f
    Tarlov's perineural, 305
  neurenteric, 303–304, 304f
  neuroepithelial, 305–306
  polar, 467, 468, 468f
  synovial, 221, 570

D

"Dead-reckoning" approach, for pedicle cannulation, 650
Dead space, in transoral closure, 52, 53f
Decompression techniques
  of carpal tunnel
    endoscopic (closed) technique, 858–859, 858f–859f
    open technique, 856–858, 856f–858f
  of cervical spine
    for cervical spondylotic myelopathy, 150–151, 152
    with laminoplasty, 228–233
    with minimally invasive laminoforaminotomy, 221–227, 224–225, 225f
    with posterior foraminotomy and diskectomy, 217–220
    for trauma stabilization, 173, 174, 175f–177f
  of craniovertebral junction abnormalities, 37
    posterior approach, 3, 7f
    ventral approach, 7f, 38–39
  for ilioinguinal neuralgia, 918–919
  lateral recess, with foraminotomy, 600, 601f, 603f
  of lumbar/lumbosacral spine
    foraminal, 604
      lateral-to-medial, 600
    in laminectomy, 587–592
    minimally invasive posterior approach, 593–599, 595f–598f
    in transforaminal lumbar interbody fusion, 643–646, 644f, 649b
  of median nerve
    in anterior interosseous nerve syndrome, 855, 856f
    in ligament of Struthers entrapment, 855, 855f
  of occipito-cervical junction, in retropharyngeal approach, 80, 80f
  of posterior fossa, 485, 489
    for Chiari I malformations, 91–95
  of radial nerve
    of posterior interosseous nerve, 867–868, 867f, 868f
    for Wartenberg's disease, 868, 868f
  for rheumatoid cranial settling, 15, 16f
  of sciatic nerve, in gluteal region, 892
  of thoracic/thoracolumbar spine
    multilevel minimally invasive, 523–526, 524f, 525f, 526b
    in thoracic laminectomy, 446f, 447, 448f, 492–495, 493f, 494f, 495f
    for trauma, 555–556
    in transforaminal lumbar interbody fusion, 643–646, 644f, 649b
  of ulnar nerve, 861–865
    endoscopic technique, 865
    simple procedure, 863, 863f, 864–865
  of vertebral bone tumors, 170
Decortication
  in decompressive thoracic laminectomy, 494, 494f
  of transverse processes, 495, 495f
Deep venous thrombosis, postoperative, 632
Degenerative disk disease, of lumbar/lumbosacral spine, 538–544
  pathophysiology of, 540–543, 541f, 542f
  transsacral approach, 680, 681f
Demyelinating disease, differential diagnosis, 154, 154f
Denis classification, of sacral fractures, 874, 875f
Denis three-column spine model, 325, 326f
Denosumab, as giant cell tumor treatment, 549
Dens
  anatomy, 112, 146
  in atlantoaxial subluxation, 16
  dysplasia, 5b
  fractures, 32
  hypoplasia, 70
  segmentation anomalies, 5b
  vertical translocation, 14–15
Dermal sinus tracts, 301–302, 301f
  excision of, 757–762
Dermoids, 156–157, 159f, 657, 759, 761f, 762
Developmental abnormalities, of the craniovertebral junction, 4t
Developmental venous anomaly (DVA), cavernous malformation-associated, 350–351
Diastematomyelia (split cord malformation), 299–301, 300f, 301f
  dermal sinus tract-associated, 757
  nonoperative treatment for, 790, 795
  sacral agenesis-associated, 796
  surgical repair, 790–795
    bony spur removal, 791–792, 791f–794f
    laminectomy, 791–792, 791f, 795
  types of, 299–300, 790
Diffuse idiopathic skeletal hyperostosis, extension injuries associated with, 327
Digastric muscle and tendon, in retropharyngeal approach, 73–74, 74f
Dimples, sacrococcygeal, 757, 759, 759f
Diplomyelia, 299–300, 300f, 790
Diskectomy. *See also* Microdiskectomy
  in cervical spine, 176
    with cervical arthroplasty, 195
    with cervical foraminotomy, 219, 219f, 220f
    incisions for, 175f, 188, 188f
    with minimally invasive laminoforaminotomy, 221, 223
    multiple-level, 188
    percutaneous endoscopic cervical (PECD), 201
    single-level, 188
    for traumatic disk herniation, 176
  lateral transthoracic approach, 359, 359f
  in lumbar/lumbosacral spine
    anterolateral retroperitoneal approach, 566–567, 567f
    far-lateral minimally invasive, 621–627, 622f, 623f, 624f
    with hemilaminectomy, 604
    minimally invasive posterior, 608–611, 608f–611f
    in minimally invasive retroperitoneal lateral interbody fusion, 418, 419f
    posterior midline approach, 572
  in thoracic/thoracolumbar spine
    with costotransversectomy, 435–437, 436f, 437f, 438f, 456f, 457, 457t
    endoscopic lateral transthoracic, 385–390
    lateral extracavitary approach, 456f, 457, 457t, 460
    lateral transforaminal approach, 458
    lateral transthoracic approach, 359, 359f
    minimally invasive, 395–399, 397f, 399b
    open, 361–364, 362f, 363f, 366f
    with midline posterior approach, 455
    minimally invasive microendoscopic, 458
    open technique, 457–458, 457f–459f
    for soft lateralized herniations, 388–389
    transfacet pedicle sparing, 456f, 457, 457t
    transpedicular, 455–460, 456f, 457f–459f, 460b
  for thoracoabdominal/retroperitoneal graft and lateral plating, 432
  transpedicular/transfacet, 456f
Disk herniation. *See also* Diskectomy; Microdiskectomy
  calcified, 161
  concomitant with cervical fracture-dislocation, 241
  implication for closed reduction, 234
  minimally invasive posterior cervical laminoforamiotomy for, 221–223, 222f

thoracic/thoracolumbar, 310–314
  evaluation of, 311–312
  pathophysiology of, 310–311
  treatment for, 312–313
Diskography, 542
Distraction-flexion injuries, of cervical spine, 239–242
  closed reduction, 239–242
    advantages/disadvantages, 239–240
    complications, 241, 242b
    indications/contraindications, 239
    key operative points in, 242b
    surgical procedure, 241
    definition, 239
Distraction fractures, thoracic/thoracolumbar, 326
Distractors, vertebral, 195, 196f
Dobhoff tubes, intraoperative placement, 54f
Dorsal approaches, to craniovertebral junction, 12, 12b
Dorsal rhizotomy. See Rhizotomy, keyhole interlaminar dorsal
Dorsal root entry zone (DREZ) operation
  caudalis, 482–484, 483f
  for dorsal spinal lipomas, 781f, 782–783, 783f
  thoracic/thoracolumbar, 480–481, 481f
"Double crush syndrome," 223
Double fascicle transfer, for musculocutaneous nerve repair, 852
Down syndrome
  atlantoaxial dislocation in, 6f
  atlantoaxial instability in, 5b
  craniovertebral junction abnormalities in, 10f
Drilling techniques
  for C1-C2 screw fixation, 126, 127, 127b
  for C1-C2 transarticular screw fixation, 119–120, 121b
  for cervical laminectomy, 213–214, 215f
  for cortical bone screw fixation, 666, 667f
  laminar, for foraminotomy, 600, 601f
  for lateral mass screw fixation, 245
  for lateral transthoracic vertebrectomy or diskectomy, 396, 396f
  for lumbar laminectomy, 588, 591f
  for lumbosacral plexus injury repair, 904
  for open-door laminoplasty, 229–230, 230f
  for thoracic laminectomy, 447, 447f
  for thoracic laminoplasty, 451, 451f
  for thoracic vertebrectomy, 364, 366f
  for transcorporeal tunnel approach, 203
  for transsacral approach, 676, 679f
Dublin's method, for atlanto-occipital dislocation measurement, 30–31, 31f
Dumbbell tumors
  definition, 807
  schwannomas, 164fk, 807, 810f, 811–812
  surgical removal of, 810f, 811–812
  treatment for, 166
  unilateral facetectomy of, 463
Duplication
  pelvic, 141
  renal, 141
Dural closure
  in myelomeningocele repair, 774, 775f
  in retropharyngeal approach to occipitocervical junction, 80

suturing techniques for, 685
in tethered cord release, 718, 718f
Dural defects
  with cord herniation, 453f
  repair of, 684–686
Dura mater incisions, in encephaloceles, 97, 98f
Duraplasty, with suboccipital craniectomy, 91, 92, 93, 94f
Durotomy
  accidental, 454
  for tethered cord release, 717, 717f
Dysphagia, craniovertebral junction abnormalities-related, 5b, 7f
Dysplasia
  cervico-oculo-acoustic, 139
  diastrophic, 144
  fibrous, 21–22, 318, 547
  oculoauriculovertebral, 139
  spondyloepiphyseal, 50, 50f–51f

E

Ear anomalies, congenital spinal anomalies-related, 139
Edwards instrumentation, for transverse process fusion, 631–632
Elderly patients
  odontoid fractures in, 129
  vertebral artery anatomy in, 88–89
Electrocardiography, in cervical spinal fusion patients, 141
Electrodiagnostic evaluation
  of lumbosacral plexus injuries, 878
  of peripheral nerve injury, 815–816
  of ulnar nerve entrapment, 823
Electromyography (EMG)
  in cervical laminectomy, 217, 217217
  in cervical radiculopathy, 223
  in cervical spondylosis, 149
  in ilioinguinal neuralgia, 918
  in lumbosacral plexus injuries, 873, 878, 903
  in lumbosacral plexus tumor surgery, 884
  in musculocutaneous nerve injury, 849
  urethral, 781
Electrophysiological monitoring/testing
  in dorsal rhizotomy, 701–702, 701f–702f, 703f
  in spinal accessory nerve surgery, 839, 841–842
Elephantiasis neuromastosa, 807
Embolization
  of aneurysmal bone cysts, 21, 545, 546f
  of giant cell tumors, 549
  of hemangiomas, 547
  of spinal tumors, 322
  of spinal vascular malformations, 348t–349t, 351–352
Embryology, of the spine, 292–293, 538, 540
  of intervertebral disks, 538, 540
  of limited dorsal myeloschisis, 785, 786f–787f
  of open myelomeningoceles, 771, 772f
  of spinal cord, 769, 770f–771f
  of spinal cord lipomas, 779–781, 780f
  of spinal deformities, 293, 293f
  of spinal vascular anatomy, 341
En-bloc resection, of chordomas, 24

Encephaloceles
  frontoethmoidal, 96
  occipitocervical, surgical treatment of, 96–99
    closure techniques, 99
    contraindications/indications, 96
    incision, 97, 97f
    with skull defects, 99
    surgical procedure, 96–99, 97f, 98f
Enchondromas
  lumbosacral, 545–546
  thoracic/thoracolumbar, 318
Enchondromatosis, 318, 546
Endoscopic techniques
  for arteriovenous malformation treatment, 348t–349t, 352
  carpal tunnel release, 858–859, 858f–859f
  decompression of sciatic nerve in gluteal region, 892
  endonasal approach
    to craniovertebral junction, 12, 37, 42
    to upper cervical spine, 57–58
  lateral transthoracic approach, 369–377
    advantages/disadvantages, 369
    closure in, 373–375, 375f
    complications, 376
    diskectomy and vertebrectomy, 385–390, 387f
    spinal canal access in, 385–387, 387f
    endoscopy port placement in, 372, 373f, 375f
    incision planning for, 371, 373f
    indications/contraindications, 369, 370t
    patient positioning for, 370, 371f
    procedure, 373
  thoracic sympathectomy, 378–384
  transnasal approaches, to craniovertebral junction, 38t
  ulnar nerve decompression or neurolysis, 865
  in upper cervical spine, 56–62
    endonasal approach, 57–58
    transcervical approach, 58–62, 59f–61f
    transoral approach, 56–57
Endovascular treatment, of vascular malformations, 348t–349t, 351–352
End-plate preparation
  for cervicothoracic anterior reconstruction, 281
  for lateral graft and plate reconstruction, 401
  for thoracoabdominal/retroperitoneal graft and lateral plating, 431
  for transforaminal interbody lumbar fusion, 644–645, 645f
Enneking staging system, for spinal tumors, 320–321, 320f–321f
Entrapment neuropathies
  of lower extremity, 886–898, 887f–889f, 891f–897f
    common peroneal nerve, 824–825, 896, 896f
    femoral nerve, 887–888, 888f, 889f
    lateral femoral cutaneous nerve, 84, 823–824, 824f, 925–927, 926f
    meralgia paresthetica, 84, 824, 925–927, 926f
    sciatic nerve, 890–893, 891f–892f, 906, 907f

Entrapment neuropathies (*continued*)
  tibial nerve, 825, 825*f*, 893–894, 893*f*–894*f*
  of upper extremity
    median nerve, 818–820, 819*f*, 820*t*
      carpal tunnel syndrome, 818, 820, 820*t*, 854, 856–859, 856*f*–859*f*
      cubital fossa entrapment, 818, 819–820
      ligament of Struthers compression, 818–819, 854, 855, 855*f*
    musculocutaneous nerve, 849, 852
    radial nerve, 821*f*, 865–868, 866*f*–868*f*
      posterior interosseous nerve syndrome, 821–822, 865, 867–868, 867*f*
      "Saturday night palsy," 821
      Wartenberg's disease, 868, 868*f*
    tarsal tunnel syndrome, 825, 825*f*
    thoracic outlet syndrome, 823, 823*f*
    ulnar nerve, 822–823, 862*f*
      distal entrapment, 862, 862*f*
      entrapment at cubital tunnel, 862–863, 863*f*
EOS imaging, of scoliois, 500, 501*f*
Ependymomas, 153
  of cauda equina (myxopapillary)
    cerebrospinal fluid dissemination of, 461
    resection of, 707–710, 708*f*, 709*b*, 709*f*
  of filum terminale, 162, 165*f*, 166, 464–465, 465*f*
  intramedullary, 155, 155*f*, 157, 158*f*
    resection of, 467, 468–470, 468*f*, 469*f*, 470*f*
Epidermoids, 156
Epidural lead and needle placement, for spinal cord stimulation, 723–728, 724*f*–726*f*
Epidural space
  abscess of, 333–338, 334*f*–338*f*
  in microdiskectomy, 584–585, 585*f*
Epidural tumors, thoracic laminectomy for, 443, 447
Epineurial repair, of peripheral nerves, 929
Erector spinae muscles, 113, 114*f*
Escherichia coli infections, 445*f*
Evoked potential monitoring. *See also* Motor evoked potentials (MEPs) monitoring; Somatosensory evoked potentials (SSEPs) monitoring
  in posterior cervical surgery, 206
Ewing's sarcoma
  lumbar/lumbosacral, 549
  thoracic/thoracolumbar, 319–320
Extended maxilotomy reconstruction, 63–69
  advantages/disadvantages, 63
  indications/contraindications, 63
  Le Fort I osteotomy in, 38*t*, 39, 63, 64, 66–67, 66*f*, 68*f*–69*f*
    with down-fracture of maxilla, 38*t*, 39, 40, 49
    with palatal split, 38*t*, 40, 49–50, 64, 66*f*, 67*f*
    single-piece, without palatal split, 63
    two-piece, with palatal split, 63
  maxilla/nasal cavity exposure in, 64, 65*f*
  palatal split in, 63, 64, 66*f*, 67*f*
  patient positioning for, 64
  preoperative planning for, 63, 63*b*
  tracheostomy in, 64
  vertical pharyngotomy in, 63, 67, 69*f*
Extended transoral approach, to craniovertebral junction, 38, 38*t*, 39, 48–51
Extension injuries, thoracic/thoracolumbar, 327, 330, 330*f*
External beam radiotherapy (EBRT), 322
Extradural meningeal cysts, 304
  with spinal nerve root fibers, 305
Extreme lateral interbody fusion retractor system, 886, 888

F

Facetectomy
  for scoliosis correction, 507, 509
  for transforminal interbody fusion, 643
  unilateral
    of dumbbell tumors, 463
    hemilaminotomy/mesial, 612
Facet joints
  cervical, 147
    in C1-C2 junction posterior approach, 107, 108, 108*f*
    C2, anatomy, 111, 111*f*
    closed reduction of
      with crown-halo traction, 234, 235*f*, 236–237, 238*b*
      with Gardner-Wells tongs, 234, 235*f*, 236–237, 238*b*
    definition, 234
    locked, 239–242
    splaying of, 182*f*
    wiring of, 183
  lumbar/lumbosacral
    anatomy and function, 570
    degeneration of, 541–542, 570
    in posterior midline approach, 573, 574*f*
Facet screw fixation, of lumbosacral spine, 669–672, 670*f*–671*f*, 671*t*
Facial deformities, Klippel-Feil syndrome-related, 139
Fascicular repair, of peripheral nerves, 930
Felty's syndrome, 13
Femoral nerve. *See also* Lateral femoral cutaneous nerve
  anatomy, 887, 888*f*
  exposure and repair, 887–888, 906, 908, 909*f*, 910*f*
Femoral nerve-to-gluteal nerve transfer, 909–9810
Ferguson and Allen classification system, for thoracic/thoracolumbar fractures, 326
Fetal surgery, for myelomeningoceles, 299
Fibrodysplasia ossificans, 144
Fifth nerve palsy, 211
Filum terminale, 165*f*
  cavernous malformations of, 162
  sectioning of, in tethered cord syndrome, 711, 712, 712*f*, 713, 713*f*, 714*f*, 716, 718
  tumors of
    astrocytomas, 162
    ependymomas, 162, 165*f*, 166, 464–465, 465*f*
    lipomas, 302
Fistulas
  arteriovenous
    clinical presentation of, 345
    dural
      dorsal, 342*f*
      microvascular treatment for, 346, 347*f*, 348*t*–349*t*
      treatment outcomes, 352, 354
    endovascular treatment for, 348*t*–349*t*, 352
    extradural, 342
    imaging of, 343–344
    perimedullary
      microvascular treatment for, 346, 350, 350*f*
      treatment outcomes, 354
    postoperative, 121
  cerebrospinal fluid, in pleural cavity, 360
Fixation techniques. *See also* Screw fixation
  atlantoaxial, 101
  C1-C2 transarticular technique, 118–122
  internal, in transverse process fusion, 631–632, 631*t*
  occipitocervical, 7*f*, 12
    dorsal, 7*f*, 9*f*, 10*f*
    rigid, 100–105
Flaps
  musculocutaneous, thoracic, 493, 494*f*, 497
  myocutaneous, for myelomeningocele repair, 775–776, 776*f*
Flexion-distraction injuries, thoracic/thoracolumbar, 326, 327, 329*f*
Fluoroscopy
  anteroposterior, for cervical arthroplasty, 195, 195*f*, 196, 197
  for facet screw fixation, 669–6670
  for image-guided screw fixation, 650–653, 651*f*–653*f*
  for transsacral approach, 676, 678*f*
Foix-Alajouanine syndrome, 345
Footplates
  for lumbar foraminotomy, 576
  for lumbar laminectomy, 588, 591*f*
  for thoracic laminectomy, 447
  for thoracic laminoplasty, 451, 452*f*, 454, 454*f*
Foramen, intervertebral, anatomy of, 576, 577*f*, 600
Foramen magnum
  abnormalities of, 5*b*
  anterior rim, in retropharyngeal approach, 76
  in Chiari malformation, 91, 92*f*
  pathologies of, 4*t*
  remnants of, 5*b*
  stenosis of, 5*b*
  surgical approaches to, 12, 12*b*
Foramen transversarium, in anterior corpectomy, 190, 190*f*
Foraminotomy
  cervical, 217–220
    advantages/disadvantages, 217
    closure, 219
    complications, 219
    concurrent with laminotomy, 229
    indications/contraindications, 217
    patient positioning for, 217
  lumbar/lumbosacral
    minimally invasive posterior, 600–603, 601*f*–603*f*, 603*b*
    open posterior lumbar, 576–578, 577*f*, 578*f*

facial deformities, 139
genitourinary defects, 141, 141f
hearing deficits, 139
pterygium colli, 138–139, 138f
Sprengel's deformity, 139, 140t, 141
thoracolumbar scoliosis, kyphosis, lordosis, 141
torticollis, 138, 138f
classification, 137–138
definition, 137
intramedullary tumor-related, 153
phenotypic features, 138, 138f
radiological evaluation, 142, 142f, 143f
treatment, 143–144
types, 137–138
Klippel-Trenauany-Weber syndrome, 345
Kyphectomy, in myelomeningocele repair, 777–779, 778f–779f
Kyphoplasty
 versus nonoperative treatment, 738–739, 739t
 versus vertebroplasty, 740
Kyphosis
 cervical
  cervicothoracic junction pedicle subtraction osteotomy for, 253–256
  congenital, 144
  diastrophic dysplasia-related, 144
  Larsen syndrome-related, 144
  in sagittal plane, 141
  as contraindication to
   cervical laminectomy, 213, 216
   posterior laminoforaminotomy, 221
 lumbar/lumbosacral, 531, 531f, 535
  proportional to pelvic incidence, 654, 655f
 myelomeningocele-related, 777–779, 777f–779f
 postoperative
  C2-C3, 107
  cervical arthroplasty-related, 198
  cervical laminectomy-related, 216
  laminectomy-related, 450, 451, 454
  posterior cervical surgery-related, 206, 209, 211
  posterior suboccipital approach-related, 84
 thoracic/thoracolumbar, congenital, 11, 141, 295–296, 296f, 297f

L

Lamina-articular process junction, in C1-C2 transarticular screw fixation, 119, 120f
Laminectomy
 cervical, 213–216
  advantages/disadvantages, 213
  for Chiari I malformation, 91–95
  closure, 210–211, 214–215
  complications, 206, 211, 215–216
  drilling technique, 213–214, 215f
  indications for, 213, 216
  lateral dissection, 210
  patient positioning for, 213, chap 31
  technique, 207, 209–210, 213–215, 214f–215f
 complications of, 450
 for diastematomyelia, 791–792, 791f, 795
 for epidural abscess, 336, 336f
 for external spinal cord decompression, 492
 for intradural extramedullary tumor resection, 461, 463f
 for intramedullary tumor resection, 467, 468, 469f
 lumbar/lumbosacral, open posterior, 587–592, 588f–591f
 for lumbosacral plexus injury repair, 904
 partial, with laminoplasty, 229
 for shunt placement, 486f, 487, 488, 490b
 for tethered cord release, 711, 712, 717, 717f
 thoracic/thoracolumbar, 443–449
  advantages/disadvantages, 443
  complications, 449, 449b
  decompressive, 492–495, 493f, 494f, 495f
  for dorsal root zone entry (DREZ) operation, 480
  indications/contraindications, 443
  minimally invasive, 448, 448f, 449f
  multiple consecutive-level, 523
  surgical procedure, 447–448, 447f, 448f, 449b, 449f
 for thoracic disk herniation, 295
 for thoracic osteomyelitis, 338
Laminoforaminotomy, posterior cervical microendoscopic, 221–227
 advantages/disadvantages, 221
 indications/contraindications, 221
 key operative steps, 226b
 patient positioning for, 223, 223f
 patient selection for, 221
 surgical technique, 223–225, 224f, 225f
Laminoplasty
 cervical, 228–233
  advantages/disadvantages, 228, 231, 232
  double-open door, 228, 231–232, 231f
  incision and exposure, 229, 229f
  indications/contraindications, 228
  laminar reclosure prevention in, 231
  open-door, 228, 229–231, 230f
  preservation of muscles attached to C2 and C7, 229, 229f, 231
 thoracic/thoracolumbar, 450–454, 454b
  expansion, 450
  for intradural extramedullary tumor resection, 461
  osteoplastic, 450
Laminotomy, 450
 for laminectomy with craniotomy footplate, 447
 for lumbosacral plexus injury repair, 904
 for spinal cord stimulator placement, 721, 721t, 723, 724, 725f
Landmarks
 of anterior cervical spine, 206
 of lateral mass quadrants, 244f, 245
 in posterior approach to cervical spine, 206, 208f
Larsen syndrome, 144
Lateral extracavitary surgical approach
 to cervicothoracic junction, 277
 to thoracic epidural abscess, 337, 337f, 338f
 to thoracolumbar trauma, 556
Lateral extraperitoneal approach, in extraperitoneal neuroectomy, 923–924, 924f
Lateral femoral cutaneous nerve
 anatomy of, 886–887, 887f, 888f, 925, 926f
 entrapment neuropathies of, 823–824, 824f
 meralgia paresthetica, 84, 824, 925–927, 926f
 in iliac crest bone graft harvesting, 800, 800f, 803, 803b
Lateral graft and plate reconstruction, 400–403, 401f, 402f, 403b
Lateral mass, as anatomic landmark, 206
Lateral mass screw fixation, of cervical spine
 C1 lateral mass-C2 pars, 123–128
  advantages/disadvantages, 124–125
  complications, 125, 127, 127b
  indications/contraindications, 123–124
  surgical procedure, 126–127, 126f, 127b
 for cervical trauma
  indications/contraindications, 178–179
  plating systems for, 182, 182f
 Magerl technique, 243–246, 244f
 for subaxial cervical spine stabilization, 284, 285f, 287f
Lateral parascapular extrapleural approach, to cervicothoracic junction, 277
Lateral plantar nerve, anatomy, 890
Lateral surgical approach, to craniovertebral junction, 12, 12b
Lateral transforaminal surgical approach, in thoracic diskectomy, 458
Lateral transthoracic surgical approach
 endoscopic, 369–377
  closure in, 373–375, 375f
  complications, 376
  endoscopy port placement in, 372, 373f, 375f
  incision planning for, 371, 373f
  patient positioning for, 370, 371f
  procedure, 373
 lateral graft and plate reconstruction following, 400–403
 minimally invasive
  for diskectomy, 395–399, 397f, 399b
  for vertebrectomy, 395–399, 398f, 399b
 thoracic/thoracolumbar
  advantages/disadvantages, 391
  complications, 394, 394b
  indications/contraindications, 391
  minimally invasive, 391–392, 391f, 392f, 393–394, 395–399, 397f, 398f, 399b
  patient positioning for, 392, 392f
Lenke classification system, for scoliosis, 503, 504f
Letterer-Siwe disease, 21, 317
Levator scapulae, anatomy, 206, 208t, 209t
Lhermitte's phenomenon/sign, 16, 147
Ligament of Struthers compression, 818–819, 854, 855, 855f
Ligamentum flavum
 anatomy and function, 147, 208t, 209t
 in cervical laminectomy, 213, 214
 in hemilaminectomy, 580, 580f
 in laminoplasty, 230
 in lumbar decompression, 612, 612f–613f, 614f
 in lumbar/lumbosacral laminectomy, 587–588, 589f, 590f
 in microdiskectomy, 584
 in transforminal interbody fusion, 644
Ligamentum nuchae
 anatomy of, 112–113, 112f, 113
 as duroplasty autograft, 92

Ligamentum nuchae (*continued*)
  in posterior cervical surgery, 206, 210*f*
  in posterior occipitocervical dissection, 86
Limited dorsal myeloschisis, 785*f*
  embryogenesis, 785, 786*f*–787*f*
  surgical treatment, 788
Lipomas
  cervical, 156, 157*f*
  of conus medullaris, 747
  of filum terminale, 302
  lumbar/lumbosacral
    classification, 746
    resectioning of, 746–752, 747*f*–751*f*
  spinal cord, 779–784
    anatomy and classification, 779
    dorsal, 779*f*, 780, 780*f*, 781–782, 781*f*–782*f*
    embryogenesis, 779–781, 780*f*
    operative outcome, 783, 785
    operative treatment, 781–783, 781*f*–784*f*
    subcutaneous, 779*f*
    terminal, 780–781, 783, 784*f*
    transitional, 780, 780*f*, 782–783, 782*f*–783*f*
Lipomyelomeningoceles, 302–303, 303*f*
  dermal sinus tract-associated, 757
  sacral agenesis-associated, 707, 796
List, Carl, 3
Localization techniques, for transforaminal lumbar interbody fusion, 643
Locked cervical facets, posterior approach to, 239–242
Longissimus muscle, anatomy, 206, 208*t*
Longus capitis muscle
  closure of, 52, 53*f*
  in transoral odontoidectomy, 44, 46*f*
Longus colli muscle
  in anterior cervical approach, 174, 176
  in cervical arthroplasty, 195
  closure of, 52, 53*f*
  in retropharyngeal approach, 75, 76*f*
  in supraclavicular approach, 265*f*, 266*f*
  in transoral odontoidectomy, 44, 46*f*
Lordosis
  cervical
    conversion into kyphosis, 209*f*
    in sagittal plane, 141
  congenital thoracic-thoracolumbar, 141, 296–297
  lumbar/lumbosacral, 552
    anterior lumbar interbody fusion for, 560, 561*f*
    measurement of, 655*f*
Low back pain, degenerative disk disease-related, 538
Lower extremity, peripheral nerves of, surgical approaches to, 886–898, 887*f*–889*f*, 891*f*–897*f*
Lumbar-lordosis mismatch, 500, 502, 503*f*, 505
Lumbar/lumbosacral spine
  anterior approaches to
    for lumbar interbody fusion
      with facet screw placement, 669
      for lumbar lordosis restoration, 560, 561*f*
      pseudoarthrosis after, 682*f*
      revision surgery after, 682*f*
      open retroperitoneal approach, 412–415, 413*f*, 414*f*, 415*f*

anterolateral approach, combined with retroperitoneal approach, 563–568, 565*f*, 566*f*, 567*f*
chondromas of, 545–546, 569–570
chordomas of, 548, 549*f*
decompression of
  foraminal, 600, 604
  in laminectomy, 587–592
  minimally invasive, 612–614, 612*f*–614*f*, 614*b*
degenerative disk disease of, 538–544
diskectomy of
  anterolateral retroperitoneal approach, 566–567, 567*f*
  far-lateral minimally invasive, 621–627, 622*f*, 623*f*, 624*f*
  with hemilaminectomy, 604
  minimally invasive posterior, 608–611, 608*f*–611*f*
  posterior midline approach, 572
facets of
  anatomy and function, 570
  degeneration of, 541–542, 570
  in posterior midline approach, 573, 574*f*
  screw fixation of, 669–672, 670*f*–671*f*, 671*t*
foraminotomy of
  minimally invasive posterior, 600–603, 601*f*–603*f*, 603*b*
  open posterior, 576–578, 577*f*, 578*f*
fusion techniques
  anterolateral retroperitoneal approach, 566–567, 567*f*
  injuries associated with, 874
  interbody fusion
    axial, 673–683, 680*f*–682*f*
    with facet screw placement, 669
    lateral transpsoas lumbar, 518, 520, 520*f*
    for lumbar lordosis restoration, 560, 561*f*
    minimally invasive retroperitoneal lateral, 416–422, 417*f*–421*f*
    pseudoarthrosis after, 682*f*
    revision surgery after, 682*f*
  minimally invasive transforminal interbody fusion, 642–649, 644*f*–648*f*, 649*b*
  for pediatric spondylolisthesis, 533–536, 535*f*
  posterior cortical bone fixation technique, 665*f*
hemilaminectomy of
  with diskectomy, 604
  minimally invasive, 604–607, 604*f*–607*f*, 607*b*
  radical, 600
  for transforaminal interbody fusion, 643
kyphosis of, 531, 531*f*, 535
  proportional to pelvic incidence, 654, 655*f*
laminectomy of, open posterior, 587–592, 588*f*–591*f*
limited dorsal myeloschisis, 785–788, 785*f*–788*f*
lipomas of
  classification, 746
  resectioning, 746–752, 747*f*–751*f*

microdiskectomy, far-lateral, 621–627, 622*f*, 623*f*, 624*f*
  far-lateral/foraminal, 615–620, 616*f*–619*f*
  minimally invasive, 621–627, 622*f*, 623*f*, 624*f*
posterior approach to
  foraminotomy, minimally invasive, 600–603, 601*f*–603*f*, 603*b*
  minimally invasive, 593–599, 595*f*–598*f*
retroperitoneal approach to
  anterolateral approach combined with, 563–568, 564*f*, 565*f*, 566*f*, 567*f*
  open, 412–415, 413*f*, 414*f*, 415*f*
rigid deformities of
  osteotomy for, 654–663, 663*f*
    pedicle subtraction osteotomy, 656*f*, 657, 658*f*, 659–660, 660*f*
    Smith-Petersen osteotomy, 654, 657–658, 658*f*, 659*f*
rigid deformities of, vertebral column resection of, 654, 658*f*, 660–662, 661*f*
spondylolisthesis and spondylolysis of, in children, 529–536
transsacral approach to, 673–683, 677*f*, 678*f*, 679*f*–682*f*
for transverse process, 628–633, 629*f*, 630*f*
transverse process fusion, 628–633, 629*f*, 630*f*
trauma, 552–557
  anatomical considerations in, 552
  classification, 553–554, 554*t*
  diagnosis, 554–555
  mechanisms of, 552–553
  treatment, 555–556
tumors, 545–551
  benign primary, 545–548
  lipoma resectioning, 746–752, 747*f*–751*f*
  primary malignant, 548–550
vertebrectomy, minimally invasive retroperitoneal, 423–430
Lumbar plexus
  anatomy of, 870, 871–872, 871*f*, 918*f*, 922*f*
  innervation of, 872*t*
  nerve sheath tumors of, retroperitoneal approach to, 882*f*, 884, 886
Lumbosacral junction, anterior approach to, 558–562
  surgical procedure, 559–562, 559*f*, 560*f*, 561*f*
Lumbosacral plexus
  anatomy, 870–873, 870*f*
  nerve sheath tumors of
    benign, 881–885, 882*f*, 883*f*
    malignant, 881, 882–883, 884*f*
  trauma, 870–880
    causative mechanisms of, 873–874
    clinical presentation of, 875–877
    management/repair strategies, 877–879, 903–911, 904*t*
      direct repair of femoral nerve, 906, 908, 909*f*
      femoral nerve to gluteal nerve transfer, 909–910
      intradural or intradural-extradural root repair, 904–905, 905*f*, 906*f*
      intradural to extradural intraplexal nerve transfer, 906, 907*f*, 908*f*

obturator to femoral nerve transfer, 908–909, 910f
for persistent foot drop, 910–911
with root avulsions, 878, 878f, 879f, 903
tumors, 881–885, 882f–884f
Lumbosacral trunk, trauma, 876, 877, 879
spontaneous recovery in, 904
Lung cancer, metastatic, 170
Lyme disease, 161
Lymphoma, 169f

M

Maffucci syndrome, 318
Magerl approach, for pedicle cannulation, 650
Magerl technique, of lateral mass screw fixation, 243–246
Magnetic resonance angiography
of arteriovenous malformations, 342–343
of cervical trauma, 173
of craniovertebral junction, 42
of craniovertebral junction abnormalities, 10
of locked facet joints, 241
Magnetic resonance imaging
of aneurysmal bone cysts, 167, 545, 546f
for anterior approach to lumbar spine, 558
for anterolateral retroperitoneal approach, 563
of arteriovenous malformations, 342, 342f, 343f
of astrocytomas, 155, 156f
of atlantoaxial subluxation, 17
of basilar invagination, 14f
for C1-C2 screw fixation, 125–126
for C1-C2 transarticular fixation, 119
for cervical arthroplasty, 194
of cervical spondylosis, 149, 151f
of cervical spondylotic myelopathy, 149, 151f
of cervical stenosis, 221, 222f
of cervical trauma, 173
of Chiari I malformation, 92f
of chordomas, 548, 549f
of congenital spinal tumors, 157, 157f
of cranial settling, 14f, 15
of craniovertebral junction, 7f, 8f–9f, 10, 42
of demyelinating disease, 154f
of dermal sinus tracts, 759, 760f
of disk herniations, 311, 455, 584, 615, 616f
of encephaloceles, 96
of ependymomas, 155, 155f
of Ewing's sarcoma, 549
for extended maxillotomy approach, 63, 63b
of fibrous dysplasia, 547
of giant cell tumors, 168f
of hemangioblastomas, 156, 157f
of hemangiomas, 547, 547f
of ilioinguinal neuralgia, 918
of intradural extramedullary tumors, 163, 164f, 165f, 461, 462f
of intramedullary tumors, 158, 467–468, 468f
in Klippel-Feil syndrome, 142, 142f, 143, 143f, 144
for lateral transthoracic vertebrectomy or diskectomy, 396
of locked facet joints, 240, 241
of lumbar/lumbosacral compression, 621, 623, 623f
for lumbar/lumbosacral decompression, 595
of lumbosacral plexus injuries, 878, 878f
of lumbosacral tumors, 545, 546f
of meningiomas, 162, 164f
of occipito-cervical junction, 22, 22f, 24
of musculocutaneous nerve injury, 849
of nerve sheath tumors, 162, 163f, 809, 882, 884f
of neurofibromas, 23, 23f, 24f
of occipitocervical junction, 71
of odontoid fractures, 130
for open posterior approach to lumbar spine, 570
of osteoid osteomas, 548
of osteosarcomas, 549
of pediatric spondylolisthesis/spondylolysis, 531–532, 532f
for pedicle screw fixation, 634, 651
of sacrococcygeal teratomas, 764
of spinal epidural abscess, 334–335, 335f
for spondylectomy, 257, 258f
of spondylodiskitis, 335f
of syringomyelia, 486, 486f
of tethered cord, 712, 712f, 716
for thoracic laminectomy, 443, 447
for thoracic pedicle screw fixation, 497
of thoracic/thoracolumbar congenital abnormalities, 291
of thoracic/thoracolumbar tumors, 315
of thoracolumbar trauma, 555
for transsacral approach, 676, 677f
of transverse atlantal ligament disruption, 31, 33f–34f
of transverse ligament injuries, 29
for vertebral cement augmentation, 740
Magnetic resonance myelography, of fixed sagittal cervicothoracic malalignment, 254
Magnetic resonance neurography
of brachial plexus injury–associated injuries, 928
of musculocutaneous nerve injury, 849
Mandibulotomy, in median labiomandibular approach, 39
Manubrium, in transmanubrial-transclavicular approach, 268
Martin-Gruber anastomosis, 854, 861
Maxilla exposure, in extended maxillotomy, 64, 65f
Maxillotomy, extended approach. *See* Extended maxillotomy reconstruction
McAfee classification system, for thoracic/thoracolumbar fractures, 326f
McCormack classification system, for thoracic/thoracolumbar fractures, 326
McCune-Albright syndrome, 21
McGregor's line, 14–15, 15f
McRae's line, 14, 15f
Mean arterial pressure (MAP)
in atlantoaxial instability–related stenosis, 113
in C1-C2 junction posterior approach, 106, 108
Medial plantar nerve, anatomy of, 890
Median labiomandibular approach, 38t, 39
glossotomy with, 48–49, 50, 50f
with/without glossotomy, 48–49
Median nerve
anatomy of, 818, 819f, 854
entrapment neuropathies, 818–820, 819f, 820t
carpal tunnel syndrome, 818, 820, 820t, 854, 856–859, 856f–859f
in elbow and forearm, 854, 855, 855f
ligament of Struthers compression, 818–819, 854, 855, 855f
Median pectoral nerve transfer, in axillary nerve repair, 848
Median tubercle C1 anterior arch, in retropharyngeal approach, 75–76, 77f
Medtronic SynchroMed II programmable pump, 731, 732f
Melanocytomas, 153
Menezes, Arnold H., 3
Meningiomas
calcified, 161
intracranial, 162
intradural extramedullary, 162, 164f, 166
of occipitocervical junction, 22, 22f, 70
of spinal cord, resection of, 464
Meningitis, dermoid cyst–related, 757, 759
Meningoceles
dorsal, 299
sacral, 304–305, 304f
Meralgia parestheticа, 84, 824, 925–927, 926f
Metastases, spinal, 320
to cervical spine, 170, 171f
epidural, thoracic laminectomy for, 443, 444f
of extramedullary tumors, 161
intramedullary spinal cord, 157
to lumbosacral plexus, 881
to spinal cord, 153
thoracic/thoracolumbar, 315
treatment for, 323
Microdiskectomy, far-lateral, 583–586, 583b, 585f, 586f
far-lateral/foraminal, 615–620, 616f–619f
paramedian posterolateral approach for, 621–627, 622f, 623f, 624f
Microendoscopic diskectomy, 458
Microforaminotomy, anterior cervical, 201
Microscopes, operating, 188, 189
Microvascular treatment, for arteriovenous malformations, 346, 348t–349t, 350, 351f
Migraine, basilar, 7f
Milling technique, in cervical arthroplasty, 196–197, 197f, 198f
Minimally invasive procedures. *See also* Endoscopic techniques
costotransvesectomy, 440–442, 441f
facet screw placement, 669–672, 670f–672f, 670t, 671t
lumbar/lumbosacral
far-lateral/foraminal diskectomy, 615–620, 616f–619f
hemilaminectomy, 604–607, 604f–607f, 607b
lumbar decompression, 612–614, 612f–614f, 614b
microdiskectomy (far lateral), 621–627, 622f, 623f, 624f

Minimally invasive procedures (*continued*)
  posterior approach, 593–599, 595*f*-598*f*
  retroperitoneal lateral interbody fusion, 416–422, 417*f*-421*f*
  transforaminal lumbar fusion, 642–649, 649*b* 644*f*-648*f*
    pedicle screw fixation with, 646–647, 646*f*, 647*f*
  lumbar retroperitoneal vertebrectomy, 423–430
    advantages/disadvantages, 423
    case example of, 428*f*, 429
    complications of, 427, 427*f*
    corpectomy with, 427
    diskectomy with, 426–427
    graft placement in, 427
    indications/contraindications, 423
    patient positioning for, 424, 424*f*
    surgical technique, 423–427
  microendoscopic diskectomy, 458
  pedicle screw placement, 650–653, 651*f*-653*f*
  posterior laminoforaminotomy, 221–227
  for spinal deformities, 518–522
    algorithm for, 518, 519*f*
    lateral transpsoas lumbar interbody fusion, 518, 520, 520*f*
    osteotomy, 520
    percutaneous pedicle screw fixation, 520–521, 521*f*
    transforaminal lumbar interbody lumbar (MIS-TLIF), 520, 521*f*
  thoracic/thoracolumbar
    thoracic pedicle screw fixation, 496
    thoracolumbar approach, 408–411, 409*f*, 409*t*
    for trauma, 556, 556*f*
  upper cervical spine, endoscopic approaches, 56–62
    endonasal approach, 57–58
    transcervical approach, 58–62, 59*f*-61*f*
    transoral approach, 56–57
Minimally Invasive Spine Deformity (MISDEF) Algorithm, 518, 519*f*
Minimally invasive spine surgery (MISS), definition of, 389
Minithoracotomy
  endoscopic, 385–390
  thorascopic, 385–390
Minithoracotomy-transdiaphragmatic approach (mini-TTA), 408–411, 409*f*, 409*t*
  for thoracoabdominal/retroperitoneal graft and lateral plating, 433–434
Monoparesis, craniovertebral junction abnormality-related, 5*b*
Morphine, intrathecal drug delivery system for, 730–737
  overdose with, 735*t*
Motor evoked potentials (MEPs) monitoring
  in costotransversectomy, 436
  effect of nitrous oxide on, 106
  effect of paralytic agents, 106
  in spinal accessory nerve surgery, 839
  in spondylolisthesis surgery, 534
  in transarticular fixation, 119
  in transforminal interbody fusion, 643
  in vascular malformation surgery, 346
Multifidus muscle, anatomy of, 206, 208*t*, 209*t*

Multiple myeloma
  cervical, 170, 170*f*
  thoracic/thoracolumbar, 318
Multiple sclerosis, 150
Musculocutaneous flaps, thoracic, 493, 494*f*
  for thoracic pedicle screw-rod instrumentation, 497
Musculocutaneous nerve, 849–853
  anatomy, 849, 850*f*
  entrapment neuropathies, 849
  injury repair, 849–853
  intercostal nerve transposition to, 914–915, 915*f*
  sensory distribution of, 849, 851*f*
Musculoskeletal anomalies, congenital, Klippel-Feil syndrome-related, 140*t*, 141
Mycobacterium tuberculosis infections, 333
Myelitis, transverse, 153
  differentiated from intramedullary tumors, 153, 154*f*
Myeloceles, differentiated from myelomeningoceles, 771
Myelography. *See also* Computed tomography myelography
  of intradural extramedullary tumors, 163
  lumbar/lumbosacral
    for anterolateral retroperitoneal approach, 563
    lumbar/lumbosacral compression, 623
Myelomeningoceles, 299
  congenital thoracic/thoracolumbar, 298–299, 299*f*
  differentiated from myeloceles, 771
  embryology of, 771, 772*f*
  lumbar, 300*f*
  prenatal repair of, 753–756, 754*f*-755*f*
  sacral agenesis-associated, 796, 797
  surgical repair, 773–779
    complications, 776–777
    dural closure in, 774, 775*f*
    with kyphectomy, 777–779, 778*f*-779*f*
    neural placode in, 773, 773*f*, 774–775, 774*f*, 775*f*, 777*f*
    segmental neural placode in, 777, 777*f*
    skin and myofascial closure in, 775–776, 776*f*
    skin incision and opening, 773, 773*f*, 774*f*, 775*f*
Myelopathy
  cervical
    cervicomedullary angle in, 15
    rheumatoid arthritis-related, 13, 16–17, 17*f*
  cervical spondylotic (CSM), 147–148, 148*f*, 149*t*
    anterior cervical diskectomy and fusion for, 186–192
    clinical presentation, 147, 148*f*, 149*t*
    differential diagnosis, 161
    imaging, 151*f*
    treatment, 150–151
  differential diagnosis of, 161
  occipitocervical junction lesion-related, 71
  vascular malformation-related, 345
Myeloschisis, limited dorsal, 785–788, 785*f*-788*f*
Myelotomy
  midline (commissural), 478–479, 479*f*
  complications, 471

of intramedullary tumors, 467, 468–469, 469*f*, 471
for shunt placement, 487–488
Myocutaneous flaps, for myelomeningocele repair, 775–776, 776*f*

N

Nasal cavity exposure, in extended maxillotomy, 64, 65*f*
Neck Disability Index, 148–149
Neck distraction test, 148
Neck pain, craniovertebral junction abnormality-related, 5*b*
Neoplastic lumbosacral plexus lesion, 881
Nerve blocks, for ilioinguinal neuralgia, 918
Nerve conduction studies, in cervical spondylosis, 149
Nerve grafts. *See also specific* nerves; Neurotization
  for peripheral nerve injuries, 816
  for spinal accessory nerve injuries, 841, 841*f*
Nerve roots, sacrifice of, as neurologic deficit cause, 258, 258*t*
Nerve root stimulation, as ilioinguinal neuralgia treatment, 920
Nerve sheath tumors, 153, 161–162
  benign, 807–812, 808*f*-809*f*, 810*f*, 811*f*
  extramedullary, 161
  of lumbosacral plexus
    benign, 881–885, 882*f*, 883*f*
    malignant, 881, 882–883, 884*f*
  malignant, 807, 811*f*
  resection of, 463–464, 464*f*
Nerve transfers
  in lumbosacral plexus, 903
  obturator-to-femoral nerves, 908–909, 910*f*
  of radial nerve, in axillary nerve repair, 848
Neuralgia
  of the genitofemoral nerve
    differentiated from ilioinguinal neuralgia, 922
    surgical treatment of, 922–924, 924*b*, 924*f*
  of the ilioinguinal nerve
    cryoblation for, 920
    decompression for, 918–919
    differentiated from genitofemoral neuralgia, 922
    nerve block treatment of, 918
    neurolysis for, 918–919
    neuromodulation treatment of, 920
    radiofrequency ablation for, 920
    surgical treatment of, 917–921
Neural placode
  in myelomeningocele repair, 773, 773*f*, 774–775, 774*f*, 775*f*, 777*f*
  of myelomeningoceles, 771, 772*f*
  segmental, 777, 777*f*
Neural tube, in myelomeningocele repair, 773
Neurapraxia, 813, 814*f*
Neurilemomas, 807
Neurocytomas, 153
Neuroectomy
  extraperitoneal, of genitofemoral nerve, 922–924, 924*b*, 924*f*
  of ilioinguinal nerve, 919

Neurofibromas, 161–162
  conventional globular, 808–809, 811
  dumbbell, 807
  of lumbosacral plexus, 881–885, 882f
  neurofibromatosis 1-associated, 881
  of occipitocervical junction, 23, 23f, 70
  pathology of, 812
  plexiform, 809, 809f, 811, 881
  surgical treatment of, 807–812, 809f
Neurofibromatosis, 161–162
  neurofibromas associated with, 881
  schwannomas associated with, 807, 881
Neurologic deficits
  congenital cervical spinal fusion-related, 143
  lumbosacral plexus trauma-related, 875–877, 876t
  myelopathy-related, 154
  nerve root sacrifice-related, 258, 258t
  spinal arteriovenous malformations-related, 342
  thoracic epidural abscess-related, 333
  thoracic/thoracolumbar fracture-related, 326
  thoracic-thoracolumbar tumor-related, 315
Neurologic evaluation, in cervical trauma, 173
Neurolysis
  of axillary nerve, 847
  of ilioinguinal nerve, 918–919
  for musculocutaneous nerve repair, 852
  of spinal accessory nerve, 839–841
  of ulnar nerve, 863–864
    endoscopic technique, 865
Neuromas, 807
  acoustic, 807
  of spinal accessory nerve, 839–840
  of sural nerve, 847–848
Neuromuscular blockade, for craniovertebral junction reduction, 44
Neurotization
  of axillary nerve, 848
  using intercostal nerves, 914–915, 915f
Neurotmesis, 813, 814f
Neurulation, of spinal cord, 292, 769, 770f–771f
Nitrous oxide, avoidance in evoked potential monitoring, 106
Nuchal ligament, anatomy of, 208t, 209t
Nuchal line, superior, 114f
Nucleus caudalis dorsal root entry zone (DREZ) operation, 482–484, 483f
Nucleus pulposus
  anatomy, 146
  in disk degeneration, 570, 584
  lumbar, 538, 539f
Nurick Disability Scale, 148, 149t, 151
Nutritional support
  postoperative, 81–82
  preoperative, in children, 42–43
NuVasive MaXcess extreme lateral interbody fusion retractor system, 886, 888

O

Obese patients, surgical table for, 615
Oblique capitis muscle, anatomy of, 206, 208t
Obliquus capitis inferior muscle, in posterior occipitocervical dissection, 86
Obliquus capitis superior muscle, in posterior occipitocervical dissection, 86
Obturator nerve
  anatomy, 887f, 888, 890
  surgical exposure of, 890
Obturator outlet approach, for iliac screw placement, 650, 652–653, 653f
Obturator-to-femoral nerve transfer, 908–909, 910f
Occipital bone, malformations of, 5b
Occipital condyles, fractures of, classification, 29
Occipitoatlantal dislocation, 32f, 100, 101f
Occipitoatlantoaxial instability, 10f
  cranial settling-related, 15
Occipitocervical junction
  anatomy, 21, 28, 101
  instability at, 100
  neural compression of, 71
  osseous anomalies of, 70
  posterior suboccipital/upper cervical exposure, 84–90
    advantages/disadvantages, 84–86
    bone exposure in, 86–89, 86f, 87f
    complications, 86–90
    indications/contraindications, 84
    patient positioning for, 84–86, 85f
    patient selection for, 84
    preoperative counseling for, 84
    soft tissue dissection in, 85f, 86, 86f
  retropharyngeal approach to, 70–78
    advantages/disadvantages, 71–72
    anatomic landmarks in, 72
    anesthesia for, 72
    anterior rim of foramen magnum in, 76
    arthrodesis with, 79–83
      complete neural decompression in, 80, 80f
      complications, 82–83
      contraindications, 79
      disadvantages of, 79
      dural closure in, 80
      indications/contraindications, 79
      postoperative care, 81–82
      retraction in, 80, 80f
    to basilar invagination, 70
    bone resectioning in, 77, 77f
    cervical fascial layers in, 82
    clival/pharyngeal tubercle in, 76–77
    digastric muscle and tendon in, 73–74, 74f
    fascial plane dissection in, 72, 73f
    hyoid bone in, 76
    hypoglossal nerve in, 74–75, 75f
    incision for, 72, 73f
    indications/contraindications, 70–71
    longus capitis muscle in, 75, 76f
    longus colli muscle in, 75, 76f
    median tubercle C1 anterior arch in, 75–76, 77f
    patient positioning for, 73f
    patient selection for, 70
    platysma muscle in, 72, 74f
    preoperative testing for, 72
    submandibular gland in, 73, 74f
    superior constrictor muscle in, 76, 77f
    superior laryngeal nerve in, 76
    tectorial membrane in, 77
    transverse cervical ligament in, 76, 77f
  rigid fixation of, 100–105
  transoral approach to, 72
  trauma, 28–36
    atlantoaxial rotatory subluxation, 29, 32
    atlanto-occipital dislocation, 28, 30–31, 32
    biomechanics of, 28
    clinical presentation, 30
    isolated fractures, 29–30
    ligamentous injuries, 28–29
    radiographic presentation of, 30–32, 31f, 32f, 34f
    transverse ligament interruption, 28–29, 31f, 33f
    treatment options, 32
  tumors, 21–27
    classification, 21
    primary benign, 21–24
    primary malignant, 21, 24–25
Odontoidectomy, transoral approaches, 38, 42–47
  indications/contraindications, 42
  preoperative craniocervical junction reduction, 43–44
  preoperative planning for, 42–43
  surgical technique, 44–47, 45f–47f
Odontoid fractures
  classification, 29–30, 129, 130f
  in elderly patients, 129
  radiographic findings in, 34f
  screw fixation of, 129–133
    advantages/disadvantages, 129–130
    anesthesia, 130
    C1 lateral mass-C2 pars screws, 123, 124f
    with cement augmentation of C2, 131, 133f
    complications, 131
    indications/contraindication for, 129
    indications/contraindications, 129
    patient positioning for, 130
    postoperative care, 131
    surgical technique, 130–131, 132f
Odontoid process
  anatomy, 111–112, 111f, 146
  fractures of. See Odontoid fractures
  tip of
    location of, 14–15
    in neck hyperextension, 28
    in transoral odontoidectomy, 45, 46f, 47f
Oligodendrogliomas, 153
Ollier syndrome, 318
Open anterolateral thoracic/thoracolumbar cordotomy, 476–477
Open costotransversectomy, 435–439
Open-door cervical laminoplasty, 228, 229–231, 230f
Open-door maxillotomy. See Extended maxillotomy reconstruction
Open lateral transthoracic approach, 356–368
  advantages/disadvantages, 361
  diskectomy or vertebrectomy after, 361–368, 362–364, 362f, 363f
  indications for, 361
Open reduction techniques
  in lateral mass fixation, 244
  posterior
    of fracture dislocations, 330, 331f
    with internal fixation, of locked facet joints, 239, 240f, 241

Open retroperitoneal approach, 412–415, 413f, 414f, 415f
Open thoracoabdominal approach, 404–407, 405f, 406f, 407f, 409f, 409t
Opisthion, in basilar invagination, 14, 15f
Oropharynx, preoperative preparation of, 42–43
Orthoses. *See also* Halo traction
   for rheumatoid cranial settling, 15
   thoracolumbar spinal, 532
   thoracolumbosacral, 567–568
Os odontoideum
   atlantoaxial dislocation-associated, 6f
   dystopic, 43f, 70
      transoral-transpalatopharyngeal resection of, 46f, 47f
   orthotopic, 70
   with unstable atlantoaxial articulation, 10f
Osteoblastomas, 22
   aneurysmal bone cyst-associated, 21
   lumbar/lumbosacral, 547–548
   thoracic/thoracolumbar, 316
Osteochondromas, thoracic/thoracolumbar, 316
Osteogenesis imperfecta, with hydrocephalus, 8f
Osteoid osteomas, 22
   lumbar/lumbosacral, 547–548
   thoracic/thoracolumbar, 316
Osteomyelitis
   thoracic epidural abscess associated with, 333
   vertebral thoracic, 338–339
Osteopetrosis, 5b
Osteophytes, 146
   posterior, 195
Osteoporosis
   as contraindication to
      cervical arthroplasty, 193
      lateral mass screw fixation, 179
      pedicle screw fixation in, 639
      rheumatoid arthritis-related, 70, 83
Osteosarcomas, 170
   aneurysmal bone cyst-associated, 21
   lumbar/lumbosacral, 549–550
   thoracic/thoracolumbar, 318–319
Osteotomy
   C7 pedicle subtraction, at cervicothoracic junction, 253–256, 255f
   for lateral transthoracic vertebrectomy, 397, 397f
   Le Fort I, in extended maxillotomy approach, 38t, 39, 64, 66–67, 66f, 68f–69f
      with down-fracture of maxilla, 38t, 39, 40, 49
      with palatal split, 38t, 40, 49–50, 64, 66f, 67f
      single-piece, without palatal split, 63
      two-piece, with palatal split, 63
   lumbar/lumbosacral, for rigid spinal deformities, 654–663, 663b
      pedicle subtraction osteotomy, 656, 656f, 657, 658f, 659–660, 660f
      Smith-Petersen osteotomy, 654, 656, 657–658, 658f, 659f
   for lumbar/lumbosacral foraminotomy, 576–577, 577f
   multiple posterior column, for scoliosis, 500
   polysegmental, 654
   Ponte, 654
   posterior wedge closing, 654
   for scoliosis correction
      pedicle subtraction osteotomy, 500, 509, 509f
      Smith-Petersen osteotomy, 507–509, 509f
   Smith-Petersen, at cervicothoracic junction, 253
   for spinal deformities, 518, 520
   three-column, for scoliosis, 500
   windowing, in endoscopic lateral transthoracic diskectomy, 386
Oswestry Disability Index (ODI), 500
"Owl's-eye en-face" approach, for pedicle cannulation, 650

P

Paget's disease, osteosarcoma associated with, 318
Pain
   atlantoaxial subluxation-related, 16, 17
   cranial settling-related, 14
   occipital, 23f
Pain management techniques
   ablative procedures
      cryoablation, for ilioinguinal neuralgia, 920
      radiofrequency ablation, for ilioinguinal neuralgia, 920
   intrathecal drug delivery system (IDDS), 730–737
   spinal cord stimulators, 720–729
Palatal split, in extended maxillotomy reconstruction, 38t, 39, 40, 49–50, 63, 64, 66f, 67f
Palmer hyperhidrosis, endoscopic thoracic sympathectomy for, 382t
Pannus formation (C1-C2), 5b
   rheumatoid, 13, 14, 16, 70
Paragangliomas, 162–163
   extramedullary, 161
   resection of, 464–465
Paralytic agents, avoidance in evoked potential monitoring, 106
Paramedian posterolateral approach, for far-lateral microdiskectomy, 621–627, 622f, 623f, 624f
Paraparesis, craniovertebral junction abnormality-related, 5b
Pars interarticularis
   anatomy, 123
   hangman's fractures of, 30
   repair of
      in far lateral/foraminal microdiskectomy, 615, 616, 617f, 618, 619f, 620
      in spondylolysis/spondylolisthesis, 533
Pectoralis muscle reflex, 147
Pedicle, thoracic, anatomy of, 497, 497f
Pedicle screw fixation. *See* Screw fixation, pedicle screws
Pelvic incidence (PI), 502, 502f, 503f, 505, 505f
   proportional to lumbar lordosis, 654, 655f
Pelvic tilt (PT), 502, 502f, 505f, 654
Pericranium grafts, for suboccipital craniectomy, 92, 93f, 94
Perineuriomas, 80

Peripheral nerves
   anatomy, 813, 814f, 929
   compressive lesions (entrapment neuropathies) of, 818–825
      anterior interosseous nerve syndrome, 820–821, 855, 856f
      common peroneal nerve entrapment, 824–825, 896, 896f
      lateral femoral cutaneous nerve entrapment, 823–824, 824f
      meralgia paresthetica, 84, 824, 925–927, 926f
      median nerve entrapment, 818–820, 819f, 820t
      in arm, 854, 855, 855f
      carpal tunnel syndrome, 818, 820, 820t, 854
      in elbow and forearm, 854, 855, 856f
      ligament of Struthers, 818–819, 854, 855, 855f
      musculocutaneous nerve entrapment, 849, 852
      pathophysiology of, 818
      posterior tibial nerve entrapment, 825, 825f
      radial nerve entrapment, 821–822, 821f, 865–868, 866f–868f
      posterior interosseous syndrome, 821–822, 865, 867–868, 867f
      Wartenberg's disease, 868, 868f
      tarsal tunnel syndrome, 825, 825f
      thoracic outlet syndrome, 823, 823f
      ulnar nerve entrapment, 822–823, 822f
      distal entrapment, 862, 862f
      entrapment at cubital tunnel, 862–863, 863f
   grafting and harvesting techniques for, 928–931, 931b
      complications of, 930–931
      donor site for, 930
      repair, 929–930
   trauma, 813–817
      classification and grading, 813, 814f, 815
      clinical assessment, 814–816
      management guidelines, 815f
      mechanisms of, 813
      pathophysiology of, 813
      reinnervation following, 813–814
      repair, 816, 929–930
   tumors of. *See* Nerve sheath tumors
Peripheral nerve stimulation, as ilioinguinal neuralgia treatment, 920
Peritoneal cavity, shunt placement in, 488–489, 490b
Peroneal nerve
   anatomy, 894, 896, 899, 900f
   surgical approaches to
      common peroneal nerve, 896, 896f
      deep peroneal nerve, 896–897, 897f
      superficial peroneal nerve, 896
Phalen's test, in carpal tunnel syndrome, 820
Pharyngotomy, vertical, 63, 67, 69f
Philadelphia collars, 32f
Plain radiography. *See* X-rays
Plantar hyperhidrosis, endoscopic thoracic sympathectomy for, 382t
Plasmacytomas
   cervical, 167, 169, 169f
   of occipitocervical junction, 25
   thoracic/thoracolumbar, 318

Plate construction
  anterior
    in anterior cervical diskectomy with fusion surgery, 190, 191f
    in cervical trauma, 177–178, 178f
    following cervicothoracic corpectomy, 282
    Caspar titanium plate-and-screw fixation, 81, 81f
  cranial, for thoracic laminoplasty, 451, 452f, 454, 454f
  lateral
    with open lateral transthoracic approaches, 365–366, 367f
    post-corpectomy graft and plate reconstruction, 400–403, 401f, 402f, 403b
    for posterior cervical stabilization, 178–183, 179f–180f, 181f–182f
    with thoracoabdominal/retroperitoneal graft and lateral plating, 431–434, 432f, 433f, 434f
  occipitocervical
    with retropharyngeal approach, 79–83
    with rigid fixation, 100–105
  posterior, in cervical trauma, 178–183, 179f–180f, 181f–182f
Pleural cavity, shunt placement in, 488, 490b
Pneumothorax, postoperative, 394
Polymethylmethacrylate (PMMA) reconstruction
  for anterior cervicothoracic reconstruction, 282
  of anterior columns, 365, 366
  in metastatic tumor treatment, 170
Polymorphonuclear leukocytes, in rheumatoid arthritis, 14
Ponticulus posticus, 107–108, 112
Posterior approaches
  atlantoaxial wiring, 109–117
    advantages/disadvantages, 109
    anatomical considerations in, 110–113, 110f–111f
    indications/contraindications, 109
    surgical technique, 113–116, 114f, 115f, 116f
  to axillary nerve, 843–848, 844f, 846f, 847f
  to cervical spine, 206–212
    advantages/disadvantages, 206
    anatomical considerations in, 206
    to C1-C2 junction, 106–108, 107f, 108f
    cervical foraminotomy and diskectomy, 217–220
    cervical laminectomy, 213–216
    closure technique, 210–211
    complications, 211
    indications for, 207t
    landmarks for, 206
    lateral mass fixation, 243–246
    for locked facets, 239–242
    patient positioning for, 206–207, 209, 209f
    surgical technique, 206–211
  cervicothoracic junction instrumentation and fusion, 283–288, 285f, 286f, 287f
    with C7 pedicle screws, 284–285, 285f, 286
    construct design challenges in, 286–287
    with lateral mass screws, 284, 285f, 287f
    length of construct, 286
    rod placement and fusion surface preparation, 285–286
    with thoracic pedicle screws, 285, 287f
    with translaminar screws, 285, 286f
  to craniovertebral junction, posterior suboccipital/upper cervical exposure, 84–90
  decompressive thoracic laminectomy, 492–495, 493f, 494f, 495f
  to lumbar/lumbosacral spine, 569–575
    advantages/disadvantages, 569
    anatomical considerations, 569–570
    foraminotomy, 576
    foraminotomy, minimally invasive, 600–603, 601f–603f, 603b
    hemilaminectomy, 579–581, 580f–582f, 604–607, 604f–607f, 607b
    indications, 569
    laminectomy, 587–592, 588f–591f
    microdiskectomy, 583–586, 583b, 585f, 586f
    minimally invasive decompression, 593–599, 595f–598f
    minimally invasive diskectomy, 608–611, 608f–611f
    operative technique, 572–574, 573f, 574f
    patient positioning for, 570–571, 571f
    radiological evaluation for, 570, 571
  sacrococcygeal teratoma resectioning, 763–768, 764f–767f
  to scoliosis correction, 500–517
    exposure and instrumentation in, 506–507
    rod rotation and vertebral body derotation, 509–511, 511f
  to spinal accessory nerve, 839, 840f
  suboccipital/upper cervical exposure, at occipitocervical junction, 84–90
    advantages and disadvantages, 84–86
    bone exposure in, 86–89, 86f, 87f
    complications, 86–90
    indications/contraindications, 84
    patient positioning for, 84–86, 85f–86f
    patient selection for, 84
    preoperative counseling for, 84
    soft tissue dissection in, 85f, 86, 86f
    vertebral artery in, 88–90, 88f, 89f
  to thoracic/thoracolumbar spine
    versus anterior approaches, 389
    decompressive thoracic laminectomy, 492–495, 493f, 494f, 495f
    laminectomy, 443–449, 444f–448f
    for thoracolumbar trauma, 556
    in vertebral column resection, 654, 656, 656f, 660–662, 661f
Posterior atlantodental interval (PADI), 15f
  in rheumatoid atlantoaxial subluxation, 17–18
Posterior interosseous nerve, anatomy, 821–822
Posterior interosseous nerve (PIN) syndrome, 821–822
  surgical treatment, 865, 867–868, 867f
Posterior ligamentous complex (PLC)
  anatomy and function, 28, 552
  integrity evaluation, 554, 554t
  role in spinal stability, 325
  in thoracolumbar trauma, 555–556
Posterior longitudinal ligament (PLL)
  anatomy and function, 146, 147, 311, 552
  in anterior cervical decompression, 176
  in anterior corpectomy, 189
  in anterior diskectomy, 189, 189f
  in disk herniations, 311
  in microdiskectomy, 585, 585f
  ossification, 311
Posterior midline approach, to thoracic disk herniation, 455
Posterior pharyngeal wall
  closure of, 54f
  in median labiomandibular glossotomy, 51f
Posterior spinal arteries, anatomy of, 341
Posterior tibial nerve entrapment, 825, 825f
Posterolateral approach
  in cervicothoracic corpectomy, 277–278, 277f–278f
  in open costotransversectomy, 435–439
Pott's disease, 356, 435, 455
Power's ratio, 30, 31f
Prenatal repair, of myelomeningoceles, 753–756, 754f–755f
Presacral approach. See Transsacral approach
Primitive neuroectodermal neoplasms, 153
Primitive streak, 292
ProDisc-C artificial cervical disk, 194, 194f
  implantation technique for, 195–197, 196f–198f
Pronator syndrome, 854
  surgical treatment, 855, 856f
Prostate cancer, metastatic, 170, 881
Proton beam therapy, for chordomas, 25, 548
Pseudoarthrosis
  anterior lumbar interbody fusion-related, 682f
  axial lumbar interbody fusion-related, 678
  C1-C2 transarticular fixation-related, 121
  pedicle screw fixation-related, 639
  transverse process fusion-related, 631
Pseudogout, 19, 19f
Pseudotumor cerebri, Chiari I malformations associated with, 95
Pterygium colli, Klippel-Feil syndrome-related, 138–139, 138f

Q

Quadriparesis, craniovertebral junction abnormality-related, 5b, 9f

R

Radial nerve
  anatomy, 821f, 865
  entrapment neuropathies, 821f, 865–868, 866f–868f
    posterior interosseous nerve syndrome, 821–822, 865, 867–868, 867f
    "Saturday night palsy," 821
    Wartenberg's disease, 868, 868f
  exposure in the arm, 865, 866f
Radial nerve transfers, in axillary nerve repair, 848
Radiation therapy
  for aneurysmal bone cysts, 545
  for chordomas, 318
  for hemangiomas, 316–317
  for metastatic tumors, 170
  for spinal tumors, 322

Radiculopathy, cervical
  minimally invasive posterior lamino-
      foraminotomy for, 221–227
  pathophysiology of, 217, 218f
  pedicle screw fixation-related, 251
  posterior foraminotomy and diskectomy
      for, 217–220
  spondylotic, 147
    anterior cervical diskectomy and fusion
        for, 186–192
    clinical presentation, 148–149
    imaging, 149, 151f
    treatment, 152
  unilateral
    percutaneous endoscopic cervical
        diskectomy for, 201
    transcorporeal tunnel approach to,
        201–205, 202f–203f, 204f
Radiofrequency ablation
  as ilioinguinal neuralgia treatment, 920
  of osteoblastoma, 316
Radioisotope (99m-technetium) bone scans,
    of thoracic/thoracolumbar tumors,
    315
Radiosurgery
  for spinal tumors, 322–323
  for spinal vascular malformations, 352
"Ramp effect," 281
Rapamycin, as chordoma treatment, 24
Reconstruction techniques
  anterior columns
    after cervicothoracic corpectomy,
        280–282, 281f
    after diskectomy and vertebrectomy,
        364–365, 367f
    of burst fractures, 327, 328f
    with cages, 388
    with endoscopic lateral transthoracic
        diskectomy, 388
    lateral plate and graft technique,
        400–403, 401f, 402f, 403b
    with polymethylmethacrylate, 365, 366
  extended maxillotomy, 63–69
    advantages/disadvantages, 63
    indications/contraindications, 63
    Le Fort I osteotomy in, 38t, 39, 40, 49, 63,
        64, 66–67, 66f, 68f–69f
    maxilla/nasal cavity exposure in, 64, 65f
    palatal split in, 38t, 40, 49–50, 63, 64,
        66f, 67f
    patient positioning for, 64
    preoperative planning for, 63, 63b
    tracheostomy in, 64
    vertical pharyngotomy in, 63, 67, 69f
  goal of, 280
  lateral graft and plate reconstruction,
      400–403, 401f, 402f, 403b
  thoracoabdominal/retroperitoneal graft
      and lateral plating, 431–434, 432f,
      433f, 434f
Rectal cancer, metastatic, 881
Rectus capitis muscle, anatomy, 113, 114f,
    206, 208t
Rectus capitis posterior muscle, in posterior
    occipitocervical dissection, 86
Recurrent laryngeal nerve
  in anterior cervical diskectomy and fusion
      (ACDF), 187, 187f
  transmanubrial-transclavicular approach-
      related injury, 269

Redlund-Johnell line, 15f
Reduction techniques
  for cervical stabilization, 174
  closed cervical
    of locked cervical facet joints, 239–242
    with traction, 234–238
      with crown halo, 234, 235f, 236–237,
          238b
      with Gardner-Wells tongs, 234, 235f,
          236–237, 238b
  of craniocervical junction
    with intraoperative traction, 44
    with preoperative traction, 43–44
  in lateral mass fixation, 244
  in pediatric spondylolisthesis, 533–534
  posterior open, for locked facet joints, 239,
      240f
Reiter's syndrome, 19
Rendu-Osler-Weber syndrome, 345
Resectioning techniques
  for cauda equina ependymomas, 707–710,
      708f, 709b, 709f
  for Ewing's sarcoma, 320
  for extramedullary spinal cord tumors, 166
  for intradural extramedullary tumors,
      461–466, 462f, 463f, 464f, 465f, 466b
  for intramedullary spinal cord tumors,
      468–475, 468f–474f
  for limited dorsal myeloschisis, 788, 788f
  pial technique, 350
  for sacrococcygeal teratomas, 763–768,
      764f–767f
  tonsillar, with suboccipital craniectomy, 91
  vertebral column
    for lumbar spinal deformity correction,
        654, 656, 656f, 657, 658f, 660–662,
        661f
    for scoliosis correction, 509, 510f
Resegmentation, of vertebral column, 292,
    540
Retinoblastomas, osteosarcomas associated
    with, 318
Retraction techniques/retractors
  in arthrodesis, 80, 80f
  in C1-C2 exposure, 107–108
  Cloward retractors, 80
  in combined anterolateral/retroperitoneal
      approach, 559, 560f
  Dingman retractors, 44, 45f, 66, 66f
  fan retractors, 373, 374f
  in odontoid screw fixation, 130–131, 132
  self-retaining retractors, 175f, 176, 210,
      210f
  Taylor-type retractors, 80, 80f
  Thompson-Farley retractors, 80
  tubular retractors, 594, 595f
    in far-lateral microdiskectomy, 621, 622f,
        623–624, 624f, 625f
    in lumbar decompression, 612, 612f,
        614b
    in lumbar diskectomy, 608, 611f
    muscle-splitting, 525, 525f, 526
    for transforminal interbody fusion, 643,
        644f
Retroarticular canal, 107–108
Retroarticular vertebral artery ring, 107–108
Retrocondylar vertebral artery ring, 107–108
Retroperitoneal approach
  anterolateral approach combined with,
      563–568, 564f, 565f, 566f, 567f

  to lumbar plexus tumors, 882f, 884, 886
  to lumbosacral plexus tumors, 882f, 884
  minimally invasive retroperitoneal lateral
      interbody fusion, 416–422,
      417f–421f
  open, 412–415, 413f, 414f, 415
Retropharyngeal approach
  to occipitocervical junction, 79–83
    anterior rim of foramen magnum in, 76
    arthrodesis with, 79–83
    complete neural decompression in, 80,
        80f
    complications, 82–83
    contraindications, 79
    disadvantages, 79
    dural closure in, 80
    indications/contraindications, 79
    intraoperative craniovertebral
        stabilization in, 80, 81f
    postoperative care, 81–82
    retraction in, 80, 80f
  to basilar invagination, 70
  bone resectioning in, 77, 77f
  cervical fascial layers in, 82
  clival/pharyngeal tubercle in, 76–77
  digastric muscle and tendon in, 73–74,
      74f
  hyoid bone in, 76
  hypoglossal nerve in, 74–75, 75f
  longus capitis muscle in, 75, 76f
  longus colli muscle in, 75, 76f
  median tubercle C1 anterior arch in,
      75–76, 77f
  superior constrictor muscle in, 76, 77f
  superior laryngeal nerve in, 76
  tectorial membrane in, 77
  transverse cervical ligament in, 76, 77f
  open, of lumbar spine, 412–415, 413f, 414f,
      415f
Retropleural approach
  for endoscopic lateral transthoracic
      vertebrectomy and diskectomy, 385,
      386–387, 387f, 388–389
  thoracic/thoracolumbar, 358, 358f,
      359–360, 362, 365f
    advantages/disadvantages, 391
    dissection and exposure, 393, 393f
    indications/contraindications, 391
    minimally invasive, 391–392, 391f,
        392f
  patient positioning for, 392, 392f
Revision surgery
  for cortical bone screw fixation, 664, 666
  following anterior lumbar interbody fusion,
      682f
Rheumatoid arthritis
  atlantoaxial rotatory subluxation-related,
      18
  clinical presentation, 13
  of craniovertebral junction, 5b, 13–19
    atlantoaxial subluxation in, 16–18
    cranial settling in, 13, 14–15, 14f, 15f, 70
    pannus formation in, 5b, 13, 14, 16, 70
    treatment outcomes, 18–19
  epidemiology, 13
  natural history, 13
  occipitocervical arthrodesis in, 83
  of occipitocervical junction, 70
  pathogenesis, 13–14
Rheumatoid factor, 19

Rhizotomy, keyhole interlaminar dorsal, for spastic diplegia, 690–706
 advantages/disadvantages, 703, 705
 anesthesia and positioning for, 696, 699, 699f, 701–702, 701f–702f
 complications, 705
 indications for, 691–692, 692f
 intraoperative neurophysiological guidance of, 701, 701f–702f, 703f
 preoperative planning for, 692–696, 693f–697f
 surgical approach, 699–703, 700f, 704f
Rib, cervical, 139, 139f, 297
Rib bone grafts
 for craniovertebral junction, 12
 with median labiomandibular glossotomy, 50
 for occipitocervical fusion, 104
 for thoracoabdominal/retroperitoneal graft and lateral plating, 431–432
Riche-Cannieu anastomosis, 854, 861
Rod rotation, in scoliosis correction, 509–514
Rotatory C1-C2 dislocation. See Atlantoaxial rotatory subluxation (AARS)
Roy-Camille technique, of lateral mass screw fixation, 243

S

Sacral agenesis, 796–798
Sacral plexus
 anatomy, 872, 872f, 873f
 trauma, 876f, 877
  root avulsions, 878
   spontaneous recovery in, 904
   surgical treatment, 904
Sacrum
 anatomy, 573
 giant cell tumors of, 548–549
 surgical exposure of, 573–574
Sagittal balance, differentiated from spinopelvic balance, 654
Sagittale foramen, 107–108
Sagittal imbalance, fixed lumbar osteotomy for
 pedicle subtraction osteotomy, 654, 656, 656f, 658f, 659–660, 660f
 Smith-Petersen osteotomy, 654, 656, 657–658, 658f, 659f
 vertebral column resection for, 654, 656, 656f, 658f, 660–662, 661f
Sagittal plane
 in scoliosis correction, 500, 503, 503f
 cervical, deformities of, 141
Sagittal vertical axis (SVA), 500, 502, 502f, 503f, 654
Sarcoidosis, differential diagnosis of, 154
"Saturday night palsy," 821
Scapula, Sprengel's deformity of, 139, 139f, 140
Schwannomas
 conventional globular, 808–809, 811
 dumbbell, 164f, 807, 810, 811–812
 of lumbar plexus, retroperitoneal approach to, 886
 of lumbosacral plexus, 881–885, 882f
 neurofibromatosis-associated, 161, 162, 807, 881
 of occipitocervical junction, 23–24
 pathology of, 812

of posterior spinal cord, 808f
 surgical treatment, 807–812
Schwannomatosis, 807
Sciatic nerve
 anatomy, 890
 surgical approaches to
  Henry's approach, 906, 907f
  intrapelvic, 890
  proximal extrapelvic, 890–893, 891f–892f
Scoliosis
 adolescent idiopathic, 293t, 502f, 503
  classification, 503, 504f, 504f
  surgical correction goals in, 503
 cervicothoracic, 141
 classification, 500, 502–503, 503f, 504f
 congenital, 293–295, 293t, 294f, 294t, 295t
  cervical spine fusion-related, 141
  cervicothoracic, 139f
  thoracic/thoracolumbar, 141
 coronal plane in, 503, 503f
 craniovertebral junction abnormality-related, 5b
 infantile, 293t
 juvenile, 293t
 Klippel-Feil syndrome–associated, 297
 neuromuscular, 293t
 open correction of, 500–517
  exposure and instrumentation for, 506–507, 507f
  with multiple techniques, 514, 514f–515f
  osteotomy
   pedicle subtraction osteotomy, 509, 509f
   posterior column osteotomy, 514, 515f
   Smith-Petersen osteotomy, 507–509, 509f
  patient positioning for, 506
  preoperative halo-gravity traction, 506
  sagittal plane in, 500, 503, 503f
  spinal alignment goals in, 503, 505–506
  vertebral column resection, 509, 510f
Scoliosis Research Society-Schwab classification system, for spinal deformity, 500, 502, 503f
Screw fixation
 anterior approach, following cervicothoracic corpectomy, 282
 of cervicothoracic junction, 285, 286f, 287f
 comparison with cortical bone screws, 664
 complications of, 634, 639
 in craniovertebral junction, 12
 facet, of lumbosacral spine, 669–672, 670f–671f, 671t
 of flexion distraction injuries, 327, 329f
 of fracture dislocations, 330, 331f
 free-hand technique, 247, 248, 249f, 250f
 iliac screws, 637–638, 637f, 638f, 639
  minimally invasive placement of
   mini-open approach with bony palpation, 650, 651
   obturator outlet approach, 650, 652–653, 653f
  image-guided technique, 247, 248–250, 251f
  indications/contraindications, 634
 lateral mass screw fixation, of cervical spine, 180, 181f, 182
  C1 lateral mass-C2 pars screws, 123–128
   advantages/disadvantages, 124–125

complications, 125, 127, 127b
   indications/contraindications, 123–124
   surgical procedure, 126–127, 126f, 127b
  for cervical trauma
   indications/contraindications, 178–179
   plating systems for, 182, 182f
  Magerl technique, 243–246, 244f
  Roy-Camille technique, 243
  for subaxial cervical spine stabilization, 284, 285f, 287f
 as lateral or transforaminal interbody fusion supplement, 520–521
 for lateral plating systems, 365–366, 367f
 for lumbar facet fixation, 669–672, 670f–671f, 671t
 lumbar screws, 634–636, 635f, 636f
 occipital-cervical, 100–105, 102f, 103f, 104f
 of odontoid fractures, 129–133
  advantages/disadvantages, 129–130
  C1 lateral mass-C2 pars screws, 123, 124f
  cement augmentation of C2, 131, 133f
  complications, 131
  indications/contraindications, 129
  surgical technique, 130–131, 132f
 in osteoporosis, 639
 for pars interarticularis repair, 533
 pedicle screws, 123, 124f, 125, 126f, 127b, 634–641
  advantages/disadvantages, 634
  after spondylectomy, 259
  C1 lateral mass-C2 pedicle, 123–128
  C7 pedicle screws, 284–285, 285f, 286
  of cervical radiculopathy, 251
  for cervical trauma, 173
  for cervicothoracic junction, 285, 287f
  with cortical bone screws, 664–668, 665f–668f
  image-guided navigation systems for, 247, 248–250, 251f
  of lateral mass, 243–246
  with lateral mass screws, 178–183, 179f–180f, 181f–182f
  S1, 637
  for scoliosis correction, 507
  thoracic/thoracolumbar, 496–499, 497f, 498f
  for transverse process fusion, 631, 631t
 placement of screws, 497–498, 498f
  biplanar fluoroscopy technique, 650
  image-guided technique, 650
  inaccurate, 248
  owl's-eye en-face approach, 650
 S1 alar screws, 636
 S1 pedicle screws, 637
 S2 alar iliac screws, 638–639
 sacral screws, 636, 637f
 for spondylolisthesis, 533, 535f
 for spinal deformities, 520–521, 521f
 surgical technique, 497–499, 497f, 498f
 thoracic/thoracolumbar, 496
  advantages/disadvantages, 496
  complications, 499
  indications/contraindications, 496
  minimally invasive screw placement, 650–653, 651f–653f
  screw-rod instrumentation, 496–499, 497f, 498f

958 Index

Screw fixation (*continued*)
    for subaxial cervical spine stabilization, 285, 287*f*
    of thoracolumbar fractures, 556*f*
    in transforaminal lumbar interbody fusion, 646–647, 646*f*, 647*f*
    translaminar screws, 123
        for cervicothoracic junction, 285, 286*f*
        for subaxial cervical spine stabilization, 285, 286*f*
    for transverse process fusion, 631, 631*t*
    in upper thoracic spine, 181*f*
Seddon classification scheme, for peripheral nerve injury, 813, 814*t*
Segmentation defects, 293–295, 293*t*, 294*t*, 296*f*
Semispinalis capitis muscle
    anatomy, 113, 114*f*, 206, 208*t*, 209*t*
    in posterior occipitocervical dissection, 86
Semispinalis cervicalis muscle, anatomy, 113
Semispinalis cervicis muscle, anatomy, 206, 208*t*, 209*t*
Sensory abnormalities, junction abnormality-related, 5*b*
Sensory nerve action potential (SNAP), 815–816
Septum resection, in split cord malformation, 791–792, 792*f*
Seromas, spinal cord stimulator-related, 727
Sharpey-type insertions, 538, 539*f*
Short Form-12 (SF-12), 148–149, 500
Short Form-36 (SF-36), 148–149
Shunts
    lumboperitoneal, 687–689
    for syringomyelia, 485–491, 490*b*
        advantages/disadvantages, 486
        complications, 490
        distal shunt placement, 488–489, 488*f*, 489*f*, 490
        indications/contraindications, 485–486
        myelotomy for, 487–488
        spinal cord exposure for, 487
    ventriculoperitoneal, for myelomeningoceles, 753, 773
Single photon emission computed tomography (SPECT), of pediatric spondylolisthesis/spondylolysis, 531, 532*f*
Skull base
    chondrosarcomas of, 25
    extended maxillotomy approach for, 63–69
Skull base approaches, to craniovertebral junction, 12
Sleep apnea, 5*b*, 43
Slip angle, in pediatric spondylolisthesis, 531, 531*f*
Smith and Robinson anterior cervical approach, 194–195, 201
"Snow cone" tumors, 471
Soft palate
    closure of, 52, 55*f*
    splitting of, in transoral odontoidectomy, 44, 45*f*
    in transoral-transpalatophayngeal approach, 38
Solitary fibrous tumors (SFTs), of occipitocervical junction, 22–23, 23*f*
Somatosensory evoked potential (SSEPs) monitoring
    in cervical laminectomy, 217217
    in costotransversectomy, 436
    in lipoma surgery, 781
    in spinal accessory nerve surgery, 839
    in spondylolisthesis surgery, 534
    in transarticular fixation, 119
    in transforminal interbody fusion, 643
    in vascular malformation surgery, 346
Somitogenesis, 292
Spasticity
    cerebral palsy-related diplegic, dorsal rhizotomy treatment of, 690–706
        advantages and disadvantages, 703, 705
        anesthesia and positioning for, 696, 699, 699*f*
        complications, 705
        indications for, 691–692, 692*f*
        intraoperative neurophysiological guidance of, 701, 701*f*–702*f*, 703*f*
        preoperative planning for, 692–696, 693*f*–697*f*
        surgical approach, 699–703, 700*f*, 704*f*
    intrathecal drug delivery system (IDDS) for, 730–737
        permanent placement procedure, 732–735, 733*f*–735*f*
Spence's rule, 34*f*
Spetzler Classification, of spinal vascular malformations, 344, 345*t*
Spina bifida occulta, 297–298
Spinal accessory nerve
    iatrogenic injury to, 836
    surgical approach to, 836–842, 842*b*
        anatomical considerations in, 838–839, 838*f*, 842*f*
        for trauma repair, 836
    tumors of, 836
Spinal cord
    compression of, Lhermitte's sign of, 147
    embryogenesis, 769, 770*f*–771*f*
    herniation of, laminoplasty for, 451, 452*f*
    intramedullary tumors, 153–160
        clinical features, 153
        differential diagnosis, 153–154
        incidence, 153
        surgical resection, 157–159, 468–475, 468*f*–472*f*
            complications, 474
            indications/contraindications, 467
        types of, 155–157
    lipomas, 779–784
        anatomy and classification, 779
        dorsal, 779*f*, 780, 780*f*, 781–782, 781*f*–782*f*
        embryogenesis of, 779–781, 780*f*
        operative outcome, 783, 785
        operative treatment, 781–783, 781*f*–784*f*
        subcutaneous, 779*f*
        terminal, 780–781, 783, 784*f*
        transitional, 780, 780*f*, 782–783, 782*f*–783*f*
    trauma, Frankel Injury Classification System of, 554, 554*t*
Spinal cord stimulators
    as ilioinguinal neuralgia treatment, 920
    implantation of, 720–729
        advantages/disadvantages, 721
        complications, 727, 727*f*, 728*f*
        device options for, 721–723, 722*f*
        epidural lead placement in, 724–726, 724*f*–725*f*
        indications/contraindications, 720–721, 721*t*
        procedure, 723–727, 724*f*–726*f*
Spinal deformities
    embryology of, 293, 293*f*
    minimally invasive correction of, 518–522
        algorithm for, 518, 519*f*
        lateral transpsoas lumbar interbody fusion, 518, 520, 520*f*
        osteotomy, 518, 520
        percutaneous pedicle screw fixation, 520–521, 521*f*
        transforaminal lumbar interbody lumbar (MIS-TLIF), 520, 521*f*
Spinal dysraphism,156, 297–298. *See also* Dermal sinus tracts
    limited dorsal myeloschisis, 785–788, 785*f*–788*f*
    occult, 302*f*, 711. *See also* Tethered cord syndrome
    open. *See* Myelomeningoceles
    surgical management of, 769–789
Spinalis muscles, 113, 114*f*
Spinal stereotactic radiosurgery (SSRS), for spinal tumors, 322–323
Spine. *See also* Cervical spine; Lumbar/lumbosacral spine; Thoracic/thoracolumbar spine
    embryological development, 538, 540
    three-column model of, 325, 326*f*
Spinopelvic balance, differentiated from sagittal balance, 654
Splenius capitis muscle
    anatomy, 113, 114*f*, 206, 208*t*, 209*t*
    in posterior occipitocervical dissection, 86
Splenius cervicalis muscle, anatomy, 113
Split cord malformations. *See* Diastematomyelia
Spondylectomy, subaxial, combined anterior-posterior approach for, 257–260
Spondyloarthropathies, seronegative, of craniovertebral junction, 19
Spondylodiskitis, imaging of, 335*f*
Spondylolisthesis
    in children, 529–536
        clinical presentation, 531
        epidemiology, 529–531
        radiological diagnosis, 530*f*, 531–532, 531*f*, 536*f*
        spinopelvic parameters in, 531, 531*f*
    classification, 529, 530*f*
    definition, 529
    dysplastic (congenital), 297, 298*f*
    operative management, 532–536
        of high-grade spondylolisthesis, 532, 534*f*, 535*f*
        of low-grade spondylolisthesis, 532
    post-laminectomy, 570
    transforaminal interbody fusion, 642–649
Spondylolysis, lumbar, in children, 529–536
    classification, 529
    definition, 529
    epidemiology, 529–531
    nonoperative management, 532
    operative management, 532–533
Spondylosis, cervical, 137
    clinical presentation, 147–149
    definition, 146, 147
    differential diagnosis, 150

evaluation, 149
  imaging studies, 149, 151f
  pathophysiology, 147–149, 148f, 149f
  treatment, 150–152
Sprengel's deformity, 139, 139f, 140, 297
Spurling's sign, 148
Stabilization
  of cervical spine trauma
    anterior, 174–178, 175f–178f
      with clamp and hook systems, 183
      combined anterior and posterior approach, 185
      with facet wiring, 183
      with interspinous wiring, 183–184, 184f
      with lateral mass fixation, 243–246
      with occipitocervical arthrodesis, 82
    posterior, 178–185, 179f–182f, 185f
    in retroperitoneal approach to occipito-cervical junction, 80, 81f
    with sublaminar wiring, 185
  endoscopic, 388
  lumbar/lumbosacral, anterolateral retroperitoneal approach, 567
  with occipitocervical arthrodesis, 82
  posterior approaches
    for cervical spine trauma, 178–185, 179f–182f, 185f
    at cervicothoracic junction, 282, 283–288, 285f, 286f, 287f
    in retropharyngeal approach to occipito-cervical junction, 80, 81f
Stab wounds, to peripheral nerves, neurotization for, 914
Staphylococcus aureus infections, methicillin-resistant, 333
Stenosis
  cervical, 146–152
    minimally invasive posterior cervical laminoforamiotomy for, 221–227
    Klippel-Feil syndrome-related, evaluation of, 143
  lumbar/lumbosacral, minimally invasive decompression of, 612–614, 612f–614f, 614b
  thoracic/thoracolumbar, laminectomy for, 443, 446f
Sternocleidomastoid muscle
  anatomy, 114f, 208t
  in supraclavicular approach, 264, 265f
  in transmanubrial-transclavicular approach, 269, 270, 270f
  in transsternal approach, 268, 269, 270, 271
Sternotomy, with transsternal approach, 269, 270–271, 271f
Stress reaction, 529
Stretch injuries, to brachial plexus, 830
Strut grafts
  alternatives to, 176
  in anterior column reconstruction, 365, 367f
  C1 anterior arch-based anchoring of, 80, 81f
  in cervical anterior stabilization, 176, 177f, 178f
  in cervicothoracic junction anterior reconstruction, 280, 281, 281f, 282
  in laminoplasty, 230, 230f
  in occipitocervical arthrodesis, 80–81, 81f

in post-spondylectomy reconstruction, 259
in thoracoabdominal/retroperitoneal graft and lateral plating, 432
Subarachnoid space, shunt placement in, 486–487, 488, 488f, 489f, 490, 490b
Subaxial Injury Classification (SLIC), 239
Subaxial instability, atlantoaxial instability-related, 18
Subcostal nerve, anatomy, 912
Subependymomas, 153
Sublaminar wiring, for cervical spine, 185
Subluxation, vertebral, Klippel-Feil syndrome-related, 143
Submandibular gland, in retropharyngeal approach, 73, 74f
Sunderland classification scheme, for peripheral nerve injury, 813, 814t
Superficial peroneal nerve, biopsy, 932–938
  anatomical considerations in, 933f
  complications, 937, 937b
  with sural nerve biopsy, 932
  surgical procedure, 933–937, 933f–937f, 937b
Superior constrictor muscle, in retropharyngeal approach, 76, 77f
Superior laryngeal nerve, in retropharyngeal approach, 76
Supraclavicular approach
  in brachial plexus surgery, 826–830
    anatomical considerations in, 826–827, 827f
    dissection techniques, 828–829, 829f
    donor nerve graft harvesting, 829–830
    incision, 828
    laceration repair, 830
    stretch injury repair, 830
  to cervicothoracic junction, 263–267, 264f–267f
Sural nerve
  anatomy, 899, 900f
  biopsy of, 899–902, 901f, 932
  neuromas of, 847–848
Sural nerve grafts
  for axillary nerve repair, 847
  harvesting techniques, 829–830
  for lumbosacral plexus injury repair, 906
Sympathectomy
  endoscopic thoracic, 378–384
    advantages/disadvantages, 378
    complications, 381, 383, 383b
    incision planning for, 379, 380f
    indications/contraindications, 378
    instrumentation for, 379b
    outcomes, 382t, 383
    patient positioning for, 379, 380f
    surgical procedure, 378–382
  iatrogenic, 411
  lumbar, 566
  via costotransvesectomy, 435, 437–439, 438f
Synkinesia, congenital cervical spinal fusion-related, 143
Syringomyelia, 306–307, 306f
  cervicothoracic, 306, 306f
  Chiari malformation-associated, 91, 92, 92f, 207, 306–307, 485
  diastematomyelia-associated, 790, 795
  intramedullary tumor-associated, 153
  lipomyelomeningocele-associated, 303, 303f

occipito-cervical junction tumor-associated, 21
pathophysiology of, 485
shunt placement for, 485–491, 490b
  advantages/disadvantages, 486
  complications, 490
  distal shunt placement, 488–489, 488f, 489f, 490
  indications/contraindications, 485–486
  myelotomy for, 487–488
  spinal cord exposure for, 487
terminal, 307
Syrinx
  ependymoma-related, 155
  hemangioblastoma-related, 156

T

"Target sign," of peripheral nerve tumors, 882f
Tarsal tunnel syndrome, 825, 825f
Tectorial membrane
  anatomy and function, 28, 112f
  in retropharyngeal approach, 77
  in transoral odontoidectomy, 45, 46f
Tenotomy, of sternocleidomastoid muscle, 138
Tension-band disruption fractures, 552–553
Teratomas, 156
  sacrococcygeal
    classification, 763, 764f
    posterior resectioning of, 763–768, 764f–767f
Tethered cord syndrome (TCS), 302
  dermal sinus tracts-associated, 301, 757, 761f
  release of
    minimally invasive technique, 716–719, 717f, 718f
    open technique, 711–715, 712f–714f, 715b
  sacral agenesis-associated, 796–797, 798
Thecal sac exposure, in lumbar diskectomy, 608, 608f, 611
Thoracic duct, in supraclavicular approach, 265
Thoracic outlet syndrome (TOS), 823, 823f
Thoracic spinal nerves, 912. *See also* Intercostal nerves
Thoracic/thoracolumbar spine
  anatomy, 493f
  anterior column reconstruction, lateral graft and plate technique, 400–403, 401f, 402f, 403b
  arteriovenous malformations
    clinical presentation, 345
    of conus medullaris, 342, 344, 344f, 345
    dural, 340, 345
      differential diagnosis, 150
    endovascular treatment, 348t–349t, 352
    intradural, perimedullary, 340
    intradural/intramedullary, 345
    microvascular treatment, 346, 348t–349t, 350
    treatment outcomes, 354
  congenital anomalies, 291–309
    dermal sinus tracts, 301–302, 301f
    diastematomyelia (split spinal cord malformations), 299–301, 300f, 301f

Thoracic/thoracolumbar spine (*continued*)
   dysplastic (congenital) spondylolisthesis, 297, 298*f*
   embryology, 292–293
   formation errors, 293, 293*f*, 294, 294*t*
   intraspinal cysts, 304–305, 304*f*, 305*f*
   Klippel-Feil syndrome, 297
   kyphosis, 141, 295–296, 296*f*, 297*f*
   lipoma of the terminal filum, 302
   lipomyelomeningoceles, 302–303, 303*f*
   lordosis, 141
   meningoceles, 299, 300*f*, 304*f*
   myelomeningoceles, 298–299, 299*f*
   neuroendothelial cysts, 305–306
   neuroenteric cysts, 303–304, 304*f*
   radiological evaluation of, 291–292
   scoliosis, 141, 293–294, 293*t*, 294*f*, 295*t*
   segmentation defects, 293–296, 293*t*, 294*t*, 296*f*
   spinal dysraphism, 297–298, 302*f*
   syringomyelia, 306–307, 306*f*
   tethered cord syndrome, 302
   of vertebral body, 293–304
  costotransversectomy, 435–439
   diskectomy via, 435–437, 436*f*, 437*f*, 438*f*
   sympathectomy via, 435, 437–439, 438*f*
  decompression in
   multilevel minimally invasive, 523–526, 524*f*, 525*f*, 526*b*
   in thoracic laminectomy, 446*f*, 447, 448*f*, 492–495, 493*f*, 494*f*, 495*f*
  dorsal root entry zone (DREZ) operation, 480–481, 481*f*
  endoscopic lateral transthoracic approach to, 369–377
  endoscopic thoracic sympathectomy, 378–384
  epidural abscess, 333–338, 334*f*–338*f*
  fractures, 552–557
   burst fractures, 326, 327, 328*f*, 552, 553*f*, 556
   Chance fractures, 326, 553
   classification, 325–326, 327*f*
   clinical presentation, 345
   comminuted, 325
   compression fractures, 326, 327, 552
   displacement/translational fractures, 553
   distraction fractures, 326
   extension fractures, 327, 330
   fracture dislocations, 325, 330, 331*f*
   pedicle screw-rod instrumentation of, 496–499, 497*f*, 498*f*
   tension-band disruption fractures, 552–553
   wedge fractures, 325, 552
  herniated disks, 310–314. *See also* Diskectomy, in thoracic/thoracolumbar spine
   evaluation of, 311–312
   pathophysiology of, 310–311
   treatment for, 312–313
  laminectomy, 295, 443–449, 444*f*–448*f*
   advantages/disadvantages, 443
   complications, 449, 449*b*
   decompressive, 446*f*, 447, 448*f*, 492–495, 493*f*, 494*f*, 495*f*
   for dorsal root entry zone (DREZ) operation, 480
   indications/contraindications, 443
   minimally invasive, 443, 448, 448*f*, 449*f*
   multiple consecutive-level, 523
   surgical procedure, 447–448, 447*f*, 448*f*, 449*b*, 449*f*
   for thoracic osteomyelitis, 338
  laminoplasty, 450–454, 454*b*
   expansion, 450
   for intradural extramedullary tumor resection, 461
   osteoplastic, 450
  open lateral transthoracic approach to, 356–368, 357*f*, 358*f*, 359*f*, 362*f*–367*f*
   advantages/disadvantages, 356
   complications, 360
   indications for, 356
   patient positioning for, 357, 357*f*
   surgical procedure, 357–360, 358*f*–360*f*
  osteomyelitis, 338–339
  thoracoabdominal approach, open, 404–407, 405*f*, 406*f*, 407*f*, 409*f*, 409*t*
  thoracoabdominal/retroperitoneal graft and lateral plating, 431–434, 432*f*, 433*f*, 434*f*
  thoracolumbar approach, minimally invasive, 408–411, 409*f*, 409*t*
  trauma, 325–332, 552–557
   anatomical considerations in, 552
   classification, 553–554, 554*t*
   diagnosis, 554–555
   mechanisms of, 552–553
   treatment, 555–556
  tumors, 315–324
   aneurysmal bone cysts, 316, 317*f*
   benign primary, 316–318
   chondromas, 318
   differential diagnosis of, 316–318
   enchondromas, 318
   eosinophilic granulomas, 317
   evaluation of, 315–316
   Ewing's sarcomas, 319–320
   giant cell tumors, 318
   hemangiomas, 316–317
   locally aggressive (malignant), 318
   malignant primary, 318–320
   metastases, 320
   multiple myeloma, 318
   osteoblastomas, 316
   osteochondromas, 316
   osteoid osteomas, 316
   osteosarcomas, 318–319
   plasmacytomas, 318
   staging systems, 316, 320–321, 320*f*–321*f*, 322*f*
   treatment, 320–323, 323*f*
Thoracoabdominal approach, open, 404–407, 405*f*, 406*f*, 407*f*
Thoracoabdominal/retroperitoneal graft and lateral plating, 431–434, 432*f*, 433*f*, 434*f*
Thoracolumbar Injury Classification and Severity Scale (TLICS), 326, 553–554, 554*t*
Thoracolumbar Injury Severity Score (TISS), 326
Thoracolumbar spinal orthosis, 532
Thoracolumbosacral orthosis, 567–568
Thoracoscopy, for endoscopic lateral transthoracic vertebrectomy and diskectomy, 385, 388–389

Thoracotomy
  lateral retropleural, 394
  for open lateral transthoracic approach, 357–358, 361
Thromboembolism, venous, 559, 562
Tibial nerve
  anatomy, 899, 900*f*
  surgical approaches to
   in ankle, 894, 894*f*
   in leg, 893–894, 893*f*–894*f*
Tinel's sign
  in carpal tunnel syndrome, 820
  in ilioinguinal neuralgia, 917
  in peripheral nerve trauma, 815, 917
Tinnitus, craniovertebral junction abnormality-related, 5*b*
Tokuhashi score, of spinal tumors, 316
Tomita score, of spinal tumors, 316
Tonsillar herniation, Chiari I malformation-related, 91, 92, 92*f*, 93
Tonsillar resection, with suboccipital craniectomy, 91
Torticollis
  cervicothoracic scoliosis-related, 141
  congenital spine anomalies-related, 138, 139
Tracheostomy
  in extended maxillotomy reconstruction, 64
  in transmandibular-median labiomandibular approach, 39
  in transoral odontoidectomy, 43
Traction injuries, to lumbosacral plexus, 874
Traction techniques
  for cervical facet joint dislocations, 234–238
  cranial skeletal, as cervical dislocation treatment, 3
  craniocervical
   intraoperative, 44
   preoperative, 43–44
  halo traction
   for cervical closed reduction, 234, 235*f*, 236–237, 238*b*, 239
   contraindication for odontoid fractures, 30
   for locked facet joint treatment, 239
   with occipitocervical arthrodesis, 82
  intraoperative, for craniovertebral junction pathology, 15
  for locked cervical facts, 239–242
Transarticular screw fixation
  of atlantoaxial subluxation, 18*f*
  C1–C2, of craniovertebral junction abnormalities, 10*f*
Transcervical approach, endoscopic, to upper cervical spine, 57–62, 59*f*–61*f*
Transcorporeal tunnel approach, to cervical radiculopathy, 201–205, 202*f*–203*f*, 204*f*
Transforaminal lumbar interbody fusion (MIS-LIF), minimally invasive, 520, 521*f*
  for adult idiopathic scoliosis, 514, 515*f*
  pedicle screw fixation with, 646–647, 646*f*, 647*f*
Transgluteal approach, to proximal extrapelvic sciatic nerve, 890, 891*f*–892*f*, 892
Translaminar approach, for facet screw fixation, 670–672, 671*t*, 672*f*

Index

Transmandibular approach, to craniovertebral junction, 39, 42, 48
Transmandibular-median labiomandibular approach, 39
Transmanubrial-transclavicular approach, to cervicothoracic junction, 268–273, 269f, 270f, 271f
Transmaxillary approach, to craniovertebral junction, 39
Transnasomaxillary approach, 39
Transoral approaches
  to craniovertebral junction, 3, 12, 12b, 37–41
    complications, 37, 38, 40
    development and history of, 37–38
    extended approaches, 38, 38t, 39, 48–51
    for intradural pathology, 40
    standard approaches, 38–39, 38t
    transmandibular-median labiomandibular approach, 38t, 39
    transmaxillary-Le Fort I osteotomy
      with down-fracture of maxilla, 38t, 39, 40
      with palatal split, 38t, 40, 49–50, 64, 66f, 67f
  endoscopic, to upper cervical spine, 58–62, 59f–61f
  in odontoidectomy, 38, 42–47
    indications/contraindications, 42
    preoperative craniocervical junction reduction, 43–44
    preoperative planning, 42–43
    surgical technique, 44–47, 45f, 45f–47f
Transoral-transpalatopharyngeal approach
  to atlas anterior arch, 45, 45f, 46f
  to basilar invagination, 42
  closure techniques, 52–55, 53f–55f
  to craniovertebral junction, 38–39, 38t, 42–47
  with median mandibulotomy. See Median labiomandibular approach
Transoral-transpharyngeal approach, to craniovertebral junction, 37
Transpalatal approach, 39
Transpedicular approach
  to cervicothoracic junction, 277
  to thoracic epidural abscess, 336, 336f, 337, 337f
Transperitoneal approach, to intrapelvic sciatic nerve, 890
Transpleural approach, in lateral transthoracic approach
  endoscopic, 385, 388–389
  open, 357–358, 362, 362f, 365f
Transsacral approach, 673–683
  advantages/disadvantages, 673
  clinical cases, 680, 680f–682f
  indications/contraindications, 674
  procedure, 676–678, 677f, 678f
  two-level presacral approach, 676, 678
Transsternal approach, to cervicothoracic junction, 268–269, 270–272
Transthoracic approach, lateral, 356–360
Transverse ligament
  anatomy, 111, 111f, 112
  normal, 33f
  in retropharyngeal approach, 76, 77, 77f
  in transoral odontoidectomy, 45
  trauma/disruption, 28–29
    classification, 31–32, 31f

radiographic appearance, 31–32, 31f, 33f–34f
    treatment options, 32
Transverse processes, decortication of, 495, 495f
Transverse process fusion, in lumbar/lumbosacral spine, 628–633, 629f, 630f
  instrumented versus noninstrumented fusion rates, 631–632, 631t
  minimally invasive techniques, 630–631
  open techniques, 628–630, 630f
Trapezius muscle
  anatomy, 114f, 206, 208t, 209t
  in posterior occipitocervical dissection, 86
Trauma. See also specific types of trauma, e.g., Fractures
  brachial plexus
    neurotization for, 914
    radiographic evaluation of, 928
    root avulsions in, 878
  lumbar/lumbosacral spine, 552–557
    anatomical considerations in, 552
    classification, 553–554, 554t
    diagnosis, 554–555
    mechanisms of, 552–553
    treatment, 555–556
  mid- and lower cervical spine, 173–185
    anterior surgical approaches to, 174, 175f–177f
      anatomic plane in, 174, 175f
      cervical plating in, 177–178, 178f
      diskectomy, 176, 177f
      incisions, 174, 175f
    initial assessment and stabilization, 173
    surgical techniques for, 173–185
  occipitocervical junction, 28–36
    atlantoaxial rotatory subluxation, 29, 32
    atlanto-occipital dislocation, 28, 30–31, 32
    biomechanics of, 28
    clinical presentation, 30
    isolated fractures, 29–30
    ligamentous injuries, 28–29
    radiographic presentation, 30–32, 31f, 32f, 34f
    transverse ligament interruption, 28–29, 31f, 33f
    treatment options, 32
  peripheral nerves, 813–817
    classification and grading, 813, 814f
    clinical assessment, 814–816
    management guidelines, 815f
    mechanisms of, 813
    pathophysiology, 813
    reinnervation following, 813–814
    repair, 816
  thoracic/thoracolumbar spine, 325–332, 552–557
    anatomical considerations in, 552
    classification, 553–554, 554t
    diagnosis, 554–555
    mechanisms of, 552–553
    treatment, 555–556
  transverse ligament, 28–29
    classification, 31–32, 31f
    radiographic appearance, 31–32, 31f, 33f–34f
    treatment options, 32
Trendelenburg's sign, 877f

Tumors
  of cervical spine
    bone tumors, 167–172
      benign tumors, 167, 168f
      malignant tumors, 167–171, 169f, 170f
      metastatic tumors, 170, 171f
    intramedullary extramedullary, 153, 161–166
      clinical features, 161
      differential diagnosis, 161
      treatment, 166
      types of, 161–163
  of craniovertebral junction, 4t
  of lumbar/lumbosacral spine, 545–551
    lipoma resectioning, 746–752, 747f–751f
    primary benign, 545–548, 547f, 548f
    primary malignant, 545, 548–550, 549f
  of occipitocervical junction, 21–27, 70
    classification, 21
    primary benign, 21–24
    primary malignant, 21, 24–25
  of peripheral nerves. See Nerve sheath tumors
  of spinal accessory nerve, 836
  of spinal cord
    intramedullary tumors, 153–160
      clinical features, 153
      differential diagnosis, 153–154
      incidence, 153
      surgical resection of, 157–159, 468–475, 468f–472f
      types of, 155–157
    lipomas, 779–784
      anatomy and classification, 779
      dorsal, 779f, 780, 780f, 781–782, 781f–782f
      embryogenesis, 779–781, 780f
      operative outcome, 783, 785
      operative treatment, 781–783, 781f–784f
      subcutaneous, 779f
      terminal, 780–781, 783, 784f
      transitional, 780, 780f, 782–783, 782f–783f
  subaxial, spondylectomy for, 257–260
  of thoracic/thoracolumbar spine, 315–324
    aneurysmal bone cysts, 316, 317f
    benign primary, 316–318
    chondromas, 318
    chondrosarcomas, 320
    chordomas, 318, 319f
    differential diagnosis of, 316–318
    enchondromas, 318
    eosinophilic granulomas, 317
    evaluation of, 315–316
    Ewing's sarcomas, 319–320
    giant cell tumors, 318
    hemangiomas, 316–317
    locally aggressive (malignant), 318
    malignant primary, 318–320
    metastases, 320
    osteoblastomas, 316
    osteochondromas, 316
    osteoid osteomas, 316
    osteosarcomas, 318–319
    plasmacytomas, 318
    staging systems, 320–321, 320f–321f, 322f
Turner's syndrome, pterygium colli associated with, 139

U

Ulnar nerve
  anatomy, 822, 822f, 861–862
  decompression of, 861–865
    endoscopic technique, 865
    simple procedure, 863, 863f, 864–865
  entrapment neuropathies, 822–823, 822f
    distal entrapment, 862, 862f
    entrapment at cubital tunnel, 862–863, 863f
  neurolysis of, 863–864
  subcutaneous transposition of, 864, 864f
  subfacial/intramuscular transposition of, 864, 864f
  submuscular transposition of, 864, 864f
  transfers, for musculocutaneous nerve repair, 852
Ultrasound
  of brachial plexus injury-associated injuries, 928
  renal, in Klippel-Feil syndrome, 141
  of sacrococcygeal teratomas, 764
University of Iowa Hospitals and Clinics, 3, 4t, 15, 37, 43, 44
Upper extremity, entrapment neuropathies of
  median nerve, 818–820, 819f, 820t
    carpal tunnel syndrome, 818, 820, 820t, 854, 856–859, 856f–859f
    cubital fossa entrapment, 818, 819–820
    ligament of Struthers compression, 818–819, 854, 855, 855f
  meralgia paresthetica, 824
  musculocutaneous nerve, 849, 852
  radial nerve, 865–868, 866f–868f
    posterior interosseous nerve syndrome, 821–822, 865, 867–868, 867f
    "Saturday night palsy," 821
    Wartenberg's disease, 868, 868f
  tarsal tunnel syndrome, 825, 825f
  thoracic outlet syndrome, 823, 823f
  ulnar nerve, 822–823, 822f
    distal entrapment, 862, 862f
    entrapment at cubital tunnel, 862–863, 863f
Upper retroarticular foramen, 107–108

V

Vascular anatomy, spinal, embryology, 341
Vascular endothelial growth factor (VEGF), 540, 541f
Vascular malformations, 340–355
  anatomy and pathophysiology, 341–342
  classification, 340, 344, 344t, 345t
  epidemiology, 340–341
  imaging, 342–344
  lumbar, 427f
  treatment, 346–353
    endovascular treatment, 351–352, 353f
    history of, 340
    microvascular treatment, 346–351, 347f, 348t–349t, 350f, 351f
    outcome, 352, 354
    radiosurgery treatment, 352
Vascular steal, 342
Velopharyngeal incompetence, transoral approach-related, 40
Venous system, of spinal cord, 341
Ventral approach, to craniovertebral junction, 12b, 37
Ventricular septal defects, Klippel-Feil syndrome-related, 141
Vertebrae
  cervical. See also Atlas (C1); Axis (C2)
    anatomy, 146–147
    C3-C7 (typical), 201
  embryology, 292–293
  lumbar, anatomy, 552
  thoracic/thoracolumbar
    "butterfly," 295, 297f
    segmentation defects, 293–295, 293t, 294t
Vertebral artery
  anatomy, 88f, 89, 110, 206, 208t, 209t
  in atlantoaxial fixation, 101
  in C1-C2 transarticular fixation, 119
  in giant cell tumors, 168f
  injury
    anterior diskectomy-related, 189f
    C1-C2 exposure-related, 106
    C1-C2 screw fixation-related, 123, 124, 126, 127, 127b
    C1-C2 transarticular screw fixation-related, 121
    pedicle screw fixation-related, 251
    ponticulus posticus-related, 112
    posterior cervical surgery-related, 211
    posterior occipitocervical junction exposure-related, 84, 88–90, 88f, 89f
    posterior suboccipital/upper cervical exposure-related, 84
    spondylectomy-related, 258, 259, 260
  in meningiomas, 166
  occlusion, atlas subluxation-related, 10
Vertebral artery ring, retroarticular or retrocondylar, 107–108
Vertebral body
  anatomy and function, 569
  complete resection of. See Spondylectomy
  congenital anomalies, 293–304
  derotation, in scoliosis correction, 509–514
    double major (Lenke type 3), 513
    double thoracic (Lenke type 2), 512–513, 512f
    main thoracic (Lenke type 1), 512
    thoracolumbar/lumbar (Lenke type 5), 513
    thoracolumbar/lumbar-major thoracic (Lenke type 6), 513–514, 514f–515f
    triple major (Lenke type 4), 513
  embryology, 540
  fractures, 185
  hemangiomas, 167
  metastatic tumors, 170
  ossification, 292–293
Vertebral bone tumors, 167–172
  benign tumors, 167, 168f
  malignant tumors, 167–171, 169f, 170f
  metastatic tumors, 170, 171f
Vertebral column
  anterolateral, anatomy, 359f
  resection
    for lumbar spinal deformity correction, 654, 656, 656f, 657, 658f, 660–662, 661f
    for scoliosis correction, 509, 510f
  resegmentation, 292
Vertebral column manipulators, 511, 511f
Vertebra plana, 167, 545–547

Vertebrectomy
  in cervical spine stabilization, 185
  for compression fractures, 364f
  lateral transthoracic
    lateral graft and plate reconstruction following, 400–403
    minimally invasive, 395–399, 398f, 399b
  lumbar/lumbosacral
    anterolateral retroperitoneal approach, 567
    minimally invasive retroperitoneal, 423–430
      advantages/disadvantages, 423
      complications, 427, 427f
      corpectomy with, 427
      diskectomy with, 426–427
      graft placement in, 427
      indications/contraindications, 423
      patient positioning for, 424, 424f
      surgical technique, 423–427
  multilevel, incisions for, 175f
  single-level, 176
  thoracic/thoracolumbar
    endoscopic lateral transthoracic, 385–390, 386f–388f
    lateral transthoracic approach, 358f, 359, 359f
    open lateral transthoracic approach, 361–362, 362f, 364–368, 364f–366f
  two-level, 177f
Vertebrobasilar insufficiency, atlantoaxial subluxation-related, 16
Vertebroplasty, 738–745
  indications/contraindications, 740
  versus kyphoplasty, 740
  versus nonoperative treatment, 738–739, 739t
  open, for aneurysmal bone cysts, 22
  for pathological fractures, 322
  surgical procedure, 740–743, 741f–743f, 743b
Vertigo
  cranial settling-related, 14
  craniovertebral junction abnormality-related, 5b
VHL syndrome, 158
Video-assisted thoracoscopic surgery (VATS), 369
Visual Analogue Scale, 148–149
Vitamin B_{12} deficiency, 0, 161
von Hippel-Lindau syndrome, 156, 158
von Recklinghausen's disease, neurofibromas associated with, 70

W

Wackenheim's line, 30, 31, 31f
Wartenberg's disease, 868, 868f
Wartenberg's sign, 823
Web neck, craniovertebral junction abnormality-related, 5b
Wedge fractures, 325, 552
Weinstein-Boriani-Biagini staging system, for spinal tumors, 321, 322f
Wildervank syndrome, 139
Wire techniques
  for atlantoaxial instability, 118
  cervical facet, 183
  interspinous, 183–184, 184f

for odontoid fractures, 119f
for pars interarticularis repair, 533
posterior atlantoaxial, 109–117
  advantages/disadvantages, 109
  Brooks and Jenkins technique, 115, 116f
  comparison with transarticular fixation, 118
  Gallie's technique, 115, 115f
  indications/contraindications, 109
  interspinous C1-C2 technique, 115–116, 116f
  surgical anatomy, 110–113, 110f–111f
  surgical technique, 113–116, 114f, 115f, 116f
  as transarticular fixation adjunct, 119, 120, 121
sublaminar, 185
Wound infections, myelomeningocele repair-related, 776
Wrong-site surgery, 211

X
X-rays
  for anterior lumbar/lumbosacral approach, 559
  for C1-C2 screw fixation, 125
  of cervical spondylosis, 149
  of cervical trauma, 173
  of craniovertebral junction abnormalities, 7f, 8, 10f
  of dermal sinus tracts, 759
  of hemangiomas, 547
  of Klippel-Feil syndrome, 142
  for lumbar/lumbosacral decompression, 595
  of lumbosacral tumors, 545
  of neurofibromas, 23
  of occipitocervical junction, 71
  of osteosarcoma, 549
  of pediatric spondylolisthesis /spondylolysis, 530f, 531
  for pedicle screw fixation, 634
  for posterior cervicothoracic instrumentation, 284
  for posterior lumbar/lumbosacral approach, 570, 571, 571f
  of sacrococcygeal teratomas, 764–765
  of scoliosis, 500, 502f
  of thoracic/thoracolumbar congenital abnormalities, 291
  of thoracolumbar trauma, 555
  for transsacral approach, 676

Z
Ziconotide, intrathecal drug delivery system for, 730–737
  overdose with, 735t
Z-plasty, 228
Zygapophyseal capsule. *See* Lateral mass
Zygapophyseal joints. *See* Facet joints